49.50

MANSON'S
TROPICAL DISEASES

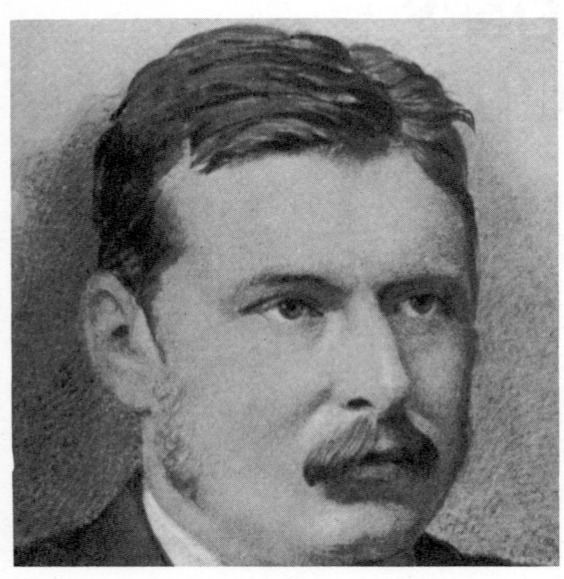

Sir Patrick Manson
GCMG, FRS (1844–1922)
Sir Patrick Manson, pioneer of tropical medicine, wrote six editions of this book between 1898 and 1921, distilling in to it, in language of classical lucidity, his immense experience and wisdom.

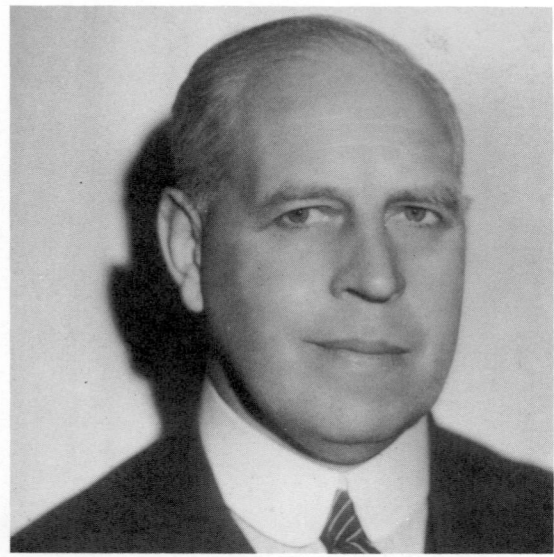

Sir Philip Manson-Bahr
CMG, DSO (1881–1966)
Sir Philip Manson-Bahr, Manson's son-in-law, prepared the next ten editions with sustained industry. By constant revision, re-writing and enlargement he kept each one abreast of the advances in knowledge of its day.

MANSON'S TROPICAL DISEASES

NINETEENTH EDITION

P. E. C. Manson-Bahr

MD, FRCP, DTM&H

Consultant Physician, Crown Agents and Overseas Development Administration. Formerly Senior Lecturer in Clinical Tropical Medicine, London School of Hygiene and Tropical Medicine; Professor of Clinical Tropical Medicine, School of Tropical Medicine and Public Health, Tulane University, New Orleans, USA; Senior Specialist, Colonial Medical Service; Vice-President of the Royal Society of Tropical Medicine and Hygiene

D. R. Bell

MB, ChB, FRCP, MFCM, DTM&H

Reader in Tropical Medicine, Liverpool School of Tropical Medicine; Honorary Consultant Physician, Liverpool Area Health Authority (Teaching); Civil Consultant in Tropical Medicine to the Royal Air Force. Formerly Consultant in Tropical Medicine, Mahidol University, Bangkok; Senior Lecturer in Preventive and Social Medicine, University of Ibadan

Baillière Tindall

LONDON PHILADELPHIA
TORONTO SYDNEY TOKYO

Baillière Tindall 24–28 Oval Road
London NW1 7DX, England

West Washington Square
Philadelphia, PA 19105, USA

1 Goldthorne Avenue
Toronto, Ontario M8Z 5T9, Canada

ABP Australia Ltd, 44 Waterloo Road
North Ryde, NSW 2064, Australia

Harcourt Brace Jovanovich Japan, Inc.
Ichibancho Central Building, 22–1 Ichibancho
Chiyoda-ku, Tokyo 102, Japan

© 1987 Baillière Tindall

Illustrations: Chapters 33 and 65 © 1987 Dr J. H. S. Pettit; Chapter 48 © 1987 Dr D. A. Warrell

First published 1898
Eighteenth edition 1982
Nineteenth edition 1987

Typeset in Great Britain by Butler & Tanner Ltd, Frome and London
Printed and bound in Great Britain by William Clowes Ltd, Beccles and London

British Library Cataloguing in Publication Data

Manson, *Sir* Patrick
Manson's tropical diseases.—19th ed.
1. Tropical medicine
I. Title II. Manson-Bahr, P. E. C.
III. Bell, Dion R.
616.9'88'3   RC961

ISBN 0–7020–1187–8

WC6
1461

Contents

Contents

Preface to the Nineteenth Edition

We have taken a new look at our readers for this edition, and tried to identify our target readership more clearly. Our main objective is to provide a fairly comprehensive manual for practising doctors in the tropics, both the clinician and the doctor faced with the wider responsibilities of the District Medical Officer, or his modern-day equivalent.

We have changed the organization of the contents to reflect this more practical approach, and readers will notice that 'Diseases commonly presenting as fever' and 'Diseases commonly presenting as diarrhoea' replace the zoological classification used in previous editions.

To continue the theme of a practical approach, we tried to ensure that we and other contributors have borne the needs of the practising doctor in mind at all times. All the main clinical sections in the book were written by practising physicians.

Although we have consigned details of life cycles and the minutiae of parasite morphology to appendices, as before, we have included sufficient information on these points in the main text to enable each chapter to stand on its own. It is now only necessary to consult the appendices if more information is needed.

And finally, a word about the appendices themselves: an enormous amount of information is to be found there, so as to adhere to the original aim of the book to provide a comprehensive source of information. We feel it was worth keeping the appendices and so save most doctors the need to buy a separate textbook of parasitology.

We warmly welcome the views and comments of our readers. If any of them cares to write to us, we promise a prompt reply.

P. E. C. Manson-Bahr
D. R. Bell

Every effort has been made to check the drug dosages given in this book. However, as it is possible that some errors have been missed or that dosage schedules have been revised the reader is strongly urged to consult the drug companies' literature before administering any of the drugs listed.

Acknowledgements

We would like to thank the following for assistance with sections of the book:

Dr V. R. Southgate—Appendix II, snails; Chapter 22, transmission, epidemiology and control of schistosomiasis.
Dr R. A. Bray—Appendix II, trematodes and cestodes.
Dr R. W. Ingle—Appendix II, crabs.
Mr A. Wheeler—Appendix II, fish.
Dr C. J. Hackett—Chapter 31.
Professor D. A. Denham—Appendix II, filariasis.
Dr P. Craig—serological diagnosis of cestodes.
Dr P. H. Rees—treatment of amoebiasis and visceral leishmaniasis.
Dr D. S. Ellis—electromicrographs in appendices.
Dr A. F. Bryceson and Professor L. Bruce-Chwatt—Chapter 1.

Many of the illustrations were provided by the Wellcome Tropical Institute Museum, courtesy Professor E. H. O. Parry. Dr H. Zaiman, the editor and the publisher of *A Pictorial Presentation of Parasites*, kindly gave us permission to use the following illustrations: Figs. 21.8, 22.25, 23.14, 23.15, 23.31, 23.38, 23.40 and 37.14. Valuable help with picture research was given by Mrs P. Dickinson, Mrs S. Aspinall and Mr C. Bracewell.

List of Contributors

S. Abdalla, LRCP, MRCS, MRCPath
Department of Haematology,
St. Mary's Hospital Medical School,
London,
UK

Haematological problems in the tropics

O. P. Arya, DTM&H, DPH, DIH, Dip. Ven.
Department of genito-urinary Medicine,
Royal Liverpool Hospital,
Liverpool,
UK

Sexually transmitted diseases in the tropics

J. W. Bailey, BSc
Diagnostic Parasitology Laboratory,
Department of Tropical Medicine,
Liverpool School of Tropical Medicine,
Liverpool,
UK

Laboratory diagnosis of parasitic diseases

E. Bertrand
Faculte de Medecine & Institut de Cardiologie,
Abidjan,
Cote D'Ivoire

Cardiovascular problems in the tropics

J. R. Billinghurst, MA, BM, FRCP
Medical and Health department,
Banjul,
The Gambia

Neurological and psychiatric problems in the tropics

P. Chaulet
Clinique de Pneumo-Pthisiologie Matiben,
Centre Hospitalier Universitaire de Beni-Messous,
Algiers,
Algeria

Tuberculosis

P. Clifford, MD, MCh, FRCS, MD (hc Karolinska
Inst. Stockholm)
formerly Department of Surgery,
Royal Marsden Hospital and King's College
Hospital,
London, UK
and Kenyatta National Hospital, Nairobi, Kenya

Cancer in the tropics

G. C. Cook, MD, DSc, FRCP, FRACP
Department of Clinical Tropical Medicine,
Hospital for Tropical Diseases,
London,
UK

Gastroenterological problems in the tropics

G. V. Gill, MSc, MD, MRCP, DTM&H
Department of Tropical Medicine,
Liverpool School of Tropical Medicine
and Arrowe Park Hospital,
Liverpool,
UK

Metabolic diseases in the tropics

L. G. Goodwin, CMG, FRCP, FRS
formerly Director of Science,
The Zoological Society of London,
London,
UK

Plant poisons

M. S. R. Hutt, MD, FRCPath, FRCP
formerly Department of Pathology,
Makerere University Medical School,
Uganda and
Department of Histopathology,
St. Thomas's Hospital Medical School,
London,
UK

Cancer in the tropics

R. P. Lane, PhD
Department of Entomology,
London School of Tropical Hygiene and Tropical
Medicine,
London,
UK

Medical entomology

D. M. Minter, PhD, BSc(Hons), MIBiol, C.Biol,
FRES
Department of Entomology,
London School of Hygiene and Tropical Medicine,
London,
UK

Medical entomology and *Medical protozoology*

M. E. Molyneux, MD, FRCP
Department of Tropical Medicine,
Liverpool School of Tropical Medicine,
Liverpool,
UK

Respiratory problems in the tropics

D. W. Mulder, MD, MSc (Epid), DTM&H
Department of Health Care and Epidemiology,
Royal Tropical Institute,
Amsterdam,
The Netherlands

Tuberculosis

J. H. S. Pettit, MD, FRCP
Department of Tropical Medicine,
Liverpool School of Tropical Medicine,
Liverpool, UK and
Department of Medicine,
National University of Malaysia,
Kuala Lumpur,
Malaysia

Dermatology in the tropics; Superficial mycoses

P. Piot, MD
Department of Microbiology,
Institute of Tropical Medicine,
Antwerp,
Belgium

AIDS in Africa

P. H. Rees, OBE, MD, FRCP, FRCP(Ed), DCMT
African Medical and Research Foundation,
Nairobi,
Kenya

Drugs

J. Riley, PhD
Department of Biological Sciences,
The University,
Dundee,
UK

Medical entomology

F. C. Rodger, MD, MCh, FRCS(Glas), DOMS
formerly Department of Ophthamology,
Princess Margaret Hospital,
Swindon,
UK and
Institute of Ophthalmology,
Aligarh University,
India

Eye diseases in the tropics

K. G. V. Smith, C.BIOL, MIBiol, FRES
Department of Entomology,
British Museum (Natural History),
London,
UK

Arthropod dermatoses, stings, bites, allergies and neuroses

M. G. R. Varma, PhD, DS, FIBiol, FRES
Department of Entomology,
London School of Hygiene and Tropical Medicine,
London,
UK

Medical entomology

D. A. Warrell, MA, DM, FRCP
Nuffield Department of Clinical Medicine,
John Radcliffe Hospital,
Headington,
Oxford,
UK

Animal poisons

S. A. Waitkins, PhD, Dip. Immun, MRCPath
PHLS Leptospira Reference Unit and
WHO/FAO Collaborating Centre for Research &
Reference on Leptospirosis,
County Hospital,
Hereford,
UK

Leptospirosis

D. Weatherall, MD, FRCP, FRCPath, FRS
Nuffield Department of Clinical Medicine,
University of Oxford,
Oxford,
UK

Haematological problems in the tropics

G. B. White, PhD
Imperial Chemical Industries PLC,
Fernhurst,
Haslemere,
UK

Medical entomology

List of plates

(Colour plates fall between pages 1198 and 1199)

Introduction
Tropical Diseases: A Manual of the Diseases of Warm Climates

Tropical Diseases by Patrick Manson MD was first published in 1898 by Cassell & Coy. It was a small book of 607 pages which fitted into an ordinary pocket and cost ten shillings and sixpence. One-third was devoted to 'Fevers'; only the causes of cholera and plague and the cause, transmission and treatment of malaria were known. Yellow fever, plague and dengue were all described and other syndromes are recognizable today, e.g. Mediterranean fever (brucellosis), Japanese river fever (Mite typhus) kala azar and negro lethargy or sleeping sickness, but their causes, transmission and treatment were unknown. Many of the important, present-day diseases of warm climates, tuberculosis, measles, infantile diarrhoea, as well as the now extinct smallpox, were not included since they were familiar to the doctors of the Western world at that time. The importance of nutritional diseases was not recognized, only one—Beriberi—the cause of which was unknown, being mentioned.

Two reprints followed in rapid succession and a second edition was published in 1900. In all, six editions had been published when Sir Patrick Manson died in 1922. The next ten editions were edited by Sir Philip Manson-Bahr, Sir Patrick's son-in-law. The book retained its size but became thicker and the number of pages rose to 900 then 1000. Four appendices were added, on Protozoology, Helminthology, Entomology and Clinical pathology. The importance of these appendices was that the book remained essentially clinical for clinicians practising often away from technical help and that technical details did not crowd out the clinical aspects. During this time *Manson's Tropical Diseases* was translated into Italian and Spanish.

Since 1966, when Sir Philip Manson-Bahr died, the importance of many communicable diseases now no longer rife in the developed world as well as nutritional diseases has become increasingly recognized and the incidence and form of cardiovascular and other diseases including cancer vary according to the environment and race. A special section has been devoted to these problems. In spite of these additions the 19th edition remains essentially a book for clinicans—although its size no longer allows it to fit into an ordinary coat pocket.

Since 1898, when *Manson's Tropical Diseases* first appeared, succeeding editions have reflected the changing nature of the subject. In the early years it was concerned exclusively with diseases of a single bacterial or parasitic cause. Now its embrace is much wider, including nutritional disorders and the peculiarly tropical aspects of cosmopolitan diseases. Most recently its contents have recognized the contributions made by altered ecology to human disease in the tropics.

SECTION I
DISEASES COMMONLY PRESENTING AS FEVER

Chapter 1
Malaria and Babesiosis

MALARIA

The name malaria is derived from the Italian *mal'aria* or 'bad air' and paludism, another word used to describe malaria, derives from the Latin 'palus' or marsh.

GEOGRAPHICAL DISTRIBUTION

In the early part of this century more than two-thirds of the world's population lived in areas where malaria was endemic, and malaria is still the most important cause of fever and morbidity in the tropical world. In tropical Africa, where it is deeply entrenched, no fewer than 373 million people live in endemic areas where *P. falciparum* is the dominant parasite, and the number of cases of clinical malaria has been estimated at between 76 and 150 million annually, the incidence showing little change over the last 20 years.[1] Outside tropical Africa 6.5 million cases were recorded in 1982.[2] There has been a sharp decline in the incidence of malaria in South-East Asia since 1977 reflecting a rapid fall in India and Sri Lanka[3] but there has been a slow increase in South and Central America.[2]

At first high hopes were held out for the world-wide eradication of the disease and by the early 1970s the population free from malaria had increased from 400 to over 1200 million. Malaria had been eradicated from the whole of Europe, most of North America including the whole of the USA, most of the Caribbean, large parts of northern and southern South America, Australia, Singapore, Japan, Korea and Taiwan.[4] However, despite some success the global eradication of malaria was not attainable for a number of reasons, including the development of insecticide and drug resistance and political and administrative difficulties. Imported malaria is becoming an increasing problem in non-endemic areas. The present distribution of malaria throughout the world is shown in Fig. 1.1.

AETIOLOGY

There are four species of malaria parasites (plasmodia) which infect man:

> *Plasmodium vivax* (vivax malaria, benign tertian (BT), tertian malaria);
> *P. ovale* (ovale malaria, ovale tertian malaria);
> *P. malariae* (quartan malaria);
> *P. falciparum* (falciparum malaria, malignant tertian (MT), subtertian (ST), pernicious malaria).

Life-cycle (Fig. 1.2)

The life-cycle of all human malaria species consists of two phases: a sexual phase (sporogony) with development and multiplication in certain female anopheline mosquitoes, and an asexual phase (schizogony) with multiplication in man.

The asexual phase in man has two parts, schizogony in the cells of the liver (pre-erythrocytic schizogony or tissue phase) and schizogony in the red cells (erythrocytic schizogony, erythrocytic phase).

Asexual phase in the human host

TISSUE PHASE

Sporozoites are inoculated by the mosquito into the host and disappear from the circulation within half an hour. Some enter the parenchymal cells of the liver where they undergo development and multiplication, known as *pre-erythrocytic schizogony*. The *tissue schizont* (Figs. I.1–3) which develops from the sporozoite enlarges and the nucleus and cytoplasm divide to form many thousands of *merozoites* which after 6–16 days

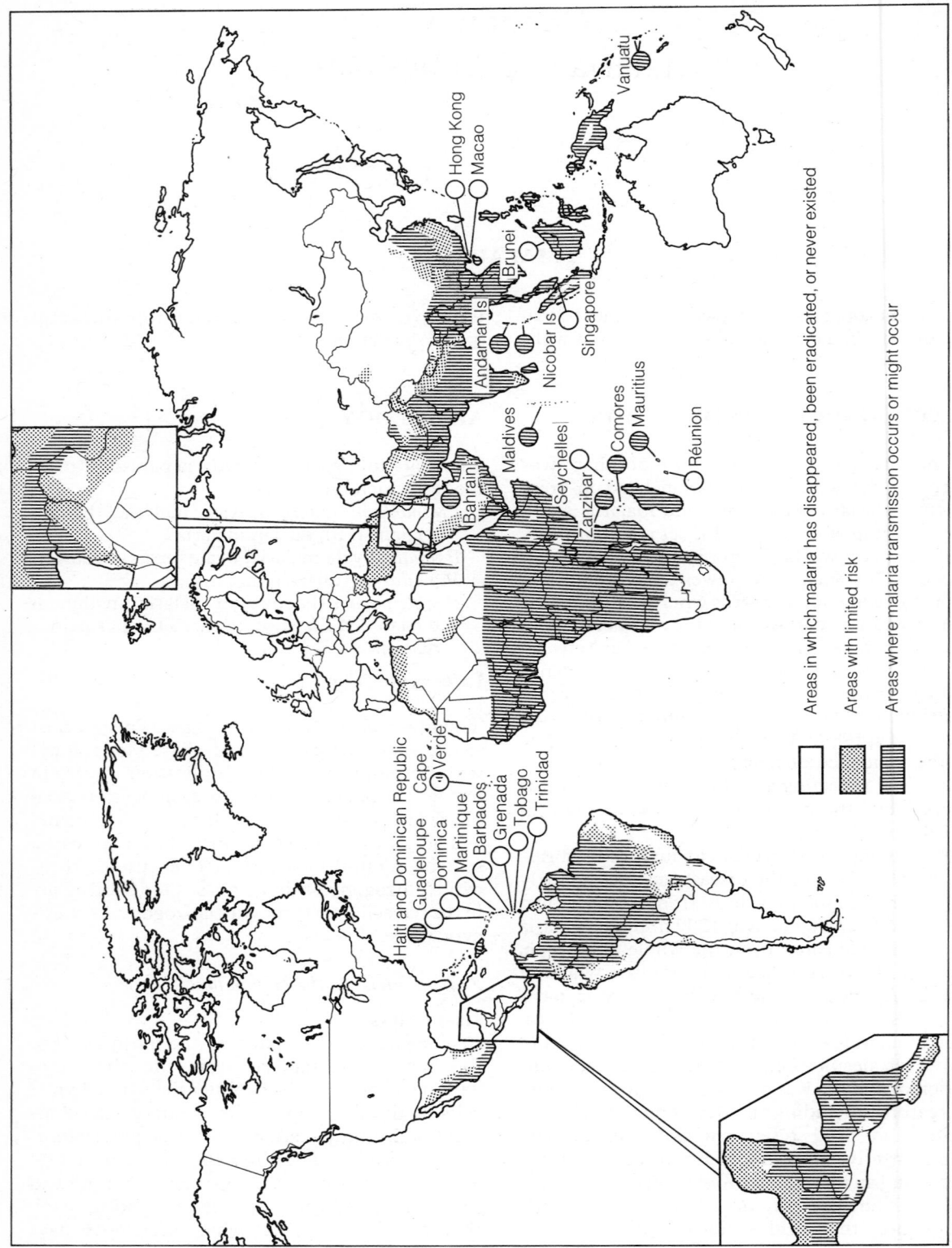

Hong Kong
Macao
Brunei
Andaman Is.
Nicobar Is.
Singapore
Maldives
Bahrain
Seychelles
Zanzibar
Comores
Mauritius
Réunion
Vanuatu

Haiti and Dominican Republic
Cape Verde
Guadeloupe
Dominica
Martinique
Barbados
Grenada
Tobago
Trinidad

Areas in which malaria has disappeared, been eradicated, or never existed

Areas with limited risk

Areas where malaria transmission occurs or might occur

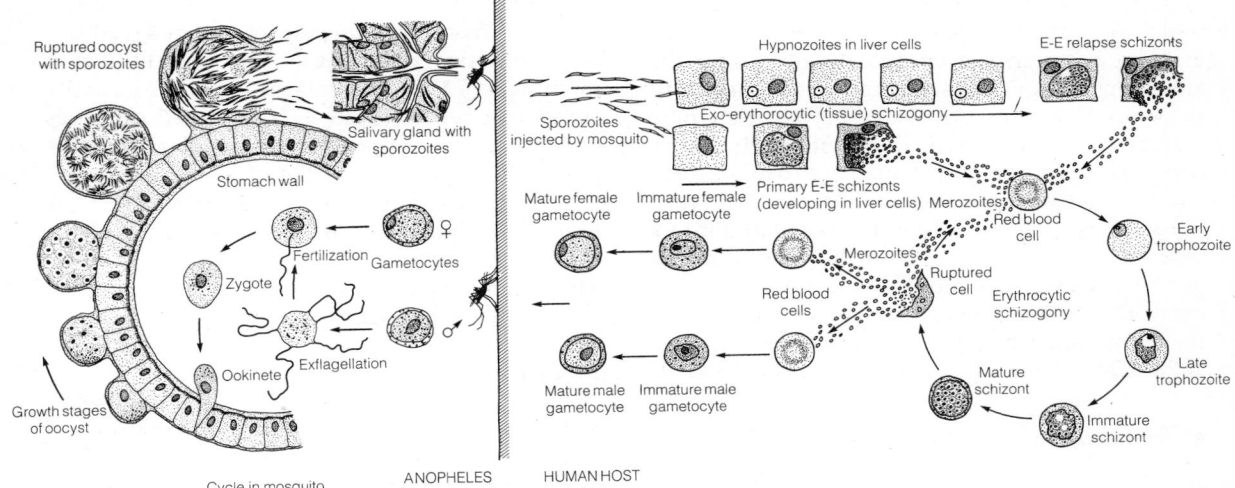

Fig. 1.2   The life-cycle of malaria parasites in the mosquito and in the human host. (After Bruce-Chwatt.[1])

rupture the liver cells and invade the circulation, where they enter red cells by a process of invagination (see erythrocytic phase). The *prepatent period* is the time from infection until the appearance of parasites in the blood and varies with the species of parasite: *P. vivax* 6–8 days, *P. malariae* 12–16 days, *P. ovale* 9 days and *P. falciparum* 5½–7 days.

EXO-ERYTHROCYTIC SCHIZOGONY[5]
(Fig. I.3, p. 1229)
In *P. vivax* and *P. ovale* malaria some of the exo-erythrocytic schizonts lie dormant and are known as *hypnozoites*. After periods of up to 250 days they become active and mature, allowing merozoites to infect red cells and give rise to an erythrocytic phase. This is the mechanism responsible for delayed prepatent periods and relapses in vivax and ovale malaria.

ERYTHROCYTIC PHASE (Fig. I.6, p. 1230)
To enter the red cell the merozoite binds to glycophorin, the major erythrocytic glycoprotein, which is specific for a particular species of parasite (see section on natural immunity, p. 12. The apex of the merozoite releases a substance which forms a deep pit in the surface of the red cell and, maintaining contact by a contact ring, the merozoite is enveloped by the red cell in a vacuole (parasitophorous vacuole) in which it is enclosed. In the red cell the merozoites develop into *ring forms* which grow in size to *trophozoites* absorbing haemoglobin leaving a pigment (*haematin*) or *haemazoin*—a combination of haemoglobin with protein which can be seen as dark granules. The trophozoite multiplies by schizogony dividing

into a number of small merozoites varying with the species to form a mature *schizont*. The merozoites are released by rupture of the red cell membrane and enter new red cells, particularly young red cells.

The erythrocytic phase, called *schizogonic periodicity*, which differs according to the species of parasite, is responsible for the febrile paroxysms. These are variable according to the species of parasite: In *P. vivax* and *P. ovale* 48 hours, *P. malariae* 72 hours and in *P. falciparum* about 48 hours. In the early stages of infection there may be several broods of parasites developing at different times so that there is no regular periodicity, but with the development of immunity the periodicity settles down and becomes regular.

GAMETOGONY
After a period some merozoites give rise to two sexually differentiated forms of *gametocytes*—male (*microgamete*) and female (*macrogamete*)—which differ in morphology in the different species of parasite. These gametocytes are taken up by female anopheline mosquitoes and they undergo further development.

Sexual phase in anopheline mosquitoes (Figs. 1.2 and I.4, p. 1229)

In the stomach of the mosquito the female mosquito forms a macrogamete and the male a microgamete. The male gamete nucleus divides and forms a number of long, slender, thread-like structures or flagellae (*exflagellation*). These enter the female gamete and fuse to form a *zygote*, which becoming mobile as an *oökinete* and penetrating between the epithelial cells lining the stomach, comes to rest on the outer surface of the stomach wall to form an *oöcyst*, of which there may be several hundreds in one stomach. In the *oöcyst* a large number of slender sporozoites form which burst out into the body cavity and enter the salivary glands ready to be inoculated into a new host at the next blood meal. The duration of the cycle in the mosquito is known as the external incubation period. It varies according to the temperature being 8–10 days at 28°C, 16 days at 20°C and cannot be completed under 15°C.

Morphology

P. vivax (Plate I.8–11)

The *ring stage* has a vacuole surrounded by a loop of thin cytoplasm and a small round nucleus. The ring enlarges after a few hours, becomes amoeboid and forms a trophozoite (Plate I.8–10) and minute grains of light brown pigment appear in the cytoplasm. The red cell enlarges and becomes pale containing tiny spots known as Schüffner's dots which stain red (Plate I.16). After 24 hours the nucleus subdivides into daughter nuclei forming a mature *schizont*, which is the *rosette* stage with eight to 24 (usually 12–18) merozoites (Plate I.11). Total duration of the stage is 48 hours.

Gametocytes appear about 5 days after the schizonts and a fully grown gametocyte occupies the whole red cell measuring 10–11 μm. The female stains bright blue and the male grey (Plate II.1).

P. ovale (Plate I.1–4)

The morphology resembles that of *P. vivax*. The red cell is oval with fimbriated edges and shows dots which stain more deeply and are called James' dots (Plate I.1–3). The rosette form contains six to 12 (usually eight) merozoites (Plate I.4). The cycle is slightly longer than that of vivax 49–50 hours.

The gametocytes resemble those of vivax but are smaller, about 9 μm, and have a lilac colour.

P. malariae (Plates I.5–7 and II.3)

Young rings are rare in the peripheral blood. Trophozoites are seen in both mature and young red cells. They are amoeboid, and *band forms* reaching from side to side of the red cell are characteristic (Plate I.6). The rosette which matures at 72 hours contains six to 12 (usually eight) merozoites (Plate I.7). The red cell does not enlarge but produces a characteristic stippling (Ziemann's dots) (Plate I.17).

Gametocytes appear after 5–23 days. The male has a large nucleus which stains pink and the cytoplasm greenish grey. The female resembles a large schizont and is spherical, about 7 μm, with a deep blue cytoplasm.

P. falciparum (Plate I.12–15)

P. falciparum attacks both young and mature red cells but invades young cells to a greater extent.[6] The rings are small (1.2 μm) and hair-like with thin cytoplasm and a prominent nucleus, which may be double, and a vacuole. Multiple infection of red cells is common (Plates I.12 and II.2). Only ring forms are found in the blood and the appearance of schizonts (Plate I.13) is a feature of serious disease, only found in non-immune persons. The red cell is unaltered in size but may show spots (Maurer's spots, Plate I.18). The rosette contains eight to 32 (usually eight to 18) merozoites (Plate I.13).

Gametocytes are elongated and crescent-shaped (crescents). They appear after 8–11 days in waves rising and falling for many weeks. If a first attack is aborted by treatment gametocytes appear in the blood in enormous numbers 10–14 days later (Plate I.14 and 15). (For a more detailed description of morphology and life-cycle see Appendix I, p. 1227.)

TRANSMISSION

Transmission by mosquitoes

In nature malaria is transmitted from man to man by female anopheline mosquitoes (only the female takes a blood meal). Only some 60 species are important vectors and are found most frequently in tropical and subtropical regions below 2000–2500 metres. There are twelve geographical zones in the world each with its own vector species (Table III. 4, p. 1406) with different habitats so that an environment which would be malarious in one area is not necessarily so in another. The most important zone is the Afrotropical where malaria is most deeply entrenched and where the major vector *Anopheles gambiae*

(Fig III. 28, p. 1413) and its sibling species occupy many different habitats and are extremely efficient vectors.

The male anopheline feeds on fruit juices and the female on blood, needing at least two blood meals before the first batch of eggs can be laid. Transmission depends upon the presence of gametocytes in the blood and their infectivity for mosquitoes. Infection is high early in the parasitaemia but falls abruptly when schizogony begins, probably because antibodies are formed. In endemic areas small children are the most prolific source of infective gametocytes. (For further details of *Anopheles* mosquitoes, their species and biology see Appendix III, p. 1413, and Table III. 4, p. 1406.)

Transmission other than by mosquitoes

Malaria can, however, be transmitted in other ways: by design or by accident, by the inoculation of blood from an infected person to a healthy person. In this way the asexual blood forms continue to develop in their own periodicities in the peripheral blood producing attacks of fever in the recipients, but pre-erythrocytic schizonts are not formed in the liver because these forms originate only from sporozoites inoculated by mosquitoes. Malaria transmitted by inoculation of blood has a shorter incubation period than sporozoite-induced infection and relapses do not occur. Nevertheless, *P. falciparum* infections transmitted in this way can be fatal.

There are three chief means by which such transmission is effected.

1 *Therapeutic inoculation*

Malaria, usually *P. vivax*, has been used in the treatment of neurosyphilis and other species have been used.

2 *Transfusion malaria*[7]

Transfusion malaria is particularly common in countries where blood donation is a commercial transaction and where blood donors come from the less affluent classes who may reside in endemic malarious areas, or who may recently have left them.

INFECTIVITY OF DONORS
Infection usually dies out in *P. falciparum* in one year, *P. vivax* and *P. ovale* in three years but *P. malariae* may remain in the blood for as long

as 50 years. *P. vivax* has been transmitted by transfusion from donors infected four years before,[8] *P. malariae* from donors infected 17 years before and *P. falciparum* was present in the blood of donors exposed 20 months to three years earlier.[9,10] The subject of transfusion malaria and other diseases has been well reviewed.[11]

CLINICAL ASPECTS OF TRANSFUSION MALARIA
Most infections occur when the blood has been stored for less than 5 days and infection with blood stored for two weeks or more is exceptional. Stored plasma is safe. Infections are frequently caused by *P. vivax* and *P. falciparum*, but *P. malariae* is also important because of its chronicity and the difficulty in detecting it. The symptoms of accidental infection with *P. falciparum* develop within 10 days, *P. vivax* 16 days and *P. malariae* 40 days, or longer. When any patient who has received a blood transfusion up to three months previously develops an unexplained fever, malaria must be suspected.

PREVENTION
Screening of donors. Examination of the blood for parasites is not usually successful but serological screening with the indirect fluorescent antibody test (IFAT) or enzyme-linked immunosorbent assay (ELISA) will show past infection, though not necessarily that the donor is infective. In non-malarious countries persons excluded from giving whole blood should include all those who have had a confirmed malarial or suspected febrile illness within a year of leaving an endemic area. Travellers not born in an endemic area who have spent only a short time in a malarious area may be accepted.

In malarious countries non-immune recipients should receive the standard three-day course of chloroquine at the time of transfusion. In chloroquine-resistant areas quinine and Fansidar should be given to recipients (see p. 31).

3 *Syringe-transmitted malaria*

Unintentional infection is common in drug addicts who share syringes and needles and some cases of *P. falciparum* infection with deaths have been recorded.

Congenital malaria

Intrauterine transmission of infection from mother to child is well established.[12] The placenta in *P. falciparum* malaria becomes heavily parasitized during the first pregnancy because it lacks the immunity possessed by the mother (see section on malaria in pregnancy, p. 25). The placenta is normally an effective barrier but congenital infection can occur without demonstrable damage to the placenta before delivery. All species of parasite may be involved. Transplacental infection is far commoner in non-immune mothers than among indigenous populations for the reason that passive immunity is transferred across the placenta to the infant who remains free of infection for some six months (see p. 15). Out of 20 Gambian mothers, 18 had high antimalarial titres and their infants also had high titres[13] but no infant had parasitaemia.

Congenital *P. vivax* and *P. malariae* infection has been reported from the UK[14] and a double congenital infection with *P. vivax* and *P. malariae* has been reported from California.[15]

PATHOLOGY

The invasion of the red cells by parasites is common to all types of malaria, and their subsequent destruction and obstruction of small vessels resulting from damage to the endothelium and consequent tissue anoxia is a feature of *P. falciparum* only. An immunopathological mechanism is responsible for some of the anaemia and for malarial nephrosis.

Fever

The pathogenesis of fever is little understood but toxic products of the parasite may release endogenous pyrogens from leukocytes. These pyrogens act on the hypothalamus to release prostaglandins which act upon the posterior hypothalamus to stimulate the sympathetic nerves to contract blood vessels and decrease heat dissipation, resulting in the classical rigor.

Blockage of small vessels and tissue anoxia in *P. falciparum*

Stickiness of the erythrocytes and adhesion to the capillary endothelium with obstruction of the small vessels ('sludging') is important but *stasis* is most important. Loss of fluid from the vessels, whilst important in some animal models, is not a major factor in human disease.

Cerebral malaria

The pathogenesis of cerebral malaria is complex and still incompletely understood. The pathological changes seen in the brain, blocking of the capillaries with parasitized red cells and necrotic lesions in the cerebral tissue, are brought about by stasis in the cerebral circulation with anaerobic glycolysis and lactic acidosis. Cerebral anoxia has not been demonstrated in man, oedema is not characteristic and the genesis of the ring haemorrhages, seen in some cases only, is not understood. The evidence for an immunopathological mechanism in cerebral malaria is poor. The cause of *coma* in cerebral malaria is unknown and cerebral oedema is no longer thought to be the cause.[16]

Anaemia (see also Chapter 58)

A rapidly increasing anaemia is a feature of *P. falciparum* malaria and severe anaemia following malaria is most commonly seen in endemic areas in young children under five years of age and in pregnant women (see p. 26). It is also seen in populations where there is unstable malaria (see section on epidemiology, p. 44), and sometimes in non-immune adults who contract malaria when it may accompany renal failure where other mechanisms may operate.

The pathogenesis of this anaemia has not been fully worked out but three main mechanisms have been suggested. Haemolysis of parasitized red cells, haemolysis of non-parasitized red cells, and dyserythropoiesis.

HAEMOLYSIS OF PARASITIZED RED CELLS
Haemolysis occurs when the trophozoites mature into schizonts which release merozoites by bursting the red cells and releasing them into the bloodstream to infect fresh red cells. This is not the only mechanism since anaemia persists longer than would be expected after waning of the parasitaemia.

HAEMOLYSIS OF NON-PARASITIZED RED CELLS
Immune haemolysis involving the adherence of circulating antigen–antibody complexes to the surface of the erythrocyte has been suggested as a cause of the severe anaemia in malaria, but although the direct antiglobulin test has been found to be positive in children with malaria in some populations, there is no evidence that this

is a cause of haemolysis of non-parasitized red cells.[17]

DYSERYTHROPOIESIS
There is increasing evidence of significant dyserythropoiesis during the acute malarial attack and impairment of marrow function has also been proposed as a mechanism for the slow recovery from anaemia following malaria. This is thought to be due to hypocellularity of the marrow and decreased iron incorporation.[18]

Blackwater fever

This is a condition characterized by severe haemolysis during an attack of malaria with massive intravascular haemolysis and haemoglobinaemia and haemoglobinuria (see section on blackwater fever, p. 19).

Thrombocytopenia

Thrombocytopenia may be caused by an immune mechanism[19] or by hypersplenism (see section on tropical splenomegaly, p. 22).

Clotting defects

Thrombocytopenia is common with a deficiency in prothrombin[20] and can cause coagulation defects.[21] As a result of blood coagulation and fibrinolysis related to the capillary lesions there can be a rapid fall in plasma fibrinogen which may be of importance,[22] but the clinical significance of disseminated intravascular coagulation (DIC) is disputed. Therapeutic measures directed towards the DIC are seldom helpful and if heparin is used may be harmful.

Hypoglycaemia and lactic acidosis

These disorders may occur in severe falciparum malaria. Red cells parasitized by mature parasites consume vastly more glucose than unparasitized ones and since they are held in abundance in deep-seated capillaries they contribute to the hypoglycaemia with anaerobic glycolysis and lactic acidosis. Hypoglycaemia may also be precipitated by quinine-induced insulin secretion.[23]

Serum potassium

The serum potassium rises during the fever as a result of red cell destruction.

Liver

In acute malaria the liver is enlarged and congested by parasitized red cells in the sinusoids and centrilobular veins, as well as by swollen parenchymal and Kupffer's cells. The organ is

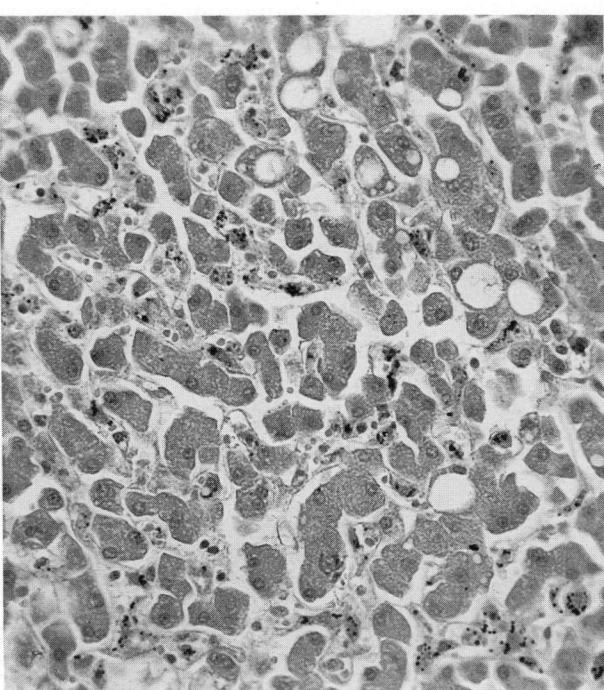

Fig. 1.3 The liver from a patient with falciparum malaria, showing cloudy swelling and fatty degeneration with intracellular malarial pigment.

soft, dark chocolate red (or yellowish and fatty) or slate grey or black from much pigment in the Kupffer's cells. Centrilobular necrosis may occur in severe falciparum infections (Fig. 1.3).

Jaundice

The pathological changes in the liver affect liver function and there is an increase in serum bilirubin and liver enzymes, although there may be little clinical evidence of liver dysfunction. The increase in bilirubin has been attributed to impairment in bilirubin transport because of reticuloendothelial blockage and disturbance of hepatocyte microvilli. Mild jaundice of both haemolytic and hepatocellular origin is common. Deep jaundice is rare although severe jaundice with liver and renal failure (hepatorenal syndrome) occurs in severe falciparum malaria.

As children in hyperendemic areas lose their inherited passive immunity they acquire repeated new infections and there is a phase of hypertrophy of macrophages in the liver and spleen, and large amounts of malarial pigment are deposited in the Kupffer's cells throughout the liver. Damage to the parenchymal cells at this stage is unusual. As immunity develops the attacks decline, the stimulation of phagocytosis decreases and the amount of pigment is reduced. Much pigment is carried away but some remains until adult life. The hypertrophy and hyperplasia of the Kupffer's cells remain and there is an increase in fine reticulin fibres in the portal tracts but a true cirrhosis does not develop. These changes lead to liver enlargement in adult life.[24]

Spleen

The spleen enlarges early in *P. vivax* and *P. falciparum* but later in quartan malaria. The size varies with the duration and degree of exposure to superinfection but it may be very large, weighing up to 800 g in the acute stage. In the acute stage it is tender and may rupture, especially during the primary attack (*P. vivax*) in non-immune persons. Infarcts occur and the pedicle may become twisted. The surface of the spleen is dark red and soft in the acute stage, congested with haemorrhages and thromboses, and sometimes with adhesions. There is reticulo-endothelial hyperplasia, the macrophages lining the sinusoids containing numerous parasitized and non-parasitized red cells. Blood flow through the spleen is impeded and hypersplenism may be one of the factors in the destruction of red cells and platelets causing anaemia and thrombocytopenia.

Kidneys

FALCIPARUM MALARIA
Renal failure occurs in falciparum malaria but is usually caused by extrarenal factors which may lead to cortical ischaemia or tubular necrosis. Immune complexes cause an acute and reversible syndrome with deposits of immunoglobulin (mainly IgM), antigen and complement in the glomerular capillaries which clear rapidly with antimalarial treatment.

QUARTAN (*P. MALARIAE*) MALARIA
The effect of *P. malariae* on the kidneys is controversial. In Nigeria a 'quartan malarial neph-

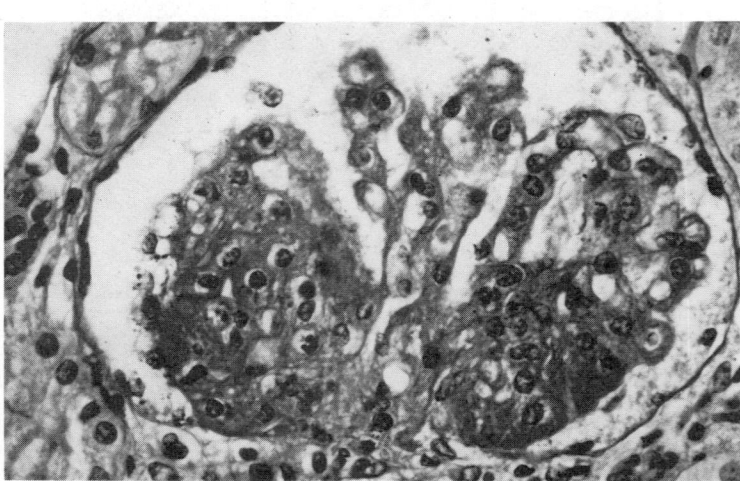

Fig. 1.4 *P. malariae*. Quartan malaria nephrotic syndrome. Glomerulus showing diffuse plexiform thickening of the capillary walls without mesangial expansion or proliferation.
(Courtesy of Professor Hendrickse.)

rotic syndrome' has been described,[25] a chronic progressive lesion with the deposition of coarse and fine deposits of immunoglobulins (IgG and IgM) containing malarial antigen in the glomerular capillary walls, which becomes irregularly thickened and twisted (Fig. 1.4). Electron micrographs show an irregular basement membrane with many lacunae. These changes do not respond to antimalarial or immunosuppressive drugs and are accompanied by persistent albuminuria, decreasing renàl function and hypertension.

Studies in other parts of West Africa have not confirmed the association of these changes with quartan malaria and suggest that the IgM is non-specific and the result of other infections (e.g. *Schistosoma mansoni*, see Chapter 22).

Central nervous system in P. falciparum

The capillaries and small vessels of the brain and meninges are congested and blocked with parasitized erythrocytes (Fig. 1.5).

Occlusion of the capillaries of the cortex is sometimes accompanied by ring haemorrhages around the blocked small vessels and petechial haemorrhages in the subcortical white matter of the cerebrum, cerebellum and brain stem; these are the so-called 'rosette' formations (Fig. 1.6).

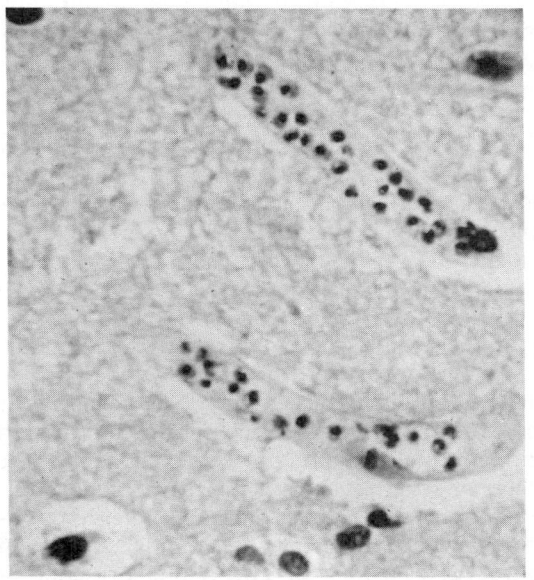

Fig. 1.5 Section from the brain of a patient with cerebral malaria, showing masses of malaria pigment in the capillaries.

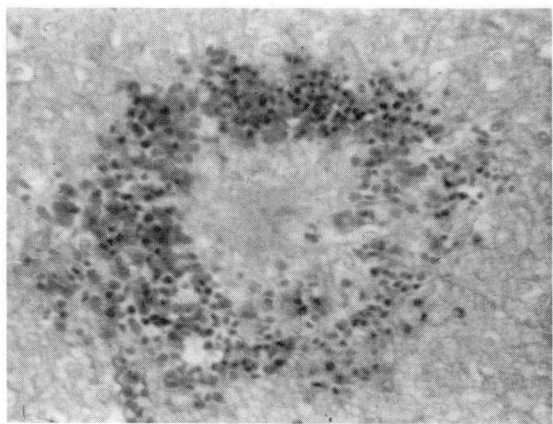

Fig. 1.6 Brain section from a patient with cerebral malaria showing the classical rosette formation caused by the extravasation of erythrocytes into the brain substance. Some of the erythrocytes appear to be parasitized.

Necrotic lesions in the mid-zonal cerebral tissue with glial reaction around an occluded capillary form the so-called 'malarial' granulomas.

Lungs

Pulmonary oedema, sometimes precipitated by fluid overload (malarial shock lung) may be found; there may also be septal oedema, endothelial cell swelling and hyaline membrane formation within the alveoli.

Other organs

At post-mortem the adrenals may be congested with haemorrhages. The *heart* is affected by the general circulatory change. The *gastrointestinal* tract may be packed with parasites in any part leading to oedema, haemorrhage and even ulceration.

Placenta

The placenta is severely affected in pregnancy. In primiparous women its function may be so impaired that abortion results and the first-born infants show low birth weights. The maternal spaces are packed with erythrocytes containing segmenting forms of the parasite and lymphoid macrophage cells loaded with parasites. There is much pigment. On the fetal side of the barrier the vessels are entirely free of parasites. In subsequent pregnancies the effect of immunity lowers the number of parasites and placental function improves (see sections on malaria in pregnancy, p. 25, and congenital malaria, p. 7).

IMMUNITY

Immunity in malaria is being extensively studied and new findings constantly reported. Immunity may be natural or acquired.

Natural immunity

This is most obvious since man is not susceptible to infection by the malaria parasites of birds or rodents and only to some of the malaria parasites of other primates, for instance *P. inui*, *P. brasilianum*, *P. eylesi*, *P. cynomolgi*, *P. cynomolgi bastianellii*, *P. simium*, *P. shortii* and *P. knowlesi*.[26, 27] It is also seen in the fact that each species of malaria parasite will develop fully only in a narrow range of invertebrate genera—the parasites of man only in *Anopheles*. The explanation of this insusceptibility of man to some animal parasites is not clear; it probably lies in differences in biochemical constitution of the various host species.

Natural immunity acts upon both the sexual and asexual erythrocytic stages as well as the tissue stages. The mechanisms involved are humoral and contain red cell factors. Natural humoral immunity is shown when tissue stages become established in the liver but are unable to infect the erythrocytes, a process that can be reversed by splenectomy, which can render certain animals susceptible to parasites to which they are normally resistant.

Natural (innate) immunity is based upon red cell factors which have been studied by epidemiological and clinical methods[28] and in vitro by the culture of *P. falciparum* parasites, although experimental results from in vitro studies should be interpreted with caution.[29]

The mechanism of natural resistance of the red cell to infection is complex. There are two possible mechanisms: cellular factors which prevent penetration and development of the parasite in the red cell (specific receptors, G-6-PD deficiency, HbF) and susceptibility of the parasitized cells to removal from the circulation by the lymphoid-macrophage system (HbS).

Specific factors preventing penetration of the red cell[29, 30]

There is a high specificity of certain parasites for the red cells of different species which involves receptors on the red cell which are recognized by the merozoites. Human red cells lacking the *Duffy* blood group are not invaded by the merozoites of *P. vivax* thus accounting for the rarity of vivax malaria in West African and American Negroes who lack this blood group.[31] *P. ovale*, however, unlike *P. vivax* can enter the red cells of Duffy-negative individuals.[32] Glycophorin A, the main human red cell membrane glycoprotein, is the main receptor for *P. falciparum* and red cells lacking this protein will not be invaded.

Sickle cell haemoglobin (HbS)

The high incidence of haemoglobin S in Africa and other parts of the world is attributed to a hypothesis of 'balanced polymorphism' in which the heterozygote, HbAS carriers, are protected against the severe effects of malaria in infancy and so have a survival advantage. Malarial parasites do not grow well in cells containing HbS because of the sickling which occurs under low oxygen tension which allows removal from the circulation by the spleen and reticuloendothelial system. Other physical mechanisms important may be a decrease in intracellular pH, deoxygenated haemoglobin, leakage of potassium and rigidity of the cell wall in cells containing HbAS.

Ovalocytosis

Ovalocytosis is a common red cell abnormality in the coastal regions of New Guinea and these red cells are resistant to penetration by *P. falciparum*.[33]

Fetal haemoglobin (HbF)

Fetal haemoglobin is found in newborn infants, hereditary persistence of fetal haemoglobin in adult life and in β thalassaemia. Newborn infants possess HbF in the blood which in conjunction with maternal antibody protects them against the effects of severe malaria. Hereditary persistence of HbF into adult life is common in Negro populations where heterozygotes carry 25% and homozygotes 100% of HbF. The presence of HbF in β thalassaemia heterozygotes has been shown to protect against falciparum malaria[34] and the number of parasites is reduced in culture in cells containing HbF.[35]

Haemoglobin C

There is no direct evidence of any protective effect in HbAC heterozygotes.

Haemoglobin E

Studies in Thailand where Hbe is common have shown no protective effect for HbAE heterozygotes.[33]

Glucose-6-phosphate dehydrogenase (G-6-PD) deficiency

There is confusing evidence of the protective effect of G-6-PD-deficient red cells against malaria but there is general acceptance that there is some protective effect.

Acquired immunity

Acquired immunity may be active or passive.

Passive immunity

Passive immunity is transferred from mother to child by IgG antibodies which cross the placenta and produce congenital or neonatal immunity which persists for up to six months of age. It is an important mechanism in hyperendemic malarious areas protecting the newborn child against severe attacks of malaria (see section on congenital malaria, p. 7).

Active immunity

Little is known about active immunity in *P. vivax*, *P. ovale* or *P. malariae* infection. It is not important in the epidemiology of these infections and apart from the nephrosis found in *P. malariae* in children there are no immunopathological effects. Acquired active immunity in falciparum malaria is stage and species specific; both humoral and cellular mechanisms are involved and act in concert. Antibodies deal with extracellular parasites, and cell-mediated mechanisms mediated by T cells with intracellular parasites. Malarial parasites are susceptible at three stages: sporozoite, merozoite and gametocyte.

SPOROZOITES

Active immunity against sporozoites is not induced since they are present in the circulation for such a short time, but artificial immunity can be produced. Antibodies to the sporozoite surface antigen prevent access to the liver cell limiting the number of sporozoites which gain access; once inside the cell the exo-erythrocytic schizont is destroyed by cytotoxic T cells.[36]

MEROZOITES

Merozoite antigens which bind to receptors on the surface of the red cells induce B cells to make antibodies which prevent the merozoites entering fresh red cells and stop them multiplying. Cellular mechanisms activate macrophages which will kill the intra-erythrocytic parasites with oxidative products.

GAMETOCYTES

Gametocytes induce antibodies in the serum which when ingested into the mosquito's stomach will prevent gamete fusion.[37]

IgG, IgA and IgM antibodies appear shortly after parasitaemia develops, the IgG persisting much longer than the others. These antibodies can be detected in sera by fluorescent, immunoprecipitation and ELISA techniques (see section on diagnosis, p. 28). Only a small proportion of IgG antibody is protective.

Role of the spleen in immunity

The spleen is all important in the adaptation of the immune process and its removal will convert an occult or mild infection to a severe one and render individuals susceptible to species of malaria to which they are normally resistant, since it traps cells and removes parasites. Its function is to form and circulate both T and B lymphocytes so that specificity for individual antigens is formed and remembered.

Short-term and long-term relapse

Immunity acts against merozoites in the blood only and prevents infection of new red cells and a continuation of illness and parasitaemia. However, in *P. vivax* and *P. ovale* infection new merozoites are released from the *hypnozoites* in the liver, which cause a long-term relapse until they are dealt with by a fresh immune response and a rise in the clinical threshold (Fig. 1.7).

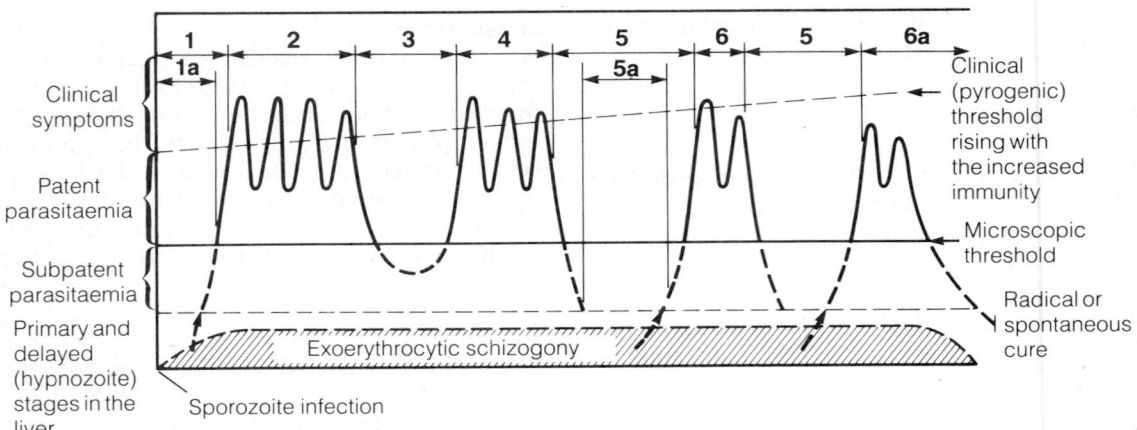

Fig. 1.7   Phases of malaria infection showing short-term and long-term relapses. 1: Incubation period. 2: Primary attack composed of paroxysms. 3: Latent period (clinical latency). 4: Short-term relapse. 5: Latent period. 5a: Parasitic latency. 6: Long-term relapse followed by parasitic relapse. 6a: Parasitic relapse.

In *P. falciparum* infection where there are no persistent liver stages a short-term relapse may occur but the infection dies out in a few months and fresh antigenic stimuli derive from new merozoites released from fresh mosquito-borne infections. In *P. malariae*, erythrocytic stages can persist safe from immune attack in internal organs for many years. Short-term relapses occur with any change in the immune response.

Antigens

Antigens important in the development of artificial immunization are present in sporozoites and the blood stages of the parasite. Anti-gametocyte antibodies developed in the vertebrate host will prevent further development in the mosquito.

Sporozoite antigens

Sporozoites possess some antigens common to the erythrocytic stages of the same species but the surface antigens which are the most important are stage and species specific.

One major protective surface antigen (circumsporozoite protein, CSP) has been identified, composed of polypeptides with a well-defined molecular weight. The DNA has been cloned and it should be feasible to produce it in quantity by DNA recombinant methods (see section on vaccination, p. 42).

Schizont and merozoite antigens

Several classes of antigens have been identified on the surface of mature schizonts in the red cell which have been located in knobs on the surface membrane of the infected red cell. Merozoite antigens have been identified which bind to the surface receptors on the surface of the red cell before entry of the parasite into the cell. A number of soluble fractions have been identified according to their resistance to heat: L (labile), R (resistant) and S (stable). S antigens characterize the strain of parasite and L antigens are related to immunity. Only S antigens appear in the blood in acute falciparum malaria and denote severity of the infection. They disappear in a few days.

Antigens of gametes, zygotes and oökinetes

These antigens induce antibodies in the vertebrate host which act against the extracellular parasites in the mosquito gut to produce 'transmission blocking immunity'.[38]

Cross immunity

There is a large amount of cross immunity between different areas and immune sera from one area (West Africa) can be effective in suppressing reaction to the parasites of another area (East Africa).[39] No difference was observed between infection developed by semi-immunes when challenged with the local Liberian strain of *P. falciparum* and strains from 400 km away.[40] However, in splenectomized chimpanzees immune human gamma globulin protected against West African falciparum but not against South-East Asian falciparum.[41]

Immunosuppression[42]

Most, but not all, immune responses can be suppressed by malaria, antibody responses more than cell-mediated responses, the newly initiated responses being most susceptible. Immunosuppression is heaviest at the time of parasitaemia and removal of parasites from the blood is attended by return to normal. The mechanism is probably by activation of suppressor T cells which affect lymphoid and non-lymphoid elements involved in immunity.

Immunosuppression plays an important part in the severity of virus (measles) and other infections to which children are especially susceptible between the ages of six months and two years, during which they show periods of heavy parasitaemia while they acquire their immunity to malaria. Immunosuppression is also important in pregnancy (see section on malaria in pregnancy, p. 25).

Effects of immunity

The newborn child is protected from infection in hyperendemic areas by transplacental transfer of protective antibodies and by immune substances in the maternal milk as well as deficiency of para-aminobenzoic acid (PABA) in the milk which is necessary for the full metabolism of the erythrocytic stages. From six months to two years of age the child is exposed to the full effects of malaria and the children acquire immunity at a high cost of recurrent illness and death, in some areas perhaps up to 50% in the first five years of life. In conditions of hyperendemic malaria the population has acquired much immunity with low parasitaemia (premunition) and low spleen rates, except in children. This leads to frequent but low sporozoite infections in the mosquitoes because they cannot pick up enough infection except from the children to form heavy infections.

A large number of non-immunes entering an endemic area will develop high parasitaemias which in turn cause the mosquitoes which feed on them to develop heavy sporozoite loads. The resulting increase in size of the infective doses may be enough to swamp the immunity of the local population causing symptomatic malaria in them and an apparent epidemic. Some adults who live apparently healthy lives in their own area may react with fever when they move to another area where the infecting doses of sporozoites are heavier.

The immunity gained can be lost if the person leaves the endemic area for a long period: students from West Africa who stay in Europe for several years may suffer severe attacks of malaria on returning to West Africa and it may be necessary for them to resort to chemoprophylaxis.

If complete eradication of malaria is not possible, as is the case at the present time in large areas of tropical Africa, the question arises whether some degree of malaria control short of eradication should be attempted. If the numbers of infective bites are reduced to the extent that holoendemic malaria becomes mesoendemic, or if drug prophylaxis on a large scale is carried out inefficiently, or breaks down, in such an area the resistance of adult persons is reduced and epidemics may be expected if conditions of transmission suddenly expand, for instance as a result of excessive rainfall or other climatic change. If, on the other hand, infection is interfered with only to the extent that fever in children is treated with just enough antimalarial drugs to prevent death and no more, and mosquito control is not attempted, their immunity is gradually built up and epidemics do not occur. Observations in East Africa[43, 44] have shown that a policy of this kind is readily accepted by the population who quickly learn to take feverish children for treatment. It entails the setting up of easily accessible dispensaries.

On the other hand, it has been said that if mosquito control short of eradication is attempted, by using modern insecticides, and if epidemics do occur, we have the means to deal with them. How far this is true in places where drug-resistant *P. falciparum* exists remains to be seen.

CLINICAL FEATURES OF MALARIA IN GENERAL

The clinical course of malaria consists of intermittent repeated courses of fever alternating with periods of freedom from any symptoms.

Incubation period

This is the number of days covering the time between infection and the first appearance of clinical signs (fever) and varies with the different species of malaria.

Prepatent period

This is the number of days between infection and the first appearance of parasites in the blood.

Fever

Malarial fever is characteristic and is usually preceded by some premonitory symptoms and consists of three stages.

1   The *cold stage* starts with shivering and rigor (chattering of the teeth and shaking of the bed) and a feeling of intense cold and lasts from one-quarter to one hour.

2   The *hot stage* follows. The feeling of cold is replaced by one of intense heat with a dry burning skin, headache, nausea and vomiting. The temperature rises up to 40–41°C. This stage lasts 2–6 hours.

3   The *sweating stage* follows. Profuse sweating soaks the bedclothes and is accompanied by a fall in temperature often to normal. The patient falls asleep and wakes feeling better but weak. This stage lasts 2–4 hours.

The whole febrile paroxysm lasts from 8 to 12 hours.

The periodic febrile response is caused by rupture of the red cell by mature schizonts and discharge of merozoites into the blood and varies with the different species of parasite. An intermittent type of fever is not present in the early stages of a primary attack since the different broods of merozoites are not synchronized.

Long-term relapse is the term used for renewal of symptoms after a long latent period and is due to release of merozoites from an exo-erythrocytic source in the liver.

Short-term relapse is the term used for a recurrence of symptoms following a primary attack caused by the survival of erythrocytic forms in the body (it is also called 'recrudescence').

CLINICAL FEATURES OF *P. FALCIPARUM* MALARIA

P. falciparum malaria is the most dangerous of the four malarial parasites. The erythrocytic stages rapidly multiply the number of parasitized cells and schizogony occurs in the deep organs.

Natural history

The natural history of falciparum malaria is very variable. In the *non-immune* a primary attack can be rapidly fatal whereas in the *immune* adult residents of an endemic area parasitaemia may be accompanied by no fever or illness. In the absence of new infection falciparum malaria dies out after two years whereas in endemic areas where reinfection regularly takes place, a comparatively healthy life can be maintained in the face of intense sporozoite attack.

Falciparum malaria in the non-immune

P. falciparum infection is characterized by fever, rapidly developing anaemia and the appearance of a number of 'pernicious' forms.

Incubation period

The incubation period varies from 9 to 14 days with an average of 12 days.

Symptoms and signs

Symptoms and signs may be very variable and are relatively slight in the first 3 or 4 days when there may be little or no fever, following which there is an onset of fever with headache, pains in the back and joints, and nausea and vomiting or mild diarrhoea, which may be so non-specific that the disease may not be suspected in people who have returned home from a short trip to an endemic area.

Primary infection

FEVER

In the primary infection the fever is irregular and shows no distinct patterns or periodicity (Fig. 1.8) but becomes intermittent in a short-term relapse (Fig. 1.9). The fever starts as a quotidian rise of temperature becoming tertian or subtertian at a later period (Fig. 1.10) when the parasite broods have synchronized, but is never so regular as in vivax malaria. Hyperpyrexia with temperature above 40°C is not uncommon. The pulse is relatively slow at first but rapid when a rigor occurs.

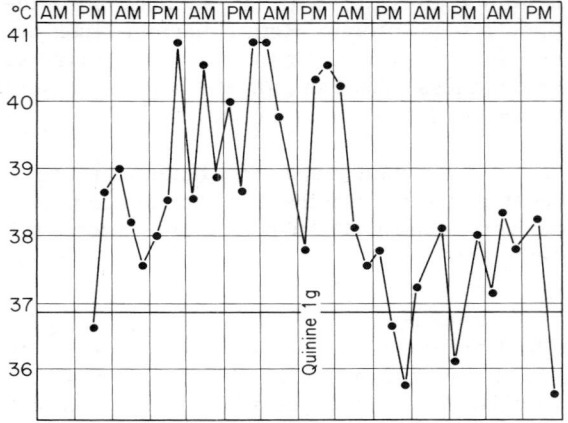

Fig. 1.8   A primary aborted attack of *P. falciparum* malaria.

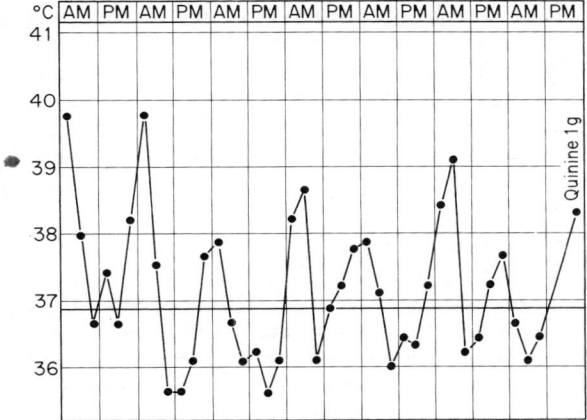

Fig. 1.9   First recrudescence ten days after a primary attack
of *P. falciparum* malaria.

The *spleen* often shows some degree of enlargement but malaria must not be excluded because the spleen is not palpable.

The *liver* becomes enlarged and there may be slight *jaundice*. The urine may contain albumin, hyaline casts and an excess of urobilinogen.

ANAEMIA

Anaemia of a haemolytic type is an important feature of falciparum malaria. It often develops early in a primary attack. There may also be a steady fall in haemoglobin and for two to three weeks after treatment has started.

In recurrent acute malaria in the non-immune (e.g. infants from six months to two years of age in hyperendemic areas) anaemia is severe and occurs with each successive bout of fever. There is no immediate reticulocytosis but complete haematological recovery follows satisfactory antimalarial treatment. Malaria is the main cause of the anaemia so widespread in this age group in hyperendemic areas. In severe falciparum malaria intravascular haemolysis with haemoglobinuria may occur. In general in falciparum malaria there is a leukopenia and monocytosis.

If treatment is not given promptly the symptoms of '*pernicious*' malaria appear quickly after 5–6 days when severe complications may develop suddenly without warning and are caused by an increase in the number of parasites in the blood.

PARASITAEMIA

Falciparum parasites may be distinguished in the blood by the presence only of rings (the presence of schizonts denotes a bad prognosis). Infections

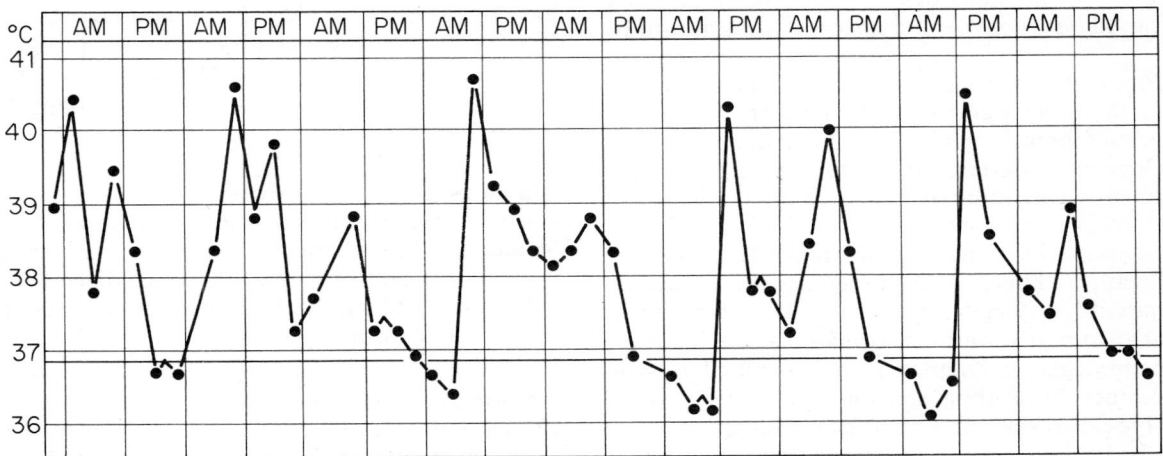

Fig. 1.10   The course of the subtertian fever in *P. falciparum* malaria.

are often heavy with more than one ring in a single red cell (Fig. 1.11 and Plate II.2). When more than 5% of the red cells are parasitized the condition is almost invariably fatal in the absence of immediate skilled treatment but cases with 30% parasitaemia have been saved with modern intensive care.

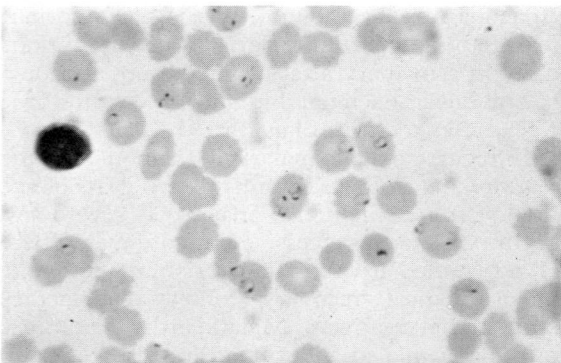

Fig. 1.11 Pernicious malaria. Heavy *P. falciparum* infection.

Parasite counts are an important feature of the management of a case of falciparum malaria. Gametocytes are often not found in primary attacks—mainly in immune and semi-immune children and in adults, usually without illness, often in the absence of other forms of parasite.

Pernicious falciparum malaria may take a number of forms: cerebral, algid, hepatorenal and gastrointestinal.

CEREBRAL MALARIA
The clinical signs of cerebral malaria are very varied but all involve some loss of consciousness.

Prodromal signs. Changes in behaviour may occur in the early stages and excitement, mania and coma follow. Any non-immune patient with falciparum malaria who shows a change in personality should be treated as cerebral malaria.

Cerebral signs. The signs are those of an encephalopathy. There may be epileptiform attacks (possibly associated with hypoglycaemia), signs of meningitis, various forms of acute insanity, hemiplegia, monoplegia and cerebellar syndromes, all leading up to a state of deep coma. Hyperpyrexia (simulating heat hyperpyrexia) is a bad sign. Cerebral malaria has a mortality rate of 20% even with good medical care. The CSF

is under pressure with an increase in lymphocytes and protein. Retinal haemorrhages are not uncommon (see Chapter 70), are a sign of vascular lesions and an indication of severity and therefore of prognostic significance.[45]

Sequelae. Permanent sequelae (hemiplegia, cerebellar ataxia and deafness) are rare and complete recovery almost invariably follows successful treatment.

ALGID MALARIA
Algid malaria is rare. It results from an overwhelming infection with collapse and peripheral vascular failure and resembles surgical shock. The skin is pale, cold and clammy, the breathing shallow, the pulse rapid and weak, and blood pressure low. The temperature is below normal. Death can follow in a few hours. Developing schizonts are often present in the peripheral blood where they are a bad sign. The cause may be failure of the suprarenals (see section on pathogenesis, p. 18), but there is recent evidence to implicate a complicating gram-negative septicaemia.

HEPATORENAL SYNDROME
Severe falciparum malaria is one of the causes of jaundice with renal failure. Although more than 50% of patients with severe falciparum malaria have raised blood urea and serum creatinine levels, the cause is usually pre-renal. In those 5–10% who have true renal failure the cause is acute tubular necrosis due to impaired renal perfusion, due either to hypovolaemia or reduction in the renal microcirculation with inadequate central blood volume. The old term 'bilious remittent fever' refers to the persistent hiccup, profuse vomiting of bile and altered blood, with watery stools, enlargement of the liver and jaundice which may be deep.

GASTROINTESTINAL SYMPTOMS
Gastrointestinal symptoms may imitate cholera (choleraic), but whether malaria can cause true dysentery is doubtful. Profuse water diarrhoea, muscular cramps and dehydration are features of the choleraic form.

PULMONARY SYMPTOMS
Cough and mild bronchitis are common in the early stages but pulmonary oedema (malaria shock syndrome) which most commonly occurs

on the second or third day after the start of treatment is a grave complication.

HYPOGLYCAEMIA

Severe recurrent hypoglycaemia may occur especially in pregnancy (see section on malaria in pregnancy, p. 26).

SPLENIC RUPTURE

Splenic rupture in acute malaria in a primary attack is rare and causes severe internal haemorrhage. There is often a short latent period; pain referred to the tip of the left shoulder is present in a small proportion of cases, with radiological changes in the left base of the lung to help in diagnosis.

Short-term relapse

Short-term relapses occur mostly up to one year, rarely up to two and very rarely up to four years after the primary infection. After the first pre-erythrocytic liver schizont there are no hypnozoite forms in *P. falciparum* so that true long-term relapses from persistent hypnozoites, as found in *P. vivax* and *P. ovale* are not found. It has been said that *stress* will provoke attacks of fever in persons with latent *P. falciparum* infection but short-term relapses were not provoked in West African volunteers by intravenous adrenaline,[46] physical stress or electroconvulsive therapy. Relapse may, however, follow trauma such as fracture of the femur or a major surgical operation or even air flights.

Falciparum malaria in the immune and semi-immune

Falciparum malaria in the immune causes little or no symptoms, although during the rainy season in a hyperendemic area occasional bouts of fever and parasitaemia lasting a day or two may occur, from which recovery occurs spontaneously. In the semi-immune in areas of unstable malaria sharper attacks occur during the period of maximum transmission and cause short periods of illness which affects the capacity to work.

Malarial cachexia is applied to a group of physical signs, the result of repeated attacks of malaria in areas where malaria is unstable. The signs are anaemia, sometimes with jaundice and enlargement of the liver and spleen. In children growth may be stunted and puberty delayed (see section on malaria in children, p. 26).

Splenomegaly

Splenomegaly is a feature of a state of semi-immunity and is responsible for the 'spleen rate' (see section on epidemiology, p. 43). Rupture of a chronically enlarged spleen from a blow on the abdomen is a recognized hazard in endemic malarious areas.

Hepatomegaly

Chronic enlargement of the liver is a not infrequent sequel of malaria which results from an increase in malarial pigment and some fine fibrosis in the portal tracts (see section on pathology, p. 10). Two major complications of falciparum malaria are blackwater fever and tropical splenomegaly.

BLACKWATER FEVER (MALARIAL HAEMOGLOBINURIA)

Geographical distribution

The geographical distribution of blackwater fever corresponds with that of holoendemic and hyperendemic falciparum malaria. Formerly it was common in areas of stable malaria where transmission is perennial and was unknown in unstable areas where the transmission season is short.

Aetiology

Blackwater fever affects only those individuals who are non- or semi-immune or those immune individuals who have lost their immunity by residence in a non-malarious area. Exposure to severe and long continued attacks of *P. falciparum* malaria is the cause (no other species are responsible) and the condition is comparable to an exacerbation of the intravascular haemolysis seen in severe falciparum malaria, although only scanty parasites may be seen in the blood.

The trigger mechanism, according to traditional views, is irregular dosage with quinine associated with exposure to cold or excessive physical exertion but there is little evidence to support this.

It is noteworthy that blackwater fever has

almost completely disappeared since the replacement of quinine by modern antimalarial drugs used for chemoprophylaxis, although there have been reports of blackwater fever after mepacrine administration.

Pathogenesis

The pathogenesis has been clarified by Maegraith.[47, 48] There is a sudden extensive intravascular haemolysis caused by an abnormal immune reaction brought about by changes in the antigenic structure of the red cell brought about by the parasite. This stimulates the production of antibodies to the red cell in an autoimmune reaction which with the addition of complement leads to haemolysis. Sensitivity to quinine may play a part. The fundamental cause of the renal failure is vascular similar to the renal shutdown found in surgical and obstetric shock and crush injury, which are reversible.

Pathology

There is a rapid *haemolysis* of both parasitized and non-parasitized red cells which may be so great that the red cell count may fall to 1×10^{12}/litre or less in a few hours. This may occur once or recur periodically at intervals of hours or days. The haemoglobin released combines with albumin to form methaemalbumin which is unable to pass the glomerular membrane and is excreted as methaemoglobin. Both conjugated and unconjugated serum bilirubin levels are raised.

Renal function

Renal function is affected at all stages of the disease with a rise in blood urea, nitrogen and creatinine, and renal failure is a common cause of death. The fundamental lesion is a renal vasoconstriction with a shunt at the junction of the cortex and medulla causing cortical and peripheral glomerular ischaemia, with marked tubular changes.[47] The combination of reduced glomerular filtration and excessive tubular reabsorption finally results in anuria.

Anaemia

Anaemia is severe. There are no changes in the red cells and malaria parasites are scanty or absent after haemolysis has begun. Because of haemoconcentration the red cell count bears little relation to the amount of blood destroyed, and the amount of haemoglobin in the serum makes estimation of the haemoglobin unreliable.

Immunity

Although the cause is thought to be an autoimmune mechanism autoantibodies cannot be detected by the antiglobulin Coombs' test. One attack of blackwater predisposes to a second. More than two attacks have been noted in 20% and 16 is the largest number recorded.

Clinical features

Natural history

The intravascular haemolysis may be slight or so severe as to lead to death from renal failure and anaemia. After recovery there is a susceptibility to further attacks and according to popular opinion in the past when a man has recovered from two attacks, the third is generally fatal.

Symptoms and signs

There is a history of residence in a holo- or hyperendemic area of several months or more, during which time there have been several attacks of falciparum malaria and a *pre-blackwater stage* may be recognized with symptoms of persistent headache, pains in the limbs and back, and ill-health in between the attacks. (Patients with high fever and marked parasitaemia do not develop blackwater fever.)

The *onset* is sudden with headache, nausea and bilious vomiting with severe pains in the loins and prostration.

Fever rises up to 39.4°C with a rigor either continuous or remittent. Occasionally there is hyperpyrexia.

Haemolysis may occur only once or be repeated every few days lasting from a few hours to several days with clear intervals.

During haemolysis the *urine* is dark red to almost black and contains methaemoglobin. There is a heavy albuminuria. On standing the urine settles into two layers: a bulky lower layer containing brown-grey sediment, in which there may be tubular casts, and an upper clearer layer. In acid urine, methaemoglobin is brown or black, and in alkaline urine, red.

Jaundice is a cardinal sign, is haemolytic in nature and moderate at first, but deepens later.

The *liver* becomes enlarged and tender and severe hepatic failure with persistent hiccup may develop and is a grave sign. The spleen is enlarged and tender.

In *moderate* cases the haemolysis may cease after the first attack, urinary flow is restored and the patient recovers.

In *severe* cases the polyuria persists, the urine becoming very dark and then more and more scanty until finally there is complete anuria and eventual death from peripheral vascular failure.

Diagnosis

Haemoglobinuria associated with fever and a rigor followed by severe anaemia, jaundice and vomiting in a patient exposed to falciparum malaria is suggestive of blackwater fever, but there are other causes of acute intravascular haemolysis which must be considered.

Quinine may induce mild haemolysis unaccompanied by fever or serious illness.

8–Aminoquinolines (primaquine) may induce haemolysis in G-6-PD deficiency and this must be excluded before a diagnosis of blackwater fever is made. Other causes of intravascular haemolysis are paroxysmal haemoglobinuria and favism. Haemoglobinuria must be distinguished from haematuria in *Schistosoma haematobium* and from heavy bilirubinuria. The liver enlargement and intense jaundice with fever may resemble Weil's disease, yellow fever or viral hepatitis.

Treatment

Treatment is directed towards renal failure and anaemia. The patient should be moved to a centre where help is available. If malaria parasites are present in the blood, an antimalarial drug should be given, chloroquine or even quinine intravenously or orally (see section on treatment of falciparum malaria, p. 33).

Renal failure

Since the renal failure is due to reversible renal anoxia correct management is very important. Renal failure must be suspected when the 24-hour output of urine falls to 400 ml and the serum creatinine rises to 12 mg/dl. Many cases can be treated conservatively by attention to fluid balance and electrolyte measures. When the blood urea reaches 170–200 mg/dl then renal dialysis must be considered.

Renal dialysis can be life-saving and if haemodialysis is not available then peritoneal dialysis must be used (see Section XVII). In Vietnam intermittent peritoneal dialysis has been continued for 120 hours and high blood urea and creatinine levels were cleared across the peritoneal membrane successfully.

Anaemia

Blood transfusion can be life-saving. If the red cell count falls below 2×10^{12}/litre, transfusion of blood, or better of packed red cells, must be given slowly with due care being paid to the central venous pressure. Care in cross-matching is essential.

Prognosis

Some cases are so mild that they are unattended with any risk. The chance of survival depends upon the number of nephrons which have escaped. Formerly, in Nigeria and Algeria the mortality was as high as 50% but the average was 25%.

Sequelae

Permanent renal insufficiency is very rare. Pigment stones may form quite soon (three weeks) after cessation of the disease.

Epidemiology

Formerly the disease occurred in non-immune (mostly expatriate) long-term residents of tropical Africa who took irregular doses of quinine and with often inadequate personal prophylaxis. More recently immune indigenous residents of the tropics, especially West Africa, who have lost their immunity by residence of two or three years in a non-malarious area or in a city where there is little or no transmission, have developed blackwater fever on return to their homes in a holo- or hyperendemic malarious area.

Control

Modern advances in the prevention of malaria and modern chemoprophylactic drugs in place of quinine have banished blackwater fever from its previous haunts and it has almost completely disappeared since 1944. With drug resistance and the reappearance of quinine as a popular drug, it may return.

TROPICAL SPLENOMEGALY (TSS, BIG SPLEEN DISEASE)

The term tropical splenomegaly syndrome was originally coined for cases of gross splenomegaly in the tropics for which no other cause could be found. Since then, one form of chronic spleno-megaly specifically related to malaria has been identified to which the term has been given. This form of splenomegaly results from an abnormal immunological response to malaria and must be distinguished from the usual splenomegaly associated with the acquisition of immunity in hyperendemic malarious areas.

Geographical distribution

TSS occurs mainly in tropical Africa, Nigeria, Sudan, Uganda, Zambia and Zaire but also in parts of New Guinea and Vietnam. It is usually found in the indigenous inhabitants of these areas but cases in Caucasian expatriates have been described from Zambia.[49, 50]

Aetiology

It is now generally accepted that malaria is intimately involved in the causation of TSS and not any one particular species is involved. There is a high malarial antibody titre in every case and the disease is found only where malaria is endemic. It occurs in only a few adults in malarious areas where the malarial splenomegaly of childhood usually regresses as immunity develops, so that some other factor is involved. This factor is an abnormal immunological response with malaria as the stimulus. Immune complexes are formed leading to stimulation of B lymphocytes and an over-production of IgM[51] from the inhibition of suppressor T cells.[52]

Pathology (for reviews see Ref. 53)

There is a massive splenic enlargement of more than 10 cm below the left costal margin. There are the following features.
1 Characteristic changes in the liver with sinusoidal dilatation, infiltration with lymphocytes and hyperplasia of the Kupffer's cells with phagocytosis of cellular debris and red cells (see Fig. 60.4(b), p. 1008).
2 Hyperglobulinaemia due to an increase in polyclonal IgM (but not IgG) with cryo-globulinaemia, a reduced C3 and the presence of rheumatoid factor without joint changes.
3 The massively enlarged spleen shows dilated sinusoids lined with reticulum cells showing marked erythrophagocytosis with lymphocytic infiltration of the pulp.
4 Characteristic blood changes. Normocytic normochromic anaemia not responsive to hae-matinics or deworming. There is a shortened red cell life-span due to sequestration in the spleen and the red cell pool is greatly increased. The reticulocyte count is raised. The plasma volume is increased caused by haemodilution and there may be lymphocytic infiltration of the bone marrow. Leukopenia and thrombocytopenia are caused by sequestration in the spleen.

Clinical features

Natural history

The condition is essentially chronic and benign although there is sometimes a severe anaemia and an increased susceptibility to secondary infection. The advanced results of portal hypertension do not develop and the condition is reversible.

Symptoms and signs

These arise during adult life. The patient complains of the enlarging spleen but otherwise few symptoms. The spleen is massively enlarged and firm (Fig. 60.4(a), p. 1008). There is a normo-chromic normocytic anaemia with leukopenia and thrombocytopenia. In advanced cases there may be wasting.

Diagnosis

There are many other causes of massive spleno-megaly in the tropics. Criteria for the diagnosis of TSS are immunity to malaria, raised serum IgM concentration, response to antimalarial drugs and hepatic sinusoidal lymphocytosis on liver biopsy (Fig. 60.4(b), p. 1008).[53]

Malarial parasites are not found in the peripheral blood. In many cases of splenomegaly in the tropics no cause may be found. Specific causes are kala-azar (Chapter 4), hepatosplenic schistosomiasis and Symmers' fibrosis (Chapter

22), post-necrotic cirrhosis of the liver (Chapter 60), thalassaemia (Chapter 58), and the obscure tropical splenomegaly in which oesophageal varices and gastrointestinal bleeding are prominent features.[54] The cardinal signs which differentiate TSS are:

a high titre of malarial antibody,

serum IgM at least two standard deviations above the local mean, hepatic sinusoidal lymphocytosis, and

a significant lowering of IgM and malarial antibody titre within three months of continuous antimalarial therapy.

Treatment

Treatment may not be necessary for patients who have adapted well to the condition but for those with disabling symptoms due to anaemia or the size and weight of the spleen in whom there is no response to chemotherapy, splenectomy may be advisable. However, it must always be followed by permanent malaria chemoprophylaxis since without chemotherapy splenectomy may be fatal.

It should be remembered that splenectomy is likely to interfere seriously with the immune processes which protect against malaria and other dangerous infections; it should not be undertaken lightly. Chemotherapy also interferes with immunity to malaria but often gives good results and should be tried before splenectomy is considered. A course of 100 mg proguanil daily has been advocated, continued for long periods, possibly for life; other antimalarials may be tried. Blood transfusion may be needed for the anaemia but with care not to overload the circulation in patients who already have increased blood volume and enlarged hearts. The response to treatment may differ in different parts of the world.

CLINICAL FEATURES OF *P. VIVAX* MALARIA (BENIGN TERTIAN, BT)

Natural history

P. vivax is a chronic relapsing infection which if untreated relapses usually for three years but can do so for eight years before dying out. Since little immunity develops there is not a great variation in the severity of the infection, which is not a fatal disease (benign tertian). The duration, number and periods of relapse vary with different strains of the parasite.

Incubation period

The incubation period is usually between 12 and 17 days but may be prolonged for 8–10 months, especially if chemoprophylaxis has been used.

Symptoms and signs

The primary attack begins with headache, pains in the back and joints, nausea and general malaise, which is more marked than in *P. falciparum*.

Fever

The fever is irregular for 2–4 days before becoming intermittent with marked swings between morning and evening. At first there is no regularity (Fig. 1.12) but after synchronization of the

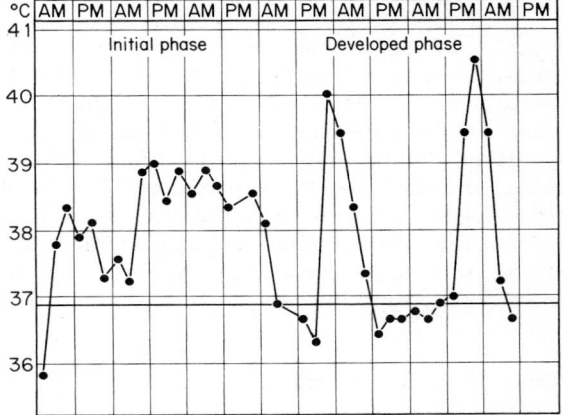

Fig. 1.12 Initial phase and development of *P. vivax* malaria.

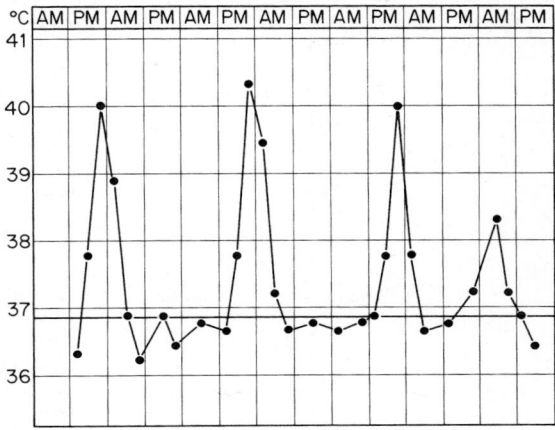

Fig. 1.13 First relapse after *P. vivax* infection, followed by spontaneous recovery.

different broods of parasites a 48-hour period (tertian) becomes established (Fig. 1.13). Paroxysms occur chiefly in the afternoon with the classical cold, hot and sweating stages, the temperature rising to 40.6°C. Exceptionally, the periodicity may be quotidian with a double infection. Although dizziness and drowsiness may occur, serious symptoms of cerebral involvement do not, and no 'pernicious' complications occur.

Splenomegaly

Enlargement of the spleen is characteristic of *P. vivax* infection and aids diagnosis. Rupture may occur as the result of an accident. The liver does not typically enlarge and there is usually no jaundice. There is only a febrile proteinuria. Haemolytic anaemia is common.

Parasitaemia

During the early phase of the primary attack parasites are scanty in the peripheral blood but are common (rings, trophozoites and schizonts) when tertian periodicity has been established. Rings may be found in the greatest number just before the rigor stage of a paroxysm. Gametocytes appear one week after the primary attack. Vivax rings can be distinguished from other species of malaria parasite by the large size of the red cell, stippling of the cytoplasm and the presence of rings, trophozoites and schizonts in the peripheral blood (Plates I.8–11 and II.1).

Long-term relapses

Long-term relapses are characteristic of *P. vivax* and *P. ovale* and are caused by activation of the hypnozoites in the liver. A single untreated attack lasts a week or more with repeated paroxysms every 48 hours. In about 60% of untreated cases clinical symptoms recur after a period of latency which varies with the strain of parasite. There are striking differences in the relapse pattern in vivax infections in different parts of the world. In some temperate parts where over-wintering or 'hibernation' must have occurred to allow the existence of the parasite to continue the incidence of vivax malaria in the past showed a peak in the spring composed of long-term relapses and delayed primary infections, and another peak in summer of new primary infections (Table 1.1).[55]

There are three different patterns: Type III has been recognized as a subspecies, *P. vivax hibernans*. Tropical strains show a short latency with frequent relapses.

CLINICAL FEATURES OF *P. OVALE* MALARIA (OVALE MALARIA)

The clinical picture resembles that of *P. vivax*

Table 1.1 Distribution of *P. vivax* Types I, II and III and characteristic patterns of infection.

Type	Incubation period	Prolonged latency	Relapses	Names of strains	Reported distribution	Transmission
I	Short, 12–20 days	No	Frequent, at short intervals	Chesson	New Guinea Vietnam West Malaysia	Perennial
II	Short, 12–20 days	Yes, 7–13 months	After one or more periods of prolonged latency	St Elizabeth Madagascar Nakhitchevan Volgograd	USA* USSR* Bulgaria* Italy* Romania* Yugoslavia* Madagascar	Seasonal
III	Long, 6–9 months	Yes, 7–13 months	After delayed primary attack or subsequent prolonged latency	Kolomenski Navoflominski	Netherlands* Sweden* Finland* USSR*	Seasonal

* With the recession of the range of *P. vivax*, strains of Types II and III have disappeared from all these areas
After World Health Organization.[55]

malaria. Relapses are much less and spontaneous recovery after a short period is usual.

Ovale parasites may be distinguished by the oval shape of the red cell (Plate I.1–4) and the dense and compact form of the trophozoites

CLINICAL FEATURES OF QUARTAN MALARIA (*P. MALARIAE*)

Natural history

This is a mild infection with a characteristic quartan (72 hours) periodicity of fever in an established infection. Although there are no hypnozoite forms in the liver to produce relapses, recrudescences may occur for periods up to 50 years due to a persisting low parasitaemia.

Incubation period

The incubation period is never less than 18 days and can be as long as 30–40 days.

Symptoms and signs

The primary attack resembles that of *P. vivax* malaria but the rigors may be more severe. After the initial attack of fever the paroxysms settle down to a quartan periodicity of 72 hours (Fig. 1.14).

Splenomegaly is frequent and may be pronounced. The liver is not usually enlarged and there is seldom jaundice.

Anaemia is less pronounced than in other forms of malaria. There are no pernicious forms. The kidneys are not involved in non-immune

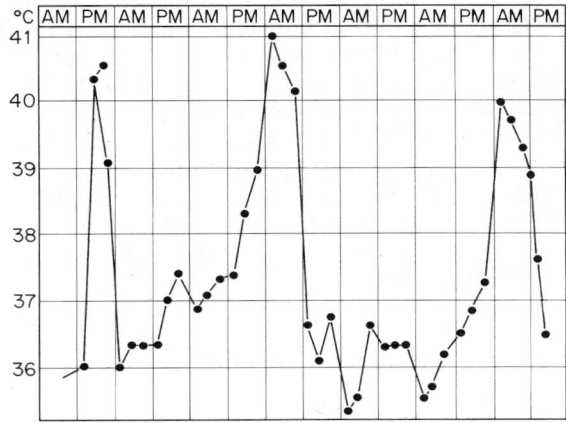

Fig. 1.14 Course of the fever in quartan malaria.

persons and quartan malaria nephrosis is confined to 'immune' children (see section on malaria in children, p. 26).

Although quartan malaria is essentially benign it may cause chronic ill-health with recurrent attacks of fever, malaise, headaches, lassitude and sweating, and in a series of non-African patients in Uganda, fluorescent antibody tests using blood heavily infected with *P. malariae* as antigen were strongly positive, although no parasites could ever be demonstrated.[56] Treatment with chloroquinine relieved symptoms and titres thereafter declined.

Parasitaemia

Quartan rings may be distinguished by the presence of rings, trophozoites and schizonts in the peripheral blood (Plate I.5–7) and the presence of 'band forms' (Plate I.6). The red cells are not enlarged and parasites are usually scanty, not more than 1% of the red cells being affected.

Recrudescences

P. malariae recrudescences are common in the first year and then follow at long intervals occurring up to 52 years later when parasites may appear in the blood with few, if any, classical symptoms.

MIXED INFECTIONS

Double infections with *P. vivax* and *P. falciparum* are common and give rise to some confusion when the ring stages of both parasites are present in the blood at the same time. Usually *P. vivax* is imposed on *P. falciparum* which suppresses it so that when the latter infection has subsided, a relapse of *P. vivax* may make its appearance after a lapse of six months, or even a year, and was commonly observed in soldiers from the Far East in both World Wars. Mixed infections of *P. vivax* and *P. malariae* which is suppressed are quite common in Sri Lanka and Malaya but *P. malariae*, although suppressed, survives longer.

MALARIA IN PREGNANCY (for treatment, see p. 34)

There is evidence of maternal immunosuppression in the second half of pregnancy which is caused by many factors: hormonal, placental and lymphocyte depression. The malaria infection itself has a marked immunosuppressive effect.

Effect on the mother

P. falciparum malaria is more hazardous in pregnancy with a high mortality affecting chiefly primigravidae, with hyperpyrexia and abortion occurring in the first trimester. A severe haemolytic anaemia with splenomegaly may develop in the second half of pregnancy which responds only to antimalarial treatment. All these effects can be prevented by chemoprophylaxis although non-pregnant women in hyperendemic areas can remain comparatively well without it. *Hypoglycaemia* has been found to be an important cause of illness and even death in pregnant patients.[23]

Effect on the fetus

In hyperendemic areas 47% of the placentas of primigravidae were heavily parasitized (see section on pathology, p. 11). There was no increase in stillbirths but the birth weight of the first-born infant was reduced, although succeeding infants were normal. Subsequent acquisition of immunity by the placenta after the first delivery accounted for this.[57] Transplacental infection of the fetus occurs only in non-immune mothers (see section on congenital malaria, p. 7).

MALARIA IN CHILDREN

P. falciparum

In children the classical features of the malarial paroxysms are not seen and the infection is usually very severe in non-immune children. The picture varies according to the degree of immunity.

Non-immune children

In primary attacks in non-immune infants and children many of the more usual features are masked. The child appears restless and drowsy and refuses food. As the temperature rises breastfed infants make frequent attempts to suckle because of thirst. Vomiting is often marked and the stools are loose. The *fever* may

be moderate but usually rises to 40°C and convulsions are common. Cerebral involvement must be suspected unless there is a rapid return of consciousness. The spleen enlarges but not for several days and the liver becomes enlarged, and jaundice is not uncommon. The very young infant may appear well in the morning and in coma by nightfall.

Semi-immune and immune children

In hyperendemic areas children, after an acquired primary infection, may show a low-grade parasitaemia with few symptoms. However, after six months as the effect of the transferred passive immunity wears off and until the age of five, the clinical attacks become severe and many die of cerebral malaria and other pernicious forms unless prompt treatment is available. After several attacks tolerance is acquired and the clinical effects become milder. Most children in hyperendemic areas in tropical Africa have enlarged spleens and livers with parasitaemia but no outward signs of disease other than anaemia, which is common and is at least partly due to malaria. In areas of unstable malaria children become stunted in growth and suffer from *malarial cachexia*.

P. vivax malaria

P. vivax is more classical in children and complications are uncommon.

Quartan malaria nephrosis (see also section on pathology, p. 10)

The *nephrotic syndrome* is associated with *P. malariae* infection in Guyana, Nigeria and East Africa[25] but not in New Guinea, Senegal or Ghana where other factors may be at work. The peak incidence is at four to five years of age. There is gross oedema, ascites, with massive proteinuria and severe hypoalbuminaemia but usually without azotaemia or hypertension. Neither antimalarial treatment nor steroids are helpful.[58,59] The prognosis is bad with eventual renal failure and death.

DIFFERENTIAL DIAGNOSIS

The differential diagnosis of malaria can be difficult since its manifestations are protean.

Two mistakes are commonly made. In early falciparum malaria (a potentially fatal condition) the possibility of malaria may not be considered because of a failure to elicit a history of travel. In the later stages an enlarged spleen may be confused with a number of conditions accompanied by splenomegaly and anaemia.

Acute falciparum malaria

The *fever* of malaria in a primary attack is not characteristic and therefore must be distinguished from a number of other conditions: virus infections, upper respiratory bronchitis, gastroenteritis, hepatitis A and arboviruses. When established and the paroxysms occur, then other febrile conditions in which rigors are prominent must be considered: bacterial septicaemia, urinary infections, gallstones and cholecystitis, kala-azar, typhoid, relapsing fever, miliary tuberculosis, amoebic liver abscess and African trypanosomiasis. (The whole subject is discussed under Fever, Chapter 56.)

Cerebral malaria must be distinguished from stroke, encephalitis and meningitis. The comatose state of falciparum malaria may be thought to be due to alcohol or diabetic coma and other toxic or metabolic states, with fatal results. Examination of the cerebrospinal fluid in a case thought to be cerebral malaria is important to exclude meningitis and relapsing fever. Minor increases in protein and cells may occur in cerebral malaria itself.

Anaemia and splenomegaly

Anaemia with splenomegaly is a presenting feature of many conditions. Chronic haemolytic anaemia of whatever cause (haemoglobinopathies), portal hypertension (*S. mansoni*, cirrhosis of the liver), kala-azar, reticuloses, leukaemia and lymphoma. Diagnosis often rests upon the exclusion of the other causes (see section on tropical splenomegaly, above) but a high titre of malarial antibody is often helpful.

DIAGNOSIS

Diagnosis entails the finding of malarial parasites in a peripheral blood smear while retrospective diagnosis can be made by serology. The most important part of establishing a diagnosis is to think of the possibility of malaria, especially in non-endemic countries to which a resident has returned after a stay in an endemic area. In these persons it is most important in every case of fever or acute illness, for which the cause is not obvious, to take a blood slide for examination and, if necessary, to start antimalarial treatment before the result is available. Since blood slides can be reported as negative even in severe cases of falciparum malaria it is important to monitor the effect of antimalarial treatment. In a non-immune person, if the temperature fails to respond to an adequately absorbed antimalarial drug after 5 days in the absence of any specific drug resistance, then the fever is not caused by malaria. In an immune individual in an endemic area, symptoms which do not respond after 24 hours' therapy are not due to malaria but some other cause.

Examination of the blood

Both thick and thin films should be prepared and examined, stained with Leishman's stain or Giemsa, which is preferable in the tropics. A rapid method is to use Field's stain (techniques of staining are described in Appendix I, p. 1237, and Appendix IV, p. 1495). Techniques of preparing blood films are described by Bruce-Chwatt.[1]

Identification of the parasites in blood films is a skill that should be acquired by everyone practising in the tropics. The presence of small rings often with a double nucleus in a thick film is normally sufficient for a diagnosis, but species identification may have to be made on a thin film which takes much longer (Appendix IV, p. 1496).

To follow the effect of treatment and to make a prognosis it is necessary to estimate the parasite count.

Parasite count

The absence of malarial parasites should not be reported until at least 200 fields of a thick film have been examined, and in doubtful cases blood films should be repeated at 4-hourly intervals.

The density of parasitaemia is measured in a thick film by counting the number of parasites and number of leukocytes in each field and, using the total white cell count, estimating the number of parasites per μl or mm^3. A convenient way of reporting is to use the following code:

+ 1–10 parasites per 100 thick fields examined;

+ + 11–100 parasites per 100 fields;
+ + + 1–10 parasites per field;
+ + + + more than 10 parasites per field.[1]

The intensity of infection is measured in a thin film in which the percentage of red cells parasitized is recorded.

Thick films give a quick diagnosis since a larger amount of blood is examined. The characteristics of the different species in a thick film can be distinguished[1] but can be more clearly distinguished in a thin film (see Fig. 1.11 and Plate II.2). Infection with *Babesia* (Fig. 1.19 and p. 48) may be mistaken for *P. falciparum* but the trophozoites characteristically show no pigment.

Serodiagnosis

Serological methods cannot replace the demonstration of parasites in the blood in the diagnosis of acute malaria but they are of value for the detection and measurement of specific antibodies, and detection of specific antigen in scanty parasitaemia with fluorescence. The main tests and the antigens used are as given in Table 1.2.

Table 1.2 Main tests and antigens used in serodiagnosis of malaria.

Test	Source of antigen	Antibodies identified
Immunofluorescence (IFAT)	Erythrocytic schizonts on a blood slide	IgG, IgM, IgA
Indirect haemagglutination (HA)	Antigen coated erythrocytes	IgG, IgM, IgA
Immunoprecipitation (gel diffusion)	Erythrocytic schizonts and soluble antigen	IgG, IgM
Enzyme-linked immunosorbent assay (ELISA)	Soluble antigens	IgG, IgM

After Bruce-Chwatt.[1]

Immunofluorescence (IFAT)

This is widely used and is suitable for diagnosis in individual patients. It is fairly specific but proper laboratory equipment is required. Antibodies are detectable within a few days of parasitaemia in a non-immune patient but low titres persist in *P. falciparum* and *P. vivax* for months or years. In *P. malariae* antibodies persist for much longer and can be useful for diagnosis between recrudescences.

Indirect haemagglutination (IHA)

The IHA test is easy to perform, requires the minimum of equipment and is suitable for the examination of a large number of sera under field conditions. Homologous antigens are best for higher sensitivity but false positives may occur. Antibodies are detectable before the infection becomes patent.

Immunoprecipitation (gel diffusion)

This test is easy to perform on large numbers of sera and a permanent record can be kept in the diffusion wells. The sensitivity is low and the test takes time but is especially useful in screening blood donors. It is also used for the detection of circulating soluble antigen (see p. 14).

Enzyme-linked immunosorbent assay (ELISA)

This test requires small quantities of antigen, is highly specific but only moderately sensitive, and less accurate than the IFAT. It is highly suitable for testing large numbers of samples under field conditions.

Radioimmunoassay

This method is used mainly for research.

Interpretation of serological tests

The early treatment of malaria in a non-immune patient produces a low level of antibody for a few weeks. With the IFAT, titres of 1/256 or above indicate recent infection, while titres of 1/20 and below are of no significance. Homologous antigens should be employed and in the absence of *P. vivax* and *P. malariae* antigen, *P. cynomolgi* (*P. vivax*) and *P. brasilianum* (*P. malariae*) or *P. fieldi* can be used.

Use of serological tests

In non-endemic areas

Serological tests should be used to screen blood donors, and exclude malaria in the diagnosis of patients with fever, anaemia, hepatosplenomegaly and the nephrotic syndrome in the absence of any parasites in the blood.

In endemic areas

Serological tests are very useful in sero-epidemiology, the establishment of age-specific indices, assessment of changes in transmission and the dilineation of foci of malaria.

TREATMENT

Drugs used in the treatment of malaria

Causal prophylactics are included under chemo-prophylaxis on p. 39. They include proguanil.

Schizonticidal drugs attack the parasite in the red cell in its asexual phase; *tissue schizonticidal* drugs act on the exo-erythrocytic or liver forms; *gametocytocidal* drugs act on the sexual forms (gametocytes) and *sporonticidal* drugs inhibit the development of oöcysts on the stomach wall of the mosquito so that no sporozoites are produced and the mosquito cannot transmit the infection.

Radical cure in the cases of *P. vivax* and *P. ovale* necessitates the use of a tissue schizonticidal drug to destroy the liver forms and prevent relapses. The action of the various drugs is shown in Fig. 1.15.

Quinine

Quinine, the oldest drug to be used against malaria, is now coming back into its own since the emergence of chloroquine resistance. It is used as quinine dihydrochloride (orally and par-enterally) and quinine sulphate (orally) in tablets of 300–650 mg or for injection 300 mg/ml. For adults the oral dose is 600 mg three times daily for 7 days.

PARENTERAL QUININE

Parenteral quinine is given intravenously. The dose is 600 mg every 8 or 12 hours in an intravenous drip of 500 ml over 4 hours.

Intramuscular quinine is usually avoided because of the danger of indolent abscesses. However, in some places, such as Thailand where drug resistance is marked, and health personnel short, it has been given successfully without abscess formation and satisfactory serum quinine concentrations were achieved.[60] It is active against the asexual forms but has no action on mature gametocytes of *P. falciparum* although it is effective against the gametocytes of *P. vivax* and *P. malariae*. It is particularly useful in cerebral and other pernicious forms of falciparum malaria where rapid clearance of the parasites is urgently needed. It is also mandatory in chloroquine-resistant malaria. The main side-effects are tinnitus, but others can occur (see Section XVII).

4-Aminoquinolines

CHLOROQUINE

Chloroquine phosphate (Aralen, Avloclor, Resochin) or chloroquine sulphate (Nivaquine) is

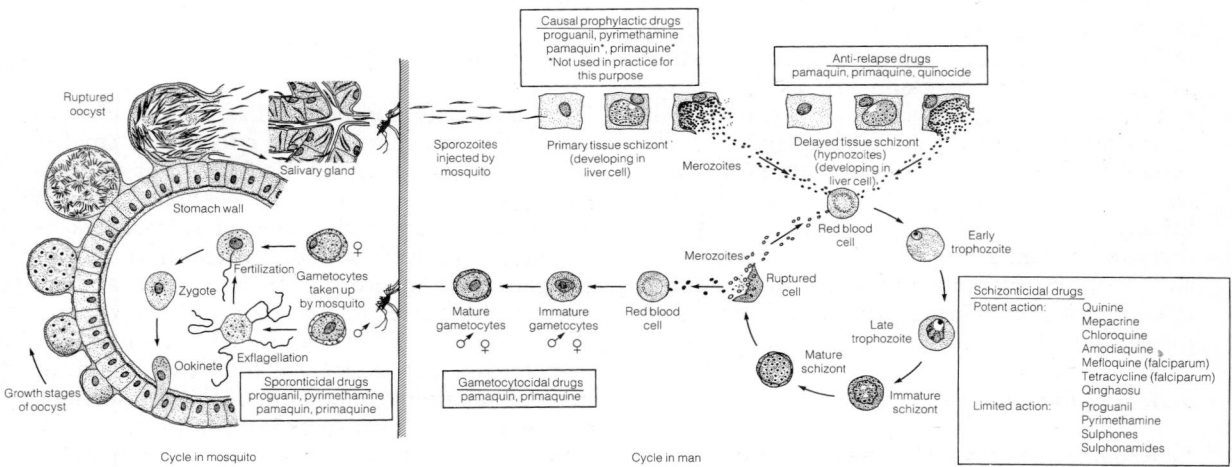

Fig. 1.15   Site of action of antimalarial drugs.

given in a total dose of 25 mg base/kg body weight over 3 days. It is given in a first immediate dose of 600 mg base (1000 mg phosphate or 800 mg sulphate) orally or half that dose parenterally.

It has a strong action on erythrocytic asexual parasites of all species and is the drug choice for acute attacks. It becomes highly concentrated in the cells of the liver and parasitized erythrocytes soon after administration. It has no action on the mature gametocytes of *P. falciparum* but does act against those of *P. vivax* and *P. malariae*. The first dose of 600 mg is usually enough for a mild attack of *P. falciparum* in a semi-immune individual. In non-immunes the first dose of 600 mg is followed after 6 hours by 300 mg, and then 300 mg daily for 2–4 days (occasionally more). The total dosage is 1500–2400 mg. It may be given in suppository form of 150–300 mg base in two to three times the oral dose. It can be given intravenously or intramuscularly in doses of 5 mg/kg base. Parenteral administration can be very dangerous in children because of the high peak blood levels achieved (see section on treatment in children, p. 34).

Side-effects are minimal (see Section XVII). Quinine and chloroquine should not be given simultaneously. Chloroquine resistance is now common and widespread (see section on drug resistance, p. 36).

AMODIAQUINE HYDROCHLORIDE (CAMOQUIN)

Amodiaquine is of great use in areas of chloroquine resistance and rapidly cleared asexual parasitaemia in Thailand where chloroquine was useless. It is given orally 600 mg followed by 400–600 mg base daily for 2–4 days to a total dose of 1.4–2.4 g. Agranulocytosis was reported from Papua New Guinea[61] and more recently, which has led to its abandonment as a chemoprophylactic drug; however, it is still used in treatment. Parenterally it has been used very successfully in severe falciparum malaria in Thailand where a loading dose of 10 mg base/kg infused intravenously over 4 hours, followed by three further infusions of 5 mg base/kg at 24, 48 and 72 hours, succeeded in the face of complete chloroquine resistance, but parasitaemia returned in half the cases.[62]

8-Aminoquinolines

Primaquine destroys the tissue forms (hypnozoites) in *P. vivax* and *P. ovale* malaria and so

is used to prevent true relapses. It is also active against the gametocytes of *P. falciparum* even in strains resistant to chloroquine and other drugs, and has been used in a single dose of 45 mg following treatment of *P. falciparum* malaria to prevent the spread of chloroquine resistance. Primaquine is given in 7.5 mg tablets—15 mg (two tablets) daily for 14 days, except in the south-west Pacific and Thailand where there is some primaquine resistance and 22.5 mg (three tablets) is given daily for 14 days. The main toxic effect is haemolysis of the red cells in G-6-PD-deficient individuals which may be dangerous in those from Asia and the Mediterranean, but not so severe in Negroes. An alternative course for these individuals is 30–45 mg primaquine once a week for eight weeks.

Dehydrofolate reductase inhibitors (proguanil, Paludrine, chlorguanide (USP))

Proguanil is no longer used in treatment. Its main action is on the liver stages of the parasite while it has less action on the erythrocytic forms but a pronounced antisporozoite activity in *P. falciparum*. It is not so effective against *P. vivax*. It is taken as 100 mg tablets by mouth; 200 mg daily is the effective chemoprophylactic dose in much of the tropical world. It causes no side-effects other than occasional heartburn.

Chlorproguanil (Lapudrine)

Lapudrine has similar properties to proguanil but persists in the blood for longer. It can be used once or twice a week as 20 mg in a single dose.

Pyrimethamine (Daraprim)

This antifolate compound has similar characteristics to proguanil but is effective in smaller doses and has a longer half-life. For chemoprophylaxis it is given once weekly in a dose of 50 mg. It is remarkably free of side-effects, is tasteless and well suited for children, but is dangerous in overdose. It has great activity against the tissue forms of *P. falciparum* and to a less extent *P. vivax*. It has a pronounced gametocytocidal effect so that the blood of persons taking pyrimethamine is non-infectious to mosquitoes. It prevents infection with *P. falciparum* malaria, except where resistance has developed. Resistance has developed in several parts of the world and there is cross resistance between proguanil and pyrimethamine.

Sulphonamides and sulphones

DIAMINODIPHENYL-SULPHONE (DDS, DAPSONE)

Dapsone has a slow schizonticidal effect. It is normally only used rarely as a chemoprophylactic, at a dose of 100 mg in combination with 12.5 mg pyrimethamine as *Maloprim* once a week. Cases of agranulocytosis have led to its greatly restricted use recently.

SULFADOXINE

Sulfadoxine has a long life (100–200 hours) in the serum. It is used in a dose of 500 mg sulfadoxine in combination with pyrimethamine 25 mg as *Fansidar*. Fansidar is less effective against *P. vivax* than *P. falciparum* and has a rare but serious side-effect in certain individuals of Stevens–Johnson syndrome or toxic epidermal necrolysis which contraindicates its use as a chemoprophylactic except under exceptional circumstances. It is used after a course of quinine in the treatment of chloroquine-resistant malaria.

Tetracycline

Tetracycline is a slow and uncertain schizonticide. It is used in non-pregnant women and adults at a dose of 1–2 g daily for 7 days following a course of quinine to prevent recrudescence of chloroquine-resistant *P. falciparum* infections.

Mefloquine

Mefloquine is a quinoline methanol drug and is highly effective as a schizonticide in chloroquine-resistant and chloroquine/pyrimethamine-resistant *P. falciparum* malaria and also against *P. vivax*. Side-effects are minimal and it is used therapeutically as a single dose of 1.0–1.5 g. It is also given in combination with Fansidar, known as *Fansimef*, in a single dose of two to three tablets. Mefloquine should not be used alone for chemoprophylaxis, but always in combination with another drug[63] to minimize the risk of resistance developing.

Qinghaosu (artemether)

Qinghaosu is the active malarial component of the Chinese herb *Artemisia annua*. It has the structure of a sesquiterpene lactone and is a very effective schizonticidal drug against chloroquine-resistant *P. falciparum* malaria and *P. vivax*.

There are two soluble derivatives: the methyl ether (*artemether*) and the hemisuccinate (*artesunate*); 900 mg of qinghaosu and 600 mg of artemether given intramuscularly in an oily solution over 3 days was highly effective against chloroquine-resistant *P. falciparum* malaria and also *P. vivax*. All three drugs have been used successfully in the treatment of cerebral malaria. Toxic effects, only found in high dosage in laboratory animals, include marrow and liver damage. Embryotoxicity has been reported in rats and mice so its use in pregnant women should be restricted to cases in which there is no alternative.[64]

Repository preparations

Cycloguanil embonate (Camolar, cycloguanil pamoate) exerts a long-term protection against *P. falciparum* and *P. vivax* up to a period of two to four months in the field. It is given as a single intramuscular injection suspended in oil of 5 mg/kg or 350 mg for a standard adult. Its use has been limited by the development of pyrimethamine- and proguanil-resistant strains which are cross resistant.

Quinidine

Quinidine is effective against *P. falciparum* and may be superior to quinine especially in Asia and Africa where strains of falciparum are more sensitive to quinidine than quinine.[65] It is given orally in a dose of 10 mg/kg (600 mg base) 8-hourly for 7 days. Intravenous quinidine gluconate has also proved more effective than quinine in the treatment of severe (cerebral) chloroquine-resistant falciparum malaria.[66] It is given as a loading dose of 15 mg base/kg in 250 ml of normal saline followed by 7.5 mg base/kg every 8 hours. ECG changes are common but there are no dysrhythmias. The blood pressure may fall during the initial infusion.

Other drugs

Other drugs which show antiparasite activity are under active development.[2] These are: phenanthrenemethanols, pyridinemethanols, triazines, acridines, pyronaridine, piperaquine, dabequine and naphthoquinones.

Clinical treatment of acute falciparum malaria

Non-immune

A primary attack of acute falciparum malaria in a non-immune individual is a medical emergency. A patient with fever who has left an endemic area, especially tropical Africa, within the incubation period of 9–14 days, and who shows no obvious cause for the fever, must be treated promptly without awaiting the result of the blood examination, unless this is available within an hour or two. If there are signs of a pernicious attack then treatment should be started immediately regardless of the result of the blood slide.

Two observations are critically important: the parasite count (see section on diagnosis, p. 27) and the sensitivity of falciparum malaria to chloroquine in the area where the infection has occurred. When in doubt quinine should be used.

Moderate or mild infections (parasite count 1/1000 RBCs or 5000/µl)

CHLOROQUINE

Adults should be given 25 mg/kg of chloroquine perorally in divided doses over a period of 3 days. Usually an adult is given 600 mg base (four tablets) followed 6 hours later by two tablets and then two tablets daily for the next 2–4 days, or longer if necessary. In cases of malabsorption or vomiting the drug can be given parenterally to adults: the first dose 300 mg base and then orally for the next 2 days. Absorption of the drug can be tested by testing the urine for chloroquine excretion (see p. 35). The parasite count should fall rapidly, becoming negative after 4 days. If this does not occur then chloroquine resistance (see p. 36) or an associated infection such as typhoid fever should be considered.

AMODIAQUINE (CAMOQUIN)

Amodiaquine is effective against chloroquine-resistant strains and should be given in a dose of 600 mg on the first day, to be followed by 400 mg daily for 2–4 days.[67, 68]

Severe and pernicious attacks

If the parasite count is over 5000/mm³ then quinine is the drug of choice since sensitivity to chloroquine cannot be assessed in time. Intra-venous quinine is the certain method of administration of the drug.

INTRAVENOUS QUININE

Quinine is given intravenously as the dihydrochloride in single doses of 10 mg/kg. In an ordinary case 600 mg is given 8-hourly in a continuous intravenous infusion lasting 2 hours. There is controversy over the dosage to be given and the use of a loading dose. To attain early a plasma quinine level of 10 mg/litre a dose of 20 mg/kg in 500 ml glucose saline over 4 hours is necessary.[69] The remaining doses, 10 mg/kg, are given every 8 hours continuously by intravenous drip.

The other view is that this dosage leads to unacceptable cinchonism and that a total daily dosage of 21.3 mg/kg given every 12 hours is adequate and no loading dose is necessary.[70] The answer would appear to be that the dosage used depends upon the area source of the falciparum malaria and that higher doses are necessary in areas of high chloroquine resistance, such as Thailand, where some degree of quinine resistance is also present and where serum quinine levels need to be maintained at 10 mg/litre (22 µmol/litre) for 6 days. In patients with hepatic failure the initial dose should be reduced and if intravenous therapy has to be continued for more than 2–3 days, the 8-hourly dose should be reduced to 7.5 mg/kg.[69] The dose needs to be only slightly reduced in renal failure as only a small proportion of the drug is eliminated in the urine.

Cerebral malaria

It is important to exclude other or associated causes of coma by an examination of the cerebrospinal fluid. The most important part of the treatment is to give intravenous quinine as described above. No other drugs should be given and steroids and heparin are positively harmful.[71] The unconscious patient needs special nursing in the sitting up position. Anticonvulsants for fits and antimicrobials for infection of the respiratory and urinary systems may be needed. *Rehydration* should be carried out with special caution in the first 24 hours and fluid output should be carefully measured because over-hydration may cause pulmonary oedema (malaria shock lung). In general, 2–3 litres of fluid are required in the first day. Parasitaemia should be monitored. When consciousness returns, quinine sulphate should be continued in a dose of 600 mg three times a day to complete 7 days' treatment.

Management of the complications of severe malaria[72]

RENAL FAILURE

The distinction between pre-renal and established true renal failure is important. Urine output, specific gravity and sodium and urea concentration with clinical assessment of the jugular venous pressure are essential. Oliguria (300 ml of urine or less in the 24 hours) suggests renal failure with a specific gravity of 1.010 or less, suggesting acute tubular necrosis. A concentrated urine with normal microscopy suggests dehydration. The oliguria should be assessed by giving 1000 ml of isotonic (0.9%) saline with the first dose of quinine (20 mg (16.7 mg base)/kg) over 4 hours, when in most cases the venous pressure will not rise above 10 cm and urine will start to flow. If the amount of urine passed in 8 hours is less than 200 ml, another 1000 ml of saline with the second dose of quinine, 10 mg/kg and a diuretic, frusemide, 80 mg should be given by intravenous injection. Patients who fail to produce more than 200 ml of urine on this regimen should be placed on a strict fluid balance regulated to the central venous pressure. Dialysis is essential (peritoneal dialysis although not as good as haemodialysis can be of great help in emergency—Chapter 72, p. 1223). If the side-effects of quinine are pronounced the dose can be reduced to 5 mg/kg every 8 hours. Parasitaemia should be carefully monitored and should fall rapidly by the end of 24 hours.

BLOOD TRANSFUSION

The red cell count may drop rapidly and continue dropping after recovery has started. It is essential to maintain the haematocrit level above 20% by transfusion of fresh blood in which both clotting factors and platelets are present.

EXCHANGE TRANSFUSION

In some cases of life-threatening falciparum malaria with parasite counts of over 30%, exchange transfusion and replacement of parasitized cells with non-parasitized cells has proved life-saving.

HYPOGLYCAEMIA

Hypoglycaemia has come to be important in severe falciparum malaria and is most common in pregnant women.[23] It appears as early as the second to third day after the start of quinine treatment but may present in early convalescence. It should be suspected when anxiety, breathlessness, sweating, convulsions or impaired consciousness develop during treatment. Prompt intravenous glucose is essential and a second attack may occur.

PULMONARY OEDEMA

The factors which cause acute pulmonary oedema during treatment are over-hydration, pregnancy, cerebral malaria, high levels of parasitaemia, acidosis and uraemia. In some patients the response to diuretics is dramatic. Patients should be nursed propped up and given oxygen.

HYPERPYREXIA

High doses of antipyretics, ice-cold sponging, fanning or a cooling blanket should be given.

JAUNDICE (HEPATORENAL SYNDROME)

Although severe jaundice is common, hepatic failure has not been seen and the treatment is that of the associated renal failure.

Treatment of semi-immune or immune individuals

Treatment of falciparum malaria in semi-immune individuals is as for a moderate or mild infection with a full course of chloroquine. Where there is some resistance, it should be followed up by three tablets of Fansidar. In immune individuals mild fever with the appearance of a few parasites in the blood can be terminated by a single dose of 600 mg chloroquine or three tablets of Fansidar, although the World Health Organization (WHO) has recommended full-dose chloroquine in such cases to minimize the emergence of chloroquine resistance.

Treatment of recrudescences

The treatment is the same as for the primary attack.

Treatment of *P. vivax*, *P. ovale* and *P. malariae*

Resistance to 4-aminoquinolines has not been reported in *P. vivax*, *P. ovale* and *P. malariae*. On the first day 900 mg of chloroquine base is given in two or three divided doses and on each of the following two days 300 mg is given in a single dose.

In order to prevent relapse in *P. vivax* and *P. ovale* the hypnozoite forms in the liver which are not affected by 4-aminoquinoline drugs must be treated with *primaquine* given in two divided doses, each of 7.5 mg (one tablet) daily for 14 days. In Thailand and the western Pacific, where larger doses are needed, 15 mg (two tablets) must be given in two divided doses daily for 14 days. *P. malariae* does not have any persistent liver stages.

Treatment in pregnancy

Acute falciparum malaria in pregnancy is especially hazardous both to the mother and the fetus. There is no evidence of teratogenic effects of chloroquine, and quinine in the doses used therapeutically does not cause abortion; in chloroquine-resistant malaria there is no alternative. Tetracycline and Fansidar are contra-indicated and *P. vivax* should be treated with a 4-aminoquinoline; suppression can be administered by a weekly dose of 300 mg until delivery when a full course of primaquine may be admin-istered. The severe anaemia found in pregnant women should be treated with antimalarials and folic acid and can be prevented by chemo-prophylaxis (see section on chemoprophylaxis in pregnancy, p. 41) and folic acid supplements in pregnancy.

Treatment in children

Children tolerate oral doses of synthetic anti-malarial drugs well, but even moderate over-dosage may be fatal. Non-immune children should receive a full curative course of treatment. If vomiting occurs within an hour of ingestion then the dose can be repeated.

Dosage for children

Age	Fraction of adult dose
Infants up to 2 years	$\frac{1}{8}$ to $\frac{1}{4}$
Children 2–6 years	$\frac{1}{4}$ to $\frac{1}{2}$
Children 6–12 years	$\frac{1}{2}$ to $\frac{3}{4}$
Over 12 years	$\frac{3}{4}$ to 1

The usual doses in uncomplicated cases are given in Table 1.3.

Table 1.3 Dosage of antimalarial drugs for oral treatment of moderately severe malaria in non-immune children according to age.*

Drug	Up to 1 year $\frac{1}{10}-\frac{1}{8}$ of adult dose	1–3 years $\frac{1}{8}-\frac{1}{6}$ of adult dose	4–6 years $\frac{1}{4}$ of adult dose	7–11 years $\frac{1}{3}-\frac{1}{2}$ of adult dose	12–15 years $\frac{2}{3}-1$ of adult dose	Regimen
Quinine	100–200 mg	200–300 mg	300–500 mg	500–1000 mg	1000–2000 mg	Daily dose to be divided into 2–3 parts continued for 7–10 days
Chloroquine	1 75 mg ($\frac{1}{2}$ tablet)	1 150 mg (1 tablet)	1 300 mg (2 tablets)	1 300 mg (2 tablets)	1 450–600 mg (3–4 tablets)	1 Initial dose
	2 75 mg ($\frac{1}{2}$ tablet)	2 113 mg ($\frac{3}{4}$ tablet)	2 150 mg (1 tablet)	2 150 mg (1 tablet)	2 225–300 mg (1$\frac{1}{2}$–2 tablets)	2 Second dose, following initial dose after 6–24 hours
	3 37 mg ($\frac{1}{4}$ tablet)	3 75 mg ($\frac{1}{2}$ tablet)	3 75 mg ($\frac{1}{2}$ tablet)	3 150 mg (1 tablet)	3 150–300 mg (1–2 tablets)	3 Daily dose for the next 2 days
Amodiaquine	1 50 mg	1 100 mg	1 150 mg	1 200–300 mg	1 400–600 mg	1 Dose for the first day
	2 50 mg	2 50 mg	2 100 mg	2 150–200 mg	2 259–400 mg	2 Daily dose for the next 2 days
Sulfadoxine + pyrimethamine	250 mg + 12.5 mg ($\frac{1}{2}$ tablet)		500 mg + 25 mg (1 tablet)		100 mg + 50 mg (2 tablets)	Single dose
Sulfalene + Pyrimethamine	Same as for sulfadoxine + pyrimethamine					Single dose

* The dosage of chloroquine and amodiaquine is expressed in terms of base. The upper limit of the adolescent dose constitutes the generally adopted adult dose. Dosages of chloroquine are adjusted for fractional use of the common formulation of the drug containing 150 mg of base per tablet. In some countries chloroquine is formulated in tablets of 100 mg of base. Mepacrine, now considered an obsolete drug, has not been included in the table.
After World Health Organization.[64]

Parenteral antimalarial treatment

Chloroquine should not be injected into infants and young children unless absolutely necessary and then the maximum dose should not exceed 5 mg/kg and must be calculated accurately according to weight. It is much safer to give the calculated dose in two tablets, each dose separated by one hour. Sudden deaths have been attributed to the parenteral administration of chloroquine in children. Quinine dihydrochloride 10 mg/kg may be given intravenously over 12 hours and repeated in 12 hours. The daily dose should not exceed 20 mg/kg. Quinine may be given by slow deep intramuscular injection only in an acute emergency with strict aseptic precautions to avoid an abscess. Children with *P. vivax* malaria will need primaquine additionally. Suitable daily doses are:

1–4 years	2.5 mg ($\frac{1}{3}$ tablet)
5–8 years	5.0 mg ($\frac{2}{3}$ tablet)
9–14 years	10 mg (1–1$\frac{1}{3}$ tablets)
15 and over	15 mg (2 tablets)

Treatment of children in endemic areas

The mother should be encouraged to treat each attack of fever, usually during the rainy season, with an antimalarial drug. Severely ill infants with cerebral malaria and heavy infections will need the treatment given to non-immune children. This method of suppression of symptoms will allow the child to maintain health during the critical period, six months to two years, during which he is acquiring immunity (see section on chemoprophylaxis in children, p. 41).

It is important to know if the antimalarial drug which is being used has been absorbed and that it has actually been administered, and if so has not been vomited. For this reason tests for excretion in the urine are necessary which can be set up without extensive laboratory equipment.

Tests for quinine and chloroquine in urine

It is sometimes important to know if these drugs have been taken by patients who are not closely supervised. The following tests are used.

For quinine in urine

TANRET–MAYER TEST

Reagent 1.45 g mercuric chloride in 80 ml distilled water added to 5 g potassium iodide in 20 ml distilled water. Add a few drops to 5 ml of filtrate of boiled and filtered urine; an immediate precipitate forms if quinine is present.

This test is also positive for chloroquine in urine.

For large amounts of quinine in urine, 20 ml urine are made alkaline with ammonium hydroxide solution and extracted with an equal amount of ether or chloroform and the extract is shaken with 3 ml of 10% sulphuric acid. A blue fluorescence, more noticeable under ultraviolet light, suggests quinine or quinidine. It can be confirmed by fluorescent emission, which occurs at 450 nm when an exciting light of wavelength 250 nm is applied, if a spectrofluorimeter is available.[73]

For chloroquine in urine

THE WILSON–EDESON TEST

A few drops of Mayer's reagent (6.8 g mercuric chloride, 24.9 g potassium iodide, 500 ml distilled water) are added to a few millilitres of urine and, if chloroquine is present, a white turbidity rapidly appears which disappears on heating but returns on cooling. This test becomes positive 12 hours after a dose of chloroquine has been taken and remains positive for 5 or 6 days after a single dose of 600 mg.[74]

THE HASKINS TEST[75]

Reagents required are a 10% solution of sodium hydroxide purified ethylene dichloride and a 0.1% solution of methyl orange in boric acid.

To 5 ml urine add 1 ml sodium hydroxide solution and 5 ml ethylene dichloride. Shake for one minute. Centrifuge if necessary to separate the layers. Draw off the ethylene dichloride layer into a clean test tube and add 0.5 ml methyl orange solution. Shake for 15–20 seconds.

The presence of a non-specific yellow colour in the ethylene dichloride layer (but not in a control urine) indicates the presence of chloroquine. It detects 2 mg/litre and the colour is intense at 10 mg/litre.

A dose of 300 mg can produce a positive result for 10 days, negative at 12 days. It is negative with a dose of 300 mg amodiaquine, and with 25 mg pyrimethamine.

LELIJFELD AND KORTMANN TEST FOR AMODIAQUINE AND CHLOROQUINE[76]

Fifty milligrams of yellowish eosin are placed in a small glass-stoppered funnel, 100 mg chloroform (reagent grade) and 1 ml N HCl are added and the mixture is shaken for a few minutes until the chloroform is light yellow as a result of solution of the eosin. The chloroform layer is allowed to separate and may be transferred to a brown, glass-stoppered bottle for storage.

The presence of chloroquine is shown if to a small test tube containing 2 ml urine, ten drops of the reagent are added and mixed by thorough shaking for a few moments, and the colour in the chloroform layer changes from yellowish to violet-red.

DRUG RESISTANCE[64]

P. falciparum malaria parasites have developed resistance to many antimalarial drugs over the last 25 years, resistance to chloroquine being the most important development. Drug resistance has been described as the ability of a parasite strain to survive and/or multiply despite the administration and absorption of a drug in doses equal to or higher than those usually recommended, but within the limits of tolerance of the subject.

Three degrees of resistance are recognized (Fig. 1.16).[77] In RI resistance parasites disappear from the peripheral blood but reappear by day 14; in RII resistance parasitaemia decreases to 25% or less of the pre-treatment level but never completely disappears, and in RIII resistance there is little or no fall in parasitaemia after chloroquine administration. Resistance has not been reported in the other malaria parasites of man.

Mechanisms of resistance[78]

Chloroquine

Chloroquine resistance arises by mutation and is stable.[79] More than one mutation is required and is the result of the parasite preventing chloroquine binding to a haemoglobin breakdown product, to form toxic complexes.[80] The spread of chloroquine resistance is helped by the possession of the biological advantages of chloroquine-resistant over chloroquine-sensitive strains.

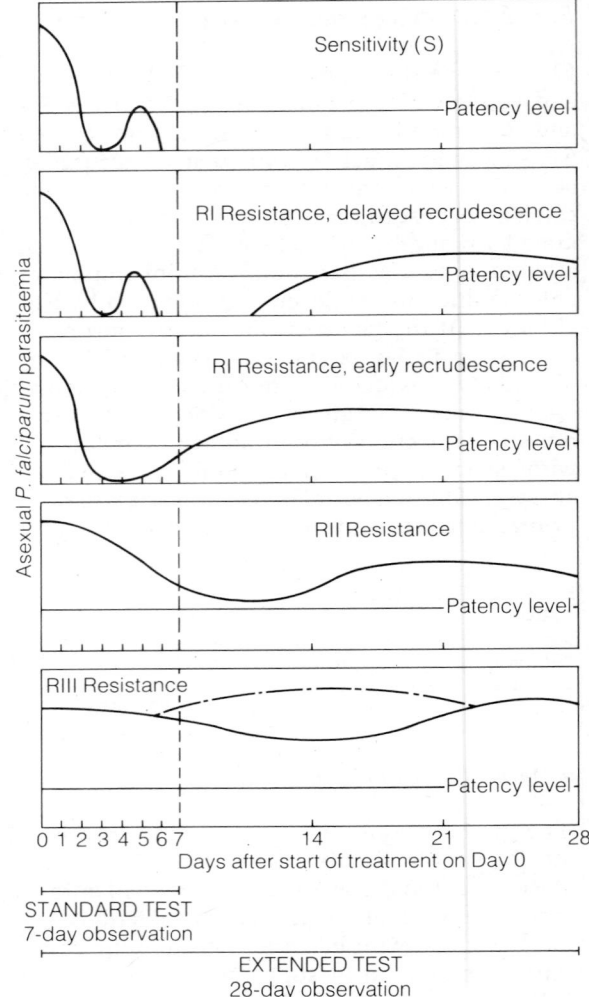

STANDARD TEST
7-day observation

EXTENDED TEST
28-day observation

—————— Patent parasitaemia may reappear by day 5 ; in sensitive (S) strains; however, it is absent on and after day 6.

—·—·— There may be an increase in parasitaemia in RIII resistance.

Note that it is not possible to distinguish between S and RI in the standard (7-day) test.

Fig. 1.16 WHO field test for response of malaria parasites to chloroquine. Diagram shows degrees of response ranging from sensitivity to high resistance. Chloroquine administered by mouth at a dose of 25 mg/kg. (From World Health Organization.[77])

Proguanil and pyrimethamine

Methods of resistance to the para-aminobenzoic acid blockers (proguanil) and antifolate drugs (pyrimethamine) comprise modification of drug transport systems, increased synthesis of blocked enzymes, increase in drug inactivating enzymes and the use of alternative pathways.[64]

Genetics of resistance

The origin of resistant strains is due to spontaneous mutations in the genetic population which are selected out under pressure of the drug. The production of drug-resistant strains is more rapid in the absence of immune defences.

Resistance to chloroquine

Resistance to chloroquine started in 1961 in South America and 1962 in Indo-China, and by 1984 had spread to much of the world (Fig. 1.17).[77] At present only parts of West Africa are apparently free. The frequency and degree of resistance tends to increase with the length of time it has been present.

Resistance to proguanil and pyrimethamine

Resistance has developed rapidly over the last 30 years and is now widespread but patchy.

Resistance to sulfadoxine–pyrimethamine (Fansidar)

Resistance to Fansidar became apparent on the Thai-Kampuchea border in the early 1980s. It is not 100% effective even in some people infected with sensitive strains. Resistance has now appeared in Burma, Malaysia and East Africa. Increasing failure rates are now apparent in Colombia and the Amazon basin.

Resistance to dapsone–pyrimethamine (Maloprim)

Resistance to Maloprim has been reported from Kenya and Tanzania.

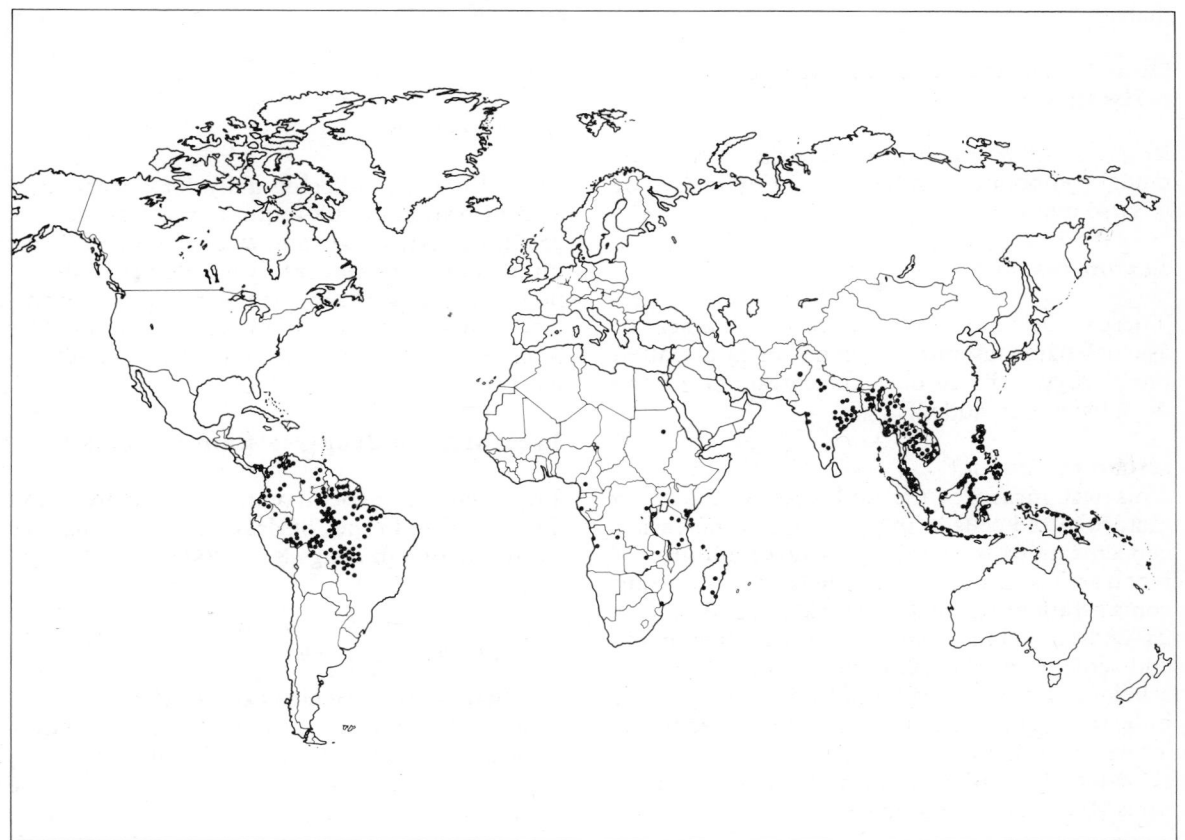

Fig. 1.17 Distribution of reported resistance of *P. falciparum* to chloroquine in 1984 according to the World Health Organization.[77]

Resistance to quinine

Reports of quinine resistance are still rare but true primary resistance has been reported from Thailand and East Africa and it has been noted that there is a steady increase in the time parasites take to disappear from the blood in East Africa after treatment with quinine.

Resistance to mefloquine

So far there is no evidence of a major problem; however, one primary mefloquine resistance case has been reported from Thailand and one from Kenya. It is probable that there is cross resistance between quinine and mefloquine. In order to prevent the development of resistance mefloquine should never be used in isolation. A combination of drugs, Fansimef, has been used, three tablets of which contain 750 mg mefloquine base, 1500 mg sulfadoxine and 75 mg pyrimethamine with 100% success in chloroquine-resistant malaria.[81]

Detection and measurement of drug resistance[64]

Response of *P. falciparum* malaria to schizonticidal compounds can be assessed by in vivo or in vitro methods.

In vitro methods

These methods are based on the development of asexual parasites into schizonts in non-clotted blood to which various concentrations of the drug have been added.

MACRO TECHNIQUE[82]
This test measures the ability of schizonts to mature in red cells in the presence of increasing concentrations of the drug. A few millilitres of blood are taken and added to vials with ascending concentrations of the drug and kept at 38.5°C for 24–28 hours. Thick blood smears are then made and schizont counts are done. Full inhibition of schizont maturation at 1 nmol/ml of chloroquine indicates chloroquine sensitivity; schizont growth at 1.5 nmol/ml indicates resistance, and schizont maturation at over 2.5 nmol/ml indicates RII or RIII resistance.

MICRO TECHNIQUE[83]
This test measures the increase in the number of ring forms and their ability to invade fresh red cells in the presence of increasing concentrations of the drug. The test is carried out on capillary blood in heparin or EDTA tubes taken from the finger and added to micro titre trays in Trager's continuous culture medium and incubated at 37.5°C for 24–26 hours. Thick films are prepared from the erythrocyte layers and the proportion of mature schizonts in the wells to which the drug has been added is compared with controls.

48-HOUR TEST
This test is similar to the micro test. It uses four times as much blood and ten times as much culture medium per well. The endpoint is assessment of invasion of the erythrocytes by parasites, as determined by examination of thin films prepared after 48 hours.

VISUAL MICRO TEST
Malaria pigment formed during maturation of rings to schizonts forms a precipitate after the addition of alkali which is visible to the naked eye and which does not occur in the presence of effective drug concentrations.

In vivo methods

Blood films are collected daily for a week after administration of chloroquine in a total dose of 25 mg/kg body weight and when possible at two-, three- and four-week intervals. However, detection of parasitaemia in a single blood film examined 7–10 days after administration of a full dose of chloroquine suggests the presence of RII or RIII resistance.

Treatment of drug-resistant malaria[84]

Treatment will depend on the area involved and the degree and types of drug resistance; usually a combination of drugs is necessary.

Areas resistant to 4-aminoquinolines but sensitive to pyrimethamine–sulpha compounds

NON-IMMUNE UNCOMPLICATED ATTACKS
Quinine (sulphate, bisulphate or dihydrochloride) 600 mg orally every 8 hours for 5 days, to be followed on the sixth day by a single dose of three tablets of Fansidar.

Amodiaquine hydrochloride (Camoquin) should be used in areas of chloroquine resistance, since although it is a 4-aminoquinoline, it has proved successful under these circumstances. Oral dosage: 600 mg at once, followed by 400–600 mg daily for 2–4 days.

SEMI-IMMUNE

A single dose of three tablets of Fansidar is given.

Areas with resistance to both 4-aminoquinolines and to pyrimethamine compounds

Quinine (sulphate, bisulphate or dihydrochloride) 600 mg orally every 8 hours for 7 days. If the patient requires intravenous quinine, the initial loading dose is 20 mg/kg in 500 ml of glucose saline to attain early the plasma levels necessary, over 10 mg/litre to inhibit the parasites. After the initial dose of quinine it is reduced to 10 mg/kg and given every 8 hours.

Areas where resistance to 4-aminoquinolines, pyrimethamine–sulpha combinations and poor response to quinine alone occurs

Quinine (sulphate, bisulphate or dihydrochloride) 600 mg orally every 8 hours for 7 days together with tetracycline 250 mg every 6 hours, or 500 mg twice daily for 7 days. Tetracycline can be given intravenously but should be avoided in pregnant women, infants and young children. Tetracycline should also be avoided in the presence of renal failure and delayed until the patient is better.

Other treatment regimens

MEFLOQUINE

Mefloquine should always be used in combination with another drug, usually Fansidar.

CHEMOPROPHYLAXIS

Chemoprophylaxis is the most important means of preventing malarial illness although personal prophylaxis must not be forgotten, especially now that drug-resistant malaria is spreading. Chemoprophylaxis may be *causal* or *suppressive*.

Causal prophylaxis

There is no true causal prophylactic since there are no drugs which will destroy the sporozoites before they enter the liver. Primaquine will destroy the liver forms after the sporozoites have entered the liver cells but, since it must be given regularly for this purpose, it is too toxic. Proguanil and pyrimethamine are active on *P. falciparum* liver forms and are used for this purpose.

Suppressive chemoprophylaxis

All blood schizonticides may be used as chemosuppressive drugs since they suppress the erythrocyte stages and do not allow an attack of malaria to develop. In the case of *P. falciparum* regular suppression will allow the infection to die out if there is no reinfection, but with *P. vivax* and *P. ovale* suppressive drugs merely suppress the erythrocytic stages and relapse will occur when the drug is stopped. This can be prevented by a radical cure which involves the use of a tissue schizonticidal drug (primaquine).

Chemoprophylaxis is necessary for all visitors to and residents of the tropics who have not lived there since infancy and so acquired immunity. Drugs should be started a week before entering the endemic area and continued for at least six weeks after leaving. Although resistance to suppressive drugs has appeared in many countries chemoprophylaxis is still essential. It is necessary to understand that no medication can be guaranteed to protect the traveller in every instance, and that a traveller developing fever after having visited a malarious area (Fig. 1.1) should seek medical attention, or if there is none available, take a full course of antimalarial treatment. A combination of one, two or more drugs may be necessary in some areas. The drugs used in chemoprophylaxis and their doses are given in Table 1.4.

Side-effects

Side-effects from drugs taken regularly for chemoprophylaxis are rare but important in that when many people are taking them, even a very small proportion showing side-effects could amount to quite a large number in the end. Side-effects which are important occur with the following drugs.

Chloroquine

Only long-term administration carries the risk of retinopathy which is present once the accumulative dose exceeds 100 g of base—a level which in the standard recommended dose for malaria suppression takes about six and a half years to

Table 1.4 Drugs used in chemoprophylaxis.

Drug	Action	Dose				Side-effects	Resistance	Remarks
		up to 2 years	3–6 years	7–10 years	Adult			
Quinine (daily)	Fair suppressive	75–150 mg	150–300 mg	300–450 mg	600 mg	Very rare	Exceptional	Association with blackwater fever. Bitter taste
Chloroquine (weekly)	Very good suppressive. Suppressive cure *P. falciparum*	50–100 mg	100–200 mg	100–200 mg	300 mg	Rare	Present and spreading to many areas	Twice weekly or once weekly. Bitter taste
Nivaquine syrup (weekly) (68 mg/one 5 ml spoonful)		1 spoonful	1½–2 spoonfuls	2–3 spoonfuls				
Amodiaquine (weekly) No longer used for chemoprophylaxis because of toxic side-effects								
Proguanil (daily) (Paludrine)	Good suppressive. Causal *P. falciparum*	25–50 mg	50–100 mg	75–150 mg	100–200 mg	Very rare	Present	Wide margin of safety. Slightly bitter
Chlorproguanil (weekly) (Lapudrine)	Good suppressive. Causal *P. falciparum*	5 mg	10 mg	15 mg	20 mg	Very rare at standard doses	Present in wide areas	No bitter taste. Danger of accidental poisoning of children
Pyrimethamine (weekly) (Daraprim)	Good suppressive. Causal *P. falciparum* and *P. vivax*	6.25–12.5 mg	12.5–25 mg	12.5–25 mg	25 mg	Rare at standard doses	Has now appeared in many areas	Caution in pregnancy and G-6-PD-deficient subjects. Not recommended for general use
Pyrimethamine + Dapsone (Maloprim)	Good suppressive	Not recommended	½ tablet	¾ tablet	12.5 mg + 100 mg (1 tablet)	Agranulocytosis	Has appeared in many areas	Not recommended for general use
Pyrimethamine + sulfadoxine (Fansidar)	Good suppressive	Not recommended	½ tablet	¾ tablet	500 mg + 25 mg (1 tablet)	Risk of Stevens–Johnson syndrome precludes its use except under the most urgent situations		Danger of Stevens–Johnson syndrome. Not recommended for general use

After Bruce-Chwatt[1] and World Health Organization.[64]

reach. Such groups should have careful monitoring of retinal function. Pruritus may be a distressing symptom, chiefly in dark-skinned people.

Amodiaquine (Camoquin)

Amodiaquine is an effective alternative to chloroquine in chloroquine-resistant areas;[68] but toxic side-effects (agranulocytosis) preclude its use as a long-term chemoprophylactic.

Fansidar

Fansidar has given rise to distressing side-effects, even after one dose. These include photodermatitis, drug fever and the most severe syndromes—agranulocytosis, Stevens–Johnson syndrome and jaundice—all of which are potentially fatal. For these reasons Fansidar should not be used for routine chemoprophylaxis.

Maloprim

After a dose of two tablets weekly, cases of agranulocytosis with deaths were reported and this dosage was discontinued. After a dose of one tablet a week only very few cases have been recorded. However, Maloprim is now no longer widely recommended for use.

What chemoprophylaxis should be taken?

Since Maloprim and Fansidar are no longer routinely recommended for chemoprophylaxis, what regimen should be followed? Chloroquine resistance is now widespread in sub-Saharan Africa and in South-East Asia. The only drugs available are Paludrine and chloroquine. Two drugs should be taken together:

> Paludrine 2 tablets (200 mg) daily
> chloroquine (Nivaquine) 2 tablets (300 mg base) weekly.

In Francophone Africa chloroquine is taken as 100 mg base daily for 6 days a week, with some success. However, the cumulative dose builds up much more rapidly and great care should be taken with this dosage. Amodiaquine should no longer be used as a prophylactic because of an unacceptably high level of agranulocytosis, perhaps as high as one in 2000. Prophylaxis should start one day before entering and last until four weeks after leaving an endemic area.

Breakthroughs must be expected and persons at risk should always have available a course of quinine (two tablets three times a day for 7 days) or three tablets of Fansidar to take if a fever, for which there is no obvious cause, develops.

P. vivax and P. ovale

For non-immune individuals subject to intense exposure to *P. vivax* and *P. ovale* radical curative treatment with 14 days of primaquine should be given during the last two weeks of the suppressive regimen.

Chemoprophylaxis in pregnancy

Chemoprophylaxis should be given to all women regardless of their state of immunity. Chloroquine is quite safe and there are no records of any fetal damage ensuing from chloroquine suppressive treatment. Paludrine is equally safe. Fansidar should not be given in the last trimester of pregnancy and probably not at all. Maloprim has not given rise to any ill-effects on the fetus but if used a folic acid supplement should be given throughout pregnancy.

Chemoprophylaxis in areas of chloroquine resistance raises difficult questions but the prevention of an acute attack of falciparum malaria outweighs all the possible dangers of chemosuppression. If these are felt to be too great then non-immune women in these areas should be advised to avoid pregnancy while resident there.

Chemoprophylaxis in children

Children of non-immune women should have chemoprophylaxis from birth; Nivaquine syrup (see Table 1.4) is a convenient way of giving chloroquine. The dosage of the drugs used is given in Table 1.4. Children of women in endemic areas have a passive immunity until the age of six months following which they are increasingly subject to malaria. The policy should be to allow these children to develop an immunity without suffering severely. Attacks of fever should be treated when they occur.

Chemoprophylaxis of immune and semi-immune people in endemic areas

Systematic chemosuppression is undertaken in pregnant women only. Mass prophylaxis of children under five is not recommended. In adults no general chemosuppression should be given.

Medicated salt

In some countries chloroquine has been added to domestic salt for widespread supply to all the inhabitants with the intention of suppressing malaria by constant dosage. In Guyana the concentration of chloroquine was 0.4%, in Iran 0.33% and in Uganda 0.38%. Parasite rates in these areas were lowered but interruption of transmission could not be claimed with certainty, though in one experiment in Tanzania this was apparently achieved.

In this form, however, chloroquine is lost by leaching during storage, especially when moisture is sealed into plastic containers, and infants and young children commonly do not receive adequate doses because they are not given salt. There is also the possibility that if strains of parasites exist which are resistant to chloroquine they could be favoured and spread as a result of this procedure. Moreover, Giglioli et al[85] have produced strong evidence that chloroquinized salt caused photo-allergic dermatitis in Guyana, similar to that described in rheumatoid arthritis and lupus erythematosus treated with high doses of chloroquine.

PERSONAL PROPHYLAXIS

It is most important to follow measures against mosquito bites since these can reduce the chance of infection and help chemoprophylaxis. Mosquito nets or screens should be used at night; long sleeves, and long trousers tucked into mosquito boots, should be worn. Antimosquito coils are very useful in the house.

IMMUNIZATION AGAINST MALARIA

Naturally acquired immunity in human malaria is slow to develop and incomplete and long-standing infections are frequent. Before introducing artificial immunization procedures it is important to know whether a vaccine involving whole live, dead or attenuated organisms or their antigens will induce a more rapidly developing and fast immunity than a natural infection. Experimental vaccination in animals has frequently induced far greater immunity than that provided by natural infection.[36]

Immunological interference with the complex cycle of malaria parasites in man and mosquitoes can be possible at a number of points: blocking of sporozoite entry into the body, prevention of growth in the liver, interruption of asexual development in the red cell, elimination of the gametocytes and prevention of their infectivity for the mosquito.

Immunization against sporozoites

Radiation-attenuated sporozoites have been used successfully to immunize mice against infection with *P. berghei*. Now identification analysis and encoding of the circumsporozoite protein of *P. falciparum* responsible for protective immunity has made possible the production of a vaccine for trial in human volunteers[4] and a recombinant circumsporozoite protein has now been produced in the bacterium *Escherichia coli* which has blocked the invasion in vitro of human hepatoma cells.[86]

Immunization against merozoites

Development of vaccines against merozoites has been hindered by the difficulty in obtaining enough parasite material and the necessity of using Freund's complete adjuvant. Trager's continuous in vitro culture has now made possible the provision of larger amounts of parasite material (Appendix I, p. 1239).

Vaccination against transmission
(induction of transmission blocking immunity)

Vaccination with exflagellated microgametes has been shown to inhibit sexual production of plasmodia in human malaria. The vaccine induces antibody which reacts after their release from red cells into the mosquito gut and agglutinates the microgametes preventing fertilization, so blocking the transmission of malaria.[87] Isolation of the surface antigens on both male and female gametes and their production by DNA recombinant technique will be necessary to produce a vaccine.

Uses of a vaccine

A *sporozoite* vaccine could be used to protect non-immune travellers and immigrants against infection but, since only a few sporozoites escaping the immune barrier can cause an infection, protection would not be 100%. A *merozoite* vaccine could help in treatment producing a rapid cure or rendering the illness less severe. A *gamete* related vaccine could be used to curb epidemics or seasonal outbreaks of malaria. A combination of all three vaccines may be possible.[4]

EPIDEMIOLOGY OF MALARIA

General factors

Natural transmission of malaria depends on the presence and relationship between three basic factors:

the *host*: vertebrate host man and invertebrate host the anopheline mosquito;
the *agent*: the malaria parasite;
the *environment*: physical, biological and socioeconomic.

These complex biological factors overlap and interreact to provide various degrees of stability and instability in the prevalence of malaria.

Factors relating to man

These include:
1 parasite rates in man, especially children;
2 recovery and mortality rates from the disease;
3 state of immunity of the population;
4 habits and living conditions of the population.

Factors relating to the parasites

These include:
1 virulence (*P. falciparum* the most, *P. malariae* the least);
2 persistence and tendency to relapse in man.

Factors relating to anophelines

These include:
1 availability of water suitable for breeding, which depends largely on climate and season, governing rainfall and temperature;
2 longevity of anophelines and the faculty of hibernation;
3 effectiveness as vectors; species vary in this and in their preferences for man as a source of blood meals;

4 dose of sporozoites inoculated at a bite in man; this can vary greatly;
5 availability of man as the donor and recipient of parasites. (For epidemoliogical zones of malaria, see Table III.4, p. 1406.)

Malaria in the human community

Endemicity is the amount and severity of malaria in an area or community.
Epidemic is a periodic or sharp increase in the amount of malaria in a community.

Estimation of malarial prevalence

To estimate the prevalence of malaria in a community a large number of people, especially infants and children, must be examined by the following methods.

SPLEEN RATE
The spleen rate is the proportion of children (aged two to ten years) in a community who have enlarged spleens. The spleen may be palpated with the child standing or lying, the examiner's hand being pressed gently against the abdominal wall until the spleen is felt or is found to be not palpable. An enlarged spleen, especially if only recently enlarged as a result of early attacks of malaria, is easily ruptured; care is therefore essential in palpation.

Measurement of the degree of enlargement is preferably made by Hackett's method (Fig. 1.18) or (less satisfactorily) by estimating the number of fingerbreadths to which it extends below the costal margin.

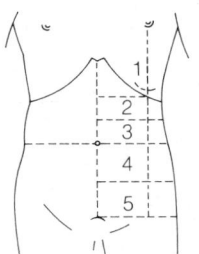 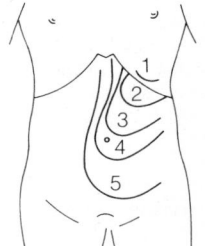

Topographical reference lines for the five classes of enlarged spleen

Projection on the surface of the abdomen of the five classes of enlarged spleen

Fig. 1.18 Classification of spleen sizes according to Hackett. A, Topographical reference lines for the five classes of enlarged spleen. B, Projection on the surface of the abdomen of the five classes of enlarged spleen.

PARASITE RATE

The parasite rate as a percentage is the proportion of persons in a given community who show malaria parasites in the blood.

The endemicity of malaria can be classified on the following basis.

1 *Hypoendemic malaria* with spleen rate of 0–10%.

2 *Mesoendemic malaria* with spleen rate of 11–50%.

3 *Hyperendemic malaria* with spleen rate consistently over 50%. The spleen rate in adults is also high.

4 *Holoendemic malaria* with spleen rate constantly over 75%. The spleen rate in adults is low; it is in this type of endemicity that the strongest adult tolerance is found.

A more general classification into stable and unstable malaria has been introduced[88] (Table 1.5).

malaria the level of immunity is high after childhood, and equilibrium is the rule.

2 *Unstable malaria*, transmitted by less efficient vectors which bite man less frequently and may be short-lived, or which exist in climatic conditions less favourable for the development of the parasites in them. Seasonal changes in the density of mosquitoes occur. Immunity in unstable malaria is not complete and fluctuates seasonally. Equilibrium is not attained in the population and epidemics therefore occur when mosquito breeding becomes seasonally prolific, usually in the summer months or after high rainfall, though (as in Sri Lanka between the two World Wars) a dry season may reduce the flow of water in rivers, leaving quiet pools favourable to the breeding of dangerous mosquitoes. The essential point of unstable malaria is lack of continuity of transmission.

Intermediate endemic forms between stable

Table 1.5 Some characteristics of unstable and stable malaria.

Characteristics	Unstable	Stable
Type of vector	Vector with infrequent man-biting habit and/or low daily survival rate	Vector with frequent man-biting habit and high daily survival rate
Environmental conditions	Not favourable for a rapid sporogonic cycle	Favourable for a rapid sporogonic cycle
Endemicity	Usually low to moderate; high endemicity may occur	Very high endemicity common; low to moderate may occur
Determining causes	Vector of low anthropophily and low to moderate longevity. Climatic conditions favourable for short periods of transmission	Vector of high anthropophily and moderate to high longevity. Climatic conditions favourable for long periods of transmission
Anopheline density (needed to maintain transmission)	High (1–10 or more bites per person/night)	Low (as low as 0.025 bites per person/night)
Seasonal changes of incidence	Pronounced	Not very pronounced, except for short dry season
Fluctuations in incidence and predominant parasite	Very marked and uneven. Most often *P. vivax* as main parasite	Not marked and related to seasons. *P. falciparum* prevalent parasite
Immunity of the population	Variable with some groups of low immunity	High, though varying in degree in different age groups
Epidemic outbreaks	Likely when climatic or other conditions suitable	Unlikely to occur in the indigenous population
Amenability to control or eradication	Not unduly difficult by imagocides and larvicides combined with chemotherapy. Daily anopheline mortality of 20–25% may be adequate for control of transmission	Very difficult to control, especially in rural areas. Eradication unlikely unless socio-economic conditions favourable. Daily anopheline mortality of at least 50% needed for a degree of control

From Bruce-Chwatt.[1]

1 *Stable malaria*, transmitted by efficient anopheline vectors breeding throughout the year which bite man frequently, are moderately long-lived and exist in climates favourable to rapid completion of the extrinsic (mosquito) life-cycle of the parasite. Reduction of temperature to about 15°C would stop transmission. In stable

and unstable occur. In order to pinpoint the epidemiological situation in any one area it is necessary to do a *malaria survey*.

Malaria survey

A malaria survey involves the collection of data

on the human host, insect vector and the environment.

HUMAN HOST

Spleen rate and parasite rate are estimated.

INSECT VECTOR

This involves identification of the species of anopheline vector, its density (number entering houses and feeding on the human population), natural infection (sporozoite rate, percentage of mosquitoes with sporozoites in their salivary glands, oocyte rate, incidence of oöcysts on the stomach walls), estimation of biting habits and longevity (see Appendix III).

ENVIRONMENTAL FACTORS

These include rainfall, temperature and humidity which affect the breeding of *Anopheles*.

Seroepidemiological surveys

Serological methods can be used to find out the natural prevalence of infection, the age specific increase in the serological profile reflecting the degree of transmission—important when control measures are to be undertaken to interrupt transmission—and to discover renewal of transmission when it was thought to have been eradicated.[89]

Mathematic models of malaria transmission

This is a complicated subject but models have been used to study the relationship between all the various factors and to test the effect of altering one or more to interrupt transmission.

Imported malaria

The problem of malaria imported into temperate regions from the tropics and subtropics has assumed large proportions. In Europe some 4000 cases were notified in 1979 which has since fallen to 3500 in 1982. *Plasmodium vivax* constituted 65% of the infections mainly contracted in India, while 25% were *P. falciparum* contracted in Africa.

P. vivax malaria is characterized by relapses and, even if a prophylactic drug has been taken regularly and for four weeks after return, relapses may occur (unless a course of primaquine has been taken) and have been known to occur up to 13 months after stopping the drug.[90] This may cause difficulty in diagnosis.

P. falciparum infection will not occur provided that the drug has been taken for four weeks after return and that the parasite is sensitive to the drug. The interval between return from the endemic area and onset of symptoms is usually between 7 and 10 days, but may be as long as one month. Any case of fever or obscure illness in a returned traveller within a month of return must be suspected as falciparum malaria, as must fever in a patient who has received a blood transfusion within the last three months. Many fatal cases have occurred because of failure to take a geographical history under these circumstances.

Airport malaria

Several cases of malaria in people working or living near airports in Europe have been caused by infected anophelines imported on aircraft surviving in a hot summer and travelling some distances, presumably on a vehicle and biting individuals often living many miles from the airport.[91]

CONTROL

The control of malaria can be achieved by action against the adult mosquitoes with insecticides, against the larvae by attacking the breeding places with antilarval measures, and by environmental control by decreasing man–mosquito contact.

The anophelines which carry malaria usually bite at night, especially about dawn and dusk. Endophilic species do so inside houses where human blood is easily available to them but some strains of well-known vectors are exophilic, biting in the open after nightfall and resting by day in vegetation; for instance, strains of *A. gambiae* in Mauritius and elsewhere.

Many species enter houses at dusk and, after a blood meal, rest on walls or ceilings, leaving at dawn.

Insecticides directed against adult mosquitoes (imagocide)

Residual insecticides (DDT and others) have been very successful in controlling malaria. They are sprayed on the inside walls of houses where the adult female anophelines come to rest after taking a blood meal. They are not killed at once but a large proportion only survive for 12–14 days and cannot pass on the infection. The development of resistance to these insecticides has limited the value of this approach.

Antilarval measures

1   Breeding places can be treated with larvicidal oil or with residual insecticides in oil or water emulsions.

2   Treatment of breeding places by draining ponds or marshes, or filling them in with earth; clearing vegetation from the edges of streams which could provide shelter for mosquito larvae.

3   The use of small fish which eat mosquito larvae, especially larvae which live chiefly near the surface, such as anopheline larvae; species used include *Lebistes* and *Gambusia*.

4   Removal of shade from the breeding places of anophelines which choose shaded water for breeding or, conversely, provision of shade to inhibit species which prefer direct sunlight. There is a difficulty, however, in that by altering shade, species may be attracted which prefer the altered conditions and these may be effective vectors.

5   Treatment of streams by intermittent flushing, provided by special siphons constructed to hold up the flow of water until the siphon is primed and discharges the dammed-up water in a turbulent and sudden gush which washes away the mosquito larvae.

Environmental measures

1   Siting of dwellings at distances of 1 km or more from collections of water or streams where anophelines can breed. Mosquitoes can travel further than this downwind but the distances suggested afford some protection. Prevailing winds at night time should be taken into consideration; so also should elevation and exposure to wind; hill tops are usually better than valleys. Formerly, in some countries, it was found useful to interpose cattle in sheds between mosquito breeding places and human habitations, so that mosquitoes which would feed on cattle would be diverted from man. Some particularly anthropophilic species, however, cannot be diverted in this way.

2   Prevention of the formation of breeding places through removal of breeding places by draining ponds and marshes and filling them in, and clearing vegetation from the edges of streams which could provide shade for the larvae.

3   Prevention of man-made malaria by filling in hollows left where earth has been extracted for the construction of railway embankments and buildings. It is important in this context that medical officers should always be consulted before such construction work is done.

Personal protection

Protection by mosquito netting is extremely important, especially for non-immune expatriates in hyperendemic areas. The windows of houses should be covered by the special metal gauze prepared for the purpose and mosquito-proofed doors may be added to existing doors so that the latter can be kept open to allow maximum air movement inside without permitting mosquitoes to enter.

Mosquito bed nets (preferably of Terylene) are also essential, but must be scrupulously maintained to avoid tearing. The net should be suspended from metal rods connecting uprights placed at the four corners of the bed and there should be no opening in the side of the net. The net should be lowered and tucked well in under the mattress before dusk and not raised until after dawn. Mosquitoes will enter a torn or badly used net which then becomes a mosquito trap.

Mosquito boots of soft leather, reaching to just below the knee, have long been advocated. Mosquitoes tend to bite under tables and chairs, and the ankles are therefore particularly vulnerable. With or without mosquito boots, long trousers or skirts are advisable in the evenings, and long sleeves also reduce the area of skin open to mosquitoes. Women who wear short skirts are obviously at a disadvantage in this respect, and even two pairs of stockings are not enough to prevent bites. Repellents such as dimethyl phthalate, however, can be useful when applied to the skin or clothes; they act for several hours, and proprietary preparations pleasant to use are generally available.

Spraying a room with a short-acting insecticide based on pyrethrum, from a 'Flit gun', is useful to clear it for a few hours, particular attention being paid to spaces beneath chairs and tables, and also to wardrobes, cupboards, bathrooms and lavatories, and to dark corners.

Control of epidemic malaria

Outbreaks of epidemic malaria brought on by unusual environmental conditions whether by abnormal rains, mass immigration of non-immunes, or war and famine can be controlled by residual insecticides plus mass chemoprophylaxis.

ERADICATION

The principles and practice of malaria eradication and its limitations are well described.[1] Plans for eradicating malaria on a world scale were drawn up by the WHO and consisted of four phases to be carried out over eight years or more.

1 *Preparatory phase:* one to two years
Identifying the problem and obtaining staff vehicles and supplies.
2 *Attack phase:* four years or more
Residual spraying aimed at the elimination of the vector and the cessation of transmission. During this time the parasite rate is determined according to age groups in samples to determine the interruption of transmission. When this falls to below 5% then all possibly infected individuals must be examined.
3 *Consolidation phase*
To mop up the remaining foci.
4 *Maintenance phase:* three years
To enter this phase there must be no evidence of malaria transmission for three consecutive years.

Results

Within 15 years of the start of the WHO campaign, malaria had been eradicated from Europe, USSR, most of the Middle East, North America, the Caribbean and large areas in the East. However, during the last decade there has been a resurgence in the disease. The causes of this failure are many: insecticide resistance and political and economic problems. The situation in tropical Africa remains unchanged and is unlikely to be affected by any eradication plan in the near future.

NON-HUMAN PRIMATE MALARIA PARASITES CAPABLE OF INFECTING MAN

P. malariae is found in chimpanzees and can infect man. *P. knowlesi* is a quotidian type parasite of *Macaca* (rhesus) monkeys in the Far East. It has been found to occur naturally in aborigines in the jungles of Malaya and some cases have occurred in Caucasian soldiers on jungle patrol. Infections were mild and not fatal.[92]

Laboratory infections of man, deliberate and accidental

Normal host	Country of origin	Species of parasite
Alouatta (howler monkeys)	Brazil	*P. simium*
Cebus, Saimiri and *Lagothrix*	Brazil	*P. brasilianum*
Macaca (rhesus monkeys)	Far East	*P. cynomolgi* *P. cynomolgi bastianellii* *P. inui*
Macaca (rhesus monkeys)	India and Sri Lanka	*P. shortii*

There is strong evidence that *P. brasilianum* was derived from human infections of *P. malariae* in the past (Appendix I, p. 1236).

BABESIOSIS (PIROPLASMOSIS)

Babesia (piroplasma) is a genus of protozoal organisms which invade and divide in red cells and cause disease in cattle, dogs, rodents and other animals. Two species can infect man: *Babesia divergens*, a parasite of cattle in the USSR and eastern Europe; and *Babesia microti*, a parasite of rodents in North America.

BABESIA DIVERGENS (B. BOVIS)

Geographical distribution

Human infection has been found only in those people whose spleens have been removed in Yugoslavia,[93] Eire[94] and Russia[95] where 27 cases have been diagnosed parasitologically and 52 serologically up to 1977.

Aetiology

B. divergens (*B. bovis*) (Fig. 1.19) is a parasite of cattle in eastern Europe and the USSR. The parasites are intra-erythrocytic rod-shaped bodies which develop to become pear-shaped and closely resemble malaria parasites except that they develop no pigment, but have a white vacuole in contrast to the pink stroma in the malarial ring. Multiple invasions of the red cell are common and the parasites divide into two and four bodies resembling a tetrad or Maltese Cross. When cultured in Trager's medium malarial parasites will develop pigment but not babesia.

mission) and then to the next host by the nymphal stage. In some species infections acquired by the nymphs are transmitted by the adult stage after a moult (transtadial passage). Man is normally infected by the nymphs.

Pathology

Babesia multiply asexually within the red cells which rupture with invasion of fresh red cells. This cycle is repeated with the major pathological features of haemoglobinàemia, haemoglobinuria, jaundice and hepatic and renal failure.

Immunity

B. divergens infects only immunocompromised

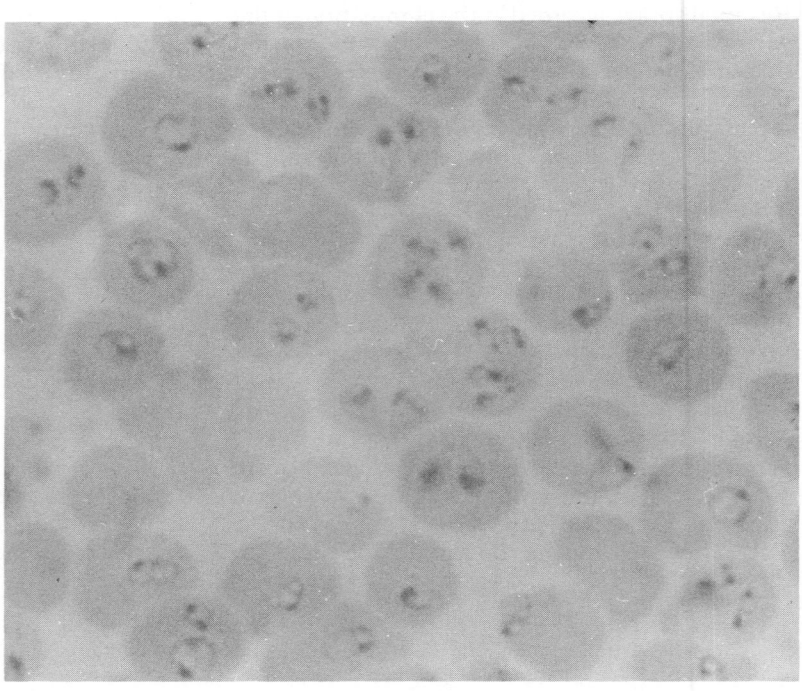

Fig. 1.19 *Babesia canis* (similar to *B. divergens*) in a blood film. (Courtesy WTIM.)

Transmission

B. divergens is transmitted by ixodid ticks of the *Boophilus* (cattle tick) species and possibly also *Ixodes ricinus* in Europe. The parasites are ingested with the blood meal, multiply in the gut epithelium and spread throughout the body. They invade the ovaries and are passed via the egg to the developing larva (transovarial trans-

individuals who have had their spleens removed and have T cell dysfunction.

Clinical features

Incubation period

This varies from one to four weeks.

Symptoms and signs

Infection with *B. divergens* results in a severe and almost always fatal infection. The onset is abrupt with high fever, chills and nausea. There is a severe haemolytic anaemia which progresses rapidly to haemoglobinuria and renal failure with jaundice.

Clinical pathology

Anaemia is severe with a high reticulocytosis and nucleated red cells in the peripheral blood. There is a marked rise in liver enzymes, blood urea and creatinine levels.

Diagnosis

The differential diagnosis from falciparum malaria and blackwater fever may be difficult but babesiosis is usually seen where there is no malarial transmission.

Parasitological diagnosis

The parasites may be seen in blood films stained with Giemsa but are usually scanty. They appear round, oval or piriform in shape or as small rings (Fig. 1.19). The distinguishing features from *P. falciparum* are the absence of pigment in the older forms and the presence of a white vacuole. Parasites may be isolated by inoculating gerbils which are susceptible.[96]

Serological diagnosis

IFAT titres up to 1/1204 have been obtained but there may be cross reactions with other babesia and malaria.

Treatment

There is no specific treatment and response to antimalarials is poor. Chloroquine 1500 mg initially by mouth with 500 mg daily for two weeks has been tried.

Epidemiology

B. divergens is an infection of animals and is infective only to humans without a spleen. Infections are sporadic since occasions when an infected tick comes into contact with a splenectomized individual are few and far between.

BABESIA MICROTI

Geographical distribution

Most cases of *B. microti* have occurred in North America on islands off the east coast of New England.[97] Cases of human babesiosis of unidentified species have been reported from California,[98] Georgia and Mexico.

Transmission

B. microti can infect people with normal T cell function and is transmitted by *Ixodes dammini* which has a wide host range, feeding readily on man, mice and voles as well as deer. It may be transmitted by blood transfusion since it has a prolonged period of parasitaemia in man.

Pathology

The pathology is similar to that of *B. divergens* though of milder degree.

Immunity

There is no evidence of T cell dysfunction in persons infected with *B. microti* and cases are mild, but in one splenectomized individual with T cell dysfunction the infection was very severe.[99]

Clinical features

Incubation period

The incubation period is one to four weeks.

Symptoms and signs

Human infection ranges from asymptomatic infections to prolonged severe illness. There is a gradual onset of fever, chills, myalgia and malaise. On examination there is often only fever but in others there is a mild to moderate haemolytic anaemia with leukopenia and sometimes hepatosplenomegaly. There is sometimes a slight rise in liver enzymes. The course of the disease is essentially benign and no fatal cases have been recorded.

Diagnosis

Parasitological diagnosis

Blood films will show scanty intra-erythrocytic parasites but tetrad forms are not seen. Small ring forms of *B. microti* are almost indistinguishable from *P. falciparum*. Parasites may be isolated by inoculating hamsters or gerbils when parasitaemia will appear in two to four weeks.

Serological diagnosis

IFAT titres are high; in one case 1/4096, without any cross reaction with other species.[99]

Treatment

B. microti infections are self-limiting but symptoms and parasitaemia may persist for some months. Chloroquine is used but its effect is difficult to judge. Quinine and clindamycin have been tried with some success.

Epidemiology

B. microti is a zoonosis with a wide range of reservoir hosts: deer, mice and voles, and is capable of infecting normal people with no T cell dysfunction. The vector *Ixodes dammini* feeds readily on man, deer and voles. Infections regularly occur along the north-east coast of New England where the environment has been allowed to revert to wilder conditions with an increase in deer and rodents. There are many inapparent infections which have been revealed by serological surveys.

Prevention

Since the tick does not transmit infection until it has been feeding in situ for at least 12 hours, regular removal of ticks will prevent infection. Blood donors from these areas must undergo serological screening for infection and anyone with a history of fever within the preceding two months must be prevented from giving blood.

REFERENCES

1 Bruce-Chwatt, L. J. (1985) *Essential Malariology* 2nd edn. London: Heinemann.
2 World Health Organization (1985) *Wld Hlth Stat.* 38, 193–231.
3 Harinasuta, T., Dixon, T. E., Warrell, D. A. et al (1982) *Southeast Asian J. trop. Med. Public. Hlth* 13, 1–34.
4 Bruce-Chwatt, L. J. (1985) *Br. med. J.* 291, 1072–1076.
5 Krotoski, W. A., Krotoski, D. M., Garnham, P. C. C. et al (1980) *Br. med. J.* i, 153.
6 Pasvol, G., Weatherall, D. J. & Wilson, R. J. M. (1980) *Br. J. Haematol.* 45, 285–295.
7 Bruce-Chwatt, L. J. (1982) *Trop. Dis. Bull.* 79, 827–840.
8 Chin, W. & Contacos, P. G. (1966) *Am. J. trop. Med. Hyg.* 15, 1.
9 Verdrager, J. (1964) *Bull. Wld Hlth Org.* 31, 747.
10 Robinson, G. L. (1966) *Br. med. J.* i, 982.
11 Bruce-Chwatt, L. J. (1974) *Bull. Wld Hlth Org.* 50, 337.
12 Covell, G. (1950) *Trop. Dis. Bull.* 47, 1147.
13 Nardin, E. H., Nussenzweig, R. S., Bryan, J. H. et al (1981) *Am. J. trop. Med. Hyg.* 30, 1159–1163.
14 Dodge, J. S. (1971) *Trans. R. Soc. trop. Med. Hyg.* 65, 689.
15 MacLeod, C. L., West, R., Saloman, W. L. et al (1982) *Am. J. trop. Med. Hyg.* 31, 893–896.
16 Looareesuwan, S., Warrell, D. A., White, N. J. et al (1983) *Lancet* i, 434–437.
17 Weatherall, D. J. & Abdalla, S. (1982) *Br. med. Bull.* 38, 147.
18 Abdalla, S., Weatherall, D. J., Wickramasinghe, S. N. et al (1980) *Br. J. Haem.* 46, 171–183.
19 Kelton, J. G., Keystone, J., Moore, J. et al (1983) *J. clin. Invest.* 71, 832–836.
20 Pannachet, P. (1967) *Ann. trop. Med. Parasit.* 61, 518.
21 Beale, P. J., Cormack, J. D. & Oldrey, T. B. N. (1972) *Br. med. J.* ii, 345.
22 Devakul, M., Harinasuta, T. & Reid, H. A. (1966) *Lancet* ii, 886.
23 White, N. J., Looareesuwan, S., Warrell, D. A. et al (1983) *Am. J. trop. Med. Hyg.* 32, 1–5.
24 Hutt, M. S. R. (1971) *Trans. R. Soc. trop. Med. Hyg.* 65, 273.
25 Hendrickse, R. G., Glasgow, E. F., Adeniyi, A. et al (1972) *Lancet* i, 1143.
26 Garnham, P. C. C. (1966) *Malaria Parasites and Other Haemosporidia.* Oxford: Blackwell.
27 Garnham, P. C. C. (1967) *Adv. Parasit.* 5, 157.
28 Luzzatto, L. (1979) *J. Am. Soc. Haematol.* 54, 961–976.
29 Pasvol, G. & Wilson, R. J. M. (1982) *Br. med. Bull.* 38, 133–140.
30 Miller, L. H., Johnson, J. G., Schmidt-Ullrich, R. et al (1980) *J. exp. Med.* 151, 790–799.
31 Mason, S. J., Miller, L. H., Shiroishi, T. et al (1977) *Br. J. Haematol.* 36, 327.
32 Mathews, H. M. & Armstrong, J. C. (1981) *Am. J. trop. Med. Hyg.* 30, 299–303.
33 Kidson, C., Lamont, G., Saul, A. et al (1981) *Proc. Natl Acad. Sci. USA* 78, 5829–5832.
34 Willcox, M., Bjorkman, A., Brohult, J. et al (1983) *Ann. trop. Med. Parasitol.* 77, 239–246.
35 Friedman, M. (1979) *Nature, Lond.* 280, 245.
36 Cohen, S. (1985) *J. R. Coll. Physns* 19, 210–212.
37 Mendis, K. N. & Targett, G. A. T. (1979) *Nature, Lond.* 277, 389–391.
38 Carter, R. & Chen, D. H. (1976) *Nature, Lond.* 263, 57–60.
39 McGregor, I. A., Williams, K. & Goodwin, L. J. (1963) *Br. med. J.* ii, 728.
40 Bray, R. S., Gunders, A. E., Burgess, R. W. et al (1962) *Riv. Malar.* 41, 199.

41 McGregor, I. A. (1965) *Trans. R. Soc. trop. Med. Hyg.* **59**, 817.

42 Weidanz, W. P. (1982) *Br. med. Bull.* **38**, 167–172.

43 Wilson, D. B. (1936) *Trans. R. Soc. trop. Med. Hyg.* **29**, 583.

44 Wilson, D. B. & Wilson, M. E. (1962) *Trans. R. Soc. trop. Med. Hyg.* **56**, 287.

45 Looareesuwan, S., Warrell, D. A., White, N. J. et al (1983) *Am. J. trop. Med. Hyg.* **32**, 911–915.

46 Bruce-Chwatt, L. J. (1963) *W. Afr. med. J.* **12**, 1.

47 Maegraith, B. G. (1948) *Pathological Processes in Malaria and Blackwater fever.* Oxford: Blackwell.

48 Maegraith, B. G. (1967) *Protozoology* **2**, 55.

49 Lowenthal, M. N. & Hutt, M. S. R. (1970) *Br. med. J.* **ii**, 262–263.

50 Bhattacharya, D. N., Harries, J. R. & Emerson, P. (1983) *Trans. R. Soc. trop. Med. Hyg.* **77**, 221–222.

51 Greenwood, B. M. & Fakunle, Y. M. (1979) *The Role of the Spleen in the Immunology of Parasitic Disease.* Basel: Schwabe.

52 Fakunle, Y. M. & Greenwood, B. M. (1976) *Lancet* **ii**, 608.

53 Fakunle, Y. M. (1981) *Clinics in Haematology* **10**, 963.

54 Nayak, N. C. (1982) In *Critical Reviews in Tropical medicine*, ed. R. K. Chandra, Vol. 1, pp. 247–273. New York: Plenum Press.

55 World Health Organization (1969) *Tech. Rep. Ser.* **433**, 19.

56 Wilks, N. E., Turner, P. P., Somers, K. et al (1965) *E. Afr. med. J.* **42**, 580.

57 McGregor, I. A., Wilson, R. J. M. & Billewicz, W. Z. (1983) *Trans. R. Soc. trop. Med. Hyg.* **77**, 232–244.

58 Gilles, H. M. & Hendrickse, R. G. (1963) *Br. med. J.* **ii**, 27.

59 Gilles, H. M. (1968) *Med. Today* **2**, 6.

60 Chongsuphajaisiddhi, T., Dauraug, V., Patch-arakessakul, V. et al (1983) *Southeast Asia J. trop. Med. public Hlth* **14**, 220–222.

61 Booth, K., Larkin, K. & Maddocks, I. (1967) *Br. med. J.* **iii**, 32.

62 Looareesuwan, S., White, N. J., Benjasurat, Y. et al (1985) *Lancet* **ii**, 805–808.

63 World Health Organization (1983) *Bull. Wld Hlth Org.* **61**, 169–178.

64 World Health Organization (1984) *Tech. Rep. Ser.* **711**, 126–127.

65 White, N. J., Looareesuwan, S., Warrell, D. A. et al (1981) *Lancet* **ii**, 1069–1071.

66 Phillips, R. E., Warrell, D. A., White, N. J. et al (1985) *New Engl. J. Med.* **312**, 1273–1278.

67 Campbell, C. C. (1983) *Am. J. trop. Med. Hyg.* **32**, 1216–1220.

68 Watkins, W. M., Sixsmith, D. G., Spencer, H. C. et al (1984) *Lancet* **i**, 375–379.

69 White, N. J., Warrell, D. A., Chanthavanich, P. et al (1983) *New Engl. J. Med.* **309**, 61–66.

70 Hall, A. P. (1985) *Lancet* **i**, 1453.

71 Warrell, D. A., Looareesuwan, S., Warrell, M. J. et al (1982) *New Engl. J. Med.* **306**, 313–319.

72 White, N. J. & Warrell, D. A. (1983) *Trop. Doc.* **13**, 153–158.

73 Clarke, E. G. C. (1969) *Isolation and Identification of Drugs*, p. 15. London: Pharmaceutical Press.

74 Wilson, T. & Edeson, J. F. R. (1954) *Med. J. Malaya* **8**, 115.

75 Haskins, W. T. (1958) *Am. J. trop. Med. Hyg.* **7**, 199.

76 Lelijfeld, J. & Kortmann, H. (1968) *Annual Report East African Institute of Malaria and Vector-borne Diseases*, p. 23.

77 World Health Organization (1973). *Tech. Rep. Ser.* **529.**

78 Leading article (1985) *Lancet* **i**, 1487–1488.

79 Rosario, V. E. (1976) *Nature, Lond.* **261**, 585–586.

80 Fitch, C. D. (1983) *Ciba Foundation Symposium* **94**, 222–232.

81 Tin, F., Hlaing, N., Tun, T. et al (1985) *Bull. Wld Hlth Org.* **63**, 727–730.

82 Rieckmann, K. J., McNamara, J. V., Frisher, H. et al (1968) *Am. J. trop. Med. Hyg.* **17**, 661.

83 Rieckmann, K. H., Sax, L. J., Campbell, G. H. et al (1978) *Lancet* **i**, 22–23.

84 Gilles, H. M., Harinasuta, T. & Bunnag, D. (1984) In *Recent Advances in Tropical Medicine*, ed. H. M. Gilles, pp. 10–15. Edinburgh: Churchill Livingstone.

85 Giglioli, G., Dyrting, A. E., Rutten, F. J. et al (1967) *Trans. R. Soc. trop. Med. Hyg.* **61**, 313.

86 Young, J. F., Hockmayer, W. T., Gros, M. et al (1985) *Science* **228**, 958–962.

87 Mendis, K. N. & Targett, G. A. T. (1981). *Trans. R. Soc. trop. Med. Hyg.* **75**, 158–159.

88 MacDonald, G. (1952) *Trop. Dis. Bull.* **49**, 569, 813.

89 Voller, A. & Draper, C. C. (1982) *Br. med. Bull.* **38**, 173–177.

90 Jopling, W. H. (1979) *Lancet* **i**, 1340.

91 Curtis, C. F. & White, G. B. (1984) *J. trop. Med. Hyg.* **87**, 101–114.

92 Chin, W., Contacos, P. G., Coatney, G. R. et al (1965) *Science, NY* **149**, 865.

93 Skrabalo, Z. & Deanovic, Z. (1957) *Doc. Med. Geogr. Trop.* **9**, 11.

94 Garnham, P. C. C., Donnelly, J., Hoogstraal, H. et al (1969) *Br. med. J.* **iv**, 768.

95 Rabinovich, S. A. (1978) *Medskaya Parazit.* **47**, 97.

96 Lewis, D. & Williams, H. (1979) *Nature, Lond.* **278**, 170.

97 Anderson, A. E., Cassaday, P. B. & Healy, G. R. (1974) *Am. J. clin. Path.* **62**, 612.

98 Scholtens, R. G., Braff, H., Healy, G. R. et al (1966) *Am. J. trop. Med.* **17**, 810.

99 Rowin, K. S., Tanowitz, H. B., Rubinstein, A. et al (1984) *Trans. R. Soc. trop. Med. Hyg.* **78**, 442–444.

TRYPANOSOMIASIS
An Introduction to Chapters 2 and 3

Trypanosomes are important causes of fever in the tropics. They have a life-cycle which involves two separate hosts, one a mammal, the other an insect. They are divided into two groups. Stercoraria and Salivaria.

Stercoraria

Development in the insect vector (triatomid bug) occurs in the posterior part of the gut (posterior station) and transmission is by faecal contamination. This group includes *Trypanosoma cruzi*, the cause of American trypanosomiasis or Chagas' disease, and *T. rangeli*.

Salivaria

Development in the insect vector (tsetse fly) is in the salivary gland (anterior station) and transmission by bite. This group includes a number of trypanosomal forms which are referred to as the *T. brucei* group and cause African trypanosomiasis or sleeping sickness.

There are a number of different forms at various stages in the life-cycle (Fig. I.23, p. 1258) of which three are important in the human context. *Trypomastigotes*, *epimastigotes* and *amastigotes* (Figure).

Trypomastigotes are long elongated slender mobile organisms 17–30 μm in length, laterally flattened with a free flagellum, attached to an undulating membrane on the body surface. There is a central nucleus and a posterior kinetoplast (Figure). They occur in the peripheral blood of the mammalian host. Multiplication occurs by longitudinal fission; the kinetoplast and nucleus divide before the cytoplasm and a new flagellum develops from the new kinetoplast. Trypanosomes may be *monomorphic* (*T. cruzi*) when all individuals possess a free flagellum and do not vary in size or shape, or *pleomorphic* (*T. brucei*) when the trypanosomes vary with regard to size and position of the nucleus and length of the flagellum (see also Appendix I, p. 1271).

Epimastigotes which are found in the insect midgut are not infective to man, but they finally change into short and stumpy *metacyclic* trypanosomes which are infective to man.

Amastigotes are intracellular round and oval forms measuring 1.5–5 μm in length without an external flagellum, and are found in the tissues of the mammalian host infected with *T. cruzi*.

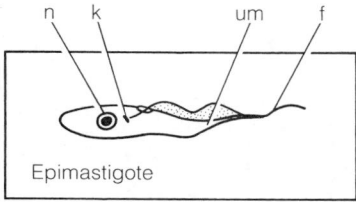

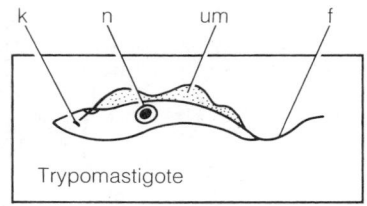

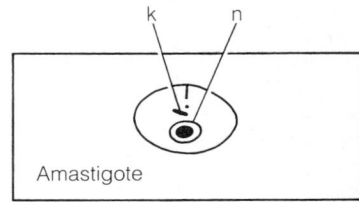

Figure Forms of trypanosome. n = nucleus, k = kinetoplast, um = undulating membrane, f = flagellum.

Chapter 2
African Trypanosomiasis

GEOGRAPHICAL DISTRIBUTION

Human sleeping sickness is found in West, central and eastern Africa between the parallels 20° north and 20° south (Fig. 2.1). Gambian sleeping sickness is found in West Africa, Zaire, southern Sudan and Uganda with the main strongholds along the Congo and Niger rivers and their main branches. Rhodesian sleeping sickness is confined to central and eastern Africa. Since the 1960s political crises and turmoil have occurred with a cycle of disorder/recrudescence so that at present Zaire has the highest incidence

in the whole of Africa and the incidence in Zambia and Uganda is on the increase. There is decreased prevalence in Nigeria and today it is only in the Benue valley that the disease is of any significance.

AETIOLOGY

African trypanosomiasis is caused by trypanosomes of the *T. brucei* group which have a life-cycle in man and in the insect vector, the tsetse fly. For morphology and structure see Appendix I, p. 1267

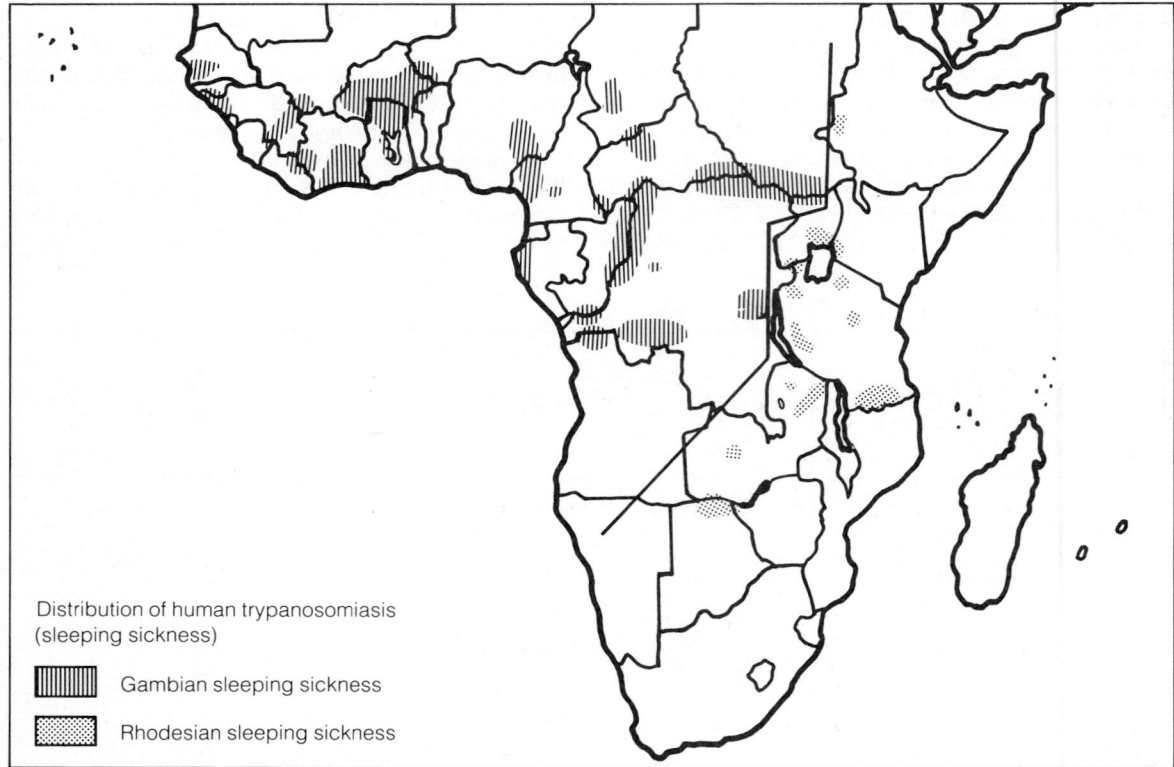

Distribution of human trypanosomiasis (sleeping sickness)

▦ Gambian sleeping sickness

▦ Rhodesian sleeping sickness

Fig. 2.1 Distribution of human trypanosomiasis (sleeping sickness). (Courtesy Department of Entomology, London School of Hygiene and Tropical Medicine.)

54

Trypanosomes are actively motile and are pleomorphic circulating in the blood of man and animals in a number of different morphological forms: long and slender (20–40 μm), intermediate short and stumpy (15–25 μm) and occasionally posterior nucleated forms (Fig. 2.2 and Plate II.6). They are covered with a surface antigenic

posterior end where they escape into the ecto-peritrophic space, migrating forwards 10–20 days after infection to the end of the anterior end of the midgut (proventricular valve). From here they proceed outwards to the tip of the labrum and return down the hypopharynx to the salivary glands.

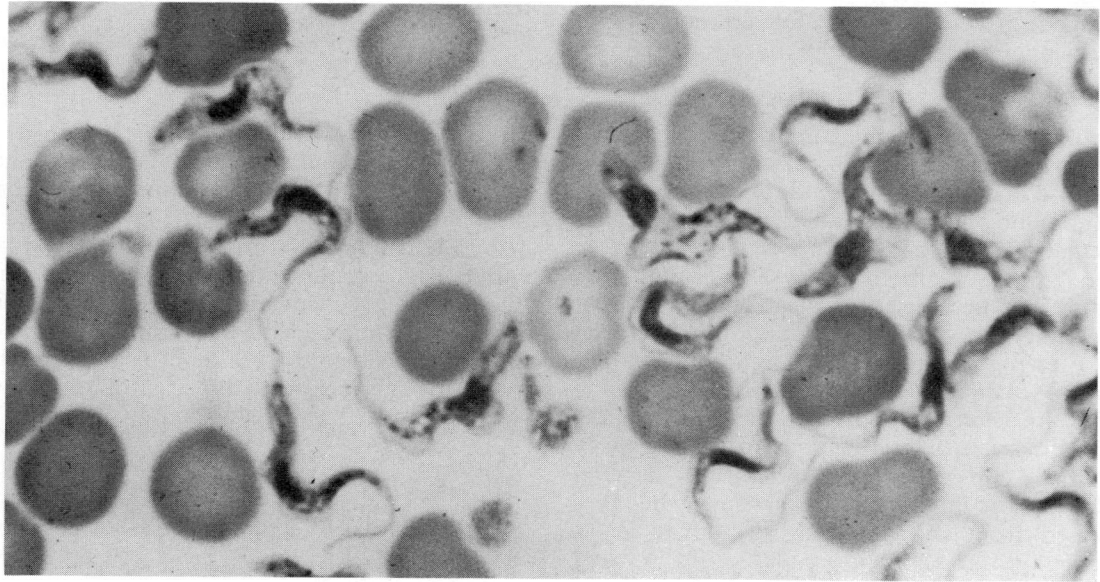

Fig. 2.2 Long, thin and stumpy forms of *T. rhodesiense* in a blood film. Posterior kinetoplast (k), nucleus (n) and flagellum (f) are arrowed. × 1400. (Courtesy W. E. Ormerod.)

coat which varies in antigenicity and is the source of the variant specific antigen (VAT) (see section on immunity, p. 60, and Appendix I, p. 1281).

Cycle in the tsetse fly (see Fig. I.30, p. 1272)

The long slender infective trypomastigote forms are taken up by both male and female flies with a blood meal. In the midgut the trypanosomes lose their antigenic coat and may take one of two possible routes.

Short-circuit route (Fig I.32,9–12, p. 1279)

The trypanosomes penetrate through the midgut wall from which they can enter the salivary glands direct.

Classical route (Fig. I.32,1–8, p. 1279)

The trypanosomes pass down the gut to the end of the peritrophic membrane until they reach its

In the salivary glands they change into multiplicative *epimastigotes* (p. 53) and then into the infective non-dividing *metacyclic* forms.

The cycle in the tsetse fly occupies a period of about one month but can be variable.

Cycle in man (Appendix I, p. 1279 and Figs. I.30, p. 1272, and I.31, p. 1278)

Man is infected by the bite of the tsetse fly with metacyclic trypanosomes which are transformed into multiplicative long slender blood forms. Short and stumpy forms are also found in the blood and tissue fluids, and this is the stage infective for the tsetse fly.

The role of the different stages is controversial and an alternative life-cycle has been postulated[1] in which 'aberrant' forms, and possible tissue forms, of the parasite are located in the ependymal cells lining the ventricles of the brain covering the choroid plexus, where they are protected from trypanocidal drugs, to re-enter the blood and cause relapses (see Fig. I.31, p. 1278).

Strains and infectivity

All trypanosomes of the *T. brucei* group are morphologically identical and were formerly thought to consist of three subspecies, based upon their infectivity for man: *T. brucei brucei* (not infective), *T. brucei gambiense* (infective) and *T. brucei rhodesiense* (infective). (Subspecific names are retained for convenience. They are not used in any geopolitical context but purely for identification purposes.)

It is now known that *T. brucei* is one species, confirmed by isoenzyme studies, in which some strains are infective and others non-infective to man and that this characteristic is not immutable.

It has long been known that human serum has a lethal effect on some forms of *T. brucei* (*T. b. brucei*) but not others (*T. b. rhodesiense*). This feature has been used in the blood incubation infectivity test (BIIT)[2] to distinguish them, but this feature is not an all-or-nothing affair. Serum-sensitive clones can undergo a change to serum resistance which then persists in subsequent variant antigenic types, indicating a way in which non-infective '*T. brucei*' can develop naturally into infective '*T. rhodesiense*' when flies infected from animals feed on human blood (Appendix I, p. 1262)

Zymodemes (Appendix I, p. 1264)

T. brucei can be classified using isoenzyme patterns.[3] The subject is complicated but analysis of these zymodemes has greatly clarified the epidemiology of the disease. A few zymodemes of *T. brucei* cause human disease in West Africa and others in East and central Africa, and mixed infections of different zymodemes circulate in both domestic and wild animal populations. Zymodeme analysis is mainly used for the study of the disease in any particular case. (For further details of the structure, life-cycle, metabolism and zymodemes, see Appendix I.)

In general, *T. b. gambiense* is a parasite adapted to man and riverine tsetse flies *Glossina fuscipes* and *G. tachinoides* which feed on man. However, in some areas the pig and some game animals (Appendix I, p. 1278) are important hosts. *T. b. rhodesiense* is a parasite adapted to wild game animals and cattle including especially the bushbuck (*Tragelaphus scriptus*) (Fig. 2.10) which lives in close contact with man and is transmitted between game animals and to man (to whom it

is not so well adapted) by the game tsetse flies, *G. morsitans*, *G. pallidipes* and *G. swynnertoni*.

TRANSMISSION

The usual method of transmission is by the bite of a tsetse fly after cyclical development or direct transmission while feeding.

Congenital transmission

T. b. gambiense

Although uncommon, congenital transmission is well documented. A case in Germany in a European child born in Hamburg, a case in France,[4] a child born in Marseilles seen at the age of two with hydrocephalus (mother had left Chad when five months pregnant), in Cameroon[5] and, more recently, a woman who was a 'healthy carrier' gave birth to a child three months after arriving in the UK from Zaire who was found to have sleeping sickness two years later.[6]

T. b. rhodesiense

Two congenital infections have been described in Zambia.[7,8]

Blood transfusion

Transmission of African trypanosomiasis by blood transfusion is rare but cases have been reported.[9,10]

Laboratory infections

Accidental infection from handling and bleeding infected rats occurs from time to time.

Transmission by tsetse flies (see also Appendix III, p. 1447)

The usual method of transmission and the only important one is by the bite of the tsetse fly in which cyclical development is the usual occurrence (see section on cycle in the tsetse fly, above). However, mechanical transmission is also a possibility.

Mechanical transmission

Duke in Uganda suggested on epidemiological grounds that mechanical transmission by *Glos-*

sina of a virulent strain of gambiense might be responsible for some epidemics and this is supported by more recent observations[11] in the Upper Volta that other biting flies, such as tabanids, could transmit in a similar manner thus accounting for trypanosomal infections acquired in areas where there were no tsetse flies (see Appendix III, p. 1445).

PATHOGENESIS

The pathogenesis of human African trypanosomiasis is not yet fully understood. Present knowledge and theory underlying the clinical, laboratory and pathological changes have been reviewed.[12] Lesions may be caused in two main ways: (1) toxic and (2) immunological.

1 Toxic

The production of a toxin by the trypanosome has been suggested but never proven. The metabolic activity of the trypanosomes leads to a high carbohydrate turnover with the accumulation of pyruvates in blood and tissue fluids and may be responsible for the inflammatory changes seen in the primary chancre, and the lesions in skeletal and heart muscle (Appendix I, p. 1271)

Destruction of the ependymal cells lining the ventricles of the brain by trypanosomes, with the release of tryptophol—an inhibitor of serotonin, the neurohormone responsible for the maintenance of sleep rhythm—has been suggested as a mechanism responsible for the disturbance of sleep rhythm in African sleeping sickness,[13] and possibly for other hypothalamic effects.

2 Immunopathological reaction[12]

An immediate hypersensitivity (Type 1) reaction may account for the pruritus and urticaria found in early cases of trypanosomiasis. Autoantibodies are produced but it is not known if these cause tissue damage. High levels of immune complexes are found but have not been shown to damage the brain or the heart. Complement activation[14] with the formation of kinins[15] could cause vascular lesions (Fig. 2.3). The dominant event in trypanosomiasis is B cell proliferation, first within the lymph glands and then in the brain which could be caused by a T cell mitogen or from interference with T lymphocyte control over B lymphocyte function (Fig. 2.3).

Immunosuppression leads to secondary infection in the late stages. The pathogenesis of the endocrine changes, impotence, amenorrhoea, obesity and more severe hypogonadism is obscure.

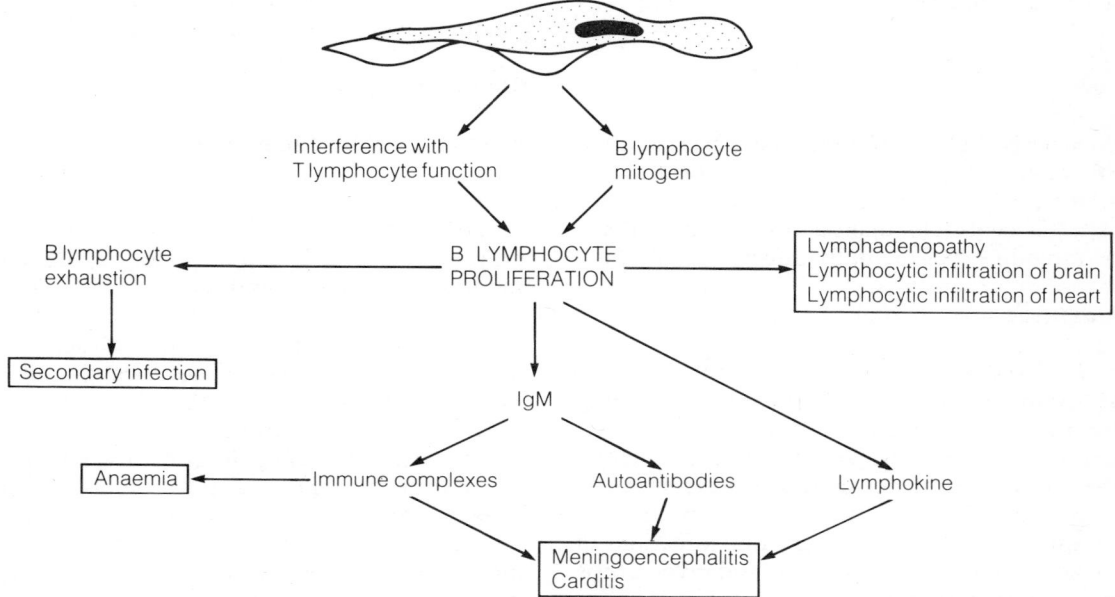

Fig. 2.3 A hypothesis suggesting a dominant role for B lymphocyte proliferation in the pathogenesis of sleeping sickness (after Greenwood and Whittle[12]).

PATHOLOGY

Few studies have appeared on the gross pathology since the review.[16] The minimum infective dose of metacyclic trypanosomes is about 300. The trypanosomes multiply in the tissue spaces at the site of the bite (chancre). There is a local inflammatory response with oedema and mononuclear infiltration. The trypanosomes then spread to the lymphatics, lymph glands and bloodstream.

Lymph glands

The lymph glands become swollen and fleshy— later hard and fibrotic. Microscopically the follicles are enlarged with prominent reactive centres and many plasma cells in the sinuses. Some cells contain Russell bodies. Trypanosomes can be demonstrated in lymph gland juice. The main feature of the pathological change is a vasculitis.

Spleen

The spleen is slightly enlarged. The malpighian follicles are few and inconspicuous. There is a general proliferation of the reticuloendothelium, congestion at the periphery of the splenic sinuses, often focal necrosis with endothelial macrophages and ingested red corpuscles. Giant cells have been observed.

Liver

The liver is slightly enlarged, there is infiltration with mononuclear cells in the periportal tracts and microscopical mononuclear cell granulomas. A specific central lobular necrosis has been demonstrated in experimentally infected monkeys.

Heart (see also Chapter 61)

In *T. b. rhodesiense* infections there is a pancarditis involving all layers of the heart including mural and valvular endocardium and the pericardium. It has been shown in experimental infection that trypanosomes are present in the interstitial tissues of the heart and especially in the endocardium.[17] In experimental infections in monkeys myocarditis is present, and myocarditis has been described in man in association with pericardial effusion.[18,19] Histologically there is a marked interstitial infiltration with plasma and morular cells with disappearance of muscle fibres and fibrosis (Fig. 61.1, p. 1012).

Similar changes may be found in *T. b. gambiense* infections.

Kidneys

There is a proliferative glomerulonephritis leading to fibrosis.

Bone marrow

The bone marrow is hypercellular with areas of gelatinous degeneration.

Lungs

The lesions in the lungs are characterized by intravascular proliferation of the reticuloendothelium which may block the capillaries with fibrosis and collapse of the alveoli.

Skin

Localized oedema due to collections of lymphocytes may be observed in the eyelids, perineum and the skin of the back.

Serous effusions

There may be serous effusions into the peritoneum, pleural cavities and pericardium.

Blood changes

Anaemia (see also Chapter 58)

Moderate and sometimes severe anaemia develops in African trypanosomiasis. Haemolysis of red cells appears to be the most important mechanism and there is a reduction in the mean red cell life-span.[20] Several mechanisms have been proposed for this haemolysis: lysins produced by the trypanosomes,[21] coating of red cells possibly with circulating immune complexes[19] and hypersplenism.

Other features include leukocytosis but with a relative neutropenia, and thrombocytopenia which is thought to be due to platelet pooling in the enlarged spleen. Thrombocytopenia is important in the pathogenesis of haemorrhage, vasoconstriction and tissue damage[22] and some cases of overt disseminated intravascular coagulation have been described in *T. rhodesiense* infection thought to be triggered by endothelial damage and haemolysis.

Other features found in the blood include autoagglutination of red cells with rouleaux formation (cold agglutinins) and a high erythrocyte sedimentation rate (ESR), low blood sugar (consumption by trypanosomes), a diminished alkali reserve, false-positive Wassermann reaction and a great increase in non-specific IgM.

All these changes revert to normal following successful treatment.

Central nervous system

Typical pathological lesions are seen only when pathogenic trypanosomes have invaded the central nervous system. No gross lesions of the nerve centres are present but there is progressive chronic leptomeningitis, especially in the Virchow–Robin space (where the pia sheathes the blood vessels and the fluid acts as lymph) and also on the vertex (Dürck's nodes).

The dura may be adherent to the skull and to the arachnoid. The brain itself is congested and oedematous, the surface smooth, with convolutions flattened by increased pressure. The consistency of the brain tissue is unaltered except for softening around any haemorrhages that may occur. The ventricles are distended with fluid. In all cases there is perivascular round-cell infiltration (perivascular cuffing) throughout the brain tissue and meninges, varying in amount

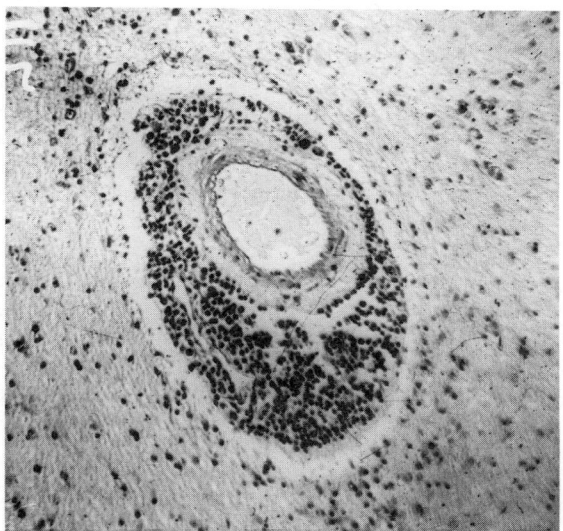

Fig. 2.4 Perivascular cuffing in the cerebral cortex due to trypanosomiasis. (Courtesy Dr A. C. Steventon.)

and in different anatomical regions (Fig. 2.4). The invading cells are glia cells, lymphocytes, the morular (Mott) and Marshalko cells (Fig. 2.5). The two latter types are degenerative plasmocytes. Morular cells stain deeply with a unilateral oval nucleus and vacuolated protoplasm. Marshalko cells are large plasma cells with a blue polar zone round the nucleus with surrounding halo and acidophilic protoplasm. The morular cells appear to play an important part in the production of IgM locally within the central nervous system in late trypanosomiasis.[23]

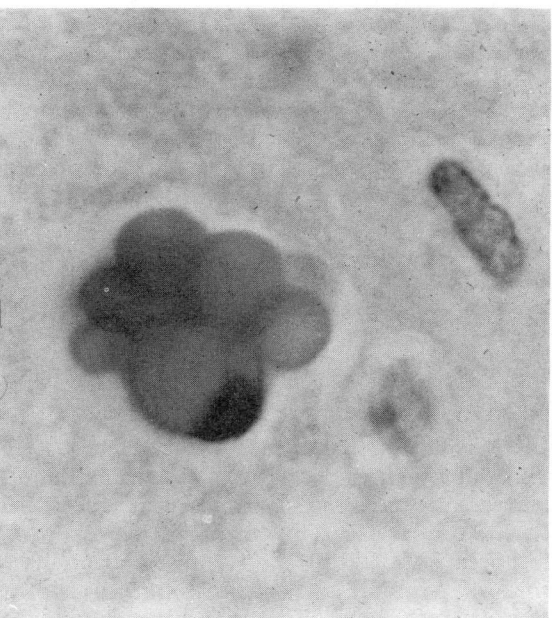

Fig. 2.5 A morular cell in the brain in cerebral trypanosomiasis.

As originally demonstrated in experimental animals and in man, in advanced cases, lesions in lymphatic glands and in brain are caused by invasion of the solid tissues by trypanosomes which have migrated from the bloodstream. In the brain they have been found mainly in the frontal lobe, pons and medulla, aggregated together in masses or nests without definite relation to blood vessels. Myelin lesions of the brain have been described.[24] The organisms also invade the cerebrospinal fluid; they enter the canal from the choroidal plexus where they congregate in active stages of division and intracellular forms have been described in the ependymal cells of the choroid plexus in mice which may represent cryptic forms of the trypanosomes.[25] (For eye complications, see Chapter 70.)

The spinal canal may even be blocked by cell proliferation. The cerebrospinal fluid in early cases is under increased pressure (30–100 cm H_2O), the total proteins being very much increased to 1 g/litre (normal 0.2 g/litre).

The cells are increased to 15–500/mm³ or more (normal 2–3) and comprise lymphocytes, mononuclears, morular cells (Fig. 2.5), eosinophils and trypanosomes.

IMMUNITY

Man is immune to infection with the common trypanosomes of big game, *T. congolense* and *T. vivax*. Although there is no direct evidence that man becomes immune after exposure to infection with *T. b. gambiense* there is no doubt that when the disease has lasted any time in a district the inhabitants exhibit a degree of resistance not seen in districts more recently invaded. There is a cyclical variation in the numbers of trypanosomes in the blood and each successive wave is associated with an antigenic change. This property is known as antigenic variation and is associated with changes in the antigens expressed on the glycoprotein surface coat of the trypomastigotes. The successive glycoprotein antigens are variant-specific surface antigens (VSSA) which produce variant antigenic types (VAT) (Appendix I, p. 1281). The host's reactions to the VATs are the basis of the immune response, the production of immune complexes, autoantibodies and immunosuppression.

Mechanism of immunity[12] (Fig. 2.3)

Trypanosomes induce depression of T and B cell responses by a mechanism that involves some kind of T suppressor cell and macrophages. There is an interference with T lymphocyte function and a great increase in B lymphocytes induced by B lymphocyte mitogens. This leads to B lymphocyte proliferation and a great increase in non-specific IgM with eventual exhaustion leading to immunodepression and secondary infection. The great increase in IgM causes immune complexes (with anaemia), and autoantibodies with the production of lymphokines cause meningoencephalitis and carditis (see pathogenesis, p. 57).

CLINICAL FEATURES

Natural history

After a tsetse bite a local lesion (common in *T. b. rhodesiense* infection) appears, to be followed by intermittent fever of variable duration, and then after a period (short, three to six months in *T. b. rhodesiense*, one to two years in *T. b. gambiense* infection) by invasion of the brain and a progressive meningoencephalitis with coma and death from intercurrent infection. *T. b. rhodesiense* causes an acute and rapidly fatal infection in contrast to *T. b. gambiense* in which infection is chronic with occasional asymptomatic cases and occasional self-cure. However, the degree of illness may be very variable and cases tolerant to both type of trypanosomes do occur forming apparently healthy carriers (see section on subclinical infection below).

Incubation period

The incubation period is two to three weeks although some cases have developed as little as 5 days after the infective bite.

Symptoms and signs

The symptoms and signs of *T. b. gambiense* and *T. b. rhodesiense* are similar except that the illness is usually chronic in *T. b. gambiense* infection with a natural duration of two to three years or more until death ensues, whereas *T. b. rhodesiense* infection runs a more rapid course and death usually occurs within a year of infection unless treatment is given.

The bite of an infected *Glossina* may be followed by a local swelling, the trypanosomal chancre (Fig. 2.6). This is more usual in *T. b. rhodesiense* and commoner in Caucasians. The trypanosomal chancre is like a large boil but is relatively painless (an important point in diagnosis) and is associated with localized lymph gland enlargement. The lesion, usually on the face or arms in *G. morsitans* transmitted and on the lower leg in *G. pallidipes* transmitted infections, soon subsides leaving a characteristic mark (of great diagnostic help), to be followed by invasion of the bloodstream.

Blood stage

The most important symptom of invasion of the blood is fever which is accompanied in Cau-

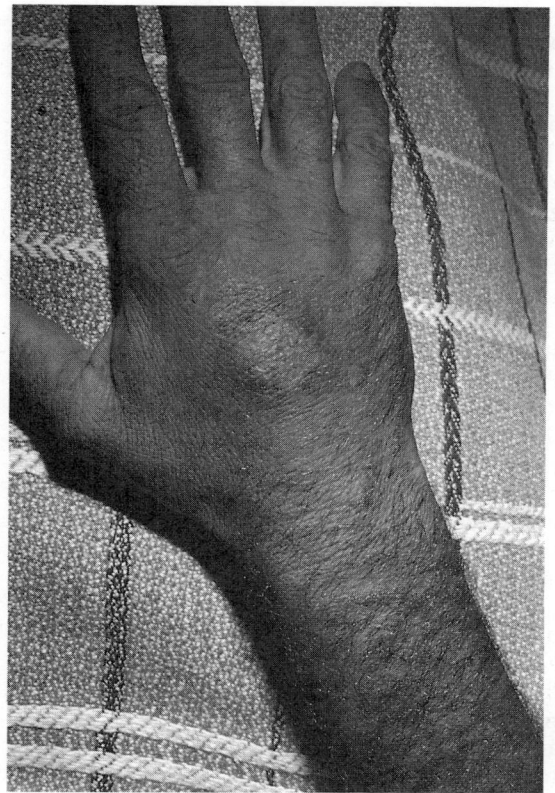

Fig. 2.6 Trypanosomal chancre due to *T. rhodesiense*. (Courtesy Dr D. M. Minter.)

casians sometimes by a peculiar type of erythema and a certain amount of connective tissue infiltration.

Fever

The onset of fever is accompanied by the appearance of trypanosomes in the peripheral blood 5–21 days after the infecting bite. A form of hyperaesthesia, known as Kérandel's sign, may be present but is uncommon: a marked tenderness on pressure over the tibiae which after a slight delay causes the patient to withdraw his limbs sharply.

The fever subsides at first, to recur at irregular periods of days or months accompanied by general malaise, severe headaches and joint pains. The bouts of fever are accompanied by waves of parasitaemia. Fever may be mild or occasionally hyperpyrexial (41°C). It may last for weeks, the apyrexial periods being prolonged or continuous without parasitaemia. As the disease

progresses the symptoms associated with the waves of parasitaemia become less frequent with the disappearance of trypanosomes from the blood, and in the later stages of the disease they are absent and the patient becomes debilitated, anaemic and feeble.

Liver

A tender enlargement of the liver is usual especially in *T. b. rhodesiense* infection.

Lymphadenopathy and splenomegaly

Lymphadenopathy may be local, most commonly involving the posterior triangle of the neck in *T. b. gambiense* infection (Winterbottom's sign, Fig. 2.7). Only one gland may be visible or there may be several. In the early stages they are soft, later becoming hard and indurated. They are usually painless and rarely suppurate.

The *spleen* is usually enlarged in the blood stages of the disease.

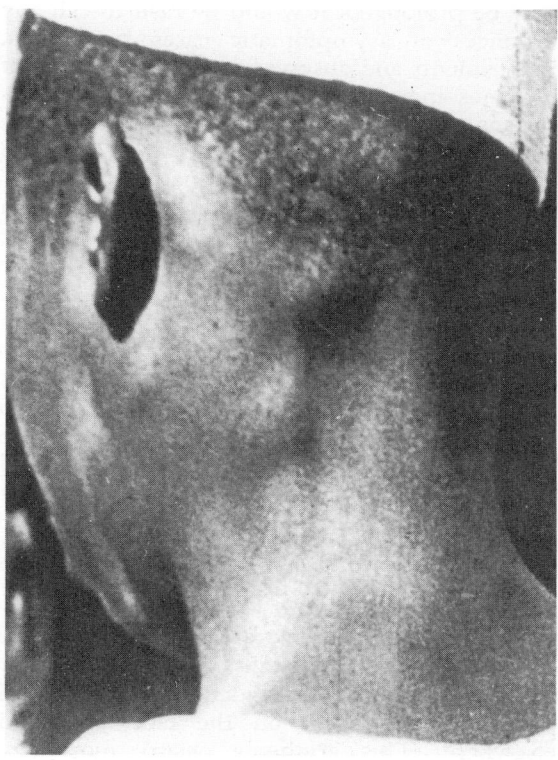

Fig. 2.7 Enlargement of the cervical lymph glands in trypanosomiasis (Winterbottom's sign). (Courtesy Dr F. Kleine.)

Blood

The blood count shows a varying degree of normocytic normochromic anaemia with a relative lymphocytosis and thrombocytopenia.

Course of the disease

In *T. b. gambiense* infection the condition of irregular fever, persistent tachycardia, debility, lymphadenopathy and anaemia may go on for months and, in some cases, years. In *T. b. rhodesiense* infection this stage does not last for more than a few months and may be as short as one month before invasion of the central nervous system takes place.

Variations in the course of the infection

Subclinical infections

In *T. b. gambiense* infections a proportion of cases may terminate spontaneously but, since this infection undergoes periods of quiescence which may be prolonged, it would be rash to call any instances of asymptomatic cases subclinical. Experiments and observations in other forms of trypanosomiasis, as well as some cases in Caucasians, justify the belief that occasionally the parasite does die out spontaneously. Observers in West Africa,[26] Katanga, Botswana,[27] Zimbabwe[28] and Zambia[29] have reported cases in which healthy Africans showed trypanosomes in the peripheral blood, but it is not known whether these infections were subsequently fatal or not. Recent methods of blood concentration which show very light infections may show these cases to be commoner, and a woman from Zaire was found to have a *T. b. gambiense* infection two years after leaving Zaire for the UK because her child born after arrival developed cerebral trypanosomiasis two years later.[6]

Unusual manifestations

SKIN RASHES

In Caucasians extensive areas of skin may be affected by a fugitive patchy, frequently annular erythema, usually most evident on the chest and back but also often on the face, legs and elsewhere. This erythema occurs most frequently in the early stages of infection. Some of the patches may be 15–30 cm in diameter, their margins fading off insensibly into the surrounding skin. This rash can be brought on by heat. Sometimes there is erythema nodosum. Itching of the skin is a feature of the early stages.

OEDEMA

Oedema of the skin and subcutaneous tissues is a feature of the early disease. Oedema of the face gives rise to the 'puffy face syndrome' (Fig. 2.8)[12] which may be due to water imbalance, and transitory localized oedema may occur on the neck, abdomen, lower eyelids and sheath of the penis.

MYOCARDITIS (see also Chapter 61)

Pericardial effusion and congestive heart failure have been described in *T. b. rhodesiense* infection[19] and mild disorders of conduction in *T. b. gambiense* infections.[30] Abnormal electrocardiograms were found in over one-third of untreated patients with *T. b. rhodesiense* infection and a useful review of the literature on the subject is given by Jones et al.[31]

OTHER FEATURES

Neuralgic pains, cramps, formication and paraesthesiae of different kinds are not uncommon; periostitis of the tibiae may occur and para-articular ossification has been described.[32] Toxic iridocyclitis and choroiditis are sometimes met with. In women endocrine dysfunction results in amenorrhoea. There is a high abortion rate and premature births, stillbirths and perinatal deaths are frequent. In men there may be impotence and in some, in the later stages, gynaecomastia or a feminine distribution of fat. The appearance known as the 'forme bouffé' is due to a myxoedematous infiltration of the subcutaneous tissue which may be mistaken for a sign of good health or obesity. There is evidence of liver dysfunction in the early stages of *T. b. rhodesiense* infection. Mild hepatocellular jaundice, alteration in liver function tests, decreased serum albumin and raised serum globulin can closely resemble findings in *P. falciparum* malaria and infectious hepatitis. Jaundice, sometimes severe enough to be mistaken for infectious hepatitis, has occasionally been the presenting sign or a prominent feature of the illness in Caucasians. Tenderness and enlargement of the liver are not uncommon in Africans in the early stage of the disease, but frank jaundice, as detected in the sclera, is unusual (about 4% in one series of cases).

Death from intercurrent disease, from rapidly developing encephalomyelitis causing convulsions, status epilepticus or coma may supervene at any stage of trypanosomiasis. Usually the case progresses into the stage known as 'sleeping sickness' which depends upon the entry of the parasite into the central nervous system.

Sleeping sickness stage (cerebral trypanosomiasis)

The terminal stage of trypanosomiasis is the result of a chronic meningoencephalomyelitis. The characteristic symptoms are those of any chronic meningoencephalomyelitis and consist of progressive mental deterioration proceeding to coma with, in some cases, localized manifestations.

In *T. b. gambiense* the interval between the start of the infection and the encephalitic stage is about two years but an interval of several years, possibly eight, may elapse. In *T. b. rhodesiense* the interval is very short, usually a few months. The average duration of this stage is from four to eight months, not infrequently less, and a course of more than a year is rare.

Generally the first indications of the oncoming of sleeping sickness are an accentuation of the debility and languor usually associated with trypanosomiasis. There is disinclination to exertion, slow shuffling gait, somnolent expression, puffiness and drooping of the eyelids and a tendency to lapse into sleep during the daytime (Fig. 2.8), contrasting with restlessness at night. The patient will walk if forced to do so with unsteady, swaying gait. There may be fibrillary twitching of the muscles, especially the tongue, tremor of the hands and, more rarely, of the legs. His speech is difficult to follow, becoming indistinct and staccato. By this time the patient has taken to bed and lies about in a corner of the hut indifferent to everything going on about him. He never spontaneously engages in conversation or even asks for food, but is still able to speak and take food if this is brought to him. If he is properly nursed there is no general wasting. So far, the striking changes are the mental and personal changes accompanying a chronic encephalomyelitis.

As the disease progresses *wasting* becomes a major feature, tremor of the hands and tongue become more marked and convulsive or choreic movements may occur in the limbs, or in limited muscular areas. Sometimes these convulsions are followed by local temporary paralyses. Sometimes there is meningismus with head retraction. There is generally intolerable pruritus, bed sores form, saliva dribbles from the mouth, the body wastes and finally the patient dies comatose or from slowly advancing asthenia. He may succumb to convulsions, hyperpyrexia, pneumonia, dysentery or other intercurrent infections.

There are considerable variations in the manifestations which may be found in any chronic meningoencephalomyelitis. Mania is not uncommon, and there may be manic depressive episodes going on to a progressive mental deterioration and idiocy. Delusions may be present.

Localized neurological signs, such as hemiplegia, facial palsy, ophthalmoplegia and men-

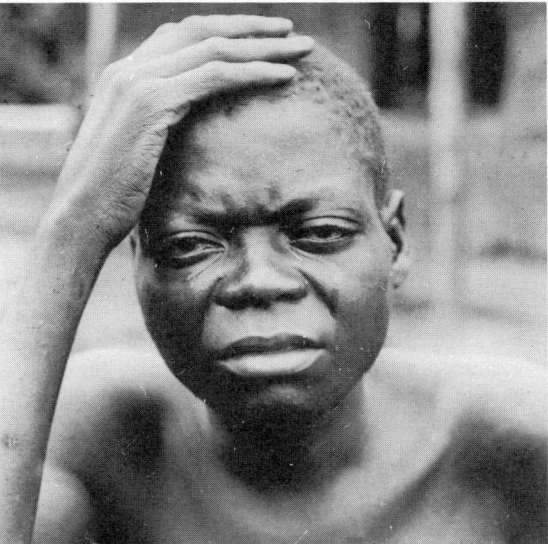

Fig. 2.9 The appearance of the patient with severe headache in the last stages of cerebral trypanosomiasis. (Courtesy Dr Cuthbert Christie.)

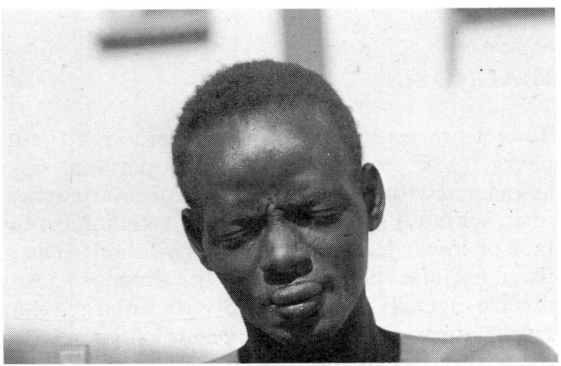

Fig. 2.8 Typical features of early cerebral trypanosomiasis with puffy lips, swollen face and sleepy vacant expression.

ingitic symptoms may occur. Persistent headache is a feature (Fig. 2.9).

In the main three principal categories of trypanosomiasis may be recognized:

1 mild with few symptoms, commonest in *T. b. gambiense* infections;
2 involving the central nervous system;
3 acute, leading to death before central nervous system symptoms develop, commonest in *T. b. rhodesiense* infections.

MORTALITY

Although spontaneous recovery may take place in the early stages of trypanosomiasis it is believed that when the disease has arrived at the stage of sleeping sickness, in the absence of treatment, death is inevitable. Many of the African villages in Senegal and The Gambia have been depopulated, and events in Zaire, Angola and Uganda bear out this estimate of the gravity of the disease in epidemic form. Many islands in Lake Victoria Nyanza have been completely depopulated. The population of the implicated districts of Uganda, originally about 300 000, was reduced in six years to 100 000 by sleeping sickness early in this century.

AFRICAN TRYPANOSOMIASIS IN CHILDREN

The occurrence of trypanosomiasis in children may point to a focus of infection near a village, although a young child may be infected anywhere while being carried on the mother's back. Even the youngest baby is susceptible.

The disease in children does not differ greatly from that in adults. The presence or absence of fever is an unreliable sign. The liver and spleen are often enlarged, but not invariably. Perhaps the main features of the illness in children are the rapid progression and the overlapping of signs associated in the adult with the 'early' and 'late' stages of the disease. Thus, cervical adenopathy and disturbances of sleep, mainly daytime somnolence, may be present soon after the onset of illness. Dullness and indifference to surroundings, disorders of reflexes and involuntary movements, including incoordination, tonic–clonic convulsions, and choreiform and epileptiform movements, are not infrequent but are more common when the disease is advanced.

Difficulty in diagnosis is the main problem since sleeping sickness is not prominent among the many causes of ill-health in African children, including malaria, anaemia, hookworm disease, malnutrition and so forth, several of which may coexist. Trypanosomes are not invariably present in the blood. Examination of the cerebrospinal fluid may provide the diagnosis and, in any case, is essential in the correct choice of treatment.

Treatment is discussed in full on p. 64. As for adults, the standard drugs are suramin, pentamidine and melarsoprol. Each is given on the basis of body weight. Children usually tolerate suramin well but if the general condition is poor the approach should be cautious, as it should be with melarsoprol. Melarsoprol has been injected into a scalp vein in the successful treatment of a baby whose cerebrospinal fluid contained trypanosomes. Although specific treatment should not be delayed, the improvement of the child's general condition is important. Vitamins, iron and perhaps chloroquine will probably be necessary.

DIFFERENTIAL DIAGNOSIS

The early accute stage of trypanosomiasis in which fever is a prominent sign must be distinguished from other causes of short-term fever: malaria (not responding to antimalarial drugs), viral hepatitis and typhoid. Later other causes of a longer-term pyrexia must be distinguished: kala-azar, tuberculosis, brucellosis, lymphoma and lymphadenoma. In the later cerebral stages syphilitic meningomyelitis, cerebral tumour, cerebral tuberculosis, chronic viral encephalitis and degenerating brain syndromes must all be considered.

DIAGNOSIS

Travel or residence in an endemic area (game parks for *T. rhodesiense*), or occupational risks associated with honey gatherers, hunters or fishermen, with a history of a painless swelling on the face or lower leg accompanied by a faint scar in these regions should suggest the diagnosis. Any fever especially if associated with enlarged cervical lymph glands (*T. gambiense*) suggests trypanosomiasis. In the late stages anyone African or Caucasian with mental symptoms who has been in an endemic area within the last two years should be checked for trypanosomal infection, so that they do not die in mental institutions of undetected cerebral trypanosomiasis.

Diagnosis may be made by finding trypanosomes in the blood, lymph gland juice or cerebrospinal fluid or by serological methods.

Examination of the blood

In early cases of *T. b. rhodesiense* infection parasites are usually, though by no means always, fairly numerous in the blood. In later cases after the febrile phase they are very difficult to find. In *T. b. gambiense* they can be found in fair numbers for a much longer time (Fig. 2.2 and Plate II.6 (see also Appendix I, p. 1261)).

Finger prick blood can be examined fresh or in thick films stained with Giemsa. In many cases prolonged search of the blood taken during pyrexial periods may be necessary and repeated slides examined. Fresh blood can be examined on a slide under a coverslip under the low power and small moving trypanosomes identified. These films can be examined much more easily if the red cells are lysed and removed; one method of achieving this is by adding aerolysin (isolated from cell free cultures of *Aeromonas hydrophila*) to the wet blood film.[33] The trypanosomes remain active for up to 60 minutes.

Concentration methods

Trypanosomes can be concentrated so that light infections can now be diagnosed. The main methods used are lysing the red cells in a large volume of blood and centrifuging, differential centrifugation when the trypanosomes collect near the buffy coat, and an anion exchange column which uses the electrical charge on the parasite to concentrate them at one end. These methods have been modified so that they can be used on finger prick blood in field conditions.

Anion exchange method (see also Appendix IV, p. 1498)

A DEAE cellulose anion exchange column can be used to separate out the trypanosomes.[34] This has been modified by developing a miniature anion exchange column (MAEC) method.[35]

Microhaematocrit buffy coat microscopy (MBCM)[36] (see also Appendix IV, p. 1497)

Finger prick blood is centrifuged in an anti-coagulated microhaematocrit tube and the tube cut 1 mm below the buffy coat to include the upper layer of red cells and 3 cm above it. The plasma and cells are expelled on to a slide and examined, preferably with dark ground illumination, at a magnification of 250.

Silicon centrifugation technique[37]

Blood is layered over silicon fluid and the red cells are lysed; it is then centrifuged and the trypanosomes are left in the supernatant fraction.

Sedimentation rate

The ESR is high in trypanosomiasis and the Westergren method is more sensitive than the Wintrobe. Sedimentation readings should be made at 10-minute intervals. The median hour rate varies from 15 to 76 mm but in untreated cases may be as high as 140 mm. The increase in ESR is closely associated with red cell clumping (auto-agglutination).

Formol gel test

This is a simple test which is usually, though not invariably, stongly positive in untreated human trypanosomiasis. It is not specific and positive reactions are also found in kala-azar, leprosy and malaria, but a positive result indicates the need for further investigation for trypanosomiasis.

Serological diagnosis

A review of serological diagnosis has been made.[38] Serological diagnosis is more useful in epidemiological surveys than for case diagnosis. The indirect fluorescent antibody test (IFAT) and enzyme-linked immunosorbent assay (ELISA) tests are used.[39–43] High titres are found in the acute stage and persist for some time after cure. The disadvantage is that the tests have to be done in a central laboratory. The indirect haemagglutination (IH) test has been used as a screening test in the field. There is a need for antigens that are stable in field conditions and appropriate in different areas. So far there is no standard antigen.

Estimation of serum IgM

Estimation of serum IgM has not been found as useful as was originally hoped since both 'false negative' and 'false positive' results are common, but a raised IgM level in an individual shows the need for further investigation.

Examination of lymph gland juice

Lymph gland puncture and examination of the aspirated lymph is the most certain method in the early stages of the disease in gambiense infections when the glands are soft before they have become sclerosed. The procedure is as follows:

1 The gland is gripped between finger and thumb of the left hand and massaged.
2 A hypodermic needle (size 14) is pushed through the skin into the substance of the gland which is then squeezed further.
3 The needle is withdrawn with a finger over the boss and its contents gently blown out on to a slide by means of a hypodermic syringe filled with air.
4 A coverslip is applied and the unstained preparation is *immediately* examined beneath the one-sixth objective. Intensely active trypanosomes are easily recognized in a positive case. They can be subsequently fixed and stained.

Gland puncture should always be reinforced by the examination of thick blood films. The glands may be unilateral or bilateral; sometimes they reach the size of a pigeon's egg and every gradation may be shown. Although the superficial glands may be easy to palpate, deeper ones may be more difficult. Three procedures for palpation are necessary: deep palpation, superficial palpation and palpation by passing the palmar surface of the hand over the neck. The glands should have the consistency of a ripe plum.

Examination of the cerebrospinal fluid (see also Appendix IV, p. 1497)

Trypanosomes may be demonstrated in the centrifuged deposit of the cerebrospinal fluid but infrequently, and in cases where they cannot be found, suggestive evidence of central nervous system involvement may be obtained by examination of the cells and estimation of the protein content. The earliest reaction from meningeal involvement is cellular and the intensity of the reaction is shown by the number and character of the cells. The presence of leukocytes indicates recent activity, whereas plasma cells, dead cells and morular cells indicate older and more chronic lesions. Any increase in the number of leukocytes above $5/mm^3$ or an increase in the protein level above the normal value for the method used indicates the possibility of a trypanosome infection in someone who has been exposed to risk.

The protein is invariably raised in cerebral trypanosomiasis and the level is an indication of the duration of the infection and the stage which the disease has reached.

A raised IgM level in the cerebrospinal fluid is more certainly indicative of trypanosomiasis, especially in late stage infections when the trypanosome itself is often difficult to find. IgM disappears slowly from the cerebrospinal fluid after treatment but, if the level is still high a year or more later and if the protein content of the fluid is also raised, the probability is that the infection has relapsed.[44]

Culture (Appendix I, p. 1318)

Trypanosomes may be isolated by culture from blood, cerebrospinal fluid or lymph and this has shown good results in experienced hands.[45,46] Positive cultures may be obtained in 5–30 days. Cultural methods have been little used in practice because of technical difficulties. However, tissue culture methods are showing promise and a culture of mammalian embryo cells in HEPES, buffered minimum essential medium with Earle's salts and heat inactivated rabbit serum has been used.[47]

Animal inoculation

Of ordinary laboratory animals the most susceptible are the guinea-pig, rat, dog and *Macaca* and *Cercopithecus* monkeys. Citrated blood, 2–10 ml, is withdrawn and inoculated intraperitoneally. The interval before the appearance of trypanosomes in the blood varies from 6 to 49 days (*T. b. gambiense* is not pathogenic in rats).

TREATMENT

Of the two drugs, suramin and tryparsamide, which have been effective in the treatment of African trypanosomiasis since the 1920s, suramin is still the choice for use in early stage infections, whether caued by *T. b. rhodesiense* or *T. b. gambiense*, although pentamidine, introduced in the 1940s, may be preferred in the latter infection. Tryparsamide, formerly so useful in late stage *T. b. gambiense* infections, became less so as resistance to it increased and is no longer available; it has been replaced by melarsoprol (Mel B, Arsobal), which has the added virtue of being effective in late stage *T. b. rhodesiense* infections which tryparsamide was not.

Suramin (Bayer 205, Antrypol)

This is given intravenously as a freshly prepared 10% solution in distilled water. The intramuscular route may be used if necessary but the injection is irritant and painful. The usual dose for an adult is 1 g (10 ml of the 10% solution) and this dose is repeated at intervals of 5–7 days until five or six injections have been given. A short and effective course in common use consists of 1 g on each of days 1, 3, 7, 14 and 21. Very rarely instances of hypersensitivity to suramin have been reported with collapse and even death, and it is wise to give a test dose of 0.1 g before the start of the main course. The full dose of 1 g should be given only to persons of good weight and in a reasonable state of health; others should receive, say, 0.25 g initially, then 0.5 g followed if there is no untoward reaction by doses of 1 g at weekly intervals. The course should be extended until a total of 5–6 g has been given. Some degree of kidney damage is common with suramin but the usual mild albuminuria is not an indication for the suspension of the drug; only if there is evidence of more severe damage, e.g. blood or casts in the urine, need there be a change of drug. Other toxic effects are infrequent but include pruritus, urticaria, papular eruption, conjunctivitis, photophobia, stomatitis, desquamation of skin and cutaneous hyperaesthesiae.

Pentamidine

Two closely related drugs, pentamidine isethionate and the French Lomidine (pentamidine methanesulphonate) are considered here together as 'pentamidine'. Pentamidine is given by intramuscular injection as a freshly prepared 10% solution in distilled water, one injection every day for 7–10 consecutive days, the dose at each injection being 3–4 mg pentamidine base/kg body weight, i.e. the usual single dose of the isethionate or of Lomidine is 150–300 mg. Since an immediate hypotensive reaction may occur patients should lie down during the injection

and adrenaline should be at hand. There are few other side or toxic effects; hypoglycaemia and diabetes have been reported as uncommon complications. Like suramin, pentamidine is effective only in the early stage of the disease before there are any signs of involvement of the nervous system.

Melarsoprol (Mel B, Arsobal)

Apart from the nitrofurazones, which are of limited use (see below), melarsoprol and its water-soluble analogue, Mel W, are the only drugs which are effective once the central nervous system has become involved. Melarsoprol is relatively toxic being liable to produce encephalopathic reactions which may be fatal; nevertheless, with attention to detail toxic effects can be minimized. The drug is issued in ampoules, ready for use, as a 3.6% solution in propylene glycol. This solution is intensely irritant and injections must be given strictly intravenously. As far as possible preliminary measures should be taken to improve the patient's general condition, e.g. the correction of anaemia by blood transfusion if needed and the use of vitamin preparations. A strict milk diet has been advocated. Patients should lie down during the injection and for 5 hours afterwards. Melarsoprol must never be used without a preliminary course of suramin to clear the blood of trypanosomes in order to avoid a Jarisch–Herxheimer reaction which occurs when large numbers of trypanosomes are killed.[48]

The usual dose recommended for each injection is 3.6 mg/kg body weight, the maximum single dose being 5 ml. One such injection is given on each of 3 or 4 consecutive days and after a rest period of one week the course is repeated. A third course of three or four injections may be given after a further rest period of one week. Such a regimen, however, may prove dangerously toxic as was the experience in East Africa in *T. b. rhodesiense* infections; workers there, and now also many in West Africa, advocate a more cautious approach, for example on days 1, 2 and 3 (or days 1, 3 and 5), 0.5 ml, 1.0 ml, 1.0 ml respectively. After a rest period of one week 2.5 ml may be given on each of the next 3 consecutive days. A further rest period of one week is followed by doses of 3 ml, 3.5 ml, 5 ml and after another week's rest the course is completed by three doses each of 5.0 ml. For children or patients who are underweight the dosage should be calculated on the basis of body weight, with similar small initial doses and a gradual increase from one-tenth of the calculated maximum dose (at 3.6 mg/kg) up to the full calculated maximum dose for body weight in the third week of treatment. Some workers are convinced of the value of a short course of suramin preceding the melarsoprol course for patients with high fever, high parasitaemia or in poor condition. Others have found steroids of value and Buyst[49] thought that a preliminary course of chloroquine helped, perhaps through its anti-inflammatory action. Warning signs of encephalopathy, such as mental excitement or twitching movements, are an indication for the suspension of treatment but this may usually be resumed with caution after a few days, during which sedation may be needed. Dimercaprol (BAL) should be given when encephalopathy occurs or is threatened, although its value is debated. Melarsoprol encephalopathies have been described as either reactive (fairly common but with a chance of recovery) or haemorrhagic (rare but almost invariably fatal).[50] As far as is practicable the use of melarsoprol should be suspended during an outbreak of influenza or other virus infection.

Melarsonyl potassium (Mel W, Trimélarsan)

This is a water-soluble analogue of melarsoprol with a similar degree of toxicity but, as it can be given by intramuscular or subcutaneous injection, it has been found useful for logistic reasons in certain circumstances in West Africa. It has given disappointing results in *T. b. rhodesiense* infections in East Africa. Further information is available.[51–53]

Diminazine (berenil)

This is another aromatic diamidine. It has proved of value in veterinary trypanosomiasis and has also been shown to be effective in the early stage of both *T. b. gambiense* and *T. b. rhodesiense* infections.[54,55] It is given by intramuscular injection as a 2% solution in 5% glucose, the dose at each injection being 2 mg/kg body weight; injections are given every day for 7–10 days. It has also been found effective when given by mouth.[56] Apart from the shorter treatment course, diminazine appears to have no advantage over suramin in *T. b. rhodesiense* infections or over suramin or pentamidine in *T. b.*

gambiense infections. Some authorities are against the use of diminazine in human trypanosomiasis because it has sometimes proved toxic in dogs and in some other animals and has undergone no formal evaluation for toxicity in man. It should be regarded as still under trial. Acute polyneuritis (Landry–Guillain–Barré syndrome) has been described after diminazine treatment for babesiosis,[57] although whether this was a direct effect of the drug was unproved.

Furacin (nitrofurazone, 5-nitro-2-furfuraldehyde semicarbazone)

This drug has cured many patients whose infections have relapsed after treatment with other drugs, e.g. melarsoprol, but its effects are uncertain and it is liable to cause polyneuropathy. Haemolysis may also be a problem in parts of Africa where glucose-6-phosphate dehydrogenase (G-6-PD) deficiency is common. It is, however, the only drug at present which offers a chance of cure when melarsoprol has failed. A stable yellow powder, it is given orally in tablet form, usually 0.5 g three or four times a day for 5–7 days. The course may be repeated after a rest period of one week and again on up to two further occasions, provided that there are intervening rest periods. Nitrofurazone should not be given to patients who are febrile; the fever should first be controlled by suramin. Patients should rest in bed and should receive a high protein diet together with thiamine. If G-6-PD deficiency is present the blood picture must be watched continuously. The heart may be affected and an increase in pulse rate may be the first sign of toxicity. Any sign of toxicity indicates immediate withdrawal of the drug. Full descriptions of the use of nitrofurazone and of its toxic effects are given by Robertson[58,59] and by Robertson and Knight.[60] Nitrofurazone has been advocated as primary therapy for trypanosomal meningo-encephalitis, i.e. instead of melarsoprol, but its use in this way is still under evaluation.

Lampit (nifurtimox)

The use of Lampit should be considered in arsenic-resistant cases. Seven out of eight melarsoprol-resistant patients were considered cured 10 months after treatment with doses used in the American trypanosomiasis, but serum IgM levels remained high.[61]

Oral treatment

Difluoromethylornithine (DFMO)

A specific irreversible inhibitor of polyamine biosynthesis previously shown to be curative in animal trypanosomiasis, this drug has been used in the Sudan to treat late stage Gambian trypanosomiasis refractory to arsenic.

A dose of 200 mg/kg once daily by mouth for six weeks was used in early cases, and 400 mg/kg once daily for five to six weeks in late stage cases.

Side-effects include diarrhoea, abdominal pain and anaemia but do not necessitate stopping the drug. Some good results have been obtained with disappearance of trypanosomes from the cerebrospinal fluid.[62]

The choice of drugs

The treatment of African human trypanosomiasis in its early and late stages may be summarized as follows:

Early stage (no central nervous system involvement)

T. b. gambiense infections	suramin or pentamidine (or diminazine)
T. b. rhodesiense infections	suramin (or diminazine)

Late stage (with central nervous system involvement

T. b. gambiense infections	melarsoprol (nitrofurazone)
T. b. rhodesiense infections	

Relapses (*T. b. gambiense* and *T. b. rhodesiense* infections)

A relapse after treatment with suramin or pentamidine should be treated with melarsoprol since it is probably due to the survival of trypanosomes within the choroid plexus where they have been found intracellularly in the ependymal cells lining the vessels in the choroid plexus.[25] A patient whose infection relapses after a course of melarsoprol should receive a second course of melarsoprol which may prove effective, but further relapses are less likely to respond to third and subsequent courses of melarsoprol, when nitrofurazone should be tried. There is some suggestion that a combination of nitrofurazone and melarsoprol is better than either drug alone in the treatment of relapses. As mentioned above in the section on serological diagnosis the presence of IgM in the cerebrospinal fluid a year or more after treatment, with a raised protein level and cell count, is a strong indication of a relapse, whereas the absence of IgM, even if protein content and cell count are raised, is against the diagnosis of a relapse.

Criteria of cure

In patients treated in the haemolymph stage of the disease there should be no clinical sign of the disease, or abnormality of blood or cerebrospinal fluid, after several examinations during two years.

In patients treated in the meningoencephalitic stage there should be no clinical signs (except perhaps of irreversible damage to the nervous system done before treatment); the cell count of the cerebrospinal fluid should fall steadily to below 5/mm³ and the protein content to below 0.3 mg/ml. Surveillance should continue for two to three years and for even longer in *T. b. gambiense* infections.

PROGNOSIS

In both *T. b. gambiense* and *T. b. rhodesiense* infections the prognosis is excellent provided that there are no signs of central nervous system involvement at the start of treatment. Suramin or pentamidine, as appropriate, will cure virtually all patients treated in the early stage of the disease. With even slight evidence of nervous system involvement the chance of cure is lessened and there is the additional risk associated with the need to use a more toxic drug, e.g. melarsoprol. However, a cure rate of some 90% is obtainable even in very advanced infections and it can, with care, be even better than this.

The first indication of a relapse after treatment is an increase in the cerebrospinal fluid cell count followed by a rise in the protein content. Such signs may not be accompanied by a deterioration in the patient's condition but complaints of tiredness, headache, fever and so forth at any time after treatment should arouse suspicion. (It should be noted that examination of the spinal fluid immediately after treatment, particularly after melarsoprol, may show a rise in cell count and protein content and a true picture may not be obtained until two or three months have elapsed.) As mentioned in the section on diagnosis, estimation of the IgM level in the cerebrospinal fluid may assist in the verification of a relapse. Indirect immunofluorescence test on the cerebrospinal fluid gives a more reliable prognosis than the cell count or protein estimation.[41] For example, the spinal fluid of most patients who subsequently relapsed remained positive in this test, whereas the reaction became negative within 18 months of successful treatment. The treatment of patients whose infections have relapsed is discussed in the section on relapses, above.

SEQUELAE

Patients treated in the early stage of the disease may be assured that there is no likelihood of future physical or mental damage. In the later stages even very marked mental impairment usually improves with treatment although recovery may not be complete, and the patient may suffer from insomnia or irritability or, very rarely, from some more serious disturbance such as paranoia or attacks of violent behaviour. Such sequelae appear to be associated only with very advanced *T. b. gambiense* infections.

EPIDEMIOLOGY

The epidemiology of African trypanosomiasis depends upon the reservoir host–vector–man relationship and the ecology that supports that connection. The bionomics and ecology of the various vector flies are dealt with in Appendix III (p. 1454) where the man–fly contact is shown to occur near watering places (palpalis group) or is occupational among groups such as hunters, honey gatherers, pole cutters, charcoal burners and now tourists entering fly-infested bush (morsitans group).

Trypanosomiasis is found in certain permanent residual foci from which it expands when conditions are favourable and to which it retreats when they are unfavourable. The infection has decreased in Nigeria but has greatly increased in Zaire, Uganda and Zambia and will almost certainly do so in the Sudan and other areas where there are social disturbances and civil war. The occurrence of these permanent foci are shown by the puzzling fact that the disease recurs time after time, with long intervals between cases, and seldom appears elsewhere in new localities in the fly belt.

Gambian sleeping sickness

Gambian trypanosomiasis is an infection of the riverine and lakeside areas of West and central Africa. It is found wherever riverine tsetse and man are in close contact, such as at river crossings, lakeside villages and waterholes frequented by man and infected flies. Fishermen are especially affected. Large epidemics have occurred in the past when man to man transmission was present. Man is the main reservoir although zymodeme studies have shown that peridomestic pigs and dogs are reservoirs in some areas of West Africa. Liberia has a low incidence of human disease but many pigs are infected with trypanosomes. The Ivory Coast has highly endemic areas with trypanosomes circulating in pigs and in the Republic of the Congo there are numerous foci of human disease but few infections in domestic animals.[63] A trypanosome enzymatically identical to a human trypanosome has been isolated from a sheep in the Republic of the Congo[62] suggesting another possible source of infection.

Kob and bushbuck have been found naturally infected in West Africa and eleven common species of antelope (bushbuck, reedbuck, waterbuck etc.) can be infected artificially with *T. b. gambiense*, but there is no evidence that this is common in nature and man remains essentially the main reservoir.

Rhodesian sleeping sickness

T. b. rhodesiense was first described in 1910 from a patient in the Zambesi region where the infection may have existed in an endemic form and whence it gradually spread northwards creating epidemics in various areas as far as Uganda, where it appeared in the early 1940s.

At present it is found sporadically in the southern part of its range and there it is not so severe a disease as in the epidemic areas further north. It is essentially an infection of antelope, particularly the bushbuck (Fig. 2.10) which has been shown to carry the trypanosomes in nature.[64] In the southern area bushbuck and man are seldom in contact with each other and the strains of *T. b. rhodesiense* are not well adapted to man. In Tanzania, where epidemics were

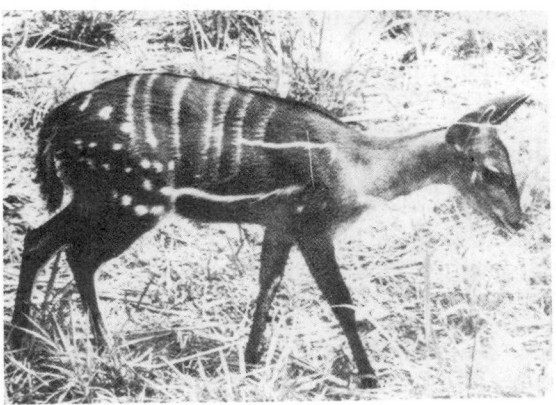

Fig. 2.10 The bushbuck, *Tragelaphus scriptus*, the reservoir host of *T. rhodesiense*.

severe in the 1920s and 1930s, man is now infected sporadically from the animal reservoir when there is triple contact between the reservoir and the fly (particularly *G. morsitans* and *G. pallipides* which show a preference for the bushbuck) and man when he goes into the bush to collect honey or to fish. The strains are well adapted to man and in exceptional circumstances can be transmitted directly from man to man by *G. morsitans* or *G. pallipides* in epidemic form in villages in Tanzania, Kenya and Uganda, and by *G. fuscipes* in Kenya causing severe disease.[27] More recently in Kenya, Uganda and western Ethiopia *T. b. rhodesiense* has become adapted to the riverine tsetse *G. fuscipes* and *G. tachinoides*. In the case of *G. fuscipes*, this may alter its habits so that it becomes peridomestic, living permanently in the rings of exotic vegetation surrounding the homesteads[65] where the cattle have been found to carry *T. b. rhodesiense*.[66]

It has been suggested that the epidemics of trypanosomiasis since the end of the last century have arisen through a conflict between two opposing ecosystems— the natural wildlife ecosystem of bush, wild animals and tsetse flies, and the artificial one composed of man, his domestic animals and cultivation.[67]

PROPHYLAXIS

Prophylactic measures are based principally on the habits of *G. palpalis*, *G. tachinoides* and other species which may transmit *T. b. gambiense*. The measures employed are so similar to those in use against *T. b. rhodesiense* and so interwoven that they must be considered together in the section on the bionomics of *Glossina* (see Appendix III, p. 1454).

Repellents

Little information is obtainable on this subject but an antimosquito cream (containing pyrethrum) has a repellent action chiefly against *G. palpalis* for 6 hours when applied to the skin, but this action is apt to be destroyed by heavy sweating with exposure to strong sunlight.[68] The most popular at present is Di-Meepol which contains dimethyl phthalate and ethylhexanediol in a non-greasy base and can be dissolved in a small amount of liquid paraffin for use in fly country. The wearing of a jacket made of wide mesh netting impregnated with a repellent (di-isopentyl malate) gave the wearer an average of 83% protection against the bites of tsetse (*G. morsitans*) over a period of 8 days.[69] The jackets had long sleeves and hoods for maximum protection. Similar jackets impregnated with other repellents, e.g. deet or permethrin, have proved effective against the bites of mosquitoes and black flies (*Simulium* spp.).

Chemoprophylaxis

Suramin is known to give protection against both *T. b. gambiense* and *T. b. rhodesiense* infections but the protection is short-lived and there is the disadvantage of the drug having to be given by intravenous injection. Pentamidine is a far better prophylactic; a single intramuscular injection of 4 mg base/kg body weight (maximum dose 300 mg) gives protection against *T. b. gambiense* infections for about six months. Its protective effect against *T. b. rhodesiense* infections is less certain. Mass pentamidine prophylaxis has been used effectively on a very wide scale for the control of *T. b. gambiense* infection, especially in the former French and Belgian African territories, although it is now acknowledged that it cannot by itself eradicate the disease. It may be of great use in special situations, e.g. for the protection of organized labour forces such as road or rail workers, or as on the Jos Plateau in Nigeria where a high risk of infection among tin miners was controlled.[70] Used in this way pentamidine isethionate causes fewer side-effects (hypoglycaemia and diabetes) than Lomidine.

Individual chemoprophylaxis for persons visiting or working in an endemic area cannot in general be recommended, particularly not for those going to the *T. b. rhodesiense* areas of eastern Africa, for there is no drug which is certainly effective for any length of time against this form of the infection. The risk to an individual of infection with either *T. b. gambiense* or *T. b. rhodesiense* is very small and, provided that no prophylactic has been given, an infection, should it occur, can usually be diagnosed easily and rapidly. On the other hand, to determine the cause of a febrile illness in someone who has received pentamidine and in particular to eliminate the possibility of trypanosomiasis can be a difficult and prolonged process.

CONTROL (Appendix III, p. 1456)

The object of any control effort in trypanosomiasis is to break the man–tsetse fly contact. This can be done by an attack on the tsetse fly by the destruction of its habitat, removal of the food supply or by killing with insecticides; or by removing man from the environment by concentration of the population in certain areas or by altering the environment on a large scale.

In the event of any of the above measures being impractical a certain amount of control can be achieved by mass chemoprophylaxis in areas where only Gambian sleeping sickness occurs.

Discriminative bush clearing along rivers and in the savannah will provide an unfavourable environment for the fly in some cases. Denial of food supply to the tsetse by destruction of the big game is not practicable because alternative sources of food are usually available. Direct insecticidal attack on the fly by spraying from the air or from the ground has been useful in some special circumstances, and is now the cheapest method for control on a wide scale (new insecticides limit the environmental damage). By far the most useful measure of control is the creation of a new environment for the population as has been done in the Anchau experiment in Nigeria. This provided a model example of the method of clearing an area of tsetse flies as well as of benefiting the population generally and of raising their standard of agriculture. Anchau became a tsetse-free corridor, linking two of the railway lines that diverge from Zaria and is some 100 km long, over 155 000 hectares in extent and with a population of 50 000. The combination of partial and barrier clearings has proved effective, but was extremely expensive.

Removal of infected populations

Trypanosomiasis has interfered with the development of one-quarter of the African continent. In part of Uganda by 1900 it was estimated to have exterminated two-thirds of the local population. To preserve the hitherto uninfected from trypanosome infection, the Government transported the entire population of the Sesse Islands and neighbouring shore of Victoria Nyanza to fly-free areas in the interior. It was hoped that, the human source of trypanosome supply being thus denied them, the tsetse flies would cease to be infective. In an emergency the infected population can be removed en masse from a trypanosomiasis area and settled in tsetse-free villages. This was successful in Tanzania between the two World Wars, but requires large areas of unoccupied land for a successful outcome, and is open to great political difficulties.[27]

For a detailed description of tsetse flies and preventive measures now in use, see Appendix III.

REFERENCES

1   Ormerod, W.E. (1979) In *Biology of the Kinetoplastida*, vol. 2, ed. W. H. R. Lumsden & D. A. Evans, London: Academic Press.
2   Rickman, L.R. & Robson, J. (1970) *Bull. Wld hlth Org.* **42**, 911.
3   Godfrey, D.G. & Kilgour, V. (1976) *Trans. R. Soc. trop. Med. Hyg.* **70**, 219.
4   Darré, H., Mollaret, P., Tanguy, Y. et al (1973) *Bull. Soc. Path. éxot.* **30**, 159.
5   Capponi, M. (1953) *Bull. Soc. Path. éxot.* **46**, 667.
6   Woodruff, A.W., Evans, D.A. & Owino, N.O. (1982) *J. Infection* **5**, 89–92.
7   Buyst, H. (1972) *E. Afr. med. J.* **50**, 63.
8   Traub, N., Hira, P.R., Chintu, C. et al (1978) *E. Afr. med. J.* **55**, 477.
9   Ferreira, F.S.C. & Menina, R.J. (1951) *Gaz. Med. Port.* **4**, 1030.
10 Pieters, G. (1951) *Ann. Soc. belge Méd. trop.* **3**, 661.
11 Laveissière, C. (1976) *Cah. O.R.S.T.O.M. Ent. Méd. Parasit.* **14**, 359.
12 Greenwood, B.M. & Whittle, H.C. (1980) *Trans. R. Soc. trop. Med. Hyg.* **74**, 716–725.
13 Ormerod, W.E. & Hussein, M.S.A. (1986) *Trans. R. Soc. trop. Med. Hyg.* **80**, 626–633.
14 Musoke, A.J. & Barbet, A.F. (1977) *Nature, Lond.* **270**, 438–440.
15 Boreham, P. (1970) *Trans. R. Soc. trop. Med. Hyg.* **64**, 394.
16 Ormerod, W.E. (1970) In *The African Trypanosomiasis*, ed. H.W. Mulligan & W.H. Potts, p. 587. London: George Allen & Unwin.
17 Poltera, A.A. (1980) *Trans. R. Soc. trop. Med. Hyg.* **74**, 706.

18 Hawking, F. & Greenfield, J.C. (1941) *Trans. R. Soc. trop. Med. Hyg.* **35**, 155.

19 Manson-Bahr, P.E.C. & Charters, A.D. (1963) *Trans. R. Soc. trop. Med. Hyg.* **57**, 119.

20 Woodruff, A.W., Ziegler, J.L., Hathaway, A. et al (1973) *Trans. R. Soc. trop. Med. Hyg.* **67**, 329–337.

21 Khaukha, G.W. & Ramasamy, R. (1981) *E. Afr. med. J.* **58**, 907–911.

22 Davis, C.E. (1982) *Acta trop.* **39**, 123–133.

23 Greenwood, B.M. & Whittle, H.C. (1973) *Lancet* **ii**, 525.

24 van Bogaert, L. (1936) *C. r. Séanc. Soc. Biol.* **121**, 1387.

25 Abolarin, M.O., Evans, D.A. Jovey, D.G. et al (1982) *Br. med. J.* **ii**, 1380–1382.

26 Ceccaldi, J. (1940) *Ann. Inst. Pasteur* 67.

27 Apted, F.I.C., Ormerod, W.E., Smyly, D.P. et al (1963) *J. trop. Med. Hyg.* **66**, 1–16.

28 Blair, D.M. (1939) *Trans. R. Soc. trop. Med. Hyg.* **33**, 729.

29 Rickman, L.R. (1974) *E. Afr. Med. J.* **51**, 467–487.

30 Bertrand, E., Sentilhes, L., Ducasse, B. et al (1966) *Méd. trop.* **25**, 603.

31 Jones, I.G., Lowenthal, M.N. & Buyst, H. (1975) *Trans. R. Soc. trop. Med. Hyg.* **69**, 388.

32 Norredam, K. & Kandelhart, E. (1971) *Ann. Soc. belge Méd. trop.* **51**, 325.

33 Pearson, T.W., Saya, L.E. & Howard, S.P. (1982) *Acta trop.* **39**, 73–77.

34 Lanham, S.M. (1968) *Nature, Lond.* **218**, 1273–1274.

35 Lumsden, W.H.R., Kimber, C.D. & Strange, E.M. (1977) *Trans. R. Soc. trop. Med. Hyg.* **71**, 421–424.

36 Murray, M., Murray, P.K. & McIntyre, W.I.M. (1977) *Trans. R. Soc. trop. Med. Hyg.* **71**, 325–326.

37 Ogbunude, P.O.J. & Magaji, Y. (1982) *Trans. R. Soc. trop. Med. Hyg.* **76**, 317–318.

38 Voller, A. (1977) *Ann. Soc. belge Méd. trop.* **57**, 273.

39 Wery, M., Wery-Paskoff, S. & van Wettere, P. (1970) *Ann. Soc. belge Méd. trop.* **50**, 613.

40 Frezil, J.L., Carrie, J. & Rio, F. (1974) *Cah. O.R.S.T.O.M. Ent. Méd. Parasit.* **12**, 111.

41 Frezil, J.L., Coulm, J. & Alary, J.C.. (1978) *Cah. O.R.S.T.O.M. Ent. Méd. Parasit.* **16**, 191.

42 Voller, A., Bidwell, D.E. & Bartlett, A. (1975) *Tropenmed. Parasit.* **26**, 247.

43 Voller, A., Bidwell, D.E. & Bartlett, A. (1976) *Trans. R. Soc. trop. Med. Hyg.* **70**, 98.

44 Whittle, H.C., Greenwood, B.M., Bidwell, D.E. et al (1977) *Am. J. trop. Med. Hyg.* **26**, 1129.

45 Weinman, D. (1960) *Trans. R. Soc. trop. Med. Hyg.* **54**, 180.

46 Weinman, D. (1963) *Bull. Wld hlth Org.* **28**, 731.

47 Brun, R., Jenni, I., Schoneneberger, M. et al (1981) *J. Protozool.* **28**, 470–479.

48 Bryceson, A.D.M. (1976) *J. infect. Dis.* **133**, 696–704.

49 Buyst, H. (1975) *Ann. Soc. belge Méd. trop.* **55**, 95.

50 Robertson, D.H.H. (1963) *Trans. R. Soc. trop. Med. Hyg.* **57**, 122.

51 Schneider, J., Leveuf, J.J. & Tanagara, S. (1961) *Bull. Soc. Path. éxot.* **54**, 345.

52 Watson, H.J.C. (1962) *Trans. R. Soc. trop. Med. Hyg.* **56**, 231.

53 Watson, H.J.C. (1965) *Trans. R. Soc. trop. Med. Hyg.* **59**, 163.

54 Hutchinson, M.P. & Watson, H.J.C. (1962) *Trans. R. Soc. trop. Med. Hyg.* **56**, 227.

55 Temu, S.E. (1975) *Trans. R. Soc. trop. Med. Hyg.* **69**, 277.

56 Bailey, N.M. (1968) *Trans. R. Soc. trop. Med. Hyg.* **62**, 122.

57 Ruebush, T.K., II. Rubin, R.H., Wolpow, E.R. et al (1979) *Am. J. trop. Med. Hyg.* **28**, 184.

58 Robertson, D.H.H. (1961) *Ann. trop. Med. Parasit.* **55**, 49.

59 Robertson, D.H.H. (1961) *Ann. trop. Med. Parasit.* **55**, 278.

60 Robertson, D.H.H. & Knight, R.H. (1964) *Acta trop.* **21**, 239.

61 Moens, F., de Wilde, M. & Ngato, K. (1984) *Ann. Soc. belge Méd. trop.* **64**, 37–43.

62 Van Nieuwenhove, S., Schechter, P.J., Declerq, J. et al (1985) *Trans. R. Soc. trop. Med. Hyg.* **79**, 692–698.

63 Scott, C.M., Frezil, J.L., Toudic, A. et al (1983) *Trans. R. Soc. trop. Med. Hyg.* **77**, 397–401.

64 Heisch, R.B., McMahon, J.P. & Manson-Bahr, P.E.C. (1958) *Br. med. J.* **ii**, 1203.

65 Willett, K.C. (1965) *Trans. R. Soc. trop. Med. Hyg.* **59**, 374.

66 Onyango, R.J., van Hoeve, K. & de Raadt, P. (1966) *Trans. R. Soc. trop. Med. Hyg.* **60**, 175.

67 Ford, J. (1971) *The Role of the Trypanosomes in African Ecology. A Study of the Tsetse Fly Problem.* London: Oxford University Press.

68 Holden, J.R. & Findlay, G.M. (1974) *Trans. R. Soc. trop. Med. Hyg.* **38**, 199.

69 Scholdt, L.L., Grothaus, R.H., Schreck, C.E. et al (1975) *E. Afr. med. J.* **52**, 277.

70 Gall, D. (1954) *Ann. trop. Med. Parasit.* **48**, 242.

Chapter 3
American Trypanosomiasis (Chagas' Disease)

American trypanosomiasis is an infection with *Trypanosoma cruzi* transmitted from animals to man by reduviid bugs.

GEOGRAPHICAL DISTRIBUTION

Human infection with *T. cruzi* is widespread in Latin America (Fig. 3.1.) where it is estimated that at least 20 million people are infected. There are eight main areas.[1]

Central America: sporadic infection with some serological evidence of infection in Texas and New Mexico[2] but little, if any, disease.

Colombia and Venezuela: widespread infection established by serological surveys but little disease and that mainly cardiopathy.

West of the Andes and northern Peru: infection widespread with little evidence of significant disease.

Southern half of Peru: high prevalence of infection with severe Chagas' disease with cardiopathy.

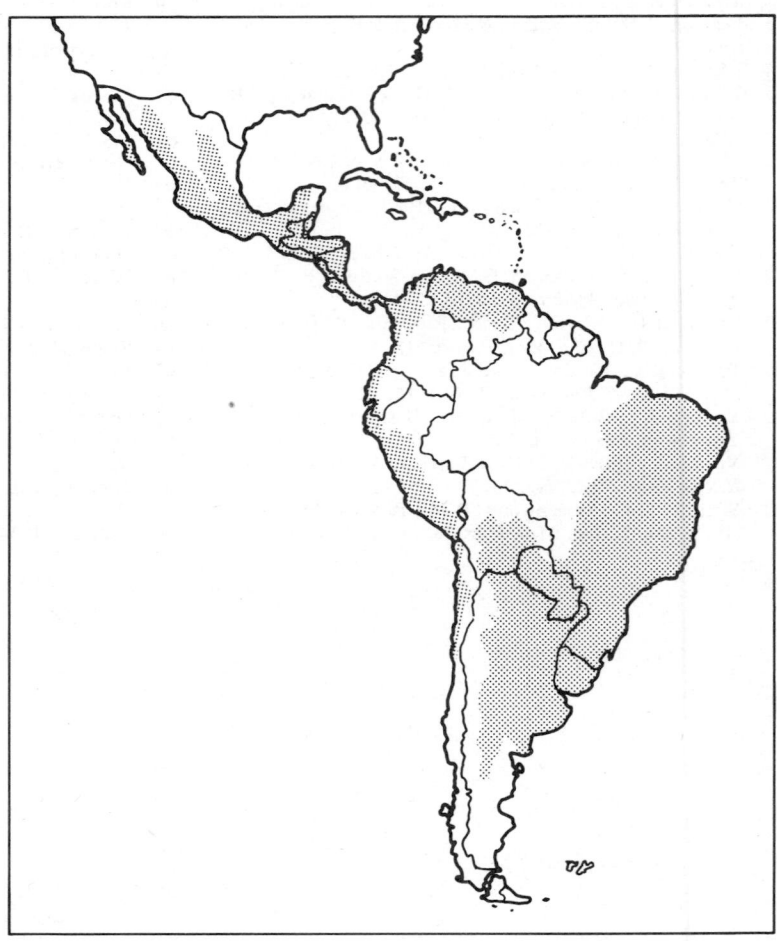

Fig. 3.1. Distribution of Chagas' disease (American trypanosomiasis).

Chile: Infection present but little disease, although there is some evidence of increasing 'mega disease'.

Northern Argentina, Paraguay, Bolivia, Uraguay and southern Brazil: the largest number of infections are found in this area with important effects on the health of the population with some cardiopathy and 'mega disease'.

The mining triangle in central coastal Brazil where infection is closely related to cardiopathy.

Pernambuco and Bahia: infection present but little associated cardiopathy or 'mega disease'.

The Amazon region is without Chagas' disease although *T. cruzi* has a wide prevalence in animals and sylvatic triatomine bugs.

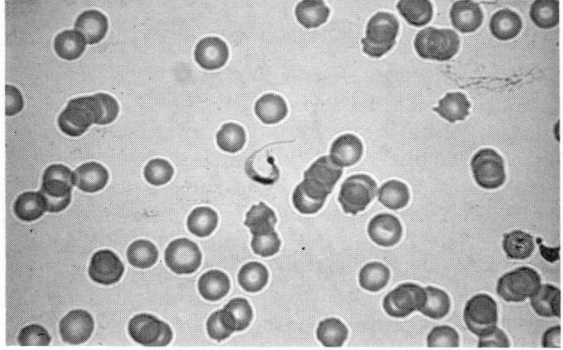

Fig. 3.2. *Trypanosoma cruzi* in peripheral blood. Note the typical 'C' shape, the large and prominent subterminal kinetoplast and the elongated central nucleus. The undulating membrane is characteristically not very obvious. (Courtesy of the Department of Medical Protozoology, London School of Hygiene and Tropical Medicine.)

Other areas in the Americas

T. cruzi infected armadillos, raccoons and opossums are found far outside the distribution of human infection especially in Louisiana and infected triatomine bugs have been found as far north as Virginia, and in Trinidad, Curaçao and Aruba[3] where serological evidence of human infection has been found, as well as in Jamaica and Belize.[4]

AETIOLOGY

The cause of South American trypanosomiasis is infection with *I. cruzi*.

T. cruzi was first described in the invertebrate vector *Panstrongylus megistus* in Brazil by Carlos Chagas in 1907 who later found it in the blood of a child. Chagas also found the trypanosome in wild animals, studied its life-cycle and described the clinical picture of the disease, later known as Chagas' disease.

In man *T. cruzi* exists in two forms, trypomastigotes in the blood and amastigotes intracellularly in the tissues. The trypomastigote form has a typical trypanosome appearance, usually C- or S-shaped, with a flagellum and a prominent posterior kinetoplast (Fig. 3.2 and Plate II.5). The amastigote is an oval- or round-shaped body with no flagellum but with a nucleus and a rod-shaped kinetoplast (see p. 53). Amastigotes are found in pseudocysts in heart muscle (Fig. 3.3) and the smooth muscle of the intestine.

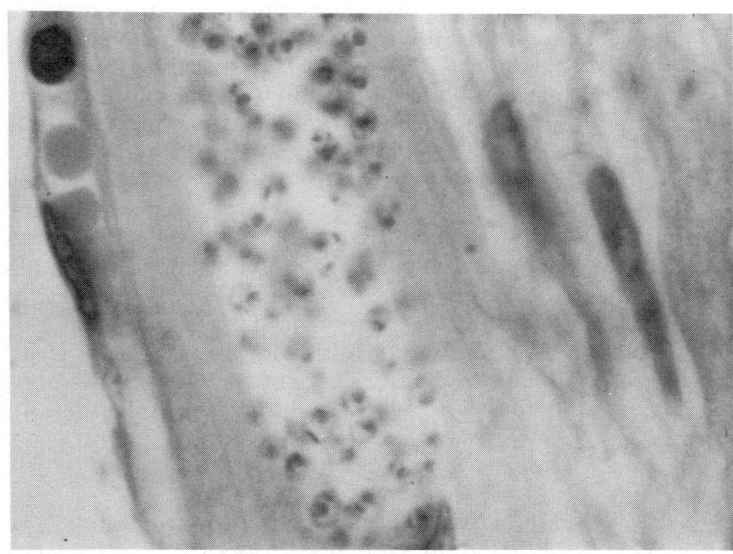

Fig. 3.3. Pseudocyst of *T. cruzi* in a cardiac muscle cell from a case of acute Chagas' disease, showing the amastigote forms. (Courtesy of The Wellcome Tropical Institute.)

Although trypomastigotes show no antigenic variation, enzyme electrophoresis has shown that there are at least three zymodemes, each found in different geographical and ecological zones. The principal zymodemes are Z1, Z2 and Z3.

ZYMODEME 1 (Appendix I, p. 1288)
Z1 exists in both domestic and sylvatic transmission cycles involving man, domestic and wild animals. It is present in Brazil and Venezuela and is associated with cardiomyopathy and not normally with mega disease.

ZYMODEME 2
Z2 has a domestic cycle only and has not been found in wild animals. It is the main zymodeme present in eastern and central Brazil and is associated with both cardiomyopathy and mega disease.

ZYMODEME 3
Z3 occurs only in sylvatic transmission cycles and is the least common zymodeme found in man.

Zymodeme analysis is of great use in determining the source of an infection and its epidemiology and has a prognostic value in determining the type of clinical disease.

TRANSMISSION

The main method of transmission is by blood-sucking bugs but other means are not uncommon: congenital, blood transfusion and laboratory infections.

Reduviid (triatomine) bugs

These are also known as 'cone nose', 'kissing' or 'assassin' bugs. Trypanosomes are ingested by bugs either in the larval or nymphal stages and, when they have passed through many stages of development in the intestinal canal after a period of 8–10 days, are passed out in the faeces as metacyclic trypomastigotes. Infection of the host takes place through the wound caused by the bite by rubbing the faeces in while scratching (see Appendix I, p. 1285, Fig. I.35, p. 1287, and Appendix III, p. 1478).

In Argentina, Brazil and Chile the common vector is the 'Vinchuca' bug, *Triatoma infestans*; in eastern Brazil, *P. megistus*; in Venezuela, Ecuador, Peru and Central America as far as 22° north in Mexico, *Rhodnius prolixus*. Many other species of the genera *Panstrongylus* and *Rhodnius* can transmit the infection to animals and bed bugs can transmit laboratory infections. Infection can also occur through ingestion of the bugs which may be important in the zoonotic cycle. (For further details of the structure, habits and identification of reduviid bugs, see Appendix III, p. 1471.)

Blood transfusion transmission (for a review, see Bruce-Chwatt[5])

In Latin America blood transfusion constitutes the second most important way of transmitting Chagas' disease. Using xenodiagnosis *T. cruzi* can be found in the blood of 60% of chronic Chagas' disease,[6] and blood is still infective when left at 6°C for 14–21 days although after more than 10 days it is considered safe. Transmission by blood transfusion can be avoided by screening blood donors using the complement fixation test (CFT), indirect fluorescent antibody test (IFAT) or enzyme-linked immunosorbent assay (ELISA). Alternatively, the addition of 0.5% solution of gentian violet (1:4000) to stored blood will eliminate *T. cruzi* after 24 hours.

Congenital transmission

Congenital transmission has been estimated to occur in 2% of deliveries to seropositive mothers and transmission via maternal milk has also been recorded. The fetus may be infected transplacentally or by inhaling amniotic fluid. There is a wide spectrum of clinical manifestations as in the adult. The fetus may be born macerated or dead,[7,8] or the newborn child may appear normal and hepatosplenomegaly or lymphadenopathy discovered on examination. A morbilliform rash may be present. Trypanosomes may be found in the blood if the phase is acute or need xenodiagnosis for demonstration. Intracranial calcification in a child with congenital Chagas' disease has been described.[9] IgM specific antibodies are diagnostic of congenital infection.

Laboratory transmission

Many cases of accidental transmission have occurred in laboratory workers, the trypanosomes entering via a needle, abrasions on the skin contaminated by infected blood, or via the conjunctiva splashed with infected fluid. All those working with *T. cruzi* should have periodic serological checks and work should only take place under conditions prescribed for dangerous pathogens.

Organ transplants

T. cruzi has been transmitted by a kidney transplant.[10]

PATHOGENESIS

Both humoral and cell-mediated immune responses are involved in Chagas' disease. Humoral antibodies appear to play little part in the pathogenesis and immune complexes are not important. A serum gamma globulin factor circulating in most patients with Chagas' cardiomyopathy which reacts with the endocardium, interstitium and blood vessels of the heart has been described.[11] EVI (endocardial-vascular-interstitial) antibody reactivity and lymphomononuclear cell infiltration are frequent in Chagas' cardiomyopathy influencing the rhythm and contractile activity of the heart.[12] Humoral antibodies keep the level of trypomastigotes in the blood to a low level.

Cell-mediated responses cause the appearance of many immune competent cells and an autoimmune mechanism is favoured to explain the degeneration in the autonomic nerve cells in the ganglia in the smooth muscle of the gut, and the ganglion cells in the heart where an antigen common to *T. cruzi* and heart muscle has been thought to be responsible for the cardiac changes in both neurons and heart muscle cells. Damage to the parasympathetic ganglia in the right atrium may lead to impaired sympathetic control with increased cardiac work and dilatation and hypertrophy. The myocardium may also be damaged directly by parasites with resulting inflammatory response and fibrosis. Chronic dilatation of the intestine and other organs is considered to be due to ganglion cell destruction and defective innervation.

A lipopolysaccharide toxin has been described which is antigenic and can damage cells causing hepatitis, myocarditis and nephropathy in mice.[13]

PATHOLOGY

Parasites may enter at the site of the bite or through the conjunctiva. The parasites multiply rapidly at the site of inoculation where they produce a focus of infiltration with leukocytes and round cells with interstitial oedema and focal lymphangitis (chagoma). The parasites are found in the trypomastigote form in the blood during the early state of dissemination but they soon enter cells of mesenchymal origin (cardiac and skeletal muscle, reticuloendothelial cells and neuroglia). In the infected cells the parasites assume the amastigote form and multiply by binary fission until the cytoplasm is filled with large numbers of amastigotes, producing an amastigote *pseudocyst* (Fig. 3.3). Since the trypanosomes do not multiply in the blood the amastigotes that are released by rupture of the pseudocyst must enter a new host cell promptly or die. This explains the difficulty in treatment of this disease since the parasite does not have to survive in the blood but rests safely in pseudocysts in various organs (see also Appendix I, p.1286).

As the pseudocysts multiply the lymphocytes, plasma cells and histiocytes of the host appear round every focus of parasite multiplication. Granulomas, sometimes containing giant cells, form with eventual fibrosis. As the cellular and humoral immune response of the host develops, parasite multiplication is suppressed and trypanosomes become very scanty in the peripheral blood. Later, even the amastigote forms become difficult to find in the tissues.

The main target organs are the muscle fibres of the heart, the smooth muscle of the digestive tract and the autonomic nerve ganglia. There is a great diminution in the ganglion cells of the right auricle and the enteric plexus of patients with chronic Chagas' disease, and it has suggested that a toxin is liberated when the pseudocysts rupture which damages the nerve cells.[14] This toxin may be a vasoactive peptide. Individuals with Chagas' disease may die in the acute phase or proceed on to a chronic phase.

Morbid anatomy

Acute Chagas' disease

The *brain* and meninges are oedematous. Microscopically there are small inflammatory foci scattered throughout the grey matter. Perivascular cuffing may also occur. Parasitization of nerve cells is extremely rare but ruptured pseudocysts in the cerebellum and basal ganglia cause death and disappearance of nerve cells.

The *heart* is flaccid and dilated. Microscopically the muscle fibres are widely separated by diffuse infiltration of mononuclear cells and proliferation of connective tissue.

T. cruzi amastigotes lie in longitudinal masses in the muscle fibres which show varying degrees of hyaline degeneration and fragmentation (Fig. 3.3). There is no cellular reaction until rupture of the muscle cell with liberation of parasites.

There is *interstitial oesophagitis* with amastigotes in the cells of the smooth muscle layers and disappearance of neurons.

The *liver* is moderately enlarged. The parenchymal cells show cloudy swelling and fatty change. Amastigotes have been reported in the Kupffer's cells.

The *spleen* is enlarged and congested but parasites are very rarely found.

OTHER ORGANS

Pseudocysts surrounded by lymphocytes may be found in the thyroid, suprarenals and gonads.

Chronic Chagas' disease

CARDIOMYOPATHY

All degrees of cardiomegaly may be found with enlargement of the right ventricle predominating. The epicardium shows areas of thickening. An apical groove between the two ventricles gives rise to a 'cor bifidum'. The intraventricular septum is hypertrophied. There is a funnel-shaped retraction of the apical wall and at the ventricular apex the myocardium is flabby with many small scars (Fig. 3.4). A *pathognomonic* cardiac change is apical aneurysms caused by thinning and bulging of the apical region of the left ventricle where there are small aneurysms, never more than 5 cm in diameter, with thin translucent walls mostly containing thrombi but rupture is rare. There are organized thrombi in the right atrium. There is no valvular or coronary artery involvement. No parasites can be seen on microscopy.

ALIMENTARY TRACT

There is an initial hypertrophy of the muscle wall followed by dilatation with megaoesophagus or megacolon (25% of patients dying of cardiomyopathic Chagas' disease also have megacolon) (Figs. 3.5 and 3.6). Microscopically

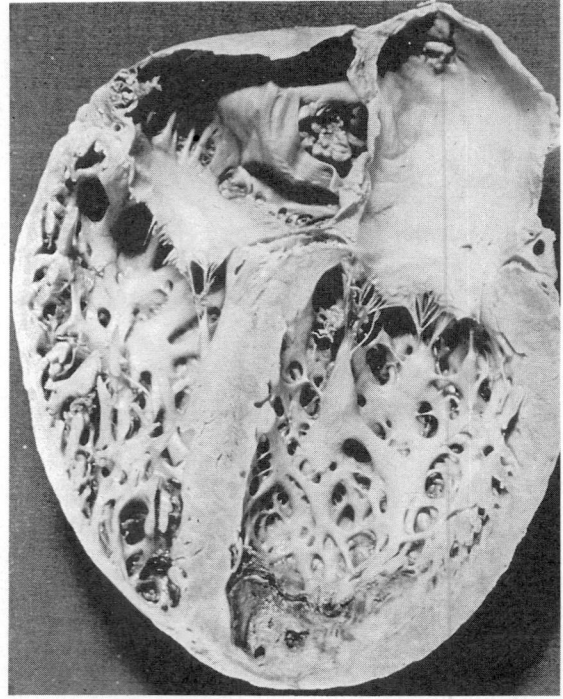

Fig. 3.4. An enlarged heart from a case of chronic Chagas' disease, showing dilatation of all four chambers and attenuation of the myocardium of the right ventricle. (Courtesy Prof. F. Koberle.)

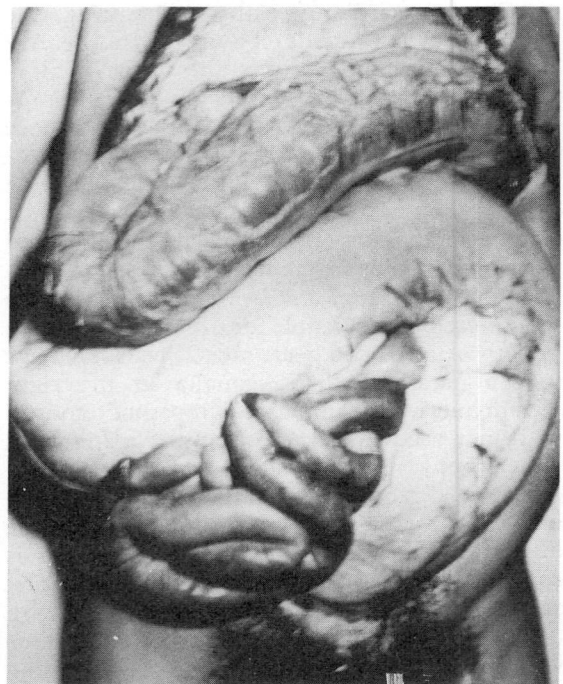

Fig. 3.5. Megacolon in chronic Chagas' disease shown at post-mortem.

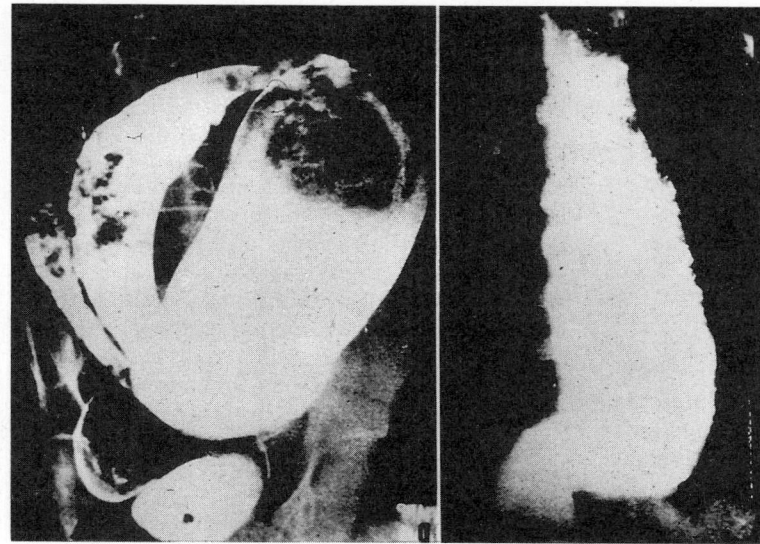

Fig. 3.6. Radiographs showing megacolon and megaoesophagus in Chagas' disease. (Courtesy Dr B. H. Kean.)

parasites are very difficult to find. The fibrous tissue is increased and the smooth muscle fibres elongate. Organs thus affected have diminished numbers of ganglion cells in the intramural plexuses.

LUNGS

These are indurated and brown with scattered brown nodules. Microscopically the alveoli contain macrophages laden with haemosiderin which are also present in the interstitial tissues. The alveolar capillaries are dilated and tortuous and there is bronchiectasis with dilatation of the larger air passages also probably caused by neurological disturbance. Hydroureter may occur.

BRAIN

The brain is involved mainly in the acute phase but chronic neurological syndromes with spastic paralysis, mental deficiency and cerebellar symptoms have been ascribed to chronic Chagas' disease.[15]

IMMUNITY

Chagas' disease is often a very chronic infection. The trypanosomes, which are intensely antigenic but show no antigenic variation (unlike African trypanosomes), possess a surface factor removable by trypsin that enables them to avoid capture by host macrophages, thus avoiding the macrophage activation system. In the absence of macrophage activation the presence of specific antibodies serves only as a vehicle to introduce more parasites into the macrophages where they replicate but, in the presence of macrophage activation, the specific antibodies direct the parasites into the mononuclear phagocytes and potentiate their intracellular destruction. These observations suggest that in vivo humoral immunity may be effective only in the presence of concomitant cell-mediated immunity.[16] Both humoral and cell-mediated immunity develop and there is a complete spectrum of host response from little or none (acute Chagas' disease) through the various manifestations of chronic Chagas' disease to a complete immunity in apparently healthy individuals with positive serological tests, and even circulating trypanosomes in very small numbers, which can only be found by xenodiagnosis, who live a normal life.

Humoral immunity

An antibody response (complement fixing, fluorescent and ELISA) develops within 30 days of infection with a resulting drop in parasitaemia (but trypanosomes can often be demonstrated by xenodiagnosis and cultural techniques for a few years after infection). There is no great increase in IgG or IgM (unlike African trypanosomiasis).

Cell-mediated immunity

Lymphocytes, macrophages and plasma cells appear round the pseudocysts within weeks and delayed hypersensitivity develops shown by an intradermal reaction developed by Mayer and Pifano using 'cruzin' prepared from cultures of *T. cruzi*.

CLINICAL FEATURES IN GENERAL

Natural history

The natural history of Chagas' disease is very variable. It can be a mild and inapparent infection and the three-year-old girl from whom *T. cruzi* was first isolated by Chagas in 1908 recently died at the age of 78, still with a patent infection and no evidence of any pathology. Most infections are inapparent. In endemic areas a significant proportion of the population show positive serology and although they are apparently healthy 30% of them may show *T. cruzi* on xeno-diagnosis, and many show electrocardiographic (ECG) changes. In Brazil in almost one-third of 2000 subjects examined the ECG was abnormal, and 9% of chest X-rays showed enlargement of the cardiac shadow.

In a small minority of patients, usually children, the infection is acute and death results from meningoencephalitis. In a much larger number, after an acute attack with recovery, or without any preceding evidence of infection, the disease proceeds to the chronic stage with the development of cardiomyopathy, megacolon or megaoesophagus. In the majority of infections persistent infection apparently causes no disability and infected persons may live out a normal life. The infection does not die out naturally, although some cases have been cured by chemotherapy.

Incubation period

In the absence of a chagoma, trypanosomes appear in the blood 14–28 days after infection and symptoms may begin.

ACUTE CHAGAS' DISEASE

Clinical features

Acute Chagas' disease is most common in the first decade of life but often escapes detection because of few symptoms, but about 10% of patients die. The first sign may be the development of a chagoma.

Chagoma

The primary lesion which develops at the site of infection is called a chagoma which results from invasion of the skin and surrounding tissues by proliferating trypanosomes. It is a local inflammatory swelling in which amastigotes multiply in fat cells and may be found anywhere on the body. When it is placed round the eye, which is the usual site, there is oedema of the eyelids and sometimes also of the malar and temporal regions, together with unilateral conjunctivitis (Romaña's sign, Fig. 3.7). It differs from the local swelling and oedema following a bug bite which resolves quickly. This stage is followed by fever and the appearance of trypanosomes in the blood some 14 days after infection. Local and generalized lymphadenopathy with amastigotes present in the lymph glands may be found.

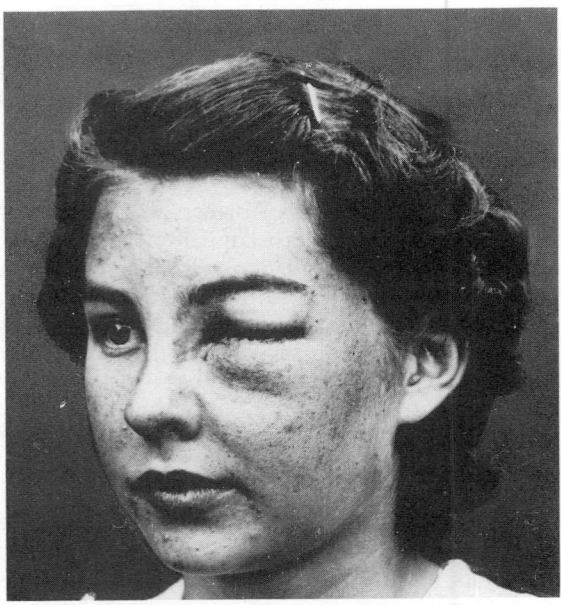

Fig. 3.7. Unilateral palpebral oedema (Romaña's sign) in Chagas' disease. (Courtesy Dr S. B. Pessoa.)

Skin

A rash may appear on the chest or abdomen consisting of sharply defined red spots, the size of a pinhead. There is no pain or itching and it fades after 7–10 days. Some children show a reaction with numerous subcutaneous painful nodules on the body (lipochagomas). There may be *hepatosplenomegaly*, cardiac arrhythmias (seen on ECG) and *myocardial* insufficiency due to an acute involvement of the heart.

Central nervous system

Although trypanosomes can be found in the cerebrospinal fluid signs of meningoencephalitis are rare.

Myxoedematous swellings

Areas of myxoedematous swelling, especially on the face (Fig. 3.8), are not uncommon in acute Chagas' disease and have led to the suggestion that the thyroid is involved. This is now doubtful and in Brazil, where Chagas made his original observations, 75% of the population normally had goitre and a cretin was found in almost every family.

ination in the early stages and later by centrifugation of clotted blood, culture, xenodiagnosis and animal inoculation.

After the acute phase the patient enters an intermediate phase which may last for the rest of his life. Trypomastigotes may occur in the blood in very low numbers and after a time become undetectable, even by xenodiagnosis. Some cases never pass out of this phase but others do and develop some of the manifestations of chronic Chagas' disease, and about 30% of chronic infections show ECG changes.

CHRONIC CHAGAS' DISEASE

Clinical features

The clinical picture varies according to the geo-

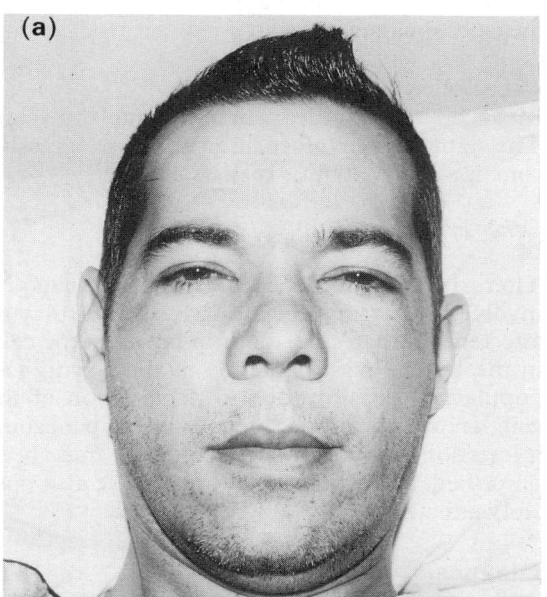 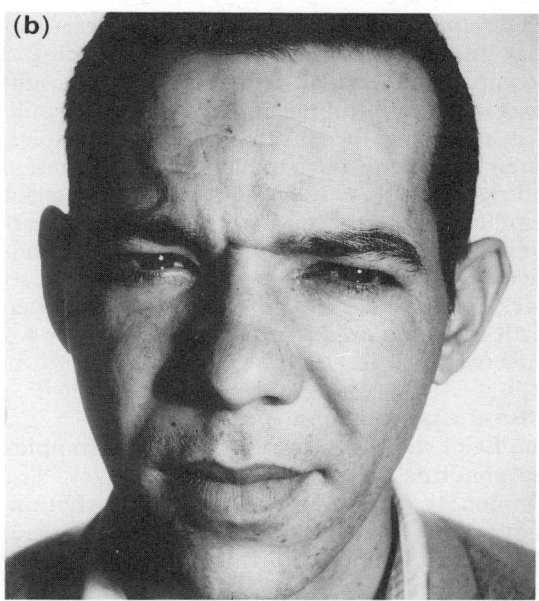

Fig. 3.8. (a) Acute Chagas' disease showing the myxoedematous swelling of the face; (b) the same patient three weeks later after subsidence of the oedema in the intermediate phase.

Blood changes

There is no anaemia but a peripheral lymphocytosis with white cell counts of 20×10^9/litre, of which 80% are lymphocytes.

Diagnosis

Isolation of trypanosomes

Trypanosomes can be found on direct exam-

graphic location. Cardiomyopathy may be the main manifestation in Colombia and Venezuela, southern Peru, central and northern Chile, whereas in northern Argentina, Paraguay and southern Brazil (São Paulo) mega disease is present and may be prominent, although cardiomyopathy is found as well. In other areas, such as Northern Peru, Pernambuco and Bahia in Brazil, *T. cruzi* infection is present with little, if any, evidence of chronic Chagas' disease (cardiomyopathy and mega disease). There is a strong correlation between the incidence of cardiomyopathy and mega disease and the different zymodemes (see section on aetiology, p. 75).

Cardiomyopathy

Chagas' cardiomyopathy manifests itself in adult life between the ages of 15 and 50. The incidence varies according to geography; in some endemic areas of disease cardiomyopathy in some form is very common. Of 3591 people examined in Chile, 1248 (35%) were infected with *T. cruzi* and 298 (23.8%) of these showed some evidence of cardiomyopathy.[17] In Venezuela serological and xenodiagnostic methods indicate that 20% of rural people are infected, of whom 50% show some heart condition, while most of the myocardial infections in rural inhabitants up to 40 years of age are due to Chagas' disease.[18]

The *clinical features* are an enlarged heart and weak muscle force with all the signs of tricuspid incompetence. Emboli from the left and right heart may cause embolism. Arrhythmias in mild cases are limited to tachycardia and extrasystoles. Later disorders of conduction are common and right bundle branch block with left anterior hemiblock is very suggestive of Chagas' cardiomyopathy. Progressive damage to the conducting nerves may produce complete heart block with Stokes–Adams attacks and sudden death in young men which is a major cause for concern in Brazil.

ELECTROCARDIOGRAPHIC CHANGES
The ECG shows widening of the QRS complex and abnormalities in the P and T waves. The commonest changes are disorders of rhythm, right bundle branch block (atrial fibrillation and left bundle branch block are rare) and left anterior hemiblock.[19]

DIFFERENTIAL DIAGNOSIS
Other cardiomyopathies resemble Chagas' cardiomyopathy, alcoholic cardiomyopathy with arrhythmias and idiopathic cardiomyopathy; endomyocardial fibrosis is rare in endemic areas. Differentiation of these cardiomyopathies in patients with positive serology is difficult.

Mega disease (mega syndromes, mal d'Engasco)

Mega disease is most prevalent in northern Argentina and southern Brazil. It affects mainly the oesophagus (megaoesophagus) and colon (megacolon). Rarely the stomach, ureters, urinary bladder and gall bladder may be involved.

MEGAOESOPHAGUS
In the early stages there may be no symptoms at all. Later there is a progressive dysphagia progressing through varying degrees until only liquids can be swallowed. Oesophagitis and regurgitation of food with aspiration pneumonia is common.

Radiology (Fig. 3.6) Barium swallow shows changes varying from cardiospasm to a greatly enlarged oesophagus resting on top of the diaphragm.

To provide extra saliva the parotid glands enlarge and combine with malnutrition to produce the 'cat face' appearance of advanced megaoesophagus.

MEGACOLON
Megacolon resembles Hirschsprung's disease. The sigmoid is involved and there is progressive constipation. Volvulus may occur.

Other organs

There is some evidence that other organs are involved. Exocrine and endocrine glands may be affected and arrested maturation of germ cells in the testicle with depletion of the Leydig cell population, possibly due to denervation of the ganglia of the pelvic plexus, or trypanosome infestation during the acute phase has been described.[20] The muscle end plates are also possibly affected.

Diagnosis

Demonstration of parasites in the blood (see also Appendix I, p. 1320)

Parasites may be shown on direct examination of wet blood films or in thick or thin stained films (Giemsa) but only in the acute phase and for a short period. In chronic infections they are very scanty and need special methods of concentration, culture or xenodiagnosis for demonstration.

Concentration methods

Typanosomes can be demonstrated in fairly

large quantities of venous blood by lysing the red cells with suitable substances, centrifugation and examining the deposit. More usually now a microhaematocrit method is used similar to that described for African trypanosomiasis (see Appendix IV, pp. 1497 and 1498).

Microhaematocrit method[21] (Appendix IV, p. 1497)

Finger prick blood is collected in four heparinized microhaematocrit tubes. The tubes are filled and sealed and centrifuged at 12 000 rev/min for 7 minutes. They are placed in a capillary tube holder on a microscope slide and the RBC/plasma junction examined under oil immersion.

Xenodiagnosis

Xenodiagnosis is the use of a triatomine bug usually *Dipetalogaster maxima* to feed on the patient's blood with examination of the bug faeces at 30, 60 and 90 day intervals. (For a detailed description see Appendix III, p. 1479).

Demonstration of T. cruzi specific antigen

Circulating *T. cruzi* specific antigen has been demonstrated experimentally using the ELISA method and may have a role to play in diagnosis of active infection.[22,23]

Demonstration of T. cruzi specific antibodies

A variety of serological tests are now available. Most antigens show cross reaction with *Leishmania donovani* and *T. rangeli*. The IFAT, indirect haemagglutination (IHA) and CFT, using a methanol extracted antigen, are used routinely. More recently an ELISA test has become available and is probably the most useful. There is also a direct agglutination test (DAT)[24] and a radioimmunoassay test.[25]

Antigens vary in specificity and a purified *T. cruzi* specific glycoprotein has been developed which does not cross react with *L. donovani* or *T. rangeli*.[26] All the immunofluorescent tests and ELISA can be performed on blood dried on filter paper.

TREATMENT

Although many thousands of compounds have been tested and in vivo activity against *T. cruzi* has been found in compounds of eight basic groups,[27] no really satisfactory drug for the treatment of Chagas' disease has yet been found. The only two effective drugs at present are nifurtimox (Lampit) and benznidazole (Radanil).

Nifurtimox (Lampit) is given orally three times a day, 8–10 mg/kg body weight daily for 60–120 days but 60 days may be just as effective.[28] Side-effects are frequent and important (see Section XVII).

Benznidazole (Radanil) is given orally, 5 mg/kg body weight daily for 60 days. Side-effects are important (see Section XVII). Chlortetracyclines and steroids should be avoided since they tend to exacerbate the infection.

Results of treatment

Both drugs remove trypanosomes from the blood during the acute phase but xenodiagnosis shows parasites still present. Serology rarely converts in chronic infections.

PROGNOSIS

The prognosis of chronic Chagas' disease is difficult. After the appearance of cardiac failure between the ages of 20 and 50 death takes place in about seven to 24 months. Many cases of chronic Chagas' infection, however, live to a good age without any symptoms and die of other causes. Nothing is known about the chances of developing cardiomyopathy or mega disease after an initial infection.

EPIDEMIOLOGY (see also Appendix I, p. 1289, and Appendix III, p. 1474)

The epidemiology of Chagas' disease depends upon the habits of the triatomine bugs and the mammalian hosts of *T. cruzi* and with most of the triatomine species described (approximately 100) reported as naturally infected with *T. cruzi*,[29] and such a variety of mammalian hosts, the epidemiology is very complex and is best understood in Venezuela, Argentina and Brazil. It is the ability to colonize human dwellings which renders triatomines important in the transmission of *T. cruzi*. Where triatomines are abundant and *T. cruzi* is present in reservoir hosts (armadillos and rodents), as in the southern

USA, there is no Chagas' disease in man because triatomines are unable to colonize the well-constructed houses. Three species in particular are important in their ability to colonize man's habitat:

> *Rhodnius prolixus* in Colombia, Ecuador, Venezuela and parts of Central America;
> *Triatoma infestans* in Argentina, Bolivia, Brazil, Chile, Paraguay, Peru and Uruguay, but spreading northwards;
> *Panstrongylus megistus* in eastern Brazil.

Less important domiciliary vectors are:

> *Triatoma dimidiata* in central and northern South America,
> *Triatoma sordida* associated with *Triatoma infestans* and
> *Triatoma brasiliensis* in the dry north-eastern Brazil.

The habits of these triatomines are described in Appendix III, p. 1474.

There are three main epidemiological situations.

1 Triatomines purely sylvatic and only occasionally infecting man, such as *Triatoma amazonica*. Palm trees are a favourite habitat especially of *R. prolixus* which lives in association with the nests of various mammals and birds in the crown of the tree (Figs. III.77, p. 1474, and III.80, p. 1477).

2 Triatomines peridomestic with bugs maintained near houses by infected opossums (*Didelphis* spp.) and rodents which have become well adapted to man. The bugs spread to the house and become domestic. Armadillos are also important reservoirs (Fig. III.76, p. 1474).

3 Triatomines purely domestic. The bugs live and hide in the cracks and crevices of the walls of adobe huts (Fig. III.78, p. 1475) and in the furniture and hangings on the walls from where they emerge at night to feed on human blood. Persons sleeping regularly in beds drawn up close to the wall establish a permanent cycle of infection with the bug population concentrated in such areas (Fig. III.79, p. 1475). The bugs also maintain themselves on chickens although they do not infect them. Domestic reservoir hosts are mainly man but domestic animals, especially dogs and cats, infected either by bite (*Triatoma infestans*) or from eating mice which eat the bugs, are also important. (For further details see Appendix III, p. 1474, and Fig. III.81, p. 1479.)

Surveys

In order to estimate the importance of Chagas' disease in any one area both the extent of transmission, the amount of infection and the effect on human health must all be studied. This can be done in surveys by vector studies studying the density of bugs and their contact with man, serological and xenodiagnostic studies to determine the amount of infection, chest X-rays, electrocardiography and barium swallow surveys to detect asymptomatic cardiomyopathy and mega-oesophagus.

CONTROL

To be successful any control scheme must involve the community.

Environmental control

Changing the environment is the most important part of any control scheme. This involves building proper houses or improving old ones so that bugs cannot infest them, or modifying them to reduce all cracks and crevices to a minimum. This is expensive and not always possible.

Vector control (see Appendix III, p. 1480)

Chemical control of the bugs has proved very successful in many countries. HCH (benzene hexachloride) is used generally applied at the rate of $2 \, g/m^2$ twice annually. Dieldrin was formerly applied but was dropped after discovery of resistance in *R. prolixus* and *Triatoma dimidiata*. Other insecticides used on an experimental scale include malathion at $2 \, g/m^2$ twice annually. Slow release formulations of normally non-persistent insecticides are promising and synthetic pyrethroids have been used. Permethrin at $0.5 \, g/m^2$ once annually and decamethrin at $0.1 \, g/m^2$ annually have given good control, although more expensive synthetic pyrethroids are competitive with HCH on a cost per house per annum scale.

Vaccines (see also Appendix I, p. 1290)

Vaccination against the disease in man is not yet practical and an important point to consider in the use of vaccines is the danger of inducing immunopathological damage with the induction of immunity since immunopathology is so important in producing the clinical manifestations of Chagas' disease.[30]

Much work has been done in animals and the production of monoclonal antibodies may identify antigens which produce protective antibody[31] and two glycoproteins have been isolated from the surface of different stages of *T. cruzi* which induced a high level of protective antibody in mice.[32]

Personal prophylaxis

Individuals may avoid infection by refusing to sleep in adobe and thatched huts. Mosquito nets must be used and the bed placed in the middle of the floor to avoid the wall, or a room not normally used for sleeping used. For all laboratory workers a recognized test with a standardized antigen (CFT, IFAT, ELISA, HA or IHA) should be performed periodically and if a positive titre is obtained xenodiagnosis should be carried out.

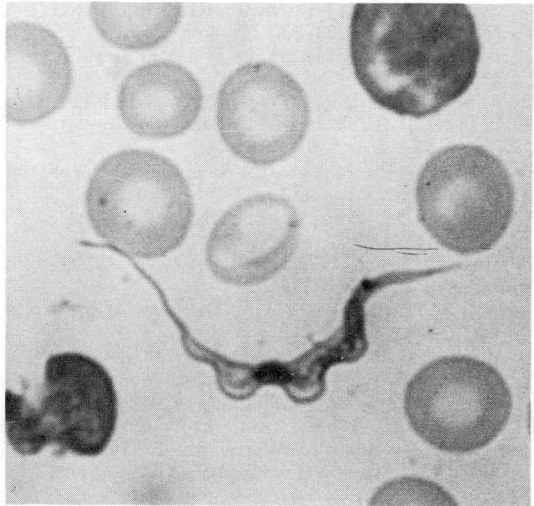

Fig. 3.9. *Trypanosoma rangeli*, Giemsa-stained bloodstream trypomastigote. Note the prominent undulating membrane, the long pointed posterior end and the size and position of the kinetoplast, in comparison with that of *T. cruzi* (Fig. 3.2). (Courtesy Dr Nestor Añez.)

HUMAN INFECTION WITH OTHER TRYPANOSOMES (*HERPETOSOMA*)

Trypanosoma rangeli (Appendix I, p. 1291)

T. rangeli, which is found in man and animals, is apathogenic to its vertebrate host but infected bugs have a shortened life-span. It is often found in man as a double infection with *T. cruzi* and this is its main importance. It is a long slender trypanosome with a long pointed end, a central nucleus and a kinetoplast some distance from the posterior end (in contrast to *T. cruzi*) (Fig. 3.9). It is found mainly in the northern states of South America (Colombia and Venezuela) often in association with *T. cruzi* with which it often shares vectors and hosts. It can be distinguished from *T. cruzi* by its morphology and development in the triatomine vector in which it undergoes anterior development, and is transmitted by the bite (Fig. I.36, p. 1293). In man it occurs as a very occult infection, rarely seen in the peripheral blood from which it can be isolated by culture (on NNN) or xenodiagnosis. The main vector is *R. prolixus*. *T. rangeli* has been isolated from a variety of mammalian hosts. In man it causes no pathology and it is most likely that it only multiplies in the invertebrate host and not in the mammalian host.

Trypanosoma lewisi – like trypanosomes

T. lewisi is a common parasite of rats to which it is harmless but becomes pathogenic when they are immunosuppressed. A few cases of human infection have been reported in Asia: a four-month-old child in Malaya ill with an intermittent fever,[33] two cases in Madhya Pradesh India with fever and with a *Herpetosoma* infection, not of rodent origin[34] and two aboriginal infections in West Malaysia[35] with an unidentified trypanosomal infection. People living in the tropics in extreme poverty may be infected with *Herpetosoma*, possibly transmitted by fleas.[1]

T. vivax

Two cases of infection with *T. vivax* have been reported in man, possibly due to some change in host immunity. There was no pathology.

REFERENCES

1 Ormerod, W. E. (1979) *Pharm. Ther.* **6**, 7–9.
2 Woody, N. C., Hernandez, A. & Suchow, H. (1965) *J. Pediat.* **66**, 107–109.
3 Downs, W. G. (1963) *J. Parasit.* **49**, 50.
4 Petana, W. B. (1978) *Bull. Pan-Am. Hlth Org.* **12**, 45.
5 Bruce-Chwatt, L. J. (1972) *Trop. Dis. Bull.* **69**, 825.

6   Schenone, H., Rubinstein, P., Knierim, F. et al (1968) *Bol. chil. Parasit.* **23,** 83.

7   Bittencourt, A. L. (1975) *Rev Inst. Med. trop. São Paulo* **17,** 135.

8   Bittencourt, A. L. (1976) *Am. J. Dis. Child.* **130,** 97.

9   Pearson, P. O., Wahlgren, M. & Bengtsson, E. (1982) *Am. J. Trop. Med. Hyg.* 449–451.

10 Chocair, P. R., Sabbage, E., Amatoneto, V. et al (1981) *Rev. Inst. Med. trop. São Paulo* **23,** 280–282.

11 Cossio, P. M., Diez, C., Szarfman, A. et al (1974) *Circulation* **49,** 13.

12 Sterin-Borda, L., Fink, S., Diez, C. et al (1982) *Clin. exp. Immunol.* **50,** 534–540.

13 Seneca, H. (1969) *Trans. R. Soc. trop. Med. Hyg.* **63,** 497.

14 Koberle, F. (1958) *Gastroenterology* **34,** 460.

15 Okamura, M. & Correa Netto, A. (1963) *Revta Hosp. Clin. Fac. Med. Univ. São Paulo* **18,** 351.

16 Nogueira, N. (1981) In *Current States and Future of Parasitology,* eds. W. S. Warren & E. F. Durall, pp. 195–207. Massachusetts: Hafferan Bros.

17 Apt, W. (1982) *Resumeres del Segundo Simposio Internazonal de Parasitologia, Santiago,* p. 53.

18 Miles, M. A. (1983) *Trans. R. Soc. trop. Med. Hyg.* **77,** 5–23.

19 Rosenbaum, M. B. & Albarez, A. J. (1955) *Am. Heart J.* **50,** 492.

20 Lamano-Carvalmo, T. L., Ferreira, A. L. & Sahao, M. A. (1982) *Rev. Inst. Med. trop. São Paulo* **24,** 205–213.

21 La Fuente, C., Saucedo, E. & Urjel, R. (1984) *Trans. R. Soc. trop. Med. Hyg.* **78,** 278–279.

22 Bongert, Z. V., Hungerer, K. D. & Galvao-Castro, B. (1981) *Mem. Inst. Oswaldo Cruz* **76,** 71–82.

23 Araujo, F. G. (1982) *Ann. trop. Med. Parasit.* **76,** 25–36.

24 Peralta, J. M., Magalhaes, T. C. R., Abreu, L. et al (1981) *Trans. R. Soc. trop. Med. Hyg.* **75,** 695–698.

25 Tarleton, R. L., Schulz, C. L., Grögl, M. et al (1984) *Am. J. trop. Med. Hyg.* **33,** 34–40.

26 Schechter, M., Voller, A., Marinkelle, C. J. et al (1984) *Lancet* **ii,** 939–941.

27 Gutteridge, W. E. (1976) *Trop. Dis. Bull.* **73,** 699.

28 Cerisola, J. A. (1977) *Pan-Am. Hlth Org. scient. Publ.* **347,** 35.

29 Miles, M. A. (1979) In *Biology of the Kinetoplastida,* eds. W. H. R. Lumsden & D. A. Evans, Vol. 2, pp. 177–196. London: Academic Press.

30 Editorial (1980) *Lancet* **i,** 466.

31 Miles, M. A., Arias, J. R., Valente, S. A. S. et al (1983) *Am. J. trop. Med. Hyg.* **32,** 1251–1259.

32 Snary, D. (1983) *Trans. R. Soc. trop. Med. Hyg.* **77,** 126–129.

33 Johnson, P. D. (1933) *Trans. R. Soc. trop. Med. Hyg.* **26,** 467.

34 Shrivavasta, K. K. & Shrivavasta, G. P. (1974) *Trans. R. Soc. trop. Immun.* **50,** 534–540.

35 Dissanaike, A. S., Ong, H. T. & Kan, S. P. (1974) *Trans. R. Soc. trop. Med. Hyg.* **68,** 494–495.

Chapter 4
Visceral Leishmaniasis

An important cause of fever in the tropics is visceral leishmaniasis (VL) or kala-azar which is a member of the protozoal genus of parasites called *Leishmania* which cause leishmaniasis, an important world disease estimated to affect 100 million people. There are two types of disease caused by *Leishmania*, one visceral leishmaniasis or kala-azar, and the other cutaneous leishmaniasis composed of Old World and New World species which are described in Section VII (diseases presenting as ulcers).

GENERAL DESCRIPTION OF *LEISHMANIA*

Leishmaniasis is caused by protozoal parasites of the genus *Leishmania* which have an intracellular (amastigote) stage in mammals and an extracellular flagellate (promastigote) stage in sandflies, which are the insect vectors.

The *amastigote* stage in the mammalian host appears as an ovoid or round body measuring 2–3 μm in length living intracellularly in monocyte, polymorphonuclear leukocyte or endothelial cells. It stains well with Giesma or Wright's stain with a pale blue cytoplasm inside a limiting membrane, and contains a relatively large nucleus which stains red and a kinetoplast consisting of a deep violet rod-like body and a dot-like basal body (Figs. 4.1 and 4.2 and Plate II.4). Amastigotes are known as Leishman–Donovan (LD) bodies.

The *promastigote* stage, which is found in both culture media and the sandfly host both being similar, has a single free flagellum arising close to

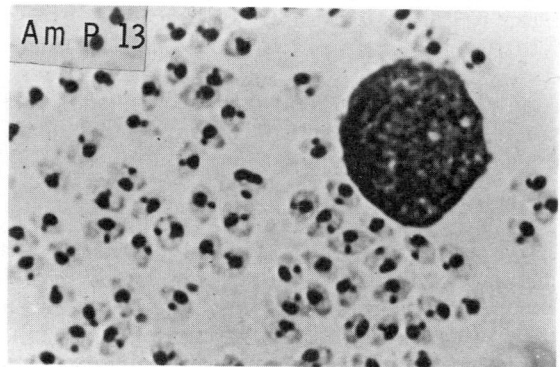

Fig. 4.2. Amastigotes of *L. donovani*.

the kinetoplast at the anterior end and possesses marked motility. The average length is 15–20 μm and the diameter 1.5–3.5 μm. The flagellum measures 15–28 μm (Fig. 4.1).

Life-cycle in the sandfly host (Appendix I, Fig. I.37, p. 1966, and Appendix III, Fig. III.19, p. 1402)

The *amastigotes* are ingested with the first blood meal of the female sandfly in which they become transformed almost immediately into *promastigotes* which multiply in the midgut and then migrate forwards to the anterior part of the thoracic midgut or 'cardia'. From here they move forward to contaminate the mouthparts to be regurgitated into the wound caused by the bite at the second blood meal. This is 'anterior development' which is followed by *Leishmania* of the subgenus *Leishmania* (Suprapylaria).

In the other subgenus, *Viannia*, development

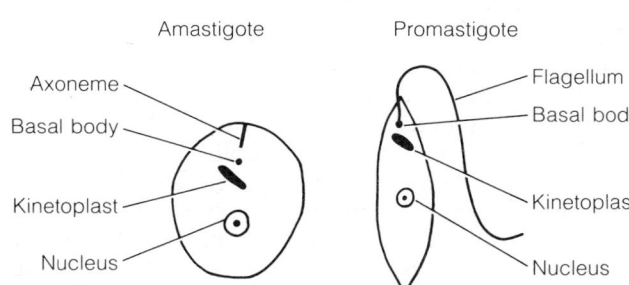

Fig. 4.1. Amastigote and promastigote forms of *Leishmania*.

in the gut includes a long period of development in the hindgut with later migration to the mid- and foregut (Peripylaria). This property is important in distinguishing the benign from the malignant forms of American cutaneous leishmaniasis.

In all cases the infection is transmitted by bite.

Development in the sandfly from the amastigote to infective promastigote stage varies from 5 to 10 days and is synchronous with the gonadotropic cycle of the host so that infections acquired with one blood meal are transmissible when the infected sandfly is ready to feed again after eggs have been laid (Appendix I, p. 1317).

In the mammalian host

After inoculation by the sandfly, either into a capillary or the dermal tissue, the promastigotes encounter macrophages which actively search them out and engulf them, tail first, by a process of invagination. The promastigote changes into an amastigote in a parasitophorous vacuole where it multiplies until the new amastigotes penetrate the cell membrane and leave the macrophage to be ingested by fresh macrophages by a process of invagination. (For morphology and structure, see Appendix I, p. 1297.)

Most leishmanial parasites normally have canine or rodent hosts and are zoonoses. Under certain circumstances they can infect man in whom they cause three main clinical types of disease.

> *Type 1*: Infection limited to the skin (cutaneous leishmaniasis).
> *Type 2*: Infection involving the mucocutaneous junction of the nose and mouth with destructive lesions (mucocutaneous, mucosal, leishmaniasis, espundia).
> *Type 3*: Infection of the reticuloendothelial system involving many viscera (visceral leishmaniasis, kala-azar).

The *Leishmania* are divided into two subgenera according to their development in the sandfly, and it is important to understand this classification since the clinical features, treatment and epidemiology all depend on it.

The two subgenera are as follows:[1]

1 *Leishmania—L.(L.)*. Development in the foregut of the sandfly (Suprapylaria)

2 *Viannia—L.(V.)*. Development in the hind- and midgut of the sandfly. (Peripylaria) (Appendix I, p. 1295, Appendix III, p. 1401, and Fig. III.19, p. 1402).

Each subgenus contains a number of complexes.

Complex	Clinical disease	Geographical area
L. (L.) donovani	Visceral leishmaniasis (kala-azar)	Old and New Worlds
L. (L.) tropica	Anthroponotic cutaneous leishmaniasis (Chapter 37)	Old World
L. (L.) major	Zoonotic cutaneous leishmaniasis (Chapter 37)	Old World
L. (L.) mexicana	Cutaneous leishmaniasis (Chapter 37)	New World
L. (V.) braziliensis	Mucocutaneous, mucosal, leishmaniasis, espundia (Chapter 37)	New World

These complexes and species cannot be distinguished morphologically although there are some differences in size and on electron microscopy (Appendix I, p. 1301), but there are cultural, biochemical (isoenzymes) and serological (excreted factor—EF) differences which correspond to different forms of clinical disease (Appendix I, p. 1263).

The association between a specific complex and the type of clinical disease caused—purely cutaneous or visceral—is not always clear.

Anthroponotic cutaneous leishmaniasis (ACL) in the western Mediterranean for instance is caused by *L. (L.) infantum*, a member of the donovani complex.[2,3]

IMMUNITY

There is a considerable variation in the immune response to infection in VL[4] and resistance to *L. (L.) donovani* infection in mice has been shown to be under genetic control.[5]

Natural immunity (see also Appendix I, p. 1302)

Some animals are completely resistant to infection and disease in man is very variable. Innate immunity in mice is controlled by the *Lsh* autosomal gene and the ability to acquire immunity is controlled by a gene close to H-2 on the major histocompatibility complex of man.[6] The finding that *L. (L.) infantum* in southern Europe may cause either cutaneous or visceral disease is relevant. A factor (possibly an antibody) is present naturally in certain sera which prevents the establishment of infection in VL, and the absence of this factor may explain the greater susceptibility of infants and young children to VL in Mediterranean areas. In VL males are four times as susceptible as females which cannot be entirely explained on environmental grounds.

Acquired immunity

Infection with all forms of leishmaniasis which is allowed to run its natural course immunizes against reinfection with the homologous strain. This immunity usually lasts for life but reinfection can occur,[7] usually many years after the first infection or after immunosuppression. In VL subclinical infections may become overt after famine or social disturbances. There is some cross immunity between different strains which is not always reciprocal. *L. (L.) major* protects against *L. (L.) tropica* but not vice versa. Cross immunity trials in monkeys confirm observations in man that neither *L. (L.) mexicana* nor *L. (L.) amazonensis* gives protection against parasites of the *L. (V.) braziliensis* complex, but recovery from infection with *L. (V.) braziliensis* and *L. (L.) mexicana* subspecies gives firm resistance to infection with any of the *L. (L.) mexicana* complex parasites. There is no cross immunity between *L. (L.) tropica* and *L. (L.) donovani*.[8]

Mechanisms of immunity

Infective promastigotes enter the body at the site of inoculation by sandfly bite where they are taken up by macrophages in which they multiply as amastigotes sheltered from the body's humoral responses. The major host response is cellular and amastigote filled macrophages are destroyed by sensitized T lymphocytes.[9] The released amastigotes are destroyed extracellularly by collagen and connective tissue responses in which necrosis sometimes plays a part. A granuloma forms with the appearance of delayed hypersensitivity (leishmanin test). What happens then depends partly upon host resistance and partly upon toxicity and immunogenicity of the parasite.[10] Host resistance in mice has been shown to be under genetic control (Appendix I, p. 1302).[5] The pattern of infection varies in different strains of inbred mice from self-healing to the uncontrolled multiplication of parasites. In both cutaneous and visceral leishmaniasis in man there is a similar wide spectrum of disease varying from anergic forms (diffuse cutaneous leishmaniasis) to a middle range of rapidly self-healing simple cutaneous lesions to hypersensitive non-healing forms (*recidiva*, *espundia*) in cutaneous leishmaniasis.[11]

In visceral leishmaniasis there is a similar spectrum, the majority of infections are self-healing and subclinical[12] and in these there is evidence that cortisone and immunosuppression therapy can activate latent leishmaniasis.[13] In the minority of cases who develop the kala-azar syndrome there is evidence of severe non-specific depression of T lymphocyte function and cell-mediated immunity through an inhibition of suppressor T cells, as evidenced by failure to develop delayed hypersensitivity to leishmanin and tuberculin until recovery, when all these functions are restored.[14] In the elimination of parasites necrosis plays a part as seen in the necrosis in certain types of cutaneous lesions and in the unusual liver necrosis reported in some cases[15].

Antigenic relationships of *Leishmania*

There is an antigenic relationship between all mammalian and lizard *Leishmania* and some mycobacteria. Adler and Adler[16] found that *L. adleri* shared antigens with *L. (L.) donovani*, *L. (V.) braziliensis* and *L. (L.) tropica*; leishmanin can be prepared from any strain of *Leishmania* as well as flagellates such as *Strigomonas oncopelti*. Common antigens are shared with mycobacteria. The antigen for the complement fixation test in kala-azar is prepared from Kedrowsky's acid-fast bacillus or tubercle bacilli.

Leishmanin test: Montenegro reaction

This skin reaction which is a measure of delayed hypersensitivity was introduced by Montenegro[17] in South America. Leishmanin is a suspension of washed promastigotes in 0.5% phenol saline (the Montenegro antigen uses Coca's fluid) in a strength of 10^7/ml and the dose is 0.1 ml intradermally (1 million organisms). The test is read after 48–72 hours and a positive result is shown by an induration of 5 mm or over which can be divided into four grades, 5–6 mm, 6–8 mm, more then 8 mm, and with blistering.[18]

Immediate sensitivity reactions have been obtained using exoantigens obtained from in vitro culture in New World cutaneous leishmaniasis.[19] Polysaccharide fractions have been used[20] and have been said to be more specific. The incidence of false-positive reactions in otherwise healthy persons varied from 1.5%[21] to 6.3%,[22] but some of these latter observations were undertaken in an area endemic for leish-maniasis. Occasional positive reactions have been noted in glandular tuberculosis,[23] lepromatous leprosy and certain mycotic infections. Equivocal results have been found in Chagas' disease but no positive reactions were elicited in Chagas' disease using antigens prepared from cultural forms of leishmania.[19] A positive leishmanin reaction shows previous exposure to leishmanial antigen of any species and indicates immunity to infection with the homologous strain which has caused the reaction. It correlates well with in vitro lymphocyte transformation.[24]

The leishmanin reaction becomes positive early in infection with *L. (L.) tropica* and *L. (L.) mexicana* and does not denote immunity to reinfection until the leishmanial lesion has completely healed. In *L. (V.) braziliensis* the test becomes positive during the active phase of the infection. In *L. (L.) donovani* it does not become positive until six to eight weeks after recovery from kala-azar.

Serological reactions

Specific humoral antibodies are found in kala-azar where agglutinating, complement-fixing and fluorescent antibodies are all used in diagnosis. Fluorescent antibodies are found in metastasizing forms of American cutaneous leishmaniasis and in some cases of *L. (L.) major* infections. In most forms of *L. (L.) tropica* and non-metastasizing forms of cutaneous leishmaniasis no antibodies can be demonstrated.

KALA-AZAR (VISCERAL LEISHMANIASIS)

Kala-azar is also known as the black sickness or fever (kala-azar), sirkari disease, burdwan fever, Dum Dum fever (after the district in Calcutta where *L. donovani* was first found in an autopsy), mard el bicha (Malta).

GEOGRAPHICAL DISTRIBUTION
(Fig. 4.3 and Appendix I, p. 1305)

Kala-azar has a worldwide distribution in the tropics and subtropics. It occurs in the Medi-

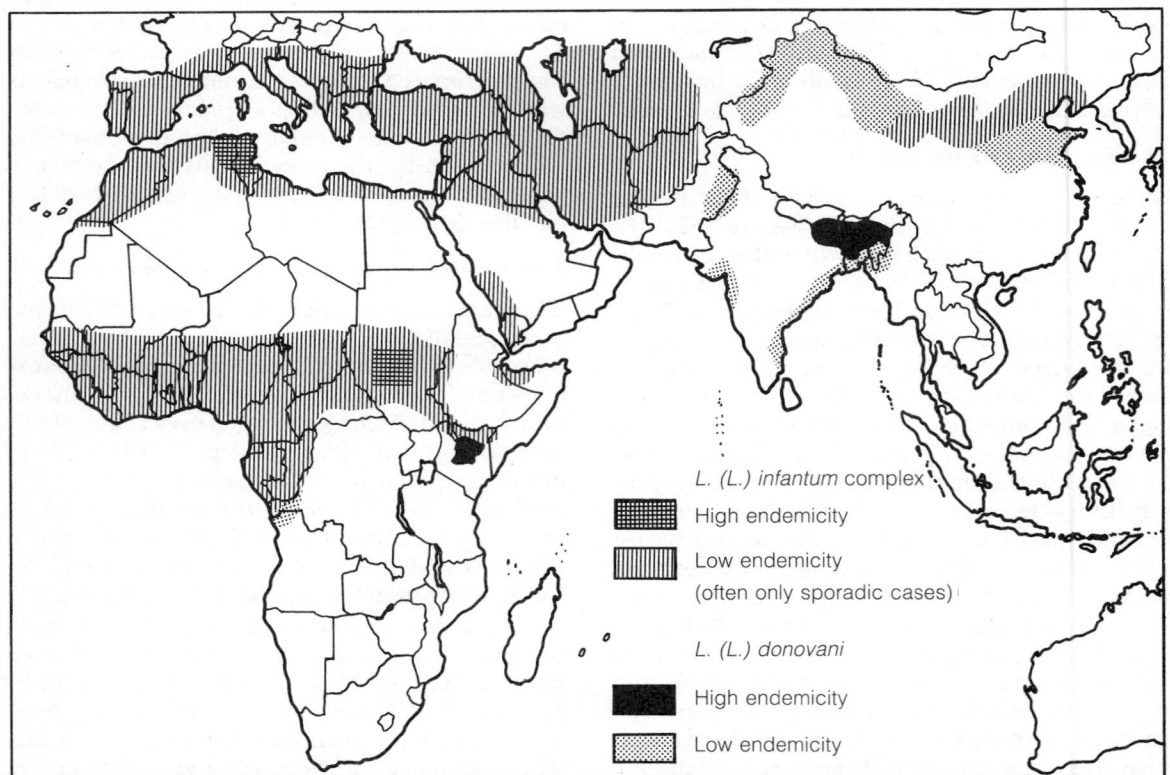

L. (L.) infantum complex

High endemicity

Low endemicity
(often only sporadic cases)

L. (L.) donovani

High endemicity

Low endemicity

Fig. 4.3.(a)   Geographical distribution of visceral leishmaniasis (kala-azar) in Europe, Africa and Asia, caused by *L. (L.) infantum* complex and *L. (L.) donovani.*

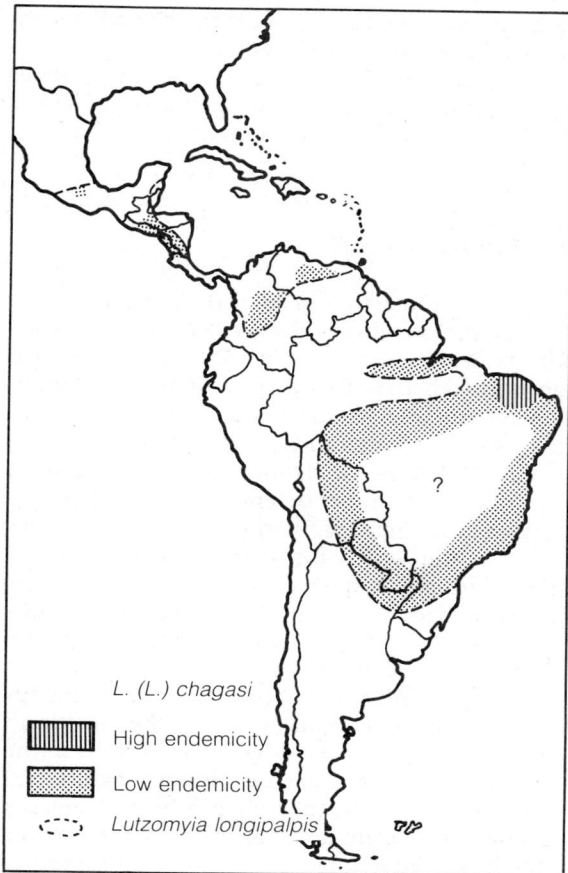

L. (L.) chagasi

▓ High endemicity

▒ Low endemicity

⌐ ⌐ Lutzomyia longipalpis

Fig. 4.3.(b) Geographical distribution of visceral leishmaniasis (kala-azar) in South and Central America, caused by *L. (L.) chagasi*.

terranean, central Asia, China, the Middle East, India, Africa and South and Central America. Recently there has been a great upsurge in the incidence, and of 400 000 cases recorded world wide in 1977, one-quarter occurred in Bihar.[25]

AETIOLOGY

Three members of the donovani complex cause kala-azar or visceral leishmaniasis (VL) (Fig. 4.3):

L. (L.) infantum in the Mediterranean area, Middle East, parts of sub-Saharan Africa and China;
L. (L.) chagasi in South America;
L. (L.) donovani in India, East Africa and parts of China.

The exact identification of the organisms responsible is still uncertain in parts of sub-Saharan Africa and China.

In the main, *L. (L.) infantum* and *L. (L.) chagasi* are infections of dogs and other canines, occasionally transmissible to man, whereas *L. (L.) donovani* is a human infection.

TRANSMISSION

Kala-azar is transmitted from one mammalian host to another including man by sandflies (*Phlebotomus, Lutzomyia*) of different species (see Appendix III and section on epidemiology, p. 107). Other much rarer methods are congenital, blood transfusion or by direct (sometimes sexual) contact or inoculation. (See also Table III.3, p. 1400, and section on Epidemiology, p. 107.)

Sandfly transmission

Following the observation that there was a correlation between the distribution of *Phlebotomus argentipes* in India and kala-azar it was found that there was a rapid development of promastigote forms in *P. argentipes*, and in 1942 kala-azar was successfully transmitted to human volunteers by the bite of *P. argentipes*.[26]

Sandflies are the principal agent of transmission in nature. They are small hairy flies with long hairy legs (Fig. III.17, p. 1397). The female sandfly feeds on blood and transmits the infection. One or more blood meals are necessary to complete the maturation of each batch of eggs. The male sandfly does not suck blood but feeds on plant juices and takes no part in transmission. Sandflies are inactive in daylight seeking shelter in dark moist places and coming out at dusk. The normal flight (more of a hop) is usually less than a metre, but sandflies can cover more than a kilometre overnight. Female sandflies feed on a variety of both warm- and cold-blooded animals and do not specially feed on man, but a few species such as *P. argentipes* in India have become domestic and depend on man. This has an important effect on epidemiology.

Breeding sites are dark damp places rich in organic matter and female flies are ready to lay eggs 3–10 days after a blood meal. The eggs are laid and larvae hatch which require high humidity to complete their development in less than three weeks, but species which live in colder climates may take up to three months. Flies emerge during the hours of darkness and mate, the female storing sufficient sperm to lay eggs at intervals throughout life, which in nature is probably rarely more than a few weeks. The life-cycle from egg to adult varies from just under one to three months.

A sandfly is infective to a new host from 5 to 10 days after the infective blood meal and remains infected for the rest of its life. Infection of a new host occurs with the second blood meal after egg laying has taken place (for further details see Appendix III, p. 1395).

Congenital transmission

Congenital transmission is rare but has been described.[27]

Blood transfusion

Kala-azar is one of the protozoal diseases that can be transmitted by blood transfusion. Amastigotes may occur in the peripheral blood in small numbers in the early stages of infection and in asymptomatic carriers who may be infective for a short period. Cases have been recorded from southern France during the incubation period and in Scandinavia where an infant was infected from blood given in an exchange transfusion from an asymptomatic donor who had previously travelled in an endemic area.

Direct contact

Since amastigotes can be demonstrated in stools containing blood and mucus and in nasal discharges, direct transmission via these routes is possible. Direct transmission by the sexual route has been described between a man with Sudanese kala-azar and his wife who had never left England.

Ingestion

Whereas predation may be of some importance in maintaining infection in carnivores and rodents there is no evidence that man can acquire infection from eating meat.

Inoculation

Transmission has been accomplished artificially to man by inoculating cultures of *L. donovani* intradermally into the skin. A nodule containing amastigotes developed at the site of inoculation. After a period of four to six months *Leishmania* were isolated on blood culture and the full-blown kala-azar syndrome developed later.[28]

Kala-azar has been contracted accidentally as a laboratory infection by accidental inoculation, usually into the finger from infected hamster spleen.

PATHOGENESIS

Infective promastigotes enter the body at the site of inoculation where they are exposed to a factor (? natural antibody) in the serum which opsonizes them so that they are ingested by polymorphonuclear leukocytes and destroyed.[29] In the absence of this factor they are taken up by macrophages in which they are sheltered from the body's immune defences and multiply to form a granuloma with an epithelioid and giant cell reaction which forms the primary lesion.[28] The immune response is cellular and varies across a wide spectrum from complete eradication of the parasites to unrestricted spread. They spread to the local lymph glands (as seen in the vervet monkey) and thence via the bloodstream in leukocytes quite early in the infection[30] to be taken up by reticuloendothelial cells in the spleen, liver, bone marrow, lymph glands and other organs. Here they elicit a granulomatous response and ultimate eradication (inapparent or subclinical infections) or continue multiplying with little host response (kala-azar syndrome), cause chronic non-healing lesions (post-kala-azar dermal leishmanoid) or an exaggerated response (mucosal lesions). The pathological consequences are determined by various immunopathological responses.

IMMUNOPATHOLOGY

Immunosuppression

Depression of cell-mediated immunity allows the development of secondary infections such as tuberculosis and bacterial infections of the bowel and lungs which are such a feature of kala-azar.

Hypersplenism

The great hypertrophy of the spleen causes hypersplenism which plays a major part in the pancytopenia by red cell destruction, pooling and sequestration of cells in the spleen.

Immunoglobulins

There is a great increase in the level of IgG and also of IgM due to polyclonal B cell activation, which may be due to secretion of a B cell mitogen or inhibition of T suppressor cells leading to an uncontrolled increase in immunoglobulin producing B cells.[31]

Complement activation

Continued consumption of complement via the classical pathway suggests immune complex formation,[32] deposits of which have been demonstrated in renal biopsies in VL.[33] Circulating immune complexes and rheumatoid factor have been demonstrated[29] which may contribute to the immune suppression found in VL.

The Coombs' direct antiglobulin test which is positive in many cases of VL[34] demonstrates the presence of complement and autoantibodies on the surface of the red cells, which may be a factor in the causation of anaemia in VL.[35] Red cell, white cell and platelet antibodies have also been demonstrated in VL[36] but these are not thought to be important factors in the severe pancytopenia which is present.

Blood changes

The blood changes are a rapidly developing anaemia and pancytopenia, all of which revert rapidly to normal following treatment with pentavalent antimony.

Anaemia

Anaemia is common, usually moderate but in children it may be severe, the red cells and haemoglobin falling to 50–60% of normal with a picture suggestive of acute haemolysis.

The anaemia is normochromic and normocytic with anisocytosis, poikilocytosis and polychromasia with a slight reticulocytosis and sometimes a few nucleated red cells in the peripheral circulation.[37]

Mechanisms for the anaemia and pancytopenia are discussed in Chapter 58.

Hypersplenism

There is a shortened life-span of the red cells with increased sequestration in the spleen,[38,39] and an increase in plasma volume.

Autoimmune haemolysis

There have been several reports of complement components [38,40] and of IgG and complement components[34] on the red cells of patients with kala-azar, but there is no direct evidence of autoimmune haemolysis in kala-azar.

Erythropoiesis

Dyserythropoietic changes are commonly found in the bone marrow of patients with kala-azar. Ferrokinetic studies have shown an increased plasma clearance of ^{59}Fe but with reduced iron incorporation into circulating red cells. This may be due to the removal of reticulocytes by the spleen.[39]

The main mechanism of anaemia in kala-azar is hypersplenism, a conclusion which is borne out by the rapid response of the anaemia to splenectomy and the absence of any anaemia in individuals who have had their spleen removed previously.

Pancytopenia

A feature of kala-azar is the *neutropenia*, often severe enough to predispose to bacterial infection although neutrophil function is normal. The cause has been studied extensively:[39] there is a shortened neutrophil survival time and sequestration of the cells takes place in the spleen.

Myeloid maturation is normal and although some white cell antibodies and immune complexes have been identified there is no evidence that these play any major role in the pancytopenia which is related to the size of the spleen and responds to splenectomy.

Thrombocytopenia

There is a fall in the platelet count in some but not all patients and the platelet count is not directly related to bleeding manifestations.[42] There is a reduced platelet survival time and sequestration takes place in the spleen[39] but platelet production is normal. Normal bleeding and clotting times are found but haemorrhagic manifestations do occur and there may be thrombocytopenia and defects in plasma prothrombin control or thromboplastin generation.

PATHOLOGY

The *spleen* in the kala-azar syndrome is often grossly enlarged. In the acute stage the capsule is smooth and the pulp increased in amount and friable, often containing massive infarcts. The enlargement is due to reticuloendothelial hypertrophy and a considerable amount of the pulp is composed of amastigotes. In more resistant cases granulomatous nodules of the Gandy Gamna type may be found with fewer parasites. In the unusual cases described from Italy there was extensive haemorrhagic necrosis.[15]

The *liver* is greatly involved. In resistant cases and in inapparent infections sarcoid-like granulomatous nodules are scattered throughout the liver. Parasites are scanty or impossible to find other than by subinoculation techniques. In the kala-azar syndrome there is little or no cellular reaction and the portal tracts contain Kupffer cells packed with amastigotes. In the unusual series of cases from Italy there were large areas of haemorrhagic necrosis resembling red atrophy in the absence of any parasites.[15]

Lymphatic leishmaniasis

The lymph glands are commonly involved in the visceral disease but are not always so associated, sometimes forming a generalized lymph gland involvement on their own. The glands are enlarged and may contain numerous parasitized histiocytes but more commonly in resistant cases there is a granulomatous picture, often with giant cells closely resembling tuberculosis with few parasites demonstrable.

The *tonsils* are commonly involved and present a similar picture. Parasites can be isolated from the tonsils in most cases of kala-azar.

Mucosal leishmaniasis

Nasopharyngeal, retropharyngeal and oral lesions are found sporadically in the Sudan and East Africa[43] and have been described from India.[44] They are found in areas where kala-azar occurs and may, or more commonly may not, be associated with visceral disease. The causative *Leishmania* is identical to that causing kala-azar.[45] Mucosal leishmaniasis is an unusual immunological response of certain individuals to infection with *L. (L.) infantum* and differs from the mucosal lesions of American cutaneous leishmaniasis (espundia) (see Chapter 37) in that there is no destruction of bone. The histology varies according to the immune response from the presence of numerous parasitized histiocytes to a granuloma containing few or no demonstrable parasites. Amastigotes are commonly found in the nasal and pharyngeal secretions and have been thought to be one method of spread.

Lungs

Although lobar pneumonia is a common secondary infection, leishmanial involvement of the lungs is more usually confined to the presence of amastigotes in macrophage cells as a part of the involvement of the reticuloendothelial system. A specific interstitial pneumonitis has been described and produced experimentally[46] caused by the activation of interstitial cells containing lipid inclusions by amastigotes.

Other organs

Parasites have been isolated at autopsy from the ventricles of the heart, the suprarenals and the parotid glands.

Renal disease

Little is known about renal involvement in kala-azar. In advanced cases the kidneys may show amyloidosis, and deposits of immune complexes in the glomeruli have been described.[33] Interstitial inflammatory foci with polymorphonuclear leukocytes have been described leading to renal failure in the late stages of kala-azar.[47]

Gastrointestinal disease

At autopsy the jejunum may be swollen with parasitized cells and small ulcerations develop from which parasites can be obtained. In five out of ten jejunal biopsies[48] parasitized macrophages were present in the villous tips and less commonly in the lamina propria and submucosa. There was a moderate inflammatory infiltrate of lymphocytes and plasma cells but there was no correlation with malabsorption.

Skin

The skin is commonly involved in kala-azar but purely cutaneous disease in the Sudan is caused by *L. (L.) major*.[45] Primary lesions occur and may be quite large (see section on clinical features, below). In fatal cases of kala-azar all levels of skin below the epidermis may contain amastigote-laden cells collected in large masses about the sweat glands and arterioles and scattered diffusely throughout the corium. Parasites can be detected in life in the dermis in a proportion of cases.[28,49] There is a close connection between these findings and the rashes associated with kala-azar (see p. 96). The pathology of post-kala-azar dermal leishmanoid is discussed on p. 105.

IMMUNITY

Natural immunity

There is a natural insusceptibility to infection which may be due to the presence of a factor (possibly a natural antibody) which prevents establishment of infection and which is absent from infants and young children in the Mediterranean who appear to be more susceptible. Men are four times as susceptible as women, which may be due to a hormonal factor.

Acquired immunity

Immunity acquired from infection is cellular and the degree of cellular immunity determines the place on the spectrum of infection from inapparent infection to overt disease. Cellular immunity is discussed in the section on pathogenesis, above.

There is an extensive depression of cellular immunity which at first may be specific but later becomes non-specific, the T lymphocytes being depressed through an inhibition of suppressor cells. This immune depression is completely reversible with successful treatment, a notable feature being the return of eosinophils with recovery. Although specific antibodies are produced humoral responses have little effect on the outcome of the infection. In areas of VL where the infection has been recently introduced the leishmanin rate is not related to age but when the infection becomes endemic then there is an increasing rate with age, so that with leishmanin rates of 60% the maximum age of incidence is in children (Fig. 4.11), suggesting that acquired immunity also has some effect on the age distribution of VL.

Once established immunity is lifelong and there are no reliable records of second attacks of VL. A naturally acquired positive leishmanin test from inapparent infection also protects against infection.

CLINICAL FEATURES

Natural history

The natural history of infection with *L. donovani* was originally thought to be a steady progression with an increasing number of parasites to death after two years unless treatment was provided. It is now clear that while this may be true of those who develop overt infection (the kala-azar syndrome) this is not true of the majority of inapparent and subclinical infections. Only 3% develop the kala-azar syndrome. Some infections may be overt but recover spontaneously after a short period of fever (see p. 98).

Incubation period

The incubation period has been determined experimentally[30] as between four and six months and clinical observations have confirmed this.[50] However, there are variations from as few as 10 days after leaving the endemic area to as long as two years,[51] two and a half, and one and three-quarter years[52] or nine years.[53] An apparently long incubation period may be due to a change in host immunity for some external reason allowing an inapparent or subclinical infection to surface and cause overt kala-azar.

Symptoms and signs

Primary leishmanioma

In a small minority of cases a primary leishmanioma may be detected as a small papule four to six months before the onset of symptoms[54-56] or have the appearance of an oriental sore[57] or be mistaken for an epithelioma (*L. (L.) infantum* may cause pure cutaneous lesions, see Chapter 37). In the main there are two types of onset: sudden with fever or chronic and insidious.

Acute onset

This is seen more usually in visitors or inhabitants of non-endemic areas. Fever develops quite suddenly of a high intermittent or remittent type but only rarely with a double rise in the 24 hours (Fig. 4.4). The fever, with sweats but without

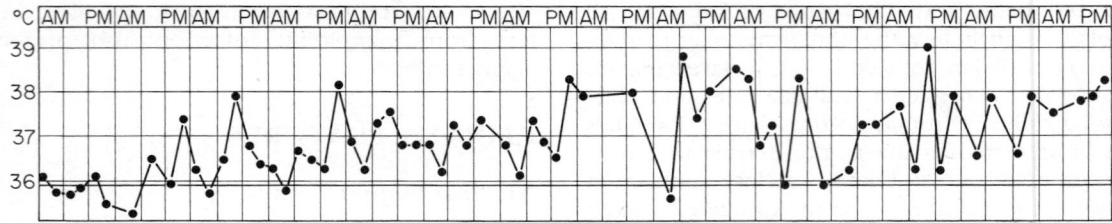

Fig. 4.4.   A 4-hourly temperature chart of a patient with kala-azar, illustrating the double rise in 24 hours.

rigors, resembles malaria and lasts for two to six weeks or longer, resisting all antimalarial therapy. Waves of fever may be separated by apyrexial periods and the spleen enlarges rapidly. A feature is that in spite of a high fever the patient remains remarkably well, ambulant and with a good appetite. An irritating *cough* in the absence of bronchitis or pneumonia is usual and *epistaxis* is common.

Chronic onset

This is commoner in endemic areas and an attack of pneumonia or dysentery may cause the patient to seek medical attention. The main symptoms are discomfort beneath the left costal margin from an enlarging spleen which may itself be felt by the patient who complains of swelling of the abdomen. Cases with a chronic onset may only be discovered by case-finding surveys.

Signs

In spite of a high fever the patient may be ambulant with a temperature of 38.9°C, unaware that he has fever. In this respect kala-azar differs from typhoid and malaria.

SPLENOMEGALY
The spleen enlarges rapidly from the onset of the illness becoming large and often reaching the right iliac fossa. In the rare acute toxic cases no spleen may be felt[58] leading to difficulty in diagnosis.

HEPATIC INVOLVEMENT
The liver is usually enlarged but not to such an extent as the spleen. Hepatic function remains good and liver function tests are usually normal. Jaundice with evidence of gross hepatocellular dysfunction is unusual and carries a grave prognosis but recovery can occur with treatment of the kala-azar. Mild jaundice is more common.

Severe liver damage with hepatic failure without jaundice was a feature of the cases described from Italy.[15] Whether cirrhosis occurs subsequent to treatment is not known.

Ascites is a late sign and usually associated with generalized oedema; the cause is either a low serum albumin, a known feature of kala-azar, or amyloid disease which can be a late complication. It responds to treatment of the kala-azar.

LYMPHADENOPATHY
Enlarged lymph glands in the inguinal and femoral regions are a common feature of the African disease but a more generalized involvement is not uncommon (see section on lymphatic leishmaniasis, below).

RENAL INVOLVEMENT
Mild proteinuria is not uncommon but kidney function is normal.[59] Gross proteinuria is not found, although a nephrotic syndrome, probably due to amyloid nephrosis complicating kala-azar and completely reversing after treatment, has been seen.

CUTANEOUS INVOLVEMENT
Obvious changes in the hair and skin are found, there is a generalized depigmentation of the skin with increased pigmentation of the palms, nail beds and mucosa. In India a characteristic earth-grey colour of the skin has given rise to the name 'kala-azar' ('black fever'). This is best seen in pale-skinned people often being missed in dark-skinned persons.[60]

Cutaneous lesions are not uncommon and may be a presenting feature of the disease. Three types can be recognized:
1 the primary lesions;
2 those occurring during the visceral disease; and
3 those occurring at any time up to 20 years after recovery from kala-azar.

Those lesions appearing during the course of

the disease are not uncommon in African kala-azar. They are numerous and polymorphic, papular, waxy or larger non-ulcerated lesions, some resembling the lesions of diffuse cutaneous leishmaniasis. They are generalized but commoner on the limbs and contain sometimes numerous but often scanty parasites. Although more common in African cases they have been described from China and resemble the cutaneous lesions found in the dog.

For the third type, see section on post-kala-azar dermal leishmaniasis (PKDL) (p. 105).

Course

Before the introduction of successful treatment some cases of kala-azar did recover but 99% of those with parasites found in the spleen or marrow progressively declined and died. Inapparent or subclinical infections are probably very common, as shown by leishmanin conversion, and it was noticeable that in Italy some cases of febrile illness which had recovered spontaneously were found to be leishmanin positive.[15]

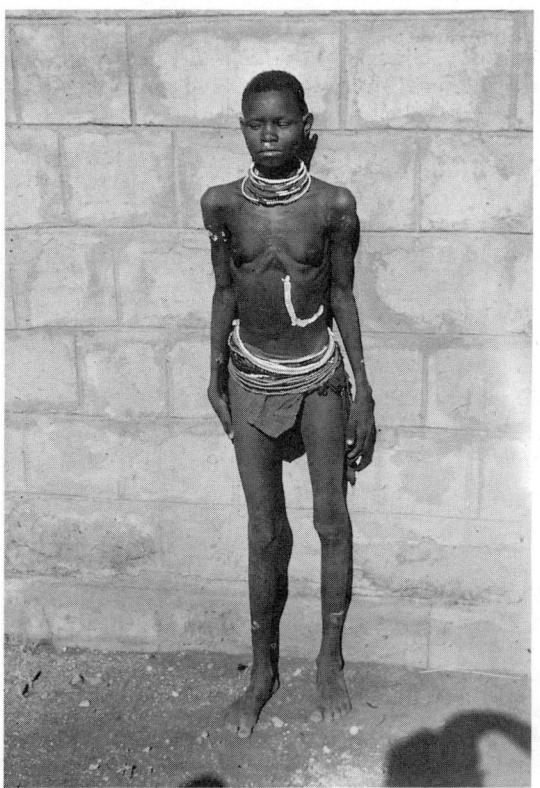

Fig. 4.5. Adult suffering from kala-azar.

In the overt case of kala-azar spells of fever and pyrexia occur for months until a low form of fever becomes persistent. Profuse sweats without rigors are common. Anaemia develops rapidly and with emaciation and gross splenomegaly produces a typical appearance (Fig. 4.5). The hair becomes dry and brittle. Oedema of the legs and haemic murmurs suggest cardiac disease. Haemorrhages are a late manifestation, and purpuric patches, petechiae, epistaxis, bleeding from the gums and vagina are found. This condition may go on for months up to one or two years when the patient is cut off by intercurrent disease, usually pulmonary tuberculosis, pneumonia or bacterial dysentery.

Parasites in the blood

Leishmania circulate in the bloodstream inside large mononuclear cells and polymorphonuclear leukocytes. They can be found from the earliest stages before any clinical signs appear[30] and have been demonstrated in 15/20 cases of kala-azar in East Africa.[61] They are also present for a period of time in inapparent infections as has been demonstrated by the recipients of blood transfusions from healthy donors in whom no signs of infection could subsequently be demonstrated, but who had travelled in an endemic area and who had positive leishmanin tests. These findings are of great importance since such persons are an excellent reservoir of infection as they form the majority of people who are infected in an endemic area, and sandflies have been infected artificially by feeding them on kala-azar patients.

Mucosal leishmaniasis

Espundia-like oral, nasal, nasopharyngeal and laryngeal lesions, with or without systemic infection, are seen in the Sudan,[43] less frequently in East Africa[28] (Fig. 4.6) and India.[44] *Oral lesions* present as nodular or ulcerated swellings of the mucosa of gum, palate, tongue or lips. *Nasal lesions* present as swelling of the nasal mucosa, but there is no destruction of the nasal septum. *Nasopharyngeal* and *laryngeal lesions* present with hoarseness, and mucosal swelling may occur. These lesions may be associated with systemic infection, may occur as a PKDL manifestation after treatment, or may occur without any systemic infection as an isolated phenomenon. All respond well to antimony therapy. The

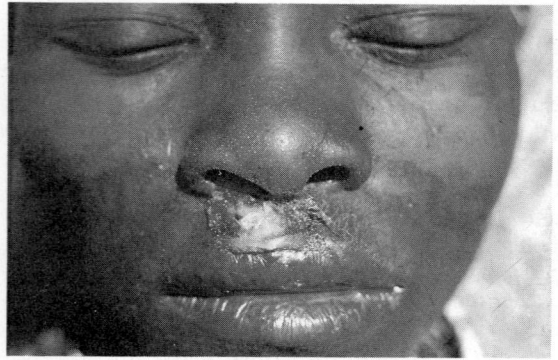

Fig. 4.6.   Mucosal lesion in kala-azar.

cause is an exaggerated or non-healing immune response.

Subclinical infections

In endemic kala-azar areas many of the inhabitants develop a positive leishmanin test although they have never had an attack of kala-azar. In the outbreak in Italy six asymptomatic individuals who had complement-fixing antibodies submitted to liver biopsy showed the presence of granulomas, in one of which *Leishmania* were demonstrated.[12] Other individuals who had recovered spontaneously after a short illness developed positive leishmanin tests suggesting that they had recovered from a leishmanial infection. Epidemiological studies have shown that such persons are immune to both naturally acquired kala-azar and experimental infection.[62] In the population of a valley in Italy the attack rate as shown by the leishmanin test was 44% but clinical illness developed in only 3% of those infected.[18] Since healthy individuals can transmit infection by blood transfusion the large number of subclinical infections is quite sufficient to maintain interhuman transmission without the presence of any animal reservoir.

Eye lesions

Retinal haemorrhages are the most frequent ocular complication of kala-azar although rare. Papilloedema has been recorded[63] and nodules may be found on the eyelids (see Chapter 70). A choroiditis causing visual disturbance may be found in association with PKDL which is reversible with treatment.

Haemorrhagic manifestations

Severe haemorrhage can be a feature of kala-azar[64] especially during epidemics. There is bleeding from the mucous membranes and a severe thrombocytopenia. Pulmonary haemorrhages have been described.[65] Immune complex deposition with disseminated intravascular coagulation is probably the cause.[66] These cases respond well to treatment.

Lymphatic leishmaniasis

Enlargement of the lymphatic glands is a feature of African kala-azar where the femoral group is especially involved. In the Mediterranean, China and elsewhere a form with generalized lymphatic glandular enlargement but without visceral involvement occurs and closely resembles tuberculosis or Hodgkin's disease. Biopsy and gland puncture will show parasites but these may be very few and the histology of granulomas and giant cell formation will suggest tuberculosis. Serology may be necessary for diagnosis. The cervical group of glands is most frequently involved and the tonsils may show granulomatous change with local cervical glandular enlargement. In these cases there may be no evidence of any systemic infection.

Neurological involvement

Delirium and confusional states may occur as in any fever but a progressive tremor of the whole body which resolved only after treatment of the leishmaniasis has been described,[67] the pathology of which is unclear.

Clinical pathology

Blood

The blood changes are anaemia, often marked, leukopenia and thrombocytopenia.

ANAEMIA
The anaemia is normocytic, normochromic with a hyperplastic bone marrow and a rapid red cell turnover.

LEUKOPENIA
There is a considerable leukopenia. The white cells are reduced to below 3×10^9/litre (3000 mm³) in 95%, below 2×10^9/litre (2000 mm³) in 75%

cases. The proportion of leukocytes to erythrocytes, normally 1 : 750, stands at 1 : 1500 or even 1 : 2000, and a complete agranulocytosis may develop in advanced cases. The differential shows a relative increase in lymphocytes with an almost complete absence of eosinophils which may return rapidly following treatment and the presence of significant numbers of eosinophils rules out the diagnosis of kala-azar.

THROMBOCYTOPENIA

The platelets are considerably reduced but bleeding and clotting times are normal.

Serum proteins

There is a marked dysproteinaemia which develops within three to six months after infection. The A/G ratio is reversed and there is a rise in polyclonal IgG up to 2.0 g/dl (Fig. 4.7).

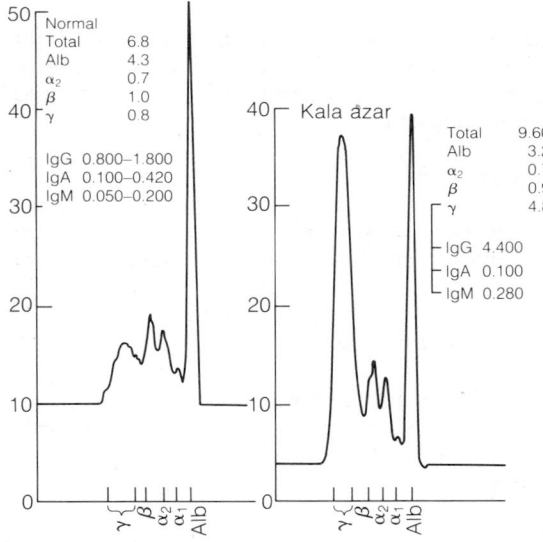

Fig. 4.7. Immunoglobulins in kala-azar.

DIFFERENTIAL DIAGNOSIS

The differential diagnosis is extensive.

Febrile period

Kala-azar should always be considered when a pyrexia of unknown origin which does not respond to antimalarial therapy is encountered. Other fevers which must be distinguished are typhoid, brucellosis, tuberculosis (with which

kala-azar is often associated), bacterial endocarditis, lymphoma and malignancies.

A striking feature of kala-azar is the remarkably clean tongue, good appetite and wellbeing which is present in spite of the fever and marked leukopenia and anaemia associated with it.

Chronic kala-azar with splenomegaly

Kala-azar, as every student of medicine knows, is an important cause of enlargement, often massive, of the spleen. Other causes, however, are hepatosplenic schistosomiasis, portal hypertension from macronodular cirrhosis, chronic lymphatic leukaemia and tropical splenomegaly (see Chapters 1 and 58). An important differential of kala-azar from portal hypertension is the absence of any gastrointestinal bleeding.

Dysproteinaemia

The dysproteinaemia with an elevated IgG is also found in lymphoma (an important differential in children), collagen diseases, leprosy, myeloma and gammopathies (where the IgG is monoclonal). A raised IgM in malaria, schistosomiasis and trypanosomiasis may also be confusing.

Unusual forms of kala-azar

Oropharyngeal leishmaniasis closely resembles oropharyngeal carcinoma, syphilis, espundia and mycotic infections. Lymphatic leishmaniasis resembles tuberculous adenitis, lymphatic leukaemia or Hodgkin's disease while the cutaneous manifestations may be mistaken for epithelioma and leprosy.

DIAGNOSIS

A diagnosis of kala-azar is based first upon a history of a visit to, or residence in an endemic area (Fig. 4.3), demonstration of parasites in spleen, bone marrow, lymph glands or material cultured from these sites, and by serodiagnosis.

Parasitological diagnosis

Parasites may be found as amastigotes in the spleen, bone marrow, liver or lymph glands or demonstrated as promastigotes on culture of these materials as well as blood.

Spleen puncture (splenic aspiration)

The practice of splenic puncture has always been controversial although it is the most reliable method of parasitological diagnosis. Originally large bore needles were used and splenic tears occurred often with disastrous results and their use has been reviewed by Kager and Rees.[68] A safer technique has been devised by Kager et al[59] which has made its use more generally possible, especially for field work in Third World countries. It is accepted that inability to cooperate, young children under the age of five, a small, soft spleen and a marked bleeding tendency are all contraindications. The practice of splenic puncture is more readily accepted by patients than marrow puncture because of its relative painlessness.

TECHNIQUE[59]
The patient lies on his back and the skin is cleaned with spirit and iodine. No local anaesthetic is necessary. A 10 ml syringe with a 21 gauge needle 31–38 mm long is inserted through the anterior abdominal wall into the anterior surface of the spleen between the midclavicular and anterior axillary lines. The patient holds his breath while the needle is in the spleen to prevent it moving and so minimize the risk of tearing. Vacuum is created immediately by suction on withdrawing the plunger, which is immediately withdrawn in a 'to and fro' movement, allowing the needle to remain in the spleen for a split second only. The syringe is withdrawn and the contents of the needle blown on to a slide and washed out into culture medium (Schneider's insect medium).[69] Smears are stained with Giemsa but Field's stain is perfectly satisfactory and easier in the field (Fig. 4.8) (see Appendix

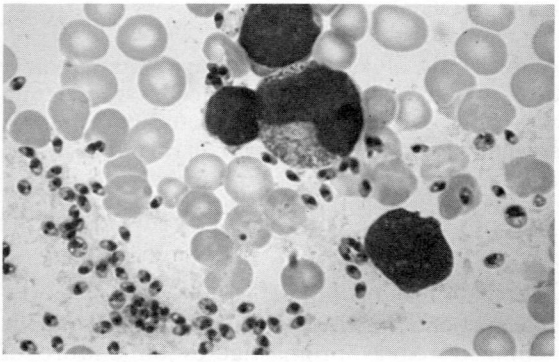

Fig. 4.8.   Splenic smear showing LD bodies.

IV, p. 1497). Amastigotes can be quantified[70] to measure the response to treatment and distinguish slow from quick responders and identify antimony-resistant cases.

It may not be possible always to have a prothrombin time performed but this does not appear to be important in the absence of an overt bleeding tendency. The patient is kept under observation for 24 hours with a half-hourly pulse rate and blood pressure for 4 hours, followed by hourly for another 4 hours.

COMPLICATIONS
Complications are pain, infection, puncture of other organs and haemorrhage. Pain is very moderate and usually temporary; infection should not occur with disposable needles and syringes, and puncture of the bowel has occurred but does not appear to matter with so small a needle.

Marrow puncture

Marrow puncture is considered safer but not nearly so accurate (Plate II.4). It is a more painful procedure than splenic puncture and is resented by many patients.

Liver puncture

This produces as good results as splenic puncture but is more dangerous and not suitable for field work.

Lymph gland puncture

This is much less accurate and depends on the presence of lymphadenopathy. Many palpable glands in the groin are unsuitable for examination.

Blood

Examination of the peripheral blood for parasites is not a diagnostic procedure although amastigotes have been demonstrated on direct blood smears both in India and East Africa. Parasitaemia was demonstrated by various methods in 15/20 kala-azar patients in Kenya.[61]

Culture media (Appendix III, p. 1321)

A good culture medium for growing *L. donovani* is Schneider's insect medium[69] but NNN medium overlayed with Schneider's medium is even better.

Hamster inoculation (Appendix III, p. 1321)

Diagnosis can be made in the absence of parasitological proof by inoculating very small quantities of material obtained from the spleen, liver, lymph gland, blood or skin. There is a delay of six months until the hamster is killed and subinoculation of a new hamster from a negative hamster has shown amastigotes after the second inoculation.

Immunodiagnosis

Diagnosis can be made in the absence of parasitological proof by the demonstration of dysproteinaemia and serologically by immunofluorescence (indirect fluorescent antibody test—IFAT), enzyme-linked immunosorbent assay (ELISA), complement fixation (CFT) and counter immunoelectrophoresis (CIEP).

Dysproteinaemia

There is a reversal of the A/G ratio with a rise in the IgG (polyclonal) up to 2.0 g/dl (Fig. 4.7). The rise is in the first six months reverting to normal within six months of cure although some dysproteinaemia was still present 10 years after infection.[71] This dysproteinaemia is responsible for the *formol gel* test which has proved useful in field diagnosis. It is relatively non-specific being positive in any condition in which the IgG or IgM is raised, such as macroglobulinaemia, multiple myeloma, and to a lesser extent in Africa, African trypanosomiasis, malaria, leprosy, hepatosplenic schistosomiasis and tropical splenomegaly.

About 5 ml of blood is drawn from a vein and allowed to clot. The supernatant serum is separated and one drop of commercial formalin (30% formaldehyde) is added to 1 ml of serum, shaken and allowed to stand. A positive result is shown by solidification with a dense white clot, like the white of a hard-boiled egg, within 20 minutes. Jellification alone is not a positive result.

Serological diagnosis

The IFAT and ELISA tests are the tests of choice but CFT and CIEP are also available.

INDIRECT FLUORESCENT ANTIBODY TEST (IFAT)
This has been the test of choice but may be superseded by the ELISA. The IFAT is the most sensitive and is group specific. An amastigote antigen is preferable to avoid cross reactions with trypanosomiasis and amastigotes of *L. enriettii* obtained from cultures of promastigotes by raising the temperature are best. Titres of 1/20 or over are significant and 1/128 diagnostic.[72] A few non-specific positive results may be found in malaria, typhoid and larva migrans. Antibodies appear early and last until six months after cure; their presence is very useful in monitoring the effect of treatment and demonstrating recrudescences and relapses.

ENZYME-LINKED IMMUNOSORBENT ASSAY (ELISA)
An ELISA test has been developed[73] which is highly sensitive and more specific than the IFAT and is the test of choice in most cases, especially where large numbers of tests are being done in field conditions on epidemiological surveys. It can be done by using the blotting paper method for collecting blood. The antigen is prepared from ultra-sonicated promastigotes of *L. donovani* and has been found to have a sensitivity of 98.4% and specificity of 100%.[74] It can be included in the routine laboratory in a district hospital.[75] ELISA antibodies persist for a long time after cure and are of no use as a test of cure.

COMPLEMENT FIXATION TEST (CFT)
This has now been largely superseded by the above tests. The antigen is prepared from Kedrowsky's acid-fast bacillus or *Leishmania*.[76] Titres of 1/10 or over are significant. Cross reactions occur with Chagas' disease, some cases of tuberculosis and leprosy. Antibodies appear in the first three months and disappear within six months of cure.

COUNTER IMMUNOELECTROPHORESIS (CIEP)
This test has proved useful being positive in 80% of early and 100% of later cases of kala-azar.[40]

Leishmanin test

The leishmanin test is of no use in the diagnosis of active kala-azar. It becomes positive six to eight weeks after recovery and remains positive for life. Positive reactions can develop spontaneously in endemic areas and are the result of subclinical infections. Such positive reactors are immune to attacks of overt disease. Leishmanin skin testing on an age and residence basis can establish the pattern of present and past infection, and the presence of macro- and microfoci leading to a knowledge of the epidemiology in that area (see section on epidemiology, below) (Fig. 4.11).

TREATMENT

General

Specific treatment with pentavalent antimonials should be started as soon as the diagnosis is established by the demonstration of the parasite, though in the absence of facilities for demonstrating the parasites it may be necessary to start treatment on clinical grounds alone. There are no contraindications to starting treatment; in general the more severe the illness and the more moribund the patient the greater the danger of delay. Severe anaemia may require transfusion but arrangements for this should not delay treatment, neither should the presence of complicating infections such as tuberculosis and malaria which should be treated synchronously. Pregnancy is not a contraindication to the prompt initiation of treatment. There are no reports of adverse effects on the fetus by pentavalent antimonials and the risks of progressive deterioration of the mother and of congenital transmission are avoided. As pentavalent antimonials are normally cleared rapidly in the urine the presence of renal failure will require observation for signs of toxicity, possible reduction of dosage and the use of shorter courses.

Apart from a good diet little supplementary treatment to the pentavalent antimonials is needed. The anaemia generally responds to successful antileishmanial treatment alone so that routine haematinics, vitamin preparations and antimalarials are not needed in the absence of specific indications. It may sometimes be necessary to transfuse the very anaemic patient at the commencement of treatment whilst awaiting the normal favourable response of the haemoglobin level, usually evident within a week or so of starting treatment.

Pentavalent antimonials (Sb^V) (see also Section XVII)

First used in the treatment of kala-azar in 1916 they remain the treatment of choice. Sodium antimony gluconate (Pentostam) and meglumine antimonate (Glucantime) are the main preparations used.

Pentostam is issued in multidose bottles in a sterile isotonic neutral solution in water so that 1 ml contains 100 mg antimony. It can be given by intramuscular or slow intravenous injection. There is usually a dull, aching pain at the site of intramuscular injection that persists for 2 or 3 hours. The standard daily dose for an adult is 6 ml (600 mg Sb^V). Dosage should probably be related more to renal function than to size so that small children may be given and need up to 20 mg Sb^V/kg (2 ml, 200 mg Sb^V, for a small child of 10 kg) whereas infections in adults usually respond to 10 mg Sb^V/kg with a normal top dose of 6 ml, though in some areas up to 9 ml is given. Both the dose used and the duration of the course vary from country to country depending on the sensitivity of the local parasite. In India a 10-day course has usually been sufficient though 30-day courses may now be necessary.[77] In China[78] where sodium stibogluconate is called *stiheike* a course consists of nine injections on alternate days or daily for six days. Elsewhere the usual course of treatment is 30 days.[79]

In Kenya it has been observed[80] that 20 mg Sb^V/kg was more effective than 10 mg Sb^V/kg, and recommendations (Table 4.1) based on 543 mg Sb^V/m^2 (400 mg Sb^V in a 20 kg child) have been made. One in six patients showed parasites after one course. Relapse rates varied from 10% to 30% in Kenya[81] where most patients who failed to respond were children under 30 kg. If parasites are still present at 30 days, treatment may be continued up to 60 days or even longer, or the amount of Sb^V given may be doubled by giving the injections 12-hourly. Antimony resistance is much less likely to occur if the injections are given 12-hourly. With higher doses than those shown in Table 4.1 side-effects may be seen.

Glucantime is much used in South America.

Table 4.1 Current recommended Pentostam dosage in Kenya.

Weight of patient (kg)	Age of patient	Daily dose of Pentostam (ml)
70	Large adult	9
60	Medium adult	8
50	18–20 years	7
40	15–17 years	6
30	11–14 years	5
20	5–10 years	4
10	2–4 years	2.5
10	2 years	2.0

The effective dose of Sb^V given is similar to that of Pentostam.

Urea stibamine is a compound of urea with ethyl stibamine (Neostibosan) used in unresponsive infections.

Alternatives to pentavalent antimonials

Although pentavalent antimonials remain the drugs of choice several other drugs may be used in infections unresponsive to Sb^V.

Diamidines

Hydroxystilbamidine was a most effective drug but is no longer marketed. Pentamidine is less effective; although the initial cure rate may be high relapses are common and side-effects include both immediate and irreversible hypoglycaemia, as well as pancreatic damage and insulin-dependent diabetes. It has been recommended[82] as 2–4 mg/kg weekly or at most thrice weekly by intramuscular or slow intravenous injection for as long as is necessary to effect a cure, often many months. Diminazene aceturate (Berenil) may be useful but the efficacy and dosage have not been fully evaluated.

Allopurinol

Allopurinol prevents the growth and division of amastigotes of *Leishmania* in culture. The active metabolite is currently under development but not yet released for clinical use. Allopurinol has been used in the treatment of antimony-resistant infections.[36] It is given orally in a dose of 16–24 mg/kg daily in three divided doses and is continued for 10 weeks although toxic effects may limit the duration.

Amphotericin B

Amphotericin B is effective but its use is limited by toxicity. A total dose of 2.0 g may be given over several weeks.

Response to treatment

Symptomatic improvement is noted within a day or so of starting treatment and certainly within a week, by which time a haematological improvement will also usually be measurable. The clearance of parasites from the spleen may be monitored by weekly splenic aspirates. The parasites may not be cleared for two or three weeks despite an early and brisk clinical and haematological improvement. Very large spleens may take several months to reduce to normal size (see section on post-kala-azar splenomegaly, below) but small spleens may become impalpable within a month of starting treatment. The haematological response may not be complete for four to six weeks. Complicating illnesses, such as pulmonary tuberculosis, should be looked for in all patients but especially if the response to treatment is delayed.

Test of cure

The test of cure is commonly defined as the absence of parasites from two successive splenic aspirates taken one week apart. Treatment can then be discontinued. Serological reactions and immunoglobulin levels revert to normal over a period of six months or so. Short-term clinical relapses (recrudescences) occur within the first six months particularly when clearance of the parasites has failed. Longer-term relapses with an interval of apparently completely normal health are unlikely to occur after two years, though episodes of PKDL may present many years later, particularly in India.

Splenectomy

Splenectomy in kala-azar has been reviewed by Rees et al.[81] Inappropriate splenectomy in kala-azar as a result of misdiagnosis continues to occur. Following splenectomy the haematological values rapidly improve with a leukocytosis up to 30 000/mm^3 or more and a thrombocytosis as a result of the removal of the effect of hypersplenism. Historically such operations have sometimes resulted in cures and splenectomy is still used very occasionally in an attempt to effect a cure in drug-resistant kala-azar. Indications for splenectomy are a huge disabling mass of spleen in a child, failure to respond to a course of antimony at full dosage (20 mg/kg/day) for at least 60 days, and no response to allopurinol. The dangers of splenectomy are great: post-splenectomy septicaemia, subsequent development of a lymphoma and loss of immunity to malaria and other infections (e.g. babesiosis). Pneumococcal vaccination may be given but is relatively ineffective after splenectomy so that it should not be relied upon alone. Penicillin prophylaxis should be maintained for three years after surgery and malaria prophylaxis continued for life if the patient resides in an endemic area.

Deaths during treatment

Deaths during treatment are uncommon. They may be due to the relentless course of the kala-azar unchecked by chemotherapy, but this is rare. Unrecognized complications such as typhoid and other septicaemias, pneumonias and tuberculosis may be important. Relatively sudden and unexplained deaths sometimes occur around the second week of treatment. They do not appear to be due to drug toxicity but perhaps are due to a phenomenon akin to the Jarisch–Herxheimer reaction. Patients should be observed carefully throughout treatment but especially at this time. Pentavalent antimonials should be stopped at the first indication of an untoward event and investigations and symptomatic treatment appropriate to the circumstances commenced. Sb^V can be restarted safely once the situation has resolved. Aspirin and other drugs containing acetylsalicylic acid should never be used in kala-azar for fear of precipitating a fatal haemorrhage. There is generally no need to treat the fever of kala-azar, indeed, a high fever may be beneficial, for amastigotes do not survive in vitro at temperatures over 40°C.

Antimony resistance

Antimony resistance may be primary from the beginning or secondary as a result of treatment. Up to 20% of cases of kala-azar may relapse on treatment with too low a dosage. Primary resistance is very rare. Secondary resistance develops during treatment following too low a dose schedule and then does not always respond satisfactorily to higher doses. It can be eliminated almost entirely by adequate dosage from the start.

Relapses

Relapse is rare if the disease is treated correctly from the start. Relapses may occur up to two years following treatment. They can be detected early by antibody titres failing to fall to negative or starting to rise.

COMPLICATIONS

The complications of kala-azar result from immunosuppression, an altered immune response developing during treatment and the effects of treatment.

Immunosuppression allows the development of pulmonary tuberculosis, a common secondary infection, which produces resistance to treatment and must be treated concurrently with the leishmaniasis. Bacterial infections such as lobar pneumonia, bacterial dysentery, measles and other infections are common causes of death in advanced cases. The altered immune response which develops during treatment results in PKDL and eye lesions, iritis and choroiditis. Sodium stibogluconate injection intravenously may result in a troublesome thrombophlebitis.

Pulmonary tuberculosis

Pulmonary tuberculosis is a common complication of untreated kala-azar. If a case of kala-azar does not respond to antimony treatment concomitant pulmonary tuberculosis should be suspected.

Cancrum oris

Cancrum oris develops in late cases of kala-azar when there is severe granulopenia. It must be distinguished from mucosal lesions and will not heal until the kala-azar has been treated successfully.

Cirrhosis of the liver

About 10% of cases of kala-azar show mild cirrhotic changes in the liver after treatment. One of the causes of persistent splenomegaly in spite of antimony treatment is portal hypertension caused by cirrhosis.

Renal amyloidosis

Renal amyloidosis presenting as the nephrotic syndrome, as well as amyloidosis of liver and spleen, can occur and resolves completely with antimony treatment.

Post-kala-azar splenomegaly

In cases where the spleen has been very large, it may not return to normal following successful treatment and in endemic areas post-kala-azar splenomegaly must be considered in the diagnosis of splenomegaly of unknown origin.

POST-KALA-AZAR DERMAL LEISHMANOID (PKDL)

This is a cutaneous form of leishmaniasis usually, but not always, following an overt attack of kala-azar.

GEOGRAPHICAL DISTRIBUTION

PKDL only occurs in endemic areas of kala-azar but not in all. It is common in India where it occurs in 20% of cases of kala-azar and less common in East Africa where 2% only show this complication. It is rare in China and unknown in the Mediterranean and Central and South America. The reasons for this distribution are unknown.

AETIOLOGY

PKDL is caused by *Leishmania* of the same zymodeme of *L. donovani* which causes kala-azar in that area. Although it usually follows an overt attack of kala-azar sometimes it appears de novo and is probably the result of an inapparent infection. In Bihar PKDL occurred in areas where transmission was continuing but not in areas where vector control had been achieved, suggesting that reinfection was necessary to cause PKDL.[83]

PATHOLOGY

The pathogenesis of PKDL is related to the immune reaction of the host. Similar skin eruptions are found during the course of kala-azar but disappear with treatment. In the majority of cases of PKDL the *Leishmania* can only be found in the skin, being absent from the viscera. In the skin they elicit a spectrum of cellular response from a tuberculoid reaction with few parasites at one end to anergic reaction at the other with many parasites and little cellular response at the other (cf. Cutaneous leishmaniasis, Chapter 37). Histologically the epithelium is thin and the sub-papillary layer oedematous, beneath which is a granulomatous mass containing macrophages with a varying number of parasites. There is an xanthomatous form with raised orange coloured

plaques which do not ulcerate.

IMMUNITY

The presence of *Leishmania* in the skin elicits a spectrum of cell-mediated response. In overt untreated kala-azar parasites can be found throughout the skin where they cause little or no cellular reaction (p. 94). With recovery of immunity which is depressed in kala-azar these parasites will elicit a response, which may be weak or strong. The degree of response can be measured by the leishmanin test which may be negative or positive (but never strongly positive). There can be a change in polarity. PKDL can appear with recovery after treatment only to disappear with relapse and to reappear again when final recovery occurs.

CLINICAL FEATURES

Natural history

PKDL occurs as a sequence to kala-azar and over 50% of the cases in India follow an attack, usually two but sometimes more than ten years previously. In quite a large proportion no previous attack of kala-azar has been recognized. In Africa the interval is much shorter and the rash appears towards the end of treatment and fades rapidly. Once established the rash may last a long time in India—up to 20 years or more.[84] The longer kala-azar has been endemic in an area the more frequent is PKDL and PKDL may be an important reservoir of *L. (L) donovani* and a source of the epidemics which can occur every 10–15 years.

Incubation period

In India this is usually two years or more, in Africa much less, from nought to nine months.

Symptoms and signs

The rash of PKDL consists of two stages: a depigmented and a nodular stage. The depigmented stage, which appears first, starts as colourless patches on the face and upper extremities where it is most marked, gradually

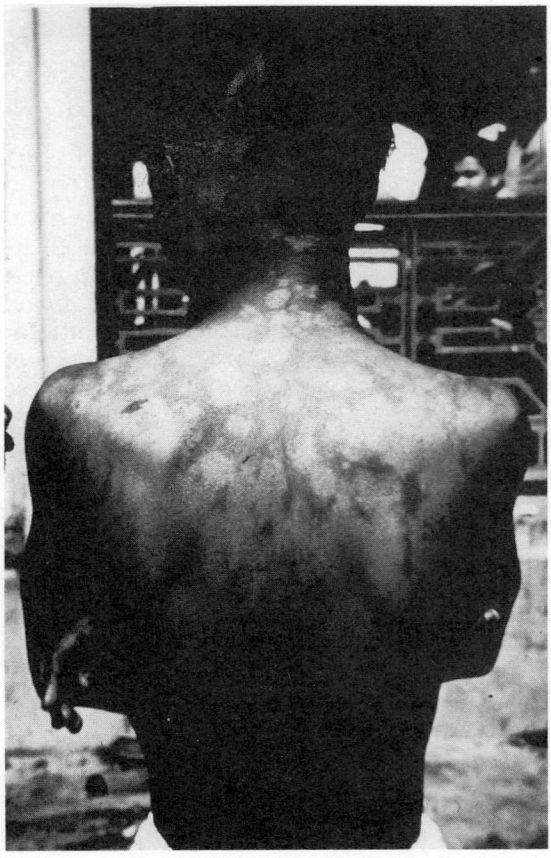

Fig. 4.9. Post-kala-azar dermal leishmanoid depigmented macular stage.

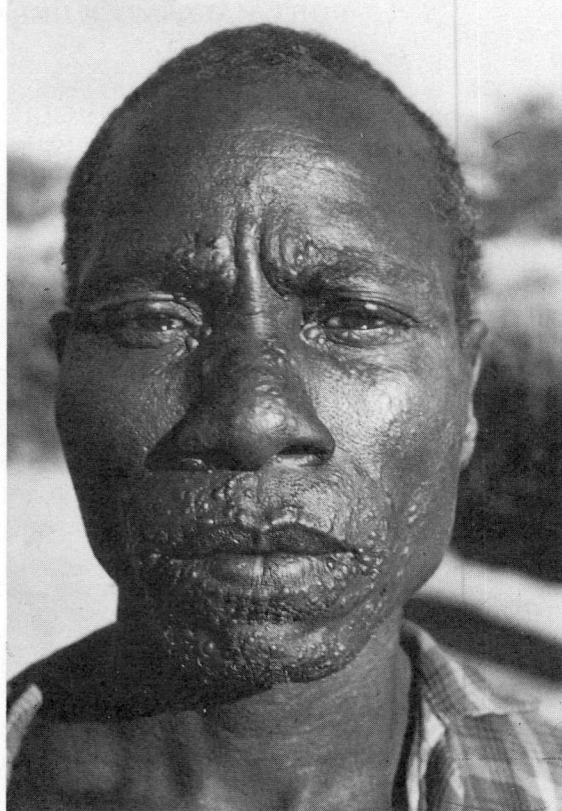

Fig. 4.10. Post-kala-azar dermal leishmanoid nodular stage.

spreading to the remainder of the body (Fig. 4.9). Minute dots gradually enlarge to irregular areas 1.25 cm in diameter which occasionally break down. The nodular stage appears later and replaces the depigmented patches. The nodules may extend to the mucous membranes and ear where they closely resemble lepromatous leprosy (Fig. 4.10).

DIFFERENTIAL DIAGNOSIS

The major differential diagnosis is from lepromatous leprosy in which acid-fast bacilli are numerous in skin smears and there is usually some evidence of nerve involvement (never in PKDL). Other conditions which can be confused are diffuse cutaneous leishmaniasis (different geographical distribution), keloids, fungus infections of the skin, leukoderma, syphilis and yaws.

DIAGNOSIS

Skin smears should be examined for amastigotes but these are usually so scanty as to be undetectable. The leishmanin test may be negative but if positive is evidence that there has been a previous attack of kala-azar, whether overt or inapparent. Serological reactions (immunofluorescence) are positive as in kala-azar even in the absence of any visceral infection. Serum proteins are normal and the formol gel test negative.

TREATMENT

The treatment is the same as for kala-azar and PKDL responds well to treatment with pentavalent antimony. When it occurs after an attack of kala-azar then a further course of antimony is required.

GEOGRAPHICAL VARIATIONS OF KALA-AZAR

Kala-azar is remarkably similar in its clinical features in all parts of the world. Minor variations are found in the frequency of PKDL (apparently absent in the Mediterranean possibly because it is a feature of *L. (L.) donovani* and not *L. (L.) infantum* infection), the presence of mucosal lesions (Africa and India), and the response to antimony treatment (some resistance to antimony is found in all areas).

EPIDEMIOLOGY AND CONTROL (see also Appendix I, p. 1305, and Table III.3, p. 1400)

Kala-azar caused by *L. (L.) infantum* and *L. (L.) chagasi* is a zoonosis with a main reservoir in dogs and wild canids found in a variety of ecosystems in a number of different habitats varying from the semiarid areas of sub-Saharan Africa to the more humid environment of Amazonia. The existence of a rodent reservoir in the Sudan is still not clear for although the parasites from rodents there were the same as those causing human disease it is not known how important these infections are epidemiologically.

Kala-azar caused by *L. (L.) donovani* is a human disease found in the crowded river valleys of eastern India and the relatively highly populated scrublands of eastern Kenya. The disease often surfaces unexpectedly as sporadic cases; changing environment and migration of peoples can cause epidemics of a disastrous nature. The reasons for this will appear in a more detailed study of the epidemiology in the various areas where kala-azar is found.

Historically the *Leishmania* causing kala-azar may be a rodent parasite which has become adapted to canids and then to man. In primary foci the parasite may circulate in rodents while secondary foci develop in canids and man. Throughout most of its geographical distribution the parasite infects man only as a dead end and maintains itself in wild and domestic canids. In India and East Africa, however, man is the only host and in the Sudan and East Africa extensive interhuman transmission takes place under epidemic conditions. In Italy observations suggest that subclinical infections in man are common and are important in the spread of kala-azar in an epidemic manner[18] and PKDL cases may provide a long-term reservoir in between epidemics.

Reservoir hosts

Canids

DOGS

The dog is the traditional zoonotic host in the Mediterranean area since it forms an excellent peridomestic reservoir developing in many cases an overt infection with a heavily parasitized skin. The parasite, which has been called *L. canis*, has been shown to be identical with *L. (L.) infantum*.[85] In Senegal a similar infection is common in dogs and the parasite has been shown to be *L. (L.) infantum*.[86] In many areas the extent of infection in dogs is more extensive in area than infection in humans, and in Senegal where canine infection is widespread human disease is absent, although isolated cases have been reported from neighbouring Gambia.[87] The significance of an isolation from a dog in Kenya[88] is not clear. The dog becomes ill 18 months to two years after infection. The illness starts with loss of hair from the ears and round the eyes giving rise to a 'spectacle' effect. It develops lymphadenopathy and splenomegaly and the whole skin becomes depilated probably because of the heavy parasitization of the dermis from which anthropophilic sandflies (*P. ariasi* and *P. perniciosus*) feed avidly with a 100% infection rate.[89] Dogs infective for about two years after infection cannot be cured but live for a few years becoming more emaciated before they die. During this time they are excellent reservoirs of infection.

There is a wide spectrum of host response, some breeds of dog being relatively resistant and only susceptible as puppies, while others such as beagles and foxhounds develop fatal infections and can act as sentinel animals. In the Mediterranean dogs are in contact with foxes in many areas.

Wild canids

FOXES

In Europe *L. (L.) infantum* infection has been found in the European fox (*Vulpes vulpes*), in southern France[90] and Italy.[91] The infections are cryptic and have been demonstrated by the subinoculation technique. In central Asia *L. (L.) infantum* is found in *Vulpes pallidi*[92] and in Brazil *L. (L.) chagasi* in *Lycalopex vetulus*[93] and *Cer-*

docyon thous in the Amazon[94] play a significant role. In other areas the significance of infections in the fennec fox[95] in North Africa is unknown.

JACKALS

Infection in jackals has been demonstrated in southern Russia and northern Iran[96] where infection in dogs and jackals coexists. Infected jackals may or may not show an overt infection. Other carnivora which have been found infected are a serval and genet cat in the Sudan[97] probably by predation on rodents.

A raccoon-dog (*Nyctereutes procyonoides*) has been found in China, the only wild animal infection found there to date.[98]

RODENTS

Leishmania have been isolated by subinoculation techniques from cryptic visceral infections of many rodents from Africa and in Europe. Most of these are not *L. (L.) infantum* but *L. (L.) major*. This applies to isolations from Kenya, and Senegal where the *Leishmania* has been found to be identical with *L. (L.) major*.[85] *L. (L.) infantum* has been isolated from *Acomys albigenes*, *Arvicanthis niloticus* and *Rattus rattus* in the Sudan.[4]

Rattus rattus may be of some importance as the only rodent so far from which *L. (L.) infantum* has been isolated worldwide: Italy,[99] Yugoslavia,[100] Iraq[101] and Brazil.[102,103] The significance of these isolations as a reservoir of human infection is not clear.

L. (L.) infantum (Fig. 4.3)

L. (L) infantum is the cause of Mediterranean kala-azar which spreads from the West along both shores of the Mediterranean and North Africa to Iran, the southern USSR and China. The main features are a zoonotic reservoir with an urban or periurban (dogs) or a rural (foxes, jackals) distribution. It is endemic, occurs sporadically and affects mainly infants, hence the name 'infantum'.

European Mediterranean (Portugal, southern Spain, southern France, Sicily, Italy, Sardinia)

The urban disease is endemic and sporadic affecting mainly infants (ponos or infantile kala-azar). It is seasonal, appearing in April but rare after November. If a child is born in October the signs of disease may be observed the following August. The reservoir is the domestic dog and the vector *P. perniciosus*. The incidence has greatly decreased in the old endemic areas of Sicily, southern Italy and Malta since malarial eradication almost eliminated *P. perniciosus*, which is a domestic or peridomestic species (Fig. III.16D, p. 1396).

The rural form occurs sporadically especially in southern France and Italy where the reservoir is the fox (*Vulpes vulpes*). The vector in France is *P. ariasi* and possibly *P. perfiliewi* in Italy.[99]

The disease is found mainly in adults and infection occurs outside the home although it can be introduced to a family from hunting dogs. Small epidemics may occur as in Italy under exceptional circumstances where many subclinical human infections can maintain the disease.[15]

North Africa

The disease is urban but rare although common in dogs. It is found in Morocco (vector *P. longicuspis*), Algeria, Tunisia and Libya (vector *P. perniciosus*) and Egypt (vector unknown)[104] where the causative *Leishmania* resembles *L. (L) major*.[105]

Eastern Mediterranean and Balkans

The disease is sporadic and urban with the reservoir in dogs. The vectors are *P. major* (Yugoslavia, Greece, Crete, Turkey, Syria, Lebanon and Israel), *P. tobbi* (Yugoslavia, Cyprus, Syria and Lebanon), *P. perfiliewi* (Yugoslavia and Rumania), *P. chinensis kyreniae* (Cyprus) and possibly *P. simici* (Yugoslavia).

Middle East

IRAN AND IRAQ

In the past the urban disease was quite common in the big cities, Teheran and Baghdad; it was urban with a dog reservoir and infants mainly affected. Now it is mainly rural with a wild canine reservoir (foxes in the north and jackals in the south). The vectors are *P. major* and *P. chinensis hupensis*. The disease in the south-western Arabian peninsula (Arabia, Southern Yemen, Aden) forms part of the Afrotropical area.

Southern USSR and Azerbaijan

The urban type of VL (dog reservoir) has disappeared from Tashkent and other cities. Two foci remain: Kzyl-Orda in Kazakhstan (Kazakh focus) and Dzhalilabad in Azerbaijan. VL is sporadic and rural, being found in areas undergoing agricultural development. The zoonotic reservoirs are the fox and jackal and the vectors: *P. caucasicus, P. chinensis, P. kandelakii, P. perfiliewei* and in the Kazakh focus: *P. smirnovi* and *P. longiductus*.[106]

East Asia and China (Fig. 4.3)

Small foci of kala-azar are found in Himalayan valleys in northern Pakistan but little is known of their epidemiology. In China where the disease has been known to occur for a long time the main endemic area is in north-east China where there appear to be two different types. In the western part kala-azar is of the classical *L. (L.) infantum* type with much canine leishmaniasis and mainly infants affected. It is thought that this represents the spread of the disease in ancient times from the West in caravans. In the eastern area there is little if any canine disease and the disease affects older patients, suggesting the recent importation of *L. (L.) donovani* by sea.[107] The vectors are *P. chinensis chinensis, P. major (wui)* and *P. alexandriae*.

Since 1958 the incidence of kala-azar has greatly decreased[78] and now the main area of kala-azar is in foci in the far west Sinkiang province where there may be a wild zoonotic reservoir, the raccoon-dog (*Nyctereutes procyonoides*) and *P. major* may be a vector.[98]

African kala-azar

Kala-azar is found in sub-Saharan Africa from the west eastwards to the Indian ocean and to the south-western tip of the Arabian peninsula which is in the Afrotropical zone. The two main endemic areas are the Sudan and East Africa.

West Africa

Here the infection is rare and sporadic and cases have come from the Hoggar,[108] Burkina Faso (Upper Volta),[109] Republic of the Congo,[110] Zaire,[111] Togo and Zambia.[112] The disease is unknown in Senegal although canine leishmaniasis is common but cases have been found in neighbouring Gambia[87] where dogs have also been found infected. In West Africa the disease appears to be of the Mediterranean type and the probable vector is *P. dubosqui*, a known vector of *L. (L.) major*.

Sudan

The parasite causing kala-azar in the Sudan and East Africa has been given subspecific status *L. (L.) archibaldi*[113] but biochemical studies do not bear this out completely and the position of the Sudanese parasites is as yet not clear. The distribution of the Sudanese disease is coincident with that of the vector *P. orientalis*, which is found from Lake Tchad in the west to the south-west corner of the Arabian peninsula. Kala-azar has been found in Lake Tchad[114] from where it extends eastwards sporadically until it becomes endemic on the flood plain of the White Nile in the south and along the Blue Nile in the north-east to the lowlands of Ethiopia (Setit Humera district and Eritrea[115]). In south-west Ethiopia and across the Red Sea in the foothills of Southern Yemen and south-west Arabia, which lie in the Afrotropical zone, the parasite is not identical to that found in the Sudan although *P. orientalis* is the vector in south-west Ethiopia and is found in the Yemen. Kala-azar affects nomad and semi-nomads who set up temporary villages on the Nile flood plain in the dry season near patches of acacia–balanites scrub which harbours the vector *P. orientalis*. Sporadic cases have the appearance of a zoonosis and *L. (L.) infantum* has been isolated from rodents (*Rattus rattus, Arvicanthis niloticus* and *Acomys albigenes*) (see p. 108). Dogs are not involved but interhuman transmission takes place causing large epidemics which occurred in the 1950s in the south when adults and all ages were affected.

East Africa

The parasite causing kala-azar in East Africa has been identified as *L. (L.) donovani*.[116] Distribution of the disease is in the main that of the vector *P. martini* from Kapoeta on the Sudan border in the west and Karamoja district in Uganda across the Northern Frontier province of Kenya to the Uebi Shebelli river in Somalia, and south to the Rift valley, the Tana river and Machakos districts in eastern Kenya. Here kala-azar is found in association with eroded termite hills (termite hill kala-azar) in microfoci[117] (Fig. III.16C, p. 1396) where *P. martini* and related species have been found to occur and from which *L. (L.) donovani* has been isolated.[30,118] Rodents do not appear to be involved and to date only one infected dog has been found,[88] the significance of which is not clear. The disease is sporadic in the northern areas but assumes epidemic proportions in areas newly occupied for agricultural settlement. Interhuman transmission occurs with epidemics lasting 10 years and 15 year intervals. The infection could be maintained in the absence of any animal reservoir in view of the great number of subclinical infections occurring (see section on subclinical infection, p. 98). During epidemics all ages may be affected but with increasing endemicity the age drops and the age group 6–14 (like India) is mainly involved.

Indian kala-azar (*L. (L.) donovani*)

Indian kala-azar has only one known reservoir which is man; efforts to find a zoonotic reservoir have so far failed[118] although leishmanial antibodies were found in the rodent *Bandicota bengalensis*. The proven vector *P. argentipes*[26] feeds solely on man and has a distribution corresponding to the disease. Although it is found in Malaya it does not bite man there and there is no kala-azar.

Indian kala-azar was highly endemic in Bengal, Bihar, Uttar Pradesh and Assam with some cases in Cape Comorin, Madras and Sri Lanka. From the end of the nineteenth century large epidemics swept these areas causing depopulation. Epidemics would occur every 15 years lasting 10 years. The last big epidemic ended in 1924 and kala-azar was reduced to a rarity following residual spraying for malaria eradication. Following cessation of the malaria campaign *P. argentipes* returned in its old numbers and since 1977 kala-azar has returned to West Bengal and Bihar and a large number of cases amounting to an epidemic have occurred. In the past kala-azar advanced slowly along the Brahmaputra valley at the rate of 160 km over seven years. Its introduction to a village could usually be traced to some individual from an infected locality. Generally, it clung to a place for six years. Houses seemed to form a 'microfocus', it was a 'house' disease and it was considered dangerous to reoccupy a house for a year. Four males are infected to one female and the age group most affected is 10–20 years.

American kala-azar (*L. (L.) chagasi*)

Kala-azar was first discovered in South America

in Paraguay in 1913 and was subsequently found to be quite common in Brazil following use of the viscerotome for the study of yellow fever. The causative agent *L. (L.) chagasi* is regarded by some as *L. (L.) infantum* introduced from Portugal and Spain, since *Lutzomyia longipalpis* (the vector) can be readily infected with Mediterranean strains of *L. (L.) infantum*,[120] but others believe *L. (L.) chagasi* to be a subspecies with minor biochemical differences indigenous to the New World, where more than one parasite may be involved.

Identified foci of infection are located in mountain regions at an altitude not usually more than 800 metres. Valleys alternate with mountain spurs and the climate is dry or only moderately humid. Kala-azar has been recorded from almost every country in South and Central America, Argentina, Brazil, Colombia, Ecuador, Guatemala, Mexico, El Salvador, French Guyana, Honduras, Surinam, Paraguay, Venezuela and the island of Guadeloupe. Incidence is greatest in the rural areas and the outskirts of some cities. The main focus is in north-east Brazil in Ceará and Bahia where it has occurred at times in an epidemic manner. The epidemiology is domestic and peridomestic involving man, dog and the sandfly *Lu. longipalpis*. The savannah fox (*Lycalopex vetulus*) is also infected but suffers severely from the infection, which does not suggest an indigenous reservoir.[49] Children mainly affected are of an age group higher than that in the Mediterranean and epidemics occur.

In the more humid Amazon region cases of kala-azar are rare but foci of human infection, infected dogs and *Lu. longipalpis* have been found and inapparent infections of a fox *Cerdocyon thous* have been found in Pará state, Amazonia, suggesting that this is the true reservoir host and that kala-azar in the Ceará Pará focus in north-east Brazil may have originally spread from this area.[121]

PREVENTION AND CONTROL

Before any methods of control can be considered an epidemiological survey must be conducted. This consists of case-finding, leishmanin skin-testing, search for reservoir hosts and vector studies.

1 Case-finding

Case-finding includes a search for overt cases of kala-azar by spleen puncture and serology

(ELISA test) to detect recent infections which may or may not become overt.

2 Leishmanin skin-testing

Leishmanin skin-testing will show past infection by age positivity studies, present infection by the rate of natural conversion and the site of infection by area studies (micro- and macrofoci). Three patterns of infection may emerge (Fig. 4.11): endemic with an increase in positivity with age, epidemic with all age groups equally affected and interrupted transmission with a sudden bulge in the later age positivity rate.

the reservoir, control of the vector, breaking the man–sandfly contact and immunization.

Control of the reservoir

As has been seen the human reservoir is important especially in an epidemic situation. Case-finding and treatment form the major components of any control scheme but because of the effect of the many inapparent infections may not succeed. In India and East Africa, however, case-finding and treatment have had a favourable effect.

Control of the canine reservoir by examining

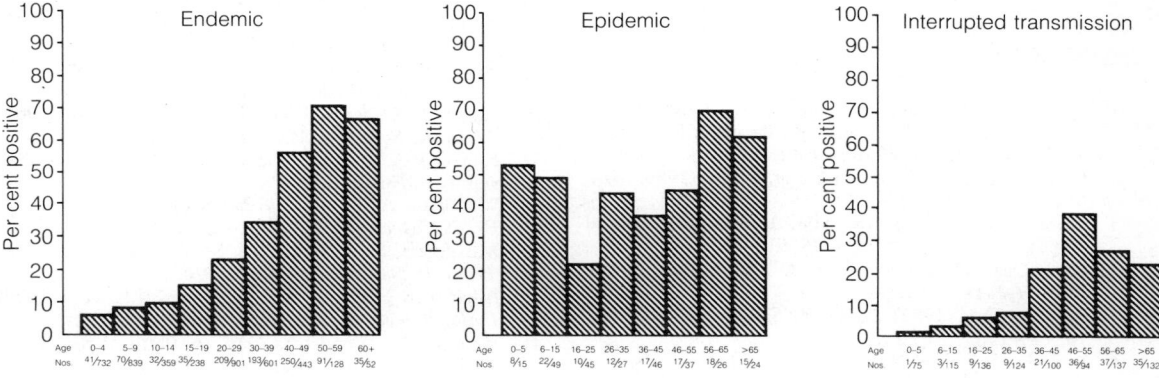

Fig. 4.11. Leishmanin positivity according to age showing three different epidemiological patterns.

3 Reservoir hosts

The importance of the human reservoir may be assessed by the rate of leishmanin conversion since apparent infections outnumber active ones by 97% to 3%. Rodent and canine reservoirs may be identified by spleen and gland smears, culture and hamster subinoculation for inapparent infections.

4 Vector studies

These involve the collection of sandflies for a long period of time since certain species may only appear at certain times of the year. Flies should be dissected for the source of blood meals and the presence of flagellates which are extremely rare (see Appendix III, p. 1403).

Control

Control may be achieved in four ways: control of

dogs with spleen and gland smears and culture, with treatment or destruction of infected dogs has been successful both in the Mediterranean and Brazil.

Vector control and breaking man–sandfly contact (Appendix III, p. 1403)

Vector control and breaking the man–sandfly contact can be done if the vector is endophilic, as in India. Cleaning up the environment around dwellings and burning houses known to be local microfoci were successful before the days of insecticides. Residual spraying of houses for malaria eradication almost completely eradicated kala-azar from India but, since this has stopped, the disease has returned. House-spraying should be repeated at six-monthly intervals. Where the vector is exophilic, as in East Africa, breaking the man–sandfly contact by siting houses away from known living and breeding places has had some success. Personal prophylaxis consists in wearing suitable clothing at sundown, sleeping off the ground and avoiding known areas of sandfly contact.

Immunization (Appendix I, p. 1303)

Since an attack of overt kala-azar as well as an inapparent infection leads to a permanent immunity a vaccine from a strain of *L. (L.) donovani* which remained limited to the skin would give good protection, but this has not yet been found, and one *Leishmania* isolated from a rodent which was tested in a field trial in East Africa[28] was later found to be *L. (L.) major* and gave no protection in the field.

REFERENCES

1 Lainson, R. & Shaw, J.J. (1986) In *The Leishmaniases in Biology and Medicine*, eds. W. Peters & R. Killick-Kendrick, Vol. 1. London: Academic Press.

2 Rioux, J.A., Lanotte, G., Pratlong, F. et al (1985) *Méd. Malad. infect.* **11**, 650–656.

3 Belazzoug, S., Ammar-Khodja, A., Belkaid, M. et al (1985) *Bull. Soc. Path. éxot.* **78**, 615–622.

4 Hoogstraal, H. & Heyneman, D. (1969) *Am. J trop. Med. Hyg.* **18**, 1091.

5 Bradley, D.J. (1982) *Trans. R. Soc. trop. Med. Hyg.* **76**, 143–146.

6 Bradley, D.J. & Kirkley, J. (1977) *Clin. exp. Immun.* **30**, 119–129.

7 Guirges, S. Y. (1971) *Ann. Trop. Med. Parasit.* **65**, 197.

8 Lainson, R. & Shaw, J.J. (1977) *J. trop. Med. Hyg.* **80**, 29.

9 Bray, R.S. & Bryceson, A.D.M. (1968) *Lancet* **ii**, 998.

10 Ridley, D.S. (1980) *Trans. R. Soc. trop. Med. Hyg.* **74**, 515–521.

11 Bryceson, A.D.M. (1972) *Essays on Tropical Medicine*, ed. J. Marshall, pp. 230–241. Amsterdam: Excerpta Medica.

12 Pampiglione, S., Manson-Bahr, P.E.C. & Guingi, F. (1974) *Trans. R. Soc. trop. Med. Hyg.* **68**, 447.

13 Broeckaert-Van Orshoven, A., Micheilsen, P. & Vandepitte, J. (1979) *Lancet* **ii**, 740.

14 Bryceson, A.D.M. (1970) *Proc. R. Soc. Med.* **64**, 1056.

15 Pampiglione, S., La Place, M. & Schlick, G. (1974) *Trans. R. Soc. trop. Med. Hyg.* **68**, 349.

16 Adler, S. & Adler, J. (1955) *Bull. Res. Coun. Israel.* **4**, 396.

17 Montenegro, D. (1924) *Am. J. trop. Med.* **4**, 331.

18 Pampiglione, S., Manson-Bahr, P.E.C., La Placa, M. et al (1975) *Trans. R. Soc. trop. med. Hyg.* **69**, 60.

19 Shaw, J.J. & Lainson, R. (1975) *Trans. R. Soc. trop. Med. Hyg.* **69**, 323.

20 Furtado, T.A. & Pellegrino, J. (1956) *J. invest. Derm.* **27**, 53.

21 Southgate, B.A. & Oriedo, B.V.E. (1967) *J. trop. med. Hyg.* **70**, 1.

22 Dostrovsky, A. & Sagher, F. (1946) *Ann. trop. Med. Parasit.* **40**, 265.

23 Correa, C. (1941) *Archos Hig. Saúde públ.* **6**, 61.

24 Tremonti, L. & Walton, B.C. (1970) *Am. J. trop. Med. Hyg.* **19**, 49.

25 Thakur, C.P., Kumor, K. & Dathak, P.K. (1981) *J. trop. Med. Hyg.* **84**, 271–276.

26 Swaminath, C.S., Shortt, H.E. & Anderson, LA. (1942) *Indian J. med. Res.* **30**, 473.

27 Lowe, G.C. & Cooke, W.E. (1926) *Lancet* **ii**, 1209.

28 Manson-Bahr, P.E.C. (1959) *Trans. R. Soc. trop. Med. Hyg.* **53**, 123.

29 Pearson, R.D., de Alencar, J.E., Romito, R. et al (1983) *J. infect. Dis.* **147**, 1102.

30 Manson-Bahr, P.E.C., Southgate, B.A. & Harvey, A.E.C. (1963) *Br. Med. J.* **i**, 1208.

31 Ghose, A.C., Haldar, J.P., Pal, S.C. et al (1980) *Clin. exp. Immunol.* **40**, 318–326,

32 Sengal, S., Aikat, B.K. & Pathania, A.G.S. (1982) *Bull. Wld Hlth Org.* **60**, 945–949.

33 Brito, T., Hoshimo-Shimutzo, S., Amato Neto, V. et al (1975) *Am. J. trop. Med. Hyg.* **24**, 9.

34 Abdalla, S.H., Kasili, F.G. & Weatherall, D.J. (1983) *Trans. R. Soc. trop. Med. Hyg.* **77**, 99–102.

35 Koech, D.K., Lyerly, W.H. Jr & Ihaa, D.W. (1982) *East Afr. med. J.* **59**, 665–670.

36 Kager, P.A., Rees, P.H., Wellde, B.T., et al (1981) *Trans. R. Soc. trop. Med. Hyg.* **75**, 556–559.

37 Kager, P.A. & Rees, P.H. (1983) MD thesis, University of Amsterdam.

38 Woodruff, A.W., Topley, E., Knight, R. et al (1972) *Br. J. Haemat.* **27**, 319.

39 Musumeci, S., D'Agata, A., Sehiliro, G. et al (1976) *Trans. R. Soc. trop. Med. Hyg.* **70**, 500.

40 Aikat, B.K., Sehgal, R.C., Mahajan, R.C. et al (1979) *Indian J. med. Res.* **70**, 592.

41 Knight, R., Woodruff, A.W. & Pettit, L.E. (1967) *Trans. R. Soc. trop. Med. Hyg.* **61**, 701.

42 Swarup-Mitra, S., Choudhury, A.K.R. & Sarkar, M. (1979) *Ind. J. med. Res.* **69**, 571.

43 Abdalla, R.F., Hadl, A., Ahmed, M.A. et al (1975) *Trans. R. Soc. trop. Med. Hyg.* **69**, 433.

44 Naik, S.R., Vinayak, V.K., Taliwar, P. et al (1978) *Trans. R. Soc. trop. Med. Hyg.* **72**, 43.

45 Abdalla, R.F. (1982) *Ann. trop. Med. Parasit.* **76**, 299–307.

46 Duarte, M.I.S. & Corbett, C.E.P. (1984) *Trans. R. Soc. trop. Med. Hyg.* **78**, 683–688.

47 Duarte, M.I.S., Silva, M.R.R., Goto, H. et al (1983) *Trans. R. Soc. trop. Med. Hyg.* **77**, 531–537.

48 Muigai, R., Shaunak, S., Gatei, D.G. et al (1983) *Lancet* **ii**, 476–479.

49 Deane, L.M. (1956) *Leishmaniasis in Brazil: Study of Reservoirs in the State of Ceará, Rio de Janeiro*. Servicio Nacional de Educacao Sanitaria.

50 Kirk, R. (1942) *Trans. R. Soc. trop. Med. Hyg.* **35**, 257.

51 Sweeney, J.S., Friedlander, R.D. & Queen, F.B. (1945) *J. Am. med. Ass.* **128**, 14.

52 Jopling, W.H. (1955) *Br. med. J.* **iii**, 1013.

53 Wright, M.J. (1960) *Br. med. J.* **ii**, 1218.

54 Mirzoian, I. (1941) *Medskaya Parazit.* **10**, 101.

55 Kirk, R. (1938) *Trans. R. Soc. trop. Med. Hyg.* **32**, 271.

56 Shiliro, G., Russo, A., Musumeci, S. et al (1978) *Trans. R. Soc. trop. Med. Hyg.* **72**, 656.

57 Cahill, K.M. (1964) *Am. J. trop. Med. Hyg.* **13**, 794.

58 Cole, A.C.E. (1944) *Trans. R. Soc. trop. Med. Hyg.* **37**, 409–435.

59 Kager, P.A., Rees, P.H., Manguyu, F.M. et al (1983) *Trop. Geogr. Med.* **35**, 125–131.

60 Das Gupta, N.N., Guha, A. & De, N. (1954) *Exp. Cell Res.* **6**, 353.

61 Chulay, J.D., Adoyo, M.A. & Githure, J.I. (1985) *Trans. R. Soc. trop. Med. Hyg.* **79**, 218–222.

62 Southgate, B.A. & Manson-Bahr, P.E.C. (1967) *J. trop. Med. Hyg.* **70**, 29.

63 Francois, J., Limbo, P., Delaey, A. et al (1972) *Bull. Soc. Opthal.* **162**, 808.

64 Maru, M. (1979) *Am. J. trop. Med. Hyg.* **28**, 15–18.

65 Veress, B., Malik, M.O.A., Satir, A.A. et al (1974) *Trop. Geogr. Med.* **26**, 198–203.

66 Blount, E.R., Hartmann, R. & Nernoff, J. (1980) *Clin. Pediat.* **19**, 139–140.

67 Chunge, C.N. Gachihi, G., Muigai, R. et al (1985) *Trans. R. Soc. trop. Med. Hyg.* **79**, 872.

68 Kager, P.A. & Rees, P.H. (1983) *Trop. Geogr. Med.* **35**, 111–124

69 Hockmeyer, W.T., Kager, P.A., Rees, P.H. et al (1981) *Trans. R. Soc. trop. Med. Hyg.* **75**, 861–863.

70 Chulay, J.D. & Bryceson, A.D.M. (1983) *Am. J. trop Med. Hyg.* **32**, 475–479.

71 Musumeci, S., Fischer, A. & Pizzarelli, G. (1977) *Trans. R. Soc. trop. Med. Hyg.* **71**, 176.

72 Martaresche, B., Dunan, S., Wuilici, M. et al (1975) *Med. Trop.* **35**, 308.

73 Hommel, M., Peters, W., Ranque, J. et al (1978) *Ann. trop. Med. Parasit.* **72**, 213.

74 Ho, M., Leeuwenburg, J., Mbugua, J. et al (1983) *Am. J. trop. Med. Hyg.* **32**, 943–946.

75 Jahn, A. & Diesfeld, H.J. (1983) *Trans. R. Soc. trop Med. Hyg.* **77**, 451–454.

76 Monsur, J.A. & Khaleque, K.A. (1957) *Trans. R. Soc. trop. Med. Hyg.* **51**, 527.

77 Thakur, C.P. et al (1984) *Br. med. J.* **288**, 985–987.

78 Wang, C.T., Wu, C.C. & He, K.Z. (1983) *J. Parasit. parasit. Dis.* **1**, 65–73.

79 World Health Organization (1982) *Document TDR/Chemleish/VL 82.3* Geneva.

80 Anabwani, G.M., Dimiti, G., Ngira, J.A. et al (1983) *Lancet* **i**, 210–212.

81 Rees, P.H., Kager, P.A., Kyambi, J.M. et al (1983) In Kager, P.A. & Rees, P.H. MD thesis, pp. 149–158. University of Amsterdam.

82 Bryceson, A.D.M. (1986) In *The Leishmaniases in Biology and Medicine*, eds. W. Peters & R. Killick Kendrick. London: Academic Press.

83 Sanuyl, E.K., Alam, S.N. & Kaul, S.M. (1979) *J. infect. Dis.* **11**, 170.

84 Sen Gupta, P.C. & Mukherjee, A.M. (1968) *J. Indian med. Ass.* **50**, 1.

85 Chance, M.L., Schnur, L.F., Thomas, S.C. et al (1978) *Ann. trop. Med. Parasit.* **72**, 533.

86 Desjeux, P., Bray, R.S., Dedet, J.P. et al (1982) *Trans. R. Soc. trop. Med. Hyg* **76**, 132–133.

87 Conteh, S. & Desjeux, P.H. (1983) *Trans. R. Soc. trop. Med. Hyg.* **77**, 298–302.

88 Mutinga, J.M., Ngoka, J.M., Schnur, L.F. et al (1980) *Ann trop. Med. Parasit.* **74**, 139.

89 Adler S. & Theodor, C. (1935) *Proc. R. Soc. B.* **116**, 516.

90 Rioux, J.A., Albaret, J.L., Houin, R. et al (1968) *Ann. Parasit. hum. comp.* **43**, 421.

91 Bettini, S., Pozio, E. & Gradoni, L. (1980) *Trans. R. Soc. trop. Med. Hyg.* **74**, 77.

92 Petrisceva, P.A. (1971) *Bull. Wld Hlth Org.* **44**, 567.

93 Deane, L.M. & Deane, M.P. (1964) *Archos Hig. Saúde publ.* **29**, 89.

94 Silveira, F.T., Lainson, R., Shaw, J.J. et al (1982) *Trans. R. Soc. trop. Med. Hyg.* **76**, 830–832.

95 Conroy, J.D., Levine, L.D. & Small, E. (1970) *Path. vet.* **7**, 163.

96 Hamidi, A.N., Nadim, A., Edrissian, G.H.H. et al (1982) *Trans. R. Soc. trop. Med. Hyg* **76**, 756–757.

97 Hoogstraal, H., van Peenen, P.F.D., Reid, T.P. et al (1963) *Am. J. trop. Med Hyg.* **12**, 175.

98 Xu, Z.B., Xiong, J., You, J.Y. et al (1982) *Chinese med. J.* **95**, 649–652.

99 Gradoni, L., Pozio, E., Gramiccia, M. et al (1983) *Trans. R. Soc. trop. Med. Hyg.* **77**, 427–431.

100 Petrovic, Z., Bordjoski, A. & Savin, Z. (1975) *Proc. 2nd. Europ. Multicolloquy of Parasitology*, Trogir.

101 El-Alhami, B. (1976) *Am. J. trop. Med. Hyg.* **25**, 759.

102 De Alencar, J.E., Pessoa, E.P. & Fontele, Z.F. (1960) *Rev. Inst. med. Trop. São Paulo* **2**, 347.

103 Lainson, R. & Shaw, J.J. (1978) *Nature, Lond.* **273**, 595.

104 Tewfik, S., Kassem, S.A., Aref, M.K. et al (1983) *Trans. R. Soc. trop. Med. Hyg.* **77**, 334–335

105 Schnur, L.F., Morsy, T.A., Feinsod, F.M. et al (1985) *Trans. R. Soc. trop. Med. Hyg.* **79**, 134–135.

106 Dergacheva, T.I. & Strelkova, M.V. (1985) *Trans. R. Soc. trop. Med. Hyg.* **79**, 34–36.

107 Leng, Y.-J. (1982) *Trans. R. Soc. trop. Med. Hyg.* **76**, 531–537.

108 Doury, P. (1957) *Arch Inst. Pasteur Alger.* **35**, 204.

109 Andre, L.J., Sirol, J., Le Vourch, C.I. et al (1978) *Med. Trop.* **38**, 435.

110 Blocher, R. (1949) *Rev. Colon Med. Chir.* **21**, 6.

111 Gigase, P., Moens, F., van Emelen, J. et al (1978) *Ann. Soc. belge. Med. trop.* **58**, 235.

112 Naik, K.G., Hira, P.R., Bhagwandeen, S.B. et al (1976) *Trans. R. Soc. trop. Med. Hyg.* **70**, 328.

113 Garnham, P.C.C. (1971) *Bull. Wld Hlth Org.* **44**, 477–489.

114 Meyruey, M. (1974) *Med. Trop.* **34**, 3.

115 Fuller, G.K., de Sole, G. & Lemma, A. (1976) *Ethiop. med. J.* **14**, 87.

116 Beach, R. & Mebrahtu, Y. (1985) *Proc. R. Soc. trop. Med. Hyg.* **79**, 445–447.

117 Wijers, D.J.B. & Mwangi, S. (1966) *Ann. trop. Med. Parasit.* **60**, 373.

118 Heisch, R.B., Wijers, D.J.B. & Minter, D.M. (1962) *Br. med. J.* **i**, 456.

119 Srivastava, L. & Chakarvarty, A.K. (1984) *Ann. trop. Med. Hyg.* **78**, 501–504.

120 Killick Kendrick, R., Molyneux, D.H., Rioux, J.A. et al (1980) *Ann. trop. Med. Parasit.* **74**, 563–565.

121 Lainson, R., Shaw, J.J., Silveira, F.T. et al (1983) *Trans. R. Soc. trop. Med. Hyg.* **77**, 323–330.

Chapter 5
Arbovirus Diseases

The diseases caused by arboviruses (*arthropod-borne viruses*) are zoonoses; that is, they are primarily infections of vertebrates other than man, and of the arthropod vectors, and can be transmitted to man. One apparent exception is o'nyong-nyong fever (ONN), of which the only known vertebrate host is man. These viruses are usually spread by the bites of arthropods, but some can also be transmitted by other means (through milk, excreta or aerosols). The arbovirus infections 'are maintained in nature principally, or to an important extent, through biological transmission between susceptible vertebrate hosts by blood-sucking insects; they multiply to produce viraemia in the vertebrates, multiply in the tissues of the insects and are passed on to new vertebrates by the bites of insects after a period of extrinsic incubation'.[1] In the same publication, however, Chumakov prefers the following definition: 'Arboviruses are zoonotic viral agents which, when circulating in the natural foci of infection, are transmitted in a more or less regular manner by arthropods, but in certain circumstances may be transmitted in other ways than by arthropods.'

Smith[2] suggests that the safest definition is that arboviruses are 'potential zoonotic viruses which cannot be otherwise classified.'

The names by which these viruses are known are of mixed origin. Some are dialect names for the illnesses they cause (chikungunya, o'nyong-nyong), some are place names (West Nile, Bwamba) and some derive from clinical characters (western equine encephalitis, yellow fever).

AETIOLOGY

Most arboviruses are spherical, measuring 17–150 nm or more, a few are rod-shaped, measuring 70×200 nm.[1] All are RNA viruses. Many circulate in a natural environment and do not infect man. Some infect man only occasionally or cause only a mild illness; others are of great clinical importance causing large epidemics and many deaths. The arboviruses of clinical importance belong to the Togaviridae, the alphaviruses, flaviviruses, the Bunyaviridae, nairoviruses, phleboviruses and other subgroups (see Table 5.1).

Alphaviruses are all transmitted by mosquitoes in nature, but in experimental work the range of mosquito species capable of transmission is larger than the known range of vectors in nature. Flaviviruses are transmitted by mosquitoes and ticks and many have been isolated worldwide from the salivary glands of bats, but only one has caused a laboratory infection in man. Some phleboviruses are transmitted by sandflies.

EPIDEMIOLOGY

Vertebrate hosts

The vertebrate hosts have been differentiated as maintenance, incidental, link and amplifier hosts.

Maintenance hosts

These 'are essential for the continued existence of the virus'.[3] They usually live in symbiosis with the viruses, without actual disease, but they develop antibody.

The maintenance hosts provisionally recognized include the following, though some have only been incriminated experimentally[4] (see footnote for list of abbreviations).

BIRDS
Prairie chicken, red-winged blackbird, blue jay, pheasant, pigeon, cardinal, sparrow, wren, grackle, wood thrush, catbird (EEE, WEE,

---

Abbreviations: EEE = Eastern equine encephalitis, WEE = Western equine encephalitis, VEE = Venezuelan equine encephalitis, SLE = St Louis encephalitis, JE = Japanese encephalitis, MVE = Murray Valley encephalitis, TBE = tick-borne encephalitis, RSSE = Russian spring–summer encephalitis, KFD = Kyasanur Forest disease, LGT = Langat virus, JUN = Junin virus, MAC = Machupo virus, LI = louping ill, POW = Powassan virus, YF = yellow fever, DEN = dengue fever, CE = Californian encephalitis, TAH = Tahyna virus, RB = Rio Bravo virus, CTF = Colorado tick fever, ONN = o'nyong-nyong virus.

Table 5.1 Arboviruses.

Virus	Geographical distribution	Transmission	Fever	Clinical form	Rash
TOGAVIRIDAE					
Alphaviruses					
*Chikungunya (CHIK)	Africa, India, South-East Asia	Mosquito	+	H	+
*Mayaro (Uruma) (MAY)	South America	Mosquito	+		+
*O'nyong-nyong (ONN)	Africa	Mosquito	+		+
*Ross River (RR)	Australia, South Pacific	Mosquito	+	Arthritis	+
*Sindbis (SIN)	Africa, Saudi Arabia, India, South-East Asia, Australia	Mosquito	+		+ (Africa only)
Mucambo (MUC)	Brazil	Mosquito	+		
Semliki Forest (SF)	South Africa, East Africa	Mosquito	+		
Ockelbo	Sweden	Mosquito	+		+
*Eastern equine encephalitis (EEE)	North America	Mosquito	+	E	
*Western equine encephalitis (WEE)	North and South America	Mosquito	+	E	
*Venezuelan equine encephalitis (VEE)	North and South America	Mosquito	+	E	
Flaviviruses					
Mosquito-borne					
*Dengue type 1 (DEN1)	Africa, Pacific, Far East, Caribbean	Mosquito	+	H	+
*Dengue type 2 (DEN2)	Far East, Trinidad, Belize	Mosquito	+	H	+
*Dengue type 3 (DEN3)	Philippines, India	Mosquito	+	H	+
*Dengue type 4 (DEN4)	Philippines	Mosquito	+	H	+
*Dengue type TH-36	Thailand	Mosquito	+	H	
Dengue type TH-SMAN	Thailand	Mosquito	+	H	
Ilhéus (ILH)	South and Central America	Mosquito	+	E	
*Japanese encephalitis (JE)	Japan, Far East	Mosquito	+	E	
Banzi (BAN)	Africa	Mosquito	+		
Bussuquara (BSQ)	South America	Mosquito	+		
*Murray River encephalitis (MVE)	Australia, New Guinea	Mosquito	+	E	+
*West Nile (WN)	Africa, India, Europe	Mosquito	+	E	+
Kunjin (KUN)	Australia, Sarawak	Mosquito	+		+
*St Louis encephalitis (SLE)	Americas	Mosquito	+	E	
Wesselsbron (WSL)	South Africa	Mosquito	+		+
*Yellow fever	Africa, South and Central America	Mosquito	+	H	
Zika (ZIKA)	Africa, South-East Asia	Mosquito	+	Lab	+
Spondweni (SPO)	South Africa	Mosquito	+		
Sepik (SE)	Australia	Mosquito	+		
*Rocio (ROC)	Brazil	Mosquito	+	E	
Tick-borne					
*Kyasanur Forest disease (KFD)	India	Ixodid tick	+	H	+
Kumlinge (KUM)	Finland	Tick	+	E	+
Langat (LAN)	Malaysia	Ixodid tick	+	E	
Louping ill	Britain	Ixodid tick	+	E	
*Omsk haemorrhagic fever (OHF)	USSR	Ixodid tick	+	H	+
*Powassan (POW)	Canada, USA	Ixodid tick	+	E	
*Tick-borne encephalitis (TBE)					
Far Eastern (Russian spring–summer encephalitis (RSSE)	USSR, Asia	Ixodid tick	+	E	
Central European	Europe and Scandinavia	Ixodid tick	+	E	
Negishi (NEG)	Japan	? tick	+	E	
Other vectors					
Rio Bravo (RB)	USA, Trinidad	? bat saliva	+	E, meningitis	
BUNYAVIRIDAE					
Bunyamwera group					
Bunyamwera (BUN)	Africa	Mosquito	+		
Calovo (CUO)	Europe	Mosquito	+		
Germiston (GER)	Africa	Mosquito	+		
Guaroa (GRO)	South and Central America	Mosquito	+		
Ilesha	Africa	Mosquito	+		
Tensaw	North America	Mosquito	+	E	

Table 5.1 (*contd.*)

Virus	Geographical distribution	Transmission	Fever	Clinical form	Rash
Wyeomyia	Central and South America	Mosquito	+		
Maguari	South America	Mosquito	+		
Bwamba group					
Bwamba (BWA)	Africa	Mosquito	+		
C Group					
Apeu (APEU)	South America	Mosquito	+		
Caraparu (CAR)	South America	Mosquito	+		
Itaqui (ITQ)	South America	Mosquito	+		
Marituba (MTB)	South America	Mosquito	+		
Murutuca (MUR)	South America	Mosquito	+		
Madrid (MAD)	Panama	Mosquito	+		
Oriboca (ORI)	South America	Mosquito	+		
Ossa (OSSA)	Panama	Mosquito	+		
Restan (RES)	Trinidad	Mosquito	+		
Nepuyo (NEP)	Central America	Mosquito	+		
Tataguine (TAT)	Nigeria	Mosquito	+		
California group					
*California encephalitis (CE)	USA, Canada	Mosquito	+	E	
Inkoo	Finland	Mosquito	+	Meningism	
*La Crosse (LAC)	USA, Canada	Mosquito	+	E	
*Tahyna (Lumbo) (TAH)	Europe, Africa	Mosquito	+		
Trivittatus	USA	Mosquito	+		
Simbu group					
*Oropouche (ORO)	South America	Mosquito	+	E	
Shuni	Africa	Mosquito	+		
Guama group					
Guama (GMA)	South America	Mosquito	+		
Catu (CATU)	South America	Mosquito	+		
Other Bunyaviridae					
Bhanja	India, southern Europe	Tick	+		
Thogoto (THO)	Africa, Mediterranean	Tick	+	E	
Nairoviruses					
Crimean–Congo group					
*Crimean–Congo haemorrhagic fever (C–CHF)	Europe, Africa, Middle East, central Asia, Pakistan	Ixodid tick	+	H	+
Hazara	Pakistan	Ixodid tick		H	
Nairobi sheep disease group					
Dugbe	Africa	Ixodid tick	+		
Ganjam	Africa, India	Ixodid tick	+		
Nairobi sheep disease	Africa, India	Ixodid tick	+		
Phleboviruses					
*Phlebotomus fever (sandfly fever) Neapolitan (SFN) Sicilian (SFS)	Africa, Asia	Phlebotomine sandflies	+		
*Rift Valley fever (RVF) (Zinga)	Africa	Mosquito	+	H	
Candiru (CDU)	Brazil	?	+		
Chagres (CHG)	Panama	*Phlebotomus*	+		
Uukuviruses					
*Hantaan virus, Puumala virus (murine virus nephropathy, MVN). Haemorrhagic fever with renal syndrome (HFRS)	China, Korea, European Russia, Scandinavia, Balkans, Europe	Contamination from rodent urine or rodent bite	+	H	
Uukuniemi	Finland, Norway, Eastern Europe	Tick	+		
ORBIVIRIDAE					
Changuinola group					
Changuinola	Central America	*Phlebotomus*	+		

Table 5.1 (*contd.*)

Virus	Geographical distribution	Transmission	Fever	Clinical form	Rash
Kemerovo group					
Kemerovo (KEM)	Europe	Tick	+		
Tribec	Europe	Tick	+		
*Colorado tick fever					
Colorado tick fever (CTF)	North America	Tick	+	HE (in children)	+
Ungrouped					
Orungo (ORU)	Central Africa and Cameroon	Mosquito	+		
RHABDOVIRIDAE					
Vesicular stomatitis group					
Vesicular stomatitis (Indiana and New Jersey)	North and Central America	*Phlebotomus*	+		
Chandipura	India, Africa	Mosquito	+		
Piry	South America	Mosquito	+		

*Of clinical importance; 2 H = haemorrhagic; E = encephalitis.
For a complete list of mosquito vectors and the arboviruses they transmit see Appendix III, Table III.6, p. 1416.

SLE), heron, egret (JE). Migrating birds can carry viruses over long distances (MVE, EEE, WEE, SLE).

RODENTS AND INSECTIVORES (VEE, KFD, LGT, JUN, MAC)
Vole, shrew, rat, *Arvicanthis*, field mouse, hedgehog, squirrel, lemming, chipmunk (European TBE, RSSE, LI), groundhog (POW), deer mouse, porcupine (CTF), sloth, small marsupials.

PRIMATES
Monkey (YF, ?DEN).

LEPORIDAE
Rabbit, hare (CE, ?TAH).

UNGULATES (CATTLE, DEER)
(?European TBE, LI).

BATS
(?RB).

MARSUPIALS, REPTILES AND AMPHIBIA
Kangaroo, snake (?EEE, WEE), lizard, alligator, turtle (?EEE).

Incidental hosts

These become infected, but transmission from them does not occur with sufficient regularity for stable maintenance. Man is usually an incidental host, often, but not always, being a dead end in the chain. Incidental hosts may or may not show symptoms. They may be necessary for the maintenance of transmission as they are the main hosts of ticks, keeping these arthropods alive in sufficient numbers to be effective carriers.

Link hosts

These bridge a gap between maintenance hosts and man (e.g. between small mammals and man by goats (via milk) in tick-borne encephalitis, and between wild birds and man by sparrows in SLE).

Amplifier hosts

These increase the weight of infection to which man is exposed, for instance pigs, which act between wild birds (especially herons) and man in JE. Dogs may also be involved.

The mode of transmission between maintenance hosts may differ from that responsible for infection of incidental hosts, including man.

The populations and characters of the vertebrate hosts and their threshold levels of viraemia are important. Small rodents multiply rapidly and have short lives, thus providing a constant supply of susceptible individuals, especially to the tick-borne viruses. On the other hand, monkeys and pigs multiply slowly, and once they have recovered from an infection with YF and JE respectively, they remain immune for life. Immunity also affects pigs in the early months of life, having been transmitted via the placenta from immune mothers, and this no doubt is a feature in other animals. African monkeys are relatively resistant to YF, but Asian and American monkeys are susceptible, probably because, unlike the African monkeys, they have not been exposed continuously for centuries to the infection. It is also possible that infection with other related arboviruses may partly immunize African monkeys (and man) against YF.

So far as is known, the only vertebrate host of ONN is man and the conditions for the spread of this infection seem to depend on the human populations involved, and the multiplicity of vector mosquitoes. In urban conditions, with a concentrated human population and prolific breeding of *Aedes aegypti* the cycle of yellow fever and dengue is also usually man–mosquito–man.

Invertebrate hosts

These include mosquitoes, sandflies and ticks and also *Culicoides* (involved in some animal viruses).

After these vectors have imbibed virus from a vertebrate in a state of viraemia, the virus undergoes an incubation period within the arthropod, known as the extrinsic incubation period. In mosquitoes this period is short: 10 days at 30°C ambient temperature and longer at lower temperatures. Mosquitoes remain infective for life without any apparent ill-effects. Their infectivity appears to increase with time after infection and their effectiveness as transmitters depends upon the frequency with which they bite.

It is also possible that arthropods, whose mouth parts are contaminated by virus in the act of feeding, could transmit the virus mechanically if they feed quickly on another animal. For instance, chikungunya virus can be transmitted mechanically by *Ae. aegypti* for 8 hours after infection.

Most arboviruses have been recovered from mosquitoes and a list of the vectors is given in Appendix III (Table III.6, p. 1416).

Ixodid ticks are involved in a closely inter-related subgroup of group B arboviruses and also in some of the other groups. Genera of ticks involved include *Haemaphysalis*, *Ixodes* and *Dermacentor* (see also Appendix III, p. 1385).

In general, mosquitoes are refractory to tick-borne viruses and ticks to mosquito-borne viruses but there may be exceptions in some conditions.[1]

TRANSMISSION

Transmission by arthropods involves several processes:

1 ingestion by the arthropods of virus in the blood (usually) or tissue fluids of the vertebrate hosts;
2 penetration of the viruses into the tissue of the arthropods, in the gut wall, or elsewhere after passing through the gut wall ('gut barrier');
3 multiplication of the viruses in the arthropod cells, including those of the salivary glands.[1]

Stage 2 and part of stage 3 represent the extrinsic incubation period of the disease.

The quantity of blood, and therefore the amount of virus ingested, seems to be important; each arthropod species must ingest a minimum quantity of a given virus before multiplication can take place. The same mosquito species can have two different thresholds for two different viruses and if one species has a low threshold, other species may have high thresholds or be completely resistant. This threshold phenomenon is extremely important in determining the efficiency of a vector and may also vitally affect the course of an epidemic.

The viruses persist in ixodid ticks for months or years and in mosquitoes for practically their whole lives, though there may be a gradual decrease of concentration of the virus with time. Viruses have been reported to persist in over-wintering mosquitoes and this could be important, for instance in *Culex tritaeniorhynchus* infected with JE, and *C. tarsalis* infected with WEE (infective by bite up to eight months).

Transstadial persistence of virus is normal in ticks and transovarial passage has been observed in some species; both are of great epidemiological importance. Transovarial passage in mosquitoes does not occur although evidence for transovarial passage of YF virus in *Ae. furcifer-taylori* has been given. Arthropods do not appear to be harmed by these infections.

Important factors in transmission by arthropods

1 Susceptibility of the arthropods to infection and ability to transmit it. There is wide variation in this.

2 Breeding habits of the arthropods and preferred habitats, whether near man and other hosts of the virus.

3 Biting habits of the arthropods; in mosquitoes whether they are anthropophilic or zoophilic, exophilic or endophilic.

4 Longevity of the arthropods, which depends to a great extent on temperature, humidity and (especially in ticks) the availability of hosts to feed on. Overwintering mosquitoes can carry virus from one year to the next—*C. tarsalis* can carry WEE for eight months.

5 Abundance of the arthropods; for mosquitoes the availability of suitable breeding places (and therefore the rainfall) is a major factor. An efficient vector may have a wide range of animals on which to feed, but if the arthropod species is abundant, and even if it bites man only

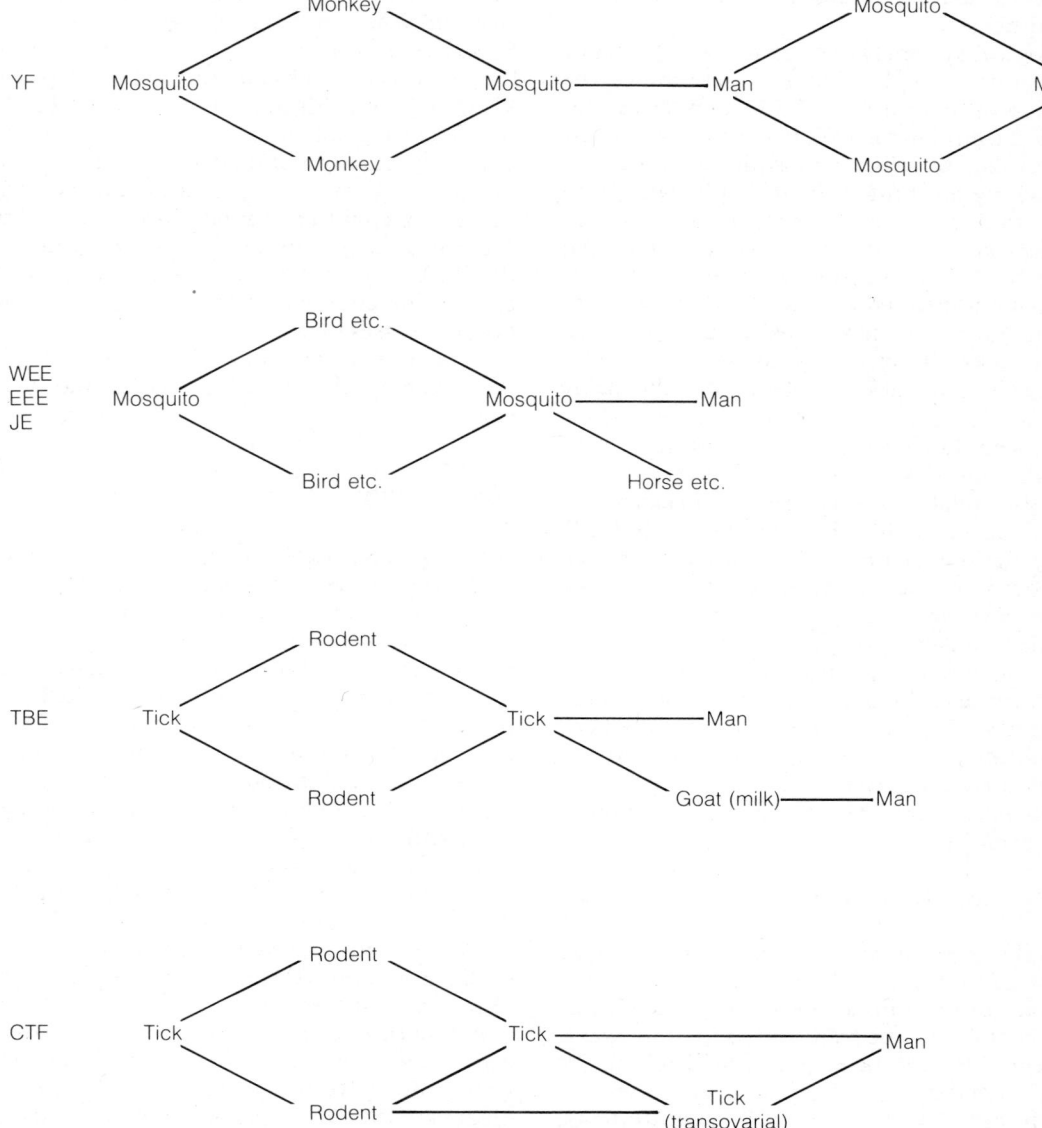

Fig. 5.1. Transmission of some arboviruses.

infrequently in the presence of other (and pre-ferred) animals, the large numbers enable it to maintain transmission to man. For instance, *C. tritaeniorhynchus*, which mostly bites birds, Bovidae, dogs and especially porcines, and only to a limited extent man, can maintain trans-mission of JE from pigs to man by sheer numbers. *C. tarsalis* feeds indiscriminately on mammals in summer, when WEE and SLE tend to occur in man and horses, but at other times it feeds on birds which carry the virus.

6 Migratory birds can help by spreading virus which is circulating in their blood or by carrying infected ticks.

7 Ecological systems are of primary importance in transmission and biocenosis determines the formation of natural foci of infection. A case in point is the circulation of YF virus among forest monkeys and tree-living mosquitoes, occasion-ally reaching mosquitoes haunting banana plan-tations raided by the monkeys, and thence reaching man and perhaps spreading from man to man by peridomestic mosquitoes. Similarly, man becomes infected with KFD when he enters the domain of infected monkeys and picks up infected ticks. Other mosquito-borne and tick-borne infections are variations on the same theme.

The mosquito-borne and tick-borne infections differ in that ticks attach themselves to ver-tebrates for relatively long periods and can there-fore overlap a viraemic phase. In the case of KFD the populations of ticks are maintained at high levels by domestic cattle, on which they feed, and the cattle are close enough to the sources of viraemia (monkeys, and possibly birds and small rodents) to maintain enough ticks to carry on the cycle in animals. Man is an intruder and though he becomes infected he is not a link in the chain. The subject is discussed in more detail in the section on KFD, p. 143.

Transmission may be represented diagramma-tically, as in Fig. 5.1.

Other factors in transmission

Although transmission of arboviruses usually takes place through the bites of arthropods, it is important to remember that some of the viruses can, exceptionally, be transmitted in other ways. European TBE can be acquired by drinking the milk of infected goats, Junin and Lassa viruses through contact with excreta of infective rodents, VEE (in cotton rats) apparently via urine or faeces infecting the nasopharynx, WEE possibly through aerosol from a patient and EEE (in pheasants) by one bird pecking another. Labor-atory infections have been reported with Kunjin virus in Australia, and others. Muroid virus nephropathy can be transmitted by aerosol from infected rodents. CTF virus is reported to have been transmitted by blood transfusion.

Many human activities encourage trans-mission of these animal viruses to man. Irrigation often promotes the breeding of enormous numbers of mosquitoes. For instance, the development of rice fields encourages *C. tri-taeniorhynchus* in Sarawak, spreading JE, and *Mansonia uniformis* and *Anopheles gambiae* in Kenya spreading chikungunya, ONN, possibly West Nile and Sindbis, and malaria. The sea-sonal cutting of old vegetation in Sarawak produces heavily polluted pools which support massive populations of culicines. The keeping of cattle, driven into marginal forest areas in India, promotes the growth and transport of ticks and the intrusion of man into forest areas lays him open to infection with yellow fever and the tick-borne diseases.

For a fuller discussion of these points the paper on epidemiology by Smith et al[5] should be con-sulted.

IMMUNITY

After a vertebrate has been infected by an arbovirus the virus probably multiplies first in the regional lymph glands where the earliest formation of antibodies also probably takes place. The antibodies are immunofluorescent (IFA), haemagglutination-inhibiting (HI), com-plement-fixing (CF) and neutralizing (N). In general HI antibodies appear early and may be long-lasting; CF antibodies appear later and may last two to five years; and N antibodies appear early and are long-lasting. But there are differ-ences; some arboviruses do not produce high titres of antibodies in man and some antibodies are short-lived or appear late.

Of these antibodies, HI and CF are important in diagnosis, but the only protective antibody is N, which is also the most specific antibody.

Arboviruses are grouped according to anti-genic characters, but after inoculation of one virus into a fresh animal, not only the hom-ologous antibodies, but also heterologous anti-bodies reacting with other viruses of the same group tend to appear. Recovery from an infection by a member of one group of arboviruses may provide some degree of resistance to a subsequent infection by another member of the same group; for instance, infection with West Nile virus may have modified the Ethiopian epidemic of YF in 1962.[6] Again, the effect of prior infection with Zika, Uganda S and other related viruses in the forest belt of Nigeria, leading to a high incidence of related antibodies, is suggested as the explanation of the absence of epidemic YF in man in that area. These related infections probably modify the disease rather than prevent infection.[7]

Active immunity in general

A person who recovers from an attack of YF possesses a solid immunity against reinfection. Neutralizing antibodies can be found as early as a few days after the beginning of the disease and are found constantly for many years in the sera of such persons. This persistence of immunity does not depend upon exogenous reinfection and the mechanism by which the antibodies are produced is not clear. It has been commented[8] that a mosquito infected with YF is not harmed by it, but continues to excrete the virus throughout life. This means a continuous release of virus, probably from epithelial cells of the salivary glands. The virus enters man (or other animals) and gains the liver and other epithelium, provoking the early antibodies in the blood, which neutralize circulating viruses. But antibodies which can be detected for so many years in man must stem from a continuing stimulus, and the sensitive cells and their progeny probably have a prophase equivalent of the virus incorporated into their genetic structure, with occasional reversion to productive development which provides the stimulus for further antibody formation. The solid and fundamental immunity probably lies at the genetic level. A degree of immunity of this kind may possibly be provided when a related virus invades epithelial cells.

Epidemics of MVE, JE and West Nile are not reported in the endemic areas of dengue, possibly because of cross protection. There seems to be an analogy with the protective effect in schistosomiasis of infection with heterologous schistosomes.

The immunology of arbovirus infections is in line with the immunological principles of virus infections in general.

Passive immunity in general

Infant rhesus monkeys and human infants born of mothers immune to YF have protective antibodies in their sera at birth which persist for several months. These immune bodies are probably transmitted via the placenta rather than in the mothers' milk, because antibodies may disappear from infant sera while they are still suckling. This passive immunity is transient. Passive immunity induced by injection of homologous immune serum, however, has been used for protection against TBE in circumstances of special risk and similar sera could be used against other infections, particularly after laboratory accidents.

CLINICAL FEATURES IN GENERAL

After the virus enters the body it reaches the lymphatic system where it multiplies and from which it is released into the blood (viraemic phase) and thence to the organs affected.

Most arbovirus infections are inapparent (producing no symptoms) or mild (producing some fever and occasionally a rash), diagnosable retrospectively by serological methods. For instance, in an epidemic of JE it was estimated that for each case of apparent disease there were 500–1000 inapparent infections. The proportions no doubt vary with circumstances.

If clinical manifestations arise after infection they do so after an intrinsic incubation period lasting from a few days to a week or more. Some arboviruses damage the endothelial lining of the capillaries increasing permeability which allows the virus to pass the blood brain barrier causing meningoencephalitis (encephalitides). Others damage the parenchymatous organs by direct damage to the cells in which they are situated, while with others damage is caused by the immune system of the host from the formation of antigen–antibody complexes and disordered complement formation which damage the renal tubules and alter the coagulation and fibrinolytic systems of the body causing haemorrhage (viral haemorrhagic fevers). There is a general pattern of biphasic illness, the first phase associated with viraemia ending when antibodies appear in the blood and the second phase when the virus is located in organs, such as the liver or brain.

The onset of clinical manifestations is nearly

always abrupt, generally occurring after the onset of viraemia. *Fever* is usual and is sometimes the only sign. In many cases the clinical manifestations last only while the virus is disseminated, recovery following without sequelae, but in other cases there is *remission*, short or long. If long, the disease is biphasic. After this *fever returns* with signs indicating localization of the virus in certain organs: albuminuria, jaundice, meningeal signs, encephalitis and myelitis. If the period of viraemia has been without symptoms and the virus becomes localized in the central nervous system, encephalitis appears late and may seem to be primary. In haemorrhagic cases there is a special risk of shock which can rapidly become irreversible unless treated promptly.

All degrees of involvement may be observed in a single epidemic, but some arboviruses cause generally mild disease, others tend to severity.

The syndromes may be grouped as follows:

1 systemic febrile diseases (Table 5.2);
2 viral haemorrhagic fevers (VHF) (Table 5.3);
3 encephalitides (Table 5.4).

SYSTEMIC FEBRILE DISEASES

This is the largest group and the mild forms of all arbovirus diseases are of this kind (Table 5.2). The course may be biphasic and the infection may go on to the more serious haemorrhagic or encephalitic forms.

Table 5.2 Systemic febrile diseases.

Chikungunya	Tahyna
O'nyong-nyong	Oropouche
Ross River fever	Rocio virus
Mayaro	Sandfly fever
Sindbis	

In addition to fever, which may suggest influenza, the following symptoms may occur:

1 *Anorexia*, with nausea and vomiting (phlebotomus fevers), or respiratory symptoms may predominate (Tahyna).
2 A *rash*, erythematous or itchy maculopapular, with congestion of the face and neck (phlebotomus), inflammation of the palate, vesicles on the feet (Sindbis), or even petechiae or more extensive haemorrhages.
3 *Conjuctivitis*, with photophobia and orbital pain (phlebotomus) or even central retinitis and chorioretinitis (Rift Valley).
4 *Epidemic polyarthritis* (Ross River in Australia).
5 *Arthralgia* (o'nyong-nyong, chikungunya) or myalgia (especially in dengue), which can be responsible for excruciating pain, sometimes so severe as to render the patient incapable of movement ('break-bone fever'); lumbar pain is also common (phlebotomus).
6 *Inflammation* and enlargement of the lymphatic glands (o'nyong-nyong, chikungunya, West Nile).
7 *Leukopenia*, which is common, and thrombocytopenia (Colorado).

DIAGNOSIS

Virological diagnosis

Blood should be taken as soon as possible after the onset of the disease, part being reserved for isolation of the virus (only useful in the first few days), and part for serological tests. Suckling mice, hamsters, guinea pigs and tissue-culture techniques are used for isolation of the virus.

If there are meningeal signs the cerebrospinal fluid may be used for isolation and is occasionally positive in TBE, CTF, JE, WEE, SLE and YF. Cells may be sedimented and examined by the fluorescent antibody technique.

After death, specimens of tissue should be taken as soon as possible, emulsified and quickly inoculated into suckling mice 1–3 days old, or adult mice, newborn hamsters, chick embryos or even guinea pigs (Junin virus). The material to be inoculated is usually treated with antibiotics, and part is kept frozen for confirmation by re-isolation of the virus.

Serological diagnosis

After infection the virus probably first multiplies in the regional lymph glands, where the earliest antibody formation also probably starts. Serological diagnosis is based on the detection of IFA, HI, CF and N antibodies and on the variations in titre found in paired sera at various stages. IFA and HI antibodies are cross reactive within the arbovirus groups, and may need confirmation by tests for N antibodies. CF antibodies are separate and distinct from N antibodies. N antibodies are usually the most specific.

If the patient has been exposed to an arbovirus of the same group as the one responsible for his illness, serological diagnosis is difficult because group antibodies are at high titre—even to some extent the N antibodies.

The gel precipitin test has been used suc-cessfully with antigens produced in cell cultures, for tests on paired sera. It has also been used to differentiate various viruses though consistently satisfactory antisera for this purpose may be difficult to obtain.

The fluorescent antibody test has been used as a reliable test for antigen in acute-phase blood clots in CTE and on post-mortem material, for instance in JE.

Some of the reagents—antigens and immune fluids—used for tests are described in World Health Organization.[1]

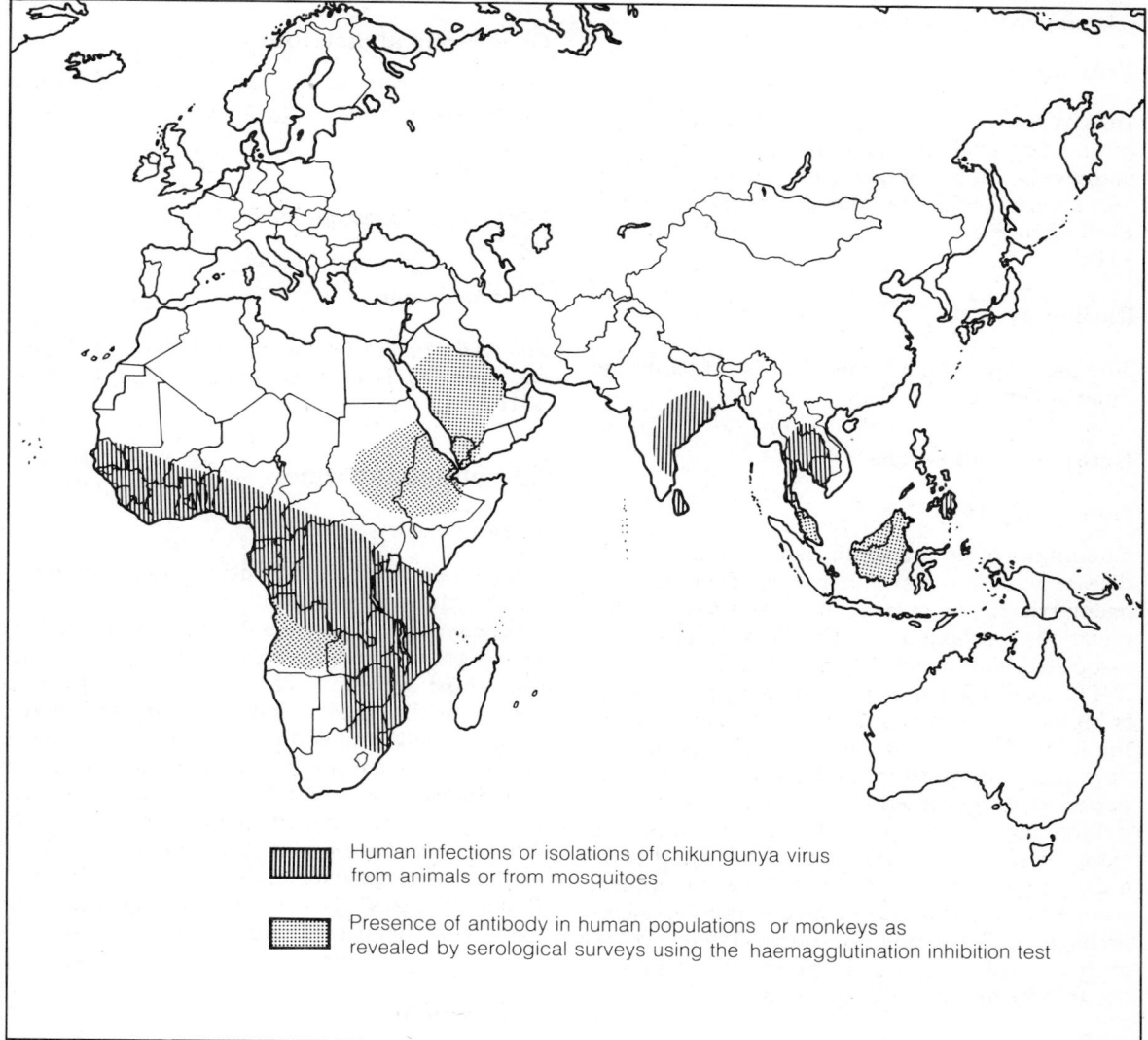

Human infections or isolations of chikungunya virus from animals or from mosquitoes

Presence of antibody in human populations or monkeys as revealed by serological surveys using the haemagglutination inhibition test

Fig. 5.2. Geographical distribution of chikungunya virus (courtesy Department of Entomology, London School of Hygiene and Tropical Medicine).

CHIKUNGUNYA (CHIK)

Geographical distribution

Antibody studies have shown that this virus is widespread in Africa and is also present in Saudi Arabia, Borneo, Malaysia, Philippines, and clinical outbreaks have occurred in many parts of Africa as well as Thailand, Cambodia, Burma, Sri Lanka and India (Calcutta, Madras, Vellore) (Fig. 5.2).

Aetiology

Chikungunya virus is an alphavirus closely related to o'nyong-nyong.

Transmission

In Africa the main vector to man is *Ae. aegypti* but a forest cycle is maintained by *Ae. africanus* and several species of *Mansonia*. In Asia the main vectors are *C. fatigans (quinquefasciatus)*, *C. tritaeniorhynchus* and *C. gelidus* (Table III.6, p. 1416).

Pathology

The pathology is not known but is probably the same as dengue.

Symptoms and signs

Natural history

Chikungunya is an acute self-limiting febrile disease with a forest and human cycle and no haemorrhagic or central nervous system complications (although in Thailand it has been associated with haemorrhagic dengue).

The *incubation period* is 2–4 days. The disease is biphasic. Onset is abrupt with severe pain in the joints and the patient prostrated. After 1–4 days the fever subsides and there is an afebrile period of 3 days when the fever returns with an itching maculopapular rash on the trunk and extensor surfaces of the limbs. After another 3–6 days the fever subsides and there is complete recovery. In Asia it is associated with mild haemorrhagic features but no shock. There are no chronic sequelae but a crippling arthralgia may occur intermittently for up to four months.

Diagnosis

Diagnosis is by paired sera for HI and N antibodies but there are cross reactions with other alphaviruses, Semliki Forest and o'nyong-nyong.

Epidemiology

There is a forest cycle involving monkeys (vervets and baboons) transmitted by *Ae. africanus* and other mosquitoes. Rodents may also be hosts since they show a transient viraemia on being inoculated with virus, while monkeys show a high viraemia.

O'NYONG-NYONG (ONN)

Geographical distribution

ONN is present in Uganda, Kenya, Tanzania and southern Sudan (Fig. 5.3).

Aetiology

ONN virus is an alphavirus closely related to CHIK.

Transmission

Anopheles funestus is the major vector but *Anopheles gambiae* is also involved (Table III.6, p. 1416).

Symptoms and signs

Natural history

ONN is an acute, self-limiting disease which is a purely human infection.

The *incubation period* is 8 days. Onset is abrupt with rigor and epistaxis; the fever settles rapidly (one-third afebrile). There is severe arthralgia involving the knees, elbows, wrists and ankles symmetrically and suffusion of the conjunctivae. On the fourth day an irritant pink maculopapular rash appears, beginning on the face and spreading to the limbs and trunk, which fades in a week. The cervical lymph glands are enlarged and the axillary and inguinal glands may also be affected. Recovery takes place within a week but joint pains may persist. There is a leukopenia with relative lymphocytosis.

Epidemiology

There is no animal reservoir and the cycle is purely man to man. Large epidemics occur when

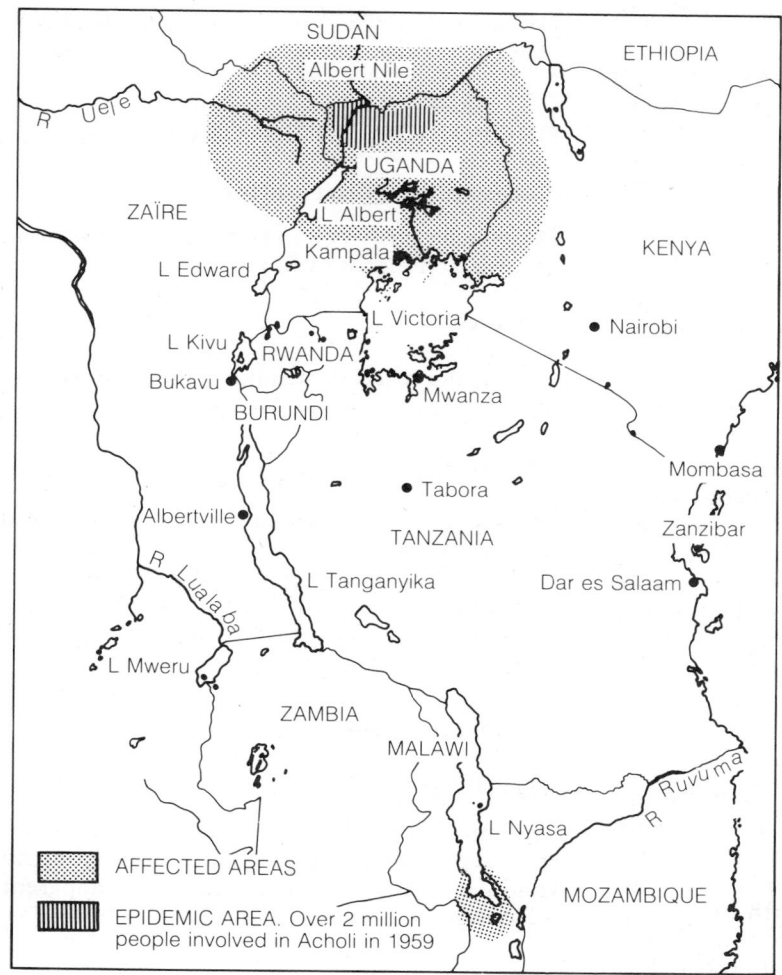

Fig. 5.3. Geographical distribution of o'nyong-nyong fever (courtesy Department of Entomology, London School of Hygiene and Tropical Medicine).

there are enough susceptible subjects, in which 70% of the population may be attacked with all the age groups affected.

Control

Wearing of mosquito nets and anti-*Anopheles funestus* measures will control the epidemics.

ROSS RIVER FEVER (EPIDEMIC POLYARTHRITIS)[9]

Geographical distribution

Ross River fever occurs annually in epidemics in northern and eastern Australia, and epidemically in Fiji, American Samoa, Cook Islands and New Caledonia. Antibody studies have shown infection to be present in New Guinea, Solomon Islands, the Moluccas and Vietnam.

Transmission

Transmission is by *Ae. vigilax* and *C. annulirostris* in Australia and *Ae. polynesiensis* in the Cook Islands. *Ae. aegypti* and *Ae. albopictus* are efficient experimental vectors (Table III.6, p. 1416, and Appendix III, p. 1424).

Pathology

Observation based on examination of joint fluids suggests that the virus multiplies in synovial cells.

Clinical features

Natural history

It is an acute self-limiting infection with arthritis lasting a week, mainly a human infection.

The *incubation period* is 3–9 days. Onset is abrupt with fever, myalgia and arthralgia. In 20% of cases there is an irritant maculopapular rash on the extremities and trunk. Knees, ankles and wrists are painful and swollen with joint effusions. Recovery occurs within a week but persistent arthritic pains may occur up to one year.

Diagnosis

HI antibodies appear in blood and joint fluid.

Epidemiology

The reservoir vertebrate hosts are unknown but wallabies are suspected. In epidemics the virus is spread from man to man and in Australia cases occur annually between summer and autumn. Explosive epidemics have occurred in Fiji, Samoa and the Cook Islands when the disease encountered a fresh non-immune population. Infection rates were 90% with 40% of the population showing clinical attacks.

MAYARO[10]

Mayaro virus causes an acute self-limiting dengue-like disease in South America. It is transmitted by *Haemagogus* mosquitoes and wild vertebrates maintain the virus in nature and amplify it. Epidemics have occurred in north and eastern South America affecting settlers along the Trans-Amazon Highway. There is a great potential for outbreaks among new immigrants and settlers opening up forested country (Table III.6, p. 1416).

SINDBIS[11]

Sindbis virus causes a self-limiting disease in South Africa with fever, diffuse papular rash and, in severer cases, vesicles on the feet from which virus has been recovered. It is transmitted by *C. univittatus*, *C. antennatus* and *C. perexiguus*. Migratory birds are involved in the spread of infection (Table III.6, p. 1416).

TAHYNA (LUMBO)

Tahyna virus causes a respiratory disease in Czechoslovakia and has been found in southern France. It is transmitted by mosquitoes (Table III.6, p. 1420).

OROPOUCHE VIRUS (ORO)[10]

Geographical distribution

Oropouche virus is a major cause of disease in the Amazon region of Brazil.

Aetiology

Oropouche virus is a member of the Simbu group of bunyaviruses (Table 5.1).

Transmission

The virus is transmitted to man as a zoonosis and thus from man to man by culicine mosquitoes, *A. serratus* and *C. quinquefasciatus*. The reservoir is sylvatic animals and ORO virus has been isolated from the three-toed sloth (*Bradypus tridactylus*) (Table III.6, p. 1420).

Clinical features

Natural history

The infection is short-lived with severe disease and aseptic meningitis in some cases[12] but no fatalities. There are a large number of inapparent infections.

Signs and symptoms

The onset is sudden with chills, headache, myalgia, arthralgia and photophobia being most common. There is a high fever which subsides rapidly although some of the patients suffer a relapse.

Diagnosis

A high level of antibody develops in the blood.

Epidemiology

The attack rate is twice as high in females as in males. The ORO virus circulates predominantly as a zoonosis in sylvatic animals but periodically is capable of causing severe urban epidemics when it is transmitted from man to man with *C. paraensis* the primary vector in these epidemics.

ROCIO VIRUS (ROC)

Rocio virus caused an outbreak in 1975 and 1976 in coastal areas of São Paulo state in Brazil. There were 825 cases with 95 deaths. It caused an illness with fever, headache and vomiting with signs of meningitis and encephalitis. The source of virus was wild birds and *Psorophora ferox* the vector (Appendix III, p. 1428).

SANDFLY FEVER (PHLEBOTOMUS FEVER, PAPPATACI FEVER)

Geographical distribution

Sandfly fever is widespread throughout the Mediterranean and Middle East, Malta, Aegean Islands, Egypt and Iran, North Africa, Red Sea and Arabian Gulf; in Asia in the Caucasus and Himalayas up to 4000 feet (Fig. 5.4).

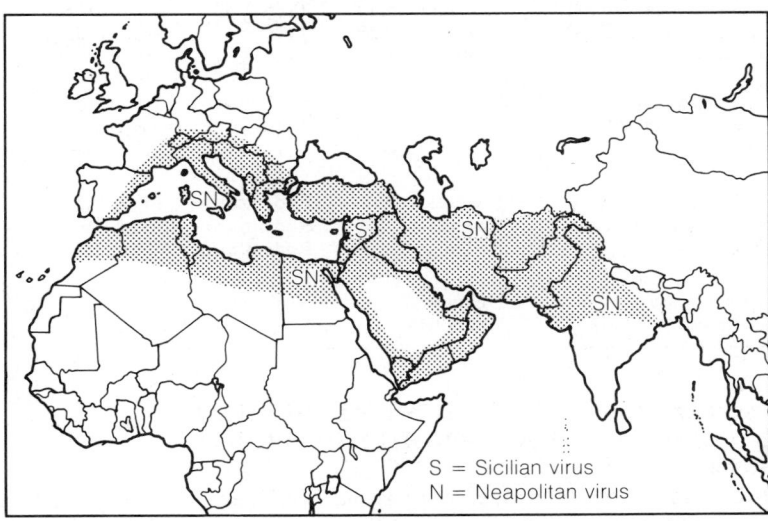

S = Sicilian virus
N = Neapolitan virus

Aetiology

The virus causing sandfly fever is a phlebovirus with eight antigenically distinct strains, only two of which—Sicilian and Neapolitan—cause human disease. The others have been isolated from insects and animals.[13]

Transmission

The sandfly responsible for transmission, *Phlebotomus papatasii* becomes infective 6 days after feeding and remains infective for life. Transovarial transmission occurs so that newly emerged sandflies are capable of transmitting infection. It is possible that a parasitic mite of the sandflies acts as a reservoir.

Clinical features

Natural history

It is an acute self-limiting disease lasting 2–4 days with complete recovery and immunity to further attacks, and no mortality.

The *incubation period* is 3–6 days.

Signs and symptoms

The onset is abrupt with high fever, congested face and neck stiffness. Ocular symptoms are marked with intense supraorbital pain and injected conjunctivae (papilloedema has been described). There is stiffness of limbs. After 3 days (2–8) the fever settles. Occasionally there is a recrudescence (saddle back fever) lasting for a

Fig. 5.4. Endemic areas of sandfly fever viruses (courtesy Wellcome Tropical Institute Museum).

day or two. There is a leukopenia. The cerebrospinal fluid (CSF) pressure is increased and there is a pleocytosis with raised protein.

Diagnosis

Paired sera for HI and N antibody tests are required. There is no specific treatment.

Epidemiology

There are no animal reservoirs. In endemic areas transmission lasts from April to October. Epidemics occur among non-immune entrants to the community, especially military forces.

VIRAL HAEMORRHAGIC FEVERS (VHF)

Viral haemorrhagic fevers are caused by a number of different viruses which may be arboviruses, arenaviruses or filoviruses. A list is given in Table 5.3. In the main these viruses cause mostly mild infections but all of them can cause severe and fatal disease with haemorrhagic manifestations, and some have caused devastating epidemics in South America and the Far East.

Other factors involved may be maturation, arrest of megakaryocytes in the bone marrow with platelet abnormalities and disseminated intravascular coagulation leading to fibrinogen depletion. Some viruses directly damage the cells of organs (e.g. hepatic necrosis in YF).

The management and immunology of viral haemorrhagic fevers is considered in general before describing each one in detail.

Table 5.3   Viral haemorrhagic fevers (VHF).

Arbovirus	Name of disease	Animal hosts	Transmission	Geographical area
Dengue virus	Dengue haemorrhagic fever (DHF)	Monkeys	Mosquitoes	Africa, Asia, America
Rift Valley fever virus	Rift Valley fever (RVF)	Various mammals	Mosquitoes	Africa
Yellow fever virus	Yellow fever (YF)	Monkeys	Mosquitoes	Africa, America
Omsk haemorrhagic fever virus	Omsk haemorrhagic fever (OHF)	Small mammals	Ticks	Asia, Siberia
Kyasanur Forest virus	Kyasanur Forest disease (KFD)	? rodents, monkeys	Ticks	Asia, India
Crimean–Congo haemorrhagic fever virus	Crimean–Congo haemorrhagic fever (C–CHF)	Small mammals	Ticks	Africa, Asia
Hantaan virus	Muroid virus nephropathy (MVN) (Haemorrhagic fever with renal syndrome) (HFRS)	Small rodents	Rodent saliva and urine	Asia, Europia, Africa
Puumala virus				
Arenaviruses				
Junin virus	Argentinian haemorrhagic fever	Rodents	Rodent urine	South America
Machupo virus	Bolivian haemorrhagic fever	Rodents	Rodent urine	South America
Lassa virus	Lassa fever	Rodents	Rodent urine	West Africa
Filoviruses				
Marburg virus	Marburg virus disease	Unknown	Nosocomial	Africa
Ebola virus	Ebola virus disease	Unknown	Nosocomial	Africa

The pathogenesis of these haemorrhagic features has been the subject of much research and may be caused by one or a combination of a number of factors. These factors are vascular damage, disorders of coagulation, immunopathology and direct damage to organs.

The viruses have a special affinity for the endothelium of capillaries and small vessels which are severely affected directly by the virus, resulting in an increased permeability. Complement activation with the formation of immune complexes which are deposited in the walls of small vessels further damages them, leading to capillary fragility (positive tourniquet test), and haemorrhage with bleeding from the mucous membranes, and even cerebral haemorrhage. Widespread haemorrhage produces hyperconcentration of the blood, hypovolaemia, hypoxia of the tissues, acidosis and hyperkalaemia which, with vomiting and dehydration, may lead to irreversible shock.

MANAGEMENT OF VIRAL HAEMORRHAGIC FEVER[14]

A case of possible VHF must be approached correctly from the start.

History

An accurate history must establish the symptoms, exact location of travel (cf. areas endemic for various VHFs) and, most important, specific contact with ill persons or their tissues and secretions and direct or indirect contact with local animals (except in the case of mosquito-borne VHF). An interval of three weeks between the last possible exposure and onset of illness rules out the diagnosis of VHF.

Symptoms

Many symptoms are non-specific but certain

specific symptoms will suggest VHF: pharyngitis, conjunctivitis, vomiting, diarrhoea, abdominal pain and, most important—haemorrhagic manifestations and shock.

Diagnosis

Rapid diagnosis is most important since it affects management of the case. Other febrile illnesses associated with shock and haemorrhage must be excluded: falciparum malaria, meningococcaemia, leptospirosis, typhus, septicaemia, plague, *Escherichia coli* septicaemia.

Extreme care must be taken in obtaining blood specimens since blood is highly infective in the first few days of viraemia. Specimens must be specially labelled so that their infectivity is clear.

Isolation

Care must be taken not to alarm the public. Although people in direct contact with patients, such as doctors, nurses and pathologists and technicians are at risk, further spread outside to the community at large does not occur except with mosquito-borne viruses.

Strict isolation, preferably under negative pressure or under a sealed tent with an anteroom where staff can don protective clothing, is necessary to protect the staff. Protective clothing includes masks and goggles. The patient should use a chemical toilet. In the case of possible mosquito-borne VHF, isolation under a mosquito net or in a mosquito-proof room is all that is necessary. Those working in the tropics will realize that much of the foregoing is impracticable. Experience has shown that *normal* barrier nursing techniques are sufficient to prevent transmission of these diseases in hospital.

Verification of diagnosis

Verification of diagnosis must first exclude other possible non-VHF causes. Specimens to be collected immediately are:

a throat swab;
a clean midstream specimen;
venous blood for antibody studies and virus isolation using a disposable needle and syringe which must be discarded in disinfectant immediately. A blood smear for malaria parasites is absolutely necessary but once fixed is safe to be examined. (See Appendix I, p. 1238.)

Convalescence

Most cases of VHF are over the infectious stage quite quickly but with arenaviruses virus can be excreted in the urine for a period of months following an attack.

Treatment

The careful management of fluid and electrolyte balance from the onset of disease is the most important facet of treatment.

Shock

Shock is a feature of many haemorrhagic fevers and the following treatment has been used for haemorrhagic dengue, and may be appropriate for other diseases leading to shock.[15] Treatment is supportive and good nursing is essential. Oxygen is useful at first. Water balance must be maintained at as near normal as possible. To restore fluids and electrolytes, infusion of 5% dextrose in half-strength normal saline, at the rate of 100 ml/kg body weight daily, is recommended. Or 10–15 ml of Ringer lactate solution/kg body weight (see below) may be infused intravenously for one hour, followed by a less concentrated electrolyte replacement fluid. Plasma or a substitute may be given to combat shock. Blood transfusion is not recommended in the hypotensive phase but may be given after recovery from shock if the patient shows signs of having had severe haemorrhage.

Hypovolaemia is usual and packed cell volume should therefore be watched; if it remains the same, or increases during replacement indicating loss of fluid to extracellular spaces, plasma should be given to maintain an adequate circulating blood volume, at the rate of 10–20 ml/kg/hour until the packed cell volume begins to decline.

In the hypotensive phase, hydrocortisone 50–100 mg daily, or aldosterone 0.1 mg/kg daily, in conjunction with the infusion fluid, may reduce mortality and sometimes has a dramatic effect. (Aldosterone raises blood pressure, conserves sodium and causes potassium to be excreted in the urine; it is therefore a rational treatment. The dose quoted is high.)

During recovery, when vascular fluid returns to the circulation, infusion of fluid should cease.

Ringer lactate solution contains approximately 131 mmol sodium, 5 mmol potassium, 4 mmol calcium, 29 mmol bicarbonate (as lactate) and 111 mmol chloride in each litre.

Some children with metabolic acidosis do not easily metabolize lactate and should therefore receive 1–2 ml/kg of 3.75% sodium bicarbonate solution intravenously every 10–15 minutes until improvement is noted.[16]

To control thrombocytopenic bleeding, transfusion of fresh human platelet concentrates is valuable. One unit of platelet concentrate is obtained from one pint of blood, and the dose used in Thai children ranged from 0.2 unit to 10 units/kg body weight.

Curative treatment

IMMUNE PLASMA

Although the efficacy of immune plasma obtained from a patient who has recovered has not yet been scientifically established, it appears to have benefited many. The immune plasma must be administered early in the illness, preferably in the first week. Later the presence of virus and naturally occurring antibody may cause the deposition of antigen–antibody complexes which in themselves cause pathological changes.

ANTIVIRAL DRUGS

Ribavirin if administered during the first week of illness has been of benefit in Lassa fever (p. 147) and Rift Valley fever (p. 134). Other possible antiviral drugs include interferon inducers.

CONTROL

Vector control

Vector control has been successful in some circumstances, for instance, during the construction of the Panama Canal when by strict discipline all collections of water capable of breeding *Ae. aegypti* (and vectors of malaria) were eliminated from the area. Similar methods were applied to cities and towns in South America under the threat of YF. When DDT was introduced, extensive use in Guyana and elsewhere soon eradicated *Ae. aegypti* and with it the threat of urban YF. In Africa, however, *Ae. aegypti* has recently shown resistance to DDT, and in some areas it is exophilic in habit, so that spraying dwellings with insecticide is ineffective. Forest mosquitoes, of course, are not susceptible to ordinary methods of spraying.

Tick control by residual insecticides has, however, achieved some success in the USSR. But the problems of vector control, especially in rural areas, are formidable.

IMMUNIZATION

Vaccines which have been developed for VHF are highly effective but are available only for YF, Rift Valley fever and Omsk haemorrhagic fever. For most other arbovirus diseases they are either experimental or can be used only in restricted groups of people, such as laboratory workers, in face of threat of outbreaks or in reservoir animals (e.g. pigs for JE), or are not yet available. The multiplicity of the viruses creates a difficulty, which may to some extent be reduced by the development of group vaccines where these give some cross protection.

Many vaccines have been developed for YF since Hindle and Aragão independently first used emulsions of organs from infected animals for that purpose. Hindle used a phenol–glycerin emulsion and later an emulsion treated with formalin after reduction of virulence by freezing.

Active immunity in YF is now provoked by vaccines consisting of virus selected by serial intracerebral passage in mice. Early vaccines were given along with specific immune human serum with the intention of preventing severe reactions, but some batches of the immune serum were found to carry the virus of hepatitis, and to cause that disease in the recipients; the method was therefore discontinued.

A more successful vaccine was derived from a highly virulent strain of YF virus isolated from an African named Asibi, in Ghana, and cultivated in vitro in mouse embryonic tissue. This procedure greatly reduced the viscerotropism of the strain without altering its neurotropism. The virus was then grown in tissue culture of minced chick embryos from which the central nervous system had been removed before mincing; after prolonged propagation in this medium it was found that neurotropism and viscerotropism were both greatly reduced, but the virus retained its antigenic properties. This was the famous vaccine 17D, still widely used and highly effective, giving protection for at least ten years, and only very rarely causing any untoward reaction. In 120 000 persons, mostly under 12 years old, vaccinated with 17D, only two developed meningoencephalitis. 17D is a live vaccine but it cannot be passed from person to person by mosquitoes.

Infants should preferably not be given YF vaccine before the age of nine months because of the somewhat greater risk of encephalitis below that age.

The French Dakar vaccine is a neurotropic virus. Of 1 880 000 persons vaccinated with this, 246 developed meningoencephalitis and 23 died.

These live vaccines all provoke active immunity, not so persistent as the immunity developed after natural infection, but nevertheless extremely effective for several years.

Immunization against YF is required by law before travellers are allowed into certain countries either for their own protection or to prevent the importation of the disease to areas where *Ae. aegypti* is present.

Apart from YF, vaccines have been produced against several arbovirus diseases, for use in animals (for instance horses) as well as in man.

Attenuated strains of VEE, Langat, West Nile and WEE viruses (some grown on chick embryo) have been developed, and the Langat vaccine may protect against Powassan, KFD and RSSE too. Strains of chikungunya, TBE, SLE, KFD, Rift Valley and CTF have been inactivated, some by formalin, and tested experimentally. For TBE the early brain vaccines gave meningoencephalitis, and were superseded by cell culture vaccines. Dengue and JE vaccines have also been devised. For various reasons these vaccines are not widely used.[17]

After vaccination against SLE, HI antibody appears in the first weeks, to a peak in the third week. CF antibody, which is more specific, appears in the second week to a peak in the second month. CF antibody was at a low titre at 18–22 months in one Florida outbreak, but neutralizing antibodies persisted; they tend to appear early.

Immunological phenomena may play a part in the pathogenesis of haemorrhagic fever and encephalitis, and this risk needs to be carefully considered in vaccinating against some arbovirus infections. Allergic encephalitis is one such risk.

DENGUE

Geographical distribution

Dengue has a worldwide tropical and subtropical distribution between 30° north and 40° south (Fig. 5.5). It is endemic in South-East Asia (types 1, 2, 3 and 4), the Pacific (type 2), West Africa (types 1 and 2), East Africa (type 2), Caribbean (types 1 and 4) and the Americas (types 2 and 3).

Aetiology

The dengue virus, a member of the flavivirus group, is an RNA virus, 17–25 mm in diameter, which can be grown in a variety of mosquitoes and tissue cultures. It possesses antigens which overlap with YF, JE and West Nile viruses and there are four serotypes (1, 2, 3 and 4), all of which can be involved in both classical dengue and dengue haemorrhagic fever. It can survive at 4°C for several weeks and −70°C for years. Dengue virus can be passed vertically in *Aedes* experimentally but the epidemiological sig-

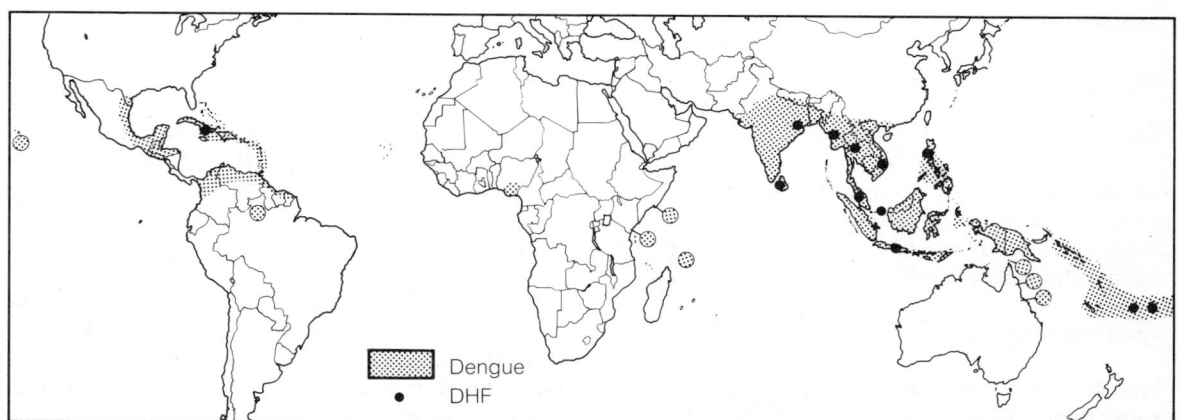

Fig. 5.5. Geographical distribution of dengue and dengue haemorrhagic fever (DHF) (courtesy Department of Entomology, London School of Hygiene and Tropical Medicine).

nificance of this is uncertain.

Transmission

Dengue is transmitted by mosquitoes (Appendix III, p. 1424). The classical type is transmitted worldwide by *Ae. aegypti* and by *Ae. albopictus* (Asia, Philippines and Japan); *Ae. polynesiensis*, *Ae. scutellaris* and *Ae. pseudoscutellaris* (Pacific Islands and New Guinea); *Ae. polynesiensis* (Society Islands) and *Ae. niveus* (Philippines) (see also Table III.6, p. 1417). Mosquitoes can be infected from the onset until the fourth day of illness and become infective from 8 to 11 days after feeding, remaining infective for life. Transovarial transmission of all four dengue viruses by *Ae. albopictus* has been demonstrated.[9]

Pathology

After inoculation the virus reaches the regional lymph glands and disseminates to the reticuloendothelial system in which it multiplies and from which it seeds the blood. In classical dengue changes can be seen in the skin where there is swelling of the endothelium of small blood vessels and perivascular infiltration with mononuclear cells.

Immunity

Immunity is antibody mediated and after recovery there is a long-standing immunity to the homologous strain but none to other serotypes or other flaviviruses although some common antigens are possessed.

Clinical features

The *incubation period* is 2–7 days.

Natural history

Classical dengue is a short-lived infection with complete recovery and is not usually fatal but under certain circumstances it can cause a severe haemorrhagic fever which can be fatal.

Symptoms and signs

The onset is sudden with high fever (40°C) which is biphasic. Severe muscle pains ('break bone fever'), headache and prostration are characteristic. After an early erythematous rash, a few days later a morbilliform or scarlatiniform rash appears beginning on the extremities, accompanied by generalized lymphadenopathy. The liver is moderately enlarged and there is a profound leukopenia. The second febrile phase lasts 2–3 days and the rash then desquamates. Convalescence is long and may be accompanied by tachycardia, general debility and often severe mental depression. Classical dengue is seldom fatal.

Diagnosis

Virus isolation in the early stages is achieved by inoculation of cell cultures: LLC-MK2 or Vero cells, cells of *Ae. albopictus*, *Ae. pseudoscutellaris*, or live mosquitoes (*Ae. aegypti*), inoculated intrathoracically and examined after 7–14 days by immunofluorescence. The type can be identified by CF or N tests or immunofluorescence with type specific monoclonal antibodies. The early stages must be distinguished from malaria and hepatitis. Chikungunya, sandfly fever and Rift Valley fever closely resemble dengue, but without the rash.

Serological diagnosis

The HI test performed on acute stage serum taken in the first 4 days and convalescent serum taken two to three weeks later will show a fourfold increase to one or more of the four serotype antigens. Neutralization tests will distinguish clearly between the four serotypes.

Treatment

The treatment is symptomatic only.

Complications

Encephalopathies have been associated with proven dengue in Indonesia.[18] Dengue haemorrhagic fever is considered later.

Epidemiology

A jungle cycle of dengue involving forest mosquitoes and wild monkeys has been postulated in Malaya and West Africa where antibodies have been found in monkeys, the significance of which is not yet clear.

Dengue fever epidemics involve many thousands of cases with attack rates of 75–80% completely disrupting the life of communities. These epidemics result from the introduction of a new serotype or the availability of a susceptible population (immigrants and young persons born since the last epidemic). These epidemics have swept up the Caribbean and eastern seaboard of the Americas and up the eastern shores of East Africa involving the islands. More recently dengue has caused vast epidemics in South-East Asia.

Control

Control of dengue rests upon vector control, mainly the domestic breeding of *Ae. aegypti* in domestic water containers. The *Aedes* index can be used to monitor the population of mosquitoes and hence foresee outbreaks and institute proper vector control. A satisfactory vaccine has yet to be developed, but for dangers, see below in section on dengue haemorrhagic fever.

DENGUE HAEMORRHAGIC FEVER (DHF)

Geographical distribution

DHF is a perennial problem in South-East Asia where it is a major cause of child morbidity and mortality. DHF has also appeared in Cuba, the Caribbean[19] and in the Pacific (Fiji). So far DHF has not been documented from Africa.

Aetiology

The cause is still not clear. Halstead[20] proposed the concept of two sequential infections with different dengue serotypes, the first infection sensitizing the patient to the second, producing a severe response which has been shown to be immunologically mediated and involving the complement system. A critical period of about six months between the two infections has been thought to be necessary. This view is supported by experience in Fiji which suffered outbreaks of dengue in 1971 and 1972 with the occurrence of haemorrhagic fever in people of all ages and in expatriates. There had been no dengue in Fiji for 30 years.[22–24] (Rosen[21] has suggested that an abnormally virulent strain of virus might be responsible.)

Pathology

The basic pathological change responsible for

DHF is increased capillary permeability leading to rapid shifts of extracellular fluid, allied to fluid depletion from decreased intake and increased loss resulting in haemoconcentration, hypovolaemia, reduced tissue perfusion and oxygenation, acidosis and widespread cellular damage leading to shock. The capillary leakage is most likely caused immunologically by the activation of complement by dengue antigen–antibody complexes which may also initiate disseminated intravascular coagulation. The *liver* shows mid-zonal hyaline or acidophilic necrosis of parenchymal liver cells and Kupffer's cells, with the appearance of Councilman lesions. The *kidneys* rarely show glomerulonephritis, probably due to immune complexes. There is a *reticuloendothelial* reaction (proliferation of lymphocytes, plasmacytoid cells and increase in phagocytosis), maturation arrest of *megakaryocytes* and hypocellularity of the bone marrow. Capillary damage results in leakage of fluid, plasma and erythrocytes into interstitial spaces and serous cavities causing pleural and peritoneal effusions, and retroperitoneal oedema. Haemorrhages are not generally severe but major gastrointestinal bleeding may appear in adolescents and adults.

Immunity

The immune status of the host is the important component which determines the development of DHF. The presence of non-neutralizing antibodies to a heterologous serotype can cause 'immune enhancement' of dengue virus growth in lymphoid cells with the release of factors increasing capillary permeability. There is a strong association of this process with a second infection on a prior exposure to another serotype or, in the case of infants, to the presence of maternal antibody to suggest that this is a cause, but it is possible that a more virulent strain might do it on its own (see section on aetiology, above).

Clinical features

On the second to fifth days of a classical dengue illness at the end of the first phase the patient deteriorates rapidly with development of the shock syndrome. Restlessness, sweating, hypotension appear and coincident with a positive tourniquet test petechiae, ecchymoses and spontaneous haemorrhages. There is tender enlargement of the liver in some cases with hypoproteinaemia, hyponatraemia, mild elevation of the liver enzymes and some nitrogen retention. The presence of disseminated intravascular coagulation is shown by the alteration in clotting factors and reduced fibrinogen. Without treatment, 50% of the patients die, but with treatment the mortality is reduced to 5% and recovery is usually rapid.

Diagnosis

A positive tourniquet test or spontaneous haemorrhages, thrombocytopenia and evidence of haemoconcentration (plus 20% or more) are the diagnostic criteria for DHF.

Serology

The CF and HI tests will be positive to all strains of dengue but neutralizing antibodies to both the primary and secondary infection will be raised, whereas to the other serotypes will be negative; thus each of the causative serotypes of dengue can be identified.[25]

Treatment

This is discussed in section on management of VHF (p. 128). Isolation of the patient is not necessary except that mosquitoes should be excluded by mosquito nets or screens. Care, however, must be taken to prevent contamination with blood in the few days of the illness during the period of viraemia.

Epidemiology

DHF in South-East Asia affects mainly indigenous young children. Adults and expatriates will develop classical dengue but escape DHF. Foreign residents living in good conditions in Bangkok with piped water tend to escape. An outbreak of DHF which started in Manila in 1963 then invaded Thailand (150 000–200 000 cases) and South Vietnam.

Control

Control measures are those applied to classical dengue fever. Immunization with vaccines presents a problem since an individual with antibodies to one serotype runs the danger of developing DHF when infected with another serotype.

RIFT VALLEY FEVER (RVF)

Geographical distribution

Rift Valley fever was first recognized in Kenya in 1931 as causing disease in sheep and man. Until 1977 it was restricted to man and domestic animals in sub-Saharan Africa with epizootics in Kenya, South Africa, Zimbabwe, Sudan, Uganda, Tanzania and Zambia. A similar virus (Zinga virus) was found to be present in West Africa (Mali, Nigeria and Zaire) and in Botswana and Mozambique but without epizootics. In 1977 RVF spread to Egypt where it caused massive epidemics and epizootics and showed a capability to spread beyond sub-Saharan Africa (Fig. 5.6).

Aetiology

RVF is a member of the genus phlebovirus of the family Bunyaviridae (Table 5.1). The virus is spherical, 90–110 nm in diameter, with a lipid envelope from which glycoprotein spikes protrude and can be found in host membrane systems. Two strains of the virus have been found: RVF and Zinga virus, which have been shown to be the same virus by the neutralization test.[26]

Pathology

The pathogenesis of RVF is still not clear but is thought to be a direct effect of the virus of increased virulence on cells, or a sensitization phenomenon similar to that seen in dengue, or some form of synergism between the virus and endemic schistosomiasis.

The pathology closely resembles that of YF. The liver is the main organ affected with midzonal hyaline changes leading to necrosis and bodies resembling the Councilman bodies of YF. The kidney tubules and spleen show toxic changes and there are haemorrhages in all the viscera. The causes of these changes are a vasculitis from viral infection of endothelial cells and antigen–antibody immune complexes. Encephalitis and extensive retinal changes may also be found.

Transmission

Transmission between the zoonotic hosts is by mosquitoes of the *Eretmapodites*, *Coquillettidiae* (Appendix III, p. 1431), *Mansonia*, *Aedes* and

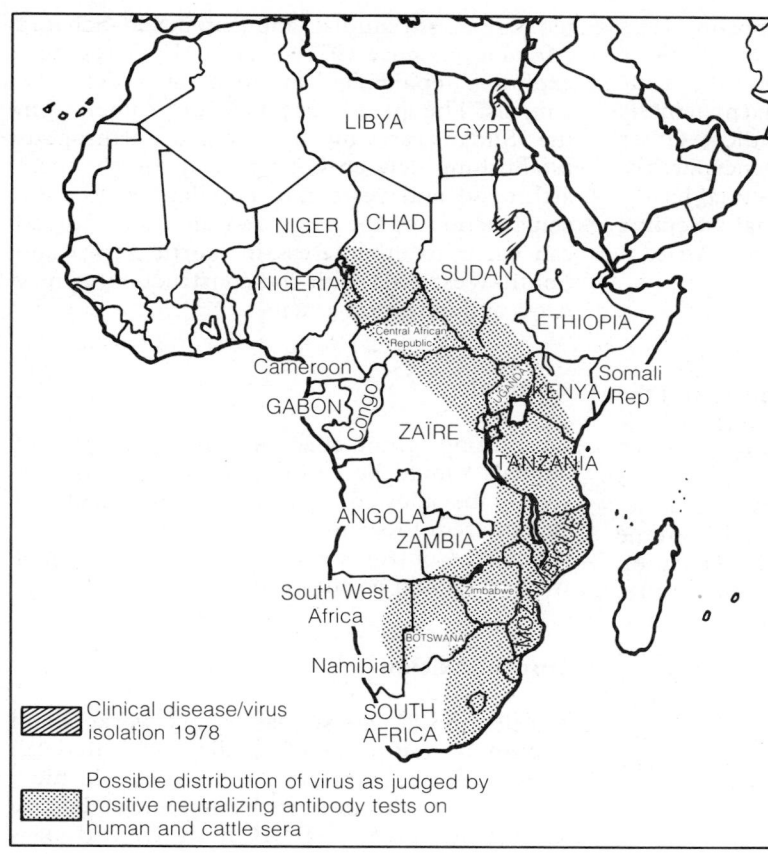

Fig. 5.6. Geographical distribution of Rift Valley fever (courtesy Department of Entomology, London School of Hygiene and Tropical Medicine).

Culex groups, (Table III.6, p. 1420, and Appendix III, p. 1424) and possibly to man by *A. caballus* and *C. theileri* in South Africa and *C. pipiens* in Egypt. Direct transmission, especially during epidemics, is by the aerosol route from infected animal tissues. Person-to-person transmission does not occur but acute phase blood as well as infected animals are highly infectious, especially in abattoirs.

Immunity

Active immunity

Immunity is antibody mediated and there is prolonged immunity to reinfection with the homologous strains after recovery. Antibodies formed are of the usual viral response (HI, CF and N). HI and CF antibodies are used in diagnosis whereas N antibodies give specificity.

Passive immunity

A passive immunity can be transferred via the placenta to the child which lasts for several months and the possession of antibodies, especially N antibodies, can be used in treatment using convalescent sera.

Clinical features

Natural history

RVF is a self-limiting disease in the great majority of infections with a short, acute febrile phase with complete recovery but, in less than 5% of cases, complications—haemorrhagic and encephalitic—can occur with fatal results.

Symptoms and signs[27]

The *incubation period* is 3–7 days. The onset is abrupt with fever, headache, joint and muscle pains and photophobia. In the majority of cases this is followed by complete recovery. In a few cases there may be recrudescence of symptoms after the initial short illness and convalescence may be prolonged. In a small proportion (less than 5% in the Egyptian epidemic) the illness is much more severe with the onset of haemorrhagic manifestations (purpura, haematemesis and melaena) and liver failure (jaundice). Other complications include meningoencephalitis, ocular involvement with retinitis, retinal haemorrhages and blindness due to retinal vasculitis and retinal detachment (South Africa,[28] Zimbabwe,[29] Egypt[30]).

Diagnosis

When cases of fever present in numbers and the three complications—haemorrhage, encephalitis and blindness—occur then there is a strong indication that these are cases of RVF, especially if associated with an epizootic in sheep and cattle. Isolation of virus within the first 7 days from the blood can be done by intracerebral inoculation into baby mice, and most kinds of cell culture. Serological diagnosis is by the HI test on paired sera, using a standard antigen from the World Health Organization.[31] Other tests are CF, agar gel diffusion, immunofluorescence and ELISA. The detection of N antibodies are diagnostic for RVF since there is no cross reaction between these antibodies and other phleboviruses.

Treatment

Cases should be managed as in all VHFs. Isolation from mosquitoes must be enforced and attendants should be protected from infected blood in the early stages. Symptomatic treatment is that of other VHFs (see p. 129). There is as yet no curative drug but laboratory experiments suggest that interferon inducers, antiviral drugs (ribavirin) or immune serum could be useful, and convalescent serum from cases of RVF who have recovered should certainly be used in severe cases.

Epidemiology

RVF is maintained in the forest in an enzootic fashion in an as yet poorly understood maintenance cycle. Rodents have been thought to be responsible but no viral isolations, only antibodies, have been found. Spectacular epizootics in domestic animals are the result of large numbers of susceptible (European) breeds of cattle and sheep, high arthropod densities and spillover from the forest cycle. Originally restricted to domestic animals and man in sub-Saharan Africa it has since 1977 spread to Egypt causing explosive epidemics in man and domestic animals. The spread was possibly by camels from the Sudan carrying infection or arthropods establishing new enzootic foci in the changing arthropod and vertebrate population after the construction of the High Aswan Dam. Spread can occur to other areas in North Africa and South-West Asia with the construction of new dams and irrigation schemes.[32,33]

Control

Quarantine is not effective but movements of animals should be controlled and sick animals should be allowed to die or recover and not slaughtered, to avoid spreading the infection in abattoirs. Control of abattoirs and vaccination of workers should be enforced.

Immunization

Vaccination of exposed laboratory workers and veterinary staff using a formalin-inactivated cell culture vaccine (expensive) should be performed.

Veterinary vaccines are the first line of defence against the spread of RVF. Both live and inactivated vaccines have been used to control the spread in animals with some success.[34]

YELLOW FEVER (YF)

Geographical distribution

Yellow fever is found in the tropical forest areas of Africa and South America (Fig. 5.7) and until early in this century caused large epidemics in the Caribbean and the subtropical and temperate regions of North America as far north as Baltimore and Philadelphia. 'Jungle' YF still occurs in Brazil and there was an outbreak in Trinidad in 1978–1979 with 18 cases and eight deaths. Many other epidemics have occurred in South America, and a large epidemic in Ethiopia was responsible for many deaths in 1960–1962, and in Senegal in 1965–1966. YF has caused fatalities in tourists, especially in West Africa, who have not been vaccinated.

West Africa was probably the original home of YF, which may have been transported to the

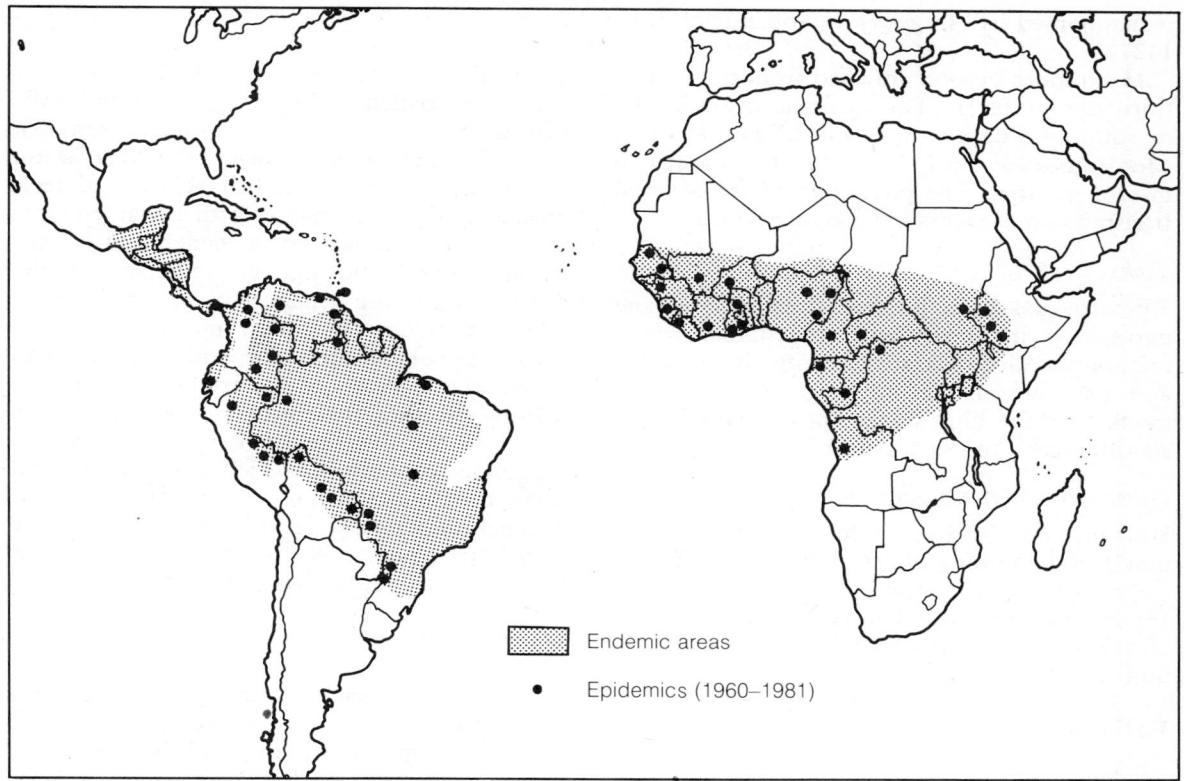

Fig. 5.7. Geographical distribution of yellow fever.

Americas by ships carrying infected mosquitoes in the post-Columbian period. YF has never been established in Europe, Asia or Australasia although potential vectors (*Ae. aegypti* in South-East Asia) abound, so that if it were introduced into Asia catastrophic epidemics could occur.

Aetiology

Yellow fever is a flavivirus (Table 5.1) 25–65 nm in size which can survive at 4°C for a month and freeze dried for many years. It can be grown on a variety of vertebrate cell cultures, chick or mouse embryo, KB or HeLa cell cultures with a cytopathic effect. There are seven strains which can infect man. Freshly isolated strains which are pantropic lose viscerotropism in the chick embryo. African strains of yellow fever possess an antigen absent from American strains and the 17D strain which is so successfully used as a live vaccine has acquired an antigen absent from the original 'Asibi' strain from which it was developed.[2]

Transmission

Mosquitoes (Table III.6, p. 1418, and Appendix III, p. 1428)

In nature YF is transmitted by mosquitoes of several genera. In the Americas the forest cycle is maintained by *Haemagogus spegazzinii* as the principal vector with *Haemagogus leucocelaenus*, *Haemagogus janthinomys* (= *falco*) and *Sabethes chloropterus* also involved. *Ae. aegypti* is responsible for urban outbreaks. Virus has also been isolated from *Ae. fulvus* in Brazil. In Africa *Ae. africanus* maintains the monkey–mosquito–monkey cycle in the forest, while *Ae. simpsoni*, which breeds close to man in the axils of plants (bananas), becomes infected from monkeys raiding the plantations, and transmits YF to man. Other *Aedes* involved in the forest cycle are *Ae. vittatus*, *Ae. luteocephalus*, *Ae. metallicus* and *Ae. taylori* from which evidence of transovarial transmission has been obtained under natural conditions in Senegal, suggesting an ideal vector for transmission among monkeys.[35] The urban cycle is maintained by *Ae. aegypti* (Appendix III, p. 1427).

Mosquitoes become infected from the first to third day of fever. The intrinsic cycle in the mosquito is 4 days at 37°C and 18 days at 18°C. Mosquitoes remain infected for life, about two to four months. The possibility of transovarial transmission has already been mentioned.

Ticks

YF virus has been isolated from *Amblyomma variegatum* in Brazil and transstadial transmission was demonstrated by infecting nymphs and passing on the infection to uninfected monkeys at the adult stage. The epidemiological significance of this is not clear.[36]

Other methods of transmission

Human blood is infective in the first 3 days of illness and handling of infected monkeys in the early stages of viraemia could cause infection. Interhuman transmission is unimportant but laboratory work with infected monkeys and mosquitoes can be dangerous.

Pathology

There is no evidence of any immune reactions influencing the pathogenesis of YF. The virus affects highly specialized epithelial or myocardial cells only; stroma cells are not involved. The changes are toxic, beginning with cloudy swelling and going on to degenerative fatty changes and coagulative necrosis. There is no inflammatory response.

Liver

Typical lesions may not be found in biopsy specimens from patients who later recover and serological evidence is necessary for diagnosis in such cases. In fatal cases, however, the liver is not shrunken; it may be reddish yellow and feels greasy. The typical lesions form a characteristic triad: microglobular fatty degeneration of epithelial liver cells throughout the hepatic lobule; dissociation of the hepatic lobule, most marked in the mid-zone (but some normal liver cells always remain around the central zone); and coagulative necrosis of the epithelial liver cells mainly affecting the mid-zone (Fig. 5.8). The nuclei of the liver cells are pyknotic and the coagulated contents of the cells stain deeply with eosin, the Councilman bodies resulting from this degeneration taking on a salmon-pink colour (Fig. 5.9). Under low power a stained section looks as if red pepper has been scattered on it.

Other organs

The lesions are variable: some degree of nephritis or nephrosis (with transient proteinuria in mild cases), adrenal lesions, lesions of the heart (fatty changes, even in the sinoatrial node and the bundle of His, corresponding with the clinical bradycardia) and lesions of the brain (perivascular haemorrhages). In the kidneys there are fatty changes with necrosis of tubular epithelium and casts in both cortex and medulla. Encephalitis was not formerly thought to be part of the picture of naturally occurring YF, but men-

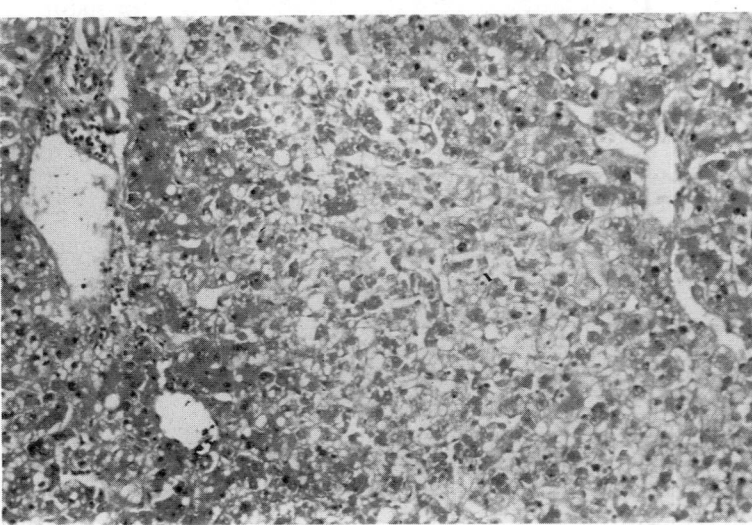

Fig. 5.8. Post-mortem appearance of the liver of a rhesus monkey with yellow fever, showing well-marked mid-zonal necrosis and minimal inflammatory changes.

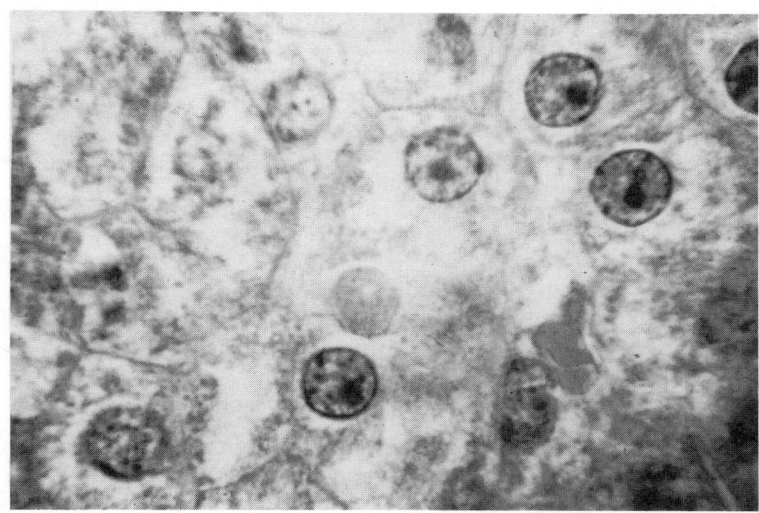

Fig. 5.9. Councilman body in the liver cell of a rhesus monkey affected with yellow fever.

ingoencephalitis was a dominant feature of the epidemic of 1960 in the Sudan and Ethiopia. Severe haemorrhages may take place in the digestive system, the internal cavities, the lungs (common), liver, spleen and kidneys. Death results from failure of the liver or kidneys or both, though cardiac damage may contribute. Patients who recover show complete replacement of lost tissue by direct regeneration and hypertrophy of surviving cells.

Immunity

Immunity is antibody mediated and lifelong immunity follows infection with YF virus. In many endemic areas where contact with virus-carrying mosquitoes is constant, i.e. near the forest, infection is common in childhood leading to a solid immunity. The immunity is antibody mediated, HF and N antibodies being found from the end of the first week of infection.

Clinical features

Natural history

In the majority of cases the infection is short and sharp with full recovery. Inapparent infections, especially in endemic areas, are common leading to the apparent freedom from infection of the indigenous inhabitants, in contrast to new arrivals, immigrants or armies. In a minority of cases and in epidemics the infection is severe with biphasic fever, jaundice and severe haem-

orrhages leading to the 'black vomit' with a high mortality. This illness was known in the eighteenth and nineteenth centuries as the 'yellow jack'.

Symptoms and signs

The *incubation period* is 3–6 days. The spectrum of infection varies from the mild abortive case (the majority) to the more severe classic case of YF (only 10–20% of cases).

Mild case

An acute febrile illness with sudden onset of fever and headache without other symptoms lasting 48 hours or less. In some other patients the headache is more severe accompanied by myalgia and slight proteinuria. The characteristic bradycardia in relation to the temperature (Faget's sign) is present and the illness may last several days with recovery.

Haemorrhagic fever

PERIOD OF INFECTION

This is the period of viraemia and lasts 3 days. There is an abrupt onset with fever up to 40°C, chills, severe headache, nausea, vomiting, abdominal pain and distressing pain in the back, loins and limbs. The patient is dehydrated with a dry tongue and foul breath. There is a yellow tint in the conjunctivae which deepens with the appearance of jaundice in the skin. Minor gingival haemorrhages or epistaxis may occur. Despite a rising temperature the pulse may decrease and Faget's sign, a falling pulse with a constant temperature or a constant pulse with a rising temperature, is present.

PERIOD OF CALM
A short period of calm follows the initial fever and in milder cases recovery may take place. This period lasts several hours to a day.

PERIOD OF RECRUDESCENCE
Viraemia is now absent and antibodies appear. The fever returns and the patient's condition deteriorates rapidly. Hepatorenal failure develops. The abdominal pain continues and the patient vomits altered blood ('coffee-ground' or 'black vomit') or fresh blood. There is melaena and diarrhoea may be present with fresh blood in the stools. Bleeding may take place from eyes, nose, mouth, bladder, rectum and other organs.

HEPATIC INVOLVEMENT
Jaundice becomes evident (but is never so deep as in relapsing fever or hepatitis) and the liver function tests deteriorate. There is no splenic enlargement.

RENAL INVOLVEMENT
There is a heavy proteinuria with a tendency to suppression of urine and granular casts and haemoglobin can be found in the urine with azotaemia.

MYOCARDIAL INVOLVEMENT
There can be hypotension and hypokinetic heart failure, and S-T segmental changes are commonly seen in the electrocardiogram. The patient may recover rapidly after a period of 3–4 days or longer over two weeks. Death occurs on the seventh to tenth day of illness. Bad prognostic signs are increasing proteinuria, haemorrhages, a rising pulse, hypotension, oliguria and azotaemia.

CENTRAL NERVOUS SYSTEM (CNS) INVOLVEMENT
Signs that the CNS is affected suggest meningitis or encephalitis and include slurred speech, nystagmus, incoordination of movements with tremor of hands and limbs, and brisk tendon reflexes. There may be convulsions and sudden death. If the patient recovers from a severe attack convalescence tends to be long but usually without sequelae. Late deaths after con-

valescence are very rare and are related to myocardial damage, cardiac arrhythmia or cardiac failure. Suppurative parotitis and bacterial pneumonia may complicate the disease.

LABORATORY FINDINGS
There is a leukopenia with thrombocytopenia and prolonged clotting and prothrombin times.

Liver. Liver enzymes (SGOT, SGPT) are elevated in jaundiced patients (but not in non-jaundiced patients) and peak between the fifth and tenth day, returning to normal by the tenth to twentieth day. There may be hypoglycaemia associated with severe liver damage.

Renal. At first the urine contains a small amount of albumin which increases on the fourth or fifth day reaching levels of 3–5 g/litre. There is biliuria.

CNS. The CSF is clear without cells but may be under increased pressure with slightly elevated protein.

Diagnosis

The diagnosis has to be made from other haemorrhagic fevers without jaundice (Lassa, Ebola, Marburg, Junin, Machupo) and with jaundice from Rift Valley fever. Other conditions which must be distinguished are falciparum malaria, louse-borne relapsing fever, infectious hepatitis and leptospirosis. A dictum worth remembering is that an epidemic of a fatal disease in which jaundice is so noteworthy as to be remarked upon is *not* one of YF but more likely relapsing fever or infectious hepatitis. Fever and heavy proteinuria is suggestive. Virus can be isolated from the blood in the first 3 days with detection of virus by ELISA.

Serological diagnosis

IFA, HI and N antibodies appear within one week of onset and CF antibodies later. Paired acute and convalescent sera showing a rising titre are diagnostic. There are cross reactions with other flaviviruses but N antibodies are specific. Background immunity in tropical populations can render serodiagnosis difficult.

Liver biopsy

Formerly the presence of Councilman bodies in

a liver biopsy was considered specific for YF but their presence in other VHFs, such as Rift Valley fever makes this no longer certain.

Management and treatment

The only isolation necessary is from mosquito bites and the patients should be nursed in a screened environment. Blood is infectious in the first 3 days. Treatment is as for other VHFs (see p. 129).

Epidemiology

There are two cycles: the forest cycle (jungle yellow fever) and the urban cycle (urban yellow fever) (Fig. III.34, p. 1427).

Forest cycle (jungle yellow fever)

AMERICA

YF virus is maintained probably in rodents (experimental infections have been recorded in the spiny rat *Proechimys dimidiatus* and *Heteromys* with persistent viraemia), maintained by *Haemagogus* mosquitoes as the principal vector. Recurrent epizootics occur in howler (*Alouatta*) monkeys who die in large numbers, starting in Panama and spreading up the east coast of Central America to Guatemala, confirming the belief recorded by Balfour in 1914 that a 'silent forest' where all the howler monkeys had died denoted the presence of YF.

AFRICA

In the forests of West, central and East Africa a jungle cycle exists as an inapparent infection in monkeys, mainly *Cercopithecus* (vervet) monkeys. Other susceptible primates with inapparent infections include colobus (important in Ethiopia), mangabeys (*Cercocebus*) and baboons (*Papio*). In East Africa some species of bushbaby (*Galago*) which are susceptible to the virus have been shown to possess antibodies in nature, suggesting that the virus may circulate in these nocturnal animals transmitted by other ectoparasites, and passed on to susceptible primates and thence to man.[37]

HUMAN INFECTION

Human infection occurs because of ecological changes created by man. In Africa by cutting down the forest and planting banana plantations, bringing monkeys into contact with *Ae. simpsoni*,

a plant axil breeder which passes the infection on to man. In the Americas humans contract the disease by engaging in woodcutting and *Haemagogus* mosquitoes bite in and around houses in forest clearings. *Sabethes* (a drought-resistant mosquito) transmits infection during the dry season (Appendix III, p. 1432).

An endemic area population will show a rising percentage of positive antibody tests with age, whereas an epidemic situation will be shown by antibodies in the older age and none in the younger age groups.

Urban cycle

When there is a high population of *Ae. aegypti*, intense transmission among humans occurs with large epidemics where there are enough non-immunes in the population, which can be brought about by immigration, or a rising number of people born since the last epidemic. Up to the early years of this century huge epidemics of this nature frequently spread throughout the Caribbean and up the east coast of North America. These epidemics of 'yellow jack' terrified the inhabitants. Similar epidemics occurred in the 'White Man's Grave' in West Africa. Once *Ae. aegypti* was controlled these epidemics became a thing of the past and no urban cases of yellow fever have been described from the Americas for the past 40 years.

However, *Ae. simpsoni* spreading up wooded valleys in an otherwise deforested environment can come into contact with man with resulting epidemics. In the Nuba mountains of southern Sudan in 1940 there was an epidemic (17 000 cases, 10% mortality rate) and in south-western Ethiopia along the Omo river in 1960–1962 (15 000–30 000 deaths, mortality rate up to 85%). In 1965–1966 in Senegal there was an epidemic mainly affecting children under 10 years with a mortality rate of 15%. Mass vaccination had been suspended in 1960.

Control

Urban cycle

Eradication and control of *Ae. aegypti* is the key to the prevention of urban YF. This includes an attack on the breeding sites in water containers and tanks and an *Aedes* monitoring system which gives an *Aedes* index of the numbers of *Aedes* mosquitoes. When this reaches a certain height an epidemic can result. In the presence of an epidemic, adult control by 'fogging' of towns and cities with insecticide will bring the epidemic to a halt. *Ae. aegypti* had been eradicated from the USA but has now returned to Louisiana, a previous hotbed of YF, in its previous numbers.

Vaccination

Yellow fever 17D is a safe, live, attenuated vaccine providing a long-lasting immunity. For purposes of certificates 10 years is considered the limit but immunity after 40 years has been documented and may be lifelong. Vaccination to YF is imperative for travellers to endemic areas and certificates are demanded for travellers from endemic areas to non-infected tropical areas. Immunity develops within 10 days after vaccination. No serious complications have been found. No consequences for the fetus have been recorded but pregnant women should avoid vaccination unless the risk from yellow fever is considered great. Infants under one year of age should not be vaccinated unless this is unavoidable, because they have a slight risk of developing encephalitis. The vaccine is prepared in chick embryos and persons sensitive to egg protein may have reactions. The French neurotropic vaccine produced in mouse brain, used in parts of Africa, has caused allergic encephalomyelitis among children. A general decline in the incidence of 'jungle' YF has resulted from the mass vaccination programme in Brazil using 17D vaccine.

OMSK HAEMORRHAGIC FEVER (OHF)

Geographical distribution

OHF occurs in the Omsk area of Siberia.

Aetiology

The virus of OHF is a flavivirus (Table 5.1) separable into two subgroups: (1) isolated from human blood and (2) isolated from *Dermacentor marginatus*. The virus can be grown on HeLa cells or chick embryos.

Transmission

The virus is harboured by ticks—*D. pictus (reticulatus)* and *D. marginatus*—with transstadial and transovarial transmission. The ticks transmit the infection to man from rodents, mainly musk-rats (Appendix III, p. 1392). The mechanism of inter-rodent transmission in nature is not known but mites may transmit the infection between musk-rats and other rodents. Infection by direct contact with musk-rat carcasses and pelts is common, and interhuman transmission occurs. There is some evidence of infection by the respiratory route.

Pathology

The pathology of fatal cases is that of VHF with haemorrhage in tissues and necrotic areas in the liver. Immunity is antibody mediated; little is known about second attacks.

Clinical features

OHF is essentially a self-limiting acute infection in the majority of cases. Little is known about the occurrence of inapparent infections.

The *incubation period* is 3–7 days.

Symptoms and signs

The onset is abrupt with fever and a papulovesicular eruption on the soft palate followed by haemorrhagic features, epistaxis, melaena and uterine haemorrhage. The fever lasts 5 days and then remits with recovery and there is a leukopenia. Sometimes the fever is biphasic recurring for 2–3 days. Complete recovery is usual with a fatality rate of 1–3%. There is no CNS involvement.

Diagnosis

Virus can be isolated from the blood in the febrile period. Serological diagnosis is made by the CF and HI tests.

Epidemiology and control

The reservoir of infection is the musk-rat and ticks. Human infection depends upon musk-rat human contact which may be via tick or the handling of musk-rat carcasses and pelts. When there is a great mortality of musk-rats then contact is greater and outbreaks occur.

Vaccination

A formalized mouse brain vaccine has been developed and should be used to protect those at risk such as trappers and water course workers.

KYASANUR FOREST DISEASE (KFD)

Local synonym: 'Monkey disease'

Geographical distribution (Fig. 5.14)

KFD was first described in 1957 in the Kyasanur Forest of Mysore (now Karnataka).[39] Small outbreaks occurred in the Shimoga district in 1958–1971 and since 1972 there have been small local outbreaks now invading North Kanara district.

Aetiology

KFD virus is a flavivirus (Table 5.1) antigenically related to TBE, Langat, OHF and West Nile viruses but there is no cross immunity. The virus can be grown in suckling mice, hamster or monkey kidney cells or HeLa cells with cytopathic effect.

Transmission

KFD virus is transmitted by the nymphal stages of ticks which have been infected in the larval stage from a rodent or monkey. The ticks are *Haemaphysalis spinigera*, *H. turturis* and *H. papuana* (*kinneari*). KFD virus is also carried by *Ixodes petauristae* and *I. ceylonensis* and has been recovered from *Dermacentor* nymphs. KFD is not normally transmitted from person to person but the blood is potentially infective up until the twelfth day (Appendix III, p. 1392).

Pathology

There are degenerative changes in the large organs. The spleen shows reduction of malpighian corpuscles and erythrophagocytosis. There is focal haemorrhagic bronchopneumonia with focal necrosis of the liver and gastrointestinal tract. The kidneys show acute degeneration of the proximal and collecting tubules. There is no encephalitis (monkeys show encephalitis and anterior horn cell damage).

Immunity

Immunity is antibody mediated. Little is known about immunity to second attacks but monkeys who recover are immune. There is no cross immunity to other flaviviruses.

Clinical features

Natural history

KFD is a fever with a vesicular eruption on the palate with in some cases meningoencephalitis and haemorrhagic manifestations. Complete recovery after a long convalescence is usual in all except 5% of cases who die. Little is known about inapparent infection but antibodies to KFD virus have been found in man and domestic animals in Kutch in north-west India.

Symptoms and signs

The *incubation period* is from 3 to 8 days after the infective tick bite. In about 20% of cases the disease is biphasic.

FIRST PHASE
The onset is sudden with malaise and fever up to 40°C by the third or fourth day. Severe conjunctivitis is a feature with a papular or vesicular eruption on the palate. There is vomiting, diarrhoea and dehydration. Myalgia in the back and calf muscles is severe. There is a general lymphadenopathy in most cases with cervical, axillary and, more rarely, epitrochlear in others. The liver may be enlarged with raised SGOT and SGPT levels but jaundice does not occur. In the majority of cases there are no haemorrhages but gastrointestinal bleeding and haemoptysis may occur. Hypotension and bradycardia are found from the ninth day lasting a week, and after 10 days the illness subsides.

SECOND PHASE
In 20% of cases, one to two weeks after the first phase, the fever returns lasting 1–7 days. There may now be symptoms of meningoencephalitis with neck stiffness, mental disturbance, tremors and giddiness lasting until the fever subsides. After recovery there is a prolonged convalescence, the patient remaining weak for some time. There is a marked leukopenia and a heavy albuminuria with casts in the urine. The CSF is normal in the first phase but shows increased protein but without cells in the second phase.

Diagnosis

KFD most closely resembles YF from which it can be distinguished by the geographical distribution (Fig. 5.14) (although at first KFD was thought to be YF) so an accurate travel history is important. Isolation of the virus from the blood up until the twelfth day in suckling mice or tissue culture, with rising antibody (IFA, HI and N) titres in acute and convalescent sera.

Treatment

Patients must be cared for in a tick-free environment and care taken in the first 12 days to avoid contamination of medical and nursing staff with blood. The treatment is as for other VHFs (p. 129).

Epidemiology

KFD virus circulates in forest rodents especially the shrew (*Suncus murinus*) but also *Rattus wroughtoni*, *R. blandfordi* and a squirrel (*Funambulus tristriatus*), maintained by larval ticks of *Haemaphysalis spinigera*, *H. turturis* and *H. papuana* (*kinneari*).

Monkeys (langur) (*Presbytes entellus*) and bonnet macaque (*Macaca radiata*) pick up larval ticks when foraging on the ground and become infected. Many die but some recover and are immune for life. When infected the monkeys show a heavy viraemia. The larvae emerge from the ground as nymphs and come into contact with man to whom they transmit the infection as a dead end infection.

Birds (grey jungle fowl and golden backed woodpecker) are important since they carry adult ticks around and spread the infection; although antibodies have been found in some, they are not thought to play any role in maintaining the infection in nature.

Amplifying mechanism[39]

Under natural conditions the contact of man and monkey with ticks is low and to raise the number of ticks to epizootic levels it is necessary to increase their numbers and the rate of infection. Monkeys provide an efficient source of infection because of their heavy viraemia, and the number of ticks is increased by man's activity in bringing cattle into the forest where they provide a good source of food for *Haemaphysalis* ticks, thus increasing their numbers. The monkeys move around the forest forming foci of infection. KFD has spread since man invaded the forest for rice cultivation, timber extraction and cattle ranching. The cut-down forest forms an interface of lantana thicket in which many species of birds nest and which is crossed by innumerable trails used by cattle, deer, ground birds and small mammals. Infection of man is basically an occupational disease contracted by males who enter the forest, and is preceded by illness and death in langur and macaque monkeys.

Control

Control is essentially a breaking of the tick–man contact. Alteration of the environment and keeping cattle out of the forest are important. Personal protection involves regular (daily) deticking of the body and repellents. A formalized vaccine has shown promising results.

Special care must be taken in undertaking post-mortems on dead monkeys found in the forest.

CRIMEAN–CONGO HAEMORRHAGIC FEVER (C–CHF)

Geographical distribution

C–CHF is found widely in Africa, Asia, USSR and Eastern Europe.

Aetiology

The virus causing C–CHF is in the Crimean–Congo group of bunyaviruses (Table 5.1).

Transmission

Transmission is by ixodid ticks of the genus *Hyalomma* in which the virus survives by transstadial and transovarian transmission (Appendix III, p. 1393). Transmission is also possible by infected blood in a hospital setting or as an epidemic in an endemic area when the exact method is not known but may be by aerosol spread.

Pathology

The pathology is that of a VHF with haemorrhagic and liver lesions.

In the *liver* there is mid-zonal necrosis with Councilman bodies, and in the *spleen*, lymphocyte depletion, necrosis of pulp, haemorrhage in kidney and other organs.

Immunity

Immunity is antibody mediated. Little is known about second attacks.

Clinical features

The disease is an acute, self-limiting infection except under epidemic conditions when the mortality may be high (30–50%). Mild and inapparent infections occur.

Symptoms and signs

The *incubation period* is 3–6 days followed by sudden onset of fever, headache, chills, myalgia and vomiting. There is a fine petechial rash and haemorrhage on the soft palate. In more than 25% severe haemorrhage on the fourth or fifth day is a feature and collapse is common. The fatality rate varies from 15% in sporadic cases to 70% in epidemics. There is a leukopenia and thrombocytopenia and occasional liver involvement. CNS complications do not occur. In Africa the haemorrhagic syndrome and death are rare.

Diagnosis

The virus can be isolated from the blood during the febrile period and antibodies measured by serological methods—CF, IH and IFAT. Failure to isolate virus from the blood in 7 days or detect antibody by the twentieth day rules out the diagnosis of C-CHF.

Treatment

Patients must be nursed in strict isolation (see p. 129) under negative pressure or in a sealed tent isolator since medical and nursing staff are susceptible to aerosol spread and blood is infectious during the febrile period. When facilities do not allow this, strict 'barrier nursing' should be enforced and staff should wear gloves and masks.

Epidemiology and control

The C–CHF virus circulates between symptomatic wild and domestic animals (sheep, goats, cattle, hares) and is transmitted to man by a *Hyalomma* tick bite. Sporadic cases occur in animal herds and small epidemics occur with interhuman spread. Secondary cases in hospital workers occur from contact with infected blood and tissues. No vaccine is yet available.

MUROID VIRUS NEPHROPATHY (MVN)[40]

Synonyms. Korean haemorrhagic fever (HFRS), epidemic haemorrhagic fever with renal symptoms (HFRS), haemorrhagic nephrosonephritis (HNN).

Aetiology

The MVN virus is a member of the Uukuvirus group of bunyaviruses (Table 5.1).[41] It is 80–115 nm in diameter. There are four antigenically distinct groups[42] each associated with a different rodent species: *Apodemus* (field mouse) (Hantaan virus), *Clethrionomys* (vole) (Puumala virus), rats from Korea, Japan and the USA, and *Microtus* from the USA.

Geographical distribution

The four antigenically distinct viruses have a worldwide distribution in China, Korea, Japan (Hantaan virus), north-eastern Asia, Scandinavia, the Balkans, Belgium and France (Puumala virus) and *Microtus*-derived virus in Alaska, eastern USA, Bolivia and India.

Transmission

No case-to-case spread has yet been recorded in man and transmission of the virus is from chronically infected rodents who excrete virus in saliva and faeces for a month and in urine for at least two years, to man. The greatest concentration is in rodent lungs and human infection is probably contracted by the aerosol route, or an environment contaminated with rodent urine, and occasionally by rodent bite.[43]

Pathology[44]

The pathogenesis of MVN is of immunological origin rather than a direct viral destructive process. Viral antigen combines with viral antibody to form complexes which trigger the classical complement pathway with destruction of platelets, activation of the coagulation and fibrinolytic systems with severe renal damage (tubular and glomurular necrosis). The vascular endothelium is a primary target of the virus and there is severe vascular damage with capillary engorgement, leakage of red cells and interstitial and retroperitoneal oedema with little or no cellular response.

The kidney shows severe renal damage with homogeneous eosinophilic tubular deposits.

Immunity

Immunity is antibody mediated and the majority of infections recover with complete immunity to reinfection. Most infections are mild or inapparent.

Clinical features

Natural history

The majority of cases develop a mild fever without nephropathy or haemorrhagic symptoms with complete recovery. Most cases of infection are inapparent. In some cases, especially the Far Eastern form, there is severe illness with haemorrhagic and renal symptoms with a 5–20% mortality.

Incubation period

The incubation period is about 14–20 days as measured from a rodent bite.[43]

Symptoms and signs

The illness may be so mild as to make diagnosis difficult but all patients have proteinuria and azotaemia and there is an erythematous rash which sometimes becomes petechial. One-fifth of the Far Eastern cases show severe features with shock, haemorrhage and gross fluid and electrolyte imbalance. The course of the disease may be divided into five phases.

1 Febrile phase (days 1–4)
The onset is abrupt with retro-orbital headache, eye pain, photophobia and mild myalgia. Gastrointestinal symptoms (abdominal pain, nausea and vomiting) are common. There is typically an erythematous rash which may become petechial on the face, neck, shoulders and upper thorax.

2 Hypotensive phase (days 5–8)
This starts about the fifth day of illness with marked proteinuria, haemoconcentration, hypotension and occasionally shock.

3 Oliguric phase (days 9–11)
This starts about the ninth day with decreased urinary output and signs of renal failure. Haemorrhagic manifestations appear with haematuria. Serious haemorrhage is unusual, but may take the form of haematemesis, melaena and cerebrovascular complications.

4 Diuretic phase (days 12–14)
The patient improves with diuresis.

5 Convalescent phase (fifteenth day onwards)
This phase is protracted, lasting up to four months. Sequelae are rare except those resulting from CNS complications.

Differential diagnosis

This includes leptospirosis (more severe muscle pain and jaundice), typhus, relapsing fever, acute nephritis, JE, TBE, other haemorrhagic fevers (Crimean–Congo and Omsk), plague and scurvy.

Diagnosis

There is an initial leukocytosis followed in the haemorrhagic phase by leukopenia and thrombocytopenia.

Serodiagnosis is the diagnostic tool.

Immunofluorescent IgM antibodies appear very early by the fifth to seventh day of illness, specific titres rising to 1/64, to fall after six to eight weeks. Other fluorescent IgG and neutralizing antibodies persist at high titre for more than three decades.

Treatment

The patient must be nursed in strict isolation (see p. 129) until convalescence. Aerosol and blood contamination of medical attendants must be avoided. In the first stages acute shock requires careful fluid balance and albumin infusions, during the haemorrhagic phase sedation and replacement of blood products, and during the renal phase careful fluid balance and electrolyte adjustment with dialysis in the most severe cases.

Epidemiology

There are three epidemiological types of infection, rural, urban and laboratory acquired, which are determined by the host species of the virus concerned.

Rural

The rural disease is widespread and patchy in the northern hemisphere. There are two types, the severe Far Eastern (Hantaan virus) associated with *Apodemus* (field mouse) and the mild northeastern European (Puumala virus) associated with *Clethrionomys* (vole). The reservoir rodents live in fields but invade houses at the beginning of winter causing peaks of disease in spring and autumn. Epidemics arise during war (especially trench warfare) and many outbreaks have occurred in the past. In the Far East endemic disease is considerable in poor countries.

Urban

The urban form, which is caused by house rats, is a mild disease of major importance in China.

Laboratory

Infections are acquired from laboratory rat colonies and are usually mild.

Control

Prevention of contact between the human population and rodents depends on improvement in living conditions. No vaccine is yet available but vaccination of targeted populations such as agricultural workers could achieve some control.

ALTAMIRA HAEMORRHAGIC FEVER

In January 1972, 22 cases of a haemorrhagic syndrome involving the skin and in some cases the mucous membranes, with melaena and bleeding from the gums and nose, occurred among some 7000 recent settlers in the Altamira region on the Trans-Amazon highway in Brazil (Altamira haemorrhagic syndrome). A further 70 cases were identified later in a larger population. Several deaths were attributed to the disease. The condition was first diagnosed as thrombocytopenic purpura; the platelet counts were very low. Attempts to isolate bacteria or a virus failed and the cause remains unknown, but it appears to have affected only recent immigrants and to be related to the abundance of black flies (Simuliidae) in the rainy season. It has been suggested that the syndrome is a hypersensitivity reaction to the bites of these flies.[45]

Arenaviruses[38]

Arenaviruses are a group numbering 13 at present of single-stranded RNA viruses 50–500 nm (110–130 nm mean) in diameter with a lipid membranous envelope, with projections on the surface and granules (arenaceus = sandy) inside the virion, all sharing certain antigenic components. They all can cause acute or persistent infections of rodents. Only four—lymphocytic choriomeningitis (LCM), Lassa, Junin and Machupo—are human pathogens. The remaining nine are Mozambique (Mopeia) and Acar from the Old World, and Tacaribe, Amapari, Flexal, Pichende, Latino, Parana and Tamiami from the New World. Tacaribe virus has been isolated from bats and mosquitoes in Trinidad; Pichende has been isolated from haemolytic anuric disease in children and healthy adults in Brazil. Lassa, Junin and Machupo are conveyed to man by contact with rodent excreta (Figs. 5.10 and 5.11).

LASSA FEVER[46]

Geographical distribution (Fig. 5.10)

Lassa fever is confined to West Africa from where it was first described in Lassa, northern Nigeria, and central Africa. Small outbreaks have occurred in Zorzor, Liberia, Panguma Tongo in Sierra Leone, and cases have occurred in various parts of Nigeria.

Serological evidence of human infection has been found in Guinea, Senegal, Mali and Zaire. It has been shown[47,48] in Sierra Leone and Nigeria that the infection occurs widely in communities as a minor illness or inapparent infection. Recent estimates suggest that there are 100 000 cases annually with 5000 fatalities.[49]

Aetiology

Lassa fever is an arenavirus which grows readily on Vero cells with cytopathic effect. Strains of virus from Sierra Leone, Liberia, Nigeria, the Central African Republic, Mozambique and Zimbabwe are serologically distinct.[50]

Transmission

Lassa fever virus is basically an inapparent infection of the multimammate mouse (rat) (*Mastomys*

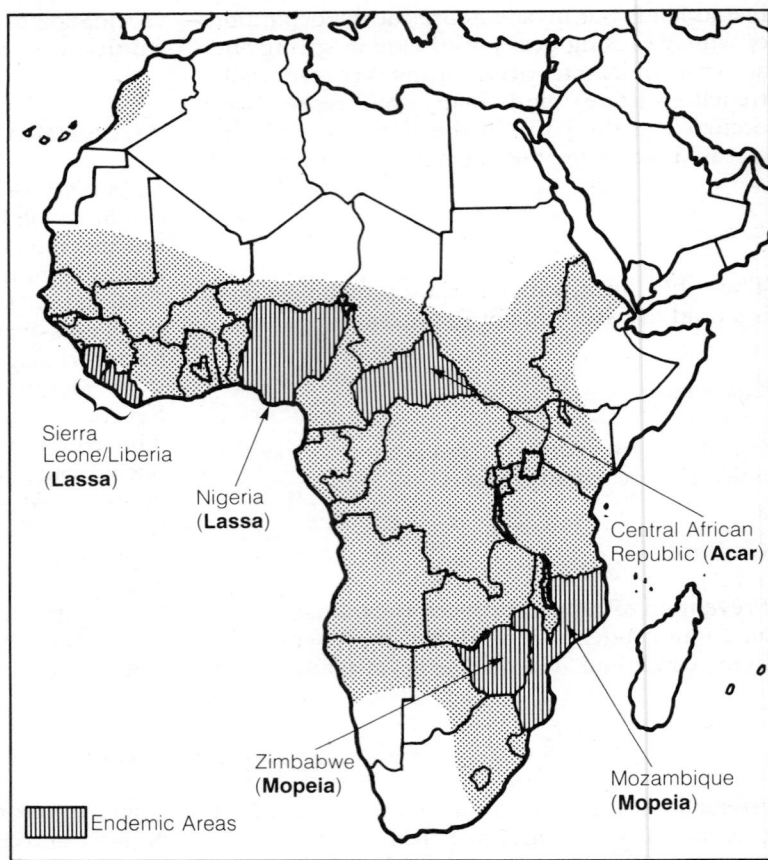

Fig. 5.10. Geographical locations of Lassa and related viruses from Africa. The stippled area represents the distribution of the single major rodent host (*Mastomys (praomys) natalensis*) in this continent (from Howard and Young[38]).

Sierra Leone/Liberia
(**Lassa**)

Nigeria
(**Lassa**)

Central African
Republic (**Acar**)

Zimbabwe
(**Mopeia**)

Mozambique
(**Mopeia**)

|||||| Endemic Areas

natalensis) from which infection spreads to man by direct contact in households, or indirect contact via food or water contaminated by rodent urine. The virus is not transmissible by aerosol in the hospital or laboratory. Nosocomial transmission occurs in a hospital setting by direct and indirect contact via blood and fomites. There is no evidence of transmission by ectoparasites or any insect.

Pathology[51]

The mechanism of the pathological changes is the same as that of other viral haemorrhagic fevers with formation of antigen–antibody complexes as well as a direct effect of the virus on capillaries causing an increase in permeability. In the *liver* there is a widespread parenchymal focal eosinophilic necrosis of hepatic cells with the presence of eosinophilic bodies resembling Councilman bodies but there is no zonal pattern of necrosis (unlike YF and RVF). The *spleen*

shows lymphoid depletion with areas of eosinophilic necrosis; the *lungs* show pleural and peritoneal effusions and focal patches of pneumonitis; and the *kidneys* focal necrosis of renal tubules. There are interstitial haemorrhages in other organs, heart and renal medulla. The *CNS* shows meningoencephalitis with oedema, congestion, neuronophagia and perivascular cuffing.[52]

Immunity

Immunity is antibody mediated and little is known about second attacks. Inapparent infections are the rule and may protect against severe infections.

Clinical features[53]

Natural history

The majority of infections take their natural

course with complete recovery without sequelae. In others, a minority, there is a severe deterioration in condition after the first week with death from haemorrhagic shock. In these cases mortality rates vary from 30% in Nigeria, 20% in Sierra Leone to 14% in Liberia.

The *incubation period* is 3–16 days, generally 7–10 days.

Symptoms and signs

The *onset* is insidious with fever which lasts 7–17 days, and malaise and pain in limb muscles. On the seventh day in severe cases there is a sudden deterioration with a severe fall in blood pressure. There is vomiting, sore throat, continuous troublesome cough with chest pains, headache and diarrhoea. The pharynx is inflamed with characteristic white or yellow patches on the tonsils and there may be ulcers with characteristic oedema of eyelids and face (an important physical sign, caused by increased capillary permeability). Occasionally there is a maculopapular rash. The blood pressure is low with a bradycardia. There is a leukopenia with albuminuria and casts in the urine. Death occurs from shock, hypotension, peripheral vasoconstriction, hypovolaemia and anuria. There are no clinical signs of meningoencephalitis.

Convalescence is from the second to fourth week with extreme weakness for several weeks and alopecia, which recovers. Deafness (20% cases) is usually reversible but may be permanent.

Differential diagnosis

At onset, Lassa fever is almost indistinguishable from other acute fevers: falciparum malaria, other VHFs, meningococcaemia and septicaemia.

The characteristic pharyngitis with white tonsillar patches and faucial oedema are important distinguishing features.

Diagnosis[54]

A detailed travel history is all-important. Laboratory diagnosis must be undertaken with precautions as for dangerous Category 4 pathogens (see p. 129). Viraemia persists well into the second week and in the urine in convalescence (up to 63 days). Isolation from the blood on Vero cell cultures can give a diagnosis within 72 hours.

The IFAT test will show antibodies by the second week, and an ELISA test is now available for the detection of both antigen and antibody allowing for early diagnosis before the development of antibody.[55] Isolation from pharyngeal secretions and from urine is also possible.

Treatment[56]

Treatment is as for VHF (see p. 129) in isolation with strict barrier nursing and with special care taken about fomites and blood and urine specimens.

Immune convalescent serum with high antibody content has been used and should be given on or before the tenth day when the treatment is very successful.[57] Possible dangers such as infection of non-Lassa patients with the serum, and the formation of antigen–antibody complexes are not met with in practice.[55] It is important that convalescent serum is obtained late in convalescence, 90–180 days after onset of illness, and it should match the strain of the virus.

Chemotherapy

Effective therapy with ribavirin has now been demonstrated.[58]

Epidemiology

The virus has been repeatedly isolated from the multimammate mouse (rat) (*Mastomys natalensis*) which is spread throughout the whole of Africa south of the Sahara. In this rodent the virus causes a chronic inapparent infection with persistent viraemia and viruria. With increasing man–rodent contact from grain stores in houses, direct and indirect infection of man occurs from food contaminated by rodent excreta or aerosol inhalation from rodent urine. Direct man-to-man spread is only found in a hospital environment where although secondary cases are common, tertiary cases are very rare. One case of Lassa fever entering a non-endemic area should not arouse the fear of an epidemic.

Control

Rodent control and decreasing man–rodent contact are the methods used. A vaccine is not yet available but the possibilities have been discussed by Clegg.[49] Surveillance of case contacts should be carried out for 21 days and any contacts developing fever isolated. Special care must be undertaken with laboratory specimens.

JUNIN VIRUS (ARGENTINIAN HAEMORRHAGIC FEVER—AHF)

Geographical distribution

The endemic–epidemic area is $100\,000\,km^2$ in the pampas north-west of Buenos Aires with a population of one million people (Fig. 5.11).

Aetiology

Junin virus can be grown on HeLa cells with a cytopathic effect or in suckling mice, and cross reacts with Machupo virus.

Transmission

Junin virus causes a chronic infection of the rodents *Calomys musculinus* and *Calomys laucha* in which it maintains persistent viraemia and viruria with virus in the saliva. The virus is transmitted to man by direct contact with rodents or indirect from contaminated food. Direct person-to-person transmission is very rare.

Pathology

There is no evidence of any immunopathological process playing a part in the pathology. The virus enters the body by the alimentary or respiratory tract and collects in local lymph glands where it multiplies, invading the reticuloendothelial system including immunocompetent cells, thus impairing the host's immune response. The virus causes capillary damage with haemorrhagic and hypovolaemic shock. There is lymphadenopathy and focal haemorrhages in many organs, especially the brain, endothelial swelling in capillaries and arterioles, focal non-zonal necrosis of the liver and renal tubular necrosis. There is some evidence of disseminated intravascular coagulation.

Immunity

Immunity is antibody mediated and little is known about second attacks.

Clinical features[59]

Natural history

Infection of man causes severe disease with a high mortality and death between the eighth and tenth day in many infections. Inapparent infection does not occur.

Symptoms and signs

The *incubation period* is 8–12 days.

There is a slow, insidious onset with chills, headache, myalgia, retro-orbital pain and nausea. This is followed by fever, conjunctival injection, oedema of face, neck and upper thorax with a petechial rash in the axilla and generalized lymphadenopathy. On the sixth to eighth day there is a sudden deterioration with haemorrhage, haematemesis, melaena, haematuria and oliguria proceeding to anuria. Pronounced *neurological* disturbances occur with tremors, psychic changes and coma. Death is caused by hypovolaemic shock. There is a heavy albuminuria with leukopenia, thrombocytopenia and altered clotting factors. Patients who recover do so when the fever falls and there is a prolonged convalescence with alopecia. Relapse may occur.

Diagnosis

Virus can be isolated from the blood during the acute febrile period. Viral antigen can be identified in cells with specific immune serum. IFAT tests on acute and convalescent sera can clinch the diagnosis.

Treatment (p. 129)

Immune plasma provided it is given within 8 days of onset is helpful. A complication is a benign febrile encephalitis four to six weeks after the onset of infection.

Epidemiology

The two main reservoir hosts *Calomys laucha* and *Calomys musculinus* live and breed in maize fields and the surrounding banks. The disease is occupational and is prevalent in rural workers, four males to one female. It occurs mainly in May when the maize is being harvested when there is a great increase in rodents and male harvesters. AHF has occurred in quite large epidemics and between 1958 and 1974 there were 16 000 cases notified.

Control

The methods are control of rodents by trapping

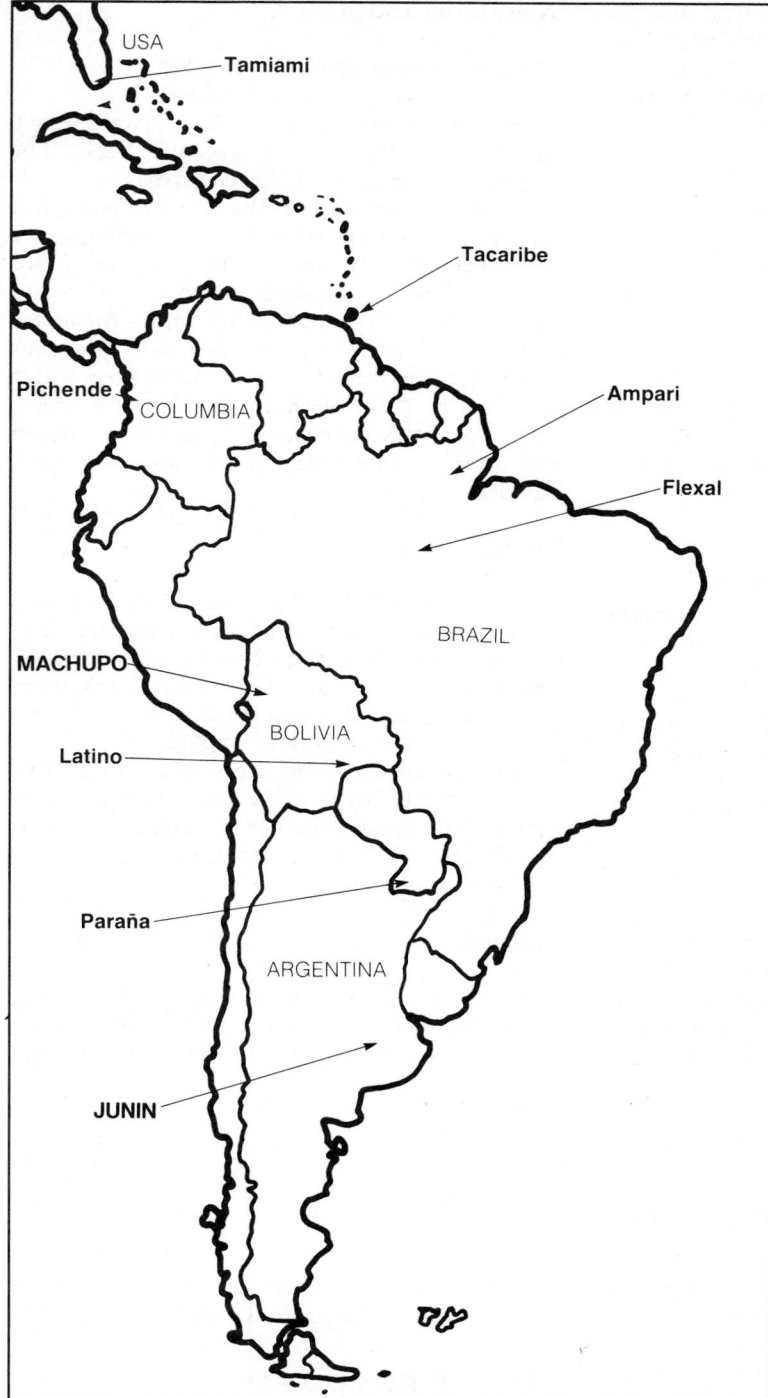

Fig. 5.11. Geographical locations of arenavirus isolates in the New World that are serologically defined as being members of the Tacaribe complex (from Howard and Young[38]).

and rodenticides and reducing man–rodent contact by mechanization of harvesting. Two types of vaccine are under trial—a formalized mouse brain vaccine and an attenuated (live) vaccine.

MACHUPO VIRUS (BOLIVIAN HAEMORRHAGIC FEVER)

Geographical distribution

Rural area in north-east Bolivia (Fig. 5.11).

Aetiology

Machupo virus is similar to Junin and Lassa fever viruses.

Transmission

The natural reservoir is the rodent *Calomys callosus* in which it causes a chronic infection with persistent viraemia and viruria. Transmission to man is by contamination of food and water by direct contact through skin abrasions. Man-to-man transmission is almost unknown except on one occasion in a non-endemic area where the index case caused five secondary cases with four deaths.

Pathology

There is congestion and interstitial haemorrhages in the gastrointestinal tract and CNS. Eosinophilic inclusion bodies are found in the Kupffer's cells of the liver. There is an interstitial pneumonia in all cases.

Symptoms and signs[60]

These are almost identical to AHF.

The *incubation period* is 7–14 days.

The onset is insidious with fever, conjunctival injection and flushing of face and neck. The disease is not so severe as AHF and many recover. In those who do not, on the sixth to tenth day there is a sudden deterioration with collapse and hypovolaemia. Haemorrhagic manifestations (30%) and neurological disturbances (50%) may occur. There is leukopenia and thrombocytopenia. This stage lasts 2–4 days and may be followed by recovery. The acute phase which lasts two to three weeks is followed by a prolonged convalescence with generalized weakness and alopecia. Inapparent infection is very rare. Relapses may occur.

Epidemiology

First recognized in 1959 in the Beni region of north-east Bolivia, it is an urban disease. The first epidemic devastated and caused the abandonment of a village. The natural reservoir, *Calomys callosus*, is found throughout the grasslands but invades houses in small towns and comes into intimate contact with man infecting him indirectly from a chronic viraemia and viruria. The disease reaches its maximum during the dry season, April to September; adult males are the most affected.

Control

Rodent control (cats and traps) in town can stop the epidemics but can do nothing about the rural rodents who are extending the endemo-epidemic area.

Filoviruses (Marburg and Ebola viruses)

Marburg and Ebola viruses are very similar in morphology but are antigenically distinct. They share no antigens with any other viruses and are classified separately as filoviruses. Virus particles are pleomorphic and appear as long filamentous U- or S-shaped particles, 2 nm long × 70–80 nm in diameter, or as circular bodies composed of an internal structure and a surface layer with numerous spikes. Multiplication is by budding from this structure. For virological studies see Johnson et al,[61] Bowel et al[62] and Pattyn et al.[63]

EBOLA VIRUS DISEASE[64]

Geographical distribution

The disease first appeared in 1976 in the equatorial provinces of southern Sudan and northern

Zaire. Epidemics have occurred and sporadic cases and serological surveys show that Ebola virus is still active in northern Zaire.

Aetiology

Ebola virus of which there are two biotypes is the cause. It is closely related but antigenically distinct from Marburg virus.

Transmission

Transmission is person-to-person by contact with a patient in the acute stage of the disease and by direct contact with blood contaminated syringes, needles and other fomites. There is no evidence of any animal reservoir or insect vectors.

Pathology

There is no evidence of any immunological mechanisms at work in the causation of the pathology. The virus is pantropic and invades cells producing necrotic lesions in all organs. The *liver* shows necrosis of single hepatocytes with fatty degeneration and necrosis at the periphery of the lobules. Eosinophilic cytoplasmic inclusions are common. The *spleen* shows atrophy and lymphocyte depletion with plasma cell infiltration. The *kidneys* show glomerular changes and focal tubular necrosis. The *heart* shows interstitial oedema and lymphocytic infiltration, and bone marrow shows degeneration of granulocyte but no change in the red cell precursors.

Immunity

Immunity is antibody mediated and there is no evidence of second attacks. Convalescent serum may help recovery.

Clinical features

Natural history

Most cases who show symptoms proceed inevitably to death but inapparent infection can occur as shown by serological surveys.

The *incubation period* is 7–14 days.

The onset is sudden with fever, severe headache, myalgia, abdominal pain and sore throat with herpetic lesions on the mouth and pharynx. There is severe conjunctival injection and gingival haemorrhages. Diarrhoea, which is a prominent feature, continues until the tenth day and measures the severity of the disease. Bleeding occurs in the majority of cases appearing towards the end of the fifth day with haematemesis and bloody diarrhoea. On the fifth to seventh day a morbilliform rash (never haemorrhagic) is visible on white but not African skins. Neurological manifestations (hemiplegia and psychosis) are common. Death occurs most commonly on the ninth day, but between the second and twenty-first day. Mortality rates vary from 50–60% in the Sudan to 80% in Zaire. There is a prolonged convalescence. There is a leukopenia at first with later an increase in granulocytes and the appearance of large cells with dark cytoplasm (virocytes) which are activated lymphocytes and lymphoblasts. Hypoproteinaemia and a raised transaminase level are present with heavy albuminuria.

Diagnosis

Diagnosis is from YF, LF and Marburg as well as other haemorrhagic fevers and a travel history is imperative. Virus can be isolated from blood by inoculation of weanling mice or guinea-pigs and then subinoculated into Vero cells. IFAT tests on paired sera show antibodies and distinguish from Marburg disease.

Treatment

The cases must be nursed under full VHF precautions (see p. 129). Anti-Ebola convalescent serum may be of help.

Epidemiology

So far there has been no evidence of an animal reservoir. The infection is conveyed from an index case to other persons by communal syringes in Zaire and mainly caused by nursing infected cases in a rural hospital environment in Sudan. Droplet infection is not a feature. There is evidence of continuing transmission in northern Zaire.

Control

Cases must be strictly isolated and nursed under conditions for Class 4 pathogens. All contact with blood, urine and other excreta must be avoided.

MARBURG VIRUS DISEASE[65]

Geographical distribution

The original cases came from workers who had handled monkeys from the Kyoga region of Uganda and serological evidence of infection has been found in monkeys in Uganda, baboons in Kenya and three monkey trappers.

Aetiology

Marburg virus is closely related but antigenically distinct from Ebola.

Transmission

The primary infections were infected by handling monkey organs and tissue cultures from vervet monkeys (*Cercopithecus aethiops*) through the intact skin by contact with infected blood. Secondary cases involved medical staff exposed to the index case from blood and in one case semen (up to 11 weeks later).

Clinical features

These are almost identical to Ebola virus disease.

Relapses occur and Marburg virus has been isolated from semen 83 days in one and 60 days in another after the onset of illness. Uveitis complicated one case[66] and virus was isolated from the anterior chamber of the eye 80 days after onset. In one laboratory infection recorded by Emond et al[67] the illness was mild and recovery complete after a long convalescence.

Diagnosis

Diagnosisis by IFAT from Ebola virus.

Epidemiology and control

There have been three outbreaks so far: first in a West German laboratory from handling infected monkeys, a second from a visitor to the Wankie park in Zimbabwe, and a third in a sugar worker in Kenya who infected the doctor who intubated him.[68] There have been 32 cases with eight deaths. Monkeys are clearly not maintenance hosts since they have fatal infections. No primary host has yet been identified but insect bites have been suggested as a factor.

ARTHROPOD-BORNE ENCEPHALITIDES

Almost all arboviruses are neurotropic in mice and are able to cause encephalitis (Table 5.4) in man although only a few do so in nature.

Transmission is by mosquito or tick bite although droplet spread can occur (VEE).

PATHOLOGY IN GENERAL

The virus enters the bloodstream from the insect vector bite and settles in the cells of the reticuloendothelial system where it replicates, causing a fever and a systemic reaction. In the majority of cases the antibody defences of the host eradicate the infection and recovery ensues after a short febrile illness. In some cases the virus enters the nervous system and invades the cells causing irreversible destruction. The pathological changes are mostly in the grey matter of the midbrain, basal ganglia, brain stem and cerebellum, where histology shows meningoencephalitis with mononuclear cell infiltration and perivascular cuffing.

CLINICAL MANIFESTATIONS

The majority of people infected develop a short, sharp febrile attack with complete recovery and immunity to reinfection. In many endemic areas a number of inapparent infections are revealed by serological surveys. In some cases the infection is biphasic and after a short period of recovery the symptoms return and signs of meningoencephalitis appear (excitability, somnolence, coma, delirium, hyperthermia and epileptiform convulsions). In some cases, especially children, spastic and flaccid paralyses which may be permanent develop.

DIAGNOSIS

Virus can be cultivated from the blood in the acute phase and antibody titres shown to be raised in convalescent sera taken 10–30 days later. A specimen of clotted blood sent on ice to the appropriate laboratory for culture and serology is necessary.

Table 5.4 Arthropod-borne encephalitides of clinical importance.

Virus	Disease	Hosts	Geographical distribution
Mosquito-borne			
(1) *Equine encephalitides*			
Alphavirus	Eastern equine encephalitis (EEE)	Wild and domestic birds, spillover to man and equines	USA, Central and South America
	Western equine encephalitis (WEE)	Wild and domestic birds, spillover to equines and man	Western North America
	Venezuelan equine encephalitis (VEE)	Wild forest rodents, spillover to equines and man	South America
(2) *Japanese B–West Nile virus complex*			
Flavivirus	Japanese B encephalitis (JBE)	Wild birds and pigs, spillover to man	Asia, Japan, Korea, Taiwan, China, Indo-China, Philippines, Thailand, Bangladesh, eastern and southern India
	St Louis encephalitis (SLE)	Passerine birds, possibly bats, spillover to equines and man	Temperate areas North America, Argentina, Brazil, Surinam, Panama, Trinidad, Jamaica
	Murray Valley encephalitis (MVE)	Birds	Australia, New Guinea
	West Nile virus	Wild birds, spillover to man	Widely distributed in Old World, South Africa and Israel
Bunyaviruses	California encephalitis (CE)		
	La Crosse (LAC)	Wild birds	North America, Canada
Tick-borne			
Flavivirus	Russian spring–summer (RSSE)	Rodents	Eastern Siberia
	European tick-borne encephalitis (TBE)	Rodents, spillover to goats and man	Eastern Europe, Scandinavia
	Powassan		Canada

Equine encephalitides (alphavirus)

Equines (horses and donkeys) are affected in an epizootic preceding an epidemic in man and act as amplifier hosts between the reservoir hosts (birds, rodents) and man.

WESTERN EQUINE ENCEPHALITIS (WEE)

Geographical distribution (Fig. 5.12)

WEE is found in Texas, Colorado, Saskatchewan and in Argentina, Brazil, Mexico and Guyana where human infections are unknown but equine epizootics occur.

Aetiology

WEE is an RNA virus 55 nm in diameter which can be cultured in tissue cultures with a cytopathic effect. Chick embryo fibroblasts are favoured.

Transmission

Transmission is by mosquitoes. *Culex tarsalis*, which feeds readily on birds, transmits the infection in the western USA, and *Culiseta melanura* in areas where *Culex tarsalis* does not occur (eastern USA) (Table III.6, p. 1417).

Immunity

Immunity is antibody mediated and protects against second attacks. Serological surveys show inapparent infections and children are most affected in epidemics.

Pathology

Pathology in fatal cases is that of a meningoencephalitis.

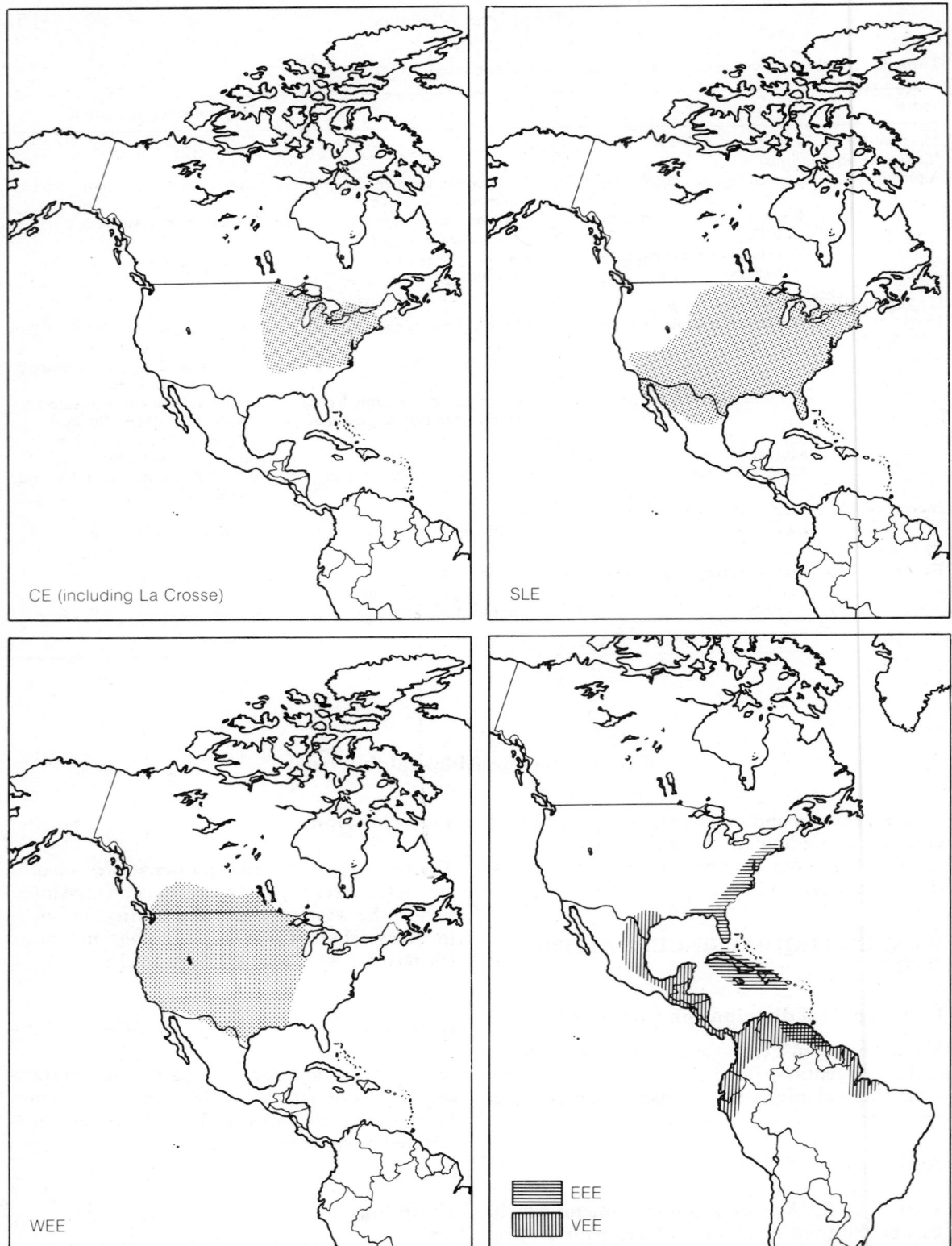

Fig. 5.12. Distribution of mosquito-borne encephalitis in the New World. CE = California encephalitis, SLE = St Louis encephalitis, WEE = Western equine encephalitis, EEE = Eastern equine encephalitis, VEE = Venezuelan equine encephalitis. (Courtesy Department of Entomology, London School of Hygiene and Tropical Medicine.)

Clinical features

The majority of infections are inapparent and most overt cases in adults recover without any sequelae but 50% of young children develop neurological complications with some permanent neurological changes. Mortality rate is 10%.

Symptoms and signs

The *incubation period* is 5–10 days.

The onset is gradual with mild fever, malaise, headache, stiff neck and drowsiness. In the minority of severe cases the fever increases with signs of CNS involvement, somnolence, coma, flaccid and spastic paralyses which recover. There is a leukocytosis in the early stages and the CSF shows a pleocytosis with increased protein in those with CNS involvement.

Diagnosis

Viral isolation in acute phase with CF and HI tests on convalescent sera.

Epidemiology

WEE virus circulates in more than 75 species of wild birds and some domestic ones. The basic transmission cycle is between *Culex tarsalis* and birds in the summer. Over-wintering of the virus may be in hibernating mammals but more likely in over-wintering mosquitoes. Epizootics in horses acting as amplifying hosts precede human epidemics. In man the highest attack rates are in infants and young males in a rural environment.

Control

Antimosquito measures are difficult in rural areas but where small towns are involved 'fogging' from the air with insecticide may terminate an epidemic. A non-neurotropic strain of virus isolated from birds has been used successfully as a vaccine but only experimentally.

EASTERN EQUINE ENCEPHALITIS (EEE)

Geographical distribution (Fig. 5.12)

EEE is found in the eastern USA (where epizootics occur in horses but human cases are rare), Mexico, Panama, Brazil, Argentina and Guyana.

Two small human outbreaks have occurred in Dominica and Jamaica, and in 1962 there was a major epidemic of 6762 cases in Venezuela, 0.6% fatal.

Aetiology

EEE virus is 50 nm in diameter and can be cultured in many tissue culture systems. There are two antigenic types, North and South American.

Transmission

Transmission is by mosquitoes; *Culiseta melanura* and *Culiseta morsitans*, *Ae. sollicitans* and *Ae. taeniorhynchus* are the main vectors but isolations of virus have been made from other mosquitoes in the field (see Appendix III, p. 1428, and Table III.6, p. 1416).

Immunity

Immunity is antibody mediated and affords protection against second attacks.

Symptoms and signs

Natural history

EEE is more severe than WEE in both horses and man. Many cases recover after a short febrile attack but in others, chiefly children and young infants, the disease is biphasic and symptoms return with CNS involvement.

The *incubation period* is 7–10 days.

The onset is gradual with fever and meningism which may resolve. However, in young children and infants the disease is biphasic and symptoms return after 1–2 days with the onset of symptoms of encephalitis. There is a leukocytosis with pleocytosis and increased protein in the CSF. Neurological sequelae occur.

Epidemiology

Transmission is maintained by birds and mosquitoes in an extensive geographical area. Infection of horses and man is accidental and in the centre of the area serological evidence of inapparent human infection can be found. EEE may cause a high mortality in birds both wild and domestic. Infection in horses is severe, most dying within a few days.

Control

Mosquito control is the only method. Vaccination is not yet available.

VENEZUELAN EQUINE ENCEPHALITIS (VEE)

Geographical distribution (Fig. 5.12)

Extensive outbreaks with human cases have occurred in Venezuela (100 000 cases in 1962 almost wiping out the equine population), Trinidad, Colombia, Brazil and Panama. The virus is now extending its area and evidence of human infection has been found in Florida.

Aetiology

VEE virus is a round particle 65–80 nm in diameter. It grows in many different cell cultures with cytopathic effect. There are a number of antigenic subtypes.

Transmission

The main vectors are *Ae. serratus* and *Ae. taeniorhynchus* and culicine species including *Culex fatigans*. Isolations have been made from about 40 other species (see Table III.6, p. 1416). *Simulium* may transmit infections and there is a possibility of man-to-man spread by droplet infection and spread among horses can occur without an insect vector.

Immunity

Immunity is antibody mediated and provides protection against second attacks. It takes therefore about 10 years to build up a susceptible population of man and equines to sustain a new epidemic.

Symptoms and signs

Natural history

Most infections are inapparent and the majority of the overt infections are mild and transient though virulence may vary in epidemics.

The *incubation period* is 2–5 days.

The onset is sudden with rigor, fever and myalgia. A sore throat and upper respiratory symptoms are a feature and diarrhoea is common (first phase lasting 1–5 days). Following a short illness recovery is complete. In some cases, and in about 4% of children under 15, the disease is biphasic and symptoms return with involvement of the CNS. Convulsions and coma and long-term sequelae, flaccid and spastic paralyses and mental depression are common. There is a leukopenia with pleocytosis and raised protein in the CSF.

Diagnosis

Virus may be isolated from the blood in the acute phase and also from the throat suggesting droplet spread. Antibody titres on paired sera are diagnostic.

Epidemiology

VEE virus circulates silently in small mammals and with a high rainfall and an increase in the number of mosquitoes and their biting, horses become infected acting as amplifying hosts. Equine cases precede human cases most commonly children in whom the disease is more severe. A high proportion of equines develop immunity so that 10 years is necessary to build up another susceptible population.

Control

Mosquito control is difficult in rural conditions and a vaccine has not yet been developed.

Japanese B–West Nile virus complex

These are all diseases caused by flaviviruses and transmitted by mosquitoes from birds, which are the main reservoir hosts.

ST LOUIS ENCEPHALITIS (SLE)

Geographical distribution (Fig. 5.12)

This is the most important arbovirus in the USA. It is widespread throughout North America but has also occurred in Jamaica and evidence of infection in birds is found in Central America, Brazil and Argentina.

Aetiology

The SLE virus is 30–40 nm in diameter and is best grown in newborn white mice but also grows on hamster and chicken kidney cell cultures. It shares antigens with Japanese B and West Nile viruses.

Transmission

The basic transmission cycle is between birds and several culicine mosquitoes. After the winter the virus is introduced by migrant birds or long-term infection of bats. The main vector to man is *Culex quinquefasciatus* in the eastern and *C. tarsalis* in the western USA. Transovarial transmission is usual (Table III.6, p. 1418).

Symptoms and signs

Natural history

Most infections are inapparent in a ratio of 100 : 1. Overt infections usually last a few days with fever and complete recovery. In a very few cases, chiefly elderly persons, CNS signs develop usually recovering rapidly with no permanent sequelae.

The *incubation period* is a few days.

Onset is sudden with fever, severe headache, followed after a few days by recovery. CNS involvement is shown by drowsiness, tremor, dysarthria and photophobia with convulsions. This lasts 10 days with complete recovery. Lymphocytosis is common. The CSF shows pleocytosis and a raised protein.

Epidemiology

C. quinquefasciatus being an urban mosquito is responsible for urban outbreaks while *C. tarsalis* in the western USA is responsible for rural outbreaks. In urban areas both sexes are affected equally but elderly people most. In rural areas males are affected more than females. Epidemics occur in the late summer and early autumn.

Control

Environmental sanitation to control *C. fatigans* in urban areas is essential. 'Fogging' with insecticides may be necessary.

JAPANESE B ENCEPHALITIS (JBE)

Geographical distribution

JBE is found in eastern Asia from Siberia to south-east India, Japan, Okinawa, Guam, Philippines and Indonesia.

Aetiology

JBE virus is 50 nm in diameter and shares antigens with SLE and MVE. It grows well on hamster and pig kidney cells and in animals and certain donkeys after intracerebral inoculation.

Transmission

Culex tritaeniorhynchus, a rice field breeder, is the main vector in north Asia and Japan; *C. pipiens* in the eastern USSR; *C. annulirostris* in Guam; *C. gelidus* in Malaysia and *C. vishnui* in India (Table III.6, p. 1417).

Pathology

In the brain there are areas of necrosis with small haemorrhages and perivascular cuffing in the grey matter most marked in the thalamus and substantia nigra. Fine calcareous particles may be seen.

Immunity

An antibody-mediated immunity protects against second attacks and builds up resistance in the population.

Symptoms and signs

Natural history

Many infections are inapparent but in about 0.2% the infection is overt and severe, reaching a mortality rate in elderly persons of up to 50%. This is the most severe of the viral encephalitides.

The *incubation period* is 4–14 days.

The onset is sudden and within 24 hours there are signs of an acute meningoencephalitis. The face and conjunctivae are suffused. There is a characteristic attitude with head retracted, arms and knees bent and shoulders pressed to the chest (Fig. 5.13). After 3 days stupor, delirium, coma and decerebrate rigidity follow. The temperature

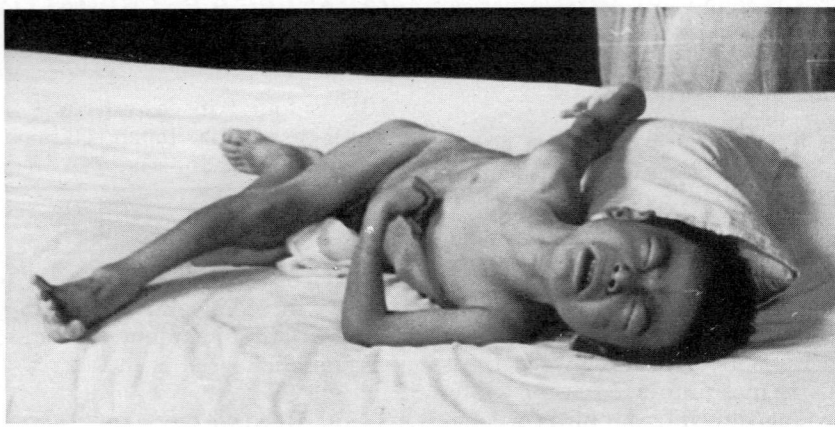

Fig. 5.13. A five-year-old boy with Japanese encephalitis.

fluctuates widely. If the acute stage is survived then recovery is slow. Upper motor neuron paralyses and extrapyramidal lesions are common. Death may occur suddenly in convalescence. Permanent sequelae, mental impairment, emotional instability, motor neuron lesions and aphasia are common. There is a leukopenia in the early stages. The CSF remains normal in half the cases and shows a pleocytosis with increased protein in the other half.

Diagnosis

HI and CF tests become positive from the third to seventh, maximum at the fortieth day. N test is positive later and remains positive for years. There are cross reactions with other flaviviral antigens. Virus can be isolated from the brain at post-mortem.

Treatment

Convalescent serum, 20 ml daily, during the first week is thought to help but is of no use when the CNS is involved.

Epidemiology

The main source of infection is the rice fields where the vector *C. tritaeniorhynchus* breeds, becoming infected from pigs or birds. Three weeks after mosquito breeding begins in the spring, virus can be found in birds and pigs but man is not involved until there is a high density of mosquitoes. The infection is amplified by pigs and conveyed to man. Birds (night heron and egrets) carry the infection from rural to urban areas. There is a seasonal summer incidence with epidemics every year in Japan where children are affected more than adults. Most cases are in children and old people but visitors of any age are affected.

Control

A formalized mouse brain vaccine is available and is given in three injections two months before the epidemic season.

MURRAY VALLEY ENCEPHALITIS (MVE)

Geographical distribution

MVE is found in Australia and New Guinea.

Aetiology

MVE is spherical, 25–35 nm in diameter. It is antigenically related to JBE. It can be cultured in hamster kidney cells, KB cells and in chick embryos with cytopathic effect.

Pathology

MVE closely resembles JBE.

Natural history

The majority of infections are inapparent in the

ratio of 700 : 1.

The *incubation period* is one to two weeks.

The signs and symptoms are the same as JBE and the overt disease is very severe with a mortality rate as high as 35%. Serious sequelae are common (residual paralyses and mental impairment).

Diagnosis

The serological diagnosis is difficult because of the presence of dengue and other flaviviruses in these areas.

Epidemiology

The virus is maintained in a cycle involving wild birds and mosquitoes. The vector *C. annulirostris* is infected from birds who carry the infection widely by migration (Table III.6, p. 1417).

WEST NILE FEVER

Geographical distribution

Serological surveys indicate that the virus is widely spread from South Africa to Egypt and Israel, southern Europe, the Middle East and south India.

Aetiology

West Nile virus is 20–40 nm in diameter. It is constructed of a nucleocapsid enclosed in a lipid containing envelope.

Transmission

The main vectors are: in Egypt, South Africa and Israel *C. univittatus* and *C. pipiens*; in Israel and France *C. modestus*; and in India *C. vishnui*. Virus has been isolated from ticks: *Ornithodorus* sp., *Dermacentor* sp., *Rhipicephalus* sp. and *Hyalomma* sp. in the USSR (Table III.6, p. 1417, and Appendix III, pp. 1389 and 1392).

Pathology

Little is known, since although deaths have occurred from meningoencephalitis no postmortems have been recorded. In monkeys encephalitic changes are present in the cerebral grey matter and the cerebellum.

Symptoms and signs

Natural history

In the great majority of cases West Nile fever is an inapparent infection; in others there is an acute dengue-like fever (for which it has often been mistaken) followed by recovery, but a few cases develop meningoencephalitis.

The *incubation period* is 3–6 days.

The onset is sudden with nausea, fever, photophobia, congested eyes and face. After 5–6 days the fever falls by lysis and there is complete recovery. In children the fever may be saddle back. There is a generalized lymphadenopathy and a maculopapular rash on the chest, shoulders, upper arms and back. In elderly patients the first phase may be followed by the development of a meningoencephalitis.

Diagnosis

The virus can be isolated from the blood in the first 6 days into suckling mice or embryonated eggs. Retrospective diagnosis with paired serum can be difficult since there is cross reaction with persons inoculated with 17D virus against yellow fever.

Epidemiology

Virus circulates widely in birds (pigeons, crows) especially in the nesting season and the young become infected with a high viraemia. The infection is spread widely by migration. *C. univittatus* is an avid feeder on birds and *C. pipiens* transmits the infection in the cooler season. Eighty per cent of the residents of Egypt show evidence of past infection. There have been epidemics of West Nile fever in South Africa and Israel.

CALIFORNIA ENCEPHALITIS (CE)

The California serogroup of viruses cause illness in the USA (Fig. 5.12). California encephalitis (CE) was the first to be isolated which frequently infects man but rarely causes clinical illness. La Crosse (LAC) virus on the other hand is an important pathogen of man. LAC virus circulates in chipmunks, tree squirrels and cottontail rabbits in a rural forest environment transmitted by *Aedes*, *Culex*, *Anopheles* and *Pso-*

rophora mosquitoes (Table III.6, p. 1419). The principal vector is *Ae. triseriatus* in which there is transovarial transmission. It causes an acute fever with encephalitic involvement mainly in children. The incubation period is 5–10 days, the onset gradual with fever, headache, neck rigidity, convulsions and coma. Permanent CNS changes are rare and the mortality less than 1%.

Tick-borne encepalitis (TBE)

RUSSIAN SPRING–SUMMER ENCEPHALITIS (RSSE) AND EUROPEAN TICK-BORNE ENCEPHALITIS

Geographical distribution (Fig. 5.14)

TBE is seasonally epidemic in scattered foci in the far eastern USSR (RSSE) and in European Russia, Austria, Hungary, Yugoslavia, Czechoslovakia and Scandinavia (European TBE). The Powassan type is found in Canada and western Ontario.

Aetiology

The virus is spherical, 20–30 nm in diameter, with a dense centre and surface membrane. It shares antigens with louping ill, Omsk haemorrhagic fever, and Kyasanur Forest disease, but not Japanese B.

Transmission (see also Appendix III, p. 1391)

The vectors are *Ixodes persulcatus* in the eastern USSR and *I. ricinus* in the West. Viral infection is maintained by transovarial transmission. Men may also become infected from drinking infected goat's milk.

Pathology

The virus multiplies in the liver before circulating in the blood, where it alters the vascular permeability and enters the brain, especially the basal ganglia and anterior horn cells of the cervical region. Histologically there is severe neuronal damage with softening and death of cells, glial proliferation, neuronophagia and lymphoid proliferation around vessels. The cervical segments of the cord, the medulla, midbrain and pons are affected

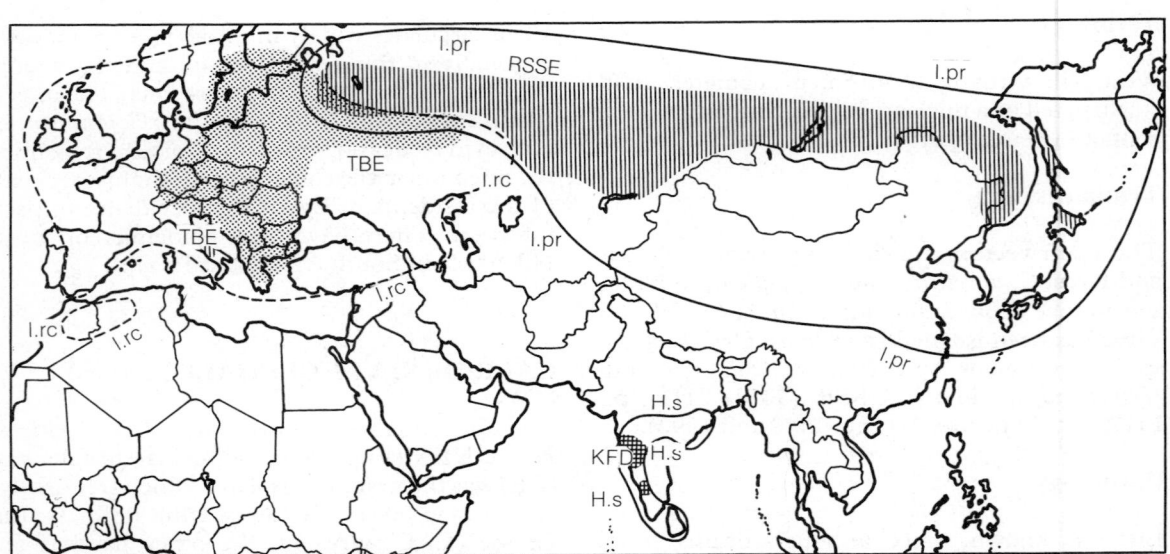

Fig. 5.14. Geographical distribution of tick-borne encephalitis—Russian spring–summer encephalitis (RSSE), European tick-borne encephalitis (TBE) and Kyasanur Forest disease (KFD)—and the main vectors. I.pr = *Ixodes persulcatus*, I.rc = *Ixodes ricinus*, H.s = *Haemophysalis spinigera*. (Courtesy Department of Entomology, London School of Hygiene and Tropical Medicine.)

Symptoms and signs

Natural history

The infection is often inapparent but when overt is severe, the Eastern (RSSE) form (30% mortality) being more severe than the European form (TBE) (3% mortality).

The *incubation period* is 8–14 days.

Onset is sudden with severe headache, fever, nausea and photophobia. In non-fatal cases the fever subsides after a week. In others the disease is biphasic and after a period of several days' recovery, the second phase develops with signs of a meningoencephalitis, which in the Eastern form is severe but in the European form mainly benign. Death comes from ascending paralysis and respiratory failure within a week of onset of the second phase. The mortality rate is higher in children. There is a leukopenia at the start with a leukocytosis at the end. The CSF shows a pleocytosis with raised protein. Residual paralyses are common involving the upper extremities and shoulder girdle.

Diagnosis

Virus can be isolated from the blood in the first week. The CF test is not so reliable as the HI and N tests.

Treatment

Hyperimmune serum used in the first week has been helpful but is of no use when meningoencephalitis has set in.

Epidemiology

The virus circulates in small wild animals, chiefly rodents, and is transmitted by larval and nymphal ticks who, when they mature, feed on larger mammals including man. The incidence of the disease is seasonal—spring and early summer—occurring in small epidemics in the Eastern USSR where it is a disease of the forest and the taiga. In Europe it is a forest disease and occurs in late spring until early autumn, and often outbreaks follow a period when voles are numerous.

Control

In some areas of the Far Eastern USSR, forests are closed to all visitors because of this infection.

Tick repellents may be of help. A formalized mouse brain vaccine is available and is used to protect laboratory workers but there are side reactions. A safe and effective vaccine is available. It is recommended for holiday makers and sportsmen in the forested areas of Europe. It is given in two doses four to six weeks apart, followed by a booster after 12 months.[69]

COLORADO TICK FEVER (CTF)

Colorado tick fever is found in the Rocky Mountain area especially in Colorado. Fever is usually biphasic and mild, sometimes with a maculopapular rash or petechiae, and sometimes causing haemorrhages and encephalitis in children, who mostly recover without sequelae. The most important hosts are the chipmunk and the golden mantled ground squirrel which infect immature ticks (*Dermacentor andersoni*). Other species of rodents may act as alternative secondary hosts for the virus.

REFERENCES

1　World Health Organization (1967) *Wld Hlth Org. tech. Rep. Ser.* 369.
2　Smith, C.E.G. (1968) *Abstr. Hyg.* **43**, 1397.
3　Smith, C.E.G. (1964) *Scient. Basis Med. ann. Rev.* 125.
4　Simpson, D.I.H. (1968) *Symp. zool. Soc. London* **24**, 13.
5　Smith, C.E.G., Heathecoat, O.H.V., Hill, M.W. et al (1970) *Trans. R. Soc. trop. Med. Hyg.* **64**, 481.
6　Pinto, M.R. (1967) *Kongressbericht über die III Tagung der Deutschen Tropenmedizinischen Gesellschaft e. V. 1967, 20–22 April*, p. 153. Munich: Urban & Schwarzenberg.
7　MacNamara, F.N., Horn, D.W. & Porterfield, J.S. (1959) *Trans. R. Soc. trop. Med. Hyg.* **53**, 202.
8　Boyd, J.S.K. (1961) *12th Annual Conference of the Indian Association of Pathologists*, 118.
9　Rosen, L., Shrover, D., Tesh, R.B. et al (1983) *Am. J. trop. Med. Hyg.* **32**, 1108–1109.
10　Pinheiro, F.P., Freitas, R.B., Travassos Da Rosa, J.F. et al (1981) *Am. J. trop. Med. Hyg.* **30**, 674.
11　McIntosh, B.M., McGillivray, G.M., Dickinson, D.B. et al (1964) *S. Afr. med. J.* **39**, 291.
12　Pinheiro, F.P., Rocha, A.G., Freitas, R.B. et al (1982) *Rev. Inst. Med. Trop. São Paulo* **24**, 246–251.
13　Tesh, R.B., Saidi, S., Gajdamovic, F. et al (1976) *Bull. Wld Hlth Org.* **54**, 663–673.
14　Center for Disease Control (1983) *Morbidity and Mortality Weekly Report* (Supplement) **32**, 2S.
15　World Health Organization (1966) *Bull. Wld Hlth Org.* **35**, 17, 74.
16　Balankura, M., Valyyasevi, A., Kampart-Sanyakorn, C. et al (1966) *Bull. Wld Hlth Org.* **35**, 51, 75.

17 World Health Organization (1966) *Wld Hlth Org. tech. Rep. Ser.* 325.

18 Sumaro, W.H., Jaha, E., Gubler, D.J. et al (1978) *Lancet* i, 449.

19 Fraser, H.S., Wilson, W.A., Thomas, E.J. et al (1978) *Br. med. J.* i, 893.

20 Halstead, S.B. (1969–70) *Yale J. Biol. Med.* 42, 350.

21 Rosen, L. (1977) *Am. J. trop. Med. Hyg.* 26, 337.

22 Editorial (1976) *Lancet* ii, 239.

23 Editorial (1977) *Br. Med. J.* ii, 1175.

24 Editorial (1978) *Asian J. inf. Dis.* 2, 112.

25 Van Tongeren, H.A.E. (1983) *Trans. R. Soc. trop. Med. Hyg.* 77, 198–200.

26 Meegan, J.M., Digoutte, J.P., Peters, C.J. et al (1983) *Lancet* i, 641.

27 Peters, C.J. & Meegan, J.M. (1981) In *Viral Zoonoses*, ed. G.W. Beran, Vol. 1, pp. 403–420. Boca Raton, Florida: CRC.

28 Van Velden, D.J.J., Meyer, J.D., Oliver, J. et al (1977) *S. Afr. med. J.* 51, 867.

29 Swanepoel, R., Manning, B. & Watt, J.A. (1979) *Cent. Afr. J. Med.* 25, 1.

30 Laughlin, L.W., Meegan, J.M., Strausbaugh, L.J. et al (1979) *Trans. R. Soc. trop. Med. Hyg.* 73, 630.

31 Shope, R.E., Peters, C.J. & Davies, F.E. (1982) *Bull. Wld Hlth Org.* 60, 299–304.

32 Meegan, J.M. (1979) *Trans. R. Soc. trop. Med. Hyg.* 73, 618.

33 Hoogstraal, H., Meegan, J.M., Khalid, G.M. et al (1979) *Trans. R. Soc. trop. Med. Hyg.* 73, 724.

34 World Health Organization (1983) *Bull. Wld Hlth Org.* 61, 261–268.

35 *Weekly Epidemiological Record* (1978) 4, 305.

36 Cornet, J.P., Huard, M., Camicas, J.L. et al (1982) *Bull. Soc. Path. Exot. Fil.* 75, 136–140.

37 Haddow, A.J. & Ellice, J.M. (1964) *Trans. R. Soc. trop. Med. Hyg.* 58, 521.

38 Howard, C.R. & Young, P.R. (1984) *Trans. R. Soc. trop. Med. Hyg.* 78, 299–306.

39 Boshell, J. (1969) *Am. J. trop. Med. Hyg.* 18, 67.

40 Fisher-Hock, S.P. & McCormick, J.B. (1985) *Abstr. Hyg. Comm. Dis.* 60, R2–R20.

41 McCormick, J.B., Palmer, E.L., Sasso, D.R. et al (1982) *Lancet* i, 765–771.

42 Schmaljohn, C.S., Hasty, S.E. & Harrison, S.A. (1983) *J. inf. Dis.* 148, 1005–1012.

43 Dournon, E., Moriniere, B., Matherson, S. et al (1984) *Lancet* i, 676–677.

44 Yang, S.H., Gu, X.S., Wang, D.Q. et al (1981) *Chin. med. J.* 94, 789–798.

45 Pinheiro, F.P., Bensabath, G., Costa, D. Jun. et al (1974) *Lancet* i, 639.

46 Monath, T.P. & Casal, J. (1975) *Bull. Wld Hlth Org.* 52, 707.

47 Fraser, D.M., Campbell, C.C., Monath, T.P. et al (1974) *Am. J. trop. Med. Hyg.* 23, 1131.

48 Arnold, R.B. & Gary, G.M. (1977) *Trans. R. Soc. trop. Med. Hyg.* 71, 152.

49 Clegg, J.C.S. (1984) *Trans. R.Soc. trop. Med. Hyg.* 78, 307–310.

50 Jahrling, P.B. (1983) *J. med. Virol.* 12, 93–102.

51 Buckley, S.M. & Casals, J. (1978) *Int. Rev. exp. Path.* 18, 97.

52 Sato, K., Ikerionun, S.E. & Katchy, K.C. (1982) *Jap. J. trop. Med. Hyg.* 10, 23–31.

53 Emond, R.T.D., Bannister, B., Lloyd, G. et al (1982) *Br. med. J.* ii, 1001–1002.

54 World Health Organization (1974) *Wkly epidem. Rec.* 41, 341.

55 Jahrling, P.B., Niklasson, B.S. & McCormick, J.B. (1985) *Lancet* i, 250–252

56 Monath, T.P. (1975) *Bull. Wld Hlth Org.* 52, 577.

57 Frame, J.D., Verbrugge, G.R., Gill, R.G. et al (1984) *Trans. R. Soc. trop. Med. Hyg.* 78, 319–324, 656–660, 761–763.

58 McCormick, J.B., Webb, P.A., Cribner, C.L. et al (1987) *N. Engl. J. Med.* (in press).

59 Elsner, B., Schwarz, F. Mando, O.G. et al (1973) *Am. J. trop. Med. Hyg.* 22, 229.

60 Child, P.L., Mackenzie, R.B., Velverde, L. et al (1967) *Arch. Path.* 83, 434.

61 Johnson, K.M., Webb, P.A., Lance, J.V. et al (1977) *Lancet* i, 569.

62 Bowel, E.T.M., Platt, G.S., Lloyd, G. et al (1977) *Lancet* i, 571.

63 Pattyn, S., Jacob, W., van der Groen, G. et al (1977) *Lancet* i, 573.

64 World Health Organization (1978) *Bull. Wld Hlth Org.* 56, 247–271.

65 Transactions Royal Society of Tropical Medicine and Hygiene (1969) *Symposium on Marburg Virus Disease* 63, 295.

66 Gear, J.J.S., Cassel, G.A., Gear, A.J. et al (1975) *Br. med. J.* ii, 489–493.

67 Emond, R.T.D., Evans, B., Bowen, E.T.W. et al (1977) *Br. med. J.* ii, 541.

68 Smith, D.H., Johnson, B.K., Isaacson, M. et al (1982) *Lancet* i, 816–820.

69 Simpson, D.I.H. & Varma, M.G.R. (1982) *Br. med. J.* 1787–1788.

Chapter 6
Other Virus Diseases

Other virus diseases common in the tropics which present as fever are measles, poliomyelitis and hepatitis.

MEASLES

GEOGRAPHICAL DISTRIBUTION

Measles has a worldwide distribution following its introduction to many countries which had been previously free, often with disastrous results, such as Fiji, Tasmania, Greenland and many tropical areas where there were isolated people without previous experience of the disease. It is one of the most important infectious diseases of the tropics and certainly the most serious of the acute infectious illnesses.[1]

AETIOLOGY

The virus, which is closely related to rinderpest and canine distemper, is a single-stranded RNA virus with a pleomorphic appearance on electron microscopy, 120–250 nm in size, consisting of two components, an outer envelope with short projections and an inner nucleocapsid of RNA and a glycoprotein. There is only one strain of virus with no antigenic variation, alterations in virulence worldwide being due to host and environmental factors. Measles virus grows slowly in human and monkey cell cultures. Viraemia occurs 4–5 days before the onset of the rash and then disappears within 24–48 hours. It can also be isolated from the throat in the coryzal stage.

TRANSMISSION

Measles is one of the most contagious infections and 90% of susceptibles will contract the disease after contact with a case. Transmission is direct from secretions of the respiratory tract by droplet spread. Cases are infectious only in the early stages when virus can be isolated from the throat. Transplacental spread does not appear to occur and, although it is possible that fetal damage may follow measles in pregnancy, this is not yet proven.

PATHOLOGY

Infection starts in the nose and throat from which, following limited multiplication, the virus spreads via leukocytes to the cells of the reticuloendothelial system, where it attacks the lymphocytes of the immune system. Further multiplication occurs preceding the viraemic phase when epithelial cells are then affected and the signs and symptoms of measles develop after an incubation period of 10–14 days. Virus multiplies in cells of the reticuloendothelial system in which it causes the appearance of large multinucleate giant cells. The target organs affected are the skin, conjunctivae, mouth, larynx, bronchial tree and gastrointestinal tract. The essential lesion is a catarrhal inflammation of the respiratory and gastrointestinal tracts, the initial inflammation of epithelial cells being rapidly followed by fatty degeneration and exfoliation of dead cells. Complete resolution is the rule with recovery, but widespread denudation of epithelium in the alimentary tract may end in mucosal atrophy.[2]

IMMUNITY

Immunity to measles is both antibody and cell mediated and following an attack of measles lasts for life. Antibodies appear with the rash and the IgM peaks at 10 days, disappearing after a month. The IgG decreases slowly over six months. Passive immunity transferred from mother to infant transplacentally lasts for the first few months of life and evidence of inapparent infection during the months of declining maternal antibody can be found in one-quarter of older children. Cell-mediated immunity (CMI) plays an important part in elimination of the virus. Because of its action on the cells of the reticuloendothelial system, measles depresses CMI, which can also be reduced simultaneously by malnutrition. This accounts for the severity of the disease in many tropical countries. A depressed CMI also reactivates tuberculosis and allows the secondary infections common in measles to develop.

CLINICAL FEATURES

Natural history

Measles is an acute self-limiting infection with recovery in the majority of cases but which in tropical populations is complicated by severe bronchopneumonia, diarrhoea, malabsorption, malnutrition, severe conjunctivitis and blindness, gangrene of limbs and death. Case mortality in the tropics is estimated to be about 5% (or even 10% in rural areas). In some village epidemics 40% of children have been known to die of measles, and the combination of whooping cough and measles is particularly dangerous.

Incubation period

The incubation period is 10–14 days.

Symptoms and signs

The onset is gradual with fever, and coryzal symptoms appear within 24 hours. Severe conjunctivitis and cough follow; this prodromal stage lasts 3–4 days. Within 3 days of onset (24 hours before the rash) *Koplik's spots* can be seen as spots of bright red colour with a small bluish white centre on the buccal mucous membrane. The *rash* (Fig.6.1) appears 24 hours later, first on the forehead and neck spreading to invade the trunk over a period of 3–4 days. The lesions are reddish maculopapular at first, becoming brown later and, in dark skins appearing totally different to lesions in pale skins, with a diffuse deep red or purple rash followed by severe desquamation

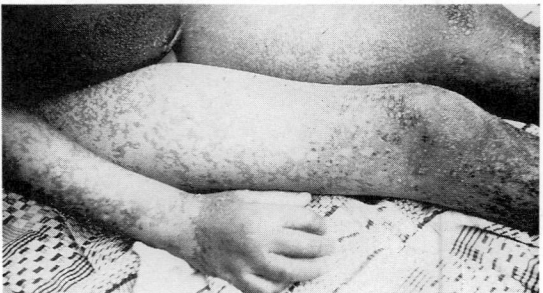

Fig. 6.1 Measles rash in an African child near the knee. In a dark skin the rash has a deep bluish colour. (Courtesy Professor D. Morley.)

2–4 days later. This may lead to patchy depigmentation and boils.

Haemorrhagic measles with purpuric rash and bleeding from mucous membranes is very rare but carries a high mortality.

Other systems

The *mouth* becomes sore interfering with sucking and eating, leading to malnutrition and cancrum oris. *Laryngitis* is common followed by bronchopneumonia which carries a high death rate. *Diarrhoea*, sometimes with tenesmus blood and mucus in the stools, leads to dehydration needing parenteral replacement to prevent death.

Nervous system

The most common nervous change is a short, generalized convulsion early in the infection from which recovery is complete.

ENCEPHALITIS

Measles encephalitis is associated with generalized convulsions, the risk increasing with age. The course is variable. Onset is 4–7 days after the rash appears (48 hours to two weeks after onset) and is shown by fever, irritability, meningism and coma. The cerebrospinal fluid (CSF) shows a moderate pleocytosis with a moderate increase in protein. Mortality can be as high as 10–15% and one-quarter of affected children are left with permanent damage. The cause of the phenomenon is most likely immunologically determined, as shown by the histological changes, perivascular cuffing, demyelination and gliosis.

Subacute sclerosing panencephalitis (SSPE)

This is caused by a persistent virus infection of the brain. It manifests itself some 5–10 years after infection with measles as a slow degenerative condition starting with personality changes, deterioration of intellect preceding signs of mental deterioration, to a state of decerebrate rigidity. Very high levels of measles antibody are found in the CSF.

Complications

CMI depression can lead to a giant cell pneumonia also seen in patients with defective CMI.

Severe ulcerative herpes of mouth and eye[3] is the result of CMI depression.

Severe conjunctivitis often associated with vitamin A deficiency causes perforation of the cornea and blindness. Measles is one of the commonest causes of blindness in the tropics (see Chapter 70).

Gangrene of the extremities may develop.

Malnutrition and measles precipitate kwashiorkor and marasmus.

Otitis media leads to mastoiditis and reduced hearing.

Measles has a major effect on development of the child.

DIAGNOSIS

The association of cough, conjunctivitis, coryza and a morbilliform rash is diagnostic but other conditions have often been mistaken for measles: tick-borne and louse-borne typhus, meningococcaemia, scarlet fever and infectious mononucleosis all have morbilliform rashes. There is a leukocytosis in the early stages followed by an inrease in lymphocytes, some of them of the Türk type.

During the prodromal period large multinucleate (giant) cells can be seen in stained smears of sputum or urine. Serological tests on acute and convalescent sera show haemagglutination-inhibiting (HI) and neutralizing (N) antibodies with a fourfold rise in titre after the initial infection.

TREATMENT

No drug is known to influence the virus.[4] The intake of food and fluid must be maintained and rehydration performed. Antibiotics are essential for otitis media, bacterial pneumonia and skin infections.

EPIDEMIOLOGY

Man is the sole reservoir of measles. The incidence of measles worldwide is diminishing in developed countries, where the mean age of onset is over 5 years. As the vaccination of infants increases, the mean age of attack rises, and unvaccinated individuals and visitors to developing countries which have no vaccination programme are at risk.

In developing countries children generally show the disease at 18–30 months and epidemics occur during the dry season when festivals and concourses of people take place. In isolated populations, such as nomads, measles may occur at any age if the last exposure was many years before. In large cities measles is endemic throughout the year; in smaller towns epidemics in children will occur every two to three years and infection will spread to the villages.

CONTROL

Both passive immunization with human immunoglobulin and active immunization with a live attenuated vaccine are highly successful.

Passive immunization

Passive immunization with human gamma globulin 0.25 mg/kg is effective if given within 5 days of exposure. Passive immunization of children on admission to hospital gave complete protection which was immediate.[5]

Active immunization

A live attenuated strain of the virus is used which gives a 98% conversion rate used under perfect conditions. Fever of moderate severity and a mild rash may occur rarely. Encephalitis is a very rare complication.

It can be given together with diphtheria, tetanus toxoid and pertussis (DPT) without losses of immunogenicity.[6] Maternal antibody is transferred transplacentally and this will inhibit the vaccine up to the age of six months. Normally vaccination is aimed at children nine months of age but vaccination at six months, despite a lower seroconversion rate, is used in areas of high risk, possibly in conjunction with a booster dose one year later. In order to eradicate the disease immunization rates of between 90% and 95% are required.

A 49% reduction in mortality in African children hospitalized with pneumonia and gastroenteritis was reported[7] when measles vaccine was given as a routine on admission. Human immunoglobulin should be given with measles vaccine to malnourished children.

Live vaccines are rapidly inactivated at room temperature and the difficulty of maintaining the cold chain is a major handicap to its use in tropical countries.

A 78% conversion rate was achieved[8] and monitoring of seroconversion rates should be a feature of all antimeasles campaigns.

An aerosol administered vaccine has been successfully developed[9] which since it can be administered by anyone with minimum qualifications by hand pump should be a great advance on previous methods of mass immunization. A heat stable vaccine is also under development.[10]

A major difficulty is that measles vaccination campaigns have to be repeated regularly and it is important that measles vaccine is incorporated into the regular health care system for rural areas along with other immunizations.

POLIOMYELITIS

GEOGRAPHICAL DISTRIBUTION

Poliomyelitis is widespread in tropical countries and epidemics are now occurring in areas where there has been some improvement in sanitation. Immigrants and visitors to these countries carry a special risk of infection since they are not immune from infection in childhood.

AETIOLOGY

Poliomyelitis is an RNA enterovirus belonging to the family *Picornaviridae*. The virion is a spherical particle 30 nm in diameter with an RNA core surrounded by an icosahedral cell with a large number of capsomeres. There are three antigenic types, 1, 2 and 3. Cross immunity between these types is minimal. Type 1 causes the major epidemics; type 2 is the least virulent and establishes itself most efficiently in the gut. A few sporadic cases of paralytic disease are caused by other enteroviruses, mainly those of the Coxsackie group. The virus grows on primary monkey kidney cells, HeLa or human amnion cell cultures. It is rapidly inactivated by dessication but is resistant to chemicals. It is inactivated below pH 3.0 and above pH 7.0 as well as by formalin, chlorine and iodine.

TRANSMISSION

Transmission is by oral or faecal excretion and infection is via the small intestinal epithelium. Droplet infection is most important in epidemic periods since the virus is most infective while in the oropharynx. The faecal/oral route is the usual method of spread in lower socioeconomic communities where infants and small children universally acquire infection.

PATHOLOGY

The main changes are in the anterior horns of the spinal cord. The route of infection is by inhalation or ingestion. The virus multiplies in the tonsils, pharynx and lymphatic follicles of the ileum from where it is rapidly excreted into the gut and appears in the cervical and mesenteric lymph glands. One to three days after infection virus can be recovered from the throat where it persists for a week and in the stools for several weeks. In overt clinical cases it enters the blood and spreads to the central nervous system (CNS) along the peripheral nerve fibres. The virus multiplies in the CNS damaging the motor neurons which are killed and removed by gliosis. Affected neurons may, however, recover. These changes are accompanied by neutrophilic infiltration and perivascular lymphocytic infiltration with the formation of granular compound corpuscles but no demyelination. A high proportion of neurons must be destroyed to cause permanent paralysis. Similar lesions may be found in the posterior columns and root ganglia.

IMMUNITY

Immunity is mediated by the intestinal epithelium preventing reinfection by the homologous strain. An attack of poliomyelitis gives permanent immunity to a second attack from the homologous strain but not to heterologous strains. Second attacks are said to be more severe.

CLINICAL FEATURES

Natural history

Most infections are subclinical and serological evidence suggests that there may be anything between 50 and 500 children infected (and mostly capable of spreading infection for a short time) for every clinically overt case. In the clinically overt infections, about 5%, the majority develop a short acute febrile illness with rapid recovery, while a minority (1%) develop paralytic poliomyelitis.

Incubation period

The incubation period is 7–14 days.

Symptoms and signs

Preparalytic stage

Injections, hard exercise before onset and other traumas are important predisposing factors.

The onset is abrupt with headache, myalgia, sore throat and fever lasting 1–3 days, occasionally a mild gastrointestinal disturbance and/or a mild aseptic meningitis. Complete recovery takes place in the majority of cases.

Paralytic stage

In those cases which go on to this stage a flaccid paralysis of muscles takes place over the next 3–5 days. The paralysis is asymmetrical—legs, arms, back, thorax and diaphragm in that order. Partial or total respiratory paralysis may occur. Sensory loss is rare but retention of urine is often associated with extensive paralysis. The mind remains clear. After a brief period muscles may recover their function over four to six weeks but after six months there is no further improvement.

Bulbar poliomyelitis

Ten per cent of paralytic cases develop cranial nerve paralysis or a combination of bulbar and spinal muscles. Soft palate, larynx and pharynx are involved with nasal voice, regurgitation of food, dysphagia and dyspnoea. Involvement of the respiratory and vasomotor centres in the medulla leads to death.

The fever usually returns to normal by the eighth day but further paralysis is always possible if there is fever. On the fourteenth day recovery begins lasting for about two months but after six months there is no further improvement. The cranial nerves recover in one month. The CSF shows a pleocytosis of 10–500 cells mm³, at first neutrophilic, later with lymphocytes predominating. The protein is raised and chloride and sugar are normal. The blood shows a neutrophil leukocytosis.

DIAGNOSIS

The triad of a preparalytic phase, asymptomatic flaccid paralysis but with mental clarity is diagnostic.

Isolation of virus

Throat swabs and faecal extract are placed into monkey kidney cell cultures where cytopathic affects are seen and the virus is typed by serological methods. There is a fourfold rise in titre of N antibodies which appear early and persist for many years, usually for life. Complement-fixing (CF) antibodies appear later, last a few years and are good evidence of recent infection in 90% of cases.

Differential diagnosis

In the early stages poliomyelitis must be distinguished from aseptic meningitis, lymphocytic choriomeningitis, leptospirosis, tuberculous and suppurative meningitis, and in the paralytic stage, from echovirus, viral encephalitides, Guillain–Barré syndrome, acute infective polyneuritis (symmetrical flaccid paralysis of all four limbs), tick paralysis and pseudoparalysis.

TREATMENT

There is no specific treatment. Bed. rest in the acute stage is important. Rehabilitation and treatment of residual paralyses is important but difficult in the rural tropics.

EPIDEMIOLOGY

Poliomyelitis is endemic where sanitation is poor and where most of the population is immunized naturally in childhood, paralytic poliomyelitis is not often seen. As standards of sanitation and hygiene improve then paralytic poliomyelitis appears where it had been almost unknown before. Where sanitation and personal hygiene are good, infection in childhood is rare and epidemics can occur affecting all ages.

CONTROL

Active immunization against poliomyelitis is very effective. The two vaccines—live attenuated virus (Sabin) and the killed vaccine (Salk)—give long-lasting immunity. Both can be used in child immunization programmes and both can be given simultaneously with triple (DPT) vaccine.

During an epidemic everyone should be immunized as soon as possible. All injections, cold operations and violent exercise should be stopped.

Control in endemic areas

In order to achieve any degree of control a high degree of immunization must be achieved in children and there are two methods of achieving this: one is to add polio vaccine to the immunization programme via the rural health delivery service, the other is to achieve much more dramatic results by a nationwide synchronized programme with three doses of oral vaccine two months apart for all children under the age of five years as recommended by Sabin.[11] This has been successful in Brazil and modified to establish control in selected areas, expanded each year until the whole country is covered (pulse immunization).[12] A start has been made in Vellore, India where 62% of the children under five received three doses of vaccine and the incidence of poliomyelitis fell dramatically.[13]

Live vaccine (Sabin)

This is the vaccine of choice. It is given by the oral route and can be administered by non-medical staff. It is given as three doses with intervals between the first and second dose of 6–8 weeks and between the second and third of six to twelve months. Since maternal antibodies are not transferred babies should start at two months of age. It can be given safely to pregnant mothers. It is the only vaccine that can be given during epidemics since its use blocks the circulation of wild polioviruses by immunizing the intestine. Oral vaccines have been associated with a small number of paralytic cases (about 1 per 3 million doses). Oral vaccine must not be given to families with young babies unless the infant is first immunized. The efficacy of the vaccine has been called into question in tropical countries where it may be affected by other intestinal viral infections or failure of the cold chain.[14]

Killed vaccine (Salk)

Killed vaccines used over a long period have eliminated paralytic poliomyelitis in some developed countries. Modern killed vaccines are extremely potent but need administration by medically trained persons and also a cold chain. However, their efficacy in tropical countries may be better than live vaccines.

HEPATITIS

Viral hepatitis is caused by at least three different viruses: hepatitis A (infectious or epidemic hepatitis), hepatitis B (serum hepatitis), hepatitis B plus delta agent and non-A, non-B hepatitis, which is caused by more than one agent.

Hepatitis A

GEOGRAPHICAL DISTRIBUTION

Hepatitis A occurs endemically in all parts of the world and infection is universal in Third World countries.

AETIOLOGY

Hepatitis A virus is an enterovirus of the Picornaviridae family. It is a small cubic virus 27 nm in diameter, stable at an acid pH and resistant to ether, chlorination and temperature up to 60°C. Its host range is man, chimpanzee and marmoset. The virus can be identified in faecal extracts by immune electron microscopy and can be cultured in primary monolayer and explant cell cultures in continuous lines of primate cells. Hepatitis A virus is shed during the incubation period as early as 9 days after exposure and during the early clinical phase, decreasing rapidly after the onset of jaundice. There is no persistence of virus and no prolonged carrier state.

TRANSMISSION

Hepatitis A virus is spread by the faecal–oral route by person-to-person contact in conditions of poor sanitation and overcrowding. In some small epidemics infection is from faecal contamination of food and water. Waterborne spread is not a major factor but food is, since it becomes contaminated by food handlers who are shedding virus in the faeces during the incubation period of the infection, and are handling uncooked food or cooked food. Inadequately cooked shellfish from polluted water is a well-known source of infection. Accidental transmission by blood is not common because of the slight degree of viraemia.

PATHOLOGY

The virus enters by the oral route and passes to the liver which is the main organ affected. There are minor small intestinal mucosal changes but hepatitis A virus damages and destroys the cells by its presence in the liver cell. There is no evidence of any autoimmune phenomenon. In *acute hepatitis* there is evidence of cell damage especially in the centrilobular region with an inflammatory reaction both neutrophil and lymphocytic, with proliferation of portal lymphoid and macrophage elements; occasionally coagulation necrosis leads to the formation of acidophilic bodies. Regeneration is complete and is associated with disruption of the liver cord pattern and proliferation of ballooned liver cells. There are all gradations of severity through to *acute fulminant* cases which can be mistaken for yellow fever where the liver undergoes acute yellow atrophy, becoming small, pale, shrunken and flabby (in yellow fever the liver is not shrunken). Histologically there is extensive necrosis, the lost liver cells being replaced by an infiltrate of neutrophils and lymphocytes.

IMMUNITY

Immunity is antibody mediated and possession of antibody to hepatitis A protects against infection with hepatitis A. This immunity is lifelong. Passive immunity can be transferred by pooled human gamma globulin and lasts for, depending on dose, up to six months.

CLINICAL FEATURES

Natural history

Infection is often subclinical and mild anicteric infections are common. There is no evidence of persistence of infection, progression to chronic liver damage does not occur and there is no persistent carrier state.

Incubation period

The incubation period is 3–5 weeks with a mean of 28 days.

Symptoms and signs

Subclinical infection

The majority of infections are symptomless but may show raised liver enzyme values.[15]

Overt infection

The onset is gradual with *anorexia* (a prominent symptom), fever, aching pain in limbs and back before the onset of *jaundice* starting about one week after onset and hepatitis A is a common cause of acute pyrexia of unknown origin in its early preicteric stages. The jaundice deepens with pale faeces and dark urine (urobilinuria precedes the jaundice by about one day) and is more pronounced than in yellow fever and other viral infections. The *liver* is enlarged and tender and there may be a slight splenic enlargement. After a few days the temperature comes down, the jaundice diminishes and complete recovery takes place. Sometimes the jaundice may last for weeks and liver scan and other procedures may be necessary to exclude other causes of jaundice. In many cases mental depression is a feature which can last for up to six months. In some cases the disease is fulminant and can be fatal even before the onset of jaundice. A high mortality has been reported in some areas in India (Indian soldiers were especially affected in the Second World War), the Middle East and North Africa, and especially in women who contract hepatitis in pregnancy (the fetus is not affected). Although jaundice may continue beyond three weeks hepatitis A infection does not progress to chronic liver disease.

DIFFERENTIAL DIAGNOSIS

Hepatitis A in its early preicteric stage is easily mistaken for falciparum malaria, infectious mononucleosis, trypanosomiasis, leptospirosis, yellow fever and other arbovirus diseases. The onset is slower, anorexia is an important sign in hepatitis A and there are no meningeal signs. Hepatitis B can only be distinguished by the longer incubation period following a history of possible parenteral infection.

DIAGNOSIS

The diagnosis is most often made by a process of exclusion and can only be made definitively by demonstrating the presence of hepatitis A antigen in the first 5 days before the onset of illness. A fourfold increase in hepatitis A IgM antibody follows, which can persist for 45–60 days and denotes recent infection. Hepatitis A IgG antibody, which appears later, persists for many years. Its presence denotes past infection and immunity to further infection (Fig. 6.2). If present in the early stages of an illness, this is not caused by hepatitis A.

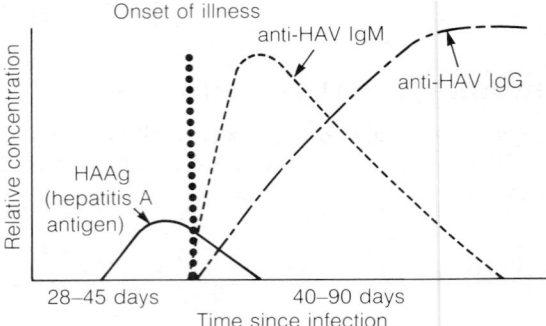

Fig. 6.2. Serological sequence of markers in hepatitis A infection. HAV = hepatis A virus.

It can be detected by radioimmunoassay and ELISA.[16] The ELISA test provides a rapid means of detecting virus in the faeces, enabling the screening of a large number of faecal specimens to detect infected food handlers, but in view of the short duration of virus excretion, this seems a foolishly wasteful application.

TREATMENT

There is no specific treatment. Abstention from alcohol for three months is advisable. Steroids may be of value in fulminant cases.

EPIDEMIOLOGY

All age groups are susceptible to infection and the highest incidence in tropical countries is in children. Visitors and immigrants from developed (where the incidence is low) to developing countries (where the incidence is high) are especially at risk. In tropical countries the peak of reported infection tends to be during the rainy season.

CONTROL

The spread of infection is controlled by simple hygienic measures and the sanitary disposal of excreta (especially the establishment of water-borne sanitation). Since faecal shedding of virus is highest during the incubation period strict isolation of patients is not a necessity, but barrier nursing and special disposal of faeces are necessary.

Gamma globulin

Normal human immunoglobulin in 0.02 to 0.12 mg/kg body weight is given intramuscularly during the incubation period and will prevent or abort an attack. It does not always prevent infection and excretion of virus. Immunoglobulin should always be given to close personal contacts of patients and to those exposed to contamination, especially travellers to tropical countries, who should always be given gamma globulin if they do not possess antibodies to hepatitis A. The immunity lasts about four months and must be given regularly for prolonged stays in highly endemic areas. No vaccine is yet available. No satisfactory standardization of immunoglobulin potency is adopted by manufacturers, and it is known that some pooled globulins—such as those from areas of low endemicity—do not possess adequate potency.

Hepatitis B

GEOGRAPHICAL DISTRIBUTION

Hepatitis B infection is found worldwide with the highest infection rates found in parts of the tropics (Fig. 6.3), West Africa and the Pacific where as many as 20% of the apparently healthy population may be carriers.

AETIOLOGY

The hepatitis B virus is a DNA virus with a complex morphology. There are three components: a large double-shelled complete virus particle of about 42 nm in diameter (formerly known as the Dane particle), small spherical particles of hepatitis B surface antigen about 22 nm in diameter, and tubular forms of surface antigen about 20 nm in diameter and many nanometres long (Fig. 6.4).[17]

The antigenic structure is complex and consists of three antigens, each of which has its equivalent antibody. They are *hepatitis B surface antigen* (HBsAg), *hepatitis B core antigen* (HBcAg) and *hepatitis Be antigen* (HBeAg).

HBsAg, formerly Australia antigen, shares a group specific antigen but contains subtype variants which can be used to determine the different geographical distributions. The antigen, which can be detected by ELISA and radioimmunoassay, has been used as a marker to demonstrate the links between hepatitis B infection, chronic liver damage and primary hepatocellular carcinoma.

HBeAg is located within the core and is a marker of the infectivity of the serum since it correlates closely with the number of virus particles. The appearance of the antigens and their appropriate antibodies can be used to determine the state of infection in any individual and to diagnose acute infection, past infection and the carrier state. The sequential appearance of the antigens and their antibodies is shown in Fig. 6.5.[18] The first to appear in the incubation period is HBsAg which survives longest to be followed later by anti-HBsAg. HBeAg appears later to be followed at an earlier stage by anti-HBcAg and anti-HBeAg which disappear earlier than anti-HBsAg (Fig. 6.5). In the persistent carrier stage HBsAg persists in the serum and is a good indicator of that state.

TRANSMISSION

The transmission of hepatitis B (unlike hepatitis A) may be by the parenteral route by blood, contaminated syringes and by hetero- and homosexual contact. Contaminated syringes are thought to contribute to the high incidence of infection in Third World countries where disposable syringes are reused on a massive scale.

Perinatal transmission from mother to infant during birth is one of the most efficient methods of hepatitis B virus (HBV) transmission and probably accounts for the high incidence of hepatitis B infection in tropical areas with the concurrent high incidence of macronodular cirrhosis and primary hepatocellular carcinoma. Case-to-case transmission among siblings is also a factor.

Blood-sucking arthropods have been thought to be important since HBsAg has been recovered from mosquitoes and bed bugs, but although there is no evidence of multiplication of virus in these insects, direct mechanical transmission is possible. Contamination of the environment with dried exudate from tropical ulcers has been suggested,[19] as also cultural procedures such as

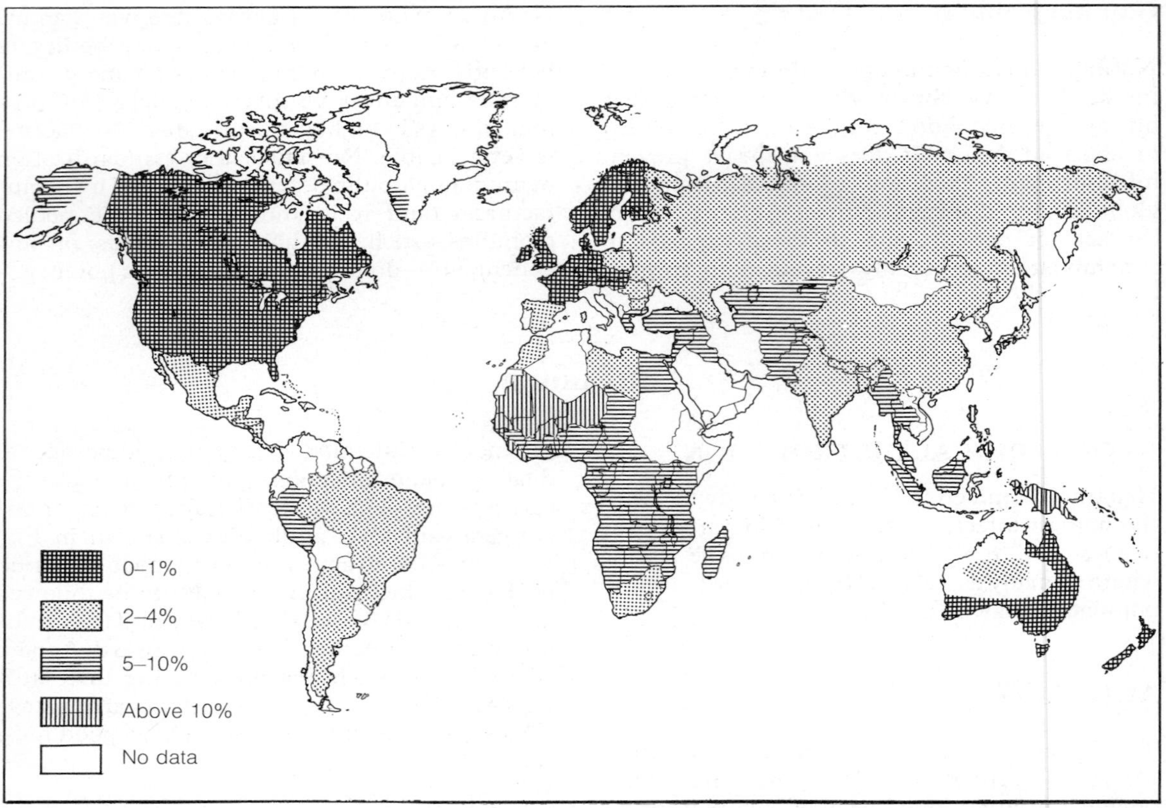

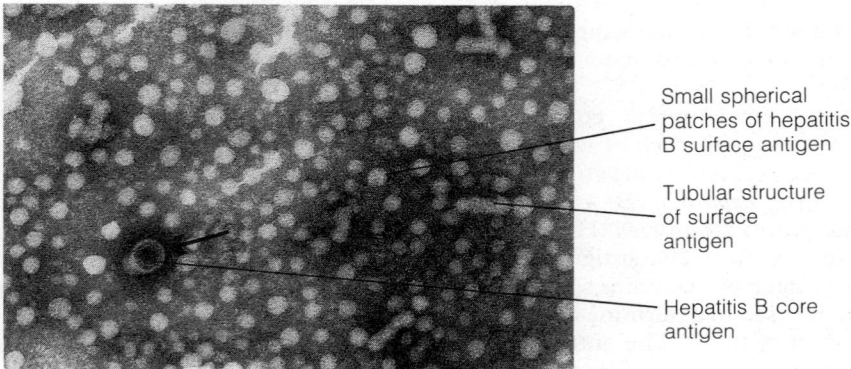

Fig. 6.3. Geographical distribution of hepatitis B.

0–1%

2–4%

5–10%

Above 10%

No data

Small spherical
patches of hepatitis
B surface antigen

Tubular structure
of surface
antigen

Hepatitis B core
antigen

Fig. 6.4. Hepatitis B core antigen. (From Zuckerman[17].)

tattooing, circumcision and tribal scarring. Virus has been introduced via the mouth but this is not a common occurrence.

PATHOLOGY

The pathogenesis of the liver changes in hepatitis

B infection is related to the immune response of the host to the structural components of the virus. In symptomless hepatitis B carriers there is no cell-mediated immunity to hepatitis B antigens, but in acute infection and chronic active hepatitis there is a cell-mediated reaction with the appearance of virus-associated antigens on

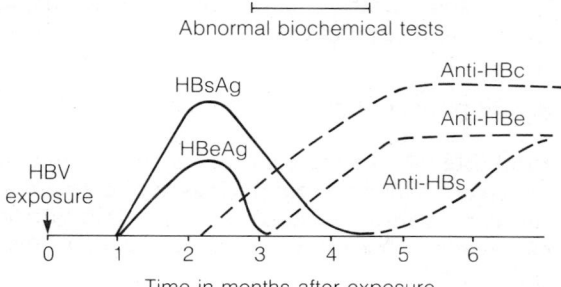

Fig. 6.5. Serological course of uncomplicated hepatitis B with recovery. (From McCallum and Zuckerman[18].)

the surface of the liver cells which are then destroyed by T lymphocytes reacting to the new antigens. In acute infection following necrosis of liver cells, the virus is removed and antigen–antibody complexes are removed by the reticuloendothelial system. T cell reaction ceases, liver necrosis stops and recovery from the acute hepatitis follows. If there is a qualitative defect in the antibody the virus is not cleared, other cells become infected to be attacked in their turn by more T cells, and immunological damage continues to chronic active hepatitis and macronodular cirrhosis.

Microscopically the liver cells vary in size and there is marked ballooning and degeneration. The cells contain two or more nuclei. Eosinophilic necrosis is most marked in the central zones and there is a focal infiltration with histiocytes, lymphocytes and plasma cells with occasional eosinophils and neutrophils, which are also found in the portal tracts.

In fulminant hepatitis there is massive liver cell necrosis most severe in the left lobe. If recovery occurs it is not clear what happens to the liver cells; some patients recover completely, others go on to macronodular cirrhosis.

An acute pancreatitis may be found involving both islet and secretory cells.

In acute hepatitis the changes caused by hepatitis B are indistinguishable under light microscopy from those caused by hepatitis A, but can be differentiated by electron microscopy and immunofluorescent techniques.

Chronic active hepatitis

Chronic active hepatitis is characterized by accumulations of lymphocytes and plasma cells in the portal tracts and in the necrotic foci scattered throughout the lobules. In the hepatic parenchyma there is 'piecemeal' necrosis and small clusters of liver cells surrounded by inflammatory cells creating 'rosettes'. Collapse and necrosis between the portal areas and the central vein has been called 'bridging necrosis'. These areas are later replaced by fibrous tissue leading on to large areas of regenerating liver cells surrounded by dense fibrous tissue (macronodular cirrhosis).

Chronic persistent hepatitis

This is characterized by a lymphocytic infiltration of the portal tracts. Hepatocellular damage is minimal and fibrosis slight or absent; it has a good prognosis but may develop into chronic active hepatitis.

A small proportion of cases maintain circulating immune complexes and may develop vasculitis or polyarteritis.

IMMUNITY

Immunity to hepatitis B is mainly cell mediated and the reaction to various parts of the virus is responsible for the liver damage. Surface antigen–antibody, core antigen–core antibody immune complexes have been found in all the recognized chronic sequelae of hepatitis B. The presence of surface antibody shows immunity to hepatitis B virus, and passive immunity can be transferred by special high-titre hepatitis B immunoglobulin which is used in special circumstances.

CLINICAL FEATURES

Natural history

Many infections are subclinical and are followed by recovery and the appearance of anti-HBsAg in the blood. Other cases do not clear the infection and the virus is integrated into the host DNA with the establishment of chronic infection and the carrier state leading to chronic active hepatitis, macronodular cirrhosis and primary hepatocellular carcinoma.

Incubation period

The incubation period is 70 days mean with a range of 50–180 days.

Symptoms and signs

The symptoms and signs of the acute phase are similar to those of hepatitis A but the illness is more prolonged, fever is less prominent and there may be joint pains and a rash in the prodromal period. The course of the illness lasts three to four weeks after which recovery occurs. In 3% of cases there is a relapse in convalescence with a return of fever and jaundice.

DIFFERENTIAL DIAGNOSIS

The jaundiced stage must be distinguished from the jaundice of acute bacterial infection, notably lobar pneumonia, and the tender liver enlargement from that found in hepatic amoebiasis and typhoid, although jaundice is less marked in these cases. Tender enlargement of the liver is also found in homozygous (SS) sickle cell disease. Numerous causes of acute haemolysis are found in the tropics, especially falciparum malaria (blackwater fever) and G-6-PD deficiency.

DIAGNOSIS

Diagnosis rests upon the detection of surface antigen, surface antibody, core antigen, core antibody, e antigen and e antibody in the serum. In the incubation period HBsAg and HBcAg are present to be followed by anti-HBcAg, both IgM and IgG. After recovery only anti-HBsAg IgG antibody is left. In the carrier state HBsAg can be detected. The presence of HBeAg is related to the degree of infection and has an unfavourable prognosis with respect to chronic liver disease.

COMPLICATIONS

Fulminant viral hepatitis

This is a serious complication which can follow, A, B, and non-A, non-B hepatitis and is common in some parts of the tropics especially Africa. It is commoner in women than men and commoner in pregnancy. Clinically a deeply jaundiced patient develops personality changes, acute maniacal behaviour or changes in consciousness. Signs of liver failure develop and the size of the liver decreases. The mortality rate is high (50–70%) and death occurs with haemorrhagic features and renal failure.

Acute pancreatitis

Viral infection of the pancreas is very common. Pancreatitis may present itself as hypoglycaemia, and is probably the cause of the chronic calcific pancreatitis found in tropical regions (see Chapter 60).

The carrier state

The carrier state has been defined as persistence of HBsAg in the serum for more than six months and becomes established in 5–10% of infected adults. In highly endemic areas in the tropics the highest incidence of carriers is in children aged between four and eight years. The carrier state is often associated with liver damage ranging from minor changes to chronic active hepatitis and cirrhosis. The persistence of hepatitis B in the population is maintained by these carriers.

Chronic active hepatitis and macronodular cirrhosis

Chronic active hepatitis is shown by the persistence of liver dysfunction with the development of the signs and symptoms of macronodular cirrhosis. Liver failure is not a feature until late in the disease.

Primary hepatocellular carcinoma
(see also Chapter 67)

An association between hepatitis B infection and hepatoma is shown by the presence of HBsAg in the blood of patients with macronodular cirrhosis and primary hepatocellular carcinoma. Primary liver carcinoma has also been found in animals infected with viruses related to hepatitis B.

TREATMENT

Interferon has a temporary inhibitory effect on virus multiplication in liver cells.

Adenine arabinoside has a significant antiviral activity against several DNA viruses and trials are in progress.

Epidemiology

The epidemiology of hepatitis B infection differs in temperate countries from tropical areas. In temperate countries the infection is blood transmitted and is found in drug addicts, homosexuals and workers in renal dialysis units. Contamination of vaccines made from human cell lines (yellow fever) has caused huge epidemics.

The cause of the high infection rate in the tropics is the high degree of perinatal transmission (see p. 174), and intersibling transmission has been shown to be of major importance in The Gambia where infection is clustered in families.[20] These factors account for the high incidence of chronic HBV carriers with the highest incidence in children between four and eight years.

CONTROL

Passive immunization (hepatitis B immunoglobulin—HBIG)

This is routinely used to protect contacts of cases. Only high titre HBIG must be used. The dose is in the range of 0.04 to 0.07 ml/kg intramuscularly and two doses should be given 30 days apart. The first dose should preferably be given within 48 hours after contamination and not more than 7 days later. It can also be used in babies born of infected mothers, given in a dose of 0.5 ml/kg within 48 hours of birth followed by monthly doses of 0.16 ml/kg for six months. This will prevent a carrier state developing and is a means of eradicating infection eventually from the population but it is more effective when combined with the vaccine (see below).[21]

Active immunization

A vaccine has been developed using surface antigen separated from the core and thus non-infective. It is obtained from the plasma of symptomless carriers.[21] The vaccine (Merck Heptavax B) is given in three doses intramuscularly first dose, second dose one month later and third dose six months later. Six months to 12 years of age: 0.5 ml each dose; adults and older children 1.0 ml. It can also be given intradermally producing a good antibody response at less cost[22] in a course of 3 × 0.1 ml injections. Complications are few—local soreness and occasionally some local swelling, and low grade fever for 48 hours; uncommonly fever, headache and malaise for 48 hours. It is not recommended for pregnant women. Studies of the use of this vaccine in high risk areas have shown that it will prevent horizontally transmitted infection and when combined with hepatitis B immunoglobulin at birth it prevents development of the carrier state.[23] In The Gambia where intersibling transmission is important this could be interrupted by the vaccination of two-month-old children.[20]

Post-exposure prophylaxis

Studies have shown that response to HBV vaccine is not impaired by the concurrent administration of HBIG and that the combination of HBV vaccine and one dose of HBIG produces immediate and sustained high levels of protective antibodies to the hepatitis B surface antigen. This combination is highly effective in preventing the HB carrier state in infants.[24]

Perinatal transmission

Maternal screening for HBsAg is recommended where available for mothers antenatally and neonates of positive HBsAg mothers given vaccine plus HBIG.

HBIG 0.5 ml is given intramuscularly within 12 hours of birth followed by 0.5 ml ($10\mu g$) of HBV vaccine intramuscularly at a separate site, followed by 0.5 ml ($10\mu g$) repeated at one and six months.

Other post-exposure prophylaxis

For adults 5 ml (0.06 ml/kg) of HBIG is given intramuscularly as a single dose within 24 hours of exposure followed by 1.0 ml ($20\mu g$) of HBV vaccine at a separate site within 7 days, repeated at one and six months.[25]

Indications for immunization[26]

Active immunization should be given to certain persons at special risk: health care personnel in contact with blood and syringes, inmates of residential institutions, sexual partners and family contacts of carriers and infants born of carrier mothers, helpers in contact with refugees from tropical countries where hepatitis B is common. Active immunization on a large scale of infants born of carrier mothers in certain tropical countries has raised the possibility of a great reduction in the carrier rate, and a reduction in the incidence of hepatocellular carcinoma.

Delta infection

GEOGRAPHICAL DISTRIBUTION

The delta agent is found all over the world. It is endemic in Italy where it was first discovered and is associated with serious liver damage. It is also prevalent among drug addicts and homosexuals. It has been found in Brazil where it causes Lábrea hepatitis or 'Lábrea black fever'.[27]

AETIOLOGY

The delta agent only acts in association with hepatitis B virus. It can cause an acute and fatal exacerbation of the disease, often leading to fulminant hepatitis.

CLINICAL FEATURES

Delta infections occur in hepatitis B carriers and are responsible for acute episodes of hepatitis sometimes called non-A, non-B hepatitis. It may cause an acute fulminant infection.[28]

DIAGNOSIS

Diagnosis is by identification of the delta marker in the blood.

Non-A, non-B hepatitis

Non-A, non-B hepatitis is found worldwide although at present it is predominantly a blood transfusion infection. Its incidence in the tropics is unknown.

AETIOLOGY

Non-A, non-B hepatitis is caused by two or possibly more agents with long- or short-term incubation periods.

CLINICAL FEATURES

The illness resembles hepatitis B, often mild, with symptomless and anicteric cases, but severe hepatitis with jaundice does occur and the infection is a significant cause of fulminant hepatitis. The infection is often followed by prolonged viraemia and a persistent carrier state with chronic liver damage in 40–50% of patients.

IZUMI FEVER

This disease of children or young adults was first described in Japan by Izumi and his colleagues in 1927, and there have been many outbreaks there since then. It also occurs sporadically.

It is probably caused by an intestinal virus; Kuroya et al[29] isolated a virus from the faeces of a patient in the acute stage, which affected young mice on intracerebral, intranasal or intraperitoneal injection; the virus spread widely in the mouse tissues. A suspension of infected mouse brain administered by stomach tube caused the typical disease in a human subject.

Neutralizing antibody has been found in human convalescent serum.

The disease is thought to be water-borne, possibly via the urine or faeces of infected rodents, or transmitted by personal contact.[30] Trombiculid mites have also been suspected on epidemiological grounds.[31]

The incubation period seems to be 5 to 13 days. Two types of illness are described, both beginning abruptly with fever and chills. In both types there is an itchy rash intermediate between scarlet fever and measles, on the trunk, face, neck and extremities, which disappears in 3 or 4 days and is followed by fine desquamation. The symptoms include joint and lumbar pains, nausea, vomiting and abdominal pain; the liver may be enlarged. The mild type lasts only a few days, but in the severe type, after the primary fever subsides there is a secondary attack, with the same characters, but with fever lasting up to two or three weeks.[32] There may even be a third febrile phase.[33]

Treatment with chlortetracycline or chloramphenicol is said to be effective.

REFERENCES

1 Morley, D., Woodland, M. & Martin, W.J. (1963) *J. Hyg., Camb.* **61**, 115.
2 Gunn (1963) Quoted by Morley et al (1963).
3 Whittle, H.C., Sandford Smith, J., Kogbe, O.I. et al (1979) *Trans. R. Soc. trop. Med. Hyg.* **73**, 66.
4 Morley, D. (1969) *Br. med. J.* **i**, 297.
5 Wesley A., Coovadia, H.M. & Watson, A.R. (1979) *Trans. R. Soc. trop. Med. Hyg.* **73**, 710.
6 McBean, A.M., Gateff, C., Manclark, C.R. et al (1978) *Pediatrics Springfield* **62**, 288.
7 Harris, M.F. (1979) *S. Afr. med. J.* **55**, 38.
8 King, B. (1978) *E. Afr. med. J.* **55**, 38.
9 Sabin, A.B., Adrediga, A.F., de Castro, J.F. et al (1983) *J. Am. med. Ass.* **249**, 2651–2662.
10 Heymann, D.L., Nakano, J.H., Maben, G.K. et al (1979) *Br. med. J.* **ii**, 99.
11 Sabin, A.B. (1980) *Bull. Wld Hlth Org.* **58**, 141–157.
12 John, T.J. & Steinhoff, M.C. (1981) *Indian J. Paediat.* **48**, 677–683.
13 John, T.J., Pandian, R., Gadomski, A. et al (1983) *Br. med. J.* **286**, 31–32.
14 Imam, I.Z. (1981) *Devl. Biol. Standard* **47**, 215–221.
15 Chang, L.W. & O'Brien, T.F. (1970) *Lancet* **ii**, 59.
16 Zuckerman, A.J. (1979) *Br. med. J.* **ii**, 84.
17 Zuckerman, A.J. (1975) *Human Viral Hepatitis.* Amsterdam: North Holland.
18 McCallum, R.W. & Zuckerman, A.J. (1981) *J. med. Virol.* **8**, 1.
19 Foster, O., Ajdukiewicz, A.B., Ryder, R. et al (1984) *Lancet* **i**, 576–577.
20 Whittle, H.C., McLauchlan, K., Bradley, A.K. et al (1983) *Lancet* **i**, 1203–1206.
21 Zuckerman, A.J. (1982) *Br. med J.* **284**, 686–688.
22 Miller, K.D., Mulligan, M.M., Gibbs, R.D. et al (1983) *Lancet* **ii**, 1454–1456.
23 Arthur, M.J.P., Hall, A.J. & Wright, R. (1984) *Lancet* **i**, 607–610.
24 Beasley, R.P., Hwang, L-Y, Lee, G.C. et al (1983) *Lancet* **ii**, 1099–1102.
25 *Morbidity and Mortality Weekly Report* (1984) **33**, 285–290.
26 Zuckerman, A.J. (1984) *Br. med. J.* **289**, 1243–1244.
27 Bensabath, G.& Dias, L.B. (1983) *Rev. Inst. Med. Trop. São Paulo* **25**, 182–194.
28 Moestrup, T., Hansson, B.G., Widell, A. et al (1983) *Br. med. J.* **286**, 87–89.
29 Kuroya, M., Yoshinari, Y., Ishida, N. et al (1954) *Jap. J. exp. Med.* **24**, 105.
30 Nishioka, K. & Morita, J. (1952) *Jap. J. exp. Med.* **22**, 333.
31 Kumada, N., Sasa, M., Miura, A. et al (1952) *Jap. J. exp. Med.* **22**, 353.
32 Nishioka, K. & Nishioka, K. (1952) *Jap. J. exp. Med.* **22**, 341.
33 Yanagishita, T., Ogawa, J. & Kimura, T. (1957) *Keio J. Med.* **6**, 35.

Chapter 7
Brucellosis and Tularaemia

BRUCELLOSIS

Brucellosis is also known as undulant fever (melitensis type), Malta fever or Mediterranean fever.

GEOGRAPHICAL DISTRIBUTION

Brucella abortus is found in temperate countries where cattle are raised extensively, especially in the USA (New Mexico and Texas) and Mexico, but also in other dairying countries of the world including Britain.

Brucella melitensis is found in those countries where the goat is extensively used, usually the hotter and drier areas; the shores of the Mediterranean, southern France, Italy, Spain, southeast and West Africa and Somalia.

Brucella suis is confined to North America where it is an important cause of disease.

AETIOLOGY

Three main species of *Brucella* infect man, *Br. abortus, Br. melitensis,* and *Br. suis.* Other species include *Br. canis,* a cause of canine abortion which caused intermittent fever and bacteraemia for four months in a 48-year-old man[1] and *Br. neotomae* of the wood rat which does not cause human illness. Brucella organisms are small, non-motile, non-spore-bearing gram-negative rods. They measure 0.6–1.5 μm in length and 0.5 μm in width and occur singly, in pairs and sometimes in fours but never in nature in longer chains. They are gram-negative, are readily stained by a watery solution of gentian violet and are best cultured in a 1.5%, very feebly alkaline, peptonized beef agar on which some time after inoculation they appear as minute clear pearly specks. After 36 hours the cultures become transparent amber and later they are opaque. No liquefaction occurs in gelatine. The individual colonies are small, round, somewhat raised discs reaching 2–3 mm in diameter about the ninth day. The optimum temperature for growth is 37°C.

Species identification

The conventional methods of species differentiation of brucellae are the need for carbon dioxide for growth, production of hydrogen sulphide, differential growth on liver agar containing basic fuchsin and thionin and agglutination by monospecific sera (Table 7.1). Only *Br. abortus* is lysed by phage.

Table 7.1 Identification of *Brucella* species.

	Br. melitensis	Br. abortus	Br. suis
CO$_2$ requirement	−	+	
H$_2$S production	−	+ 4 days	+ 5 or more days
Growth on thionin	+	−	+
Growth on basic fuchsin	+	+	−
Monospecific agglutination			
Br. abortus	−	+	+
Br. melitensis	+	−	−

TRANSMISSION

Viability of organisms

Br. melitensis remains viable for up to 37 days in both fresh and salt water, in dried soil for 43 days and in damp soil for 72 hours. Exposure to the sun greatly reduces the survival time. It is resistant to gastric juice.

The normal process of ice-cream and cheese making does not destroy *Br. melitensis.*

Br. abortus can survive in butter up to 142 days and has been isolated from ice-cream which had been frozen for one month. It is susceptible to gastric juice.

Br. suis has been isolated from hog carcases after 21 days of refrigeration.

180

Transmission to man

Direct interhuman transmission is extremely rare, perhaps only occurring via the urine or blood transfusion. No case of brucellosis in nursing infants of infected mothers has been recorded. Brucellosis is transmitted to man via infected milk, via the respiratory tract or ocular route or by direct contact. It now appears that the respiratory route is probably the main portal of entry.[2]

Br. melitensis. Infection is usually acquired via infected goats' milk, since *Br. melitensis* is not destroyed by the gastric juice. Since the pasteurization of milk was introduced the infection has virtually disappeared from Malta. In the Mediterranean and Africa, the respiratory tract is the main portal of entry from inhalation of dust contaminated by the large number of organisms shed in the placentae of infected goats.

Brucella abortus. Milk is an important source of infection, despite the fact that *Br. abortus* is destroyed by gastric juice in vitro. Infection via the respiratory tract from contaminated air is probably also common, as is direct contact in the case of veterinarians. Aerosol spread and entry via the eye is responsible for laboratory infections.

Brucella suis. Direct contact is the method of infection, since the disease occurs in farm workers and meat packers who are infected through abrasions in the skin in contact with infected hog carcases.

Insect vectors

Mosquitoes and blood-sucking flies can be experimentally infected and remain so for 4 or 5 days. Isolations of *Brucella* have been made from mosquitoes in the southern USSR, but transmission by this method is not proven.

PATHOLOGY

The pathology of brucellosis is discussed by Spink.[3]

A significant feature of brucellosis is the location of the organism intracellularly. Brucellae enter the body and localize in the regional lymph glands where they proliferate and may cause necrosis. The bacteria invade the bloodstream and are carried in leukocytes to those areas where there is abundant reticuloendothelial tissue, the liver, spleen, lymph glands and bone marrow, where they become localized, mainly in the mononuclear cells (Fig. 7.1). The basic and characteristic tissue response consists of monocytes and large phagocytes which form granulomas, especially in the liver, spleen, marrow and lymph glands. Granulomas consist of epithelioid

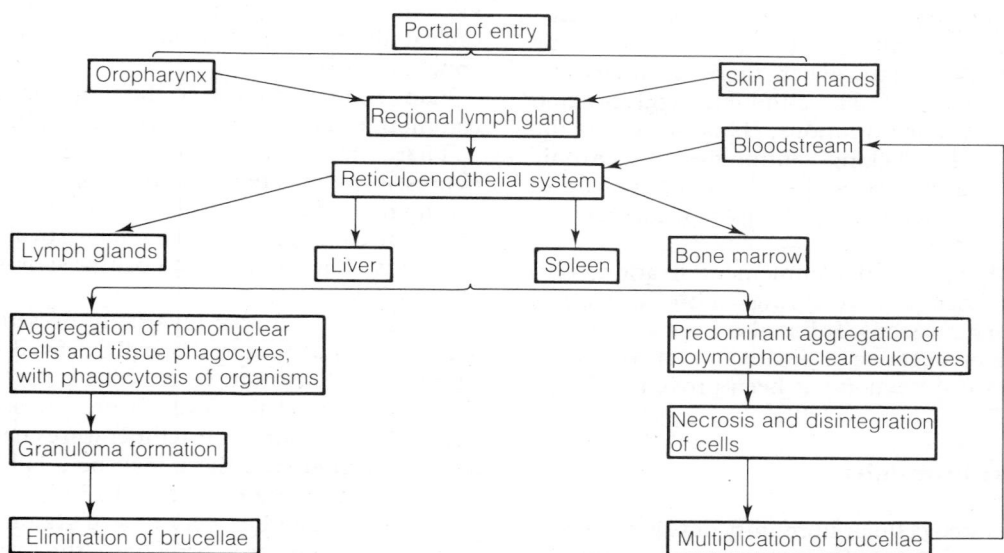

Fig. 7.1 The fate of *Brucella* organisms in the human body.

cells, lymphocytes and giant cells. These granulomas, which disappear rapidly on recovery from the infection, have been used in diagnosis especially by liver and bone marrow biopsy. Rarely there is necrosis and abscess formation. Caseous granulomas in the lung are a feature of *Br. suis* infections.

It is believed that *Brucella* endotoxin is responsible for most of the signs and symptoms of brucellosis but that tissue hypersensitivity is responsible for the granulomas.[3] The *Brucella* organisms are responsible directly for the metastatic lesions which may cause abscesses in the bones (especially the vertebrae), bacterial endocarditis and meningitis.

IMMUNITY

Some immunity results from an attack of brucellosis but second attacks do occur. The immune response of the host is both humoral and cellular.

Humoral immunity

Agglutinin, precipitin and opsonin antibodies appear in the blood towards the end of the first two weeks and persist for a long time. The primary response is an increase in IgM (agglutination reaction) followed later by a secondary response with an increase in IgG and IgA (anti-human-globulin, Coombs' test). In primary acute infections the IgM (agglutination) antibodies are present in high titre and a prozone phenomenon is seen when there is no agglutination below 1/100, although agglutination occurs at higher dilutions. This is due to the presence of 'blocking' antibodies. In chronic infections and in persons with past exposure to infection, only IgG and IgA antibodies are present.

Antiglobulin and complement fixation (CF) tests are often positive during health,[4] as in many veterinary surgeons. It has also been shown that they can be negative or positive in low titre even when active infection has been proved by blood culture.[5]

Cellular immunity

Well-marked cellular immunity develops, shown by a positive brucellin reaction of the skin and a granulomatous reaction in the tissue to the presence of intracellular *Brucella*. This is responsible for the pathological changes found in the liver, spleen, lymph glands and bone marrow.

CLINICAL FEATURES

Natural history

Brucellosis is usually a self-limiting disease and 50% of cases recover their health in one year.[3] The death rate of untreated brucellosis is about 2%. Death is usually due to bacterial endocarditis.

Incubation period

The incubation period is usually one to three weeks, but occasionally several months. The onset may be sudden, as in the malignant or undulating type, or insidious, as in the intermittent type.

Symptoms and signs

Weakness, fatigue, chills and sweats are usual. Profuse nocturnal sweating so that the night-clothes and bed-linen have to be changed several times during the night is typical.

Anorexia, loss of weight and headache are common and pain in the back of the neck is sometimes associated with *Brucella* spondylitis. There may be pain in the back and abdominal pain associated with a tender enlargement of the liver and spleen. Pain in the right iliac fossa caused by mesenteric gland adenitis may mimic appendicitis.

Pains in one or more of the larger joints, are common, usually without signs of arthritis.

There may be nervousness and mental depression associated with insomnia.

Patients with brucellosis present with a multitude of complaints but characteristically have few signs. The commonest positive sign is fever.

Fever. Fever is almost invariably present in an active case and bacteriologically proved disease rarely occurs without fever. The most characteristic feature of the fever in brucellosis is the peculiar behaviour of the temperature chart (Fig. 7.2). In a mild case there may be a ladder-like rise through a week or 10 days to 39 or 40°C and then through another week or so a gradual fall to normal. In mild cases, which are the exception, the fever which is of continued or remittent type

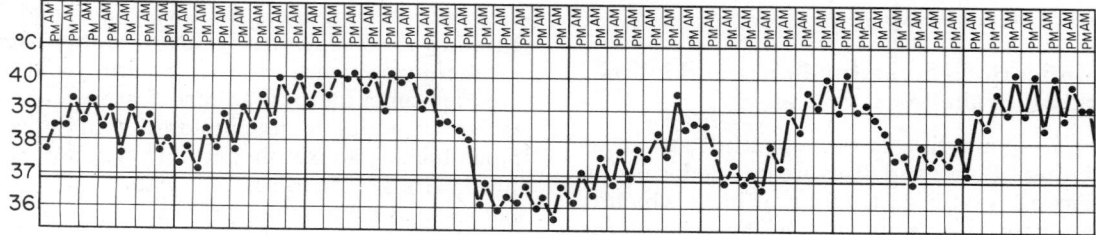

Fig. 7.2 A typical temperature chart from a case of undulant fever.

disappears without complication in about three weeks. Usually after a few afebrile days the fever returns and runs a similar course, the relapse being in its turn followed by another afebrile period and so on during several months. This is the 'undulant' type of fever, from which the disease was named 'undulant fever'.[6] The peak of the temperature curve occurs towards midday or early afternoon, which distinguishes it from typhoid and other continued septic fevers, in which this takes place towards night time.

In other cases a continued fever persists for one, two or more months—the 'continued' type.[6]

Although usually remittent or continuous, the fever sometimes has intermissions. The swinging temperature chart may then suggest bacterial endocarditis or malaria. The fever in untreated cases persists for an average of about four months but the range extends from three weeks to more than two years.

Splenomegaly. This is found in almost half the patients[3] and is a good indicator of the continuing activity of the disease. The spleen is tender and firm and seldom extends beyond 5–6 cm from the costal margin. Occasionally in *Br. melitensis* infection the spleen may be greatly enlarged and *Brucella* can be isolated in pure culture from it.

Lymphadenopathy. Lymphadenopathy is common. The cervical and axillary glands, which are most often involved, are soft, discrete and slightly tender.

Hepatomegaly. Hepatomegaly is much less frequent than splenomegaly. When enlarged the liver is tender. Jaundice occurs rarely.

Tenderness over the spine. This is common and cases of suspected brucellosis should always be examined by heavy percussion over the spine.

Skin. An unusual skin manifestation has been reported[7] in which skin papules are scattered over the body. The papules are granulomas from which *Br. melitensis* can be cultured.

Chronic brucellosis

Of patients with *Br. abortus* 80% recover completely within a year with antibiotic therapy.[3] A minority of patients who have continued ill-health will show definite evidence of localized disease, such as spondylitis, meningoencephalitis, cholecystitis, bone lesions or radiculoneuritis. A small number show persistent ill-health without any signs of disease and are subject to severe headaches, mental depression, nervousness and vasomotor dysfunction. It is probable that these individuals have a hypochondriacal background and brucellosis accentuates this instability and causes further symptoms.

Clinical differences between *Br. abortus*, *Br. melitensis* and *Br. suis*

On the whole *Br. abortus* infections are much milder and run a shorter course than *Br. melitensis* and prolonged pyrexial cases lasting many months are not as common as in *Br. melitensis*. On the other hand *Br. abortus* infection may be very persistent, lasting over a year or more. *Br. suis* infections may be severe and fatal, suppurating complications are more frequent and a chronic state of debility ensues more frequently if proper treatment is not given.[3]

Blood changes in brucellosis

The white cell count is usually normal, but a leukopenia is common in chronic cases. A normochromic, normocytic anaemia may also be present. This may be contributed to by marrow depression or haemolysis.

COMPLICATIONS

Complications involving bones and joints (surgical brucellosis)

Brucella spondylitis is very painful and incapacitating.[8] Bones and discs are invaded, causing osteomyelitis with destruction of bone which is replaced by granulation tissue. The symptoms are similar to those of a herniated disc with root pain, and it may be difficult to distinguish *Brucella* spondylitis of the spine from tuberculosis, except that in brucellosis repair proceeds along with bone destruction which can be seen on the X-ray as osteoporosis with osteosclerosis. Rarely an epidural abscess may form.

Suppuration may occur in the larger joints, especially the hip joint. Osteomyelitis of the long bones is occasionally seen.

Cardiovascular complications

Bacterial endocarditis usually develops on a valve previously damaged by congenital or acquired disease.

Hepatic complications

Most patients develop granulomatous lesions in the liver parenchyma. Hepatic enlargement may be accompanied by jaundice.[9] Cirrhosis has been claimed to follow severe necrotizing hepatitis due to brucellosis.[10] Cholecystitis may appear in association with hepatitis.

Hypersplenism

Hypersplenism with leukopenia, thrombocytopenia and haemorrhage is a rare complication. Haemolytic anaemia has also been recorded in association with splenomegaly and *Brucella* were recovered from the spleen.[11]

Genitourinary complications

Orchitis and epididymitis are not uncommon. *Brucella* are excreted in the urine over a long period of time and chronic pyelonephritis has been reported.

Neurobrucellosis

Neurological complications of brucellosis may appear at the onset of the illness, during con-valescence or long after the fever[12] and may be caused by *Br. melitensis*, *Br. abortus*, or *Br. suis*.

A meningomyelitis may occur with spinal features; leptomeningitis is an early feature and may lead to an adhesive arachnoiditis with signs of spinal block and xanthochromic cerebrospinal fluid;[13] *Brucella* meningitis is liable to be misdiagnosed as tuberculous or viral meningitis.[14]

Diffuse progressive encephalitis, often associated with optic, VIth and VIIIth nerve lesions, may occur and meningoencephalitis as well as subarachnoid haemorrhage, neuritis and myelopathy have been described.[15]

Transient episodes including aphasia, dysarthria, paralyses, tinnitus, deafness, visual disorders and epileptiform convulsions can all occur.[16] The organisms are not usually recovered from the cerebrospinal fluid, in which agglutination tests are negative.

A neuropsychiatric form of the disease is well known.[17]

Hypersensitivity reactions

Veterinary surgeons who are especially exposed to infection may become sensitized to the products of *Brucella* and develop hypersensitivity reactions, such as skin rashes and fever, when exposed to infected animals and their excretions. Erythema nodosum may be a symptom of *Brucella* infection.

DIAGNOSIS

Differential diagnosis

The differential diagnosis of brucellosis may be difficult in the early stages when it has to be distinguished from typhoid, tuberculosis and other causes of prolonged fever such as reticulosis.

Chronic *Br. melitensis* infection can closely resemble kala-azar with fever, splenomegaly and hypersplenism and where both infections are endemic both can coexist in the same patient.

Brucella spondylitis closely resembles tuberculous or typhoid osteitis and may only be distinguished by the evidence of repair (osteosclerosis) alongside destruction (osteoporosis) which can be seen on radiological examination.

Other localized manifestations of brucellosis may be confused with a multitude of conditions and brucellosis should be considered in the diagnosis of uveitis, acute choroiditis, orchitis and epididymitis.

Isolation of *Brucella*

Blood culture

The organism may be recovered from the blood as early as the second day of fever; 5–10 ml should be drawn and distributed into several flasks of broth. The broth should be incubated for at least 24 hours and for as long as 26 days. Subcultures should be made on trypsin agar slopes. Cultures of blood clot sometimes give better results. The clot is macerated and transferred to crystal violet tryptose broth (bactotryptose 20 g, bactodextrose 1 g, sodium chloride 5 g, *p*-aminobenzoic acid 100 mg, crystal violet 0.1% aqueous solution 1.4 ml, distilled water 1000 ml) in a screw-capped vial. The medium is adjusted to pH 6.9 and incubated at 35°C under CO_2 tension for 4–7 days. The culture is then streaked on a solid medium consisting of bactotryptose agar containing 1 ml of 0.1% aqueous crystal violet. Inoculations are made once a week for three weeks and the plates incubated for 4 days.

Isolation from urine

This is much more difficult to achieve. The urine must be a catheter or mid-stream specimen obtained after the fifteenth day.

Isolation from bone marrow

Br. abortus has been isolated from the bone marrow when blood cultures are sterile.

Isolation from tissues

Brucella may be isolated from excised lymph glands, bone and lung but not from liver. Material can be inoculated into guinea-pigs whose blood is then examined for a rise in agglutination titres to *Brucella*.

Biopsy of liver and marrow may show non-caseating granulomas which are not specific but may be suggestive.

Immunodiagnosis

Antibodies can be demonstrated by agglutination, CF and anti-human-globulin (Coombs') tests, by radioimmunoassay and by enzyme-linked immunosorbent assay (ELISA).

Agglutination

Agglutinating antibodies appear in the blood after the second week of the disease and persist for a long time.

Specificity. Cross reactions occur with *Br. tularensis* and *Vibrio cholerae*. Heterologous titres are lower than homologous, and heterologous antibodies can be removed by absorption. Persons immunized with cholera vaccine will show a raised titre of *Brucella* agglutinins, especially if they have had previous *Brucella* infection, but these decrease rapidly with time. A properly standardized antigen may be prepared from any species of *Brucella* and the test can be carried out by tube or rapid slide agglutination, using Castañeda's antigen.[18] By estimating titres before and after treatment of the serum with mercaptoethanol the level of IgG and IgM antibodies can be determined separately.

Prozone phenomenon. Blocking antibodies may prevent agglutination in dilutions below 1/100 and may be obviated by testing dilutions up to 1/10 240. Blocking antibodies may be found in the sera of patients who have had active disease for a number of years and patients whose sera show either a low titre or no agglutination should be tested with anti-human-globulin serum.

Interpretation of the test. Low titres of 1/20 to 1/80 are often found in patients without evidence of brucellosis or in healthy persons. Active brucellosis is most likely to be associated with a titre of above 1/100. When a properly standardized antigen is used the great majority of patients with bacteriologically proved disease will have titres of 1/160 to 1/320. A diagnosis of brucellosis cannot be established on the titres alone since many healthy people connected with animal husbandry may show a significant titre of *Brucella* agglutinins in their blood.

Rapid slide agglutination test. A rapid slide agglutination test using standard antigens as supplied to veterinarians has been used very successfully in the field for the diagnosis of brucellosis, and compared very favourably with the standard agglutination test.[19]

Complement fixation test

The CF test measures IgG antibodies and should be performed in combination with the anti-human-globulin test.

Anti-human-globulin (Coombs') test[20]

Brucella organisms incubated with the patient's serum are washed free of serum and exposed to anti-human-globulin (Coombs'). Agglutination follows if there has been significant antibody binding. The advantages of this test are that blocking antibodies are overcome and that the test measures only IgG antibodies so that differentiation can be made in association with the agglutination test between acute (IgM and IgG) and chronic (IgG and IgA only) cases. Two types of antibody response can be distinguished: chronic cases and those persons regularly exposed to *Brucella* antigen, such as veterinary surgeons, where the direct agglutination test is either weakly positive or negative but the anti-human-globulin test is positive to a high titre, and acute cases, where the direct agglutination test is positive to a high titre, but who show later a marked reduction in all types of antibody over a period as long as 12 months or more.[21]

Radioimmunoassay

A radioimmunoassay method to determine the levels of specific anti-*Brucella* IgM, IgG and IgA immunoglobulin has been devised[22] which avoids the difficulties with blocking or non-agglutinating antibodies and can demonstrate IgM antibody associated with acute, or IgG and IgA antibodies with chronic *Brucella* infection. It can also help eliminate the diagnosis of brucellosis by showing the absence of any antibodies.

ELISA

An ELISA test has been developed[23] which distinguishes acute cases with elevated IgM from chronic cases with high IgG in the absence of IgM. Cross reactions can occur with yersiniosis.[24]

Interpretation of serological reactions

Interpretation of serological reactions in chronic brucellosis can be very difficult. Occupationally exposed people, such as dairy farmers, veterinarians and abbattoir workers, develop high titres of antibody without illness, and these antibodies may persist for years. If the agglutination, mercaptoethanol complement fixation and anti-human-globulin tests are all positive and there is occupational exposure then a diagnosis of chronic brucellosis can be made. If these tests are negative, then brucellosis can be excluded with a high degree of certainty.

Brucellin (melitine) test

A polyvalent antigen prepared from all three species of *Brucella* and standardized by nitrogen content has been used to measure delayed cutaneous hypersensitivity. The test is used in just the same way as the tuberculin test. A positive reaction denotes exposure to or infection with brucellosis at some time in the past and is useful for epidemiological purposes. A negative reaction may be useful in individual cases to exclude infection.

TREATMENT

On the whole *Br. abortus* infection is more amenable to treatment than *Br. melitensis*.

Tetracycline

Tetracycline is the antibiotic of choice and this or chlortetracycline or oxytetracycline should be given in a dose of 500 mg four times daily by mouth for 21 days. Using this regimen 90% of 32 cases of acute brucellosis recovered.[3] The temperature approaches normal by the fourth or fifth day. The course should be repeated within six to eight weeks if a relapse occurs.

Streptomycin and tetracycline

A combination of streptomycin 1 g daily intramuscularly with 500 mg tetracycline four times daily by mouth for 21 days is the most widely recommended therapy. It can be supplemented by moderate doses of sulphonamide.

Sulphonamides

Sulphonamides alone are not so effective and have no effect on the course of bacterial endocarditis due to *Brucella*.

Trimethoprim and sulphamethoxazole (co-trimoxazole)

Results of co-trimoxazole treatment in acute brucellosis have been very encouraging.[25,26] Disappearance of symptoms within 48 hours and normal temperatures within the first week have been found. Dosage is two tablets 12-hourly for four weeks. When used in 30 cases there was no response in two, relapse in four, but cure in 24.[27]

Rifampicin

With rifampicin 300 mg at 12-hourly intervals for 16 days temperatures returned to normal in an average of 6 days and there were no relapses after 12 months.

Combination chemotherapy with rifampicin and tetracycline

The best results with brucella endocarditis and chronic brucellosis are obtained with this combination. Treatment (rifampicin 600 mg daily, tetracycline 500 mg 8-hourly) should be continued for six to 12 weeks.

Steroids

Steroids administered in combination with antibiotics to acutely ill patients have a dramatic effect and improvement may be noticed in 24 hours. The mechanism of this favourable action is not understood but is similar to the effect of steroids on patients severely ill with typhoid fever.

Steroids may be administered in the form of ACTH gel 25 IU intramuscularly every 6 hours or 100 mg hydrocortisone intravenously every 8 hours for 72–96 hours.

Hypersensitivity reactions may be treated by desensitization with Castañeda's antigen in gradually increasing doses.

EPIDEMIOLOGY

Brucellosis is essentially a zoonosis and is contracted from animals.

Brucellosis in animals

Brucellosis in goats. The Mediterranean Fever Commission demonstrated that the goat was the reservoir of brucellosis on the island of Malta, the infection being transmitted to man through the milk. Goats are infected in many parts of the world. Under natural conditions the goat harbours only *Br. melitensis* and the most susceptible animal is the young goat, especially during the first pregnancy. Little illness is caused and healthy animals may shed large numbers of organisms in the milk for a considerable time. The organisms are located in the reticuloendothelial tissues of the pregnant uterus, kidney and mammary gland and infection of man is from the milk and products of conception.

Brucellosis in sheep. Natural infections of sheep are caused by *Br. melitensis*, but *Br. abortus* has also been recovered from them. They are more resistant than goats but the pregnant young ewe is quite susceptible. Organisms are rarely excreted in the urine or for longer than one or two months in the milk.

Brucellosis in cattle (Bang's disease). Brucellosis in cattle is primarily due to *Br. abortus*, but *Br. melitensis* can also infect them. The most susceptible animal is the pregnant heifer and the organism lodges in the uterus and causes abortion. Organisms also lodge in the supramammary lymph glands and are shed in the milk for a long time. Man is infected from milk and the products of conception.

Brucellosis in pigs. All species of *Brucella* can infect pigs. There are two strains of *Br. suis*: the American strain, which produces abundant hydrogen sulphide and is highly infective for man, and the Danish strain, which produces little or no hydrogen sulphide and is not infective for man. Natural infections with *Br. melitensis* and *Br. abortus* have also been found. The pregnant sow is not especially susceptible and the infection is spread by the semen of the boar. Infection of man is mainly from handling pig meat.

Brucellosis in other animals. Brucellosis has been found in horses and rarely in dogs. Strains have been isolated from reindeer and susliks (rodents) in the USSR and from caribou in North America. Camels are not uncommonly infected and serological evidence of infection has been found in eland and wild rodents in East Africa. Guinea-pigs may be used to isolate *Brucella* from suspected material in the laboratory. Strains of *Brucella* differing from the classical strains have been isolated from the desert wood rat (*Neotoma lepida*) and called *Brucella neotomae*.

Age and sex distribution

Brucellosis is predominantly a disease of adult males, which suggests a connection with occupation. Unlike young animals, children show a comparative resistance to the disease and, although the infection rate in children may be high, the morbidity rate is low. The physiological and metabolic factors responsible for this resistance are not known.

Occupation

Brucellosis is a disease of farmers, dairy-men, herdsmen, meat-packers, veterinary surgeons and laboratory workers. Not more than 10% of the cases of brucellosis in North America are due to drinking unpasteurized milk.[3] In the Mediterranean area the greatest prevalence of *Br. melitensis* is the season of lowest rainfall, explained by the birth of kids in the spring and the greater consumption of goats' milk during the summer months.

Veterinarians show a high incidence of infection though they do not necessarily manifest illness, but may exhibit an extreme degree of hypersensitivity to *Brucella* antigen.

Meat-packers may acquire both *Br. abortus* and, in the USA, *Br. suis* infection which appears intermittently, involving several patients at a time, suggesting intermittent exposure to a contaminated environment.

Among farmers and ranchers it is a common practice for families to drink unpasteurized milk. In areas of high endemicity, such as parts of the Mediterranean and Africa, a considerable proportion of the inhabitants show serological evidence of past infection.

PREVENTION

In endemic areas all milk and milk products should be sterilized by boiling or pasteurization and all cheese should be made from pasteurized milk.

Meat-packers must be protected by gloves when handling carcases. Farmers should be suitably garbed when dealing with the products of conception, which must be destroyed.

The eradication of brucellosis from herds is a major problem and must be tackled on a government scale.

Prophylactic vaccination

Vaccination of man against *Brucella* infection using killed vaccines has proved a complete failure.[28] A vaccine derived from the protein–polysaccharide complex from the cell wall of S forms of *Brucella* has been prepared which creates less sensitivity problems than the previous live 19-BA vaccine. The dose of 1.0 to 2.0 mg caused no marked general reactions and a high percentage of seroconversions.[20] Vaccination is useful for persons at high risk.

TULARAEMIA

Tularaemia is a specific infectious disease of rodents caused by *Francisella (Pasteurella) tularensis* and is transmitted from these animals to man by the bite of infected blood-sucking insects, by the handling of infected animals or by the ingestion of infected water. It is also known as deer fly fever; Pahvant Valley plague; rabbit fever; Ohara's disease; yatobyo (Japan) or lemming fever.

GEOGRAPHICAL DISTRIBUTION

Tularaemia occurs as a human infection in three main geographical areas, North America, Europe, USSR, and to a lesser extent Japan.

AETIOLOGY

Fr. tularensis is a small non-motile gram-negative organism measuring 0.3–0.7 µm in length; when stained in the tissues it gives an appearance of being surrounded by a capsule. Though normally occurring as a rod-like structure, it frequently assumes a coccus shape. It stains best in tissue preparations with Giemsa stain, but in smears from cultures it shows up well with aniline gentian violet. On account of their small size some of the organisms pass through the coarser bacterial filters. There are two types, type A with a 5–7% mortality, associated with a rabbit reservoir and a tick vector, and type B which is less virulent and associated with rodents.

Cultural characteristics

The organism is difficult to culture. It will not grow on plain agar or in bouillon but will produce an abundant growth on serum–glucose–cystine agar. The cystine medium is inoculated with the heart blood of an infected animal or a small piece of liver or spleen is rubbed on the surface and allowed to remain in contact with the medium. Growth appears about the third day and flourishes luxuriantly in subcultures without the addition of fresh animal tissue. To ensure the primary growth it is necessary that a piece of animal tissue be added to the medium. Fermentation of glucose, laevulose, maltose and glycerine occurs with acid formation.

Composition of cystine agar. Cystine agar consists of beef infusion agar, having a pH of 7.6, to which 0.02% of cystine is added. It is then sterilized for 15 minutes in a steam sterilizer and subsequently incubated for 24 hours to ensure sterility. Cultures of *Fr. tularensis* are very infectious and should be handled with great care.

TRANSMISSION

Fr. tularensis is transmitted in nature by a large variety of routes of which there are three main ones: among rodents by water, to carnivores by ingestion from eating rodents and to birds and larger animals by ticks, biting flies and mosquitoes. Man acquires the infection by direct contact from skinning rabbits, by ingestion from eating them as food and from tick and horse fly bites. It can also be easily acquired in the laboratory.

Water-borne infection

The infection is maintained among rodents mainly by water. The water is contaminated by dead animals and excreta and large numbers of rodents may be infected and die in this way.

Ingestion

Carnivora are infected chiefly from the consumption of sick, infected rodents which are easy to catch.

Insects

Ticks can act as vectors and are very suitable, since the nymph stages feed on small rodents and when they become adult feed on larger mammals including man, thus transmitting the infection from rodents in an efficient manner. The infection is also transmitted transovarially through the egg, and this is a method by which the infection is maintained through the winter.

Dermacentor andersoni (wood tick), *D. variabilis*, *D. occidentalis*, *Ixodes ricinus* and *Haemaphysalis leporispalustris* (rabbit tick) can all transmit the infection. *Dermacentor andersoni* is particularly important in the USA and *Fr. tularensis* is found in the intestinal lumen in the cells of the gut wall in the body fluids and in the faeces. The organism can also be transmitted by biting fleas, the deer fly (*Chrysops discalis*) as well as the stable fly (*Stomoxys calcitrans*), the bed bug (*Cimex lectularis*), the squirrel flea (*Ceratophyllus acutus*), the rabbit louse (*Haemodipsus ventricosus*), and the mouse louse (*Polyplax serratus*) can all transmit the infection, and maintain it in rodents. Four species of mosquito, *Aedes* and *Theobaldia* have been shown to transmit *Br. tularensis* under experimental conditions, and in Sweden *Aedes cinereus* does so in nature. Mosquitoes transmit the infection to birds.

PATHOLOGY

Fr. tularensis can enter the body by one of three main routes.

1 The respiratory route via the tonsil.
2 Intestinal canal from ingestion.
3 Cutaneous route by insect bite or direct contact.

Since the disease is rarely fatal the pathology is best seen in infected animals. The pathological appearances of infected guinea-pigs and rabbits at autopsy much resemble those of plague. In an experimentally infected guinea-pig there is haemorrhagic oedema at the site of inoculation, with blood-stained peritoneal exudate and diffusely enlarged spleen in which characteristic small necrotic foci can be found. Similar lesions may be detected in the liver. On microscopic section of these organs a dense infiltration with polymorphonuclear cells can be found but the organisms can only be detected with difficulty. In the spleen of the mouse, on the other hand, little or no leukocytic response occurs and when stained with Twort's light-green neutral red stain *Br. tularensis* can be demonstrated in large numbers. In the few recorded cases of autopsy in man nodules have been found in the lung and spleen.

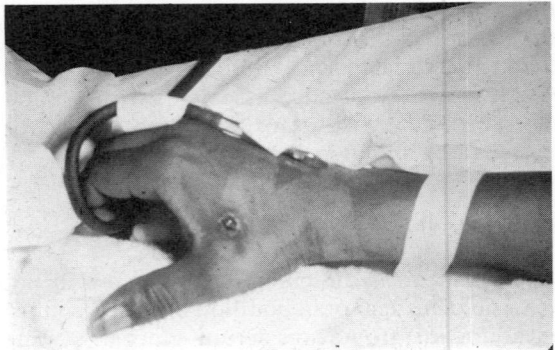

Fig. 7.3   An ulcer on the hand in tularaemia. (Courtesy WTIM.)

IMMUNITY

There is apparently a long-lasting immunity in man and there is no record of a second generalized attack, though a local reinfection may occur. Agglutinating antibodies appear in the serum in the second week and reach their maximum between the fourth and eighth weeks, when there is a gradual fall, but they may persist for up to 11 years. Serum antibodies can be used in diagnosis but cross reactions occur with *Br. melitensis* and *Br. abortus* (23% of tularaemia sera cross react with *Br. melitensis* and *Br. abortus* and 35% of *Br. melitensis* and *Br. abortus* with tularaemia). In 13% of cases of tularaemia the serum agglutinates *Proteus* OX19 in a dilution of 1:80 or over.

Skin sensitivity can be demonstrated by an intradermal test employing a suspension of killed organisms.

CLINICAL FEATURES

The disease in man presents in a number of ways dependent upon the route of infection. The incubation period is 1–10 days.

Cutaneous (ulceroglandular) form

Local cutaneous disease results from infection from the bite of an infected tick or fly or direct contact of the skin with an infected source. An inflamed papule develops at the site of infection, which becomes pustular with a necrotic centre. This separates, leaving a punched-out ulcer (Fig. 7.3) which is replaced by a scar on healing. There is a painful enlargement of the local lymph glands which may suppurate after one or two months and may remain enlarged for two or three months. There are general signs of infection with fever and prostration.

Ophthalmic (oculoglandular) form

The site of entry of infection is the conjunctival sac, which is usually involved unilaterally. There is itching, lacrimation, photophobia and pain in the eye with swelling of the preauricular, parotid, submaxillary and cervical lymph glands. The eyelids become swollen and the conjunctiva red and covered with small discrete nodules and grey exudate. Punched-out ulcers develop and last for two or three weeks, after which there is recovery. Suppuration of the glands is common. Dacryocystitis and corneal ulcers occur, and permanent impairment of vision may follow.

Oral and abdominal form

This follows infection by ingestion of infected meat. There is a necrotizing pharyngitis with abscesses on the roof of the mouth, fever, enlargement of local lymph glands and sometimes abdominal pain, vomiting and diarrhoea. Peritonitis may develop.

Typhoid (septicaemic) form

This form may arise primarily from infection via the respiratory route or as a late result of a local infection. The onset is sudden with severe headache, vomiting, chills and fever. Myalgia and arthralgia are common. The initial rise in temperature is above 40°C, with generalized weakness, aching, prostration, sweats and loss of weight. The fever may show an initial rise followed by remission and a secondary rise or a continuous course lasting usually 10–15 days, and rarely three or four weeks. Petechial, roseolar, papular and pustular rashes may appear. In one-half of the cases pulmonary symptoms develop. A slightly tender enlargement of the spleen is found in one-third of cases. There is a moderate polymorphonuclear leukocytosis of $12–15 \times 10^9$/litre.

Pleuropulmonary form

Pulmonary involvement may follow the other forms. There are dyspnoea, malaise, chills and pleuritic pain. Milder forms resemble atypical pneumonia and may last up to one month. There may be pleurisy, effusion, pneumonic consolidation or lobular bronchopneumonia with abscess, gangrene and cavitation in severe cases. There is an associated enlargement of the bronchial and mediastinal glands.

Subclinical infections

Subclinical infections are common and serological tests recently showed that in Sweden up to 23% of the population has been infected, the infection being subclinical in as many as 32% of those with positive reactions.[30]

Complications

Complications have been reported: peritonitis, persistent ascites, appendicitis and intestinal haemorrhage in the oral and abdominal forms. Pericarditis, osteomyelitis and meningitis have all been recorded.

Course

Except in the severe forms the disease is not usually fatal. In one-third of cases recovery is slow, the debilitating effect may be very marked and lassitude may persist for months. The mean duration of fever in untreated cases is 26 days and adenopathy may last for three or four months.

Although tularaemia is not usually fatal, in a series of severe untreated cases there was a mortality rate of 62% in pulmonary and 20% in typhoidal forms of the disease.

Fr. tularensis may remain dormant intracellularly in the body for years.

DIAGNOSIS

The differential diagnosis of the local form must be made from plague, tick typhus and rat bite fever. The diagnosis is made by isolation of the organism from the patient's ulcer or gland juice obtained by aspiration and inoculated into guinea-pigs, mice or rabbits, from whose tissues the organism may be isolated on special media as described. The organisms are rarely present in the blood. Serological diagnosis may be made using agglutination tests with cultures of *Fr. tularensis* or the spleens of infected mice in a formalinized citrate suspension. Cross reactions with undulant and typhus fevers may occur as described previously.

TREATMENT

Streptomycin is specific for the infection and extremely effective. One gram intramuscularly daily for 7 days will terminate the infection. The patient should be kept in bed for a time after subsidence of the fever and convalescence should be prolonged. More recently tetracycline 250 mg four times daily for two weeks has been preferred. The inflamed glands should not be incised.

EPIDEMIOLOGY

Tularaemia is essentially a rural infection and has a varying epidemiology according to the area in which it occurs. There are nine main ways in which outbreaks of human infection can occur.[31]

1 Vector-borne: by ticks and tabanid flies.
2 Trapping: from the skins of infected rodents, musk-rats and rabbits.
3 Hunting: from the consumption of rabbit meat.
4 Water-borne: from the water of streams infected by dead rats, well water infected by mice and field voles.
5 Agricultural: from working in haystacks contaminated by field voles and mice.
6 Domestic: laboratory infections.
7 Use of grain and other products contaminated by mice.
8 Processing of agricultural products.

9   Trench and foxhole outbreaks in wartime.

The origin of human outbreaks is invariably natural infections of different species of wild mammals.

Natural infections

Fr. tularensis occurs as a natural infection of wild rodents, especially rats, field mice, hares and rabbits. It has an extremely wide host range and many other species of animals as well as birds can be infected. A complete list of natural infections has been given by Burroughs et al.[32] Natural infections occur in the following areas.

  USA: wandering shrew, grey fox, dog, cat, various ground squirrels (Pirote, Wyoming, Beechey's and Columbian), chipmunk, beaver, wood rat, white-footed mouse, meadow mouse and varieties (Sawatch and Tule) of musk-rat and brown rat (*Rattus norvegicus*), varying hare, jack rabbit, black-tailed jack rabbit, cotton-tail rabbit, sheep, calves, ruffed grouse, sharp-tailed grouse, bobwhite quail and horned owl.

  Canada: Richardson's ground squirrel, Osgood's white-footed mouse, Drummond meadow mouse, varying hare, white-tailed jack rabbit and Franklin's gull.

  Sweden: lemming and varying hare.

  Central Europe: rabbit and hare.

  USSR: introduced musk-rat, little ground squirrel, steppe lemming, water rat, continental vole, large water vole, house mouse and long-tailed field mouse.

  Asia Minor: continental vole, house and harvest mouse.

  Japan: local rabbit.

North America

In North America the most important reservoir of infection is the jack rabbit, hares and their relatives. The infection is found in Wyoming and Montana in streams contaminated by dead beavers, which have been found in large numbers. Man acquires the infection as a hunter from skinning rabbits, and preparing carcases for cooking and also after tick and deer fly bites (*Chrysops discalis*). Occasionally contact with sheep is the source of infection. The disease is most prevalent during the months of June, July and August.[33]

Europe

In Sweden the lemming and varying hare are the main reservoirs and tularaemia is known as 'lemming fever'; it is caused by contact with infected water contaminated by the bodies and excreta of lemmings. Outbreaks have occurred in peasant women who go barefoot in summer and are bitten by numerous mosquitoes (*Aedes cinereus*). In Austria, Czechoslovakia and Poland the rabbit and hare are the main reservoirs and in France the infection has become much more common since the introduction of hares from central Europe for sporting purposes. In northern Europe cases occur from July to October and in southern Europe from June to August.

USSR

In Russia the water rat and introduced muskrat, which spread widely in the Ukraine after the disturbance caused by the great tank battles of the Second World War, are the main reservoirs, and there was a great increase in the number of human infections after the war. In central Asia *Microtus* and *Arvicola* are the predominant rat hosts.

PREVENTION

Prevention depends upon avoidance of the circumstances leading to infection in the various endemic areas. Rabbits should not be skinned without gloves and sick rabbits should not be eaten. Cooking destroys the infection, as does prolonged freezing. Experimental work in the laboratory with *Fr. tularensis* must be undertaken with great caution.

REFERENCES

1   Blankenship, R.M. & Sanford, J.P. (1975) *Am. J. Med.* **59**, 424.
2   Editorial (1983) *Lancet* (1983) **ii**, 1180.
3   Spink, W.W. (1956) *The Nature of Brucellosis*. Minneapolis: University of Minnesota Press.
4   McDevitt, J.G. (1970) *J. Hyg, Camb.* **68**, 173.
5   Poole, P.M. (1975) *Postgrad. med. J.* **51**, 433.
6   Hughes, M.L. (1897) *Mediterranean, Malta or Undulant Fever*. London: Macmillan.
7   Gee-Lew, B.M., Nicholas, E.A., Hirose, F.M. et al (1983) *Arch. Dermatol.* **119**, 56–58.
8   Lowbeer, L. (1948) *Am. J. Path.* **24**, 723.

9 Rossmiller, H.R. & Ensign, W.G. (1948) *Cleveland Clin. Q.* **15**, 184.

10 McCullough, N.B. (1951) *Pub. Hlth Rep. Wash.* **66**, 205.

11 Weed, L.A., Dahlin, D.C., Pugh, D.G. et al (1952) *Am. J. clin. Path.* **22**, 10.

12 Nelson-Jones, A. (1951) *Lancet* **i**, 495.

13 Sahadevan, M.G., Mahinder Singh, Joseph, P.P. et al (1968) *Br. med. J.* **iv**, 432.

14 Mugerwa, R.D. & D'Arbela, P.G. (1976) *E. Afr. med. J.* **53**, 266.

15 Fincham, R.W., Sahs, A.L. & Joynt, R.J. (1963) *J. Am. med. Ass.* **184**, 269.

16 Spink, W.W. & Hall, W.H. (1949) *Trans. Am. Clin. Climat.* **61**, 121.

17 Spink, W.W. (1959) In *Textbook of Medicine*, eds. R.L. Cecil & R.F. Loeb, 10th edn, p. 226. Philadelphia: W.B. Saunders.

18 Spink, W.W. & Anderson, D. (1952) *J. Lab. clin. Med.* **40**, 593.

19 Cox, P.S.U. (1968) *Trans. R. Soc. trop. Med. Hyg.* **62**, 521.

20 Kerr, W.R., Coghlan, J., Payne, J.D.H. et al (1966) *Lancet* **ii**, 1181.

21 Coghlan, J. & Weir, D.M. (1967) *Br. med. J.* **ii**, 269

22 Parratt, D., Nielsen, K.H. & White, R.G. (1977) *Lancet* **i**, 1075.

23 Sippel, J. E., El-Madry, N.A. & Farid, Z. (1982) *Lancet* **ii**, 19.

24 Granfors, K. & Toinanen, A. (1982) *Lancet* **ii**, 669.

25 Farid, Z., Hassan, A., Wahab, M.F.A. et al (1970) *Br. med. J.* **iii**, 323.

26 Lal, S., Modawal, K.K., Fowle, A.S.E. et al (1970) *Br. med. J.* **iii**, 256.

27 Rigatos, G.A., Polyzos, A.K. & Kappos-Rigatou (1975) *Münch. Med. Wschr.* **117**, 961.

28 World Health Organization (1964) *Wld. Hlth Org. tech. Rep. Ser.*, 289.

29 Vershilova, D.A., Dranovskaya, E.A. & Karinskaya, G.A. (1982) *J. Microbiol. Epidemiol. Immunol.* **10**, 59–65.

30 Dahlstrand, S., Ringertz, O. & Zetterburg, B. (1971) *Scand. J. infect. Dis.* **3**, 7.

31 Pavlovsky, E.N. (1966) *Natural Nidality of Transmissible Diseases*. Urbana, Ill: University of Illinois Press.

32 Burroughs, A.L., Holdenfeld, R., Longanecker, D.S. et al (1945) *J. Infect. Dis.* **76**, 115.

33 Cummings, H.S. (1937) *Bull. Off. int. Hyg. pub.* **29**, 2532.

Chapter 8
Typhoid Fever (Enteric Fever)

Typhoid, a common cause of fever, is worldwide in its distribution wherever sanitary conditions are poor and is particularly prevalent throughout the tropics. In Africa *Salmonella typhi* is predominant, while paratyphoid A occurs in eastern Europe, the USA, the Far East and India. Paratyphoid B is found in Europe and is responsible for 20% of the cases in North America. Paratyphoid C is found in Guyana and also eastern Europe.

AETIOLOGY

Enteric fever is caused by *Salmonella typhi, S. paratyphi A, S. paratyphi B (S. schottmülleri)*, and *S. paratyphi C (S. hirschfeldii)*.

Salmonella are gram-negative flagellated, non-sporulating, facultative, anaerobic bacilli that ferment glucose. They grow well on ordinary media and form pale, colourless colonies on Mac-Conkey's medium since they do not ferment lactose (non-lactose fermenters). They may be distinguished from each other by biochemical reactions involving certain sugars (Table 8.1) and by their antigenic structure.

Antigenic structure

Salmonella have a somatic (O) antigen situated on the surface of the organism which is a lipo-polysaccharide and group specific. The flagellar (H) antigen situated in the flagellae is a protein and species specific. The Vi (K envelope) antigen is a polysaccharide which forms an envelope surrounding the surface of the organism protecting the O antigen from bactericidal agents. It is related to invasiveness and the effectiveness of vaccines. *S. typhi* produces an endotoxin which forms the outer portion of the cell wall and is composed of the released O antigen, a lipo-polysaccharide and lipid A which contributes to the pathogenesis of typhoid fever.

Bacteriophage typing

Bacteriophage typing can identify more than 80 stable strains of *S. typhi* and identify their source from a particular geographic area or carrier, which is a valuable tool for tracing sources of infection.

Antigen analysis

S. typhi (group D), *S. paratyphi A* (group A), *S. paratyphi B* (group B) and *S. paratyphi C* (group C) can be identified by the O group antigen and by the presence of Vi antigen which is only found in *S. typhi* and *S. paratyphi C*.

Table 8.1 Biochemical characteristics of *S. typhi* and *S. paratyphi*.

Species	Glucose	Mannitol	Xylose	D-Tartrate	Mucate
S. typhi	A	A	V	A	V
S. paratyphi A	+	+	−	−	−
S. paratyphi B	+	+	+	−	+
S. paratyphi C	+	+	+	+	−

A, acid, no gas. V, variable reaction. +, acid and gas. −, no reaction.

SALMONELLA TYPHI INFECTION

TRANSMISSION

S. typhi only affects man and the source of infection is another infected human being excreting bacilli in the faeces, urine or other secretions. Typhoid has been transmitted congenitally when neonates are affected.

Source of infection

Patients

The typhoid patient excretes bacilli in the faeces and urine for about a month. Infected vomit and pus from abscesses are also sources.

Carriers

Three per cent of cases of typhoid fever become carriers and the rate increases with age and the prevalence of gallbladder disease.

CONVALESCENT CARRIER

The convalescent carrier passes bacilli in the excreta for up to six months after an attack of typhoid.

CHRONIC FAECAL CARRIER

The chronic faecal carrier outnumbers urinary carriers by ten to one and continues to pass bacilli intermittently for at least one year after infection. Women are carriers more frequently than men, the gallbladder and bile ducts being the source of infection. In *Schistosoma mansoni* infection the organisms (*Salmonella typhi* and *S. paratyphi A*) live inside the adult worms and create a carrier state (see Chapter 22) which does not cease until the schistosomiasis has been treated.

CHRONIC URINARY CARRIERS

Chronic urinary carriers are caused by infection of the renal pelvis and are much less common except in areas where the incidence of *Schistosoma haematobium* is high (Egypt). The organisms live inside the adult worms (see Chapter 22) and in this case urinary outnumber faecal carriers by seven to one.

Typhoid may be transmitted by water, food or, more rarely, direct ano-oral transmission.

Water-borne transmission

S. typhi can survive for several weeks in fresh water (also in salt and brackish water), ice, dust, dried sewage and on clothing. It does not survive in raw sewage for longer than a week. It can also survive and multiply in milk and milk products.

Food

Food can be infected by water used to wash and keep it fresh and improperly sealed cans can be infected by water used to cool them during manufacture. Food can be infected by carriers who handle it and by fomites, dust and probably flies.

Shellfish are important sources of infection since they filter polluted water and by concentrating the organism render an ineffective dose effective by concentrating a large number of organisms in their bodies.

Ano-oral transmission

Direct transmission was thought to be the method in camps occupied by prisoners from areas where typhoid was endemic with a high carrier rate, and epidemics occurred even with good sanitation and a protected water supply.

Portal of entry

The major route of entry is via the intestinal tract for which a sufficiently high infective dose is necessary.

Infective dose

Infectivity is directly related to the size of dose of organisms. The ingestion of 10^5 organisms caused disease in 25% and 10^9 in 95% of volunteers. With an increase in the size of dose the incubation period decreases but the severity of the disease is not affected. Strains that do not possess the Vi antigen are less infective. The size of infective dose is decreased by the simultaneous ingestion of bicarbonate.[1] A gastric acidity of less than pH 2 kills most organisms, and patients with achlorhydria on antacid therapy or who have had a gastrectomy need much smaller doses to develop disease.

PATHOLOGY

Early stages (incubation period)

The portal of entry is the gastrointestinal tract. The typhoid bacilli attach themselves to the tips of the villi in the upper intestinal tract which they invade directly or multiply before doing so. Stool cultures become positive for several days after infection, becoming negative, only to become positive again later in the disease. The organisms pass to the intestinal lymph follicles and the mesenteric lymph glands, and via the systemic circulation to the liver and spleen where they are filtered out by the reticuloendothelial cells. Typhoid bacilli multiply in the mononuclear phagocytic cells of the lymph glands, lymph follicles, liver and spleen, but cause only slight changes in these organs and there are no clinical symptoms.

Clinical phase

When the number of organisms has built up sufficiently, depending on the strain and host response, they leave their intracellular habitat in the lymph glands and pass via the thoracic duct into the general circulation with the production of clinical symptoms. During this phase of bacteraemia the organisms may invade any organ but most commonly the liver, spleen, bone marrow, gallbladder and Peyer's patches of the terminal ileum where they are taken up and multiply in mononuclear phagocytic cells which are the macrophages or *typhoid cells* (Fig. 8.1), so charac-

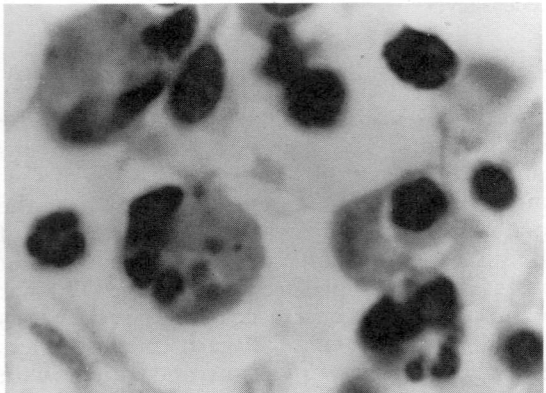

Fig. 8.1   Typhoid cell. (Courtesy WTIM.)

teristic of the disease which when aggregated form *typhoid nodules* (Fig. 8.2). Typhoid nodules are most commonly found in the Peyer's patches, mesenteric lymph glands, liver, spleen and bone marrow but also in the parotid glands, kidneys

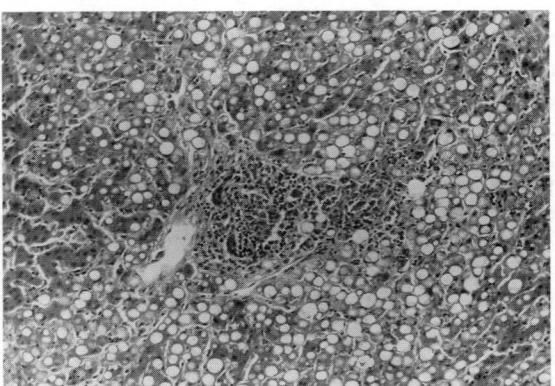

Fig. 8.2   Typhoid nodule in portal tract of liver. (Courtesy WTIM.)

and testes. The main pathological changes are found in the intestinal tract.

Intestinal tract

The main changes are found in the lower ileum but there may be extensive large intestinal involvement similar to that in shigellosis. In the lower ileum there are a series of changes in the Peyer's patches.

Hyperplasia occurs during the first week of illness involving most of the Peyer's patches and lymph follicles of the caecum but also other lymphatic tissue in the intestine. These tissues become infiltrated with mononuclear cells, and typhoid nodules are common. If the hyperplasia does not resolve *necrosis* occurs after 7–10 days (first week) or clinical symptoms followed by *sloughing* of the mucosa during the second week, and *ulceration* during the third week forming typhoid ulcers (Fig. 8.3) which, following the

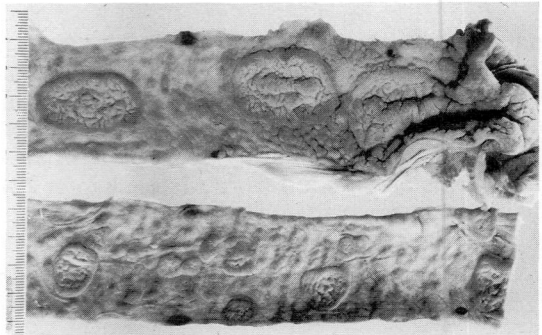

Fig. 8.3   Typhoid ulceration of the small intestine. (Courtesy WTIM.)

shape of the Peyer's patches are oval in shape situated in the long axis of the bowel on the side opposite to the mesentery. These ulcers occupy the lower third of the ileum. There is some peritoneal exudate and during the period of sloughing (second week) a blood vessel may be eroded and *haemorrhage* occur. *Perforation* into the peritoneal cavity may occur during the period of ulceration (third week).

Lymph glands, spleen and liver

The *mesenteric lymph glands* are swollen with macrophage and reticuloendothelial cells becoming soft with areas of focal necrosis. The *spleen* is acutely enlarged, red, soft and congested containing typhoid nodules but in holoendemic malarial areas the presence of pigment renders the colour grey. The *liver* is enlarged and typhoid nodules result from hypertrophy and hyperplasia of the Kupffer's cells (Fig. 8.2). Cloudy swelling of the hepatocytes and focal necrosis are found. The *gallbladder* may rarely show cholecystitis. Chronic cholecystitis is rare in tropical areas and gallbladder carriers are rare in the Chinese in Hong Kong.[2]

Heart

The myocardium shows non-specific necrosis with degenerative changes in, and fatty infiltration of, the heart muscle cells.

Kidneys

The kidneys most commonly show swelling and degeneration of the proximal tubular epithelium. Pyelonephritis and pyelitis with persistent structural damage have been described.[3] Glomerulonephritis and the nephrotic syndrome can occur.[4]

Lungs

The lungs show bronchitis and pneumonia of a granulomatous nature is found in many patients. Lung abscess and empyema are not uncommon.

Central nervous system

Changes are rare but encephalopathy with ring haemorrhages, capillary thrombi, perivascular demyelination, transverse myelitis and Guillain–Barré syndrome can occur. Pyogenic meningitis has been described.[5]

Skeletal muscle

Skeletal muscle characteristically shows Zenker's degeneration, a hyaline degeneration of muscle fibres in the abdominal wall and thighs.

Focal lesions

Typhoid abscesses may occur almost anywhere; osteomyelitis, brain abscess and abscess of the spleen (Fig. 8.4) and liver (Fig. 8.5) have all been reported, the exudate in these cases being polymorphonuclear and not mononuclear.

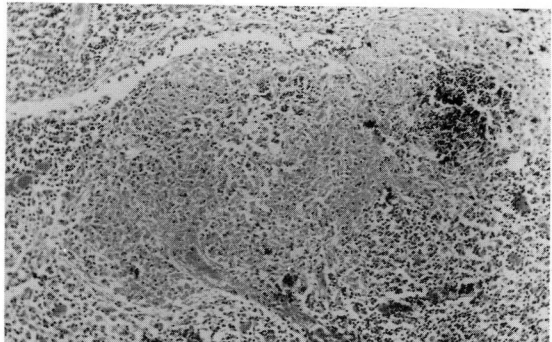

Fig. 8.4 Typhoid abscess in spleen. (Courtesy WTIM.)

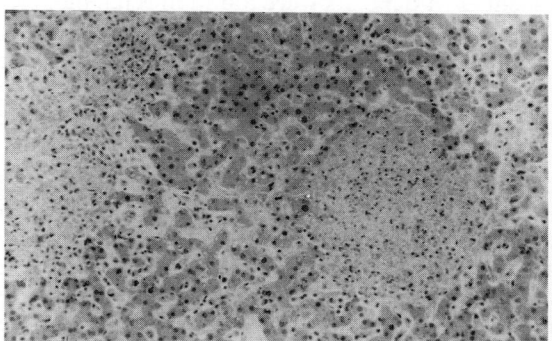

Fig. 8.5 Typhoid abscess in liver. (Courtesy WTIM.)

PATHOGENESIS

The pathogenesis of the lesions found in typhoid is not clear.

Endotoxin

Endotoxin injected into volunteers caused fever, chills, anorexia and sometimes vomiting[1,6] which rapidly declined and the reaction became progressively less after repeated injections,[6] and it is unlikely that this endotoxin is responsible for the symptoms of typhoid which are long and drawn out. Endotoxin may act in another way by stimulating macrophages. The macrophages produce substances called monokines which can cause cellular necrosis, fever and other changes found in typhoid fever. Endotoxin may stimulate the macrophages to release substances locally causing necrosis in the lymphatic tissue and liver, and systemically to cause fever and other manifestations of typhoid.

Other mechanisms

Disseminated intravascular coagulation (DIC)

DIC is unusual in typhoid but local DIC can be demonstrated by laboratory tests not uncommonly and may cause the central nervous system changes found.

Immune complexes

Circulating immune complexes may be responsible for the heavy proteinuria found in typhoid as well as glomerulonephritis (nephrotyphoid). Mild glomerular changes with immunofluorescent IgM deposits were found in renal biopsies which disappeared with recovery.[7]

IMMUNITY

Naturally acquired typhoid confers considerable immunity and second attacks are unusual in endemic areas where children are mainly attacked. Second attacks do occur and in one outbreak 11 men who had suffered typhoid five months previously had second attacks. There was, however, a significant diminution in the attack rate in previously infected persons.[8] Experimental infection also offered some protection to subsequent challenge[1] which was not dependent upon the level of O, H or Vi antibody. The immune response is both humoral and cellular.

Humoral immune response

Secretory IgA in the intestine may determine whether penetration of the mucosa occurs.

Specific antibodies

The earliest antibody response is a rise in the somatic O (IgM) antibody titre. The flagellar H (IgG) antibody develops more slowly and persists longer as do Vi antibodies. O antibody protects against the effects of injected endotoxin but H and Vi antibodies are not protective in any way.

Cellular immune response

The major feature of typhoid is activation of macrophages and phagocytosis as a defence mechanism. These macrophages play an important part in defence but the mechanism in typhoid is as yet not clear.

It may be that an opsonizing antibody formed against an antigen facilitates phagocytosis by macrophages which have been activated by a lymphokine formed in response to a bacterial antigen, but none of these processes has been defined or identified in typhoid.

CLINICAL FEATURES

Natural history (classical untreated case)

After the ingestion of typhoid bacilli there may be a temporary slight diarrhoea. When the incubation period (7–14 days) has been passed there is onset of fever which sometimes, but not always, increases stepwise with headache, malaise and other symptoms. After the first week the fever becomes sustained during the second week and the patient becomes toxic. The fever starts to subside during the third week by lysis (Fig. 8.6) when classical perforation and haemorrhage can occur. By the end of the fourth week the temperature returns to normal except where focal abscesses have formed, and relapses most commonly occur at this stage.

Incubation period

The incubation period is usually between 7 and 14 days but can be as short as 3 or as long as 60 days, depending on the size of the infecting dose.

Symptoms and signs

The *onset* is gradual but may be sudden especially in paratyphoid with shivering and rigor. *Headache* is a common early symptom accompanied by malaise, anorexia, pains in the limbs and insomnia. *Epistaxis* is common, less so in paratyphoid. *Abdominal pain* is diffuse and the normal bowel function is disturbed with either diarrhoea or constipation. *Cough* and chest discomfort are usual. *Nerve deafness* is common during the first week.[4]

The patient is toxic with a dry uncomfortable mouth and is thirsty. The facies is characteristic (typhoid facies) with flushed cheeks and a general apathy but there is no prostration. Meningism is not uncommon and slight jaundice occurs in the more toxic patients.

The *temperature* is invariably raised and may

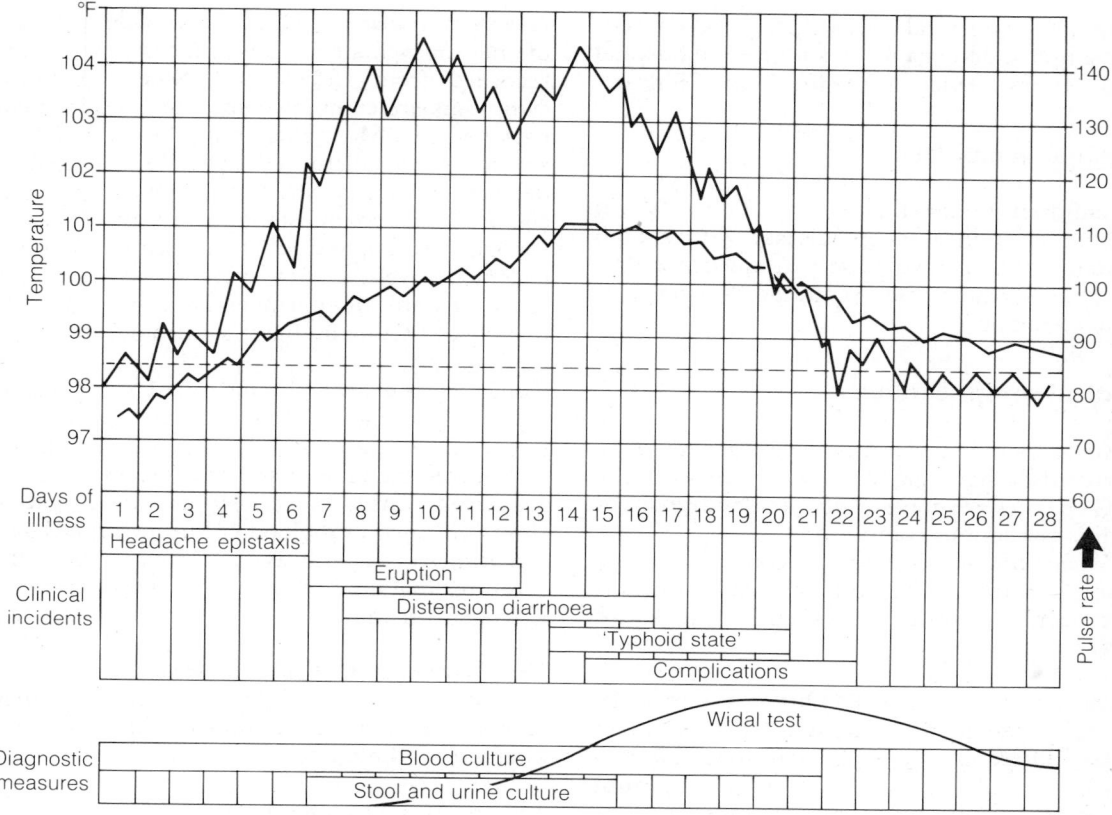

Fig. 8.6 Classical pattern of typhoid fever. (Courtesy WTIM.)

mount in a steplike fashion in the first week but this classical pattern is uncommon. It may reach its peak in the first 24–28 hours and after a period of continued fever begin to remit at night and terminate by lysis (Fig. 8.6). The fever is frequently atypical and may assume any form.

The *pulse* is slow and a relative bradycardia is considered a classical sign but is now less common. The *abdomen* is mildly distended and 'uncomfortable' being slightly tender on palpation, especially in the lower quadrants. The *spleen* is enlarged in 20–70% of cases[9] at some stage in the illness, sometimes as early as the second or third day, in other cases not until the second or third week or even later; rarely it may become palpable only after the fever has settled. Splenomegaly is of little use as a sign in diagnosis in holoendemic malarious areas where most young people have an enlarged spleen. *Rose spots* are hardly ever seen in dark-skinned people. They appear about the seventh to tenth day and vary considerably in number, size, shape and dis-

tribution. There may be only two or three on the abdomen, or the body and limbs may be covered. In 90% of cases the rash is on the trunk and the spots are of a pale colour, slightly raised, round or lenticular and fade on pressure. In dark-skinned people they are darker than the surrounding skin. A more profuse eruption occurs in paratyphoid A.

Liver involvement with jaundice and evidence of hepatocellular and cholestatic changes is not uncommon. The *stool* is characteristic in about 25% of cases being loose and pale ('peasoup' stool). The *chest* invariably shows a marked bronchitis and lobar consolidation will be found in some cases. The *mental condition* is one of apathy (typhoid facies) but stupor and coma are infrequent (see section on neuropsychiatric complications below). Meningism is common.

Atypical cases

Many cases are atypical and ambulant and do not

resemble the classical disease. They may present as a simple diarrhoea or be admitted to hospital for a perforated ulcer as the first sign of illness.

Typhoid in children

In children under five in the Third World typhoid is often a severe disease with a high mortality. The presentation is frequently atypical with diarrhoea and vomiting. Meningitis is not uncommon.

Medical complications

Cardiovascular. Myocarditis occurs in a minority of patients. There may be no symptoms and the ECG changes are non-specific. In children myocarditis is a serious complication.

Venous thrombosis appears commonly as a minor thrombosis of the calf vein. Major thromboses occur (rarely) in the femoral and subclavian veins.

Typhoid lobar pneumonia. This is a rare complication seen in the second to third week of illness. There are signs of lobar consolidation, but the typical symptoms and rusty sputum of pneumonococcal pneumonia are absent. The incidence is 1–2%.[4] A haemorrhagic pleural effusion which grew *S. typhi* has been reported, as has empyema.

Haemolytic anaemia. This is a well-recognized complication. In Hong Kong it is often associated with glucose-6-phosphate dehydrogenase deficiency or haemoglobinopathy.[10] Severe haemolytic anaemia occurred in 2% of cases[4] but despite detailed investigation the cause may not be found, although in some cases Coombs' test is positive and the haemolysis may be the result of an autoimmune phenomenon.

A *haemolytic–uraemic* syndrome may be found in severe typhoid fever associated with DIC.[11]

Renal. One-quarter of typhoid patients excrete *S. typhi* in their urine at some point. Transient proteinuria is due to immune complex-mediated glomerulonephritis which may present as renal failure or a nephrotic syndrome (nephrotyphoid) often associated with *Schistosoma haematobium* infection (see Chapter 22). A suppurative typhoid pyelonephritis with extensive renal damage may occur.

Neuropsychiatric complications. A wide spectrum of neuropsychiatric disturbances have been recorded from India[12] and Nigeria.[13] These symptoms are commoner in patients from poor backgrounds. Most commonly the level of consciousness is disturbed with disorientation, delirium or coma which are grave prognostic signs. Other manifestations are fits, parkinsonism, schizophrenic states with catatonia, encephalomyelitis, transverse myelitis with spastic paraplegia, peripheral and cranial neuropathy and Guillain–Barré syndrome.

Typhoid meningitis. Found in 1% of cases[4] typhoid meningitis occurs mainly in children under five years of age. The picture is that of a pyogenic meningitis and typhoid may not be suspected until bacteriological investigation shows *S. typhi* in a blood culture. *S. typhi* may sometimes but not always be recovered from the cerebrospinal fluid which is otherwise typical of a pyogenic meningitis.

Peripheral neuropathy. Peripheral neuropathy of the 'burning feet' type may occur, which responds to large doses of vitamin B complex after two to three weeks.

Pharyngitis and suppurative parotitis. These are found in 1–3% of cases.

Liver. Asymptomatic typhoid hepatitis is common with elevation of the liver enzymes.

Jaundice. This occurs in a minority of patients.

Cholecystitis. Acute cholecystitis is commoner in women than men and may occur in patients who have not had a clinical attack of typhoid fever. Severe upper right-sided abdominal pain with jaundice develops and a positive Murphy's sign.

Chronic cholecystitis may occur months to years later when *S. typhi* is isolated from the stones or bile.

Surgical complications

The two main surgical complications are intestinal perforation and haemorrhage.

Intestinal perforation. This occurs in 3–4% of cases and is responsible for 25% of the deaths. The classical signs of perforation are rare. Much commoner is the atypical variety which occurs in the seriously ill toxic patients. The first signs may be the appearance of the free fluid in the peritoneal cavity, the disappearance of bowel sounds and vomiting. Diminished liver dullness and the demonstration of gas in the peritoneal cavity by X-rays are valuable signs. A pelvic abscess may form. Perforation may occur in a patient on chloramphenicol therapy, in which case the bowel contents are sterile, producing only a localized area of adherent bowel and pus.

Other intestinal complications can occur such as paralytic ileus, acute intestinal obstruction from adhesions, and adherent and twisted loops of bowel.

Intestinal haemorrhage. This occurs in 2–8% of cases and is usually seen between the fourteenth and twenty-first days of illness. There may be several small bleeds or a massive silent haemorrhage. The complication is signalled by an increase in pulse rate, a fall in blood pressure and the development of shock.

Genitourinary complications. These include typhoid orchitis in convalescence. Pyelitis is common in typhoid and is rarely recognized.

Skeletal system. This is affected by typhoid arthritis which may affect the ankle and hip joints. Typhoid osteomyelitis of the long bones is rare. Typhoid spine is rarer than is thought and is usually confused with brucellosis and tuberculosis. It may occur many years after an attack of typhoid although rarely after chloramphenicol. Zenker's degeneration of muscle affects especially the muscles of the abdominal wall and the thighs. Clinical, biochemical and histological evidence of severe muscle involvement causing typhoid polymyositis was observed in four patients; all reversed on treatment with chloramphenicol.[14]

Typhoid abscesses. These may occur anywhere, especially in the spleen[15] and breast.[16]

LABORATORY FINDINGS

The white cell count is $5–6 \times 10^9$/litre (5000–6000/mm³), but may range from 1.2 to 20×10^9/litre (1200/mm³ to 20 000/mm³) if there are complications. The erythrocyte sedimentation rate (ESR) is raised and the platelets reduced. Serum enzymes are raised and the bilirubin is about twice normal.

DIFFERENTIAL DIAGNOSIS

Typhoid fever is the second commonest cause of fever in the tropics lasting more than a few days and should be considered in all cases of fever of whatever duration. The blood should be examined for malaria parasites, and a white cell count and blood culture done. When the fever has lasted for three weeks the differential diagnosis narrows to kala-azar, amoebic liver abscess, tuberculosis, bacterial endocarditis, brucellosis, hidden pus, lymphoma and collagen diseases.

DIAGNOSIS

The five cardinal signs of typhoid are fever, low pulse–temperature ratio, the characteristic toxaemia, splenic enlargement and rose spots. The presence of the first three should arouse strong suspicion and other signs—abdominal distension, pea soup stools and intestinal haemorrhage should confirm the diagnosis. Rose spots are hard to see in dark skins; they may not appear until the temperature has fallen. White skins are apt to show spots as the result of mosquito bites and a heat rash.

Isolation of the organism

The organism may be isolated from the blood, bone marrow, stool, urine and bile.

Blood culture. In the early stages of the illness blood culture is the most conclusive diagnostic method and should be employed in all suspected cases during the first 7–10 days and in relapses. However, a positive blood culture may be obtained at any stage in the illness. The blood should be cultured in bottles containing bile salts (0.5% sodium taurocholate).

Clot culture.[17] This is superior in the isolation of *S. typhi* from early cases since the use of normal serum instead of the patient's serum enhances the chances of isolating the organism. Positive cultures may be obtained in less than 24 hours by culturing clots free from the patient's serum in streptokinase broth (15 ml of 0.5% bile salt broth containing 100 units of streptokinase per ml) put up in 100 ml bottles containing slopes of Wilson and Blair's medium.

Marrow culture. This is a most sensitive method of isolating *S. typhi*. It has proved reliable in China and was positive in 95% of patients as compared with 43.3% with blood culture in Peru.[18]

Faecal culture. *S. typhi* and the paratyphoid bacilli may be isolated from the faeces throughout the illness but most frequently during the second and third weeks. Cultivation of the organisms from the faeces in all stages of the disease is now successful in about 75% of cases by employing the brilliant green enrichment method, tetrathionate broth or Wilson and Blair's agar medium for concentrating the bacilli. Stools may be sent through the post in meat broth in which the organisms remain viable for many days.

Some positive findings from stool culture are open to misinterpretation and the case may be one of an enteric carrier suffering from some other illness.

Rectal swab culture. This is not as accurate as culturing 1 g of stool but is more convenient for use as a routine measure on admitting febrile patients into hospital.

Urine. Bacilluria occurs after the fourteenth day in about 25% of cases. It is intermittent and morning specimens should be examined daily for a week when other methods have proved unsuccessful. The positivity rate increases greatly in areas where *Schistosoma haematobium* is endemic.

Bile. Bile may be examined by culturing duodenal aspirate collected by a duodenal string capsule (Enterotest).

Other sites

Culture of skin snips of rose spots has also been quite successful. *S. typhi* has been isolated from cerebrospinal fluid, peritoneal fluid, mesenteric lymph glands, pharynx, tonsils and abscesses.

Serological diagnosis

Serological tests are of limited value in diagnosis. The Widal test has been in use for a long time but is not very satisfactory.

Widal test

O antibody rises early but falls quickly and a fourfold increase in the absence of recent immunization is indicative of active infection. However, it is only group specific. H antibody appears later but persists for a long time after immunization. It may not be possible to wait to allow sequential specimens of serum to be examined and diagnosis on one specimen is usually not possible. The presence of Vi antibody does not necessarily mean active infection.

Immunofluorescence

Immunofluorescence using whole *S. typhi* organisms as antigen has been developed[19] but is neither very specific nor sensitive.

Diazo reaction in urine

In the absence of laboratory facilities the diazo reaction of the urine is of great value.[4] the test is a red coloration given by the froth of the urine of typhoid patients when mixed with the diazo reagent and is caused by the presence of a substance containing a phenol ring formed by the putrefaction of protein in the intestine.

The diazo reagent is made up from two stock solutions, A and B. *Stock solution A:* sulphanilic acid 0.5 g, concentrated hydrochloric acid 5 ml and distilled water 100 ml. *Stock solution B:* sodium nitrite 0.5 g, distilled water 100 ml.

Mix 40 parts of A with 1 part of B. Solution A is stable. Solution B must be made up fresh every three weeks and kept at 4°C.

A quantity of diazo reagent is mixed with an equal quantity of an early morning specimen of urine and a few drops of 30% ammonium hydroxide are added.

The mixture is shaken and a positive reaction is a red or pinkish coloration of the froth. The diazo reaction is positive in typhoid in 80% of the cases between the fifth and fourteenth day of illness, not usually as early as the second or later than the twenty-first day of clinical illness. False-positive reactions in non-typhoid patients are about 5% and positive reactions may also be found in pulmonary tuberculosis, measles and typhus.

Diagnosis of carriers

The diagnosis of a carrier depends on the isolation of *S. typhi* or *S. paratyphi* from the faeces or urine and in view of the intermittent nature of excretion at least six consecutive examinations should be made before the result is declared negative. Examination of the aspirated bile is invaluable, or the stool may be examined after 200 mg of calomel followed by a saline purgative.

The presence of Vi agglutinins in a dilution of over 1/10 is valuable as a screening measure.

TREATMENT

The patient can be treated in a general hospital with good nursing care and barrier nursing. Care should be taken with the disposal of urine and faeces. The diet should be light and nutritious and the fluid and electrolyte balance attended to. Antibiotic treatment may have to be started before a definite diagnosis is available, on suspicion only, especially if the patient is ill.

Chloramphenicol

Chloramphenicol is the drug of choice and is more effective than ampicillin and co-trimoxazole in reducing the duration of fever and symptoms.[20] It is most effective when given orally. Since it is bacteriostatic and not bactericidal early treatment may not lead to eradication since the immune defences of the body have not developed and relapse may occur. It must be given in adequate doses for a period of time. A loading dose is no longer considered necessary and shorter courses are now given than previously recommended, 8 mg/kg 4-hourly for 5 days may be adequate in patients who are not severely ill but, if fever persists at the end of 5 days, then the drug must be continued for another 5 days.[21,22] This treatment should reduce the temperature to normal with relief of symptoms within 3–4 days. Many authorities maintain the administration of chloramphenicol for 7–10 days after defervescence but shorter courses can be just as effective and are more economical, an important advantage in the Third World.

Combined treatment with chloramphenicol 500 mg and tetracycline 500 mg 6-hourly for 3 days followed by 250 mg chloramphenicol and 250 mg tetracycline 6-hourly for 12 days may reduce the carrier rate and can be used in mild uncomplicated cases.

Other drugs

Because of the possibility of toxicity of chloramphenicol and the development of drug resistance other drugs have been used.

Ampicillin

Ampicillin has been used in doses of up to 200 mg/kg daily but the failure rate and relapse is high.

Amoxycillin

Amoxycillin compares well with chloramphenicol and is an effective alternative for the treatment of typhoid in a dose of 1 g 6-hourly for 14 days[23] while 2 g a day for 21 days gave better results than chloramphenicol with no carriers and a 2% relapse rate.[24]

Co-trimoxazole

A dose of two tablets twice a day until defervescence and for 7 days afterwards has proved successful[25,26] producing a more rapid clinical improvement but a slower defervescence than chloramphenicol.

Toxic crises

In severe cases a toxic crisis with central and peripheral circulatory failure and mental derangement may develop, probably due to a large scale destruction of typhoid bacilli and release of large amounts of typhoid endotoxin. This complication may be eliminated by using a combination of steroids and chloramphenicol. For the other toxic effects of chloramphenicol see Section XVII.

Resistance[27]

Chloramphenicol-resistant *S. typhi* began to appear in 1962; in 1972 a major epidemic of chloramphenicol-resistant typhoid was reported from Mexico where 80% of the isolates were resistant and in 1975 from South Vietnam where 60% were resistant.[28] Drug resistance is mediated by a plasmid R factor (resistance factor) and chloramphenicol should only be used for severe cases.

Steroid therapy

The immediate effect of steroids is dramatic in very toxic and ill patients. Steroids can be given early in the infection and where there are minimal intestinal symptoms. They should be avoided during the third week of the illness. Hydrocortisone, 200 mg, should be given at once parenterally followed by 15 mg prednisone three times daily for the first day, 10 mg three times a day the second day, 5 mg three times a day on the third day, 5 mg twice on the fourth day and 5 mg on the fifth day.

Relapses

Relapse accompanied by a return of fever and a positive blood culture may occur on the average 5 days after recovery from an attack but rarely later than two weeks. Rarely a chronic relapsing form may be found lasting for many months, especially following treatment with insufficient doses of chloramphenicol. Relapses are seldom more severe than the original attack[9] but can be of the utmost severity. The general relapse rate is higher after chloramphenicol but a relapse rate of only 4% was found in patients who had chloramphenicol for 12 days after defervescence of the fever.[29] Relapses are common with associated schistosomal infection. A relapse is treated in the same way as the primary attack.

Post-treatment check

When the patient has recovered the urine and stools must be cultured until three negative cultures have been obtained before discharge from medical supervision is allowed.

Treatment of carriers

Faecal carriers. The convalescent carrier is easier to treat than the chronic carrier. Six of nine convalescent carriers were cured by a combination of tetracycline and chloramphenicol used as in treatment of a normal case.[4] Chronic carriers must be treated with a prolonged course of treatment.

Ampicillin has been used successfully, 500 mg 6-hourly for at least 14 days, but a course for as long as six weeks has been necessary.

Trimethoprim with sulphamethoxazole given for one month as in treatment of a case of typhoid cleared one out of four carriers, but the remaining three cases had chronic cholecystitis.[30]

Since either the gallbladder or the biliary tract may be the source of the chronic infection where there are gallstones or a lesion of the gallbladder, the only chance for successful eradication of the typhoid infection is cholecystectomy. Since the deep bile passages are often involved the common bile duct should always be drained.

Urinary carriers. These should be treated in the same way as chronic faecal carriers and if *Schistosoma haematobium* infection is present this must also be treated.

Treatment of complications

Intestinal perforation

The treatment of intestinal perforation is subject to argument. Huckstep[4] found that the mortality rate of conservative treatment with gastric suction, intravenous fluid and electrolyte replacement with antibiotic treatment was 27%, whereas under the conditions in which he was working the surgical mortality was 80–100%. More recent observers doubt the wisdom of conservative treatment and where skilled surgery is available surgical treatment of patients with perforated ulcers is now generally agreed to be indicated. Wedge excision of the ulcer or segmental resection of the ileum has been recommended.[31]

Acute cholecystitis

Acute cholecystitis should be treated conservatively on the lines of intestinal perforation.

Intestinal haemorrhage

Massive intestinal haemorrhage can be treated with blood transfusion and supportive care. Small haemorrhages may not need transfusion. Most cases recover.

PROGNOSIS

In developed countries most cases in an epidemic will be diagnosed early and have a very low fatality rate. In Third World countries many patients will be treated on an outpatient basis and have a low mortality while inpatients in these countries will be severely ill and have a higher mortality.

EPIDEMIOLOGY

In developed countries most cases of typhoid are sporadic. Large epidemics occur due to contaminated water supplies or food contaminated by polluted water, such as in 1964 in Aberdeen where corned beef was contaminated by cooling water at the factory in Argentina. *Milk* and *ice cream* infected by a carrier can cause small epidemics. In Third World countries where there are so many convalescent and sick carriers the chronic carrier is less important. The incidence is highest in the dry season when water supplies are concentrated but may peak at the onset of the rains when organisms are flushed into streams and wells. Any temporary camp put up in the tropics to house refugees or prisoners of war is almost bound to develop typhoid in epidemic proportions, because if the inmates have come from an area where there is a lot of typhoid, the number excreting organisms can lead to spread from unclean fingers, even in the presence of clean water and good sanitation.

Age

The age-related incidence varies. In some countries (Iran and Africa) typhoid is an infection of children and there are many cases under two years of age. In epidemics all age groups are affected.

PREVENTION AND CONTROL

Immunization

Evidence accumulated in two World Wars and subsequently shows that TAB vaccination provides some degree of protection; that this protection is only partial has been shown in volunteers who developed protection against moderate doses of organisms, but not against larger doses.

TAB vaccine is associated with more side-effects and an acetone inactivated *S. typhi* is now the vaccine of choice.

Primary immunization. Adults and children over 10 years are given 0.5 ml subcutaneously with a second dose four to six weeks later and a third dose of 1.0 ml six to twelve months later. Children under 10 receive half the adult dose. A booster dose every three years is recommended. Volunteer studies suggest that the protection provided lasts 12 years.

Intradermal vaccination is just as effective and gives fewer reactions; 0.1 ml is given intradermally at the same intervals. A single injection of vaccine has been found to confer a substantial degree of immunity not significantly different from that obtained with two doses[32, 33] (see Chapter 71).

Travellers to endemic areas should drink only treated or bottled water. *S. typhi* is killed by heat at 58°C, iodination and chlorination. Food must be heated uniformly for several minutes. Travellers should avoid eating uncooked vegetables and unpeeled fruit that has not been thoroughly washed with chlorinated water. Shellfish should not be eaten uncooked.

PARATYPHOID (ENTERIC) FEVER

AETIOLOGY

Paratyphoid fever is caused by a number of species of *Salmonella*: *S. paratyphi A*, *S. paratyphi B* (*S. schottmülleri*), *S. paratyphi C* (*S. hirschfeldii*), *S. typhimurium* and *S. cholerae-suis*. Almost any *Salmonella* can at times cause an enteric-like fever.

TRANSMISSION

S. paratyphi A is exclusively a human infection, the others are of animal origin. Transmission to man is by food and meat pies and ice creams are the usual source vehicles.

CLINICAL FEATURES

The paratyphoid A and B organisms are less invasive and more irritant to the intestinal tract than *S. typhi* so that there is usually an initial attack of diarrhoea and vomiting before the invasive stages. The incubation period is shorter and the disease milder. Ambulant cases are commoner than in typhoid but the carrier stage is shorter. In paratyphoid A duration of the fever is longer than in typhoid. Although there are less likely to be complications, relapses are more common.

In paratyphoid B lymphoid follicles of the whole of the intestinal tract may be involved including the stomach, colon and rectum. Jaundice, venous thromboses and suppurative lesions are commoner.

PARATYPHOID C

Paratyphoid C as observed by Giglioi[34] in Guyana is a septicaemia in which the intestinal tract may not be specially involved. Complications such as arthritis, abscess formation and cholecystitis are common while fixation abscesses from intramuscular injections may occasionally contain a pure culture of the bacillus. The mortality of the series of 92 patients was 38%.

The treatment is as for typhoid fever. Most cases of enteric fever are so mild as not to need any treatment. As with all *Salmonella,* antibiotic treatment tends to increase the likelihood of increasing the carrier rate.

REFERENCES

1 Hornick, R. B., Greisman, S. E., Woodward, J. E. et al (1970) *New Engl. J. Med.* **283,** 686.
2 McFadzean, A. J. S. & Ong, G. B. (1966) *Br. med. J.* **i,** 567.
3 Belzer, M. (1965) *J. Urol.* **94,** 23.
4 Huckstep, R. L. (1962) *Typhoid Fever and other Salmonella Infections.* Edinburgh: Livingstone.
5 Vaizey, J.M. (1959) *E. Afr. med. J.* **36,** 65.
6 Greisman, S.E. & Hornick, R.B. (1973) *J. Infect. Dis.* **128,** 265.
7 Sitprija, V., Pipatanagul V., Boonpucknavig, V. et al (1974) *Ann. intern. Med.* **81,** 210–213.
8 Marmion, D.E., Naylor, G.R.E. & Stewart, I.D. (1953)
9 Marmion, D.E. (1952) *Trans. R. Soc. trop. Med. Hyg.* **46,** 619.
10 McFadzean, A.J.S. & Choa, G.H. (1953) *Br. med. J.* **ii,** 360.
11 Basty, H. (1974) *Acta med. iran.* **17,** 131.
12 Breakey, W.R. & Kala, A.A. (1977) *Br. med. J.* **ii,** 357.
13 Osuntokun, B.O., Badimosi, O., Ogunnemia, K. et al (1972) *Archs Neurol. Psychiat.* **27,** 7.
14 Naidoo, P.N. & Yan, C.C. (1975) *S. Afr. med. J.* **49,** 619.
15 Martinez-Vasquez, J.M., Pahissa, A., Tornos, M.O. et al (1977) *Br. med. J.* **i,** 1323.
16 Barrett, G.S. & MacDermot, J. (1972) *Br. med. J.* **ii,** 627.
17 Thomas, J.V., Watson, K.C. & Hewstone, A.S. (1954) *J. clin. Path.* **7,** 50.
18 Guerra-Caceres, J.G., Gotuzzo-Herencia, E., Crosby-Dagnini, E. et al (1979) *Trans. R. Soc. trop. Med. Hyg.* **73,** 680.
19 Das, K.K. & Sant, M.U. (1972) *J. Postgrad. Med.* **18,** 123.
20 Snyder, M.J., Gonzalez, O., Palomono, S. et al (1976) *Lancet* **ii,** 1175.
21 Rowland, H.A.K. (1961) *J. trop. Med. Hyg.* **64,** 101.
22 Rowland, H.A.K. (1961) *J. trop. Med. Hyg.* **64,** 143.
23 Pillay, N., Adams, E.B. & North-Coombes (1975) *Lancet* **ii,** 333.
24 Scragg, J.N. & Rubidge, C.J. (1975) *Am. J. trop. Med. Hyg.* **24,** 860.
25 Farid, Z., Hassan, A., Washab, M.P.A. et al (1970) *Br. med. J.* **ii,** 323.
26 Kamat, S.A. (1970) *Br. med. J.* **ii,** 605.
27 Editorial (1973) *Lancet* **i,** 1008.
28 Meyruey, M.H., Goudineau, J.A., Berger, P.M. et al (1975) *Rev. Épid. Méd. soc. Santé publ.* **23,** 345.
29 El Ramli, A.H. (1950) *Lancet* **i,** 618.
30 Brodie, J., MacQueen, I.A. & Livingstone, D. (1970) *Br. med. J.* **iii,** 318.
31 Welch, T.P. & Martin, N.C. (1975) *Lancet* **i,** 1078.
32 World Health Organization (1966) *Bull. Wld Hlth Org.* **34,** 211.
33 Ashcroft, M.T., Singh, B., Nicholson, C.C. et al (1967) *Lancet* **ii,** 1056.
34 Giglioi, G. (1929) *Trans. R. Soc. trop. Med. Hyg.* **23,** 335.

Chapter 9
Toxoplasmosis

Toxoplasma is a parasite of cats and other felines which are infected from eating rats, mice and other rodents. In man it can cause fever and other clinical syndromes.

GEOGRAPHICAL DISTRIBUTION

Toxoplasmosis infection is distributed worldwide. It is a common cause of 'opportunist' infection in immunosuppressed subjects.

AETIOLOGY

Toxoplasmosis is caused by a coccidian parasite *Toxoplasma gondii* which has a sexual cycle (schizogony) and gametogony (isosporan phase) in the intestinal epithelium of the definitive host, the domestic cat, and an asexual cycle (toxoplasmic phase) in man in which endozoites (tachyzoites) parasitize cells, especially of the reticuloendothelial system forming 'pseudocysts' in the acute stages and cystozoites (bradyzoites) forming 'tissue cysts' in the chronic stage.

Life-cycle

Feline host (enteric or isosporan phase)[1,2]

Oöcysts ingested by the cat release *sporozoites* which enter the epithelial cells lining the intestine where they undergo *schizogony* to form *schizonts*. These form *microgametes* and *macrogametes* which fuse to form a *zygote* which develops into an *oöcyst* which is passed out in the stool. It then sporulates, forming two *sporocysts*, each with four *sporozoites*, in 3 or 4 days and is ready to infect another host. In this cycle the prepatent period from infection to oöcyst shedding is 20–30 days. Oöcysts continue to be shed for 7–20 days in primary infections but not in reinfections, except when the cat is young.[3]

Cats may also be infected by ingesting *cysts* in the infected meat of prey animals. The *cystozoites* released from the cyst enter the intestinal epithelial cells to undergo schizogony in the enteric cycle. In this case the prepatent period is about 5 days.

Intermediate or prey host (toxoplasmic phase)
(man)

Ingested oöcysts release the sporozoites which enter macrophages in the tissue in which they multiply as *endozoites* (toxoplasmas) forming pseudocysts, the walls of which contain no parasite material. These cells rupture releasing the endozoites to infect new macrophages.

Endozoites are curved or crescent-shaped organisms 4–6 μm × 2–3 μm in size with one end rounded. With Giemsa stain they appear blue with a red or purple nucleus. They are seen enclosed in pseudocysts which are macrophages containing up to 100 endozoites (Fig. 9.1). As immunity develops the endozoites change their form and become *cystozoites* which are elongated sporozoite-like forms enclosed in a true or tissue

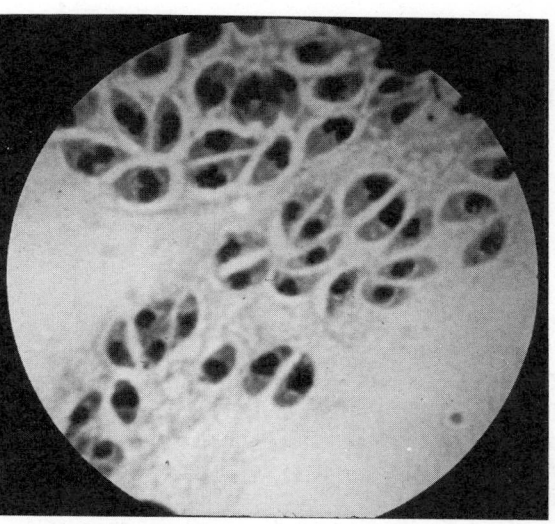

Fig. 9.1 Endozoites in peritoneal exudate from a mouse.

207

cyst, the walls of which are composed of host tissue which shields them from the immune defences of the host. Each tissue cyst contains thousands of cystozoites (Fig. 9.2). These cysts can lie dormant for the whole of the host's life and can resist normal and refrigeration temperatures (destroyed by one hour at 50°C) and gastric juice. On being ingested by a cat the cystozoites enter the intestinal epithelial cells where they undergo schizogony and follow the enteric cycle. If the tissue cysts are ingested by another intermediate or prey host they enter macrophages and follow the toxoplasmic cycle as above. Parasites can be transmitted transplacentally in the toxoplasmic phase.

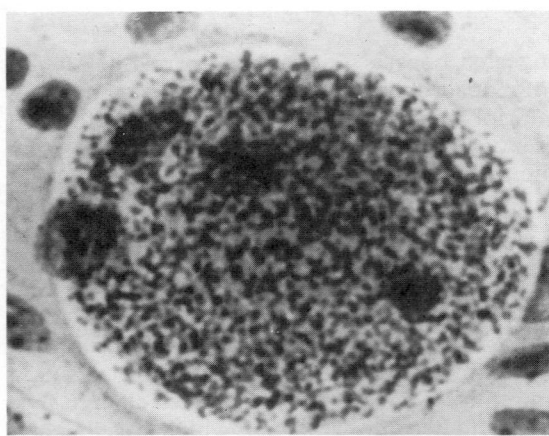

Fig. 9.2 Cystozoites in a tissue cyst in mouse brain.

TRANSMISSION

Transmission is by the ingestion of oöcysts from faecally contaminated soil, ingestion of 'tissue cysts' in the flesh of intermediate hosts, transplacental (congenital), blood transfusion or organ transplant.

Cats

Cats become infected at about four weeks of age from faecally contaminated soil, acquiring a primary infection. They shed oöcysts in the faeces for 7–20 days following which they become immune. Kittens are the most important source of infection and can shed oöcysts for longer periods after reinfection. Human infec-

tion from eating tissue cysts in the undercooked flesh of intermediate host animals is well documented and the relative importance of the two sources of infection is a matter for conjecture. Oöcysts are well preserved in soil which is moist and shaded but not if exposed to the sunlight and desiccation. Beneath houses raised on stilts oöcysts can remain infective for 24–98 days.[4] Contact with infected soil is more important in human infection than direct contact with cats.

Intermediate hosts

Human infection may be acquired from eating tissue cysts in undercooked pork, mutton and beef.[5] Clusters of cases have arisen from eating pork,[6] hamburgers[7] and mutton.[8] Handling and dissection of diseased animals (rats) is also a route of infection.

Congenital transmission

Infection takes place via the placenta only when the mother acquires the infection for the first time during the first four months of pregnancy.[8] Maternal antibodies when present protect the fetus. At birth the child's antibody titre will be the same as the mother's but the baby will have no IgM antibody as this cannot cross the placenta. The child's antibody titre will fall to nothing in six months if the fetus is not infected. The risk of infection is only one or two per 10 000 pregnancies and is highest where there is an annual 3–5% seroconversion rate in the population. At a higher rate most women in the 20–30 years age group are already immune and the chance of infection in pregnancy is correspondingly less. Infection may be acquired from blood transfusion[9] or from organ transplants, liver,[10] kidney[11] and heart.[12]

PATHOGENESIS

In the initial stages of infection the crescent-shaped endozoites (Fig. 9.1) invade and multiply in nucleated cells of all types of tissue but especially macrophages of the reticuloendothelial system which they destroy causing focal necrosis. Nests of endozoites are produced forming 'pseudocysts' which rupture and spread the infection. As the immune defences of the host build up the toxoplasma parasites are walled off forming 'tissue cysts' containing large numbers of cystozoites, which are found in the brain and muscles.

PATHOLOGY

Three pathological processes are at work to produce the lesion: in acute toxoplasmosis the direct action of the endozoites on the cells causes necrosis and there is also a type III antigen–antibody reaction between host antibody seeping through vessel walls and reacting with parasite antigen to cause intravascular thrombosis and infarction. In the chronic stage tissue cysts rupture to release cystozoites which elicit a type IV reaction with round cell infiltration, granuloma formation and tissue necrosis.

Acquired toxoplasmosis

Acute stage

Lymphadenopathy. The commonest changes are found in the lymph glands with clumps of weakly staining histiocytes around the follicles and occasionally inside them. Necrosis is not a feature and the clusters of histiocytes are not specifically recognizable unless stained serologically. Large reticular cells containing debris are found but the parasite is very rarely seen.

Encephalitis. Toxoplasmic encephalitis may be found in immunosuppressed adults with large areas of cerebral necrosis due to infarction following thrombosis of small vessels. Glial nodules are few or absent but parasites are more numerous than in the congenital form.

Chronic stage

Tissue cysts remain dormant in the tissues until they rupture and the cystozoites are destroyed forming small granulomas.

Congenital toxoplasmosis

Early in pregnancy toxoplasmosis may cause fetal death or miscarriage. Later a live child may be born who may die in the first few weeks of life with generalized toxoplasmosis or later develop choroidoretinitis and serious involvement of the brain followed by intracerebral calcification.

Acute generalized toxoplasmosis (found in immunosuppressed subjects)

This is characterized by lesions in the heart, liver, lungs and brain.

Heart. Parasites enter the heart muscle cells forming pseudocysts often with little or no cellular response.

Lungs. Lungs show a toxoplasma atypical pneumonia with endozoites and mononuclear cells in the bronchioles and congestion in the alveoli.

Liver. There are large areas of necrosis with giant cells and extramedullary haemopoiesis and jaundice.

Brain. There is encephalitis with necrosis of brain cells from invasion by endozoites and small scattered infarcts. Periaqueductal and periventricular necrosis results from parasitization of the ependymal cells with endozoites with consequent inflammation and formation of small ependymal ulcers. The aqueduct of Sylvius becomes blocked with resultant hydrocephalus. Endozoites are numerous in lesions in the brain and lungs in subjects where cell-mediated immunity has been suppressed when dormant tissue cysts are reactivated.

Chronic infection

Brain. The presence of tissue cysts containing cystozoites which rupture causes tissue necrosis, granuloma formation with the formation of microglial nodules, gliosis and later calcification.

Chorioretinitis. Similar changes in the retina cause choroiditis. These changes in brain and retina produce the tetrad of signs and symptoms of congenital toxoplasmosis: convulsions, intracerebral calcification, hydrocephalus and chorioretinitis.

IMMUNITY

Immunity to toxoplasmosis is both humoral and cellular.

Humoral immunity

In the acute stage IgG antibodies (measured by

the dye, complement fixation (CF) and specific immunofluorescence tests) reach their maximum two months after infection and persist, probably for life. IgM antibodies (measured by specific immunofluorescence and enzyme-linked immunosorbent assay (ELISA) tests) appear before IgG antibodies and disappear before the IgG antibodies reach their peak. These antibodies clear endozoites from the blood but tissue cysts containing cystozoites remain unaffected in the brain and muscle.

Cellular immunity

Cellular immunity is the basis of immunity in chronic infection and can be transferred by lymphocytes.[13] In man this immunity is lifelong and is due to the persistence of tissue cysts in the body from which cystozoites escape from time to time, only to be destroyed by the host's cellular immune system; but this periodic challenge serves to reinforce the immune response and so maintain immunity.

CLINICAL FEATURES

Acquired toxoplasmosis

Natural history

After a primary infection the vast majority of toxoplasma infections are symptomless and inapparent. It is estimated that 30% of the human race is infected, varying in different localities from 5% to 90%. An overall 3% seroconversion rate annually in the population indicates the extent of inapparent infections. In some susceptible individuals and in those who are immunocompromised from whatever cause, an acute symptomatic infection develops. This may be mild and self-curing or more severe causing acute generalized toxoplasmosis. In women who are infected for the first time in the first four months of pregnancy the fetus may become infected (see section on congenital toxoplasmosis, below).

Incubation period

It is difficult to determine this with any accuracy but where the source of infection has been traced as after the consumption of semi-cooked meat it has been 10–12 days.[7]

Signs and symptoms

GLANDULAR TOXOPLASMOSIS
This is the commonest form of symptomatic toxoplasmosis. It often presents as a localized, painless lymphadenopathy with or without fever. Less common is a generalized lymphadenopathy with chronic illness and splenomegaly. Toxoplasmosis is important in the differential diagnosis of this syndrome (see section on differential diagnosis, below). There may or may not be fever, rash, hepatitis with jaundice and arthralgia. Pericarditis has been described.[14]

GENERALIZED TOXOPLASMOSIS
This is usually mild except in immunocompromised people in whom there may be a severe febrile illness, prostration, rash and many organs affected.

ENCEPHALITIS
This presents as fever and convulsions with xanthochromic cerebrospinal fluid under pressure with a raised protein count and mononuclear pleocytosis.

CHORIORETINITIS
This is uncommon in acute cases. When it does occur it resembles the congenital form.

INAPPARENT INFECTION
In the vast majority of infections tissue cysts lie dormant in the brain or muscle, only detectable by the presence of specific IgG in the serum, but these cysts may be the source of severe disease in immunocompromised people.

Laboratory findings

The blood count shows a normal or slightly reduced white cell count with lymphocytosis, monocytosis and sometimes atypical cells. A normochromic normocytic anaemia develops during prolonged illness.

Congenital toxoplasmosis

About 60% of babies infected in utero are asymptomatic at birth; of the others, the child may be born prematurely, stillborn or die shortly after birth. Some live to show signs of congenital toxoplasmosis later in life, usually chorioretinitis or cerebral disease.

Signs and symptoms

GENERALIZED TOXOPLASMOSIS

Some children are born jaundiced with a papular or purpuric rash. There may be hepatosplenomegaly with ocular manifestations, nystagmus and strabismus. Other manifestations are anaemia, lymphadenopathy, pneumonia, cataract and optic atrophy.

CHORIORETINITIS (OCULAR TOXOPLASMOSIS) (see also Chapter 70; Plate VI.3)

Chorioretinitis occurs both in acquired toxoplasmosis, where it is focal, and in congenital toxoplasmosis, where it is generalized and found in 90% of cases, eventually causing blindness.

CEREBRAL TOXOPLASMOSIS

Toxoplasmosis has a severe effect on the central nervous system where it causes the tetrad of signs known as 'Sabin's tetrad': internal hydrocephalus, chorioretinitis, convulsions and cerebral calcification. Associated with these signs may be microcephalus, mental retardation, spastic paralysis, impaired vision, deafness and psychomotor disturbances.

DIAGNOSIS

Differential diagnosis

Glandular toxoplasmosis can resemble many conditions including glandular tuberculosis, lymphoma, Hodgkin's disease, leukaemia, African trypanosomiasis, visceral leishmaniasis and glandular fever.

Generalized toxoplasmosis can resemble septicaemia and other severe febrile conditions.

Cerebral toxoplasmosis in immunocompromised persons can resemble viral encephalitis and cerebral tumour.

Isolation of toxoplasma

This is difficult and not always practical. Endozoites may be seen in tissue impression smears stained with Giemsa stain and in sections stained with haematoxylin and eosin. Fluorescent antibody stains may identify parasites as also can electron microscopy. Endozoites will be found in acute and cystozoites in chronic infections.

Animal inoculation and culture

Tissues or the buffy coat of centrifuged blood may be inoculated intraperitoneally into white mice or a cell culture. Endozoites can be seen in the peritoneal fluid after 4–18 days.

Serology

Owing to the persistence of IgG and the existence of so many inapparent infections it is essential to measure both IgG and IgM specific antibodies. Interpretation of results is difficult. IgG antibodies may be measured by the dye test,[15] CFT, indirect haemagglutination, indirect fluorescent antibody test, latex agglutination, direct agglutination and Indian ink immunoreaction.[16] IgM specific antibodies may be measured by IgM assay[17] and an ELISA test.[18]

Usually several tests are employed but the dye test is still prominent for IgG.

Interpretation

In principle IgG titres show past infection and any titre of IgM means recent acute infection. IgM antibodies develop first during the acute period and disappear after peaking of the IgG level. IgM does not cross the placenta but if it leaks across then it has a half-life of 3–5 days. In diagnosis it is important to distinguish early infection with positive IgM but low IgG titres from chronic infection with high IgG titres and no IgM. In congenital toxoplasmosis it is important to distinguish between passive transfer of antibodies from the mother to the fetus (no IgM) and actively acquired antibody (IgM present) caused by infection in utero. In pregnant women suspected of infection IgM levels should be estimated at three-weekly intervals when rising titres are significant. In women at risk of having a toxoplasma infected infant any titre of IgG high or low will indicate that she is protected and that the fetus is free of infection. IgM antibody in the cord blood is diagnostic of active infection but is only present in 25% of infected infants.[19] If there is no IgM in the cord blood then IgG levels must be followed up and if they show a tenfold fall in three months then the child is not infected; if they remain constant or rise, then he or she is.

TREATMENT

Indications for treatment are active clinical disease (positive antibody titres by themselves do not need treatment) in the adult, ocular lesions and congenital infection in all cases, regardless of symptoms.

Pyrimethamine sulphonamide combination

Pyrimethamine (Daraprim) 75 mg daily is given for 3 days followed by 25 mg daily for four to six weeks. (Children: 2 mg/kg daily for 3 days followed by 1 mg/kg daily for four to six weeks.)

Sulphadiazine is given 500 mg four times daily (children 25 mg/kg) for four to six weeks.

Sulphamethoxazole pyrimethamine combinations are not so effective. Marrow depression can be countered with folinic acid 3–10 mg daily. Treatment is only effective against endozoites and not tissue cysts and should be continued until signs of activity have ceased.

Spiramycin

This is less toxic and is recommended in pregnancy as well as acquired cases. The dosage is 500–750 mg four times daily for adults, and for children, 50–100 mg/kg twice daily for four to six weeks. These two treatments may be used alternately.

PROGNOSIS

Most acute cases, acquired or congenital, recover. Immunosuppressed individuals do not do so well. When a woman acquires toxoplasmosis during pregnancy, abortion should be considered. If a woman has had one infected infant then further children will be free of toxoplasmosis.

EPIDEMIOLOGY

In most human communities the prevalence of toxoplasma antibodies is high and at one time exposure to infected meat was thought important. Now it has been shown that *young cats* are the most important shedders of oöcysts at their first infection (1- to 2-year-old cats are immune) and that faecally contaminated soil is the source of infection (see section on transmission, above).

In humid tropical areas houses on stilts are important and people who associate with cats under these circumstances have a greatly increased prevalence of antibody.

CONTROL

Control of infected cat faeces and soil is the most important control measure. Limiting of the cat population and a house construction programme are other measures. The aim is to prevent congenital toxoplasmosis and this could be done by testing for antibody early in pregnancy. Those with no antibody should be urged to avoid contact with cats, and treatment provided if seroconversion occurs.

REFERENCES

1 Frenkel, J.K., Dubey, J.P. & Miller, N.L. (1971) *Sci., Washington* **167**, 893.
2 Hutchinson, W.M., Dunachie, J.F., Sim, J.C. et al (1970) *Br. med. J.* **i**, 142.
3 Dubey, J.P. & Frenkel, J.K. (1974) *Vet. Path.* **11**, 350
4 Ruiz, A. & Frenkel, J.K. (1977) *J. Parasitol.* **63**, 931–932.
5 Work, K. (1971) *Acta path. microbiol, scand., B suppl.* **221**, 51.
6 Weinman, D. & Chandler, A.H. (1954) *Proc. Soc. exp. Biol. Med.* **87**, 211.
7 Kean, B.H., Kimball, A.C. & Christensen, W.N. (1969) *J. Am. med. Ass.* **6**, 1002.
8 Desmonts, G., Couvreur, J., Alison, E. et al (1965) *Rev. fr. Étud. clin. Biol.* **10**, 952.
9 Siegel, S.E., Lunde, M.H., Gelderman, A.H. et al (1971) *Blood* **37**, 388.
10 Anthony, C.W. (1972) *J. Am. med. Women. Ass.* **27**, 601–603.
11 Reynolds, E.S., Wallis, K.W. & Pfeifer, R. (1966) *Archs intern. Med.* **4**, 401.
12 Stinson, E.B., Bieber, C.P., Griepp, R.B. et al (1971) *Ann. intern. Med.* **74**, 22–36.
13 Frenkel, J.K. (1967) *J. Immunol.* **98**, 1309.
14 Kean, B.H. & Kimball, A.C. (1965) *Ann. intern. Med.* **62**, 786.
15 Sabin, A.B. & Feldman, H.A. (1948) *Science, N.Y.* **108**, 660.
16 Safar, E.H., Azab, M.E. & Osman, Z.M. (1984) *Trans. R. Soc. trop. Med. Hyg.* **78**, 169–172.
17 Fleck, D.G. & Kwantes, M. (1980) *PHLS Monograph*, No. 13. London: HMSO.
18 Payne, R.A., Isaac, M. & Frances, J.M. (1982) *J. clin. Path.* **35**, 892–896.
19 Desmonts, G. & Couvreur, J. (1975) *Infection of the Fetus and Newborn*, eds. S. Krugman & A.A. Gershon. New York: Liss.

Chapter 10
Rickettsial (Typhus) Fevers

GEOGRAPHICAL DISTRIBUTION

The human rickettsial diseases are widely distributed but are divisible into different forms, some of which are adapted to a local arthropod host and have a local distribution.

AETIOLOGY

Rickettsiae are very small bacteria with a gram-negative bacterial-like cell wall and internal structure with a DNA genome. They are obligatory intracellular parasites possessing endotoxins similar to those of gram-negative bacilli. Morphologically they appear as small bacilli or cocci and coccoid forms in dense masses are common (Fig. 10.1). They stain well with Giemsa, red with Castañeda and red with the surrounding cell wall blue with Macchiavello's stain.

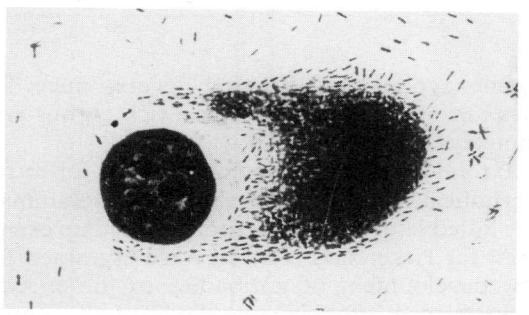

Fig. 10.1 *Rickettsia prowazeki* in a cell from the peritoneal surface of the spleen of a gerbil.

NATURAL HISTORY

Rickettsiae are normally inhabitants of the alimentary tract of insects and *R. pediculi* is an extracellular intestinal parasite which is harmless to its host, the body louse. In lice and fleas rickettsiae parasitize the intestinal cells, multiplying in the epithelial cells of the gut, which they distend and rupture, to appear in large numbers in the faeces. This infection can kill the louse, which does not transmit infection by bite but by direct contamination from the faecal contents.

In ticks, rickettsiae are dispersed in a more widespread manner invading all cells and their nuclei, especially the ovary, so that infection is transmitted hereditarily by bite. In mites rickettsiae invade the body cavity of the adult mite and are transmitted hereditarily by the larval stages of the mite which infect via the salivary glands. Ticks and mites form permanent reservoir hosts while lice and fleas do not since the infection is not transmitted hereditarily.

All rickettsiae, except louse-borne typhus and trench fever, are zoonoses. They may be divided into three main groups and two minor ones (see Table 10.1).

1. Typhus group.
2. Spotted fever group.
3. Scrub typhus group.
4. Q fever.
5. Trench fever.

The different species of rickettsiae may develop in other than their usual vectors. *Rochalimaea quintana, Rickettsia prowazeki, R. mooseri, R. conori, R. rickettsi, R. akari, R. tsutsugamushi (orientalis)* and *Coxiella burneti* all multiply in the haemolymph of the body louse (*Pediculus*) and can be passaged through lice by intracoelomic inoculation, though after a certain number of passages *R. orientalis* ceases to multiply in the stomach of the louse. All the rickettsiae except *R. orientalis* and *R. quintana* multiply or survive in the haemolymph of the mealworm (*Tenebrio molitor*) and in the tick *Ornithodoros moubata*. All except *R. tsutsugamushi* and *R. rickettsi* can be passaged repeatedly from louse to louse by rectal inoculation. *R. conori* is pathogenic to lice and causes severe damage to the mucosa of the stomach and death within 3–7 days.[1] Using immunofluorescence antibodies to *C. burneti* have been demonstrated in the sera of mice inoculated with pools of fleas and mites from an endemic area,[2] and complement-fixing antibodies to the spotted fever group were also found in mice inoculated

Table 10.1 Rickettsial diseases.

Group	Rickettsia	Clinical disease	Transmission	Host	Geographical area
1 Typhus group	*R. prowazeki*	Louse-borne typhus (epidemic typhus)	Body louse (*P. humanus*)	Man	Worldwide
	R. prowazeki var. *mooseri*	Murine typhus (flea-borne typhus)	Flea	Rodents	Scattered foci worldwide
	R. canada	RMSF-like disease	Tick	?	Georgia, USA
2 Spotted fever group	*R. rickettsi*	Rocky Mountain spotted fever (RMSF)	Ixodid tick	Rodents Dog	Western hemisphere
	R. conori	*Fièvre boutonneuse* African tick typhus	Ixodid tick	Rodents Dog	Mediterranean littoral, Africa, India
	R. siberica	Siberian tick typhus (Asian tick rickettsiosis)	Ixodid tick	Long-tailed suslik	East and central Siberia
	R. australis	Queensland tick typhus	Ixodid tick	Marsupials	Queensland
	R. akari	Rickettsialpox	Mouse mite	Mouse	USA, USSR, South and central Africa
3 Scrub typhus group	*R. tsutsugamushi* (*orientalis*)	Scrub typhus (mite typhus)	Larval trombiculid mite		Asia, Australia, New Guinea, Pacific Islands
4 Q fever	*Coxiella burneti*	Q fever	? ticks and direct transmission	Mammals	Worldwide
5 Trench fever	*Rochalimaea* (*Rickettsia*) *quintana*	Trench fever	Body louse (*P. humanus*)	Man	Eastern Europe, Africa, Mexico, South America

with pools of arthropods from both endemic and non-endemic areas for human rickettsiosis. Both *C. burneti* and spotted fever group antigens have been demonstrated by immunofluorescence in arthropod smears from endemic and non-endemic areas, suggesting a wide distribution of these organisms in nature.[3]

ISOLATION AND CULTURE

All rickettsiae grow readily on the chorioallantoic membrane of fertile egg, or preferably in the yolk sac, and duck eggs are highly suitable. They do not kill the embryo but produce round prominent foci visible 5 days after inoculation and develop completely in 7 or 8 days. They also grow in tissue culture and in a medium of minced chicken embryo with a mixture of guinea-pig or rabbit serum and Tyrode's solution. Rickettsiae may be isolated by inoculation of material into animals. Guinea-pigs are used for murine, epi-

demic typhus and spotted fevers, mice for *R. akari* and north Queensland tick typhus and monkeys for *R. conori*.

Ground or whole blood clot is used for intraperitoneal inoculation of animals. The animals are killed later and the peritoneal exudate examined for rickettsiae. The sera are examined for the development of antibodies to the specific rickettsiae. Rickettsiae may be adapted to mice by intranasal passage or to eggs by yolk sac inoculation to allow for the study of the morphology and the preparation of antigens. None of the species can readily be cultivated on solid media. Practically pure strains of *R. prowazeki* can be obtained by intrarectal injection of lice (Weigl's method).

DIFFERENTIATION OF RICKETTSIAE

Rickettsiae may be differentiated by their behaviour in guinea-pigs and by serological reactions.

Neill–Mooser reaction

This is a distinctive reaction in guinea-pigs inoculated with blood or material infected with rickettsiae. In a positive reaction a redness and swelling of the scrotum appears and typical typhus lesions are found in the scrotum in the endothelial lining of the tunica vaginalis, whose cells are swollen and filled with rickettsiae. Some strains of rickettsiae give this reaction more strongly than others. It is nearly always positive with *R. rickettsi* and *R. mooseri* but in only 70% of cases with *R. prowazeki* and is usually negative with *R. conori*.

Serological reactions

Specific rickettsial antisera are prepared in guinea-pigs and used to identify unknown strains by agglutination, CF and fluorescent tests.

Pathological differences

Rickettsiae conveyed by lice and fleas are characterized by invasion of the endothelium and mesothelium, producing distension of the cytoplasm of the host cells without affecting the nuclei, while in guinea-pigs they cause proliferative endangiitis without thrombonecrosis. In typhus-infected lice and fleas the rickettsiae are intracytoplasmic, inhabiting the lining cells of the gut and are not hereditarily transmitted. The spotted fever group conveyed by ticks is characterized by thrombonecrosis of arterioles and venules and in human tissue rickettsiae invade smooth muscle cells as well as endothelium, mesothelium and histiocytes. In tissue cultures a massive infection of nuclei takes place. In infected ticks the rickettsiae are intranuclear as well as intracytoplasmic and invade nearly all types of cells, features which serve to distinguish the spotted fever group. They are hereditarily transmitted.

Rickettsiae may also be differentiated by the serological reactions induced in the mammalian host.

Weil–Felix reaction (Table 10.2)

The Weil–Felix reaction uses the strains of *Bacillus proteus* known as OX2, OX19 and OXK, which are agglutinated by the sera in rickettsial fevers. The typhus fevers can be classified serologically as follows:

OX19 type   Vectors: louse and flea
OXK type   Vector: mite
Indeterminate   Vector: tick

Cross reactions may occur with *B. proteus* infections, undulant fever, relapsing fever, tularaemia and rat bite fever, especially with the OXK strain.

Table 10.2 Differentiation of rickettsial infections by serology.

Rickettsiosis	Complement fixation[a]			Weil–Felix reaction[b]		
	Typhus	Rocky Mountain spotted fever	Q fever	OX19	OX2	OXK
Group 1						
Primary epidemic typhus	+ + +	O	O	+ + +	+	O
Brill–Zinsser disease	+ + +	O	O	O or + + +	O	O
Murine typhus	+ + +	O	O	+ + +	+	O
Group 2						
Rocky Mountain spotted fever	O	+ + +	O	+ + +	+ + +	O
Tick typhus	O	+ + +	O	+ + +	+ + +	O
Rickettsialpox	O	+ + +	O	O	O	O
Group 3						
Scrub typhus	O	O	O	O	O	+ + +
Q fever	O	O	+ + +	O	O	O

After Murray.

[a] + + + = titres of 1/40 to 1/1280; O = titres less than 1/5.
[b] + + + = titres of more than 1/160; O = titres of 1/4 or less.

Specific rickettsial agglutination and CF tests

Rickettsiae are obtained as antigenic material from yolk sac cultures treated with ether or from mouse lung suspensions centrifuged and treated with kieselguhr. Agglutination tests are left at 37–40°C for 18 hours and read by the naked eye. CF tests are done in the usual manner. Rickettsial agglutinins appear earlier than OX19 antibodies. Complement-fixing antibodies appear later.

Specific rickettsial tests are of value in the diagnosis of laboratory infections in previously vaccinated individuals in whom the Weil–Felix agglutinin response is less vigorous. Specific rickettsial antigens are also needed for the differential diagnosis of murine and epidemic typhus and the spotted fever group, which all show a rise in the OX19 agglutinins. With highly purified washed antigens from yolk sac cultures it is possible to differentiate epidemic from murine typhus and Rocky Mountain spotted fever. The differential diagnosis of rickettsial infections by serology is shown in Table 10.2.[4]

Specific toxin–antitoxin tests in mice can also be used to demonstrate a protective effect with homologous immune sera.

Indirect fluorescent antibody tests (IFAT) can be used to diagnose typhus cases retrospectively since they show a group-specific response in the sera of patients convalescent from typhus fevers. An IFAT using rickettsiae cultured in yolk sacs was able to differentiate between Rocky Mountain spotted fever and typhus at a titre of 1/80 or over without any cross reactions between groups.[5] Specific serological and active immunization tests have shown antigenic differences in *R. orientalis* in contrast to the antigenic homogeneity in *R. prowazeki*. There are three main antigenic variants of *R. orientalis* and there is no cross immunity relationship with the other rickettsiae. These differences are important in the preparation of vaccines.

1   TYPHUS GROUP

Louse-borne typhus fever (epidemic typhus)

This form of typhus is variously known as true exanthematic, historic or classical typhus and tabardillo (Mexico); its chronic form is Brill's (Brill–Zinsser) disease or recrudescent epidemic typhus.

GEOGRAPHICAL DISTRIBUTION
(Fig. 10.2)

The classical form of typhus used to be distributed worldwide and has constituted the most important disease in world history. In the Middle Ages it was widespread in Europe and it was especially prevalent in Ireland during the Great Famine of 1845–1847. Between 1917 and 1923 there were 30 000 000 cases with over 300 000 deaths in Russia and Europe. It has been reported from every country in Europe; the last great wave was in 1933–1934 in the Soviet Union and throughout Europe, including Spain and Portugal. During the Second World War typhus occurred in eastern Europe and Italy where an epidemic was halted in 1943 for the first time with DDT and other insecticides. Epidemic typhus can be found in the temperate highlands of the tropics over 1600 m. It has been found in the North-West Frontier province of Pakistan, the Himalayas, Afghanistan, China, Manchuria, Mongolia, Indonesia, the Philippines, Hawaii, north-east Australia and Japan. Typhus is endemic in Ethiopia; epidemics have crossed the Sahara and occurred south of it.

In South America louse-borne typhus is a problem of residents in the Andean highlands where it is endemic. In Africa over the last seven years the greatest number of cases have been reported from Burundi, Ruanda (where major epidemics occurred in the 1970s) and Ethiopia (7000–17 000 cases annually[6]). In Europe the disease is present as Brill–Zinsser disease (see p. 222) and in the eastern USA as a zoonosis in flying squirrels occasionally transmitted to man.

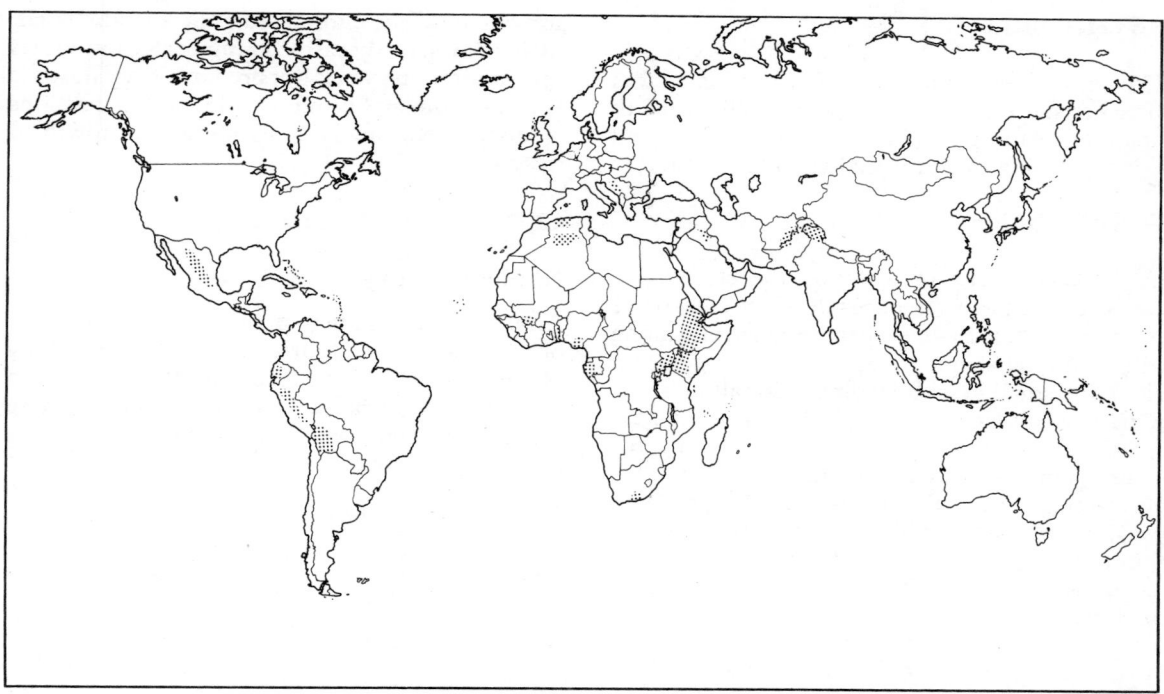

Fig. 10.2   Present-day endemic foci of louse-borne typhus (*R. prowazeki*). (Courtesy Department of Entomology, London School of Hygiene and Tropical Medicine.)

TRANSMISSION

Body louse (*Pediculus humanus*) (see Appendix III, p. 1468)

In the great majority of cases transmission is from man to man via the body louse. Only the body louse transmits typhus. The head louse (*P. capitis*) and the crab or pubic louse (*Phthirus pubis*) do not transmit the disease.

The rickettsiae which are abstracted from the blood of a case of typhus multiply in the epithelial cells of the gut which become distended and rupture, so that rickettsiae appear in large numbers in the faeces. The disease is then transmitted by the faeces through abrasions in the skin (made by scratching) or ocular conjunctiva. The louse can die of the rickettsial infection if infected during the first 10 days of illness. Rickettsiae can be transmitted by louse saliva and the lice themselves can be infected by eating the faeces of infected lice. Lice are infected for life but there is no transovarial transmission and the eggs remain free of rickettsiae. Man is the only source of infection but *R. prowazeki* has been isolated from flying squirrels in the USA[7] where it exists as a zoonosis.

Ticks

Although *R. prowazeki* has been isolated from ticks[8] there is no evidence of tick transmission in nature.

Other methods of transmission

Airborne

Airborne infection through inhalation of dried louse faeces in fomites can be important in hospitals and crowded conditions. Louse faeces kept at room temperature remain infective for 66 days.

Blood

Blood samples taken during the first 10 days may infect attendants. Blood transfusion from a donor in the incubation stage has been known to transmit the disease.

Laboratory

Laboratory infections in workers with *R. prowazeki* can occur and the organism must be treated as a dangerous pathogen in laboratories.

PATHOLOGY

The basic lesion is the result of disseminated foci of rickettsial infection of the endothelial cells of small vessels in the skin, brain, liver, heart and kidney causing disseminated vascular lesions.

Vascular lesion

In the early phase of infection the endothelial cells are killed as a direct result of the rickettsiae and their toxins. Platelet thrombi form and along with endothelial hypertrophy and proliferation block the small vessels leading to small infarcts. A perivascular response of polymorphonuclear leukocytes and monocytes is followed by macrophages, lymphocytes and plasma cells later. This perivascular infiltration is responsible for *typhus nodules* (Fig. 10.3) which can be found in the skin, myocardium, liver and other viscera, and the brain where they are commonest in the medulla and basal ganglia but may also be found in the cortex. These changes are a direct result of the rickettsiae and their toxins but later with the appearance of antibody, immune mechanisms may play a part.

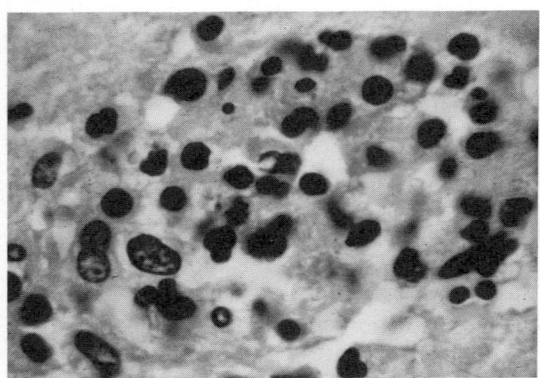

Fig. 10.3 Typhus or Wohlbach's nodule.

Other pathological changes

Perivascular lesions in the portal system of the liver, focal interstitial vascular lesions in the kidney and an interstitial type of pneumonia.

IMMUNITY

The immunity following infection is solid and long-lasting but is not sterile since the rickettsiae are not entirely eliminated, but remain latent (Brill–Zinsser disease). Humoral antibodies appear after one week but are not rickettsiostatic and the cellular immunity which also develops is more important in controlling the growth of rickettsiae.

CLINICAL FEATURES

Natural history

An untreated case may proceed rapidly to death on the twelfth to fourteenth day after a long sustained fever or may recover after the second week by crisis or rapid lysis. In milder cases there is a mild shorter fever and inapparent infections must be common.

Incubation period

This varies between five and 23 days with an average of 12 days.

Symptoms and signs

Classical typhus is rarely seen nowadays because most cases where medical attention is available rapidly respond to treatment. The following description applies to untreated typhus fever. Louse-borne typhus is characterized by a high sustained fever, severe headache and prostration.

Early phase

Vague malaise and headache may precede the onset which is abrupt with *fever* (Fig. 10.4), severe headache and prostration, pain in the back and limbs with nausea and vomiting. The fever rises rapidly in 2 days to 40°C and remains there until death or the twelfth to fourteenth day, with some scarcely perceptible morning remissions.

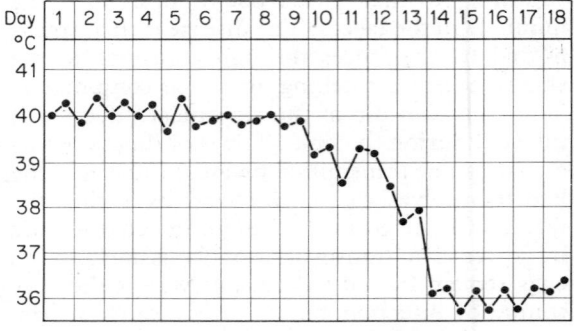

Fig. 10.4 Temperature chart of a case of typhus fever (untreated).

Other signs

The face becomes congested, the conjunctivae suffused with photophobia. The patient is stuporose with a drunken look not seen in any other infection, except perhaps plague. The patient is drowsy, often delirious, with insomnia (coma vigil). The mouth is foul and the tongue coated, with sordes on the lips. The urine contains albumin with an increase in chlorides and urea, and in severe cases haematuria may occur. The spleen is usually enlarged and palpable. An unproductive cough with few physical findings is common.

Rash

The rash which is so characteristic of typhus may appear as early as the third day but more usually on the fifth day. It starts on the abdomen and

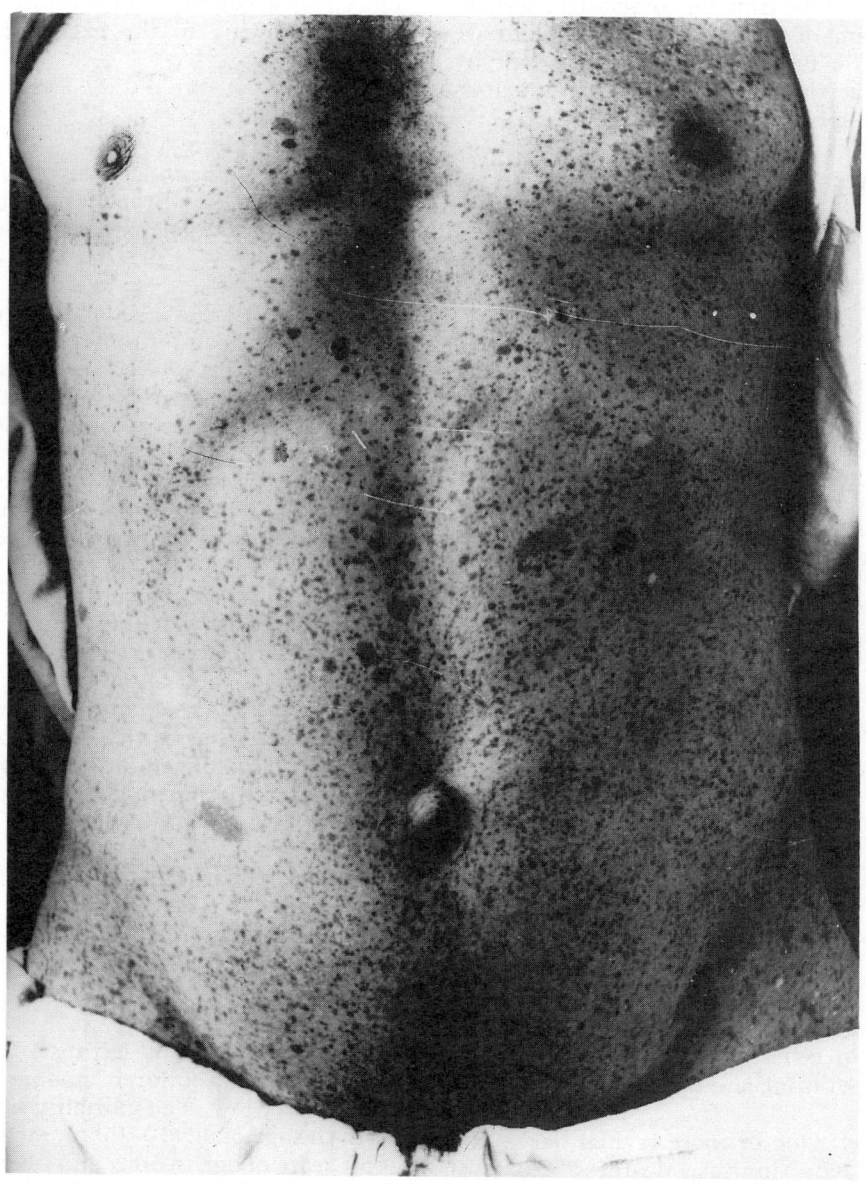

Fig. 10.5 Typhus rash in the second week showing the typical distribution. The dark-coloured areas are petechial; the lighter-coloured, discrete areas disappear on pressure.

inner aspect of the arms, spreading over the chest, back and trunk and involves the face only in severe cases. It is absent in 10% of cases. The rash (Fig. 10.5) consists of roseolar macules with fine, irregular, dusky mottling underlying the epidermis, best described as 'subcuticular mottling'. Usually it becomes petechial and may then be seen on the palms of the hands and soles of the feet. It is rarely bright red and sometimes haemorrhagic. In dark-skinned people the typhus rash may be difficult to discern and thorough cleansing of the skin and a good light are necessary. The rash may be made evident by partial compression with a tourniquet, such as the band of a sphygmomanometer.

Other features

General

There is a profound mental lethargy and the patient sinks into the 'typhus' state. The expression becomes dull and vacant and the face has an earthy hue which has been called 'facies typhosa'. At this stage the skin emits an odour which has been compared to that of mice (not everyone is capable of smelling this but some experienced physicians have been known to diagnose typhus by the smell before seeing the patient). A slow, muttering delirium supervenes during the second week.

Pulmonary. Signs of bronchitis appear with the rash but radiology reveals no pneumonitis.

Cardiac. At first the pulse : temperature ratio is low but increases at the end of the first week. An increasingly rapid pulse indicates a poor prognosis. The blood pressure is low.

Jaundice. Jaundice may be present in some cases but is never marked but raised transaminases may appear early.

Neurological

Cortical irritation. Meningism is not uncommon. The cerebrospinal fluid is under pressure with an increase in cells. Muscular twitchings and incontinence of urine and faeces are common.

Cranial nerves. One or more cranial nerves are usually affected, tinnitus, deafness (80% of cases), dysphagia and dysphonia being the main effects.

Laboratory findings

Oliguria, proteinuria and nitrogen retention are common. The white cell count which is reduced in the early stages rises later, mostly in large monocytes. Eosinophils are rare. The haemoglobin is raised from haemoconcentration.

Course

The classical course of the disease is seldom seen nowadays owing to the excellent response to treatment.

Complications

Secondary infections. These are common in untreated cases. Bronchopneumonia, otitis media, suppurative parotitis and noma are common.

Thromboses. Thrombosis of the femoral vein is not uncommon, and thrombosis of the large and small arteries may lead to gangrene of the extremities, toes, scrotum and hemiplegia. Gangrene of the lung is a complication of typhus bronchopneumonia.

Neurological. Hemiplegia or monoplegia from typhus nodules in the brain has been reported.

Relapsing fever. Relapsing fever is frequently seen in association with typhus fever and this superadded infection is serious.

Convalescence. Marked improvement takes place after the fever has settled but recovery is slow and may be prolonged for two to three months.
　Thrombocytopenia may occur in convalescence with purpura.

Alopecia. Loss of hair on the scalp and legs is common.

PROGNOSIS

Mild cases of typhus lasting 10 days are frequently seen in children amongst whom mortality is very low. The mortality rate is moderate up to the age of 40 (10–15%), rapidly increasing at 50 years of age to 50% and over the age of 50 few survive if untreated. Some relapses have been recorded. Deep coma, severe hypotension and tachycardia with a falling body temperature are signs of a poor prognosis.

DIFFERENTIAL DIAGNOSIS

Typhoid fever. Differentiation is based upon the onset and course of the fever and in the time of appearance and characteristics of the rash. Typhus has a rapid onset, the fever rapidly reaches a high sustained level and the rash appears earlier (fifth day).

Measles. Malignant measles in the tropics may closely resemble typhus. Koplik's spots are important and the upper respiratory tract is heavily involved.

Viral haemorrhagic fever. Dengue and other forms of VHF may closely resemble typhus. In dengue the patient is not so ill, joint pains are prominent and the suffusion of the face is not so marked.

Other conditions. Purpura, cerebrospinal meningitis and relapsing fever have all to be considered.
Other forms of typhus must be distinguished serologically and by the presence in some of an eschar.

DIAGNOSIS

Isolation of rickettsiae

Rickettsiae may be isolated from blood and other tissues in the first 5 days of fever. Ground blood clot and tissues are inoculated intraperitoneally in male guinea-pigs which are then observed for signs of fever from 6 to 10 days later. The Neil–Mooser reaction (see p. 215) is slightly positive (in contrast to murine typhus). Rickettsiae may also be isolated by inoculation of the yolk sacs of embryonated eggs. Rickettsiae isolated may be distinguished by specific rickettsial agglutination tests (see p. 216).

Serology

The *Weil–Felix reaction* (Table 10.2) is highly diagnostic. Titres against the OX19 strain rise rapidly towards 1/500 towards the end of the fever reaching a maximum in the third and fourth weeks then declining, remaining at 1/50 to 1/100

for weeks or even months. Moderately severe cases show high titres, but in the severest cases titres are low.

Immunofluorescence

The IFAT is the test of choice and is used to distinguish primary epidemic typhus from the recrudescent Brill–Zinsser disease. In typhus the IgM response is early and there is no IgG; in Brill–Zinsser disease there is an IgG response from the start.[9] Antibodies persist for many years. Differentiation between louse-borne and murine typhus can be made with specific a CF test or absorption type IFAT.

Specific rickettsial agglutination tests and skin biopsy

In countries where typhus is endemic the titre of normal persons may be above 1 in 100 and after antityphus inoculation agglutinins often appear in low titre. Specific rickettsial agglutinins appear at the same time and follow the same course. Complement-fixing antibodies appear a little later. Skin biopsy for the identification of the rash has proved particularly useful. Sections show lesions resembling periarteritis nodosa. The petechiae in the skin are due to thrombosis of the smaller vessels.

Modified typhus

In people who contract typhus after having received typhus vaccine the disease is greatly modified with headache, a few days' fever and transient rash. There is a negligible mortality.

TREATMENT

On admission the patient should be bathed with soap and water or a 1% solution of lysol. His clothes should be promptly disinfested by heat. The patient and hospital garments should be carefully dusted with 10% DDT delousing powder on admission and once a week until discharge. After these measures no quarantine is required. Nursing is of great importance. Stuporose patients and those in coma should be moved from side to side to prevent bedsores. If the temperature rises above 40°C cold sponging is indicated. Fluids should be administered in adequate quantities, at least 1500 ml per day.

Barbiturates must be avoided and delirium or restlessness treated with diazepam, paraldehyde or chloral hydrate. In severely ill and toxic patients steroid therapy should be given concurrently with antibiotics, prednisone 40 mg at once followed by 20 mg at intervals of 6 hours for 12 hours.

Fluid and electrolyte balances must be carefully maintained.

Antibiotics

Louse-borne typhus is very susceptible to tetracycline and chloramphenicol. No other antibiotics are effective. There is no evidence yet of any resistance.

Tetracycline

Doxycycline (Vibramycin). The long-acting doxycycline is the treatment of choice. A single 200 mg dose in adults and 100 mg in children is effective without any relapses.[10]

Tetracycline hydrochloride (Achromycin). This is given orally 25–50 mg/kg body weight daily in four, three or two divided doses. Care should be taken in newborn infants but the short course of tetracycline necessary is not a serious problem with young children or pregnant women. Intravenous tetracycline is given 0.5 g every 6–12 hours with a maximum of 2.0 g daily.

Chloramphenicol. Chloramphenicol is given orally, 50 mg/kg for children and 75 mg/kg for children daily in four, three or two divided doses.

Results

The fever settles within 48 hours and the patient rapidly recovers.

Relapse

Since the antibiotics are rickettsiostatic and not rickettsicidal relapses may occur, but provided that antibiotics are continued until 48 hours after the fever has settled relapses are rare and respond to the same treatment as before.

BRILL-ZINNSER DISEASE

A mild form of typhus was originally described in New York by Brill in 1898 among the Jewish population. The infection was introduced by immigrants from south-east Europe who were all born abroad. Brill's disease is a late recrudescence of long dormant infection occurring sometimes as late as 30 years after leaving an endemic area in persons free from lice, and *Rickettsia* infected glands have been excised from two asymptomatic patients who had emigrated from Poland 20 years previously. Brill's disease has initiated epidemics and constitutes the main reservoir of infection in interepidemic periods in eastern Europe.[11] The disease may be differentiated from epidemic typhus by the presence of IgG antibodies at the start of the infection.

EPIDEMIOLOGY

Man is the only reservoir of infection but *R. prowazeki* has been isolated from flying squirrels (*Glaucomys volans*) in the USA[7] and cases of epidemic typhus (ten a year) have occurred whose origin can only be from these animals.[12] Antibodies have been found in the blood of people living in association with flying squirrels.

Epidemics can occur whenever a population becomes louse infected, the source of infection being Brill–Zinnser disease or a case of typhus from a neighbouring area. Louse-borne typhus is a disease of poverty and dirt and its presence denotes low economic standards. In Europe and North Africa it was frequent in the winter and spring months when heavy clothing afforded an excellent opportunity for lice breeding but, during the last 40 years, the disease has disappeared from these areas. In highland areas in the tropics epidemics appear during the wet winter months of the year.

PREVENTION AND CONTROL (see also Appendix III, p. 1470)

The basis for the control of epidemic typhus is louse control and immunization. In dealing with epidemics where case reporting has been good and the number of cases small, residual insecticides should be applied to all contacts. Where the infection is known to be widespread the application of residual insecticides to all persons in the community is indicated. Ten per cent DDT powder for delousing can be applied by a powder duster. The DDT powder is sprayed down the opening of the neck and up the trousers in men and skirts in women. The lethal effect of DDT on lice lasts for more than two weeks and if it is impregnated as an emulsion on clothes for more than four weeks. Where resistance to DDT has been developed by the lice then other residual insecticides must be employed such as 1% malathion dust. A single dose of doxycycline to each member of the affected population will stop an epidemic immediately.[13]

IMMUNIZATION

Killed vaccine probably reduces the incidence of the disease in exposed persons and reduces the mortality to practically zero. A formalin-killed tissue culture vaccine made from *R. prowazeki* should be administered subcutaneously in two doses each of 1 ml separated by an interval of 10–14 days, followed by a booster dose of 1 ml at the beginning and in the middle of the typhus season. The use of egg yolk vaccine should be avoided in persons sensitive to egg protein. Living vaccine of the E strain will produce immunity for up to five years but febrile reactions are common.

Laboratory personnel working with epidemic typhus rickettsiae should be immunized regularly with killed vaccine, as should doctors, nurses and health personnel working with typhus patients.

Murine typhus (flea typhus)

GEOGRAPHICAL DISTRIBUTION

Murine typhus (endemic typhus, shop typhus) is of worldwide distribution (Fig. 10.6). It is especially endemic in certain areas such as North America, Mexico, India, Pakistan, Queensland and Malaya (shop or urban typhus) and infected rats have been found in the Mediterranean area.

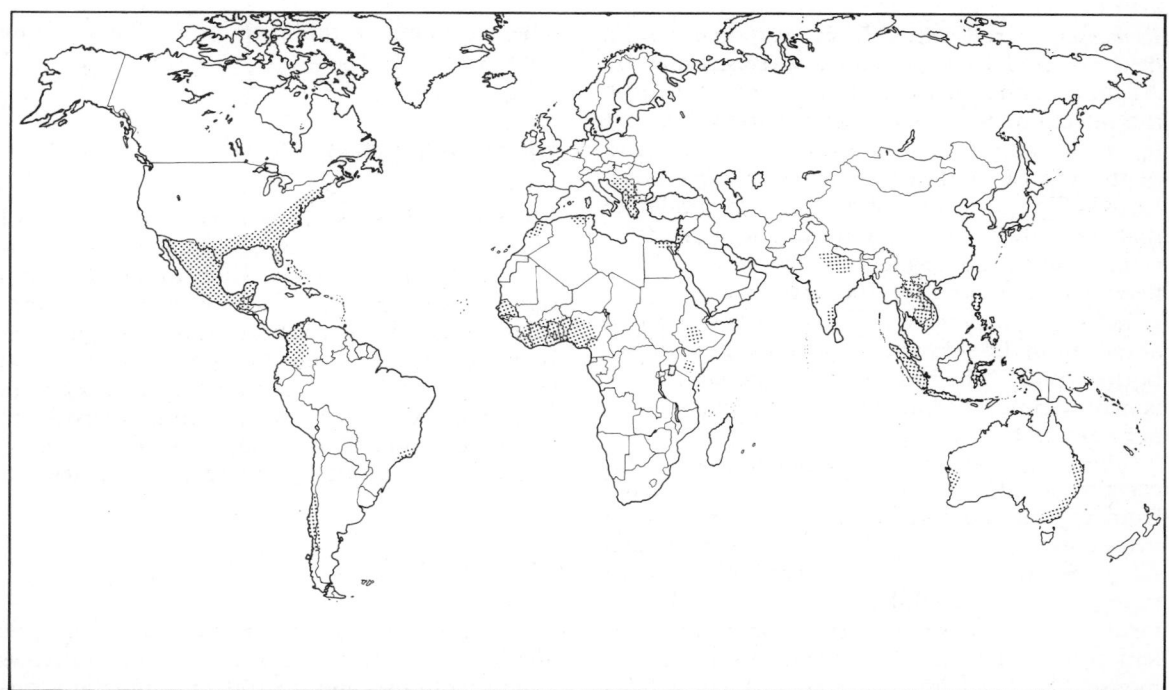

Fig. 10.6 Geographical distribution of flea-borne (murine) typhus (*R. mooseri*). (Courtesy Department of Entomology, London School of Hygiene and Tropical Medicine.)

AETIOLOGY

R. mooseri, which is closely related to *R. prowazeki*, is an infection of rodents and is a more primitive disease than *R. prowazeki*, from which it may be differentiated by a more strongly positive Neill–Mooser reaction and by specific rickettsial agglutination tests.

R. mooseri seems to have undergone two mutations, changing both its vertebrate and invertebrate host, to evolve into *R. prowazeki*. In Mexico a type of typhus exists which may be regarded as intermediate between the murine and louse-borne types. The more recent origin of epidemic typhus is shown by the fact that *R. mooseri* is harmless to the flea, whereas *R. prowazeki* causes death of the louse, to which it is less well adapted. It is probable that endemic (murine) typhus may be converted into epidemic (louse-borne) typhus which may be maintained in interepidemic periods by rats in this manner.

TRANSMISSION (Appendix III, p. 1482)

R. mooseri is transmitted from rat to man by the flea *Xenopsylla cheopis* and also sometimes by *X. astia*, neither of which insects are harmed by the infection. *R. mooseri* is transmitted from rat to rat by the rat louse (*Polyplax spinulosa*) and by the tropical rat mite (*Bdellonyssus (Liponyssus) bacoti*). The cycle in these insects is similar to that described in the louse. The rickettsiae remain alive and virulent in the faeces of the flea for 40 days and for 100 days in vacuo. The rickettsiae enter man from faecal infection of abrasions in the skin after scratching, as in louse-borne typhus. The brown rat (*Rattus norvegicus*) is mainly concerned in temperate climates and is not harmed by the infection.

There is evidence in Shanghai that under certain conditions rickettsiae can be converted from the rat–louse–rat cycle via the rat flea to man–louse–man cycle.[14] The armadillo and field rats in South America are susceptible to murine typhus and intracellular strains of rickettsiae virulent for mice sometimes become non-virulent and extracellular after passage through the mouse flea (*Leptopsylla segnis*) which is susceptible to *R. mooseri* and which although it does not bite man may be responsible for airborne infection from the heavy accumulation of infected faeces on the fur of the rat.[15]

Trombiculid mites, *Ascoschoengastia indica*, have been found naturally infected with murine typhus[16] in Malaysia. The mites were taken from house rats and sewer rats (*Rattus norvegicus*).

CLINICAL FEATURES

The symptoms and signs closely resemble those of louse-born typhus but are much milder in every respect. The mortality rate in untreated cases is very low, about 1.5%.

DIAGNOSIS

Murine typhus cannot be differentiated from louse-borne typhus by the IFAT, but by specific rickettsial agglutination tests and by its non-epidemic nature.

TREATMENT

The treatment is the same as for louse-borne typhus.

EPIDEMIOLOGY

Murine typhus is a zoonosis and the most important feature in its occurrence is the residence of human beings, such as dockers and brewery workers, in areas where rats abound, such as grain stores and breweries. Cases occur in small numbers fom time to time and the seasonal incidence remains constant, the majority of cases occurring in summer and autumn. Negroes are less susceptible than Caucasians and the incidence is twice as high in males as in females.

CONTROL

The flea population should be reduced by the application of 10% DDT to rat runs, burrows and harbourages and the rodent population controlled by warfarin and rat-proofing of grain stores (see Chapter 27).

2 SPOTTED FEVER GROUP (TICK TYPHUS)

The spotted fever group of rickettsial fevers are zoonoses transmitted by ixodid (hard) ticks which are the true reservoirs of infection. Larval ticks are infected from feeding on small mammals, such as rodents with rickettsaemia, which on developing into adults, transmit the infection to their maintenance hosts—dogs, deer, bear and wild cats or other mammals according to the geographical area. The rickettsiae which are ingested by the larval ticks invade every cell in the body, especially the ovary and salivary glands. They remain infected for life and infection is transmitted hereditarily through the egg and by bite via the salivary gland. Man who is infected by adult ticks is a dead-end infection, taking no part in transmission of the disease. Tick typhus has a worldwide distribution and occurs in the New World (American tick typhus) and Old World (fièvre boutonneuse, African tick typhus, Indian and south Asian tick typhus, Siberian and north Queensland tick typhus). (For morphology and life cycle of *Ixodid* ticks see Appendix III, Figs. III.8, p. 1386, III.13, p. 1390, and III.12B, p. 1388.)

American tick typhus

American tick typhus is caused by *Rickettsia rickettsi* and occurs in North America (Rocky Mountain spotted fever) and in Central and South America.

ROCKY MOUNTAIN SPOTTED FEVER (RMSF)

Geographical distribution (Fig. 10.7)

Geographically there are two main groups: western RMSF and eastern RMSF.

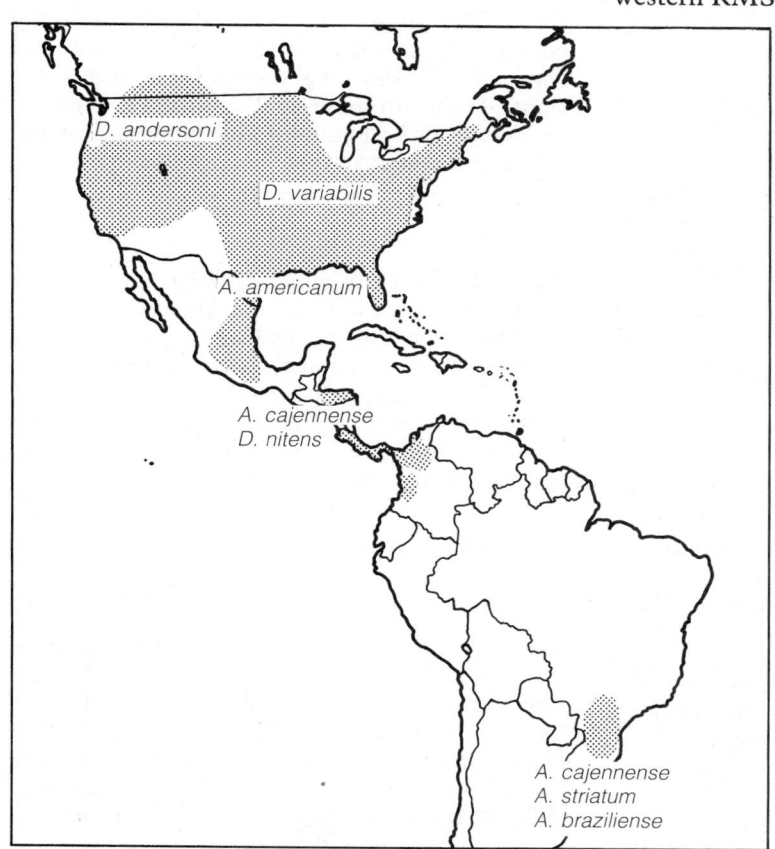

Fig. 10.7 Geographical distribution of Rocky Mountain spotted fever (*R. rickettsi*). (Courtesy Department of Entomology, London School of Hygiene and Tropical Medicine.)

Western Rocky Mountain spotted fever

Western RMSF is found in the western states of the USA, Idaho, Oregon, Washington, Montana (Bitter Root Valley), Wyoming, Utah, Colorado, Oklahoma, Texas and New Mexico.

Eastern Rocky Mountain spotted fever

Eastern RMSF has spread widely in recent years from eastern British Columbia, Alberta and Saskatchewan eastwards to involve nearly the whole of the eastern USA.

Aetiology

RMSF is caused by *Rickettsia rickettsi*, a member of the spotted fever group which shares minor antigens with the typhus group and contains both mild and virulent strains but is responsible for all the spotted fevers in the New World.

Transmission (see also Appendix III, p. 1392)

Western RMSF

The main tick responsible for transmission is the wood tick *Dermacentor andersoni* (Rocky Mountain wood tick), the natural maintenance hosts of which are the Rocky Mountain goat, sheep, black bear, badger and lynx. The larval ticks feed upon ground squirrels and woodchuck from which they become infected. After feeding on infected blood there is a period of 12 days during which the rickettsiae multiply and all stages of the tick larva, nymph and adult of both sexes are efficient intermediary hosts. In endemic areas the proportion of infected ticks is one in 296.

Eastern RMSF

The main transmitter is the dog tick, *Dermacentor variabilis* (American dog tick), the maintenance hosts of which are the dog which carries the adult ticks into suburban gardens where they infect man. Other maintenance hosts from which rickettsiae have been isolated or in which antibodies have been found, include cottontail rabbits, grey and red foxes, opossums, raccoons and deer. The larval stages are infected from the meadow mouse, *Microtus pennsylvanicus*.

South, central and eastern USA

Amblyomma americanum (lone star tick) is the vector and the reservoir of infection is the pocket gopher (*Geomys brevipes dutcheri*).

Rhipicephalus sanguineus (the brown dog tick) may also transmit infection in Texas and northern Mexico.

Pathology

In contrast to most other forms of tick typhus there is no primary eschar. *R. rickettsi*, in contrast to other rickettsiae, invades the nuclei of the endothelial cells of the blood vessels, where they may be found in considerable masses, as well as the cell cytoplasm and other tissues. The endothelial cells are destroyed and the rickettsiae escape into the bloodstream and establish other foci. This vascular damage results in mural thrombi (Fraenkel's nodules), perivascular infiltration and gangrene. There is usually a well-marked skin rash, bronchopneumonic consolidation and subserous petechial haemorrhages. Similar lesions including microinfarcts are found in the brain. The myocardium shows cloudy swelling and the spleen is enlarged and firm. The lymphatic glands are generally enlarged. Focal necrosis of the hepatic cells and congestion of the renal cortex are found. Constant lesions in man and animals are haemorrhages in the genitalia and gangrene of the prepuce and scrotum.

Immunity

Immunity develops which is short-lived and not sterile. Relapses and second attacks occur and the protection afforded by Cox type tick vaccines is only partial and short-lived. The mechanism is not clear; antibodies develop which are not protective and cellular immunity is probably involved. Immune complexes play a part in the severe vascular lesions found in RMSF.

Clinical features

Natural history

Man is very susceptible to RMSF and inapparent infections do not apparently occur. However, the infection can be very variable, being so mild that the patient remains ambulant, or so severe that death occurs within 3–6 days after onset. The mortality rate of untreated RMSF varies from 90% in the Bitter Root Valley of Montana to under 20% in the eastern USA.

Incubation period

The incubation period is 3–7 days, the shorter the period the more severe the disease.

Symptoms and signs

There may be a history of tick bite but there is no eschar. Prodromal symptoms of anorexia, irritability and feverishness are rare. The *onset* is sudden with severe headache, chills, fever, severe muscular pains in the back and legs and arthralgia. With these are prostration, nausea and vomiting.

FEVER

By the second day the fever rises to 39.4–40°C and by the fifth to 40.6–41.7°C, a level at which hyperthermia develops and is a serious sign. A typhus-like condition ensues with intense headache, conjunctival injection, photophobia and meningeal irritation.

RASH (Fig. 10.8)

The rash appears characteristically around the fourth but can be delayed up to the seventh day. It appears as small rose coloured macules resembling measles but in 2–3 days becomes darker red or purplish and around the fourth day after the onset petechial, becoming confluent and haemorrhagic, especially on the more dependent

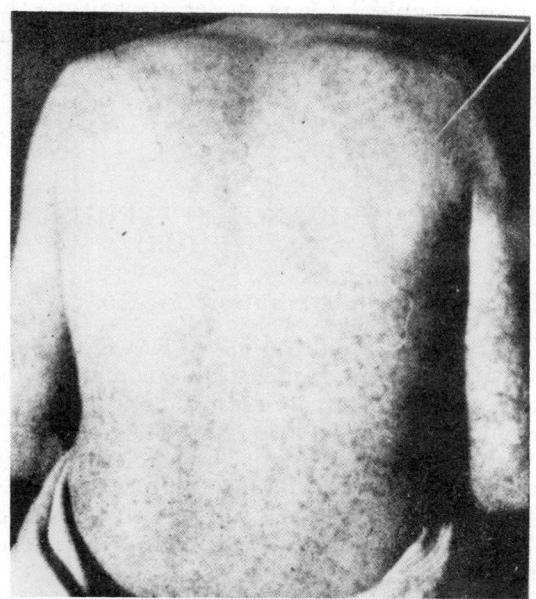

Fig. 10.8 The rash of Rocky Mountain spotted fever.

parts of the body. The rash starts peripherally round the wrists and ankles spreading to involve the palms and soles and the rest of the body, even the mucous membranes. During the third week as the fever settles desquamation sets in and the eruption fades often leaving a few pigmented spots.

CARDIOVASCULAR SIGNS

The pulse : temperature ratio at first normal, later increases. Hypotension develops and the increased vascular permeability results in decreased intravascular fluid, hypovolaemia and general and pulmonary oedema. The electrocardiogram shows minor S–T changes. Gangrene of the toes, fingers, ears and genitalia may occur from circulatory insufficiency. Thrombosis of large vessels causes gangrene of a limb or hemiplegia. Haemorrhages from the nose, genitourinary tract and kidney may occur. Disturbed clotting mechanisms have been found[17] and platelet counts are low. Disseminated intravascular coagulation may occur.

NEUROLOGICAL SIGNS

Involvement of the central nervous system is shown by insomnia, restlessness, stupor and coma. Convulsions, tremors and other movements may occur. The cranial nerves may be involved with transient deafness common. Electroencephalographic changes can persist for many months.

OTHER ORGANS

Liver. The liver is usually enlarged and the spleen enlarged, firm and tender. During the second week jaundice may occur. The serum enzymes are increased and the prothrombin time prolonged.

Kidney. The urine is scanty and contains albumin and casts. Oliguria and nitrogen retention are common in severe cases and tubular necrosis may supervene with prolonged hypotension.

The white cell count is increased with a lymphocytosis in the early stages.

Course

In fatal cases death occurs 9–18 days after onset. With recovery convalescence is prolonged. Relapses may occur with insufficient treatment.

Complications

Secondary bacterial infection, broncho-pneumonia, parotitis and otitis media are rare.

Differential diagnosis

The most important differential diagnosis is from measles and meningococcaemia. Measles has marked respiratory symptoms and signs. A skin biopsy can be stained for meningococci. The IFAT using specific rickettsial antibody can give a quick diagnosis. Cerebral malaria can be excluded by blood examination. Other typhus fevers can be differentiated by specific rickettsial agglutination tests. Isolation of rickettsiae (see p. 214) takes time and can only be done from the blood in the very early stages.

Serology

Antibodies may be demonstrated during the second week. The Weil–Felix is of the indeterminate type (Table 10.2) showing agglutination against OX19 and OX2 strains. Louse-borne and other typhus fevers may be distinguished by specific rickettsial agglutination or CF tests.

Treatment

No quarantine measures are necessary. Owing to the potential severity of the disease immediate antibiotic therapy should be instituted on suspicion.

Antibiotic therapy

Tetracycline hydrochloride 2 g daily in two or four divided doses is given for 6 days, doxycycline 200 mg daily for 6 days. Response is rapid in a suspected case with a fall in the temperature within 48–72 hours.

Supportive therapy may be necessary for the serious cardiovascular and blood clotting abnormalities. Serious toxic cases can be helped greatly by a short course of steroids.

Epidemiology

Western RMSF. This occurs in valleys near the foothills in sharply defined zones. The adult ticks rest on tall grass lining the game paths and tracks and attach themselves to large mammals passing (including man). Ramblers, hunters and visitors to national parks are at risk. Attacks of RMSF tend to occur during the spring when the ticks are most numerous.

Eastern RMSF. In the eastern USA, RMSF is a 'backyard' disease occurring in suburban areas. Infected adult ticks are brought into the house and garden on domestic dogs.

Control

Control measures are based upon tick control and prevention of tick bites. Tick control may be obtained in some areas by spraying the woodsides and pathsides with DDT once or twice a month during the tick season. Tick bites may be prevented by avoiding notorious areas in spring and summer and wearing protective clothing. The shirt must be tucked inside the trousers and socks or high boots should be worn outside over trousers. An important precaution is to remove the clothes and search for ticks twice daily since ticks will only transmit the infection after some hours to a day in situ. Ticks should be removed with forceps gently so that they are not crushed and the mouthparts maintained intact. Contact between the ticks and skin, especially the fingers, must be avoided. Dogs should be regularly deticked. The haemolymph of attached ticks can be examined for rickettsiae and if positive the person should be kept under surveillance for fever for 14 days. If fever develops then a full antibiotic course must be given. *Vaccines* against RMSF have not proved useful.

SOUTH AMERICAN TICK TYPHUS (SÃO PAULO TICK TYPHUS)

Geographical distribution (Fig. 10.7)

In Central and South America RMSF is found in Mexico (fiebre manchada), Colombia (fiebre petequial), Brazil (fiebre macuculosa, São Paulo typhus).

In *Colombia* RMSF is found on the Tobia river, a tributary of the Rio Negro, in a narrow valley of the Magdalena basin at an altitude of 700–1400 m. A second endemic zone exists north and west of the Villeta river at 500–1500 m.

In *Brazil* RMSF is common in Minas Gerais state.

Aetiology

The same prototype *R. rickettsi* is the cause.

Transmission

In Colombia the tick vectors are *Amblyomma cajennense* and *Dermacentor nitens*. In Brazil the tick vectors are species of *Amblyomma, A. cajennense, A. striatum* and *A. braziliense*. The

mammalian reservoirs are the opossum, domestic and wild dog, wild rabbits and the agouti.

Clinical features

These are in general similar to RMSF of North America, except that there is a transition from north to south from the classical type without an eschar to Brazil where an eschar is present and the disease resembles fièvre boutonneuse of the Old World.

Old World tick typhus

The commonest forms of Old World tick typhus are fièvre boutonneuse and African tick typhus with local epidemiological variations. The other forms are of local importance, Indian and south Asian tick typhus. Siberian tick typhus and Queensland tick typhus.

FIÈVRE BOUTONNEUSE

Geographical distribution (Fig. 10.9)

Fièvre boutonneuse occurs throughout the Mediterranean littoral and many other districts

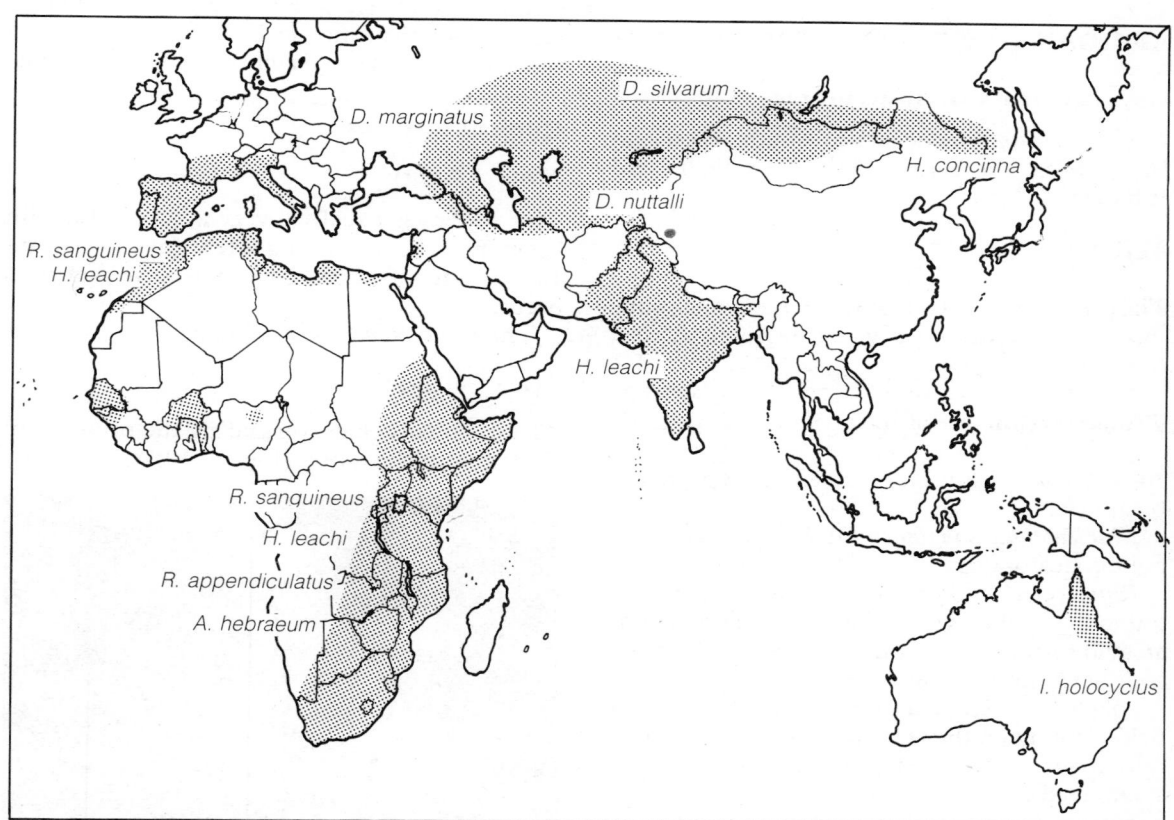

Fig. 10.9 Geographical distribution of Old World tickborne typhus fevers. (Courtesy Department of Entomology, London School of Hygiene and Tropical Medicine.)

in southern France, Italy, Portugal, Spain, Greece, Roumania and the Crimea.

Aetiology

The causative rickettsia is *R. conori*. There may be local variations and one *R. israeli* has been described from Israel.

Transmission

The vector is the dog tick, *Rhipicephalus sanguineus*, which is maintained on the dog which is susceptible and constitutes a reservoir host since its blood can be infective to man and monkeys. A rodent reservoir has not been excluded and it was noted that fièvre boutonneuse almost completely disappeared from southern France when the rabbit was exterminated by myxomatosis but returned when the rabbit returned. *R. conori* could be connected with the rabbit or rabbit flea.[18]

AFRICAN TICK TYPHUS (TICK FEVER)

Geographical distribution (Fig. 10.9)

African tick typhus occurs in South, West and East Africa, the Sudan, Eritrea, Somalia and Ethiopia.

Aetiology

The causative rickettsia is *R. conori* of which subspecific status has been given in South Africa, *R. conori* var. *pijperi*.

Transmission (see also Appendix III, p. 1392)

In Africa the tick vectors are either dog ticks or bush ticks.

Rhipicephalus sanguineus (dog tick) is a cosmopolitan tick of dogs.

Rhipicephalus appendiculatus (a bush tick) is found in shrubby wooded grassland and veld, is an avid man biter and the main vector of typhus contracted in the bush.

Amblyomma hebraeum (the South African bont tick) is found on the veld. *R. conori* can be transmitted for several generations. The immature stages feed avidly on man.

Haemaphysalis leachi (a dog tick) is a widely distributed dog tick which transmits urban cases of tick typhus. Transmission can occur from contamination of the skin and eyes from infected ticks crushed while deticking dogs, as well as by bite.

Reservoirs of infection are not known but immature ticks feed on birds and small mammals while adults feed on large wild and domestic animals. Dog ticks maintain the infection in dogs.

Rickettsiae have been isolated from, and antibodies found in, rodents in Kenya.[19]

AFRICAN TICK TYPHUS AND FIÈVRE BOUTONNEUSE

Pathology

Fatal cases are rare and limited to the old and very young. The findings are similar to those of RMSF except for the presence of a primary eschar.

Immunity

All ages and both sexes are susceptible and second attacks can occur. There is an apparent racial immunity since in East Africa almost no cases have ever been diagnosed in rural Africans.

Clinical features

Natural history

Tick typhus is usually a very mild disease with spontaneous cure, lasting a few days to a week. Inapparent infections have not been shown to occur.

The *incubation period* is 5–7 days.

Symptoms and signs

Tick typhus is characterized by the presence of an eschar (tache noire) (Fig. 10.10).

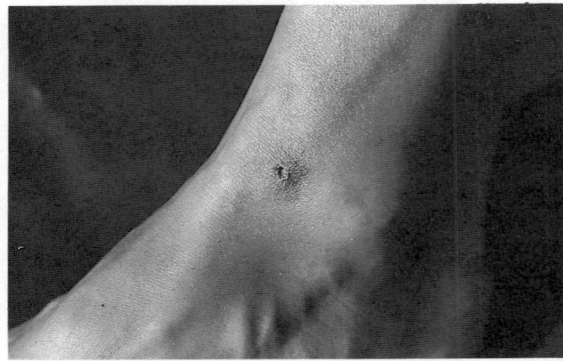

Fig. 10.10   The primary eschar in African tick typhus.

A *primary eschar* precedes the onset and is present at the onset of fever. The eschar (the portal of entry of infection), which is painless, consists of a small ulcer 2–5 mm in diameter with a black necrotic centre and a surrounding pink areola. The regional lymph glands are enlarged. The eschar is usually situated at the site of the tick bite which is on the lower part of the leg, the back or axilla. When it is situated on the head it may be very difficult to find because of the hair, but can be suspected by the regional adenitis in the occipital region. Rarely there may be no eschar.

Fever. The onset is sudden with headache and sometimes neck stiffness.

Rash. A mild maculopapular rash appears on the fifth day but may be very faint. It involves the whole body including the soles of the feet and palms of the hands. In severe cases it becomes haemorrhagic. In South Africa it is frequently absent.

Other system involvement is rare. The electrocardiogram may show inverted T waves and there may be breathlessness.

Unusual forms. There may be no eschar or rash and this can give difficulty in diagnosis.

Course

The course is usually mild. Fever abates in the second week. In some cases the infection can take a severe course with high fever, delirium, stupor and coma with central nervous system involvement and marked disorder of liver and kidney function. These cases occur in infection transmitted by dog ticks rather than bush ticks.[20]

Complications

Gangrene of the scrotum, fingers and toes is rare.

Differential diagnosis

The most important differential diagnosis is from measles, cerebrospinal fever and typhoid. In measles there are marked respiratory symptoms, in cerebrospinal meningitis the cerebrospinal fluid will be abnormal and in typhoid the onset is much slower, there is no eschar, and the patient is much more ill. The eschar must be differentiated from an infective lesion with regional adenitis developing on a tick bite.

Diagnosis

Rickettsiae are seldom isolated.

Serology

The disease gives an indeterminate reaction and in most cases the Weil–Felix shows a higher titre to the OXK strain than the OX19. Specific rickettsial antibodies can be demonstrated against the homologous strain.

Treatment

Many cases resolve without treatment. Tetracycline used as for RMSF is very successful.

Epidemiology

There are two main epidemiological types: 'urban' and 'bush'.

Urban type

In the Mediterranean only the urban type is found. It is also found in sub-Saharan Africa. The disease is a 'backyard infection' contracted from dog ticks (*Rhipicephalus sanguineus, H. leachi*) brought into the house by dogs from the surrounding area.

Bush type

In sub-Saharan Africa as well as the urban type the disease is contracted as a bush infection from bush ticks (*Rhipicephalus appendiculatus, A. hebraeum*) in areas removed from human habitation in game parks, hunting areas where game wardens, hunters and tourists are infected, and it is a 'safari disease'.

Control

Ticks may be avoided by sleeping raised above the ground in the bush, avoiding lying on grass and avoiding contact with dogs in the home. Regular deticking of dogs is essential. In prevention of the bush form daily deticking of the person while travelling in endemic areas is highly successful since the tick takes several hours to transmit the infection. Ticks should be sought for at the waist line when a belt is worn, in the groins and round the genitals. It is important to remove the tick without crushing it since the infection can be transmitted by contamination. Gentle traction or the previous application of 0.6% pyrethrin in methyl benzoate or of camphorated phenol to the skin makes detachment easier.

INDIAN AND SOUTHERN ASIAN TICK TYPHUS

A mild sporadic form of typhus has been found in the Kumaon Hills in the North-West Frontier of Pakistan and other cases have been reported from Lucknow and the Simla Hills. Hoogstraal[21] states that tick typhus in Asia includes boutonneuse fever, Siberian tick typhus and *R. conori. R. siberica* and a number of new strains whose infectivity for man is not known have been isolated from West Pakistan.[22] Antibody studies in Nepal have shown the absence of epidemic and murine typhus but the presence of both mite and tick typhus.[23]

SIBERIAN TICK TYPHUS

A tick-borne rickettsial disease (*R. r. siberica*) has been reported from east and central Siberia. It is a mild form with a primary eschar, headache and rash.

It is transmitted in western Russia and central Europe by *Dermacentor marginatus*, western Siberia by *D. silvarum*, the Far East by *Haemaphysalis concinna* and central and eastern Siberia, central Asia and Tibet by *D. nuttalli*, the maintenance host of which is the long-tailed suslik which when present in the environment denotes the presence of tick typhus.[24] Rickettsial complement-fixing antibodies have been found in farm animals.[25]

NORTH QUEENSLAND TICK TYPHUS

A mild form of rickettsial disease has been described in north and to a lesser extent in south Queensland. It causes a syndrome resembling boutonneuse fever. Although it is related to this group it can be differentiated by specific rickettsial serological tests; the *Rickettsia* has been named *R. australis*. The vector is *Ixodes holocyclus* and rickettsial complement-fixing antibodies have been found in bandicoots, kangaroo rats and bush-tailed opossums. There is an eschar with regional adenopathy, a rash and a typhus-like course.

Rickettsialpox (vesicular rickettsiosis)

GEOGRAPHICAL DISTRIBUTION (Fig. 10.11)

Rickettsialpox has been described from eastern USA, in New York[26,27] where it was formerly much more common, and other cities, from Francophone Central Africa[28] as '*rickettsiose vesiculeuse*' and as vesicular rickettsiosis from the USSR and South Africa.

AETIOLOGY

Rickettsia akari belongs to the spotted fever group and possesses common antigens with *R. rickettsi* but is distinct from other Old World tick-borne rickettsiae being most closely related to *R. australis. R. akari* can infect mice with death on the ninth to thirteenth day and guineapigs in which it produces a scrotal reaction. It grows readily in the yolk sac of chick embryos.

TRANSMISSION

R. akari is a natural infection of both house mice and field mice and is transmitted by the mouse mite *Allodermanyssus sanguineus*.[27] *Bdellonyssus bacoti*, another murine ectoparasite, can transmit in the laboratory. The infection is transmitted to man by contact with mice and their ectoparasites. The mouse mite transmits the infection either by bite or faecal contamination.

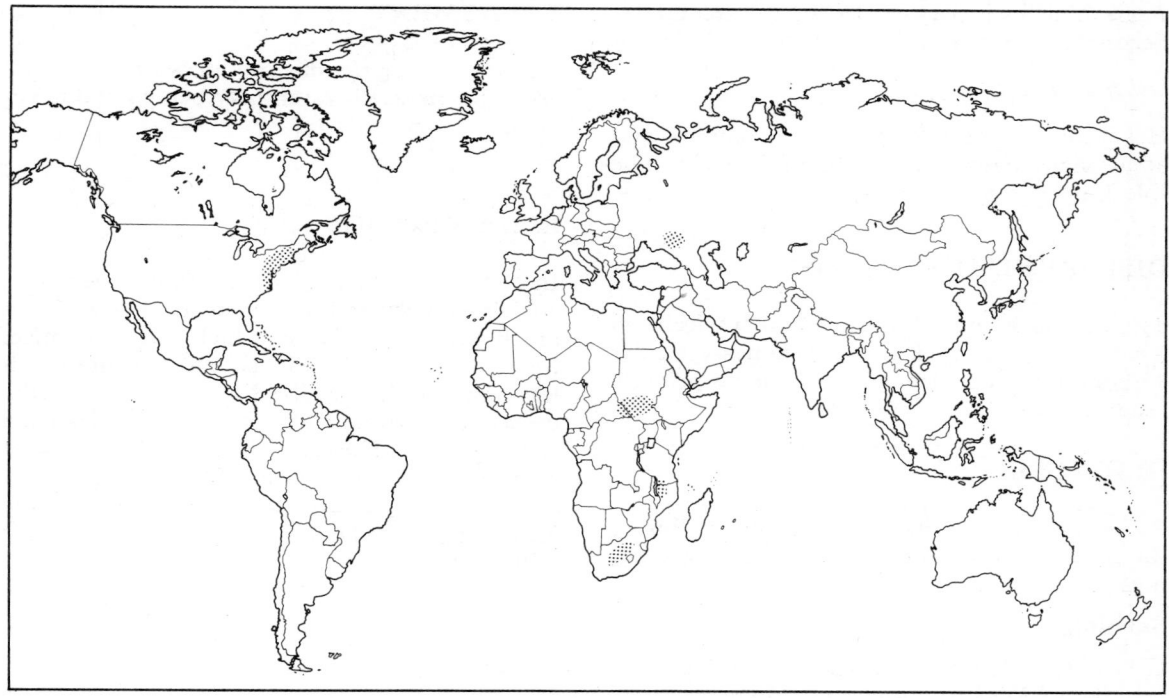

Fig. 10.11 Geographical distribution of rickettsialpox (*R. akari*).

PATHOLOGY

R. akari is extracellular, intracytoplasmic and intranuclear. A primary lesion or *eschar* forms at the site of attachment of the mite and the rickettsiae invade the endothelial cells of small vessels which become necrotic with thrombosed perivascular infiltration and small haemorrhages. The sebaceous glands and hair follicles may be involved.

Rash. A rash follows generalized spread with similar changes in the small vessels and necrosis of the epithelial cells forming an intraepidermal vesicle.

IMMUNITY

Little is known about immunity or the occurrence of second attacks.

CLINICAL FEATURES

Natural history

A primary eschar forms at the site of the mite attachment which is followed a week later by generalized spread with fever, other signs and a generalized pox-like rash which subsides after another week, the patient invariably recovering.

The *incubation period* is 7–9 days.

Symptoms and signs

Eschar. The initial lesion forms an eschar which starts as a deep-seated papule enlarging to become a vesicle 5–15 mm in diameter with a reddened areola. The fluid at first clear becomes cloudy and the vesicle shrinks to form a black eschar. The regional lymph glands are enlarged.

Onset. One week after the appearance of the eschar the onset is sudden with fever, chills, sweating, muscular pain and prostration.

Rash. The rash is constant appearing on the second day of fever consisting of sparse maculopapular spots up to 8 mm in diameter, becoming vesicular and drying up in a few days to form black crusts which are shed leaving some discoloration. The rash is general but is absent from the palms and soles and mucous membranes.

Fever. The fever rises to 41°C on the second day becoming remittent to fall by lysis after 1–7 days.

Other symptoms

Headache and neck stiffness are common and occasionally nausea, vomiting and vertigo. The spleen may be palpable.

DIFFERENTIAL DIAGNOSIS

The diagnosis must be made from varicella in which the whole pock lesion becomes vesicular without a black centre, and there is no primary lesion.

DIAGNOSIS

Rickettsiae can be isolated from the blood during the fever by inoculation into mice and guinea-pigs.

Serology

CF and specific rickettsial agglutination tests are positive to *R. akari* antigen but there are cross reactions with RMSF. The Weil–Felix is negative.

TREATMENT

Tetracycline 2 g per day produces a rapid recovery. The disease is essentially benign and never fatal.

EPIDEMIOLOGY

In New York where it was first described rickettsialpox occurred in tenement houses with much garbage pollution which attracted mice. Since the 1950s the disease has become much less common. In the USSR and South Africa the disease has a feral reservoir. *R. akari* has been isolated from *Microtus* in Korea suggesting that field mice are also hosts. The infection may appear in new suburbs where house mice come into contact with field mice and there is a change in the environment.

CONTROL

Antimite measures (DDT) and antimouse measures (garbage clearance) will control spread.

3 SCRUB TYPHUS (MITE TYPHUS)

GEOGRAPHICAL DISTRIBUTION
(Fig. 10.12)

Scrub typhus is indigenous in Japan, South Korea, Formosa, the Pescadores, the Philippines, Hong Kong, Yunnan province in China, extensive areas in Indo-China, northern Thailand, Burma, Malaya, India (Madras, Simla Hills, Bombay, Bihar, Punjab), in the south-east province of Sri Lanka, the Maldive Islands, the Andaman and Nicobar Islands, Sumatra, Java, Bornea, northern Celebes, Papua New Guinea and islands off the coast, New Britain, Bougainville, New Georgia, the northern New Hebrides, Queensland and north-eastern Australia. The geographical range also extends from south-eastern Siberia to west of the Indus river and possibly also Tibet, Nepal, Afghanistan and Eastern Iran. There are also pockets in the Pakistan Himalayas. Scrub typhus may occur anywhere where the ecological factors for its presence are operative, namely the presence of rodent hosts and the trombiculid mites.

AETIOLOGY

The cause is *Rickettsia tsutsugamushi* (*R. orientalis, akamushi, nipponica*) which grows well in the yolk sac of embryonated eggs (from hens which have not been fed with antibiotics) and tissue culture. It readily infects white mice which die in 12 days and guinea-pigs, but strains vary widely in their infectivity. There are at least four antigenic groups and only the homologous strain can provide the appropriate antibodies but there are also heterologous antigens and all strains provoke OXK agglutinins in man.

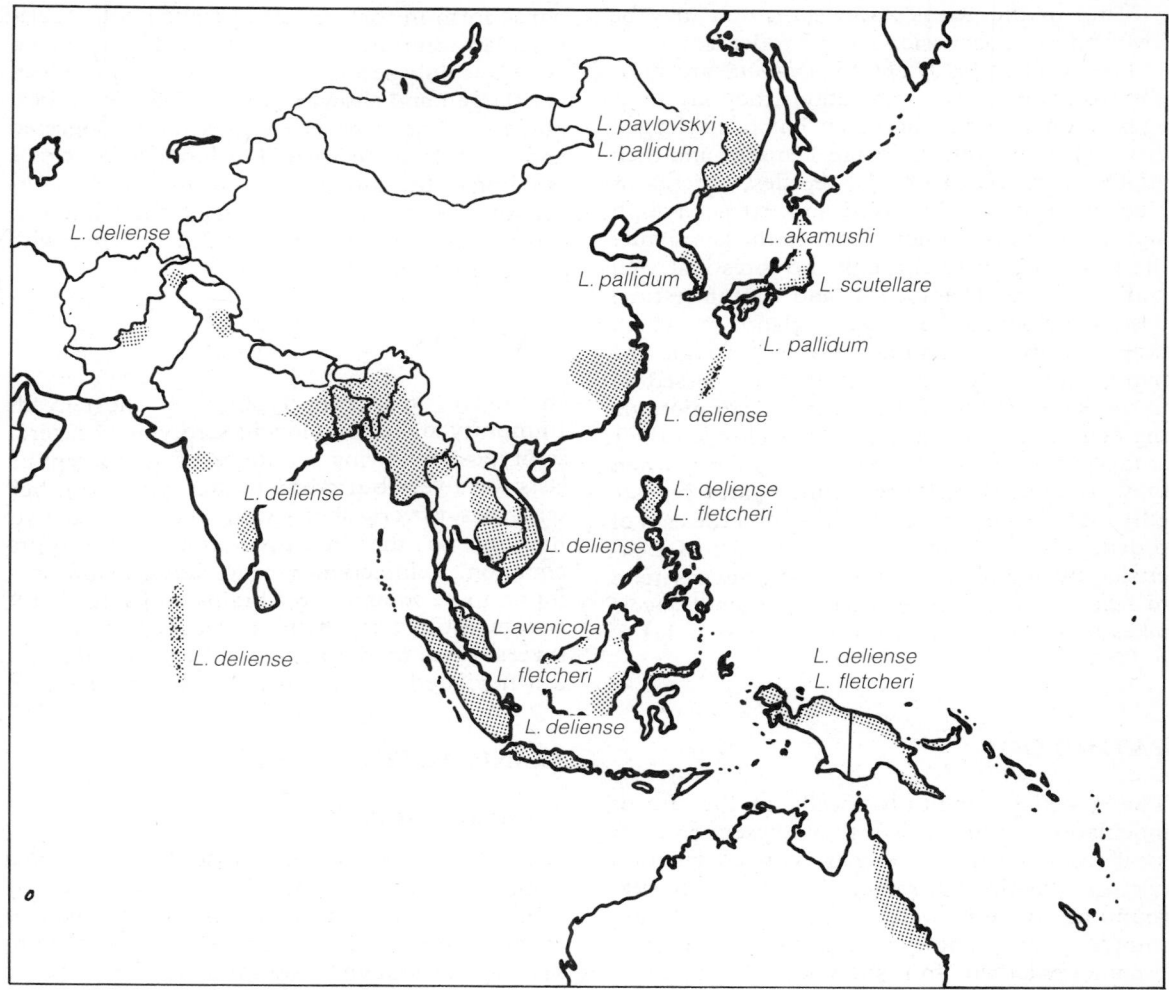

Fig. 10.12 Geographical distribution of scrub (mite-borne) typhus (*R. tsutsugamushi* (*orientalis*)). (Courtesy Department of Entomology, London School of Hygiene and Tropical Medicine.)

TRANSMISSION (see also Appendix III, p. 1383)

R. tsutsugamushi is a zoonotic infection of rodents transmitted by larval mites (genus *Leptotrombidium*), the adults of which are trombiculid mites (genus *Trombicula*), and are not parasitic. Each strain of rickettsia is transmitted by a different mite and has a different host. The mite is both a reservoir and a vector and the infection is transmitted by bite and transovarially. Because of transovarial transmission a site can remain infected for long periods in the absence of an infected host.

Leptotrombidium akamushi is the vector in the classical areas of the disease, in Japan in the cultivated plains of rivers (Fig. III.5, p. 1383).

Leptotrombidium deliense is the main or an important vector over most of the distribution of the disease from coastal Queensland in the east through Papua New Guinea, the Philippines and China (Fig. III.4, p. 1383).

Other vectors are:

L. fletcheri, an important vector in Malaysia, Borneo, New Guinea and the Philippines.

L. avenicola on the sandy beaches of Malaysia.

L. pallidum in limited areas of Japan, Korea and Russia.

L. pavlovskyi in Siberia and Russia.

L. scutellare in the Mount Fuji area of Japan.

Mites of the genus *Ascoschoengastia* may be involved in transmission among rodents.

The adult mites (*Leptotrombidium*) are non-parasitic and live on vegetation; they lay their eggs on the ground where they hatch; six-legged larvae (Kedani mite or 'patau') emerge and then attach themselves to birds, reptiles, rodents or man upon which they feed and extract lymph and tissue fluids but not blood. In the larval mite the rickettsiae pass through the intestinal wall and enter the haemocoele and extraintestinal tissues including the salivary glands in which they multiply, remaining viable through the nymph and adult stages until they are passed on to the larval mites of the second generation via the egg. The larval mites do not cling to their animal hosts for more than 3 or 4 days, when they drop off. Rickettsiae are inoculated repeatedly into the same patch of skin upon the ears of rodents and this facilitates the uptake of rickettsiae by uninfected mites which always tend to feed upon the same place. The whole cycle takes about 40 days in the tropics (Fig. III.6, p. 1384).

PATHOLOGY

The rickettsiae multiply locally at the site of inoculation, from which they disseminate. A local lesion forms an eschar with coagulation necrosis affecting the epidermis, corium and surrounding tissues, well delineated by a surrounding line. The lymph glands in the area become enlarged and show central necrosis. There is general lymph gland enlargement. The rickettsiae have a predilection for the vascular endothelium and cause intravascular and perivascular lesions in the smaller blood vessels, especially in the skin, myocardium, lungs and brain.

Endovascular lesions with thrombosis and haemorrhage are marked in the lungs and there is a perivascular infiltration with monocytes, plasma cells and lymphocytes with focal oedema. In the myocardium there is an interstitial invasion of monocytes and focal necrosis; in the lungs the walls of the alveoli become thickened and the alveolar spaces are filled with serum and red cells.

In the brain there is a focal perivascular reaction with neuroglial proliferation, monocytic infiltration and focal necrosis. The 'typhus nodules' in mite typhus differ from those of the louse-borne form in that the chief change is the perivascular infiltration; the intima of the blood vessels is only secondarily involved. The spleen is enlarged and shows septic changes with focal necrosis. The liver is enlarged and congested and shows focal necrosis. The kidneys show pale swelling of the cortex and a narrow zone of congestion. There is an effusion of fluid into the tunica vaginalis and generalized oedema with haemorrhage into the tissues.

IMMUNITY

Immunity in scrub typhus is short-lived. Immunity to the homologous serotype (of several serotypes) following an attack of scrub typhus lasts for a year but cross immunity to the other serotypes is very short-lived, only one to two months, so that multiple attacks are quite common. Reinfection with *R. tsutsugamushi* was found to be common in a highly endemic area.[29] Serum antibodies which persist for from one to several years do not appear to be protective and cell-mediated mechanisms play the major role.[29]

CLINICAL FEATURES

Natural history

Scrub typhus is a severe disease. Following on a mite bite an eschar develops to be followed by high fever and prostration with a rash. Involvement of the central nervous system, myocardium and clotting system follows and the mortality rate varies according to locality from 0 to 30% in untreated cases.

The *incubation period* is 4–10 days during which the primary eschar develops.

Symptoms and signs

Eschar. The mite bite usually passes unnoticed but there may be a pricking sensation and the mite or mites can be seen through a strong magnifying glass with their heads buried in the skin. When the patient becomes conscious of pain and tenderness in the lymphatic glands of the groin or axilla inspection of the skin will reveal an eschar. The eschar is usually situated about the genitals or armpits. It is a small (2–4 mm), round, dark, tough, firmly adherent eschar with a necrotic centre surrounded by a painless, livid red areola. Sometimes there may be just a papule which develops and disappears during the incubation period and may therefore not be seen. Occasionally two or three eschars are discovered and eschars were found in 82%[30] and in 48%[31] of cases of scrub typhus in Vietnam.

Although a line of tenderness can be traced to the local lymphatic glands no lymphangitic cord can be made out but the regional lymph glands become enlarged and tender.

Onset. The onset is sudden with severe frontal and bitemporal headache, anorexia and chills alternating with flushes of heat.

Fever. Fever of a continued type develops mounting over a period of 6 days to 40°C or 40.6°C. Associated with this is conjunctival injection, and photophobia with half-closed, watery, glistening eyes.

Bronchitis. Bronchitis is severe with a harassing, dry, bronchial cough.

The pulse : temperature ratio is low.

Lymphadenopathy. Lymphadenopathy is characteristic. Observers in Burma describe generalized lymphadenopathy as present in 90% of cases. The glands are noticeably palpable in the posterior triangles of the neck, sometimes so pronounced as to give a bull-neck appearance. The enlargement of the posterior occipital glands may be the cause of occipital pain in association with neck rigidity.

Rash. About the sixth or seventh day the eruption of large, dark red papules appears. It is usually maculopapular or sometimes papular or macular. It lasts 3 or 4 days and is found mainly on the trunk, upper arms and thighs, sometimes extending to the face, hands and feet, which occurred in 35% of cases.[30]

Spleen. The spleen is moderately enlarged.

Other systems

Central nervous system. Involvement of the central nervous system may appear during the second week. Apathy gives way to meningoencephalitis, delirium, restlessness, stupor, coma, muscular weakness, coarse tremors and convulsions. The cranial nerves are involved, and nerve deafness, papilloedema, congestion of retinal vessels and, less commonly, dysarthria and dysphagia may develop.

Myocardium. Systolic murmurs, ectopic beats, occasional cardiac enlargement, transient gallop rhythm and electrocardiogram abnormalities—inversion of T waves and prolongation of the P–R intervals—may occur. Heart failure is rare but the blood pressure may fall with cyanosis, shock and general oedema. Gangrene is rare.

Renal. Renal insufficiency is common but failure rare. There is a diuresis with recovery.

Clotting mechanisms. Disseminated intravascular coagulation has been described by Chernof[17] and the coagulation time increases but haemorrhages are rare although melaena can occur.

Course

By the end of the second week, sooner or later, according to the severity of the case, the fever begins to remit by lysis and to become normal after a few days. The eschar develops into a sharp-edged deep ulcer which, after separation of the crust, begins to heal during the second week and the lymphadenopathy subsides.

Clinical variations

The constitutional symptoms may be very slight although there is a well-marked extensive eschar; or the fever may be severe and complications set in. The duration of the disease may vary from one to four weeks but three weeks is an average. Relapses do not occur in the untreated case.

Mild cases of scrub typhus are not uncommon and a combination of diagnosis by isolation of the organisms, antibody titration by IFAT and Weil–Felix showed that scrub typhus was responsible for 23% of all febrile illnesses on an oil palm estate in Malaya. The clinical syndrome whether mild or severe was difficult to distinguish from other infections since eschars, rashes and lymphadenopathy were uncommon.[32]

Complications

Parotitis, melaena, coma, mania, cardiac failure or oedema of the lungs may all end in death. Pregnant women contracting scrub typhus mostly abort and die.

Sequelae

Eye sequelae are found in 98% of cases especially

enlargement of blind spots, contraction of visual fields and scotomas. Non-specific involvement of the cochlear system was found in 11% during convalescence and deafness may persist for months. Long-term sequelae did not develop in soldiers who survived scrub typhus in the Second World War.

Laboratory findings

An early leukopenia becomes a leukocytosis later in the disease. Jaundice is rare but serum transaminase levels may be elevated. Albuminuria is common and nitrogen retention may be found.

DIFFERENTIAL DIAGNOSIS

The classical picture of eschar, rash and fever is easy to diagnose but cannot be distinguished from tick-borne rickettsias other than by serological means. Where eschar and rash are absent then differentiation must be made from other severe fevers—falciparum malaria (which may coexist), typhoid, viral haemorrhagic fevers and cerebrospinal meningitis. Points in diagnosis are lymphadenopathy and splenomegaly in typhus.

DIAGNOSIS

Rickettsiae may be isolated from the blood in the early stages by grinding up blood clot with normal saline, centrifuging at low speed and inoculating 0.3 ml of supernatant fluid intraperitoneally into mice. The mice die 10–16 days later when rickettsiae can be demonstrated in peritoneal smears.

Serology

Antibodies appear during the second week and last until long after recovery. The Weil–Felix shows agglutination to the OXK proteus strain (see p. 215 and Table 10.2), but a rise in OXK antibodies was found in only 47% of cases.[32] Specific rickettsial agglutination and CF tests to rickettsial antigens are positive. The IFAT is the test of choice; and IgM response is good in primary infections but is suppressed in reinfections; a fourfold rise in titre is the criterion for diagnosis; titres of 1/40 appear at the end of the first week and a fourfold rise with maximum titres follows by the end of the second week.

TREATMENT

Tetracycline drugs are specific. A single dose of 200 mg doxycycline followed 4–5 days later by a second dose will eliminate all early relapses. Tetracycline hydrochloride should be given as 2 g per day in three or four divided doses until the fever has settled for 48–72 hours. If treatment is instituted in the first 3 days relapses are likely.

Treatment of complications

Falciparum malaria and scrub typhus may coexist in the same patient and the possibility should be considered in patients with falciparum malaria who are not responding to antimalarial therapy. Severe cases of scrub typhus should be carefully watched and electrocardiograms taken for signs of myocardial failure. Where inversion of the T waves has occurred than a prolonged convalescence must be ensured. Myocardial failure must be treated with complete bed rest and digitalization and diuretics.

EPIDEMIOLOGY AND CONTROL

Scrub typhus may occur anywhere where the ecological factors for its presence are operative, namely the presence of rodent hosts and the trombiculid mites. The larval mites live and feed upon 'maintenance' hosts.

Maintenance hosts

Maintenance hosts comprise some 20 species of rats, tree shrews and several species of birds which can disseminate the infected mites. In Japan the mites (*L. akamushi*) live and feed on rice rats and quail. In Upper Burma the Yunnan buff-breasted rat (*Rattus flavipectus yunnanensis*) and Assamese tree shrew (*Tupai belangeri versurae*) have been found naturally infected with rickettsiae.[33] Larval trombiculae are also found in large numbers on the ears of the maintenance hosts, the field vole (*Microtus montebelloi, Mus jerdoni, R. rattus rufescens, R. norvegicus, R. agrarius, R. jalorensis* and in the Imphal district *R. bullocki*. In the forests around Kuala Lumpur the main hosts are three giant rats, *R. mulleri, R. sabanus* and *R. bowersi*. In Jarak Island in the Malacca Straits, *R. r. jaraki* and

R. argentiventer form the main hosts. The rat-mice cycle is kept up in these rodents and in towns in Malaysia, for instance Kuala Lumpur, the infection is transmitted from the jungle rats to the Malayan house rat (*R.r. diardi*) and in the far east of the USSR rickettsial antibodies have been found in cattle.[34]

The rickettsiae passage between the 'reservoir' hosts (rodents) and the mites. The numbers of mites are built up by successive generations infected with rickettsiae in 'mite' or 'typhus' islands until there is a spillover into man, who is an 'incidental' or casual host. Although many species of rodents and other small mammals can become infected with rickettsiae,[35] it has yet to be demonstrated that they constitute a reservoir of infection. They provide a measure of rickettsial prevalence in trombiculids which may not feed on man, so that rates of rickettsial isolations from mammals and their antibody prevalence rates can be used as an indicator of the level of endemicity and the risk to man.[36]

Epidemiology

There is a wide variation in infection rates and mortality in man which is not dependent on the virulence of the local strain of rickettsiae but on the number of organisms in the mites. It is recorded that in South Bat Island in the Purdy group off Papua New Guinea, which is uninhabited by man, there is a population of rats saturated with *R. tsutsugamushi* and infested with larval mites (*L. deliense*). In 1944, 26 of 41 sailors contracted scrub typhus there in 46 days and two died.

Scrub typhus occurs in scrubby terrain associated with man's modification of the vegetation and also in forest, glacial slopes and semidesert. In the Pakistan Himalayas there are ecological islands of appropriate fauna of rodents and ectoparasites in some of which scrub typhus has been demonstrated and from which, in spite of isolation, the infection may have spread to form new endemic areas.[37] In endemic foci the infection evolves slowly and different species of mites and rodents are concerned over a period of years. Manmade activities may introduce scrub typhus to new areas or increase its endemicity if already present. In Malaya and South-East Asia the areas of highest endemicity have been largely manmade by deforestation, as in abandoned rubber plantations overgrown with rank kunai grass known as 'lalang' (Malaya and Papua New Guinea) and in weed-covered waste patches on the outskirts of large towns, such as Calcutta, Bombay, Rangoon, Mandalay, Singapore and Kuala Lumpur, where scrub typhus is a backyard disease.

Endemic areas may also be developed on the edges of virgin forest where they form the hedgerow type of endemic centre.

In Japan man acquires mite typhus in 'yudokuchi', which means poisonous places. These areas, which have been known for centuries, occur chiefly along the banks of big rivers in the southern island of Honshu.

There is a seasonal incidence of scrub typhus carried by *T. akamushi* from May to October, but an epidemiological variant known as 'winter scrub typhus' or 'shichito fever' carried by *L. scutellare* is also found. Outbreaks of scrub typhus may be of various types. It is explosive in people who visit a 'yudokuchi' for the first time, when all the cases will occur in 10–12 days, or the outbreak may be followed by a rapid decline consequent upon occupation and clearance of the site. Sporadic cases may occur following occasional visits to a 'yudokuchi' from an uninfected site. There may be a delayed epidemic consequent upon subsequent use of a 'yudokuchi' as a latrine or recreation area. Lastly, cases may occur repeatedly following upon occupation, abandonment and reoccupation of an infected camp site.[38]

Prophylaxis and control

Control is based upon regulation of the environment and antimite measures. Chemoprophylaxis can be used but immunization is of little value. The environmental features which produce infection must be identified in different districts and known endemic areas, which are often localized to relatively small geographical regions such as second degree growths in deforested areas, should be avoided. Prospective camp sites may be prepared by cutting all vegetation level with the ground and burning it. After thorough clearing the ground dries in two to three weeks, killing the mites. More immediate occupation can be achieved by spraying with dieldrin or gammexane (BHC). Antimite measures consist in the use of miticides and repellents (Appendix III, p. 1384).

Dibutyl phthalate (DBP) is lethal to mites which are killed when walking on impregnated cloth, and 58 g of DBP or dimethyl phthalate

(DMP) will treat two sets of tropical uniform. Fingers are dipped into the fluid and rubbed lightly over the cloth. DBP and DMP will resist up to eight washes in cold water and wading through rivers. Five per cent emulsion of DBP or DMP in 2% soap emulsion is effective as a repellent. A mixture of benzyl benzoate and DBP is effective.

Chemoprophylaxis

A weekly 200 mg oral dose of doxycycline proved highly effective in preventing scrub typhus in volunteers and could be a very successful prophylactic taken in conjunction with malaria prophylaxis in highly endemic areas.[39]

4   Q FEVER (QUERY FEVER)

GEOGRAPHICAL DISTRIBUTION

Q fever (Nine Mile fever, Balkan grippe, Red River fever of Zaire) has a worldwide distribution with varying epidemiology throughout (Fig. 10.13).

AETIOLOGY

Q fever is caused by *Coxiella burneti*, a minute (0.2 μm) endospore-like rickettsia which is very resistant to adverse conditions. It can withstand heat (60°C for 30–60 minutes), can survive for weeks in blood clot at normal temperatures and can withstand desiccation and 0.5% formalin for 4 days. In nature it exists in the 'smooth form' or phase 1 and changes on adaptation to chick embryos to the 'rough form' or phase 2. It causes characteristic pathological effects in monkeys, mice and guinea-pigs. There is a well-defined febrile reaction during which the blood is infective for guinea-pigs. Mice inoculated intraperitoneally show enlargement of the liver and spleen with characteristic histological changes. In sections and smears of infected mouse liver and spleen, large numbers of rickettsiae occur in relatively large intracytoplasmic colonies. Flu-

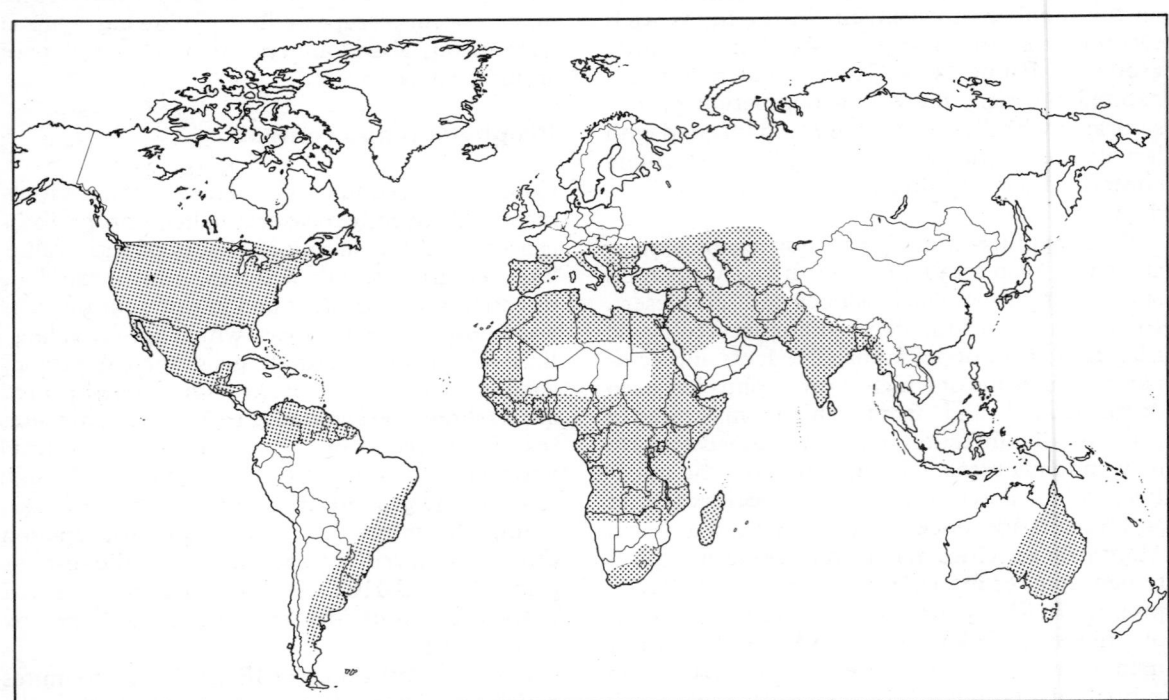

Fig. 10.13   Geographical distribution of Q fever.

orescent microscopy is of special value in estimating the number of rickettsiae in yolk sac cultures.

C. burneti can be cultivated on minced chicken embryo, reaching its maximum growth during the second week. When 8- or 9-day embryos are inoculated numerous rickettsiae are visible in membranes removed after 6 days and incubated at 34°C.

TRANSMISSION

C. burneti is maintained in nature in small wild animals by ticks which introduce the infection into domestic flocks and herds, in which further dissemination is direct from one animal to another as well as by ticks. Since *C. burneti* is excreted in milk, placental tissues and amniotic fluid, it is transmitted by milk, placental products, faeces and aerial dust. Man may be infected by ticks (in the western USA) or more usually by airborne infection from infected animals and by handling meat products, milk or placentas, or by drinking infected milk. It is a common laboratory infection and must be handled with special precautions in laboratories.

PATHOLOGY

C. burneti is a cytoplasmic parasite and develops in the histiocytes of the spleen and the Kupffer's cells of the liver. The infected cells swell and cause enlargement of these organs. The basic lesion is a granuloma sometimes with a cleared central area, the so-called 'doughnut' granuloma, and in some cases liver biopsy has shown focal lesions where there is eosinophilic necrosis of the sinusoid walls with a granulomatous appearance and occasional multinucleate giant cells. A frequent finding in fatal cases is interstitial pneumonitis. In cases of endocarditis there are vegetations on the affected values. The pathology is described by Whittick.[40]

IMMUNITY

Immunity in Q fever is fast and lifelong. Recovery from natural infection in both man and animals confers complete immunity to reinfection which is both humoral and cellular.

Humoral

Complement-fixing antibodies develop against the polysaccharide antigen of both phase 1 and phase 2 organisms. Phase 1 antibodies are protective and organize the destruction of phase 1 organisms by macrophages.[41] They appear later and rise more slowly than phase 2 antibodies and are indicative of chronic infection (e.g. endocarditis). Phase 2 antibodies are indicative of acute infection but are not protective. They appear during the first week, rise to a peak at three to four weeks and fall slowly to a low titre after 24–36 months.

Cellular

Cell-mediated immunity is the critical factor in the development of protective immunity. Its presence is demonstrated by the appearance of delayed hypersensitivity as shown by the skin test.[42]

CLINICAL FEATURES

Natural history

C. burneti infection is a zoonosis, the full cycle is complex and the natural history is not well understood since the organism has been isolated from many insects, mosquitoes, ticks, chiggers, lice and flies and many wild and domestic animals. Man is usually infected by inhalation and develops a very varied clinical picture.

The *incubation period* is 14–26 days.

Symptoms and signs

Q fever may present as a fever, pneumonitis, hepatitis, pericarditis,[43] a condition resembling glandular fever[44] or probably most commonly an inapparent infection.

Fever

This fever is known in America as 'nine mile fever' from the Nine Mile Creek in the Rocky Mountains. The course and duration vary considerably. There may be a rapid defervescence after 6–9 days or the course may be protracted to the third or fourth week and the temperature falls by lysis. There is no rash except in the form described as Red River fever of Zaire. There is severe headache, shivering and even rigors, photophobia, anorexia and pain in the back and legs. There is often splenomegaly and a tender enlargement of the liver.

Pneumonitis

Pulmonary involvement is varied but is mild, and self-limiting. It is shown by a dry cough with crepitations in the lungs. Radiology shows single or multiple homogeneous segmental densities usually apparent in the lower lobes resembling a typical virus pneumonia which can last for as long as two months.

Hepatitis

Hepatic involvement is found in about 30% of cases and resembles viral hepatitis. The liver becomes enlarged and focal granulomas may be seen on liver biopsy. Jaundice is rare and the liver function tests are usually normal.

Endocarditis

Endocarditis is a serious manifestation. It may come on from two to 20 years after the original infection and is commonest where artificial valves have been inserted. Often there is no history of previous valvular disease. The disease resembles subacute bacterial endocarditis but with negative blood cultures.

Glandular fever

A glandular fever-like syndrome may occur with pharyngitis, fever and headache, an absolute lymphocytosis and occasionally cervical lymphadenopathy and splenomegaly. There may be additional signs of pericarditis and myocarditis.

Inapparent infection

Serological surveys have shown evidence of past infection in farm workers who have had no previous illness.

DIFFERENTIAL DIAGNOSIS

Q fever has to be distinguished from typhoid, atypical virus pneumonia, ornithosis, glandular fever, toxoplasmosis, viral hepatitis and subacute bacterial endocarditis; all varied conditions because of the wide variation in the clinical features of Q fever.

DIAGNOSIS

Serology

Acute infection is diagnosed by a fourfold rise in phase 2 antibody in two specimens of blood taken at 10 and 14 days. The presence of both phase 1 and phase 2 antibodies is indicative of chronic infection and high titres (>1/200) are found in endocarditis.

Isolation of organisms

C. burneti may be isolated from the blood early in the infection by inoculating blood into guinea-pigs and demonstrating rickettsiae in peritoneal smears or by the appearance of antibodies in their sera. Organisms may be demonstrated on heart valves by fluorescent antibody staining.

TREATMENT

Uncomplicated Q fever is usually self-limiting and responds well to tetracycline or doxycycline or chloramphenicol with disappearance of the fever in 36–48 hours. In endocarditis antibiotic therapy must be prolonged for many months and is not always successful. A regimen of tetracycline plus clindamycin has been found effective.[45]

EPIDEMIOLOGY

Reservoir in nature

It has been suggested[46] that *C. burneti* originated as a commensal inhabitant of ticks and that they may constitute a permanent reservoir since transovarial passage of the organism has been demonstrated in *Dermacentor andersoni*, *Ornithodoros* and *Hyalomma* species. Natural infections of rodents have been found in nature and *C. burneti* has been isolated from a gerbil (*Meriones*) in Morocco, a rabbit in North Africa and from the brown rat, house mouse, vole and marmot (*Spermophilus leptodactylis*) in Transcaspia. In East Africa Heisch has found it in a rodent, *Lemniscomys striatus*. In the Salt Lake City region the rabbit and chipmunk have been found infected. In Australia the natural reservoir in Queensland is the bandicoot (*Isoodon torosus* or *I. obesulus*) and rickettsiae have been isolated from a tick, *Haemaphysalis humerosa*, an ectoparasite of the bandicoot and opossum. In Russia it is claimed that infection is also found in birds such as field sparrows, redstart, wagtail, pigeon, domestic hen, swallow, buzzard and magpie, and in their mites. The infection is maintained in nature by ticks and *C. burneti* has been demonstrated in the following ticks: *Rhipicephalus sanguineus* in Arizona, *Hyalomma savignyi* in Spain, *Hyalomma mauritanicum* in Algeria, *Haemaphysalis excavatum* in Morocco, *Haemaphysalis punctata* from sheep in Zimbabwe and *H. dromedarii* from bulls in Egypt. The cattle tick, *Boophilus annulatus microplus*, maintains the infection in cattle in Australia and transmits it to man.

Human infection

When ticks are involved in human transmission cases are few and sporadic. Farm workers are commonly affected by direct transmission when they are in contact with sheep at lambing time or with sheep which abort. There is a high incidence in those whose work takes them to farms where they are exposed to direct infection, rural postmen, agricultural machinery salesmen and those in contact with agricultural workers, such as village barbers and grocers. Where direct transmission is involved outbreaks may be explosive and involve a number of individuals. Abattoir workers are at risk.

VACCINATION

Vaccination is very effective and should be given to all high risk groups such as laboratory workers and heavily exposed groups, such as farm workers in endemic areas, and milk and meat handlers.

Phase 1 organisms must be used as polysaccharide phase 1 antigen and is an efficient immunizer. One dose (0.5 ml containing 30 μg of inactivated phase 1 *C. burneti* organisms) is given subcutaneously and gives good protection.[47] Only seronegative and skin test negative persons are immunized and the development of protective immunity is monitored by the appearance of antibodies and delayed hypersensitivity measured by the skin test (diluted vaccine intradermally). Reactions in seronegative and skin test negative persons are minimal.

PREVENTION AND CONTROL

Control of the infection on a community basis rests upon the control of the disease in domestic animals either by immunization or treatment. Milk from goats, sheep and cows must be pasteurized. Calving and lambing in endemic areas should be confined to an enclosed area which can be decontaminated. Immunization is the most effective control measure for the individual.

5 TRENCH FEVER (WOLHYNIAN FEVER, FIVE-DAY FEVER)

GEOGRAPHICAL DISTRIBUTION

Trench fever occurred in epidemic form in both World Wars; in 1914–1918 on both eastern and western fronts and in 1942–1943 on the eastern front. Studies have shown its presence in Mexico, North Africa and eastern Europe, wherever louse-ridden populations exist.

AETIOLOGY

Rochalimaea (Rickettsia) quintana is a small gram-negative bacillus which lives extracellularly in the cuticular margin of the epithelium of the midgut of lice (not intracellularly as does *R. prowazeki*). It has been suggested[48] that it is a transformation from mild inter-

epidemic typhus to a milder labile type resulting from environmental conditions which affect both the human and louse hosts.

TRANSMISSION

Lice become infected by feeding on infected humans. They do not die but remain infected for about a year. It is not certain whether they transmit by bite or faecal contamination but *R. quintana* has been found in clean lice fed on humans infected with contaminated louse faeces.[49]

PATHOLOGY

Little is known because the disease is not fatal.

IMMUNITY

There is little immunity. Rickettsiae may persist in the blood of carriers for months or years.[50] Single or multiple attacks may occur, sometimes as late as eight years after infection.

CLINICAL FEATURES

Natural history

Trench fever is a self-limiting disease but is very variable; there are many inapparent and mild infections as well as relapsing forms.
  The *incubation period* is 10–30 days.

Symptoms and signs

The *classical 'quintana' type* ('febris quintana') is not the commonest. The onset is sudden with headache, fever, prostration and hyperaesthesia of the skin and pain in the back and lower limbs ('shin bone fever'). The fever is intermittent every 4 or 5 days ('febris quintana'). In the majority of cases there is a *rash,* a macular eruption of rose red spots lasting for a variable period. Other forms are commoner: a single acute febrile attack of 3–4 days' duration, single or multiple relapses over one to two months and a severe 'typhoidal' type with sustained fever. Inapparent infections are common and large numbers of carriers exist.

DIFFERENTIAL DIAGNOSIS

Except in epidemic form trench fever is difficult to diagnose from other fevers. The relapsing form must be distinguished from louse-borne relapsing fever which along with louse-borne typhus occurs in louse-ridden populations.

DIAGNOSIS

Rickettsiae can be isolated from the blood by culture on blood agar in a carbon dioxide rich atmosphere or by feeding clean lice on the patient and transmitting it to mice or monkeys. Specific rickettsial agglutination tests are positive.

TREATMENT

Tetracyclines are specific as for louse-borne typhus fever.

EPIDEMIOLOGY

No animal reservoir is known although the infection can be transmitted to monkeys. A close relative, *R. vinsonii* has been isolated from voles. Human carriers, of which there are many, are the reservoir, the carrier state lasting for a long time. The infection breaks out when louse-infected people are gathered together (prisons, camps, refugees) in unhygienic conditions.

CONTROL

Control measures against lice, as in louse-borne typhus fever (see p. 222), are effective. Immunization is not effective.

REFERENCES

1 Weyer, F. (1953) *Z. Hyg. Infekt. Frankh.* **137**, 419.
2 Burgdofer, W. (1970) *Am. J. trop. Med. Hyg.* **19**, 1010.
3 Rehacek, J., Zupanc Icova, M., Kovakova, E. et al (1975) *J. Hyg. Epidem. Microbiol. Immunol.* **19**, 329.
4 Murray, E.S. (1977) *Infectious Diseases,* ed. P. Hoeprich, 2nd edn., p. 794. New York: Harper & Row.
5 Philip, R.N., Casper, E.A., Ormsbee, R.A. et al (1976) *J. clin. Microbiol.* **3**, 51.
6 World Health Organization (1982) *Bull. Wld Hlth Org.* **60**, 159–164.
7 Bozeman, F.M., Masiello, S.A., Williams, M.S.E. et al (1975) *Nature, Lond.,* **255**, 545.
8 Burgdofer, M., Ormsbee, R.A., Schmidt, M.L. et al (1973) *Bull. Wld Hlth Org.* **48**, 563.
9 Murray, E.S., O'Connor, J.M. & Gaon, J.A. (1965) *J. Immunol.* **94**, 734.
10 Huys, J., Freyens, P., Kahiyigi, J. et al (1973) *Trans. R. Soc. trop. Med. Hyg.* **67**, 718.
11 Gaon, J.A. & Murray, E.S. (1966) *Bull. Wld Hlth Org.* **35**, 133.
12 Ackley, A.M. & Peter, W.J. (1981) *South med. J.* **74**, 245–247.
13 Krause, D.W., Perini, P.L., McDade, J.E. et al (1975) *E. Afr. med. J.* **52**, 421.
14 Raynal, J.H., Dournier, J. & Velliot, E. (1939) *Chin. med. J.,* **56**, 11.
15 Farnang-Azad, A., Traub, R. & Wisseman, C. (1983) *Am. J. trop. Med. Hyg.* **32**, 1392–1400.
16 Gispen, R. (1950) *Documenta neerl. indones. Morb. trop.* **2**, 23.
17 Chernof, D. (1964) *New Engl. J. Med.* **270**, 1042.
18 Le Gac, P. (1974) *Bull. Soc. Path. éxot.* **67**, 261.
19 Heisch, R.B., McPhee, R. & Rickman, L.R. (1957) *E. Afr. med. J.* **34**, 459.
20 Gear, J.H.S., Muller, G.B., Martins, H. et al (1983) *S. Afr. Med. J.* **63**, 807–810.
21 Hoogstraal, H. (1967) *Am. Rev. Ent.* **12**, 337.
22 Robertson, R.G. & Wisseman, C.L. Jr (1973) *Am. J. Epidem.* **97**, 55.
23 Brown, G.W. et al (1981) *Trans. R. Soc. trop. Med. Hyg.* **75**, 586–587.

24 Lipink, S.I. et al (1983) *Meditsinghaya Parazitologiya i Parazit. Bologni.*

25 Yastrebov, V.K., Mikhailov, A.K. & Shipynov, N.V. (1968) *Zh. Mikrobiol. Epidem. Immunobiol.* **45**, 98.

26 Huebner, R.J., Jellison, W.L. & Pomeranz, C. (1946) *Pub. Hlth Rep. Wash.* **61**, 1677.

27 Huebner, R.J., Stamps, P. & Armstrong, G. (1946) *Pub. Hlth Rep. Wash.* **61**, 1605.

28 Le Gac, P. & Giroud, P. (1951) *Bull. Soc. Path. éxot.* **44**, 413.

29 Bourgeois, A.L., Olsen, J.G., Fang, R.C.Y. et al (1982) *Am. J. trop. Med. Hyg.* **31**, 532–540.

30 Fang, R.C.Y., Lin, W.P., Chao, P.S. et al (1975) *Trop. Geogr. Med.* **27**, 143.

31 Berman, S.J. & Kundin, W.D. (1973) *Ann. intern. Med.* **79**, 26.

32 Brown, G.W., Robinson, D.M. & Huxsoll, D.L. (1976) *Trans. R. Soc. trop. Med. Hyg.* **70**, 444.

33 Mackie, J., Davis, G.E., Fuller, H.S. et al (1946) *Am. J. Hyg.* **43**, 195.

34 Somou, G.P., Shubin, F.N., Kiryanov, E.A. et al (1973) *Zh. mikrobiol. Epidem. Immunobiol.* **2**, 62.

35 Harrison, J.L. & Audy, J.R. (1951) *Ann. trop. Med. Parasit.* **45**, 186.

36 Muul, I., Liat, L.B. & Walker, J.S. (1975) *Trans. R. Soc. trop. Med. Hyg.* **69**, 121.

37 Traub, R., Wisseman, C.L. & Ahmad, N. (1967) *Trans. R. Soc. trop. Med. Hyg.* **61**, 23.

38 Audy, J.R. (1968) *Red Mites and Typhus.* University of London Heath Clark Lecture. London: Athlone Press.

39 Twartz, J.C. et al (1982) *J. infect. Dis.* **146**, 811–818.

40 Whittick, J.W. (1950) *Br. med. J.* **i**, 979.

41 Abinanti, F.R. & Marmion, B.P. (1957) *Am. J. Hyg.* **66**, 173–195.

42 Kazar, J. et al (1984) *Acta virol.* **28**, 134–140.

43 Grist, N.R. & Ross, C.A. (1968) *Br. med. J.* **i**, 119.

44 Eshchar, J., Waron, M. & Alka, W.J. (1966) *J. Am. med. Ass.* **195**, 390.

45 Turck, W.P.G. et al (1976) *Q.Jl Med.* **45**, 193–217.

46 Marmion, B.P., Stewart, J., Barber, H. et al (1954) *Lancet*; **i**, 1288.

47 Marmion, B.P., Kyrkov, M., Worswick, D. et al (1984) *Lancet* **ii**, 1411–1414.

48 Weyer, F. (1949) *Zentbl. Bakt. Parasitkde,* **153**, 115.

49 Varela, G., Fournier, R. & Mooser, H. (1954) *Revta. Inst. Enferm. trop. Mex.* **14**, 39.

50 Mohr, W. & Weyer, F. (1964) *Dt. med. Wschr.* **89**, 244.

Chapter 11
Bartonellosis

Alternative names. Oroya fever, Guaitara fever, Carrión's disease, Verruga peruviana.

GEOGRAPHICAL DISTRIBUTION

The disease occurs between the ninth and sixteenth parallels south latitude at an altitude of 800–3000 m in certain narrow valleys (quebradas) of the western slopes of the Andes in Peru, Ecuador, Colombia, Chile and also in Guatemala (Fig. 11.1). *Bartonella*-like infections associated with febrile anaemia or dermal nodules have been reported from Thailand, Sudan, Niger, Pakistan and the eastern USA but their relationship to *Bartonella bacilliformis* is not clear.

AETIOLOGY

Bartonella bacilliformis occurs in two forms: one is a rod-shaped slightly curved gram-negative bacillary organism, $2\,\mu m \times 0.5\,\mu m$, staining well with Giemsa, often in branching rods and chains but never crossed, which occurs in a large proportion of the red cells (Fig. 11.2) during Oroya fever. The other is a rounded body about $1\,\mu m$ or less in diameter, usually oval or pear-shaped and containing chromatin granules. Some occur singly or end-to-end in pairs or chains. V forms probably represent dividing organisms; Y-shaped forms are also not uncommon.

They are difficult to detect in fresh blood; phase-contrast microscopy has shown that they are feebly motile in fresh blood.[1] When dried

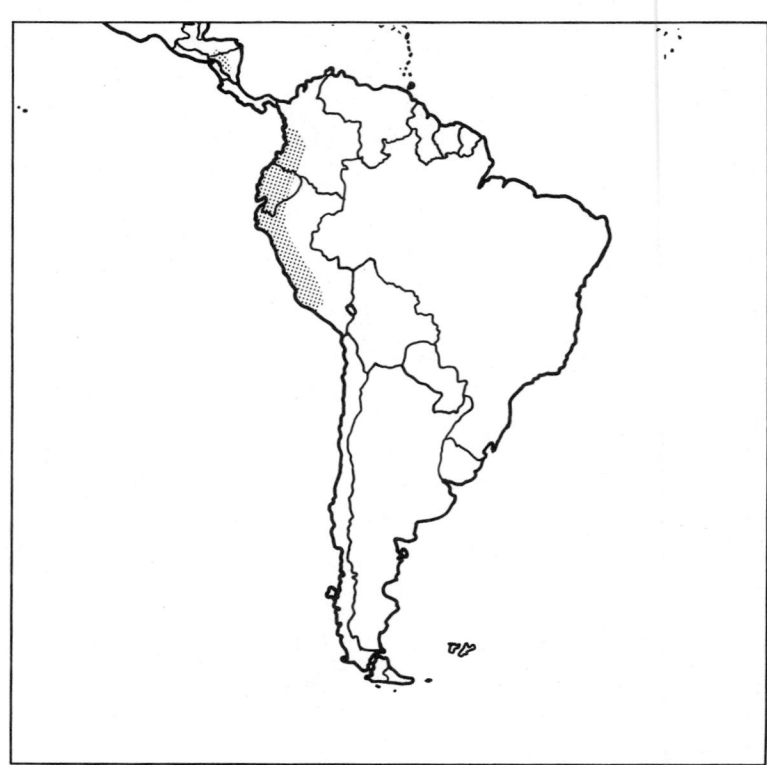

Fig. 11.1 Geographical distribution of bartonellosis.

246

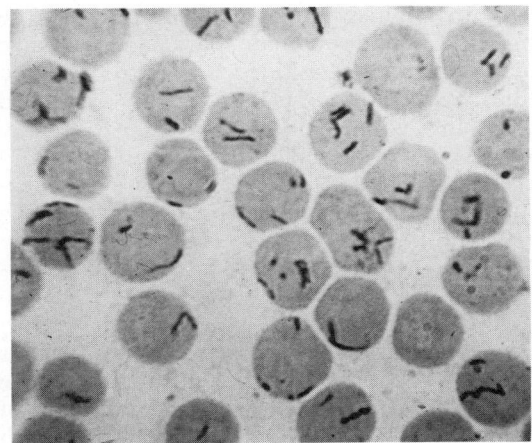

Fig. 11.2 *Bartonella bacilliformis* in blood.

films are 'shadowed' with palladium and examined by bright field microscopy it is found that the organisms lie in depressions; by electron microscopy lashing flagella are visible, each with a diameter of 20 nm, in bundles of up to 10 flagellae for each organism.

Intravenous injection of *Bartonella bacilliformis* into macaca monkeys causes irregular fever and anaemia, while the organisms can be demonstrated in the blood cells. Intradermal inoculation into the supraorbital tissues gives rise to verrugous nodules. From the morphological point of view *Bartonella* and *Rickettsia* have resemblances, since both are minute, pleomorphic, gram-negative and intracellular. Barton considered them protozoal but Noguchi regarded *Bartonella* as a bacillus.

Cultural characteristics

Bartonella was first cultured on solid media in citrated blood, sent in cold storage from Lima to New York, of patients with Carrión's disease. It is an obligatory aerobe and grows best at low temperatures on blood agar media. Battistini's method of culture is simple. A small drop of blood from the finger of the patient is withdrawn into serum-agar or Noguchi's *Leptospira* medium. The end is sealed in flame and the whole placed in the incubator at 28°C. Colonies are visible in 5 or 6 days. *B. bacilliformis* is also readily cultivated in the allantoic fluid of the developing chick embryo at 25–28°C. The growth is rapid and abundant and the cultivated bodies are 0.6–1.6 μm in length. The agar slant

method devised by Zinsser for cultivation of rickettsiae is preferred.[2]

TRANSMISSION

Although *Bartonella* can be transmitted experimentally to monkeys and grey squirrels (*Citellus tridecemlineatus*) no animal reservoir has yet been demonstrated in nature. After inoculation of grey squirrels the organism could only be recovered for the first 24–48 hours and the animals were asymptomatic.[3]

Bartonella-like (*Haemobartonella muris*) bodies are found in the blood of healthy mice and certain rodents; they cannot be cultured and exist as a latent infection. They are transmitted by rat lice and after splenectomy cause an acute fatal anaemia resembling Oroya fever. A similar anaemia occurs in the dog after splenectomy when infected with *Bartonella canis*. Verruga can be conveyed by inoculation to puppies and rabbits and *Bartonella* occurs as a natural infection in native American Indian dogs.[4]

Human reservoir

It is probable that the main reservoir consists of a number of asymptomatic human cases in whom the blood contains *Bartonella*. *Bartonella* was cultured from seven of 81 students and three of the seven were completely asymptomatic, and in the verruga zone 10–15% of people have been shown to be chronic carriers with positive blood cultures.[3] *B. bacilliformis* can be seen in the endothelial cells of cutaneous verruga nodules so that cases of verruga can act as a source of infection.

Sandfly transmission (Appendix III, p. 1401)

It was thought the vector was a sandfly, *Lutzomyia verrucarum*,[4] and further evidence incriminating *L. noguchii* and *L. verrucarum* was obtained when insects were collected in a verruga district of Peru and sent to New York, where they were ground up in saline and injected intradermally into monkeys.[5] Only sandflies were found to contain *Bartonella* and *L. verrucarum* is now regarded as the only proven vector, though an outbreak of Oroya fever in the Mantaro valley of Peru has been described in the absence of *L. verrucarum*.[6] In the Narino department of south-western Colombia the habits of *L. colombianus* are so nearly like those of *L. ver-*

rucarum that it may be a vector in this area. *L. noguchii* and *L. peruensis* are also suspected as vectors.

The *Bartonella* adhere to the midgut in moderate numbers after feeding on infected patients and blood and *Bartonella* have been found occasionally on the proboscis of wild-caught sandflies suggesting that transmission may be mechanical.

PATHOLOGY

Red blood cells

The aetiological agent invades red blood cells in which it multiplies causing destruction of the cells with a rapid and extreme blood destruction. In severe cases the blood count may drop in three or four weeks to 500 000/mm³. The anaemia is typically normocytic and hypochromic. This destruction of the red cells is due to an intravascular haemolysis since 50% of labelled erythrocytes were found to have a half-life of 6 days. However, those red cells which survived this period had a normal survival rate. Normal erythrocytes injected into patients in the febrile anaemic phase behaved similarly, but red cells from a patient with verruga peruana survived normally, suggesting that they had acquired the property of resistance to the haemolytic process after cessation of the febrile stage.

There is an associated polymorphonuclear leukocytosis with an absence of eosinophils.

Reticuloendothelial system

The organisms invade the cells of the reticuloendothelial system causing reticuloendothelial hyperplasia in the lymph glands, Kupffer's cells of the liver and histiocytes in the spleen, bone marrow, kidneys, adrenals, pancreas, thyroid and testes. They also parasitize the endothelial lining cells of the blood and lymph vessels which may be so distended by clusters of the parasites that the infected cells may be detected on low-power microscopic examination.[5] Marked changes are present in the liver, spleen and bone marrow. In the liver, areas of degenerative and central necrosis are found around the hepatic veins. In the centre of the necrotic areas a yellow pigment resembling haemosiderin is present in abundance. The spleen is invariably enlarged and contains necrotic areas with pigment.

The malpighian bodies are not affected. The lymphatic glands contain large macrophage endothelial cells studded with rod-shaped bodies. *B. bacilliformis* is found in closely packed masses in swollen endothelial cells, especially those of the lymphatic glands, spleen, liver and intestines. The bone marrow shows proliferation, necrosis and marked phagocytosis of the large endothelial cells.

Verruga stage

The verrucous eruption is a sequela to the lesions in the reticuloendothelial system. Primarily the pathological changes consist in proliferation of the endothelium of the lymphatic channels which become obstructed by plasma cells and fibroblasts, but the structure is much more vascular than that of yaws which it otherwise resembles. The capillary blood vessels become dilated so that the granulomatous tumours are vascular, almost cavernous and apt to bleed profusely. A feature of the pathological histology is the formation around the blood vessels of nodules of angioblasts characteristic of the disease. *B. bacilliformis* is seen in considerable numbers in the endothelial cells of cutaneous verruga nodules, but distension of the cells is less than that seen in Oroya fever cases. *Bartonella* bodies may be found in blood corpuscles after prolonged search.

IMMUNITY

Recovery from the disease in any of its forms confers lasting immunity and it has been shown that immunity to *Bartonella* infection is rapidly acquired but bears no relation to the presence of specific agglutinins in the blood.[7] Passage from the Oroya fever to the verruga stage, which is a change in the host–parasite relationship resulting from the development of immunity, is accompanied by a diminution of symptoms. It was shown that graduated inoculation of verrugous material induces an artificial immunity.[5] In monkeys infected with verruga, splenectomy reverses the process and produces Oroya fever.

Serum antibodies which agglutinated the organism in titres from 1/10 to 1/80 have been found in the sera of patients in both the Oroya and verruga stages.[7] Cross reactions occurred with *B. proteus* OX19, OXK and OX2. A strong agglutinating serum can be prepared for testing cultures of *B. bacilliformis*.

Prophylactic inoculation with formolized suspension of *B. bacilliformis* resulted in partial immunity so that any subsequent attacks of Oroya fever were modified.[7]

CLINICAL FEATURES

Natural history

Bartonellosis presents a varied clinical picture ranging from a large number of asymptomatic carriers to the non-fatal verruga peruana, to the severe and often fatal Oroya fever.

Symptoms and signs

Two forms of the disease are apparent as Oroya fever and verruga peruana.

Oroya fever

The incubation period of Oroya fever is about three weeks. Its onset is insidious and is marked by malaise, soon followed by a rapidly developing anaemia and an irregular remittent pyrexia, associated with very severe pains in the head, joints and long bones. The bone pains are probably connected with disturbances in the haemopoietic system. Very often the initial fever is like that of malaria. The most severe types resemble fulminating typhus and are known as 'the severe fever of Carrión'. The liver and spleen are enlarged and tender and there is a generalized lymphadenopathy, and a characteristic anaemia develops with a tendency to macrocytosis with nucleated red cells and a high reticulocytosis with a variable leukocytosis. In the febrile phase most of the red cells contain numerous bacilliform organisms. Death rate varies from 10% to 40%, the end coming within two or three weeks of the onset of the disease. A terminal delirium is often noted. In those cases which proceed to the verruga stage the fever may last three to four months. Often there is a secondary infection with *Salmonella typhimurium*, which may prove fatal.

Verruga peruana stage (*localized bartonellosis or eruptive stage*)

The period of incubation subsequent to the development of Oroya fever is 30–40 days but where the initial fever is absent it is at least 60 days. Although verruga is usually a sequel of Oroya fever it may arise spontaneously and inde-

pendent of Oroya fever. The initial stages are characterized by peculiar rheumatic-like pains together with fever, the pains being like those of yaws only more severe. As in yaws the constitutional symptoms subside on the appearance of the skin lesions. The eruption may be sparse or abundant, discrete or confluent. Some granulomas may fail to erupt, others may subside rapidly and others may continue to increase and then after remaining stationary for a time gradually wither, shrink and drop off without leaving a scar.

Two types of eruption are seen, miliary and nodular. The miliary eruption (Fig. 11.3), not

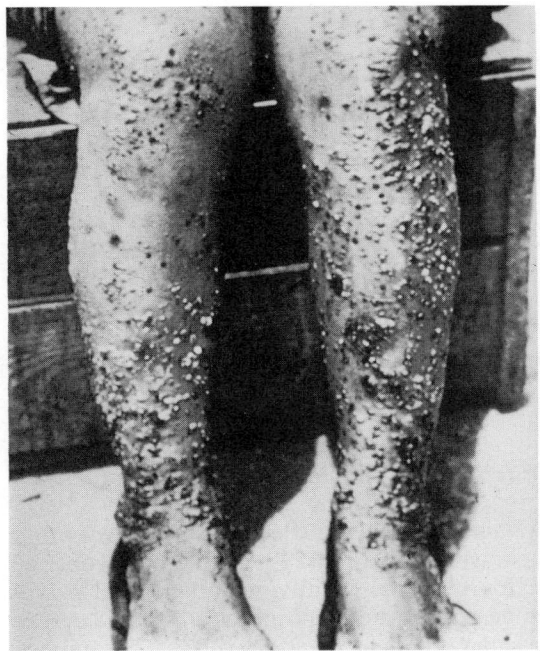

Fig. 11.3 Verruga-like eruption in bartonellosis. (Courtesy Dr P. D. Marsden.)

exceeding the size of a small pea, is found most abundantly on the face and extensor aspect of the extremities, less commonly on the trunk. A pink macule first appears, later darkening and becoming nodular. The verruga artificially produced in monkeys by injection of *Bartonella* bodies is bright cherry pink. These nodules, which are flat or somewhat pedunculated, are vascular and may develop on mucous surfaces in the mouth, oesophagus, stomach, intestine, bladder, uterus and vagina; hence the dysphagia which is a common symptom, and occasional haematemesis, melaena, haematuria and bleeding from the vagina.

The Oroya and verruga stages frequently coexist and relapses of both the fever and the eruption may occur.

The nodular eruption (Fig. 11.4) which is rarer is more chronic than the miliary. Individual lesions may grow to the size of a pigeon's egg and may become strangulated and a source of danger from haemorrhage. This type does not invade the mucous membranes and is usually confined to the regions of the knees and elbows. It appears in crops and lasts two to three months. The mortality rate from verruga is practically nil.

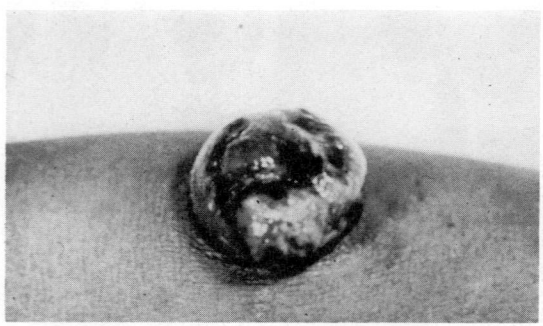

Fig. 11.4 Giant nodule on the arm caused by bartonellosis. (Courtesy Dr P. D. Marsden.)

Neurobartonellosis[8]

Bartonella may invade the brain in large numbers in parasitized red cells. The pathological changes are found in the ependyma and choroid plexus, the vessels of the meninges and in the neurons. Vascular changes include venous thrombosis, adventitious haemorrhage and characteristic glio-epithelial verrucomas.

Clinically, nervous system involvement occurs during the haemolytic phase, the cerebral form presents as meningoencephalitis with or without convulsions and has a high mortality. The spinal form which is less common presents as spastic or flaccid paralysis which may leave permanent disability, and the neuronal forms appear during the verruga stage arising from granulomas in the spinal or cranial nerves; these resolve with little or no disability. The cerebrospinal fluid shows raised protein with a pleocytosis and numerous intracellar *Bartonella*. Treatment is that of the systemic disease.

DIAGNOSIS

B. bacilliformis can be seen in the red cells on blood examination in the acute febrile stages and in smears from the verrugas. The organisms can be cultured from the blood on appropriate media. Serology is of no use.

TREATMENT

Chloramphenicol is the antibiotic of choice. The fever subsides in 48 hours and there is a rapid return of the blood to normal.[9] The dose is 4.0 g daily in four divided doses for 5 days. Other antibiotics are also effective including penicillin, tetracycline, streptomycin or co-trimoxazole.

COMPLICATIONS

Salmonellosis is the most frequent complication occurring in 40–50% of cases of Oroya fever. Salmonella infection is shown by a worsening of the patient's condition and a recurrence of fever with gastrointestinal symptoms.

Other complications are thromboses, pleurisy, parotitis and meningoencephalitis; transitory arthralgia may precede the eruption.

DIFFERENTIAL DIAGNOSIS

The Oroya fever stage must be distinguished from malaria, typhus, typhoid and acute haemolytic anaemia of various causes. The verruga stage may resemble yaws or secondary syphilis. Other conditions are multiple warts and fatty tumours (Dercum's disease). Single lesions may resemble fibrosarcoma or angioma.

EPIDEMIOLOGY

History

It is probable that this disease existed in certain Andean valleys in north-west South America in pre-Columbian days. Many thousands died of this fever during the reign of the Inca Huayna Capac and it is possible that Pizarro's men also suffered from it.

The earliest account of this disease was that of Gago de Vadilla in 1630. In the 1870s when the central railway was being constructed from Lima to Oroya in Peru a severe epidemic broke out among the construction workers resulting in 7000 deaths. In 1906 out of 2000 men employed on tunnel work 200 perished. In 1885 a medical student, Carrión, inoculated himself with blood from a verruga nodule and died from Oroya fever, from which experiment Peruvian physicians concluded that verruga and Oroya fever were different stages of the same disease.

Present status

A considerable outbreak occurred in the Guaitara valley in southern Colombia near the Ecuador boundary in 1936 mainly in the valleys of the Mayo, Sambingo, Pacual and Juanambu tributaries of the Rio Patia. The latest outbreak with 200 deaths was in 1959 and occurred between January and April in the city of Anco which lies at 2400 m above sea level in the valley of the Mantaro river in the Peruvian Andes.[6] It has again become a serious problem in Peru following completion of the malaria eradication programme and the cessation of spraying.[10]

The range of the infection is singularly limited and is confined to certain narrow valleys and ravines, the inhabitants of neighbouring places being exempt.

The disease is acquired only at night and a single night's residence in an endemic area may be sufficient. During the outbreak in the 1870s on the central railway in Peru infection could be avoided by leaving the endemic area before nightfall. The disease is most prevalent from January to April when the streams are in flood, the air hot, still and moist, malaria epidemic and insect life abundant.

Control

Control of the vector sandflies is easily obtained with DDT and sandflies have been eradicated from human habitations.[11]

REFERENCES

1 Peters, D. & Weigand, R. (1952) *Z. Tropenmed. Parasit.* **3**, 313.
2 Weinman, D. J. & Pinkerton, H. (1938) *Proc. Soc. exp. Biol. Med.* **37**, 596.
3 Herrer, A. (1953) *Am. J. trop. Med. Hyg.* **2**, 645.
4 Townsend, C. H. T. (1913) *J. Am. med. Ass.* **19**, 1717.
5 Pinkerton, H. & Weinman, D. J. (1937) *Proc. Soc. exp. Biol. Med.* **37**, 587.
6 Herrer, A., Blancas, F., Cornejo-Ubillus, J. R. et al (1959–60) *Revta med. exper.* **13**, 27.
7 Howe, C. (1943) *Archs intern. Med.* **72**, 147.
8 Trelles, J. O. (1973) In *Tropical Neurology*, ed. J. D. Spillane, p. 387. Oxford: Oxford Medical Publications.
9 Urteaga, B. & Payne, E. H. (1955) *Am. J. trop. Med. Hyg.* **4**, 507.
10 Herrer, A. (1979) Personal communication.
11 Hertig, M. & Fairchild, G. B. (1948) *Am. J. trop. Med.* **28**, 207.

SECTION II
DISEASES COMMONLY PRESENTING AS DIARRHOEA

Diarrhoea is almost universal in the tropics where it is a major cause of morbidity and mortality in children and morbidity in adults. Acute infective diarrhoea may be caused by vibrios, bacteria, viruses, protozoa and helminths, and the function of the small bowel may become so deranged as to lead to malabsorption (see also Chapter 57, and Tables 60.3, p. 1000, and 60.4, p. 1002).

Acute infective diarrhoea (Chapter 12)
  Aetiology
  Pathogenesis
  Management (rehydration, adjunct therapy)
  Sequelae

Diarrhoea caused by vibrios (Chapter 13)
  O group 1 *V. cholerae* vibrios (cholera)
  Non-O group 1 *V. cholerae* vibrios
  Non-O group vibrios

Diarrhoea caused by bacteria (Chapters 14 and 15)

Bacteria causing diarrhoea (Chapter 14)
  Toxigenic *Escherichia coli*
    Enterotoxic *E. coli* (ETEC) (traveller's diarrhoea)
    Enteropathogenic *E. coli* (EPEC) (acute gastroenteritis of infants)

Shigella sp.
Clostridium (pigbel)
Yersinia enterocolitica
Campylobacter

Non-typhoidal *Salmonella* and food poisoning (Chapter 15)

Diarrhoea caused by viruses (Chapter 16)
  Rotavirus
  Norwalk virus

Diarrhoea caused by protozoa (Chapter 17)
  Giardia lamblia (giardiasis)
  Entamoeba histolytica (amoebiasis)
  Balantidium coli (balantidiasis)
  Coccidial enteritis (isospora, sarcocystis, cryptosporidium)

Diarrhoea caused by helminths (Chapter 18)
  Capillaria philippinensis (capillariasis)

Tropical malabsorption syndrome (tropical sprue) (Chapter 19)

Chapter 12
Acute Infective Diarrhoea

Acute infective diarrhoea is a major problem in the Third World where it accounts for an enormous mortality and morbidity, particularly in children under the age of three and is an important cause of malnutrition.[1]

AETIOLOGY (see also Table 60.3, p. 1000)

Acute infective diarrhoea may be caused by any one of a number of pathogens.

Vibrios

O1 group *V. cholerae*, non-O1 group *V. cholerae* and non-O group vibrios *V. parahaemolyticus*, *V. fluvialis*, *V. damsella* and *V. hollisae*.

Bacterial

Enterotoxic and enteropathogenic *Escherichia coli*, *Shigella* sp., *Yersinia enterocolitica*, *Campylobacter* and *Clostridium*.

Viral

Rotavirus, Norwalk virus and enteroviruses.

Protozoal

Giardia lamblia, *Entamoeba histolytica*, *Balantidium coli*, and *Isospora*.

The mix of pathogens varies from country to country and rotavirus is commoner in children especially in more developed countries. The four commonest pathogens encountered in Bangladesh were *E. coli* (20%), rotavirus (19%), *Campylobacter* (14%) and *Shigella* sp. (12%).[2] Protozoa are not uncommon causes, *G. lamblia* and *E. histolytica*, while *Cryptosporidium* is increasingly recognized as a pathogen.

Helminthic

Capillaria philippinensis is an unusual cause of acute diarrhoea in the western Pacific.

PATHOGENESIS OF ACUTE DIARRHOEA (see also Chapter 60, p. 1000)

The enteropathogens may be divided into three broad groups, those which act through an enterotoxin (enterotoxic), those which are enteropathogenic and act through a cytotoxin and those which produce no toxin and in which the cause of the diarrhoea is obscure.

Enterotoxic (*V. cholerae* (O1), enterotoxic *E. coli* (ETEC), *Clostridium welchii* and some *S. dysenteriae* 1)

This group is exemplified by cholera (see Chapter 13) where an enterotoxin from the organism operates on the small intestine by means of cyclic AMP (cAMP) and the transport of water and electrolytes across the villi of the small intestine is reversed so that they are actually secreted rather than absorbed. In these diarrhoeas there is an extremely watery stool with no blood or mucus (secretory diarrhoea).

Enteropathogenic (*Shigella*, *Campylobacter*, enteropathogenic *E. coli* (EPEC))

In this group, which acts through a cytotoxin, there is invasion of the lining of the bowel with the appearance of blood and mucus in the stools, and the large bowel is also affected (dysentery). As a result of the formation of immune complexes reactive arthritis (Reiter's syndrome), large joint arthropathy and a severe haemolytic uraemic syndrome are rare complications.

MANAGEMENT OF ACUTE DIARRHOEA

The main aim in management is to restore the hydration of the body after dehydration since this can lead rapidly to acidosis, shock and death. The degree of dehydration can be rapidly assessed from the loss of elasticity in the skin folds of the dorsum of the hand or the abdomen and the degree of sunken eyes. Estimation of the amount of rapid weight loss can also help. Rehydration may be accomplished by the oral or parenteral route.

Oral rehydration

Glucose can enhance sodium absorption by the small bowel and an electrolyte and glucose solution can correct acidosis and dehydration.[3]

Oral rehydration salt (ORS) is obtainable in packets from UNICEF or can be made up locally, containing sodium chloride 3.5 g, sodium bicarbonate 2.5 g, potassium chloride 1.5 g and glucose 2.0 g, each packet to be mixed with one litre of potable water. A sugar/salt solution is as effective and another method is a plastic spoon with a measure at each end for glucose in one and salt in the other, to be added to a measured quantity of water; this has proved cheap and reliable.* Molasses can be used instead of sugar.

Rice water has been used as a rehydration fluid in Singapore and Bangladesh.[4] In cases where there is difficulty in swallowing, ORS can be given by nasogastric tube. In adults 250 ml of ORS solution should be drunk every hour until symptoms subside. In infants the ORS solution should be made up differently: sodium chloride 2.3 g, sodium bicarbonate 3.3 g, potassium chloride 2.6 g and glucose 2.0 g per litre. The fluid should be given in 8 oz bottles, 8 oz/hour for the first 2 hours, to be followed by 8 oz of water during the third. The 3-hour cycle to be repeated until hydration is normal.[5]

Simple sugar/salt solution (SSS)[6] (see also Chapter 72, p. 1223)

Sucrose can replace glucose and a simple solution can be made from locally obtained products for oral rehydration where the complete ORS (WHO) is not available.

SSS. Sodium chloride (salt) 3.5 g/litre and sucrose (sugar) 30 g/litre accompanied by adequate potassium supplementation in children can be used by untrained village personnel.

An ORS containing both glucose and glycine has been shown to be significantly better than a

solution containing glucose and electrolytes only.[7]

Parenteral rehydration

ORS therapy can fail in a proportion of cases because of severe vomiting or glucose–galactose malabsorption and in severe dehydration with shock the parenteral route must be used.

Intravenous rehydration (see also Chapter 72, p. 1223)

There are a number of solutions available.

IN ADULTS

Dacca solution (5-4-1). Sodium chloride 5 g, sodium bicarbonate 4 g, potassium chloride 1 g per litre to which should be added 2 ml of 50% glucose.

Acetate solution. Sodium chloride 5 g, potassium chloride 1 g, sodium acetate 6.5 g per litre plus 2 ml of 50% glucose.

Hartmann's solution (lactated Ringer's solution). Sodium chloride 6.2 g, potassium chloride 0.4 g and sodium lactate 2.3 g per litre plus 2 ml of 50% glucose.

In severe dehydration these must be given in a rapid infusion amounting to 10% of the admission weight over 1–2 hours.

The major signs of dehydration, sunken eyes and inelastic skin, should be monitored regularly. The measuring of fluid intake and output is best achieved by use of a 'cholera cot' which is a bed with a hole in the middle under the patient's buttocks with a plastic bucket underneath to collect the daily excreta (see Fig. 13.2). The total fluid lost is replaced plus 500 ml daily. Every attempt should be made to prevent the blood pressure falling to maintain urine excretion.

Maintenance phase

ORS therapy should be used when some recovery has occurred but if this is not possible then maintenance phase solutions must be used intravenously.

Maintenance phase solutions

Adults. Sodium chloride 500 ml of normal saline, potassium chloride 15 ml of 1 mEq K^+ per ml,

---

* A special spoon, with a measure at each end to measure the correct amount of sugar and salt, can be obtained from the Institute of Child Health, 30 Guilford Street, London WC1N 1EH.

sodium bicarbonate 50 ml of 7.5% sodium bicarbonate. Add these to 435 ml of 5% glucose.

Infants. Sodium chloride 333 ml of normal saline, potassium chloride 15 ml of 1 mEq K^+ per ml, sodium bicarbonate 33 ml of 7.5% sodium bicarbonate and add to 619 ml of 5% glucose.

Adjunct therapy

Adjunct therapy consists in the use of antimicrobial, antimotility and antisecretory drugs. In general infants with non-cholera diarrhoea can be managed with oral therapy alone but if there is dysentery then antimicrobial drugs will shorten the course and lessen the severity of the disease.

Antimicrobial drugs

Many antimicrobial drugs have been used: tetracycline, streptomycin plus sulphonamides, trimethoprim/sulphamethoxazole combinations (TSM). TSM in adults with an experimental ETEC infection reduced the severity and duration of the diarrhoea[8] and every traveller to the tropics will agree with Du Pont et al[9] that this approach is very successful. Other specific indications for antimicrobial drugs are cholera (tetracycline), *G. lamblia* (metronidazole) and *E. histolytica* (metronidazole).

Antimotility drugs

These drugs are not recommended in Third World countries where invasive enteropathogens are common since they can have an adverse effect on the course of infection.[10]

Antisecretory drugs

Loperamide, which has an antisecretory effect against cholera toxin, has been tested with acute infective diarrhoea in infancy but has been found to be ineffective.[11] Another study showed that loperamide reduced the duration of diarrhoea and could be a useful adjunct in treatment in well-nourished children, especially if the response to ORS was slow, but warned against its use in malnourished populations.[12]

Absorbents such as kaolin and charcoal are thought to act by binding enterotoxin but in practice these have had little effect in controlled studies.

Control of diarrhoeal diseases

This is important and can be effective. The principles are the provision of clean water to reduce the infection from drinking polluted water but, more importantly, to allow regular washing to improve personal and environmental hygiene so that interfamilial faecal–oral transmission of infection is prevented. Supplementary feeding programmes have been used to assist this process but it is doubtful if they keep it under control.[13]

SEQUELAE

Secondary hypolactasia

In acute infections of the small intestine there is damage to the brush border of the enterocyte with depression of the disaccharidases, especially lactase. This leads to lactose intolerance which is often a clinical problem resulting in a recurrent diarrhoea following an acute infective diarrhoea. Avoidance of milk and milk products is necessary until complete recovery of the enterocyte (see Chapter 19). Cow's milk intolerance can be precipitated in infants by toxigenic *E. coli* infection and it may be very difficult to distinguish between the two.

Tropical enteropathy and malabsorption

Repeated bacterial and viral infections of the small intestine are important causes of tropical enteropathy and malabsorption[14] by damaging the enterocyte and causing the intestinal environment leading to these two conditions.

Folate malabsorption

Malabsorption of folate found in children with chronic diarrhoea[15] is an important cause of failure to thrive and this reinforces the impression that treatment with folic acid improves malnourished children with diarrhoea.

REFERENCES

1 Chen, L.C. & Scrimshaw, N.S. (1983) *Diarrhoea and Malnutrition: Interactions, Mechanisms and Interventions.* New York: Plenum.
2 Stoll, B.J., Glass, R.I., Huq, I.M. et al (1983) *Br. med. J.* **285**, 1185–1188.
3 Cash, R.A., Forrest, J.H., Nalin, D.R. et al (1970) *Lancet* **ii**, 549.

4   Wong, H.B. (1981) *Lancet* **iii**, 102–103.
5   Nalin, D.R. (1976) *Lancet* **ii**, 958.
6   Clemens, J.D., Ahmed, M., Butler, T. et al (1983) *J. trop. Med. Hyg.* **86**, 117–122.
7   Nalin, D.R., Cash, R.A., Rahman, M. et al (1970) *Gut* **11**, 768–772.
8   Black, R.E., Levine, M.M., Clements, M.L. et al (1982) *Rev. infect. Dis.* **4**, 540–545.
9   Du Pont, H.L., Reves, R.R., Galindo, E. et al (1982) *New Engl. J. Med.* **307**, 841–844

10 Levine, M.M. (1982) *Med. Clinics N. Am.* **66**, 623–638.
11 Owen, J.R., Boradhead, R., Hendrickse, R.G. et al (1981) *Ann. trop. Paediatr.* **1**, 135–141.
12 Diarrhoeal Study Group UK (1984) *Br. med. J.* **289**, 1263–1267.
13 Feachem, R.G. (1983) *Bull. Wld Hlth Org.* **61**, 967–979.
14 Cook, G.C., Kajubi, S.K. & Lee, F.D. (1969) *J. Path.* **98**, 157.
15 Tomkins, A.M., Madi, K. & Ogilvie, B.M. (1978) *Proc. nutr. Soc.* **37**, 10A.

Chapter 13
Diarrhoea Caused by Vibrios

Vibrios are minute organisms 1.5–2 μm in length by 0.5–0.6 μm in breadth which inhabit an aquatic, in many cases a marine, environment in which they are associated with crustacea, binding to their chitinous coats for protection. They possess H and O antigens and are divided into two main groups by the O antigen. The group which possesses an enterotoxin causes a secretory diarrhoea and cholera is characterized by a special O1 antigen and is termed O group 1 *V. cholerae*, while the others which do not possess this antigen are called non-O group 1 *V. cholerae*, or formerly non-agglutinating (NAG) or non-cholera vibrios, *V. parahaemolyticus*, *V. fluvialis*, *V. mimosa* and *V. hollisae*[1-3] which with slight exceptions do not produce an enterotoxin.

O GROUP 1 *V. CHOLERAE* VIBRIOS (CHOLERA)

GEOGRAPHICAL DISTRIBUTION

Cholera occurs endemically in India, Pakistan, Bangladesh, Afghanistan and many parts of the Far East. In the past cholera was endemic in the Yangtze valley in China. Epidemics occur periodically in the Middle East and in Africa and major pandemics spreading to almost all the world have occurred in the past. Classical cholera caused by *V. cholerae* is limited to the Indian Pakistan subcontinent while the El Tor vibrio is responsible elsewhere. Isolated countries, such as the Andaman Islands and Australia and New Zealand, have escaped.

AETIOLOGY

Discovery of *Vibrio cholerae* (the comma bacillus)

Snow[4] with his famous Broad Street pump experiment first demonstrated the importance of water in the spread of cholera. The cholera vibrio was first discovered by Koch in Egypt in 1883; this he confirmed in Calcutta in 1884 by finding it in every case of the disease examined. His observations have since been abundantly confirmed. Rogers recounted that in India, many years before Koch, Surgeon-Major Macnamara suggested that cholera was due to living organisms spread by water.

Description of the cholera vibrio

The cholera vibrio is a very minute organism, 1.5–2 μm in length by 0.5–0.6 μm in breadth—about half the length and twice the thickness of the tubercle bacillus. It is generally curved like a comma, hence its name. After appropriate staining, flagella can be distinguished at each end or at one end only—sometimes one, sometimes (though less frequently) two. These flagella, though of considerable length—from one to five times that of the body of the bacillus—are difficult to see in ordinary preparations owing to their extreme tenuity. They are not always present during the entire life of the parasite. They impart very active spirillum-like movements. The individual bacilli, when stained, show darker parts at the ends or at the centre. Sometimes in culture two or more bacilli are united, in which case an S-shaped body is the result; several bacilli may thus be united, producing a spirillar appearance. The cholera vibrio is easily stained by watery solutions of fuchsin or by Löffler's method, dried cover glass films being used. It is gram-negative. The vibrio grows best in alkaline media at a temperature of 30–40°C. Growth is arrested below 15°C or above 42°C; a temperature over 50°C kills the vibrio. Meat broth, blood serum, nutrient gelatine and potato are all suitable culture media. It multiplies rapidly without curdling in milk; it dies rapidly in distilled water; it survives longer if salt is added to the water and survives for up to 285 days in sea water.

V. cholerae (O1) has two biotypes, classical *V. cholerae* and El Tor *V. cholerae*. Each type is divided into three serotypes by their O antigen, Inaba, Ogawa and Hikojima. O1 *V. cholerae* can be distinguished from non-O1 cholera and other vibrios by agglutination tests for their O antigen and by biochemical tests (Table 13.1). The classical strain can be differentiated from El Tor by a haemagglutination test and by its ability to haemolyse the red cells of sheep and goats.

Since the early 1970s classical *V. cholera* has largely been displaced from its homeland in Bangladesh and epidemics and pandemics have been caused by the El Tor biotype, but more recently it has made a comeback and the classical biotype is replacing El Tor in Bangladesh[5] and Africa.

Differentiation of toxic and non-toxic vibrios and of classical and El Tor *V. cholerae*

Biochemical tests

These are shown in Table 13.1.

Agglutination test

This can be done on fresh stools as well as cultures and is necessary before the actual diagnosis of cholera can be made. The method used is an agglutination test with a pure O high-titre serum against a living or formolized suspension of the vibrio. A boiled suspension must not be used since for the preparation of pure O sera, sus-

Table 13.1 Differentiation of vibrios from closely allied species.

	Oxidase test	Oxidase fermentation		Utilization of amino acids			String test
		Oxidation	Fermentation	Lysine	Arginine	Ornithine	
Vibrio	+ + + +	+	+ (no gas)	+	−	+	+
Aeromonas	+ + + +	+	+ (gas ±)	−	+	−	±
Pseudomonas	+ +	+	−	±	±	±	−
Plesiomonas	+ +	−	−	+	+	+	

El Tor vibrio

In 1905 a haemolytic vibrio was isolated from the dead bodies of Mecca pilgrims at the quarantine camp at El Tor in Egypt. In 1961 this variety of cholera spread from an endemic focus in the Celebes and by 1965 had invaded 23 countries, among them countries from which cholera had been absent for many decades. In 1970 El Tor cholera had spread to the Middle East, the USSR and Africa south of the Sahara.

The El Tor vibrio belongs to the same serological group as *V. cholerae* but many strains show antigenic instability. It is haemolytic but this is not a constant feature. El Tor biotypes are resistant to group IV cholera phage and to polymyxin B. They agglutinate chicken erythrocytes and may produce haemolysin. El Tor is a hardier strain than classical cholera. It persists longer in man in the carrier state and in nature, surviving well on prepared foods and living longer in water, and has replaced the classical strain in its homeland, the Ganges riverine system.

pensions of *V. cholerae* are used from which the H antigen has been removed by prolonged boiling. Sera are prepared in rabbits against O antigens of the Inaba, Ogawa and Hikojima subgroups which will contain agglutinins, not only against the main O antigen, but also against the subsidiary antigens characteristic of each of the subgroups. Formol suspensions are satisfactory and for preliminary diagnosis in the field rapid slide agglutination with O sera of a titre of 1/4000 diluted to 1:50 or 1:100 can be used, but results should be confirmed by tube agglutination. Agglutination tubes should be placed in a water bath at 52°C and a preliminary reading made at the end of 2 hours. For the confirmation of rough or partially rough variants of *V. cholerae* a high-titre serum prepared against a rough strain should be employed. Tests should be carried out with suspensions in 0.4–0.5% sodium chloride.

Haemagglutination reaction

The technique of a haemagglutinating test for the identification of cholera vibrios has been described.[6] The O antigens of vibrios are absorbed on to human, rabbit or sheep red cells and are tested against increasing dilutions of homologous serum. Incubation at 36°C for one hour and standing for one hour at room temperature gives the best results when the slide method is used. One drop of each serum dilution and one drop of antigen are mixed on excavations on a slide and then rocked. Visual clumping appears rapidly with homologous antigens and agglutination is complete within 15 minutes.

Bacteriophages

About 14 races of bacteriophage which lyse the cholera vibrio have been isolated. They are known as A–N. Of these only A and N are selective and act upon the true cholera vibrios only.

TRANSMISSION[7,8]

Cholera is transmitted from man to man by the oral route. No animal reservoir is known except that vibrios may be maintained in salt water shellfish under certain circumstances. The dose of infection is important and may be water-borne, food-borne or person to person (faecal–oral).

Infective dose

The infective dose is high in healthy adult males with normal gastric acidity. Large doses were necessary to produce diarrhoea in 50% of adult volunteers.[9] Lower doses are infective in the presence of achlorhydria or prior neutralization of the gastric juice and achlorhydria is found in association with malnutrition in poor countries so often affected by cholera, and with the smoking of *Cannabis indica*.[10]

Water-borne transmission

Transmission by water may be primary through drinking water or secondary by the use of water to irrigate or freshen foods. Infection acquired from drinking water has always been accepted as the main method of transmission. The source of the water may be rivers, wells, tanks or aquatic reservoirs. Snow[4] demonstrated the importance of water with his Broad Street pump experiment but did not discount other methods, and doubts have been cast as to the importance of water as the main method of transmission. Concentrations of *V. cholerae* in surface water have always been found to be below the necessary infective level and the incidence of cholera in communities with protected wells, and those without has shown no differences. However, vibrios can survive in sterilized spring and well water for up to one year, and in sea water for over nine months.[11] The use of polluted water to irrigate and freshen vegetables is undoubtedly important in the spread of cholera.

Aquatic reservoirs

V. cholerae has frequently been isolated from wells, rivers and tanks in India in the absence of cases of cholera or faecal contamination. The existence of a permanent aquatic reservoir offers an explanation for the permanent endemic foci of cholera in Bangladesh and formerly the Yangtze river in China.

Vibrios have also been isolated from brackish estuarine and salt water in more temperate areas. Most of these vibrios have been non-toxic strains but toxic strains have been isolated and El Tor vibrios were recently established as endemic in salt water in Kiribati[12] and the Louisiana Gulf coast.[13] Vibrios can adsorb on the chitin and multiply in chitinous shellfish, such as crab, shrimp and zooplankton and thus survive and form a permanent aquatic reservoir.

Food-borne

Most documented occurrences of food-borne cholera are the result of contamination of food by polluted water. Vibrios survive longer in non-acidic and sterilized (cooked) foods and boiled rice, and milk and milk products are important in the spread of cholera. The addition of salt to fresh fruit and boiled rice makes them excellent propagating material.

Shellfish

Vibrios adsorbed on to the chitin of shellfish are protected from the gastric juice[14] and have been responsible for outbreaks of cholera in Kiribati,[12] Louisiana and Italy.[15]

Person-to-person transmission (faecal–oral)

Person-to-person transmission has usually been

discounted in the spread of cholera but analysis of epidemics can provide an alternative explanation to many epidemics.[8] Cholera will spread amongst members of a household 2 days after the index case and this is more common in poor, less cleanly households than in those more wealthy. Poor living conditions are associated with outbreaks of cholera. The recent spread of cholera in the dry desert areas of Chad and northern Cameroon in connection with feasts and festivals was in accordance with this method of transmission.[16] Hospital cases of cholera are not important, since they are immobile and are in relatively clean conditions.

Sweat

V. cholerae was viable after seven weeks in sweat[17] and these findings are relevant to the spread of cholera in arid climates. Sweat was thought to be the method of transmission among South African miners undergoing heat acclimatization.[18]

Soil

Cholera vibrios can survive in soil and multiply in earth worms which may die.[19] The relevance of this to transmission is not known.

Sewage

Most people in cholera areas do not produce sewage and *V. cholerae* is rarely found in sewage. Sewage is of little importance in transmission.

Carriers

The source of infection in cholera is carriers. The prevalence amongst the healthy population is under 1% in normal periods but rises rapidly during the cholera season, especially among children, who are the main source of infection.[20]

Acute carriers

Acute carriers are important in the maintenance and transmission of cholera. They occur following asymptomatic or mild cases, which outnumber symptomatic cases by five or ten to one and more in the case of El Tor vibrios. The duration of the acute carrier state is 1–8 days but longer with the El Tor strain.

Chronic carriers

A chronic carrier is one who excretes vibrios for more than three weeks[21] but the chronic carrier state is rare and the vibrios are 'rough' and probably non-pathogenic[22] and chronic carriers play little part in maintenance of the infection in nature.[23] The vibrios are maintained in the gallbladder.

International spread

The presence of relatively large numbers of asymptomatic infections makes wide dissemination of the organism possible within one or two weeks. Chronic carriers who cannot be detected prolong the duration of possible spread. Uncontrolled migration and pilgrimages introduce infection into a country. In some countries widespread smuggling has contributed to the international spread of cholera.

PATHOGENESIS

Cholera is not a systemic infection and the vibrios are confined to the small intestine in which they multiply rapidly. They do not invade the mucosa or enter the portal system, nor do they damage the mucosa or affect its ability to absorb (but see below, section on cytotoxin).

Enterotoxin

The cholera vibrios secrete a toxin (enterotoxin)[24,25] which is a simple protein molecule with no carbohydrate or lipid and with a molecular weight of more than 90 000. Each molecule contains one subunit B, molecular weight 27 000, and four subunits A, each with a molecular weight of 14 000. Subunit B binds to the surface receptors of the enterocyte (which is a ganglioside, a complex type of lipid found in cell membranes) and this allows subunit A to enter the enterocyte where it acts as a hormone impostor to activate adenyl cyclase, increases greatly the amount of cyclic AMP (cAMP), which accumulates in the enterocyte and inhibits the absorption of sodium chloride. cAMP also stimulates secretion of sodium chloride and bicarbonate causing a net secretion of large amounts of fluid and electrolytes into the intestinal lumen.[25] This results in the copious secretory diarrhoea of cholera with an isotonic fluid very low in protein with a mean bicarbonate concentration approximately twice and a potassium concentration four times that of plasma. The results are hypovolaemia, hyponatraemia and hypokalaemia. Glucose does not interfere with the cAMP effect on the intestine but stimulates salt and water absorption on its own.[26]

Cytotoxin

A *Shigella*-like cytotoxin is produced by some strains of *V. cholerae* which may be responsible for some of the symptoms of cholera (occasional blood and mucus in the stools).[27]

PATHOLOGY

Rigor mortis occurs early and persists for a considerable time. Curious movements of the limbs may take place in consequence of post-mortem muscular contractions. On dissection, the most characteristic pathological appearances in cholera are those connected with the circulation and with the intestinal tract.

If death occurs during the algid stage the surface presents a shrunken and livid appearance. All the tissues are abnormally dry. The muscles are dark and firm; sometimes one or more of them are ruptured, evidently from the violence of the cramps during life. The right side of the heart and the systemic veins are full of dark, thick and imperfectly coagulated blood which tends to cling to the inner surface of the vessels. Fibrinous clots extending into the vessels may be found in the right heart. The lungs are usually anaemic, dry and shrunken, occasionally congested and oedematous. The pulmonary arteries are distended with blood, the veins empty. The liver is generally loaded with blood; the gallbladder full of bile; the spleen small. Like all the other serous cavities the peritoneum contains no fluid, its surface being dry and sticky. The inner surface of the bowel has generally a diffuse rosy-red, occasionally an injected appearance. There is a large amount of fluid in the gut lumen with varying amounts of the characteristic rice-water material and occasionally blood. The mucous membrane of the stomach and intestine is generally pinkish from congestion or there may be irregular arborescent patches of injection here and there throughout its extent.

On microscopical examination of the contents of the bowel during the acute stage of the disease the cholera vibrio, in most cases, may be demonstrated. Usually it is in great abundance, occasionally in almost pure culture in the upper part of the small intestine and duodenum, but it may be very scarce in the large gut. Sections of the intestine show the vibrio lying on and between the epithelial cells of villi and glands.

The vibrios are confined almost entirely to the gastrointestinal canal, mainly to the lumen. The tissue changes are explained by dehydration of the tissues and by haemoconcentration and low blood pressure, which result in temporary ischaemia.

Marked renal and suprarenal changes are found in those who have died in the stage of shock.[28] The kidneys show patchy ischaemia of the cortex with medullary congestion and there may also be necrosis of the cortical tubules. It is thought that cortical vasospasm is responsible for the complete cessation of urinary secretion. In a histochemical examination of the suprarenal glands it was concluded that depletion of the lipoid material from the cortex may be associated with increased liberation of cortical hormones, so that the suprarenals may play an active part in the symptomatology of cholera.

IMMUNITY

Natural immunity

There is a great variation in susceptibility since not everyone exposed to infection becomes infected and of those who do the majority are asymptomatic and only a minority develop disease which can be severe and fatal.

In endemic areas cholera is basically a problem in children under 10. In non-endemic areas there is little or no age variation. The resistance in older persons is related to the level of vibriocidal antibody in the serum; the higher the level the more likely is the infection to be asymptomatic. Infection is dose related and is affected by the acidity of the gastric juice. In volunteers it was found that the larger the dose the shorter the incubation period if the infection was symptomatic. The simultaneous administration of bicarbonate profoundly increased the chance of infection.[9] Vibrios survived much longer in the gastric juice of those with achlorhydria than with normal gastric juice and there was a preponderance of blood group O in cholera patients.[20]

Acquired immunity

As far as is known acquired immunity in cholera is entirely humoral. Cholera vibrios live in the intestinal canal where they produce toxin; they do not circulate in the body. However, humoral antibodies are produced along with copro-antibodies. The antibodies may be of importance in the defence of the body against multiplication of the vibrios in the gut if they come into contact with them after being produced in the intestines (coproantibodies) or excreted into the intestinal lumen from the circulation.

The antibodies which are formed are both antitoxic and antibacterial.

Immunity following infection

Second attacks of cholera are not uncommon but infected volunteers were highly resistant to homologous and heterologous challenge.[29] How long this immunity persists is not known. High levels of serum antibody do not protect completely from the disease but as seen above they are generally associated with some resistance to infection, probably by means of coproantibody.

Cholera enterotoxin

Cholera enterotoxin is antigenic and IgG neutralizing antibodies develop during clinical cholera, but since purified toxoid fails to provide protection against challenge the immune mechanism is almost certainly not antitoxic.[29] A method of detecting these antibodies has been developed[30] which uses their power to neutralize cholera toxin. The supernatant fluid of a vibrio culture serves as antigen which is standardized and matched against test sera by double diffusion agar technique.

Antibacterial antibodies

Recent experiments with volunteers have suggested that the predominant immune mechanism in cholera is antibacterial[29] and the antibodies which develop include agglutinins, vibriocidal antibodies and coproantibodies. Vibriocidal antibodies appear early and persist for many weeks[24] and require complement for their demonstration. They increase in the serum of man during exposure to cholera and after immunization.

Coproantibodies (IgA) are the most important

antibodies in protection and appear in the absence of serum antibodies along the entire gut. They decline soon after they are formed and disappear in three months. They could be of great importance in immunization against infection since they could be induced by live avirulent oral vaccines.

Immunoglobulins

Changes have been described in the immunoglobulins in 12 patients with classical cholera, 10 with El Tor, and volunteers given cholera lipopolysaccharide (LPS) or phenolized vaccine.[31] All cholera patients showed an increase in IgA and IgM. All sera gave precipitation reactions and showed neutralizing activity. There were higher precipitin titres in the cholera patients. IgG is involved in antitoxic activity and IgM and IgG in vibriocidal activity in which IgM predominates. IgA and IgG are found in the stools of monkeys infected with cholera and IgA plays a major part in the mechanism of immunity within the bowel via coproantibody.[32]

CLINICAL FEATURES

Natural history

Most cholera infections are asymptomatic resulting in an acute carrier state with or without a short attack of diarrhoea, but in a minority of cases depending on the size of dose and immune response of the host, infection results in the rapid onset of an acute secretory diarrhoea with loss of fluid and electrolytes from the body and death from dehydration or a rapid recovery and rapid return to health.

The *incubation period* is 3–6 days.

Symptoms and signs

Description of the average case

The onset is sudden. When florid cholera sets in as a painless diarrhoea, profuse watery stools at first faecal in nature pour one after the other from the patient. Quickly the stools lose their faecal character, becoming colourless, or rather like thin rice or barley water, later containing small white flocculi in suspension. Enormous quantities of this material are generally passed. Presently vomiting, also profuse, at first perhaps of food, but very soon of the same rice-water material, supervenes. Agonizing cramps attack the extremities and abdomen; the implicated muscles stand out like rigid bars or are thrown into lumps from the violence of the contractions (due to depletion of chlorides and hypocalcaemia affecting the neuromuscular junction). The patient may rapidly pass into a state of collapse. In consequence, principally of the loss of fluid by the diarrhoea and vomiting, the soft parts shrink, the cheeks fall in, the nose becomes pinched and thin, the eyes sunken, and the skin of the fingers shrivelled like a washerwoman's (Fig. 13.1). The surface of the body becomes cold, livid and bedewed with a clammy sweat; the urine and bile are suppressed; respiration is rapid and shallow; the breath is cold and the voice is sunk to a whisper. The pulse soon becomes thready, weak and rapid; then, after coming and going and feebly fluttering, it may disappear entirely.

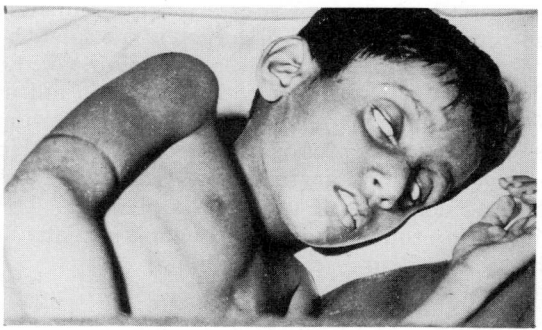

Fig. 13.1 Dehydration and collapse in cholera.

The surface temperature sinks several degrees below normal, 33.9–34.4°C, whilst that in the rectum may be several degrees above normal, 38.3–40.6°C. The blood pressure is low. The systolic may register 50 mmHg but is frequently unregistrable. The patient is now restless, tossing about uneasily, throwing his arms from side to side, feebly complaining of intense thirst and of a burning feeling in the chest; severe muscle cramps caused by hyponatraemia or hypokalaemia are a common feature. Although apathetic, the mind generally remains clear but sometimes the patient may wander or may pass into a comatose state.

This, the 'algid state' of cholera, may terminate in one of three ways—in death, in rapid convalescence or in febrile reaction.

When death from collapse supervenes it may do so at any time from 2 to 30 hours from the commencement of the seizure, usually in from 10 to 12. On the other hand, the gradual cessation of vomiting and purging, the reappearance of the pulse at the wrist, the increase of blood pressure and the return of some warmth to the surface may herald convalescence. In such a case, after many hours' absence, secretion of urine returns, and in a few days the patient may be practically well again. Usually, however, a condition known as the 'stage of reaction' gradually supervenes on the algid stage.

Anuria is accompanied by congestion of the mucous membranes and conjunctivae, malar flush, delirium and gradual increase in depth and rate of respiration. Recovery is marked by the passage of a few millilitres of turbid, highly coloured urine and this is followed by a 'critical diuresis' resembling that seen in some cases of acute glomerulonephritis.

Renal failure in cholera has been compared to anuria following crush injuries. The blood urea is invariably raised and may reach 350 mg. Anuria may persist for 50 hours and the patient may yet recover. When the patient passes one litre of clear urine in 24 hours the danger of relapse has usually passed. According to the modern school of physiological thought the main factor is *renal anoxia*.

The importance of charting the amount of urine, hour by hour, day by day, in the reactionary stage of cholera cannot be overemphasized. These data are essential if threatened anuria is to be successfully combated.

When the patient enters the reaction or cholera typhoid stage, the surface of the body becomes warmer, the pulse returns, the face fills out, restlessness disappears, urine is secreted and the motions diminish in number and amount becoming bilious at the same time. Coincidently with the subsidence of the more urgent symptoms of the algid stage and this general improvement in the appearance of the patient, a febrile condition of greater or less severity may develop. Minor degrees in this reaction generally subside in a few hours; but in more severe cases the febrile state becomes aggravated, and a condition in many respects closely resembling typhoid fever, 'cholera typhoid', ensues.

Hyperpyrexia is an occasional, though rare, occurrence in cholera. In such cases the axillary temperature may rise to 41.7°C and the rectal temperature perhaps to 42.8°C. These cases also are almost invariably fatal.

In cholera there is a considerable variety in the character of the symptoms and in their severity, both in individual cases and in different epidemics. It is generally stated that the earlier cases are the more severe, those occurring towards the end of the epidemic being on the whole milder.

Ambulatory cases occur during all epidemics, characterized merely by diarrhoea and malaise.

Cholera sicca

A very fatal type is known as 'cholera sicca'. In these cases though there is no, or very little, diarrhoea or vomiting, collapse sets in so rapidly that the patient is quickly overpowered as by an overwhelming dose of some poison.

For the effects of cholera on the eye, see Chapter 70.

Complications

The common complications are persisting enteritis, diarrhoea, corneal ulcers, cholecystitis and abortion in pregnant women. Pneumonia is common in the colder countries but rare in hot ones. Gangrene of the extremities, penis and scrotum, formerly observed, is seldom seen nowadays. Cerebrovascular accidents may occur in the elderly.

Clinical pathology

Loss of fluid and salts

The total loss of fluid may exceed 10 litres in 24 hours. The salt content of the stools in the rice-water stage is about 0.5–1%. There is considerable loss of alkaline bases in stools which disturbs the osmotic balance and leads to acidosis. The vomits are usually less in volume than the stools and in contrast they are acid and contain a lesser amount of salt.

Blood changes

The loss of fluid may be more than 60% in fatal cases. The plasma specific gravity is elevated. There is haemoconcentration with red cell counts of 6×10^{12}/litre and over. Leukocytosis is usual in cholera, the counts being 20×10^9/litre in some. The percentage of neutrophil leukocytes is increased to 80% or over, compared with the normal 68%, while the number of lymphocytes is diminished. This increase is more than can be accounted for by the concentration of the blood. The protein content of the blood is increased in the acute stage of cholera.

Blood urea

There is a definite rise of blood urea in all patients from the time of onset of the attack. The urea increases progressively but falls fairly rapidly in patients during recovery. In the acute stage it varies from 28 to 125 mg/dl with an average of 62 mg (compared with the normal of 15–35 mg).

Circulatory failure

The profound circulatory failure which is such a feature of cholera is not of central but of peripheral nature. The loss of body fluid is, of course, a factor but the distribution of the blood plays a much more important role in the circulatory changes which occur. The arteries and capillaries are empty and the veins engorged in the splanchnic area. The effective circulatory volume of the blood is very much reduced. There is a fall in blood pressure as the result of loss in circulating fluid, the systolic pressure being often 70 mmHg or lower on admission to hospital. In severe cases there is no measurable diastolic pressure. The circulation time is lengthened owing partially to the increased viscosity of the blood.

Sequelae

Sequelae are rare and usually limited to debility. Cholera in pregnancy usually leads to abortion. The prognosis of cholera is especially bad in opium addicts.

DIFFERENTIAL DIAGNOSIS

Differential diagnosis of food poisoning from cholera is based upon the violent and distressing vomiting which precedes the diarrhoea of food poisoning, the severity of the pain and the greenish, offensive nature of the stools. The urinary flow is never suppressed, whilst the axillary temperature is raised. Enterotoxic strains of *Escherichia coli* which cause 'non-vibrio cholera' and *V. parahaemolyticus* infections can produce a very similar picture.

Algid or choleraic subtertian malaria may

simulate true cholera very closely (see Chapter 1). Acute bacillary dysentery may occasionally be so sudden and severe in its onset as to resemble cholera. Acute trichinosis is distinguished by leukocytosis and pronounced eosinophilia. Children suffering from cholera sometimes develop hyperpyrexia with cerebral manifestations which may be mistaken for meningitis.

DIAGNOSIS

During the height of the epidemic the diagnosis of cholera is generally easy; the profuse rice-water discharges, shrivelled fingers and toes, feebly husky voice, cramps and suppression of urine, together with the high rate of mortality, are generally sufficiently distinctive. But in the first cases of some outbreaks of diarrhoea which may or may not turn out to be cholera and the true nature of which, for obvious reasons, it is important to determine, correct diagnosis is not so easy. Control measures should be applied if the clinical evidence is suggestive without waiting for bacteriological confirmation.

In the first place stools should be examined microscopically. If vibrios are present in large numbers they may be detected by their scintillating rotatory movements in hanging-drop preparations or by their characteristic shape in faecal films stained by carbol fuchsin. They may be diagnosed in the field with a McArthur microscope and dark field and identified by rapid slide agglutination (see p. 260). Rectal swabs are useful for diagnosis especially in an epidemic.

In an autopsy on a suspected case of cholera at least two sections of the small gut, each about 13 cm in length—one just above the ileocaecal valve and the other in the middle of the ileum—should be ligated, cut off, dropped into sterile saline and sent to a bacteriological laboratory for examination as soon as possible.

Identification of cholera vibrios

It is important that vibrios be identified correctly before making a diagnosis and there are a number of related vibrios which can only be distinguished from cholera by serological, agglutination, haemagglutination tests and the ability to haemolyse red cells. (For details a textbook of bacteriology should be consulted.)

Identification in the field

It is important that stool samples are collected in the field before treatment with an antimicrobial drug, and are transferred to the laboratory for identification in the correct manner.[33]

Collection of specimens

Stool samples are collected before any antimicrobial treatment has been given with a sterile no. 36 or no. 28 catheter, a glass rod or by means of a rectal swab directly and not from a pan which could be contaminated. The specimens so obtained should then be transported to a laboratory in special transport media if this is not close at hand.

Transport media

Transport media which also act as enrichment media may be:
1 alkaline sea salt fluid (Venkatraman Ramakrishnan (VR) medium);
2 Cary–Blair medium;
3 taurocholate–tellurite–peptone medium.

Positive slide agglutination

Vibrios may be tested with polyvalent cholera diagnostic serum in the field on a slide to give a provisional diagnosis before submitting them to more positive identification.

Isolation from water

Vibrios have been isolated from water by collecting 200 ml in screw-capped bottles to which 20 ml of a solution of 10% peptone and 5% sodium chloride were added. The pH was raised to 9 with N/1 sodium chloride, thymol blue being the indicator. After incubation overnight 2 ml amounts were added to 10 ml quantities of peptone water and after 6 hours one drop was placed on Aronson's medium. Several litres of water can be filtered through kieselguhr-impregnated filter paper. This is subsequently folded and placed in bismuth sulphite enrichment medium and incubated. It has been suggested that the fluorescent antibody technique could be used for the rapid detection of *V. cholerae* in water after concentrating the vibrios on membrane filters in the usual way.[34]

Serological tests

There are many laboratory tests for cholera.[35] Serological tests at present are useful only for retrospective diagnosis and may be of little value in a vaccinated or exposed population. They are, however, useful in measuring the results of vaccination.

Antibodies may be measured by a vibriocidal test, agglutination or haemolysis inhibition.

The vibriocidal test[36] is the most sensitive and has been used on paired sera of patients suspected of cholera and in surveys to determine the level of past experience and the current immune status of a community.

Antitoxin levels may be determined by a mouse protection test or by agar gel double diffusion technique against the supernatant of a vibrio culture.

Neutralizing antibodies may be determined by inoculating an isolated rabbit intestinal loop with the test sera and cholera enterotoxin.

TREATMENT

The aim of treatment is to restore the fluid and electrolyte balance of the body and remove the vibrios from the intestinal canal.[37]

Antimicrobial drugs

The administration of antimicrobial agents to which vibrios are sensitive shortens the duration of diarrhoea and the excretion of vibrios in the stools.

Good results were obtained with a mixture of dihydrostreptomycin, sulphadiazine and sulphamerazine, but streptomycin-resistant vibrios appeared shortly after the widespread application of the drug.

Tetracycline and chloramphenicol are equally effective whether administered orally or intravenously, causing a very rapid reduction in the number of vibrios in the stools. To ensure freedom from bacteriological relapses 500 mg of the drug should be administered about 3 hours after admission and then every 6 hours for 3 days. Tetracycline is valuable in the treatment of subclinical cases and carriers. Purging with magnesium sulphate has disclosed that some persons continue to harbour *V. cholerae* after such treatment.

Doxycycline in a single adult dose of 300 mg is as effective as tetracycline and has the advantage of a single dose treatment as well as being less expensive.[38]

Erythromycin is also effective but should be held in reserve in case tetracycline-resistant vibrios appear.

A combination of trimethoprim (10 mg/kg) and sulphamethoxazole (50 mg/kg) to a daily maximum of 390 mg trimethoprim and 1600 mg sulphamethoxazole (four tablets) in two equal doses for 4 days (not less) eliminated the vibrios,[39] and a single intramuscular injection of 2 g of sulphormethoxine has proved successful; it is circulated through the enterohepatic system.[40]

Dehydration and electrolyte replacement

Cholera patients require immediate replacement of fluid and electrolytes and correction of the acidosis even, if possible, before admission to hospital. Thereafter the fluid balance is maintained by replacing the fluid lost during treatment.

Methods of oral and parenteral rehydration in the management of acute infective diarrhoea are described in Chapter 12.

Maintenance phase

The measurement of the excreta is facilitated by the 'cholera cot' which is a bed with a hole in the middle under the patient's buttocks and a calibrated plastic bucket placed underneath to collect the excreta (Fig. 13.2). The total fluid lost is replaced plus 500 ml daily. Anuria often occurs and every effort must be maintained to re-establish the blood pressure. Promethazine chlorotheophyllinate 25–50 mg checks the vomiting.

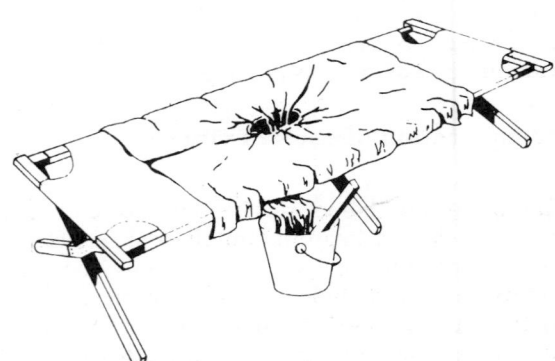

Fig. 13.2　A cholera bed.

Children

The treatment of cholera in children is more difficult. The initial fluid requirement cannot be calculated on the basis of plasma specific gravity and body weight so that the initial fluid requirement must be judged clinically. Acidosis and potassium deficiency may be of greater importance. A single replacement solution with which acidosis is corrected at the same time is used. A solution containing less sodium, such as half-strength Darrow's solution (see Chapter 72), is preferred nowadays to the Dacca solution.

Mortality rate

The death rate for cholera was always high. In former days in India it was seldom less than 70%. In the decade ending 1908 it was 54.2% in Indian and 78.5% in British troops in India. With improved methods of treatment it has declined considerably and cholera has now become one of the most effectively treated diseases. When treatment procedures are properly applied deaths are extremely rare. In children case fatality rates remained at 15–20% until the single replacement solution was used, when the rate fell to 0.6% in a series of 300 children under the age of 10 years.

Convalescence

A patient should not be discharged from treatment control unless there have been three negative stools or at least 3 days of treatment with an effective antibiotic at a dosage of 500 mg every 6 hours. Neither procedure guarantees the absence of vibrios in the body.

Carriers

Oral streptomycin,[41] tetracycline and long-acting sulphonamides have all been used with varying success in the treatment of carriers. Chemotherapy of carriers and contacts is used in the management of an epidemic.

Management of an epidemic

The basis of management in the short term is the treatment of cholera cases, carriers and contacts. Vaccination of the population is not useful during an epidemic.

The treatment of cholera cases should be organized (preferably in advance of arrival of the epidemic) in temporary hospitals built in the bush of temporary materials and on cholera beds. The provision of intravenous and oral fluids is arranged on a mass basis before the epidemic arrives. Proper attention to this organization reduces the mortality from 30% to 1%.

Treatment of carriers and contacts

Mass chemotherapy of contacts and carriers has been undertaken with varying success. Tetracycline failed to eradicate cholera and mass chemotherapy is not justified.[42] On the other hand adequate tetracycline therapy can prevent cholera.[43] Long-acting sulphonamide (sulphadoxine) given to those who develop diarrhoea and direct contacts of cases can reduce the infectivity of persons and reduce the severity of clinical manifestations.[44] Both sulphadoxine (one dose) and tetracycline in divided doses for 3 days reduced the transmission of cholera among family contacts and chemoprophylaxis can be of limited usefulness in highly endemic areas.[38]

EPIDEMIOLOGY

Cholera may be endemic or epidemic.

Endemic cholera

True endemic areas of cholera are found in Bangladesh (and historically in the Yangtze valley in China and, at the present time, certain parts of Asia and Africa and an area in the south-eastern USA.[13] The definition of an endemic zone is difficult but has been described as one in which the total number of months with absence of cholera cases does not exceed 30 in 32 years or one in which a break of five or more months in the incidence of cholera does not take place. These endemic areas are related to certain water systems near the coast at low level and are densely populated.[45]

In the endemic areas temperature and relative humidity are the main determining factors. In January when relative humidity is low and the temperature at its lowest, cholera is at its lowest ebb to rise with the temperature until the monsoon sets in in May or June. Rogers believed that the condition necessary for the spread of cholera in India was a relative humidity of over 40% and that by watching the climatic conditions the annual incidence of cholera and the onset of epidemics could be foreseen so that steps could be taken in time to lessen its spread.

Mechanisms of maintenance of infection in endemic zones[23]

Four mechanisms are possible.
1　Maintenance in an animal reservoir (none has ever been shown).
2　Maintenance in chronic carriers in the population (these are rare and probably excrete non-pathogenic vibrios.
3　Continuous transmission of vibrios in the community at low level (stool cultures have shown long periods without any carriers or many different phage types of vibrios).
4　Maintenance of *V. cholerae* in aquatic reservoirs (see p. 261), which is probably the main reservoir of infection in endemic cholera from which infection can be introduced to the population from eating inadequately cooked seafood. This may be called primary transmission. Secondary transmission occurs from man to man by contaminated water, food or some other faecal–oral route.[23]

Epidemic cholera

Epidemic cholera can arise in areas where primary transmission is not possible but where secondary transmission occurs because of poor sanitation and hygiene.

Spread of cholera

Cholera follows the great routes of human intercourse and is conveyed by man from place to place. In India and Arabia during religious gatherings hundred of thousands of people used to be collected together under highly insanitary conditions, as at the Hardwar and Mecca pilgrimages. Cholera broke out among the devotees who, when they separated and proceeded home, carried the disease along with them, infecting the people of places they passed through. The Hedjaz has for the past 100 years been the point of relay of cholera in its progress from the Far East towards the West. During that period there have been more than 27 outbreaks. In India cholera spreads from its home in lower Bengal over the northern, western, central and southern provinces in a series of waves of two to four years' duration. Cholera never travels faster than a man

can travel but, in modern times owing to the increased speed of locomotion and the increased amount of travel, epidemics advance more rapidly and pursue a more erratic course than they did formerly. On the other hand isolated countries such as the Andaman Islands, Australia and New Zealand have so far escaped. An epidemic of considerable virulence occurred in Celebes (Indonesia) in 1938. Cholera broke out in Bengal in 1947 and in the autumn months an epidemic of considerable proportions raged in the Delta of Egypt. Centres of less importance are Burma and the Philippines.

Pandemics

From a study of the great pandemics it can be concluded that cholera has reached Europe by three distinct routes:
1　via Afghanistan, Iran, the Caspian Sea and the Volga river;
2　via the Persian Gulf, Syria, Asia Minor and Turkey in Europe; and
3　via the Red Sea, Egypt and the Mediterranean. The world incidence since 1923 is well described by Swaroop and Pollitzer.[45]

El Tor cholera

The cholera of the great pandemics of the past was caused by the classical *V. cholerae*. Since the 1970s the epidemics and pandemics have been caused by the El Tor vibrio which shows considerable epidemiological differences from classical cholera. The El Tor vibrio is a tougher organism, creates a wider spectrum of disease with more mild cases and a higher carrier rate. Classical cholera is thought to be spread mainly by water but El Tor cholera spreads more by person-to-person contact, clothes and sweat in overcrowded conditions, during which a high rate of infection builds up until practically the whole population are carriers. The disease spreads in the dry season in large epidemics.[46]

　In 1961 El Tor cholera spread from an endemic focus in the Celebes and by 1965 had invaded 23 countries, among them countries from which cholera had been absent for many decades. El Tor cholera spread as far as Iran and the USSR. In 1970 El Tor cholera spread again as far as the southern part of the USSR and North Africa and appeared for the first time in the twentieth century in Africa south of the Sahara, where it is now endemic in West Africa and has occurred in the southern Sudan, Uganda, Kenya, Zimbabwe, Angola and Mozambique. It has reached Europe and the Pacific Islands and is endemic on the Gulf coast of Louisiana in the southern USA. El Tor cholera has been spread by land often by smugglers and by sea by small coastal vessels.

CONTROL OF CHOLERA

It is now practical to distinguish between primary and secondary transmission and the long-term aim should be to prevent primary transmission by removal of contaminated seafood from the diet or thorough cooking. Most control measures are aimed at preventing secondary transmission but without much success[8] and the methods used to date have been quarantine, control of water supplies and sanitation. Prophylactic vaccination has not proved adequate.

Quarantine

Quarantine can never be an efficient protection against the introduction of cholera since cholera carriers may be intermittent excretors. The tendency of cholera caused by the El Tor vibrio to create endemic foci in various parts of the world is of great importance. It is due to the existence of carriers and to the fact that vaccines in use at present do not confer a sufficient degree of immunity to protect a community in the absence of adequate environmental sanitation and other anticholera measures. Early and reliable reporting of cholera is a moral and legal obligation for every state.

Sanitation

Long-term control has been achieved with a combination of improved water supplies and sanitation.

Control of cholera can only be obtained by the investigation and surveillance of all enteric and diarrhoeal diseases and the construction of sanitation facilities to keep pace with social and industrial development and with the growth of tourism and trade. During the great religious festivals the sanitary condition of the devotees must be looked after as far as possible, special care being given to provide them with good drinking and bathing water.

Water supplies

For chlorination the usual residual free chlorine is 1–2 parts in 5 million or 2.7–5.4 kg of bleaching powder per 5 million litres. Potassium permanganate at a dilution of 1:500 000 (faint purple colour) kills cholera vibrios in a short time. This dilution is obtained by adding 454 g to each 250 000 litres. In a well of 9000 litres the amount would be 15 g. The mixture should be made in a bucket first and thoroughly mixed with the well water.

Prophylactic vaccination

The immunity produced by vaccination does not seem to be very persistent, lasting at the maximum for three or four months.

Most workers are now sceptical as to the role of vaccination and the WHO have now stated that international certificates of vaccination are not necessary for travel. Three main types of vaccine are used:
1 agar-grown phenol-killed (Kasauli);
2 formol-killed freeze-dried (Walter Reed);
3 phenol-killed grown on casein hydrolysate (Haffkine).

Vaccines prepared with classical vibrio strains are effective against both classical and El Tor biotypes. WHO requirements for cholera vaccine are 4000 million organisms/ml but it has been recommended that no vaccine should contain less than 8000 million per ml.

The usual dose is 0.5 ml of 4000×10^6 each of killed cholera vibrios of Inaba and Ogawa serotypes followed 7–28 days later by 1 ml of the same. An El Tor component is not necessary. Undesirable reactions have been observed among adults from endemic areas who have circulating antibodies and among those who have had repeated booster doses. Intradermal injections of 0.1 ml should be considered for boosters as they are less reactogenic (Chapter 71). Cholera may be combined with TAB vaccine as TABCho vaccination. Since vaccination can hardly be considered as satisfactory with the vaccine employed at present, oral vaccination has again become of interest, especially after its success in poliomyelitis. If an organism with strong immunogenicity could be found with no tendency to become virulent, oral vaccination might well become an efficient form of control using live vaccines.

Cholera toxoid vaccines have proved to be of no practical value.

Vaccination with two doses of parenteral vaccine gives 50% protection for three months and reduces the incidence of symptoms but not the severity. The protective effect probably relies on short-lived IgA coproantibody secreted in the bowel. The larger the dose of vibrios reaching the small intestine the greater the susceptibility, the shorter the incubation period and the more severe the symptoms. Gastrectomized people are at greater risk but previous experience of live organisms and parenteral vaccine all exert some effect.

NON-O GROUP 1 *V. CHOLERAE* VIBRIOS

GEOGRAPHICAL DISTRIBUTION

Cases of gastroenteritis caused by non-0 group 1 *V. cholerae* vibrios have been reported from the USA[47] and Italy.[48]

AETIOLOGY

Non-O group 1 *V. cholerae* vibrios are associated with a marine environment and are attached to crustacea, especially oysters.

TRANSMISSION

Because of their association with crustacea, infection is acquired from eating raw seafood, especially oysters.

PATHOLOGY

Non-O group 1 *V. cholerae* do not produce an enterotoxin except on rare occasions[47] and the pathology of the diarrhoea is not clear.

CLINICAL FEATURES

The *incubation period* is half an hour to 5 days.

Symptoms and signs

The illness caused consists of a short self-limiting attack of gastroenteritis lasting from one hour to 5 days. Fever, abdominal cramps and diarrhoea with, on very rare occasions, blood and mucus in the stools (cytotoxin-producing strains).

TREATMENT

All the strains isolated were sensitive to tetracycline, chloramphenicol, kanamycin and cephalothin.[47]

NON-O GROUP VIBRIOS

Non-O group vibrios are part of the bacterial flora of plankton and chitinous copepods in a marine environment. They possess an enzyme, chitinase, which allows them to be absorbed on to the chitinous surfaces.[49] They can be cultured on thiosulphate–citrate–bile salt (TCBS) medium and haemolytic strains are pathogenic to man.

Vibrio parahaemolyticus

GEOGRAPHICAL DISTRIBUTION

V. parahaemolyticus is a common cause of summer diarrhoea in Japan and is common in Malaysia,[50] Calcutta and Bangladesh.

AETIOLOGY

V. parahaemolyticus can be isolated by the same media and methods as for cholera vibrios (see p. 267) but can be distinguished from *V. cholerae* by the large characteristic green colonies on TCBS in contrast to the yellow sugar-forming colonies of *V. cholerae*.

TRANSMISSION

It is transmitted by ingestion of raw shellfish in most cases but can also cause local infection of abraded skin which has been in contact with sea water.

PATHOLOGY

An enterotoxin is produced which causes watery diarrhoea but some strains produce a heat-stable cytotoxin which renders them invasive and causes the dysenteric form. The cytotoxin is closely allied to Shiga toxin.[27]

CLINICAL FEATURES

There are two main forms, one a secretory diarrhoea (some cases of traveller's diarrhoea are caused by *V. parahaemolyticus*) and the other a dysentery with blood and mucus in the stools.

The *incubation period* in the secretory diarrhoea form is 20–24 hours and shorter in the dysenteric form—2–3 hours. In both forms there are diarrhoea, abdominal cramps, vomiting and fever and the illness lasts about 3 days.

Cutaneous infection

Some cases of infected abrasions following contact with sea water have been due to these organisms.

TREATMENT

V. parahaemolyticus responds to tetracycline. Rehydration therapy is seldom necessary.

Other non-O group vibrios

Other non-O group vibrios are *Vibrio damsella*, *V. hollisae*, *V. fluvialis*, *V. alginolyticus*.

V. damsela is an important pathogen of the damsel fish and has been isolated from infected wounds acquired in salt or brackish water.[51]

V. hollisae caused diarrhoea and abdominal cramps and in one case bloody diarrhoea in people who had eaten raw shellfish.[51]

V. fluvialis has been isolated from cases of gastroenteritis.[51]

V. alginolyticus has been found to be important in acute diarrhoea in man.[52]

REFERENCES

1 Blake, P.A., Weaver, R.E. & Hollis, D.G. (1980) *Ann. Rev. Microbiol.* **34**, 341–367.
2 Davis, S.R., Fanning, R., Madden, J.M. et al (1981) *J. clin. Microbiol.* **14**, 631–639.
3 Lee, J.V., Shread, P., Furniss, A.L. et al (1981) *J. appl. Bacteriol.* **50**, 73–94.
4 Snow, J. (1849) *On the Mode of Communication of Cholera.* London.
5 Samadi, A.R., Shahid, N., Eusof, A. et al (1983) *Lancet* **i**, 805–807.
6 Felsenfeld, O., Freeman, L. & Moorig, V.L. (1955) *Am. J. trop. Med. Hyg.* **4**, 318.
7 Feachem, R.G. (1981) *Trop. Dis. Bull.* **78**, 865–880.
8 Feachem, R.G. (1982) *Trop. Dis. Bull.* **99**, 1–47.
9 Hornick, R.B. et al (1971) *Bull. N.Y. Acad. Med.* **47**, 1181.
10 Nalin, D.R., Levine, M.M., Rhead, J. et al (1978) *Lancet* **ii**, 859.
11 Pollitzer, R. (1959) *Cholera.* Geneva: World Health Organization.
12 McIntyre, R.C., Tira, T., Flood, T. et al (1979) *Lancet* **i**, 311.
13 Shandera, W.X., Hafkin, B., Martin, D.L. et al (1983) *Am. J. trop. Med. Hyg.* **32**, 812–817.
14 Nalin, D.R. (1976) *Lancet* **ii**, 958.
15 Baine, W.B., Mazzotti, M., Greco, D. et al (1974) *Lancet* **ii**, 1370.
16 Merson, M.M., Black, R.E., Khan, M. et al (1980) In *Cholera-related Diarrhoeas: Molecular Aspects of a Global Health Problem*, eds. O. Ouchterlong & J. Holmgren, pp. 34–35. Basel: Karger.
17 Dodin, A. & Felix, H. (1972) *Bull. Acad. natn. Med.* **156**, 845–852.
18 Isaacson, M. & Smit, P. (1979) *Prog. Water Tech.* **ii**, 89.
19 Nalin, D.R., Robbins-Browne, R., Levine, M.M. et al (1980) *Proc. 11th Int. Cong. Chemotherapy and 19th Int. Conf. Antimicrobiol Agents and Chemotherapy*, eds. J.D. Nabon & E. Grassi, pp. 936–937. Washington: American Society of Microbiology.
20 Sen, R., Sen, D.K., Chakrabarty, A.N. et al (1968) *Lancet* **ii**, 1012.
21 Bart, K.J. & Mosley, W.H. (1970) *Lancet* **ii**, 47.
22 Sigel, S.P. et al (1980) *Infect. Immunol.* **28**, 681–687.

23 Miller, C.J., Feacham, R.G. & Drascar, B.S. (1985) *Lancet* i, 261–263.

24 Finkelstein, R.A., Sobocinski, P.Z., Atthasampunna, P. et al (1966) *J. Immunol.* **97**, 25.

25 Carpenter, C.C.J. (1971) *Am. med. J.* **71**, 50–51.

26 Cash, R.A., Forrest, J.H., Nalin, D.R. et al (1970). *Lancet* ii, 549.

27 O'Brien, A.P., Chen, M.E. & Holmes, R.K. (1984) *Lancet* i, 7708.

28 De, S.N. (1961) *Cholera: Its Pathology and Pathogenesis.* Edinburgh and London: Oliver & Boyd.

29 Levine, M.M., Hoover, D., Berquist, J. et al (1979) *Trans. R. Soc. trop. Med. Hyg.* **73**, 3.

30 Felsenfeld, O. (1959) *Abstr. Rep. 1st Sci. Ass. Microbiol. India*, 8.

31 Felsenfeld, O., Felsenfeld, A.D., Greer, W.E. et al (1966) *J. infect. Dis.* **116**, 329.

32 World Health Organization (1969) *Wld Hlth Org. tech. Rep. Ser.* 414.

33 World Health Organization (1974) *Guidelines for the Laboratory Diagnosis of Cholera.* Geneva.

34 Chibrikova, E.V., Schurkina, I.I., Tabskov, P.K. et al (1962) *Zh. Mikrobiol. Epidem. Immunobiol.* **33**, 9.

35 Felsenfeld, O. (1964) *Bact. Rev.* **28**, 72.

36 Finkelstein, R.A. (1962) *J. Immunol.* **89**, 264.

37 World Health Organization (1967) *Wld Hlth Org. tech. Rep. Ser.* 352.

38 De S., Chaudhuri, A., Dutta, P., et al (1976) *Bull. Wld Hlth Org.* **54**, 177.

39 Gharagozloo, R.A., Naficy, K., Mouin, M., et al (1970) *Br. med. J.* iv, 281.

40 Bougrade, A., Duchessin, M., Kadio, A. et al (1972) *Med. Afr. noire* **19**, 93.

41 Forbes, G.I., Lockhart, J.D.F., Robertson, M.J. et al (1968) *Bull. Wld Hlth Org.* **39**, 381.

42 Bencic, C., Wittaksono, H., Hondro, S. et al (1976) *Trop. Doctor* **6**, 2.

43 McCormack, W.M., Choudhury, A.M., Jahangir, N.A. et al (1968) *Bull. Wld Hlth Org.* **38**, 787.

44 Baylet, R. & Diop, S. (1973) *Bull. Soc. Path éxot.* **66**, 54.

45 Swaroop, S. & Pollitzer, R. (1954) *Bull. Wld Hlth Org.* **12**, 311.

46 Felix, H. & Dodin, A. (1981) *Bull. Soc. Path. éxot. Filialis* **74**, 17–30.

47 Morris, J.G. Jr., Wilson, R., Davis, B.R. et al (1981) *Ann. intern. Med.* **44**, 656–658.

48 *Morbidity and Mortality Weekly Report* (1981) **30**, 374–375.

49 Kaneko, T. & Colwell, R. (1975) *Appl. Microbiol.* **29**, 269.

50 Jegathesan, M. & Paramasiuan, T. (1976) *Am. J. trop. Med. Hyg.* **25**, 201.

51 Morris, J.G. Jr, Wilson, R., Hollis, D.G. et al (1982) *Lancet* i, 1294–1297.

52 Carpenter, C.C. J. (1979) *New Engl. J. Med.* **300**, 39.

DIARRHOEA CAUSED BY BACTERIA
An Introduction to Chapters 14 and 15

Bacteria may secrete an enterotoxin causing a secretory diarrhoea with no cellular exudate or a cytotoxin causing dysentery with a cellular exudate and blood and mucus in the stool. Some secrete a mixture of both.

Organism	Secretory diarrhoea (enterotoxin)	Dysentery (cytotoxin)
Toxigenic *E. coli*	+ +	−
Enterotoxic *E. coli* (ETEC)		
Enteropathogenic (EPEC)	−	+ +
Shigella spp.	+ in early stages	+ +
Clostridium welchii (C)	−	+ +
Yersinia enterocolitica	+	+
Campylobacter	+	+
Non-typhoidal *Salmonella*	+	+ +
Bacterial food poisoning	+ +	−

Chapter 14
Bacteria Causing Diarrhoea

TOXIGENIC *ESCHERICHIA COLI* (ENTEROTOXIC AND ENTEROPATHOGENIC)

Toxigenic *E. coli* consists of two groups, entero-pathogenic (EPEC) and invasive, and entero-toxic (ETEC) and non-invasive.

GEOGRAPHICAL DISTRIBUTION

Toxigenic *E. coli* has a worldwide distribution and is an important cause of acute gastroenteritis in infants and traveller's diarrhoea in adults.

AETIOLOGY

Enteropathogenic *E. coli* (EPEC) produces a heat-stable cytotoxin almost identical to *Shigella* toxin and is invasive. Enterotoxic *E. coli* (ETEC) is non-invasive and produces a heat-labile entero-toxin almost identical to cholera toxin. Any one strain may produce one or more of these toxins.

TRANSMISSION

Infection is acquired by the oral route by eating contaminated food and less frequently by con-taminated water.

PATHOLOGY

EPEC, being invasive, causes damage to the mucosa with a local reaction of poly-morphonuclear leukocytes followed by micro-abscesses and ulcers. ETEC enterotoxin produces a similar effect to cholera toxin with reversal of the transfer of electrolytes and excretion of fluid into the bowel (see p. 262) but no mucosal changes.

CLINICAL MANIFESTATIONS

The majority of infections are short, self-limiting infections lasting 2–3 days causing traveller's diarrhoea in adults and acute gastroenteritis in infants. EPEC infections cause dysentery with bloody diarrhoea, tenesmus and marked fever. The stool contains red cells and pus cells, and the haemolytic uraemic syndrome has been reported (see p. 283). ETEC infections cause a secretory watery diarrhoea with cramps, nausea and vomit-ing without any blood or pus in the stools.

TREATMENT

The treatment is rehydration where necessary (see Chapter 12) and adjunct therapy including antibiotics where sensitive strains exist.

Traveller's diarrhoea (turista)

GEOGRAPHICAL DISTRIBUTION

Traveller's diarrhoea occurs worldwide but affects especially travellers to the Third World from temperate countries. No country is exempt and many names have been given to this form of diarrhoea; in Mexico it is called turista and this has proved a popular name. Shipboard diarrhoea is of a similar nature.

AETIOLOGY

Traveller's diarrhoea is most commonly caused by ETEC[1] in travellers of high socioeconomic status such as athletes, businessmen, diplomats and western tourists. Residents of Third World countries develop diarrhoea of a different aeti-ology: EPEC, rotavirus, Norwalk virus, *Cam-pylobacter*, *Shigella*, *Giardia*, non-O group 1 *V.*

cholerae and non-O group vibrios especially *V. parahaemolyticus*,[2] although these can also cause traveller's diarrhoea.

TRANSMISSION

Infection is acquired from eating food which has been contaminated by human hand; less usually from drinking water.

PATHOLOGY

Pathology is according to the type of organism causing the infection. ETEC produces pathological effects the same as cholera, while with EPEC and *Shigella* the pathology is that of dysentery.

CLINICAL FEATURES

Natural history

Traveller's diarrhoea is a self-limiting infection lasting 2–3 days, usually recovering without treatment.

The *incubation period* is short and the onset is within 48–72 hours after entering the country (in distinction to *Shigella* which does not appear until three weeks or more later). After a period of three weeks in the new environment further attacks are unlikely.

Symptoms and signs

The attack usually begins abruptly with mild abdominal colic and diarrhoea but in more severe cases there may be fever, chills, vomiting and pains in joints and muscles. Profuse diarrhoea and consequent dehydration leads to thirst and dehydration. The diarrhoea, particularly in a hot climate and in infants, can lead quickly to water depletion and heat stroke when so much fluid is lost by sweating, as well as by the bowel. The attack is usually over in a day or two but may last a week. The patient is little the worse for it, regaining intestinal stability and appetite very quickly.

DIFFERENTIAL DIAGNOSIS

Traveller's diarrhoea appears during the first three weeks after arrival in a country and usually there is only one attack in each location. Dysentery appears later after arrival at any time and there can be more than one attack.

DIAGNOSIS

Diagnosis is made on the characteristic history and symptoms. The stools must be examined for *Giardia* and cultured for *Shigella* and pathogenic *E. coli* but this takes time. The presence or absence of pus cells and red cells is important since this can affect treatment. An important point is that if trophozoites of *E. histolytica* are found in the stools they may be harmless commensals as they have been prevented from encysting by their rapid transit through the bowel and may not be the cause of the symptoms.

TREATMENT

In mild cases no treatment is necessary other than maintaining a good fluid intake using sweetened water and drinks. Alcohol must be avoided. Antimotility drugs such as Lomotil do have a soothing effect but are not recommended in Third World countries where they can have a deleterious effect since invasive pathogens are common. Kaolin and charcoal have been recommended to absorb toxins but actually have little effect. In severe cases rehydration therapy may be necessary and an oral rehydration solution (ORS) with glucose should be used (see Chapter 12, p. 256).

Drug treatment

Streptotriad (sulphodiazine) is sometimes very effective in ETEC infection. It should be given as two tablets twice daily until the diarrhoea stops. However, it should be given with caution since it encourages the development of drug-resistant enterotoxic strains.

Tetracycline is also very effective when the ETEC strain is sensitive; 250 mg four times a day should be given but not to pregnant women or children.

Drug prophylaxis

The use of drug prophylaxis is controversial and is useful only in those cases caused by ETEC which is tetracycline- and streptomycin-sensitive.

Streptotriad one tablet twice daily is undoubtedly effective.[3]

Doxycycline 100 mg daily was highly effective in preventing traveller's diarrhoea.[4]

Co-trimoxazole (Septrin) two tablets a day is highly effective.

Neomycin sulphate 375 mg twice daily may also be given.[5]

Drug prophylaxis must not be continued for more than three weeks and is only useful in travellers of high socioeconomic status, such as athletes, in whom peak physical fitness is required and in businessmen and diplomats, since indigenous inhabitants of Third World countries suffer from diarrhoea caused by other pathogens.

Personal prophylaxis

Personal prevention is paramount but is not easy to achieve. Care on the choice of food and drink, avoiding food which has not been thoroughly cooked and water which has not been boiled or sterilized with sterilizing tablets, even for cleaning the teeth. Fruits without thick skins or vegetables should not be eaten raw since they may have been grown fertilized with human manure.

Acute gastroenteritis of infants

This is one of the commonest diseases of young indigenous children in the Third World and is a major cause of mortality and morbidity.

AETIOLOGY

The commonest causes are EPEC, ETEC, rotavirus, *Campylobacter* and *Shigella*.

TRANSMISSION

The infection is acquired by mouth from faecal–oral contamination from the hands of mothers and foods prepared for weaning and, most important, the use of infant foods which are made up with contaminated water and administered in contaminated feeding bottles.

PATHOLOGY

The pathogenesis and pathology is described on p. 276.

SYMPTOMS AND SIGNS

The main effect on the infants—usually under the age of one year—is a severe diarrhoea with vomiting often leading rapidly to severe dehydration and death.

DIAGNOSIS

Examination of the stool is important, since the presence of red cells and pus cells will show an invasive organism is present (EPEC, *Shigella*, *Campylobacter*), while a watery stool will show that the cause is ETEC or rotavirus. The stool should be examined for glucose with a Clinistix and for fat using the Sudan dye. The presence of both glucose and fat suggests rotavirus.

TREATMENT

Treatment consists of rehydration (see Chapter 12) using oral rehydration with ORS or in severe cases parenteral rehydration.

Antibiotics

Where the pathogen is invasive with red cells and pus cells in the stools then an antibiotic is indicated (see Chapter 12, p. 257).

EPIDEMIOLOGY

Children

The age incidence of the various pathogens differs: two to 15 months for rotavirus and two to four years for *E. coli*. Many infants have six to eight episodes of acute diarrhoea per year and the morbidity and mortality are considerable.

The degree of infection rests upon certain protective factors; the gastric juice protects against all but a heavy inoculum, malnutrition can affect its secretion and achlorhydria is genetically controlled. Acute diarrhoeal diseases are endemic when the causes may be varied but epidemics occur when only one pathogen is present. Rotavirus, *E. coli* and *Shigella* are commonest in the hot weather while *Campylobacter* shows no variation.

Adults

Causes are similar to those in children except that rotavirus is seldom found. Traveller's diarrhoea (*E. coli*) occurs mainly in non-indigenous adults.

CONTROL

Breast milk

Breast milk contains substances which prevent the growth of *E. coli* and contain secretory IgA antibodies against *E. coli* and rotavirus;[6] the presence of these is short-lived but there is a continuing antiviral factor of unknown type. The practice of breastfeeding also prevents infection from contaminated artificial feeds.

Sanitation

In a heavily contaminated environment the provision of clean water does not have as much effect as was hoped, probably because water is obtained from many sources and the contaminated environment causes a high degree of oral–faecal transmission via food.

SHIGELLOSIS (BACILLARY DYSENTERY)

GEOGRAPHICAL DISTRIBUTION

Shigella spp. cause disease all over the world but the incidence and prevalence of infection are much greater in Third World countries where *S. dysenteriae* is the main pathogen, while *S. flexneri* and *S. sonnei* are more important in developed countries.

AETIOLOGY

Shigella spp. comprise four serogroups: *S. dysenteriáe*, *S. flexneri*, *S. boydii* and *S. sonnei*. Each group contains a number of serotypes except for *S. sonnei* which has only one. They can be differ-

entiated by biochemical and serological differences (Table 14.1).[7] *Shigella* spp. differ from *E. coli* in that they are non-motile, do not ferment lactose and are invasive.

TRANSMISSION

Man is the only host of *Shigella* except for some primates who are not important in the transmission chain. Methods of transmission are person to person, water, food (milk and ice cream) and flies.

Person-to-person transmission

This is the most important method of trans-

Table 14.1 Differentiation of *Shigella* spp. (after Keusch[7]).

	S. dysenteriae	*S. flexneri*	*S. boydii*	*S. sonnei*	*E. coli*
Ferments:					
Glucose	−	−	+	+	+
Lactose	−	−	−	− (late +)	+
Mannitol	−	+·	+	+	+
Grows on:					
Lysine decarboxylase	−	−	−	−	+
Ornithine decarboxylase	−	−	−	+	+
Motility	−	−	−	−	+
Gas from glucose	−	−	−	−	+
Serogroup	A	B	C	D	
	(serotypes 1–10)	(serotypes 1–6)	(serotypes 1–15)	(1 serotype)	

mission and accounts for the frequency of household cases in the family after the index case. *Shigella* is one of the 'gay diseases' being transmitted among homosexuals by anal–oral contact.

Water-borne

Community wide epidemics of water-borne shigellae have occurred when the water supply has been contaminated by sewage and on ships from contaminated water. Shigellae can survive for 3 days in salt water but generally they do not survive well in the environment.

Food

Shigellae can survive in various foods and have been recovered from milk products in optimum conditions after 30 days. Hospital epidemics have occurred from contaminated milk and ice cream.

Flies

The peak incidence of shigellosis correlates with the peak incidence of fly infestation in tropical countries and Shigellae have been isolated from the feet, vomit and faeces of flies which become contaminated after settling on dysenteric stools.

Source and dose of infection

Infective dose

Compared with cholera vibrios and *Salmonella* the infective dose of *Shigella* is very small so that if only a few survive the gastric juice they are still infective. As few as 10–100 viable *S. dysenteriae* organisms can produce symptomatic disease;[8] with *S. flexneri* and *S. sonnei* 10 000 organisms are necessary.[9] The source of infection may be symptomatic patients or carriers.

Symptomatic patients

Under epidemic conditions in dry desert countries where large collections of people are herded together in camps without adequate sanitation the presence of dysenteric stools in the open and numerous flies maintains a high level of infection. Stools may also contaminate fomites. Intense sunlight and heat destroy the dysentery bacilli so that if the stools dry up they will become sterilized.

Carriers

Carriers are important in more settled conditions and are either mild or convalescent cases who remain infective for a short period of time, usually a week or two only, or more chronic carriers who excrete shigellae intermittently over several months and who may be difficult to detect because of this. *S. dysenteriae* carriers tend to persist much longer than *S. flexneri* and tend to be ill, whereas *S. flexneri* carriers are usually well. The carrier state may occur in people without any history of dysentery. Chronic long-term carriers are important in epidemiology especially if they are food handlers. Detection is by repeated examination of the stools of food handlers.

PATHOGENESIS

Shigellae cause disease by their 'invasiveness', a capacity to invade and destroy the epithelial cells of the large intestine. All shigellae possess an exotoxin which has enterotoxic, cytotoxic and neurotoxic properties. This entotoxin is most manifest in *S. dysenteriae* and to a less extent in the other shigellae.[10]

The *enterotoxin* produces a secretory effect on the intestine similar to that produced by cholera toxin and is responsible for the watery (secretory) diarrhoea but whether by the same mechanism is uncertain.[11]

The *cytotoxin* binds to the cell surface and is transported to the cell interior where it inhibits protein synthesis[12] causing cell necrosis and dysentery.

The *neurotoxin* may be responsible for neurological complications in children but not in adults.

PATHOLOGY

The large bowel and sometimes the lower part of the ileum are affected. *S. dysenteriae* and some *S. flexneri* cause a severe acute colitis, while *S. sonnei* and *S. boydii* produce much milder lesions.

Acute colitis

The shigellae invade the epithelial cells of the mucosa where the primary lesions are in the solitary follicles. Here they multiply in the submucosa and lamina propria. The crypts become distorted and necrotic forming microabscesses which coalesce and spread to form ulcers. Long segments of the colon become covered by a large greyish membrane. Bleeding occurs from the ulcers giving rise to the 'red currant' jelly stools. Other lesions include small discrete nodular lesions with yellow crusted pock-like ulcers and small clearcut ulcers with well-defined edges, like those found in amoebic dysentery. (In shigellosis the whole mucosa is involved whereas in amoebiasis there are usually areas free of inflammation in between the ulcers.)

In *S. sonnei* and *S. boydii* and some *S. flexneri* infections there is a general catarrhal inflammation of the large bowel without haemorrhage except for a few flecks of blood in the stools.

Diarrhoea and dysentery

Two different types of diarrhoea are found in shigellosis; one a secretory diarrhoea found in the early stages of disease and which may be the only form found in mild infections, a result of the enterotoxic effect of the exotoxin, and the other a true dysentery with blood and mucus in the stools—the result of the cytotoxic effect.

The mesenteric glands may be enlarged and shigellae have been recovered from them in severe infections. In prolonged cases the bowel wall may become paper thin but perforation is rare. A late result may be a patchy chronic ulceration of the bowel but shigellae are not a cause of ulcerative colitis. Bacteraemia is very rare and the extraintestinal manifestations associated with *S. dysenteriae* infection have an immunological or toxic basis.

Immunopathological effects

There are a number of complications, the results of the formation and deposition of immune complexes: a leukaemoid reaction of the blood[13] proceeding on to a haemolytic-uraemia syndrome with or without disseminated intravascular coagulation with a severe microangiopathic haemolytic anaemia, thrombocytopenia, renal lesions[13] and loss of protein from the gut ulcers; Reiter's syndrome with conjunctivitis and urethritis resulting from the deposition of immune complexes in the joints with the production of a sterile arthritis, and destructive joint lesions[15]— 80% of these patients have the HLA-B27 tissue type. Other rarer complications are urticaria, rose red spots similar to typhoid spots,[16] infection of skin wounds and corneal ulceration,[17] vulvovaginitis,[18] appendicitis, splenic abscess, and in children meningitis, cerebral lesions and peripheral neuropathy.

IMMUNITY

There is no evidence of any natural immunity.

Acquired immunity

There is evidence of some acquired immunity. In the Second World War in North Africa before the appearance of sulphonamides, dysentery always broke out in troops freshly arrived from Britain but thereafter the incidence was sporadic. It seems therefore that some degree of immunity was acquired in spite of the fact that so many types of bacilli were identified there.[19] Infection with any one of these gave some protection against the others but the immunity was not solid and second attacks of dysentery are not uncommon.

Humoral antibodies

Antibodies to the lipopolysaccharide O antigen and neutralizing antibodies to the cytotoxin develop.

Haemagglutinating antibodies are found in the serum in over 60% of *S. dysenteriae* type 1 infections within 10 days of infection and persist for several months. An antibody response has been demonstrated by enzyme-linked immunosorbent assay (ELISA) specific to the lipopolysaccharide O antigen with elevated IgG antibodies lasting as long as 180 days.[20] Neutralizing antibodies to the cytotoxin were used in the past for treatment (dysentery antiserum). They were not bactericidal but neutralized the cytotoxin with a beneficial clinical effect.

Coproantibodies

Little is known about the formation of coproantibodies but local coproantibody must be important since a live streptomycin-dependent *S. flexneri* oral vaccine has been used extensively in Yugoslavia which gave measurable protection.[21]

CLINICAL FEATURES

Natural history

Shigellosis is essentially a self-limiting disease and the clinical features vary from a short attack of watery diarrhoea lasting a few days to a severe dysentery with severe colonic damage causing death. Asymptomatic infections are not uncommon and can result in the carrier state.

Incubation period

The incubation period is between 2 and 7 days with a median of 5 days.

Symptoms and signs

The clinical effects depend upon the amount and proportions of the enterotoxin and cytotoxin in the toxin produced by the infecting organism. Most of the severe cases are caused by *S. dysenteriae* 1 and some strains of *S. flexneri*. *S. sonnei* and other *S. flexneri* strains cause only a mild illness, the main symptoms being a watery diarrhoea with no blood but some tenesmus lasting a few days. *S. sonnei* can cause a rapidly fatal infection in infants.

In the more severe cases caused by *S. dysenteriae* 1 and some *S. flexneri* the onset is more abrupt and the stools soon come to consist of little save bloodstained mucus. Griping and tenesmus may be severe with distressing dysuria. Fever is high and there may be a rigor. The face is pinched and the expression anxious; the patient may even become delirious and mentally confused. There is marked thirst.

Fulminating and gangrenous attacks are almost invariably due to *S. dysenteriae* 1. The onset is abrupt with chills or smart rigor, vomiting and rapid rise of temperature. The stools soon become excessively frequent, 20–60 in the day and are mucoid or mucopurulent with blood and occasionally sloughs of mucous membrane. Toxaemia is a feature as a result of absorption of the exotoxin.

The cheeks are flushed, the expression anxious, the pulse rapid and the tongue coated and yellow or dry and brown. Abdominal distension and hiccup occur. Muscular cramps and oliguria may develop as a result of dehydration due to loss of fluid, with dry shrivelled skin, collapsed veins, low blood pressure and peripheral failure of circulation. The urine contains albumin and granular casts and there may be retention of nitrogen. The patient is restless and may die in uraemic coma.

If the intestinal mucosa is extensively ulcerated there may be such loss of protein that hypoproteinaemia develops; this is always serious and may be fatal.[22]

Perforation with peritonitis may occur though it is rare. It demands immediate laparotomy. On the other hand chronic peritonitis may occasionally develop with effusion of serum into the peritoneal cavity and distension of the abdomen, tenderness and perhaps dullness in the flanks, flatulence, vomiting and colicky abdominal pain. This is accompanied by polymorphonuclear leukocytosis. The treatment is not surgical.

A choleraic form has been described in which the onset is acute with collapse and profuse watery stools, later containing blood. This form is usually fatal.

There is a moderate polymorphonuclear leukocytosis which in a substantial minority of cases leads to a leukaemoid reaction 5–10 days after the onset of the illness[13] which may precede the haemolytic uraemic syndrome described below. Sonnei infection in infants may be so severe that death results from toxaemia before any diarrhoea and with very little evidence of bowel symptoms.

SEQUELAE

Post-dysenteric colitis (irritable bowel syndrome)

In some cases loose stools persist for some time after recovery. Any dietetic indiscretion or period of tension will bring on an attack of diarrhoea with some colicky abdominal pain. The stools are loose but contain no blood; shigellae are never isolated from the stools and barium enema and sigmoidoscopy reveal no lesions. This usually clears up after a period of six months but can lead on to a permanent irritable bowel syndrome.

Granular proctitis

A granular proctitis limited to the lower part of the rectum with the passage of blood and mucus in the stools can be diagnosed by protoscopy. It usually responds well to a steroid enema.

Stricture of the colon

Stenosis of the large bowel may follow a severe attack of *S. dysenteriae* dysentery and was not uncommon in the First World War when there was no adequate therapy. Megacolon occurs rarely.

COMPLICATIONS

Perforation

This is rare since the inflammation is confined to the mucosa. When it occurs the prognosis is bad.

Haemorrhoids

Haemorrhoids are common as a result of straining at stool and rectal prolapse may occur especially in malnourished children with dysentery.

Joint complications

Reiter's syndrome

This is a polyarthritis involving mainly the smaller joints with conjunctivitis, uveitis, mouth and penile lesions and a skin rash (keratoderma blennorrhagica) involving the palms of the hands and soles of the feet; 80% of patients are HLA-B27 tissue type. Reiter's syndrome can be progressive with destruction of the joints resulting in crippling disability.

Large joint arthropathy

A symmetrical sterile arthritis involving the large joints, mainly the knees and ankles, may occur in convalescence. The synovial fluid contains *Shigella* agglutinins in high titres. Prognosis is good with little disability.

Haemolytic-uraemia syndrome

The haemolytic-uraemia syndrome is an immune complex disease found in 13% of *S. dysenteriae* 1 infections. After a stormy and toxic onset with initial improvement, 7–10 days after onset there is a leukaemoid reaction with a severe haemolytic anaemia, thrombocytopenia, glomerulonephritis with uraemia and loss of protein from ulcers in the large bowel.

Other complications

Other complications are parotitis, and in children peripheral neuropathy. Effort syndrome may occur in adults.

DIAGNOSIS

Differential diagnosis

Differentiation has to be made from other causes of acute diarrhoea, cholera, toxigenic *E. coli*, *Campylobacter* and amoebiasis (Table 14.2). Other causes are dysenteric *Schistosoma mansoni* (eosinophilia and ova in stools), ulcerative colitis (chronic course) and carcinoma of the colon and rectum. *Shigella* dysentery tends to be an acute, short, self-limiting infection and the diagnosis is made by stool examination, stool culture or rectal swab.

Stool examination

In the early stages of the choleraic forms there may be just a watery stool but soon blood appears. The red currant jelly appearance of the stool and the exudate are characteristic. Macroscopically the stool consists almost entirely of blood and mucus with little or no faecal material (red currant jelly). In the exudate there is a preponderance of polymorphs which constitute over 90% of the cells intermingled with red cells. Macrophages are also present which since they are large and often contain red cells can be confused with *Entamoeba histolytica* trophozoites; however, they are non-motile, hyaline and contain vacuoles, fatty granules, red cells and even leukocytes. A further confusion is that in cyst passers trophozoites of *E. histolytica* may appear in the stools alongside the exudate of *Shigella* dysentery and thus confuse the issue. These trophozoites do not usually contain red cells. For the differentiation from *E. histolytica* infection, see Table 14.2.

Isolation of organisms

It is often difficult to isolate organisms in practice so a negative stool culture should by no means rule out the diagnosis of shigellosis. Shigellae are delicate organisms and stools should be cultured fresh. Rectal swabs are very useful. The stools can be preserved for transport in buffered 30% glycerol saline. Cultures can be made on both

Table 14.2 Differential diagnosis between *Shigella* (bacillary) and amoebic dysentery.

Bacillary dysentery	Amoebic dysentery
Acute disease with tendency to epidemic spread. 'Lying-down dysentery'	A chronic endemic disease. 'Walking dysentery'
Incubation period short: 7 days or less	Incubation period long: 20–90 days or more
Onset acute	Onset insidious
Pyrexia common	Pyrexia rare unless complicated
Complications: toxic arthritis, eye complications	Complications: hepatic and other abscesses, amoebiasis of skin, perforation
Tenderness over whole abdomen, more marked over sigmoid	Tenderness local, mostly over sigmoid, thickening of sigmoid, transverse colon and caecum
Ulcers on free edge of transverse folds of mucous membrane, distributed transversely to long axis of gut	Ulcers begin as small abscesses of submucosa in long axis of gut; flask-shaped
Ulcers serpiginous with ragged undermined edges communicating with other ulcers; bases of granulation tissue. Rarely perforate	Ulcers oval, regular, involving all coats; bases of black necrotic tenacious sloughs (Dyak-hair sloughs). Not uncommonly perforate
Mucous membrane hyperaemic and inflamed. Bowel wall not thickened	Mucous membrane not inflamed. Bowel wall thickened
Stools scanty in quantity but very frequent; bright blood red, gelatinous viscid mucus, odourless, 'red currant jelly'	Stools, faeces mingled with blood and mucus, offensive, smelling of decomposing blood. Generally copious
Tenesmus very severe	Tenesmus not usual
Stools, microscopic picture: numerous discrete red cells; polymorphs abundant, some macrophages. Few bacteria visible	Stools, microscopic picture: red cells numerous and in clumps; polymorphs and macrophages scanty. Large numbers of motile bacilli. *E. histolytica* trophozoites containing ingested red cells present
Leukocytosis present in early stages	Leukocytosis 10 000–25 000, with 70% polymorphs

MacConkey's and Salmonella–Shigella (SS) media. Suspected *Shigella* colonies are inoculated on to Kligler's iron agar, motility–indole–urea medium and Simmons' citrate medium. Accurate diagnosis can be made with specific agglutinating and specific typing antisera.

Serological diagnosis

Serology is not of much use. Agglutinins may appear 6–12 days after onset but often fail to appear. Haemagglutinating antibodies appear in 60% of *S. dysenteriae* infections within 10 days of infection and persist for months. An ELISA test demonstrated IgA, IgM and IgG antibodies specific to the lipopolysaccharide antigen of *S. dysenteriae* 1 from 10 days after infection lasting for 180 days.[20]

Sigmoidoscopy

Sigmoidoscopy is not justified in the acute stages when it can be dangerous. Proctoscopy can be very useful. In severe cases necrotic mucous membrane shows as a greyish or green membrane due to coagulation necrosis with areas of haemorrhage and intense inflammation. Bloodstained mucus or mucopus is present. In less severe cases

the mucosa bleeds readily and there are irregular superficial ulcers with mucopus. There may be small discrete nodular lesions with yellow crust, pock-like ulcers or small cleancut defined ulcers. In more chronic cases the ulcers resemble those of ulcerative colitis scattered over apparently normal mucosa.

TREATMENT

Treatment is based on three main lines: general, rehydration therapy and antimicrobial drug therapy.

General

The patient need not be nursed in full isolation but all stools should be disposed of in antiseptic utensils. Except in the mildest cases the patient should be confined to bed. For the first day or so no food should be given but ORS must be freely available because thirst develops rapidly as fluid is lost. Later the diet should be light and food should be taken in small amounts at short intervals until the patient's hunger demands satisfaction.

The patient may need a sedative such as

diazepam. For severe abdominal pain tincture of opium (0.6 ml) gives great comfort[23] but should be used sparingly in case it delays passage along the bowel. A hypodermic of morphine sometimes may be needed, but only if an antispasmodic has failed to give relief.

Rehydration therapy

Rehydration therapy may be needed since dehydration can occur rapidly with the choleraic forms. For oral and parenteral rehydration see Chapter 12, p. 256.

Antimicrobial treatment

Antimicrobial drugs shorten both the course of the clinical illness and convalescent excretion of the organism when an absorbable drug to which the isolate is sensitive is used.

Drug resistance

Over the last 25 years the problem of drug resistance has become severe and sulphonamides are no longer of much use. In India the commonest resistance pattern was resistance to ampicillin, chloramphenicol, streptomycin, sulphadiazine and tetracycline.[24] Resistance is due to a transferable factor composed of DNA, called a plasmid, which is rapidly transferable through all the *Shigella* strains and other gram-negative bacilli and has been disseminated round the world. There are three main different types of plasmid resistance and strains isolated from Central America, South-East Asia and Africa can be identified by their resistant plasmids.[25]

Choice of drug

When antimicrobial drugs were first introduced sulphonamides were very successful but now are of little use. The main drugs of choice are ampicillin, tetracycline (not in children), trimethoprim–sulphamethoxazole(Bactrim, Septrin), nalidixic acid and furazolidone.

The sensitivity pattern of the organisms isolated locally must be tested ideally. Therapy in an individual case is started before the results are available. In many hospitals in the tropics, of course, there are no facilities for sensitivity testing.

Ampicillin. The dosage is 500 mg four times daily for 5 days for adults and 100 mg/kg per day in four divided doses for children.

Tetracycline. The dosage is 500 mg four times daily for adults (not in children) for 5 days.

Trimethoprim–sulphamethoxazole. Two tablets should be given twice daily for 5 days for adults, and one to two tablets twice daily for children (two to five years).

Nalidixic acid. The dosage is 55 mg/kg in four divided doses per day for 5 days. (It should not be given to women in the first three months of pregnancy or patients with damage to the central nervous system or reduced hepatic function.) It may give a false-positive test for sugar in the urine.

Furazolidone. The dosage is 100 mg four times daily for 5 days; it is useful in ampicillin-resistant cases.

Chloramphenicol. This may be effective in some tetracycline-resistant strains.

Response to treatment

Where the organism is sensitive to the drug the response is rapid. In Nicaragua there is evidence that where *E. histolytica* trophozoites and colonic abscesses are found the disease is much more serious and does not respond to treatment until antiamoebic drugs, such as metronidazole, are used.[26]

Test of cure

Bacteriological tests of cure include three negative rectal swabs or faecal cultures examined a few days after the end of treatment. For food handlers six or even 12 negative bacteriological examinations are desirable.[27]

Treatment of carriers

Carriers are easily treated if the organism is sensitive to one of the antimicrobial drugs.

Treatment of complications

Granular proctitis. This is best treated with steroid enemas.

Haemolytic-uraemia syndrome. Peritoneal or haemodialysis will save some patients.

EPIDEMIOLOGY

Infection occurs year round with an increase in the summer in temperate areas with an increase in the fly population. The disease spreads rapidly in epidemics after being introduced to a concentration of people, such as in army camps, concentration, prisoner of war and refugee camps where sanitation is defective.

Adults are chiefly affected under these conditions but where the infection is endemic then infants and children account for the majority of cases and *Shigella* accounts for 10% of diarrhoeal disease in children in tropical areas.

CONTROL

Personal prevention consists of avoiding food (cooked or uncooked) which may have been contaminated by flies or the hands of infected persons and strict attention to kitchen hygiene and personal hygiene, such as washing the hands in soap and clean water after defecation. In homes and public lavatories fresh clean water should be available alongside the lavatory pan and in kitchens washing facilities should be close at hand. Cooks and food handlers should be fully instructed and subject to discipline. They must be suspended from work if suffering from diarrhoea and examined before returning to work.

Public prevention is the responsibility of the public health, hospital, military or other authorities, who should supply wholesome water, supervise food and markets, provide for disposal of human and animal wastes and suppress flies.

Immunization with an oral streptomycin-dependent strain has been used in Yugoslavia with some success.

CLOSTRIDIUM WELCHII (PERFRINGENS) INFECTION (PIGBEL, DARMBRAND, ENTERITIS NECROTICANS)

GEOGRAPHICAL DISTRIBUTION

Clostridium welchii (*perfringens*) infection is prevalent in New Guinea[28] where it causes 'pigbel' in the highlands and is an important disease. It also occurred in Germany after the Second World War where it caused 'Darmbrand' in malnourished people[29] and has been found in China[30] and Uganda.[31]

AETIOLOGY

Clostridium welchii (*perfringens*) type C is the cause. This organism is widely distributed in soil and in the stools of asymptomatic carriers and pigs and produces an exotoxin which is responsible for the manifestations of the disease.

TRANSMISSION

Infection is acquired by the oral route from infected pig meat. Although carriers are common there is no evidence for human-to-human transmission.

PATHOGENESIS

The exotoxin produced by *C. welchii* type C is readily destroyed by trypsin. A diet which consists of 90% sweet potato, low protein intake and is associated with the presence of trypsin inhibitors reduces the amount of trypsin available, which allows production of the toxin to proceed unabated[32] causing a severe necrotizing enteritis. Other factors in the causation are the presence of *Ascaris* infestation (with possible trypsin inhibitors) and dietetic factors which allow bacterial colonization of the small intestine.

PATHOLOGY

Enteritis necroticans is a segmental disease. The jejunum is mainly affected but the duodenum and occasionally the ileum and colon may be affected. Segments of the jejunum may be affected varying from a few centimetres to the whole length of the bowel. The outer coat of the bowel is covered with seropurulent exudate, the underlying wall being green and necrotic extending throughout the whole thickness of the bowel. The wall may become thin and perforate. Microscopically the bowel wall shows oedema, haemorrhage and polymorphonuclear infiltration. The mesenteric lymph glands are enlarged and later there may be histological evidence of healing and fibrosis.

IMMUNITY

There is little immunity but antitoxic antibodies are formed and these have been used successfully in immunization to control human disease.

CLINICAL FEATURES

Natural history

Pigbel is an acute infection varying from a short attack of diarrhoea with recovery to a rapidly fatal necrotizing enteritis. The mortality rate may be as high as 85%.

Incubation period

This is usually 48 hours but varies from 24 hours to one week after eating the infected material.

Symptoms and signs

Following a meal of pig meat there is fever followed by vomiting, abdominal pain and distension, and bloody diarrhoea with tarry stools. Dehydration, toxaemia and shock follow. The progress of the case varies; some cases are fulminating and die within 24 hours while others may be so mild as to suggest an attack of gastroenteritis. Examination of the abdomen usually reveals a palpable thickened segment of small intestine. A neutrophil leukocytosis is present.

DIFFERENTIAL DIAGNOSIS

Differential diagnosis is from acute gastroenteritis, food poisoning, peritonitis, acute intestinal obstruction, acute pancreatitis, acute amoebic colitis, liver abscess and abdominal sickle cell crisis.

DIAGNOSIS

The organism *C. welchii* (*perfringens*) type C can be demonstrated in the stool and small bowel contents with fluorescein-stained antibody.

Culture is also possible but difficult to interpret in an area where the carrier rate is 50–100%.

Straight X-ray of the abdomen may show gaseous distension and fluid levels.[33]

TREATMENT

Medical treatment with nasogastric intubation, intravenous fluids and electrolyte replacement is required.

Antimicrobial drugs

These have been used with benefit: chloramphenicol, ampicillin and penicillin in normal dosage.

Antiserum

Type C antitoxins have been found useful.

Surgical treatment

The indication for operation is persistent toxicity and evidence of intestinal obstruction. Resection of the affected bowel is the operation of choice but a bypass operation is thought to carry a lower mortality rate.[34] The mortality rate in these cases is high, between 15% and 85%.

SEQUELAE

In recovered patients jejunal stenosis may occur with subacute intestinal obstruction, fistulae and malabsorption.

EPIDEMIOLOGY

In Papua New Guinea pigbel is associated with pig feasts every few years when many pigs are slaughtered under unhygienic conditions and eaten partly raw. In Uganda the disease is not epidemic but sporadic. Males predominate since only they partake in feasts. Asymptomatic human infections are common but play no part in the epidemiology.

CONTROL

Clostridial toxoid prepared from type C cultures has proved successful[35] in immunization and a disease which has a high mortality is now largely preventable.

YERSINIA ENTEROCOLITICA

GEOGRAPHICAL DISTRIBUTION

Y. enterocolitica infection is worldwide but is becoming of greater importance in some tropical areas although it is still uncommon in Asia.[36]

AETIOLOGY

Y. enterocolitica is a small gram-negative coccobacillus which grows well on agar containing bile salts, is oxidase negative, does not ferment lactose and grows best at 25°C. The organism has a lipopolysaccharide endotoxin in its cell wall which produces an enterotoxin resembling that of *E. coli* (see p. 276) which is probably responsible for the diarrhoea, but the organism is also enteropathogenic and causes ulceration.

PATHOLOGY

Y. enterocolitica attacks the ileum, caecum and mesenteric lymph glands. The ileum becomes acutely inflamed with ulceration, and polymorphs appear in the stool. A feature is the presence of white nodules like tubercles in the ileocaecal region and mesenteric lymph glands. In some cases infection is followed by arthralgia and erythema nodosum of immunological origin.

TRANSMISSION

The natural reservoir of infection is farm animals, pigs, goats, dogs and cats. Man is infected from drinking water or food contaminated by animal faeces or fomites. Man-to-man transmission is extremely rare.

CLINICAL FEATURES

Natural history

The infection is a short-term self-limiting diarrhoea and is rarely diagnosed.

The *incubation period* is 4–10 days.

Symptoms and signs

The onset is with fever, abdominal pain and diarrhoea which varies from semisolid to watery or bloody stools. The abdominal pain is confined to the right lower quadrant.

COMPLICATIONS

Some patients develop arthritis or erythema nodosum and septicaemia can occur in immunodepressed persons.

DIAGNOSIS

Y. enterocolitica infection closely resembles acute appendicitis from which it must be distinguished since operation makes the condition worse. The organism can be isolated from the stool with difficulty and enrichment techniques are necessary. *Y. enterocolitica* can be identified by finding non-lactose-fermenting colonies giving an acid reaction without gas or hydrogen and urease positive.

Serology

Serology can be of use in differentiating the infection from acute appendicitis. There is a rise in agglutinin titres in paired sera; cross reactions are found with *Brucella*, *Vibrio* and *Salmonella*.

TREATMENT

Y. enterocolitica is sensitive to streptomycin, tetracycline, chloramphenicol and co-trimoxazole but resistant to the penicillins. Many cases are self-limiting and do not require antibiotic treatment.

EPIDEMIOLOGY

Since the reservoir is domestic animals infection is clustered in families or in groups of people sharing the same food or water. Spread through the community does not occur.

CAMPYLOBACTER

GEOGRAPHICAL DISTRIBUTION

Campylobacter is an important cause of enteritis the world over in both developed and Third World countries.

AETIOLOGY

Campylobacter jejuni, the cause of *Campylobacter* enteritis, is a motile oxidase- and catalase-positive curved gram-negative rod resembling a vibrio. It is a member of a large group of organisms and there are many serotypes but only *C. jejuni* and *C. intestinalis* have caused disease in man. It grows anaerobically on special media[35] which differentiates it from vibrios which are aerobic. Many strains of *C. jejuni* produce a heat-labile enterotoxin which is immunologically related to the enterotoxin of *V. cholerae* and enterotoxin *E. coli*[38] and has been prepared in purified forms.[39] So far no cytotoxin has been isolated but *C. jejuni* is also invasive.

TRANSMISSION

C. jejuni is an inhabitant of the gastrointestinal tract of a wide variety of wild and domestic animals and can be transmitted by animal to person, person to person, food, milk or water.

Animal to person. Pets are an important source of infection.

Person to person. An infected mother can transmit the infection to her children and epidemics can occur in children's hospitals and nurseries. *C. jejuni* is an important cause of infantile diarrhoea (see p. 278).

Food. Poultry is an important source of infection and food handlers are infected in this way similar to *Salmonella* except that *C. jejuni* does not multiply.

Milk. Raw milk has been responsible for some outbreaks.

Water. C. jejuni is commonly found in contaminated surface water and water-borne transmission is important in Third World countries.

PATHOLOGY

C. jejuni affects both the jejunum and ileum and the large bowel.

C. intestinalis can cause bacteraemia and a toxic shock syndrome and not enteritis.[40]

C. jejuni causes a secretory diarrhoea by reason of the enterotoxin. It is also invasive and causes large bowel ulceration with bloody diarrhoea (dysenteric form). Systemic infection is not uncommon and blood cultures taken at onset of the infection reveal *Campylobacter* bacteraemia although no metastatic lesions are found.

C. pyloridis has been suggested as a cause of duodenal ulcer (see Chapter 60).

IMMUNITY

Little is known about immunity. Second attacks of *C. jejuni* enteritis occur. IgA, IgM and IgG antibodies can be detected in 90% of patients suffering from *C. jejuni* enteritis[41] which appear and decline in the usual pattern of an acute infection. Poor antibody responses are found in prolonged infections.

CLINICAL FEATURES

Natural history

C. jejuni is an acute short-lived infection. Asymptomatic cases are very common and are the source of carriers but these do not become chronic. Most symptomatic cases present as an acute secretory diarrhoea lasting 2–3 days. Some develop dysentery with bloody diarrhoea and show a longer course.

The *incubation period* is 2–10 days, usually about 5.

Acute diarrhoea

The onset is sudden with abdominal pain and a secretory watery diarrhoea. There is little fever and no vomiting. After 2–3 days the diarrhoea disappears. In infants dehydration may be severe.

Dysenteric form

The onset is sudden with fever and severe abdominal pain resembling acute appendicitis or acute cholecystitis. The diarrhoea is bloody and resembles *Shigella* infection or ulcerative colitis. Proctoscopy or sigmoidoscopy may show ulcerative lesions in the rectum which on biopsy resemble *Shigella* infection.

DIAGNOSIS

The differential diagnosis is from cholera, ETEC and viral enteritides in the secretory diarrhoeal form and from *Shigella* infection, ulcerative colitis and other dysenteries in the dysenteric form.

Diagnosis is made by direct smear examination of the stool using 1% aqueous basic fuchsin which diagnosed 94% of cases and proved superior to culture (see Chapter 57, p. 938).[42] Isolation of the organism can be done by culture on special medium anaerobically.[37]

Serology is not of much use but has been employed in detecting carriers.

TREATMENT

Severe cases of acute secretory diarrhoea, especially in children, will need rehydration (see Chapter 12). The dysenteric form requires antimicrobial therapy. *Erythromycin* is specific, 500 mg three times daily for 5 days. *Doxycycline* 100 mg twice daily for 5 days is an alternative.

COMPLICATIONS

A reactive arthritis following the infection is found in about 1–2% of cases as in other bacterial diarrhoeas.

A haemolytic uraemic syndrome has been reported following *C. jejuni* infection similar to that found in *Shigella*.[43]

EPIDEMIOLOGY

The epidemiology resembles that of *Salmonella* except that the organism does not multiply in food or milk. *Campylobacter* enteritis is a zoonosis. The reservoir of infection is in wild and domestic animals. Contact with animals or animal products is an important feature of the epidemiology. Contact with animals includes pets and handling poultry. Poultry is the major source of *C. jejuni* infection in many countries. In Third World countries *C. jejuni* is an important cause of infantile gastroenteritis and is transmitted from person to person (see p. 289). Waterborne epidemics may be large and important in tropical countries.[44]

CONTROL

Control is similar to that of *Salmonella* with control of food hygiene and processing of animal products. Detection and treatment of carriers is important in control of children's infections. No protective vaccine is available.

REFERENCES

1 Rowe, B., Taylor, J. & Bettelheim, K. (1970) *Lancet* **i**, 1.
2 Ryder, R.W., Oquist, C.A., Greenberg, H. et al (1981) *J. infect. Dis.* **144**, 442–448.
3 Steffen R. & Gesell, O. (1981) *J. trop. med. Hyg.* **84**, 239–242.
4 Sack, R.B. et al (1984) *Am. J. trop. Med. Hyg.* **33**, 460–466.
5 Kean, B.H. & Waters, S.R. (1959) *New Engl. med. J.* **261**, 71.
6 Hanson, L.A., Ahlstedt, S., Carlsson, B. et al (1978) *Acta Paed. Scand.* **67**, 577–582.
7 Keusch, G. (1982) *Crit. Rev. trop. Med.* **1**, 77–108.
8 Levine, M.M., Du Pont, H.L., Formal, S. et al (1973) *J. infect. Dis.* **127**, 261–270.
9 Du Pont, H.L., Hornick, R.B., Dawkins, A.T. et al (1969) *J. infect. Dis.* **119**, 296–299.
10 Keusch, G.T., Grady, G.F., Takeuchi, A. et al (1972) *J. clin. Invest.* **51**, 1212–1218.
11 Flores, J., Grady, G.F., McIver, J. et al (1974) *J. infect. Dis.* **130**, 374–379.
12 Keusch, G.T. (1981) In *Receptor Mediated Binding and Internalisation of Toxins and Hormones*, ed. J. Middlebrook & L. Kohn, pp. 85–110. New York: Academic Press.
13 Rahaman, M.M., Alum, A.K. & Islam, M.R. (1974) *Lancet* **i**, 1004.
14 Koster, F., Levin, J., Walker, L. et al (1978) *New Engl. J. Med.* **298**, 927–933.
15 Calin, A. & Fries, J.F. (1976) *Ann. intern. Med.* **84**, 564–566.
16 Barrett-Connor, E. (1969) *Am. J. trop. Med. Hyg.* **18**, 555–558.
17 Roper, D.L. (1979) *Arch. Ophthalmol.* **97**, 888–889.

18 Murphy, T.V. (1979) *Pediatrics, Springfield* **63**, 511–516.

19 Boyd, J.S.K. (1957) *Trans. R. Soc. trop. Med. Hyg.* **51**, 471.

20 Lindberg, A.A., Haeggman, S., Karlsson, K. et al (1984) *Bull. Wld Hlth Org.* **62**, 597–606.

21 Mel, D.M., Arsic, B.L., Nicolic, B.D. et al (1968) *Bull. Wld Hlth Org.* **39**, 375.

22 Fairley, N.H. (1961) In *Recent Advances in Tropical Medicine*, ed. N.H. Fairley, A.W. Woodruff & J.H. Walters, 3rd edn. London: Churchill.

23 Rowland, H.A.K. (1967) *Med. Today* **1**, 29.

24 Arora, D.R., Midha, N.K., Ichhpujani, R.L. et al (1982) *Ind. J. med. Res.* **76**, 74–79.

25 Frost, J.A., Vandepitte, J., Row, B. et al (1981) *Lancet* **ii**, 1074–1076.

26 Vijil, C. (1971) *Lancet* **ii**, 823.

27 Christie, A.B. (1968) *Br. med. J.* **ii**, 285.

28 Murrell, T.G.C., Roth, L., Egerton, J. et al (1966) *Lancet* **i**, 217.

29 Zeissler, J. & Rassfield-Sternberg, L. (1949) *Br. med. J.* **i**, 267.

30 Shann, F., Lawrence, G. & Pan, Jun-Di (1979) *Lancet* **i**, 1083.

31 Musoke, L.K. & Sekabunga, J.G. (1972) In *Medicine in a Tropical Environment*, ed. A.E. Shapes, J.W. Kibukamusoke & M.S.R. Hutt, p. 395. London: BMA.

32 Lawrence, G. & Walker, P.D. (1976) *Lancet* **i**, 125.

33 Bassett, D. (1966) *Papua New Guinea med. J.* **i**, 267.

34 Smith, F. (1969) *Aust. NZ J. Surg.* **38**, 199.

35 Lawrence, G., Shann, F., Freestone, D.S. et al (1979) *Lancet* **i**, 227.

36 Butler, T., Islam, M., Islam, M.R. et al (1984) *Trans. R. Soc. trop. Med. Hyg.* **78**, 449–450.

37 Simmons, N.A. (1977) *Br. med. J.* **ii**, 707.

38 Ruis-Palacios, G.M., Torres, N.R., Ruis-Palacios, B.R. et al (1983) *Lancet* **ii**, 250–253.

39 Klipstein, F.A. & Enger, R.F. (1984) *Lancet* **i**, 1123–1124.

40 Van der Zwan, J.C. (1984) *Lancet* **i**, 449.

41 Kaldor, J., Pritchard, H., Serdell, A. et al (1983) *J. clin. Microbiol.* **18**, 1–4.

42 Park, C.H., Hixon, D.L., Dolhemus, A.S. et al (1983) *Am. J. clin. Path.* **80**, 388–390.

43 Chamovitz, N.B., Hartstein, A.I., Alexander, S.R. et al (1983) *Pediatrics, Springfield* **71**, 253–256.

44 Rogol, M., Sechter, I., Falk, H. et al (1983) *Eur. J. clin. Microbiol.* **2**, 588–590.

Chapter 15
Non-typhoidal *Salmonella* and Food Poisoning

NON-TYPHOIDAL *SALMONELLA*

GEOGRAPHICAL DISTRIBUTION

Salmonellae are found throughout the animal kingdom and cause human disease all over the world.

AETIOLOGY

Salmonellae are gram-negative non-spore-bearing bacilli which grow well on ordinary media and do not ferment lactose on Mac-Conkey's medium (non-lactose fermenters), although a strain of *S. typhimurium* has been found which does ferment lactose resembling *Escherichia coli*. They possess group specific somatic O antigens which divide *Salmonella* into a number of groups labelled A to Z and species specific flagellar H antigens indicating a number of serotypes. The somatic O antigen forms part of the *endotoxin* which is responsible for tissue damage and an *enterotoxin* is also produced which is responsible in part for the diarrhoea. There are a large number of different serotypes responsible for human salmonellosis which vary in different parts of the world. In the main, six types are responsible for most human disease. These are *S. typhimurium*, *S. enteritidis*, *S. thompson*, *S. newport*, *S. dublin* and *S. cholerae-suis*.

TRANSMISSION

Source of infection

Salmonella infects either animals or man. The main sources of infection are domestic poultry products (chickens, ducks, turkeys) and eggs (duck eggs especially), pigs and cattle. Animals become infected from the environment or food contaminated by other animals and transmit the infection among themselves during transport, while being held for market or at the abattoir.

Workers at abattoirs and food handlers become infected and transmit the infection.

Carriers

Half the symptomatic patients pass salmonellae in the stools for two weeks after onset and few remain positive for one month. A small number continue for longer, especially young infants. Chronic carriers who excrete organisms over one year are extremely rare.

Schistosomiasis and the carrier state

Adult schistosomes harbour salmonellae in their bodies where they are immune to the host's defence mechanisms. From here the *Salmonella* organisms invade the systemic circulation from time to time causing recurrent bacteraemia and a carrier state.

Infective dose

The infective dose varies widely for different *Salmonella* serotypes; 10^5–10^6 bacilli are normally required to produce symptomatic infection in adults. However, asymptomatic infection and some epidemics can be caused by lower doses. Achlorhydria from antacids, gastric surgery or drugs renders individuals more susceptible. In neonates the infective dose is lower because a reduced gastric acidity caused by frequent milk feeds favours infection but actual disease is less common since mothers secrete O and H antibodies in the milk which acts protectively in the gut. The incidence of *Salmonella* enterocolitis is also much reduced in breastfed infants because they are not exposed to the risks of bottle feeding.

Route of transmission

The route of transmission can be food, direct

human to human by faecal–oral contact or by other methods. Water-borne infection is rare.

Food

Food is the most important means of transmission. Commercially processed poultry is the commonest source in many 'developed' countries and eggs, meat, meat products, unpasteurized milk and milk products are also commonly to blame. Food may be contaminated at source; for instance, eggs infected from the hen's ovary or infected on laying passing through the cloaca, or during preparation when the working surface may be contaminated by one carcase and all the other carcases become infected.

Animals

Pets, dogs, cats, birds, turtles are all routes of infection.

Direct man-to-man transmission

Faecal–oral contact plays a large part in spreading infection in institutions such as children's and old people's homes. Neonates may be infected at birth and give rise to cross infection in an infants' ward. Since *Salmonella* can be found in the respiratory tract aerosol transmission is possible.

Other methods

Flies, cockroaches, other insects and contaminated medicines have all transmitted infection.

PATHOLOGY

The salmonellae localize and multiply in the ileum and colon where they may be adversely affected by the normal bowel flora, and antibiotics which inhibit the normal flora may reduce the dose of *Salmonella* necessary for infection. *Salmonella* does not cause disease when the organisms are localized to the lumen and they must penetrate the mucosa to cause symptoms. Salmonellae in proximity to the microvilli cause them to degenerate together with the apical cytoplasm of the enterocyte. The bacilli then enter the cells and multiply within cytoplasmic vacuoles. Epithelial damage results with increase in

the cell turnover and the bacilli reach the lamina propria where there is a tissue response involving polymorphonuclear leukocytes and macrophages. In overwhelming infections the chief finding is an acute colitis with abundant mucus on the surface of a hyperaemic colon and subserosal haemorrhagic effusions on the peritoneal surface of the ileum. Visceral involvement of the pancreas and renal tubules may result from shock. However, ulceration is rare and inflammation of the lamina propria with accompanying smooth muscle spasm is probably responsible for the abdominal cramps and tenesmus. The immune response keeps the salmonellae localized, although transient bacteraemia is fairly common in *Salmonella* food poisoning.

Mechanism of diarrhoea

Diarrhoea is more of a feature in non-typhoidal *Salmonella* infection than typhoid infection. Invasion of the lamina propria is essential for the production of diarrhoea and although an *enterotoxin* is produced by *Salmonella*, activation of the adenyl cyclase system (see Chapter 12) may be caused by a different mechanism to that of *V. cholerae*, involving the production of prostaglandins by the polymorphonuclear leukocytes in the lamina propria which activate the adenyl cyclase system and cause secretory diarrhoea.

Intestinal lesions

The organisms are normally confined to the small intestine but colonic involvement is not uncommon[1] when the colon shows changes closely resembling ulcerative colitis. The small intestine shows minimal changes with histological changes in the lamina propria.

Metastatic lesions

Abscesses may occur in any organ or tissue; these are polymorphonuclear leukocyte abscesses. Cholecystitis and meningitis may occur.

IMMUNITY

Humans ingest *Salmonella* organisms relatively frequently and the result is determined by the infective dose (see p. 292), the virulence and invasiveness of the organism and host resistance.

Virulence and invasiveness of the organism

The virulence and invasiveness varies with the serotype. The ability to multiply in the intestine is affected by the presence of normal bacterial flora and the administration of an antibiotic which inhibits this flora allows the salmonellae to persist and increase in numbers in the intestine.

Host resistance

Salmonellae are cleared from the body by cellular and humoral mechanisms. Opsonins formed by the polymorphonuclear leukocytes enable macrophages to ingest the bacteria and destroy them. Immunity following an infection is not long-lasting and second attacks occur. These defence mechanisms are affected by a number of factors, age and the presence of certain diseases.

Age

Neonates and the elderly have a much higher rate of infection. This accounts for a high incidence of *Salmonella* infection in nurseries and old people's institutions.

Associated diseases

A large proportion of cases of hepatic cirrhosis, collagen diseases, leukaemia, lymphoma and other neoplasms in which there is immunosuppression have associated *Salmonella* bacteraemia. Two other conditions in which special mechanisms are at work are sickle cell anaemia and bartonellosis.

SICKLE CELL ANAEMIA (SS)
In individuals with SS who commonly develop bone infarcts and osteomyelitis the causative organism is usually a *Salmonella*. This may be due to the destruction of the spleen which results from splenic infarcts in childhood reducing the amount of serum components necessary for opsonization of the organisms (see Chapter 58).

BARTONELLOSIS
The acute haemolytic phase of bartonellosis (see Chapter 11) is complicated by *Salmonella* bacteraemia in nearly half the cases. This is due to deficient opsonizing capacity associated with defects in the alternative complement pathway.

CLINICAL FEATURES

Natural history

Asymptomatic infection is common and most symptomatic cases follow a mild to moderate self-limiting course of fever, abdominal pain and diarrhoea lasting 3–5 days followed by complete recovery. Serious illness occurs chiefly in the very young and old or in association with some other disease. But some apparently healthy adults do suffer from serious invasive disease without obvious predisposing cause.

Incubation period

A period of 8–48 hours is necessary for the organisms to multiply in the bowel and lamina propria to cause symptoms so that the incubation period is 8–24 hours with a range of 8–48 hours (longer than in staphylococcal food poisoning—3 hours).

Symptoms and signs

Salmonella enteritis

The onset is sudden with colicky abdominal pain and diarrhoea. Nausea and vomiting are not prominent features. The *abdominal pain* is variable in intensity and often severe and colicky. *Diarrhoea* may be a few loose stools or severe with the stools containing mucus and often blood tinged. *Fever* is prominent ranging from 38°C to 39°C but can be higher.

On examination, the abdomen shows hyperperistalsis with mild to moderate tenderness and rebound tenderness (suggesting acute appendicitis). The illness usually subsides naturally within 5 days but rarely continues for as long as two weeks. Continuation for longer should suggest an alternative diagnosis or a complication.

Children

Children suffer symptoms for longer and diarrhoea is more prominent. Dehydration is more severe than in adults and infants may develop a rapidly fatal necrotizing enteritis.

Salmonella septicaemia

This is especially common with *S. choleraesuis*. Septicaemia complicates a small number of cases of any *Salmonella* infection and presents with fever, rigors and metastatic lesions. Rose spots and splenomegaly may develop but typhoidal symptoms are absent. Septicaemia is commonly associated with an associated schistosomal infection (see Chapter 22).

Salmonella colitis

Salmonella infection of the colon is unusual and when it occurs is usually caused by an animal *Salmonella*. Bloody diarrhoea denotes colonic involvement and the clinical picture resembles that of a *Shigella* infection or an ulcerative colitis. *Salmonella* infection and ulcerative colitis may coexist. It is essential to treat the associated *Salmonella* infection with an antibiotic as well as the ulcerative colitis and to culture the stools in exacerbations. In infants a *Salmonella* septicaemia may cause rapid death with only slight histological evidence of colonic involvement.

Laboratory findings

The leukocyte count is usually normal but some patients may show a moderate leukocytosis.

Stools do not contain pus cells although smears from mucoid flecks will show some polymorphonuclear leukocytes.

Stool culture

Early in the illness stool culture will always yield salmonellae which persist for two weeks.

COMPLICATIONS

Endocarditis

Salmonella endocarditis causes a rapid and extensive destruction of the valves with perforation. This should be suspected when bacteraemia recurs after treatment. *S. typhimurium* and *S. choleraesuis* are the main organisms responsible.

Mycotic aneurysm

Salmonella can infect any abnormality of the aorta and persistent fever following infection in a known case of aortic aneurysm should raise suspicion. Atherosclerotic aneurysms of the abdominal aorta or iliac vessels or prosthetic valves and grafts may all be infected. Normal arteries are very rarely affected.

Localized infection

Salmonella abscesses may present in any organ or tissue.

Central nervous system

Salmonella meningitis affects neonates and children under two years of age. Premature, immune-deficient and obstetrically injured infants are most at risk. Cerebral and subdural abscess may occur and salmonellae can be recovered from the cerebrospinal fluid.

Osteomyelitis

Any bone may be affected but the diaphysis and epiphysis of the long bones are most frequently involved. Vertebral lesions are not uncommon with the disc spaces attacked early and bone structures later. Mediastinal and paravertebral abscess may occur.

Arthritis

Pyogenic arthritis from haematogenous spread involves the knees, shoulders, hips and sacroiliac joints and occurs most commonly in children. Reiter's syndrome may occur in male adults.

Abscesses

Salmonella is one of the commonest causes of splenic abscess but is rare.

DIFFERENTIAL DIAGNOSIS

Salmonella enteritis must be distinguished from staphylococcal food poisoning, acute appendicitis and other acute diarrhoea diseases caused by *Shigella*, enterotoxic and enteropathogenic *E. coli*, *Vibrio parahaemolyticus*, *Yersinia enterocolitica* and *Campylobacter jejuni*.

Staphylococcal food poisoning has a much shorter incubation period of about 3 hours (range 1–6 hours) and there is no fever. Acute appendicitis will show local rebound tenderness, the bowel sounds may be absent and there is a polymorphonuclear leukocytosis. The other acute diarrhoeal diseases can be distinguished by stool culture. The presence of leukocytes in the stools is of little help.

Salmonella septicaemia must be distinguished from other septicaemias.

DIAGNOSIS

Salmonellae can be isolated from the stools in the early stages. Stool culture is more reliable than rectal swab; 4–5 g of stool should be cultured in an enrichment medium before being plated out on MacConkey's medium, and the non-lactose fermenters picked off and identified by biochemical and O group serotyping.

TREATMENT (see also Chapter 57, p. 939)

Acute enteritis

Antibiotics are of no assistance in the treatment of acute enteritis; none have been proved to help and all prolong the carrier state by suppressing the normal bowel flora.

Bacteraemia

Cases with septicaemia require antibiotic therapy. *Chloramphenicol* is the drug of choice; dosage should be as in typhoid fever: 50 mg/kg daily in four divided doses for up to 14 days. *Amoxycillin* or *ampicillin* is preferable for long-term treatment and in cases where the organism is sensitive to these drugs doses of 100 mg/kg daily in four divided doses should be given. *Salmonella* endocarditis requires high dose long-term treatment with ampicillin.

Treatment of chronic carriers

Chronic biliary carriers should be treated in the same way as typhoid carriers (see Chapter 8, p. 204). Cholecystectomy combined with an antibiotic is often successful.

EPIDEMIOLOGY

There are three epidemiological patterns.
1 An explosive epidemic following a communal meal at a gathering at which infected food is served.
2 Isolated cases over a wide area traceable to some central source from which food has been distributed.
3 Institutional outbreaks localized to certain institutions and persisting for a long time.

CONTROL

Control is based on the detection of carriers in food handlers and workers in food factories and personal hygiene in institutions. Detection and control of *Salmonella* infection in food animals is important and heat treatment or pasteurization of animal feeds has reduced the infection in many places. The main control measure is the maintenance of proper food hygiene standards, and the strict segregation of cooked and uncooked foods.

OTHER TYPES OF FOOD POISONING

Toxins formed outside the body

STAPHYLOCOCCAL FOOD POISONING

Aetiology

Staphylococcus aureus, most often phage types II and IV produce a powerful enterotoxin—a water-soluble low molecular weight protein which remains stable after boiling for 30 minutes.

Transmission

Transmission is by contaminated food.

Source of infection

Humans are the most important source of infection. The hands of persons involved in the preparation of food are responsible. Only minor skin lesions are present and occasionally nasal carriers have been implicated.

Animals can excrete *S. aureus* in fresh milk contaminated by a mastitis.

Vehicle of infection

Cooked food is the vehicle since it best supports the growth of staphylococci. Ice cream, cheese and processed foods are all common sources. Food left out after processing allows the enterotoxin to be produced within 4–5 hours at 30°C, which is then preserved by deep freezing and is present when the food is thawed out and reheated to cause poisoning. The contaminated food is odourless and apparently quite fresh.

Pathology

Enterotoxin has no local effect on the gastrointestinal tract and can produce symptoms when injected parenterally.

Clinical features

Incubation period

The incubation period is 3 hours (range 1–6 hours) after eating the contaminated food. This period is influenced by the amount of enterotoxin present.

Symptoms and signs

Increased salivation is followed by nausea, vomiting, abdominal cramps and diarrhoea. In severe cases there is rapid dehydration and shock. There is no fever. The duration is normally very brief (5–6 hours) but symptoms can last for several days. Death only occurs in the very young, old and debilitated persons.

Differential diagnosis

The short incubation period and absence of fever distinguishes staphylococcal food poisoning from other bacterial causes. It can resemble ciguatera and other fish poisoning (see Chapter 48, p. 894).

Diagnosis

Gram staining of suspected food will show staphylococci in large numbers.

Treatment

In severe cases with shock and dehydration, rehydration with parenteral fluids is essential (see Chapter 12, p. 256).

Prevention

Enterotoxin is not formed at temperatures below 6.7°C and the best preventive is rapid refrigeration of all perishable food after preparation. Reheated foods must not be allowed to remain for long periods after reheating.

OTHER ORGANISMS

Bacillus cereus and *Citrobacter* species produce an enterotoxin during sporulation. *B. cereus* is most commonly implicated in contaminated rice foods. *Clostridium botulinus* toxin arises in improperly canned foods and leads to oculomotor and skeletal muscle paralysis.

OTHER TOXINS

Non-bacterial toxins may cause an attack of food poisoning after contamination of food. Heavy metals, *ciguatera* and *scrombrotoxic* (see Chapter 48) fish poisoning, and mushroom poisoning (see Chapter 49).

Toxins formed inside the gastrointestinal tract

Bacterial food poisoning by an enterotoxin produced in the intestinal tract is found with a number of species of bacteria. *Salmonella, V. cholerae* group (see Chapter 13), enterotoxic *E. coli* (see Chapter 14) and a cytotoxin with *Clostridium welchii (perfringens)* (C) (pigbel see Chapter 14).

REFERENCE

1 Mandal, B.K. & Mani, V. (1976) *Lancet* **i**, 1129.

Chapter 16
Diarrhoea Caused by Viruses

Viral diarrhoea is an important cause of morbidity and mortality in infants and is caused most commonly by rotavirus but occasionally by Norwalk and enteroviruses.

ROTAVIRUS

GEOGRAPHICAL DISTRIBUTION

Rotavirus has a worldwide distribution but is an important cause of diarrhoea in underdeveloped countries.[1,2]

AETIOLOGY

Rotavirus is a spherical RNA virus 70 nm in diameter with an inner and outer capsid. The virus appears as a wheel with spokes radiating from a hub. Rotavirus can be found in non-diarrhoeal stools but is much more common in the stools of children with diarrhoea. There are many animal species with similar viruses. Human rotavirus has been shown to cause diarrhoea in experimental newborn animals while adult human volunteers showed little or no disease.

TRANSMISSION

Transmission can be water-borne from water contaminated by human or animal faeces or by faecal–oral contact from cases. Carriers, especially adult carriers, can be important in the production of infection.

PATHOLOGY

Rotavirus particles can be demonstrated in enterocytes of children and there is subsequently a blunting of villi, increase in crypt death and flattening of the epithelial cells and an increase in inflammatory cells.

Diarrhoea

Diarrhoea is of the secretory type resulting from a disordered electrolyte and water transport in the small bowel (see Chapter 12). There is a net secretion of water, sodium and chloride but the sodium loss is not reversed with glucose as it is in cholera and enterotoxic *Escherichia coli*. In some cases an 'invasive' diarrhoea with blood and leukocytes in the stool has been described.[3]

Malabsorption

Changes in the bowel mucosa result in reduced disaccharide activity and children with rotavirus infection show sugar malabsorption during the illness with an increase in reducing substances in the stools (important in diagnosis).

IMMUNITY

Passive immunity

The low incidence of infection in infants under three months of age suggests that some immunity transferred from the mother and breastfeeding provides added protection.

Acquired immunity

Acquired immunity is short-lived. Antibodies appear with infection and recurrent infection is needed to restimulate their production. In underdeveloped countries this is common and the maximum incidence is in infants from 6 to 12 months and most adults show antibodies, although their stools are negative.

CLINICAL FEATURES

Natural history

Most infections are subclinical and there is a spectrum of disease ranging from inapparent and mild infection through an acute self-limiting illness lasting 3–8 days to a severe gastroenteritis with dehydration and death.

Incubation period

The incubation period varies from 1 to 5 days but is usually less than 48 hours.

Symptoms and signs

The onset is abrupt, and fever and vomiting are prominent with watery diarrhoea. The vomiting stops within the first 2 days after onset. In developing countries a substantial proportion of children develop dehydration and rotavirus is second only to cholera in causing dehydration. Most cases resolve within 10 days but in some cases the diarrhoea persists for another three weeks, probably because of secondary malabsorption. Virus is shed in the stools, frequently continuing for 10 days and sometimes three weeks after the onset.

COMPLICATIONS

Respiratory infection is common and some association with Henoch–Schönlein purpura and haemolytic uraemia syndrome in children has been shown.

Malabsorption

Lactose malabsorption commonly occurs during and following the illness and this may be countered by reducing the lactose intake.

DIFFERENTIAL DIAGNOSIS

The characteristic early vomiting and fever help to distinguish rotavirus infection from bacterial diarrhoea and cholera.

DIAGNOSIS

Virus in the stools

Electron microscopy of a watery suspension of stool will show virus particles. Rotavirus can be demonstrated in the stools by an enzyme-linked immunosorbent assay (ELISA) technique.[2]

Reducing substance in the stools

Because of lactose malabsorption reducing substances may be demonstrated in the stool by Clinistix.

Serology

Antibody may be detected in the serum as soon as the third day of illness reaching a peak after 14–21 days. The antibodies may be detected by complement fixation or ELISA tests.

TREATMENT

Rehydration is the most important measure.

Oral rehydration should be instituted (see Chapter 12). Although the loss of fluid is not reversed by glucose, glucose or sucrose may be used. During the diarrhoea children should continue to receive breast milk and with artificial feeding the lactose intake should be reduced to one-third to one-half during the early part of the disease.

EPIDEMIOLOGY

Rotavirus is a disease of infants. The infection is commonest from the age of six to 12 months and both sexes are equally affected. By the age of two years nearly all children show serum antibody. Adults in contact with cases occasionally develop diarrhoea and a small proportion of adult traveller's diarrhoea is caused by rotavirus. Rotavirus diarrhoea has a seasonal incidence occurring throughout the year but with a preponderance in winter.[2]

CONTROL

Control can be achieved by preventing faecal–oral contact and by clean water supplies.

VACCINE

A live oral attenuated bovine rotavirus strain has shown some protection in volunteers[4] and the development of cultural methods for rotavirus makes a vaccine possible.

NORWALK VIRUS

GEOGRAPHICAL DISTRIBUTION

Norwalk virus is distributed worldwide and seroepidemiological studies have shown the presence of infection in Bangladesh, Ecuador and the Philippines.

AETIOLOGY

Norwalk virus is a small RNA virus 27 nm in size.

TRANSMISSION

Transmission is principally by the faecal–oral route.

PATHOLOGY

Although virus particles have not been demonstrated in the mucosa the proximal small bowel shows broadening and blunting of the villi with some cellular infiltrate which reverts to normal within two weeks. Brush border enzymes are affected and malabsorption of fat and xylose has been found even during asymptomatic infection.

IMMUNITY

A short-term resistance to reinfection develops but little is known of the mechanism or duration.

CLINICAL FEATURES

Natural history

Norwalk virus produces a short-term mild diarrhoeal disease and there is a majority of symptomless inapparent infections.

The *incubation period* averages 48 hours.

Symptoms and signs

Vomiting, watery diarrhoea and fever cannot be distinguished from other viral diarrhoeas.

DIAGNOSIS

Diagnosis is made by electron microscopic examination of the stool and by an increase in Norwalk antibody during the course of the illness.

TREATMENT

Most diseases are mild and self-limiting and treatment is seldom required. When needed oral rehydration therapy (see Chapter 12) should be used.

EPIDEMIOLOGY

Norwalk virus primarily affects older children and adults in camps and collections of young people.

REFERENCES

1 Walker-Smith, J.A. (1978) *Archs Dis. Child.* **53**, 355.
2 Saha, M.R., Sen, D., Datta, S.P. et al (1984) *Trans R. Soc. trop. Med. Hyg.* **78**, 818–820.
3 Clemens, J.D., Ahmed, M., Butler, T. et al (1983) *J. trop. Med. Hyg.* **86**, 117–122.
4 Vesikari, T., Isolauri, E., Delem, A. et al (1983) *Lancet* **ii**, 807–811.

Chapter 17
Diarrhoea Caused by Protozoa

A number of protozoa may cause diarrhoeal disease.

Amoebiasis (*Entamoeba histolytica*) *E. polecki, Dientamoeba fragilis*)

Giardiasis (*Giardia lamblia*)
Balantidiasis (*Balantidium coli*)
Coccidial enteritis (*Isospora belli, Sarcocystis, Cryptosporidium*

AMOEBIASIS

GEOGRAPHICAL DISTRIBUTION

Amoebic infection has a worldwide distribution being found in arctic, temperate and tropical countries. It is more prevalent in tropical areas where invasive amoebic infection is common. The presence of pathological zymodemes in the tropics and poor sanitation is responsible for this state of affairs.

AETIOLOGY

Entamoeba histolytica is a protozoon which normally lives and multiplies in the contents of the large intestine in man but can under certain conditions invade the tissues and can spread from the bowel to the liver, lungs, brain, skin and other organs. *E. histolytica* is present in two forms: *trophozoites* and *cysts*.

The *trophozoite* (10–40 µm) has a characteristic nucleus (2.8–4.5 µm), a small central karyosome and peripheral chromatin in the form of fine granules (Figs. 17.1a, 17.8a and I.12,1 and Appendix I, p. 1244). The cytoplasm has two zones: an outer with a clear ectoplasm and an inner with a granular cytoplasm enclosing food vacuoles containing ingested red cells in the pathogenic strains. The trophozoites, which multiply by binary fission, are actively motile and in wet preparations move by thrusting out pseudopodia from the ectoplasm into which the other contents of the cell flow.

Cysts

The fully formed cyst (Figs. 17.1b, 17.8c and I.12 and Appendix I, p. 1244) has a greenish refractile appearance in the fresh state, is smaller (9.5–17.5 µm) than the trophozoite and more compact. The nucleus divides by mitosis to produce two and then four *nuclei* which have the same characteristics as the nucleus of the trophozoite though they are smaller. Each nucleus has a central karyosome and peripheral chromatin granules. The cyst wall is tough and within it are one or more *chromatoid bodies*—oval bars stained black with iron haematoxylin and in the early stages glycogen, staining brown with iodine.

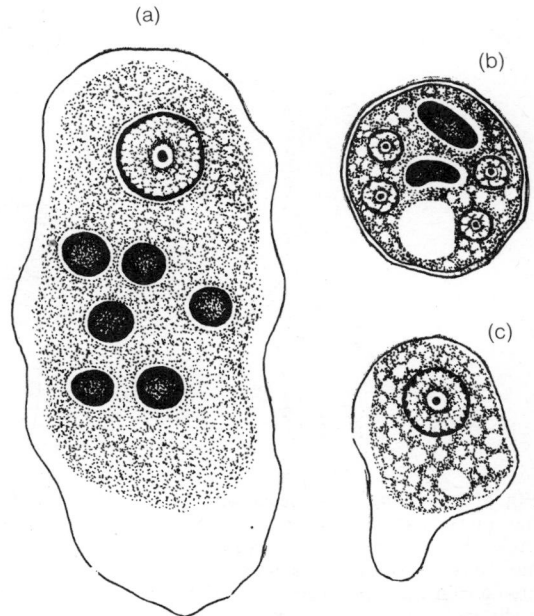

Fig. 17.1 *Entamoeba histolytica.* (a) Trophozoite containing ingested red cells. (b) Cyst with four nuclei. (c) Precystic stage.

Life-cycle (Fig. 17.2)[1]

The trophozoites inhabit the crypts of the caecum and first part of the colon where they feed on mucus and its contents and probably live in symbiosis with the intestinal bacteria. As they pass down the colon and the faecal material becomes drier the conditions are less favourable and the trophozoites protect themselves by encysting, influenced by the right bacterial flora. In the process of encystation the trophozoites discharge undigested food and condense into a spherical mass, the *precystic stage*, with a tough wall and a single nucleus (Figs. 17.1c and 17.8g). Cysts are usually found without trophozoites in the faeces of infected persons not suffering from diarrhoea but trophozoites can be demonstrated after a purge has been given. Cysts are never found in metastatic lesions in the liver or other organs; only haematophagous trophozoites are found in such lesions. Cysts are ingested and pass through the stomach to encyst in the small intestine whence they travel down to the caecum. The 'minuta' forms of *E. histolytica* are non-

pathogenic. *E. hartmanni* is a distinct species and is smaller than *E. histolytica*, the trophozoites measuring under 10 μm and the four nucleate cysts 3.8–8 μm. It never invades the tissues (see Appendix I and Table I.2, p. 1243).

VIRULENCE

E. histolytica infection is commonly present without producing any lesions in the bowel and these amoebae are known as 'non-invasive' or non-pathogenic amoebae. In other cases the amoebae have a capacity to invade the bowel and produce lesions; these are known as 'invasive' or pathogenic amoebae. There are a number of strains of amoebae, most of which are 'non-invasive'.

Enzyme electrophoresis has shown that there are 22 zymodemes of *E. histolytica* distributed on a geographical basis of which only nine are invasive and have been isolated from cases of intestinal ulceration or hepatic disease (Fig. I.13, p. 1246). Only a few of these are common and

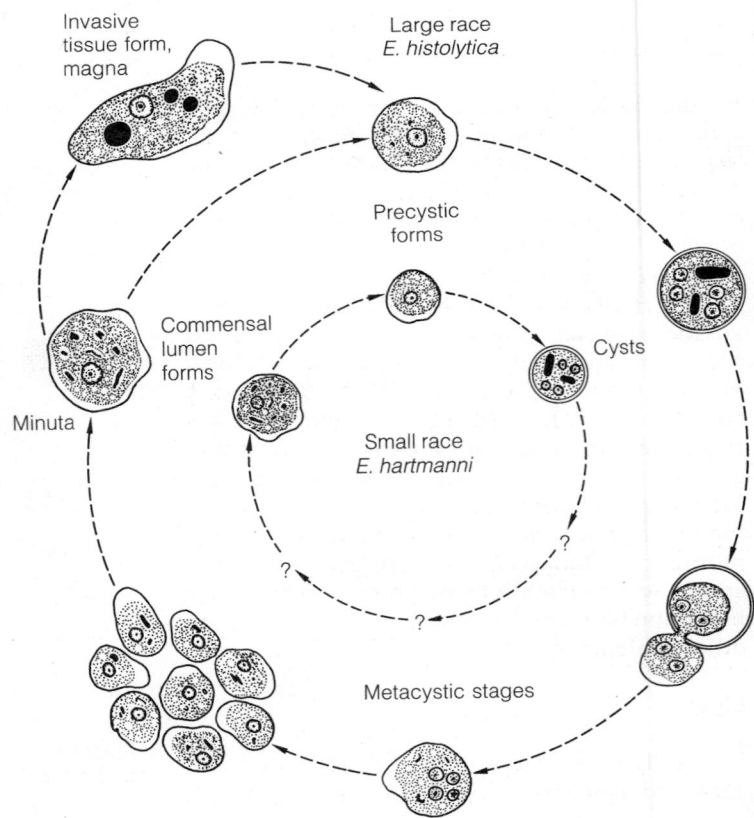

Fig. 17.2 Human entamoebae with four nucleate cysts. The inner circle shows the life-cycle of small race *E. hartmanni*; question marks indicate unknown metacystic stages. The outer circle shows the life-cycle of the large race *E. histolytica*, with tissue phase (invasive forms) outside the normal circle. Arrows indicate the course of development. (After Hoare.[1])

one zymodeme has been shown to be responsible for all the amoebic disease in India (see Appendix I, Fig. I.14, p. 1247).[2] Invasiveness correlates with the position of a phosphoglucomutase band on starch gel electrophoresis.[3,4]

Invasive strains do not lose invasiveness in culture and even in asymptomatic infection show some evidence of invasion as shown by positive serological responses by the host.[5] Cysts produce trophozoites with the same invasive or non-invasive characteristics when infecting a new host. This explains why there are so many cyst passers in whom the presence of cysts in the stool is of no pathological significance unless they are of a pathological strain.

Other factors affecting the ability of *E. histolytica* to invade the bowel and produce disease may be *diet* with an excess of cholesterol and carbohydrate in the diet[6] and frequency of infection linked with rapid transmission, as in Durban.[7]

TRANSMISSION

Source of infection

Animal hosts of *E. histolytica* include monkeys, dogs, cats, pigs and rats. Infected dogs and cats do not excrete cysts and are therefore not infective. Transmission from animals to man is exceedingly rare and man-to-man transmission is the rule.

Cyst passers

Cysts are the only infective form; trophozoites are destroyed by the gastric juice and patients with acute amoebic colitis are not infectious to others. The cysts are passed in the faeces of healthy carriers or cyst passers. The cysts are extremely resistant to external environmental conditions. They can remain viable in refrigeration at 4–8°C for several days, in cool faeces for 12 days or more and in cool water for several weeks. They can be passed through cockroaches and the intestines of filth flies and have been recovered from their vomit. They can resist 1/2500 mercury bichloride, 5% hydrochloric acid or 0.5% formalin for 30 minutes and 1/500 potassium permanganate for 24–48 hours. Cysts are killed by desiccation and heating to above 50°C and deep freezing below −5°C, 1/20 cresol for 30 minutes and 5% acetic acid at 30°C in 15 minutes. They are killed by superchlorination and iodine. Coagulation and sand filtration are necessary for the treatment of water supplies.

Route of transmission

Infection by cysts occurs most frequently by direct person-to-person transmission or contamination of food. Water-borne transmission is unusual.

Person-to-person transmission

Cysts are passed from person to person by fingers soiled with faeces either directly into the mouth or by food which is not cooked after handling. In West Africa where young children are commonly infected their mothers are found to be excreting cysts and the common practice of manual feeding of children affords ample opportunity for infection if the fingers are contaminated.

Food

Food may be contaminated when being grown and uncooked vegetables are a common source of infection especially if they are grown on ground fertilized by human excreta.

Water-borne

Water-borne transmission is unusual. Contaminated water contains cysts which can live in water for several days, even two weeks. Infection from small contaminated bodies of water such as waterholes and unprotected wells may well occur in underdeveloped countries. Water-borne epidemics have been described in the USA and Japan but considerable doubt has been cast as to the cause of these epidemics and bacterial dysentery in which commensal trophozoites are passed in the stools may have led to the mistaken diagnosis of amoebic colitis.[8]

Homosexual transmission

There is strong evidence of male homosexual transmission, 21.5% of whom were found to be infected, with a strong association with oro-anal sex.[9] But all zymodemes isolated from homosexual men have been non-pathogenic and eradication of the amoebae did not improve moderate inflammatory histopathology in the rectum. There is no evidence to suggest that *E. histolytica* is a pathogen in homosexual men.[10]

NATURAL HISTORY

Infection with *Entamoeba histolytica* runs a very varied course. It may be a completely asymptomatic intestinal infection or a severe amoebic colitis (amoebic dysentery) which can be acute and self-limiting or run a more chronic course. Extraintestinal infection (extraintestinal amoebiasis) may occur with abscesses in the liver or other organs such as the lung, brain, pericardium or skin.

1 *Intestinal amoebiasis*: amoebic colitis, non-dysenteric colitis, amoeboma and amoebic appendicitis. Acute dysenteric symptoms are sometimes accompanied by a tender and enlarged liver; in this condition there is thought to be no actual invasion of the liver by amoebae, and it is best referred to as non-specific hepatomegaly which does not involve any assumption as to its exact aetiology. Complications and sequelae of intestinal amoebiasis are perforation, peritonitis, haemorrhage, intussusception, post-dysenteric colitis and stricture.

2 *Extraintestinal amoebiasis*: hepatic liver abscess and cutaneous. Complications of liver abscess are rupture or extension, bacterial infection, haematogenous spread to other organs. Involvement of other organs (lung, brain, spleen, etc) may occur without manifest liver involvement.

Intestinal amoebiasis (amoebic colitis)

PATHOLOGY

The results of infection are varied and five different forms of *E. histolytica* infection may be distinguished: the symptomless cyst passer, the cyst passer with intestinal disturbance, frank amoebic colitis and mild chronic amoebiasis, with or without disturbance in the function of the colon (Fig. 17.3).

When *E. histolytica* invades the tissues of the intestine the lesions are most often found in the caecum and ascending colon or the sigmoid; the appendix may be involved and ulcers have exceptionally been found in the lower ileum. In fulminating necrotizing amoebic dysentery the whole colon may be full of ulcers with extensive destruction in its whole length (Figs. 17.4 and 60.1, p. 1002).

The early lesions are minute ulcers in the mucous membrane; they are flask-shaped in that the neck of the ulcer is much narrower than the deeper part (Fig. 17.5a). The margins are rolled and the edges are undermined; the ulcers are capped with dense yellow or even black sloughs. Trophozoites can be found in the depths of these ulcers where they can be seen as rounded bodies with a single nucleus in the submucosa with little or no surrounding cellular reaction (Fig. 17.5b). The mucous membrane between ulcers is usually normal and, if secondary bacterial infection does not take place, there is little evidence of inflammation. The process is essentially one of necrosis with lysis of cells rather than inflammatory response.

The vessels at the base of the ulcer become thrombosed but the ulcerative process may extend down to arterioles and severe or even fatal haemorrhage may occur. Some ulcers pass through the muscular layers, perforating the bowel wall or rendering it so thin that bowel contents can seep into the peritoneal cavity, giving rise to peritonitis or local peritoneal abscess.

In chronic cases polypoid tags may project into the lumen of the gut. When healing takes place, cicatricial pigmented scars mark the sites of former ulcers.

An amoeboma, or amoebic granuloma, may result from repeated invasion of the colon by *E. histolytica*, with superadded pyogenic infection. Amoebomas are found in the caecum (40%), rectosigmoid junction (20%) and ascending, transverse or descending colon. Granulation tissue is formed with the presence of lymphocytes, plasma cells and eosinophils. Fibrous tissue is formed later. There is remarkably little inflammation; most of the swelling is due to oedema. Amoebae are scanty and difficult to demonstrate. Radiology reveals coning of the caecum, a filling defect, narrowing of the bowel and the appearance of a stricture. All these features disappear rapidly with treatment. The fluorescent antibody test is positive, often in high titre. The amoeboma may become very large, forming a hard swelling very difficult to differentiate clinically from carcinoma. Cases have been recorded in which the diagnosis of carcinoma has been contradicted by examination of tissues after death.

Experimentally produced amoebic dysentery

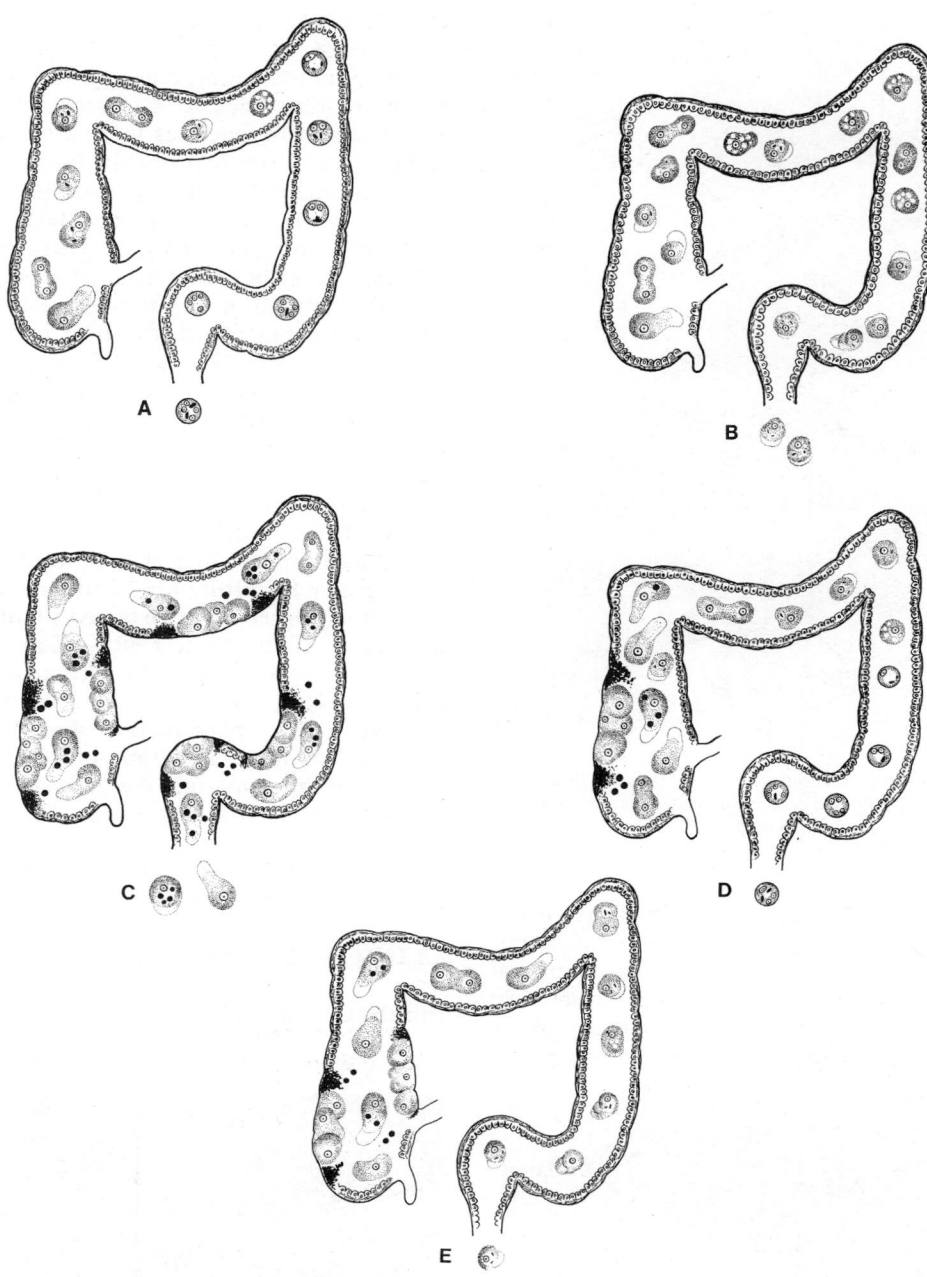

Fig. 17.3 The correlation between forms of *E. histolytica* in the stools and clinical forms of amoebiasis. A, Symptomless carrier with bowels functioning normally. Trophozoites (minuta and precystic forms) in the lumen of the ascending and transverse colon and cysts in the descending colon. The carrier passes formed stools with cysts. B, Carrier with intestinal disturbance. Trophozoites (minuta and precystic forms) in the lumen throughout the large bowel. The patient passes loose stools with small amoebae. C, Frank amoebic dysentery. Trophozoites invading the entire wall of the large bowel (ulceration) and ingesting red blood cells. The patient passes fluid stools with haematophagous amoebae. D, Mild or chronic amoebiasis. Haematophagous trophozoites and lesions restricted to the proximal sector of large bowel; the distal section is functioning normally. The patient passes formed stools with cysts. E, Mild or chronic amoebiasis. Haematophagous trophozoites restricted to the proximal sector of large bowel; function of colon disturbed. The patient passes semifluid or soft stools with small amoebae.

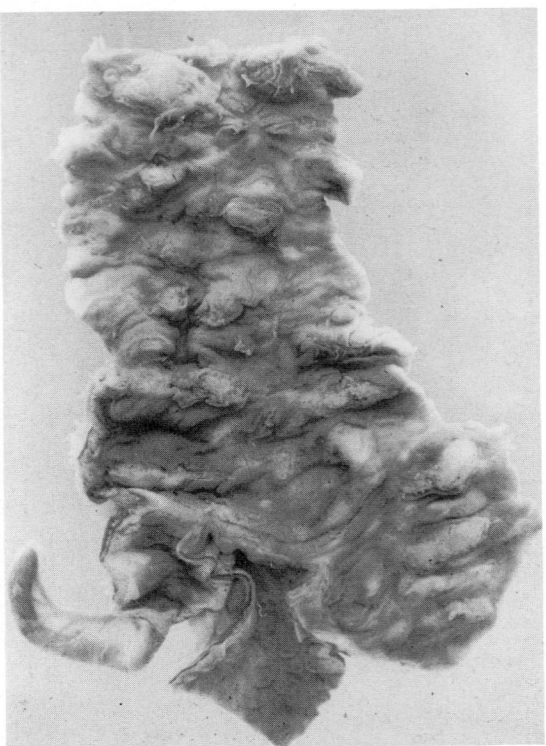

Fig. 17.4 Amoebic ulceration of the terminal ileum and caecum showing typical ulceration. (Courtesy Dr Sandosham.)

in kittens and dogs differs essentially from the disease in man. When introduced into the rectum of the animal, the amoebae produce a superficial excoriation within 2 or 3 days and the lesions are more generalized than in man. Cysts are never found and chronic ulceration does not occur.

IMMUNITY

There is no indication that any one human race has more resistance to *E. histolytica* than any other; such differences as there are in incidence and severity are more probably due to differences in environmental conditions and diet.

There is no evidence that one attack of amoebic dysentery protects against subsequent attacks; infection does not protect against superinfection. Normal commensal *E. histolytica* does not make parenteral contact with the host and therefore does not provoke the formation of antibodies. But invasive *E. histolytica* can provoke the formation of persisting antibodies, though these are not obviously protective. Antigenic differences between strains have, however, been demonstrated by complicated techniques.

One of these antibodies is an immunoglobulin (gamma globulin) which can immobilize *E. histolytica* grown in culture for 24 hours, but the titre is low and the serum to be tested should be used undiluted. With this test 88% of patients with amoebic liver abscess, 90% with acute amoebic colitis and 78% with chronic amoebic colitis were positive; 18% of persons free of amoebic infection were positive. The immobilization factor is apparently transmissible via the placenta from a positive mother to her fetus, as judged by tests on cord blood.

For serological tests involving antibodies, see section on diagnosis (p. 313).

CLINICAL FEATURES

Incubation period

The incubation period of acute amoebic colitis is

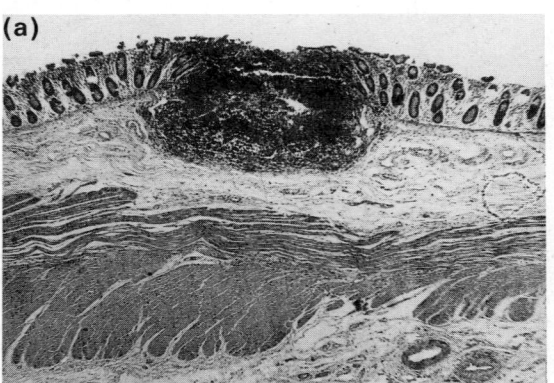
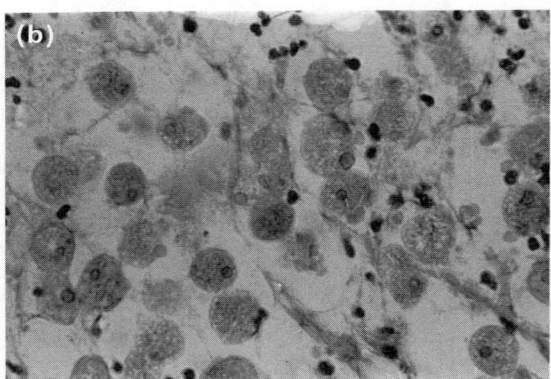

Fig. 17.5 (a) Low power view of early amoebic ulcer in the large intestine. (Courtesy WTIM.) (b) Trophozoites of *E. histolytica* in section from base of rectal ulcer. (Courtesy Dr B.H. Kean.)

8–10 days but is often impossible to calculate, since the patient may have had a latent infection with commensal amoebae until precipitated into dysentery by some other factor, possibly an intestinal infection with pathogenic organisms such as shigellae or schistosomes, or possibly malaria or other debilitating conditions such as a low protein diet. Persistent heavy superinfection may conceivably be a factor.

Symptoms and signs

The *onset* is usually insidious, except in fulminating cases (see below) with abdominal discomfort, a mild windy looseness of the bowels or frank diarrhoea in recurring bouts, not necessarily with blood or excessive mucus. Tenderness may develop over the caecum, simulating appendicitis, or the transverse colon, simulating peptic ulcer, or more commonly the sigmoid colon. In more severe cases there may be tenesmus.

In *mild* cases the patient is generally well nourished, sometimes even constipated, more often passing only a few dysenteric motions each day. Trophozoites are scanty on direct faecal smear and few ulcers, or none, can be seen at proctoscopy.

In *moderately severe* cases there is some deterioration in the general condition but not enough to force the patient to bed. Dysenteric stools number five to 15 each day and trophozoites are numerous on direct smear. There are typical amoebic ulcers in the rectal mucosa. Africans in Durban are often incapacitated with bloody diarrhoea, pain and tenderness, but with surprisingly little constitutional disturbance; this contrasts strongly with the condition in severe bacterial dysentery when the patient is acutely ill, toxic and dehydrated.

Severe amoebic colitis. This may occur at any age. In Nigeria children often show this form in which the onset is relatively sudden as a result of extensive, fulminating, necrotizing amoebic colitis and which is commonly fatal. The patient is ill and toxic with poor general nutrition, extreme asthenia, fever and more or less dehydration with depletion of electrolytes sometimes amounting to shock, with muscle cramps. The complexion may be muddy. Hiccup is a bad sign. There is meteorism, vomiting, dysuria, tenesmus or even total incompetence of the anal sphincter; the patient may pass over 15 motions in the day though, exceptionally, there may be no

diarrhoea. The rectal mucosa is severely damaged with confluent ulcers and haemorrhages. Peritonitis is a common complication, with ileus. In this condition proctoscopy is contraindicated.

The faeces usually contain much dark and altered blood and blood-streaked mucus or even gangrenous sloughs; there are usually but not always abundant trophozoites containing ingested red cells.

In uncomplicated amoebic colitis continuous pyrexia is unusual; fever may be intermittent. There is usually moderate leukocytosis of 10–25×10^9/litre, with 70% polymorphonucleocytes.

Chronic amoebic colitis. There is no such entity as chronic amoebic colitis. Post-dysenteric ulcerative colitis (see below) is rare and eventually subsides. More usually colonic symptoms after an attack of amoebic colitis are due to an irritable bowel or psychoneurosis.

Amoeboma. An amoeboma can produce a tumour of the caecum, transverse colon, sigmoid or rectum and may cause acute intussusception (especially when in the caecum). It may rarely lead to intestinal obstruction. Differentiation from carcinoma can be difficult even by radiography and cysts or trophozoites may not be found in the faeces. Clinically an amoeboma can be mistaken for a growth of the intestine; surgical removal without antiamoebic drugs is likely to be fatal.[11] Medical treatment alone is effective. Amoebae can invade a tumour and antiamoebic treatment will reduce such a tumour but will not cause it to disappear; this suggests carcinoma.

DIFFERENTIAL DIAGNOSIS ☞

Three mistakes are made in diagnosis of amoebic colitis.

The first mistake is to regard amoebic colitis as responsible for the irritable bowel syndrome or 'colitis' especially if *E. histolytica* cysts are found in the stool as well as numerous psychosomatic symptoms. There are some individuals who are convinced they have amoebic disease in spite of all evidence to the contrary.

The second mistake is to miss the possibility of invasive amoebiasis in the differential diagnosis of carcinoma of the colon or rectum (amoeboma) and ulcerative colitis.

The third mistake is not to consider the possibility of amoebiasis in the diagnosis of long continued low pyrexia and ill-health.

Amoebic infection may coexist with other diseases such as *Shigella* dysentery, typhoid, schistosomiasis, ulcerative colitis and carcinoma.

The finding of trophozoites of *E. histolytica* in the stools is not absolute proof that amoebiasis is the cause of the patient's illness, while the finding of cysts is a strong indication for an alternative diagnosis since cysts are rarely found in the stools of patients with amoebic colitis.

Acute amoebic colitis may resemble acute appendicitis very closely with abdominal pain and tenderness over the caecum. In acute appendicitis there is more systemic upset and antiamoebic treatment will settle acute amoebic colitis very quickly.

Other causes of dysentery

In *Shigella dysentery* the onset is more acute, there is more systemic upset and the stool contains polymorphonuclear leukocytes (see Table 14.2, p. 284). In some cases with a double infection, treatment with tetracycline will be effective for both.

In *Schistosoma mansoni dysentery* the rectum is more granular on proctoscopy and ova of *S. mansoni* can be found in rectal snips. In endemic schistosomal areas where ova, ulceration of the colon and haematophagous trophozoites are found then it is usually the amoebic infection which is responsible for the symptoms.

Other rarer causes of dysentery are *Balantidium coli* (see p. 327), *Trichuris* (see Chapter 21) and tuberculous ulceration of the colon.

Ulcerative colitis

Non-specific ulcerative colitis is easily confused with amoebic colitis when trophozoites may be found in the stools. In these cases the amoebic infection must first be treated and a lack of response will indicate the true diagnosis.

Post-dysenteric ulcerative colitis (see below) is more difficult to separate from ulcerative colitis but there will be a history of severe amoebic colitis and serology will be positive.

Amoeboma

Amoeboma of the colon and stricture must be distinguished from carcinoma. If a biopsy is possible, this will settle the diagnosis; if not,

amoebic serology must be used and, if positive, a therapeutic trial instituted when an amoeboma will respond with surprising rapidity. In all cases of carcinoma of the bowel, if there is the slightest possibility of an amoebic infection then a serological test must be performed before laparotomy.

COMPLICATIONS

Death may result from exhaustion, haemorrhage, perforation or liver abscess (see below). The commonest fatal complication is perforation of the bowel, leading to peritonitis. Perforation may occur during sigmoidoscopy but apart from such trauma the bowel contents may leak or seep through the bowel wall, resulting in localized inflammatory masses or abscesses or generalized peritonitis. In the first two the prognosis is good but generalized peritonitis is more common and dangerous.

General peritonitis may be of two types. In the first, which is rare, perforation occurs in the course of only moderately severe dysentery or in patients who appear to be well controlled by treatment. The onset is abrupt with severe abdominal pain and board-like rigidity of the abdominal muscles. In this type laparotomy is indicated as the bowel wall can be repaired. In the second type the peritonitis is a complication of severe amoebic ulceration of the colon, though it may occur rarely in patients in whom there is no history and no clinical evidence of dysentery. In such patients there is usually a slow onset of abdominal distension, pain not being marked and rigidity being slight. Hiccup is a bad sign and vomiting is even more significant. Rebound tenderness suggests peritoneal irritation but is not a certain sign of peritonitis; nor is slight distension.

Haemorrhage from erosion of a blood vessel by an amoebic ulcer may be serious and urgent, requiring immediate blood transfusion and energetic antiamoebic measures.

Intussusception is possible (usually caecocolic) and pain is then severe with a sausage-shaped mass in the course of the colon and an empty right iliac fossa. Specific treatment should be given but resection should not be delayed too long.

Post-dysenteric ulcerative colitis may follow a severe attack of amoebic colitis which has been treated and although the colon remains damaged amoebae are absent. The mucosa appears red and oedematous with superficial erosions but no ulceration. Treatment is difficult and anti-amoebic treatment of little use. Left to itself it will gradually resolve. Massive necrosis of the colon is rare[12] and megacolon has been reported.[13]

Stricture of the colon may develop; rectal stricture, though rare, can follow acute amoebic dysentery or even chronic infection in which dysentery is not prominent. It must be differentiated from the stricture of lymphogranuloma venereum and from malignant disease.

The *skin* around the anus or round the stoma of a colostomy may be extensively ulcerated (Figs. 17.6 and 17.7). Such distressing and unnecessary ulceration should never occur if physicians and surgeons are alive to the possibility of amoebic infection. Treatment with antiamoebic drugs is dramatically successful, but the sequelae remain.

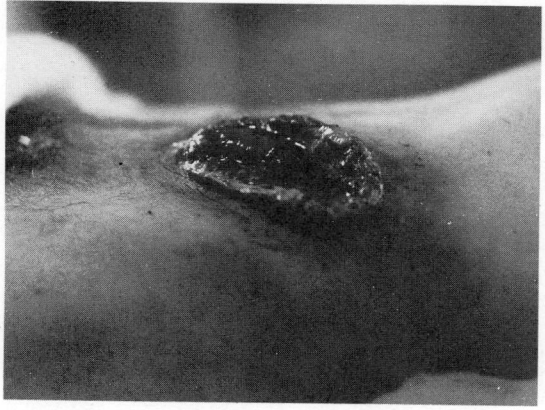

Fig. 17.6 Amoebic skin ulceration surrounding a colostomy opening in a patient with amoeboma of the colon.

Anogenital amoebiasis is one of the commonest forms of the infection seen in Papua New Guinea. The appearance may resemble that of a squamous carcinoma. Lesions of the penis in men and vaginitis and cervicitis in women are common in this area.

Rare complications include involvement of the prostate and balanitis with granuloma which may be very destructive but which respond to treatment. The vulva and vagina are sometimes infected directly from the bowel.

DIAGNOSIS

The first step in diagnosis is to have the disease in mind and to ask patients with abdominal symptoms if they have travelled in the tropics or other endemic areas. Complaints of recurrent diarrhoea, 'haemorrhoids' or rectal bleeding should raise suspicions. Diagnosis of amoebic dysentery depends upon the history, symptoms and signs, endoscopic examination of the lower bowel and especially upon the recognition of *E. histolytica* trophozoites in the stools or other materials, but certain other tests are useful. Trophozoites are found in the faeces of patients with amoebic dysentery, but they can usually be produced in cyst passers if a simple purgative is given.[14] They tend to appear in intermittent showers and examination of three specimens at intervals of a week is better than examination of three specimens on consecutive days.[11]

Examination of the stool (see Appendix IV, p. 1489)

The faeces must be collected in a receptacle free from disinfectant and examined fresh. The stool

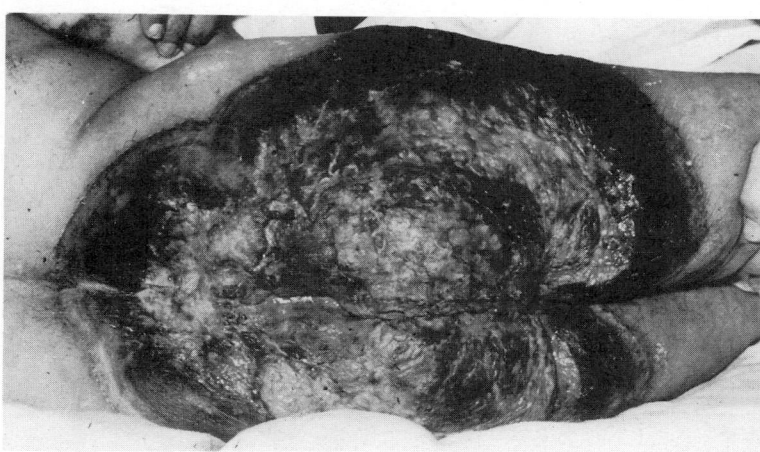

Fig. 17.7 Amoebic ulceration of the skin over the sacrum, coccyx and perineum. (Courtesy WTIM.)

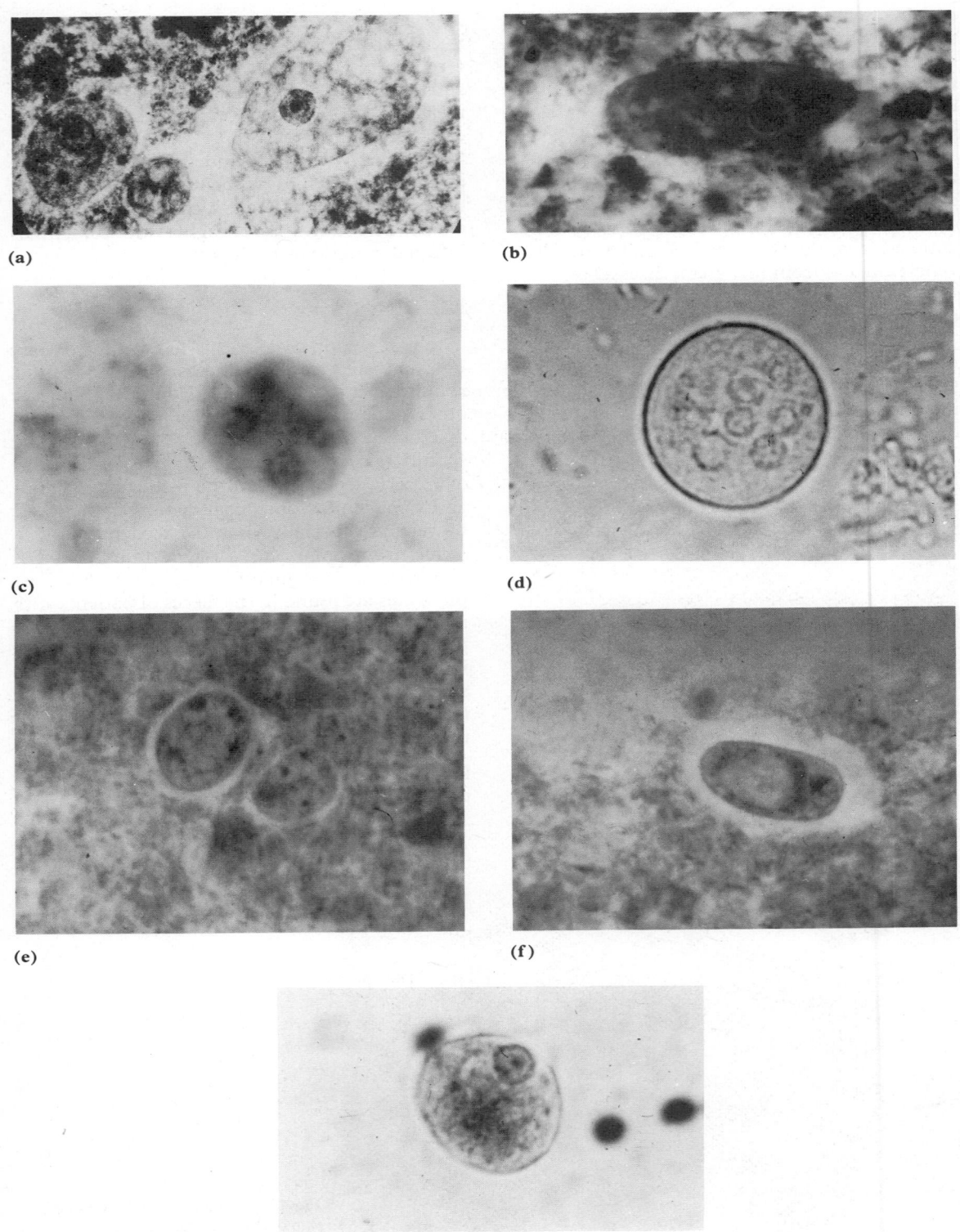

passed in acute amoebic colitis has a typical appearance. The faecal matter is loose and glutinous with stringy mucus. The blood is dark and semifluid and mixed in the mucus. There is a characteristic odour which is not faecal. A portion of the bloodstained mucus must be chosen and compressed on to a slide on a warmed stage, covered with a coverslip and examined for trophozoites. Active trophozoites tend to be found in clumps. They may be found on one evacuation and not in the next. They remain alive in the faeces for a few hours but become distorted in the presence of urine, but they 'round up' and stop moving in 15 minutes on exposure to cold.

Trophozoites of *E. histolytica* have a clear, faintly greenish, transparent body several times the diameter of a red cell; when stained by eosin they are seen to be refractile with a distinct ecto- and endoplasm (Fig. 17.8a). They are actively motile and usually elongated producing a single blunt pseudopodium into which the endoplasm flows so rapidly that the ectoplasm may not be apparent until the amoeba slows down. The important feature is that they contain ingested red cells and without these any amoeboid organism should not be diagnosed as *E. histolytica*.

Large motile macrophages such as are found in other forms of diarrhoea have been mistakenly diagnosed as *E. histolytica*. *E. coli* has much more sluggish movements, the ectoplasm is not clearly defined and is extensively vacuolated with the vacuoles containing bacteria, yeasts and other debris (Figs. 17.8b and I.15, p. 1248).

The presence in the stool of blood, pus or mucus should be noted. Aggregations of red cells, disintegrated intestinal epithelium and Charcot–Leyden crystals may be present but there is no characteristic exudate which is typical of amoebic dysentery (apart from an exudate which contains actively motile trophozoites containing ingested red cells). The cellular characters are no different from those of mucous colitis

and other chronic lesions of the bowel. On the other hand, the exudate in acute bacterial dysentery is diagnostic (Chapter 14). Trophozoites of *E. histolytica* may be found in a stool whose characters are typical of bacterial dysentery; in such a case the bacterial dysentery may be the cause of the patient's illness.

Cysts are more likely to be found in the faecal parts of the stool than in mucus. They have four nuclei (Figs. 17.8c and I.15, p. 1248, and Appendix IV, p. 1491). Concentration methods such as zinc sulphate centrifugal flotation or formol ether concentration methods are used (see Appendix IV, p. 1490). A drop of Gram's iodine to the final preparation shows up the nuclei. Cysts of *E. coli* have eight nuclei and do not usually contain chromatoid bodies (Fig. 17.8d and Appendix IV, p. 1491). Cysts of *E. histolytica* and *E. hartmanni* may be confused; both have one to four nuclei but if the mean diameter of several cysts is above 10 μm they are probably *E. histolytica* and, if below, *E. hartmanni*. For differential characters of amoebae see Table I.4, p. 1248.

If desired, thin fixed smears can be made for more careful examination by placing the slide in Schaudinn's fixative for 30 minutes before staining with Gomori's trichrome stain or Heidenhain's iron haematoxylin.

Faeces which cannot be examined fresh may be preserved in merthiolate–iodine–formalin (MIF) or polyvinyl alcohol.[15]

Culture

E. histolytica may be cultured on special media[16] or axenically in a diphasic medium.[17] Although culture can be of use in diagnosis its main use is for the production of large numbers of trophozoites for the production of antigen or enzyme analysis for the identification of invasive zymodemes. In the series of 535 cases of amoebic dysentery recorded by the former editor of this

---

Fig. 17.8   Identification of amoebae in stools.

Trophozoites
(a) *E. histolytica*: actively motile. Size 10–40 μm. Clear outer ectoplasm. Inner granular endoplasm with ingested red cells.
(b) *E. coli*: sluggishly motile. Size 20–30 μm. Ectoplasm not defined, contains bacteria, yeasts, etc. but *no* ingested red cells.
Cysts
(c) *E. histolytica*: size 9.5–17.5 μm. Four nuclei. One or more chromatoid bodies.
(d) *E. coli*: size 10–30 μm. Eight nuclei. No chromatoid bodies.
(e) *Endolimax nana*: size 6–12 μm. Two to four nuclei. No chromatoid bodies.
(f) *Iodamoeba bütschlii*: size 7–15 μm. One nucleus. One refractile body and one large glycogen mass staining with iodine.
Precystic form
(g) *E. histolytica*. (Courtesy Dr J. Tatz.)

book, Sir Philip Manson-Bahr, 509 were diagnosed by microscopic examination of faeces, and the remainder by demonstration of amoebae in scrapings from amoebic ulcers. Amoebic lesions were demonstrated in material obtained from 234 of 258 sigmoidoscopies.

Histological diagnosis may be difficult but fluorescent staining (see below) is of great help in this connection.

In partly healed amoebic dysentery lesions may be distinguished as pinpoint oval or circular pits, irregularly disposed. The bowel surface may be peppered with them and the term 'pig skin' appearances has been applied to them. They can persist even after treatment. Occasionally solitary ulcers resembling carcinoma are seen in the rectum, even as long as 20 years after the primary infection.

Radiology

Radiology is not much help in uncomplicated amoebiasis but can be valuable in detecting perforation and by barium enema such conditions

as stricture, amoeboma and intussusception, though this is unwise in the presence of severe dysentery. There may be large filling defects (Fig. 17.9) in the ascending and transverse colon which disappear rapidly with antiamoebic treatment.

Endoscopy

Endoscopy by proctoscopy or (better) sigmoidoscopy is called for when the stools are negative, to obtain material for examination, to assess the results of treatment or to differentiate from other possible diseases of the lower bowel. Amoebic ulceration also occurs in the sigmoid and rectum, though it is most common in the caecum and ascending colon. No preparation of the patient is needed apart from defecation and the examination is best done in the knee–chest position; it is uncomfortable for the patient but need not be painful. The appearances may be normal even when lesions are present elsewhere in the bowel, so that normal endoscopic appearances do not exclude active amoebic colitis. The

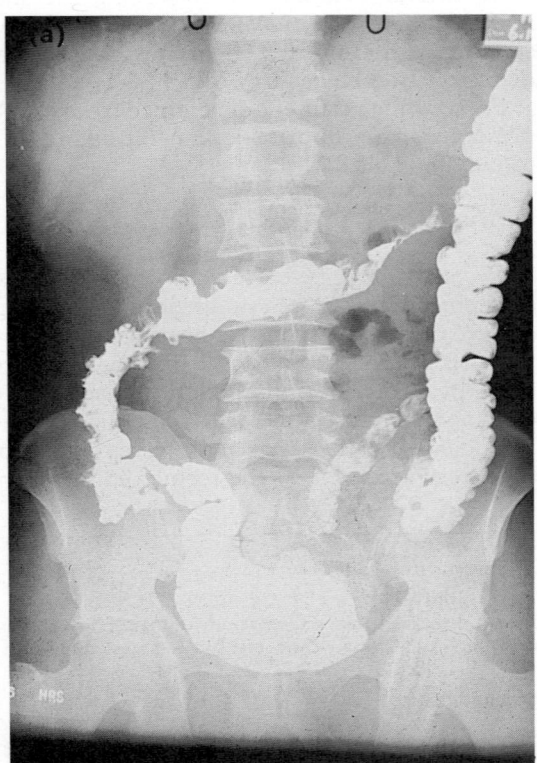
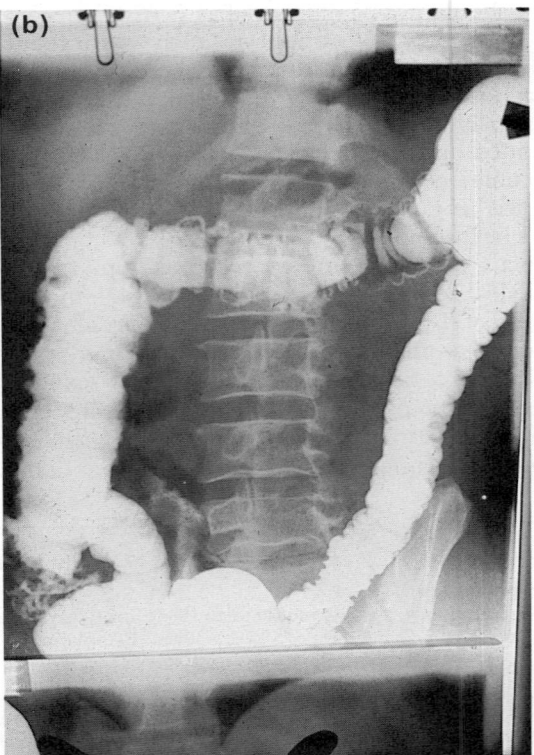

Fig. 17.9 Barium enemas showing an amoeboma of the large bowel: (a) before treatment; (b) after 7 days' treatment with metronidazole.

commonest findings when the rectum is involved are small submucous haemorrhages covered with flecks of bloodstained mucus in which trophozoites can be found. Less commonly ulcers are found. The ulcers are usually shallow, covered with yellowish exudate and up to 2 cm or more in diameter. The edges are raised and undermined with some local hyperaemia though the mucous membrane between ulcers is usually normal. In large ulcers grey sloughs may be found and in these severe cases great care is necessary in manipulating the sigmoidoscope as the bowel wall is very friable. The normal tone of the sphincter may be abolished. Material from ulcers is best removed for examination by a glass pipette, a Volkmann spoon or a pair of bronchial biopsy forceps.

Endoscopy alone cannot be relied upon to distinguish amoebic ulceration from ulcerative colitis or bacillary or bilharzial dysentery. It is always essential to identify the parasite and if *E. histolytica* cannot be found in material from ulcers, repeated examination of faeces is called for. The presence of *Schistosoma* eggs in the faeces or biopsy material is not proof that the ulcers or the symptoms are due to bilharzia.

Immunodiagnosis

Immunodiagnostic tests are of most help in the diagnosis of amoeboma and amoebic liver abscess but are of less help in the diagnosis of acute amoebic colitis. The tests in use are the fluorescent antibody test (FAT), gel diffusion (GD) test, cellulose acetate membrane precipitin (CAP) test, counterimmunoelectrophoresis (CIE) and enzyme-linked immunosorbent assay (ELISA). The complement fixation test (CFT) and indirect haemagglutination (IHA) have now largely been superseded.

Fluorescent antibody test (FAT)

The FAT uses an insoluble antigen. Titres higher than 1/160 are significant and over 1/256 very suggestive of invasive amoebiasis.[18] This test is very sensitive with a low specificity, with a 20% false-positive rate, especially in other liver diseases (hepatitis etc). It remains positive for long after successful treatment and is of little use as a test of cure. It is useful as a screening test to be followed by more specific tests, such as the GD or CAP tests. It is useful in sero-epidemiological studies[19] and can be used to

identify amoebae in tissue sections which can be scanned rapidly and more effectively than by conventional staining.[20] It can identify species of amoebae in tissues by specific fluorescent staining.

Gel diffusion (GD) test[21]

The GD test uses soluble antigen and is still a useful immunological test. Results are either positive or negative and a positive test means past or present invasion of the tissues. It is commonly positive in acute amoebic colitis and post-dysenteric colitis and always positive in amoebic liver abscess. It does not indicate whether the infection is light or heavy but a negative reaction almost completely excludes amoebic invasion of the tissues. One disadvantage is that it takes 24–48 hours to perform and it is positive in 15% of Africans with other diseases.

Cellulose acetate membrane precipitin (CAP) test[22]

The CAP test uses a soluble antigen which is simple to perform and gives results in about 4 hours. The membranes used in the test may be pre-treated with antigen and stored for several months. It is highly specific with no false positives and slightly more sensitive than the GD test. It becomes negative three months after recovery but a positive result can persist after successful treatment indicating past rather than present infection, whereas the GD test shows a close correlation with the presence or absence of active infection.

Counterimmunoelectrophoresis (CIE)

The CIE is easy to perform and a result can be given in under an hour. A negative CIE excludes amoebic liver abscess. It can also be used to detect amoebic antigen in stools or aspirated pus.[23]

Enzyme-linked immunosorbent assay (ELISA)

An ELISA test is the most sensitive and shows the greatest changes in antibody titre. Titres persist for the longest time so that it is of little use as a test of cure. Amoebic antigen may be detected in stools or pus.[24]

Latex agglutination test[25]

A simple latex agglutination test is available as a

commercial kit (Serameba) which has been evaluated and found to be reliable.[26] In clinical practice, for the differential diagnosis of invasive amoebiasis it is usual to do a screening test with the more sensitive FAT and test the positive reactions with the less sensitive but more specific GD or CAP tests.

TREATMENT

Invasive amoebiasis should be regarded as an exception to the general rule that, in a parasitic disease, parasitological proof of the diagnosis must be obtained before the start of treatment. With the introduction of metronidazole, which is virtually free from serious toxic effects, a therapeutic trial may be justified in view of the frequent difficulty in finding and recognizing *E. histolytica*. The severer forms of amoebic dysentery can resemble ulcerative colitis and an amoebic abscess may be difficult to differentiate clinically from a hepatoma or a hydatid cyst. In cases of doubt treatment for amoebiasis should be given first so that disasters such as the use of steroids for amoebic 'ulcerative colitis' are avoided.

Drug treatment

Drugs used in the treatment of amoebiasis may be amoebicides acting at all sites (metronidazole, tinidazole), indirect amoebicides acting in the lumen and wall of the bowel (tetracycline) or direct acting amoebicides acting in the lumen of the bowel (diloxanide furoate).

Imidazoles

Metronidazole and other imidazoles have now almost completely replaced emetine and other more traditional remedies in the treatment of invasive amoebiasis. Metronidazole (Flagyl) may be given as a single daily dose of 1.4 g for 3 days, care being taken to give the tablets slowly with a sweetened drink to reduce vomiting. In Mexico 2 g daily of metronidazole or other imidazoles has been found effective and is given for 5 days.[27]

Tinidazole is also given as a daily single dose of 2 g and is given for 3 days. Metronidazole may be given in a dose of 800 mg three times daily for 5 days but this may be less effective than single dose administration. Nearly all reports of failure of metronidazole to cure have been with three

times daily regimens. Although it seems sensible to eradicate the parasite from the lumen of the bowel there are some doubts as to the value of treatment with luminal amoebicides, particularly in endemic areas where luminal infections are probably self-limiting and reinfections almost inevitable.[28]

Nitroimidazoles should be used cautiously in pregnancy. They should not be used for cyst passers but if a pregnant woman is ill with invasive amoebiasis, particularly with severe dysentery or liver abscess, their use may be life-saving and less fraught with danger than alternatives, such as emetine.

Luminal amoebicides

The imidazoles are so well absorbed that their luminal action is poor in comparison to their tissue action.

8-Hydroquinolines have been used and were widely sold for the treatment of traveller's diarrhoea but because of the association with subacute myelo-optic neuropathy (SMON) in Japan should no longer be used for this condition. However, Diodoquin and clioquinol are still used as luminal amoebicides and used like this have never caused SMON.

Diloxanide furoate (Furamide). If a luminal amoebicide is needed, diloxanide furoate is safe and reasonably effective; thus an imidazole (tissue amoebicide) and, if need be, diloxanide furoate (luminal amoebicide) should be all that is necessary to treat all forms of amoebiasis, though in certain circumstances it may be necessary to fall back on the older preparations.

Diphetarsone (Bémarsal) is a useful pentavalent arsenical luminal amoebicide. It is given by mouth in a dose of 30 mg/kg twice daily for 10 days.

Other drugs

Emetine hydrochloride is a tissue amoebicide, acting in the wall of the bowel and in the liver. It is no longer made in the UK. The dose was 60 mg daily by intramuscular or deep subcutaneous injection for 10 days. While under treatment the patient must be kept in bed since the drug is cardiotoxic and the heart must be monitored electrocardiographically when the T wave will become inverted but return to normal after treatment.

Another drug that has been used is chloroquine for liver involvement in a dose of 150 mg (base), twice daily for 15 days, always given in combination with another drug.

Treatment of amoebic peritonitis

In the first type of peritonitis, which is rare, with a clearcut history of perforation, surgical repair with an omental patch gives a good result.

In the second type with a leaking bowel or liver and a friable colon a conservative approach is the only one. Antibiotics of the tetracycline group and other antibiotics are sometimes used with tissue amoebicides and may be life-saving, especially if damage to the colon is such that a bacterial peritonitis or septicaemia threatens. Patients showing early signs of peritonitis should be given metronidazole (1.4 g single daily dose) or a similar imidazole, if necessary intravenously, if there is evidence of paralytic ileus. Tetracycline or another broad-spectrum antibiotic should also be given. Nasogastric suction and the maintenance of fluid balance by the intravenous route will be essential. Probably the main cause of death in such patients is septicaemic shock. Metronidazole will have a dual action on both the amoebae and on gram-negative anaerobic bacteria from the gut. It may be necessary to resort to injections of emetine though the potential cardiotoxicity of emetine in a patient who may be already in shock should be recalled.

Treatment of cyst passers

Attitudes towards the treatment of cyst passers have changed. Cysts of non-invasive strains of *E. histolytica* do not need treatment and a group of cyst passers followed for nine months showed that all lost their cysts spontaneously.[28] Most cyst passers certainly in temperate countries probably excrete non-invasive strains.

Test of cure and course

Three negative stools and a negative GPD test are a mark of cure. Stools should be examined monthly after this as the reappearance of cysts usually means a return of a symptomatic infection. Sometimes patients suffer a number of apparent relapses of the intestinal infection and reinfection may be the cause so that the environment and other members of the household should be examined for possible sources of infection.

EPIDEMIOLOGY

Amoebiasis is strongly associated with slum conditions, bad sanitation, poverty and ignorance and probably with the general state of health and nutrition of the people; this is true of both actual amoebic dysentery and symptomless infection. In the Durban area the incidence and severity of the infection at all ages is greatest in the urban slum area where the Africans live on a diet largely deficient in protein. In the rural areas, on the other hand, where conditions and diet are better, the infection in Africans is usually mild or symptomless.

Though living in unsanitary conditions, Indians in the urban environment of Durban are much less subject to amoebic dysentery than Africans, and Europeans least of all. It is unlikely that differences of virulence of strains are responsible, but even though sanitary conditions are probably the main factor there may be other influences not clearly known. Certainly diet seems to be important.

It has sometimes been suggested that amoebic dysentery is almost confined to adults and that it is more common in men than in women. In the Durban area, however, where the general load of parasites is very heavy, amoebic dysentery and its complications are often seen in children; the same is true of Egypt, Ghana and Nigeria, as well as elsewhere. For instance, Olatunbosun[29] reported 15 children who died of acute invasive amoebiasis and came to autopsy in Lagos. One had a cerebral abscess, several had liver abscesses, several peritonitis and two intussusception but the others had no extraintestinal lesions. All had bronchopneumonia and most were anaemic. Fulminating amoebiasis in children was reported in Nigeria by Lewis and Antia[30] and in Lagos, 60% of all outpatients suffering from acute amoebic dysentery were children.[31] Most of the mothers were cyst carriers. Indeed, pregnancy seems to predispose to amoebic dysentery. In a survey of villages in The Gambia,[32] where sanitation was non-existent, over the period of a year nearly the whole population (98.3%) was infected with *E. histolytica*. Infection rates were lowest inland and highest near the coast; there was a sharp rise in prevalence at the beginning of the rainy season. More females than males were passing cysts; infection in children was common. Attempts to find cysts in the environment—water, soil, food, flies and so forth—were unsuccessful, even though sensitive culture methods were used.

PREVENTION

Control measures effective for enteric bacterial infections are also effective for amoebiasis. A safe and adequate water supply and sanitary disposal of sewage and refuse afford good protection. Ordinary chlorination of water cannot be relied upon to kill cysts and, although hyper-chlorination will do so, it is expensive and gives an objectionable taste and is therefore impracticable.

Filtration is necessary but cysts can pass sand filters if the filtration rate is high. Water likely to contain cysts should therefore be treated with a coagulant, allowed to settle before sand filtration at not more than 30 litres/1000 cm^2/minute and then chlorinated to at least 1 p.p.m. residual chlorine. Metal microfabric is often used to remove particulate matter from water but even such fabric with the smallest aperture (23 μm) will not prevent cysts from passing.[33] For personal protection where safe water is not supplied to the community, water should be boiled or treated by approved domestic measures.

Cysts can live in water (or faeces) for several days, few remaining alive after two weeks. Putrefaction damages them and desiccation kills them at once. A high temperature is more lethal than a low temperature, though deep freezing kills them at once, and at body temperatures they die within a few days.[34] People who live in endemic areas should therefore be careful in the selection of foods, especially those bought from street vendors. Cooking kills the cysts but foods commonly eaten uncooked, such as tomatoes, salads, strawberries and others grown close to the ground and possibly fertilized with human faeces, should be avoided or thoroughly washed in safe water.

Kitchen hygiene practices which minimize the risk of exposure should be instituted and facilities for hand washing by cooks should be installed. All these measures should be taught to and understood by food handlers.

Travellers in endemic areas who stay in hotels have been advised to use water from the hot water taps for drinking, tooth-brushing, washing dishes and cups etc., because water at 50°C kills cysts in 5 minutes. A rough test is that if the water is too hot for the hand to tolerate it is almost certainly harmless.[35] This reasoning applies also to bacterial diseases and to traveller's diarrhoea.

Cysts have been found in the vomit and faeces of flies (which also carry them on their feet) and in the droppings of cockroaches. These pests should be suppressed and food should be protected from them. Cyst passers who are food handlers should normally be treated but if there are a large number of them the cysts should be identified as to whether or not they are of an invasive strain of *E. histolytica*.

Amoebic infection of the liver (amoebic hepatitis, amoebic liver abscess)

'Amoebic liver abscess continues to provide the greatest pitfall in clinical tropical medicine.'[36]

The commonest *metastatic complication of amoebiasis* is hepatic amoebiasis or liver abscess. Other tissues and organs may be involved and amoebiasis of the lung, amoebic pericarditis by direct extension, amoebic abscess of the brain and other organs, spleen, psoas muscle, buttocks and thigh by systemic spread.

GEOGRAPHICAL DISTRIBUTION

Amoebic liver abscess is commonest in areas of intense infection, such as Natal, India and Mexico. It may rarely be found in persons who have never been to the tropics.[37]

Expatriates living in endemic areas may be more liable to liver abscess than the indigenous people, but the latter are certainly prone: 500–600 cases each year in Durban.[38] Children do not escape and many abscesses have been found in them before and after death in both Nigeria and Durban. Expatriate children rarely develop liver abscess, perhaps because they live in good sanitary conditions. Amoebic liver abscess seems to be particularly common in some ship stewards and kitchen staff who are well nourished.[16]

PATHOLOGY

The trophozoites reach the portal system via the portal veins from the bowel and the pathological process is one of necrosis by lysis at the centre of the lobules. A form of 'amoebic hepatitis' with amoebae among the liver cells without any necrosis[39] is now no longer thought to exist,[40] and so-called amoebic hepatitis is as Rogers originally described—a very early stage of liver abscess in which a number of small necrotic foci (or abscesses) form which, if not treated, tend to enlarge and coalesce into one or more big abscesses. The abscesses may be single (65–75%) or multiple (25–35%) and the right lobe is affected four times as often as the left.

As liver abscess develops the liver enlarges and in the early stages contains grey, ill-defined globular necrotic patches up to 2.5 cm in diameter. These necrotic patches liquefy and coalesce, forming the characteristic ragged abscess cavities full of viscid, chocolate-brown (anchovy sauce) thick pus which contains disorganized liver tissues and clots or streaks of blood (Fig. 17.10). The pus is sometimes greenish from bile. Trophozoites of *E. histolytica* can often be found in the pus after drainage of the abscess for a few days and they are present in large numbers in the walls of the abscess cavity. Cysts are never found. The abscess can become secondarily infected with pyogenic organisms, especially if open operation is performed (which is contraindicated); in this case trophozoites tend to disappear.

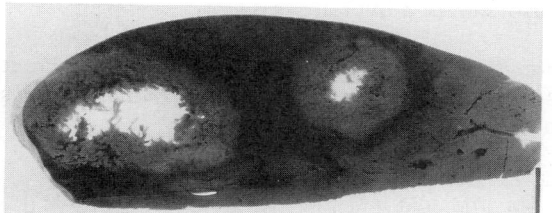

Fig. 17.10 Multiple liver abscess from a case of acute amoebic colitis.

Histologically, three zones can be recognized: a centre containing yellow or grey opaque material that is amorphous and necrotic and contains no leukocytes; a median zone of stroma and a shaggy outer fibrinous wall invaded by trophozoites which are clustered in the fibrin next to viable liver tissue. The surrounding liver is oedematous and infiltrated with chronic inflammatory cells (Fig. 17.11).

Liver abscesses may be single or multiple and are usually (but not invariably) found in the right lobe. Multiple abscesses have been misdiagnosed as metastatic carcinoma, the correct diagnosis

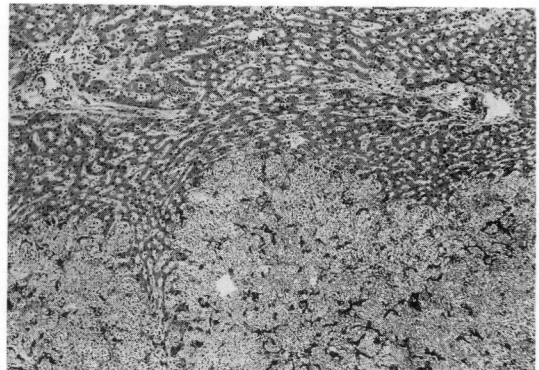

Fig. 17.11 The structure of miliary amoebic liver abscess containing *E. histolytica*.

having been made only when histological examination revealed trophozoites in the abscess walls. A single abscess may attain great size.

An abscess in the right lobe tends to push up the right cupola of the diaphragm and this can be seen on the radiograph, providing an important point in diagnosis. As an abscess approaches the surface of the liver, adhesions are commonly formed with the surrounding organs; they may prevent the abscess from bursting into the peritoneal cavity. Apart from the peritoneal cavity an abscess may burst into the pleural cavity or the lung itself, though pleural adhesions may prevent general spread. An abscess (usually in the left lobe) may infect the pericardium, with all the serious effects of that condition.

Liver abscesses may become encysted with thick fibrous walls and the contents may eventually become cheesy or cretified until the cyst contracts. Calcified abscesses can sometimes be found by radiography and must be differentiated from hydatid cysts or calcified suprarenals.

CLINICAL FEATURES

Natural history

The natural history of amoebic liver abscess is one of gradual progression with increasing size until it ruptures or the patient dies of inanition. Sometimes it will heal spontaneously and calcified abscesses have been seen on radiology in the liver with no previous history of hepatic amoebiasis.

Incubation period

Liver abscess may occur after a long period, perhaps many years after the patient left the endemic area, and the importance of asking a patient who has an enlarged liver if he or she has been abroad cannot be overemphasized. In this, as in so many other cases in which tropical diseases may be involved, it is imperative to ask the question: 'Where have you been?' The explanation of this long latent period may be that the infection persisted without symptoms until some stimulus provoked multiplication of the entamoebae, or that the original infection induced hypersensitivity and that reinfection provoked the reaction. Steroid therapy for some other condition may also be the stimulus.

Symptoms and signs

There is a great variety in the symptoms from few to many and severe. Males outnumber females by eight to one. The patient has usually resided in the tropics for some time but may have left many years before; however, a liver abscess can be contracted after quite a short visit. In about half the cases there is a history of dysentery in the previous month but often there is no history of any previous dysentery.

Amoebic hepatitis. The early stages of amoebic liver abscess present with a low-grade fever and right hypochondrial tenderness. The liver is enlarged and tender and there is a leukocytosis.

These symptoms and signs respond dramatically to antiamoebic treatment.

Amoebic liver abscess. When a larger abscess has formed, the symptoms and signs are more marked. The onset may be gradual or acute, with pain in the right hypochondrium or chest, and intercostal tenderness to pressure between the ribs. The pain is continuous and may be worse on breathing or referred to the right shoulder. There can be great loss of weight and wasting.

Fever. Fever is usual with profuse sweating and sometimes rigors and often resembles that of typhoid, though it may be periodic rather than continuous (Fig. 17.12). However, the patient may be completely afebrile.

Abdomen. The liver is enlarged and tender but if the abscess is deeply situated tenderness may be absent.

Chest (Fig. 17.13). There are usually signs at the base of the right lung with cough and X-ray evidence of a raised diaphragm. There may be visible swelling with oedema over the right lower ribs and a sharp tap on the right lower chest is extremely painful. Abnormal physical signs in the right lower chest should always lead to the suspicion of a liver abscess.

Jaundice. Jaundice is uncommon and when it occurs is usually mild, but deep jaundice does not exclude a liver abscess.

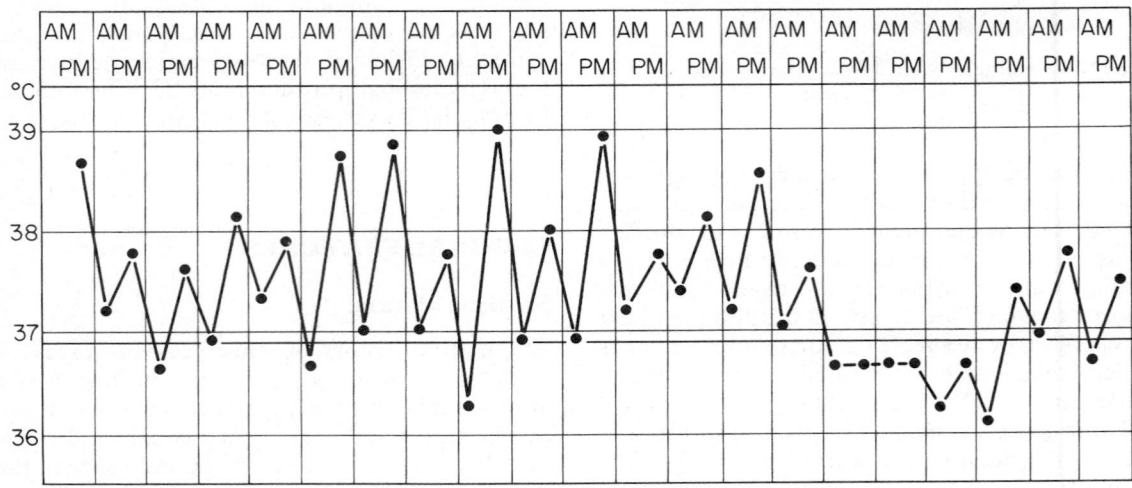

Fig. 17.12   Typical temperature chart for a patient with amoebic liver abscess.

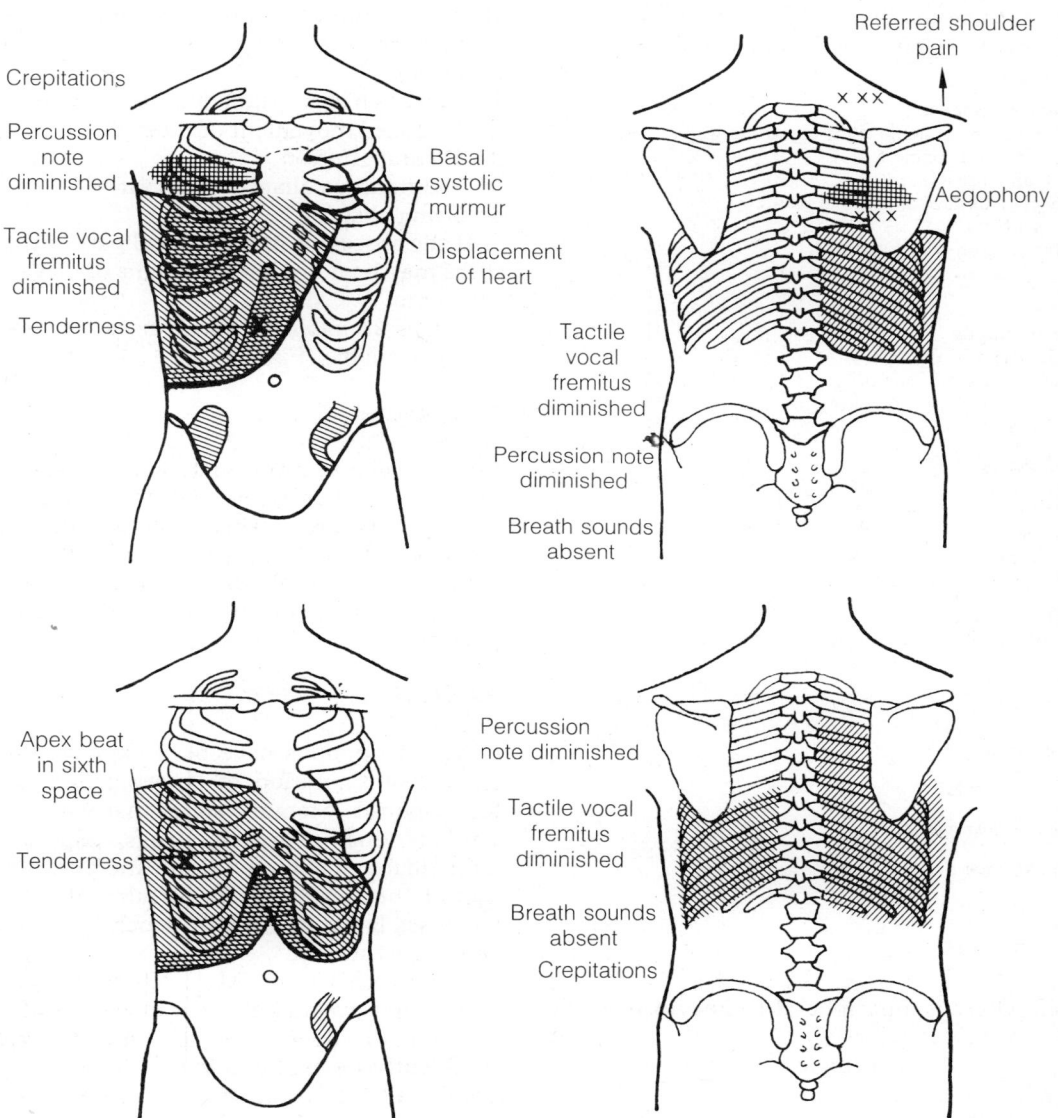

Fig. 17.13 Physical signs of amoebic liver abscess. *Above*, abscess in the right lobe and *E. histolytica* cysts in the faeces. The patient was cured by aspiration. *Below*, hypertrophy of the left lobe and *E. histolytica* cysts in the faeces. The patient was cured by aspiration of 1.8 litres of sterile pus.

Unusual manifestations which can confuse the diagnosis are hepatocellular and cholestatic jaundice and hepatic coma.

The previous administration of corticosteroid drugs may produce fulminant liver disease.

The features found in 764 cases of amoebic liver abscess seen in Thailand were as follows.[41] (Figures are given as percentages.)

Presenting symptoms

Fever and pain at the right costal margin	82
Fever without pain	13
Abdominal mass	3
Others (jaundice, abdominal pain, dysentery)	2
Referred pain (right shoulder)	28

Signs

Fever	97
Hepatomegaly	91
Tenderness of the liver	95
Jaundice (usually slight)	32
X-ray, raised right diaphragm	85
Leukocytosis	87

Site of abscess

Right lobe	87
Left lobe	8
Both lobes	5
Single cavity	94

Pus

Reddish-brown	89
Creamy or yellowish green	11

Recovery of E. histolytica

From pus	11
From stool	14

Rupture of abscess	27
Pulmonary amoebiasis	3
Pleural effusion	9

DIAGNOSIS

Blood. There is a peripheral leukocytosis in the range $15–35 \times 10^6$/litre with 70% polymorphs. A normocytic hypochromic or normochromic anaemia is usual.

Liver function tests. These are variable. The serum bilirubin is not usually raised and the transaminases and alkaline phosphatase only slightly raised. Rarely the alkaline phosphatase is markedly elevated.

Stool. Trophozoites and cysts are usually absent from the stools.

Radiological findings

Anteroposterior and lateral views of the chest will show elevation of the diaphragm with 'tenting' and immobility of the right dome (Fig. 17.14) with restriction. Many cases of liver abscess are missed because they often present as pulmonary cases and five radiological signs are important.[42]

1 Elevation of the right dome of the diaphragm.
2 Reduced movement of the right dome.
3 Pleural effusion.
4 Pulmonary collapse, often early.
5 Lung abscess.

If the abscess is in the central part of the liver there may be no pulmonary signs or elevation of the dome.

Isotope scanning of the liver is very helpful where available (Fig. 17.15).

Ultrasound

Where available ultrasound is the most valuable method of identifying and localizing a liver abscess.[43] In areas where sophisticated equipment is not available aspiration of the abscess with Lipiodol replacement or induction of a pneumoperitoneum to outline the right diaphragm[44] are all of value.

Aspiration

Different opinions have been expressed on the subject of aspiration of amoebic liver abscess for diagnosis. Stamm[11] states that with modern serology and non-toxic drugs, aspiration is unjustifiable for purely diagnostic purposes and should be reserved for treatment of large abscesses liable to burst or which fail to resolve on drug treatment.

On the other hand, McLeod et al[38] argue that aspiration is called for if there are signs of pus in or about the liver. It is safe and the liver can confidently be explored with a long, wide-bore needle. The decision whether or not to explore is a matter of clinical judgement, but when signs of abscess are present, delay in aspiration and evacuation of the pus can lead to prolonged illness and serious complications.

For aspiration deep local analgesia usually suffices, but nervous subjects should have a general anaesthetic. If there are localizing signs, such as a tender spot, a fixed pain, localized oedema, localized pneumonic crepitus, pleuritic

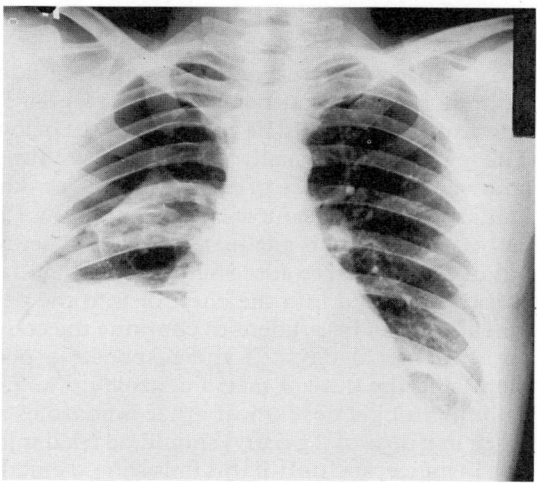
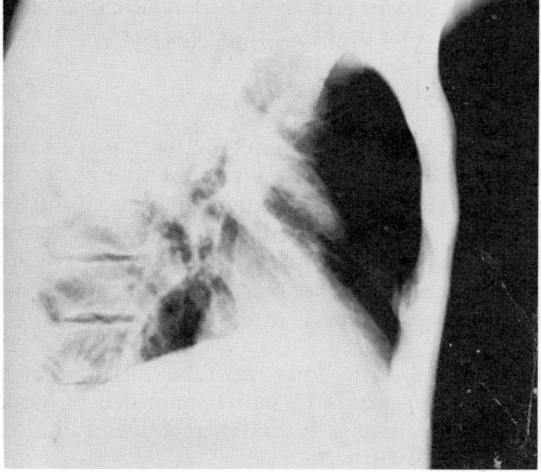

Fig. 17.14   Anteroposterior (left) and lateral (right) views of amoebic liver abscess showing tenting of the diaphragm.

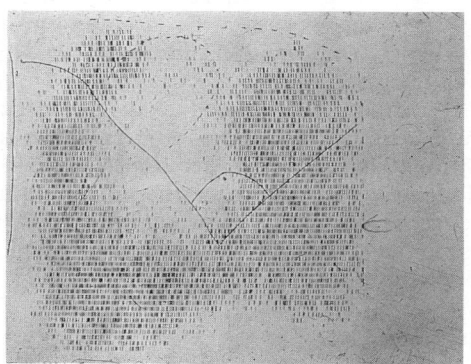

Fig. 17.15   Radioisotope scan from a patient with an amoebic liver abscess.

or peritoneal friction, these should be taken as indicating, with some probability, the seat of the abscess and the most promising spot for exploratory puncture. If no localizing sign is present, the needle should first be inserted in the anterior axillary line in the eighth or ninth interspace, but not more than 9 cm deep—the distance of the inferior vena cava from any part of the chest wall in an adult is 10 cm. This is because most liver abscesses are situated in the upper and back part of the right lobe. The needle swings when the liver is engaged and, as it does so, it should be pushed gently forward. The operator knows when he is in the abscess cavity because the needle is felt to pass into space. The syringe should then be affixed and aspiration commenced. Effusion of serum into the pleural cavity immediately near the abscess sometimes occurs.

Examination of pus

Typical amoebic pus is 'anchovy sauce' coloured but may be white. It is odourless unless secondarily infected. It should always be cultured to see that it is sterile. To demonstrate trophozoites is not easy, but several methods may be used.

Direct examination

To obtain trophozoites from hepatic pus the last part of the aspirate is collected and left until a sediment forms. Trypsin is added to digest the debris and the preparation is centrifuged. The deposit is examined for trophozoites, which may be found in 90% of abscess pus. Trophozoites may also be obtained from the wall of a liver abscess by needle biopsy at the time of aspiration. Trophozoites may also be demonstrated by immunofluorescence,[20] immunoelectrophoresis[23] and ELISA.[24]

Immunodiagnosis

Most serological tests are of great value in the diagnosis of liver abscess. The CFT is positive in 100%,[45] the IHA in 100%,[46] the GD test in 96%[21] and the ELISA is most promising. The FAT gives some false-positive results. Most serological tests remain positive long after successful treatment and are of little value in assessing cure.[47] The best test of cure is the GD test.

Differential diagnosis

Amoebic hepatitis and amoebic liver abscess are often missed because they are not thought of in differential diagnosis in non-endemic countries and since they mimic serious and untreatable conditions, but are eminently responsive to treatment in their own cases, a therapeutic trial with an antiamoebic drug is often used.

Amoebic hepatitis. This must be distinguished from *viral hepatitis* in which jaundice is more marked, the liver less tender and liver function tests more disturbed.

Fever. Other causes of fever with sweats and wasting must be distinguished: malaria, typhoid, kala-azar, pyaemia and bacterial endocarditis.

Amoebic abscess. Amoebic abscess is a space-occupying lesion of the liver and must be distinguished primarily from *hepatoma* which is common in the same areas as liver abscess. The necrotic centre of a hepatoma may resemble pus but there is accompanying cirrhosis and the jaundice is much deeper with greatly deranged liver function tests. However, a therapeutic trial with antiamoebic drugs should always be tried before the patient is condemned to death with a hepatoma. Other space-occupying lesions are *hydatid cyst*, which is not tender, empyema of the gallbladder with deep jaundice and tenderness.[36]

Lung conditions. The signs at the base of the right lung with cough and blood-streaked sputum suggest a right lower lobar pneumonia or pleural effusion. A liver abscess should always be thought of if a right basal pneumonia fails to respond to antibiotics. Lung abscess can be formed by spread through the diaphragm or blood spread and closely resembles a bacterial lung abscess. Often a therapeutic trial is necessary.

Sub-diaphragmatic abscess. The liver is not tender and the right dome of the diaphragm is obscured.

Solitary pyogenic liver abscess. The pus will be white with a well-marked odour and contain staphylococci or other organisms.

TREATMENT

Most abscesses respond to metronidazole without aspiration although if the response is slow aspiration should be considered (see below). The patient will usually feel better within 24 hours of the first dose of metronidazole or other imidazole. A 3-day course of metronidazole 1.4 g daily (single dose) is adequate for most abscesses but in the very large abscesses or those that have already ruptured into the chest or into the peritoneum it may be prudent to continue the course for a further 3 days. If the response is poor, increasing the dose of metronidazole up to 2.4 g daily in a single dose (most other imidazoles are given in a dose of 2 g daily) should be tried in the first instance, and only if this fails should emetine be resorted to.

There is usually no need to combine another tissue amoebicide, such as chloroquine, with imidazole preparations used in large single doses daily. Such combinations increase the risk of toxicity with no increase in cure rate. If a luminal amoebicide is to be used diloxanide furoate should be given in a dose of 0.5 g three times daily for 10 days. Most patients with liver abscess no longer have a patent luminal infection at the time of presentation and what evidence there is does not suggest a role for luminal amoebicides in preventing subsequent relapse.[28]

Aspiration

If the abscess is large and the patient very ill aspiration is indicated although very large abscesses may resolve on drug therapy alone. Aspiration produces a more rapid alleviation of the condition. Any indication of impending rupture, such as into the peritoneal cavity, is an indication for aspiration.

Open drainage

Open drainage is normally completely contra-indicated and in the past led inevitably to secondary infection and death. However, if the pus is very thick and cannot be aspirated or the abscess is secondarily infected or rupture has occurred, then it should be done. Laparotomy should be performed and a drain inserted, always connected to an underwater seal and should be removed as soon as possible. If there is a complete perforation into the peritoneum laparotomy and aspiration with peritoneal toilet is necessary.

An antibiotic as well as an antiamoebic drug is necessary. Aspiration of the left lobe of the liver is usually only possible with a laparotomy to direct the aspiration under direct vision or where the abscess is very deep and cannot be located through the right chest.

PROGNOSIS

The prognosis is usually excellent. Relapse may occur in some cases.

COMPLICATIONS

Spread to the lung: pleural effusion

A pleural effusion may develop in the right pleural cavity in association with a liver abscess in the upper part of the right lobe of the liver. A liver abscess may rupture into the right pleural cavity causing pleurisy, effusion or empyema. The development of this is often insidious but may be sudden with marked pain and shock. The right side is invariably involved and the signs are those of pleural effusion but enlargement of the liver may suggest the diagnosis. The pleural cavity may contain pus of the anchovy sauce kind and trophozoites may be found in it.

Amoebic lung abscess

Amoebic infection of the lung may be secondary by direct spread through the diaphragm or primary by haematogenous spread.

Direct spread

The condition presents as a right basal pneumonia which does not respond to antibiotics. The sputum often suggests amoebiasis with small haemoptyses or quantities of reddish brown material sometimes containing trophozoites. The right diaphragm is raised and the lung is consolidated or contains an abscess. A hepatobronchial fistula may develop which drains the abscess successfully. Occasionally an amoebic abscess of the lung is 'coughed up' with the production of amoebic pus from the bronchial tract.

Haematogenous spread

Haematogenous spread with lung involvement in the absence of liver involvement can occur but is rare. There may be single or multiple abscesses or areas of consolidation. The sputum may contain trophozoites but these are probably *E. gingivalis* if they do not contain red cells.

Amoebic infection of the lung may lead to bronchiectasis but responds well to antiamoebic treatment with metronidazole and, when there is an associated liver abscess, this should be aspirated.

Amoebic peritonitis (see also p. 315)

An amoebic liver abscess not uncommonly ruptures into the peritoneal cavity either suddenly or by gradual leaking. If sudden, the picture is that of acute peritonitis with shock, followed by distension and signs of free fluid. Treatment is surgical with plasma or blood for shock. Thereafter the standard antiamoebic treatment is indicated, together with tetracycline. In some cases there are local collections of pus which should be drained.

Amoebic pericarditis

Amoebic pericarditis is usually associated with abscess in the left lobe of the liver; it is rare. One type presents a pericardial rub or a clear effusion with radiographic signs of pericarditis. This indicates that the underlying liver abscess is near the pericardium; if the abscess is drained and standard treatment given the pericardial lesion resolves. Rupture of an abscess into the pericardium may be fatal in a few hours. There is pain and respiratory distress, and signs of pericardial effusion develop; it may lead to tamponade. There are also signs of the liver abscess. Diagnosis is confirmed by aspiration of characteristic pus from the pericardium; differentiation from purulent pericarditis due to bacteria is obviously important. A negative GD test excludes amoebiasis as a cause of pericarditis. Treatment is urgently needed and is often successful. Aspiration or drainage of the pericardium and of the liver abscess is called for, together with specific antiamoebic treatment and antibiotics if bacterial infection occurs. Diuretics may be indicated. Late results may include constrictive pericarditis which may require pericardectomy. The indication for low salt diet and diuretics are the same as for other pericardial disease.[48]

Other complications

Abscesses have been found in the spleen, the psoas muscle, the buttocks (sometimes connected with a pararectal abscess and secondarily infected by bacteria) and the thigh. These conditions respond well to metronidazole.

Other rare complications of liver abscess are rupture into various hollow abdominal organs—stomach and colon—which may be followed by severe haemorrhage. The abscess may communicate with the biliary system, when the liver pus is heavily stained with bile. The liver abscess itself, usually bacteriologically sterile, may become infected by bacteria, in which case the patient tends to become toxic and the fever does not settle; the pus changes in character. Treatment is with antibiotics in addition to antiamoebic drugs and aspiration. Surgical drainage may be needed if these measures fail.

Amoebic infection of the urinary tract has been described but authentic cases are rare. Trophozoites cannot live long in urine but if they have access to the urinary passages and are passed out quickly they may be recognizable. They may possibly gain access directly via the urethra, or via a fistula with the intestine, or by extension of a liver abscess into the kidney, or by blood or lymphatic spread. Care should be taken that haematophagous macrophages are not mistaken for trophozoites. Cysts do not occur in urine.

Amoebic abscess of the brain

Amoebic abscess of the brain is an uncommon complication, usually, but not always, associated with a liver abscess. The abscess which is usually in the frontal lobe is silent, being found almost always at autopsy. Occasionally it may produce pressure symptoms and should be suspected in any patient with liver abscess who shows signs of mental deterioration. There is no meningitis, the diagnosis is made by aspiration through burr holes in the absence of a CT (computed tomographic) scan. Response to antiamoebic drugs is very poor and the condition is usually fatal.

GIARDIASIS (*GIARDIA LAMBLIA*)

GEOGRAPHICAL DISTRIBUTION

Giardia infection is distributed worldwide in both the developed and underdeveloped world.

AETIOLOGY (see also Appendix I, p. 1255)

G. lamblia lives in the upper part of the small intestine particularly the duodenum. The *trophozoites* (Fig. 17.16A and B) resembles a half pea split longitudinally and measures 12–18 μm in length. The ventral surface has a concave sucking disc with a raised ridge at its anterior end and the posterior extremity tapers into a fine tail terminating in two flagella. The oval nuclei are in the anterior end and the flagellate swims rapidly swaying from side to side (Fig. 17.17). *Giardia* reproduces by binary fission.

The *cyst* (Fig. 17.16C) is formed in the lower bowel and may occur in large numbers in the stools. It is oval, measuring 10.5 × 7.4 μm. The body becomes rounded and there are at first two nuclei dividing into four in a mature cyst. In

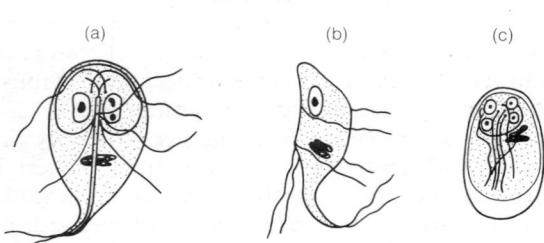

Fig. 17.16   *G. lamblia*. A, Trophozoite full view. B, Trophozoite lateral view. C, Cyst.

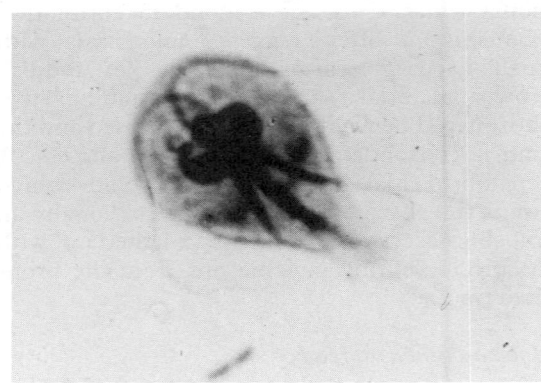

Fig. 17.17   *G. lamblia*. Trophozoite. (Courtesy WTIM.)

iodine solution it stains faint yellowish brown (Fig. 17.18). Cysts remain viable at 21°C in water for 8 days and in stored water at 8°C for up to 5 weeks. They can resist the concentration of chlorine normally present in tap water. They are killed at 50°C and by 2% iodine solution (five drops to one litre) allowed to stand for 30 minutes. *Giardia* may be cultured on Diamond's medium[17] modified by omitting the autoclave step and sterilizing by membrane filtration.

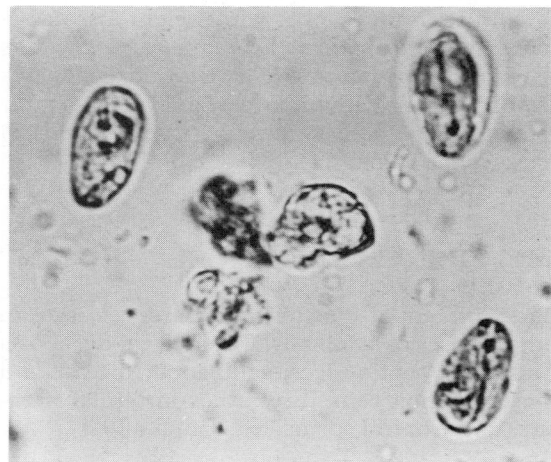

Fig. 17.18 *G. lamblia.* Cysts in the stool. (Courtesy WTIM.)

TRANSMISSION

Man is the usual source of infection although mammals, such as dogs, beavers and musk-rats, can become infected and excrete cysts.

The source of infection is children who excrete large numbers of cysts (adults excrete few cysts). Transmission is by faecal–oral contact, food contaminated by food handlers or faeces, or contaminated water.

Faecal–oral route. This is the usual method of transmission in endemic tropical areas where family infection is the rule. There is a high rate of infection in homosexuals.

Food. Vegetables can be contaminated from fertilizer made from human excreta or by food handlers in the market.

Water-borne transmission. This is responsible for outbreaks of giardiasis in temperate countries from clean mountain streams contaminated by hikers, beavers or musk-rats, and in tap water as in Leningrad. The 'hill diarrhoea' of India was probably water-borne *Giardia* infection.

PATHOLOGY

Susceptibility to infection is increased by achlorhydria, cannabis[49] and the possession of blood group A,[50,51] chronic pancreatitis, protein energy malnutrition and certain immune deficiency states, such as lack of IgA,[52] hypogammaglobulinaemia and AIDS (see Chapter 68).

The trophozoites are normally found in the mucus adherent to the mucous membrane of the duodenum and jejunum where they attach to the mucosal cells by means of the sucker disc.

Mucosal invasion has been documented but is infrequent and does not correlate with the severity of clinical manifestations.[53] Interference with the function of the enterocyte and a decrease in the level of disaccharidases is the most important factor. In experimental *Giardia* infection[54] blunting of the villi develops in the first two weeks accompanied by a decreased level of disaccharidases due to a direct toxic effect of the trophozoites on the brush border. Electron microscopy shows damage to the microvilli at the site of attachment. Later changes in the mucosa may be caused by cytopathic sensitized T cells as in graft versus host disease.[54] T lymphocytes are involved in the final clearance of the infection and there is an increase in the number of mucosal lymphocytes. The severity of the morphological changes in the mucosa correlates with the severity of symptoms in some patients[55] but not in all. In those cases associated with malabsorption the presence of circulating antibody[56] suggests immunological damage, and histological changes similar to those found in tropical malabsorption develop, ranging from crypt elongation to total villous atrophy. The gallbladder and bile ducts are occasionally invaded without any symptoms but it is probable they have moved there as a result of preoperative procedures.

Malabsorption

The mechanism of malabsorption in *Giardia* infection is not yet clear. Disturbance of intestinal mobility, and luminal competition for substrates have been suggested, but the mechanism is probably the same as in tropical sprue; the parasite alters the small intestinal environment so that it is colonized by enterobacteria[57] causing malabsorption.

IMMUNITY

In endemic areas giardiasis is so common that most children become infected early during childhood. The first infection is symptomatic but the infection which is common in young children is rare in older children and adults, suggesting that an efficient immunity develops. The mechanism of such an immunity is as yet not clearly understood. The immune response involves both antibody and T cells. Circulating antibody has been demonstrated[56] and T cell-mediated immunity is responsible for eradication of the infection. IgA may be involved, since IgA-deficient persons are especially susceptible to infection and anti-IgA antibody has been demonstrated on the surface of *Giardia* trophozoites.[58]

CLINICAL FEATURES

Natural history

There is a wide spectrum of disease and spontaneous eradication of the infection is the rule. About 20% of infections are symptomatic and in most cases cause an acute diarrhoeal illness subsiding after one or two weeks. In a small number of patients bowel disturbance persists but the symptoms and passage of cysts do not continue for more than three months. Rarely patients may remain infected and symptomatic for many years.[59] Under 10% of cases develop clinical malabsorption with weight loss and lethargy.

The *incubation period* is usually about two weeks but may be as long as several months.

Symptoms and signs

Diarrhoea is the main symptom. It is usually worse in the morning, often explosive, usually offensive and with pale, almost white stools, but without blood or pus.

Weakness, abdominal pain, nausea, anorexia and failure to thrive in children are important symptoms.

Dyspepsia with *Giardia* infection resembles hepatic dysfunction with dull upper epigastric pain, marked nausea and flatulence suggesting gallbladder disease.

Malabsorption

Malabsorption of D-xylose and fat is common and malabsorption of vitamin B_{12} was found in 50% of all patients.[55] However, serum folate levels were normal, anaemia did not occur and calcium levels were normal. In more advanced cases giardia infection with malabsorption resembles tropical sprue with weight loss, lassitude and fatty stools. The important point is that malabsorption caused by *Giardia* disappears after treatment with metronidazole, and not after tetracycline, whereas tropical sprue responds to tetracycline alone.

DIFFERENTIAL DIAGNOSIS

The differential diagnosis of giardiasis is from other causes of small bowel diarrhoea, dyspepsia caused by peptic ulcer, gallbladder disease and malabsorption caused by other intestinal parasites and tropical sprue (see Chapter 19).

DIAGNOSIS

Trophozoites can be demonstrated in fluid and samples obtained from the jejunum and cysts in the stools.

Stool examination

Cysts are not always present in the stools and treatment should be given in suggestive cases even when the stools are negative, when a good response is obtained. Stools are examined by the formol ether concentration method (see Appendix IV, p. 1490). They were positive in 85% of symptomatic cases[55] but in another series only in 50%. In other cases the diagnosis can be made by examination of jejunal aspirate or mucosal smears from a jejunal biopsy.

Jejunal aspirate

The 'string test' (enterotest) is used in which a string with a small weight is swallowed to which the trophozoites in the jejunum adhere and can be shown on microscopical examination.

Jejunal biopsy

Mucosal impression smears from a biopsy will show trophozoites.

Immunodiagnosis

In some cases, especially with the malabsorption syndrome, immunodiagnosis is of great help. A fluorescent antibody test[56] and a gel diffusion test[60] are available and an ELISA test should be of great use.[61]

TREATMENT

The drug of choice is one of the imidazole drugs.

Imidazoles are effective treatment if given in large single doses daily.

Metronidazole and tinidazole are given in a single dose of 2.0 g[55] or as 2.0 g to be followed by a second dose one week later.

Mepacrine is not so satisfactory. It is given in a dose of 100 mg three times daily for 10 days. It was 91% effective with one course and 95% with a second.[55]

Alcohol should be avoided because of the Antabuse effect with imidazoles and milk and milk products avoided because of the associated alactasia. Relapses are rare but can occur up to six months after treatment. Frequent relapses should call to mind a possible IgA deficiency.

EPIDEMIOLOGY

Giardiasis may be endemic, sporadic or epidemic.

Endemic

Children under three years of age are three to four times more frequently affected than adults and excrete larger numbers of cysts. In rural areas of the tropics *Giardia* is a family infection passed round by faecal–oral infection from hand-feeding in poor hygienic conditions. Under these conditions it is an infection of young children related to poor personal hygiene, poverty and poor sanitation.

Sporadic

Sporadic infection is acquired by travellers and *Giardia* is quite a common cause of traveller's diarrhoea (see Chapter 14).

Epidemic

Epidemics of water-borne giardiasis have occurred in the USA[62] and institutional outbreaks occur in mentally retarded children's homes transmitted faeco-orally.

CONTROL

Water can be protected from infection by super-chlorination and clean water; proper disposal of excreta and clean hands will prevent transmission.

BALANTIDIASIS (BALANTIDIAL DYSENTERY)

GEOGRAPHICAL DISTRIBUTION

Balantidium coli is a common parasite of pigs worldwide. Human infection is sporadic in temperate areas of the world and cases have been recorded from many countries. In some areas of the tropical and subtropical world there is a high prevalence: New Guinea,[63] Venezuela, Brazil, southern Iran[64] and Georgia in the southern USA.

AETIOLOGY

Balantidium coli is a common parasite of pigs, wild boar, sheep, horses, cats, dogs, guinea-pigs and monkeys. Although *B. coli* from man can be transmitted to pigs, the pig parasite has so far not been transmitted to man. *B. coli* is a large ciliated protozoon which exists in two forms, one *trophozoites*, the other a *cyst*.

The *trophozoite* is oval in shape, 30–200 μm long × 40–60 μm wide, and various races are recognized by their size. The body is clothed with a thick covering of cilia (Figs. 17.19 and 17.20). There is a large kidney-shaped *macronucleus* with close by a small *micronucleus*. The protoplasm contains two contractile food vacuoles. At the anterior end there is a *peristome* which leads into a *cystostome* or mouth, and at the posterior end an anus or *cytopyge*. Trophozoites are not normally found in formed and semiformed stools.

The *cyst* is ovoid 40–60 μm long (Figs. 17.21 and 17.22) and is passed in the faeces. It contains the parasite of which there may be two which may be seen moving within the cyst, inside which the parasite loses its cilia. The life history is not yet completely known.

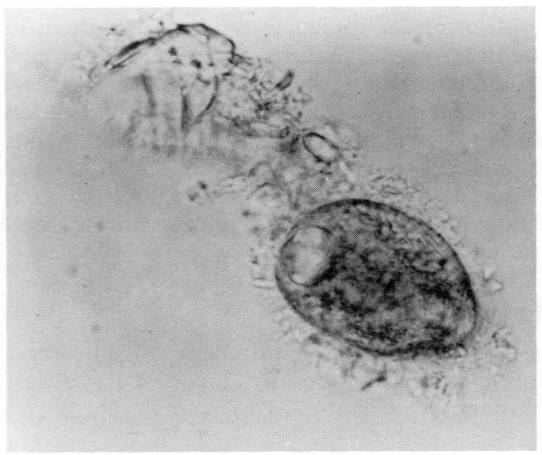

Fig. 17.19 *B. coli*. Trophozoite showing cilia and contractile vacuole. (Courtesy Dr J.S. Tatz.)

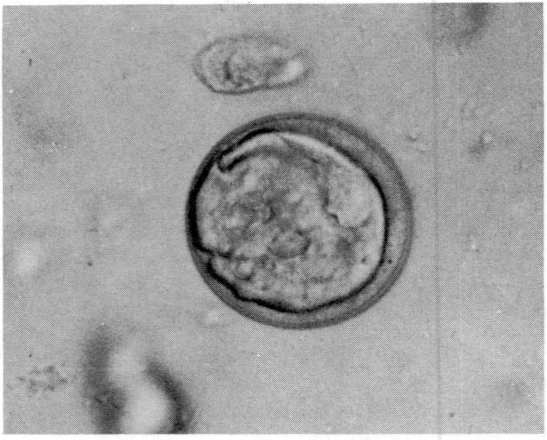

Fig. 17.21 *B. coli*. Cyst in stool. (Courtesy Dr R. A. Shooter.)

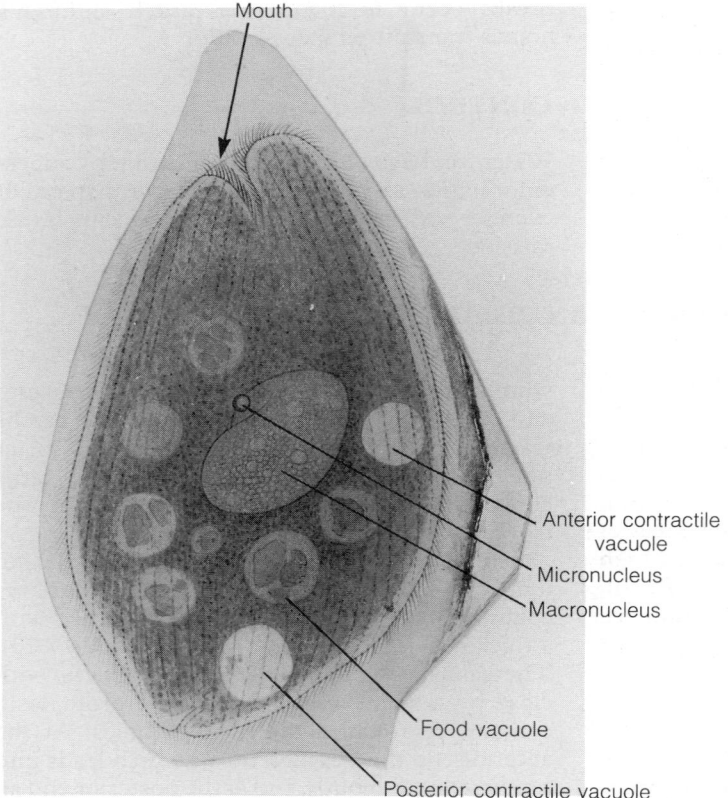

Mouth

Anterior contractile vacuole

Micronucleus

Macronucleus

Food vacuole

Posterior contractile vacuole

Fig. 17.20 *B. coli*. Trophozoite.

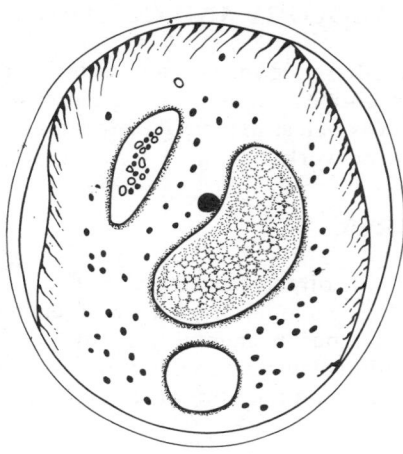

Fig. 17.22   *B. coli*. Cyst (× 1200) showing nuclei, remains of cilia and posterior contractile vacuole.

TRANSMISSION

Infection is from cysts and pigs are the main source. The route is faecal–oral by direct contact from hands infected with pig faeces. Water-borne transmission can occur from water contaminated by pig faeces.[65]

IMMUNITY

Little is known about immunity but second attacks can occur and antibodies are used in diagnosis.

PATHOLOGY

In man *B. coli* is probably always a tissue invader. The cysts exist in the small intestine and the trophozoites pass into the large intestine where they burrow into the mucosal surface and set up colonies. It is probable that lytic action helps in this process as hyaluronidase is produced by *B. coli*.[66]

Both gross and microscopic pathology closely resemble that of amoebic infection. Ulcers are found with rounded base and wide neck and cellular infiltration round the base. Trophozoites are found in large numbers in exudates on the surface, congregated in the follicles and embedded in the tissues forming the base of the ulcers. They invade the submucosa and the muscular coat and even enter the lumen of blood vessels and lymphatics and have been found in the mesenteric lymph glands. The early lesions appear as minute haemorrhages, then later as ulcers and abscesses. In advanced cases the colon may be a mass of ulcers throughout its length, resembling those of amoebic dysentery.

CLINICAL FEATURES

Natural history

There is a wide spectrum of disease, and many cases are asymptomatic; in Venezuela 80% of infections have no symptoms,[67] other infections frequently disappear spontaneously, whereas others develop dysentery with blood and mucus in the stools which may be fulminating and fatal.

The *incubation period* is unknown.

Symptoms and signs

The onset may be gradual or sudden. There may be constipation, abdominal pain and weight loss or there may be diarrhoea with blood and mucus in the stools. Fulminating infections lead to perforation of an intestinal ulcer and balantidial peritonitis.[68] Chronic symptoms may persist for years.

COMPLICATIONS

Liver abscess containing numerous trophozoites has been reported[67] and many balantidial liver abscesses have been mistaken for amoebic liver abscesses.

Vaginitis and *urinary tract* infection have been found.[69]

DIFFERENTIAL DIAGNOSIS

Amoebic colitis, *Shigella* dysentery and ulcerative colitis must all be distinguished. This is done by stool examination.

DIAGNOSIS

Trophozoites are found in 90% of mucoid and bloody stools while cysts are found in semiformed and formed stools by concentration techniques (see Appendix IV, p. 1490) (Fig. 17.21). *B. coli* may be cultured in media with bacteria used for *E. histolytica*.

Immunodiagnosis

A fluorescent antibody test is available.[70]

TREATMENT

Tetracycline is the treatment of choice; 2 g is given daily for 10 days.[71]

    Metronidazole has been very effective[72] but in other hands has been disappointing; 1.2 g is given daily for 7 days and 750 mg daily for children.

    Paromomycin (Humatin) 50–100 mg/kg is given daily for 5 days.[73]

EPIDEMIOLOGY AND CONTROL

In areas where pig/man contact is intimate, such as New Guinea, there is a high prevalence of infection as well as in mental institutions in many parts of the world.

CONTROL

Control of direct faecal–oral infection is by improving personal hygiene and encouraging hand washing in mental institutions. Super-chlorination of water supplies is important where pigs can contaminate the water supply.

ENTAMOEBA POLECKI INFECTION

GEOGRAPHICAL DISTRIBUTION

The majority of cases reported in man have been from Papua New Guinea but the parasite is found worldwide.

AETIOLOGY

The taxonomic status of *E. polecki* is controversial. It closely resembles *E. histolytica* and cannot be distinguished enzymatically.[74] It occurs in both trophozoites and cyst form.

TRANSMISSION

E. polecki is common in monkeys and pigs and is transmitted via the cysts from pig or monkey to man. Man-to-man transmission may occur.

Clinical features

Almost all cases are asymptomatic but heavy infections are associated with intestinal symptoms, including diarrhoea, anorexia, abdominal pains and cramps.

DIAGNOSIS

Uninucleate cysts in the stools are the main feature and the persistence of uninucleate cysts in the absence of quadrinucleate cysts should lead to a suspicion of *E. polecki*.

TREATMENT

Most drugs are ineffective. *Metronidazole* 750 mg three times daily followed by *diloxanide furoate* (Entamide) 500 mg three times daily for 10 days was successful.[75]

DIENTAMOEBA FRAGILIS INFECTION (see Appendix I, p. 1251)

D. fragilis is only known in the trophozoite stage. It is non-invasive but a low-grade eosinophilia with vague abdominal symptoms from intestinal irritation may occur with heavy infections. *Paro-* *momycin* 500 mg three times daily for 5–7 days has proved effective. Other drugs have not been evaluated.

COCCIDIAL ENTERITIS

Isosporiasis (*Isospora belli*)

Isospora belli has a worldwide distribution but is most prevalent in South America and Africa. It is rarely reported from man.

AETIOLOGY

The cause is *Isospora belli*, a coccidian parasite which has two cycles in the epithelial mucosa of the only host known, man. One cycle is sexual with sporogony and the other asexual with schizogony.

Life-cycle (see also Appendix I, p. 1241)

Infection occurs from ingestion of ripe oöcysts. The oöcyst is ovoid with a thin translucent wall containing two sporocysts each containing four crescent-shaped sporozoites (Fig. I.13,2, p. 000). These sporulated oöcysts encyst in the small intestine to invade the epithelial cells where they form trophozoites.

Asexual cycle (schizogony). The trophozoites mature into schizonts with the formation of merozoites. The host cell ruptures and the merozoites invade fresh cells to start the cycle all over again.

Sexual cycle (sporogony). The merozoites develop into multicellular male gametocytes and unicellular female gametocytes. The male gametocytes rupture forming male microgametes which fertilize the female macrogametes to form immature oöcysts (Figs. 17.23 and I.11,1,

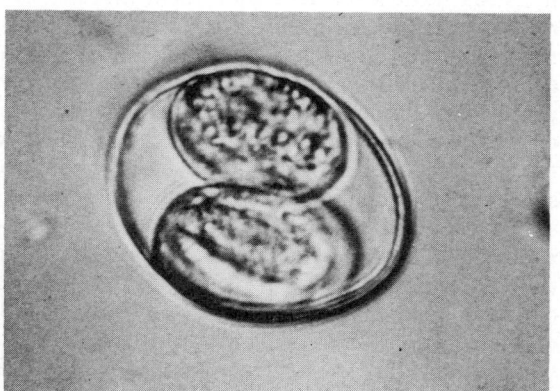

Fig. 17.23 Oöcyst of *Isospora belli* in stool.

p. 1241) which are then discharged into the lumen of the bowel and passed out in the faeces where they sporulate after 48 hours and become infective (Fig. I.11,2, p. 1241).

TRANSMISSION

Transmission is by the faecal–oral route.

PATHOLOGY

Little is known of the mechanism by which such lesions as have been described are produced. In the patients described by Brandborg et al[76] pathology varied, but none had a normal intestinal mucosa and in some the changes were patchy. In one case the villi- were flattened, the crypts elongated with inflammatory infiltration of the lamina propria.

IMMUNITY

Little is known about immunity but immunological deficiency predisposes to enteritis.

CLINICAL FEATURES

Natural history

Most infections are asymptomatic; any symptomatic ones are self-limiting, lasting two to three weeks but rare cases last many months with malabsorption.

Incubation period

In experimental infections symptoms developed one week after infection and oöcysts were recovered from the stools 9–15 days after ingestion.

Signs and symptoms

Most infections are asymptomatic but a minority may lead to disease. It is an important infection in immunosuppression disease (e.g. acquired immunodeficiency syndrome (AIDS)). Diarrhoea, abdominal colic, weight loss and mild malabsorption can all occur. In the rare cases of severe malabsorption patients may be ill for much longer.

Laboratory findings

There may be a mild peripheral eosinophilia.

DIAGNOSIS

Oöcysts which are immature appear irregularly in the faeces and need concentration techniques to demonstrate them, or duodenal intubation and intestinal biopsy. *I. belli* oöcysts are elongated ovoids (20–33 × 10–19 μm), tapered at the end with a smooth double layered hyaline wall (Figs. 17.23 and I.11,1 and 2, p. 1241). They can be distinguished from the sporocysts of *Sarcocystis*

bovihominis and *suihominis* by their smaller size and absence of sporozoites when freshly passed in the stool.

TREATMENT

Combined therapy with pyrimethamine and sulphadiazine for seven weeks as in toxoplasmosis is curative. Co-trimoxazole (trimethoprim 80 mg, sulphamethoxazole 100 mg) two tablets 6-hourly for two to three weeks has also been found effective.

Epidemiology

So far as is known man is the only host. Close contact between humans is necessary for transmission and *Isospora* infection occurs in homosexuals and patients with AIDS.[77] (See also Chapters 60 and 68.)

Sarcosporidiosis. 1   Intestinal sarcocystosis (formerly *Isospora hominis*)

Sarcocystis is a coccidian parasite with two hosts. In the intermediate (prey) host it forms muscle cysts (sarcocysts) containing cystozoites; in the definitive (predator) host it undergoes sporogony in the intestinal mucosa.

Man can be either the definitive host (intestinal sarcocystosis) for some species, or the intermediate host for others with the formation of sarcocysts in muscles (see section on muscle sarcocystosis, below).

GEOGRAPHICAL DISTRIBUTION

Distribution in cattle and pigs is 100% in some areas, is worldwide but few cases have been diagnosed in man.

AETIOLOGY

Intestinal sarcocystosis in man is caused by two species (formerly known as *Isospora hominis*): *Sarcocystis bovihominis* (specific to cattle) and *Sarcocystis suihominis* (specific to pigs).

LIFE-CYCLE (see also Appendix I, p. 1242)

S. bovihominis and *S. suihominis* have an intermediate stage as sarcocysts in the cardiac muscle and oesophagus of cattle and pigs. The sarcocysts are ingested by the prey host (man) and burst, liberating numerous cystozoites which penetrate the intestinal epithelium to the subepithelial tissues where they undergo schizogony, forming further sarcocysts. After a period some merozoites become differentiated and enter cells of the intestinal mucosa where they form macro- and microgametocytes. The microgametocytes multiply into a number of microgametes which escape into the gut lumen and the macrogametocyte enlarges to form a macrogamete which is fertilized by a microgamete from the lumen, to form an oöcyst containing two sporocysts. The oöcyst ruptures and infective sporocysts, each containing four sporozoites surrounded by a tough membrane, are passed out in the faeces where they are infective. The sporocyst of *S. bovihominis* is 13.1–17 μm × 7.7–10.8 μm, and of *S. suihominis* 12.6 × 9.3 μm.

On ingestion of the free sporocysts by the intermediate hosts (cattle and pigs) the sporozoites are released and enter vascular endothelial cells in which they multiply by repeated schizogony forming numerous merozoites. After about a month these merozoites enter muscle cells, secrete a cell wall, multiply and develop into sarcocysts containing a large number of cystozoites. The sarcocysts remain dormant until eaten by the definitive (predator) host.

TRANSMISSION

Transmission is by eating undercooked beef and pork.

PATHOLOGY

Little is known about pathology in man. Cases from Thailand have been described with segmental eosinophilic or necrotic enteritis.

IMMUNITY

Nothing is known about immune processes in man.

CLINICAL FEATURES

Natural history

Although some symptomatic cases have now been described it is thought that most infections are asymptomatic and symptoms are dose related:

Incubation period

In experimental infections symptoms have started 3–6 hours after ingestion of infected beef followed 14–18 days later with the passage of sporocysts and abdominal symptoms.

Symptoms and signs

In experimental human infections vomiting took place after eating the meat, followed by abdominal pain, anorexia, nausea, bloating and diarrhoea associated with passage of sporocysts. In Thailand intestinal obstruction has followed segmental enteritis, needing segmental resection of the bowel. Apart from severe cases there is a self-limiting mild diarrhoea.

Diagnosis

The sporocysts are scanty in the faeces and need concentration techniques for their demonstration. Mature sporocysts can be found from the ninth day after infection and may be differentiated from those of *I. belli* by the presence of four sporozoites and their larger size: *S. bovihominis* 13.1–17 μm × 7.7–10.8 μm, *S. suihominis* 12.6 μm × 9.3 μm.

TREATMENT

There is no specific treatment.

EPIDEMIOLOGY AND CONTROL

Wherever raw or semicooked beef and pork are eaten, as in Thailand, then infection may be found.

Control is by cooking beef and pork or deep freezing which destroys the sarcocysts.

Sarcosporidiosis. 2   Muscle sarcocystosis

Man is acting purely as an intermediate host and there is no intestinal infection.

GEOGRAPHICAL DISTRIBUTION

Sarcocystosis in the muscles of man has been so rarely described that little is known about the distribution.

AETIOLOGY

In about 40 human cases the sarcocysts present resembled those found in the local monkeys:[78] *Macaca fascicularis* in South-East Asia, *Macaca mulatta* in India and *Cercopithecus talapoin* in Africa and Europe. In three cases in human heart muscle the cysts resembled *S. bovicanis*. *S. lindemanni* is no longer an entity.

TRANSMISSION

Little is known about transmission but the oral–faecal route from close contact with non-human primates is most likely.

PATHOLOGY

Most sarcocysts elicit little inflammatory response and measure up to $100 \times 325 \mu m$. Each cyst contains many cystozoites measuring $7-16 \mu m$ in length. Inflammation follows upon death of the cyst probably caused by an antigen–antibody reaction. There is an infiltration with neutrophils, eosinophils and lymphocytes with subsequent appearance of plasma cells and fibrosis. Vasculitis is commonly present.

IMMUNITY

Little is known about immune processes but antibody-mediated immunity keeps schizogony at bay and necessitates the formation of cysts.

CLINICAL FEATURES

Natural history

Most cases are asymptomatic and signs and symptoms only follow death of the cysts.

Signs and symptoms

Localized painful muscular swellings 1–3 cm in diameter and lasting 2–4 days are often accompanied by slight fever, bronchospasm and eosinophilia. A case has been reported in which intermittent swellings of arms and legs was associated with a progressive muscular weakness and paraesthesiae of hands and feet. There was an eosinophilia of 40% and muscle biopsy showed sarcocysts (Fig. 17.24) and radiology showed faint shadows in the leg muscles.[79]

DIAGNOSIS

Diagnosis is by muscle biopsy. Differentiation has to be made from toxoplasma cysts and *Trypanosoma cruzi*. Cystozoites are PAS (periodic acid–Schiff) positive. Serology is of no value.[80]

TREATMENT

Treatment is usually unnecessary although steroids will eliminate the symptoms of muscle swellings.

EPIDEMIOLOGY AND CONTROL

Little is known about the epidemiology but contact with non-human primates must be important and shared feeding places or closer contact with them should be avoided.

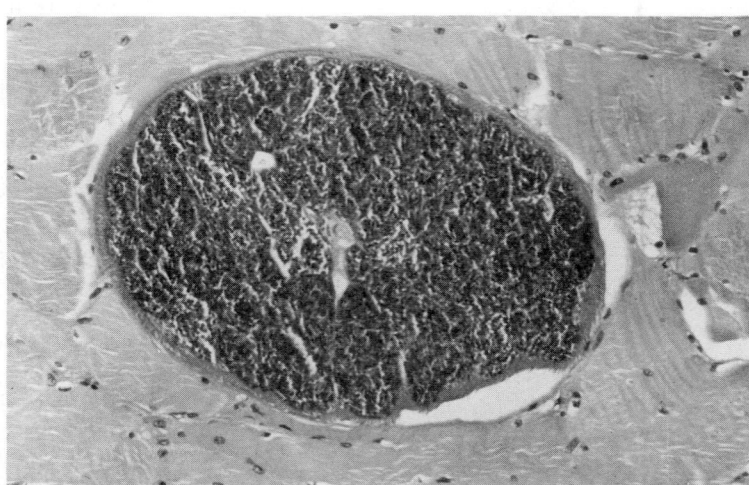

Fig. 17.24 Sarcocyst in human muscle. Cyst border and striatid membrane covering thousands of cystozoites. (Courtesy Dr S.B. Lucas.)

Cryptosporidiosis

GEOGRAPHICAL DISTRIBUTION

Cryptosporidiosis is widely distributed in the tropics where it affects two groups of people: children who are immunologically normal and adults suffering from AIDS in central and East Africa. In children it is an important cause of acute diarrhoeal disease and heavy infections are found in Costa Rica[81] and Bangladesh.[82]

AETIOLOGY

Cryptosporidium contains about 11 named species found in 12 different hosts. There appears to be little host specificity and *Cryptosporidium* species from man can infect calves, mice and rats. *Cryptosporidium* is a coccidian parasite with a life-cycle which is extracellular in the mucoid material on the surface of epithelial cells of the bowel.

Life-cycle (see also Appendix I, p. 1242)

Asexual cycle

An oöcyst ingested with the food liberates sporozoites which attach themselves to the epithelial

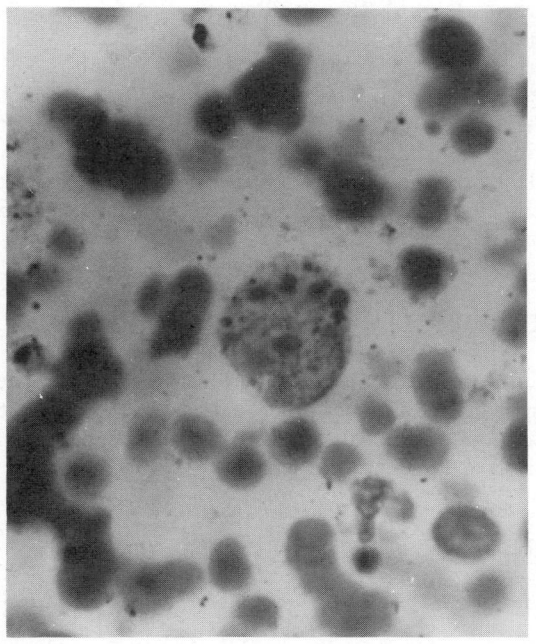

Fig. 17.25 Schizont of *Cryptosporidium* in stool.

cell. The nuclei divide to form schizonts which when fully grown measure 7 μm across, each containing eight nuclei (Fig. 17.25). The schizont divides into eight merozoites, each of which forms a new schizont.

Sexual cycle

Merozoites form gametocytes of both sexes when fertilization takes place to form an oöcyst (Fig. 17.26) containing four masses of cytoplasm, each of which becomes a sporozoite. Many oöcysts liberate their sporozoites while still in the host causing autoinfection and possibly massive parasitism. The oöcysts pass out in the faeces where they are infective to a new host.

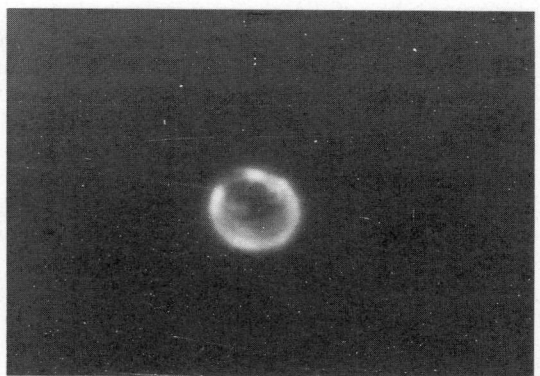

Fig. 17.26 Oöcyst of *Cryptosporidium* in stool stained with phenol auramine. (Courtesy G. Nichols.)

TRANSMISSION

Cryptosporidiosis is mainly a zoonosis and transmission is by the oral–faecal route from calves and other animals through contamination of food. Person-to-person infection is important and household studies have shown outbreaks of cryptosporidiosis in household contacts of infected persons and in children attending day nurseries.[83]

PATHOLOGY

In experimental infection numerous parasites are found in the brush border of the villi of the small intestine but are also present throughout the whole intestine and can be found in rectal biopsies. Penetration of the intestinal epithelial cells is only found in immunocompromised individuals.

IMMUNITY

Little is known about immunity but since the infection is self-limiting and most heavy in young children and calves it must be controlled by immune reactions.

CLINICAL FEATURES

Natural history

Although originally recognized as a cause of illness in immunocompromised individuals it is now apparent that cryptosporidiosis is an important cause of diarrhoea in immunologically normal persons.[83] In the majority of infections it causes symptoms, usually a mild self-limiting diarrhoea but in children this can be severe with dehydration. In immunocompromised individuals it causes a chronic intestinal infection with malabsorption and weight loss causing 'slim disease' in homosexuals infected with AIDS, and is a common cause of death in heterosexual African AIDS.

Incubation period

Symptoms begin one to two weeks after contact with infected calves.

Symptoms and signs

Symptoms vary from a self-limiting acute diarrhoea to severe dehydration. In Costa Rica the diarrhoea ranged from mild to severe with numerous watery stools and severe dehydration.[81] In some children the diarrhoea became chronic causing severe malnutrition. In other cases the onset was with fever and nausea followed by abdominal cramps and diarrhoea which persisted for 14 days. Immuno-compromised patients commonly have a severe secretory diarrhoea leading to wasting and malabsorption.[77]

DIAGNOSIS

The oöcysts are ovoid in structure, 5–6 μm in size and with Giemsa stain blue with reddish and purple corpuscles. They can be differentiated from yeasts by Kinyoun's cold acid fast stain when the oöcysts stain red and the yeasts green.

Oöcysts can best be demonstrated by coverslip flotation using Sheather's sugar solution and staining with one of two stains: a modified Ziehl–Neelsen's technique using hot carbol fuchsin[84] or a carbol (phenol) auramine stain[85] with which the oöcysts fluoresce when examined under oil immersion and an incident light fluorescence microscope (Fig. 17.26), or a safranin–methylene blue stain (see Appendix IV, p. 1500). Oöcysts appear in the stools 56 hours after onset of symptoms, remaining numerous for 4 days, then decreasing to none after the twelfth day.

TREATMENT

There is no specific treatment.

EPIDEMIOLOGY

Cryptosporidiosis is now recognized as a common cause of diarrhoea worldwide. In Third World countries it is a common cause of diarrhoea in children in urban areas. In Costa Rica children were affected from the age of one year upwards and the incidence of infection was highest in the warm humid months, May–June, when child-to-child infection was possible.[81]

In adults infected with heterosexual AIDS in Africa, cryptosporidiosis is a common opportunistic infection in the final stages, causing death from a massive infection with severe diarrhoea and malabsorption. (See also Chapters 60 and 68.)

CONTROL

Contact with calves, in whom infection is widespread, should be avoided and care taken with hygiene in schools and day nurseries where children are collected together.

REFERENCES

1   Hoare, C.A. (1957) *Trans. R. Soc. trop. Med. Hyg.* **51**, 304.
2   Sargeaunt, P.G., Baveja, U.K., Nanda, R. et al (1984) *Trans. R. Soc. trop. Med. Hyg.* **78**, 96–101.

3   Sargeaunt, P.G. & Williams, J.E. (1978) *Trans. R. Soc. trop. Med. Hyg.* **72**, 164–166.
4   Sargeaunt, P.G. & Williams, J.E. (1978) *Trans. R. Soc. trop. Med. Hyg.* **72**, 519–521.
5   Jackson, T.F.H.G., Gathiram, V. & Simjee, A.E. (1985) *Lancet* **i**, 715–718.
6   Neal, R.A. (1968) *Eighth International Congress on Tropical Medicine & Malaria*, Teheran, p. 244.
7   Powell, S.J., McLeod, I., Wilmot, A.J. et al (1966) *Lancet* **ii**, 20.
8   Boyd, J.S.K. (1961) *J. trop. Med. Hyg.* **64**, 1.
9   Phillips, S.C., Mildran, D., William, D.C. et al (1981) *New Engl. J. Med.* **305**, 603–606.
10 Goldmeier, D., Price, A.B., Billington, O. et al (1986) *Lancet* **i**, 641–644.
11 Stamm, W.P. (1970) *Lancet* **ii**, 1355.
12 Essenhigh, D.M. & Carter, R.L. (1966) *Gut* **7**, 444.
13 Faegenburg, D., Chiat, H., Mandel, P.R. et al (1967) *Am. J. Roentg.* **99**, 74.
14 Woodruff, A.W. & Bell, S. (1967) *Trans. R. Soc. trop. Med. Hyg.* **61**, 435.
15 Hennessey, E.F. & Elsdon-Dew, R. (1967) *Med. Today* **1**, 25.
16 Robinson, G.L. (1968) *Trans. R. Soc. trop. Med. Hyg.* **62**, 285.
17 Diamond, L.S. (1968) *J. Parasit.* **54**, 1047–1156.
18 Stamm, W.P., Ashley, M.J. & Bell, K. (1976) *Trans. R. Soc. trop. Med. Hyg.* **70**, 49.
19 Mathews, H.M. (1981) *Laboratory Management* **19**, 55–62.
20 Parelkar, S.N., Stamm, W.P. & Hill, K.R. (1971) *Br. med. J.* **i**, 212.
21 Powell, S.J., Maddison, S.E., Wilmot, A.J. et al (1965) *Lancet* **ii**, 602.
22 Stamm, W.P. & Phillips, E.A. (1977) *Trans. R. Soc. trop. Med. Hyg.* **71**, 490.
23 Mahajan, R.C. & Ganguly, N.K. (1980) *Trans. R. Soc. trop. Med. Hyg.* **74**, 300–302.
24 Grundy, M.S. (1982) *Trans. R. Soc. trop. Med. Hyg.* **76**, 396–400.
25 Morris, M.N., Powell, S.J. & Elsdon-Dew, R. (1970) *Lancet* **i**, 1362.
26 Stamm, W.P., Ashley, M.J. & Parelkar, S.N. (1973) *Trans. R. Soc. trop. Med. Hyg.* **67**, 211.
27 Perches, A., Nieves, M., Landa, L. et al (1976) In *Chemotherapy of Liver Abscess in Amoebiasis*, eds. B. Sapulveda & L.S. Diamond. Inst. Mex. del Seguro Social, Mexico.
28 Nanda, R., Baveja, V. & Anand, B.S. (1984) *Lancet* **ii**, 301–303.
29 Olatunbosun, D.A. (1965) *Trans. R. Soc. trop. Med. Hyg.* **59**, 72.
30 Lewis, E.A. & Antia, A.U. (1969) *Trans. R. Soc. trop. Med. Hyg.* **63**, 633.
31 Nnochiri, E. (1968) *Parasitic Disease and Urbanization in a Developing Country*. London: Oxford University Press.
32 Bray, R.S. & Harris, W.G. (1977) *Trans. R. Soc. trop. Med. Hyg.* **71**, 401.
33 Upton, A.J. (1969) *Trans. R. Soc. trop. Med. Hyg.* **63**, 542.
34 Dobell, C. (1919) *The Amoebae Living in Man*. London: Bale Sons and Danielsson.
35 Neumann, H.H. (1970) *Lancet* **i**, 420.
36 Walters, J.H. (1970) *Trans. R. Soc. trop. Med. Hyg.* **64**, 220.
37 Wright, R. (1966) *Br. med. J.* **i**, 957.
38 McLeod, I.N., Powell, S.J. & Wilmot, A.J. (1966) *Br. med. J.* **ii**, 827.
39 Doxiades, T. (1964) *J. Am. med. Ass.* **187**, 719.
40 Powell, S.J. (1969) *Med. Today* **3**, 48, 85.
41 Harinasuta, T., Bunnag, D., Jaroonvesama, N. et al (1968) *Eighth International Congress on Tropical Medicine and Malaria*, Teheran, p. 258.
42 Middlemiss, H. (1964) *Trans. R. Soc. trop. Med. Hyg.* **58**, 197.
43 Vicary, F.R. (1977) *Gut* **18**, 386.
44 Ellman, B., McLeod, I.N. & Powell, S.J. (1965) *Br. med. J.* **ii**, 740.
45 Robinson, G.L. (1972) *Trans. R. Soc. trop. Med. Hyg.* **66**, 435.
46 Kessel, J.F., Lewis, W.P., Pasquel, C.M. et al (1965) *Am. J. trop. Med. Hyg.* **14**, 540.
47 Krupp, I.M. & Powell, S.J. (1971) *Am. J. trop. Med. Hyg.* **20**, 421.
48 Wilmot, A.J. (1962) *Clinical Amoebiasis*. Oxford: Blackwell.
49 Nalin, D.R., Levine, M.M., Rhead, J. et al (1978) *Pediatrics* **ii**, 859–862.
50 Barnes, G.L. & Kay, R. (1977) *Lancet* **i**, 808.
51 Paulsen, O. (1977) *Lancet* **ii**, 984.
52 Ament, M.E. & Ruben, C.E. (1972) *Gastroenterology* **62**, 216.
53 Wolfe, M.S. (1975) *J. Am. med. Ass.* **23**, 1362.
54 Gillon, J., Althamery, D. & Ferguson, A. (1982) *Gut* **23**, 498–506.
55 Wright, S.G., Tomkins, A.M. & Ridley, D.S. (1977) *Gut* **18**, 343.
56 Ridley, M.J. & Ridley, D.S. (1976) *J. clin. Path.* **29**, 30.
57 Tomkins, A.M., Wright, G.S., Drasa, B.S. et al (1978) *Gut* **17**, 397.
58 Briaud, M., Morichau-Beauchant, M., Matuchansky, C. et al (1981) *Lancet* **ii**, 358.
59 Alp, M.N. & Hislip, I.G. (1969) *Aust. Ann. Med.* **18**, 232.
60 Vinayak, V.K., Jain, P. & Naik, S.R. (1978) *Ann. trop. Med. Parasit.* **72**, 581–582.
61 Haralabidis, S.T.H. (1984) *Ann. trop. Med. Parasit.* **78**, 295–300.
62 Moore, G.T., Cross, W.M., McGuire, D. et al (1969) *New Engl. J. Med.* **281**, 402.
63 Radford, A.J. (1973) *Med. J. Aust.* **i**, 238–241.
64 McCarey, A.G. (1952) *Br. med. J.* **i**, 629.
65 Walzer, P.D., Judson, F.N., Murphy, K.B. et al (1973) *Am. J. trop. Med. Hyg.* **22**, 31.
66 Tempelis, C.H. & Lysenko, M.G. (1973) *Exp. Parasit.* **6**, 31.
67 Wenger, F. (1967) *Kasmera* **7**, 433.
68 Correa Henao (1947) Quoted by Isaza Mejia, G. (1955) *Antiquoia Med.* **5**, 488.
69 Isazar Mejia, G. (1955) *Antiquoia Med.* **5**, 488.
70 Zaman, V. (1965) *Trans. R. Soc. trop. Med. Hyg.* **59**, 80.
71 Hoekenga, M.T. (1953) *Am. J. trop. Med. Hyg.* **2**, 271.
72 Garcia-Laverde, A. & Bonilla, L. (1975) *Am. J. trop. Med. Hyg.* **24**, 781.
73 Sotolongo, F., Otero, R. & Argudin, J. (1966) *Revta cub. Med. trop.* **18**, 103.
74 Sargeaunt, P.G. (1984) Personal communication.
75 Salaki, J.S., Shirey, J.L. & Strickland, G.T. (1979) *Am. J. trop. Med. Hyg.* **28**, 190–193.
76 Brandborg, L.L., Goldberg, S.G. & Breidenhach, W.C. (1970) *New Engl. J. Med.* **283**, 1306.

77 Whiteside, M.E., Barkin, J.S., May, R.G. et al (1984) *Am. J. trop. Med. Hyg.* **33**, 1065–1072.

78 Beaver, P., Gadgil, R.K. & Morera, P. (1979) *Am. J. trop. Med. Hyg.* **28**, 819–844.

79 Mandour, A.M. (1965) *Trans. R. Soc. trop. Med. Hyg.* **59**, 432.

80 Markus, M.B. (1978) *Adv. vet. Sci. comp. Med.* **22**, 159.

81 Mata, K., Bolanos, H., Pizarro, D. et al (1984) *Am. J. trop. Med. Hyg.* **33**, 24–29.

82 Rahaman, A.S.M.H., Sanyal, S.C., Al-Mahmud, K.A. et al (1984) *Lancet* **ii**, 221.

83 Navin, T.R. (1985) *Eur. J. Epidemiol.* **1**, 77–83.

84 Garcia, L.S., Bruckner, D.A., Brewer, T.C. et al (1983) *J. clin. Microbiol.* **18**, 185–190.

85 Nichols, G. & Thom, B.T. (1984) *Lancet* **i**, 735.

Chapter 18
Diarrhoea Caused by Helminths

Intestinal capillariasis is caused by two species of *Capillaria*. *Capillaria philippinensis* causes a local but important disease in the South China Sea and *Capillaria hepatica*, a common parasite of rats, only infects man very occasionally and is unimportant.

CAPILLARIA PHILIPPINENSIS

GEOGRAPHICAL DISTRIBUTION

The disease is known from the South China Sea, the west coast of Luzon in the Philippines and the coast of Thailand.

AETIOLOGY

Capillaria philippinensis resembles *Trichuris trichiura* and is a slender nematode, the male 2.1–3.7 mm and the female 2.6–4.9 mm long. The male spicule has a long sheath without spines, the female vulva is distant to the oesophagus.

Life-cycle[1]

The eggs (45.5 μm × 21 μm) are of two types: one with flattened bipolar plugs which are passed out in the stool, unembryonated, to be ingested by freshwater fish in which they hatch and locate in the intestinal submucosa ready to be eaten by the definitive host; the other type is thin-shelled and embryonated which hatches in the intestine of the host and reinvades the bowel, building up the parasite load by autoinfection, as in *Strongyloides* infection. The normal life-cycle is probably a bird–fish cycle[2] and man acquires the infection from eating raw fish.

TRANSMISSION

Infection is contracted from raw fish which is followed by autoinfection.

PATHOLOGY

The adult *Capillaria* are found in the crypts of the small intestine partially embedded in the mucosa but also free in the larynx, oesophagus, stomach and colon. They cause little inflammation and up to 40 000 worms have been recovered at autopsy. The worms cause severe changes associated with malabsorption, flattening of the villi and atrophy of the crypts of Lieberkühn.[3]

IMMUNITY

Little is known of the mechanism which enables such heavy infections to be built up by autoinfection. Little immune response seems to be invoked.

NATURAL HISTORY

Capillariasis is a progressive infection lasting for years. The worm load builds up with autoinfection leading to severe symptoms and malabsorption.

CLINICAL FEATURES

The incubation period is unknown.

Symptoms and signs

The symptoms and signs are those of severe

malabsorption and protein-losing enteropathy. The first symptoms are diffuse abdominal pain and borborygmi to be followed later by watery diarrhoea with numerous sprue-like stools daily and malabsorption of sugars and fats. In more advanced cases there is weight loss, generalized muscle weakness and severe peripheral oedema. Progressive loss of weight leads to cachexia and death. Patients who recover from one attack usually suffer several relapses and some symptoms for as long as three years.[4]

DIAGNOSIS

The differential diagnosis is from *Strongyloides* and other causes of malabsorption, postinfective and parasitic (*Giardia, Fasciolopsis buski*). The diagnosis is made by finding eggs, larvae or adults in the stool. The eggs must be distinguished from those of *Trichuris* (Fig. 21.9, p. 422, and Plate III.18) and the thin-walled embryonated egg of *Strongyloides* (which is not found in the stool).

TREATMENT

This involves removing the worms and replacement therapy.

Drug treatment

Mebendazole is the drug of choice. It is given in a dose of 400 mg daily for 10–30 days. Thiabendazole can also be used, 25 mg/kg body weight daily for one month, continuing on alternate days up to six months.[5]

EPIDEMIOLOGY

The disease is found in small epidemics around estuaries and rivers in the fishing villages where the migratory fish which travel up the rivers from salt water are caught and eaten. There are three species of fish: *Eleotris melanosoma* (birut), *Hypseleotris bipartita* (bagsit) and *Ambassis miops* (bagsan) which can all be infected experimentally and pass the infection to monkeys. The disease is contracted by the human population because of their predilection for eating raw fish.

CONTROL

The prevalence of the disease has been greatly reduced when the habit of eating raw fish has been discontinued.

CAPILLARIA HEPATICA

This worm is a relatively common parasite of rats and other mammals. Spurious human infections have been recorded when eggs of *C. hepatica* have appeared in the faeces. In genuine infections eggs do not appear in the stools. At least 10 cases of genuine infection have been recorded.[6]

The pathological and clinical picture is that of an acute or subacute hepatitis with eosinophilia and there may be dissemination of the adults and eggs to the lungs and other viscera.[7] The diagnosis is made on liver biopsy or at post-mortem.

A case of severe *C. hepatica* has been successfully treated with prednisone, disophenol and pyrantel tartrate (veterinary anthelmintics).[8]

REFERENCES

1 Cross, J.H., Banzon, T. & Singson, C. (1978) *J. Parasit.* **64**, 208–213.
2 Cross, J.H. & Basaca-Sevilla, V. (1983) *Trans. R. Soc. trop. Med. Hyg.* 77, 511–514.
3 Fresh, J.W., Cross, J.H., Reyes, V. et al (1972) *Am J. trop. Med. Hyg.* **21**, 169–173.
4 Watten, R.H., Beckner, W.M., Cross, J.H. et al (1972) *Trans. R. Soc. trop. Med. Hyg.* **66**, 828–834.
5 Whalen, G.E., Rosenberg, E.B., Strickland, G.T. et al (1969) *Lancet* **i**, 13.
6 Faust, E.C. & Russell, P.F. (1964) *Craig and Faust's Clinical Parasitology*, 7th edn. Philadelphia: Lea & Febiger.
7 Otto, G.F., Berthrong, M., Appleby, R.E. et al (1954) *Bull. Johns Hopkins Hosp.* **94**, 319.
8 Periera, V.G. & Franca, L.C.M. (1983) *Trans. R. Soc. trop. Med. Hyg.* 77, 1274–1275.

Chapter 19
Malabsorption in the Tropics

In order to understand the mechanisms of malabsorption in the tropics it is necessary to know the structure and functions of the jejunal mucosa and the variations that may be found in a tropical environment caused by genetic or infective influences.

STRUCTURE AND FUNCTION OF THE JEJUNAL MUCOSA

The mucosa of the jejunum is lined with intestinal villi, 0.1–0.25 mm long numbering 10/mm² of mucosal substance. Normally they are finger-like with shallow crypts and no ridges. The villi are lined with columnar cells or enterocytes[1] which have a well-defined brush border of microvilli which contain the disaccharide enzymes. Absorption of carbohydrates depends upon these disaccharides, especially lactase, which is responsible for the hydrolysis of lactose.

Glucose, lactose, xylose, iron and water-soluble vitamins are absorbed to a certain extent proximally but mainly in the ileum which also absorbs vitamin B_{12}.[1] Fat is digested as the triglyceride in emulsion in the lumen and the emulsifying system is dependent on a triple combination of fatty acid bile salt and monoglyceride. There are many influences, genetic and parasitic, which may affect the integrity of the mucosa and cause disturbance of function and malabsorption.

Structure and function of the jejunal mucosa in the tropics

The jejunal mucosa of people living in the tropics differs from that in temperate areas. Finger-shaped villi are rare and leaf-shaped villi common. Ridges are common and convolutions rare. This has given rise to the condition known as tropical enteropathy (TE).

TROPICAL ENTEROPATHY (TE) (see also Chapter 60, p. 1001)

GEOGRAPHICAL DISTRIBUTION

TE is almost universal among the inhabitants of tropical countries; Uganda, central Africa, Nigeria, Thailand, south India, Bangladesh, Pakistan and in the western hemisphere, Puerto Rico, Haiti and Peru.[2]

AETIOLOGY

Many causes have been suggested for these jejunal changes but the most likely cause seems to be repeated bacterial and viral infections involving the small intestine.[3] Immune response to antigens derived from pathogens causing gut infections may damage the enterocyte and produce enzyme deficiencies causing TE and malabsorption.[4]

PATHOLOGY

With increasing degrees of damage the intestinal villi assume a 'leaf', 'ridge' or 'convoluted' pattern. In the tropics the normal pattern of most apparently healthy individuals is leaf- or ridge-shaped in contrast to the finger-shaped villi of temperate areas.

Histologically there is a reduction in the height of the villi and an increase in depth of the crypts with an increase in cellular infiltrate in the lamina propria and in the number of leukocytes between the epithelial cells.[5]

CLINICAL FEATURES

Most people with TE are asymptomatic but abnormal D-xylose tests and flat blood glucose curves after oral dosage are common in indigenous people.[6-8] Vitamin B_{12} absorption takes place much more slowly.[9] Folate depletion is associated with monosaccharide malabsorption possibly from changes in the enterocyte and may cause megaloblastic anaemia. Whether TE is the precursor of tropical malabsorption is still not clear but the relative absence of tropical malabsorption from Africa where TE is common suggests that it is not.

EPIDEMIOLOGY

TE is associated with lower socioeconomic groups in tropical countries. Expatriates living under similar conditions also rapidly develop the same changes. They can avoid it by living in Western style in places such as embassies.[8]

TREATMENT

Removal from the environment leads to a rapid restoration of the mucosa to normal.

Causes of malabsorption in the tropics are as follows (see also Table 60.3, p. 1000).
- Hypolactasia
- Parasitic
  - *Giardia lamblia* (see Chapter 17)
  - *Strongyloides stercoralis* (see Chapter 21)
  - Capillariasis (see Chapter 18)
  - *Fasciolopsis buski* (see Chapter 22)
  - Intestinal coccidiosis (isosporosis) (see Chapter 17)
- Pancreatic calcification (see Chapter 60)
- Malnutrition (see Chapter 45)
- Intestinal tuberculosis (see Chapter 45)
- Primary/Mediterranean intestinal lymphoma (see Chapter 67)
- Postinfective tropical malabsorption (tropical sprue, TS)

HYPOLACTASIA (see also Chapter 60, p. 1001)

Hypolactasia due to a low small intestinal lactase concentration may be primary, specifically in lactase but with the other disaccharidases normal, or secondary to damage to the brush border of the enterocyte which occurs after small intestinal infection, and in postinfective tropical malabsorption.

PRIMARY ADULT HYPOLACTASIA

At birth lactase is present in the jejunum in high concentration in all ethnic groups but in those groups with adult hypolactasia concentrations fall in the first four to five years of life, so that the vast majority of the world's adult population, which includes nearly all the indigenous populations of the tropics, has a low concentration of intestinal lactase with malabsorption of lactose which is under genetic control.[10] Most Negroes, Asians and South Americans are lactase deficient and lactose malabsorbers[11] whereas northern Europeans, African pastoralists (Masai and cattle-owning tribes) and populations in the north-west of the Indian subcontinent are not lactase deficient and can drink milk.

Symptoms and signs

Although all lactase-deficient individuals may not develop symptoms, those who do develop nausea, bloating, abdominal pain and diarrhoea after eating foods containing lactose. These symptoms are dose dependent in contrast to cow's milk allergy (see below); 50 g of lactose produces symptoms in 70–80% of malabsorbers whereas 10–15 g of lactose or half a pint of milk will produce symptoms in only 30–60%.[12]

Diagnosis

No morphological changes are found on biopsy and other disaccharidases are normal in distinction to secondary hypolactasia. Proof may be obtained by observing the results of withdrawal and later reintroduction of lactose from the diet or by a lactose tolerance test. Other methods are the detection of hydrogen in the breath after a lastose load[11] or detection of reducing substances in the stool with Clinitest tablets. Almost all lactose malabsorbers will develop diarrhoea, borborygmi, abdominal pain and bloating after taking 50 g of lactose.

Treatment

Milk and all products containing milk should be removed from the diet. This results in complete cure. Aspirin has been suggested as helpful because of its prostaglandin inhibitory properties.

SECONDARY HYPOLACTASIA

Secondary depression of small intestinal disaccharidases occurs after severe damage to the enterocyte. This may occur in tropical malabsorption, viral and bacterial infections of the small intestine (see Chapters 1, 9, 14 and 16) and in severe kwashiorkor (see Chapter 45) where lactose intolerance introduces problems in treatment.

Diagnosis

As well as the methods used in primary hypolactasia jejunal biopsy will show morphological changes and there will be a deficiency of other disaccharidases.

COW'S MILK ALLERGY

Cow's milk allergy is an allergy to the protein in cow's milk and must be distinguished from hypolactasia. It occurs in infants, disappearing by the age of two years. The disease can occur in breastfed infants whose mothers drink cow's milk but disappears when the mother gives up this practice.

TROPICAL MALABSORPTION
(POSTINFECTIVE TROPICAL MALABSORPTION, TROPICAL SPRUE (TS))
(see also Chapter 60, p. 1001)

Because of differences in views on aetiology the name tropical sprue (TS) will be used.

GEOGRAPHICAL DISTRIBUTION

Although tropical enteropathy is present widely throughout the tropics, tropical sprue (TS) is not correlated with its presence, especially in Africa where TE is common but TS is rare.

TS occurs mainly in South-East Asia, especially India and Nepal, but is also found in south China, Vietnam, Indo-China, Indonesia, Philippines, Sri Lanka, Burma and Mauritius. A few cases have come from Fiji and some from the northern Mediterranean (south Italy). In the western hemisphere TS occurs in the Caribbean, Puerto Rico and Haiti (but not Jamaica[13]) and was formerly present in the southern USA, Central America, Guyana and Queensland. Until recently it was thought to be absent from Africa but patients with all the features of malabsorption responding to tetracycline have been reported from Zimbabwe[14] and elsewhere.[15] However, TS is extremely rare in Africa and is unlike the typical cases seen in Asia. There are also variations in the clinical picture of TS between the Old and New Worlds, anaemia being a more prominent feature in the New World.

AETIOLOGY

TS is defined as a syndrome, occurring among residents of or visitors to the tropics, of diarrhoea with malabsorption of two or more substances.

The cause of malabsorption in TS is a change in mucosal pattern of the small intestine which affects both structure and function and is responsible for the malabsorption of all nutrients, fat, protein, carbohydrate, vitamins and even water. The loss of these nutrients results in steatorrhoea, loss of weight, anaemia, hypoproteinaemia, tetany and other deficiency states, both of minerals and vitamins. The causes of these mucosal changes are controversial and there are two main lines of thought: one infective, the other a chronic deficient intake triggered off by some mechanism.

Infective (postinfective malabsorption)

This school[16] thinks that the cause is primarily infective. An acute infection (viral, bacterial or parasitic) sets off a chain of events in which pathogens subsequently damage the enterocyte and an increase in a tropic hormone, enteroglucagon, causes small intestinal stasis with bacterial overgrowth of enterotoxin producing coliform organisms[17] which can cause mucosal damage,[18] and viral agents have been found in the stools in TS.[19] Folate depletion increases the mucosal damage and the whole process can be terminated by tetracycline and folic acid.

Nutritional (tropical sprue)[20]

Dietary factors

Dietary factors have been suggested as being causal in the tropical sprue syndrome, by its occurrence in areas where unsaturated fats predominate in the diet and its absence from the predominantly maize-eating areas of Africa where saturated fats are in use. The unsaturated fatty acids may discourage the bacteria normally resident and allow the growth of coliform bacteria.

The relations between TS, folate and vitamin B_{12} are complex[21] and patients with TS rapidly become depleted of both substances with secondary changes in the gastrointestinal mucosa, bone marrow with megaloblastic anaemia and occasionally the nervous system. Malabsorption of vitamin B_{12} is not due to vitamin-binding bacteria damage to the intrinsic/B_{12} complex, but damage to the ileal mucosal receptors is thought to be the cause. In long-standing TS, patients show gastritis depressing gastric secretion and consequently defective intrinsic factor secretion. The position with folate is less clear. Impaired hydrolysis of polyglutamate and impaired absorption of its digestive product, folic acid, may be responsible but the jejunal crypts can obtain the necessary folate by an alternative pathway. TS can occur against a background of low dietary folate and administration of folic acid rapidly reverses the megaloblastic changes in the crypt cell nuclei with improvement in morphology. Loss of nutrients from the gut may also be important. Dehydration, hyponatraemia and hypokalaemia are extremely common in the more severe cases of TS.[22] Excessive loss of albumin via the intestine (protein-losing enteropathy) occurs in a proportion of cases[23] and folic acid may also be lost in a similar manner.[24]

TRANSMISSION

TS was originally thought to be transmitted by water but the agent which triggers off the condition is spread by the oral–faecal route in poor environmental conditions and TS is common in hippies in whom hepatitis is also common.

PATHOLOGY

Intestinal lesions

The chief lesions originally described by Bahr[25] and finally confirmed by jejunal biopsy[26] are found in the villi of the jejunum and ileum. Under a binocular microscope the villi are leaf-like (as opposed to finger-like) with ridges and convolutions. Microscopically the changes may be graded into five grades (Fig. 19.1). The villi become broadened and fused together. The enterocytes stain poorly and are reduced to low columnar or cuboidal types with an increase in the number of mitotic figures in the cells lining the crypts which become greatly shortened, indicating a rapid turnover or a failure of maturation. The enterocytes are vacuolated with grossly abnormal microvilli on electron microscopy. Goblet cells are numerous and the fundi of Lieberkühn's follicles are distended, the interstitial tissues being infiltrated with lymphocytes and plasma cells. These changes may be reversed rapidly with folate and vitamin B_{12} but may persist after antibiotics alone, even though vitamin B_{12} absorption has returned to normal.

Other organs

In advanced cases at post-mortem the body is grossly emaciated. The skin is dry with irregularly scattered areas of pigmentation and some petechial haemorrhages. There is brown atrophy of the heart. The marrow is hyperplastic (megaloblastic) or pale and hypoplastic. Osteoporosis and osteomalacia may be present.

Pathophysiology

In the early stages of TS, malabsorption of glucose, fat, B_{12} and folate occur and after four months there is a fall in serum B_{12} and folate with some anaemia.[27] Folate deficiency and megaloblastic anaemia do not always occur.[28] Subacute degeneration of the cord has occurred in very chronic cases.[29] In severe cases serum calcium, magnesium and some fat-soluble vitamin concentrations are reduced. The prothrombin index is prolonged.

Fat absorption

The mechanisms for the failure to absorb fat are not clearly understood and have been inad-

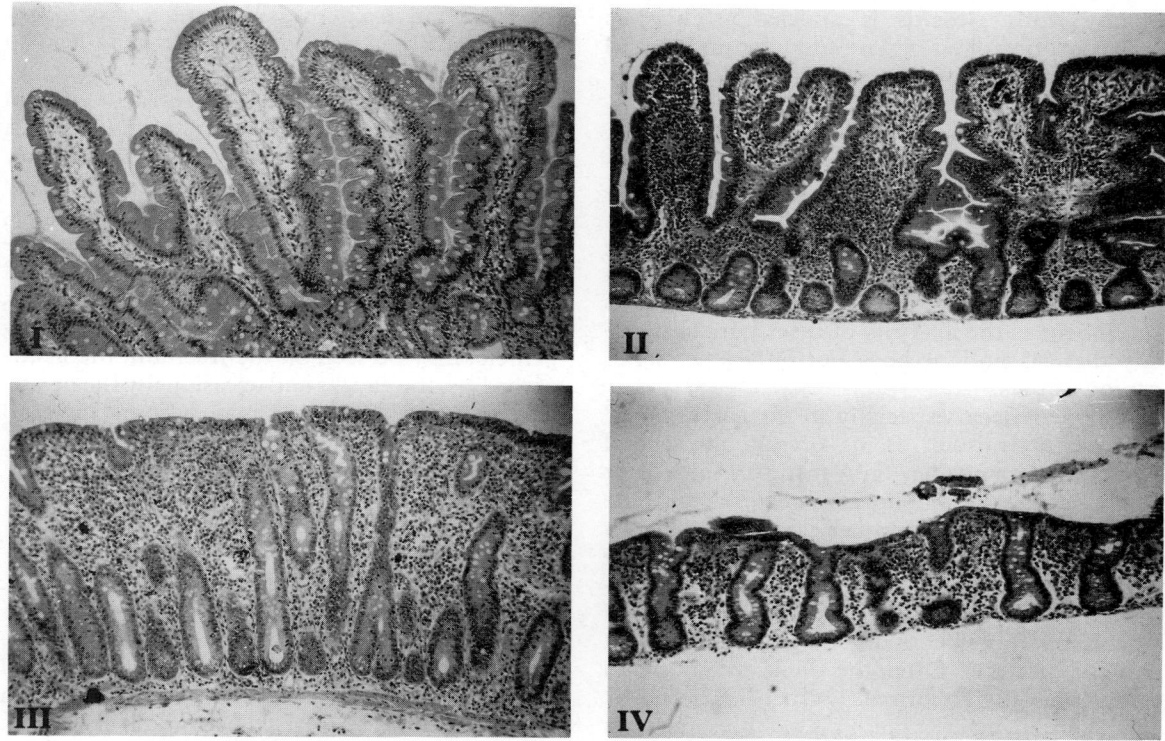

Fig. 19.1 Jejunal biopsies showing tropical sprue, grades I, II, III and IV. The villi are broadened and fused, the epithelial cells columnar or cuboid. There are numerous goblet cells and interstitial infiltration with lymphocytes and plasma cells. (Courtesy Dr D. S. Ridley.)

equately studied. Bile salt deconjugation does not take place in TS in the small intestine as it does in the 'blind loop' syndrome.[30]

CLINICAL FEATURES

Natural history

TS is very variable in its course from self-limiting infection to a long drawn out chronic disease leading to emaciation and death. Manifestations of TS in the Caribbean with an emphasis on anaemia are different to those of TS in India where diarrhoea and loss of weight are more apparent leading to doubts as to whether the two syndromes have the same cause.

Incubation period

This is not usually determinable. Symptoms and signs do not appear until about three months after arriving in an endemic area. In epidemics

of TS in India the incubation period was 5–6 days.[3]

Symptoms and signs

There are two very different forms of TS.

1 The most usual form seen now has an acute onset, runs a short self-limiting course and remits on leaving the endemic area. The main features are recurrent diarrhoea, steatorrhoea and weight loss.

2 The other, much rarer now, but seen in endemic areas in India, has a slow insidious onset, runs a slow very chronic progressive course lasting up to 20 years, with emaciation, anaemia and osteoporosis.

1 Usual form. The onset is sudden with an acute attack of diarrhoea which persists on and off with abdominal distension and colic gradually progressing on to steatorrhoea. There is no anaemia, hypoalbuminaemia, oedema or neuropathy while glossitis is unusual.[32] There is malabsorption of fat, xylose and vitamin B_{12}, and jejunal biopsy shows the lesions of TS.

2 Classical TS. The onset is slow and insidious. The diarrhoea and wasting persist and in adults there is a sore tongue (glossitis) with ulceration, anaemia, muscle cramps from hyponatraemia, osteoporosis, marked loss of weight and wasting with emaciation.

Diarrhoea is the commonest symptom and is prominent in the majority of cases but occasionally there is no diarrhoea but only pale, solid, copious stools.

The diarrhoea, especially in the early stages, may be intermittent, being present for several weeks then remitting, only to return at a later stage. Repeated remissions and relapses continue for months or years. In other cases the diarrhoea may persist throughout the course of the disease with little or no remission. The stools in established cases are pale, fermenting, acid and foul smelling and may contain a large amount of fat and float in water. Often the stools are not noted to be especially abnormal. Dyspepsia caused by carbohydrate malabsorption is troublesome with feelings of weight, oppression and gaseous distension after eating. The abdomen may feel like a drum and borborygmi roll through the bowel (Fig. 19.2).

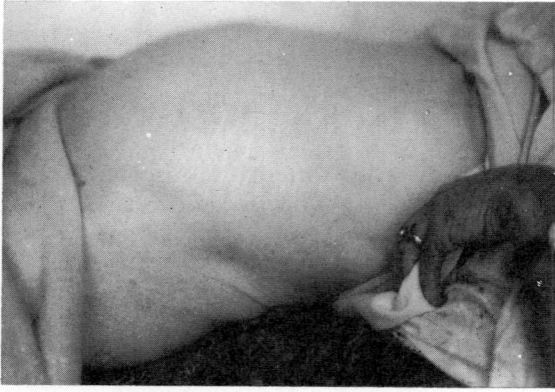

Fig. 19.2   TS abdomen, showing intense meteorism.

Anorexia, nausea and *vomiting* are often prominent in the early stages but may persist or appear at any stage.

Loss of energy and lassitude are important symptoms and may be marked. Mental and physical fatigue and emotional irritability are common and may overshadow the other symp-toms and end in a depressive state. *Loss of weight* is invariable and considerable and may lead to emaciation in a chronic case.

Glossitis and *stomatitis* are the result of vitamin B_2 deficiency and the mouth lesions, though painful, are very superficial and vary in intensity from day to day. During an exacerbation the tongue looks red and angry; superficial erosions, patches of congestion and perhaps minute vesicles appear on its surface, particularly about the edges and tip. Patches of superficial erosion, sometimes covered with an aphthous-looking pellicle, may be seen on the fraenum, the inside of the lips, the cheeks and occasionally the palate. The pharynx and uvula may become raw and sore.

CLINICAL PATHOLOGY (Table 19.1)

Steatorrhoea, the result of malabsorption of fat, is found in 95% of patients. The stools of TS are characterized by their light colour and excessive size and they may be five or six times the normal amount. They are pale and frothy and although bile pigments are present they contain excess fat; microscopic examination frequently shows fat globules. Normally, neutral fats in the faeces are in the proportion of 1 to 2 fatty acids; in pancreatic disease this ratio is reversed to as high as 15 to 1, while in TS more splitting of fat takes place and the proportion of neutral fats to fatty acids is 1 to 3 or 1 to 5. In fat balance tests in which the patient is given a fixed diet of 50 g daily for several days, TS patients do not retain the normal amount of fat (90% of the ingested fat), the figure being less than 85%. With an intake of 50 g of fat daily the steatorrhoea ranges between 6 and 25 g of fat a day and an excretion of more than 10 g a day establishes the presence of steatorrhoea.

Anaemia is almost invariable in classical TS but is not so marked in the milder forms seen today. It is more prominent in TS seen in the western hemisphere. Deficiencies of iron, vitamin B_{12} and folic acid all play a part. Crystalline folic acid absorption differs from the natural absorption from green vegetables; the serum folate falls rapidly and FIGLU (form-iminoglutamic acid) appears in the urine after 20 g of histidine. The Schilling test is affected before the level of serum vitamin B_{12} and the absorption of vitamin B_{12} given with intrinsic factor is decreased.

Table 19.1 The clinical pathology of tropical sprue.

	Normal	Tropical sprue
Serum		
Albumin	4.0–5.2 g/100 ml	Diminished
Carotene	0.06–0.4 mg/100 ml	Diminished
Calcium	7.0–10.5 mg/100 ml	Diminished
Cholesterol	150–250 mg/100 ml	Diminished
Potassium	3.5–4.7 mmol/litre	Diminished
Magnesium	1.7–2.0 mmol/litre	Diminished
Folate	3.5–8.5 ng/ml	Diminished
Vitamin B$_{12}$	150–850 pg/ml	Diminished
Iron	50 μg/100 ml	Sometimes diminished
Total iron binding capacity	Less than 300–400 μg/100 ml	Sometimes increased
Tolerance tests		
D-Xylose (25 g orally)	Urinary excretion 4–5 g or greater in 5 hours	Diminished (normal in pancreatic deficiency)
Glucose (100 g orally)	35 mg rise in fasting plasma level	'Flat curve'
Vitamin A (0.22 g/kg of oily solution containing 60 000 units/g (2 mg β-carotene))	Rise of at least 50 May units in 3–8 hours	Diminished
Stool fat		
Chemical determination (100 g/day)	5 g/day	Increased
[131]I-Triolene (3-day collection)	Up to 4%	Increased
[131]I-Oleic acid (3-day collection)	Up to 4%	Increased

There is a progressive fall in haemoglobin and the marrow, which is normoblastic in the early stages, shows some degree of megaloblastosis after two months and frank megaloblastic change after four months.[33] The blood picture of a fully developed case of tropical sprue is a megaloblastic macrocytic (cells varying from 7.8 to 8 μm) anaemia with a normal white cell count or leukopenia associated with a relative lymphocytosis. Blood crises may occur and are characterized by a rapid fall in haemoglobin and red cells.

An associated iron deficiency is often found in women and in cases of TS in India where iron deficiency is common. The serum iron is low and the total iron-binding capacity is high. In a group of Indian patients the serum iron was half that of a control group and stainable iron was never found in the marrow even in the presence of gross megaloblastic change.[34]

Subacute combined degeneration of the cord may occur and mild neuritic signs are common; occasionally a peripheral neuropathy resembling beriberi develops which responds to thiamine.

Carbohydrate malabsorption is responsible for a flat glucose tolerance curve and low D-xylose absorption. There is strong evidence of a persistent deficiency of intestinal lactase in tropical sprue even when the malabsorption has apparently been cured.[35] This deficiency can be demonstrated by a flat lactose tolerance curve, intestinal hurry after a lactose barium meal and the breath hydrogen test when the time of the appearance of hydrogen in the breath after oral lactulose is significantly prolonged.[11] (See also Chapter 60, p. 1001.)

Electrolyte and salt malabsorption may cause sodium deficiency in advanced cases of TS with low blood pressure, signs of peripheral circulatory failure and the oedema which occasionally occurs in sprue and which is due in part to salt depletion.

Calcium deficiency can cause tetany and a positive Trousseau's sign although osteoporosis is not found in tropical sprue.

Low serum potassium causes flaccidity of the muscles, reduced tendon reflexes and electrocardiographic changes with occasional arrhythmia.

Hypoproteinaemia causes muscle wasting and occasionally generalized oedema with a low serum albumin.

Vitamin A deficiency is shown by the skin, which is dry, often with marked follicular hyperkeratosis. A high incidence of xerosis of the conjunctivae is related to a poor vitamin A intake of the population. Vitamin B deficiency is responsible for the glossitis and cheilosis, and angular stomatitis is seen in 20% of cases of acute TS.

Vitamin C deficiency can produce scorbutic phenomena; petechial haemorrhages, noticeable on the thighs and legs, formerly occurred in patients fed on milk and disappeared on the administration of adequate amounts of vitamin C. Small subcutaneous haemorrhages are common in atrophic cases of TS. Amino acid excretion in the urine of TS patients is decreased.[36] Porphyrinuria can occur as in pellagra.

Evidence of *disordered pituitary–adrenal function* as shown by a low blood pressure, delayed water excretion and low output of 17-keto and ketogenic steroids in the urine is common. The basic lesion is a functional depression of pituitary in the unstimulated state and the pathogenesis is obscure.[6]

Amenorrhoea and menstrual disturbances are extremely frequent in women with advanced TS. Symptoms of TS become exacerbated during pregnancy. There may be premature labour with death of the fetus or the infant may be born with various deformities—spina bifida and incomplete ossification of the calvarium, suggesting deficiences of vitamins A, B and D.

TS in children

Children are rarely affected but in epidemics in south India they frequently develop an illness identical to that in adults with chronic diarrhoea, weight loss and nutritional and electrolyte disturbances found in TS. The illness differs in that it is relatively unresponsive to treatment and in many cases persists for several months.[37]

Course

The disease often appears to be self-limiting but in some villages in India up to one-third of those affected died.[34] Expatriates may recover spontaneously after return to a temperate climate but once the disease has been present for a year or more it is persistent. Intestinal atrophy consequent on TS may ensue and the patient's absorptive mechanisms are permanently impaired. Slight irregularities in the quality or amount of food, chill, fatigue and other trifling causes suffice to bring on dyspepsia accompanied by flatulence and diarrhoea. These cases may linger on for years. Usually they improve during the summer in temperate climates, getting worse during the winter and spring or during cold weather. Ultimately these patients die from general intestinal atrophy, diarrhoea or some intercurrent disease.

Radiology

The radiological changes are those of a deficiency or malabsorption pattern.

The mucosal folds of the small intestine are reduced in number and are irregular in width and spacing, with thick transverse barring seen on X-ray and giving an appearance of 'stacked coins'. Peristalsis is disordered and in advanced cases the mucosal folds may be entirely absent.[38]

DIAGNOSIS

Any patient with chronic or recurrent diarrhoea who is residing or has resided in an endemic area who has lost a considerable amount of weight should be considered as probably suffering from malabsorption.

DIFFERENTIAL DIAGNOSIS

It is important to distinguish TS from malabsorption caused by *Giardia* (see Chapter 17) and strongyloidiasis (see Chapter 21) since malabsorption associated with these parasites will not respond to tetracycline but, in the case of *Giardia*, only to metronidazole.

Other causes of malabsorption are gluten-sensitive enteropathy, not common in the tropics and responding only to a gluten-free diet, and secondary or primary hypolactasia. In chronic pancreatitis neutral fats predominate in the stool and the diastatic index of the urine is increased. Intestinal tuberculosis and lymphosarcoma of the mesenteric glands will show signs elsewhere. Whipple's disease, intestinal lipodystrophy, can be distinguished by biopsy, and gastrojejunocolic fistula and blind loop syndrome by radiology. Where the megaloblastic anaemia is marked, other causes of megaloblastic anaemia need to be considered—pernicious anaemia (very rare in the tropics) and nutritional megaloblastic anaemia (see Chapter 58). In neither of which are signs of malabsorption present. Pellagra has a distinct rash and no signs of malabsorption.

The diagnosis of TS is made by finding evidence of malabsorption as shown by steatorrhoea, reduced D-xylose and carotene absorption, diminished serum folate and vitamin B_{12} (Table 19.1). Confirmation can be obtained by small bowel biopsy.

TREATMENT

The object of treatment is to correct the bacterial contamination of the bowel and restore the deficiencies caused by malabsorption. This is done by the administration of broad-spectrum antibiotics, vitamins, proteins and electrolytes.

Tetracycline 2 g daily for two to three weeks will improve the vitamin B_{12} absorption and reduce the steatorrhoea to normal in 5 days in about half the cases.[24] Folic acid is specific in many cases and should be commenced directly the diagnosis has been established. It is given in doses of 10 mg three times daily for 10 days, followed by 10 mg twice daily for 10 days and then 5 mg once daily as a maintenance dose for the duration of stay in an endemic area. Vitamin B_{12} should be given in conjunction with the folic acid to prevent the onset of cord changes and should be given intramuscularly once weekly in doses of 1 mg.

The progress of the case will be measured by the degree of steatorrhoea, the glossitis, haemoglobin level, body weight and intestinal absorptive capacity as measured by the D-xylose and carotene tests. If there is evidence of other vitamin deficiences these should be corrected by the appropriate vitamin. Electrolyte abnormalities should be corrected and calcium administered as calcium gluconate intravenously if tetany is present.

In severe cases of anaemia blood transfusion may be necessary.

No special diet is necessary any longer. If there is hypoproteinaemia then a high protein diet should be given.

Results of treatment are variable. Most cases of mild tropical sprue treated early recover completely although a long-term follow-up of antibiotic therapy showed that not all cases were cured and that there was a high rate of relapse or recurrence.[39] Most cases improve rapidly on antibiotics and folic acid. In south India half of the patients treated with antibiotics alone for two or three weeks showed some improvement in steatorrhoea but in only one-fifth did the fat excretion return to normal.[24]

Long-term antibiotic treatment for a number of months has produced some improvement in intestinal function. Vitamin B_{12} and folic acid have the greatest effect on the anaemia but folic acid alone has arrested the diarrhoea in some cases and produced considerable improvement in alimentary function. In other cases little or no effect is noted. In cases of TS of long duration permanent damage may be suffered by the absorptive apparatus and atrophic changes in the small bowel may persist into old age. These individuals show permanent signs of malabsorption and develop diarrhoea if careful attention is not paid to their diet.

Prognosis

Response to treatment is often rapid and some patients notice an improvement in 2–3 days. In more chronic cases most patients show improvement within three months of treatment and tests of intestinal absorption and mucosal changes will have improved. Most patients are completely cured. The relapse rate is not known.

Convalescence

In many cases of TS the intestinal defect persists although the symptoms of malabsorption have disappeared. If possible, TS patients ought not to return to the tropics if they are aged over 50. Young adults usually recover completely. If they do return to a hot climate a maintenance dose of 5 mg of folic acid daily is recommended.

EPIDEMIOLOGY

Tropical sprue occurs both endemically and epidemically. It is endemic throughout India, South-East Asia and the Far East, including northern Australia, as well as the tropical and subtropical areas of South and Central America.

Atmospheric temperature has no influence for sprue originates at high altitudes in Sri Lanka and the Himalayas.

Epidemic TS is present today in many parts of India where 13 epidemics have been recorded.[34] In the Second World War TS behaved in Burma like an epidemic disease[40] with an incubation period and a seasonal incidence; a large epidemic occurred in India in 1960–1961.[5] The disease has disappeared in the last 20 years from many of its old haunts. In Singapore and Sri Lanka it has disappeared since the introduction of deep refrigeration. Both sexes are affected but children are rarely attacked. All races may be attacked and the indigenous inhabitants of the East are commonly affected.

In east India the TS season lasts from March to September with a peak incidence in June, coinciding with the fly season. In epidemics the disease starts in a village with a few cases and then spreads through the community over the next three to four years with a clustering in space and time and a concentration in some houses, others being unaffected. There used to be residences in Bombay and Sri Lanka which were notorious for the incidence of TS and were known as 'sprue houses'. The disease is apt to occur in one or more members of a family.

REFERENCES

1   Booth, C.C. (1965) In *Symposium on Advanced Medicine*, ed. N. Compston. London: Pitman Medical.
2   Cook, G.C. (1980) *Tropical Gastroenterolgy*, p. 271. Oxford: Oxford University Press.
3   Cook, G.C., Kajubi, S.K. & Lee, F.D. (1969) *J. Path.* 98, 157.
4   Wright, S.G. (1978) *J. R. Soc. Med.*, 71, 910.
5   Baker, S.J., Ignatius, M., Mathan, V.I. et al (1962) In *Intestinal Biopsy*, Ciba Foundation Study Group No 14, ed. G. Wostenholme & M.P. Cameron, p. 84. London: Churchill.
6   Baker, S.J., Mathan, V.I. & Joseph, I. (1962) *2nd Wld Congr. Gastroent.*, 4.
7   Banwell, J.G., Hutt, M.S.R. & Tunnicliffe, R. (1964) *E. Afr. med. J.* 41, 46.
8   Lindenbaum, J., Kent, I.H. & Sprinz, H. (1966) *Br. med. J.* ii, 1157.
9   Kajubi, S.K. & Okel, R.M. (1973) *Afr. J. med. Sci.* 4, 403.
10 Cook, G.C. (1973) In *Intestinal Deficiencies and their Nutritional Consequences,* ed. B. Borgström, A. Dahlqu-
ist & L. Hambraeus, p. 52. Uppsala: Almquist & Wiksdall.
11 Cook, G.C. (1978) *Br. med. J.* ii, 238.
12 Bayliss, T.M. et al (1975) *New Engl. J. Med.* 292, 1156–1159.
13 Da Costa, L.R. (1972) *Am. J. digest. Dis.* 17, 105.
14 Thomas, G. & Clain, D. (1976) *Gut* 17, 877.
15 Moshal, M.G., Hift, W., Kallichurum, S. et al (1975) *J. trop. Med. Hyg.* 78, 2.
16 Cook, G.C. (1984) *Lancet* i, 721–723.
17 Tomkins, A.M., Drason, B.S. & James, W.P.T. (1975) *Lancet* i, 59.
18 Klipstein, F.A., Enger, R.F. & Short, H.B. (1978) *Lancet* ii, 342.
19 Mathan, M., Mathan, V.I., Swaminathan, S.P. et al (1975) *Lancet* i, 1068–1069.
20 Booth, C.C. (1984) *Lancet* i, 1018.
21 Editorial (1980) *Lancet* i, 290.
22 Black, D.A.K. (1946) *Lancet* ii, 671.
23 Vaish, S.K., Ignatius, M. & Baker, S.J. (1965) *Q. Jl Med.* 34, 15.
24 Baker, S.J. & Mathan, V.I. (1967) quoted by Baker (ref. 34).
25 Bahr, P.H. (1915) *A Report on Sprue in Ceylon.* London: Cambridge University Press.
26 Shiner, M. (1956) *Lancet* i, 17.
27 O'Brien, W. & England, N.W.J. (1966) *Br. med. J.* ii, 1157.
28 Sheehy, T.W., Wallace, D.K. & Legters, L.J. (1965) *J. Am. med. Ass.* 94, 1069.
29 Booth, C.C. & Mollin, D.L. (1964) *Am. J. digest. Dis.* 9, 770.
30 Bevan, G., Engert, R. & Klipstein, F.A. et al (1974) *Gut* 15, 254–259.
31 Baker, S.J. & Mathan, V.I. (1968) *Am. J. clin. Nutr.* 21, 984.
32 Tomkins, A.M., James, W.P.T., Cole, A.C.E. et al (1974) *Br. med. J.* iii, 380.
33 O'Brien, W. (1967) In *Tropical Medical Conference*, ed. J.H. Walters. London: Pitman Medical.
34 Baker, S.J. (1967) In *Tropical Medicine Conference*, ed. J.H. Walters. London: Pitman Medical.
35 Gray, G.M., Walter, W.M., Jr & Colyer, E.N. (1968) *Gastroenterology* 54, 552.
36 Satwekar, K. & Radhakrishnan, A.N. (1965) *Clin. chim. Acta* 12, 394.
37 Mathan, V.I., Joseph, S. & Baker, S.J. (1969) *Gastroenterology* 56, 556–570.
38 Paterson, D.E., David, R. & Baker, S.J. (1965) *Br. J. radiol.* 38, 181.
39 Pickles, F.R., Klipstein, F.A., Tomasini, J. et al (1972) *Ann. intern. Med.* 76, 203.
40 Leishman, A.W.D. (1945) *Lancet* ii, 813.

SECTION III
HELMINTHIC DISEASES

Chapter 20
Filariasis

Filariasis is caused by infection with slender, elongated worms which are called filarial worms because of the hair-like physique of the adult forms. Table 20.1 summarizes their salient identifying characteristics. They can conveniently be divided into groups according to the normal habitat of the adult worms in this way:

1 Lymphatic filariasis:
   Wuchereria bancrofti
   Brugia malayi
   Brugia timori

2 Subcutaneous filariasis:
   Onchocerca volvulus
   Loa loa
   Mansonella streptocerca
   Dracunculus medinensis

3 Serous cavity filariasis:
   Mansonella perstans
   Mansonella ozzardi

4 Other (unclassified) species

We shall deal with these different groups of diseases separately because although the parasites within each group may show similarities there is a great difference between the groups.

Table 20.1 Filaria worms which cause filariasis in man.

Adult form	Tissue	Microfilaria form	Tissue	Invertebrate vector
Wuchereria bancrofti	Lymphatics	Mf bancrofti	Blood[a]	Mosquito spp.
Brugia malayi	Lymphatics	Mf malayi	Blood[a]	Mosquito spp.
Brugia timori	Lymphatics	Mf timori	Blood[a]	Mosquito spp.
Loa loa	Connective tissue	Mf loa	Blood[a]	*Chrysops* spp.
Onchocerca volvulus	Skin	Mf volvulus	Skin	*Simulium* spp.
Mansonella perstans	Serous membranes	Mf perstans	Blood	*Culicoides* spp.
Mansonella ozzardi	Serous membranes	Mf ozzardi	Skin and blood	*Simulium* spp. and *Culicoides* spp.
?	?	Mf bolivarensis	Blood	?
Mansonella streptocerca	Skin	Mf streptocerca	Skin	*Culicoides* spp.
Dirofilaria spp.	Lung and subcutaneous tissues	—	—	Mosquito spp.
Meningonema peruzzi	Subarachnoid space	Mf peruzzi	Cerebrospinal fluid	?
Dracunculus medinensis	Subcutaneous tissues	Larval *D. medinensis*	External water	*Cyclops*

[a] Exhibit periodicity.

1 LYMPHATIC FILARIASIS
Bancroftian filariasis (*Wuchereria bancrofti*)

GEOGRAPHICAL DISTRIBUTION

W. bancrofti is distributed throughout the tropical regions of Asia, Africa, China, the Pacific and the Americas[1–4] (Fig. 20.1). The nocturnally periodic form occurs indigenously in almost every tropical and subtropical country in a very widespread but focal distribution pattern. It has disappeared from North America and Australia and from some islands in the Caribbean, and has greatly diminished in the last 25 years in the Americas, especially Brazil. It continues to be of great importance in the growing towns of Asia where it is increasing in prevalence. The rural form adapted to anopheline mosquitoes occurs commonly in East and West Africa, where it is

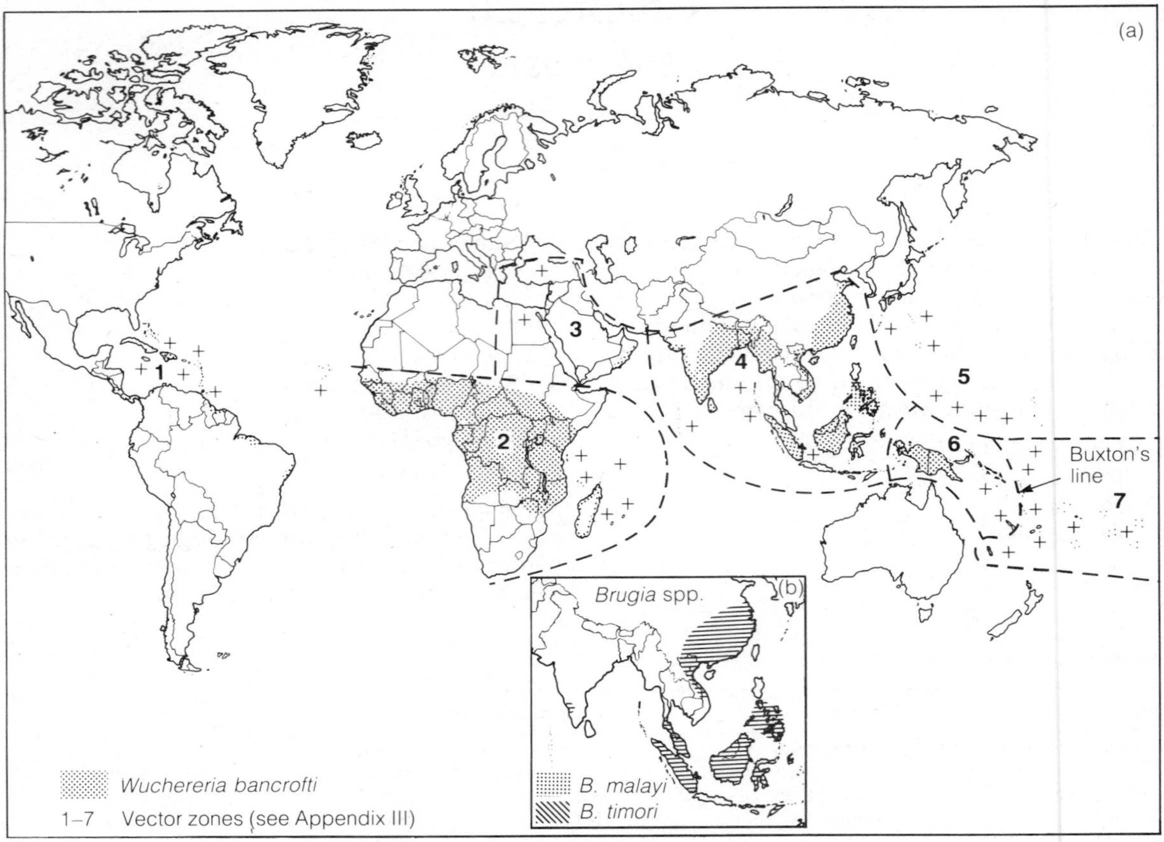

Fig. 20.1 Geographical distribution of lymphatic filariasis. (a) Bancroftian filariasis (aperiodic Bancroftian filariasis zone 7 east of Buxton's line). Zones: 1, neotropical; 2, afrotropical; 3, middle eastern; 4, oriental; 5, western Pacific; 6, Papuan; 7, southern Pacific. (b) Inset: Brugian filariasis. (Based on *Lymphatic Filariasis*, Report of WHO Expert Committee, 1984.) See Table III.5, p. 1407.

the only form, South-East Asia, South America and Papua New Guinea. The diurnally subperiodic form is restricted to the South Pacific area where it is transmitted by day-biting mosquitoes as a rural infection. Two small communities in the Nicobar Islands have been found to have diurnally subperiodic *W. bancrofti* infection, possibly due to ancient migrations from South-East Asia.

A nocturnally subperiodic form is found in jungle areas of Thailand.

AETIOLOGY

Adult *W. bancrofti* are thread-like white worms. The male (4 cm × 0.1 mm) is coiled, with a corkscrew-like tail and two spicules, the larger measuring 500 μm. The female (6.5 cm × 0.2–2.8 mm)

has a tapering anterior end with a rounded swelling (Figs. 20.2, II.61 and II.62, p. 1364). The adults lie coiled together in lymphatic vessels and glands where they can be separated with difficulty.

The eggs lie in the upper uterus enclosed in

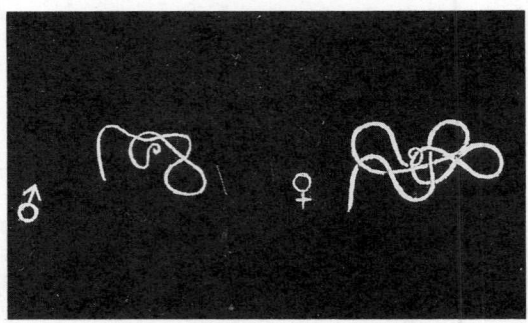

Fig. 20.2 Adult male and female *W. bancrofti*.

a chorionic membrane which becomes a sheath when the microfilariae are born, viviparously (Fig. II.63, p. 1364). The microfilariae are sheathed and measure $280 \times 7 \mu m$ (Fig. II.65, p. 1365). There is a clear cephalic zone (Figs. 20.3 and II.73,2, p. 1371). At one-fifth of the

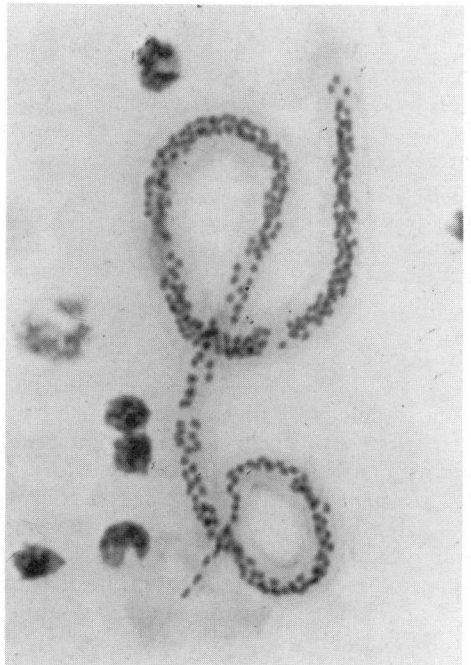

Fig. 20.3 Microfilaria of *W. bancrofti*.

length from the head is a V-shaped patch known as the 'anterior V spot' and a short distance from the tail is the 'posterior V spot'. There is no terminal nucleus as in *B. malayi*. The microfilaria (mf) of *W. bancrofti* can easily be distinguished from mf *Loa loa* in dried blood smears where mf *Loa loa* shows a characteristic attitude (Fig. 20.28, p. 388). (For a full description of morphology, see Appendix II, p. 1364.) *W. bancrofti* is one species composed of three distinct strains according to the periodicity of the microfilariae in the peripheral blood.

Periodicity of microfilaraemia

Nocturnally periodic

This form is adapted to transmission by night-biting mosquitoes. The microfilariae are absent from the peripheral blood during the day when they rest in the arterioles of the lungs. They appear in the peripheral blood at night, to reach maximum numbers between 22.00 and 02.00 hours. Periodicity is a biological rhythm inherent in the microfilariae but influenced by the circadian rhythm of the host which involves changes in the oxygen tension between venous and arterial blood by day and night and changes in the body temperature which occur every 24 hours (see Appendix II, p. 1365, and Fig. II.66, p. 1366).

Diurnally subperiodic

This strain is adapted to transmission by day-biting mosquitoes. The microfilariae are present in the blood by day and night but in greater numbers during the day.

Nocturnally subperiodic

Microfilariae are found in both day and night blood but in greater numbers at night.

Life-cycle (Fig. II.67, p. 1367)

The adult worms, male and female, live in the lymphatics where they can survive for 10 to 18 years. Living larvae (microfilariae) are produced from ova in the double uterus of the female worm and sheathed microfilariae (Fig. II.63, p. 1364) begin to appear in the peripheral blood six months to one year after infection. But in light infections, presumably because the male and female worms have failed to find each other, microfilariae may never be produced at all. The microfilariae remain in the arterioles of the lungs during the day and emerge at night (nocturnally periodic) when night-biting mosquitoes are most active (22.00 to 01.00 hours). Microfilariae (which can persist for 5–10 years in the absence of reinfection) undergo three stages of development in the insect host (culicine or anopheline mosquitoes) to form infective larvae (Figs. II.68, II.69 and II.70, p. 1368), which are injected by the female mosquito while feeding (Fig. II.71, p. 1369). The infective form makes its way to the nearest lymph glands where it becomes adult in three months to one year. (For a complete description of the life cycle and development in the insect vector, see Appendix II, p. 1367.)

TRANSMISSION

W. bancrofti is transmitted by various species of mosquitoes and Table III.5 (p. 1407) gives a complete list of these vectors. Complete development can occur in a wide variety of mosquitoes which are not vectors in nature and species which are vectors in one area may not be so in other areas because of behavioural or genetic differences.

The *nocturnally periodic form* is transmitted by night-biting mosquitoes and *Culex quinquefasciatus* and *Aedes aegypti* serve worldwide to transmit the urban infection. The rural form is adapted to anopheline mosquitoes and is transmitted by *Anopheles gambiae* and *A. funestus* in East and West Africa, and other anophelines in South-East Asia, South America and Papua New Guinea.

The *diurnally subperiodic form* in the Pacific is transmitted by day-biting mosquitoes of the *Aedes kochi* and *Aedes scutellaris* and *Aedes vigilax* groups (for full details see Table III.5, p. 1407).

There is no other method of transmission. Congenital transmission does not occur. Microfilariae can be transmitted by blood transfusion and will circulate in the recipient's blood for up to 33 days, during which time they maintain their periodicity but they do not develop into adult worms. Congenital microfilaraemia has been reported[5] but is of little significance (see section on immunity).

PATHOLOGY

Following an early period of vigorous responsiveness described in early filariasis a spectrum of disease develops (Fig. 20.4).[6] On one hand are people with no signs of infection or disease and asymptomatic persons with microfilaraemia (microfilaria carriers) and, on the other, those who develop signs of responsiveness against adult worms with fever and who develop chronic pathology later. In the case of tropical pulmonary eosinophilia (TPE) there is a vigorous immune response directed against the microfilariae with consequent pathology (see p. 371).

The damage to the lymphatic vessels is mediated by an immune response to the presence of the adult worms. Why this response is episodic or intermittent is not known but it may be related to the bursts of metabolic activity of the worms, or to the release of immunologically provocative substances by worms which have sustained mechanical trauma. Successive bouts of lymphangitis inevitably lead to more and more fibrosis of the lymphatic vessels and the formation of lymphatic hypertension. This in turn leads to the formation of dilated and tortuous collateral lymphatics and the apparent development of 'new vessels'—almost certainly the result of hypertrophy of small pre-existing channels.

Reactions around the microfilaria are probably the cause of the tropical pulmonary eosinophilia syndrome.

Pathology of early filariasis

The early stages of filarial infection have been described in American soldiers in the Pacific[7] and in human volunteers infected with *B. malayi* and *B. pahangi*.[8,9] The earliest changes occur four weeks after infection and involve the regional lymph glands. Studies in cats[10,11] have shown that pathological changes in the lymphatics and lymph glands are the result of an immunological reaction by the host. Within 4 days of the infective larvae reaching the lymphatics there is a marked cell-mediated response in the regional lymph gland followed by an antibody-mediated response in the afferent lymphatics caused by an antimacrofilarial antibody. This response is the cause of the local lymph gland enlargement in early filariasis. After the infective larvae migrate down the lymphatics considerable changes take place with a great increase in diameter and the formation of large tortuosities. These changes rapidly revert to normal following death of the worm from macrofilaricidal drugs. Disturbance of the lymph flow with lymphoedema results only when a strong resistance to reinfection has developed with the appearance of an anti-microfilarial antibody. The acute inflammatory changes induced by these processes are first an infiltration of polymorphonuclears, histiocytes and many eosinophils with a few lymphocytes in

Fig. 20.4 Spectrum of clinical manifestations of lymphatic filariasis in endemic areas (after Otteson[6]).

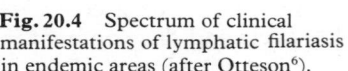

None   Asymptomatic microfilaraemia   Filarial fever   Chronic pathology   Tropical pulmonary eosinophilia

and around the lymphatics, followed later by death of the adult worm with epithelioid granuloma and foreign body giant cells. Dead worms calcify or become lysed and surrounded by fibrosis. Lymphatic abscesses may form at the site of dead and degenerating worms. The lymphatics are finally obliterated by fibrosis and microfilariae disappear from the blood.

Secondary infection

The role of secondary streptococcal infection in the production of lymphoedema has long been argued. Elephantoid changes have been produced in cats only after secondary infection with beta-haemolytic streptococci which induced excess collagen tissue affecting the lymphatic vessels and glands severely.[12] Early in the infection lymphatic function is affected by changes following the action of the antimicrofilarial antibody; this is shown by attacks of lymphangitis, lymphadenitis, funiculitis, orchitis and filarial fever, all of which are reversible with filaricidal drugs. Later, as a result of secondary streptococcal infection and the deposit of collagen, the lymphatics are permanently destroyed by fibrous obliteration which causes elephantiasis, a process which is not reversible (Fig. 20.5). Adult worms may be found in lymphoedematous tissues, especially the breast, and can be dissected out of enlarged lymphatic glands.

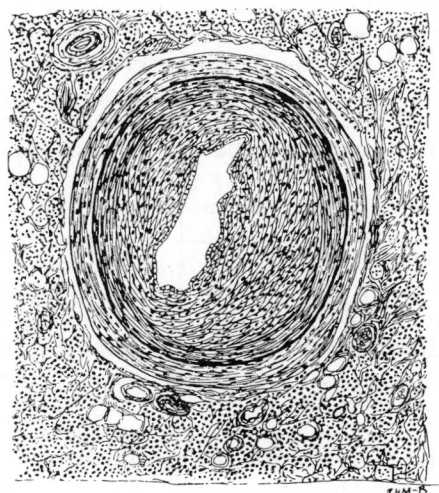

Fig. 20.5 Occlusion of the lymphatic vessels in lymphatic filariasis by proliferation of the endothelium.

Chyluria

The same pathology as that described in the lymph vessels draining the limbs and genitalia may also develop within the abdominal cavity. When lymphatic hypertension affects the small intestine lymph varices will contain the milky lymph, called 'chyle'. Varices filled with chyle may then rupture into the renal pelvis and 'chyluria' is the result. The urine is milky or pink due to an admixture of blood and the urine may closely resemble a strawberry milk shake (Fig. 20.7, p. 360).

Lymph scrotum

Lymphatic hypertension affecting the scrotum may result in the formation of countless intradermal dilatations of lymph vessels. When these rupture the patient develops a diffuse weeping of lymph from the scrotum which makes it extremely vulnerable to secondary infection.

Hydrocele

This is among the commonest manifestations of *W. bancrofti* infection. It usually follows inflammation surrounding worms which are lying in the lymphatics of the spermatic cord, presenting as episodes of funiculitis.

Late filariasis: elephantiasis

Elephantiasis is the result of long-standing lymphatic hypertension. The lymphoedema fluid acts as a tissue culture medium for connective tissue cells and encourages proliferation of the cellular elements of the skin and subcutaneous tissues.

IMMUNITY

Little is known about immunity in lymphatic filariasis other than the immunopathological effects on the lymphatics and its influence on the development of elephantiasis (see section on pathology). In many endemic areas a large proportion of the population show varying degrees of microfilaraemia without any evidence of filarial disease and some people never develop a patent infection or show any signs of disease. Adult persons not previously exposed to infection react more vigorously to infection than those who have been exposed since childhood and the clinical picture of early filariasis in such people is different.[161]

Humoral immune mechanisms directed against adult worms are responsible for the damage to the lymphatics and eventually clear the microfilariae from the blood, which accounts for the fall in microfilaraemia with age (see section on epidemiology). Cellular immune mechanisms are responsible for the death of microfilariae which occurs in some people and is responsible for tropical eosinophilia (see p. 371).

CLINICAL FEATURES

Natural history

In endemic areas people become infected early in life and develop microfilaraemia reaching a peak between 15 and 20 years of age, decreasing in later life, so that older people show little or no microfilaraemia. Most people with microfilaraemia show no signs or symptoms of disease at any time. In others, signs of filarial disease develop in early adult life. Early features are attacks of fever, lymphangitis and funiculitis. Hydrocele and obstructive lymphatic disease develop later. Persons who enter the endemic area from non-endemic areas in adult life develop signs of disease much earlier, as in the American marines in the Pacific in the Second World War,[7] often within nine months after entering the endemic area.

Incubation period

The incubation period is from five to 15 months but adult worms have been recovered on biopsy within three months after exposure.[7]

Symptoms and signs

Early filariasis

The onset is accompanied by painful swelling of the scrotal contents, arms or legs, and the commonest signs encountered are funiculitis, epididymitis, orchitis and scrotal oedema. Swelling of the inguinal, femoral or epitrochlear lymph glands is common followed by lymphangitis and filarial fever.

FILARIAL FEVER ('ELEPHANTOID FEVER', 'MUMU' IN SAMOA, 'WANGANGA' IN FIJI)

Filarial fever is an acute recurrent fever with headache, malaise, chills, rigors and sweating and it may closely resemble malaria. It recurs irregularly often continuing for many years after leaving the endemic area and may come on for the first time as long as 20 years after leaving the tropics. It is usually accompanied by symptomatic lymphangitis and other early signs of filariasis but may occur as fever alone. The cause is still open to doubt, perhaps the result of an immunological reaction in the dilated lymphatics or secondary streptococcal infection (see section on pathology, above). The former view is supported by the excellent response of the fever and other early signs of filariasis to filaricidal drugs, as well as the great reduction in 'fever' which has followed mass chemotherapy campaigns. The latter explanation is favoured by the often good response of filarial fever to antibiotics.

FILARIAL LYMPHANGITIS AND LYMPHADENITIS

Acute lymphadenitis and lymphangitis are characteristic of Bancroftian and Malayan filariasis. The onset is acute, involving a single gland or group of glands within the inguinal, axillary, cervical or epitrochlear regions. This is accompanied by fever; 6–8 hours later retrograde (centrifugal) lymphangitis starts in the glands and spreads peripherally. The lymphatic trunks become painful and cord-like with characteristic red streaks running down the arms or legs. The distal affected limb becomes swollen and oedematous during the attack which may continue for several days accompanied by the fever. The oedema takes several weeks to disappear and tension in the inflamed area may be relieved spontaneously by a lymphatic discharge from the surface of the skin. Lymphangitis may be confined to the groin glands, testis, spermatic cord (endemic funiculitis) or abdominal lymphatics. When an extensive abdominal varix ruptures, symptoms of peritonitis rapidly develop and may be fatal (abdominal filariasis).

The lymphadenitis and lymphangitis often recur several times a year. Some individuals may have one or two attacks only while others may continue with numerous ones. The attacks are most frequent during adulthood and become less frequent in later life as signs of obstructive filariasis develop.

FILARIAL FUNICULITIS AND EPIDIDYMITIS

Lymphangitis of the spermatic cord gives rise to funiculitis which has been called 'endemic funiculitis'. It is usually accompanied by filarial fever and orchitis. Fluid aspirated from the tunica vaginalis is cloudy and contains a number of polymorphonuclear cells and occasional red cells, together with microfilariae. The acute symptoms last a few days but recur at intervals. In sections dead and calcified adult filarial worms blocking the vasa efferentia causing extensive fibrotic change are found and it is possible, although not yet fully proved, that this may result in sterility. The end result is a thickened spermatic cord.

FILARIAL ORCHITIS
The onset is sudden with pain radiating to the groin and tenderness of the testis which may swell to twice its usual size with a boggy feeling on palpation. The skin of the scrotum may become red and swollen. Orchitis is associated with filarial fever, and recurrent attacks lead sooner or later to hydrocele.

FILARIAL ABSCESS
Many abscesses in the tropics are ascribed to filariasis without reason. Filarial abscesses must be distinguished from tropical pyomyositis in which the abscesses are deep within the muscles of the arms and legs (see Chapter 69).

Filarial abscesses develop within superficial lymphatics on the limbs or scrotum and at first the symptoms resemble an attack of lymphangitis but the pain and swelling continue, to be followed after some weeks by rupture and a discharge of pus. Pus may be sterile or contain bacteria. Fragments of dead adult worms may be discharged.

Chronic obstructive filariasis

LYMPH GLAND ENLARGEMENT
Great enlargement of the lymphatic glands with fibrotic changes is common in chronic filariasis. The glands (groin glands usually but, in the Pacific, epitrochlear glands) are enlarged to 5–7.5 cm in diameter and may form permanent 'tumours'. On section they resemble an unripe pear, the central portion being fibrotic and the peripheral, glandular. They may contain numerous coiled up adult worms.

Varicose groin glands (Fig. 20.6) are frequently associated with lymph scrotum, chylocele or chyluria. As a rule the patient is not aware of the existence of the varicosities until they are large. Then a sense of tension or an attack of lymphangitis draws attention to the area

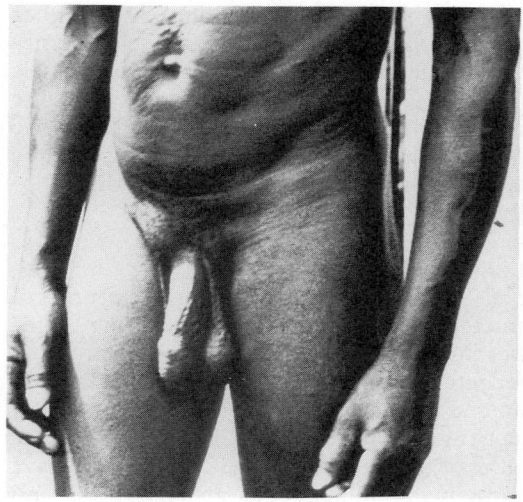

Fig. 20.6 Varicose groin glands. (Courtesy Dr D. Price.)

where soft swellings are discovered. These swellings may be of insignificant size or they may be as large as a fist. They may be noted in both or only one groin and affect the inguinal or femoral glands alone or together.

THICKENED LYMPHATIC TRUNKS
After the initial swelling and inflammation of lymphangitis have subsided a line of induration remains. On excising this thickened tissue and dissecting it, minute cyst-like dilatations of the lymphatics have been found containing live or dead adult filariae (but this surgical treatment is *not* recommended).

LYMPH SCROTUM
The scrotum is thickened and the lymphatic varicosities in the skin are discharging serous, serosanguineous or milky fluid. Many cases have an associated inguinal or femoral adenopathy.

HYDROCELE
Recurrent attacks of filarial orchitis lead sooner or later to hydrocele. This condition in some endemic areas very commonly accompanies elephantiasis of the scrotum and is used as one of the indicators of filarial disease amongst populations. The walls of the sac are thickened and may contain calcified remnants of adult filariae. The hydrocele fluid is clear, straw-coloured and may contain microfilariae. Filarial infiltrations of the cords vary in size, form and number. There

may be one small single nodule or a number strung to thickened lymphatic vessels. Sometimes lymphatic obstruction affects the vessels so as to cause lymphangiectasis and lymphatic varicoceles. It may, however, cause cystic dilatation or 'lymphocele'. The spermatic veins are often the seat of chronic thrombophlebitis.

CHYLURIA AND LYMPHURIA

Filarial chyluria results from rupture of obstructed and dilated small intestinal lymphatics into the urinary tract so the chyle no longer returns to the blood via the thoracic duct. Prolonged chyluria may result in the loss of fat in the urine amounting to 15% of the lymphatic drainage of the gut. Prolonged chyluria will have the same metabolic effect as malabsorption and cause considerable loss of weight with vitamin, electrolyte and other deficiencies. The protein loss in lymphuria may lead to oedema secondary to hypoalbuminaemia.

Loss of lymphocytes in prolonged chyluria may lead to low lymphocyte levels which when associated with immunosuppression from drugs may encourage opportunist infections.[13] Chyluria appears sometimes without warning but often starts with pain in the back and aching sensations about the pelvis and groins, probably caused by distension of the pre-existing varix. Retention of urine from the presence of chylous or lymphatic clots may be the first indication of trouble. The patient then suddenly becomes aware that he is passing milky urine which may be pink or red (Fig. 20.7); sometimes it is white in the morning and red in the evening or vice versa. It may change from chylous or lymphous. Chyluria is likely to occur for the first time, or as a relapse, in pregnancy or after childbirth. The presence of blood is caused by the rupture of small blood vessels into the dilated lymphatics when microfilariae may appear in urine passed during the night only.

CHYLOCELE, CHYLOUS ASCITES, CHYLOUS DIARRHOEA

Chylocele is not unusual in the tropics. A fluctuating swelling of the tunica vaginalis which does not transmit light and which is associated with lymph scrotum or with varicose groin glands, chyluria or microfilaraemia, would suggest chylocele. Steatorrhoea may occur owing to involvement of the mesenteric lymph glands and may proceed to chylous diarrhoea.

PHYSICAL CHARACTERISTICS OF CHYLOUS URINE (Fig. 20.7)

Chylous urine is milky in appearance owing to suspended fat particles. If it is passed into a glass and allowed to stand it will coagulate and separate after a period of hours into three layers. At the top is a cream-like pellicle, at the bottom scanty reddish sediment and in the middle a mass of milky or reddish-white urine. Microscopically the deposit contains red blood cells, lymphocytes, granular fatty matter, epithelium and urinary crystals and, in some cases, microfilariae. If ether or xylol is shaken up with chylous urine the fatty particles dissolve and the urine becomes relatively clear. On evaporation of the ether the fat may be recovered.

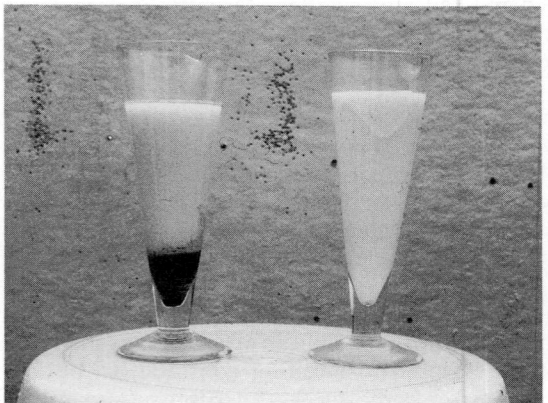

Fig. 20.7 Lymphatic filariasis. Chyluria—milky urine with sedimented blood.

ELEPHANTIASIS AND LYMPHOEDEMA

Swelling of the distal parts of the body appears during acute attacks of filarial lymphangitis and consists of pitting oedema which at first subsides completely. After each attack oedema increases and subsides more slowly until it finally becomes permanent. The oedema eventually ceases to pit and after a period of time becomes firm. When the skin becomes chronically thickened it can be called elephantiasis and this is associated with hypertrophy of the subcutaneous tissues. The skin may become verrucose and nodular and cover extensive hypertrophy and fibrous hyperplasia of the subcutaneous tissues.

In 95% of cases the lower extremities, either one or both, alone or in combination with the scrotum, or arms are affected. The foot and ankle only, the foot, leg and thigh may each or all be involved, and more rarely the breast (Fig. 20.8), vulva and circumscribed portions of the integuments of the limbs or trunk.

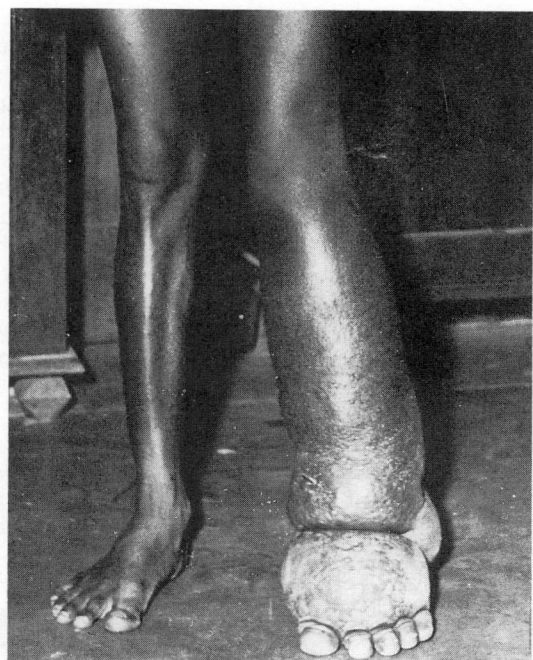

Fig. 20.9 Lymphatic filariasis. Elephantiasis of the leg. (Courtesy Dr C. J. Hackett.)

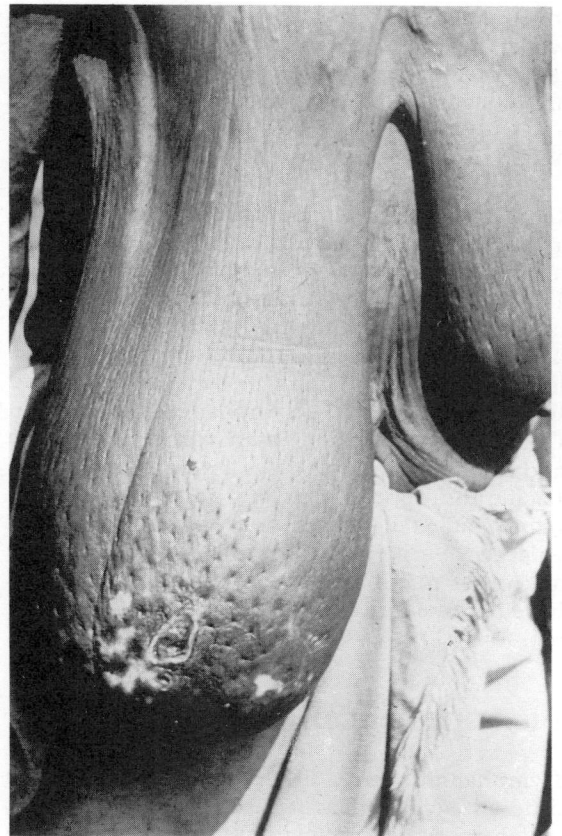

Fig. 20.8 Lymphatic filariasis. Lymphoedema of the breast.

ELEPHANTIASIS OF THE LEGS (Fig. 20.9)

This usually, though by no means always, is confined to below the knee. After frequent attacks of fever and lymphangitis the swelling may attain enormous dimensions, the leg attaining a circumference of almost a metre in advanced cases. Deep fissures develop in the elephantoid tissue and maceration with repeated trauma and poor healing lead to ulceration. Patients with elephantiasis are less likely to have microfilaraemia than those without. If microfilariae are present the density will be lower than that found in the corresponding age group without elephantiasis.

ELEPHANTIASIS OF THE SCROTUM (Fig. 20.10)

Elephantiasis of the scrotum may attain an enormous size and the largest recorded weighed

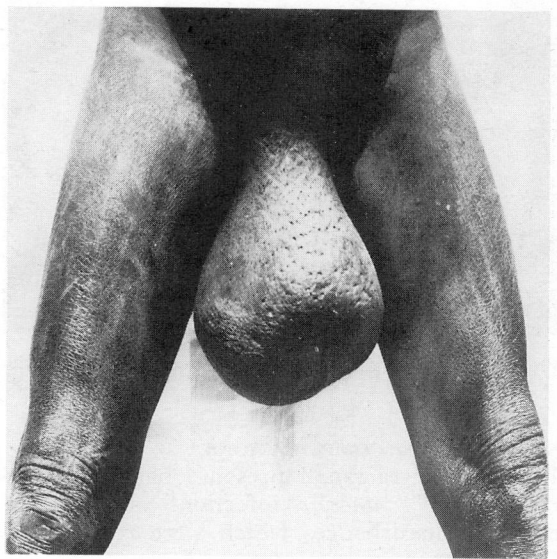

Fig. 20.10 Lymphatic filariasis. Elephantiasis of the scrotum. (Courtesy Dr J. Benfield.)

102 kg. Even small degrees of elephantiasis may reduce fertility by raising the temperature of the testes.

FILARIAL ARTHRITIS

This form of arthritis is not uncommon in areas endemic for filariasis. The condition runs a benign course affecting usually the knee joint but the ankle may be involved. The joint, which becomes painful, warm and tender, is indistinguishable from other forms of arthritis. Effusions into the joint may be creamy[14] but do not contain microfilariae. Microfilaraemia is present in every case and rapid cure follows treatment with diethylcarbamazine (DEC). The cause may be a lymphatic fistula into the synovial sac from lymphangiectasia and stasis in the popliteal lymphatics.[15]

OCULAR FILARIASIS

Adult worms may invade the orbit giving rise to a unilateral proptosis (Fig. 20.11) or the anterior chamber of the eye causing iridocyclitis, keratitis or glaucoma (see Chapter 70, p. 1166).

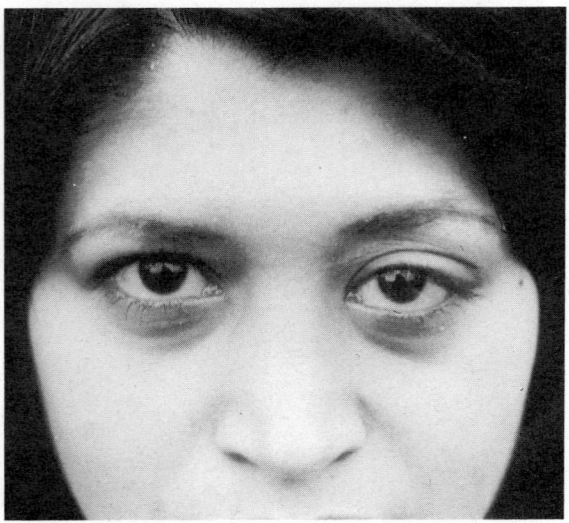

Fig. 20.11 Lymphatic filariasis. Unilateral proptosis of the left eye.

NEUROLOGICAL COMPLICATIONS

Increased intracranial pressure has been described in *W. bancrofti* infection[15] and psychoneurotic disturbances which were relieved by DEC.[17,18]

CARDIAC COMPLICATIONS

An unusual case has been described[18] in which a haemorrhagic pericardial effusion containing microfilariae but without microfilaraemia cleared rapidly following treatment with DEC.

RENAL COMPLICATIONS

Renal biopsies in some cases of glomerulonephritis associated with filariasis have shown a diffuse mesangial proliferative glomerulonephritis with C3 deposition in the glomeruli which has been produced in cats experimentally infected with *B. pahangi*.[20] These changes are suggestive of an immunological cause.

Variations in the clinical picture

In *W. bancrofti* infection in East Africa there is a high proportion of hydroceles but elephantiasis of the legs and scrotum is relatively uncommon. In West Africa elephantiasis is rare and hydrocele not common although microfilaria rates of 40–50% are recorded in some areas. In India the lesions are mainly hydrocele and funiculitis and little lymphoedema or lymphangitis is seen. In China the main lesions are hydrocele, chyluria and elephantiasis of the legs and scrotum. In the Pacific the upper limbs and breasts were commonly affected, elephantiasis was gross and enlarged lymph glands were common but these and other manifestations of lymphatic filariasis have become rare as a result of successful control measures.

DIFFERENTIAL DIAGNOSIS

Lymphangitis and filarial fever have to be differentiated from acute bacterial lymphangitis, which spreads centripetally from the periphery towards the lymph glands, and from other causes of recurrent fever with rigors, septicaemia, malaria, relapsing fever, relapsing typhoid, tuberculosis, pyelonephritis, liver abscess and gallstones.

Varicose groin glands. These must be distinguished from hernias for which they are often mistaken. This can be done by observing that they are not tympanitic on percussion; that though pressure causes them to diminish they do so slowly and without the sudden dispersion accompanied by gurgling, as in hernia; that there is a relatively slight or absent impulse on coughing and that they subside slowly when the patient lies down and return slowly when the erect posture is resumed. The diagnosis is strengthened by the coexistence of lymph scrotum, chyluria or chylous hydrocele or by the presence of microfilariae in the blood. They also have to be differentiated from 'hanging groins' of onchocerciasis which are folds of atrophic lax skin containing enlarged glands.

Filarial glandular enlargement. This has to be distinguished from other causes of lymphatic glandular enlargement, especially in the inguinal region, chronic infection of the feet (the inguinal glands are usually enlarged in people who wear no shoes), tuberculous adenitis, lymphogranuloma inguinale, reticuloses, lymphoma and leukaemia.

Filarial orchitis, endemic funiculitis and hydrocele. These have to be distinguished from encysted hydrocele, lipoma, spermatocele, gonococcal epididymitis, tuberculous epididymitis, *Schistosoma haematobium* infection of the cord, strangulated hernia and suppuration of the spermatic cord. A non-filarial epidemic funiculitis has been described from Sri Lanka.[21] It is difficult to distinguish filarial from non-filarial infection but in endemic areas of filariasis hydrocele is accepted as an indicator of filarial disease.

Chyluria. This must be distinguished from other causes of lymphatic obstruction in the abdomen, especially tuberculosis.

Elephantiasis. Microfilaraemia is usually absent in cases of filarial elephantiasis so it is often impossible to prove the filarial origin of these cases. Filarial (*W. bancrofti*) elephantiasis must be distinguished from other causes of elephantiasis.

Endemic elephantiasis is caused by silica particles in the soil destroying the lymphatic system of the legs (see Chapter 44). This occurs in elevated areas where there is no filariasis and is confined to the lower limbs, the scrotum and genitals escaping. Lymphangiography shows destroyed lymphatic channels.

Other filarial causes. Onchocerciasis causes usually only scrotal oedema. *Loa loa* does not cause elephantiasis.

Elephantiasis in leprosy caused by destruction of the inguinal lymph glands is associated with other signs of lepromatous leprosy.

Elephantiasis nostras is an uncommon cause of elephantiasis due to repeated streptococcal infections of the feet.

Surgical causes are ablation of the inguinal and femoral glands.

Milroy's disease is a congenital absence or insufficiency of the lymphatic channels found mostly in young women in temperate countries.

Elephantiasis of the scrotum with a large hydrocele must be distinguished from scrotal hernia which is not translucent to light.

DIAGNOSIS

The diagnosis is made by finding sheathed microfilariae in the blood. Microfilaraemia is not a good measure of diagnosis of filarial disease since microfilarial density does not correlate with disease severity and microfilariae may be present only in the early stages. In lymphatic filariasis microfilariae do not appear until at least nine months after exposure. Microfilaria rates peak in the 15–19 year age group in endemic areas but, in the late stages of filarial disease, microfilariae cannot be found in the blood. The absence of microfilaraemia does not exclude filarial disease, nor does its presence in an endemic area denote it.

Microfilariae can persist in the blood for three weeks after transfusion and live after the death of the adult worm for 6–18 months.

Microfilariae may be detected in the blood by direct examination, by counting chamber and by membrane filter techniques.

Direct examination

Twenty microlitres of blood are taken from finger prick or ear lobe and spread as a thick film. After drying it is simultaneously dehaemoglobinized and stained, usually with a Romanowsky stain, such as Giemsa. A special stain is needed to demonstrate the sheaths. (See also Appendix IV, p. 1494.)

Counting chamber

The disadvantage of this test is that venous blood is usually used but $100\,\mu l$ of blood obtained by finger prick is the method preferred in Tanzania.[22]

Membrane filter (see Appendix IV, p. 1494)

Relatively large amounts of blood may be filtered through either a Millipore or Nucleopore membrane filter with a great gain in sensitivity of diagnosis. The filter may be examined fresh or stained in the usual way for microfilariae.[23–25] Several refinements have been developed since Bell's original description of the method.

Centrifugation (See also Appendix IV, p. 1494)

Knott's method used 1 ml of blood diluted in 9 ml of distilled water and 1 ml of commercial formalin. The suspension is shaken, centrifuged and the deposit examined for microfilariae.

Diethylcarbamazine provocative test

Nocturnally periodic microfilariae may be demonstrated in the blood in the daytime by the administration of a small dose of diethylcarbamazine which flushes the microfilariae from the lungs into the peripheral circulation; 80% of cases with nocturnal microfilaraemia were detected by this test.[26] This allows surveys for nocturnally periodic filariasis to be carried out in daylight hours. The blood should be examined 15 minutes after an oral dose of 6.0 mg/kg or 45–60 minutes after 2.0 mg/kg[27] and after 90 minutes for *B. malayi*.[28] This test is of no use in subperiodic filariasis.[29] Care must be taken in areas where both lymphatic filariasis and onchocerciasis are found together, lest a severe Mazzotti reaction occurs.

Blood changes

Lymphatic filariasis does not cause anaemia but there is a moderate eosinophilia in early cases (33–50% of Wartman's cases[6] averaged 850/mm³). In the later stages there is no eosinophilia.

Lymphangiography

Lymphangiograms are not specific in filarial lymphoedema, and show dilatation and tortuosity of the lymphatic trunks in the legs with filling of the collaterals and dermal backflow.[30] The inguinal lymph glands are increased in number and size, containing filling defects with tortuous afferent but minute efferent vessels. In chyluria diffuse sacculated collateral lymphatics may be seen bypassing the iliac and paraortic glands and a concentrated plexus of dilated lymphatics is found adjacent to the renal pelvis[31] (Fig. 20.12). Hypaque injected subcutaneously in the foot followed by xeroradiographs gives clear pictures

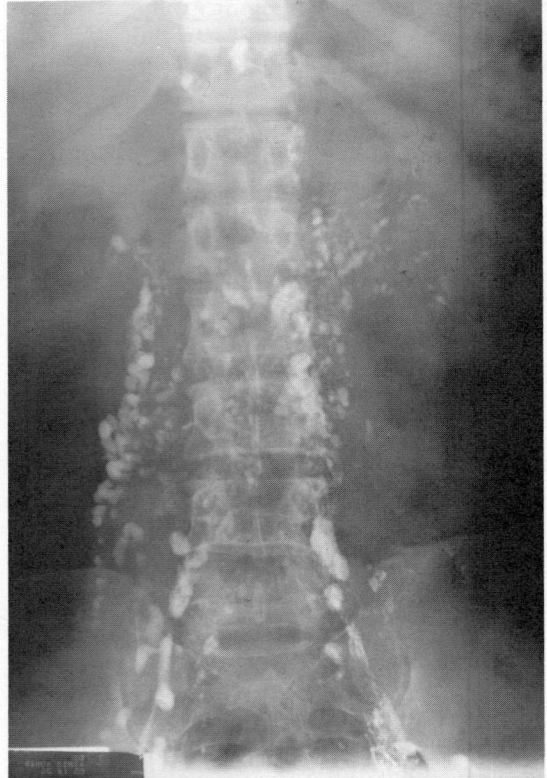

Fig. 20.12 Lymphangiogram from a case of chyluria showing dilated collateral renal lymphatics.

of lymphatics and glands and can be repeated frequently.[32]

Filarial elephantiasis usually shows other signs of filarial disease such as lymphatic glandular enlargement, hydroceles and elephantiasis of the scrotum to distinguish it from endemic elephantiasis (see Chapter 44). There is usually no microfilaraemia but antimicrofilarial antibodies are present (see section on serodiagnosis, below).

Serodiagnosis

Filarial antigens are complex and differ with the different stages of the life-cycle. The detection of filarial antigens is being investigated but tests are not yet available routinely. Serological tests are used to detect filarial antibodies but are not yet species specific and so may cross react with other helminths.

Antimicrofilarial antibodies (filarial fluorescent antibody test (FAT))

Antimicrofilarial antibodies are directed to the cuticle or sheath. They are not detectable in the presence of microfilaraemia (see section on immunity) but are found when the host reaction against microfilariae is high and microfilariae are not circulating as in TPE. *B. pahangi* microfilarial antigen is used and the cytoplasmic antigen is exposed by sonication of the microfilariae so that when any antibody is present the results are not affected by the presence of circulating microfilariae.[33] Antibodies can be found in about one-quarter of filarial subjects, mostly those with lymphatic obstruction.[34] Although useful in the diagnosis of some cases of elephantiasis, in long-standing cases antibodies may be undetectable. Cross reactions occur with *Ascaris* (85%) and *Strongyloides* (60%) and occasionally with other tissue-invasive helminths.

Antiadult antibodies

Antiadult antibodies are found in a titre of 1 in 8 or more in all filarial subjects but not in controls but there is no correlation with the clinical state.[34]

Enzyme-linked immunosorbent assay (ELISA)

An ELISA test using antigens derived from adult *Litosomoides carinii* and *Setaria cervi* has been developed[35] which detected 83% of symptomatic cases of filariasis while only four out of 40 asymptomatic carriers and one of 50 controls were positive. Cross reaction occurs with *Strongyloides*. This is now the test of choice. The test has very little practical value in endemic areas.

Complement fixation test (CFT)

The CFT uses as antigen a 1% alcoholic extract of *Dirofilaria immitis*.[36] It is positive in about one-quarter of cases of Bancroftian filariasis. There is a considerable cross reaction with *Ancylostoma*, *Schistosoma* and *Strongyloides* infections, but it is almost always positive in cases of the tropical eosinophilia syndrome which is its main application.

Haemagglutination

Haemagglutinating antibodies may be present when complement-fixing ones are absent but this technique has never been shown to be of any practical value.

Skin test (intradermal reaction)

The intradermal test using an antigen prepared from *D. immitis* is now little used. It is an immediate hypersensitivity reaction which detects antibodies. Cross reactions occur with intestinal helminths and other filariae which vitiates its use both for individual diagnosis and epidemiological surveys. Under certain conditions it may have limited epidemiological applications.

TREATMENT

The treatment of filariasis consists of chemotherapy directed against the adult worms (macrofilaricidal) and against the microfilariae (microfilaricidal), combined with symptomatic treatment to relieve the damage caused by the reaction of the body to the destruction of adult worms.

Chemotherapy

Macrofilaricidal drugs

Suramin (Antrypol) has a lethal action on adult *W. bancrofti* and also some effect on microfilariae but it is no longer used for this infection because of its toxic effects (see section on onchocerciasis, p. 383). Diethylcarbamazine (see below) *does* have macrofilaricidal effects in *W. bancrofti* and is the only drug in widespread use for this purpose.

Microfilaricidal drugs

Microfilaricidal drugs are used in mass chemotherapy for the control and eradication of filariasis by removing the human reservoir of infection. They are also used in the treatment of clinical filariasis since they control the signs of filarial disease. They are specific in TPE.

Diethylcarbamazine citrate (DEC) (Hetrazan, Banocide, Notézine) is a microfilaricidal agent also capable of killing adult *W. bancrofti*, *B. malayi* and *B. timori* worms.[37] It can be administered in tablets or in low doses in medicated salt (see section on control, below). The dose required to prevent and remove clinical manifestations is the same as that required to kill adult worms. It is not known whether DEC acts against the infective stages and so could be used prophylactically.

Furapyramidone has been used in China where it is reported to have both macrofilaricidal and microfilaricidal action.[38]

Metriphonate (trichlorphon) is a good microfilaricidal agent and is used in a dose of 10–15 mg/kg every 14 days for five to 16 doses. It is useful in campaigns directed against both *S. haematobium* and *W. bancrofti*. It is also macrofilaricidal in a proportion of cases.

DEC exerts no direct lethal action on the microfilariae but modifies them so that they are engulfed by phagocytes and thereby removed from circulation. In closed cavities such as hydroceles the microfilariae are not affected. The dose is 6 mg/kg body weight daily in three divided doses after meals for two or three weeks. The normal adult dose is 150–200 mg three times a day. The microfilariae rapidly disappear from the blood but may reappear after six months if adult worms are not killed. *B. malayi* is more susceptible to treatment with DEC than *W. bancrofti*.

Reactions to DEC are commoner in Malayan filariasis and in microfilaria carriers. They are of considerable significance in mass treatment. In the main reactions are of two types:[39]

1 General reactions, with headache, malaise and anorexia, with or without fever, occurring on the second day of treatment and subsiding by the sixth day when further drug therapy is safe. In mass treatment a large proportion of the population suffers causing considerable disruption.

2 Local reactions with painful swelling of lymph nodes, retrograde lymphangitis, abscess, suppuration or lymphoedema occurring in a smaller proportion of people, usually those with signs of disease with or without microfilaraemia.

Minor reactions are abdominal pain, diarrhoea, urticaria and provocation of asthmatic attacks in those with bronchial asthma.

Scrotal tumour

Although surgical treatment of elephantiasis has proved unsuccessful, the surgical removal of the grossly elephantoid skin and scrotal tissues with preservation of the penis and testicles has proved very worthwhile and many patients have been very grateful for this operation.

Symptomatic treatment

Recurrent lymphangitis and filarial fever

Treatment should consist of analgesic/antipyretic, elevation of the affected part, followed by the application of an elastic bandage if necessary.

DEC has also proved to be very effective in the treatment of the early manifestations of filariasis including filarial fever and lymphangitis. Where filarial control measures are applied, as in Tahiti, these early manifestations of filarial disease rapidly disappear from the population.

Lymph scrotum

Lymph scrotum should be kept scrupulously clean but is otherwise best left alone.

Chyluria

A full course of DEC followed by bed rest usually leads to remission.

Chylocele, hydrocele

Chyloceles and hydroceles should be treated surgically along conventional lines but a full course of DEC should be given to eradicate the parasites.

Elephantiasis

The lymphoedema must first be reduced by prolonged firm bandaging and further swelling prevented by permanent support of the tissues. An intermittent positive pressure apparatus (Flowtron, Huntley Medical, Luton, England), such as used in the treatment of non-filarial lymphoedema, has proved very effective in the reduction of oedema.

KNOTT'S METHOD OF BANDAGING

The patient is put to bed and firm bandaging is started from the foot upwards. Sponge rubber is used to protect the tissues. The bandages are removed every day and replaced a little tighter. Results are sometimes good even in the largest legs. Fluid is eliminated from the tissues and people who could hardly walk because of the size of their legs may become active again. After the swelling has been reduced a spiral elastic stocking may succeed in preventing recurrence.

Chemotherapy

DEC may prove useful, as with the case of *B. timori* (see p. 370).

EPIDEMIOLOGY

The nocturnally periodic form of *W. bancrofti* contains two epidemiologically distinct forms. Of widest distribution is the strain adapted to urban mosquitoes of the *Culex pipiens* and *C. sitiens* groups and *Aedes aegypti*. This form has increased greatly in incidence in the expanding tropical cities where environmental sanitation is poor, contaminated stagnant water abounds and containers are used to store water used in the absence of piped water supply.

Rural Bancroftian filariasis is adapted to anopheles mosquitoes, *A. gambiae* and *A. funestus* in Africa and other anophelines in South-East Asia, South America and Papua New Guinea.

The diurnally subperiodic form of *W. bancrofti* is found in the Pacific east of Buxton's line (Fig. 20.1) and is transmitted by day-biting mosquitoes of the *Aedes kochi*, *Ae. vigilax* and *Ae. scutellaris* groups. It is a rural infection dependent upon the coconut, in the husks of which the vectors breed (Table III.5, p. 1408).

The importance of Bancroftian filariasis may be assessed either by parasitological criteria of infection or by how much disease is produced.

Microfilaria rate

Most infected people exhibit microfilaraemia and the 'microfilaria rate' is the percentage of the population found to be carrying microfilariae in the peripheral blood. Microfilaria rates start in the 1–4 year age group and rise to a peak in the 15–20 year age group. The subsequent rise is not proportional to the rise in age and rates fall to almost nil in advanced age.

Disease rate

The disease rate is the percentage of the population exhibiting signs of filarial disease—recurrent fever, recurrent lymphangitis, hydrocele and chyluria. Hydrocele in many areas is the main marker for the disease. The *endemicity rate* is the percentage of people who show evidence of filarial infection with either microfilaraemia or disease and may be expressed in a community, as shown in Table 20.2.[41]

CONTROL

The control of filariasis rests on two methods: chemotherapy and vector control.[42]

Mass chemotherapy with diethylcarbamazine

Mass treatment produces an immediate reduction in the microfilaria level in the population. There is no known animal reservoir outside Malaya. It has been successful on a small scale in Tahiti[43] where a quick reduction in the number of adult filariae has been obtained, and in West Africa. It is applicable to both urban and rural areas and has a beneficial effect by curing acute symptoms and thus diminishing the danger of pathological lesions. Partial control of microfilaraemia has been obtained with cooking salt medicated with DEC.[44]

Success depends upon obtaining good cooperation from the population which is often difficult to achieve with large communities. The whole population must be treated since it is not possible to identify all the microfilaria carriers at one examination. Reactions may be severe,

Table 20.2 Classification of epidemiological types of microfilariasis.

Type	Microfilarial prevalence	Microfilarial density	Clinical signs	Comments
1	+ + + +	+ + + +	+ + + +	Normal situation, stable intense transmission
2	+ + + +	+ + + +	+	Relatively recent importation of filariasis
3	+	+	+ + + +	Emigration of young, clinically unaffected people; old people with clinical signs, often amicrofilaraemic, remain in area
4	+	+	+	Normal situation, stable low-level transmission

particularly in Malayan filariasis and where there is a heavy microfilaraemia (see p. 370).

DEC is used in divided doses of 6 mg/kg once a month for 12 months.[45] Low doses of the drug have been incorporated in popular foods in a strength corresponding to a daily intake of 50–100 mg per person. DEC is stable on boiling and autoclaving. Mel W has been used in a single dose in mass chemotherapy but there have been some deaths, which make it unsuitable for control purposes.

Long-term mass chemotherapy has been effective in preventing the development of new cases of filariasis with advanced pathology.[43,46] In the early stages of the campaign there is a dramatic reduction in the incidence of early filarial disease such as filarial fever, lymph gland enlargement, lymphangitis and abscesses.[47] Failure to interrupt transmission may be due to primary treatment failure, secondary microfilaraemia recurring after treatment during the prepatent period, and new infections.[48] Weekly spaced doses of DEC before the transmission season have been used to great effect and are more acceptable than intensive courses of DEC. The addition of levamisole 2.5 mg/kg in a single oral dose before the first dose of DEC gave a much more rapid decrease in the level of microfilaraemia.[49] In Samoa *Ae. polynesiensis* is able to ingest and concentrate microfilariae from ultralow density microfilaria carriers after mass chemotherapy.[50]

Vector control

Adult mosquito control in towns is desirable on general grounds. Larvicidal control does not depend on the cooperation of the local population. However, vector control is slow to affect the prevalence of filariasis in a population. The number and longevity of the vectors must be reduced to a very low level for many years before transmission is interrupted owing to the long life of the adult worms. Prolonged insecticide applications aimed at control may give rise to insecticide resistance.

Since the vectors of filariasis can be classified into four general groups—*Anopheles*, *Aedes*, *Mansonia* and the *Culex pipiens* complex—the diversity in the bionomics of these species calls for different control measures. Control of *Anopheles* can be undertaken as part of an antimalarial campaign, by spraying houses with DDT or dieldrin. Control of *Aedes* may be undertaken by house or aerial spraying. Villages may be protected from *Aedes* by controlling breeding places within a perimeter of 100 m because of the short flight range of the species. Local breeding places can be controlled by village hygiene, such as was developed by Amos in Fiji. Control of the *C. pipiens* complex has failed because of the development of resistance to DDT. Larval control campaigns have been of limited effectiveness.

Combined methods

A programme using both methods combined will certainly reach its goal more rapidly than a single method but it depends upon the epidemiology of the infection in each area, the resources of the country and the personnel available.

Personal prophylaxis

In nocturnally periodic Bancroftian filariasis mosquitoes bite at night so that sleeping under a mosquito net or in a screened room provides very good protection. Prophylaxis with DEC has not generally been successful, but following some experimental work with monkeys[51] DEC 200 mg twice daily for three days every month, or 100 mg once a week has been suggested.

Malayan filariasis (*Brugia malayi*)

GEOGRAPHICAL DISTRIBUTION
(Fig. 20.1)

Brugia malayi is confined in distribution to South and South-East Asia from India in the west to Korea in the east (Fig. 20.1).

AETIOLOGY

The cause of Malayan filariasis is *Brugia malayi*. The genus *Brugia* contains eight species. Only *B. malayi* and *B. timori* cause infection in man although *B. pahangi* has been transmitted to man experimentally. *B. malayi* adults are practically identical with *W. bancrofti* and the females are indistinguishable. The microfilaria of *B. malayi* is sheathed, measures 200–250 × 5–6 μm and can be distinguished from mf *W. bancrofti* by the two isolated nuclei at the tip of the tail and the absence of nuclei in the cephalic space (Figs. 20.13, II.72, p. 1370, and II.73,3, p. 1371) (for further information see Appendix II). The life-cycle is similar to that of *W. bancrofti* but the period of maturation of the adult worm in the human body is much shorter.

B. malayi consists of two forms: nocturnally periodic and nocturnally subperiodic. The *nocturnally periodic* form is an infection of rural populations and has a focal distribution in Asia: in rural areas of Sri Lanka (from where it has now almost disappeared), Thailand, Malaysia, Vietnam, China, South Korea, Borneo and Indonesia. It is a parasite of man and no natural infections have been found in animals.

The *nocturnally subperiodic* form is a zoonosis and is a natural infection of a variety of animals. It is found in Malaya along the Pahang and Perak rivers, in Thailand and on Palawan Island in the Philippines.[52]

PATHOLOGY AND IMMUNITY

See Bancroftian filariasis, p. 356.

CLINICAL FEATURES

Natural history

The natural history is similar to that of *W. bancrofti* although the clinical picture is somewhat different. Symptoms begin earlier (sometimes within one month or less) and lymphoedema of the legs is a prominent and early symptom.

Incubation period

The incubation period is shorter than in *W. bancrofti*. Microfilariae have been found in the blood of a child aged three and a half months and high microfilaria rates are found in children below the age of five years.

Symptoms and signs

There are few symptoms apart from bouts of fever and lymphangitis which occur with greater

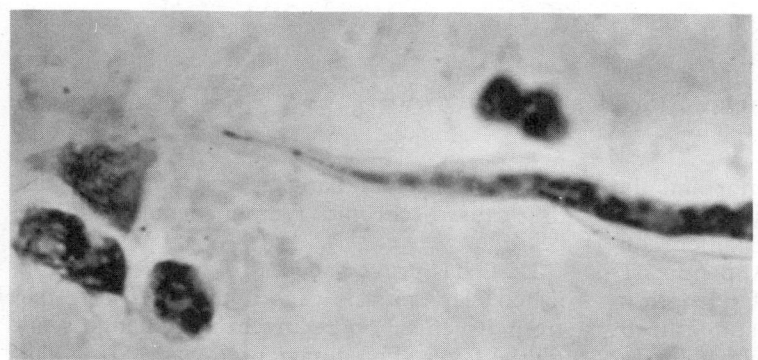

Fig. 20.13 Mf *B. malayi* showing two isolated nuclei in the tip of the tail.

TRANSMISSION

The *nocturnally periodic* form is transmitted by a number of different vectors, open swamp species of *Mansonia* (*Mansonioides*) of the *M. dives* and *M. uniformis* groups, and anophelines of the *A. barbirostris* and *A. hyrcanus* groups.

The *nocturnally subperiodic* form is transmitted by shade swamp *Mansonia* (*Mansonioides*) of the *M. dives* and *M. uniformis* groups (see Table III.5, p. 1409).

frequency than in Bancroftian filariasis. Lymphatic abscesses are common and are associated with inguinal and axillary adenopathy. Lymphoedema is confined to the legs below the knees and the arms below the elbows, and gross elephantiasis is uncommon. Hard, cord-like lymphatic vessels form with hard lymph gland enlargement. The genitourinary system usually escapes but hydrocele is not common. Chyluria is almost unknown.[53] Previously uninfected migrants who enter an endemic area show a more or less typical but more rapid course and develop episodic attacks of lymphangitis and fever after a few months. Elephantiasis tends to develop in such people more often and sooner; lymphoedema may develop after six months and elephantiasis one to two years after arrival.[54]

DIAGNOSIS AND TREATMENT

See Bancroftian filariasis, p. 363.

EPIDEMIOLOGY

The *nocturnally periodic* strain is found in association with coastal rice fields and also amongst forest aboriginals. The *nocturnally subperiodic* form is found in rural villages and plantations along the lower reaches of major rivers in swamp forest where it is a zoonosis.

Microfilaria rates. Microfilaraemia develops early, often under five years of age, and reaches 40–50% in adult life.

Disease rates. Lymphangitis and filarial fever are found in up to 50% of people in some areas whereas the elephantiasis rate is low at 2–3%. Hydrocele is not common and cannot be used as a reliable indicator of disease.

Mosquito infection rates. In Malaysia it is recognized that the majority of larval filariae in wild caught *Mansonia* (*Mansonioides*) mosquitoes are of avian or mammalian origin.

CONTROL

Mass treatment with DEC has been used in the control of Malayan filariasis but has had to sometimes be suspended because reactions to DEC are commoner and more severe than in Bancroftian filariasis (see p. 365).

Timorian filariasis (*Brugia timori*)

Timorian filariasis is found in Timor and the eastern Flores Islands in south-east Indonesia. It is nocturnally periodic. The adults differ morphologically from *B. malayi* (see Appendix II) and the microfilariae are longer with a length to width cephalic space of about 3 : 1, and a sheath which does not stain bright pink with Giemsa. The vector is *Anopheles barbirostris* which breeds in rice fields and readily bites man. The clinical pattern is similar to that of *B. malayi* and acute recurrent lymphangitis with filarial abscesses in the lymphatic trunks are a major feature. Subsequent scars over thickened hard, cord-like lymphatics are a mark of the disease. Elephantiasis is minimal. The parasite is very sensitive to DEC and mass treatment combined with vector control should be very effective. A mass chemotherapy campaign using small doses of DEC in cooperation with the villagers after a health education campaign has been shown to reduce the microfilaria rate, as well as decreasing the

incidence of lymphangitis and abscesses, and has caused chronic lymphoedema to disappear.[55]

DEC has proved successful in treating established elephantiasis caused by *B. timori* apart from its effect on recurrent lymphangitis and filarial fever. The dosage used was 300 mg daily in three divided doses for 10 days with as many repeated courses as are necessary.[40] In most cases the swelling resolved in one year.

ENZOOTIC BRUGIA INFECTION

Three cases of zoonotic *Brugia* infection have been reported from Colombia, South America. An unknown *Brugia* species has been found in a cervical lymph gland—so far the only *Brugia* species in man known from this continent.[56]

Tropical pulmonary eosinophilia (TPE, occult filariasis)

GEOGRAPHICAL DISTRIBUTION

Tropical pulmonary eosinophilia is found most commonly in South-East Asia but has also been reported from other areas where filariasis occurs, notably the east coast of Africa and Brazil. The salient features are asthma-like symptoms associated with a high eosinophilia.

AETIOLOGY

TPE was first described by Meyers and Kouwenaar[57] from Indonesia. Its filarial origin was clarified by Lie Kan Joe[58] and Beaver.[59] Which species of filaria causes TPE is still a matter for discussion since there is no microfilaraemia and adult filariae are inaccessible. The microfilariae found in the tissues of patients in South-East Asia have been of the *B. malayi* type, while those in India and Curaçao resembled *W. bancrofti*. Some observers have thought that filariae of animal origin were responsible and experimental infection of man with *B. pahangi* produced all the symptoms and signs of TPE.[60] It is probable that any species of lymphatic filaria in the appropriate host could produce TPE but observations of specific reaginic IgE antibodies have shown that hypersensitivity to microfilariae of human origin is mainly responsible.[61]

TRANSMISSION

The filariae responsible are transmitted in the same way as *W. bancrofti* and *B. malayi*.

PATHOLOGY

TPE is the result of an immunological hyper-responsiveness on the part of the host which effectively clears all microfilariae from the blood, mostly in the lungs. It is mediated by IgG antibody, the asthmatic symptoms resulting from allergic responses mediated through specific IgE antibodies bound to lung mast cells.[6] The acute phase is caused by an antibody-dependent mechanism while the chronic phase which is marked by pulmonary fibrosis may result from a type III delayed hypersensitivity response caused by an increase in or inadequately suppressed pulmonary lymphocyte reaction.[6]

This immunological hypersensitivity is found only in certain hosts and is probably of genetic origin since the majority of cases are found in persons of Indian origin. In the *acute phase* microfilariae are destroyed with the production of typical lesions in the lymph glands,[62] lung,[63] liver[64] and spleen.

The enlarged lymph glands show a pronounced hyperplasia of the lymph follicles and reticular cells; many yellowish grey nodules 1–2 mm in diameter are scattered throughout the gland tissue and consist of large aggregations of eosinophils in the centre of which microfilariae or remnants may be found, surrounded by hyaline material known as Meyers–Kouwenaar bodies. Epithelioid granulomas with foreign body giant cells may be seen. In the lungs the alveoli are filled with eosinophils, sometimes with microfilariae inside them. The nodules, which are up to 5 mm in diameter, are also found in the liver and spleen. Microfilariae tend to be more numerous in the spleen. The nodules in the lungs and liver may be few or many and microfilariae may be almost impossible to demonstrate. Most lesions in these situations consist of epithelioid granulomas with foreign body giant cells and varying numbers of eosinophils, microfilariae and Meyers–Kouwenaar bodies. In the *chronic* phase fibrosis takes place in the lungs with increase in the interstitial tissue and restriction of airflow through the small bronchi.

IMMUNITY

The immune response as has been described is a type I and type II response against microfilariae of one or more species. Recurrent attacks occur due either to reinfection or a return of microfilariae to the peripheral blood.

CLINICAL FEATURES

Attacks of respiratory symptoms of an asthmatic nature occur, often associated with fever and splenomegaly. There is a tendency to relapse, eventually proceeding on to pulmonary fibrosis.

Incubation period

Little is known about the incubation period but it is probably the same as that of the species of filaria responsible.

Symptoms and signs

The onset is with cough, lassitude, dyspnoea on exertion and asthma, especially at night, occasionally associated with haemoptysis. Associated symptoms may include fever and splenomegaly. In advanced cases the lungs undergo multifocal fibrotic changes.

Lung function tests show a restrictive abnormality in 70% and an obstructive one in 30% of cases.

Radiology of the chest shows changes in 20% of cases. In these there is a disseminated mottling most marked in the mid- and lower zones consisting of small nodules up to 5 mm diameter, many fine linear shadows which clear rapidly following treatment with DEC (Fig. 20.14).

Lymphadenopathy. In one form the lymph glands are chiefly affected and there may be generalized lymphadenopathy with the glands showing the typical picture of TPE.

Cardiac complications. TPE may be associated with cardiomyopathy[65] and raises the possibility that the eosinophils were damaging the myocardium. There is a geographical coincidence between TPE and endomyocardial fibrosis in India. Occasionally pericarditis and pericardial effusion may occur[66] and bilateral eosinophilic pleural effusions have been described.[67]

Neurological complications. TPE may occasionally present with complications of a focal neurological nature. Aphasia, disorientation, double vision and facial palsy without any neurological signs which responded within two weeks of DEC therapy were reported by Ravindran.[68]

DIAGNOSIS

Since microfilariae cannot be demonstrated in the blood recourse must be had to serology. There is a universal increase in antimicrofilarial antibody titre, often to a very high degree in all serological tests (see p. 365). The *Dirofilaria immitis* CFT is virtually always strongly positive. It is not possible to consider the diagnosis of TPE with negative serology. Lung or lymph gland biopsy may show typical histology.

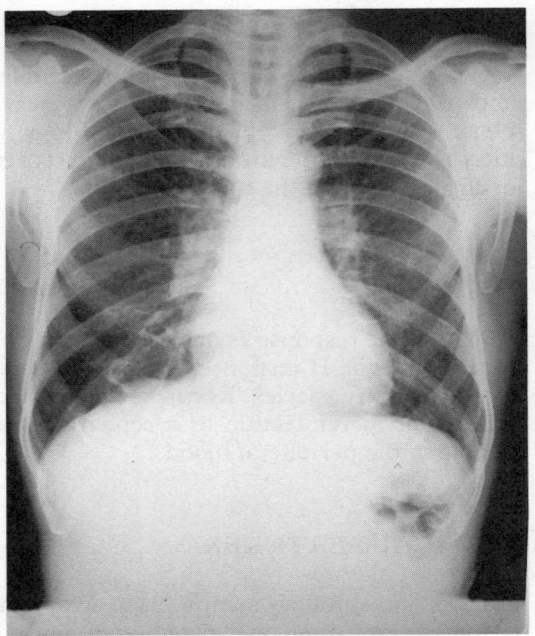

(a)

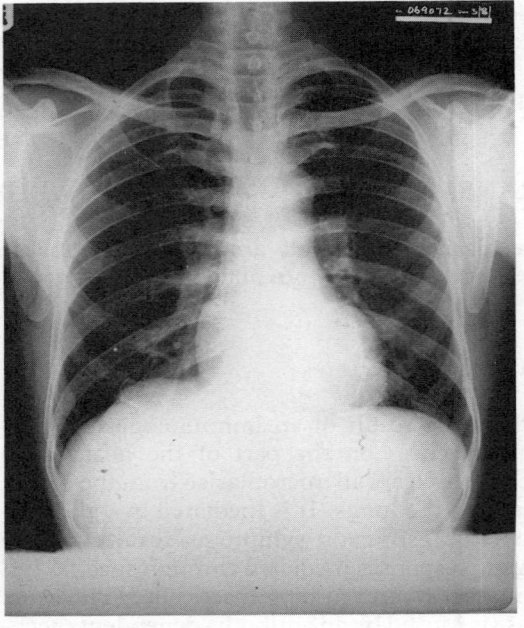

(b)

Fig. 20.14   Radiological changes in the lungs in TPE before (a) and after (b) treatment with DEC.

DIFFERENTIAL DIAGNOSIS

Differentiation has to be made from bronchial asthma, pulmonary tuberculosis, miliary tuberculosis, allergic disease from inhaled dust (farmer's lung), pulmonary aspergillosis, eosinophilic lung reaction to drugs, eosinophilic leukaemia, and other helminthic infections with a tissue stage, *Ascaris*, *Ancylostoma*, *Strongyloides*, trichinosis, *Schistosoma mansoni* and *S. japonicum*. In all these, serology is the diagnostic tool although cross reactions in some of the tests with *Strongyloides* may cause trouble (see p. 437). Confusion may also arise with visceral larva migrans (VLM) caused by *Toxocara* and differentiation may be difficult since serology may cross react (see p. 415).

TREATMENT

DEC is very effective in treatment and is used in the same dosage as in *W. bancrofti*. There is a relapse rate of 20% and some cases may need two or three treatments. Relapse can occur any time up to six months after treatment. In chronic cases fibrotic changes may be irreversible.

EPIDEMIOLOGY

There is a seasonal incidence depending on the country. About 90% of cases occur in people of Indian origin. Males are affected more than females and the maximum incidence is at 20–30 years of age. The natural history of the untreated disease is not really known. In some patients symptoms may remit spontaneously after a few months. In others, the disease progresses to permanently disabling pulmonary fibrosis.

2   SUBCUTANEOUS FILARIASIS

Subcutaneous filariasis in humans is caused by two filariae: *Onchocerca volvulus* (onchocerciasis) and *Loa loa* (loiasis).

Onchocerciasis

GEOGRAPHICAL DISTRIBUTION

Human onchocerciasis is found in both the Old and New Worlds but about 95% of all cases are in Africa.

New World. Important foci exist in Mexico, Guatemala, Venezuela and the upper Orinoco basin (Fig. 20.15) from where the infection has spread to northern Brazil in Roraima[69] and in Colombia where a new focus is well established,[70] and more recently in Esmeraldas province in Ecuador.[71]

Old World. In Africa the infection occurs south of the Sahara in a wide belt stretching from west to east (Fig. 20.16). The northern boundary of this zone coincides roughly with 15° north and runs from Senegal to Ethiopia. Small foci exist in the north of the Sudan along the Nile and in the Yemen. The southern limit starts at 14° south in Angola and runs west and south to the Cholo district of Malawi at 17° south, extending into Tanzania at latitude 12° south where important foci are found in the Usambara mountains, Mahenge, Rovuma and Morogoro. More recently a new focus has been found in Macha in Zambia at 25° south.[72]

AETIOLOGY

Human onchocerciasis is caused by *Onchocerca volvulus*. The adults are slender, white worms; the male $2.5\,\text{cm} \times 0.2\,\text{mm}$ and the female $35–70\,\text{cm} \times 0.4\,\text{mm}$ (Fig. 20.17). Both male and female worms live in subcutaneous nodules or free in the subcutaneous tissues. The female is ovoviviparous, producing microfilariae.

The microfilariae are sheathless, $300 \times 0.8\,\mu\text{m}$, with a sharply pointed recurved tail (see Figs. 20.18 and II.73,1, p. 1371). Microfilariae are found free in the fluid within nodules but are mainly found in the dermal layer of the skin

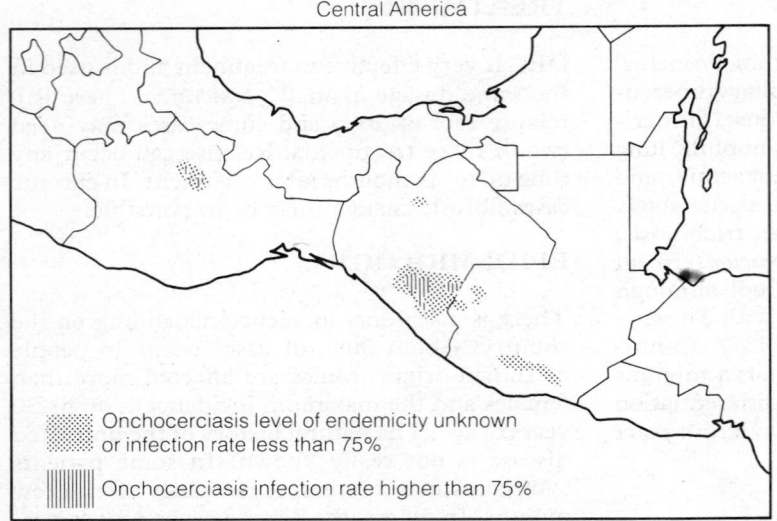

Central America

Onchocerciasis level of endemicity unknown or infection rate less than 75%

Onchocerciasis infection rate higher than 75%

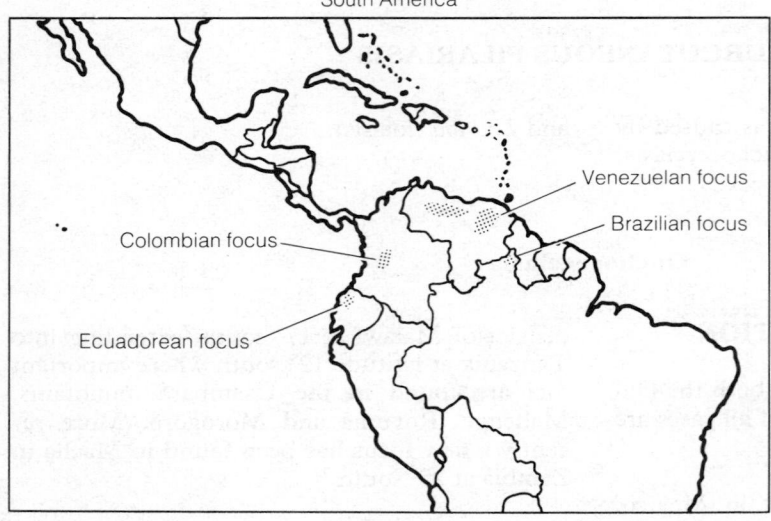

South America

Venezuelan focus

Brazilian focus

Colombian focus

Ecuadorean focus

Fig. 20.15 Geographical distribution of New World onchocerciasis. (Courtesy Department of Entomology, London School of Hygiene and Tropical Medicine.)

(Fig. 20.22, p. 377) spreading centrifugally from where an adult lies either in the nodule or free in the tissues. Microfilariae do sometimes appear in the blood and are also found in the eye in heavy infections. They may sometimes be found in the urine, sputum and cerebrospinal fluid, especially after treatment. They are occasionally found in ascitic fluid.

The microfilariae of *O. volvulus* are morphologically indistinguishable throughout the range of the parasite. Microfilariae from the upper Orinoco basin in Venezuela vary in measurement and enzyme structure from the African strain[73] and in West Africa there are at least four different patterns of acid phosphatase distribution on isoenzyme analysis, and significant differences between forest and savannah strains.[74,75]

There is such a degree of onchocerca–simulium adaptation that there is incompatibility between parasite strains and vectors from different geographical areas. There are at least six different onchocerca–simulium complexes in West Africa.[76] The main African differentiation is into three strains: a forest strain with low ocular pathogenicity, a humid savannah zone

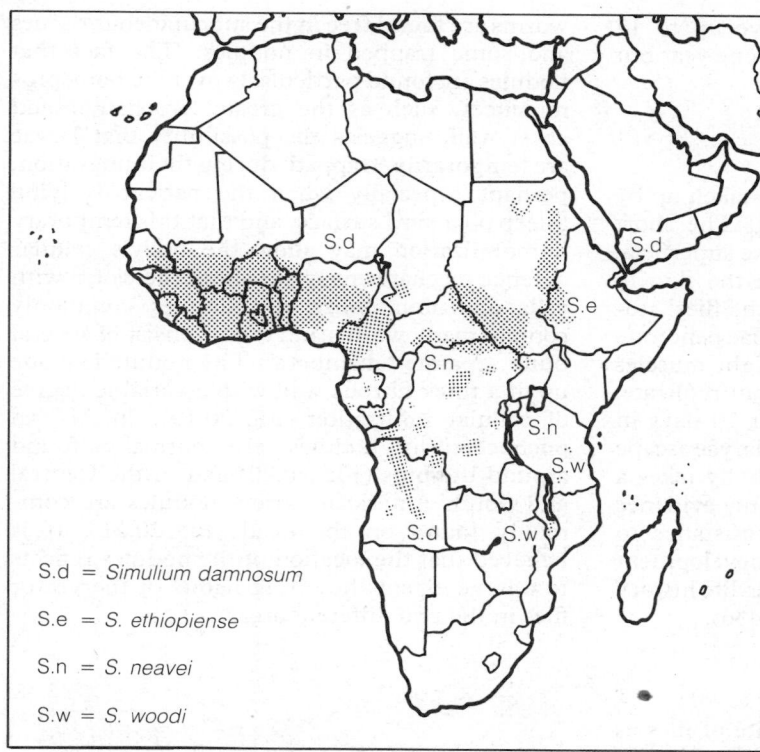

S.d = *Simulium damnosum*

S.e = *S. ethiopiense*

S.n = *S. neavei*

S.w = *S. woodi*

Fig. 20.16 Geographical distribution of Old World onchocerciasis.

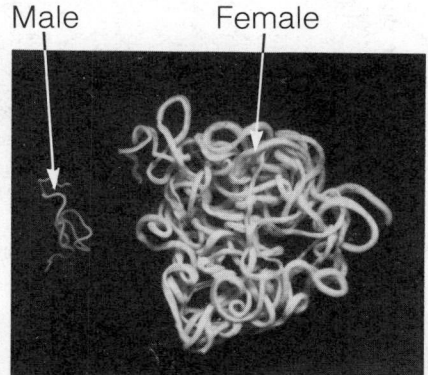

Male   Female

Fig. 20.17 Adult *Onchocerca volvulus*, male on left, female on right.

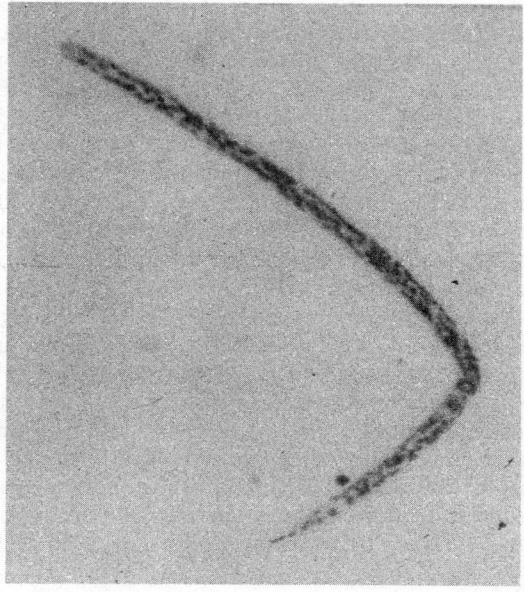

Fig. 20.18 Mf *Onchocerca volvulus*, more than 275 μm long, no sheath, cephalic space longer than twice the width of the body.

strain with moderate disease and a dry savannah zone strain with high pathogenesis and a high rate of blindness.

Many related but different onchocerca parasites are found in animals, especially bovids, but *O. volvulus* has only been found in man and the gorilla, although it has been transmitted experimentally to the chimpanzee. A new microfilaria bolivarensis has been described from human blood in the onchocerciasis area of the Orinoco basin[77] which is smaller than mf volvulus and more readily invades the blood, but these differences are not constant.[73]

Adult onchocerca worms can live up to 17 years. Most microfilariae die within one year but some may live for up to three years.

Life-cycle

Microfilariae present in the skin are taken up by the *Simulium* vector when feeding. The short proboscis of the flies is prone to cause superficial injury allowing the microfilariae in the skin to contaminate the blood and so into the flies' stomachs. In the stomach the microfilariae penetrate the stomach wall, migrate to the flight muscles where they develop further but do not replicate, and reach the proboscis after about 10 days in favourable circumstances. Infective larvae escape from the proboscis when the female fly takes a second blood meal. There is now some evidence that infected flies develop some resistance to reinfection (for a description of the development in the fly, see Appendix II; and for the life history of *Simulium*, see Appendix III, p. 1436).

TRANSMISSION

Transmission is normally by the bite of flies as described and the only other method of transmission of the infection reported is congenital transmission. One in 20 babies born in heavily infected areas have microfilariae in the skin soon after birth. This may be due to transplacental transmission of the microfilariae from blood, especially after treatment of the mother with DEC or transplacental passage of infective forms when the adults may become established in newborn infants.[78] These findings are of obvious importance to those assessing the interruption of transmission in eradication schemes.

Simulium flies can only breed in well-oxygenated water because their larvae have an obligatory aquatic state development. They require a high oxygen tension and the disease is associated therefore with relatively fast running water, such as in rivers and streams. The presence of the vectors of this blinding disease near to rivers in Africa has given onchocerciasis the name 'river blindness' (see Appendix III, p. 1436).

PATHOLOGY

The infective larva migrates through the subcutaneous tissues from the bite site and develops into an adult worm in about one year. Some worms are found free in the subcutaneous tissues and some trapped in nodules. The fact that nodules are found particularly over the bony prominences, such as the greater trochanter and chest wall, suggests the possibility that larvae are temporarily 'trapped' during their migration, perhaps especially when the patient is lying asleep on a hard surface, and that this temporary immobilization may allow the body's cellular defence mechanisms to surround the worm with cells and immobilize it. Nodules commonly contain many worms and often consist of several quite separate 'chambers'. The nodule is made up of a thick fibrous wall with a variable degree of cellular infiltration (Fig. 20.19). In African onchocerciasis nodules are normally found around the hips (Fig. 20.20) and in the Central and South American variety nodules are commonly found on the head (Fig. 20.21). It is believed that the location of the nodules reflects to a large extent the biting habits of the vector flies in the two different areas.

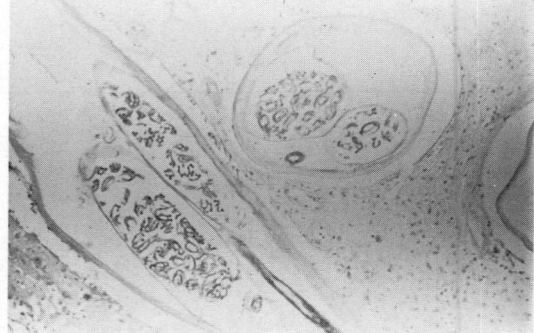

Fig. 20.19 *Onchocerca volvulus*: adults in subcutaneous nodule. (Courtesy Dr H. Zaiman.)

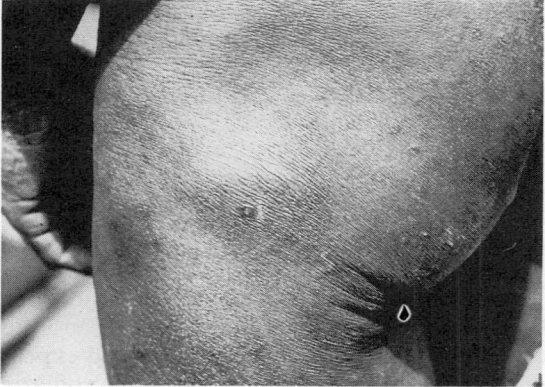

Fig. 20.20 Onchocercal nodule on the iliac crest surrounded by atrophied skin.

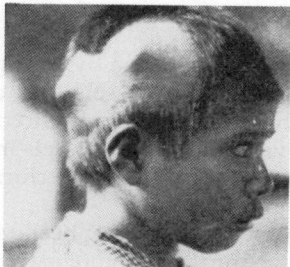

Fig. 20.21 Onchocercal nodule on the scalp of a Mexican patient.

Worms normally take about 11 months to mature and for the female to start producing microfilariae. At this time symptoms first appear in the form of itching and microfilariae can be found in the skin at about the same time (Fig. 20.22). For this reason the incubation period and prepatent period are commonly the same.

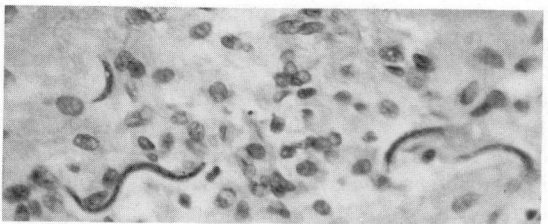

Fig. 20.22 Microfilariae of *O. volvulus* in subcutaneous tissue.

Microfilariae are found in largest numbers adjacent to the nodules and become progressively less in number the further away from the nodule the skin specimen is taken for examination.

The nodules themselves may occasionally undergo lipomatous transformation (Fig. 20.23).

The main significant pathology arises from the reaction to dead microfilariae in the skin and the eyes. In the skin the condition is called onchodermatitis; the basic lesion is the cellular reaction to the dead microfilariae. Immunological mechanisms are at work and include type I intermediate hypersensitivity reaction,[79] type II delayed hypersensitivity reaction[80] and immune complex formation.[81] The result is immune complex formation followed by complement activation and mobilization of immunocompetent cells and probably occurs in that order, as in the case of the granulomatous reactions surrounding schistosome eggs in the tissues (see Chapter 22).

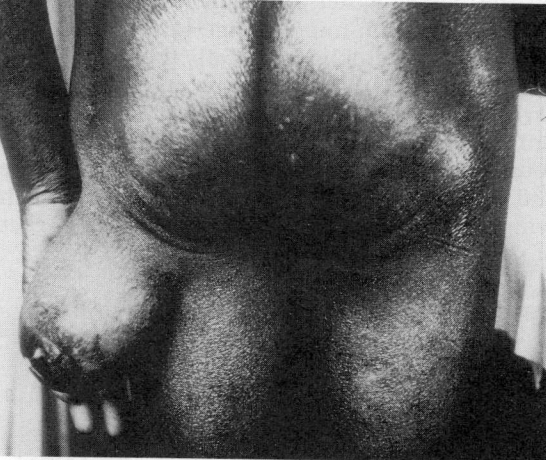

Fig. 20.23 Lipomatous transformation of an onchocerca nodule (oncholipoma). (Courtesy Dr D. Bell.)

This basic focal inflammatory lesion is responsible for the pathology seen in the skin, the lymph glands and the eyes, although the posterior ocular lesions have a different aetiology.

Skin changes

The earliest skin changes are the development of foci of inflammation surrounding dead microfilariae. Histological appearances are often of 'microabscesses'. Between the focal lesions the skin is commonly oedematous but shows no other significant pathological changes.

Later in the evolution of the disease there is an increasing amount of destruction of the elastic tissue and the skin tends to form redundant folds. There may be loss of pigment in those with pigmented skin, especially in African cases, in the pretibial region. The histological appearance of the skin in advanced cases closely resembles that of normal skin in very old subjects, i.e. presbyderma. The most advanced changes are seen in patients with very high microfilarial densities. Densities of < 50 mf/mg are often associated with few pathological changes and minimal or entirely absent subjective complaints.

Lymph glands (onchocercal lymphadenitis)

The regional lymph glands are usually enlarged in response to a significant microfilarial load in the distal skin because the lymph glands are responsible for removal of the rubbish liberated by the death, either spontaneous or following treatment, of the microfilariae in the skin. The glands enlarge and histologically there are foci of inflammation surrounding the microfilariae in early cases and cellular atrophy, followed by fibrosis in late cases. Enlarged glands are surrounded by skin with marked loss of elastic tissue and the 'hanging groin' effect develops in which lymph glands appear to be enfolded in a pocket of skin (Fig. 20.24).

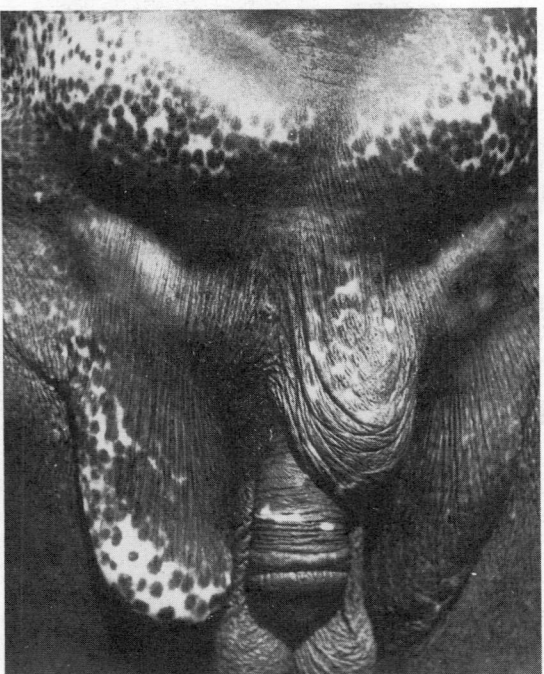

Fig. 20.24 Depigmentation of skin and hanging groin in onchocerciasis. (Courtesy Dr S.G. Browne.)

Hernia

This is a definite complication of onchocerciasis[82] and takes the form of direct inguinal hernia or femoral hernia. The scrotum is often involved.

Elephantiasis

Minor elephantiasis of the scrotum may occur in heavily infected cases but the most usual effect on the genitalia is an unusually pendulous rather than elephantoid scrotum. Minor changes in the lower limb also occur mainly in the form of thickening of the skin around the ankles. Chronic lymphoedema and true elephantiasis, as seen in lymphatic filariasis, do not occur.

Eye lesions

Microfilariae enter the eye by passing along the sheaths of the ciliary vessels and nerves from under the bulbar conjunctiva directly into the cornea and via the nutrient vessels into the optic nerve, and via the posterior perforating ciliary vessels into the choroid.[83,84]

In the past there have been serious disagreements about the pathological effects on the eye due to onchocerciasis mainly concerning the posterior segment but the following views are now widely accepted.[85]

Dead microfilariae in the cornea and ciliary body give rise to foci of inflammation. The earliest effect in the cornea itself is the development of small foci of cellular inflammation developing around demised microfilariae. These cause the characteristic 'snowflake keratitis' and are potentially wholly reversible lesions. The major pathology of the anterior chamber is caused by the development of vascular infiltration of the cornea in response to dead microfilariae, the infiltrates taking the form of leashes of blood vessels passing into the cornea from the anterior chamber and conjunctiva resulting in a cellular organization of the cornea. This conversion of the cornea into connective tissue initially takes place from each side and from below and eventually results in complete organization and opacification of the cornea (further descriptions are given in Chapter 70, p. 1153).

Inflammation surrounding microfilariae which have died in the ciliary body gives rise to multifocal iritis, the formation of posterior synechiae and the development of secondary cataract.

The genesis of posterior ocular lesions is more obscure and is dealt with in Chapter 70 (p. 1152).

With the exception of punctate keratitis the ocular lesions of onchocerciasis are 'irreversible' in the sense that they will not resolve after specific anti-onchocercal chemotherapy. It has been suggested that concomitant vitamin A deficiency may aggravate the damage done to the eyes by onchocerciasis, although the mechanism is obscure.

IMMUNITY

There is no good evidence of immunity to reinfection in the case of onchocerciasis and in endemic areas the numbers of microfilariae, and by inference the numbers of adult worms, commonly rise slowly throughout life. Immune reactions to the dead microfilariae apparently are entirely responsible for the development of early skin and eye lesions although the destruction of elastic tissue in the skin may be due to 'toxin' produced by the microfilariae.

Immunosuppression

It may be that very heavy infections with *Onchocerca volvulus* produce generalized depression of the immune system although this is still largely conjectural. Lepromatous leprosy may be twice as common in some areas where onchocerciasis is highly endemic than in other areas where the disease is not found.[86] The mechanism of this suggested immunosuppression is not known.

CLINICAL FEATURES

Natural history

Onchocerca volvulus is a long-lived parasite and can live for as long as 17 years in the absence of any transmission (microfilariae did not disappear from the skin until 17 years after the eradication of *Simulium neavei* from the Kodera valley in western Kenya). The infection follows a varying number of courses as described in the section on pathology above but, after many years in older people, the adult worms and microfilariae eventually succumb to the immune processes and only the signs of burnt out disease remain, with no microfilariae or adult worms to be found. Onchocerciasis does not kill the individual but only cripples him from itching skin and blindness. Onchocerciasis is an important cause of blindness in Africa and Central America and these people succumb to other infections and often die from starvation. In areas where infections are light the presence of onchocerciasis in the community can pass unnoticed until actively searched for by skin snips. These people have no idea that they are infected and often the administration of one tablet of DEC reveals an extensive prevalence in the community.

Incubation period

The time between the inoculation of infective larvae and the first appearance of microfilariae in the skin is commonly 15–18 months with extremes of 10–20 months. Symptoms start when the microfilariae appear in the skin about 15–18 months after infection.

Symptoms and signs

Onchocerciasis may produce no symptoms at all where transmission is light. Many onchocerciasis areas have remained undiscovered until skin snips in symptomless inhabitants have shown the presence of onchocercal infection.

Patients presenting with clinical onchocerciasis fall into two categories. Those with recent relatively light infections present with a pruritic skin rash; these are children living in endemic areas and adults, often expatriates, who come to live there without previous exposure to infection. Those with heavy infections of long duration present with deteriorating vision or gross skin manifestations.

Skin symptoms and signs (onchodermatitis)

In light, recently acquired infections an adult female worm, usually impalpable, is present

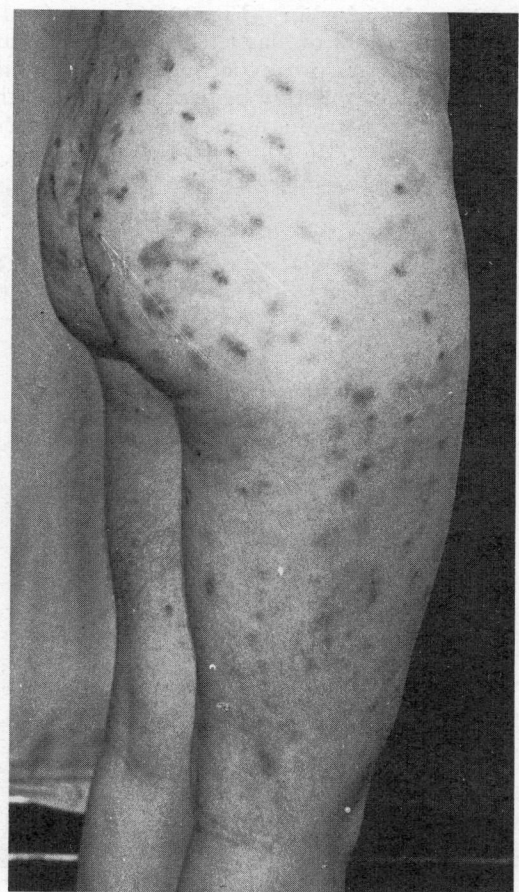

Fig. 20.25 Onchodermatitis.

around the limb girdle on the affected side. Microfilariae from these worms then invade the skin of the anatomical quarter and produce the characteristic lesions. The main symptom is pruritis ('gale filarienne', filarial itch) with a rash composed of numerous small circular raised discrete papules 1–3 mm in diameter which are red on a white skin (Fig. 20.25) and are usually confined to one anatomical quarter of the body or on the back in a 'butterfly' distribution on the buttocks. Microfilariae are present in small numbers in these cases. In the indigenous inhabitants of areas of high endemicity the skin shows gross scarring. In Africa the skin lesions are commonest over the lower limbs but may cover the whole body. There is a thickening of the skin owing to subcutaneous oedema and this produces the characteristic 'peau d'orange' effect which is often associated with lymph gland enlargement, especially in the groins. Later there is a heavy lichenification and thickening of the skin (xeroderma or lizard skin) (Fig. 20.26) and finally atrophy with loss of elasticity and a premature aged appearance (presbyderma). In these cases microfilariae can readily be demonstrated in the skin, often in enormous numbers, except in burnt

out 'presbyderma' where they have disappeared from the skin.

In Central America gross skin changes are less marked than elsewhere even when microfilariae are abundant, but some people, especially children, may show angry reddish-mauve lesions on the face ('erisipela de la costa') and adults may show a thickened smooth white face giving a leonine appearance ('mal morado').

Depigmentation ('leopard skin', LS)

In long-standing onchocerciasis patchy depigmentation of the skin is found, usually in the pretibial regions, but also in the groins (Fig. 20.24) and over the iliac crests. This has been called 'leopard skin' (LS) and is distinct from onchodermatitis. No microfilariae can be found in skin snips and often there is no evidence of active onchocerciasis. The cause of LS is controversial; it is invariably associated with long-standing onchocerciasis, repeated bites from *Simulium* in hyperendemic areas and the presence of multiple palpable onchocercal nodules on the body.[87] In one area in Nigeria 26.4% of all the people examined showed LS and its presence was used to assess the distribution of onchocerciasis[88] but there is no correlation between the incidence of LS and the density of microfilariae in the skin, and there is a marked difference in incidence in different onchocerciasis areas between the forest zone (36%) and the savannah zone (4.3%).[89] Other factors have been considered: black fly saliva and toxins[87] and depigmentation from repeated *Simulium* bites without onchocercal infection of that part of the skin has been recorded.[90]

Other marked clinical features (lymphadenopathy, hernia, hanging groins) are described in the section on pathology, above.

Nodules

Nodules which are usually situated in the lower half of the body in African onchocerciasis (Fig. 20.20) when situated on the head may erode the skull and cause epilepsy (Fig. 20.21). The Nakalanga syndrome in Uganda is pygmy dwarfing, resulting from pituitary damage,[91] though by what mechanism is as yet unknown.

Lungs

A few cases of pulmonary infiltrates resembling

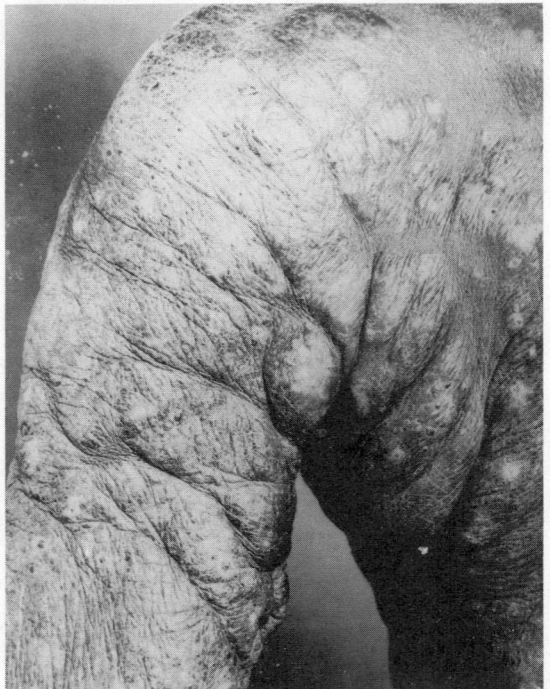

Fig. 20.26 Lichenification of the skin in long-standing onchocerciasis (lizard skin). (Courtesy Dr P.W. Hutton.)

TPE were encountered in an onchocerciasis area in West Africa.[92]

Arthritis

Two types of arthritis may occur: a monoarthritis affecting the large joints—usually the hip or the knee where nodules are close to large joints—and an acute arthritis with microfilariae in the synovial effusion has been described. Deep-seated pain in the hip is a common symptom in onchocerciasis, presumably due to an adult worm sited close to the hip joint. This pain disappears rapidly on treatment with DEC. The other form is a polyarthritis resembling rheumatoid arthritis caused by immune complexes, which does not respond to DEC.

Other symptoms

Many ill-defined symptoms may be associated with onchocerciasis but not always demonstrably on a causal basis until treatment of the infection removes the symptoms.

Vague *muscle pains*, backache and symptoms of 'myositis' may occur.

Giddiness and dizziness are common symptoms in some areas, often associated with scarring of the ear drum but microfilarial involvement of the drum has never been shown.

Sowda

Sowda from the Arabic for black or dark, is a localized form of onchocerciasis common in the Yemen[93] but also found in the northern Sudan and the savannah in Nigeria. It has recently been described in Guatemala.[94]

Sowda is the result of a strong immune response on the part of the host (see section on pathology, above) in contrast to African onchocerciasis. The infection is localized usually to one limb but both legs, an arm or the trunk may be involved. Itching is first noticed in the leg below the knee which spreads up to the sacroiliac joint. The involved skin becomes swollen and darkened and covered with scaling papules. The regional lymph glands (usually groin glands) become greatly enlarged. Microfilariae are extremely difficult to find in skin snips but the Mazzotti test is positive.

Pathological changes in the skin and glands are characteristic. In the skin the changes are the same as in African onchocerciasis but are more severe and the dermis is more severely damaged. The lymph glands show follicular hyperplasia (in contrast to follicular atrophy in African onchocerciasis).[95] The condition responds well to treatment.

Laboratory findings

The most marked finding is a peripheral eosinophilia in the blood. Except in the most advanced and burnt out cases there is often a marked eosinophilia of 4×10^9/litre or more. Symptomless onchocerciasis revealed by a peripheral eosinophilia is a common finding in expatriates from West Africa who are undergoing a post-tour 'check'.

DIFFERENTIAL DIAGNOSIS

The pruritic onchodermatitis (filarial itch) must be distinguished from infection with *Mansonella streptocerca*, in which the lower limbs are rarely affected; scabies, where the typical burrows and mites can be found between the fingers; insect bites which come on early after residence in the tropics; prickly heat; contact dermatitis; and sycosis cruris, a chronic low-grade bacterial infection of the legs.

In heavy infections of long standing the skin changes must be differentiated from tertiary yaws, superficial mycoses, leprosy and chronic eczema.

DIAGNOSIS

The diagnosis is made by demonstrating microfilariae of *O. volvulus* in skin snips (see Appendix IV, p. 1493). Skin snips (two to four) should be taken from the thighs, buttocks and iliac crests in African cases and from the scapula, buttock and face regions in American cases. After cleaning the skin with spirit and allowing to dry, a small needle or entomological pin is slipped under the epidermis which is raised and sliced off with a safety razor blade, removing a small piece of skin 2–3 mm in diameter and 0.5–1 mm deep. The Walser corneoscleral punch enables the operator to take snips rapidly and almost painlessly, but the instrument is expensive (about £60), needs frequent resharpening and there are disquieting doubts about the efficacy of cold sterilization in glutaraldehyde. The snip itself, which should be bloodless, is placed in physiological saline and examined after 20–30 minutes in a wet state under the microscope. Teasing the skin is unnecessary. It has been shown that about 20% of the microfilariae only will be detected in this way. About 80% will emerge if the snip is incubated in saline in a covered microlitre plate for 12–24 hours. The microfilariae must be distinguished from *M. streptocerca* in Africa and *M. ozzardi* in South America which, although found in the blood, can appear in skin snips contaminated by blood (Figs. 20.41 and II.73,6, p. 1371). The portions of skin can be weighed and the density of microfilariae per milligram calculated. Large numbers of skin snips may be collected and examined later in a base laboratory using microtitration plates. To detect low density microfilarial concentration in the skin may need many skin snips and more than six are not usually tolerated. Skin snips can be taken in the field, preserved in ethanol and subjected to collagenase digestion,[96] but this results in only a 20% increase in yield over the incubation method and is difficult to justify.

Mazzotti test[97]

This test consists of observing the reaction to a test dose of DEC 50 or 100 mg by mouth. The reaction is against the microfilariae killed by the DEC. When microfilariae are present in the skin there is a reaction starting 2–24 hours later with intense pruritus, the appearance of a rash (or an acute exacerbation of a rash if present) which can be unpleasant, and in cases with a heavy skin load of microfilariae causes microfilaraemia and microfilariuria with fever, lymphadenopathy, arthropathy and, in some cases, death.[98] This test must always be preceded by the examination of skin snips for microfilariae and is contraindicated in heavily infected individuals and in those in whom the eye is suspected of being involved. The Mazzotti reaction is also a complication of treatment and care must be taken (see section on treatment, below). A Mazzotti patch test using a topical application of DEC has been devised which can detect low concentrations of microfilariae without the disadvantage of the full Mazzotti test.[99]

Serological tests

Serological tests are useful in cases with few or no microfilariae in the skin and CFT titres bore an inverse ratio to the mean number of microfilariae/mm^2 of skin[100] and individuals with the highest microfilarial counts had the lowest titres against onchocercal antigen with immunofluorescence.[101]

Immunofluorescence

The filarial FAT is the test of choice and since it is those cases who exhibit few or no microfilariae in the skin who need to be diagnosed it is useful as a screening test. Titres up to 1.256 are common.

ELISA test

An ELISA test using a crude soluble antigen from adult *O. volvulus* has been developed in Guatemala[102] and shows promise. It is highly sensitive in low density infections and 81.4% of infected individuals showed titres of more than 1 : 160 and only 2.6% less. Cross reactions with intestinal helminths occurred in 17.4% of helminthic infections tested (especially *Strongyloides*).

Skin test

Immediate hypersensitivity skin tests are of some use in detecting people exposed to onchocerciasis and using a microfilarial antigen tests were positive in 85% of persons infected with onchocerciasis.[103]

Conclusion

If no microfilariae are detected in the skin or eyes and the Mazzotti test is negative then the individual is not infected with onchocerciasis.

TREATMENT

Three drugs are used in treatment although other drugs have some effect.

1   *Diethylcarbamazine (DEC)*
This is given orally, induces destruction of the microfilariae by the host's immune system but does not kill adult worms. The disadvantages are side-effects, notably the Mazzotti reaction (see above).

2 *Suramin (Bayer 205)*

Suramin, which is given intravenously weekly, kills adult worms but has many severe side-effects, e.g. peripheral neuropathy, renal damage, exfoliative dermatitis and a fatal diarrhoea.

3 *Ivermectin*

This is a new drug given orally in a single dose, kills microfilariae slowly and avoids the Mazzotti reaction. It appears to be the drug of choice.

Diethylcarbamazine (Hetrazan, Banocide, Notézine)

Diethylcarbamazine is given in lightly infected cases to remove the microfilariae from the skin, but has to be given repeatedly over many years to give any benefit. In areas of light to moderate endemicity a great number of persons carrying *O. volvulus* have no symptoms and are in no need of treatment; in fact if they are treated the natural host–parasite relationship will be upset and subsequent reinfections may be symptomatic. If fibrosis and scarring of the skin is advanced these processes can only be arrested. To forecast reactions a small dose should be given at first: day 1, 50 mg; day 2, 50 mg three times a day; day 3, 100 mg three times a day; and from day 4 onwards 250 mg three times a day. The traditional course of 2 mg/kg body weight three times a day for three weeks is unnecessarily long: 7 days' treatment will kill all the microfilariae. There is no evidence that prolonged or repeated courses kill the adult worms. As the adult worms are not killed after DEC treatment, the microfilariae will return and reach half the previous concentration within one year and reach the pre-treatment level in one to three years.[104] Symptoms return after a period of three to six months. If there is a severe reaction to treatment this may be controlled by steroids. Antihistaminics are of little use. Prednisolone should always be given during treatment of patients with eye involvement, but high doses inhibit the microfilaricidal effect.

The only justification in using DEC to treat onchocerciasis nowadays is in mild symptomatic cases which do not justify the hazards of suramin and when ivermectin is unobtainable. To avoid recurrent Mazzotti reactions treatment has to be repeated every one to four weeks and continued for years.

Reactions to diethylcarbamazine

In heavily infected cases collapse, dyspnoea, vertigo and even death may occur, as in the Mazzotti reaction. These reactions are caused by the invasion of the blood and internal organs by microfilariae. Among neurological complications vertigo and mild parkinsonism with microfilariae in the cerebrospinal fluid have been recorded.[105] The eyes may show a brief exacerbation of watering, with photophobia and itching. Symptomatic relief occurs in 24–48 hours while clearance of microfilariae from the anterior chamber takes one to three weeks. Prednisolone will prevent and remove the cardiovascular and lymphatic manifestations of severe reactions but does not prevent pruritus or skin rash. A weekly suppressive dose of 200 mg of DEC may keep the eyes free from infection but may produce regular itching after each dose.

Suramin (Antrypol, Bayer 205)

Suramin, which acts on both the microfilariae and adult worms, is a potentially dangerous drug and great care should be taken in using it in a disease which is not fatal. Involvement of the eyes is an indication for suramin treatment.

Traditionally microfilariae were first removed from the skin by a course of DEC, but the rationale for this is difficult to see, especially as suramin itself is slowly microfilaricidal. Suramin should be given intravenously once a week in doses (for a 60 kg subject) of 0.2 g, 0.4 g, 0.6 g, 0.8 g, 1 g, 1 g.[106] This can be relied upon to kill adult worms. In addition, almost all of the microfilariae in the skin and eyes will be killed.

The side-effects of suramin used in onchocerciasis are of three types. Those due to the drug include tenderness of the palms of the hands and soles of the feet; polyuria and increased thirst; tiredness, anorexia and malaise; exfoliative dermatitis; and ulceration of the mouth and tongue. Those due to death of the adult worms include urticaria and swelling of the affected part; extrusion of adult worms; deep abscesses; and painful immobilization of the hip joints caused by the adult worms round the joint capsule with pain referred to the knee from this source. Effects due to death of the microfilariae begin immediately after the start of treatment and include: itching of the skin; dermatitis with papular and vesicular eruption followed by desquamation; pyrexia; bronchitis; iritis; and swelling with pain and limitation of movement of fingers, wrists, ankles and knees, all possibly caused by the deposition of immune complexes. The indications for stopping suramin are gross albuminuria, diarrhoea, fever and exfoliative skin changes.

Ivermectin

Ivermectin is an avermectin derived from *Streptomyces avermitilis*. Discovered in 1982[107] it has a strong but slow microfilaricidal action; a single dose of 50–200 μg/kg orally reduced the skin microfilariae by 90% in one week and a year afterwards the microfilarial counts were still low.[108] Yearly treatments will keep the microfilarial counts at a low level and prevent progressive tissue damage. Ivermectin may be suitable for mass treatment and reduce the transmission of the disease. However, toxicity remains a danger and it could be a danger if it crosses the blood–brain barrier.

Other drugs

Metriphonate (trichlorphon)

This drug has been found effective against microfilariae[109] but has no advantages over DEC and is not a recommended treatment.

Benzimidazole derivatives: mebendazole plus levamisole

Mebendazole stops the development of the embryos in onchocerciasis.[110] It is given in conjunction with levamisole when the combination is both microfilaricidal and embryostatic. Microfilarial counts fall slowly and the effects last for six months. Mebendazole is given in a dose of 30 mg/kg daily in divided doses for three weeks. Levamisole is given 2.5 mg/kg twice in the first week and then weekly for three weeks, starting one week before the mebendazole, but the need for prolonged and repeated courses makes this combined treatment highly impractical.

Nodulectomy

Nodulectomy has limited use as many worms are present outside nodules, but it should be used whenever nodules are on or near the head since this can reduce the incidence of blindness. Mass denodulization has been used in Guatemala to control the disease but has not been so successful as was first hoped for.

Suppressive treatment

If the patient cannot tolerate suramin or if early reinfection is unavoidable, weekly suppressive doses of diethylcarbamazine (50 mg) may be given. A series of reactions decreasing in severity will occur and after about six weeks the dosage can be increased to 200 mg which can be continued as long as desired and which will keep the skin free from microfilariae and the eyes protected from microfilarial invasion, and eliminate a source of infection for *Simulium*.

EPIDEMIOLOGY

The main single factor influencing the extent of human infection is the infective density of the *Simulium* vectors. This depends on the size of the *Simulium* population, number of infective flies, concentration of infective larvae in these flies, longevity of female *Simulium*, seasonal variation in numbers and the distance of human dwellings from the breeding grounds. The only host is man and once infected he is infective to flies for many years. The duration of patent infection lasts as long as 17 years. Human host factors to be considered are occupation, seasonal migration, changes in habits of the human population, attraction to the flies of different age, sex and racial groups and social and economic changes in the human population.

Epidemiology of African onchocerciasis

Ninety-five per cent of all human onchocerciasis infections are found in Africa. African *Simulium* consist of the *S. damnosum* and *S. neavei* complexes (see Fig. 20.16).

S. damnosum complex

The *S. damnosum* complex is composed of a number of species (Table 20.3) associated with large rivers and small streams and the *Simulium* can breed anywhere where there is an adequate velocity of water (60–250 cm/s), adequate food supplies and suitable attachment sites existing at depths not greater than 14 cm below the water surface. *S. damnosum* has been known to fly 300 km for breeding purposes to invade new areas and establish new colonies during the rainy season.

Table 20.3 Principal vectors of onchocerciasis in Africa.

Species	River type	Form (and zone) of onchocerciasis			Notes
		Severe (dry savannah)	Moderate (humid savannah)	Benign (forest)	
Simulium damnosum complex					
S. sirbanum	Large	+ + +	+	−	Trans-African
S. damnosum	Large	+ + +	+ +	−	Trans-African
S. soubrense A	Large	−	+ + +	+ +	West Africa
S. soubrense B	Large	−	+ + +	+ +	West Africa
S. squamosum	Small	−	+ +	+ + +	West Africa
S. yahense	Small	−	+ +	+ + +	West Africa
S. sanctipauli	Large	−	+	+ + +	West Africa
S. kilibanum	Upland	−	−	+ + +	East Africa
Simulium neavei complex					
S. ethiopiense	Upland	−	−	+ + +	Ethiopia
S. neavei	Upland	−	−	+ + +	Zaire, Uganda (Kenya)
S. woodi	Upland	−	−	+ + +	Tanzania, Malawi

SUDAN SAVANNAH (DRY) (VECTORS: *S. DAMNOSUM, S. SIRBANUM*)

S. damnosum and *S. sirbanum* are found in the river valleys of the West African savannah where they cause intense onchocercal infection among the population along the banks. In the dry season they are found near the banks of the streams where the humidity is sustained so that transmission is seasonal and in the dry season.

Hyperendemic infection begins in childhood as early as the first year of life. In the Red Volta district the fly infection rate is 13% and the microfilaria rate 38% under 10 years, 90% under 20 years and 100% over 20 years. There is no decrease in the microfilaria rate with age and microfilaria rates are higher in males than females.[111] In many parts more than 50% of the inhabitants show signs of disease; 30% have impaired vision and 4–10% are blind. In some villages of Burkina Faso (Upper Volta) and Ghana the percentage of blindness reaches 13–55%.[112] The greatest incidence of blindness is usually found in adult males who form the backbone of the labour force and, as their life is not shortened, they remain a burden to the community. Mass blindness can reduce the efficiency of a primitive agricultural community to below survival level and large areas of suitable agricultural land along the large rivers have been abandoned as a result of onchocerciasis.

Hydroelectric schemes entail the construction of large dams and inundate up river breeding places of *Simulium* but create new sites down-stream and in the spillways of the dams. Small earth dams invariably create new breeding places.

HUMID SAVANNAH (*S. SOUBRENSE, S. SQUAMOSUM* AND *S. YAHENSE*)

In the humid savannah transmission is perennial and the disease is not so severe, microfilarial densities are moderate and eye lesions rare, with blindness rates seldom above 3% in the over-five year age group.[89]

FOREST ZONE (*S. SQUAMOSUM, S. YAHENSE, S. SANCTIPAULI, S. KILIBANUM*, AND THE *S. NEAVEI* COMPLEX)

The main features governing the distribution of *S. neavei* are the existence of perennial streams containing a suitable crab host and sufficient forest cover for the adult stages. Vectors of the *S. neavei* group have a restricted flight range and are confined to forests and bush-lined streams. *S. neavei* is not a strong flier and the maximum recorded flight is 29 km from the nearest breeding place. It is unable to migrate from one focus to another except through forest galleries. It is thus a good candidate for eradication from a river system as was achieved at Kodera in western Kenya. Infections in *S. neavei* transmitted onchocerciasis are light and go mostly unnoticed by the local population. Blindness is very rare except in Kasai in Zaire where there is a high blindness rate with many nodules.

Epidemiology of Central and South American onchocerciasis (see Fig. 20.15)

Following the first discovery of onchocerciasis in Guatemala by Robles in 1915 there has been controversy over whether the infection was indigenous or introduced. It was suggested that the parasite had been imported into Central America by slaves from Jamaica or the Sudanese servants who accompanied the French troops of the Emperor Maximilian. However, it has been shown[113] that the American species did not develop well in African *Simulium* and the close adaptation of *O. volvulus* to *S. ochraceum* implies an association of more than 400 years.

In Venezuela and Colombia the infection may well have been introduced by the slaves imported in the Spanish era to pan the rivers for gold. There appear to be two different varieties of onchocercal disease, one found in Guatemala and Mexico with numerous nodules frequently on the head, considerable eye involvement but mild onchodermatitis, which is probably indigenous, and another found in Venezuela, Colombia and Ecuador resembling the African savannah type with few or no nodules, gross skin changes, lymphatic gland enlargement and 'hanging groins', which may well have been imported.

Mexico and Guatemala

The principal vectors *S. ochraceum* and *S. metallicum* breed in small streams at altitudes between 500 and 1500 m. *S. callidum* breeds in large rivers as well as small streams and has a greater range. All these species breed the year round but peak production is in the dry season. The main zone of transmission lies between 750 and 1500 m where the coffee plantations are located. Transmission is confined to the dry season. Infections are heavy in the *S. ochraceum* areas, there are many head nodules and eye involvement is common. Dermatitis is not severe and the skin presents a thickened, smooth, white appearance of the face called 'mal morado'.

Venezuela, Colombia and Ecuador

In Venezuela there are two main areas, one in the coastal region and the other in the south bordering on Brazil and across the border in Amazonia. In coastal Venezuela *S. metallicum* is the vector and onchocerciasis is mild. In the south and in Amazonia in the Roraima focus, *S.*

limbatum and *S. oyapockense* (formerly reported as *amazonicum*) are vectors. The Yanomama Indians are affected, the skin lesions are severe and lymph gland enlargement and 'hanging groins' common. In the western Andes in Colombia, where *S. exiguum* is the vector, lesions are mild but in Esmeraldas province in the Andes in Ecuador where the two main racial groups Chachilla (Indians) and Negroes are equally infected, the severe effects of the disease, skin depigmentation, lymphadenopathy and 'hanging groins' are found exclusively in Negroes.[71]

CONTROL

Combined control methods are those aimed at both the vector and the human host. Campaigns against the parasite are based on nodulectomy and chemotherapy. None of the older drugs is used for mass chemotherapy owing to an unacceptably high rate of side-effects, but ivermectin holds great promise for the future.

Vector control measures

In order to carry out vector control it is necessary to understand the biology of the vectors in each area. In Africa larvicides have been used mainly, though adulticides have been employed also. DDT employed as a larvicide can control *S. damnosum*, but failure can be caused by lack of control of breeding sites in small tributaries. Adulticides have been applied to resting places of *S. damnosum* by dispersion from aircraft and this has been successful in some cases where additional treatments are provided. An extensive campaign supported by the World Health Organization to eradicate *Simulium* from the Volta river basin is now under way in West Africa based on aerial applications of the organophosphate insecticide temephos to breeding sites using helicopters. Results have been good but reinvasion is a problem since *Simulium damnosum* can fly up to 300 km from its breeding sites.

S. neavei has been entirely eradicated from Kenya by larvicidal treatments, except for a small focus on the Uganda border. Transmission has been completely interrupted and no new cases of onchocerciasis have been reported in any of the districts since the elimination of the vector.

Control of the vector species of Simuliidae in the Americas is confined to Mexico where larvicidal control on a yearly basis has produced a marked reduction in the density of the adult vector population.

Where control has been achieved the results can be amazing. *Simulium* control along the Victoria Nile in 1952 was followed by a spectacular uncapitalized development and previously untenable land was transformed into a major producing area of food and cash crops.

Mass nodulectomy

This has been conducted thoroughly and efficiently in Mexico and Guatemala for the past 30 years and it has greatly reduced the incidence of severe ocular complications. However, patients from whom all palpable tumours have been removed still harbour large numbers of microfilariae which have given rise to heavy infections in *Simulium* fed on them. Still, as a means of preventing blindness, it has a lot to recommend itself.

Personal prophylaxis

A weekly dose of 100–200 mg of DEC will not necessarily prevent infection but will prevent a heavy infection developing. If infection occurs a full course of treatment can be given on leaving the endemic area.

ZOONOTIC ONCHOCERCIASIS

Two species of *Onchocerca*, *O. gutturosa* worldwide and *O. dukei* in Africa commonly infect bovids. *O. gutturosa* infection of man has been reported from Manitoba and Saskatchewan,[114] Illinois[115] and the Crimea.[116] All these cases presented as fibrous nodules on the wrist containing adult worms. No microfilariae were demonstrated.

Loiasis (filariasis caused by *Loa loa*)

GEOGRAPHICAL DISTRIBUTION

Human loiasis is confined to the rain forest and swamp forest areas of West Africa and central Africa from 8° north to 5° south of the equator from the Gulf of Guinea eastwards to the Great Lakes. It is especially common in Cameroon and on the Ogowe river. Its distribution includes the coastal plain and follows the course of the Congo river and its tributaries to a point about 1500 miles from the mouth (Fig. 20.27). It is also found in the southern Sudan between the Bahr al-Ghazal and Congo rivers between latitudes 4° and 6° north and longitudes 27° and 31° east. More recently *Loa loa* has been found to be the cause of 'Kampala eye worm' in Uganda, where the simian parasite may be responsible[117] and Ethiopia.[118]

AETIOLOGY

Loiasis is caused by *Loa loa*, a filarial worm which lives in the connective tissues of man. The adult *Loa loa* is a semitransparent filiform and cylindrical worm, the male measuring 3–3.4 cm × 0.35–0.43 mm, and the female 5.7 cm × 0.5 mm (see Figs. II.80, II.81 and II.82, p. 1376). The microfilaria is sheathed and similar in size (298 × 7.5 μm) and structure to mf bancrofti from which it may be impossible to distinguish in fresh blood. In stained films, however, it assumes a stiff angular attitude, the nuclei of the central column of cells are larger and less deeply stained, and the cephalic end of the column more abruptly terminated (Figs. 20.28 and II.73,4 and 5, p. 1371). The sheath does not stain with Giemsa.

By special staining methods a large genital cell at the beginning of the posterior third is a marked feature. Mf loa takes up 1/5000 methylene blue in 10 minutes, more rapidly than mf bancrofti. *Loa loa* in man is adapted to a day-biting *Chrysops* fly and is diurnally periodic. Microfilariae appear in the blood between the hours of 08.00 and 20.00. This periodicity is not easy to change but changes gradually when a patient moves round the world (see also Appendix II, p. 1377). Human *Loa loa* must be distinguished from simian *Loa loa* which is adapted to night-biting *Chrysops* and is nocturnally periodic.

Life-cycle

The adult worm lives in the subcutaneous tissues travelling round the body, where it may be seen crossing the conjunctiva of the eye (Fig. 20.29

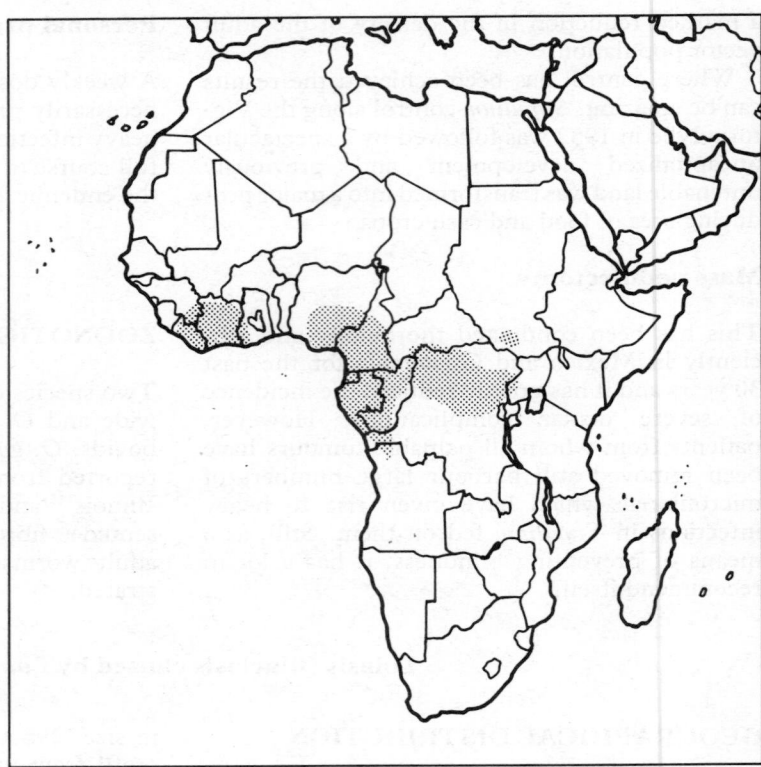

Fig. 20.27 Geographical distribution of *Loa loa*. (Courtesy Department of Entomology, London School of Hygiene and Tropical Medicine.)

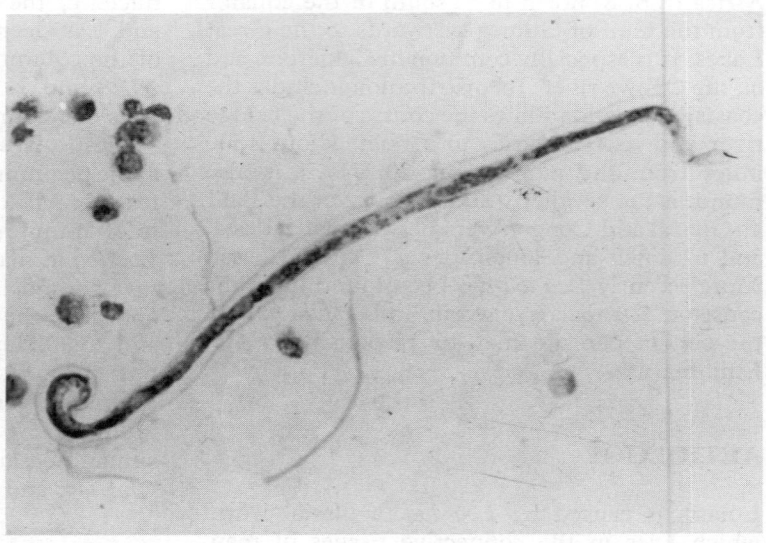

Fig. 20.28 Mf *Loa loa*, more than 250 μm long, sheath loosely applied.

and Plate VI.3) or appear under the skin (Fig. 20.30). Microfilariae appear in the blood during the day where they are taken up by day-biting *Chrysops* and develop in the thoracic muscles and fat body of the *Chrysops* in 10 days to appear at the root of the proboscis, the sheath of which they pierce and emerge on the skin of the human host from which they disappear

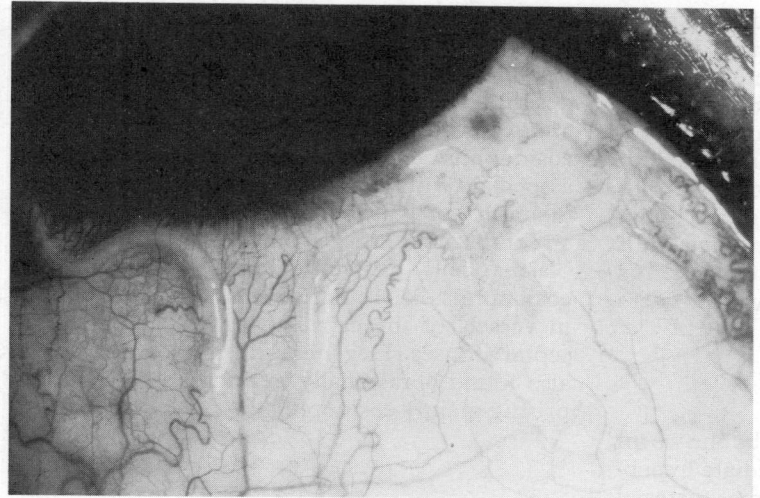

Fig. 20.29   Adult *Loa loa* beneath the conjunctiva. (Courtesy Dr J. Anderson.)

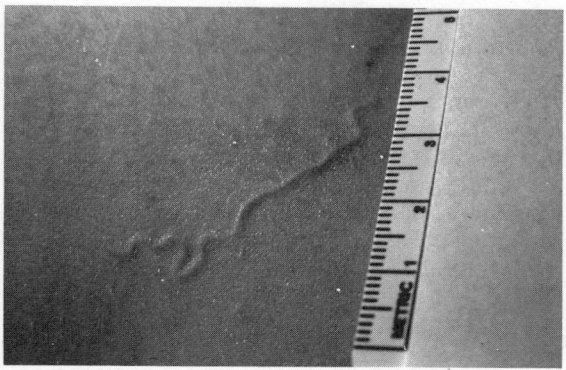

Fig. 20.30   Adult *Loa loa* under the skin. (Courtesy Dr P.G.P. Manson-Bahr.)

rapidly by burrowing into the skin, where they migrate along the fascial planes. (For morphology and development of *Loa loa* and mf *Loa loa*, see Appendix II, Fig. II.83, p. 1377.)

TRANSMISSION

Human *Loa loa* is transmitted by day-biting *Chrysops* flies of the forest canopy, *C. silacea* and *C. dimidiata*. In the southern Sudan and East Africa *C. distinctipennis* and *C. longicornis* are the vectors and *C. zahrai* in the Cameroon highlands (Fig. III.49, p. 1444).[119]

In Ethiopia the vector is *C. streptobalius*.[118] A larger simian parasite (*Loa loa papionis*) occurs in mandrills, has a nocturnal periodicity and is transmitted by night-biting tree-top *Chrysops*— *C. langi* and *C. centurionis*.[119] Simian *Loa loa*

may be transmitted to man in Uganda where human *Loa loa* infections are light and cause a conjunctival granuloma, known as the Owen–Hennessey granuloma or 'Bung eye' (see Chapter 70, ocular loiasis). (For morphology and bionomics of *Chrysops*, see Appendix III, p. 1439, and Fig. III.47, p. 1439.)

PATHOLOGY

After the larva has entered the human body through the bite of a *Chrysops*, development is slow and maturity is not attained until a year or longer, although in monkeys it is about four months. The parasite lives and moves around in the fascial layers from which the microfilariae are liberated, travelling up the lymphatics to the bloodstream where they lodge in the lungs. Many patients with classical symptoms have no microfilariae in the blood, presumably due to the failure of the male and female worms to find each other. It is impossible to estimate the number of adult worms present in any given infection and whereas one particular *Loa* may show itself about the eye or elsewhere it is only one of many.

During the period of growth and development in man *Loa loa* makes frequent excursions through the subdermal connective tissues. It has been noticed very often beneath the skin of the fingers and it has been excised from under the skin of the back, from above the sternum, the left breast, the lingual fraenum, the loose skin of the penis, the eyelids, the conjunctiva, the anterior chamber of the eye and the scalp.

The parts most frequently mentioned are the

eyes and, although the worm may attract more attention in this situation, it does seem as though it has a decided predilection for the eye and its neighbourhood. A patient of Manson's once stated that the average rate at which a *Loa* travelled was about 2.5 cm in two minutes. Both Manson and others have observed that warmth seems to attract them to the surface of the body. Chesterman in Zaire reported finding live adult worms in 10% of all cases operated on for hernia and elephantiasis, while cretified worms were frequently encountered.

Calabar swellings

Calabar swellings, which are caused by the worm in its wanderings, are a type I immediate hypersensitivity reaction to the antigenic material released by the developing or adult worm. Recurrent swellings on the arm or leg (Fig. 20.31) may

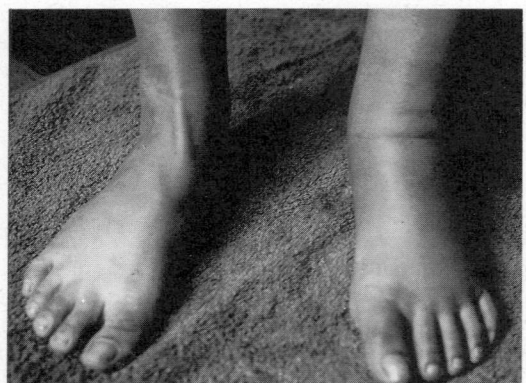

Fig. 20.31 Calabar swelling of the left foot.

cause permanent induration of the fascia and connective tissues round the tendon sheaths forming cyst-like swellings resembling ganglia which cause pain on movement. Dying worms under the skin may cause a chronic abscess followed by a granulomatous reaction and fibrosis. In one patient who had manifested these swellings over a period of seven years all adult filariae appeared to die out at the same time and were discharged in a calcified state from minute chronic abscesses, which appeared on the hands, arms and legs.

Whether alive or dead this worm evokes a high eosinophilia of 30–40% and an eosinophilia is common in expatriates who have resided in endemic areas in Nigeria, Zaire and Cameroon.

Lymphadenopathy

Changes in the lymph glands have been described in patients with loiasis. These changes are expansion of the sinuses by histiocytes and eosinophils and atrophy of lymphoid follicles associated with fibrosis of capsule and trabeculae, dilatation of lymphatic vessels in both capsule and trabeculae, and a prominent infiltration with plasma cells, Russell bodies, mast cells and eosinophils. Microfilariae of *Loa loa* were located in vessels of the capsule, trabeculae and periseptal sinuses. Degenerating microfilariae were also found occasionally in microabscesses comprising mainly eosinophils.[120]

IMMUNITY

An immunity develops in the inhabitants of endemic areas since active immature worms are often seen in children but seldom in adults, while microfilaraemia is found chiefly in adults. The mechanism of this immunity is not understood and adult worms can be very numerous in the inhabitants of endemic areas where they are well tolerated.

The numbers of microfilariae appear to be controlled by a humoral immune response and high antimicrofilarial antibody titres are a feature of loiasis, very high titres being found in the absence of microfilariae from the blood. In patients with a high microfilaraemia a suppression of the immune response exists allowing a high number to circulate.[121] Patients with numerous adult worms and high microfilaraemia do not appear to suffer ill-effects but can react very severely to DEC. A type I (reaginic) hypersensitivity response is responsible for the calabar swellings and it is noteworthy that patients with a large number of adult worms do not suffer from calabar swellings but only from the migrating adults which they often do not notice unless they cross the eye.

CLINICAL FEATURES

Natural history

The adult worms are very slow to mature (one year or more) and are long-lived, up to 17 years, and so can continue to cause symptoms many years after leaving the endemic area. They are usually harmless causing occasional calabar swellings and appearances under the conjunctiva of the eye, becoming calcified when they die.

Incubation period

Owing to the long period of immaturity and the delay in the appearance of microfilariae in the blood (up to seven years), the incubation period between infection and the appearance of symptoms may be very long. In some cases calabar swellings appear between one and two years after entering or visiting the endemic area but in many cases the parasite does not show itself until three or four years have elapsed. In one case an adult was extracted from the eye 17 years after the host had left Africa.

Symptoms and signs

Expatriates of any race are more troubled than the indigenous inhabitants who show a considerable tolerance to the presence of many worms. The migration of the adult worm usually causes no symptoms, being noticed in a mirror when it appears under the conjunctiva of the eye (Fig. 20.29 and Plate VI.3) or under the skin (Fig. 20.30) where it may pass unnoticed, appearing and disappearing within 10–15 minutes, leaving no trace behind. In the eye, however, there may be pain associated with swelling and tumefaction (Fig. 70.12, p. 1166) of the eyelids. Should a *Loa loa* wander into the area of the glottis or urethra the consequences are serious and great pain may be caused. The death of an adult worm may cause a localized abscess in the groin or axilla or a calcified worm may appear on X-ray. The immature and adult worms often cause transient oedematous swellings, called calabar swellings.

Calabar swellings

The swellings are about 10 cm in diameter or more, painless, though somewhat hot both objectively and subjectively, not pitting on pressure and usually disappearing in about 3 days. They come suddenly and disappear gradually and occur in any part of the body. They may irritate slightly but the skin maintains its normal colour. One swelling occurs at a time but recurs at irregular intervals and perhaps for years after

the patient has left the endemic area. In some instances the swellings seem to be due to rubbing provoked by the irritation of a *Loa* just under the skin (Fig. 20.30). In the hand or forearm they may give rise to a sense of powerlessness or soreness as if the part had received a blow. They never suppurate. The effects of temperature upon these swellings is important. During the hot summer months they are frequent but in the cold weather distinctly uncommon. For ocular loiasis, see Chapter 70 (p. 1166).

Unusual manifestations

CEREBRAL MANIFESTATIONS
Loa loa is the most frequent filarial invader of the central nervous system. Kivits[122] and Toussaint and Davis[123] have described cases of meningoencephalitis with choroidoretinitis and microfilariae in the cerebrospinal fluid. Browne[124] described transient hemiparesis in a woman in Zaire who had been infected for 25 years. Schofield[125] has described peripheral nerve involvement.

Another form of severe cerebral complication follows treatment with DEC of heavily infected cases of loiasis with numerous microfilariae in the blood.[126]

LYMPHOEDEMA
Solid oedema of one leg persisting for six weeks has been observed in a European from West Africa who had been affected for a number of years and hydroceles have also been reported. However, it is always difficult to exclude a double infection with *W. bancrofti*.

ARTHRITIS
Acute arthritis with effusion (many microfilariae of *Loa loa* were in the joint fluid) of the left knee, followed by the left ankle and right knee, has been reported in a heavy *Loa loa* infection.[127] X-ray examination showed calcified *Loa loa* adults in the periarticular soft tissues; all symptoms cleared following diethylcarbamazine treatment and an anti-inflammatory drug.

Other manifestations

Urticaria and dermatitis with pruritus are sometimes found in *Loa* cases. However, double infections with *O. volvulus* are difficult to exclude. Multiple intramuscular abscesses and even infections of the hip joint have been recorded.

An adult worm in the wall of the bowel has caused intestinal obstruction[128] and glomerulonephritis has been described,[129] possibly from obstruction of the small vessels of the kidney by microfilariae.

DIFFERENTIAL DIAGNOSIS

Calabar swellings. These may resemble the transient swellings produced by other migrating parasites, *Gnathostoma* and myiasis, in which the reactions are more severe, the reaction being more intense and lasting longer. In myiasis the maggots do not migrate.

Skin manifestations. Other helminths may migrate under the skin in the larval stage. Subcutaneous *Loa loa* causes little or no reaction, is usually single and only appears transiently for a few minutes. *Strongyloides* (larva currens) moves slowly, causes a marked reaction with intense irritation and multiple tracks which lasts 10 hours. Hookworm (cutaneous larva migrans) hardly moves, causes one or more lesions with an intense pruritic reaction and swelling and lasts for many weeks. Guinea-worm is a much larger worm and can be palpated under the skin. In the eye *Loa loa* is subconjunctival and much larger than *Toxocara* which may appear in the anterior chamber.

DIAGNOSIS

Microfilaraemia

Microfilariae are found in the blood more commonly in adults than children. They are absent in early (up to seven years after infection) and single sex infections. The sheathed microfilariae (Figs. 20.28 and II.73,5, p. 1370) can be demonstrated in the blood between 10.00 and 14.00 hours either in a thick drop of 20 ml or by one of the concentration methods described in Appendix IV (p. 1494). The DEC provocation test is of little use. In old thick drop preparations *Loa loa* and *B. malayi* have a shrunken appearance while other microfilariae do not. This is due to the greater permeability of the cuticle in the former which permits faster drying and more

rapid staining. *W. bancrofti* becomes shorter and its width identifies it. Other microfilariae do not shrink in the same manner.

Eosinophilia

Eosinophilia is present in high degree in all cases of recent infection. A symptomless eosinophilia in an expatriate from West Africa may be due to loiasis as well as onchocerciasis or a *Mansonella perstans* infection.

Immunodiagnosis

There is no specific test of *Loa loa* as all filarial infections are cross reactive. Humoral antibodies are almost always present in high titres and can be demonstrated by the CFT, indirect fluorescent antibody test (IFAT) or ELISA.

CFT

The CFT is positive in 85% of loiasis[35] and becomes positive one to three years after infection reverting to negative after seven years.

IFAT

The filarial FAT is the test of choice and is positive in high titres especially in the absence of microfilaraemia.

ELISA

The ELISA test will probably be the test of choice since it may become species specific.

TREATMENT

Diethylcarbamazine

Diethylcarbamazine rapidly immobilizes the microfilariae which are destroyed in the liver.[130] It also unmasks the adult parasites which are recognized as foreign and destroyed by the body's own defences. The developing worms are most susceptible and the older ones less so.

The dose is 2–3 mg/kg body weight three times daily up to 600 mg daily for 21 days. The results are excellent and the macrofilarial drugs used in other forms of filariasis are not necessary.

During treatment there is often fever, malaise, swelling of joints, joint pains and pruritus. If there is a heavy infection with microfilariae—1000/20 mm³ or more—there is a great risk of encephalitis, which may be due to toxic material from the worms killed by treatment or to 'clumping' of microfilariae in the small blood vessels. Severe headache is a sign of this complication and purpura has been seen. The treatment of these heavy infections is difficult because of severe reactions. Treatment with DEC may start with very small doses but even these may be unacceptable. Brumpt[131] suggested exchange transfusion but apheresis (repeated removal of the buffy coat with the microfilariae) and return of the blood to the patient followed by DEC has been successful.[132]

Care must be taken also where patients with loiasis are also infected with *O. volvulus* and who are liable to develop severe skin reactions. Steroid and antihistaminic drugs are of little value in dealing with reactions during treatment of *Loa loa* infections. Adult worms should not be removed surgically from the eye since they are so easily killed with DEC.

Mebendazole

Low dose mebendazole has been used as a treatment for loiasis; 100 mg three times daily for 45 days has been shown to cause a slow drop in the microfilariae count avoiding Mazzotti type reactions.[133]

EPIDEMIOLOGY (see Appendix III, Fig. III.49, p. 1444)

Man is the only host of human *Loa loa*. Although it can be transplanted to monkeys and infect them, and even hybrids of human and simian *Loa* bred,[134] it is unlikely that natural transmission to monkeys occurs since day-biting *Chrysops* do not feed on them and night-biting *Chrysops* would not transmit the diurnal human form, but it is possible that in Uganda, where *Loa loa* infections are very light, the simian parasite is involved.

The main vectors which maintain the infection in man in nature are female *Chrysops silacea* and *C. dimidiata*. These live in the forest canopy and are attracted down mainly by dark colours and woodsmoke.[135] They need the forest canopy to rest on and lay eggs in wet mud in swamps and river edges below the forest trees. Transmission takes place during the long wet season (April to December) by *C. silacea*, although *C. dimidiata* is absent during the heavy rains (June to October). At certain seasons the risk of transmission is great and at others negligible. In the Bahr al-Ghazal some transmission is maintained on the edge of the forest zone into the edge of the savannah by *C. distinctipennis* and *C. longicornis* which are vectors of only secondary importance. To a less extent in the Cameroon highlands grassland area *C. zahrai* can transmit naturally.[119] The only feasible vector in Ethiopia is *C. streptobalius*.[118]

Houses built on hills at the level of the forest canopy and buildings in plantations which provide cover for flies from the forest are particularly places where human infections are acquired.[119]

CONTROL

Environmental control

Houses and camps should be sited away from the forest edge and swamps. Light-coloured clothing should be worn and smoke prevented.

Vector control

Control of *Chrysops* has not been achieved to any degree. The larvae can be destroyed in the mud in which they live with suspensions of dieldrin and a whole year's crop may be destroyed at any one time since they need several months for development. However, this method has not proved practical at the present time.

Personal prophylaxis

Individuals may avoid being bitten by wearing light-coloured clothing and the frequent application of an insect repellent will reduce the risk of bites.

Chemoprophylaxis

Duke[136] has shown that in monkeys DEC may act as a prophylactic by killing young immature worms. The effective dose in man is 5 mg/kg daily for 3 days each month. A course of radical treatment should precede this procedure.

Mansonella (Dipetalonema) streptocerca

GEOGRAPHICAL DISTRIBUTION
(Fig. 20.32)

Originally described from Ghana, *M. strep-tocerca* is found in West Africa especially in Ghana and Zaire.

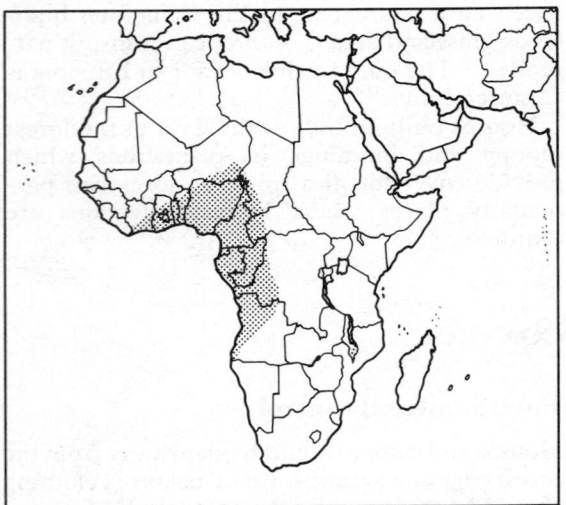

Fig. 20.32 Geographical distribution of *M. streptocerca*. (Courtesy Department of Entomology, London School of Hygiene and Tropical Medicine.)

AETIOLOGY

Adult streptocercae are thin sinuous worms, the male 17×0.05 mm, and the female 27×0.075 mm. They inhabit the dermis of the upper thorax and shoulders. The microfilariae, $180–240\,\mu$m $\times 2.5–5.0\,\mu$m in size, are unsheathed and also inhabit the dermis. They have a characteristic pattern of nuclei posterior to the clear cephalic space with four oval nuclei followed by seven to 10 smaller, more rounded, nuclei and an oval round terminal nucleus in a characteristic curved posterior portion of the worm producing the 'walking stick handle' or 'shepherd's crook' tail. These features distinguish them from mf volvulus and mf perstans (Figs. 20.33, II.73,8, p. 1371, and II.79, p. 1375).

TRANSMISSION

M. streptocerca is transmitted by a midge, *Culicoides grahami* (see Appendix III).

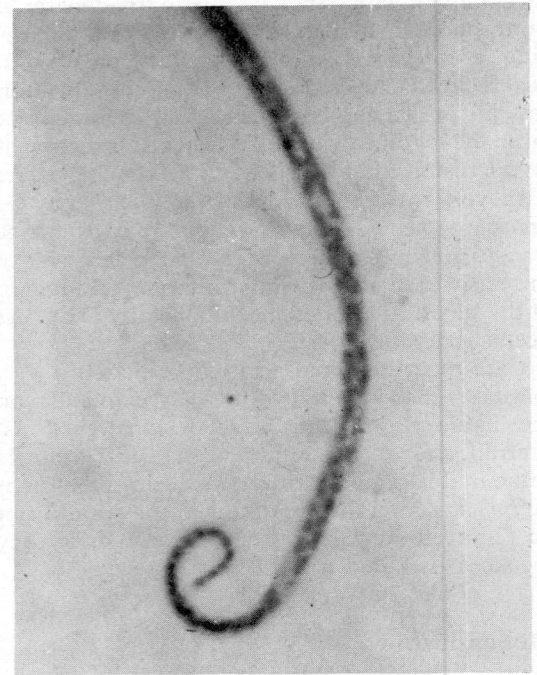

Fig. 20.33 Mf *M. streptocerca*, less than $250\,\mu$m long, tail bent into a crook shape.

PATHOLOGY

In many cases no pathology is caused but reaction against dead adult worms and microfilariae produces similar changes to those found in onchocerciasis but less severe. The eye is not affected. Papules form around dead adult worms and obstructive lymphadenitis with a reaction around a dead adult worm composed of an immune complex of IgE and filarial antigen has been seen.[137]

IMMUNITY

There is little or no reaction against live worms but, following DEC treatment, reactions are similar to those found in onchocerciasis.

CLINICAL FEATURES

The incubation period is three to four months. Those persons with symptoms have an itching dermatitis most marked over the thorax and shoulders. The skin is thickened and there are hypopigmented macules. The axillary lymph glands are enlarged.

DIFFERENTIAL DIAGNOSIS

Diagnosis must be made from onchocerciasis and leprosy. The unsheathed microfilariae of *M. streptocerca* can be found in skin snips. They are not so mobile as those of *O. volvulus* and when stained assume the characteristic 'walking stick handle' shape (Figs. 20.33 and II.79, p. 1375).

The Mazzotti reaction is positive and since DEC kills the adult worms around which quite large papules form it can be distinguished from the reaction in onchocerciasis.

TREATMENT

DEC kills both microfilariae and adults and is given in the same dosage as for onchocerciasis for 3 weeks. Since both adult worms and microfilariae are killed the chances of a cure are excellent and not nearly so difficult to achieve as in onchocerciasis.

EPIDEMIOLOGY

Similar microfilariae are found in the skin of chimpanzees but whether *M. streptocerca* is a zoonosis has not been established. In some parts of the endemic area up to 90% of the inhabitants are infected.

Dracunculiasis (guinea-worm)

GEOGRAPHICAL DISTRIBUTION

Old world

Dracunculus medinensis is a natural infection of the dog, horse, cow, wolf, leopard, polecat, monkey and baboon. In man the current distribution includes much of West Africa, parts of East Africa and western India (Fig. 20.34). A few relatively small foci are reported to exist in the Punjab area of Pakistan and in Iran, Saudi Arabia, Yemen and possibly Iraq. In the past there were foci in Eritrea, Republic of Guinea and north-western Liberia. Recently a small focus has been found in northern Kenya.

New World

In North America *D. medinensis* is a natural infection of the fox, silver fox, raccoon, mink and

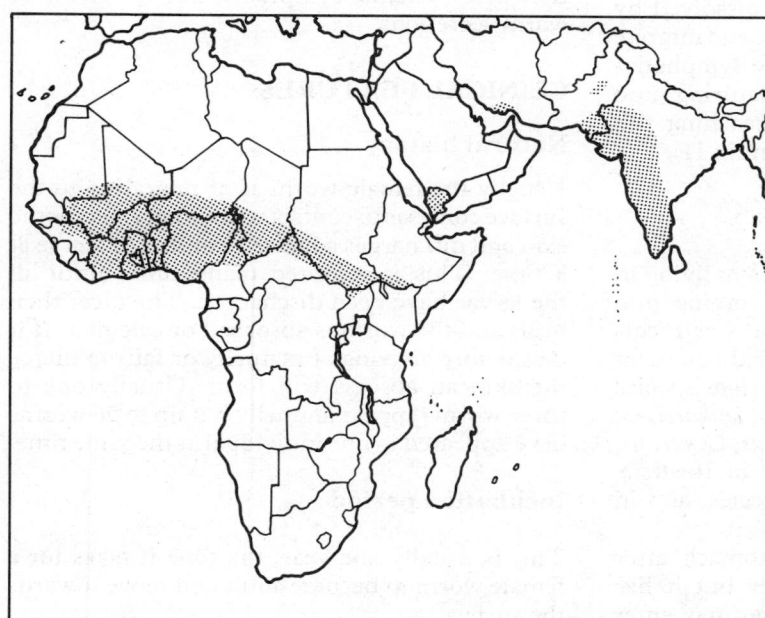

Fig. 20.34 Geographical distribution of *Dracunculus medinensis* (guinea-worm). (Courtesy Department of Entomology, London School of Hygiene and Tropical Medicine.)

dog. In man it was formerly said to occur in a limited part of Brazil, Curaçao, Demerara and Surinam. Calcified worms have been seen on X-ray in indigenous North Americans,[138] probably of zoonotic origin.

AETIOLOGY AND LIFE-CYCLE
(Fig. II.88, p. 1379)

The guinea-worm (*Dracunculus medinensis*) has an adult stage in the human host and a larval stage in *Cyclops*, a crustacean which lives in fresh water. The female *D. medinensis* is a large worm up to 60 cm in length which lives in the connective tissues (Figs. II.84 and II.85, p. 1378). The male is small, 1.2–2.9 cm long, which dies after copulation and is absorbed by the female. When the double uterus is full of embryos (Fig. II.86, p. 1378) the female worm is drawn towards those parts of the body in contact with water and 90% migrate to the legs and feet especially behind the outer malleolus where it penetrates the skin and extrudes the uterus through the head, and discharges the larvae into the water (Figs. 20.35 and 20.36). The larvae, which measure 500–750 μm (Fig. II.87, p. 1379), can live for 6 days in clean and two to three weeks in muddy water, are swallowed by a *Cyclops* which actively chases them. In the body of the *Cyclops* they undergo two moults and reach the infective stage in 14 days (Fig. II.89, p. 1380). When the *Cyclops* is swallowed by man it is dissolved by the gastric juice and the larvae escape and migrate to the subcutaneous tissues via the lymphatics which they reach in 43 days, maturing into worms in three to four months, reaching full development in one year (see Appendix II).

TRANSMISSION

The infection is transmitted by *Cyclops* living in fresh water which is infected by coming into contact with infected persons via small collections of water or step-wells in arid countries used for drinking and washing. *Cyclops* species involved are *Cyclops quadricornis*, *C. leukarti*, *C. hyalinus* and allied species *C. strenuus*, *C. viridis*, *C. coronatus*, *C. bicuspidatus* and, in the true tropics, *C. multicolor* and other species, and in Nigeria *C. nigerianus*.

Normally infection is via the stomach after ingestion of *Cyclops* infected water but it has been suggested that infected *Cyclops* may enter the vagina and be destroyed by the acidity, releasing larvae which make their way to the retroplacental region in pregnant women.[139]

PATHOLOGY

The female guinea-worm lives in the connective tissue of the limbs and trunk where she causes no harm until approaching maturity. When mature she migrates downwards to the lower limbs in the vast majority of cases, on the dorsum or sole of the foot (Fig. 20.35), occasionally the scrotum but rarely the arms or back except in water carriers where the back may be a characteristic site, and the head or the eye where it can cause loss of the eye. The main pathological effects are caused by death of the worm which causes a sterile abscess, which when secondarily infected results in cellulitis, but chills, fever and local painful swellings commonly precede the emergence of the worm. Guinea-worms have been found coiled in a hernial sac and retroplacentally causing bleeding in pregnancy.

IMMUNITY

There is no acquired immunity, reinfection is common, one or two worms usually appearing every year. Dead worms often elicit an acute inflammatory reaction with suppuration and often a type I immediate hypersensitivity reaction with systemic symptoms, due to release of worm secretions.

CLINICAL FEATURES

Natural history

Usually the female worm after migrating to the surface comes into contact with water, pierces the skin and discharges a limited number of larvae at a time. This is repeated many times until all the larvae have been discharged. The ulcer then heals and the worm is absorbed or calcified. If it dies before arriving at maturity or fails to pierce the skin an abscess will form. Usually one to three worms appear annually but up to 56 worms have appeared in one individual at the same time.

Incubation period

This is usually one year, the time it takes for a female worm to become adult and move towards the surface.

Symptoms and signs

Guinea-worm ulcer

The first sign is when the worm pierces the skin. There is a burning sensation so that the affected individual wishes to bathe his leg in water. The dermis becomes elevated and a blister develops (Fig. 20.35). If the limb is placed in water the

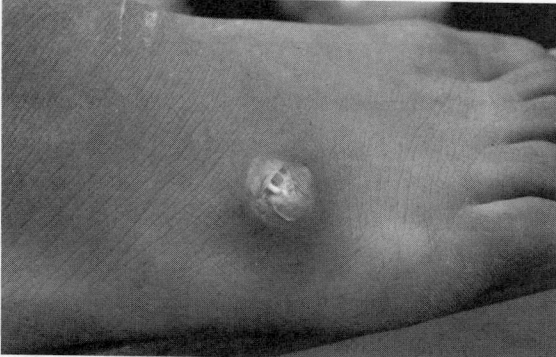

Fig. 20.35 A guinea-worm blister.

blister ruptures to reveal a small superficial erosion 1.25–1.8 cm in diameter. At the centre of the erosion is a small hole from which the head of the worm may be seen protruding which, if covered with water, projects a clear tube—the uterus—about 1 mm in diameter which fills with an opaque fluid which discharges into the water (Fig. 20.36). Examination of the fluid under low power reveals many *Dracunculus* larvae coiled up which straighten out and then move jerkily about. If the cold water is reapplied after about an hour the process will be repeated until the uterus has been exhausted. Provided there is no

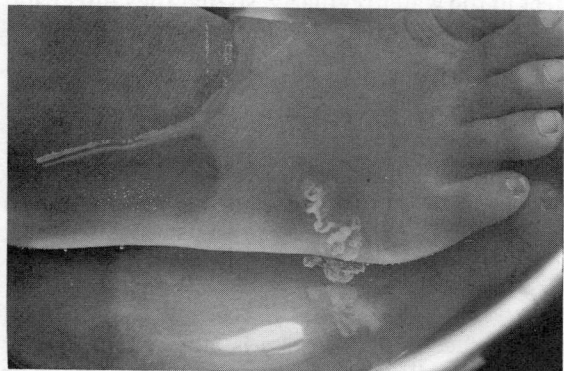

Fig. 20.36 A guinea-worm discharging larvae into water.

secondary infection the ulcer heals spontaneously and no scar is left.

General symptoms

General symptoms may appear at the beginning when the blister forms; urticaria, nausea, vomiting, asthma, giddiness and fainting. These symptoms may be due to an anaphylactic type I immediate hypersensitivity reaction to the secretions (toxins) of the guinea-worm.

Complications

Abscess formation

Sterile subcutaneous abscess may be due to a premature death of the female worm or attempts to remove the worm manually which then breaks and discharges into the subcutaneous tissues. The abscess forms a deep-seated fluctuant swelling not communicating with the exterior except in the case of manual removal. Should this become secondarily infected then a spreading cellulitis may develop, often involving the whole limb.

Arthritis and synovitis

Joints and tendons may become involved with the spread of cellulitis. The joints mainly involved are the knee, ankle and the Achilles and hamstring tendons. Joint effusions may be serous or purulent but bony ankylosis is rare. The Achilles and hamstring tendons frequently become contracted.

Abdominal pain

Another site for appearance of the adult worm is the peritoneal cavity with abdominal pain.

Guinea-worm can be an extremely disabling disease which seriously affects the production of farmers at an important stage of agriculture.

Laboratory findings

There is a peripheral eosinophilia.

DIAGNOSIS

Examination of the ulcer and the application of cold water makes the diagnosis. If the worm cannot be seen it may be palpated under the skin. Dead calcified worms are easily seen on radiological examination.

Serology

Although antibodies are produced which can be demonstrated by immunofluorescence, serology is of no practical use.

Intradermal test

An immediate hypersensitivity intradermal test using ether extracted dried adult worm is available producing a positive wheal 2–3 cm in diameter after intradermal injection of 0.25 ml, but again is of little clinical use.

TREATMENT

The rapid removal of the worm cannot be achieved without chemotherapeutic help; otherwise it ruptures on attempts to remove it with disastrous results, abscess formation and cellulitis.

Traditional methods (Fig. 20.37)

This uses a slow method of extraction. The protruding part of the worm is attached to a matchstick which is twisted a small amount each day until the worm has been removed.

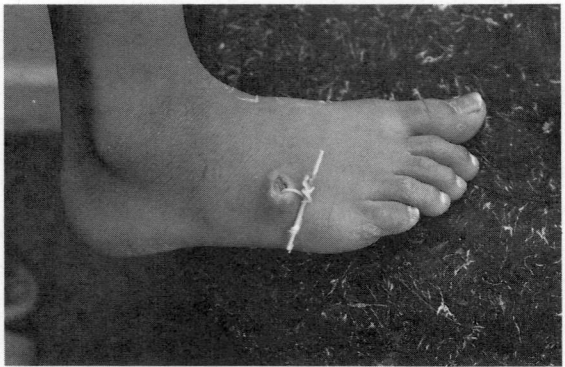

Fig. 20.37   The traditional method of removal of guinea-worms.

Chemotherapy

Chemotherapy acts by reducing the inflammation and allowing the worm to extrude naturally or allow itself to be removed easily without rupture. Three drugs have been used, all with the same result:[140]

> *niridazole*, 25 mg/kg daily for 10 days;
> *metronidazole*, 400 mg daily for 10–20 days or 30–40 mg/kg, three times daily for 3 days;
> *thiabendazole*, 50 mg/kg daily in two divided doses for 3 days.

Mebendazole has not been so successful.

The worms may be extruded naturally or extracted manually within one to two weeks. Fresh worms can emerge after treatment has been started since chemotherapy does not kill immature worms.

EPIDEMIOLOGY

Although guinea-worm is mainly a human infection it is not usually regarded as a zoonosis, but in America it has been found in the silver fox (*Vulpes fulva*), the raccoon (*Procyon lotor*) and the mink (*Mustela vision*), and in Africa and Asia it is widespread among carnivora.

The incidence of guinea-worm is associated with contact with small sources of water in pools and wells in semi-arid countries. In the Sahel in some areas over half the adult farmers are incapacitated during the peak season of agricultural work, because of the emergence of worms, and since the incubation period is one year, regular annual infections are contracted during the brief wet season when scant sources of surface water are available. In wetter areas transmission occurs towards the end of the dry season when water supplies are limited to a few stagnant pools. In India guinea-worm infection is associated with 'step-wells' which the inhabitants enter via a series of steps and immerse their feet in the water regularly, so that they infect and are infected regularly from the same source.

CONTROL

It would be quite possible to eradicate guinea-worm since improvement to the water supplies would remove the necessity to use surface water or wells. Much can be done in control.

Wells. All wells should have walls built around the surface so that access is stopped and water has to be collected by drawing up with a rope or pumped up.

Anticyclops measures. Cyclops can be removed from wells by means of an organophosphorus compound, temephos, administered in slow-release granules.[141] This is harmless to man.

Personal prophylaxis

Boiling or chlorination of drinking water will prevent infection as will sieving the water through tightly woven cloth. Two layers of ordinary shirting material are adequate.

3   SEROUS CAVITY FILARIASIS

Serous cavity filariasis is caused by two species of *Mansonella* (mansonelliasis): *Mansonella perstans* and *Mansonella ozzardi*.

Mansonella (Dipetalonema) perstans

GEOGRAPHICAL DISTRIBUTION
(Fig. 20.38)

M. perstans is widely distributed throughout central Africa in man and chimpanzee. In Zaire, Nigeria, Ghana, Sierra Leone, Ivory Coast, Zambia and Uganda a high proportion of the inhabitants in some areas are infected. It is also found in the New World, in Venezuela, Trinidad, Guyana, Surinam, northern Argentina and Amazonia.

AETIOLOGY

Adult worms are seldom seen since they live in

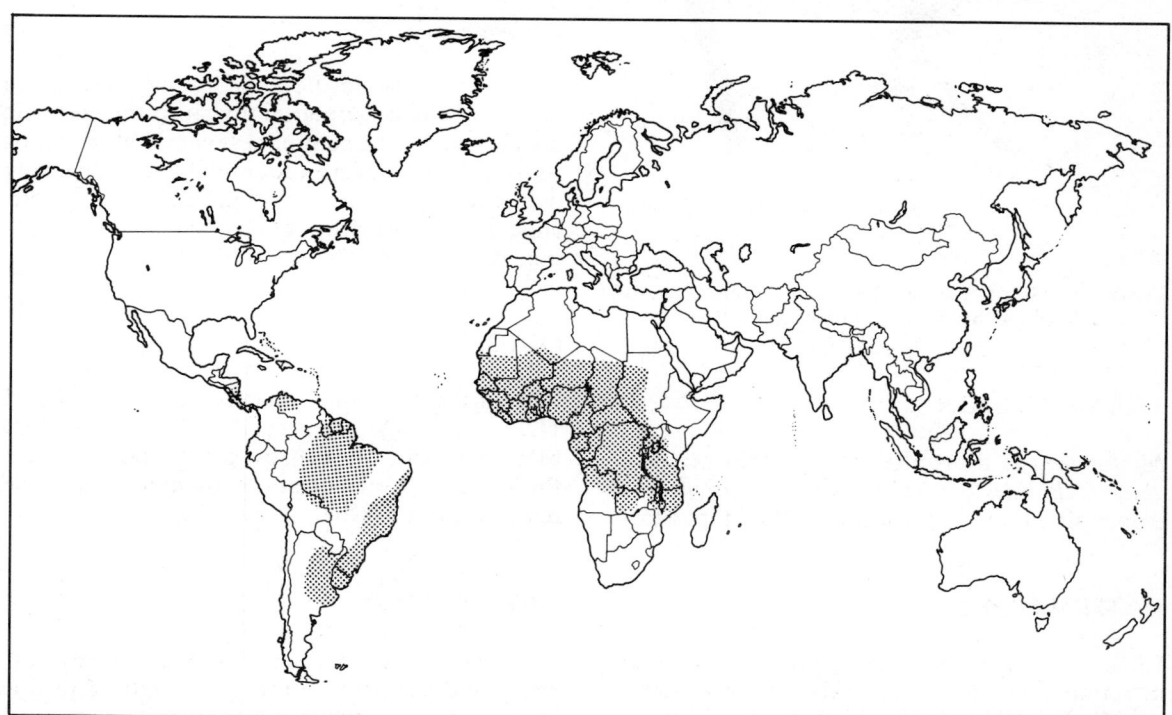

Fig. 20.38   Geographical distribution of *M. perstans*. (Courtesy Department of Entomology, London School of Hygiene and Tropical Medicine.)

serous cavities (pleural and peritoneal), mesentery, peri-renal space, retroperitoneal space and pericardium. Occasionally they have been found in subcutaneous cysts. They are cylindrical worms, the male (4–5 cm × 0.06 mm) is smaller than the female (7.8 cm × 0.12 mm). The microfilariae (200 × 4.5 μm) are unsheathed and possess the power of elongation and contraction so that they vary in measurements and forms (90–110 × 4 μm). Mf perstans is smaller than mf bancrofti and the caudal end is blunt with a terminal nucleus (Figs. 20.39, II.73,7, p. 1371, II.77 and II.78, p. 1375) which distinguishes it from mf ozzardi which has a sharp tail, and mf streptocerca which has a hooked tail. They are non-periodic and circulate in the blood in equal numbers by day and night and can survive in the circulation after transfusion for three years. They are frequently seen in the cerebrospinal fluid.

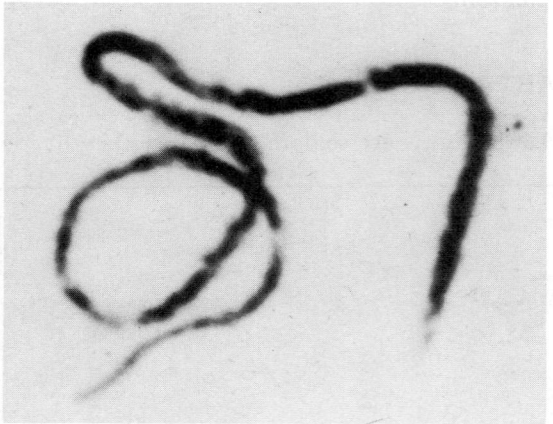

Fig. 20.39 Mf *M. perstans*, less than 250 μm long, tail straight with a prominent terminal nucleus.

TRANSMISSION

M. perstans is transmitted by midges *(Culicoides)*, *Culicoides grahami* and *C. austeni* (see Appendix III, p. 1435, and Fig. III.44, p. 1435).

PATHOLOGY

Little is known about the pathology since the infection is symptomless in the vast majority of infections. Pathological changes may be produced by an immune response in certain individuals: a symptomless eosinophilia, pleuritis,

abdominal pain, pruritus and transient skin swellings and a low IgE titre.[142]

IMMUNITY

In the majority of cases the parasite is well tolerated but, in the patient described by Almauina et al,[142] the side-effects after treatment were a type III hypersensitivity reaction and included circulating immune complexes, complement and alternative pathway activation.

CLINICAL FEATURES

The natural history of *M. perstans* is a symptomless infection persisting throughout the life of the host. In a few cases there may be a reaction and adult worms are killed. The incubation period is unknown.

Symptoms and signs

Symptoms are commoner in expatriate Europeans than in the indigenous people.

Eosinophilia

A symptomless eosinophilia found during the course of a check-up after a visit to the endemic area is usually the commonest sign. Other symptoms are quite severe abdominal pain, especially over the hepatic area,[143,144] pericarditis,[145] pleuritis, severe pruritus and subcutaneous swellings resembling calabar swellings.

DIAGNOSIS

The unsheathed microfilariae (Figs. 20.39 and II.73,7, p. 1371) are recovered easily from the blood and can be seen by direct staining on a thick film. Concentration methods may be necessary (Appendix IV, p. 1494).

TREATMENT

No treatment is necessary for symptomless carriers. In those with symptoms thought to be due to *M. perstans* treatment should be instituted with caution because of reactions. *Mebendazole* is the drug of choice, given orally, 100 mg twice daily for 30 days;[146] it may be combined with levamisole 300 mg daily for one week.[147]

EPIDEMIOLOGY

In Africa *M. perstans* is found commonly in chimpanzees and gorillas and is a zoonosis. It also occurs in other areas in the absence of the large apes and is a purely human infection in large areas of its range, and an infection rate of 50% is not uncommon. Little can be done in the way of control.

Mansonella ozzardi

GEOGRAPHICAL DISTRIBUTION
(Fig. 20.40)

Mansonella ozzardi is found in the New World in two main areas:

1 Mexico, Panama, Colombia, Venezuela, Surinam, French Guyana, Peru, Brazil, Bolivia and Argentina;

2 in the Caribbean, Puerto Rico, Antigua, Guadeloupe, Nevis, Dominica, Martinique, St Lucia, St Vincent, Trinidad, Turks Islands and Haiti.[4]

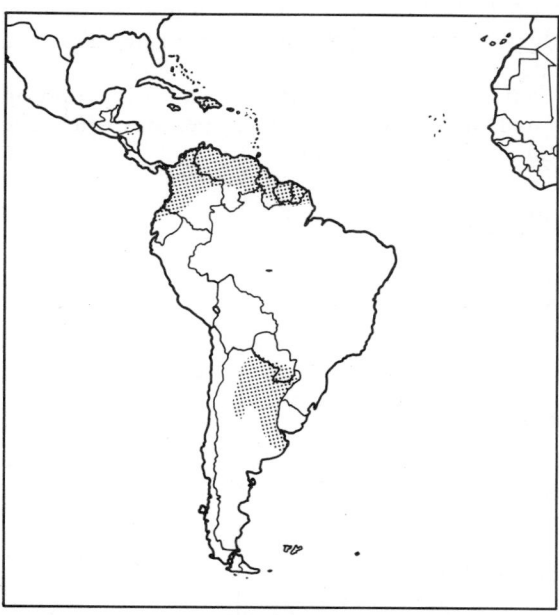

Fig. 20.40 Geographical distribution of *M. ozzardi*. (Courtesy Department of Entomology, London School of Hygiene and Tropical Medicine.)

AETIOLOGY

The male *M. ozzardi* is 24–28 mm long with a coiled tail and one spicule; the female is 32–51 mm × 0.13–0.16 mm and has a vulva 0.76 mm from the anterior extremity. They are seldom seen but have been found in the peritoneal cavity. The microfilariae, 207–232 × 3–4 μm, are unsheathed and closely resemble mf perstans but have a sharp tail (Figs. 20.41 and II.73,6, p.1371). They are non-periodic and since they can be found in the blood and the skin must be distinguished in South America from mf perstans and mf volvulus by the characteristic pointed tail. They can survive following transfusion of infected blood for over two years. Although there are two biological groups of *M. ozzardi* patterns of acid phosphatase[148] and ultrastructural studies[149] have shown no differences between the two.

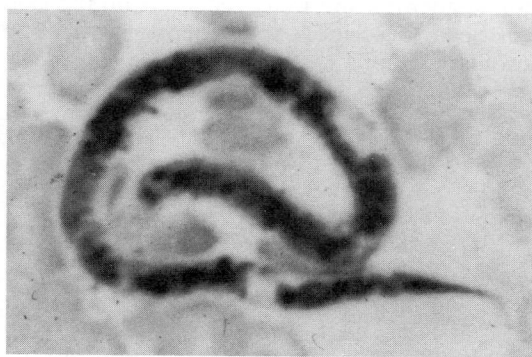

Fig. 20.41 Mf *M. ozzardi*, less than 250 μm long, nuclei not to tip of tail.

TRANSMISSION

M. ozzardi consists of two biological forms—one *Simulium* transmitted and the other *Culicoides* transmitted.

Simulium transmitted type is found on the South American mainland mainly in Amazonia where it is transmitted by black flies of the *Simulium amazonicum* group.[150]

Culicoides transmitted type is found in the Caribbean where it is transmitted by midges *Culicoides furens*[151] in St Vincent and Antigua, and possibly *C. paraensis* in St Vincent, and *C. phlebotomus* in Trinidad.[150] (See also Appendix III, p. 1436).

PATHOLOGY

Most infected people are completely symptomless and no pathology has been described.

IMMUNITY

Little is known about immunity but the prevalence increases with age suggesting that there is little acquired resistance. All races are susceptible.

CLINICAL FEATURES

Joint pains, headaches, coldness of the legs, inguinal adenitis and itchy red spots on the skin have been described in patients with high microfilaraemia.[152]

DIAGNOSIS

The unsheathed microfilariae (Figs. 20.41 and II.73,6, p. 1371) are found in the peripheral blood on direct examination. They can also be found in skin snips where they can be confused with *O. volvulus*.[153]

TREATMENT

There is no response to DEC. No drug is known to have activity.

EPIDEMIOLOGY

M. ozzardi is a human infection although it has been transmitted to a patas monkey.

Simulium transmitted M. ozzardi is found in villages along the banks of the Amazon but is less common along its tributaries. Prevalence rates can be very high, varying from 15.6% to 84.6%.[154] The infection is commoner in men than women and the microfilaria rate rises with age.

Culicoides transmitted M. ozzardi is found on small islands and occurs near beaches where the *Culicoides* abound.

4   OTHER SPECIES

Other species of filaria which may infect humans are *Dirofilaria species* (dirofilariasis) and *Meningonema peruzzi*.

Dirofilariasis

Dirofilariasis in man is caused by three different dirofilariae which are normally parasites of dogs, cats and wild canids. There are two types.

Pulmonary dirofilariasis caused by *Dirofilaria immitis*, a parasite of dogs.

Subcutaneous dirofilariasis caused by *Dirofilaria tenuis*, a parasite of the raccoon, and *Dirofilaria repens*, a parasite of dogs and cats.

PULMONARY DIROFILARIASIS[155]

Geographical distribution

Most pulmonary dirofilarial infections have been reported from the USA.[156–158]

Aetiology

The cause is *Dirofilaria immitis*, normally a parasite of the heart of dogs. The adult worm inhabits the right ventricle of the dog where it occurs in large coiled masses. Only immature *D. immitis* worms have been found in the lungs of man. They are 100–350 μm in diameter with a thick multilayered cuticle projecting inwards to form prominent internal longitudinal ridges. Microfilariae circulate in the blood of dogs but have not been found in man.

Transmission

Transmission is by mosquitoes: *Culex quinquefasciatus*, *C. annulirostris* and *Aedes aegypti*. In man the parasite develops only partially in the right ventricle of the heart before being swept into the pulmonary artery. Immature worms are usually found. Adult worms containing microfilariae have been found but never circulating microfilariae.

Pathology

The worm causes solitary pulmonary nodules limited to the periphery of the lungs. They show a central area of necrosis surrounded by a granulomatous zone. A single worm, usually necrotic but sometimes calcified, occupies the lumen of the artery.

Clinical features

Most patients are asymptomatic and 'coin lesions' are detected in the lungs on routine radiography. These nodules are well defined and are usually thought to be malignant. When present symptoms can include cough, haemoptysis and chest pain.

Diagnosis

Diagnosis can only be made by biopsy. There is no peripheral eosinophilia and serology is of no help.

Treatment

The only treatment is surgical excision.

SUBCUTANEOUS DIROFILARIASIS

Geographical distribution

Subcutaneous dirofilariasis has been found in the USA, Asia, Africa, Europe and South America.

Aetiology

D. tenuis normally lives in the subcutaneous tissues of the raccoon. *D. repens* lives in the subcutaneous tissues of dogs and cats. *D. tenuis* males are 40–48 mm × 190–260 μm and the females 80–130 mm × 190–260 μm. *D. repens* resembles *D. tenuis* but is greater in diameter. Microfilariae circulate in the blood of raccoons and dogs but not of man.

Transmission

Transmission is by mosquitoes.

Pathology

In man, an abnormal host, subcutaneous nodules are formed consisting of a coiled degenerating worm surrounded by granulomatous tissue containing epithelioid cells, giant cells, histiocytes and eosinophils.

Clinical features

Lesions occur in many parts of the body but most commonly in the conjunctiva (*D. repens*), scrotum, breast, arm and leg. The nodules are occasionally slowly migrating.

Diagnosis

Diagnosis is by biopsy. The worm can be distinguished from other dirofilariae by size and structure of the cuticle. There is no peripheral eosinophilia.

Treatment

Treatment is by surgical excision.

Meningonema peruzzi

Cases of encephalopathy with microfilariae in the cerebrospinal fluid have been described from Zimbabwe[159] which have been shown to be caused by *Meningonema peruzzi*, a filarial parasite which normally occupies the subarachnoid space of cercopithecus monkeys.[160] The microfilariae resemble those of *M. perstans* but have an inconspicuous sheath. Microfilariae of *O. volvulus* may also appear in the cerebrospinal fluid during treatment with DEC.

Treatment with DEC caused the microfilariae to disappear in these cases with relief of symptoms.

REFERENCES

1 Hawking, F. (1976) *Trop. Dis. Bull.* **73**, 937.
2 Hawking, F. (1976) *Trop. Dis. Bull.* **73**, 967.
3 Hawking, F. (1977) *Trop. Dis. Bull.* **74**, 649.
4 Hawking, F. (1979) *Trop. Dis. Bull.* **76**, 693.
5 Raghavan, N.G.S. (1958) *Bull. natn Soc. Mal. mosq. Dis.* **6**, 147–154.
6 Otteson, R.E.A. (1984) *Trans. R. Soc. trop. Med. Hyg.* **78**, Suppl., 9–18.
7 Wartman, W.B. (1947) *Medicine, Balt.* **26**, 333.
8 Edeson, D.F.B., Wilson, T., Wharton, R.H. et al (1960) *Trans. R. Soc. trop. Med. Hyg.* **54**, 229.
9 Dondero, T.J., Mullin, S.W. & Balasingham, S. (1975) *S.E. Asian J. trop. Med. publ. Hlth* **3**, 569.
10 Schacher, J.F. & Sahyoun, P.F. (1967) *Trans. R. Soc. trop. Med. Hyg.* **49**, 588.
11 Denham, D.A. & Rodgers, R. (1975) *Trans. R. Soc. trop. Med. Hyg.* **69**, 173.
12 Bosworth, W. & Ewert, A. (1977) *Trans. R. Soc. trop. Med. Hyg.* **71**, 21.
13 Date, A., Chandy, M. & Pulimood, B.M. (1983) *Trans. R. Soc. trop. Med. Hyg.* **77**, 112–113.
14 Salfield, S. (1975) *Med. J. Aust.* **i**, 264.
15 Das, G.C. & Sen, S.B. (1968) *Br. med. J.* **ii**, 27–29.
16 Collomb, H., Camerlynck, P., Dumas, M. et al (1969) *Bull. Soc. Path. éxot.* **62**, 907.
17 Kenny, M. & Hewitt, R. (1950) *Am. J. trop. Med. Hyg.* **30**, 895.
18 Carayon, A., Collomb, H. & Sankale, M. (1959) *Bull. Soc. med. Afr. noire Lang. fr.* **4**, 299.
19 Reddy, G.S. & Balasundram, S. (1977) *J. Indian Med. Ass.* **68**, 125.
20 Au, A.C.S., Denham, D.A., Draper, C.C. et al (1980) *Trans. R. Soc. trop. Med. Hyg.* **74**, 674–675.
21 Power, S. (1946) *Lancet* **i**, 572.
22 McMahon, J.E., Marshall, T.F. de C., Vaughan, J.P. et al (1979) *Ann. trop. Med. Parasit.* **73**, 457–464.
23 Chularek, P. & Desowitz, R.S. (1970) *J. Parasit.* **56**, 6, 23.
24 Tanaka, H. & Shibuya, T. (1980) *Jap. J. exp. Med.* **50**, 393–394.
25 Nathan, M.B. et al (1982) *Ann. trop. Med. Parasit.* **76**, 339–345.
26 Wijeyaratne, P.M. Singha, P., Verma, O.P. et al (1982) *Trans. R. Soc. trop. Med. Hyg.* **76**, 387–391.
27 McMahon, J.E. (1982) *Tropenmed. Parasit.* **33**, 28–30.
28 Russel, S., Sundaram, R.M., Chandrasekharan, A. et al (1975) *J. commun. Dis.* **7**, 59.
29 Weller, P.F. & Otteson, E.A. (1978) *Trans. R. Soc. trop. Med. Hyg.* **72**, 31.
30 Cohen, L.B., Nelson, G.S., Wood, A.M. et al (1961) *Am. J. trop. Med. Hyg.* **10**, 843.
31 Cahill, K.M. & Kaiser, R.L. (1964) *Trans. R. Soc. trop. Med. Hyg.* **58**, 356.
32 Rodgers, R., Davis, R. & Denham, H.A. (1975) *J. Helminth.* **49**, 31.
33 Hedge, C.E. & Ridley, D.S. (1956) *Trans. R. Soc. trop. Med. Hyg.* **71**, 304.
34 Grove, D.I. & Davis, R.S. (1978) *Am. J. trop. Med. Hyg.* **27**, 508.
35 Tandon, A., Srivavast, A.A.K., Saxena, R.P. et al (1983) *Trans. R. Soc. trop. Med. Hyg.* **77**, 439–441.
36 Ridley, D.S. (1956) *Trans. R. Soc. trop. Med. Hyg.* **50**, 255.
37 Goodwin, L.G. (1984) *Trans. R. Soc. trop. Med. Hyg.* **78**, 1–8.
38 Jing, W.X. et al (1983) *Jingsu med. J.* **9**, 17.
39 Partono, F., Purnomo & Soewarta, A. (1979) *Trans. R. Soc. trop. Med. Hyg.* **73**, 536.
40 Partono, F. (1985) *Trans. R. Soc. Med. Hyg.* **79**, 44–46.
41 Lagraulet, J., Barsinas, M., Fagneaux, G. et al (1973) *Bull. Soc. Path. éxot.* **66**, 139.
42 World Health Organization (1967) *Wld Hlth Org. tech. Rep. Ser.*, 359.
43 Laigret, J., Kessel, J.F., Bambridge, B. et al (1966) *Bull. Wld Hlth Org.* **34**, 925.
44 Hawking, F. & Marques, R.J. (1967) *Bull. Wld Hlth Org.* **37**, 405.
45 Laigret, J., Kessel, J.F., Malaide, L. et al (1965) *Bull. Soc. Path. éxot.* **58**, 895.
46 Marshall, C.L. & Yasukawa, K. (1966) *Am J. trop Med Hyg.* **15**, 934.
47 Burnet, G.F. & Mataika, J.U. (1964) *Trans. R. Soc. trop. Med. Hyg.* **58**, 545.
48 Mahoney, L.E. & Kessel, J.F. (1971) *Bull. Wld Hlth Org.* **45**, 35.
49 Temu, S.E. & McMahon, J.E. (1981) *Trans. R. Soc. trop. Med. Hyg.* **75**, 835–836.
50 Bryan, J. & Southgate, B.A. (1967) *Trans. R. Soc. trop. Med. Hyg.* **70**, 39.
51 World Health Organization (1984) *Tech. Rep. Ser.*, 702.
52 Wilson, T. (1961) *Trans. R. Soc. trop. Med. Hyg.* **55**, 107.
53 Dondero, T.J., Bhattacharya, N.C., Black, H.R. (1976) *Am. J. trop. Med. Hyg.* **25**, 64.
54 Partono, F. (1984) *Trans. R. Soc. trop. Med. Hyg.* **78**, 9–12.
55 Partono, F., Pornomo, Soewarta, A. et al (1984) *Trans. R. Soc. trop. Med. Hyg.* **78**, 370–372.
56 Kozek, W.J., Reyes, M.A., Ehrman, J. et al (1984) *Am. J. trop. Med. Hyg.* **33**, 65–69.
57 Meyers, F.M. & Kouwenaar, W. (1939) *Geneesk Tijdschr. Ned.-Indië* **79**, 853.
58 Lie Kian Joe (1962) *Am. J. trop. Med. Hyg.* **11**, 646.
59 Beaver, P.C. (1970) *Am. J. trop. Med. Hyg.* **19**, 181.
60 Buckley, J.J.C. & Wharton, R.H. (1961) *J. Helminth. Syph.* **17**, 1.
61 Otteson, R.E.A., Neva, F.A., Paranjape, R.S. et al (1979) *Lancet* **i**, 1158.
62 Bras, G. & Lie Kian Joe (1951) *Documenta neerl. indones. Morb. trop.* **3**, 289.
63 Danaraj, T.J. (1959) *Archs Path.* **67**, 15.
64 Webb, J.K.G., Job, C.K. & Gault, E.W. (1960) *Lancet* **i**, 835.
65 d'Abrera, V. St. E. (1958) *Med. J. Malaya* **12**, 559–562.
66 Singh, M.M., Sharma, S.K. & Patney, R.M. (1974) *Indian Heart J.* **26**, 261–263.
67 Boornazian, J.S. & Fagan, M.J. (1985) *Am. J. trop. Med. Hyg.* **34**, 473–475.
68 Ravindran, M. (1979) *Br. med. J.* **ii**, 1262.
69 Rassi, M.H., Castillo, H., Hernandex, I. et al (1977) *Bull. Pan. Am. Hlth Org.* **11**, 41.
70 Ewert, A., Corredor, A., Lightner, L. et al (1979) *Am. J. trop. med. Hyg.* **28**, 486–490.
71 Guderian, R.H., Swanson, D., Carillo, D.R. et al (1983) *Tropenmed. Parasit.* **34**, 149–154.
72 Beaver, P.C., Hira, P.R. & Patel, B.G. (1983) *Trans. R. Soc. trop. Med. Hyg.* **77**, 162–166.

73 Botto, C., Arango, M. & Yarzabal, L. (1984) *Tropenmed. Parasit.* **35**, 167–173.

74 Braun-Munziger, R.A. & Southgate, B.A. (1977) *Bull. Wld Hlth Org.* **55**, 569.

75 Omar, M.S. & Garms, R. (1981) *Tropenmed. Parasit.* **34**, 259–264.

76 Duke, B.O.L., Lewis, D.J. & Moore, D.J. (1966) *Ann. trop. Med. Parasit.* **60**, 318.

77 Godoy, G.T., Orihel, G. & Volca, N. (1980) *Am. J. trop. Med. Hyg.* **1**, 250–261.

78 Nelson, G.S. Personal communication.

79 Donnelly, J.J., Rockey, J.M., Bianco, A.E. et al (1983) *Ophthal. Res.*

80 Bartlett, A., Turk, J., Ngu, J. et al (1978) *Trans. R. Soc. trop. Med. Hyg.* **72**, 372.

81 Steward, M.W., Sisley, B., Mackenzie, C.D. et al (1982) *Clin. exp. Immunol.* **3**, 1–11.

82 Nelson, G.S. (1958) *Trans. R. Soc. trop. Med. Hyg.* **52**, 272.

83 Rodger, F.C. (1959) *Trans. R. Soc. trop. Med. Hyg.* **53**, 141.

84 Neumann, E. & Gunders, A.E. (1973) *Am. J. Ophthal.* **75**, 82.

85 Anderson, J. & Fuglsang, H. (1977) *Trop. Dis. Bull.* **74**, 257.

86 Prost, A., Nebout, M. & Rougemont, A. (1979) *Br. med. J.* **i**, 589–590.

87 Browne, S.G. (1960) *Trans. R. Soc. trop. Med. Hyg.* **54**, 325.

88 Edungbola, L.D., Oni, G.A. & Aiyedun, B.A. (1983) *Trans. R. Soc. trop. Med. Hyg.* **77**, 303–309.

89 Anderson, J., Fuglsang, H., Hamilton, P.S.J. et al (1974) *Trans. R. Soc. trop. Med. Hyg.* **68**, 209.

90 Fuglsang, H. (1983) *Trans. R. Soc. trop. Med. Hyg.* **77**, 881.

91 Raper, A.B. & Ladkin, R.G. (1950) *E. Afr. med. J.* **29**, 339.

92 Mahoney, J.L. (1982) *S. Afr. med. J.* **61**, 50–52.

93 Fawdry, A.L. (1957) *Trans. R. Soc. trop. Med. Hyg.* **51**, 253.

94 Schwartz, D.A., Brandling-Bennett, A.D., Figueroa, M. et al (1983) *Acta trop.* **40**, 383–389.

95 Connor, D.H., Gibson, D.W., Neafie, R.C. et al (1983) *Am. J. trop. Med. Hyg.* **32**, 123–137.

96 Schultz-Key, H. & Karam, M. (1984) *Trans. R. Soc. trop. Med. Hyg.* **78**, 157–159.

97 Mazzotti, L. (1959) *Revta Inst. Salubr. Enferm. trop. Méx.* **19**, 1.

98 Bryceson, A.D.M., Warrell, D.A. & Pope, H.M. (1977) *Br. med. J.* **i**, 742.

99 Stingl, P., Ross, M., Gibson, D.W. et al (1984) *Trans. R. Soc. trop. Med. Hyg.* **78**, 254–258.

100 MacRae, A.A., Anderson, R.I. & Fazen, L. (1977) *Am. J. trop. Med. Hyg.* **26**, 658.

101 Buck, A.A., Anderson, R., Colston, A.C., Jr et al (1971) *Bull. Wld Hlth Org.* **45**, 353.

102 Ricardo Lujan, L., Collins, W.E., Stanfill, P.S. et al (1983) *Am. J. trop. Med. Hyg.* **32**, 747–752.

103 Hashiguchi, Y., Kawabata, M., Guillermo, Z.F. et al (1979) *Trans. R. Soc. trop. Med. Hyg.* **73**, 543.

104 Duke, B.O.L. (1957) *Trans. R. Soc. trop. Med. Hyg.* **51**, 37.

105 Duke, B.O.L., Vincelette, F. & Moore, P.J. (1976) *Tropenmed. Parasit.* **27**, 123.

106 Rougemont, A., Taylefors, B., Ducam, M. et al (1980) *Bull. Wld Hlth Org.* **58**, 917–922.

107 Aziz, M.A., Diallo, S., Diop, I.M. et al (1982) *Lancet* **ii**, 171–173.

108 Awadzi, K., Dadzie, K.Y., Schulz-Key, H. et al (1984) *Lancet* **iv**, 921.

109 Salazar Mallen, M., Gonzalez Barranco, D. & Jurado Mendoza, J. (1971) *Ann. trop. Med. Parasit.* **65**, 393.

110 Awadzi, K., Schultz-Key, H., Howells, R.E. et al (1982) *Ann. trop. Med. Parasit.* **76**, 459–473.

111 Nelson, G.S. (1966) *Helminth. Abstr.* **35**, 311.

112 World Health Organization (1966) *Wld Hlth Org. tech. Rep. Ser.*, 335.

113 De Leon, J.R. & Duke, B.O.L. (1966) *Trans. R. Soc. trop. Med. Hyg.* **60**, 735.

114 Ali-Khan, Z. (1977) *Ann. trop. Med. Parasit.* **71**, 469.

115 Beaver, P.C., Horner, G.S. & Bilos, J.Z. (1974) *Am. J. trop. Med. Hyg.* **23**, 595.

116 Azarova, N.S., Miretsky, O.Y. & Sonin, M.D. (1965) *Medskyya Parazit.* **34**, 156.

117 Nnochiri, E. (1972) *E. Afr. med. J.* **49**, 198.

118 White, G.B. (1977) *Trans. R. Soc. trop. Med. Hyg.* **71**, 161.

119 Duke, B.O.L. (1961) Patrick Buxton Memorial Prize Essay, London School of Hygiene and Tropical Medicine.

120 Paleologo, F.P., Neafie, R.C. & O'Connor, D.H. (1984) *Am. J. trop. Med. Hyg.* **33**, 395–402.

121 Orlando, G., Galli, M. & Lazzarin, A. (1982) *Boll. Inst. Sieroterapico, Milan* **61**, 258–261.

122 Kivits, M. (1952) *Ann. Soc. belge Méd. trop.* **23**, 235.

123 Toussaint, D. & Davis, P. (1965) *Archs Ophthal.* **74**, 470.

124 Browne, S.G. (1954) *J. trop. Med. Hyg.* **57**, 229.

125 Schofield, F.D. (1955) *Trans. R. Soc. trop. Med. Hyg.* **49**, 588.

126 Downie, G.C.B. (1966) *Jl R. Army med. Corps* **112**, 46.

127 Bouvet, J.P., Thrizol, M. & Auduier, L. (1977) *Acta trop.* **34**, 281.

128 Negesse, Y., Lanoi, E., Neafie, C. et al (1985) *Am. J. trop. Med. Hyg.* **34**, 537–546.

129 Pillay, V.K.G., Kirch, E. & Kurtzman, N.A. (1973) *J. Am. med. Ass.* **225**, 179.

130 Woodruff, A.W. (1951) *Trans. R. Soc. trop. Med. Hyg.* **44**, 479.

131 Brumpt, L.C. (1966) *Bull. Soc. med. Hôp. Paris* **177**, 1049.

132 Muylle, L. et al (1983) *Br. med. J.* **287**, 519–520.

133 Van Hoegaerden, M. & Flocard, F. (1985) *Lancet* **i**, 1278.

134 Duke, B.O.L. (1964) *Ann. trop. Med. Parasit.* **58**, 390.

135 Duke, B.O.L. (1955) *Ann. trop. Med. Parasit.* **49**, 260.

136 Duke, B.O.L. (1963) *Ann. trop. Med. Parasit.* **57**, 82.

137 Meyers, W.M., Connor, D.H., Marman, L.E. et al (1972) *Am. J. trop. Med. Hyg.* **21**, 528.

138 Spiers, R.E. & Baum, A.H. (1953) *J. Kansas med. Soc.* **54**, 553.

139 St George, J. (1975) *Ann. trop. Med. Parasit.* **69**, 383.

140 Kale, O.O., Elemile, T. & Enahoro, F. (1983) *Ann. trop. Med. Parasit.* **77**, 151–157.

141 Rao, C.K., Kumar, S., Jain, M.L. et al (1982) *J. commun. Dis.* **14**, 36–40.

142 Almauina, M., Galli, M., Rizzi, M. et al (1984) *Trans. R. Soc. trop. Med. Hyg.* **78**, 489–491.

143 Stott, G. (1962) *J. trop. Med. Hyg.* **60**, 107.

144 Wiseman, R.A. (1967) *Trans. R. Soc. trop. Med. Hyg.* **61**, 667.

145 Gelfand, M. & Wessels, O. (1964) *Trans. R. Soc. trop. Med. Hyg.* **58**, 552.

146 Wahlgren, M. (1982) *Ann. trop. Med. Parasit.* **76**, 557–559.

147 Maertens, K. & Wery, M. (1975) *Trans. R. Soc. trop. Med. Hyg.* **69**, 359.

148 Nathan, M.B. (1983) *Trans. R. Soc. trop. Med. Hyg.* 77, 141.

149 Kozek, W.J. & Raccurt, C. (1983) *Tropenmed. Parasitol.* **34**, 38–53.

150 Shelley, A.J. & Shelley, A. (1976) *Ann. trop. Med. Parasit.* **70**, 213.

151 Buckley, J.J.C. (1934) *Trans. R. Soc. trop. Med. Hyg.* **28**, 1.

152 Batista, D., Oliveira, W.R. & Rabello, V.D. (1960) *Rev. Inst. Med. trop. São Paulo* **2**, 281.

153 Moraes, A.P. (1976) *Trans. R. Soc. trop. Med. Hyg.* **70**, 16.

154 Kozek, W.J., d'Alessandro, A., Juan Silva, H. et al (1982) *Am. J. trop. Med. Hyg.* **31**, 1131–1136.

155 Ciferri, F. (1982) *Am. J. trop. Med. Hyg.* **31**, 302–308.

156 Jung, R.C. & Espenan, P.H. (1967) *Bull. Wld Hlth Org.* **37**, 405.

157 Beaver, P.C. & Orihel, T.C. (1965) *Am. J. trop. Med. Hyg.* **14**, 1010–1029.

158 Pacheco, G. & Schofield, H.L. (1968) *Am. J. trop. Med. Hyg.* **17**, 180.

159 Duke, D.C., Gelfand, M., Gadd, K.G. et al (1968) *Cent. Afr. med. J.* **14**, 21.

160 Orihel, T.C. (1973) *Am. J. trop. Med. Hyg.* **22**, 596.

161 Partono, F. (1982) *S.F. Asian J. trop. Med. publ. Hlth.* **13**, 275–279.

Chapter 21
Soil-transmitted Helminths

These are intestinal nematodes part of whose development takes place outside the body in the soil.

Soil-transmitted nematodes are of great importance in the health of many populations in Third World countries where the frequency of infection is a general indication of the local level of development of hygiene and sanitation. These nematodes are usually found as multiple infections and measures against and treatment of one closely affect the others. They may be divided into three types according to their life-cycle.

TYPE 1 DIRECT

Embryonated eggs are passed which hatch and reinfect within 2–3 hours by being carried from the anal margin to the mouth and either do not reach the soil or, if they do, do not require a period of development there. This group includes *Enterobius vermicularis* (pinworm) and *Trichuris trichiura* (whipworm).

TYPE 2 MODIFIED DIRECT

Eggs are passed out in the stool which require a period of development in the soil before being ingested, where they hatch, releasing larvae which penetrate the mucous membrane of the stomach and enter the circulation to reach the lungs, passing up the respiratory tract to enter the oesophagus and reach the intestine where they become adult. These include *Ascaris lumbricoides* (roundworm) and *Toxocara canis* (the *Ascaris* of the dog).

TYPE 3 PENETRATION OF THE SKIN

In this group eggs are passed out in the stools to the soil where they hatch into larvae which undergo further development before they are ready to penetrate the skin and reach the circulation and lungs which they penetrate to enter the respiratory tract, and move up to enter the oesophagus and reach the small intestine where they become adult. *Ancylostoma* (hookworm) and *Strongyloides stercoralis* belong to this group but differ in that *Strongyloides* larvae are passed in the stool and autoinfection can occur at the anal margin, or independent development take place in the soil where it can exist in the absence of any further cycle through man.

TYPE 2 MODIFIED DIRECT (*Ascaris, Toxocara*)
Ascaris

GEOGRAPHICAL DISTRIBUTION

Ascaris lumbricoides (roundworm) is one of the commonest and most widespread human infections. Possibly one in four of the world's population is infected. It occurs in Asia, Central and South America, Europe, Africa and North America.

The prevalence of *Ascaris* varies in different parts of the world. In China and South-East Asia it is highly prevalent. In the Central Asian Republics of the USSR it is common in humid areas. In Central and South America the average rate of infection is 45% and in parts of Africa 95%. In Europe it is low in the north and light to moderate in the south. In the southern USA it is moderate.

AETIOLOGY AND LIFE-CYCLE
(Fig. 21.1)

Ascaris lumbricoides (Fig. 21.2) is a comparatively large worm (female 20–25 cm × 3–6 mm; male

Ascaris lumbricoides

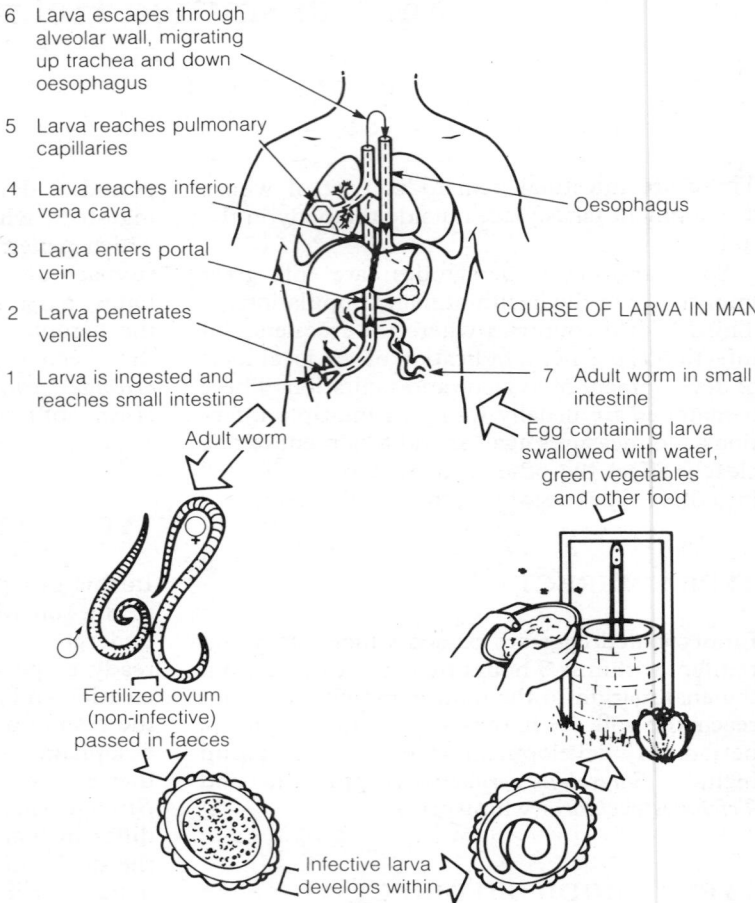

6   Larva escapes through alveolar wall, migrating up trachea and down oesophagus

5   Larva reaches pulmonary capillaries

4   Larva reaches inferior vena cava

3   Larva enters portal vein

2   Larva penetrates venules

1   Larva is ingested and reaches small intestine

Oesophagus

COURSE OF LARVA IN MAN

7   Adult worm in small intestine

Egg containing larva swallowed with water, green vegetables and other food

Adult worm

Fertilized ovum (non-infective) passed in faeces

Infective larva develops within ovum

Fig. 21.1 Life-cycle of *Ascaris lumbricoides* (roundworm). (Courtesy WTIM.)

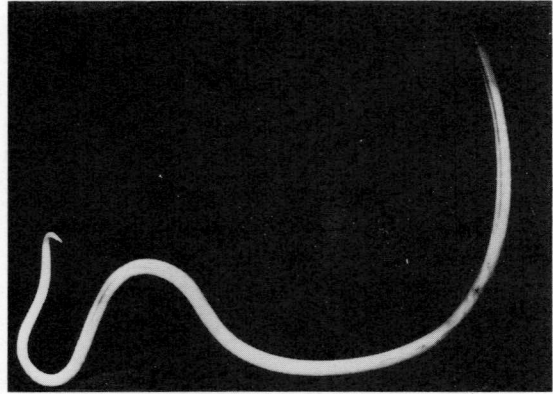

Fig. 21.2   Adult *Ascaris* worm (roundworm). (Courtesy WTIM.)

15–31 cm × 2–4 mm) which inhabits the small intestine (the morphology is described in Appendix II). Eggs (Fig. 21.3) are laid in the small intestine and are passed out as immature ova containing no segmented or differentiated embryo. In damp soil an embryo develops at 36–40°C in two to four months (at the optimum of 25°C in three weeks) which lies coiled up in the egg undergoing one moult before being hatched as an infective second stage rhabditiform larva in the small intestine when the egg is swallowed (Appendix II, p. 1347, and Fig. II.35, p. 1348). Here the rhabditiform larva penetrates the mucous membrane, enters the bloodstream reaching the lungs via the right heart where it cannot pass through the lung capillaries, so that

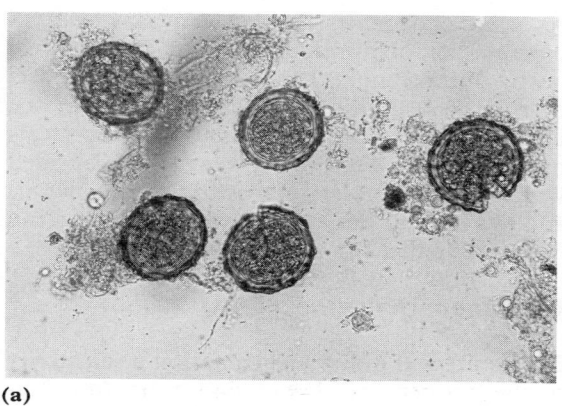

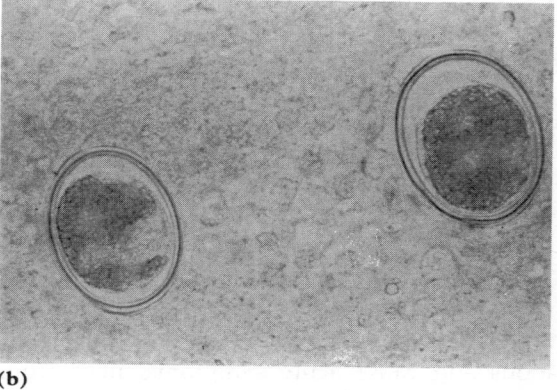

(a)

(b)

Fig. 21.3 Eggs of *Ascaris lumbricoides* (roundworm). (a) Fully formed, fertile, in stool (courtesy WTIM). (b) Decorticated from liver abscess (courtesy Dr M. L. Chu).

it burrows through the alveolar wall to enter the respiratory tract. From here it is carried up the trachea to the larynx, where it crawls over the epiglottis and enters the oesophagus, is swallowed a second time to reach the small intestine. The whole process takes 10–14 days during which time the larva moults twice, the fourth moult taking place between the twenty-fifth and twenty-ninth day. Larvae may reach the intestine as early as the fifth day. In man the period from infection to the first passage of ova in the stool is from 60 to 70 days.

Ascaris suum

Ascaris suum is almost indistinguishable from human *Ascaris* and man is not a normal host but *Ascaris* pneumonia is common in pigs and a proportion of similar respiratory troubles in people associated with pigs may be due to *Ascaris suum*. Although *Ascaris suum* can infect man, he is not its normal host, double infections may occur and eosinophilic granuloma of the bowel may be caused by *Ascaris suum*.

TRANSMISSION

Infection is acquired from the ingestion of eggs from contaminated soil usually by children when playing around the house situated in suitable soil.

PATHOLOGY

Pathology may be caused by migrating larvae or adults.

Migrating larvae (*larval ascariasis*)

Migrating larvae cause symptoms from their actual physical presence and the immune reactions they elicit.

Ascaris pneumonia

Damage to the lungs occurs during the migration of larvae on their way to the intestine. A 'Loeffler's syndrome' may be produced with fever, cough, sputum, asthma, eosinophilia and radiological pulmonary infiltration. In 1956 it was concluded that the majority of cases of Loeffler's syndrome were due to larval ascariasis.[1] Segments of fourth stage larvae can be seen in the bronchioles associated with infiltration with polymorphonuclear and eosinophilic leukocytes with scattered Charcot–Leyden crystals usually associated with lysed eosinophils.

Other organs

Small areas of necrosis with eosinophils may be found in the liver.[2] Migrating larvae have been recovered from aspirated gastric juice and sputum. If the larvae reach the general circulation they may cause localized symptoms resembling those of visceral larva migrans caused by *Toxocara canis*. Larvae may wander into the brain, eye or retina[3] causing granulomas simulating *Toxocara canis*. In small children ascariasis is frequently associated with *Toxocara*. Hundreds of larvae have been removed from a swelling in the neck (but see lagochilascariasis, p. 418).

Adult worms

Adult worms by themselves cause little pathology in their normal habitat (small intestine). Heavy infections can cause intestinal colic which is the most important complaint. Aggregate masses of worms may cause volvulus, intestinal obstruction (Fig. 21.4) or intussusception.

Wandering ascarids

Wandering ascarids may reach abnormal situations and cause acute symptoms: ileus from mechanical obstruction, perforation of the bowel in the ileocaecal region, acute appendicitis from a worm blocking the lumen, diverticulitis, gastric or duodenal trauma, blocking of the ampulla of Vater with pancreatic necrosis, blocking of the common bile duct with obstructive jaundice, entry into the liver parenchyma and liver abscess, invasion of the genital tract and oesophageal perforation.

Ascaris liver abscess

Ascaris liver abscess is caused by female *Ascaris* worms migrating up the common bile duct into the liver where they die releasing the eggs. Histologically there is a granulomatous reaction round the dead worm with release of the eggs which can be demonstrated in the abscess as smooth, oval bodies from which the outer coat has been digested (Fig. 21.3b). In some parts of the world *Ascaris* liver abscess is commoner in young children than amoebic abscess.

Peritoneal lesions

Granulomatous masses may form around the eggs released from female worms which have escaped into the peritoneum and mimic tuberculous peritonitis.[4] An eosinophilic granuloma of the bowel may be caused by *A. suum*.

Biliary ascariasis

Biliary ascariasis is not uncommon in the Philippines where 20% of patients treated surgically for biliary disease are found to have live or dead *Ascaris* worms in the biliary tract[5] and in South Africa where it is common in children.[6] The symptoms are acute onset of right upper abdominal pain sometimes with fever and jaundice from recurrent cholangitis. Adult worms may be demonstrated on plain radiographs, by barium meal or by intravenous cholangiography. At postmortem cholangitis or liver abscess may be found. Good results follow anthelmintic treatment after the acute symptoms have subsided with supportive treatment. Adult worms, larvae and ova may all initiate stone formation and can be found in the core of many bile duct stones.[7]

Immunopathological effects

Many infected individuals manifest a sensitivity to the antigens of *Ascaris* and entry to a laboratory where worms are being dissected is enough to cause conjunctivitis, urticaria and asthma. The skin of these people is extremely sensitive to minimal doses of *Ascaris* antigen and gives an immediate hypersensitivity reaction often with urticaria and erythematous lesions.

The passage of adult worms in sensitive persons may give rise to intense anal pruritus, vomiting of worms and oedema of the glottis.

It has been postulated that the high serum IgE levels found in *Ascaris* might inhibit the development of ordinary asthma but this has been shown not to be the case.[8]

Indirect effects

Microorganisms may be carried by adult worms on their migration from the bowel and a relationship between *Ascaris* infection and the incidence of poliomyelitis has been shown.

Nutritional relationships

Ascariasis may contribute to protein energy malnutrition. From calculations in an experimental study in man[9] it has been estimated that in children infected with 13–40 worms approximately 4 g of protein are lost per day from a daily diet containing 35–50 g of protein. Kwashiorkor has been associated with *Ascaris* infection from the time when it was first recognized as a nutritional syndrome. *Ascaris* infection may contribute to vitamin A deficiency and children suffering from night blindness have shown rapid improvement in their eye symptoms within a few days of therapeutic elimination of the worms. Infected children have also been shown to excrete a significantly lower amount of vitamin C after a test dose of ascorbic acid. *Ascaris* can also adversely affect normal growth.

IMMUNITY

Man acquires only a partial immunity to reinfection and animals can be protected using extracts of adults and larvae.[10] The main immune reaction is humoral and directed against the migrating larval stage. The reaction to adult worms in unusual locations is cellular.

Larval migratory stages

The antigens which elicit antibodies are released at the moulting period between the second and third larval stages when there is a great increase in IgE. A further response is elicited in the bowel between the fourth and fifth stages, at which time there may be a marked loss of worm burden and this may be a regulatory mechanism in natural infections.

Adult stage

Adult worms in the bowel elicit no response but when they wander into the tissues the response is cellular and results in a granuloma. Immediate hypersensitivity to adult *Ascaris* antigens develops in some people.

CLINICAL FEATURES

Natural history

Most *Ascaris* infections are symptomless but heavy infections in childhood give rise to symptoms. These heavy infections are controlled by immunity, or by diminished exposure, so that adults show much lighter infections, although reinfection can occur throughout life.

Incubation period

The incubation period from infection with swallowed eggs to the first appearance of eggs in the stools is 60–70 days. In larval ascariasis pulmonary symptoms occur 4–16 days after infection.

Symptoms and signs

Light infections do not usually cause symptoms though a single adult worm can cause a liver abscess or block the common bile duct. Acute manifestations are roughly proportional to the number of worms harboured and serious disorder may be caused when the burden amounts to 100 worms or more.

Larval ascariasis

ASCARIS PNEUMONIA

During the migratory stages the larvae cause a pneumonitis 4–16 days after infection with fever, cough, sputum and radiological infiltration of the lungs. There is a high eosinophilia and larvae can be found in the sputum or gastric juice, especially if a quantity is collected, digested with trypsin and centrifuged. Seasonal attacks of *Ascaris* pneumonia have occurred in Saudi Arabia following the onset of spring rains and the restarting of transmission.[11] The pneumonitis is of short duration, about three weeks (in contrast to tropical pulmonary eosinophilia which lasts for many months). There may be asthma which can be so intense as to cause status asthmaticus[2] and the liver may become involved, becoming enlarged and tender.

GENERAL SYMPTOMS

Larvae on reaching the general circulation may cause symptoms similar to those of *Toxocara canis*. Neurological disorders including convulsions, meningism and epilepsy, palpebral oedema, insomnia and tooth grinding during the night may occur. When the larvae wander into the brain they cause granulomas presenting as small tumours in the eyes, retina or brain.

Adult ascariasis

The main manifestation of adult ascariasis is small bowel obstruction (Fig. 21.4) which usually occurs in children and as many as 1000 worms have been removed from one patient. Gastrointestinal discomfort, colic and vomiting are quite common.

MIGRATORY ADULT WORMS

Adult worms tend to migrate when their environment is disturbed. In the presence of tetrachlorethylene, anaesthetics or fever they migrate and wander into the bile ducts, ampulla of Vater, appendix, perineal sinuses and Eustachian tubes. They can cause volvulus and gangrene of the bowel, intestinal perforation and peritonitis, acute pancreatitis, suppurative cholangitis, liver abscess, acute cholecystitis and obstructive jaundice.

It is important for these reasons not to give

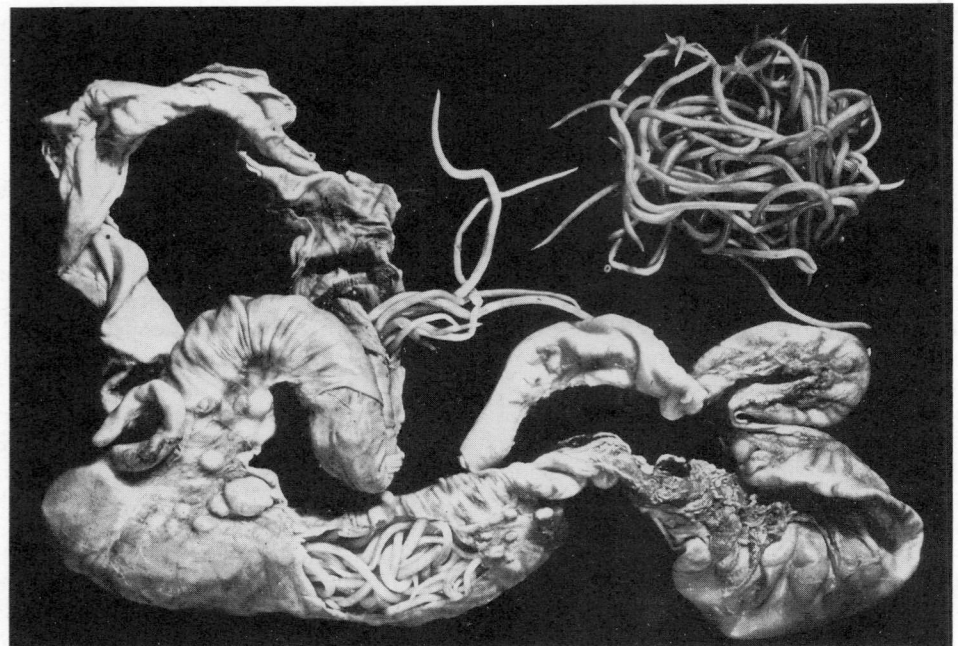

Fig. 21.4   Impacted mass of adult *Ascaris* worms in the small intestine causing fatal intestinal obstruction.

tetrachlorethylene when there is a possibility of *Ascaris* infection and to deworm children when they are ill and febrile or before giving an anaesthetic.

DIAGNOSIS

A diagnosis can be made from the passage of worms in the stool or by finding eggs in the stool.

Fertile eggs are oval and measure about $60 \times 45\,\mu$m. The shell is transparent, is surrounded by an outer mamillated shell stained by bile pigments and contains an unsegmented embryo (see Figs. 21.3a and II.41, p. 1362, and Plate III.7 and 8).

Unfertile eggs are longer and narrower ($90 \times 40\,\mu$m), have a thinner shell, more irregular outer covering (Plate III.9) and are found in about two-thirds of infections either due to a shortage or absence of males. In male infections no eggs are passed in the stool.

Decorticated eggs are usually found in ectopic sites where they have had the outer shell removed and present as smooth oval objects (Fig. 21.3b).

Eosinophilia

In larval ascariasis there is a high eosinophilia but in adult infections there is little or none. If a high eosinophilia occurs in adult infections then an associated *Toxocara* or *Strongyloides* infection must be suspected.

Adult worms

Sometimes the passage of an adult worm will be reported and cause distress. The size and shape will distinguish it from other worms which may be noticed by patients, especially tapeworms.

Radiography

X-ray examination 4–6 hours after an opaque meal displays the worms as cylindrical filling defects or as string-like shadows produced by the opaque substance which the worms have swallowed.

Serological diagnosis

Specific antibodies have been detected in persons infected with *A. lumbricoides* and both the complement fixation and precipitin tests have been utilized for the detection of infection. Hypersensitivity to *Ascaris* is well recognized and cutaneous tests have been used in man as diagnostic aids. There is a lack of correlation between the immunological reaction and the presence of eggs in the faeces, but in pigs the incidence of positive reactions increases with the severity of the pathology produced by the migrating parasites.[12] Since there is much cross reactivity with other helminthic antigens, immunodiagnosis is of little help in *Ascaris* infections, either adult or larval.

DIFFERENTIAL DIAGNOSIS

The syndrome of pulmonary symptoms, radiological lung infiltration and hypereosinophilia are common to a number of helminthic and other infections.

Larval ascariasis must be distinguished from *Toxocara*, hookworm, *Strongyloides*, schistosomiasis and tropical pulmonary eosinophilia (TPE). Essentially, larval ascariasis is a short-term illness lasting two to three weeks with a rapidly falling eosinophilia.

Toxocara (see p. 414). Often associated with *Ascaris*, *Toxocara* causes the visceral larva migrans (VLM) syndrome which persists for many months with a persistently high eosinophilia, and lung symptoms are not prominent. Wandering *Toxocara* larvae cause almost identical lesions of the brain and eye as *Ascaris* and can now be diagnosed by specific serological tests.

Hookworm (see p. 424). The invasive stage of hookworm lasts two to three months, subsiding gradually, ova being found in the stool from 42 days onwards. It may be preceded by a localized eruption on the legs (ground itch).

Schistosomiasis (see Chapter 22). The invasion stage of schistosomiasis (Katayama syndrome) lasts two to three months. There is usually splenomegaly and specific serology is available for diagnosis.

Tropical pulmonary eosinophilia (TPE) (see p. 371). TPE may closely resemble *Ascaris* pneumonia. It occurs mainly in adults (*Ascaris* in children), has a much longer duration and specific filarial serological tests will be positive (older tests using less specific antigens did cross react with *Ascaris*). It responds rapidly to diethylcarbamazine.

Other eosinophilic lung syndromes. Pulmonary aspergillosis, drug reactions and eosinophilic leukaemia all last much longer.

TREATMENT

Treatment is effective only against the adult worms. Although the vast majority of *Ascaris* infections cause few, if any, symptoms it is easy to treat and it is wise to treat any established infection especially if the egg count is high (see Appendix IV).

Albendazole. A single dose of 400 mg will remove *Ascaris* worms in practically every case but cost may preclude its use.[14]

Pyrantel pamoate (Combantrin). This is also extremely effective against *Ascaris*. However, it does not have such a broad spectrum and is less effective against the other helminths. It is given as a single dose of 10 mg/kg body weight. It can be cheaper.

Levamisole. This is less effective against hookworm and is not effective against pinworm. For *Ascaris* it is given as a single dose of 4 mg/kg. It has been used successfully in mass treatment.

Mebendazole. This is active against *Ascaris* but has to be given 100 mg twice daily for 3 days, an obvious disadvantage.

Piperazine compounds. These have now largely been superseded. Piperazine citrate (Antepar) is given as a single 4 g dose but may cause ataxia ('worm wobble').

Tetrachlorethylene. Often used in the past, tetrachlorethylene has little place in treatment of any helminthic infection because it causes *Ascaris* worms to migrate and cause intestinal obstruction, but it is still used in treating hookworm where cost is the first consideration.

Treatment of complications

Whenever possible a trial of medical treatment should be given prior to surgical intervention. Intestinal obstruction may often resolve with medical treatment. The worms are paralysed with piperazine and intravenous fluids are given and the bowel is rested. Liquid paraffin may help to lubricate the paralysed worms and assist their expulsion into the large bowel where they can do no harm. If surgery is necessary the worms should be paralysed first if time permits so that at operation it may be possible to milk the worms from the small bowel into the large bowel without opening the lumen of the gut. If this fails, it will be necessary to open the gut and remove the worms or, especially if there is evidence of ischaemia, to resect the obstructed length of gut together with the enclosed worms.

If time permits it is wise to treat ascariasis before any elective surgery, particularly abdominal surgery.

EPIDEMIOLOGY

Ascaris eggs develop best in shady, damp soil and it is mainly a family infection since the soil around the house is seeded regularly from the droppings of small children who play on infected soil, infect others and reinfect themselves by mouth from contaminated fingers. The prevalence and intensity of infection is highest in the younger age groups and highest in preschool children who are the principal agents in the spread of infection. Other agents for spreading infection widely may be dung beetles and cockroaches which can ingest and excrete viable eggs.

The soil remains infective for a long time and eggs can still be infective after 10 years in the soil and caused *Ascaris* pneumonia in volunteers.[15] *Ascaris* eggs are destroyed by direct sunlight and temperatures above 45°C. Where faeces are used as agricultural fertilizer infection is common in agricultural workers but in overcrowded towns of non-industrial societies with poor hygiene prevalence may be higher in urban than rural communities. In most damp areas of the tropics and subtropics transmission is perennial but in drier areas (notably parts of Arabia) transmission is limited to the short rainy season in the spring, and this may produce short outbreaks of spring *Ascaris* pneumonia in adults.

CONTROL

Control must be based on a combination of personal hygiene, proper disposal of faeces, health education and mass treatment.

Environmental control

Basic environmental measures include safe disposal of human excreta, prevention of soil contamination round the houses by building a non-soil base, exposing agricultural fertilizer to the sun and composting it to increase the temperature above 45°C which will destroy the eggs.

Health education

Health education should be based on what the people need to know, what they can do for themselves and what motivates them to participate actively. This will need a preliminary sociological survey to determine how the programme should be developed.

Mass treatment

Mass treatment has been very successful. The objective is not to eliminate infection entirely but to reduce the worm loads. The target is the young children and mass treatment of the community does not produce significantly better results than selective treatment of children. In Japan a prevalence rate of 49% in 1949 was reduced to 5.3% in 1964. In this campaign as the prevalence decreased, the dose frequency was reduced from twice or three times a year to once or twice.

In the Philippines periodic mass treatment is given three times a year at four-month intervals for three years. Broad-spectrum anthelmintics are used: pyrantel pamoate (Combantrin), albendazole, mebendazole, flubendazole and levamisole have all been used with success. Because of its broad spectrum of action albendazole is now the drug of choice but much will depend upon cost.

Toxocariasis

Toxocariasis in man is the result of infection with the dog *Ascaris*—*Toxocara canis*—which does not undergo normal development in man but is arrested at the larval stage causing toxocariasis, visceral larva migrans (VLM) or ocular toxocariasis.

GEOGRAPHICAL DISTRIBUTION

Toxocara canis infection in dogs has a worldwide distribution and infection rates vary from 2% to 90%.

Visceral larva migrans (VLM), which was first described in the southern USA,[16] has been recognized mainly in the southern and eastern USA but also in Europe, the Caribbean, Mexico, Hawaii, the Philippines, Australia, South Africa and possibly eastern Europe.

Ocular toxocariasis (granulomatous ophthalmitis) first described in the USA[17] has been recognized in many parts of the world and serological surveys have shown many cases of ocular toxocariasis in Britain.[18]

AETIOLOGY

Toxocara canis is a roundworm infection in dogs. The morphology resembles that of *Ascaris lumbricoides* (see Appendix II, p. 1348), the males being 4–6 cm long and the females 6.5–10 cm long. The eggs, which are pitted superficially, measure $85 \times 75 \mu m$ being larger than those of *Ascaris*. They are not found in man but only in dog faeces and contaminated soil.

Life-cycle

In the dog the life-cycle is similar to that of *Ascaris* in man except that transplacental infection of the puppies takes place in pregnant bitches and the puppies born with a patent infection shed numerous eggs from birth. In contrast adult dogs excrete few eggs. dogs are infected by ingesting the eggs from soil or as puppies at birth so that the whole cycle may be maintained in a small flat without any access to the outside.

In man, who is not the normal host, the eggs hatch in the stomach and second stage larvae penetrate the mucosa to enter the circulation via the mesenteric vessels reaching the intestinal viscera and liver where they are held up in the capillaries, but may pass into the general circulation through the lungs and end up in the brain, eye and other organs. In these organs as well as the liver the larvae are eventually held up and destroyed by a granulomatous reaction which blocks their further migration and causes pathology. In the human host the larvae do not grow or moult but can remain alive for as long as 11 years, as has been shown experimentally.

TRANSMISSION

The main source of infection is puppies which excrete large numbers of eggs. Infection is acquired by children playing in contaminated soil or in playgrounds as in *Ascaris* infection and is encouraged by the habit of earth eating (pica). Direct infection from handling puppies is also important.

PATHOLOGY

The pathology depends upon the density of infection. In heavy infections in childhood the syndrome of visceral larva migrans (VLM) is produced whereas lighter infections cause ocular toxocariasis found in later life.

Visceral larva migrans

In heavy infections in children the second stage larvae, which are $450 \mu m \times 16$–$20 \mu m$ in diameter, are arrested mostly in the liver where they cause few or many miliary lesions.[19] These lesions are composed of granulomas which can be seen as white subcapsular nodules the size of millet seeds. Other sites are the lungs, kidneys, heart, striated muscle, brain and eye. Microscopically the granulomas contain a centre of closely packed eosinophils and histiocytes surrounded by larger histiocytes with pale vesicular nuclei sometimes arranged in a palisade-like manner. Occasionally there is an atypical multinucleate giant cell. Living second stage larvae may sometimes be demonstrated in recent granulomas but more usually only the remains can be seen. Less commonly they reach the lungs or brain where similar lesions can be seen.

Ocular toxocariasis

In the eye the granulomatous reaction forms a large subretinal mass with a superimposed patch of choroiditis which can closely resemble a retinoblastoma (for further details see Chapter 70).

IMMUNITY

In the abnormal host (man) the larvae elicit both a humoral and cellular response. Antibodies are formed which cause a quantitative rise in immunoglobulins which is mostly IgG but also IgM (the globulin may be so elevated that a positive formol gel test can be shown) and IgE, and there is a peripheral eosinophilia. The larvae themselves elicit a cell-mediated granulomatous response causing the granulomas so typical of the infection. In the dog immunity to reinfection develops so that adult dogs pass few or no eggs.

CLINICAL FEATURES

Natural history

Following infection from ingested eggs which hatch in the stomach the larvae migrate to the liver where they may be arrested or continue and reach other organs. In most cases the larva is destroyed without causing any trouble but in some cases it can survive for many years, and on its wanderings may eventually cause a lesion. Unless the infection is heavy and the VLM syndrome is produced most cases of infection never cause any trouble. Heavy infections cause VLM which can be self-limiting or can cause death in a few cases. Lesions in the eye can cause severe loss of vision and even complete loss of sight in the affected eye.

Incubation period

No incubation period can be determined but in heavy infections (VLM) is similar to that of *Ascaris*. In light infections many years may pass before the ocular granuloma presents iself.

Symptoms and signs

There are two main clinical presentations: VLM and ocular toxocariasis (granulomatous ophthalmitis).

Visceral larva migrans[20]

This is seen most commonly in younger children. The child becomes unwell with an enlarged liver, fever and asthma. There is a marked hypereosinophilia and there can be pulmonary signs (radiological mottling), cardiac dysfunction, nephrosis, neurological lesions (fits, epilepsy, pareses and transverse myelitis). There is a great increase in the serum globulin and the eosinophil count is raised $10–20 \times 10^9$/litre. In many urban areas where lead paint is used this is ingested with the soil with the habit of pica and signs of lead poisoning may accompany VLM (blue lines on the gums and anaemia).

PROGRESS

Most cases of VLM recover naturally after two years but some die and post-mortem will reveal extensive lesions in the liver and sometimes the brain.

Ocular toxocariasis[21]

The retinal lesion presents as a solid retinal tumour often at or near the macula. In the early stages it is raised above the level of the retina and closely mimics a retinal neoplasm. Later when the acute phase has subsided the lesion remains a clearcut circumscribed area of retinal degeneration. Formerly these lesions were designated tuberculous, exanthematous or neoplastic. If the lesion is central the visual acuity is reduced or central vision may be lost (see Chapter 70).

Strabismus due to macular damage is often the presenting symptom. Low-grade iridocyclitis with posterior synechiae may develop and progress to general endophthalmitis and detachment of the retina. The second stage larva may rarely be seen with a slit-lamp microscope in the anterior chamber of the eye. Secondary glaucoma may result.

DIFFERENTIAL DIAGNOSIS

VLM must be distinguished from other migrating helminths, larval ascariasis (much shorter duration), strongyloidiasis (much longer duration), tropical pulmonary eosinophilia (pulmonary symptoms more marked and found in adults).

Ocular toxocariasis must be distinguished from a retinal tumour (retinoblastoma) and other causes of choroiditis (toxoplasmosis). All cases of retinoblastoma in children should have a serological test to exclude toxocariasis.

DIAGNOSIS

Demonstration of larvae

This is very difficult and seldom achieved. Larvae or portions of degenerate larvae may be seen at the centre of the granuloma in liver biopsy or post-mortem material. A larva has been demonstrated in the cerebrospinal fluid[22] in a case of meningitis.

Liver biopsy may show a granuloma containing many eosinophils which can be suggestive but which must be distinguished from a *Schistosoma mansoni* granuloma. In biopsy and post-mortem material *Ancylostoma braziliense* and *Ancylostoma caninum*, which usually invade the skin, can occasionally enter man via the intestinal tract and form granulomas in the viscera. Autoinfection with *Strongyloides* may cause a similar picture. Immunofluorescent staining of histological sections may be necessary to differentiate them.

Serology

The difficulty with serological diagnosis has always been to obtain an antigen specific to *Toxocara* second stage larvae which does not cross react with other tissue helminths. A specific antigen has been obtained from the secretory/excretory products of second stage *Toxocara canis* larvae which is both sensitive and specific.[23] It has been used in an enzyme-linked immunosorbent assay (ELISA) test[24] which is now the test of choice, but human A and B blood group substances share similarities with parasite derived antigen which has raised some doubts as to the specificity of the test.[25]

ELISA[18]

A strong positive result is greater than 1.5 times screening level.

Other tests which have been used are passive haemagglutination and immunofluorescence. A radioallergosorbent test (RAST) has been used to detect larva specific IgE.[26] The skin sensitivity test has been abandoned.

TREATMENT

Two drugs are used in treatment: diethylcarbamazine and thiabendazole.

Diethylcarbamazine (DEC)

This is the drug of choice. DEC is given orally 3 mg/kg body weight three times daily for 21 days.

Thiabendazole

Thiabendazole is given orally 50 mg/kg body weight daily in three divided doses for 7–28 days depending upon the tolerance shown to the drug.

In VLM the high eosinophilia may persist for months after clinical cure which is shown by subsidence of the fever and hepatomegaly. Once overcome, relapses do not occur and second infections are unlikely. In ocular toxocariasis the addition of steroids may be needed (see Chapter 70). Loss of vision can be arrested but lost vision not restored.

EPIDEMIOLOGY

T. canis is a common inhabitant of adult dogs and puppies. Puppies are infected by second stage larvae in utero and are born with established intestinal infections. The puppies excrete eggs on to the ground which are ingested by small children along with *Ascaris* and *Trichuris* ova and, in urban areas in the USA, lead products found in old paint. Toxocariasis is often associated with *Ascaris* and *Trichuris* infection and in urban areas with signs of lead poisoning. The commonest age of infection is around two and a half years and the infection is patent from about three to five years of age. It is uncommon at a later age unless an unusual habit of dirt-eating is present, as in mental defectives. Ocular toxocariasis is found at a later age. A statistical association between the incidence of *Toxocara* infection as shown by skin sensitivity tests and poliomyelitis and epilepsy has been shown.[27] This is probably due to the introduction of the viral agents from the intestine by the migrating second stage larvae.

CONTROL

Control rests upon control of infection in dogs, especially puppies, which are the main agent of infection and regular treatment of dogs and bitches as well as newborn puppies with anthelmintics is essential when there are children in the house. Dogs should be denied access to sandpits in the back yard and playgrounds.

Lagochilascariasis

GEOGRAPHICAL DISTRIBUTION

Lagochilascariasis is a rare infection of man, who is an accidental host. Cases have been described from South and Central America and the Caribbean.[28]

AETIOLOGY

Lagochilascaris minor is a parasite of the opossum (see also Appendix II, p. 1348). The adult worms live in cavities in the submucosa of the small intestine and eggs containing infective larvae pass out in the stool where they are ingested by mice and other small mammals. The larvae hatch in the intestine and migrate to skeletal muscle where they mature and wait to be ingested by the definitive host, the opossum.

TRANSMISSION

Man becomes infected either by ingesting eggs from the soil or eating the intermediate host. A case reported from Tobago was thought to have acquired the infection through eating the raw meat of the manakou opossum.

PATHOLOGY

In man, *Lagochilascaris* causes subcutaneous abscesses on the head and neck and lesions in the nasopharynx. The tonsils and lymphoid tissue are replaced by granulomatous tissue containing epithelioid granulomas with larvae and eggs. Abscesses form in the neck which discharge pus.

CLINICAL FEATURES

Early symptoms are recurrent tonsillitis, a feeling of worms crawling at the back of the throat and even discharge of small white worms from the mouth. Tender tumours which swell and eventually burst discharging pus and worms form in the cervical region.

DIAGNOSIS

Adult worms can be recognized by a longitudinal furrow along the lateral line (see Appendix II).

TREATMENT

Most anthelmintics are ineffective but levamisole was curative in one case.[28]

TYPE 1　DIRECT *(ENTEROBIUS, TRICHURIS)*
Enterobiasis (oxyuriasis, threadworm, pinworm)

GEOGRAPHICAL DISTRIBUTION

Enterobius vermicularis has a worldwide distribution.

AETIOLOGY

The adult *Enterobius vermicularis* worms (Figs. 21.5 and II.54, p. 1359) are small and white with a double bulb oesophagus and a mouth surrounded by a cuticular expansion and the skin is transversely striated. The female (9–12 mm) has a long, pointed tail and a slit-like vulva in the anterior quarter of the body (Fig. II.54A, p. 1359). The male, which is much smaller (2.5 mm), has a posteriorly curved third and a blunt caudal

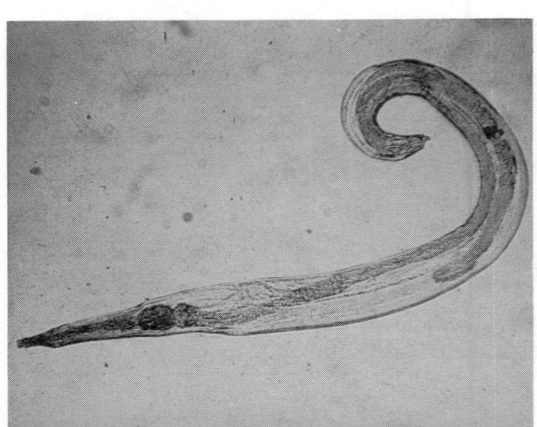

Fig. 21.5 Adult *Enterobius vermicularis* (pinworm, threadworm).

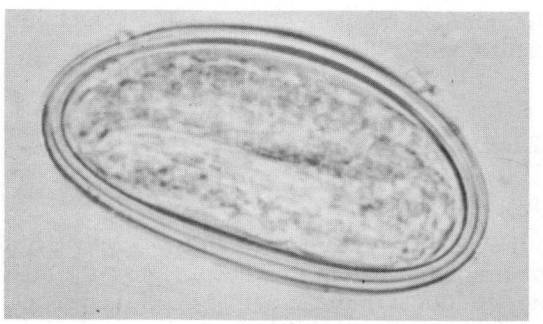

Fig. 21.6   Egg of *Enterobius vermicularis*, as laid partially embryonated.

extremity (Fig. II.54B and C, p. 1359). The egg (Fig. 21.6 and Plate III.19) measures 50–54 × 20–27 μm and has a characteristic shape flattened on one side. It is almost colourless with a bean-shaped double contour shell containing a fully formed embryo.

Life-cycle (Fig. 21.7)

There is no multiplication inside the body. The mature female has a duration of life of 37–93 days and when the ovary is full of eggs she migrates down to the anus from which she emerges to lay

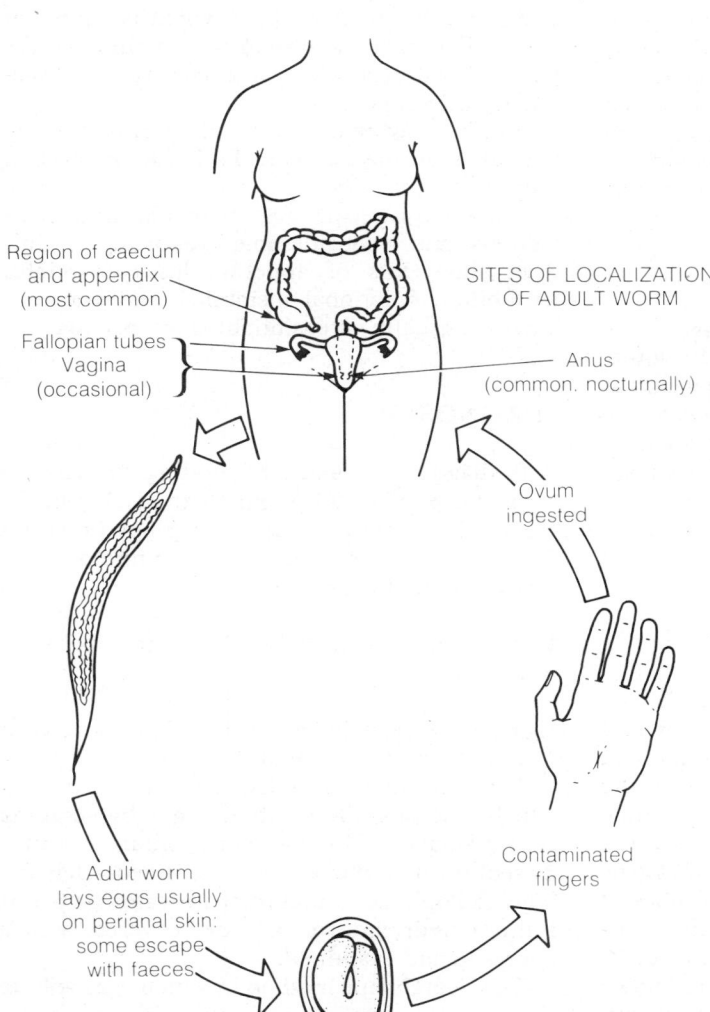

Enterobius (oxyuris) vermicularis
Pinworm

Region of caecum and appendix (most common)

Fallopian tubes Vagina (occasional)

SITES OF LOCALIZATION OF ADULT WORM

Anus (common. nocturnally)

Ovum ingested

Contaminated fingers

Adult worm lays eggs usually on perianal skin: some escape with faeces

Fig. 21.7   Life-cycle of *Enterobius*. (Courtesy WTIM.)

the eggs on the perianal skin and on the perineum. The eggs which are ingested in faecal material lodged under the fingernails hatch in the stomach and larvae emerge which rapidly grow to 140–150 μm in length. They pass through the intestine to the caecum and appendix where they invade the glandular crypts and mature. The whole cycle takes between two and four weeks.

TRANSMISSION

There are four possible ways of transmission; the commonest is by direct transmission from the anal and perianal region to the mouth by fingernail contamination and by soiled night-clothes. A second way is by exposure to viable eggs on soiled bed linen and other contaminated objects in the environment. A third way is via the mouth or nose from contaminated dust in which embryonated eggs have been found. The fourth way is by retroinfection[29] in which eggs hatch on the anal mucosa and larvae migrate up the bowel.

PATHOLOGY

The adult worm lives in the upper part of the large intestine, especially the caecum and lower ileum, where minute ulcerations may develop at the site of attachment of the adult worms to the caecal and appendiceal mucosa. At times haemorrhages occur and secondary infection causes ulcers and submucosal abscesses. Symptoms are caused when gravid females migrate out of the anus on to perianal skin to deposit eggs, where they cause pruritus.

Ectopic lesions

Occasionally *Enterobius* is found in the female genital organs and more rarely in the ear and nose. Rarely worms can invade the abdominal cavity and cause pinworm granulomas of the liver,[30] ovary, kidney, spleen and lung. Chronic pelvic peritonitis has been described.[31] The route by which *Enterobius* gains access to these organs is not clear but may be via the fallopian tubes or haematogenous spread. Direct infection following abdominal operations may also occur. The granuloma which forms around the female and eggs consists chiefly of lymphocytes with few eosinophils and no giant cells. Four cases of eosinophilic granuloma of the large bowel and omentum have been ascribed to *Enterobius*.[32]

CLINICAL FEATURES

Natural history

In the majority of infections *Enterobius* lives out its normal lifespan in the caecum and appendix, migrates down to the anus and deposits its eggs, and the larvae re-establish themselves in the host causing little or no symptoms.

Symptoms and signs

Pruritus ani is the main symptom and varies from a mild itching to acute pain which is mainly at night. The pruritus provokes scratching of the perianal region resulting in excoriation and secondary infection.

Vulvitis may be caused by pinworms entering the vulva causing a mucoid discharge and *pruritis vulvi*.

General symptoms are insomnia and restlessness, and a considerable proportion of children show loss of appetite, loss of weight, irritability, emotional instability and enuresis. There is usually no eosinophilia or anaemia.

DIAGNOSIS

The diagnosis is made by finding the characteristic eggs (Fig. 21.6 and Plate III.19) in the faeces (5% only), perianal scrapings or swabs from under the fingernails, or from finding adult worms round the anus, usually at night.

Faecal examination (see also Appendix IV, p. 1493)

Eggs are present in the faeces of no more than 5% of infected individuals.

A Cellophane swab has been devised with which it is possible to obtain eggs by scraping the perianal area. Enclosed in a container, it may be sent through the post and examined at leisure. The Cellophane is mounted in water or 0.1 M sodium hydroxide on a slide, covered with a coverslip and examined.

The Scotch tape method in which eggs adhere to a sticky surface is very popular (see Appendix IV).

TREATMENT

The whole family must be treated to avoid reinfection. Chemotherapy must be combined with education and personal hygiene aimed at preventing autoinfection. Although it is simple to effect a temporary cure, eradication may prove difficult because of reinfection from the contaminated environment or from asymptomatic members of the same household. Eradication may necessitate repeated courses of treatment for up to a year or more.

Chemotherapy

Albendazole is the treatment of choice, as a single oral dose of 400 mg or 10–14 mg/kg for children.

Mebendazole is as effective in a single oral dose of 100 mg.

Pyrantel pamoate (Combantrin) 10 mg/kg may be given as a single oral dose repeated every six weeks until the environment is clear.

During treatment it is important to prevent reinfection. The child must sleep in cotton drawers and gloves and the fingernails must be kept short and scrubbed. Other members of the family or school should also be treated.

EPIDEMIOLOGY

Enterobiasis is worldwide in distribution and is a group infection, commoner in children than adults. It occurs in family groups or institutions, such as asylums and schools, especially under crowded conditions. When one infection is found it is likely that there are others. Although it is a human infection, chimpanzees, gibbons and marmosets can all be infected.

Trichuriasis (*Trichuris trichiura*) (whipworm)

GEOGRAPHICAL DISTRIBUTION

Trichuris trichiura is a worldwide infection. It is estimated that 755 million people in the world are infected.[33]

AETIOLOGY

Trichuris trichiura is a greyish-white worm often slightly pink which lives in the caecum and appendix. The male (30–45 mm long) has an attenuated anterior portion containing a cellular oesophagus which is half as long again as the thicker posterior portion, and a caudal extremity curved through 360° with a single spicule in the sheath which is studded with spines (Figs. 21.8 and II.56,1, p. 1361). The female (30–35 mm long) has the posterior half occupied by a stout uterus packed with eggs (Fig. II.56,2 and

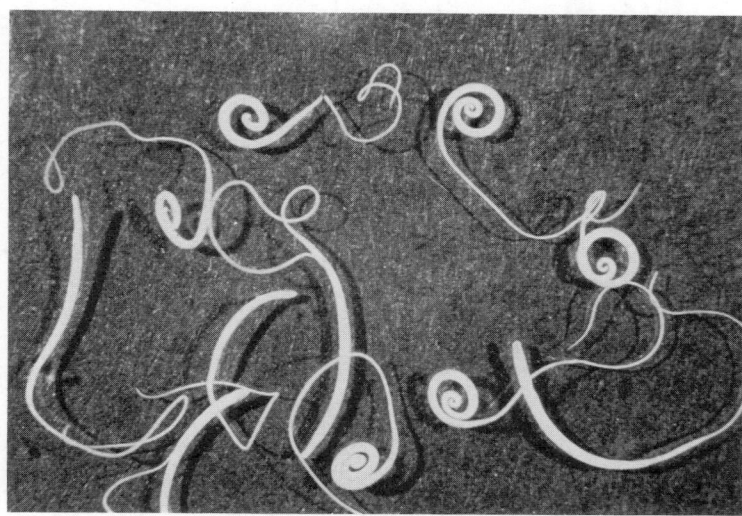

Fig. 21.8 Adult *Trichuris* worms (whipworms), male and female. (Courtesy Dr H. Zaiman.)

3, p. 1361). The egg (50 × 22 μm) is brown with a characteristic band-shape and a single shell with a plug at each end and contains a single embryo (Fig. 21.9 and Plate III.18).

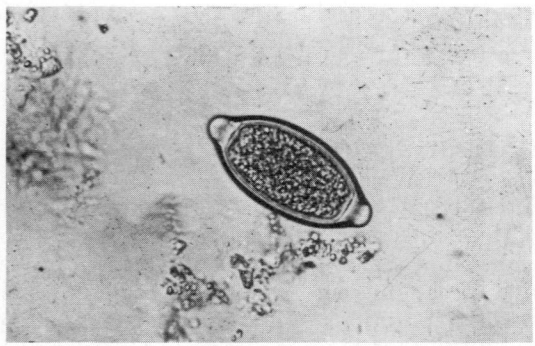

Fig. 21.9   Egg of *Trichuris*. (Courtesy WTIM.)

Life-cycle (Fig. 21.10)

The worms live in the caecum where they maintain their position by transfixing a superficial fold of mucosa and lie embedded in mucus between the intestinal villi. The egg is laid unsegmented and embryonation takes at least 21 days. It can withstand low temperatures but not desiccation. Infection is direct from stale faeces. The egg hatches after being swallowed in the intestine where the shell is digested by the intestinal juices and the larva emerges in the small intestine where it penetrates the villi and develops for a week until it re-emerges and passes to the caecum and large intestine, where it attaches itself to the mucosa and becomes adult.

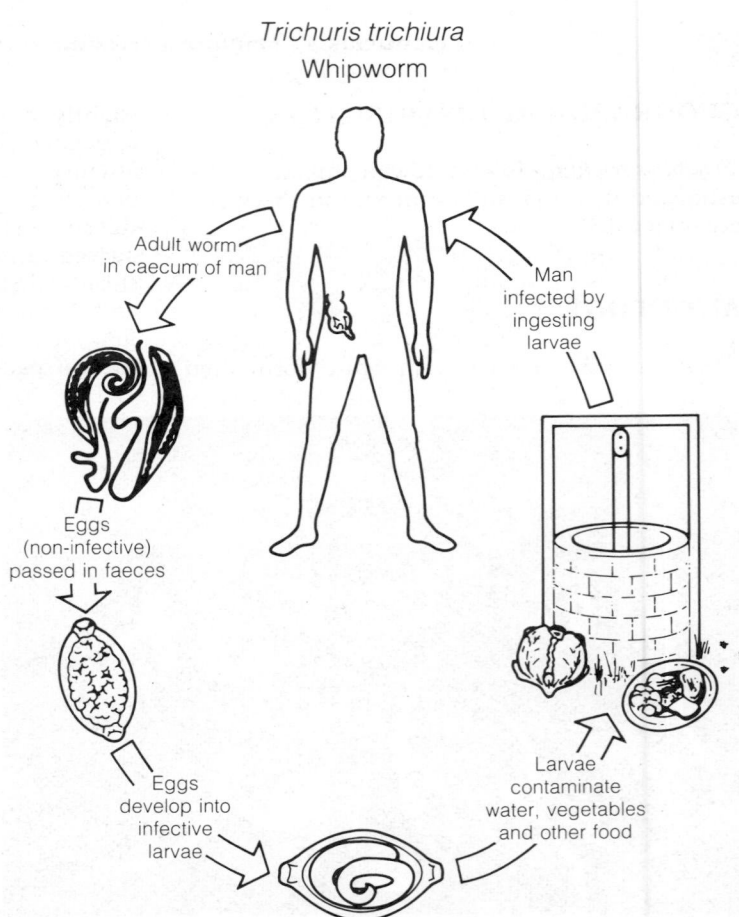

Fig. 21.10   Life-cycle of *Trichuris*.
(Courtesy WTIM.)

TRANSMISSION

Transmission is direct from mature eggs to the mouth via fingers contaminated from infected soil.

PATHOLOGY

When there are only a few worms there is little damage but with heavy infections the worms spread throughout the large bowel to the rectum. They cause haemorrhages, mucopurulent stools and symptoms of dysentery with rectal prolapse.[34]

Trichuris is frequently associated with *Ascaris* and hookworm and a secondary infection with *Entamoeba histolytica* causes further ulceration.

CLINICAL FEATURES

Natural history

In the vast majority of infections which are light, the worms live harmlessly in the caecum and appendix but when the infection is heavy (more than 10 000/g of faeces) there can be marked symptoms and signs.

Incubation period

The prepatent period from the ingestion of eggs to the appearance of eggs in the stool is 60 days.

Symptoms and signs

In light infections there are no symptoms but when associated with *Ascaris* or hookworm mild symptoms occur. Epigastric pain, vomiting, distension, flatulence, anorexia and weight loss may occur.[35] Pain in the epigastrium and right iliac fossa is common.[36] When associated with *Entamoeba histolytica* or *Balantidium coli*, symptoms are highly aggravated and dysenteric symptoms occur. Anaemia and low serum albumin is more pronounced in double infections with *Trichuris* than in amoebic infections alone.[37] There is usually no eosinophilia which, if pronounced, usually denotes a concurrent *Toxocara* infection with which it is often associated.

Trichuris dysentery

In heavy infections as seen in the southern USA,

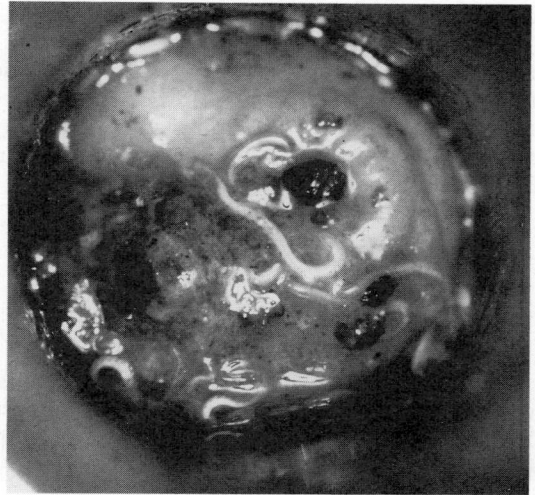

Fig. 21.11 Proctoscopic view of *Trichuris* worms causing dysentery.

infection may extend from the caecum to the rectum and there may be quite a severe dysentery with blood and mucus in the stools and prolapse of the rectum (Fig. 21.11). These infections, which are often associated with amoebiasis, respond well to anthelmintic treatment.

DIFFERENTIAL DIAGNOSIS

In severe infection the clinical picture may resemble hookworm disease, acute appendicitis or amoebic dysentery.

DIAGNOSIS

The diagnosis is made by finding the characteristic eggs in the stool (Fig. 21.9 and Plate III.18) by direct smear or by concentration methods (see Appendix IV). An egg count (see Appendix IV) will reveal the degree of infection and 30 000 eggs/g of stool or more is a heavy infection[34] which would indicate the presence of several hundred worms and the production of symptoms.

Proctoscopy in cases of dysentery will show numerous worms attached to the mucosa which is reddened and ulcerated where they are responsible for the dysentery.

Radiological appearances

In some cases a 'honeycomb' appearance of the small bowel has been seen with the appearances of Crohn's disease with deformity of the bowel most marked in the proximal colon but also in the ileum and appendix.

TREATMENT

Mebendazole is the drug of choice. A single oral dose of 600 mg will reduce the egg count by over 85% and is just as good as the standard dose of 100 mg twice daily for 3 days.[38]

Albendazole is equally effective.

EPIDEMIOLOGY

Trichuris trichiura is primarily a human infection but *Trichuris suis* of pigs is indistinguishable from the human species and can infect man. There is an increased incidence of *Trichuris* infection in people handling pigs.

Trichuris infection is common in areas of high rainfall, high humidity, dense shade and poor sanitation and contaminated soil. The greatest prevalence is in children of primary school age who pollute the soil around the house and who develop heavy worm burdens. *Trichuris* infection is often associated with *Ascaris* and *Toxocara*, the epidemiology of which is similar.

Control is the same as that for *Ascaris*; avoidance of soil pollution and periodic mass chemotherapy.

TYPE 3　PENETRATION OF THE SKIN (*ANCYLOSTOMA, STRONGYLOIDES, TRICHOSTRONGYLUS*)

Ancylostomiasis (hookworm)

Hookworm disease (ancylostomiasis) caused by two hookworms *Ancylostoma duodenale* and *Necator americanus* is an extremely common infection and in many cases the nematodes, which are often present in huge numbers attached to the small intestine, from which they suck blood and protein, cause disease (hookworm anaemia, hookworm disease).

GEOGRAPHICAL DISTRIBUTION

The hookworm occurs in all tropical and subtropical countries.[39]

A. duodenale is essentially a parasite of southern Europe, the north coast of Africa, northern India, north China and Japan. It was introduced by migration into Paraguay around 3000 BC by Japanese fishermen[40] and is the predominant hookworm in coastal Peru and Chile. It has been introduced into Western Australia and into areas where *N. americanus* is the predominant human hookworm, southern India, Burma, Malaya, the Philippines, Indonesia, Polynesia, Micronesia and Portuguese West Africa.

N. americanus is the predominant hookworm of central and southern Africa, southern Asia,

Melanesia and Polynesia. It is widely distributed in the southern USA, the islands of the Caribbean, Central America and northern South America where it was introduced by slaves from Africa.

AETIOLOGY

Two species of hookworm, *Ancylostoma duodenale* and *Necator americanus*, infect man.

Ancylostoma duodenale

A. duodenale is a small cylindrical white, grey or reddish-brown (from ingested blood) thread-like worm (Fig. II.38, p. 1351). Both male and female worms have a buccal capsule containing two pairs of teeth (Fig. II.40, p. 1352) (cf. *N. americanus*) for attaching to the small intestinal mucosa. The male ($0.8–1.1 \times 0.4–0.5$ cm) has a copulatory bursa at the rear end consisting of an umbrella-like expansion of the cuticle (Fig. II.39A, p. 1351). The female ($1–1.3 \times 0.6$ cm) is slightly larger and has the body cavity occupied by the ovary and coiled uterine tubes packed with eggs. The vulva is in the posterior third of the body. The maximum egg output occurs 15–18 months after infection; the interval between infection and final disappearance of eggs from the stool with death of the worm averages six years. The female produces 25–35 000 eggs each day and some 18–54 million during its lifetime. (For full morphological description, see Appendix II.) The eggs (50–60 μm × 35–40 μm) are elliptical with a transparent shell and when freshly laid contain two to four segments (blastomeres) (see Figs. 21.12 and II.41, p. 1352).

p. 1353) which are free-living and have a bulbed oesophagus. They feed avidly on bacteria. The larva moults on the third day and the oesophagus disappears on the fifth day, the larva becoming elongated and fully developed at 20–30°C. It then moves away from the faeces into the soil and moults to form a *filariform* (infective) larva (Fig. II.46a, p. 1353) which has a simple muscular oesophagus and a protective sheath. The larva moves towards oxygen and cannot survive in

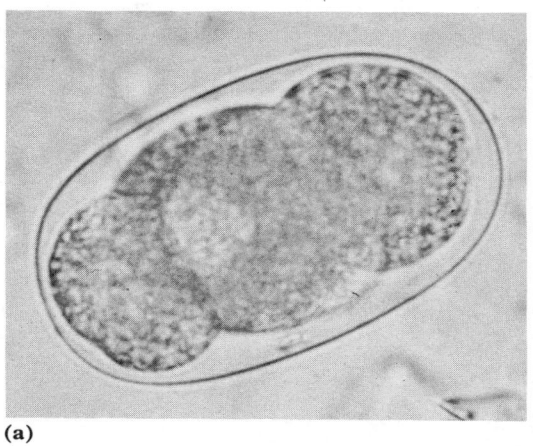
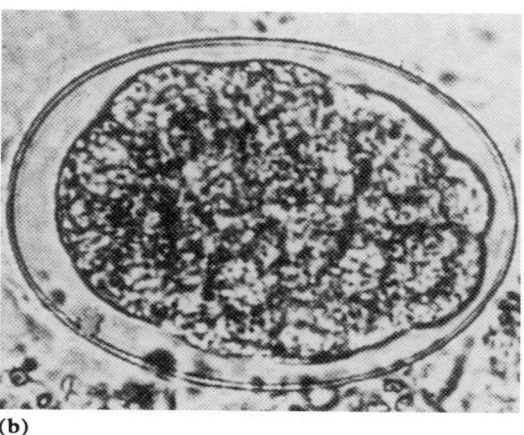

(a)   (b)

Fig. 21.12   Hookworm eggs. (a) Immature egg showing developing larva (courtesy Dr J. S. Tatz). (b) Mature egg (courtesy WTIM).

Necator americanus

N. americanus closely resembles *A. duodenale* but it is shorter and slenderer (0.9–1.1 × 0.4 cm) and can be distinguished from *A. duodenale* by the position of the vulva in the female which is in the anterior third of the body (Fig. II.43, p. 1352) and the buccal capsule which is smaller than that of *A. duodenale*, has cutting plates instead of teeth (Fig. II.45, p. 1353). The egg is slightly larger than that of *A. duodenale* (64–75 × 36–40 μm). The female necator lays 6000–20 000 eggs daily and has a life duration on average of five years.

Life-cycle (Fig. 21.13)

The eggs are deposited into the lumen of the intestine containing two, four or eight blastomeres and are passed out in the faeces where, if deposited in damp shaded soil, they hatch into *rhabditiform* (first stage) larvae (Fig. II.46b,

water. The larvae are most numerous in the upper 2.5 cm of soil but can ascend from deeper layers. Protected from desiccation they can live in warm damp soil for two years. Direct sunlight, drying, or salt water are fatal. When the filariform larva comes into contact with the skin of the host it penetrates it and enters the bloodstream reaching the lungs on the third day. Breaking through the alveoli it enters the bronchioles, moves up the trachea, down the oesophagus to the stomach and small intestine. During this migration the third moult takes place and the buccal capsule is formed. It arrives in the intestine on the seventh day and a fourth moult takes place, the buccal capsule assumes the adult form and the worm attaches itself to the mucosa of the small intestine, where they can be seen at post-mortem as small thread-like structures each containing a small red lining of ingested blood. In three to five weeks it becomes sexually mature and the female produces fertile eggs. Adult worms live from one to nine years and produce 30 000 eggs per day (necator 9000 eggs per day).

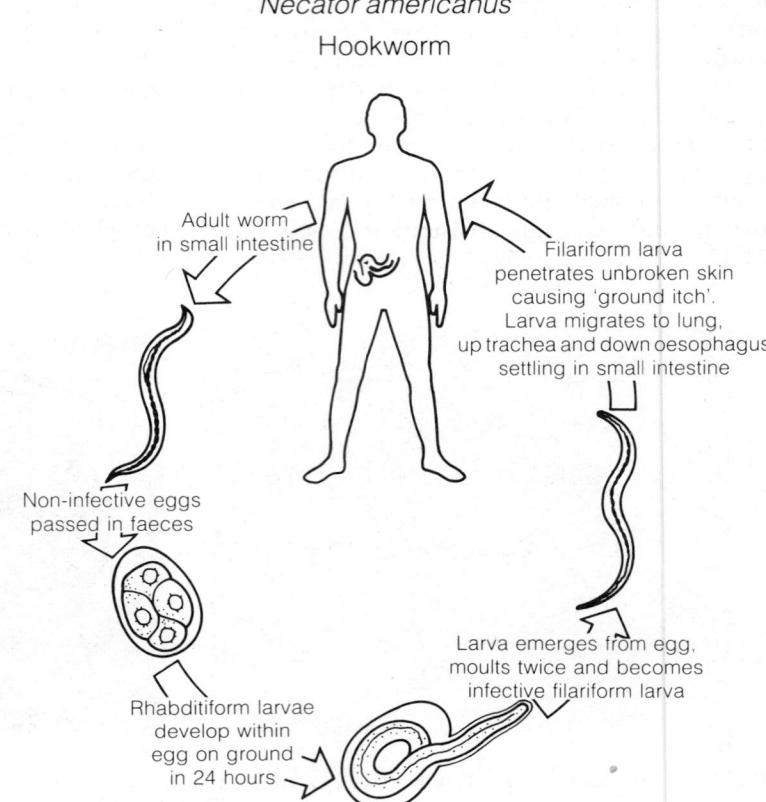

Necator americanus
Hookworm

Adult worm
in small intestine

Filariform larva
penetrates unbroken skin
causing 'ground itch'.
Larva migrates to lung,
up trachea and down oesophagus
settling in small intestine

Non-infective eggs
passed in faeces

Larva emerges from egg,
moults twice and becomes
infective filariform larva

Rhabditiform larvae
develop within
egg on ground
in 24 hours

Fig. 21.13 Life-cycle of hookworm.
(Courtesy WTIM.)

The life-cycles of *Ancylostoma* and *Necator* are similar except that:
1 *A. duodenale* can infect via the mucous membrane of the mouth as well as the skin.
2 *N. americanus* infects only through the skin.
3 Migrating larvae of *N. americanus* grow and develop in the lungs, whereas those of *Ancylostoma* do not.

The migrating infective filariform larvae of *A. duodenale* are arrested in their development and migrate to the mammary gland where they are excreted in the milk and infect the child.[42] Third stage infective filariform larvae of *N. americanus* have been found in the milk but none of the infected mothers were found to have infected babies.[43]

TRANSMISSION

Infection is normally acquired via the skin (or mouth) from *filariform* (infective) larvae in the soil contaminated by human faeces. However, other methods of transmission which are comparatively unimportant have been suggested:
1 Through eating uncooked meat containing the larvae of *A. duodenale* which have migrated into the muscles of the animal where they can survive for 26–34 days.[41]
2 Via human milk (hypobiosis as in *A. caninum* in puppies).

PATHOLOGY

Ancylostoma causes pathology at three stages of the infection (the first two caused by larval hookworm usually seen only in expatriates who receive a primary infection).
1 Vesiculation and pustulation at the site of entry (ground itch). This is usually mild or absent in the tropics except in expatriates.
2 Asthma and bronchitis during migration through the lungs with small haemorrhages into the alveoli and eosinophilic and leukocytic infiltration.

3 *Established infection* seen in the inhabitants of endemic areas leading to hookworm anaemia and hookworm disease.

Hookworm anaemia

The classical anaemia of hookworm infection is a hypochromic microcytic anaemia, the relationship of which to hookworm infection has long been debated. The main theories which have been put forward as to the causation of anaemia are chronic blood loss and depletion of iron stores with deficiency of iron intake and toxic factors.

Hookworms have been shown to produce active suction impulses 120–200 times per minute and evidence indicates that the hookworm is indeed an habitual blood-sucker or needs serum.[44] The blood loss has been estimated as 0.03 ml/day/worm in *N. americanus* and 0.15 ml/day/worm in *A. duodenale* infections.[44] There is a significant relationship between the level of haemoglobin and the worm burden, which depends upon the level of iron stores in the body.[45] Hookworm anaemia is of the iron deficiency type and responds dramatically to iron salts by mouth and also to removal of the hookworm burden, but after a much longer period. Light infections may cause anaemia where the iron intake is deficient and anaemia may also be caused in spite of the presence of an adequate iron intake, provided that the worm burden is heavy enough. A folate deficiency may be present masked by the severe iron deficiency anaemia and become overt only when this has been corrected.

Little is known about the anaemia which develops in light primary infections. It may be related to that which develops in pups infected with *A. caninum* and be of immunological origin.

HYPOPROTEINAEMIA

Loss of protein is an important feature of hookworm anaemia which is a cause of protein-losing enteropathy and the oedema of hookworm disease which does not respond to diuretics.[46] The protein loss, which is in excess of the red cell loss and is closely related to the hookworm load, is caused by a limited capacity for albumin synthesis as well as loss caused by anaemia and other factors such as liver disease.

Hookworm enteropathy

There have been conflicting reports on the role of hookworm in tropical malabsorption states. Structural abnormalities of the villi reverting to normal after deworming have been shown in Puerto Rico[47] and India,[48] but no changes were reported from Africa.[49] It has been suggested that it is the associated hypoalbuminaemia which is the cause of the enteropathy.

Pathological anatomy

In fatal cases the pathological changes are those of severe anaemia. There is plenty of fat in the usual situations. The appearance of plumpness is further increased by a greater or lesser amount of general oedema. There may be effusion in one or more of the serous cavities. The heart is dilated and flabby. The liver is fatty and the kidneys and all other organs pale.

If the post-mortem examination has been made within an hour or two of death the ancylostomes in numbers ranging from a few dozen up to many hundreds will be found attached by their mouths to the mucous surfaces of the lower part of the duodenum, jejunum and perhaps the upper part of the ileum. If the examination has been delayed for some time the parasites will have loosened their hold and are then found in the mucus coating the bowel. Many small extravasations of blood, some fresh, others of long standing, are seen in the mucous membrane and a minute wound in the centre of each extravasation represents the point at which a hookworm had been attached. Old extravasations are indicated by punctiform pigmentation. Occasionally streaks or large clots of blood are found in the lumen of the bowel and severe melaena may occur in children. The hookworms secrete some anticoagulant substance and may move from spot to spot, thereby increasing the damage and blood loss. The worms themselves may be seen in situ to show thin red streaks from fresh red blood in the intestinal canal; at other times they will be iron grey owing to the deposition of haemosiderin granules in the intestine.

IMMUNITY

Although many heavy infections can be found, light infections are more usual in endemic areas and the worm burden does not increase with age, suggesting that some method of controlling the worm burden is operating.

Dogs develop a partial protective immunity

towards *A. caninum* which in endemic areas can cause a 50% mortality from anaemia in early life. Pups that survive to adult life retain only minimal intestinal infection. After a single infection with 1000 irradiated *A. caninum* larvae a significant immunity can be demonstrated by worm counts following challenge with unirradiated larvae[50] but there was no evidence of protective immunity in a volunteer repeatedly exposed to infection with *A. duodenale*[51] and no evidence of protective immunity in a field study.[52] Primary infections in man may cause fever, eosinophilia and a moderate anaemia, even when the infection is light. Such light infections do not cause symptoms of anaemia in the indigenous inhabitants of endemic areas, suggesting that a partial immunity has developed. Immediate hypersensitivity develops in hookworm infections and a skin test using an antigen prepared from *N. americanus* larvae has been used in Venezuela to indicate both prevalence and load of hookworm infection.[53] Fluorescent antibody titres rise with primary infections and then decline but there is no correlation between titres and worm loads and cross reactions occur with *Strongyloides*.

CLINICAL FEATURES

Natural history

After the establishment of adult worms in the intestine at an early age in children exposed to infection, as soon as they can crawl the females start to lay eggs. The number of eggs passed bears a direct relation to the number of female worms. The higher the worm load the greater the blood loss so that where iron intake is satisfactory then up to 100 worms may cause no symptoms. With worm loads of 500–1000 then significant blood loss and anaemia will result, even in the presence of an adequate iron intake. It has been suggested that the freedom from hookworm anaemia shown by the African population of South and central Africa is due to the use of iron cooking pots which is also responsible for haemosiderosis, whereas in East Africa where aluminium pots are mostly used, haemosiderosis is not found but hookworm anaemia is common. Light infections last the lifetime of the host causing no trouble but in a minority and, in some areas a large minority, symptoms result from heavy infections.

Incubation period

In larval ancylostomiasis symptoms appear one to two weeks after the primary infection and in established infection eggs appear from the forty-second day onwards after infection.

Symptoms and signs

Larval hookworm

This is usually seen in a primary infection, most usually in non-immune expatriates. It is not so common or so marked as in *larval ascariasis*.

At the site of entry of the infective larvae there is a 'ground itch', which consists of an irritating vesicular rash limited to the exposed portion of the body, usually the soles of the feet or the hands. After one or two weeks pulmonary symptoms develop with a dry cough and asthmatic wheezing. Fever and a high degree of eosinophilia are found. These symptoms gradually disappear and ova of hookworm can be seen on or about day 42 after infection. The whole episode is self-limiting, lasting not more than two or three months.

Light infection (100 worms or under)

The main effects of light infections may be seen in Europeans and other expatriates who have arrived recently in an endemic area. The practitioner in the tropics should always be on the lookout for these cases, especially in children. Minor degrees of anaemia induce a tendency to fatigue and lassitude and digestive disturbances are common. Any of these symptoms in the presence of an eosinophilia should lead to the suspicion of infection.

Established infections in indigenous people

The essential symptoms of ancylostomiasis are connected with progressive iron deficiency anaemia associated with gastric and intestinal dyspepsia but not wasting. An early symptom is epigastric pain or discomfort which may be relieved by food and may be mistaken for duodenal ulcer. Although many people who suffer from irregular abdominal pain may show hookworm ova in the stools it does not necessarily follow that hookworm infection is the cause of the abdominal pain.

The taste may be perverted, some patients

exhibiting and persistently gratifying an unnatural craving for such things as earth, mud or lime (pica or geophagy). The stools may contain blood and frank melaena may occur in children. The occult blood test is always positive in the stools in cases where symptoms are caused by hookworm.

When the iron deficiency anaemia develops then symptoms of anaemia occur. The mucous surfaces and the skin become pale. The face is puffy and the feet and ankles swollen and there may be generalized oedema caused by the hypoalbuminaemia. There is lassitude, breathlessness, palpitations, tinnitus and vertigo, mental apathy, depression and liability to syncope. There is often koilonychia. There is a high output failure and haemic murmurs can be heard over the heart, which is seen to be enlarged on radiographic examination. Hookworm anaemia is a common cause of heart failure in the tropics and may easily be confused with rheumatic carditis. Ophthalmoscopic examination may reveal retinal haemorrhages. An irregular fever may be found in any severe anaemia.

The anaemia is typical of iron deficiency (see Chapter 58). The haemoglobin is reduced to a greater degree than the red cell count. The mean corpuscular volume is decreased and the mean corpuscular haemoglobin concentration may fall to as low as 22. The red cells show microcytosis and severe hypochromia. The serum iron is greatly reduced and the total iron-binding capacity of the serum greatly raised, indicating that iron stores are very low. There is no marked poikilocytosis or leukocytosis, although there may be an eosinophilia of 7–14%. The serum albumin is reduced in heavy infections. Because of the persistent anaemia, growth and development become stunted in children.

The rate of progress varies in different cases. In some a high degree of anaemia and even death may result within a few weeks or months of the appearance of the first symptoms. More frequently the disease is chronic, ebbing and flowing or slowly progressing through a long series of years. Prolonged exposure in the European has led to the production of the 'poor white', stunted in both mental and physical capacities.

DIFFERENTIAL DIAGNOSIS

In countries where hookworm infection is endemic, eggs may be found in the stool in any number of conditions which are not causally related. In these conditions an egg count is essential to determine the worm load (see below). Light infections in expatriates associated with moderate eosinophilia and mild anaemia must be differentiated from other helminth infections: *Schistosoma mansoni*, *Fasciola hepatica* and other liver flukes and *Strongyloides*. The epigastric pain associated with hookworm infection may suggest duodenal ulcer or pancreatitis and any patient from an endemic area with epigastric symptoms who has hookworm ova in the stool should be treated, since in many cases the symptoms will disappear without the need for any further investigation.

Severe hookworm anaemia must be distinguished from other iron deficiency anaemias, and generalized anasarca from kwashiorkor and the nephrotic syndrome.

DIAGNOSIS

The diagnosis is made by finding eggs in the stool (Fig. 21.12). Rhabditiform larvae may be found in stale stools and be mistaken for *Strongyloides* in which larvae only and not eggs are found in the stool (see Appendix IV, p. 1492, and Appendix II, Fig. II.53, p. 1358). The eggs may be confused with those of *Trichostrongylus* which are more translucent and smaller. In light infections concentration methods are necessary, such as zinc sulphate concentration, formol ether or the Kato smear (see Appendix IV). The worm load can be estimated by an egg count (Stoll egg count method, see Appendix IV). Since ancylostoma lays an average 25 000 eggs per day the number of eggs in a gram of stool multiplied by the daily stool weight in grams divided by 25 000 will give the estimated worm load. An egg count of 2500/g is significant and will be associated with symptoms. Less then 25 worms is insignificant while 500 to 1000 worms invariably cause disease.

Other diagnostic tests

Barium meal studies will not reveal the worms but radiological abnormality of the duodenum is closely related to haemoglobin levels in hookworm patients.[54] Serological diagnosis is not practical since there are so many cross reactions with other helminths.

TREATMENT

Treatment consists of elimination of the parasites and treatment of the anaemia if present. Treatment of the anaemia is the first priority but there is no reason why both objectives should not be proceeded with concurrently if non-toxic anthelmintics are used. Suggestions in the past that one drug might be best for one species and another for the other do not apply to modern drugs. Light asymptomatic infections are often best left untreated, especially if reinfection is probable.

Treatment is usually directed against the adult stages but there is evidence that albendazole in a single dose of 400 mg is active against the preintestinal larval stages of *N. americanus*.[55]

Elimination of adult parasites

In the past it was necessary to examine posttreatment stools for 48 hours and examine any worms passed to determine whether the infection in the area was *A. duodenale* or *N. americanus*, since the latter was much more resistant to treatment. With the more modern drugs this is no longer necessary. It is not necessary usually to remove all worms but to reduce the worm load significantly. The drug of choice is albendazole.

Albendazole. This is effective against both *A. duodenale* and *N. americanus*. A single dose of 400 mg will produce an 80% reduction in egg count and 200 mg daily for 3 days will give 100% cure. It is also highly effective against *Ascaris* and is therefore especially suitable for mass treatment.[13]

Mebendazole. A regimen of 100 mg twice daily for 3 days is highly effective against both *A. duodenale* and *N. americanus*.

Levamisole. A single dose of 150 mg orally or 2.5 mg/kg body weight is less effective against *N. americanus*.

Pyrantel pamoate (Combantrin). A single dose of 10 mg/kg body weight is given.

Bephenium hydroxynaphthoate (Alcopar). This has now largely been superseded but a single dose of 5 g will eradicate *A. duodenale* but three or more consecutive doses are necessary for *N. americanus*.

Tetrachlorethylene. The sole advantage of tetrachlorethylene is that it is cheap. It has to be given in a high dosage, 6 ml, which is relatively toxic and is now little used because of the danger with concurrent *Ascaris* infection.

EPIDEMIOLOGY AND CONTROL

The only reservoir of infection is man and the propagation of hookworm infection depends upon an adequate source of infection in the human population, the deposition of eggs in a favourable environment for extrinsic development of parasite, appropriate conditions of the soil (moisture and warmth) to allow larvae to develop and suitable conditions for the infective larvae to penetrate the skin. In many tropical and subtropical countries transmission is perennial but in cooler and drier climates transmission may take place in the warmer or wet seasons. In some temperate climates local environmental conditions may allow transmission, as in the Cornish tin-mines in the past and in the Rand in South Africa today. Cultural and agricultural practices such as the use of human faeces for fertilizer provide good opportunities for infection.

The methods which are employed to determine the amount of hookworm in a community are determination of the *prevalence* and *intensity* of infection by stool surveys and egg counts from which the worm burden can be calculated. These surveys will show whether the infection in the community is low grade, moderate or severe. Soil pollution in the area must also be studied and filariform larvae of hookworm can be demonstrated in soil by the Baermann method[39] or they can be cultured (see Appendix IV). Studies of the nutritional level of the community, especially the haemoglobin level, must also be undertaken.

The basis of prophylaxis and control is the provision of proper sanitary arrangements for the disposal of faeces. This was the basis of the hookworm campaigns originally organized in the southern USA by the Rockefeller Foundation. However, the success or failure of these campaigns depended upon health education and the correct use of latrines, and campaigns have often failed because this was not achieved.

Faecal contamination of the soil must be prevented and promiscuous deposition of faeces about huts, villages and fields must be forbidden. The Chinese plan of storing faeces for months in large cemented watertight pits is a good one since if the *Ancylostoma* larvae are kept in pure faeces they die in the absence of air and earth. After storing in this manner valuable fertilizer is secured for the agriculturist. In the tropics the larvae rarely survive longer than six to eight weeks and do not wander outside a 10 cm radius, but can migrate to the surface from a depth of 90 cm.

After the provision of latrines, intensive mass treatment in America has been found most effective; however, mass treatment campaigns have failed in most of the tropics. The provision of cheap shoes to prevent infections has failed because they are not worn where they are most needed, that is at home.

The fortification of a staple diet with iron salts has been suggested as a measure to build up the iron stores of the population in areas where hookworm infection is heavy and the dietary iron intake barely sufficient.

Mass treatment

With the availability of more effective non-toxic modern drugs, given as a single dose, mass treatment campaigns become a real possibility and by regularly reducing the worm load may greatly increase the haemoglobin level and health of the people. The only obstacle at present is the cost of the drugs.

Cutaneous larva migrans (creeping eruption, sandworm, plumber's itch, duckhunter's itch)

Cutaneous larva migrans is a cutaneous eruption resulting from exposure of the skin to the infective filariform larvae of non-human hookworms (*Ancylostoma braziliense*, *A. caninum*) and *Strongyloides* of the nutria and raccoon. The infective larvae cannot complete their normal life-cycle in the human host but persist under the skin without developing further where they cause cutaneous larva migrans.

GEOGRAPHICAL DISTRIBUTION

Creeping eruption occurs in most warm humid tropical and subtropical areas, being especially common in the southern USA, along the coast of the Gulf of Mexico and Florida. It is also common on the coasts of West, South and East Africa, South-East Asia, India, Malaysia, Sri Lanka and Thailand.

AETIOLOGY

Ancylostoma braziliense (see Appendix II, p. 1352) is the hookworm of dogs and cats. It is smaller than *A. duodenale* (female 1 cm and male 8.5 mm long), the internal pair of ventral teeth are smaller and the dorsal rays in the copulatory bursa are distinctive (Fig. II.42). The eggs are indistinguishable from those of human hookworms. The life-cycle is similar to that of *A.*

duodenale but man is an unsuitable host and the third stage larva does not enter the bloodstream but wanders under the skin causing cutaneous larva migrans.

A. caninum is the dog hookworm. Its life history is similar to that of *A. braziliense*.

Strongyloides. Filariform larvae of *S. stercoralis* can re-enter the skin as part of autoinfection around the anus and buttock where they cause larva currens, a rash rather like that of cutaneous larva migrans.

Strongyloides myopotami (nutria) and *Strongyloides procyornis* (raccoon) all produce similar lesions in the human host[56] in which they cannot complete their normal life-cycle. The lesions are more persistent.

TRANSMISSION

Infection is acquired from damp contaminated soil through the skin of that part of the body in contact with the soil (foot, abdomen).

PATHOLOGY

The filariform larvae are unable to penetrate below the stratum germinativum of human skin where they form a tunnel with the corium as a floor and the stratum granulosum as a roof. Local eosinophilia and round cell infiltration occurs round the tunnel which may persist for months. Rarely the larvae reach the lungs where they cause transitory pulmonary symptoms and eosinophilia and may be recovered from bronchial washings. They do not mature in the intestine.

IMMUNITY

Little is known about immunity. There is no protective immunity and people can be infected more than once.

CLINICAL FEATURES

Natural history

The larvae wander under the skin and can persist for months before they eventually die.

Incubation period

Symptoms start immediately after penetration of the skin, a matter of a few hours only

Symptoms and signs

There is a red itchy papule at the site of entry which becomes elevated and vesicular. The larvae move several millimetres to a few centimetres each day and leave tunnels which become dry and crusted. The track is linear and twists and turns (Fig. 21.14). It causes an intense pru-

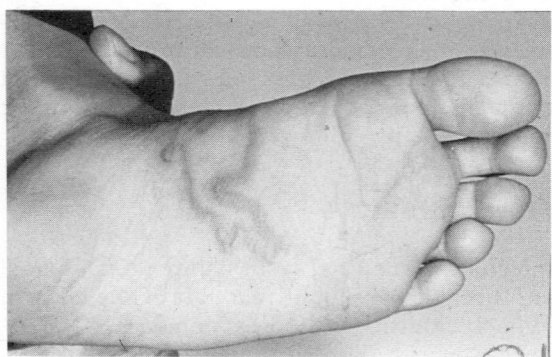

Fig. 21.14   Cutaneous larva migrans (*A. braziliense*).

ritus and the skin is scratched and becomes secondarily infected. The lesions may be single or multiple. The commonest sites are the hands and feet with *A. braziliense* but the abdomen is often infested in plumber's itch and the lesions may be very numerous indeed (Fig. 21.15).

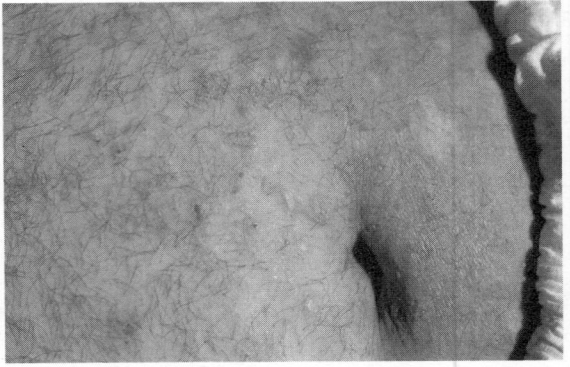

Fig. 21.15   Multiple burrows of cutaneous larva migrans (creeping eruption).

The lesions produced by non-human hookworms (cutaneous larva migrans) are well defined, move very slowly and persist for months. There is little surrounding flare and the track is indurated. In contrast the lesions produced by *Strongyloides* (larva currens) are less well defined, have a red flare on the outside, move much more rapidly and persist for a few hours only.

DIAGNOSIS

Creeping eruptions can be caused by *Strongyloides stercoralis* (larva currens, see p. 433), *Gnathostoma spinigerum* (see Chapter 24), *Cutaneous myiasis* (*Hypoderma bovis* and *Hypoderma lineatum*, see Chapter 51), warble fly maggots (*Gasterophilus*, see Chapter 51), cutaneous *Fasciola hepatica* (see Chapter 22).

The diagnosis is clinical. *Ancylostoma* larva migrans is usually situated on the foot or toe (Fig. 21.14) and lasts for months, moving very slowly. *Strongyloides* (larva currens) is situated on the buttocks and trunk and lasts for hours only, moving comparatively quickly. Non-human *Strongyloides* is usually situated on the trunk and abdomen and can persist for many months. *Loa loa* causes no cutaneous reaction and appears and disappears in a matter of minutes. There is usually no eosinophilia but if there is then internal migration of the larvae can be suspected. It is not possible to retrieve the larva since it is invariably in advance of its track and impossible to isolate. There are no serological tests.

TREATMENT

Thiabendazole is the drug of choice. It is given in a dose of 25 mg/kg twice daily for 5 days. A further 5 days' treatment may be necessary after 2 days' rest.[57] Itching should cease in 24 hours and the rash disappears in 10 days.

Strongyloides responds better to treatment than hookworms. Other dosage schedules are 50 mg/kg as a single dose weekly until the lesions disappear.[58,59]

Topical thiabendazole[60] is given by grinding up a 0.5 g tablet with 5 g of petroleum jelly and applying liberally over the track of the worm daily for 5 days.

Mebendazole is sometimes effective given in a dosage of 100 mg three times daily for 7 days.

Metriphonate can be given topically: 10% in petroleum jelly and covered with plastic over the worm tracks, left on overnight.

EPIDEMIOLOGY

The source of infection is soil contaminated with dog and cat faeces underneath beach houses on stilts, exposure taking place when people crawl underneath to repair facilities (plumber's itch) or bathe with bare feet and walk along the sand above the high water mark (sandworm) or expose themselves to mounds contaminated by nutria and raccoons in the marshes (duckhunter's itch). In subtropical countries exposure is commonest during the summer months and early autumn.

CONTROL

Little can be done to control dogs and cats but infection can be prevented by wearing sandals above the high water mark and protective clothing when underneath houses in hot areas.

Strongyloidiasis

GEOGRAPHICAL DISTRIBUTION

Strongyloides stercoralis has a worldwide distribution in the tropics and subtropics. It is highly prevalent in parts of tropical Brazil, Colombia and South-East Asia. In temperate climates it is not uncommon in inmates of institutions, such as mental hospitals, prisons and in mentally retarded children's homes. It has become a serious problem in individuals receiving suppressive treatment.

AETIOLOGY

Strongyloidiasis is caused by *Strongyloides stercoralis* (see Appendix II), a nematode worm which has two forms, one parasitic and the other free living. There are three developmental forms: adult, rhabditiform larva and filariform (infective) larva.

Life-cycle (Fig. 21.16)

There are two life-cycles in which reproduction takes place: an internal sexual cycle involving parasitic worms and an external sexual cycle involving free-living worms.

Internal sexual cycle

The adult female parasitic worm (2.5 × 0.034 mm) tapers anteriorly and ends in a conical tail. There is an oesophagus occupying a quarter of the body which has two bulbs divided by a constriction. The vulva lies in the posterior third of the body and there is a prominent uterus containing 50 eggs (50–58 × 30–34 μm) (Fig. II.52,1, p. 1357). The male exists but disappears from the bowel soon after oviposition and eggs can be produced parthenogenetically (as happens with *S. ratti*). The eggs hatch immediately in the bowel into male and female rhabditiform larvae which pass out in the faeces to continue the external sexual cycle.

External sexual cycle

The free-living rhabditiform larvae (Fig. II.52, 2, p. 1357) develop into free-living adults which copulate in the soil and produce eggs. The free-living forms have a double bulbed muscular oesophagus. The free-living female is smaller (1 × 0.05 mm) than the parasitic female, the vulva lies posteriorly and the uterus contains eggs measuring 70 × 40 μm (Fig. II.52,4, p. 1357). The male form measures 0.7 × 0.035 mm (Fig. II.52, 3, p. 1357). The rhabditiform larvae produced by both parasitic and free-living forms are indis-

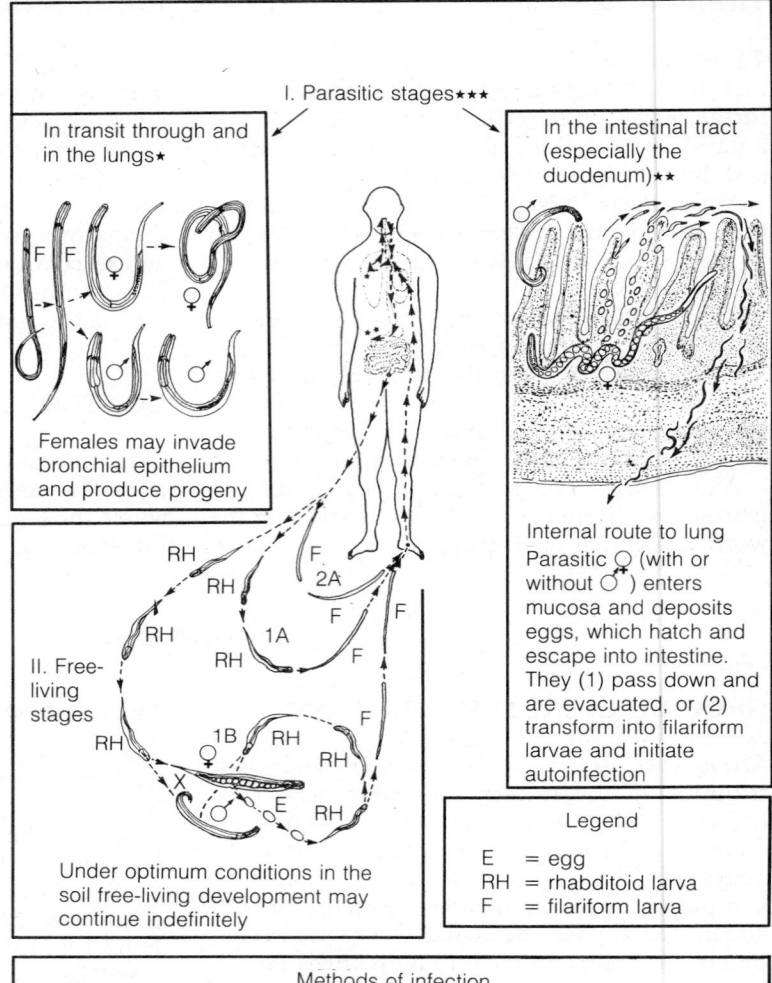

Fig. 21.16 Life-cycle of *Strongyloides stercoralis*.

tinguishable and develop into filariform (infective) larvae (Figs. 21.17 and II.52,5, p. 1357) which can remain alive in the soil for many weeks.

Infection and autoinfection

Under unsuitable conditions the external sexual cycle may be omitted and the filariform larvae infect the definitive host via the skin or buccal mucosa as in *Ancylostoma* or *Necator*. The larvae travel up to the lungs, enter the bronchi, cross over the glottis and pass to the small intestine where they mature into parasitic adults.

Autoinfection

Autoinfection, which results in multiplication in the host indefinitely, arises in one of two ways. The filariform larvae do not pass out in the stools

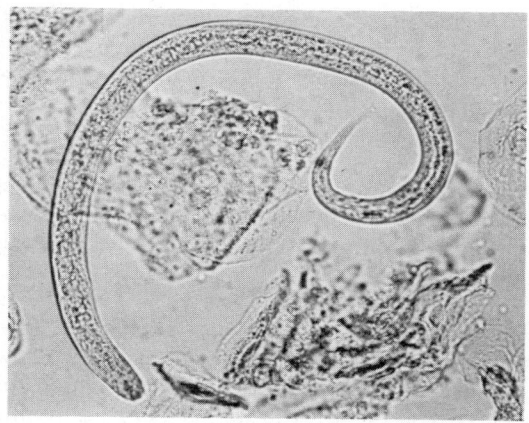

Fig. 21.17 *Strongyloides stercoralis*. Rhabditiform larva in stool. (Courtesy Dr J. S. Tatz.)

bur reinvade the bowel or skin. The other way is when the filariform larvae lodge in the bronchial epithelium and produce further progeny. Auto-infection leads to a build up in the body of the population so that the worms can maintain themselves in the absence of any further infection from an external source, and results in the intermittent recurrence of symptomatic episodes. In the case of any breakdown in the immune defences a rapid increase in the worm burden results in hyperinfection.

PATHOLOGY

The pathogenic effects begin with the entry of the infective larvae into the skin. The filariform larvae cause petechial haemorrhages at the site of invasion accompanied by intense pruritus, congestion and oedema. The larvae migrate into cutaneous blood vessels and are carried to the lungs. In the lungs they enter the alveoli and pass up the respiratory tree where they may be delayed by the host response, become adults and invade the bronchial epithelium. Passing through the lungs the young worms may cause symptoms resembling those of broncho-pneumonia with some lobular consolidation.

When they have become lodged in crypts of the intestine the females mature and invade the tissues of the bowel wall but rarely penetrate the muscularis mucosae, and move in tissue channels beneath the villi, where the eggs are deposited. The eggs hatch out and first stage larvae work towards the lumen of the bowel and are passed out in the faeces.

In heavy infections the first stage larvae, instead of passing out in the faeces, develop in the bowel, bore into the wall of the duodenum and jejunum and develop to the adult stage, producing ova, while encysted in the bowel. From the bowel they spread throughout the lymphatic system to the mesenteric lymph glands and can enter the general circulation and be found in the liver, lungs, kidneys and gallbladder wall. The ileum, appendix and colon are sites of reinvasion and here the worms cause granulomas with a central necrotic area often containing a degenerate larva. The mesenteric glands may be similarly affected. The lungs may show abscesses and the liver may be enlarged with small pinpoint larval granulomas. The larvae may carry micro-organisms and an overwhelming septicaemia caused by *Escherichia coli* has been caused in this way. In light infections jejunal biopsy has shown oedema, cellular infiltration and eosinophilic infiltration of the mucosa with partial villous atrophy.[61] At post-mortem, ulceration and atrophy of the mucosa are seen with numerous adult worms in the wall of the duodenum and jejunum. At times filariform larvae fail to break out of the alveoli, gain access to the general circulation and can invade the brain, intestine, lymph glands, liver, lungs and, rarely, myocardium.

TRANSMISSION

Infection is acquired originally from contaminated soil from free-living filariform infective larvae. Once established further infection may be acquired from the bowel or anal skin from parasitic infective larvae. The transmission of *Strongyloides* through the milk has been demonstrated in several animal species and it is possible that this occurs in man.

IMMUNITY

An immunity to reinfection develops in most individuals after a primary infection and the *Strongyloides* adults and larvae are confined to the small intestine and the worm load is controlled. Immunity is both antibody and cell mediated.

Humoral antibody-mediated immunity is elicited by the secretions of the infective larvae with a type I response, an eosinophilic tissue response and a peripheral eosinophilia often with urticarial rashes. Antibodies are produced which cross react with many other helminths including filariae.

Cell-mediated immunity is elicited by adult and larval worms in the tissues, which are localized and destroyed by a cell-mediated granulomatous reaction. If cell-mediated immunity is depressed for any reason, such as immunodepressive states or drugs, then a generalized hyperinfection results causing massive strongyloidiasis.

CLINICAL FEATURES

Natural history

In the majority of cases a small population of adult worms maintains itself in the small bowel for many years (30 or more) in the absence of any further infection from the outside causing recurrent symptoms when filariform larvae enter the perianal skin, and cause a recurrent rash (larva currens) sometimes associated with urticaria. In a small minority of cases the defences of the body break down and a generalized severe infection ensues.

Incubation period

The prepatent period from infection to the appearance of rhabditiform larvae in the stools is one month.

Symptoms and signs

The vast majority of infections in endemic areas are symptomless. When for various reasons the number of strongyloides present in the intestine increases then symptoms develop.

Diarrhoea. Watery mucous diarrhoea may develop, the degree of which depends on the intensity of the infection, its duration and the ability of the host tissues to encapsulate the worms. Frequently diarrhoea alternates with constipation.

Strongyloides enteropathy. Malabsorption of fat and vitamin B_{12} with chronic diarrhoea[61] and protein-losing enteropathy with malabsorption,[62] which were all rapidly reversed by anthelmintic treatment, have been described and the mechanism suggested is a hypersensitivity reagin-like reaction with the liberation of his-

tamine and increased capillary permeability and oedema of the lamina propria.[61] In massive strongyloidiasis the lacteals of the small bowel may be so involved that their obstruction causes malabsorption.

Hypereosinophilia. When autoinfection takes place, hypereosinophilia and pulmonary symptoms resembling tropical pulmonary eosinophilia may occur.

Skin rashes. These are of two types. One, occurring around the anus and anywhere on the trunk, is a linear eruption (larva currens) in which the larvae migrate under the skin causing an itching rash with a larval track which is not indurated and has a red flare at the edge which moves quite rapidly, disappearing in a few hours (Plate VI.4) in contrast to the more indurated and persistent track of non-human hookworm (cutaneous larva migrans). The second form is urticaria caused by allergy to the larvae penetrating the skin in an individual who has already been sensitized. The creeping type of eruption, which is seen mainly in infections from Indo-China and was common in prisoners of war in the Far East in the last war, can last for 30 years or more.

Massive strongyloidiasis. In persons debilitated by disease, malnutrition or serious illness, especially in institutions, serious illness and sometimes death may result from massive invasion of the tissues by strongyloides.[63] Treatment with immunosuppressive drugs for lymphoma and other conditions may produce the same result.[64] First stage larvae develop in the duodenum and jejunum, bore into the bowel wall, become adult and produce ova. In this way the number of strongyloides is immensely increased and infective larvae invade the tissues and circulate, causing massive strongyloidiasis. There is a severe diarrhoea, often with malabsorption, oedema, liver enlargement and paralytic ileus. In these cases encephalopathy is common and pyogenic meningitis with strongyloides larvae in the meninges has been described.[65,66] Fatal bowel infarction has occurred.[67] Prompt treatment with thiabendazole will save some of these patients.

Laboratory findings

Towards the end of the early stage of infection there is a high leukocytosis up to 25×10^9/litre and an eosinophilia of $10–12 \times 10^9$/litre is characteristic. Later when the infection is chronic there is a moderate eosinophilia which may persist for years. In generalized massive strongyloidiasis the eosinophilia disappears and is an indication of a poor prognosis.

DIFFERENTIAL DIAGNOSIS

Strongyloidiasis must be differentiated from other tissue invading helminths: *Ascaris*, ancylostomiasis and liver flukes. Disseminated strongyloidiasis may closely resemble tropical pulmonary eosinophilia, especially since serology cross reacts (see Chapter 20). Larva currens resembles cutaneous larva migrans but in distinction from it in larva currens the rash is situated mainly round the buttocks and on the trunk, lasts only a few hours and may occur intermittently for many years.

DIAGNOSIS

Only adults or rhabditiform larvae (Fig. 21.17) appear in the stools or duodenal drainage. They can be demonstrated by the formol ether method or cultured in charcoal at 26°C for a week (see Appendix IV, p. 1492).

The differentiation of the rhabditiform larvae from hookworm and *Trichostrongylus* is shown in Fig. II.53 (p. 1358) and Appendix IV (p. 1492). Radiological diagnosis is not much used but the appearances have been described by Louisey and Barton.[68]

Serology

There is considerable cross reaction with other helminths and filariae. The filarial complement fixation test (CFT) is positive in 45% of larva currens[69] and in 65% of acute cases but may be negative in massive strongyloidiasis. A sensitive ELISA test is also in use, but its specificity is not yet defined.

Immunofluorescence. The filarial fluorescent antibody test cross reacts and is sometimes useful in diagnosis. An indirect fluorescent antibody test (IFAT) using *Strongyloides* antigen with cross reacting antibodies absorbed with a 1/10 saline dilution of *Dirofilaria immitis* showed no cross reactions with filariasis and titres of 1/20 were significant.[70]

TREATMENT

Strongyloides should usually be treated whether or not the infection is giving rise to symptoms. It should especially be looked for and treated in immunosuppressed patients, for example those on steroid therapy. Both thiabendazole and mebendazole are effective. Massive strongyloidiasis responds very effectively.[71] Thiabendazole is effective in a dose of 25 mg/kg twice daily for 3 days. Mebendazole 100 mg three times a day for 7 days has proved moderately effective, but two to four weeks' treatment is needed to achieve high cure rates. Albendazole, 400 mg once or twice daily for 3 days, will probably prove to be the drug of choice.

EPIDEMIOLOGY

Man is the most important host of *Strongyloides* but dogs and chimpanzees have been found infected with strains indistinguishable from those of man. Larvae are unable to survive temperatures below 8°C or above 40°C or desiccation. Strongyloidiasis thrives in conditions of overcrowding on damp soil in tropical conditions such as rural villages in South-East Asia. It was very common amongst prisoners of war in Burma and Indo-China in the Second World War, but it may also become established in deep mines in cold climates.

CONTROL

Control methods are the same as for hookworm: prevention of contact with the soil by wearing shoes and control of excreta.

Strongyloides fülleborni

GEOGRAPHICAL DISTRIBUTION

Strongyloides füllerborni is widely distributed in monkeys and in Pygmies in Zaire and Zambia in forested areas. In Papua New Guinea human infection is widely distributed in western Papua New Guinea, along the Fly river and in the eastern highlands in forested areas.[72]

AETIOLOGY

Strongyloides fülleborni can be distinguished from *S. stercoralis* by the prominent vulvar lips, narrowing behind the vulva and a prominent oesophagus. Eggs are passed in the stool in contrast to *S. stercoralis* and resemble those of hookworm for which they are commonly mistaken. There may be two strains of the parasite, one in Africa and the other in Papua New Guinea. The life-cycle is similar to that of *S. stercoralis*.

TRANSMISSION

Transmission is similar to that of *S. stercoralis* from contaminated soil; although in infants the route has not been determined, transmission via the placenta or milk has been suggested.

PATHOLOGY

Pathology as far as is known, is similar to that of *S. stercoralis*; although heavy populations may build up without ill effect in infants abdominal symptoms with oedema may result causing 'swollen belly' sickness, probably from protein loss.

SYMPTOMS AND SIGNS

In most cases there are no symptoms at all; 24% of Pygmies in Zaire were found to be passing ova[73] and very heavy infections were found without any evidence of disease. In infants in New Guinea 'swollen belly' sickness is characterized by respiratory distress, abdominal distension, generalized oedema and variable disturbance of gastrointestinal function.[74]

DIAGNOSIS

Ova resembling hookworm can be demonstrated in the stool and distinction from hookworm ova made by culturing the stool to obtain adults and then identify them.

TREATMENT

Thiabendazole and mebendazole are effective as used in *S. stercoralis* infection. Plasma infusions to correct hypoproteinaemia may be necessary.

EPIDEMIOLOGY

S. fülleborni is a zoonosis infecting monkeys and apes in tropical Africa where it is common in human populations in the rain forest. Although it is a zoonosis interhuman transmission may occur[75] and 24% of Pygmies have been found infected.[73] In Papua New Guinea infection, which is abundant in children from three to five years old, is rare in adults; there it is confined to mainly forested areas in western New Guinea, along the Fly river and in the eastern highlands which suggests a zoonosis, although no animal host has been identified.

Trichostrongyliasis

GEOGRAPHICAL DISTRIBUTION

Normally a parasite of sheep and goats, human infection with *Trichostrongylus* is widespread in central Africa, Egypt and in Asia in India, Assam, Indonesia and Japan.

AETIOLOGY

Three species can infect man: *Trichostrongylus colubriformis*, *T. orientalis* and, more rarely *T. probolurus*. The female worm (5–8 × 0.07 mm) is slender and pink with a posterior vulva (Fig.

II.50A, p. 1356); the male (4–5 × 0.07 mm) has bilobed copulatory bursa and two spicules (Fig. II.50B, p. 1356). The mouth is unarmed. The parasites are situated in the duodenum and jejunum where they are not attached to the bowel but are a half to a third buried in mucus. The eggs, which have a transparent hyaline shell, resemble those of hookworm but are larger (85 × 115μm), are passed in the stool in the morula stage and are remarkably resistant to desiccation and cold. The life-cycle is similar to that of hookworm but they do not migrate through the lungs. Adults mature in the intestine within 25–30 days.

TRANSMISSION

Infection is acquired through the skin or mouth from contaminated food or drink.

PATHOLOGY

Little is known about pathology and none has been observed, even in individuals with high egg counts.

SYMPTOMS AND SIGNS

These are few but mild anaemia and general ill-health may result.

DIAGNOSIS

Diagnosis is made by finding eggs in the stool and adults after treatment.

TREATMENT

Levamisole is the drug of choice and is given as a single oral dose of 2.5 mg/kg. Thiabendazole is less effective.

EPIDEMIOLOGY

T. colubriformis is a parasite of sheep and goats and is common in some areas where sheep and goats are kept and up to 70% of the inhabitants may be infected.

T. orientalis is common among people who look after donkeys and goats and the use of human excreta as fertilizer in Asia is responsible for the high level of infection.

OTHER NEMATODES FOR WHOM MAN IS NOT THE NORMAL HOST

Trichinosis (*Trichinella spiralis*)

GEOGRAPHICAL DISTRIBUTION
(Fig. 21.18)

Trichinosis has a worldwide distribution and is important as an infection of man in Europe and the USA. It is less important in the tropics but occurs in both East and West sub-Saharan Africa. It is an important cause of disease and death in the Arctic where polar expeditions have died as a result of trichinosis.

AETIOLOGY

Trichinella spiralis occurs in two forms: adult and cystic.

The adult *Trichinella spiralis* (Fig. II.58, p. 1362) is a white worm just visible to the naked eye which inhabits the small intestine. The male

(1.6 × 0.04 mm) has a cloaca situated posteriorly between two caudal papillae. The female (3–4 × 0.06 mm) has a vulva in the anterior fifth, an ovary in the posterior half of the body and a coiled uterine tube in the anterior portion.

Life-cycle (Fig. 21.19)

The female lives for 30 days and is viviparous. The eggs (20μm) live in the upper uterus and the larvae (100 × 6 μm) break out, living free in the uterine cavity. One female produces more than 1500 larvae. The larvae, which emerge as early as 4–7 days after infection, continue to be produced for four to 16 weeks. They make their way via the lymphatics and blood circulation to the right heart and lungs where they enter the arterial circulation and reach striated muscle where they encyst.

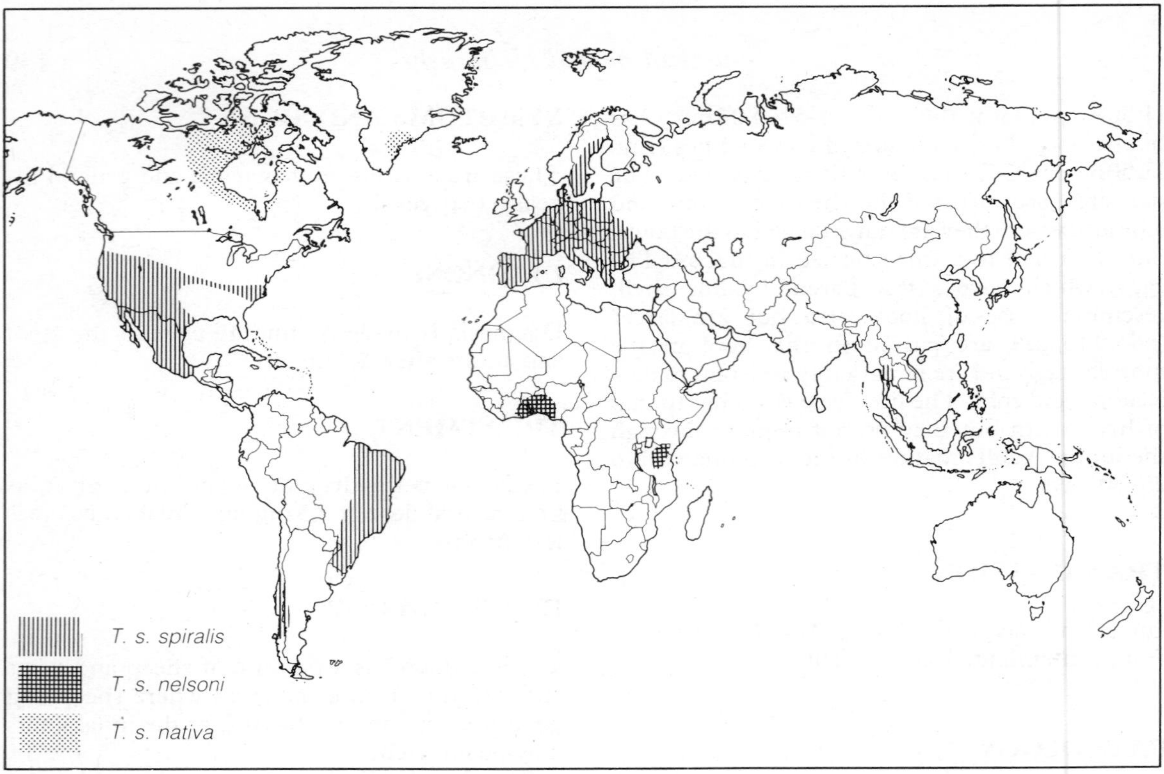

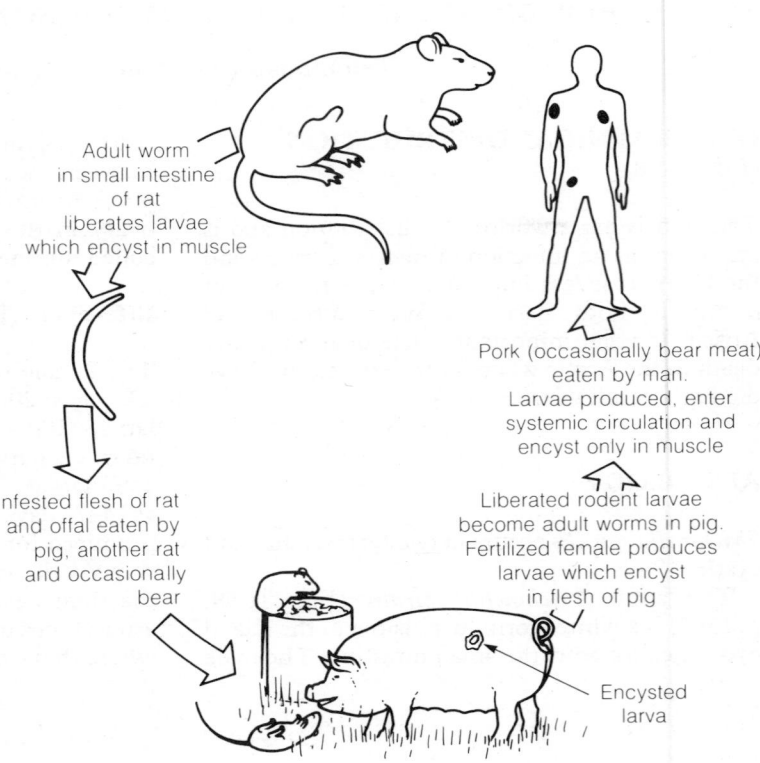

Fig. 21.18 Geographical distribution of trichinosis.

Legend:
- T. s. spiralis
- T. s. nelsoni
- T. s. nativa

Trichinella spiralis

Adult worm
in small intestine
of rat
liberates larvae
which encyst in muscle

Pork (occasionally bear meat)
eaten by man.
Larvae produced, enter
systemic circulation and
encyst only in muscle

Infested flesh of rat
and offal eaten by
pig, another rat
and occasionally
bear

Liberated rodent larvae
become adult worms in pig.
Fertilized female produces
larvae which encyst
in flesh of pig

Encysted
larva

Fig. 21.19 Life-cycle of *Trichinella spiralis*.

Cystic stage

The cyst is formed by the larva encapsulated by the host tissue. The capsule is an adventitious ellipsoidal sheath with blunt ends resulting from cellular reaction around the tightly coiled larva (Fig. 21.20). The long axis parallels that of the muscle fibres and host amino acids nourish it so that it can remain alive for many years. In man calcification may take place after six months and lead to death of the larva. When consumed by a carnivorous host the cysts are digested in the stomach and after encysting the larvae, which are resistant to gastric juice, invade the duodenal and jejunal mucosa where they penetrate the columnar epithelium and develop into adults after 36 hours. The period between infection and the encysting stage in the muscles is 17–21 days.

Species and strains of *Trichinella*

Trichinella spiralis contains three subspecies which can infect man. They are indistinguishable morphologically but vary in their host specificity and can be distinguished enzymatically.[76]

Trichinella spiralis spiralis of temperate regions with domestic pigs the source of human infection.

Trichinella spiralis nativa of the Arctic regions; a parasite of carrion feeding carnivores; polar bears and walruses are the main sources of human infection.

Trichinella spiralis nelsoni in Africa and southern Europe in wild carnivores with wild pigs the source of human infection.

T. s. nativa is very resistant to freezing and *T. s. nelsoni* and *T. s. nativa* have a low infectivity for domestic pigs and rats.

TRANSMISSION

Transmission is by mouth from eating undercooked meat.

T. s. spiralis

Human infection is acquired from eating undercooked pork from infected pigs. The pigs are infected from eating raw garbage or perhaps from eating rats which themselves become infected from garbage.

T. s. nativa

Human infection is acquired from eating bear meat (the top predator), polar bear in the Arctic and brown bears in sub-Arctic regions of the USSR and North America. Walrus meat can also be infective. Polar explorers have died as a result of eating polar bear meat.

T. s. nelsoni

Human infection results from eating bush-pig or wart-hog meat which are infected themselves from carrion.

PATHOLOGY

The capsule of the infective larva is digested in the intestine since it is resistant to the gastric juice and penetrates the duodenal and jejunal mucosa where the amount of trauma and irritation depends upon the number of larvae. This will cause the symptoms of the *enteric phase*.

After 5–7 days the worms mature and the females discharge larvae to the tissues causing symptoms of the *migratory or invasive* stage. Later the larvae encyst causing symptoms of the *encystment* stage. Larvae only encyst in striated muscle but travel through the brain and heart muscle where they are unable to encyst.

Striated muscle

Larvae after travelling through the circulation encyst in muscles of the diaphragm, masseters, intercostals, laryngeal, tongue and ocular muscles. At first there is a basophilic degeneration of the muscle fibres followed by formation of a hyaline capsule around the larva with an inflammatory infiltrate of lymphocytes and a few eosinophils (Figs. 21.20 and II.60, p. 1363). Foreign body giant cells may be present. The infiltrate subsides and fat is deposited at the poles and after six months calcification takes place, eventually leading to death of the larva.

Brain

Larvae migrate through the brain and meninges causing leptomeningitis, granulomatous nodules in the basal ganglia, medulla, cerebellum and perivascular cuffing in the cortex. They can be

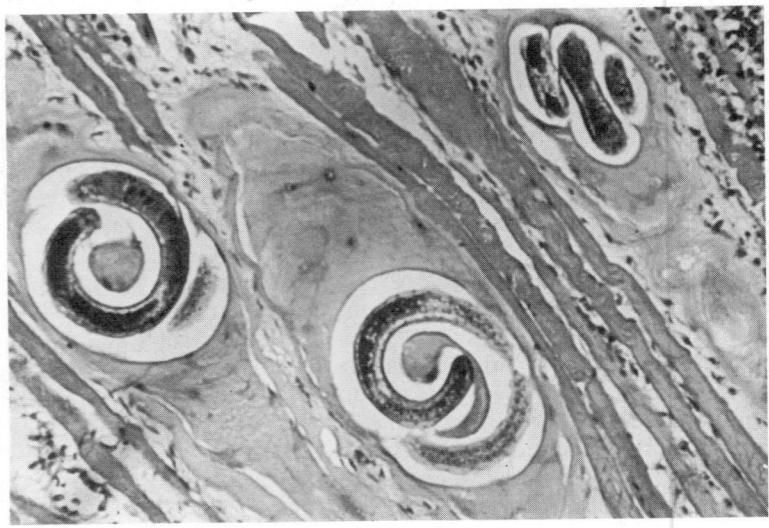

Fig. 21.20 Larva of *T. spiralis* in muscle.

found in the cerebrospinal fluid with a raised cell count and increased protein.

Heart

The larvae cause considerable damage on passage through the myocardium, cellular infiltration and necrosis with subsequent fibrosis of the myocardial bundles.

IMMUNITY

Natural immunity

Natural immunity is confined to cold-blooded animals with a temperature below 37°C.

Aequired immunity

A well-marked immunity to reinfection develops after the first infection but it is necessary for the infective larvae to develop through to the adult stage before immunity is produced, which is both antiadult and antilarval. Cell-mediated immunity is largely responsible but humoral antibodies develop.[77] Immunized mice respond rapidly to challenge infections with an inflammatory reaction in the bowel and the elimination of adult worms. Cellular immunity can be transferred by cellular elements and diminished by corticosteroids, adrenalectomy and whole body irradiation.

A type I hypersensitivity reaction is responsible for most of the pathology of the migratory or invasive phase, fever, oedema, rash, hypereosinophilia and tissue damage. Immune complexes are not apparently important. Humoral antibodies develop and are used in diagnosis. Cellular immunity is responsible for sealing off the cysts during the stage of encystment. Both immediate and delayed hypersensitivity can be demonstrated by skin tests.

CLINICAL FEATURES

Natural history

Trichinosis is a self-limiting infection lasting in light infections two to three weeks and in heavy infections at the most two to three months. Except in heavy infections mortality is low. Light infections are often asymptomatic and routine examination of diaphragms at autopsy have shown a significant number containing calcified cysts in endemic areas.

Incubation period

From eating infected meat the development of symptoms of the enteric phase is up to 7 days after infection and for the migratory phase from 7 to 21 days.

Symptoms and signs

The symptomatology depends upon the level of infection and can be related to the number of larvae per gram of muscle. Light infections (subclinical) up to 10 larvae, moderate 50 to 500 larvae and severe and possibly fatal infections more than 1000. In symptomatic cases symptoms develop in three stages: enteric (invasion of the intestine) phase, migration of the larvae (invasive phase) and a period of encystation in the muscles.

Enteric phase

Irritation and inflammation of the duodenum and jejunum where the larvae penetrate causes nausea, vomiting, colic and sweating, resembling an attack of acute food poisoning. There may be a maculopapular skin rash and in a third of the cases symptoms of a pneumonitis occur between the second and sixth day lasting about 5 days.

Migratory (invasion) phase

The cardinal symptoms and signs of this phase are severe myalgia, periorbital oedema and eosinophilia. There is difficulty in mastication, breathing and swallowing due to the involvement of the muscles and there may be some muscular paralysis of the extremities. There is a high remittent fever with typhoidal symptoms, splinter haemorrhages under the nails and in the conjunctivae and blood and albumin in the urine. Characteristically there is a hypereosinophilia from the fourteenth day which decreases after a week and persists at a lower level. An absence of eosinophilia denotes a poor prognosis. The lymph glands may be enlarged as well as the parotid and submental glands. Occasionally there is splenomegaly. In severe cases there may be subpleural, gastric and intestinal haemorrhages.

MYOCARDIAL COMPLICATIONS

Myocardial complications are frequent and may lead to congestive heart failure four to eight weeks after infection; between the second and fifth week sudden death from dysrhythmia or congestive heart failure with peripheral oedema may occur. Pericardial effusion is common. Most cases recover completely but a few continue with chronic cardiac disability.

NEUROLOGICAL COMPLICATIONS

During the passage of larvae through the central nervous system symptoms of meningitis, meningoencephalitis and focal cerebral lesions may develop. Ocular disturbances, diplegia, deafness and a syndrome resembling motor neuron disease, epileptiform attacks and coma may occur in very heavy infections.

Encystment phase

This is the third stage and may be severe. There may be cachexia, oedema and extreme dehydration. During the second month after infection there is a decrease in muscle tenderness, fever and itching subside and congestive heart failure may appear. Damage to the brain may persist with protean neurological signs which may clear up later or persist. Gram-negative septicaemia from organisms introduced by the larvae,[78] permanent hemiplegia[79] and Jacksonian epilepsy 10 years after an attack of trichinosis have been described.

Prognosis

Death is unusual except in cases of heart failure when it occurs during the sixth and seventh week from exhaustion, heart failure, pneumonitis, peritonitis or nephritis. Persistent leakage of larval antigen leads to a continued low eosinophilia and circulating antibody with positive serology and immediate and delayed hypersensitivity.

DIFFERENTIAL DIAGNOSIS

Trichinosis resembles many conditions: typhoid, encephalitis, myositis and tetanus; with the association with a high eosinophilia it closely resembles the tissue stages of schistosomiasis (Katayama syndrome), hookworm, *Strongyloides* and other helminthic infections. Trichinosis may also resemble collagen disorders such as periarteritis nodosa and acute rheumatoid arthritis.

DIAGNOSIS

Diagnosis is made by demonstrating larvae and by serology.

Demonstration of larvae

Larvae have been isolated from the peripheral blood in the early stages of the migration phase by mixing blood with dilute acetic acid and centrifuging. Larvae may be demonstrated in muscle by trichinoscopy.

Trichinoscopy

This can only be used when the encystment phase has started from 7 days after infection onwards. Samples (1 cm^2) of deltoid, biceps, gastrocnemius or pectoralis major are digested with 1% pepsin and 1% hydrochloric acid for several hours at 37°C, filtered or centrifuged and the number of larvae per gram of muscle estimated. Larvae can also be seen on muscle pressed between two slides which is more useful in the first three weeks of the disease.

Xenodiagnosis can be performed by feeding diaphragmatic tissue to uninfected albino white rats and examining them one month later.

Biochemical tests

In the acute phase there are serum enzyme changes with a rise in the creatine phosphokinase, lactate dehydrogenase and myokinase levels.[80]

Serology

Circulating antibody can be detected as early as two weeks in heavy infections and three to four weeks in lighter infections. Titres fall markedly after one to two years but decrease before this. The bentonite and latex (BFT and LFT) tests, IFAT and ELISA tests are now used. The antigens used are larval antigens originally extracted in Coca's fluid or an acid-soluble protein fraction—Melcher antigen[81]—but more refined antigens are becoming available.

BFT and LFT

The BFT and LFT are tests of choice. Bentonite and latex particles are added to trichinella extract and glycerine solution. The reagents are stable and the tests are easily and quickly performed. They detect antibody during the acute stage of the disease[82,83] becoming positive about day 15. A titre of 1:5 is diagnostic.

Immunofluorescence (IFAT)

The IFAT becomes positive in high titre from two to three weeks after infection falling to a lower level after three months.

ELISA

The ELISA has proved most useful, being very sensitive.

TREATMENT

Treatment is directed against the larvae and against the immune reaction they invoke.

Larvicidal

Mebendazole. Prolonged oral high dosage with mebendazole has proved effective. A dose of 20 mg/kg body weight 6-hourly for two weeks has proved larvicidal and may have to be repeated.[84]

Immunosuppression

In severe life-threatening infections the immune response must be controlled and prednisone 20 mg three times daily is given, initially reducing and finally discontinuing over a period of two to three weeks. Some cases are resistant to prednisone. Old calcified larvae do not need any treatment.

EPIDEMIOLOGY (Fig. 21.21)

Man is not the normal host of *T. spiralis* and becomes infected only after eating raw or undercooked flesh. The usual type, *T. s. spiralis*, found in Europe and North America is an infection of the black and brown rats by which it is propagated. These rats are cannibalistic and may be eaten by domestic pigs which infect man when he eats raw or undercooked pork. This type is common wherever uncooked sausage is eaten, especially in Germany and other areas of the world to which Germans have gone, for example, North America and Chile.

Clinical illness is most likely to occur when sausage prepared from a single heavily infected pig is eaten by a family or community. Where the meat has been diluted by uninfected meat then the disease is mild or subclinical. In the USA two outbreaks occurred in 1956 and one in 1957[85] and a severe epidemic occurred in England in Liverpool in 1953. Under the conditions developed by man for raising and fattening pigs, garbage which contains unsterilized pig scraps and other trimmings is the commonest

Temperate zone: *T.s. spiralis*

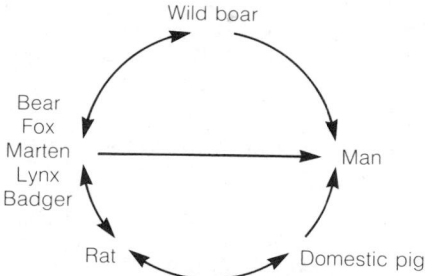

Africa: *T.s. nelsoni*

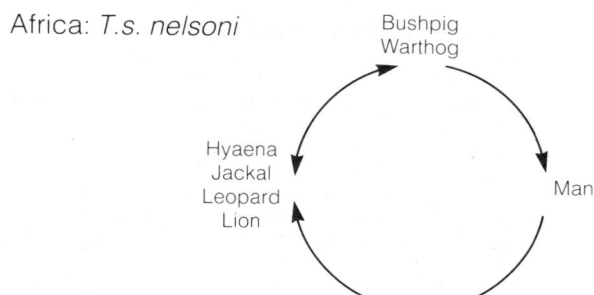

Arctic: *T.s. nativa*

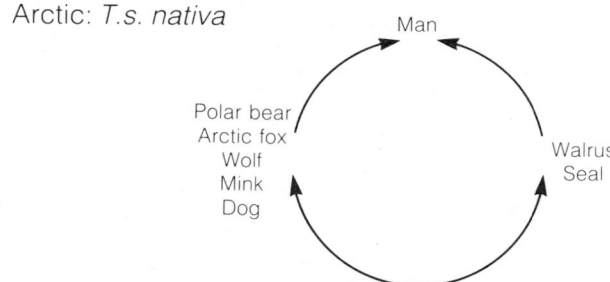

Fig. 21.21 Epidemiology of *T. spiralis*.

source of infection in pigs in the USA at the present time. Another possible source is the ingestion of faeces of other infected animals, mice, rats, foxes and other pigs at a time when mature larvae are becoming established in the intestinal wall.[86] The majority of infections are symptomless and Link[87] has estimated 350 000 new infections in the USA yearly, of which only 16 000 produced symptoms. It is estimated that subclinical trichinosis can be demonstrated in 20% of the population in the USA and 1% in England by digestion of material obtained at autopsy.

T. s. nativa is found mainly in Alaska and the northern regions of the world.[88] Here trichinosis is found in the white whale, walrus, hair seal, tree squirrel, black and white polar bear, dog, wolf, fox and wolverine. The polar bear, which is at the top of the Arctic food pyramid, is usually heavily infected and is the usual source, along with the black and brown bear, of human infections. Bear meat is eaten as a luxury and as an essential food in polar regions and whole expeditions have died of trichinosis after eating polar bear meat. Two epidemics have been reported from Alaska as a result of the consumption of black bear meat.[89] In 1947 an epidemic occurred in Greenland with 300 cases and 33 deaths caused by eating walrus meat.

T. s. nelsoni is found in Africa south of the

Sahara where it has been described from East Africa[90] and Senegal.[91] The infection is found in bush pigs (*Potamochoerus porcus*) and in the lion, leopard, cheetah and hyena. Man is infected when he eats the bush pig; domestic pigs are not infected.

PREVENTION

The main method of prevention is thorough cooking of all meat and regular meat inspection by means of trichinoscopy of all pork. Effective treatment of pork may be instituted by means of refrigeration. Storage of pork in deep freeze units at $-18°C$ to $-15°C$ is effective. The cysts are destroyed by storage at $-15°C$ for 20 days, $-20°C$ for 10 days, $-25°C$ for 6 days and immediately by quick freezing at $-37°C$.[92]

Cooking of all garbage will prevent the infection of pigs and dressed pork may be irradiated by cobalt-60 or caesium-137, which kills the cysts. In the Arctic and sub-Arctic regions bear meat should be avoided.

REFERENCES

1 Loeffler, P. (1956) *Archs. int. Allergy* **8**, 54.
2 Beaver, P.C. & Danaraj, T.J. (1958) *Am. J. trop. Med. Hyg.* **7**, 100.
3 Parsons, H.E. (1952) *Archs Ophthal.* **6**, 799.
4 Reddy, C.R.M., Rao, D.V., Sarma, E.N.B. & Swamy, G.M.N. (1975) *J. trop. Med. Hyg.* **78**, 146.
5 Horrilleno, E.G., Limbo, D.M., Eufemio, G.G. et al (1964) *J. philipp. med. Ass.* **40**, 40.
6 Louw, J.H. (1974) *S. Afr. J. Surg.* **4**, 219.
7 Batu, A., Myint, S., Myint, A. et al (1975) *Trans. R. Soc. trop. Med. Hyg.* **69**, 167.
8 Carswell, F., Meakins, R.H. & Harland, P.S.E.G. (1976) *Lancet* **ii**, 706.
9 Venkatachalak, P.S. & Patwardhan, V.N. (1953) *Trans. R. Soc. trop. Med. Hyg.* **47**, 169.
10 Williams, J.F. & Soulsby, E.J.L. (1970) *Exp. Parasit.* **26**, 290.
11 Gelpi, A.P. & Mustafa, A. (1967) *Am. J. trop. Med. Hyg.* **16**, 646.
12 Soulsby, W.J.L. (1957) *Br. vet. J.* **113**, 439.
13 Bassily, S., El-Masry, N.A., Trabolksi, B. et al (1984) *Ann. trop. Med. Parasitol.* **78**, 81–82.
14 El-Masry, N.A., Trabolski, B., Bassily, S. et al (1983) *Trans. R. Soc. trop. Med. Hyg.* **77**, 160–161.
15 Brudastov, A.N., Lemelev, V.R., Kholmukhamedov, S.K. et al (1971) *Med. Parazit. (Mosk.)* **40**, 165.
16 Beaver, P.C., Snyder, C.H., Carrera, G.M. et al (1952) *Pediatrics, Springfield* **9**, 7.
17 Wilder, H.C. (1950) *Trans. Am. Acad. Ophthal.* **55**, 99.
18 Ree, G.H., Voller, A., & Rowland, H.A.K. (1984) *Br. med. J.* **288**, 628–629.
19 Dent, J.H., Nichols, R.L., Beaver, P.C. et al (1956) *Am. J. Path.* **32**, 777.
20 Beaver, P.C. (1969) *J. Parasit.* **55**, 3.
21 Woodruff, A.W. (1970) *Br. med. J.* **3**, 663.
22 Wang, C., Huang, C.Y., Chan, P.H. et al (1983) *Lancet* **i**, 423.
23 Bisseru, B. & Woodruff, A.W. (1968) *J. clin. Path.* **21**, 449.
24 Savigny, D.H., Voller, A. & Woodruff, A.W. (1979) *J. clin. Path.* **32**, 284.
25 Smith & Gradoni (1984).
26 Brunello, F., Genchi, C. & Falangiani, P. (1983) *Trans. R. Soc. trop. Med. Hyg.* **77**, 280.
27 Woodruff, A.W., Bisseru, B. & Bowe, J.C. (1966) *Br. med. J.* **i**, 1576.
28 Botero, D. & Little, M. (1984) *Am. J. trop. Med. Hyg.* **33**, 381–386.
29 Schuffner, W. (1944) *Munch. Med. Wschr.* **31**, 411.
30 Daly, J.J. & Baker, G.F. (1984) *Am. J. trop. Med. Hyg.* **33**, 62–64.
31 Pearson, R.D., Irons, R.P. & Irons, R.P., Jr (1981) *J. Am. med. Ass.* **245**, 1340–1341.
32 Shiraki, T., Otsuru, M., Kenmotsu, N. et al (1974) *Jap. J. Parasit.* **23**, 125.
33 Muller, R. (1975) *Worms and Disease. A Manual of Medical Helminthology.* Heinemann, London.
34 Jung, R. & Beaver, P.C. (1952) *Pediatrics, Springfield* **8**, 548.
35 Wolfe, M.S. (1978) *Clinics in Gastroenterology* **7**, 201–217.
36 Swartzwelder, J.C. (1939) *Am. J. trop. Med.* **19**, 437.
37 Gilman, R.H., Davis, C. & Fitzgerald, F. (1976) *Trans. R. Soc. trop. Med. Hyg.* **70**, 313.
38 Kan, S.P. (1938) *Am. J. trop. Med. Hyg.* **32**, 118–122.
39 Faust, E.C. & Russell, P.F. (1964) *Craig and Faust' Clinical Parasitology*, 7th edn. Philadelphia: Lea & Febiger.
40 Manter, H.W. (1967) *J. Parasit.* **53**, 3.
41 Schad, G.A., Murrell, K.D., Fayer, R. et al (1984) *Trans. R. Soc. trop. Med. Hyg.* **78**, 203–204.
42 Schad, G.A., Chowdhury, A.B., Dean, C.C. et al (1973) *Science* **180**, 502.
43 Setasurban, P., Punsri, P. & Muennoo, C. (1980) *S.E. Asian J. trop. Med. Publ. Hlth* **11**, 535–583.
44 Roche, H. & Layrisse, M. (1966) *Am. J. trop. Med. Hyg.* **15**, 1031.
45 Foy, H. & Kondi, A. (1960) *Trans. R. Soc. trop. Med. Hyg.* **54**, 419.
46 Brumpt, L.C. & Ho Thi Sang (1955) *Bull. Soc. Path. éxot.* **48**, 46.
47 Sheehy, T.W., Meroney, W.H., Cox, R.S. et al (1962) *Gastroenterology* **42**, 148.
48 Burman, N.N., Sehgal, A.K., Chakravarti, R.N. et al (1970) *Indian J. med. Res.* **58**, 317.
49 Gilles, H.M., Watson-Williams, E.J. & Ball, P.A.J. (1964) *Q. Jl. Med.* **33**, 1.
50 Miller, T.A. (1965) *J. Am. vet. med. Ass.* **146**, 41.
51 Ball, P.A.J. & Bartlett, A. (1969) *Trans. R. Soc. trop. Med. Hyg.* **63**, 362.
52 Shin, H.K. (1969) *Korean J. Publ. Hlth* **6**, 230.
53 De Hurtado, I. & Layrisse, M. (1968) *Am. J. trop. Med. Hyg.* **17**, 72.
54 Rowland, H.A.K. (1966) *Trans. R. Soc. trop. Med. Hyg.* **60**, 481.
55 Cline, B.L., Little, M.D., Bartholomew, R.K. et al. (1984) *Am. J. trop. Med. Hyg.* **33**, 387–394.

56 Little, M.D. (1965) *Am. J. trop. Med. Hyg.* **14**, 1007.
57 Miller, M.J. & Maynard, G.R. (1967) *J. Can. med. Ass.* **97**, 860.
58 Katz, R., Ziegler, J. & Blank, H. (1965) *Archs Dermat.* **91**, 420.
59 London, I.D. (1965) *Sth med. J., Nashville* **58**, 1026.
60 Harland, P.S.E.G., Meakins, R.H. & Harland, R.H. (1977) *Br. med. J.* **ii**, 792.
61 O'Brien, W. (1975) *Trans. R. Soc. trop. Med. Hyg.* **60**, 69.
62 Laudanna, A.A., Polack, M., Betarello, A. et al (1973) *Revta Inst. Med. trop. São Paulo* **15**, 222.
63 Bras, G., Richards, R.C., Irvine, R.A. et al (1964) *Lancet* **ii**, 1257.
64 Rogers, W.A. & Nelson, B. (1966) *J. Am. med. Ass.* **195**, 685.
65 Wilson, S. & Thompson, A.E. (1964) *J. Path. Bact.* **87**, 169.
66 Owor, R. & Wamukota, W.A. (1976) *Trans. R. Soc. trop. Med. Hyg.* **70**, 497.
67 Ali-Khan, Z. & Seemayer, T.A. (1975) *Trans. R. Soc. trop. Med. Hyg.* **69**, 473.
68 Louisey & Barton (1971) *Radiology* **98**, 535.
69 Gill, G.V. & Bell, D.R. (1979) *Br. med. J.* **ii**, 572.
70 Dafalla, A.A. (1972) *J. trop. Med. Hyg.* **75**, 109.
71 Cahill, K.M. (1967) *Am. J. trop. Med. Hyg.* **16**, 451.
72 Ashford, R.W., Wall, A.J. & Babon, A.D. (1981) *Ann. trop. Med. Parasit.* **75**, 269–279.
73 Pampiglione, S. & Riccardi, M. (1971) *Parassitologia* **13**, 257.
74 Ashford, R .W., Vince, J.D., Gratten, M.J. et al (1979) *Papua New Guinea med. J.* **22**, 120–135.
75 Pampiglione, S. & Riccardi, M.L. (1972) *Parassitologia* **14**, 329.
76 Flockhart, H.A., Harrison, S.E., Robinson, A.R. et al (1982) *Trans. R. Soc. trop. Med. Hyg.* **76**, 541–554.
77 Larsh, J.E. (1967) *Am. J. trop. Med. Hyg.* **16**, 1123.
78 Punya Gupta, S., Courodmitree, C. & Siriyadhan, P. (1969) *J. med. Ass. Thailand* **52**, 281.
79 Spink, W.W. (1935) *Archs intern. Med.* **56**, 238.
80 Hennekeuser, H.H., Pabst, K., Poeplau, W. et al (1968) *Dt. med. Wshr.* **93**, 865.
81 Melcher, L.R. (1943) *J. infect. dis.* **71**, 31.
82 Anderson, R.I., Sadun, E.H. & Schoenbeckler, M.J. (1963) *J. Parasit.* **49**, 642.
83 Kagan, I.G. (1960) *J. infect. Dis.* **197**, 65.
84 Levin, M.L. (1983) *Am. J. trop. Med. Hyg.* **32**, 980–983.
85 Dauer, C.C. & Davids, D.G. (1959) *Publ. Hlth Rep. Wash.* **74**, 715.
86 Zimmerman, W.J., Hubbard, E.J. & Matthews, J. (1958) *J. Parasit.* **44**, 34.
87 Link, V.B. (1953) *Publ. Hlth Rep. Wash.* **68**, 416.
88 Rausch, R. (1953) *Publ. Hlth Rep. Wash.* **68**, 533.
89 Maynard, J.E. & Pauls, E.P. (1962) *Am. J. Hyg.* **76**, 252.
90 Forrester, A.T.T., Nelson, G.S. & Sander, G. (1961) *Trans. R. Soc. trop. Med. Hyg.* **33**, 503.
91 Onde, M. & Carayon, A. (1968) *Bull. soc. med. Afr. noire Lang. fr.* **13**, 332.
92 Kagan, I.G. (1959) *U.S. publ. Hlth Rep.* **74**, 159.

Chapter 22
Trematode Infections

Trematodes are parasites of man and other animals which can be divided into two classes: schistosomes, which have a mammal as a definitive host with a snail as an intermediate host; and hermaphroditic flukes, which have mammals as definitive hosts, snails as first intermediary host, and crustacea, fish or vegetation as second intermediary hosts. They are important parasites in the tropical world, and their life-cycle is intimately bound up with the life-style, culture and feeding habits of tropical populations.

SCHISTOSOMIASIS

Schistosomiasis is the name given to a group of diseases which affect more than 200 million people in 73 countries of the world.[1] Four main species are responsible for human infection: *Schistosoma haematobium*, *S. mansoni*, *S. japonicum* and *S. intercalatum*. Three other species occur much less commonly: *S. mekongi*, *S. mattheei* and *S. bovis*. The main details of the commonest worms are given in Table 22.1.

GEOGRAPHICAL DISTRIBUTION
(Fig. 22.1)

S. haematobium is confined to Africa and the Near and Middle East, *S. mansoni* is found in Africa, Saudi Arabia, the Yemen, South America and the Caribbean, while *S. japonicum* is confined to the Far East. *S. intercalatum* is found in man only in limited foci in West and central Africa: Zaire, Congo, Central African Republic, Gabon, Cameroon and Nigeria. It is spread by the movements of labourers and nomads.

MORPHOLOGY AND LIFE-CYCLE OF SCHISTOSOME WORMS

The adult schistosome worms, both male and female, live in the mesenteric, portal or vesical veins of the vertebrate host and the life-cycle consists of alternate generations each with its own host, the adult worms inhabiting vertebrates and the two larval stages, miracidium (hatches from egg and invades snail) and cercaria (leaves the snail and invades the mammalian host) freshwater snails specific to each schistosome species. A feature of the life-cycle is that multiplication takes place in each host so that it is very difficult to break the cycle.

Less common schistosomes found in man

Other schistosomes may occur in man but are of little importance since they have zoonotic hosts.

S. mattheei

S. mattheei is a parasite of sheep and cattle, goats, horses and wild game in south-east and central Africa. Terminal spined eggs (Fig. 22.3e) are found in the urine and stools. The snail vector is of the *Biomphalaria* genus.

S. bovis

S. bovis is a parasite of sheep and cattle in East and central Africa. Terminal spined eggs (Fig. 22.3f) are found in the urine. The snail vector is of the *Bulinus* genus.

Table 22.1 The main schistosomes infecting man.

Species	Size	Egg	Site in man	Snail vector	Hosts	Geographical distribution
S. haematobium	Male 10–15 × 0.75–1.0 mm Female 20–26 × 0.25 mm	In urine, rarely stool. 140–170 × 40–70 μm. *Not* acid fast. Terminal spine Figs. 22.3c and 22.21	Vesical veins. Occasionally veins of rectum and portal system	Genus *Bulinus*	Man most important. Rarely baboons and monkeys	Most of Africa, Near and Middle East (Iraq), Mauritius
S. mansoni	Male 6–13 × 1.0 mm Female 7–17 × 0.25 mm	In stool. 115–175 × 45–70 μm. Acid fast. Lateral spine Figs. 22.3a and 22.22	Inferior mesenteric and portal venous system	Genus *Biomphalaria*	Man most important. Also baboons, rodents, raccoons	West, central and East Africa, Angola, Middle East, Saudi Arabia, Yemen, Madagascar, South America, Caribbean
B. japonicum	Male 12–20 × 0.5–0.55 mm Female 12–28 × 0.3 mm	In stool. 70–100 × 50–65 μm. Acid fast. Small lateral knob Figs. 22.3b and 22.23	Superior and inferior mesenteric and portal venous system	Genus *Oncomelania*	Mainly a parasite of water buffalo, dogs, cats, rats, pigs, horses, goats and other mammals. Also infects man	Japan, China, Philippines, Celebes
S. intercalatum	Male 11–14 × 0.3–0.4 mm Female 10–14 × 0.15–0.18 mm	In stool. 140–180 × 30–50 μm. Acid fast. Terminal spine Figs. 22.3d and 22.24	Mesenteric and portal venous system	Genus *Bulinus*	Man only in nature. Other animals experimentally only	Zaire, Gabon, Cameroon
S. mekongi	Male 6–15 × 0.5–0.55 mm	In stool. 30–55 × 50–65 μm. Small lateral knob	Superior mesenteric and portal veins	*Tricula aperta*	Dogs	Laos and Thailand

S. haematobium-like schistosome in India[2]

A schistosome with terminal spined eggs similar to those of *S. haematobium* is found in a small focus in Maharashtra state, India. Transmission occurs at a low level maintained by the intermediate host, the freshwater limpet, *Ferrissia tenuis*.

S. japonicum-like schistosomes in Thailand, Laos and Malaysia

A number of japonicum-like schistosomes have been found in Thailand, Laos and Malaysia forming a complex of related species, all with zoonotic hosts and causing mostly subclinical infections in man.

Section III. Helminthic Diseases

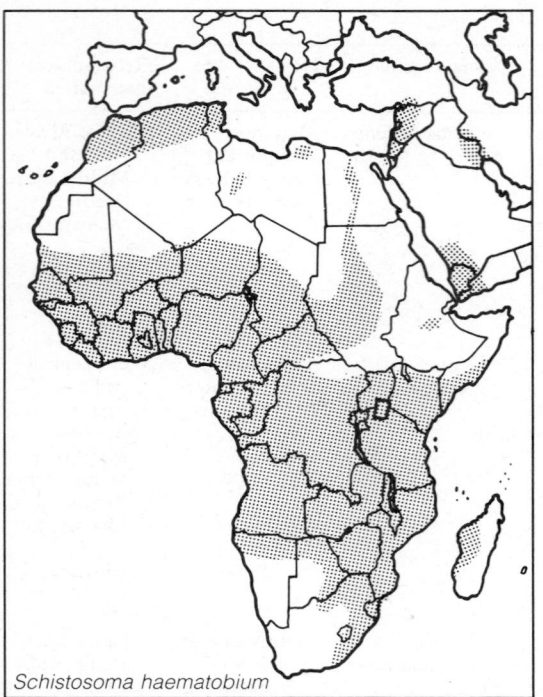

Schistosoma haematobium

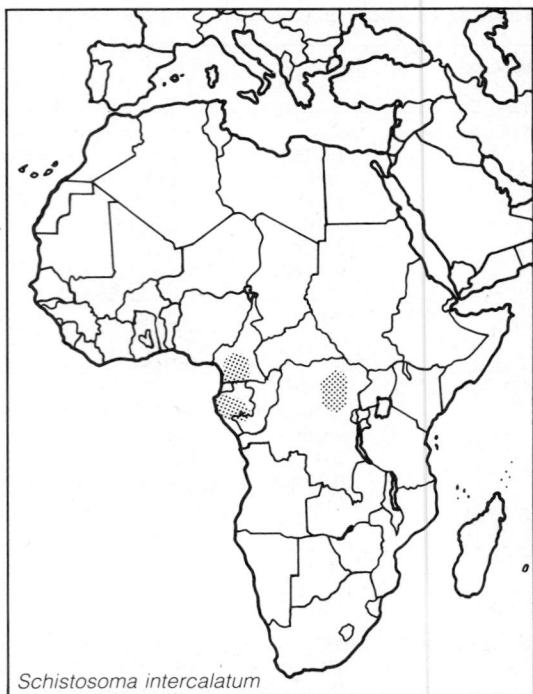

Schistosoma intercalatum

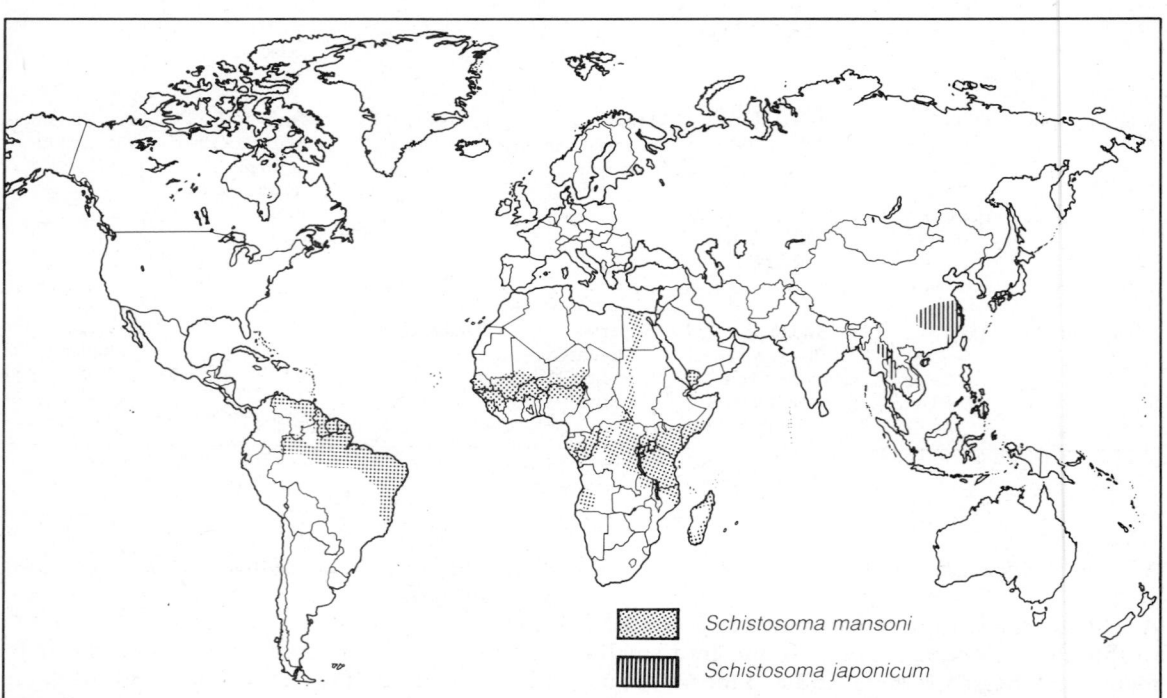

Schistosoma mansoni

Schistosoma japonicum

Fig. 22.1 Geographical distribution of schistosomiasis. (Courtesy Dr V. R. Southgate.)

S. mekongi

S. mekongi is a parasite of dogs in Laos and Thailand. Eggs are similar to those of *S. japonicum* but can be distinguished by being smaller and rounder. The snail host is *Tricula (Lithoglyphopsis) aperta*. Infections in man are mostly subclinical and asymptomatic.

S. japonicum-like schistosomes in Peninsular Malaysia

Schistosomes have been found among the Orang Asli (aboriginals). Evidence of infection is mostly serological and eggs are found in the liver, rarely in the stools. Natural infections have been found in *Rattus mulleri*. The snail vector is *Robertsiella kaporensis*.[3]

S. mansoni-like schistosome in northern Thailand

An *S. mansoni*-like schistosome has been found in northern Thailand. Eggs are not found in stool or rectum but in the submucosa of the large bowel.[4]

Morphology

Adult

The adult worm (male and female, Figs. 22.2 and II.13–II.15 p. 1333) has a prehensile *oral sucker* surrounding the mouth anteriorly and a *ventral sucker* on the ventral surface with which it attaches itself to the wall of the vessel in which it lives. The *mouth* near the anterior extremity leads to an *oesophagus* and thence to the *gut* which divides into two *caeca* which reunite and end blindly, there being no anus. Food consists of blood. Excretion of waste products is performed by two longitudinal canals opening posteriorly and fed by connecting tubules. The male reproductive organs consist of *testes* dorsal and posterior to the ventral sucker which discharge through *a genital pore* posterior to the ventral sucker. The male worm is flat and leaf-like and is folded to form a *gynaecophoric* canal which enfolds the slender female for almost its entire length. The female reproductive organs consist of *ovary* in the posterior half of the body from which an oviduct passes forward to the *uterus* which contains the eggs, and opens at the genital pore posterior to the ventral sucker so that the genital pores of both male and female face each other. (See also Fig. II.13, p. 1333.)

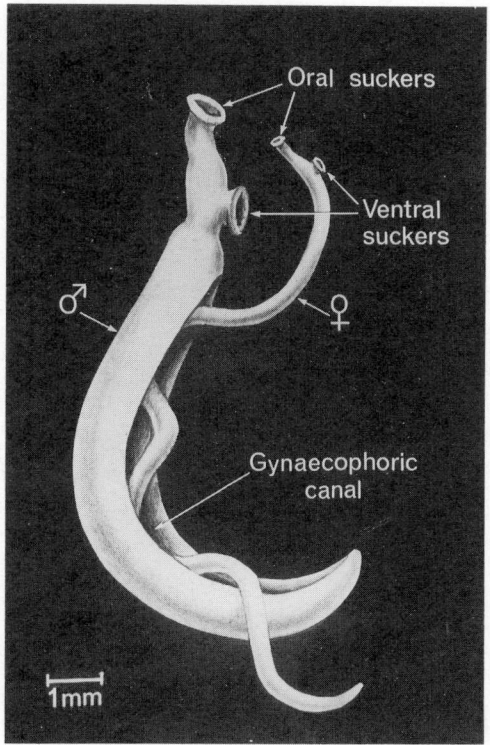

Fig. 22.2 Male and female schistosomes. (Courtesy WTIM.)

Egg

Schistosome eggs are round or oval with one spiny appendage, the size and shape varying according to species (Figs. 22.3, 22.21–22.24 and Plate III.11, 12 and 13). Each fertilized female lays many eggs each day: *S. haematobium* 500–1000, *S. mansoni* 250–400, *S. japonicum* 1500–3000. The eggs of *S. mansoni* are released singly while those of *S. japonicum* and *S. haematobium* are released in groups. Each egg contains a ciliated miracidium which matures in 6–10 days and may remain alive for up to three weeks after being laid; its movements may be seen under the microscope in a fresh preparation, and is the mark of a live egg. Most eggs die if they do not soon reach fresh water but *S. japonicum* eggs can survive outside the body for 80 days in cold, moist conditions thus allowing them to overwinter. Schistosome eggs secrete histiolytic enzymes which help passage through the tissues and an antigenic protein (soluble egg antigen) which is responsible for much of the pathology. Eggs of *S. mansoni*, *S. japonicum* and *S. inter-*

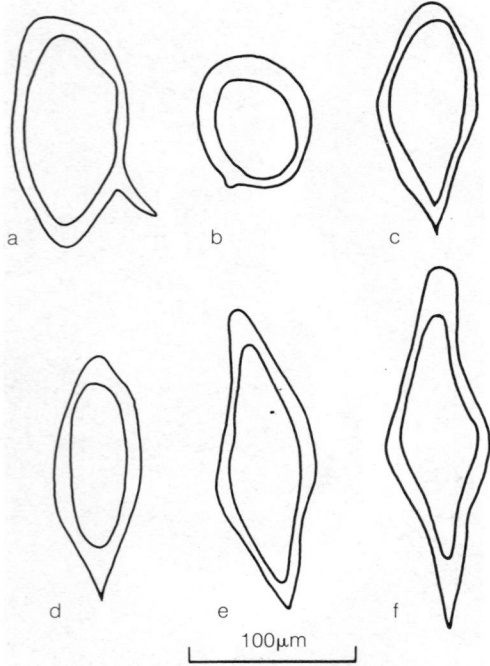

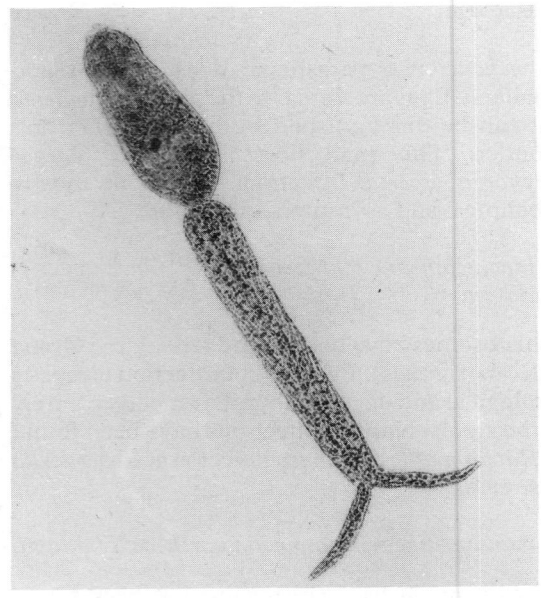

Fig. 22.3 Eggs of *Schistosoma* spp. (a) *S. mansoni;* (b) *S. japonicum;* (c) *S. haematobium;* (d) *S. intercalatum;* (e) *S. mattheei;* (f) *S. bovis.*

Fig. 22.4 Schistosome cercaria. (Courtesy Dr O.D. Standen.)

calatum are acid fast with Ziehl–Neelson stain but *S. haematobium* eggs are not acid fast.

Miracidium (Fig. II.17, p. 1334)

Miracidia are ovoid, about 160 μm long and swim with cilia attached to epidermal plates. They are viable only in fresh water and swim away from the bottom towards the light at the surface of the water where they attach themselves to any snail penetrating the tissues by means of a pair of cephalic glands. They will only develop further in species of snail to which they are specifically adapted. Snails can be infected by multiple miracidia.

Cercariae (Figs. 22.4 and II.18, p. 1335)

Cercariae are unisexual and fish-like with a pear-shaped head and a *forked tail*, 400–600 μm in length with one oral and one ventral sucker, a mouth, oesophagus and a pair of short caeca. Two pairs of glands in front of the ventral sucker secrete enzymes to penetrate the skin of vertebrates, and four pairs behind to help attachment to the skin. Maximum conditions for

shedding of cercariae are strong sunlight and a water temperature of 25–30°C; a snail may shed 300–500 cercariae daily in daylight in *S. haematobium* and *S. mansoni*, but only up to 20 in *S. japonicum* at night. Cercariae may survive up to 72 hours (average 48 hours) in fresh water but lose their infectivity after 12 hours.

Cercariae of *S. mansoni* and *S. haematobium* move vertically, swimming upwards and sinking back down passively; *S. japonicum* cercariae collect in the surface film where they remain. The cercariae attach themselves to their definitive host by the ventral or oral sucker and penetrate the skin within 3–5 minutes, shedding their tails. Only about 40% of cercariae which penetrate the skin will become adult, depending on the host's immunity.

Schistosomule

The schistosomule is the tailless cercarial body which forms after entry into the tissues. It changes its membrane covering so that it can survive in a saline environment and its metabolism changes to anaerobic glycolysis. After remaining in the tissues it migrates to the lungs over 3–6 days developing into an adult in one to four weeks, forming an immunologically tolerant covering membrane.

Snails (intermediate host)

The snail intermediate hosts of *S. haematobium* are of the *Bulinus* genus (Fig. 22.5), of *S.*

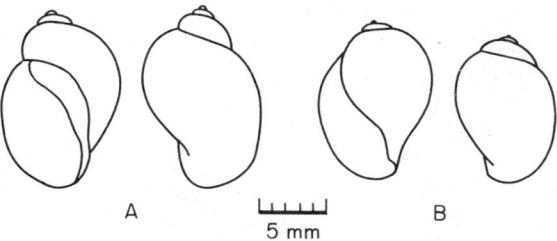

Fig. 22.5 Snails of the *Bulinus* genus hosts of *S. haematobium*. A, *Bulinus truncatus* group. B, *Bulinus africanus* group.

mansoni, the *Biomphalaria* genus (Fig. 22.6) and of *S. japonicum*, the *Oncomelania* genus (Fig. 22.7) and can be recognized by the shape of their shells. Strains of the species of schistosomes which infect man vary in their ability to infect

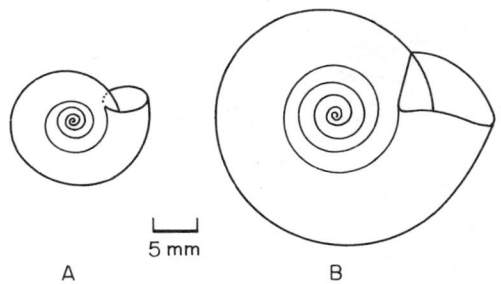

Fig. 22.6 Snails of the *Biomphalaria* genus hosts of *S. mansoni*. A, *Biomphalaria alexandrina*. B, *Biomphalaria glabrata*.

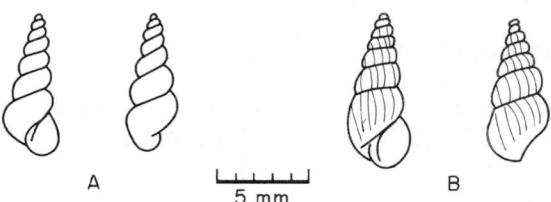

Fig. 22.7 Snails of the *Oncomelania* genus hosts of *S. japonicum*. A, *Oncomelania hupensis nosophora*. B, *O. h. hupensis*.

snail hosts. Some schistosomes easily infect snails of one geographical area but fail to infect, or infect with difficulty, the same snails from a different area. *Bulinus* and *Biomphalaria* snails live in fresh water, are hermaphroditic and non-

operculated. Those of the genus *Oncomelania* are unisexual, operculated, amphibious and adapted to live on land. A full list of species of snail hosts involved is given in Appendix II (Tables II.2–II.5, pp. 1336–1337).

Life-cycle (Fig. 22.8)

The eggs from an adult female in the definitive mammalian host are passed into fresh water via the urine or stools according to species of schistosome where they hatch into the first larval stage—a *miracidium*—which then enters the intermediate host *snail*, in certain species of which, specific to each species of schistosome, it forms a large number of *sporocysts* which, after a period of four to seven weeks, emerge from the snail as the second larval stage—*cercariae*. Cercariae can live in the water for 48–72 hours during which time they must find a new mammalian host or die. On reaching a new host the cercaria penetrates the skin in a few minutes to become a *schistosomule* which enters the lymphatics or veins to pass through the right heart and lungs, from where some pass into the circulatory system to reach the mesenteric vessels, while others may pass directly through the diaphragm to reach the liver and portal system. Growth into adult form takes place in the liver where paired worms may be found after 26 days. Most worms leave the liver when they are mature and mated and migrate to the mesenteric veins (*S. mansoni, S. japonicum* and *S. intercalatum*) or the veins of the vesical plexus (*S. haematobium*).

The period from penetration by the cercariae to egg laying is 30–40 days or more. The mated worms move as far as possible forward towards the fine terminal vessels where the female leaves the male and, progressing to the smallest vessel, deposits her eggs, retracting after having done so (Fig. 22.9). The eggs escape from the venules into the tissues, those of *S. haematobium* largely into the wall of the bladder but occasionally into the large bowel; those of *S. mansoni, S. japonicum* and *S. intercalatum* largely into the wall of the lower bowel. Many pass through the mucosa to be excreted in urine or faeces but some remain trapped in the tissues where they give rise to a tissue reaction. Some eggs of all species are usually also found in the genital tract, liver, lungs, central nervous system and other organs. The eggs alone are responsible for most of the pathological effects of infection.

Adult schistosomes can live for long periods

Schistosoma mansoni

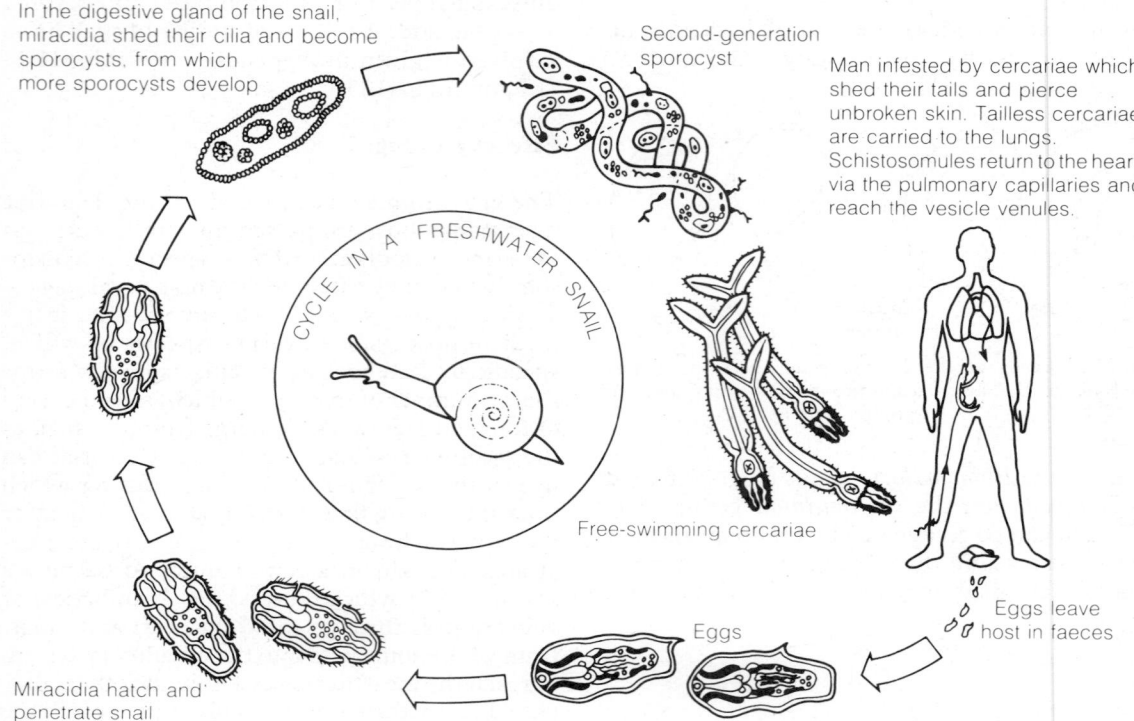

In the digestive gland of the snail, miracidia shed their cilia and become sporocysts, from which more sporocysts develop

Second-generation sporocyst

Man infested by cercariae which shed their tails and pierce unbroken skin. Tailless cercariae are carried to the lungs. Schistosomules return to the heart via the pulmonary capillaries and reach the vesicle venules.

CYCLE IN A FRESHWATER SNAIL

Free-swimming cercariae

Eggs

Eggs leave host in faeces

Miracidia hatch and penetrate snail

Fig. 22.8   Life-cycle of *S. mansoni*. (Courtesy WTIM.)

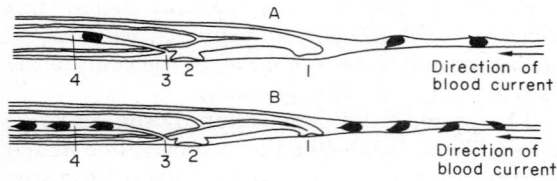

A

Direction of blood current

B

Direction of blood current

Fig. 22.9   The deposition of eggs by *S. mansoni* (A) and *S. haematobium* (B) in the blood vessels and their passage to the exterior. 1, Anterior sucker. 2, Posterior sucker. 3, Vaginal orifice. 4, Uterus with contained eggs.

and viable *S. mansoni* infections have been found 30 years and 18–20 years after leaving an endemic area.[5] The average duration of life is much less and the mean life-span has been estimated as 3.3 years.[6]

TRANSMISSION

Transmission of schistosomiasis requires three conditions.

1   A source of infection for the contamination of fresh water with human or animal urine or faeces containing schistosome eggs.

2   The presence in the water of the right species of snail in which miracidia hatched from the eggs are capable of producing cercariae which can infect man.

3   Human contact with water by bathing, wading or washing in it or drinking.

Source of infection

Man is the main source of infection, children who pass large numbers of eggs being the main source.

Animal hosts

Although *S. haematobium* has (though rarely) been found in baboons, monkeys and rodents in Africa, these animals are probably not important as reservoir hosts, and man is the main host. Many primates are susceptible to experimental infection.

   S. mansoni has been found in baboons; some

may have been infected from human sources, but some baboon communities can maintain the infection among themselves. Baboon faeces containing eggs and reaching a stream in Tanzania have certainly caused infection in persons bathing in the water.[7] On Guadeloupe rats, *Rattus rattus,* have a particularly high prevalence (about 60%) of *S. mansoni* in freshwater mangrove swamps, forest lakes and ponds, whereas in running water transmission sites the prevalence varies between 3% and 20% in rats—here man is the most important host. Interestingly, the schistosome populations in the various foci can be distinguished by the chronobiological pattern of cercarial emergence: where man is the main host peak emergence occurs at about 11.00 hours, where *Rattus rattus* is the main host peak emergence is about 17.00 hours.[8] *Rattus norvegicus* does not act as a host for *S. mansoni* on Guadeloupe. Calves and sheep have been infected experimentally, with both *S. mansoni* and *S. intercalatum,* passing viable eggs in their faeces, a finding which may be epidemiologically important. In parts of South Africa, *S. mattheei,* a parasite of cattle and sheep, is known to infect man and it is clear that *S. mattheei* will hybridize with *S. haematobium.*[9] *S. japonicum* is known to have a very wide natural definitive host range. Mao and Shao[10] note that in some endemic areas *S. japonicum* is known to infect at least 31 species of mammal belonging to five orders. Variation in definitive host specificity is known to occur with different strains of *S. japonicum*; for example, the Taiwan strain is pathogenic for animals but not for man. In southern Laos the snail (*Tricula aperta*) is not amphibious so the epidemiology of *S. mekongi* is very different from that of the classical *S. japonicum.*

Interestingly Appleton and Eriksson[11] discovered apparently viable *S. mansoni* eggs in the faeces of a grey headed gull and a spurwing goose. They concluded that the birds probably ingested the eggs with human faeces and there are obvious epidemiological implications if this phenomenon is more common than hitherto realized especially considering the distances birds migrate within South Africa.

Snail hosts

Specific snail hosts are necessary, of the *Bulinus* genus for *S. haematobium* and *S. intercalatum,* the *Biomphalaria* genus for *S. mansoni* and the *Oncomelania* genus for *S. japonicum.* (For a com-plete list of species and distribution, see Appendix II, Tables II.2–II.5, p. 1336–1337.)

Factors relating to snails

These factors are multiple, acting together rather than individually.

Composition of the water. Generally the snail hosts of schistosomes infecting man require fresh water, although some populations have been found in habitats on the coastal plain of Tanzania with high concentrations of chlorides.[12] Calcium is important because it is a major constituent of the shell and evidence suggests that some molluscs, for example *Biomphalaria pfeifferi,* absorb calcium directly from the surrounding water.[13] The main body of evidence in the literature shows that the molluscan fauna is either non-existent or at the best poor in acidic waters, for the presence of calcium has been shown to be important for both growth and fecundity as well as shell formation.[14] The alkaline and calcium-rich waters of Surinam and Venezuela are highly suitable for *Biomphalaria glabrata,* whereas the acid (pH 4.5–5.5) waters devoid of lime in Guyana are not, and schistosomes are not found there.[15]

Temperature. Temperature is an important factor in both the life history, i.e. growth, fecundity and mortality, and distribution of freshwater snails. For example, the optimum temperature for *Biomphalaria pfeifferi* is about 25°C.[16] The high temperatures found in otherwise suitable habitats on the coastal plains of Tanzania and South Africa possibly explain the absence of *Biomphalaria pfeifferi.*[16,17] At 18°C *Bulinus globosus* can only just maintain a population, and above 39°C snails die. There is little or no transmission of human schistosomiasis above an altitude of 1800 m where the water temperatures are too low.

Light. In general the snails are not found in heavily shaded water which may explain the absence of the disease from heavily forested areas. The presence of light is essential for photosynthesis and the growth of plants, so it is probable that lack of light removes an important food resource of snails and substratum for the deposition of eggs. Thus, there is a strong argument for covering irrigation canals or putting the water into pipes whenever possible. Numerous *Bulinus* spp. have been bred in the laboratory for many generations in almost total darkness, but population growth was restricted. *Biomphalaria* have been recovered from the bottom of Lake Victoria at a depth of about 12 m, where the light cannot possibly have been strong.

Habitat. Muddy channels favour snails and mud absorbs molluscicides as well as encouraging vegetation, which is why concreted channels, which can be cleared, have been constructed for irrigation. Still or slow-flowing water is preferred by snails, as in ponds, dams, lakes, irrigation canals and slow streams or rivers. Appleton[18] estimated the upper limits of tolerance for *Biomphalaria pfeifferi* and *Bulinus* sp. to be about 0.3 m/sec. Snails browse on the microflora and decaying vegetation, so higher plant life is not necessarily essential. However, ecological studies have shown that there is a correlation between some plants and certain species of snail; for example, *Bulinus rohlfsi* in Lake Volta, Ghana increased in huge numbers alongside the proliferation of floating masses of vegetation, in particular, *Ceratophyllum demersum*. Some snails (e.g. *Biomphalaria alexandrina*) prefer permanent and stable habitats such as drains leading from canals; *Bulinus truncatus* prefers large canals. Seasonal small pools are much used for washing and bathing and watering cattle; they are the centres of intense transmission. A good example of such transmission sites are the laterite pools in The Gambia where *Bulinus senegalensis* is an important host.

Season. Though there are irregular population changes independent of climate, most snail populations fall during the rainy season, to increase in the drier warmer months after the rains (for instance in East Africa). Where water temperatures are more stable some snail populations show no seasonal trends; the greatest stability is found in *Oncomelania quadrasi* in the Far East. Some water bodies completely dry up during the dry season, and such habitats are occupied by species capable of aestivation. For example, *Bulinus senegalensis* is able to aestivate for six to seven months[19] and periods of five to eight months have been recorded for *Bulinus nasutus*, and *Bulinus globosus*. Usually, only a relatively small percentage of the total snail population survives desiccation, but on emergence from aestivation the snails possess at least twice the breeding activity of non-aestivated snails. *Oncomelania* (which is operculated) hibernates in cold weather in Asia. Interestingly, it is possible for aestivating snails to maintain a viable parasite infection which may be of epidemiological significance.

Predators. Ducks eat snails and so do the large (non-vector) snails *Marisa cornuarietis* and *Thiara granifera*, which also compete for food, and certain species of fish, e.g. *Tilapia melanopleura* and *Clarisa* sp. *Marisa cornuarietis* has been used quite effectively in the Caribbean in reducing the population of *Biomphalaria glabrata*, as a predator of ova and juveniles but primarily as a competitive feeder. There is some concern that widespread introduction of *M. cornuarietis* into Africa could result in damage to rice cultivation.

Snail egg masses. These can be carried on the feet of water birds and infect other bodies of water.

Factors relating to the release of cercariae and infection of man

Age of snails. Generally young snails are more susceptible to infection than old snails, although the reverse obtains in certain genetic stocks of *Biomphalaria glabrata*.

Infection. The number of cercariae produced by a snail depends upon many factors, such as the level of compatibility of host and parasite, the age, size and nutritional status of the host and the number of miracidia to which the snail has been exposed. Also, the number of cercariae produced will vary between snails within a population and in individual snails at different times post infection. At the upper end of the scale *Biomphalaria glabrata* will produce around 3000 per day and over 100 000 during the course of an infection. At the lower end *Oncomelania quadrasi* will produce on average as few as 15 cercariae of *S. japonicum* per day. *Oncomelania* spp. are much smaller than *Biomphalaria* spp. Infected snails are more susceptible than uninfected snails to adverse conditions.

Season. Depending upon intermediate host and habitat, active transmission can take place either over a long period or can be more intense over a shorter period. Rainfall and temperature are two important physical factors affecting transmission patterns. For example, in The Gambia the

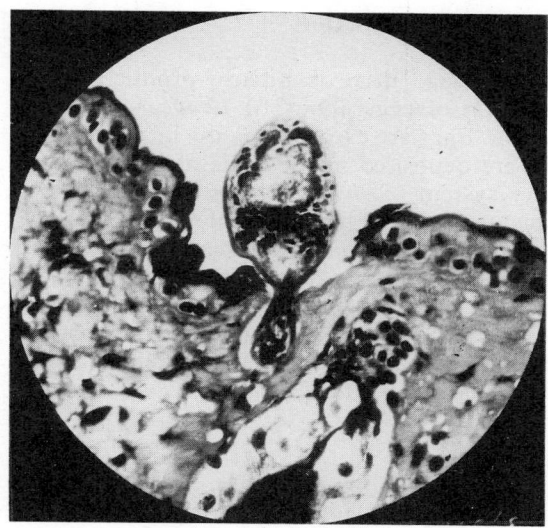

Fig. 22.10 Cercarial penetration in schistosomiasis. (Courtesy Dr O. D. Standen.)

depressions on the laterite plateau fill with water during the wet season. These depressions are inhabited by *Bulinus senegalensis*, a species capable of withstanding prolonged desiccation and an excellent host for *S. haematobium* and *S. bovis*. The temporary pools serve as washing and bathing places and are used for watering cattle and during their existence transmission is intense. During the dry season the pools dry up and there is no transmission. *Bulinus jousseaumei* and *Biomphalaria pfeifferi* tend to be found in the small streams leading into the main river. During the rainy season these tributaries become swollen and turbulent and the snail populations are severely reduced, but at the end of the rainy season the streams drop in level, the velocity is reduced and the remaining snails start breeding with increasing temperature, especially where patches of slack water occur. Human water contact occurs again during this period giving rise to dry season transmission of schistosomiasis. This example serves to illustrate that active transmission patterns can vary within a limited geographical area where climatic conditions are similar for all of the foci.

Time of day. Light is the main stimulus causing the release of cercariae of both *S. haematobium* and *S. mansoni*. Under natural conditions the pattern of cercarial emission of *S. mansoni* from *Biomphalaria glabrata* corresponds to the curves for temperature and intensity of illumination, commencing at about 09.00 hours and peaking around 15.00 hours and subsequently declining. Slight variations exist with different isolates of *S. mansoni* and *S. haematobium* on the peak and length of the shedding period but the general pattern remains the same. However, an interesting situation occurs on Guadeloupe where two chronobiologically distinct strains of *S. mansoni* coexist. One strain follows the usual course as seen in *S. mansoni* elsewhere, but the other peaks in the evening at about 19.00 hours. It is known that rats are an important reservoir host and the later peak shedding period coincides with a high activity period for rats. Similarly, the peak shedding period for *S. japonicum* tends to occur during the evening and this coincides with maximum activity of many of the reservoir hosts.

Velocity of water. Velocity of water is an important factor affecting infectivity of cercariae. Sentinel animals placed in water containing equal numbers of cercariae but at varying velocities have shown that peak infectivity occurred when the velocity was about 30 cm/s;[20] below this fewer cercariae make contact with the host, and above this the cercariae which make contact tend to be swept away.

PATHOLOGY

The stages of schistosomiasis are: invasion, maturation, established infection and late stage. In general, since the main agent of pathology is the egg, the heavier the infection, the greater the pathology and morbidity. Light infections cause little pathology and morbidity, while very heavy infections can cause death.

Invasion

In this stage the cercariae penetrate the skin or mucous membrane (Fig. 22.10), usually taking less than 15 minutes, and acting by a combination of cercarial muscular action and glandular secretion. Once through the horny layer of the skin the schistosomules enter the dermis and hypodermis where they probably remain for 4 or 5 days before entering the lymphatic system and thence the veins, the right heart and the lungs. After that their progress is not clearly known, but they reach the liver, where, presumably, they mature.

In unsensitized persons the reactions to the first invasion by these embryo parasites are mild, with only slight inflammatory reactions in the skin, lungs and liver (occasionally with cough, bloody sputum or even asthma), but after repeated exposures the skin shows itchy papules and local oedema. This cercarial dermatitis may be quite marked and may indicate the date of infection. It is usually worse in infections with bird and animal schistosomes, which do not mature. In an endemic area, however, the local people often show no local skin reaction but in new visitors the reaction may be marked, especially after reinfection. The absence of this reaction, for instance in Africans, may be a reflection of passive immunity derived from the mother, followed by active immunity in childhood.

Maturation

This begins two to eight weeks after infection; males and females couple and eggs are produced. The young couples of *S. mansoni* and *S. japonicum* descend the portal vein against the stream, reaching the mesenteric veins in the intestinal walls, where the main egg-laying takes place (Fig. 22.9). *S. haematobium* probably also matures in the liver, though this has not been demonstrated, and the adult worms find their way, by some process not understood, to the veins of the genitourinary organs.

Katayama fever

The characteristic pathological manifestation in this stage in moderate and heavy infections is an acute febrile reaction with hypereosinophilia lasting for several days or weeks (Katayama fever) which is most marked in *S. japonicum*, less marked in *S. mansoni* and almost completely absent in *S. haematobium* infections. It occurs at the time when egg production is commencing. Katayama fever is the result of a cross reaction between egg and worm antigens with antibody levels rising rapidly to meet the antigenic stimulus with the formation of antigen–antibody immune complexes, acute serum sickness and glomerulonephritis.[21] IgA, IgG and IgD are all normal but IgM is raised in Katayama fever indicating recent active stimulation of immunological systems.[22]

Established infection

In this stage there is intense production and excretion of eggs about 10–12 weeks after infection. Eggs are excreted via the urine or faeces and are deposited in the walls of the genitourinary system (*S. haematobium* but occasionally *S. mansoni*), the rectum and colon (*S. japonicum*, *S. mansoni* and *S. intercalatum* but occasionally *S. haematobium*). Eggs are also deposited in the liver (*S. mansoni* and *S. japonicum*), lungs (*S. mansoni* and *S. japonicum*), genital organs, central nervous system and almost all the organs of the body at one time or another.

Schistosomal granuloma

There is no proof that living adult worms in the veins set up any inflammatory reaction. Dead worms, however, do cause some reaction. The egg is the main cause of the pathological changes found in schistosomiasis. Schistosomal egg antigen (soluble egg antigen, SEA) is the primary element which leads to the formation of the granuloma. The egg stimulates first an eosinophilic reaction followed by a secondary granulomatous response which is the result of delayed hypersensitivity. The eggs set up an inflammatory reaction with epithelioid, plasma and giant cells surrounded by loose fibrous tissue (Figs. 22.11, 22.12 and 60.31, p. 1004). These granulomas or tubercles may coalesce and the eggs calcify causing changes in the walls of the bladder in urinary tract schistosomiasis (*S. haematobium*) and the large bowel in intestinal schistosomiasis (*S. mansoni*, *S. japonicum*) although eggs do not usually calcify in the intestine. With *S. japonicum* these changes occur earlier and to a greater extent as the result of a greater number of eggs. The *liver* is especially involved with granuloma formation around the eggs and a coarse periportal fibrosis (Symmers' fibrosis, *hepatosplenic schistosomiasis*). The lungs may be involved in the same process, *cardiopulmonary schistosomiasis* (*S. mansoni* and *S. japonicum*) and also the central nervous system (*S. japonicum*).

In *S. mansoni* infection granulomas form round single eggs, there are few plasma cells and polymorph abscesses are rare. In *S. japonicum*, on the other hand, the number of eggs in the tissues is very large and early massive lesions form round the egg masses indicating high

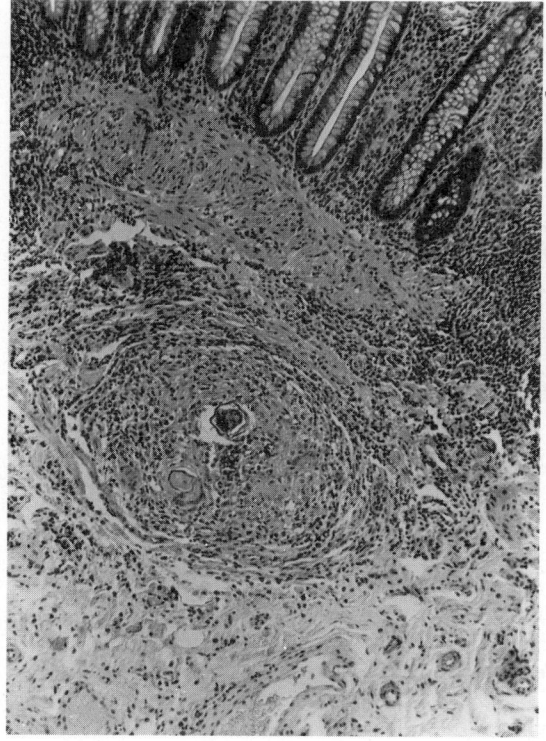

Fig. 22.11 Schistosomal granuloma (*S. mansoni*) of bowel. The structureless mass at the centre is an egg.

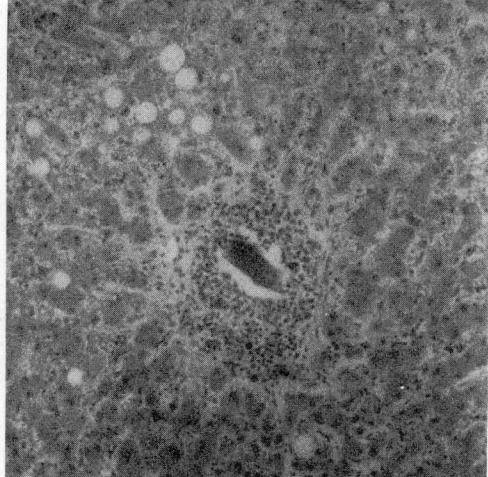

Fig. 22.12 Schistosomal granuloma in liver (*S. mansoni*). The structureless mass at the centre is an egg. (Courtesy Dr B. H. Kean.)

antigen concentrations, there are large numbers of plasma cells and necrotic lesions suggesting immune complex formation.

Hepatosplenic schistosomiasis

HEPATOMEGALY

Hepatomegaly is a well-marked sign of *S. mansoni* and *S. japonicum*. The hepatic changes usually begin insidiously but may be acute in some cases. Eggs trapped in the liver venules cause proliferation of the vascular endothelium with endophlebitis and the formation of granulomas, and fibrous tissue is increased in the portal spaces. The circulation through the granulomas is arterial so that although the blood flow remains normal there is a shift between the arterial and portal circulation, the portal flow being reduced to 20% and the arterial flow raised to 80% causing portal circulatory obstruction with relatively normal liver function.

SPLENOMEGALY

The increase in hepatic presinusoidal pressure leads to an increase in splenic venous pressure with congestive splenomegaly and, in addition, there is a proliferation of the lymphoid follicles and germinal centres as a result of increased T cell production from immunological activity and splenic hyperplasia. Histologically there is distension of the venous sinuses and a hypercellularity reflecting the *hypersplenism* which is a feature of hepatosplenic schistosomiasis. A giant cell lymphoma of the spleen may occur.[1]

SYMMERS' PIPE-STEM FIBROSIS (CLAY PIPE-STEM CIRRHOSIS) (Fig. 22.13)

This is a periportal fibrosis without any significant destruction of the liver cells which is the result of a chronic perisinusoidal inflammation leading to fibrosis caused by the deposition of eggs. There is broadening and lengthening of the portal areas which can be seen macroscopically to resemble the stem of a clay pipe (Fig. 22.13). It is most commonly seen in *S. japonicum* infection where the onset is most rapid and prevalence higher because of the large number of eggs deposited. In *S. mansoni* it occurs where infections are most heavy, such as the Nile Delta (Egyptian splenomegaly) and in Brazil where strain differences may be important[23] but is rare in the rest of Africa. It is not seen in pure *S. haematobium* infections.

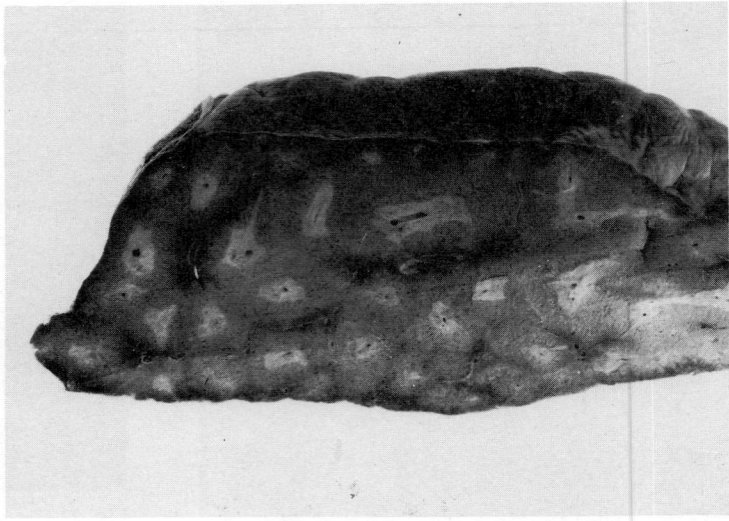

Fig. 22.13 Hepatosplenic schisto-somiasis. Symmers' pipe-stem fibrosis. (Courtesy WTIM.)

Intestinal schistosomiasis

Intestinal schistosomiasis is caused almost entirely by *S. japonicum, S. mansoni* and *S. intercalatum.* Although the rectum is involved in 70% of *S. haematobium* infections, the eggs are usually dead and cause no pathology. However, lesions in other parts of the colon and appendix are not uncommon and are usually polypoid.[24] The incidence and type of lesions produced vary greatly from region to region. Ova are widely distributed throughout the large bowel in the submucosa and muscle without any obvious lesions. The colon may become thickened and the mucosa granular with yellow pinpoint elevations surrounded by an area of hyperaemia which may ulcerate with the formation of shallow ulcers most commonly seen in *S. japonicum.* Lesions are commonest in the rectosigmoid area but the rectum frequently appears quite normal.

POLYPOSIS OF THE COLON
The incidence of polyposis is regional. In *S. mansoni* it is found in 20% of cases in Egypt[25] but not in Brazil[26] or in other areas of Africa. In *S. japonicum* polyposis is quite common. There may be fatal intestinal haemorrhage or excessive protein and iron loss.[27, 28]

BILHARZIOMA
Granulomatous masses known as *bilharziomata* may occur in the intestinal wall causing intestinal obstruction or massive tumours resembling Burkitt's tumour. Bilharziomata have been reported from the Sudan,[29] Uganda[30] and islands in Lake Victoria.[31]

Peritonitis

Schistosomal tubercles composed of granulomas surrounding ova may be spread over the peritoneum closely resembling tubercles, and ova of *S. haematobium* were present in large numbers of such tubercles spread generally over the surface of the lungs and peritoneum, although they were absent from the stools and urine.[32]

Appendix

The appendix frequently contains ova of *S. mansoni* and *S. haematobium* without any evidence of pathology, but subserosal nodules may be found in the appendix and neighbouring caecum where they can cause stenosis and obstructive appendicitis.

Urinary tract schistosomiasis

S. haematobium is the sole cause of urinary schistosomiasis although ova of *S. mansoni* were found in the urine of 15% of patients in St Lucia where there is no *S. haematobium* infection,[33] and bladder lesions in which only the ova of *S. mansoni* could be demonstrated have been described.[34] The eggs cause mucosal and submucosal granulomatous lesions of the bladder and ureters. Small papules form on the bladder mucosa which go on to ulceration and polyp formation or fibrose with the formation of 'sandy patches' and eventually in some cases calcification of the entire bladder wall and a contracted bladder. When the granulomas are situated in the submucosa of the ureters or near the ureteric openings, or where there are massive polypoid lesions which obstruct the openings, there is disturbance of the normal ureteric peristaltic movements and an *obstructive uropathy*.

HYDRONEPHROSIS (OBSTRUCTIVE UROPATHY)

Two forms of hydronephrosis are found; one occurs during the early stages of infection in young people as a result of granulomatous changes in the ureteric walls, which is completely reversible with treatment and causes no lasting renal damage; the other develops as a result of long continued infection in older people, the result of fibrotic strictures and bacterial infection with severe cortical destruction and renal failure. This form does not reverse with treatment. However, renal failure from this cause is not thought to be a common end result of *S. haematobium* infection.

CANCER OF THE BLADDER (see also Chapter 67)

There is a high geographical correlation between the incidence of bladder cancer and those areas where the prevalence of *S. haematobium* is high, where in contrast to elsewhere 73% of cases of bladder cancer are below the age of 50 and the cancer is a squamous cell carcinoma[35] in contrast to a transitional cell type. Carcinogens have been suggested as an explanation. *Tryptophan* is found in high concentration in the bladder in patients with schistosomal cancer and this substance may be produced as a result of defective metabolism of the adult worm. *Nitrosamines* have also been suggested as a carcinogen. There is a high level of nitrosamines in the urine associated with heavy bacteriuria[36] which, acting for a long time as a carcinogen, results in the malignant change.[37] (See Chapter 67)

Cardiopulmonary schistosomiasis

PNEUMONITIS

An allergic larval pneumonitis occurs during the migration of the schistosomules through the lungs during their migration after infection and is associated with a peripheral eosinophilia.

Another form of pneumonitis (verminous pneumonia) is seen following antischistosomal treatment when dead and dying *S. haematobium* worms lodge in the lungs as emboli. Transient chest X-ray shadows are very often seen, but resolve without harm as the worms are consumed by phagocytic cells.

SCHISTOSOMAL COR PULMONALE (see also Chapter 61)

Schistosomal cor pulmonale may be seen in the three main schistosomal infections but is commonest in *S. mansoni* and *S. japonicum*. Ova or adult worms bypass the portal system in established hepatosplenic schistosomiasis and reach the systemic venous system where they are trapped as they pass through the lungs in the small pulmonary arterioles, where they cause a granulomatous reaction and after prolonged deposition and in considerable numbers cause obliterative endarteritis, pulmonary hypertension and corpulmonale (Fig. 61.2, p. 1013). Histologically typical intra- and para-arterial granulomas are seen in the lungs. In Brazil cor pulmonale due to *S. mansoni* was found in 15% of patients with Symmers' fibrosis brought to autopsy, and active pulmonary arteritis was present in 90%.[26] Elsewhere than in Brazil and Egypt schistosomal cor pulmonale due to *S. mansoni* is rare.

Central nervous system

Ova of the three main species of schistosomes can be found in the brain and spinal cord in digest preparations but significant lesions are rarer. Lesions result from the deposition of eggs in the small arterioles with infarction and granulomatous lesions.

CEREBRAL LESIONS

Cerebral lesions are almost invariably caused by *S. japonicum* possibly because the small size of the eggs allows for easier passage to different places. In the brain lesions are diffuse or localized with large granulomas containing ova. A localized granuloma in the cerebellum caused by *S. mansoni* has been described.[38]

SPINAL CORD LESIONS

S. mansoni is the commonest cause of spinal cord lesions although *S. haematobium* is responsible for some. The lesions, which are localized, may be extra- or intramedullary granulomas and cause a transverse myelitis or involve the cauda equina. Occasionally an adult worm may enter a spinal artery where it either blocks the artery with local necrosis or steadily deposits eggs.

Renal schistosomiasis

GLOMERULONEPHRITIS

Renal lesions are common in *S. mansoni* infections and in some parts of the world as many as a quarter show renal lesions of some kind.[39] There is a high prevalence of glomerulonephritis with antigen–antibody immune complex deposits in the glomeruli. The renal lesion is of the membranoproliferative type with focal mesangial thickening and occasional capsular adhesions with crescent formation. These changes do not reverse with treatment.

NEPHROTIC SYNDROME

This is seen in *S. mansoni* and *S. haematobium* infections and is usually associated with *Salmonella* infection.[40] Some cases show interstitial lesions, the result of *Salmonella* pyelonephritis, while the majority show proliferative glomerular lesions with minimal basement membrane changes. Diffuse granular deposits of IgG and IgM in the glomerular mesangial wall suggest immune complexes. These changes are reversible with treatment of both the *Salmonella* and schistosome infections.[40, 41]

AMYLOID

Renal amyloidosis was found in 10 of 60 cases of schistosomal nephropathy.[42]

PYELONEPHRITIS

Pyelonephritis is caused by chronic bacterial infection secondary to urinary schistosomiasis and is associated with *S. haematobium* infection in Egypt[43] but not in sub-Saharan Africa.[44]

Male genital tract

The penis, prostate and seminal vesicles may be involved in *S. haematobium* infection.

PENIS

In the early stages polyps may form in the penile urethra and the prostatic urethra becomes swollen. Later superficial ulcers develop which heal by fibrosis leading to urethral stricture with secondary infection, periurethral abscesses and fistulae with calculi. Elephantoid hyperplasia of the penis and scrotum can occur.

PROSTATE

In the early stages ova are deposited in the interstitial tissue, submucosa and muscular coats with prostatic enlargement. Ova escape in the secretions with haemospermia. Later fibrosis occurs with diminution in size and adherence to the base of the bladder, often with calcification.

TESTES

The testes frequently contain ova of *S. haematobium* and, more rarely, *S. mansoni*. Destruction by granulomatous lesions has been described[45] but this rarely leads to loss of fertility. Funiculoepididymitis may develop accompanied by a small hydrocele as a result of fibrosis.

Female genital tract

The uterus is rarely involved but the cervix, vagina and vulva may be seriously affected by *S. haematobium* (*S. mansoni* infection has been described from Puerto Rico and Brazil).[46] The *cervix* may show extensive warty granulomatous masses closely resembling carcinoma but there is no connection between the two. The *vulva* and *vagina* may show sandy patches, nodules, ulcers, leukoplakia and granulomatous masses. Vesicovaginal fistulae may develop. Involvement of the fallopian tubes may lead to sterility.

Other organs

Using the digest method eggs of *S. haematobium* and *S. mansoni* can be found in almost any organ[47, 48] but usually in the absence of any histological changes.

Pancreas

The pancreas is involved occasionally in *S. mansoni*, *S. japonicum* and *S. haematobium*.[30] In *S. mansoni* ova are found deposited in the pancreas and can cause significant fibrosis. The ova may be seen in various stages of degeneration in the interlobar and parenchymal tissues with focal or diffuse fibrosis and parenchymal atrophy. Adult schistosome worms may be found in the venules in the pancreas and surrounding tissues. Pancreatic involvement does not usually cause symptoms in life but advanced pancreatic involvement in the late stages of hepatosplenic disease can cause pancreatic dysfunction. Glycosuria associated with *S. mansoni* has been known to resolve on antischistosomal treatment. Pancreatic calcification has been found in association with *S. haematobium*.[49]

Gallbladder

Adult *S. mansoni* worms have been found in the subserosal venules and eggs with surrounding granulomatous reaction in all layers of the gallbladder.[50]

Skin

Both *S. mansoni* and *S. haematobium* may cause skin lesions. Nodules in the skin with *S. mansoni* eggs in granulomas[51] and warty irregular vegetations and papules containing *S. haematobium* ova surrounded by a granulomatous reaction were found on the abdomen and round the umbilicus originating from adult worms in the paraumbilical plexus.[52] Ova have been found in tumours of the vocal cord and an ulcer on the lip thought to be syphilitic.

Association of *Schistosoma* and other infections

Salmonella infections

Chronic persistent bacteraemia with *Salmonella* is not uncommon in patients infected with the three main schistosomes and with *S. intercalatum*.[53] *Salmonella* can colonize the intestinal tract of the adult worms or they can attach themselves to the covering tegument where they are spread diffusely and multiply freely. This is probably the result of an immunological tolerance on the part of the schistosome worm because of shared antigens.

Hepatitis B

Patients with hepatosplenic schistosomiasis show hepatitis B surface antigen rates four times those of populations without schistosomiasis. The morbidity of hepatitis B in populations infected with schistosomiasis is unusually severe compared with non-infected populations.[54]

Anaemia in schistosomiasis (see also Chapter 58)

S. mansoni and S. japonicum

Some degree of anaemia is common in *S. mansoni* and *S. japonicum* infections, the mechanism varying according to the stage of the infection. In the early stages, a mild normocytic nor-

mochromic anaemia may develop, possibly of immunological origin, with a shortening of the red cell life-span and compensatory marrow hyperplasia.[55] In the established disease, the ova in passage through the bowel wall lead to the formation of ulcers and polyps resulting in considerable blood loss from the colon,[56] leading to iron deficiency. In advanced hepatosplenic schistosomiasis with portal hypertension and oesophageal varices, bleeding increases the loss of iron. Splenomegaly may also lead to hypersplenism with varying degrees of pancytopenia.[57] Liver failure may lead to prolongation of the prothrombin time with bleeding.

S. haematobium

Urinary blood loss has been estimated at 2.6–12.6 ml (0.6–37.3 mg iron) daily[58] and in northern areas of Kenya urinary schistosomiasis is associated with a considerable degree of anaemia[59] but may not be the only cause; *S. haematobium* is not thought to be an important cause of anaemia[60] in most places.

S. intercalatum

Reaction to the deposition of eggs in the tissues is less than in *S. mansoni* so that less pathology is caused. The eggs are deposited in the mesenteric venules of the intestine where the lesions are situated. Hepatomegaly is common and may be severe and egg granulomas occur in the liver. However, hepatosplenic schistosomiasis is not seen in pure *S. intercalatum* infections.

IMMUNITY

Natural immunity

All races, ages and both sexes are susceptible to infection.

Acquired immunity

A well-developed immunity develops in schistosomiasis and is shown by the acquisition in adult life in endemic areas of almost complete immunity to reinfection. Most adult inhabitants of endemic areas who are infected from an early age possess a striking immunity and show few signs of infection (passing few or no eggs). They can remain unharmed when exposed to doses of cercariae which will kill non-immune people. The immunity acquired is protective against both schistosomules and adult worms but, when directed against ova, causes the distinctive pathology which is characteristic of the disease.

Schistosomules

A protective immunity develops against infection so that the number of schistosomules reaching adult life is reduced but there is no effect on those adult worms that survive.

The mechanisms against the cercariae and schistosomules are twofold. First there is an antibody-dependent cell-mediated cytotoxic mechanism which is dependent upon eosinophils and IgG. IgG brings the eosinophils into contact with the schistosomules to which they bind, when degranulation and release of lytic agents from the eosinophil cause destruction of the schistosomule.

A second mechanism involves IgE and macrophages. IgE immune complexes bind to the macrophages attached to the schistosomule and release their lysosomal enzymes which destroy it. Other schistosomules are destroyed during their migration by an as yet unknown mechanism.

Adult worms

Adult worms evade the immune response by adapting their cuticle by covering it with host-like antigens. Adult schistosomes transferred surgically from infected monkeys to the portal systems of normal monkeys provide the major stimulus to immunity against challenge by cercariae, but they are not themselves affected by this immunity and they lay their eggs normally. But if adults from mice (and other hosts) are transplanted into monkeys, the 'mouse' adult worms do not begin to produce eggs until some weeks later, presumably until they have become adapted to the new host. Moreover, if 'mouse' adult worms are transferred to monkeys which have previously been immunized against mouse body tissues, the 'mouse' worms are killed within 24–44 hours. This suggests that worms which have lived in mice have incorporated mouse antigens into their cuticular tissues and that these antigens are attacked by the antimouse antibodies of the monkeys and the worms are destroyed. The mouse antigens appear to be located on the surface of the worms and this incorporation of host antigens to the surface of the parasites probably explains why the original

'monkey' schistosomes escape the consequences of the immunity they themselves engender.[61,62]

This concomitant immunity is important in the epidemiology and severity of disease. A strong immunity to superinfection is acquired by the end of the first decade of life after which the worm burden is lost exponentially with a half-life of several years.[63] Heterologous immunity may be important in experimental infections in mice with *S. bovis* and *S. mattheei* and *S. rodhaini* and *S. mansoni*.[64] Infection with *S. bovis* or *S. mattheei* reduced the expected egg load of subsequent challenge with *S. mansoni* by 74% and 85% respectively and a similar response was observed in monkeys. Cross resistance has been demonstrated in the baboon between *S. mansoni* and *S. haematobium*.[65] This suggests that natural zooprophylaxis may be important in the human infection. In some areas man is continually exposed to infection with 'animal' schistosomes and perhaps the severity of *S. mansoni* infections in Brazil and Egypt is in part due to the absence of concomitant transmissions of bovine schistosomes.

Unisexual infection can produce some resistance and inoculation of irradiated cercariae can also do so. Cattle vaccinated with irradiated schistosomules develop a large number of adult worms which produce few or no eggs but which protect the animal against challenge from any number of normal cercariae. These facts suggest the possibility of protective heterologous vaccines.[66] *S. mansoni* infections in mice suppress the immune response to *Plasmodium berghei* and *Salmonella*.

Adult worm antigen (circulating soluble antigen—CSA) is present in the gut of the adult worm and has been demonstrated in the plasma of patients with both *S. mansoni* and *S. haematobium*[67] which, together with free antigen–antibody complexes, is of relevance to the pathology of Katayama fever and the nephrotic syndrome. The presence of CSA can also be used as a marker of living adult worms in the body. Adult worms themselves cause little or no pathology.

Eggs

Eggs (SEA) induce a strong immune response which is mainly cell mediated and is responsible for the egg granuloma so characteristic of the pathology of the disease. The granuloma, at first large and florid, later decreases in size and is modulated by an antigen-specific suppressor T lymphocyte response as well as other factors, such as antibodies and immune complexes. Genetic factors are thought to be involved in the extent of modulation.[68]

Immunosuppression

Various forms of immunosuppression have been reported. Cell-mediated responses were impaired by schistosome antigens suppressing the production of histamine from basophils,[69] the adult antigen only being involved.[70]

Immunopathological results

Schistosome dermatitis

The allergic dermatitis which occurs on first exposure to cercariae penetrating the skin is part of the first mechanism of immune response, an antibody-dependent cell-mediated cytotoxic mechanism involving eosinophils and IgG.

Katayama fever

Katayama fever, which occurs about six weeks after a primary infection at a time when egg deposition is commencing and large numbers of eggs are being deposited, is due to circulating large-sized immune complexes involving both CSA and soluble egg antigen (SEA) causing a serum sickness-like disease.

Immune complex lesions

Circulating immune complexes are responsible for glomerulonephritis and the nephrotic syndrome (see p. 468).

Granulomatous lesions

All the granulomatous lesions causing the main pathological effects of schistosomiasis in many organs, including the liver, are due to the immune response generated by eggs.

Other factors affecting the immune response

The nutritional status of an animal influences the infection. In experimental *S. mansoni* infection the number of worms developing in animals on a deficient diet is usually greater than in animals on a normal diet. Rats deficient in vitamin A have

less resistance to *S. mansoni* than normal rats and a diet deficient in cystine, selenium and vitamin E has a profound effect in increasing the severity of *S. mansoni* infection in mice.

In experimental work, however, protein deficiency has a deleterious effect on *S. mansoni* causing it to produce fewer eggs and more abnormal eggs than in animals normally fed. The abnormal eggs may be more readily absorbed in animals deficient in protein and may more readily stimulate a granulomatous reaction; rats in this condition develop fibrosis of the liver more readily than normal rats.

Human patients who have moderate nutritional deficiency and are infected with *S. mansoni* derive no benefit from a high protein diet alone, but when they are treated they respond more rapidly than usual. Treatment is less effective in vegetarians than in non-vegetarians.

Effect of treatment on immunity

Immunity persists after treatment, an important factor when considering mass treatment; 60% of patients resisted reinfection for at least one year after treatment, the resistance increasing with age.[71]

CLINICAL FEATURES

Schistosomiasis mansoni (intestinal schistosomiasis caused by *S. mansoni*)

Natural history

This is very variable and in general the disease is less serious in East Africa than in Egypt and South America. Many asymptomatic cases are found passing a few ova in the stools who appear to live an apparently normal life; others have vague abdominal pains, while others develop the complication of hepatosplenic schistosomiasis and eventually die from the complications of portal hypertension. In non-immune individuals a heavy primary infection can result in serious illness and death.

Incubation period

Cercarial dermatitis, which is common in non-immunes, arises and subsides in 24 hours after exposure. The toxaemic phase develops 15–20 days after exposure and eggs appear in the stool 40–55 days after infection.

Signs and symptoms

The infection can be divided into five stages.
1　The stage of invasion.
2　The toxaemic and hypersensitive phase.
3　The acute intestinal disease.
4　The stage of chronic irreversible effects:
　　a chronic intestinal form;
　　b hepatosplenic form;
　　c cardiopulmonary form.
5　The rare development of lesions in the nervous system, heart and skin.

THE STAGE OF INVASION
This stage includes cercarial dermatitis (swimmer's itch), itchy papules and surrounding oedema) arising within 24 hours and receding within a few days. This suggests a high density of cercariae. It also includes migration and development of the schistosomules and symptoms may start as early as 2 or 3 days after infection with fever, pulmonary symptoms (cough), eosinophilia and moderate splenomegaly. This is rare and probably represents a very early hypersensitive reaction. It is seen in Europeans but not Africans.

THE TOXAEMIC PHASE
This stage is most marked in primary infections in non-immune individuals. It develops 15–20 days after exposure with a typhoid-like illness, hepatomegaly, splenomegaly, eosinophilia, lymphadenitis and sometimes dysentery (especially in Brazil). This is the Katayama syndrome, which is seen in both *S. mansoni*, where it is less severe, and in *S. japonicum*. It starts insidiously with fever for a few weeks, resembling the fever of typhoid or brucellosis. The patient feels ill and sometimes becomes troubled with an urticarial eruption, with wheals and swelling of soft tissues about the eyes, prepuce and scrotum. The spleen and liver are slightly enlarged and there is eosinophilia, an important diagnostic feature. Cough may be troublesome. Electrocardiographic changes with inversion of the T waves over the left precordial leads sometimes occur. In one series of both European and African patients, the prepatent period varied from 9 to 87 days, most had swimmer's itch, cough, weight loss and eosinophilia but urticaria was rare. Half the patients had diarrhoea and

liver tenderness but only 10% splenomegaly. Several had mental symptoms suggesting some encephalopathy. *S. mansoni* ova appeared in the stools between 40 and 50 days after exposure, the shortest 34 and longest 97 days. Drug treatment was effective only after eggs had appeared in the stools.[72] Heavy primary infection in non-immune individuals can be fatal as it was in the Second World War in West Africa and still is in immigrant labour on large irrigation schemes in the Sudan. In these cases steroid treatment can be life-saving and excellent results have been obtained with steroids combined with anti-schistosomal drugs.[73]

The Katayama syndrome is usually mild and transient, including the eosinophilia, which is an important pointer. In Africa eosinophilia should always be regarded as possibly bilharzial and efforts should be made to find eggs, though they may not be found in the prepatent period.

In the stage of completion of maturation the main features are lassitude, fever, headache, backache, generalized pain, anorexia, loss of weight, occasional vomiting and diarrhoea. Eosinophilia is almost constant. The intradermal reaction does not become positive until four to six weeks after exposure. The intensity of symptoms depends upon the worm load.

ACUTE INTESTINAL PHASE
The acute intestinal disease is a result of the deposition of eggs in the wall of the bowel. It may begin suddenly about 40–55 days after infection. Dysentery is prominent with fever, weakness, anorexia, loss of weight and abdominal tenderness; it may last six to 12 months. Intestinal schistosomiasis may be present in a patient suffering from amoebic or bacillary dysentery and the diagnosis of bilharzial dysentery should not be made without excluding other more likely causes, especially in Africa where multiple infections are common. Bilharzial dysentery may be more common in South America.

CHRONIC INTESTINAL DISEASE
In chronic intestinal infection there may be little or no symptoms and in endemic areas the majority of infected individuals have intestinal infections without any symptoms or bowel disturbance.

In the stage of established disease there may be a chronic catarrhal state with swollen granular and haemorrhagic mucous membrane and numerous eggs in the mucosa and submucosa, especially of the rectum. Polyps and papillomas form, not only in the rectum but also in any part of the colon or even, rarely, in the small intestine. The polyps vary in size from a few millimetres and are dusky red, blue or rosy. They may ulcerate.

Localizing symptoms in *S. mansoni* infection occur in rather less than half the cases and consist of abdominal pain, sometimes diarrhoea or even dysentery, or even constipation. Other causes of dysentery should always be looked for even if eggs are found.

Sigmoidoscopy shows no abnormality in the majority of cases. In the others small submucous haemorrhages are followed by small yellow elevations of the mucosa, more rarely ulcers and polyps. These lesions usually show ova in a rectal snip which, however, may be positive in the absence of any visible mucosal changes.

Intestinal granulomatosis and polyposis. This is common in Egypt and the Middle East and is accompanied by severe chronic bloody dysentery with protein-losing enteropathy,[27,28] weight loss and anaemia. Lesions in the descending colon are recognized by barium enema, sigmoidoscopy and colonoscopy when numerous large pedunculated polyps can be demonstrated which may result in complete or partial obstruction of the bowel. The lesions are reversible with treatment[74] but permanent obstruction may develop. Bowel perforation is rare. Localized bowel granulomas may cause intussusception or rectal prolapse. Granulomatous masses may be present generally over the abdominal peritoneum. The bowel lesions may closely resemble Crohn's disease or ulcerative colitis.

Hypertrophic osteoarthropathy. This complication occurs in a few patients with intestinal disease, especially polyposis. It is manifested by arthritis in several large joints and clubbing of the fingers without the pulmonary features associated with other causes of the condition. It is reversible after treatment of the schistosomiasis.

HEPATOSPLENIC SCHISTOSOMIASIS

Hepatosplenic schistosomiasis with portal hypertension occurs in those areas where infections are heavy and there is a heavy egg load. In most cases the evidence of hepatosplenic disease is the presence of a firm enlargement of the liver[75] with or without splenomegaly which, in the Caribbean and South America, is used as a marker for the disease. This hepatomegaly is usually symptomless but in well-developed cases the clinical features of hepatosplenic schistosomiasis are those of portal hypertension with relatively normal liver function and an enlarging spleen which may reach enormous proportions (Fig. 22.14). Liver function is preserved but tests may show deterioration with the onset of ascites or after haematemesis. Oesophageal and gastric varices may bleed repeatedly and are a cause of death, haematemesis occurring in one-third of all cases. The enlarged spleen leads to hypersplenism with anaemia, leukopenia and thrombocytopenia. A raised IgG distinguishes it from tropical splenomegaly (raised IgM). In the later stages when there is ascites, there is a reduction in serum albumin leading sometimes to general anasarca.

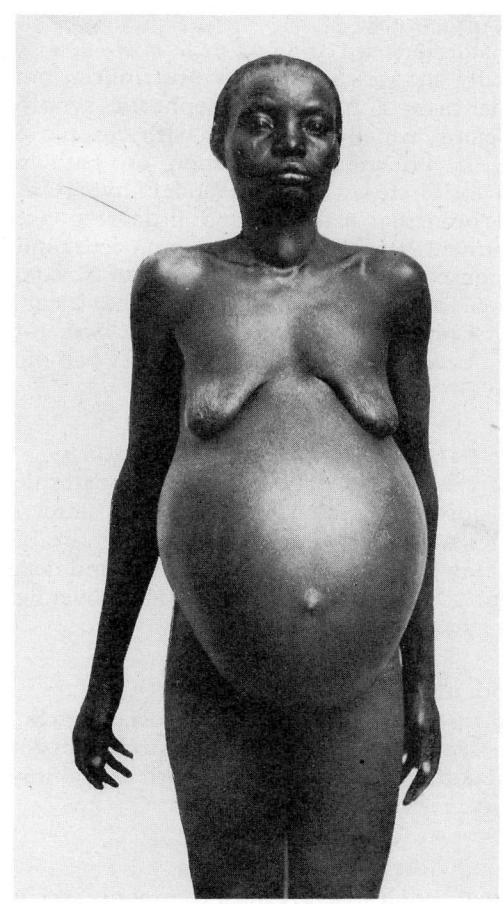

Fig. 22.14 Hepatosplenic schistosomiasis. (Courtesy Dr S. C. Jones.)

CARDIOPULMONARY SCHISTOSOMIASIS (see also Chapter 61)

Cardiopulmonary schistosomiasis is much rarer in *S. mansoni* than in *S. japonicum* infection and is always associated with the hepatosplenic form. The features are of an increasing cor pulmonale with pulmonary hypertension, dyspnoea, cyanosis often with finger clubbing, raised jugular venous pressure, accentuated second pulmonary sound and right heart strain with right ventricular preponderance and peaked P waves in lead 2 on electrocardiography. Chest radiographs show mottling caused by the enlarged small pulmonary arteries with right heart enlargement. A rare manifestation of pulmonary schistosomiasis has been described: a solitary pulmonary nodule formed by a cavity surrounded by fibrosis with sclerosing endarteritis containing eggs of *S. mansoni*.[76]

RENAL LESIONS

Renal lesions are common in *S. mansoni* and are usually shown clinically by proteinuria, but in some cases a full-blown nephrotic syndrome develops, usually associated with chronic *Salmonella* infection (see section on pathology, above). There is a high incidence of hypertension and bronchial asthma[77] and little response to treatment. Renal amyloidosis can occur, and its response to treatment is poor. Ova of *S. mansoni* can be found in the urine, and bladder lesions in which only ova of *S. mansoni* have been found have been described (see section on pathology, above).

CARCINOMA OF THE LIVER AND HEPATITIS B

There is an association between hepatosplenic schistosomiasis and hepatitis B infection. Patients with this double infection more often develop jaundice, intractable ascites and hepatic failure.[54] An association with primary liver hepatoma has not been confirmed.

ENDOCRINOLOGICAL LESIONS

S. mansoni infection has been associated in South America with dwarfism and impairment of gonad function, gynaecomastia and with sexual immaturity.

NEUROLOGICAL COMPLICATIONS

Spinal cord lesions are most commonly seen in *S. mansoni* infection. The schistosomal granuloma may be extra- or intramedullary and cause a transverse myelitis of acute or chronic onset which may show spontaneous improvement or unremitting deterioration.[78] Cauda equina lesions may also occur. There is a peripheral eosinophilia, complement-fixing and other antibodies in the blood and antibodies specific to both adult worms and ova in the cerebrospinal fluid with a lymphocytic pleocytosis and raised protein.[79] There is no consistent response to treatment but antischistosomal drugs and high dose prednisone, as well as surgery, are recommended.[78] The granulomas themselves always regress with antischistosomal chemotherapy, but the cord may not recover, presumably due to ischaemic damage. *S. mansoni* lesions in the brain are rare but have caused epilepsy.

Morbidity due to S. mansoni infection

The general effects of *S. mansoni* infection are difficult to assess and the effect of the disease on the rate of growth, onset of menstruation and nutritional status is regarded in South Africa as less than expected. In expatriate and Caucasian children resident in tropical Africa failure to thrive and a falling off in achievement in school should lead to a check for *S. mansoni* infection when eosinophilia, positive serology or the presence of a few ova in the stool will lead to treatment with a great improvement in health. Surveys of the effect of infection in the indigenous population have shown that there is a high incidence of colicky abdominal pain and bouts of diarrhoea with blood, with a small proportion showing enlargement of the liver and/or spleen. Studies on the output of work in infected communities have shown no clearcut results owing to the number of variables.

Mixed infections

In those parts of Africa where both *S. haematobium* and *S. mansoni* are prevalent, mixed infections are not rare (60% in parts of the Nile Delta, 22% in European patients in Zimbabwe). *S. mansoni* eggs may be found in large numbers in the faeces of patients in whom *S. haematobium* infection has gone so far as to produce calcification of the bladder, dilatation of the ureters and hydronephrosis. *S. haematobium* eggs are quite often present in faeces. Haematospermia may occur and eggs of either *S. haematobium* or *S. mansoni* may be present in the spermatic fluid.

Granulomas in the peritoneum can simulate tuberculosis.

Granulomatous masses, due to either *S. haematobium* or *S. mansoni*, can be found in association with the colon and even with the small intestine. In the colon they tend to be sausage-shaped. They can lead to obstruction or even volvulus.

Schistosomiasis haematobium (urinary schistosomiasis caused by *S. haematobium*)

Natural history

In general *S. haematobium* is a mild infection which is usually symptomless or manifests itself by recurrent painless haematuria. Among people living in an endemic area almost all children are infected at an early stage and macroscopic haematuria is common and microscopic haematuria almost universal. The urinary tract may be affected in adolescents, 30% of whom in some areas will show hydronephrosis or hydroureter. These abnormalities usually resolve naturally without permanent damage and, as age increases, the number of eggs passed falls in number until in late adult life no eggs are passed, and there are no signs of infection except for some scarring of the bladder. In some cases, however, complications develop with chronic renal infection, bladder abnormalities and carcinoma. The morbidity caused by urinary schistosomiasis is open to question but it is not a significant cause of death in most endemic areas.

Incubation period

The incubation period is difficult to determine but after the cercarial dermatitis which may occur a few hours after exposure, symptoms may arise from two months to over two years after infection, although mature eggs are passed 30–40 days after infection.

Symptoms and signs

In light infections there are usually none at all, the infection being detected on routine examination of the urine. Symptoms and signs vary in non-immune visitors and the inhabitants of endemic regions. Cercarial dermatitis and Katayama fever (see p. 458) do not occur in the indigenous inhabitants and are rare in non-immunes. The main symptoms and signs result from lesions of the bladder and ureters. These are haematuria, temporary or permanent hydronephrosis, chronic bacteriuria, pyelonephritis with renal failure and bladder changes.

HAEMATURIA

A painless haematuria is the first sign of *S. haematobium* infection, appearing especially towards the end of micturition, the so-called terminal haematuria. If the urine is allowed to stand minute blood clots may settle to the bottom and microscopical examination will show the characteristic terminal-spined eggs (Figs. 22.15 and 22.21). Haematuria is often disregarded by African children in endemic areas where it is almost universal and boys tend to regard it as a natural physiological phenomenon, the counterpart of menstruation in girls. It may last for months or even years but tends to decrease so that older adults do not suffer from haematuria.

Pain is usually absent, but may take the form of a dull sense of oppression in the suprapubic or perianal region, or there may be scalding on micturition. *Frequency* and *urgency* of micturition are early symptoms and there may be

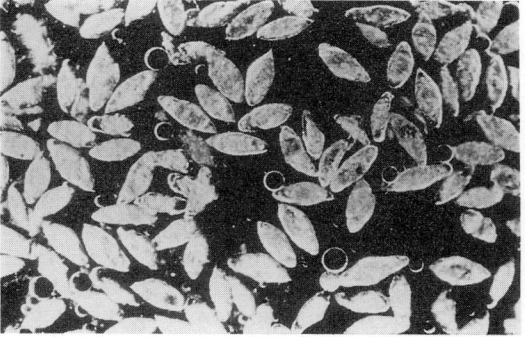
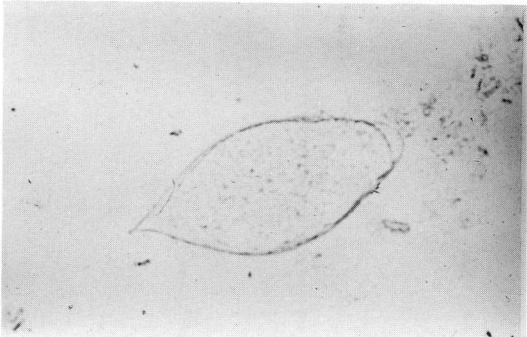

Fig. 22.15 *S. haematobium* eggs in urine.

rectal symptoms with the passage of blood and mucus.

RENAL EFFECTS

The effects on the renal tract vary in different geographical areas and are somewhat controversial. They are hydronephrosis and hydroureter (temporary or permanent), chronic bacteriuria and pyelonephritis with cortical destruction of the kidney, and extensive bladder changes.

Nephrotic syndrome. A nephrotic syndrome has been described in association with pyelonephritis and also with *Salmonella* infection[41] but is not common.

Temporary hydronephrosis and hydroureter. In the acute stage of urinary schistosomiasis hydronephrosis is the result of ureteric obstruction by lesions which interfere with the smooth muscle of the ureteric wall which, with disturbance of the ureterovesical sphincter, obstructs the flow of urine with ureteric reflux. The hydroneph-

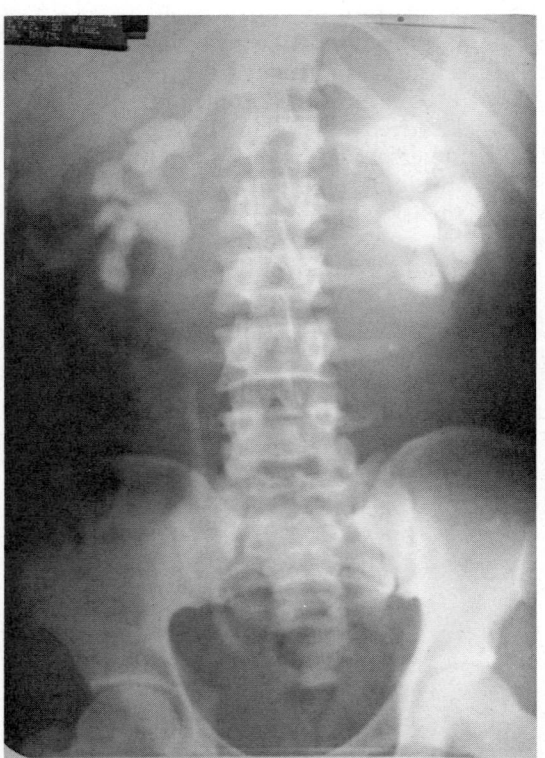

Fig. 22.16 Bilateral hydronephrosis in *S. haematobium* infection, reversible by treatment.

rosis is often bilateral with hydroureter most marked in the lower third of the ureter (Fig. 22.16) and disappears with treatment. It is common in many areas and in East Africa 30% of symptomless young adults may show these changes. In a small longitudinal study of infected children in Nigeria, observed for up to 74 weeks, nodular filling defects of the bladder, dilatation of the ureters and hydronephrosis resolved after adequate treatment,[80] and in Durban these lesions often regress.[81] The long-term effect of such changes on renal function is not yet clear but in Tanzania hydronephrosis and non-functioning kidneys are found in 10% of all adults, and there is indirect evidence that they can cause the death of numbers of young people.

Permanent hydronephrosis. Permanent hydronephrosis is due to atonicity of the ureters and in some cases fibrous strictures.

Chronic bacteriuria and pyelonephritis. Rates of 5% in young boys with asymptomatic disease and higher in symptomatic infections have been found in some surveys, but others have failed to demonstrate any association of bacterial infection and urinary schistosomiasis. Coliform bacilli and occasionally *Salmonella* are the usual cause. Bacteriuria cannot be cured without treatment of the schistosomiasis; as a result pyelonephritis is common in Egypt[43] but not in sub-Saharan Africa.[44] It has been suggested that the high infection rate in Egypt is associated with instrumentation such as cystoscopy.

Renal failure. In some areas renal failure is a common complication but renal failure was a rare cause of death in South Africa.[81] The variation from place to place is probably related to differing intensities of infection.

EFFECTS ON THE BLADDER

There are marked cystoscopic changes, calcification of the bladder and carcinoma.

Cystoscopic changes. The cystoscopic changes seen in *S. haematobium* are characteristic. In the early stages there are small well-defined haemorrhagic areas which are a sign of activity to be followed later by yellow nodules containing dead ova. Later ulcers may form. Small raised papules develop into small papillomas which may break off and be excreted in the urine. In late burnt out cases typical 'sandy patches' are formed which

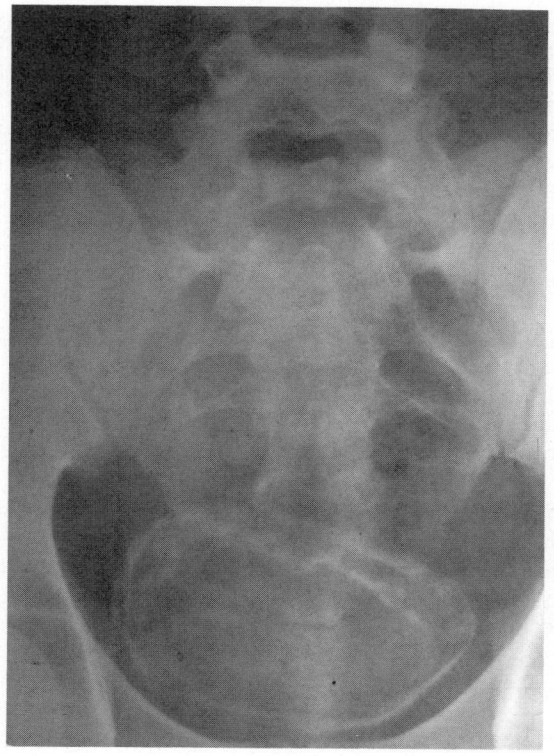

Fig. 22.17 Calcification of the bladder in late *S. haematobium* infection.

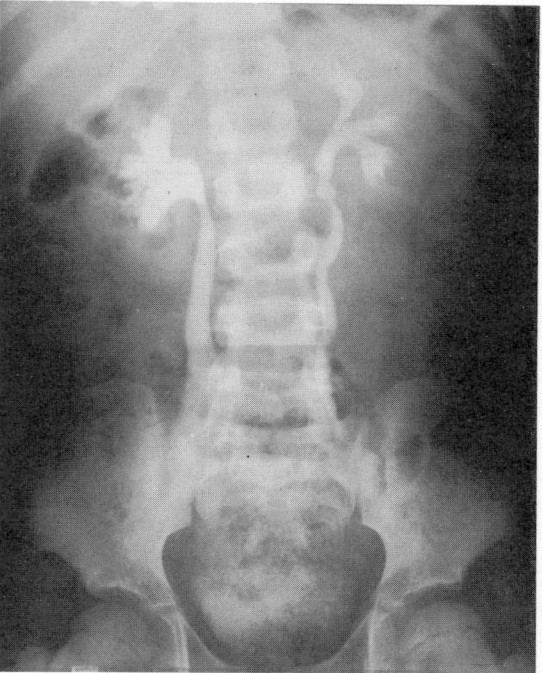

Fig. 22.18 Dilated ureters, calcified bladder and hydronephrosis caused by *Schistosoma* infection. (Courtesy Dr D. M. Forsyth.)

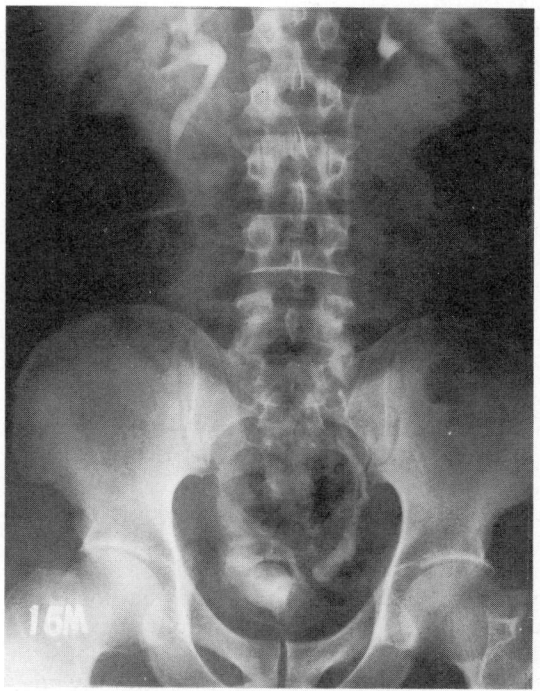

Fig. 22.19 Bladder stone caused by *S. haematobium*. (Courtesy Dr D. M. Forsyth.)

represent areas of fibrosis and are permanent and a sign of past infection.

Calcification of the bladder. Calcification of the bladder (Figs. 22.17 and 22.18) producing a 'fetal head' appearance is common in established infection but is reversible with treatment,[82] disappearing in old age. The appearance is due to calcification in dead eggs, not calcification of the bladder tissues, and a calcified bladder is not made rigid in this way.

Contraction of the bladder. The bladder may hypertrophy, dilate or contract when marked frequency of micturition is found and the only treatment may be surgical. The cause is fibrous thickening of the bladder wall. Retention with overflow may occur.

Bladder stone. Renal calculi do not occur but bladder stones containing ova of *S. haematobium* may be found (Fig. 22.19). The aetiological role of schistosomiasis in bladder stone formation is unproven.

Carcinoma of the bladder. Carcinoma of the bladder shows itself as gross haematuria with bladder irritation, weight loss and metastases in the inguinal, femoral and peritoneal lymph glands. It occurs after a period of 10–20 years in the third and fourth decades of life. It is typically of squamous cell type.

ECTOPIC DISEASE

Male genital tract. Urethral stricture, fistulae and elephantoid penile changes are accompanied by a sense of urethral discomfort and impotence. Prostatic involvement will cause frequency of micturition, impairment of the urinary stream, pain and discomfort on micturition and coitus, or constipation. Haemospermia is accompanied by sterility. The prostate will at first be enlarged and later small with small fluctuant cysts.

Female genital tract. Fibrosis of the ovaries with sterility is uncommon, but tubal lesions may cause sterility. The cervical and vaginal lesions give rise to bloody discharge and on inspection the lesions closely resemble carcinoma of the cervix, but no evidence of any connection of schistosomiasis with carcinoma of the cervix has been found.[83]

Pulmonary. Pulmonary involvement, which is not as common as in *S. mansoni* infection, can lead to congestive heart failure and cor pulmonale. There is widespread obliteration of pulmonary arterioles and a rise in blood pressure with hypertrophy of the right ventricle. The predominating symptom is dyspnoea. On radiography the enlargement of the right side of the heart is evident, often with diffuse and fine mottling of the lungs due to bilharzial tubercles which resemble miliary tubercles. Schistosome eggs may, rarely, be found in the deposit of sputum digested with 4% potassium hydroxide and centrifuged.

Nervous system. S. haematobium can affect the spinal cord, forming a granuloma containing the characteristic eggs, which compresses the cord, giving rise to symptoms and signs of transverse myelitis or radiculitis of the cauda equina. Eggs have also been found in the brain, accounting for epileptic symptoms. In these conditions the complement fixation test (CFT) is strongly positive and the circumoval precipitation test (COPT) in the cerebrospinal fluid is positive.

Skin. Ova deposited in the skin give rise to lesions consisting of the ova surrounded by granulomatous reaction and eosinophils leading to raised nodules or papules, which have been found in many areas. Soft warty vegetations and papules were found on the abdomen, especially round the umbilicus, where they originated from adult worms in the paraumbilical veins[52] and in the scrotum after Barlow's deliberate self infection[84] and in the perineum.

Skeletal manifestations. Skeletal rarefaction with scoliosis and fractures of the long bones may occur in heavy infections from excessive loss of phosphate and defective calcification resulting from renal tubular damage.

Unusual sites. Ova were present generally over the pleural surface of the lungs and peritoneum in an unusual case[32] although they were not found in the stools or urine. Appendicitis due to the accumulation of eggs has been reported.

General effects of *S. haematobium* infection

In non-immune individuals, especially expatriate Caucasians, the allergic manifestations of early infection may be prominent with tiredness as the chief symptom. On a community basis morbidity due to *S. haematobium* is difficult to assess.[85] Significant disease is found to occur even in lightly infected individuals, and infected adults show more permanent features of pathology in the urinary tract than children, suggesting progressive disease. Studies on a Gambian community suggest that urinary schistosomiasis may be a significant cause of mortality.[86]

Schistosomiasis intercalatum (caused by *S. intercalatum*)

Natural history

S. intercalatum infection causes a much milder disease than *S. mansoni* although it involves the large intestine and liver. Many asymptomatic cases occur and surveys have shown 5–25% of the population infected in some areas.

Incubation period

The incubation period is similar to *S. mansoni*.

Symptoms and signs

On the whole symptoms are slight. A toxaemic stage has been noted in the early stages but is mild and rare. The symptoms of established disease are intestinal: episodes of abdominal pain, mainly in the left iliac fossa, together with bloody diarrhoea and tenesmus. Granulomas, polyps and schistosomal tumours may occur in the colon and upper rectum.

Sigmoidoscopy shows a sandpaper appearance with minute haemorrhages and polyps may be seen occasionally. The rectal mucosa is friable and contains numerous ova. *Rectal biopsy* shows oedema and ulceration of the mucosa with little inflammatory reaction and a striking absence of cellular reaction.[87]

Hepatic involvement. S. intercalatum has a weak antigenic stimulus and hepatic granulomas are never situated outside the portal triangle and are smaller than those of *S. mansoni*. The spleen and liver may be enlarged but there is no hepatosplenic schistosomiasis. Granulomas may be found in the ovaries and adnexa.[88]

Pulmonary manifestations. These are absent.

Other features. Abortion in the third month of pregnancy has been noted.

Schistosomiasis japonicum (Far Eastern schistosomiasis caused by *S. japonicum*)

Natural history

S. japonicum causes a much more severe disease than the other schistosomes, probably because a much larger number of ova are released into the bowel and liver. The disease affects the intestine and although some infections are asymptomatic, many suffer a severe disease with fever, hepatosplenic and cerebral lesions, eventually resulting in death.

Symptoms and signs

Of the American troops affected during the Second World War 10–40% were asymptomatic.[89] There are three stages.

FIRST STAGE

This occurs soon after infection (30–40 days) as a marked Katayama syndrome, fever with urticaria, angioneurotic oedema, abdominal pain and cramp, cough and hypereosinophilia (60% or more). There may be diarrhoea. A fulminating type with sudden onset has been described in which abdominal rigidity is a marked feature.

SECOND STAGE

The second phase is characterized by bloody diarrhoea (dysentery), emaciation, hepatic (12–

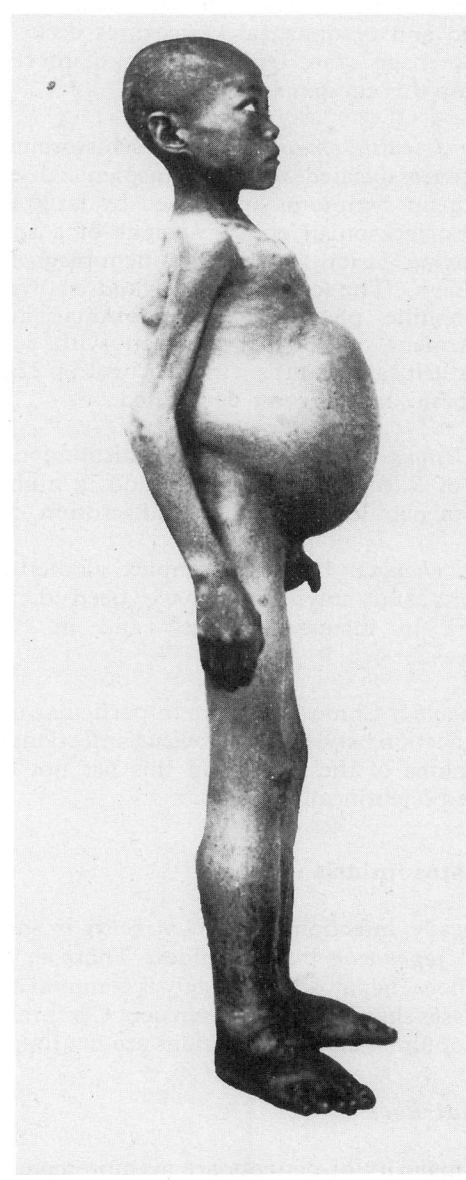

Fig. 22.20 Terminal stages of schistosomiasis japonicum. (Courtesy Dr J. A. Thomson.)

16%) and splenic enlargement (2–8%) with severe pain in the right hypochondrium and cough. This stage may resemble typhoid fever.

THIRD STAGE
The third stage occurs from three to five years after infection. Hepatosplenic schistosomiasis develops with Symmers' pipe-stem cirrhosis, with ascites and oedema of the limbs, anaemia and dysentery. Cardiopulmonary disease may develop. Superficial abdominal veins are distended and oesophageal varicosities occur but haemorrhage is rare. Only a *minority* of infections develop this complication.

Cerebral schistosomiasis. Cerebral schistosomiasis is often associated with hepatosplenic disease. The main symptoms are caused by large local lesions: jacksonian epilepsy, signs of a space-occupying lesion, often with hemiplegia and blindness. The cerebrospinal fluid shows an eosinophilic pleocytosis. Hypopituitarism or impairment of gonadal function with sexual immaturity and dwarfism may occur (Fig. 22.20). The bones may become decalcified.

Skin lesions. Skin lesions are not uncommon and eggs of *S. japonicum* can be found in multiple pruritic papules on the chest and scrotum.

Renal changes. Immune complex glomerulonephritis and amyloidosis have been demonstrated in infected rabbits[90] and in chimpanzees.[91]

Carcinoma. Chinese workers in particular claim a connection between *S. japonicum* infections and carcinoma of the colon, but this has not been proved scientifically to date.

Schistosomiasis mekongi

Clinically infection with *S. mekongi* is similar to *S. japonicum* but is milder. There is mild diarrhoea, hepatosplenomegaly is common and a few cases show portal hypertension. Cerebral and cardiopulmonary complications are not found.

S. mattheei

The majority of patients are asymptomatic but mild bloody diarrhoea with cramp-like abdominal pain occurs with mild hepatosplenomegaly and mucosal granulomatous lesions on sigmoidoscopy.

S. bovis

Most patients are asymptomatic but haematuria has been noted.

DIFFERENTIAL DIAGNOSIS

Katayama fever

Katayama fever can be clinically confused with typhoid fever, but there is never eosinophilia with typhoid. Fever and eosinophilia occur in several other invasive helminthic infections including tropical eosinophilia, visceral larva migrans, trichinosis and liver flukes. A geographical history, a search for ova, serology and the relatively transitory nature of Katayama fever will help to distinguish it.

Schistosomiasis may cause such diverse symptoms that it is not suspected as a cause of disease, especially in non-immune persons. Patients with either *S. mansoni* or *S. haematobium* have been diagnosed at times as having peptic ulcer, cholecystitis, hepatitis, pancreatitis and appendicitis—only to be cured when a light infection with schistosomiasis has been discovered after a long search. Conversely, all sorts of conditions have been ascribed to schistosomiasis just because a concurrent infection has been discovered in an endemic area where schistosomiasis is common.

S. haematobium

Haematuria can be confused with the painless haematuria of early tuberculosis of the kidney, papilloma and carcinoma of the bladder and the ectopic lesions as cancer of the genital tract or tumour of the spinal cord.

S. mansoni

S. mansoni may present with vague abdominal symptoms suggestive of peptic ulcer, pancreatitis or dysenteric conditions such as Crohn's disease, amoebiasis, tuberculosis, intestinal polyposis and ulcerative colitis. Hepatosplenic schistosomiasis must be distinguished from other causes of portal hypertension as well as kala-azar, leukaemia, thalassaemia and tropical splenomegaly but hepatosplenic schistosomiasis is remarkable for the retention of good liver function until the very late stages.

DIAGNOSIS

Travel to or residence in an endemic area with a blood eosinophilia should arouse suspicion of schistosomiasis. A definitive diagnosis is made by examination of the urine, stool, rectal or bladder biopsy for eggs, and by serological tests.

Examination of the urine

The important diagnostic features are the presence of microscopic haematuria and terminal-spined eggs (Fig. 22.21 and Plate III.11).

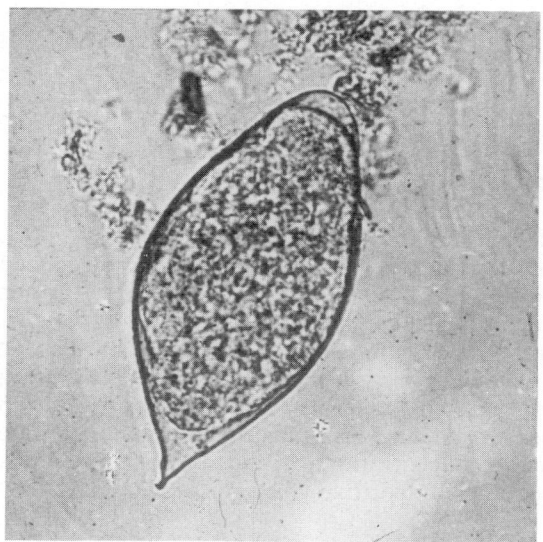

Fig. 22.21 Egg of *S. haematobium*. (Courtesy WTIM.)

Microscopic haematuria

Red cells are always present in the urine in active urinary schistosomiasis. Detection of blood by the dipstick method is extremely useful in detecting infected people in a community in mass examinations.[92]

Eggs

Eggs of *S. haematobium* are passed in the urine with a peak output between 10.00 hours and 14.00 hours. There is no advantage in making the patient exercise beforehand or in examining the last part of the urinary stream. Several specimens should be examined before pronouncing a negative result. The eggs are sought either in the centrifuged deposit or by filtration (see Appendix IV, p. 1493, for details).

Egg counts. The egg count should be done to measure the intensity of infection, and is essential in surveys or drug trials. Counts of less than 100 eggs/10 ml are light; 100–400/10 ml moderate and over 400/10 ml heavy infections. In some cases it may not be possible to find eggs in the urine.

Cystoscopic diagnosis

Cystoscopy will show evidence of past or present disease in the absence of ova in the urine. Sandy patches denote past infection while haemorrhages and papules denote active infection and bladder biopsy will show ova.

Stool

The eggs of *S. mansoni* (Fig. 22.22 and Plate III.12), *S. japonicum* (Fig. 22.23 and Plate III.13), *S. intercalatum* (Fig. 22.24) and sometimes *S. haematobium* are passed in the stool. Direct smear is the least sensitive method and a sensitive concentration technique must be used on several occasions if light infections are not to be missed.

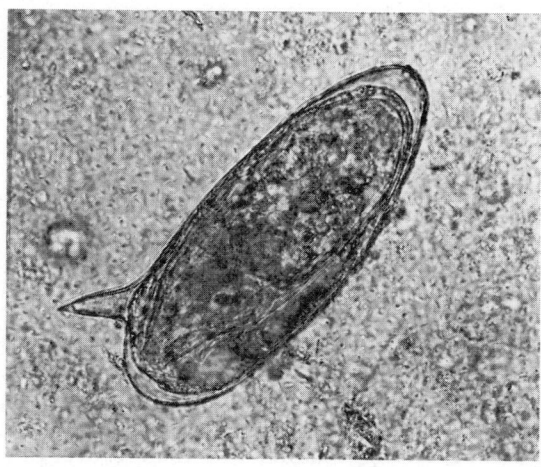

Fig. 22.22 Egg of *S. mansoni*. (Courtesy Dr O.D. Standen.)

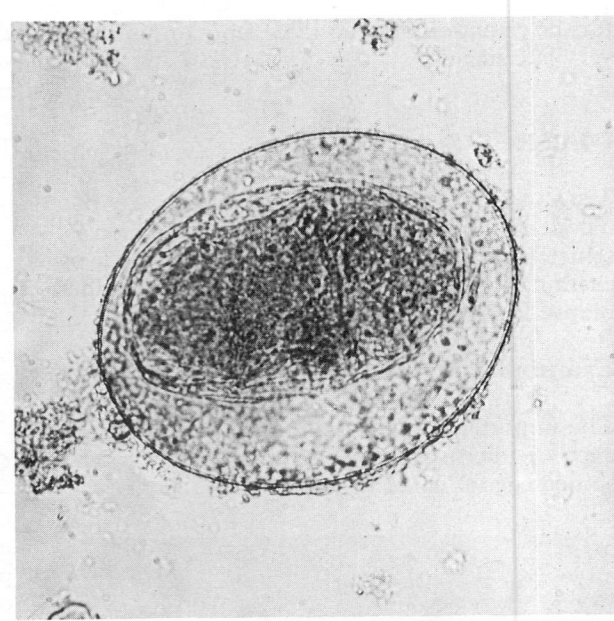

Fig. 22.23 Egg of *S. japonicum*. (Courtesy WTIM.)

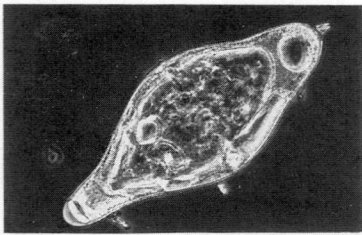

Fig. 22.24 Egg of *S. intercalatum*. (Courtesy Dr V.R. Southgate.)

Direct smear

A small portion of stool is emulsified in saline and examined microscopically. The average weight of stool in a direct smear preparation is 2–4 mg. It is easy to see how egg outputs of even 100 000/day could be missed using this method.

Concentration methods

Concentration methods are described in Appendix IV, p. 1490. The most commonly used ones are the Kato thick smear and its modifications, formol ether concentration and filtration and the egg count method of Bell[93] or Stoll (see Appendix IV, p. 1491). Egg counts less than 100 eggs/g denote light, 100–400/g moderate, and over 400/g heavy infections.

Rectal snips

Rectal snips are used for the diagnosis of *S. mansoni* and *S. japonicum*, although blackened dead eggs of *S. haematobium* are by no means uncommon in rectal snips and are a sign of past and not active infection. Through a proctoscope a portion of mucous membrane is teased off using a curette and examined as a squash preparation between two slides. This method is as accurate as the concentration methods but one method is occasionally positive when the other is not.

Bladder biopsy

A portion of the bladder mucosa obtained through a cystoscopy may be examined in the same way.

Viability of eggs

Eggs continue to be passed for years after curative treatment but are dead. Dead eggs usually mean a healed infection and their viability can be tested as follows. Under direct microscopy the flame cells may be seen to move in the miracidium when formed. Blackened structureless eggs are dead. The best test for viability is the miracidiascope.

Miracidiascope

This relies on the addition of fresh water to the eggs and waiting for them to hatch. Urine or 5 g of faeces is strained through a sieve to remove the coarse material. The fluid is allowed to stand and when the sediment has settled the supernatant fluid is discarded and warm tap water added to it in a conical glass against a dark background. The miracidia can easily be seen moving around with a hand lens.

Congo red test

Congo red has been used to test the viability of *S. mansoni* eggs. Live miracidia inside eggs as well as outside stain light blue, whereas dead ones stain red. Immature eggs containing undeveloped miracidia were not stained.[94]

Serology

Serological tests are more useful in *S. mansoni* and *S. japonicum* than in *S. haematobium* but there is no species specificity. They are useful in diagnosis of both apparent and inapparent infections. Many tests are available: enzyme-linked immunosorbent assay (ELISA), immunofluorescence, CFT, slide flocculation, plasma card, precipitin, haemagglutination, Cercarienhüllenreaktion, miracidial immobilization and COPT. The antigens used may be egg antigen or the gut-associated polysaccharide adult antigen. The main disadvantage of serological tests is their inability to distinguish between past and present infection. Antigen-detecting tests are still in their infancy.

Enzyme-linked immunosorbent assay

The ELISA test uses soluble egg antigen. It is highly sensitive (92–100% in *S. mansoni* and mixed infections) and highly specific reaching 100% positive with infection intensities of 160 eggs/g.[95] It becomes positive before eggs appear in the stool, and in all persons who had been in contact with infected water and not passing eggs without any symptoms, specific ELISA antibodies were present and no false negatives were found.[96] However, how far non-human schistosomes can elicit positive ELISA tests is not yet known. Antibodies are measured as a multiple of an accepted level and reported as 1.0, 1.5 or 2.0 and over times the screening level. But the level

bears no relationship to the intensity of infection. It is of no use as a test of cure since the levels of antibody do not fall after treatment for a number of years.

Immunofluorescence

An indirect fluorescent antibody test (IFAT) using either gut-associated adult or cercarial antigen[96] is a practical sensitive test much used up till now as a preliminary screen in sero-epidemiological surveys using dried blood on filter paper. It is not much used in clinical work because of cross reactions with animal schistosomes. False negatives can occur in long-standing infections. A titre of 1/16 or over is significant. It is of no use as a test of cure and has largely been superseded by the ELISA test.

Complement fixation test

This has now been superseded by the ELISA test.

With either cercariae or adult worms it is highly sensitive, will detect infection long before the worms are mature and can become positive within three weeks of exposure. Titres are usually between 1/20 and 1/60 but fall in long-standing infections. It is of no use as a test of cure. It is not species specific and becomes positive after exposure to non-human schistosomes as well as showing 100% cross reactivity with trichiniasis (but not vice versa), *Fasciola hepatica* and unisexual infections which are harmless to man.

Cercarienhüllenreaktion (CHR)

In this test a membrane is formed round cercariae immersed in immune serum but not in control serum. The test can be valuable in the diagnosis of present and recent infections when eggs cannot be found in urine or faeces. The test becomes positive 40–70 days after infection and negative five to seven months after successful treatment; it can be used as an index of cure. IgG is involved.

Circumoval precipitin test (COPT)

The COPT depends upon the formation of precipitates round the schistosome eggs immersed in dilutions of sera from infected persons; these are antigen–antibody complexes formed by secretions and excretions of the living miracidia in the eggs and specific antibodies in the sera.

Slide flocculation tests

Antigens prepared from excretions and secretions of the adult worms are sensitive and specific for the slide flocculation tests. One antigen is prepared from the cercarial material adsorbed on to crystals of lecithin–cholesterol, and with this the test is sensitive. In this test the antigen is allowed to fall on a drop of inactivated serum, the slide is rotated for 2 minutes and the result is read under the microscope. In the cercarial slide flocculation test IgG and IgM are concerned.

Plasma card tests

For the plasma card test cards coated with plastic on which a drop of plasma from a finger puncture has been placed are used with an antigen solution containing charcoal powder as a visualizing agent. The cards can be dried after the test and filed as records.

Intradermal test

The intradermal test using adult worm or cercarial antigen has now largely been discarded as it denotes exposure to any species of schistosome whether human or animal and is of no use in endemic regions where there is a high background of positivity.

Other tests

Other tests are being developed. Of particular interest are those depending on the detection of antigen rather than antibody, since they may determine whether the infection is active or not.[97] Free antigen–antibody complexes may be detected in early active infections and can be developed to act as useful diagnostic tests.[98]

Summary of serological tests

The ELISA is the test of choice for diagnosis both of light infections and for screening returned travellers. The COPT and CHR are the tests of choice for test of cure.

Radiological examination

In *S. haematobium* infections of the bladder, calcification is relatively late. Some eggs die in the mucosa and in fibrous tissue in the bladder wall; they die and calcify and X-ray shows a thin line of calcification round the whole bladder, sometimes very dense around mounds of granulation tissue, and extending to the lower ureters, the seminal vesicles or even the posterior urethra. Calcification does not usually involve the muscle coat though in rare cases it may do so.

The ureters may be either narrowed or dilated with hydroureter, hydronephrosis or filling defects in the ureters and bladder (large filling defects are a feature of severe disease in Nigeria). It is not certain that such lesions are progressive; they may regress with treatment but a radiologically non-functioning kidney does not regress.[60]

In *S. mansoni* infection when eggs cause ulceration of the mucous membrane healing takes place by fibrosis and subsequent crops of eggs may become entombed, producing granulomas or polyps which can be demonstrated radiologically by barium enema, appearing as multiple small filling defects, mostly in the sigmoid. They may even produce symptoms of obstruction and be indistinguishable radiologically from carcinoma.

Oesophageal varices can also be demonstrated radiologically but gastric varices are more difficult.

Portal venography to demonstrate the state of the portal vein and collateral circulation and the site of any obstruction can be carried out by injecting 30 ml of contrast material through a wide bore needle rapidly into the spleen and taking serial films in rapid succession.

X-ray examination of the chest may help in the diagnosis of cor pulmonale. For instance, fluoroscopy often shows pulsation of the pulmonary artery and enlargement of the right ventricle. Pulmonary angiography and cardiac catheterization, however, demand special techniques. The easiest way of making a presumptive diagnosis of cor pulmonale is by electrocardiography.

The radiological changes in *S. japonicum* infection are very similar to those in *S. mansoni* infection.

TREATMENT

The introduction of orally administered single dose antischistosomal drugs has brought the possibility of mass chemotherapy within reach as well as made the treatment of individual infections cheap and simple, without the need for admission to hospital. Niridazole, hycanthone, lucanthone and trivalent antimony compounds have now all been superseded. Praziquantel, oxamniquine and metriphonate have replaced them and are so successful that light infections proven parasitologically or serologically can all be treated safely, as well as heavier infections, especially in children in endemic areas. But in many endemic areas it is neither practical nor economic to treat light infections, unless as part of an attempt to control transmission. Most people with light infections will come to no harm.

Praziquantel (Biltricide, Droncit)

Praziquantel is active against all species of schistosome: *S. haematobium*,[99] *S. mansoni*,[100] *S. japonicum*,[101] *S. intercalatum*[102] and *S. mekongi*.[103] It is the drug of choice where available and where expense is not too much of a problem. The dose is 40 mg/kg in a single dose given after the evening meal to avoid dizziness; 2 × 20 mg/kg divided doses given 4–6 hours apart is just as effective.[104] In *S. japonicum* larger doses are necessary: 60 mg/kg given in two divided doses in one day[105] is necessary but side-effects of abdominal pain and vomiting are common.

Oxamniquine (Vansil, Mansil)

Oxamniquine is effective only against *S. mansoni*, especially strains from West Africa and Brazil. It is just as effective as praziquantel but cheaper. The dose is 15 mg/kg in a single dose, but in East and central Africa 60 mg/kg divided into three or four doses, each of 15 mg/kg should be given over 2–3 days. It should be given after the morning and evening meal; drowsiness and dizziness are the most important side-effects, but generalized convulsions occasionally occur.

Metriphonate (Bilarcil, trichlorphon)

Metriphonate is an organophosphate compound effective only against *S. haematobium*. It blocks the worm's acetylcholinesterase and paralyses it, causing irreversible 'lung shift'. The dose is 10 mg/kg; three doses at two-week intervals are necessary. Side-effects are minimal although the plasma cholinesterase drops temporarily. Its main asset is its low cost.

Other drugs: Oltipraz

Oltipraz has proved highly effective against all three species of schistosomes but has been withdrawn because of side effects.

Complications of treatment

Modern drugs have made it possible to treat cases even where there is considerable evidence of liver damage but heavily infected cases may develop 'verminous pneumonia' following 'lung shift' of the dead worms (see p. 461). This comes on within a week or two of treatment with the development of asthma and pulmonary infiltrations. Symptoms and signs disappear within a few days.

Test of cure

Egg excretion is usually interrupted by the end of the second week after treatment. A measure of egg excretion (stool or urine) at around the fourth week will indicate how effective treatment has been. Some dead eggs may continue to be shed for a time but the overall excretion of eggs will have dropped considerably if the drug has been effective. Microscopic examination will show whether the egg has the morphology of a recently laid egg or alternatively a hatching test may be performed. Although an interruption in egg excretion is observed it may be only temporary, notably in *S. mansoni* treated with niridazole. If an absolute cure is the aim, further examination of stool, urine, rectal snips and serology should be carried out three months after treatment. If treatment has been given on the finding of an eosinophilia and recent definite exposure, in an attempt to kill the worms before egg deposition starts, it will be useful to follow the eosinophil count. It may well rise during the first four weeks after successful treatment of an early or established infection but it will then steadily decline to normal levels.

Treatment of complications

S. haematobium

Many of the urological abnormalities that can be

demonstrated by radiology are reversed when the worms are eradicated. No surgical treatment for obstructive uropathies and similar lesions should be contemplated until after a trial of chemotherapy and subsequent reassessment. Even bladder calcification may resolve at least partially. Persistent haematuria after treatment raises the possibility of carcinoma. Orthodox surgery, such as colocystoplasty,[107] for patients whose bladder capacity is reduced to below 300 ml, with symptoms, can be considered.

S. mansoni

There has been concern that the simultaneous chemotherapeutic death of many worms may lead to clinical deterioration and doubts that treatment could usefully change damaged tissues. However, it is probably always worthwhile to attempt to cure an infection if there are complications due to the parasite. Egg deposition is prevented and progression halted and often there is considerable clinical improvement. Proliferative rectal lesions may resolve in the same way as the proliferative bladder lesions of *S. haematobium* but in debilitated patients with schistosomal polyposis, endoscopic surgical removal of the polyps is indicated.[108]

Neurological lesions, especially cord compression, may sometimes be treated on suspicion rather than absolute parasitological proof, though in the absence of improvement it will often be necessary to resort to surgery without delay. Pulmonary and portal hypertension often improve surprisingly and remarkably after chemotherapy. If haematemesis complicates portal hypertension, transfusions of fresh blood, often massive, are required. Oesophageal compression with a Sengstaken–Blakemore tube is not without its dangers and vasopressors are of limited value. Emergency surgery is hazardous but as a recurrence of bleeding is probable elective surgery should be considered, though it is difficult to be certain of its value. Given satisfactory liver function (albumin 3.2 g/dl or more), no jaundice, no ascites and a prothrombin time that is normal or near normal, an end-to-side portacaval anastomosis is satisfactory.

It is necessary to deworm the patient during the operation. A trivalent antimonial is given, the worms are flushed along the portal vessels and filtered out in the portal vein.[109] An alternative is to treat the patient prior to surgery and bring egg deposition to a halt at the earliest possible

moment. Most shunt operations do not require removal of the spleen and because of adhesions splenectomy is often difficult. If the spleen is removed, however, it should be remembered that if the patient is returning to an area of malaria transmission, antimalarials must be taken for the rest of life, whatever the previous immune status.

Injection sclerotherapy using modern fibreoptic instruments has rendered portocaval shunt operations almost obsolete in some centres.

Salmonella septicaemia complicating schistosomiasis cannot be cured by antibiotics alone. The *S. mansoni* or *S. haematobium* infection must also be treated.

S. japonicum

No reversal in the permanent fibrotic changes of hepatosplenic schistosomiasis can be expected but the cerebral lesions will subside and clear without the need for surgical intervention.

EPIDEMIOLOGY

Schistosomiasis is primarily a rural disease although it does occur in some towns and cities. Transmission depends on a variety of factors.
1 Contamination of fresh water with human/animal urine or faeces containing viable schistosome eggs.
2 The presence in the water of snails susceptible to infection by miracidia hatched from those eggs and capable of producing cercariae infective to man. Water temperature, rate of flow, acidity or alkalinity and content of organic matter conducive to snail growth are important factors.
3 Human contact with water containing living cercariae, from fishing, bathing, washing, playing and drinking. Also, the timing of water contact activities often coincides with peak cercarial shedding and peak urinary output. Many studies have shown that children are particularly important because they are attracted by water and pass the greatest number of eggs within the population. Usually, children aged between five years and 15 years fall into this category.

The introduction of greatly increased human populations in irrigation areas enhances greatly the chance of infection. There is a great need for sociocultural implications to be assessed and public health measures to be planned prior to irrigation schemes being built. Bousfield[110] showed that the migration of infected people from the north-east to the south of Brazil caused the spread of schistosomiasis from its original focus. Interestingly, the parasite has adapted to another snail host in the south, *Biomphalaria tenagophila*. In the vicinity of Lake Sibaya in South Africa the fear of crocodiles and hippopotami are important factors in transmission because the villagers tend to use the small shallower habitats, favoured by *Bulinus globosus* (the host for *S. haematobium*) and not *Biomphalaria pfeifferi* (the host for *S. mansoni*); hence the explanation for the mean prevalence of 72% for *S. haematobium* and absence of *S. mansoni*. An increase in development of the area would undoubtedly result in a decline of the crocodile and hippopotamus populations and would allow the utilization of deeper water favoured by *Biomphalaria pfeifferi* and increase the chances of initiating a transmission cycle of *S. mansoni*.[111] In Zanzibar *S. haematobium* infection is highly focal: in good areas wells, running streams or piped water are available as water supplies and prevalence for *S. haematobium* is about 30%;[112] in bad areas only a few virtually stagnant streams or pools are available and infection rates reach almost 100%. In these areas the infection is not only common, it is also heavy in individual patients.

In Iraq schistosomiasis is a disease of fishermen and gardeners as well as agricultural workers, but is a social rather than an occupational disease, heaviest in poor conditions. Studies in Brazil have demonstrated that prevalence, intensity and rate of splenomegaly are significantly higher in the environs of the town rather than in the central area and this is considered to be due to the social differences between the populations living in the two areas.

Small dams or pools are dangerous in that they attract both bathers and snails, which may be introduced as eggs on the feet of water birds. The shores of lakes, especially near inflowing streams which are likely to be contaminated with human excreta, are also dangerous. Studies on the shores of Lake Volta have shown that the greatest density of infected snails is close to the shoreline.

Irrigation is a major factor in transmission and is likely to increase as water conservation schemes, agricultural programmes and generation of hydroelectric power all become desirable. In well-maintained irrigation canals, however, snails do not thrive, but with poor management, poor drainage channels with night storage dams and temporary pools, conditions suitable for the multiplication of snails exist. These factors have been responsible for the increase of *S. haematobium* and *S. mansoni* infections observed in many irrigation areas.

In the Gezira plain of the Sudan extensive irrigation over vast areas, over 8000 square kilometres, has led to an increase in the prevalence of schistosomiasis. A series of papers on the Blue Nile Health Project has been published,[113] which gives the latest information on a comprehensive approach to the prevention and control of water-associated diseases in irrigated areas of the Sudan.

In Egypt the changes in the relative frequencies of the snail populations is reflected in changes in the parasite populations, and the recent increase of *S. mansoni* has important public health implications since hepatosplenic schistosomiasis caused by *S. mansoni* is more difficult to treat and is associated with more morbidity and mortality than urinary schistosomiasis.

Recent studies by Wilkins et al[114] in The Gambia suggest that the sequence of events with regard to immunity and infections differs from that envisaged by Bradley and McCullough.[63] Wilkins et al[114] believe that the worm burdens in children are in a dynamic state and that the decline in intensity and prevalence of infection in children in their second decade of life is due to the rate of acquisition being less than the rate of loss. However, an epidemiological role for concomitant immunity is not ruled out,[114] because the prevalence of infection is greater in adult males than in females, although adult females appear to have more exposure to infection. Hence, they suggest that protective immunity might be more important in adult life than in childhood in The Gambia but add that the epidemiological role of protective immunity may not be the same in all foci.

Infection is strongly influenced by social and religious practices in relation to contact with water. In Egypt females may have more frequent contact with water than males, in washing clothes and utensils. However, water contact studies in Malumfashi, Nigeria showed that males were involved in 98% of activities involving contamination and exposure,[115] hence accounting for the marked male predominance of *S. haematobium* infection. Peak water contact activity often occurs during the warmer part of the year when snail populations are often at peak densities. Such social influences are important.[116]

PREVENTION

Active transmission of schistosomiasis relies on infected people utilizing and contaminating water resources which harbour freshwater snails capable of transmitting the disease. Generally, prevention depends upon limiting the human water contact and contamination of the environment with schistosome ova. These objectives can be achieved through improvements of living standards and more specifically by chemotherapy and snail control, and may be listed accordingly.

1 Treatment of infected persons (though this leaves the question of animal reservoirs unsolved, especially important with *S. japonicum*). A variety of effective drugs now exists for the treatment of schistosomiasis, praziquantel being particularly effective in a single oral dose. With improvements in quantitative parasitological diagnostic techniques it is now possible to identify those members of a community passing most eggs and therefore most likely to suffer from disease symptoms. Usually school children fall into this category, and one approach has been to use targeted chemotherapy against those heavily infected thereby reducing morbidity and prevalence within a community. In the Gezira, Sudan, praziquantel was used for mass treatment in villages with prevalence rates of more than 40%; in villages with a lower prevalence rate only infected persons were treated (selective population chemotherapy), resulting in a marked reduction (50% to 11%) in prevalence in one year.

2 Provision of latrines, especially at work places connected with irrigation canals. The ventilated pit latrines are an improvement on the usual pit latrines used in developing countries, but it is generally considered that this approach will only affect transmission patterns in the long term.

3 Provision of properly constructed and controlled bathing places for children, which can be kept free from snails. Such protected swimming baths have been suggested to prevent indiscriminate bathing in infected water.

4 Siting of villages well away from snail-bearing irrigation canals and, if possible, other snail-bearing waters. This may not be possible if the waters are ponds forming the only water supplies for the people.

5 Provision of piped water or properly constructed wells that are maintained and positioned in sites which are more convenient than the infected sites. However, it has been demonstrated in some countries, for example St Lucia and Zimbabwe, that piped water supplies should be supplemented by laundry facilities and showers if a marked reduction in water contact patterns using the traditional sites is to be seen. It should be noted that schistosome cercariae can pass in small numbers through conventional sand filters[117] and through metal microfabric Mark 1 (apertures 35 μm), though they are almost completely held back by microfabric Mark 0 (aperture 23 μm).[118]

6 Destruction of snails utilizing chemical, environmental and biological methods.

7 Education of the people.

8 Reduction of contact with snail-bearing water by covering irrigation channels or by conveying irrigation water in concrete channels above ground level as in various schemes in Morocco. The provision of foot and cart bridges are also helpful in reducing water contact.

9 Advances continue to be made on the characterization of schistosome antigens with the overall aim of developing a vaccine against the disease. Field trials using cryopreserved schistosomula attenuated through radiation (live vaccine) have demonstrated that intensity of *S. bovis* infections and therefore morbidity, can be reduced in cattle. If a vaccine is developed then logistic problems of delivery will have to be overcome.

Personal prophylaxis

Personal prophylaxis on the part of non-immune visitors can be practised by remembering that any fresh water, whether rivers, lakes or dams, is potentially infective south of the Sahara at altitudes below 5000 feet. Crossing rivers at fords where the population washes clothes and gossips should be avoided. Protective clothing is not much use except that rubber boots which are easily dried off may offer some protection.

CONTROL

Improved understanding of the epidemiology of schistosomiasis, the development of simple quantitative diagnostic techniques, and the development of better, safer drugs have been central to the development of new strategies for control. The primary objective of most control programmes is to reduce morbidity within the infected population. Disease symptoms are caused by eggs deposited in tissues; therefore the elimination or reduction of adult worms will reduce the chances of morbidity developing. There is evidence that certain age classes within a community (e.g. 10–14 year olds) are more likely to be passing more eggs than other age classes, but within an age class there is considerable variation in worm loads. This recognition of the variability of worm loads has led to several different control approaches within endemic populations. Selective population chemotherapy relies upon identification, then treatment, of infected people. Selective group treatment is really a variant of selective population chemotherapy, and relies upon treating the age classes with peak prevalence, intensity and morbidity, either as a group or all of those infected. Targeted chemotherapy concentrates upon treating those individuals with high levels of egg output who are at the greatest risk of developing disease symptoms. Each approach is not mutually exclusive to any other, and in some situations it may be desirable to utilize a combination. It is recognized that after chemotherapy transmission will continue, albeit at a lower level than pre-treatment, and that the rate of reinfection will vary in different individuals. It is accepted that re-treatment schedules will have to be implemented. In some situations chemotherapy campaigns can be supported by well-planned snail control programmes, and depending upon transmission sites and transmission patterns will determine the type of snail control, i.e. blanket mollusciciding, focal mollusciciding or slow release formulations.

Macdonald[118] evaluated the various control measures by relating them to the life-cycle of the schistosomes, pointing out that in such an infection, in which sexual pairing takes place and in which there is an intermediate host, the numbers of potentially pathogenic worms are enormously increased by the large numbers of eggs discharged each day by a single pair of adult worms, that they are again enormously increased if the eggs reach fresh water in which there are many snails of species susceptible to the infection, because each miracidium which develops in a snail gives rise to hundreds of cercariae. From a mathematical analysis of factors bearing on infection he argued that reduction in the numbers of miracidia will not significantly reduce the numbers of invasive cercariae. This argument is flawed, however, as there are many situations when the snail population has a low infection rate, when the limiting factor in cercarial pro-

duction must obviously be the number of miracidia rather than the number of snails. More recently, the Macdonald model has been modified to take into account the efficiency of the miracidium in host location.[120] It was shown that if miracidia are inefficient hunters, then the resulting model is very sensitive to perturbations, such that a small change in snail numbers will cause appreciable changes in percentage of snails infected and result in attainment of threshold (the point at which schistosomiasis ceases to be endemic). On the other hand, if miracidia are efficient the model is less sensitive to perturbation and threshold and is more difficult to reach.

Snail control

Two general strategies for snail control are in current use: focal control and area control. The former approach is employed where transmission is limited to particular foci, and area control is used where transmission is widespread, such as throughout an irrigation system. Mollusciciding is particularly suited to areas where transmission is seasonal and confined to relatively small habitats such as are found in the Yemen Arab Republic. It is also useful in parts of larger water bodies, for example, Lake Volta, Ghana where transmission is focal; in countries, such as Egypt and Sudan where extensive irrigation is used for agriculture and population density is high, mollusciciding has been shown to be an important part of the control strategy. Mollusciciding in the majority of habitats is unlikely to result in the complete eradication of snails, especially as snails have such a remarkable reproductive potential and therefore ability to recover from damaged populations. Consequently, mollusciciding must be continued for long periods to be effective. Knowledge of the biology of the life-cycle of the snail is also relevant to the timing of mollusciciding. In Egypt, for instance, *Bulinus truncatus*, abundant in large canals and less abundant in drains, can double its population in 14–16 days in March and its highest death rates are in midsummer. *Biomphalaria alexandrina*, on the other hand, is most abundant in drains and less so upstream; it reaches its maximum abundance in the presence of the water hyacinth, *Eichhornia crassipes*, doubling its population in 14–16 days in March, with its highest death rates in summer.

A single area-wide treatment with molluscicide in April is therefore recommended; during the rest of the year search for isolated foci of snail breeding and individual treatment of those foci will be effective in control.

Efforts have been made towards using non-chemical methods, i.e. biological control for reducing the incidence of snail-borne disease. One of the theoretically ideal methods is to replace the vector snail with another species which is resistant to the parasites but has a higher intrinsic rate of natural increase due to a higher growth rate, better utilization of food resources, longer life-span, etc. *Helisoma duryi*, a member of the family Planorbidae, has been the subject of many laboratory and some field experiments and apart from *Biomphalaria glabrata*, it seems to suppress most species of *Bulinus* and *Biomphalaria*. Nevertheless, further experiments to examine the influence of *H. duryi* on intermediate hosts will be required to elucidate the nature of the competitive interactions, to find out under which conditions/biotypes the competition may act and to establish that the snail does not have any adverse effects on crops, such as rice or indeed transmit any harmful parasites to man or domestic animals before it is used on a wider scale as a biological competitor.

The large snail *Marisa cornuarietis* eats the egg masses of snails and competes with other species for food. *Marisa* was originally used in Puerto Rico, but more recently has been used in a manmade lake in Tanzania. Prior to the release of *Marisa* the dam held thriving populations of *Biomphalaria pfeifferi*, *Bulinus tropicus* and the melaniid *Melanoides tuberculata*, but after 24 months the three pulmonate species had been eliminated; only *Melanoides tuberculata* remained at the same population density as originally recorded. Detailed laboratory experiments have shown that the predatory behaviour of *Marisa* is an extremely plastic phenomenon that may be influenced by environmental factors, as well as age, genotype and the physiological state of the snail. *Marisa* is not, so far as is known, an intermediate host of any important parasite.

Several species of mollusc-eating fish have been studied as biological control agents, including *Tilapia melanopleura*, *Clarisa* sp. and *Serranochromis* sp. but more data regarding their effectiveness are required. Other developments include the discovery that rediae of echinostomes will devour the sporocysts of schistosomes. The results of small scale field trials show that to be effective an abnormally high infection rate (70%)

must be maintained, so as yet these methods are of limited practical use.

Molluscicides

Details of molluscicides and the role of molluscicides in schistosomiasis control can be referred to in a World Health Organization publication.[121]

Control of snail intermediate hosts by molluscicides is an effective means of reducing transmission of schistosomiasis, but it is usually used alongside other methods such as chemotherapy and environmental control. Control by molluscicides is expensive; application must often be frequently repeated and requires supervision.

Niclosamide (Bayluscide) is highly toxic to snails, their eggs and to schistosome cercariae and can be handled safely: its disadvantages are its high cost and its lethal effects on fish and other organisms. It is the compound which is currently used in large scale control operations and is available as either a wettable powder containing 70% active ingredient or as an emulsion concentrate with 25% active ingredient.

Although *Frescon* is the most active molluscicide known, the compound has not fulfilled its early promise and is no longer available.

Sodium pentachlorophenate is highly effective against aquatic and amphibious snails and their eggs, and has been widely used with success, but it is irritating and potentially dangerous to the handler; its activity may be reduced by bright sunlight. Pentachlorophenol is widely used in China and copper pentachlorophenate in Venezuela.

Copper sulphate (and other copper compounds) is active at low pH and is somewhat less toxic to fish than some molluscicides; it is safe to handle but is absorbed by solid and organic material and its toxicity to snails and their eggs is variable in the field. It corrodes equipment. It is readily available and now substantially cheaper than other synthetic compounds. A new exciting development in the application of using copper based molluscicides is the development of the slow release method. Basically, the copper compounds are mixed in glass which itself is soluble in water and thereby releases the copper at a controlled rate. The advantage of this development is that application is less expensive in terms of human resources. Field trials in Zambia and Zimbabwe using slow release methods have yielded encouraging results.

Other molluscicides include organo-tin and lead compounds, dinex (a dinitrophenol), carbamates, 3-trifluoromethyl-4-nitrophenol (TFM), nicotinanilides and some plants, endod (*Phytolacca dodecandra*), *Jatropha* spp. and *Ambrosia maritima*.

The interest, search for and use of plant molluscicides is based upon the hope that they may prove cheaper and more readily available than synthetic compounds. The use of natural, indigenous materials has attractions over the use of expensive, imported, synthetic compounds. This area of study has been admirably reviewed by Kloss and McCullough.[122] Many studies, including field trials, have been carried out on *Phytolacca dodecandra* in Ethiopia. The berries are used as the major traditional laundry soap, the active principle being several derivatives of oleanolic acid of triterpenoid saponin. It has the disadvantage of not being lethal to egg masses of snail hosts at molluscicidal concentrations but it is lethal to other organisms, such as tadpoles, frogs and more importantly fish. However, to date well over 1000 plant species have been screened for molluscicidal activity and it seems likely that research in this field will expand. However, there are still major problems related to working out the cost effectiveness of such compounds, finding their chronic toxicity and the developing snail control programmes in rural areas using local resources and collecting comparable data.

Application of mass chemotherapy

In Brazil mass chemotherapy of the whole population was given wherever prevalence exceeded 20%; between 5% and 10% the entire 7–18 years age group was treated and where it was less than 4% only the positive individuals.[123] A combination of mass chemotherapy and control of transmission by molluscicides has been used in varying proportions in different programmes.

In Brazil chemotherapy, coupled with health education, has achieved significant results;[123] in Egypt chemotherapy combined with focal molluscicidal control has had considerable success against *S. haematobium*.[124]

Vaccines

Vaccination has achieved some success in cattle in which worm loads have been reduced using irradiated cercarial vaccine. Heterologous immunization using non-human schistosomes from animals and hybrid worms as living vaccines has had some success in monkeys,[125] but since the major defence mechanism of the body is the schistosomal granuloma which is responsible for pathology, work along these lines obviously bristles with difficulties.

SWIMMER'S ITCH (CLAM-DIGGER'S ITCH, CERCARIAL DERMATITIS)

This is a condition caused by penetration of schistosome cercariae into the human skin after release from their snail intermediate hosts in shallow waters (usually lake shores, rice fields or even sea shores). The schistosome cercariae which cause swimmer's itch are mainly parasites of birds but a few are parasites of mammals; the cercariae are usually immobilized after penetrating the skin, although a few may possibly survive in the deeper tissues for some time.

Swimmer's itch is found in many parts of the world—the Americas, Europe, Africa and Australasia. The cercariae have been described under the names *Cercaria elvae*, *C. ocellata*, *C. herini* and others. The adult worms include *Gigantobilharzia sturniae*, *Trichobilharzia* spp. (from black swans and silver ducks). *Schistosomatium douthitti* (from rodents), *Austrobilharzia* spp. (from the silver gull) and *Schistosoma spindale* (from water-buffalo). Snails involved include *Lymnaea stagnalis*, *L. undussumae*, *Pyragus australis*, *Polypylis hemisphaerula* and doubtless many others.

The initial exposure to these cercariae only elicits a mild response, but subsequent exposures cause a reaction to certain cercarial antigens resulting in itching, formation of macules and eventually large papules. The papules are often accompanied by erythema, oedema and intense pruritus. The symptoms can arise within a day of bathing in infected water. Application of 5% copper sulphate is said to relieve the itching, and 2% methylene blue to prevent bacterial infection. The intradermal and complement fixation tests become positive. Systemic complications with evidence of hepatocellular damage, cough, fever, myalgia and abdominal pain were noted in Vietnam in two outbreaks of schistosome dermatitis where there was no *S. japonicum* infection.[126]

HERMAPHRODITIC FLUKES

Flukes are comparatively large fleshy parasites which live in the biliary tract (liver flukes), intestinal canal (intestinal flukes) or lung (lung flukes) of the vertebrate host. They are zoonotic infections which have a life-cycle involving a vertebrate host and two intermediate hosts. The adult fluke lives in the vertebrate host (man or animal) and lays its eggs which pass out into water where they hatch into *miracidia* which enter the first intermediate host, a snail, in which they develop to form *cercariae*; these leave the snail to enter a second intermediate host, a fish, crustacean or aquatic vegetation, on or in which they encyst as *metacercariae*. The flesh or vegetation is then eaten by a vertebrate and an adult infection is established (Table 22.2).

1   LIVER FLUKES

The liver flukes, *Fasciola hepatica* (and *F. gigantica*), *Clonorchis sinensis* and *Opisthorchis*, *Dicrocoelium dendriticum* live in the intrahepatic bile ducts where, in contrast to schistosomes, the pathological effects are caused by the adult flukes and not the eggs.

Fasciola hepatica and *F. gigantica*

GEOGRAPHICAL DISTRIBUTION

Fasciola hepatica is distributed worldwide and is especially prevalent in sheep-rearing areas. Human infections are sporadic and rare but minor local epidemics have occurred in England,[127] France, Cuba and Germany from eating watercress.

Fasciola gigantica occurs primarily in cattle in Africa and overlaps with *F. hepatica* in small areas of East and South Africa and western Asia. Human infections have been reported from central Africa, Uzbekistan, Vietnam and Hawaii.

AETIOLOGY

Fasciola hepatica is a large fleshy fluke 2.3–3 × 1.5 cm broad, pale grey in colour with dark borders. It is broadly leaf-shaped with a distinct cephalic cone at the anterior end (Fig. 22.25). The egg (Fig. 22.26) is operculated 130–140 × 63–90 μm, ovoid, brown and bile-stained.

Fasciola gigantica is larger, up to 7.5 cm in length and less broad with a less distinct cephalic cone. The egg is slightly larger and of a different shape to *F. hepatica*. There are oral and ventral suckers and an ovary placed anterior to the testis in the posterior end of the body.

Life-cycle (Fig. 22.27)

The life-cycle involves snails of certain species and aquatic vegetation. The adult fluke lives in the biliary passages where the eggs are laid in the immature stage and are evacuated in the faeces. After maturing in water for 9–15 days at 22–25°C the miracidia escape from the eggs and invade snails of many species of *Lymnaea* (Table 22.2). In the snail intermediate host the mother sporocyst is followed by first and second generation rediae and blunt-tailed cercariae which leave the snail and swim about in the water before encysting as metacercariae on aquatic plants where they are viable for long periods in a moist environment, and are viable at −2°C to −10°C but are killed at −20°C. The metacercariae are ingested by mammals eating the vegetation or drinking from the bottom of contaminated pools. The metacercariae excyst in the duodenum, migrate through the intestinal wall into the peritoneal cavity, penetrate Glisson's capsule of the liver and traverse the parenchyma to the biliary passages.

The incubation period between infection and the development of the adult flukes is about three to four months.

Table 22.2 Trematode flukes which can infect man.

Adult fluke	Morphology	Egg	Site	Vertebrate hosts	First intermediate host	Second intermediate host	Geographical distribution	Clinical features
LIVER FLUKES								
Fasciola hepatica (Fig. 22.25)	Large leaf-shaped, 2–3 × 1.5 cm	130–140 × 63–90 μm (Fig. 22.26)	Biliary tract	Sheep, cattle, man	Freshwater snails: Lymnaea truncatula, L. viridis, L. viator, L. bulimoides, humilis, columella, Lymnaea tomentosa. Land snail: Practicoella gresicola and possibly Bulinus sp.	Aquatic vegetation: Watercress	Europe, western Asia, highlands South Africa Far East South America North America Caribbean Australasia	Transient hepatic disturbance with jaundice and fever
Fasciola gigantica	Larger, up to 7.5 cm long		Biliary tract	Sheep, cattle, other herbivores and man	Fully aquatic lymnaeid snails		Africa and South America	
Dicrocoelium dendriticum	Small, 1.5 × 2 mm	40 × 25 μm	Biliary tract	Herbivorous animals	Land snails: Theba carthusiana Zebrina detrita Helicella candidula H. itala Cepaea nemoralis Helix vulgaris Eulota lantzi E. rubens	Brown ants: Formica fusca F. rufibarbis Proformica nasuta Catagliphis bicolor C. aenescens	Cosmopolitan in animals. Human cases in Europe, Near East, Africa and China	Dyspepsia and hepatomegaly with eosinophilia
Clonorchis sinensis (Fig. 22.28)	10–25 × 2.5 mm	20–30 × 15–17 μm (Fig. 22.29)	Biliary tract	Man, dog, pig, cat, mouse, camel, badger	Freshwater snails: Bythinia (Parafossarulus) manchouricus B. fuchsiana Additional: B. longicornis Assiminea lutea Melanoides tuberculatus	Carp species: Most important Golden carp (Carassius auratus) Ctenopharyngodon idella Mylopharyngodon aethiops Cultur recurviceps and more than 80 other species plus some freshwater shrimps (see Appendix II)	China, Taiwan, Indo-China, Korea, Japan — South China	Recurrent cholangitis with jaundice, pancreatitis and cholangiocarcinoma

Table 22.2 (continued).

Adult fluke	Morphology	Egg	Site	Vertebrate hosts	First intermediate host	Second intermediate host	Geographical distribution	Clinical features
Opisthorchis tenuicollis (*felineus*)	8–11 × 1.5–2 mm	30 × 12 μm	Biliary tract	Dog, cat, pig, man	*Bythinia leachi.* An additional host is *Bythinia tentaculata*	Freshwater fish: Tench, ide, barbel, roach	Eastern Europe, USSR and India	Recurrent cholangitis
Opisthorchis viverrini	8–11 × 1.5–2 mm	30 × 12 μm	Biliary tract	Civet cat, cat, dog, man	*Bythinia funiculata, B. siamensis, B. goniomphalus, B. laevis*	Freshwater fish: *Cyclochalicthyus siaja Hampala dispar Punitus orphoides P. goniomotus P. poctozyron Labiobarbus lineatus Osteochilus* spp.	North-East Thailand	Recurrent cholangitis

INTESTINAL FLUKES

Adult fluke	Morphology	Egg	Site	Vertebrate hosts	First intermediate host	Second intermediate host	Geographical distribution	Clinical features
Fasciolopsis buski (Fig. 22.35)	3 cm × 12 cm × 2 mm	130–140 × 80–85 μm (Fig. 22.36)	Small intestine	Pig and man	Freshwater snails: *Segmentina hemisphaerula S. trochoideus Hippeutis umbilicalis H. cantori*	Aquatic vegetation: Water calthrop (*Trapa natans*) *T. bicornis T. bispinosa* Water chestnut (*Eliocharis tuberosa*) Water bamboo (*Zigania aquatica*) Water hyacinth (*Eichornia crassipes*)	China; India and Taiwan Taiwan South China; Chekiang and Canton Taiwan. Also Assam, Malaysia, Borneo and Burma	Chronic diarrhoea, preprandial pain, oedema of face and trunk, malabsorption
Heterophyes heterophyes (Fig. 22.39)	Small 1–1.7 × 0.3–0.7 mm	20–30 × 15–17 μm	Small intestine	Man, rat, fox, dog, wolf, jackal	Brackish water snails: *Pirinella conica Cerithidea cingulata Tympanotonus micropterus*	Freshwater fish: Mullet (*Mugil cephalus*) Minnow (*Gambusia affinis*) Goby (*Acanthogobius* sp.) *Tilapia nilotica* and sp. of *Liza, Tridentiga, Glossoglobus* and *Therapon*	Middle East; Far East; Japan; Egypt	Diarrhoea and preprandial pain

Species	Adult size	Egg size	Habitat	Definitive host	First intermediate host (snail)	Second intermediate host / source	Geographical distribution	Symptoms
Metagonimus yokogawai	1.1 × 0.42–0.7 mm	27 × 16 μm	Small intestine	Man, cat, dog, rat, pig, pelican	Freshwater snails: *Semisulcospira libertina*, *Thiara granifera*	Freshwater fish: *Plecoglossus altivelus* (ayu), *Carassius auratus* (golden carp), *Cyprinus carpio* (common carp), *Zacco temminckii*, *Photimus steindachneri*, *Acheilognathus lanceolata*, *Pseudorasbora parva*, *Tribolodon taczanouski*	Korea, Formosa and Japan. Balkan states. Common in Far East	Occasionally temporary abdominal pain and watery diarrhoea
Gastrodiscoides hominis	5–8 × 3–5 mm	150–170 × 60–70 μm	Large intestine	Many herbivores	Freshwater snail: *Helicorbis coenosus*	Aquatic plants	Assam, Bangladesh, Malaya, Thailand, Philippines, Indonesia	Diarrhoea in heavy infections
Echinostoma lindoensis	1 cm × 1 mm	83–116 × 58–69 μm (Fig. 22.41)	Small intestine	Man, rat, pig and other mammals	Freshwater snails: *Amnis sarasinorum*, *Gyraulus convexiusculus*	Freshwater snail: *Vivipara javanica* Freshwater mussels: *Corbicula lindoensis*, *C. subplanta*, *C. celebensis*, *C. javanica*	Japan, Philippines, Indonesia, Malaya	Mostly symptomless. Heavy infections: diarrhoea, abdominal pain and eosinophilia
Echinostoma malayanum	1 cm × 1 mm	83–116 × 58–69 μm	Small intestine	Man, rat, pig and other mammals	Freshwater snail: *Lymnaea leuteola*	Snails: *L. leuteola*, *G. convexiusculus*, *Indoplanorbis exustus* Fish: *Barbus stigma*	Malaya, Thailand, India, Sino-Tibetan border	Mostly symptomless. Heavy infections: diarrhoea, abdominal pain and eosinophilia
Euparyphium ilocanum	1 cm × 1 mm	83–116 × 58–69 μm	Small intestine	Man, rat, pig and other mammals	Snails: *Gyraulus convexiusculus* (Philippines and Indonesia) *G. prashadi* and *Hippeutis umbilicalis* (Philippines)	14 Species of snail: *G. prashadi*, *Vivipara burranghina*, *Planorbis umbilicatus*, *V. rudipellis*	Philippines, Celebes, Indonesia	Mostly symptomless. Heavy infections: diarrhoea, abdominal pain and eosinophilia

Table 22.2 (continued).

Adult fluke	Morphology	Egg	Site	Vertebrate hosts	First intermediate host	Second intermediate host	Geographical distribution	Clinical features
LUNG FLUKES *Paragonimus westermani* (Fig. 22.42)	8–20 × 5–9 mm Cuticular spines singly spaced. Ovary simply branched (4–6 lobes)	90 × 55 μm (Fig. 22.43)	Cystic cavities in lungs	Wild and domestic felines	Freshwater snails: *Semisulcospira libertina* (optimum host)	Crab: *Eriocheir japonicus* (main host in Japan) Crayfish: *Cambaroides japonicus*	Japan	Pulmonary symptoms, cough and haemoptysis. Cerebral complications. Occasionally eggs in skin
					S. extensa *S. multicincta* *S. gottschei* *S. nodiperda* *S. cancellata*	Crabs: *Eriocheir sinensis* (main host in China) *Geothelphusa dehaani* *G. obtusipes* *Sinopotamon denticulatus* *Candidopotamon rathbuni* *Sesarma dehaani* *Sesarmops sinensis* Crayfish: *Cambaroides similis* *C. dauricus, C. schrenki* *Procambarus clarkii*	China and Korea	Pulmonary symptoms, cough and haemoptysis. Cerebral complications. Occasionally eggs in skin
					Thiara granifera	Crab: *Potamon myazakii*	Taiwan	
					Brotia asperata	Crabs: *Parathelphusa grapsoides* *P. mistio* *Sundathelphusa philippina*	Philippines	
					Melanoides tuberculata	Crabs: *Potamon smithianus* *Parathelphusa degasti* *Parathelphusa* sp.	Thailand	

Species	Morphology	Size	Habitat / Development	Other hosts	Freshwater snail	Crabs	Distribution	Symptoms
Paragonimus myazaki	Cuticular spines singly spaced. Ovary profusely branched		Lungs	Crab eating mammals, wild boar and marten as paratenic hosts		Crab: Geothelphusa dehaani	Japan	
Paragonimus heterotremus	Cuticular spines singly spaced. Ovary profusely branched		Lungs		Brotia costula	Crabs: Parathelphusa maculata Potamon cognatus	Thailand, Laos and Malaya	Pulmonary signs. Cerebral involvement and migratory subcutaneous swellings
Paragonimus szechuanensis (skrijabini)	Cuticular spines in groups. Ovary profusely branched		Does not develop to maturity. Immature flukes only. No eggs		Freshwater snail: Tricula humida	Crabs: Sinopotamon denticulatus	China	Immature flukes only which migrate through body. Subcutaneous swellings (cutaneous larva migrans). Eosinophilic granuloma in brain. Cerebral lesions. Hepatic lesions
Paragonimus hueitungensis	Cuticular spines single spread. Ovary profusely branched		Does not develop to maturity. Immature flukes only. No eggs		Freshwater snail: Tricula cristella	Crabs: Sinopotamon denticulatus S. joshueiense Isopotamon sinense I. papilionaceus	China	Migratory subcutaneous swellings. No ova laid. Pulmonary signs not marked. No cerebral involvement
Paragonimus tuanshenensis	Cuticular spines single spread. Ovary profusely branched		Lungs		Freshwater snail: Oncomelania chiui	Crab: Sinopotamon denticulatus	China	Pulmonary symptoms. No cerebral symptoms or subcutaneous swellings
Paragonimus compactus	Cuticular spines in groups. Ovary simply branched	Smaller, 75 × 48 µm	Lungs				India	Pulmonary symptoms only

Table 22.2 (continued).

Adult fluke	Morphology	Egg	Site	Vertebrate hosts	First intermediate host	Second intermediate host	Geographical distribution	Clinical features
Paragonimus africanus	Cuticular spines in groups. Ovary simply branched	67–113 × 42–56 μm	Lungs	Mongoose (Crossarchus obscurus) and Atilax paludinosus. Dog, cat and African drill (Mandrillus leucophaeus)	Freshwater snail: Potadoma freethii	Crabs: Sudanautes africanus S. ambryi, Liberonautes latidactylus (S. pelii)	Cameroon and Zaire	Mild pulmonary symptoms. No radiological signs. No cerebral lesions. Retroauricular cysts
Paragonimus uterobilateralis	Double uterus. One on each side		Lungs	African civet cat (Viverra civetta)		Liberonautes latidactylus	Nigeria	Pulmonary symptoms only
Paragonimus mexicanus (peruvianus)			Lungs	Cats	Freshwater snails: Pomiatopsis lapidaria Aroapyrgus costaricensis	Crabs: Pseudothelphusa chilensis Psychophallus tristani Potamocarcinus magnus	Central and South America	Pulmonary signs and cerebral complications
Paragonimus caliensis Paragonimus ecuadorensis			Lungs					

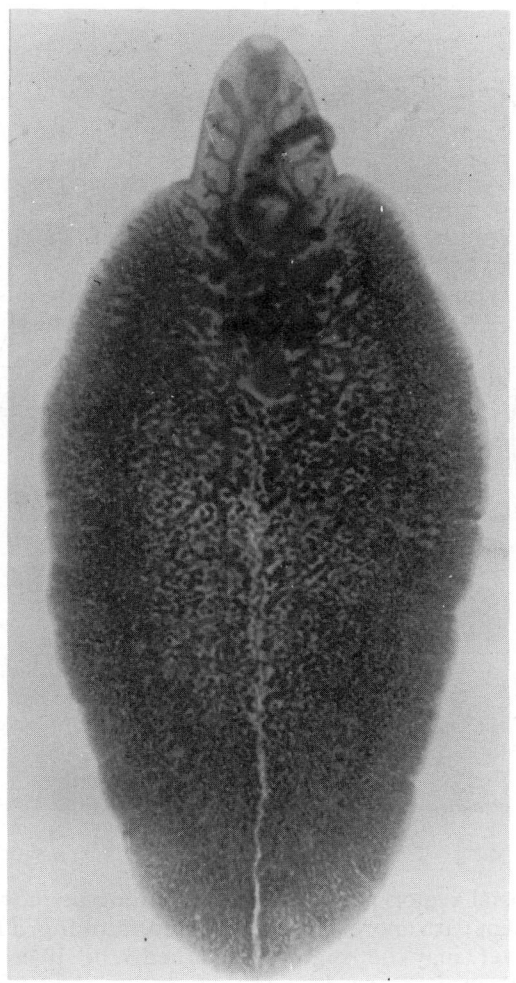

Fig. 22.25   Adult *F. hepatica*. (Courtesy Dr H. Zaiman.)

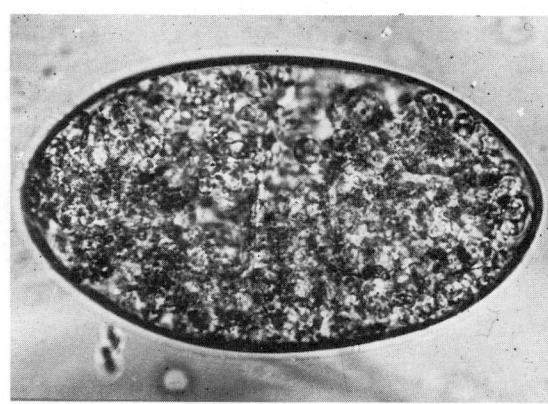

Fig. 22.26   Egg of *F. hepatica*. (Courtesy WTIM.)

TRANSMISSION

Transmission is by lymnaeid snails (Table 22.2). Man acquires the infection as the result of eating raw watercress or sucking grass on which metacercariae have encysted from contamination of the water by sheep.

PATHOLOGY

The pathological effects are caused by the adult fluke. In the invasion stage symptoms are caused during penetration of the intestinal wall and migration across the peritoneum and entry into the liver. In the phase when mature flukes are being established there may be marked destruction of liver tissue, subcapsular haematoma and, rarely, intra-abdominal haemorrhage. Haemobilia may cause significant blood loss in heavy infections. Small necrotic foci and micro-abscesses in the liver have been described.[128] Most patients recover spontaneously with evacuation of the worms via the intestinal tract or calcification[127] when parenchymal regeneration occurs but scar tissue may form.

In the chronic phase the flukes live in both the hepatic and extrahepatic ducts where they can cause inflammation and obstruction with epithelial hyperplasia and fibrosis round the ducts and new duct growth. Mechanical obstruction may lead to cholangitis, cholecystitis and gallstones. Fibrosis of the portal tracts with compression of the adjacent liver cells has been described[129] but an association with portal hypertension and ascites is as yet unproven. The migrating larvae on their journey to the liver may be trapped in ectopic foci and flukes have been recorded from the blood vessels, lungs, subcutaneous tissues, ventricle of the brain and orbit.[130]

IMMUNITY

Little is known about immunity. Most human infections are transitory and the flukes are evacuated via the intestinal tract or killed and calcified.

CLINICAL FEATURES

Natural history

Most human infections are very light and tran-

Fasciola gigantica and Fasciola hepatica

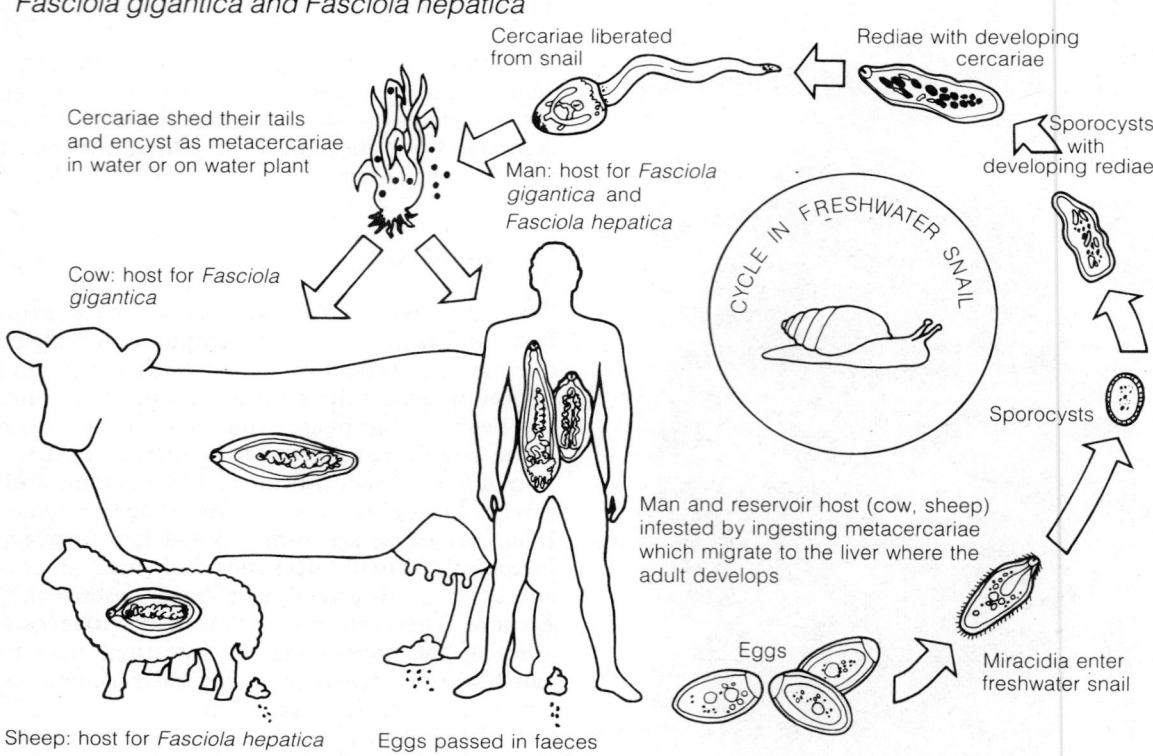

Fig. 22.27   Life-cycle of *F. hepatica* and *F. gigantica*. (Courtesy WTIM.)

sitory but some cause symptoms during the early stages and then recover spontaneously. In chronic infection liver complications may develop which can be severe. In the migrating stages larvae may become trapped in the skin (cutaneous fascioliasis) as well as some other organs.

Incubation period

The period between ingestion of the infective material and symptoms is very short but if symptoms do not develop then eggs will not appear in the stools for three to four months.

Signs and symptoms

Acute phase

After a short period of dyspepsia there may be an acute illness, the main feature being an enlarged tender liver, fever and a high eosinophilia. There is a dragging cramp-like pain in the right sub-

costal region aggravated by coughing or movement with anorexia, headache and vomiting. The fever may be slight or marked, the liver is enlarged and tender and there is a marked eosinophilia. Urticaria and dermatographia may be present; usually these signs subside over a period of one year. In more severe cases recurrent fever, hepatic enlargement and jaundice may lead to prostration and wasting. In the cases described from Liverpool[131] there were recurrent bouts of obstructive jaundice with fever, vomiting and severe anorexia and anaemia from haemobilia. In the acute phase there is a leukocytosis of $12–40 \times 10^9$/litre with 40–80% eosinophils. Pulmonary infiltrates with eosinophilia were described in the acute phase.[132] Haemobilia may cause melaena and anaemia, and the stool may contain occult blood in lesser infections.

Chronic phase

In the chronic phase there may be no symptoms but there may be right upper quadrant pain, fever and vomiting from cholangitis and gall-stones may develop. Eosinophilia and deranged liver function tests may be found.

Cutaneous fascioliasis

Cutaneous fascioliasis caused by migrating larval flukes has been observed in South America, France and Iraq, usually in association with hepatic fascioliasis. Reddish-brown, round or oval, subcutaneous nodules appear on the abdomen, which migrate and are pruritic and painful. Biopsy shows eosinophilic infiltration and tunnels with necrotic walls, in which the parasite may or may not be present.

Halzoun

Although *F. hepatica* is not the usual cause of halzoun (see section on pentastomiasis, Chapter 24), eating infected raw sheep's liver may lead to young adult worms attaching themselves to the pharyngeal mucosa where they can cause bleeding and neck oedema.

DIAGNOSIS

Differential diagnosis

Fever, hepatomegaly and eosinophilia may be found in schistosomiasis, opisthorchiasis and clonorchiasis. In the early stages *Fasciola hepatica* may resemble viral hepatitis. Attacks of right subcostal pain with fever and jaundice may suggest cholangitis and gallstones.

Spurious infections

Eggs may be ingested from food contaminated by animals and pass through the bowel unchanged. Their appearance in the stool is transitory and must not be confused with a genuine infection.

Eggs (Fig. 22.26)

Eggs are often scanty and need concentration methods to demonstrate them. Duodenal aspiration and the string test may produce eggs when direct stool examination is negative.

Serodiagnosis

Antibodies appear early and diagnosis can be made during the acute stage of the infection when there are no eggs in the stools. Complement fixation, immunodiffusion, haemagglutination, immunoelectrophoresis and immunofluorescent tests are all available. Immunofluorescence has given reliable results with positive titres of 1/100 but counterimmunoelectrophoresis (CIE) has been recommended as the test of choice since it is sensitive and can be used as a test of cure. Antibodies with other tests persist for two or more years after cure but with diminishing titres. Cross reactions occur with *Paragonimus* and schistosomiasis but a more specific cuticular adult antigen is available which cross reacts only with *Fasciola gigantica*.[133] A skin test using *F. hepatica* antigen demonstrates exposure to infection[134] but does not distinguish between active and past infection.

TREATMENT

Praziquantel is not as effective in fascioliasis as in other fluke infections; this has been blamed on the inability of the drug to penetrate the fluke's thick integument. It is given in an oral dose of 20 mg/kg daily for 3 days.[135] Success has been claimed with *bithionol* used in the past in an oral dose of 30–50 mg/kg every alternate day for 10–15 days, and *emetine hydrochloride* 40 mg by subcutaneous injection daily for 7–10 days, and metronidazole 1.5 g daily for 13–21 days.[136]

EPIDEMIOLOGY

Fasciola hepatica is associated with the keeping of sheep and cattle and human infection occurs where these animals are allowed to contaminate watercress beds and other edible vegetation.

CONTROL

Preventing access of all animals to commercial watercress beds and control of the source of water used to irrigate the beds are necessary.

Dicrocoelium dentriticum

This is a common parasite of sheep and other herbivores which only rarely infects man.

GEOGRAPHICAL DISTRIBUTION

The fluke is common in sheep and other herbivores in Europe, Turkey, North Africa and parts of Asia. It is less common in North and South America. A closely related fluke *D. hospes* occurs in West Africa. Only 100 cases have been recorded in man in Europe, the Near East, Africa and China.

AETIOLOGY

The fluke measures 15×2 mm. The egg is brown and thick-shelled with a large operculum and measures $40 \times 25 \, \mu$m.

LIFE-CYCLE (see Fig. II.12, p. 1329)

The life-cycle is unusual in that water is not necessary. The eggs do not hatch in water but are ingested by land snails of various species (Table 22.2) in which development takes place, cercariae leaving the snail by migrating to the respiratory chamber to agglomerate in large numbers in the slime balls cemented by mucus which are left as the snail crawls along. A second intermediate host, the brown ant, *Formica fusca* and *F. rufibarbis*, and other ants (Table 22.2)

ingest the slime balls and the metacercarial stages develop in the ants which are then ingested by sheep and other animals on grass.

TRANSMISSION TO MAN

Transmission is accidental by swallowing infected ants.

PATHOLOGY

The pathology is similar to that of *F. hepatica*.

CLINICAL FEATURES

Only some 100 cases have been described. The symptoms and signs are similar to those of *F. hepatica*: chronic constipation, dyspepsia and an enlarged liver with eosinophilia.

DIAGNOSIS

It is important to exclude spurious infections (eggs in the faeces) which are caused by eating infected liver.

TREATMENT

Praziquantel in one oral dose of 50 mg/kg is effective.[135]

Clonorchiasis (*Clonorchis sinensis*)

Clonorchis sinensis, *Opisthorchis tenuicollis* and *O. viverrini* (see section on opisthorchiasis, below) are related liver flukes which have intermediate hosts in snails and in freshwater fish. Human infection is the result of the cultural habit of eating raw fish.

GEOGRAPHICAL DISTRIBUTION

Clonorchis sinensis is found endemically in Japan, Korea, all of China except the north-west, Taiwan and Indo-China. There is no evidence that *Clonorchis* infection has become established

outside the endemic zones. Cases from Hawaii and California are infected from imported, frozen or pickled fish.

AETIOLOGY

Clonorchis sinensis (Figs. 22.28 and II.3, p. 1324) is a reddish fluke, spatulate, tapering anteriorly and semi-transparent, measuring $10–25 \times 2.5$ mm. It has a smooth cuticle and an oral and ventral sucker. The egg (Fig. 22.29) (Plate III. 5) measures $20–30 \times 15–17 \, \mu$m. It is operculated, yellow-brown and one of the smallest

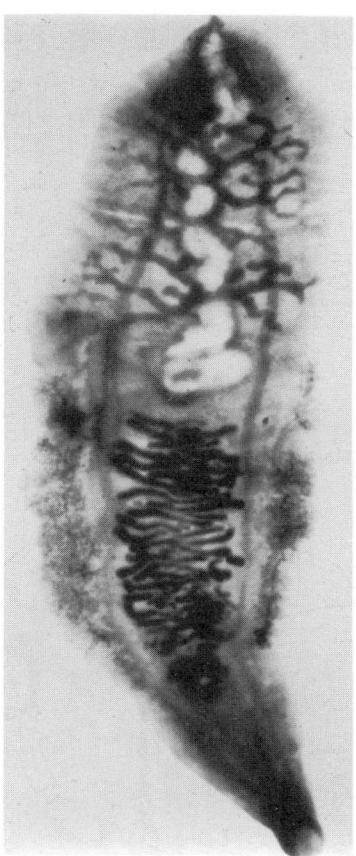

Fig. 22.28   Adult *C. sinensis.*

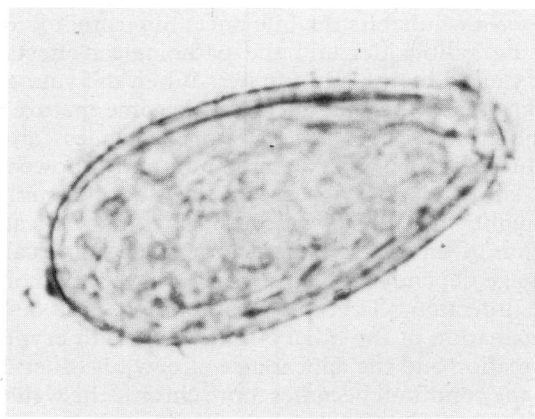

Fig. 22.29   Egg of *C. sinensis.*

trematode eggs found in man (to be distinguished from *Heterophyes* and *Metagonimus*). The eggs are passed out into fresh water where they hatch into *miracidia* which penetrate snails of the *Bythinia (Parafossarulus) manchouricus*, *Bythinia fuchsiana* and *Bythinia longicornis* species (Fig. 22.30).

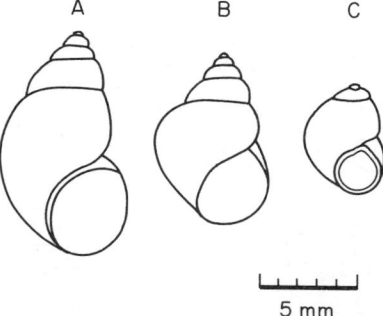

5 mm

Fig. 22.30   A, *Bythinia (Parafossarulus) manchouricus*. B, *Bythinia fuchsiana*. C, *Bythinia longicornis*.

LIFE-CYCLE (Fig. 22.31)

In the snail, development into *sporocysts* and then *rediae* takes three weeks and *cercariae* are discharged into the water. The cercariae (Fig. 22.32), which have blunt tails, measure 450–550 μm × 100–120 μm, swim to attach themselves to more than 80 species of fish (see Table 22.2 and Appendix II, p. 1325). The most important species are members of the carp family, *Carassius auratus* (golden carp), *Mylopharyngodon aethiops*, *Ctenopharyngodon idella*, and *Cultur recurviceps*. In China, freshwater shrimps may also be important. In the fish the cercariae shed their tails and encyst as *metacercariae* under the scales or in the flesh of the fish. These cysts can withstand a temperature of 50–70°C for 15 minutes and are situated under the scales in carp, but in the flesh in other fish, so that domestic animals which eat offal whole become infected, whereas man who removes the scales may not. The metacercarial cysts possess a capsule which is protective against the gastric juice so that when the fish are eaten half raw or pickled in soy sauce they pass through the stomach to the duodenum, where they are digested by the succus entericus near the ampulla of Vater. The metacercarial cysts discharge *adolescercariae* which attach themselves to the mucosa and develop into young flukes, maturing in 26 days when they ascend the bile duct by positive chemotaxis, although 95% may be destroyed on the way. In the bile ducts the flukes grow as large as the calibre of the ducts where they can live for up to 26 years.[137] Egg production is heavy in the cat—2400 eggs daily—and 21 000 adult worms have been found at autopsy in man.

TRANSMISSION

Man is infected by eating raw fish containing the metacercarial cysts in vinegar, sunomono, or covered with salted soybean paste, sashimi.

Clonorchis sinensis

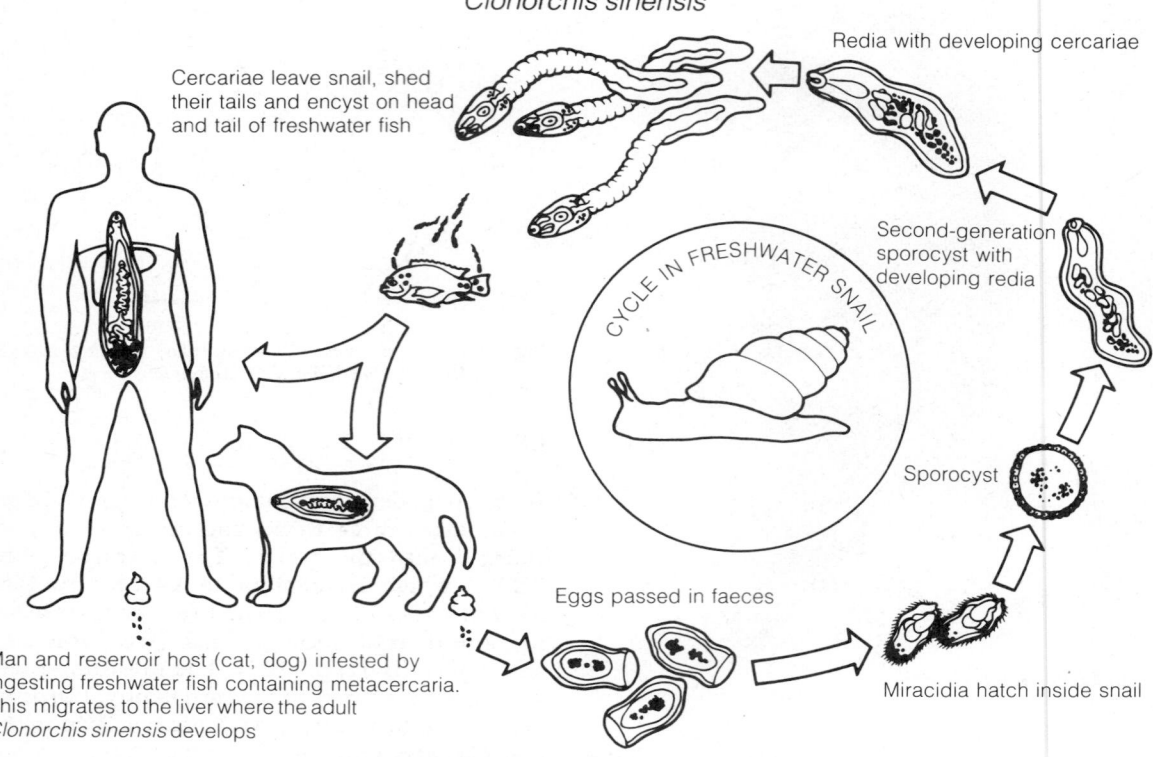

Cercariae leave snail, shed their tails and encyst on head and tail of freshwater fish

Redia with developing cercariae

CYCLE IN FRESHWATER SNAIL

Second-generation sporocyst with developing redia

Sporocyst

Eggs passed in faeces

Miracidia hatch inside snail

Man and reservoir host (cat, dog) infested by ingesting freshwater fish containing metacercaria. This migrates to the liver where the adult *Clonorchis sinensis* develops

Fig. 22.31 Life-cycle of *C. sinensis*. (Courtesy WTIM.)

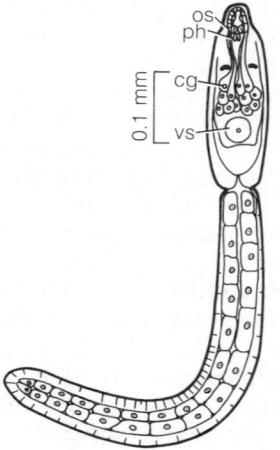

Fig. 22.32 Cercaria of *C. sinensis* (note unforked tail). os = oral sucker, ph = pharynx, cg = cephalic secretory gland, vs = ventral sucker.

PATHOLOGY

C. sinensis inhabits the bile ducts but cannot live in the gallbladder and the pathological effects are caused by the adult flukes. When the young flukes reach the bile ducts and become mature, proliferative and inflammatory changes are induced in the biliary epithelium and followed by encapsulating fibrosis of the ducts. Hsu[138] thought that this was caused by mechanical action of the flukes. The degree of pathological change depends on the intensity and duration of the infection. There is proliferation and desquamation of the biliary epithelium with crypt formation and the appearance of new bile ducts. As the condition becomes more chronic the walls of the ducts become infiltrated with eosinophils and leukocytes. The smaller portal vessels become fibrosed with associated dilatation of the portal vein and increased portal pressure. There is fibrous formation around eggs which infiltrate the hepatic parenchyma.[139] The bile ducts with thickened walls expand into cavities and diverticula a centimetre or more in diameter in which large numbers of parasites may be found (Fig. 22.33).

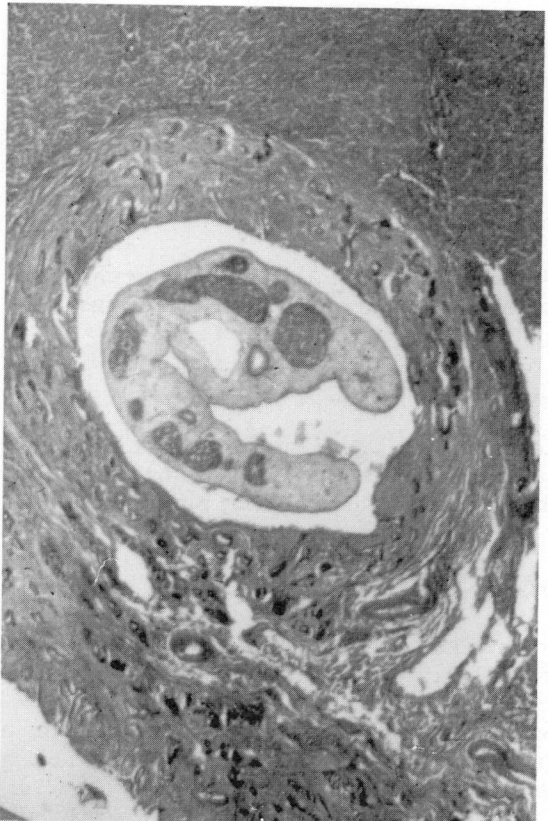

Fig. 22.33   Cross-section of an adult *C. sinensis* lodged in an intrahepatic bile duct.

parasites, and sometimes the parasites themselves, escape into the intestine. Changes have been described in the pancreas, spleen, kidneys and adrenals in all of which adult flukes may be found.[140] Changes in the pancreas may include atrophy of Langerhans' cells. Splenomegaly was present in 22–40% in one series of autopsies.[141] Secondary infection, usually due to *Escherichia coli*, causes cholangitis, cholangiohepatitis, pyelophlebitis and abscesses, but in most infections no serious complications are found.

Jaundice may occur owing to bile retention from intrahepatic bile duct strictures. Gallstones may form round dead worms and eggs. Worms present in the pancreatic duct may give rise to clinical symptoms of acute pancreatitis with raised enzyme levels.

Clonorchiasis and carcinoma of the liver

Clonorchis infection is associated with bile duct carcinoma as distinct from hepatocellular carcinoma of the liver seen so commonly in other countries (see Chapter 67).

Adenomatous hyperplasia of the bile duct epithelium is associated with adenocarcinoma of the liver[142] which occurs most commonly in males aged 36 and over. The carcinoma may be a polypoid adenocarcinoma or an anaplastic carcinoma arising from the bile duct epithelium, and the adenomatous tissue in the wall of the bile duct or a mixture of both types.[142] The tumours are predominantly adenocarcinomas but the anaplastic type resembles a primary liver cell carcinoma. Clonorchiasis is an important cause of primary adenocarcinoma of the liver in man.[140] A high incidence of nitroso compounds in the diet has been suggested as interacting with liver fluke to produce bile duct carcinoma, since this has been achieved experimentally.[143]

Cirrhosis of the liver

Although micronodular cirrhosis and biliary cirrhosis have been described there is no evidence that *Clonorchis* infection plays any role in causation.

One thousand worms may be lethal but the mean intensity of infection in endemic areas is 100–200 flukes. The diverticula communicate with the bile ducts along which the eggs of the

IMMUNITY

Little is known about immunity and clinical observation of patients suggests that acquired immunity does not develop. Some infections are light, others heavy, but since the incidence of infection rises steadily with age to a peak incidence between 30 and 50 years of age there is little evidence of concomitant immunity, such as is seen in schistosomiasis.

CLINICAL FEATURES

Natural history

The majority of infections are asymptomatic and in areas of high endemicity up to 50% of the population may be infected with light infections (under 100 flukes) and in Japan where 60–80% of all infections are light[144] it is not possible to assess the effect. Infection lasts a long time, up to 24 years. Moderate infections (100–1000 flukes) may cause some symptoms and heavy infections (over 1000 flukes, 10 000 ova/g) cause serious disease. Heavy infections cause recurrent cholangitis, pancreatitis and death with cachexia and ascites after a number of years, or cholangiocarcinoma may supervene and cut life short.

Incubation period

Symptoms may begin with the entry of immature flukes into the biliary system 26 days after ingestion of contaminated raw fish.

Symptoms and signs

In heavy infections there is an acute stage.

Acute stage

Malaise, low-grade fever and eosinophilic leukocytosis with an enlarged tender liver and right subcostal pain herald the infection, but it is difficult to diagnose since ova do not appear in the stools until three to four weeks after onset of symptoms. In light and moderate infections there is little or no acute phase and, although 80% of infections were associated with vague gastrointestinal symptoms, a control group of uninfected people showed the same symptoms.[145]

Chronic stage

Recurrent acute cholangitis. This is the main symptom complex associated with the chronic stage. It presents as recurrent fever with rigors and jaundice, leading to suppurative cholangitis with *E. coli* infection. Abscesses form in the liver which need surgical attention. (See also section on recurrent pyogenic cholangitis, Chapter 60.)

Gallstones. These are common.

Pancreatitis. There may be recurrent acute pancreatitis with abdominal pain and a raised serum amylase. Hypoglycaemia has been recorded as a complication and is not uncommon.[146]

Jaundice. This may occur during the early stages with acute cholangitis but in the later stages more permanently from intrahepatic bile duct strictures. Jaundice may also be caused by temporary impaction of masses of flukes in the common bile duct.

Terminal phase. In the terminal phase chronic diarrhoea with peripheral oedema, ascites and cachexia develop.

Night blindness. Night blindness from vitamin A deficiency associated with jaundice is not uncommon.

Pulmonary symptoms. Haemoptysis without any radiological signs of lung disease or eggs in the sputum has been recorded.

Clinical pathology

Eosinophilia is not a feature of the chronic stage but liver function tests may show cholestatic changes with a raised alkaline phosphatase.

DIAGNOSIS

In the acute stage the differential diagnosis is from the early stages of other flukes, schistosomes and nematode infections, including visceral larva migrans. In the chronic stage the main difficulty is to assess the role of possible *Clonorchis* infection in recurrent cholangitis with fever, rigors and jaundice due to recurrent pyogenic cholangitis, gallstones and cholecystitis. Later micronodular and biliary cirrhosis must be differentiated. The diagnosis is made by finding the eggs of *Clonorchis* in the stool or duodenal aspirate. The eggs, 20–30 × 15–17 μm (Fig. 22.29 and Plate III.5) resemble those of heterophyid flukes but are differentiated from them by their more prominent opercular shoulders and a small spine-like process at the end opposite to the operculum. Other opisthorchid eggs are very similar.

Concentration methods. These are usually necessary and a variation of the ether sedimentation method (see Appendix IV) has been found useful.[147] McIlwaine buffer pH 4.0 and 0.5% Tween 80 with 0.01% Merthiolate as a preservative is used with the ether sedimentation method and increases recovery values for eggs up to 90–100% in small amounts of sediment.

Egg counts. Stoll's egg counting method (see Appendix IV, p. 1491) is used and <1000 eggs/g are considered lightly infected and >1000 eggs/g heavily infected. Faecal egg counts as a measure of intensity of infection are unreliable[148] and obviously so when jaundice is present, when bile passage obstruction prevents eggs from reaching the gut.

Duodenal aspirations. Recovery of eggs from duodenal aspirate will help distinguish *Clonorchis* from *Heterophyes heterophyes*, the eggs of which are not found in the duodenum. A strong solution of magnesium sulphate injected into the duodenum paralyses the sphincter of Oddi and contracts the gallbladder which expels bile and eggs into the duodenum.

Percutaneous cholangiography. This can show the flukes as small curved filling defects within dilated bile ducts or as mounds attached to the duct walls. The biliary ducts may show both strictures and dilatations.[149]

Serology. Serology is not very reliable.

Antigens. Fat-free antigens are prepared from adult flukes and have been found to be useful.[150] IFAT, CIE and CFT are all available, the IFAT and CIE being the tests of choice.

The CFT becomes positive 20 days after infection and stays positive as long as there is an active infection. It gives titres up to 1/200 which, since they decrease after cure, can be used as a test of cure.

TREATMENT

Drug treatment

Praziquantel is the drug of choice in treatment. Three oral doses, each of 25 mg/kg given in one day, were highly effective[151] but since these doses are impractical in the field a single dose of 40 mg/kg is sufficient for lighter infections, but moderate infections must be given 2 × 30 mg/kg, and heavy infections 3 × 25 mg/kg in the 24 hours.[152]

Other drugs have been used: hexachloroparaxylene (Hetol), which is no longer available, was satisfactory and bithionol (Bitin) 30–50 mg/kg orally on alternate days for two to three weeks has also been successful. Other drugs used have been emetine hydrochloride and pentavalent antimony.

Surgical treatment

When there is diffuse suppurative cholangitis the treatment is surgical; the gallbladder is opened and the bile ducts washed out to remove the plug of dead flukes; suitable antibiotics are administered. The bile ducts have been washed out in this way to remove the flukes with good effect in cases in which there is no suppuration.

PROGNOSIS

The prognosis is good in light infections and patients do not die from the disease. In heavy long-standing infections serious impairment of liver function occurs with death in many cases.

EPIDEMIOLOGY

Clonorchiasis is a zoonosis with a reservoir mainly in dogs and cats which in Japan are the major hosts where 45% of cats and 20% of dogs are infected.[153]

Human infection

Man is infected by eating raw fish, a custom in many Eastern countries.

Fish culture in ponds which contain many snails is responsible for the high incidence in Kwantung province, Canton and Chaochoufu where infection rates in some villages are 40–100%.[139] On the east coast of Vietnam infection rates run at 50% of the population. The incidence of infection is highest in the older age groups and is maximum at 30–50 years. In some parts of China children under 15 have the highest incidence.

CONTROL

Health education towards changes in eating habits and avoiding raw and improperly cooked fish has had some success in China. The meta-cercariae are killed by freezing at −10°C for 5 days or salting in a 10% saline solution, but

heavily salted fish must not be eaten on the first day of salting. Other methods of preservation such as pickling or cold smoking are ineffective.

Opisthorchiasis

Opisthorchiasis is caused by infection with two very similar flukes: *Opisthorchis tenuicollis (felineus)* and *Opisthorchis viverrini.*

GEOGRAPHICAL DISTRIBUTION

O. tenuicollis is found in eastern Europe and the USSR and occasionally India. *O. viverrini* is found in north-eastern Thailand where 25% of the population are thought to be infected[154] and it is an infection of public health importance. An opisthorchid type of fluke has been described from Ecuador[155] where 32% of 214 people and 3% of dogs in one village were found infected.

AETIOLOGY

The fluke, which shows only minor morphological differences from *C. sinensis*, lives in the intrahepatic bile ducts and pancreas and has been found in the lung. It measures 8–11 × 1.5–2 mm. The egg (Plate III.4) which measures 30 × 12 μm, is slenderer than the egg of *C. sinensis.*

LIFE-CYCLE

The life-cycle is the same as that of *C. sinensis* with a definitive mammalian host and two intermediate hosts, a snail and freshwater fish. *O. tenuicollis* has a reservoir host in wolverine, dog, cat and pig, a snail host *Bythinia leachi* (Fig. 22.34), fish hosts, tench (*Tinca tinca*), ide (*Leuciscus idus*), barbel (*Barbus barbus*) and roach

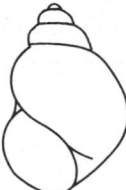

Fig. 22.34 *Bythinia leachi,* molluscan host of *Opisthorchis felineus.*

(*Rutilus rutilus*). *O. viverrini* has as reservoir hosts civet cat, cat and dog, snail hosts, *Bythinia funiculata, B. siamensis, B. goniomphalus* and *B. laevis*, and fish hosts. *Cyclochalicthyus siaja* is the most important species; others are *Puntius orphoides* and *Hampala dispar* (Table 22.2).

PATHOLOGY

Opisthorchid flukes are relatively non-pathogenic. They lodge in medium and large intrahepatic bile ducts where they cause similar changes to *C. sinensis.*

IMMUNITY

Clinical observation of patients suggests that little immunity develops.[156]

CLINICAL FEATURES

Opisthorchiasis is a benign infection and most patients are asymptomatic.

SYMPTOMS AND SIGNS

An *acute syndrome* with fever, myalgia, skin eruptions, right subcostal pain, hepatomegaly and hypereosinophilia has been described, but is rare.

Chronic infections. Light infections are asymptomatic but in moderate and heavy infections there may be symptoms similar to those of *C. sinensis* with recurrent cholangitis. Cholangiocarcinoma is associated with opisthorchid infection in Thailand.[157]

DIAGNOSIS

Stool examination may show eggs (Plate III.4) which must be distinguished from those of *C.*

sinensis and *Heterophyes*. Filtration of duodenal aspirate is more sensitive than faecal examination.[158] Overcrowding of worms may be responsible for low egg counts which are not a good measure of intensity of infection[148] and there is a natural tendency for egg counts to drop in the course of the disease.

Serodiagnosis

Immunoelectrophoresis gives positive results when egg counts are more than 10 000/g.[159]

TREATMENT

Praziquantel is the treatment of choice and a single dose of 40 mg/kg cured 95.8% of patients as measured by a single faecal sample.[160] *Albendazole* in a dose of 100 mg/kg twice daily for 3

days gave an average 81.5% worm reduction after four months in hamsters.[161]

EPIDEMIOLOGY

In endemic areas prevalence rates rise steadily from youth to reach a maximum at 50 years of age.

CONTROL

O. viverrini infection has been controlled in north-eastern Thailand by a combination of selective chemotherapy and health education. Praziquantel 40 mg/kg was given to stool-positive cases once a year for three years along with health education and sanitation which reduced the reinfection rate by 50%, while with treatment only the pre-treatment infection rate had returned in one year.[162]

2   INTESTINAL FLUKES

Intestinal flukes are zoonoses which accidentally infect man. All have two intermediate hosts: one a snail and the second aquatic vegetation in the case of *Fasciolopsis buski* and *Gastrodiscoides hominis*, and freshwater fish or molluscs in the

case of *Heterophyes heterophyes*, *Metagonimus yokogawai* and *Echinostoma*. Pathology is caused by the adult flukes except where eggs are carried to ectopic sites.

Fasciolopsis buski (giant intestinal fluke)

Fasciolopsis buski is normally a parasite of pigs which constitute the reservoir of infection.

GEOGRAPHICAL DISTRIBUTION

F. buski is found in China, India (Assam), Malaysia, Sumatra, Borneo, Thailand and Burma. In China 5% and in Assam 50% of the population may be affected and it is estimated that there are 10 million human infections in east Asia.

AETIOLOGY

F. buski is the largest human trematode measuring 3 cm × 12 mm × 2 mm thick (Figs. 22.35 and II.1, p. 1323) and lives in the small intestine, rarely the stomach. It is flesh-coloured and has an oral and a ventral sucker. The egg (Fig. 22.36

and Plate III.1) is large, operculated and yellow, measuring 130–140 × 80–85 μm. Eggs are found in large numbers in the faeces and each fluke can lay 25 000 a day.

LIFE-CYCLE (Fig. 22.37)

The life history is similar to that of *F. hepatica* with one stage in freshwater snails and the other as metacercariae on freshwater plants. The eggs hatch after three to seven weeks in the water and the miracidia develop in freshwater snails, *Segmentina hemisphaerula*, *Hippeutis umbilicalis* and *Hippeutis cantori* (Far East) and *Segmentina trochoideus* (India) (Table 22.2 and Fig. 22.38). In the snail sporocysts are formed which develop into redia and daughter redia to produce *cercariae* (the whole cycle in the snail takes two months). The cercariae, which are blunt-tailed, oval and

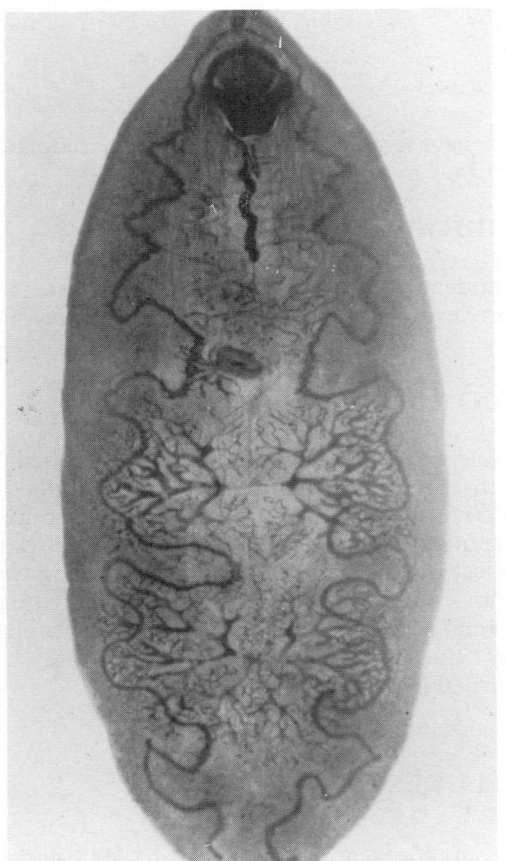

Fig. 22.35 Adult *F. buski*. (Courtesy WTIM.)

Fig. 22.36 Egg of *F. buski*. (Courtesy WTIM.)

Fasciolopsis buski

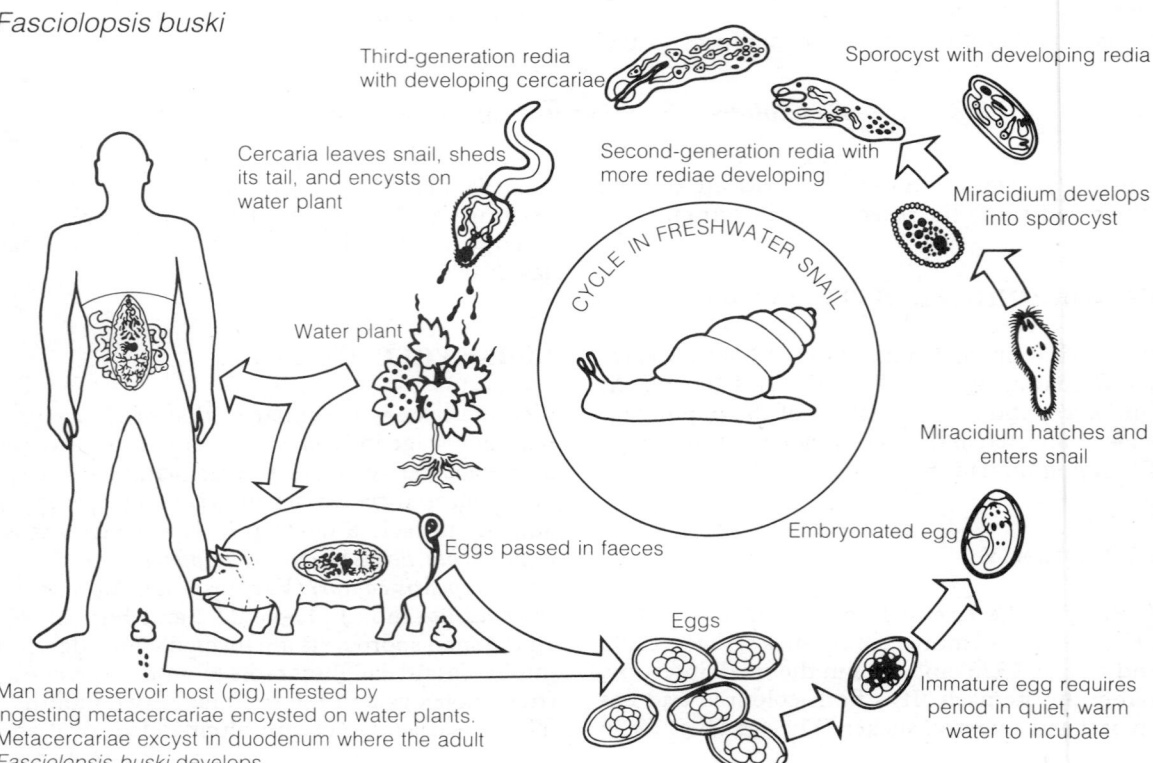

Third-generation redia with developing cercariae

Sporocyst with developing redia

Cercaria leaves snail, sheds its tail, and encysts on water plant

Second-generation redia with more rediae developing

Miracidium develops into sporocyst

CYCLE IN FRESHWATER SNAIL

Water plant

Miracidium hatches and enters snail

Eggs passed in faeces

Embryonated egg

Eggs

Immature egg requires period in quiet, warm water to incubate

Man and reservoir host (pig) infested by ingesting metacercariae encysted on water plants. Metacercariae excyst in duodenum where the adult *Fasciolopsis buski* develops

Fig. 22.37 Life-cycle of *F. buski*. (Courtesy WTIM.)

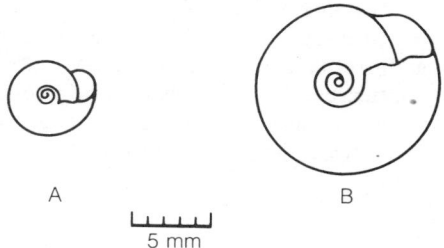

Fig. 22.38 Molluscan hosts of *F. buski*. A, *Segmentina hemisphaerula*. B, *Hippeutis cantori*.

short-lived, encyst as metacercariae on fresh-water plants; those important to man are the water calthrop (*Trapa natans*) in China, *T. bicornis* in India and Taiwan and *T. bispinosa* in Taiwan; the water chestnut (*Eliocharis tuberosa*) in south China, the water bamboo (*Zigania aquatica*) in Chekiang and Canton, and the water hyacinth (*Eichhornia crassipes*) in Taiwan. On ingestion by pigs or man the cysts pass through the stomach and excyst in the duodenum where the young flukes attach themselves to the intestinal wall becoming mature in 90 days. The adult flukes are relatively short-lived, the life-span not exceeding six months. The whole cycle from passage of egg through the snail and water plants until new adults are laying eggs is approximately five months.

TRANSMISSION

Transmission is from pig to man or man to man. People tear off the outer layers of the plant with the teeth before eating them. Often the plants are grown in ponds fertilized by human and pig excreta.

PATHOLOGY

Pathology is caused by the adult fluke. At the site of attachment, usually the mucosa of the duodenum or jejunum but in heavy infections the pylorus, ileum or even colon, the flukes cause inflammation, ulcerative and secretory changes. The number of flukes varies from a few up to 1000–2000. The pathological results are usually considered to be toxic or allergic but are more likely the result of hypoalbuminaemia secondary to malabsorption or a protein-losing enteropathy. Studies have shown some impairment of absorption of vitamin B_{12} and lowered serum B_{12} levels.

IMMUNITY

Little is known about immunity. Since the life of the adult fluke is about six months, reinfection must be very common to keep the levels of infection up in the community, in which all ages are infected. Infections may be light or heavy but what controls the level is unknown. Spontaneous cure occurs after six months away from an endemic area when all the flukes will have died off.

CLINICAL FEATURES

Natural history

The clinical features vary with the level of infection; most light infections are asymptomatic but in heavy infections (500 flukes or more) abdominal symptoms predominate with oedema of the face and body. Death is rare and follows cachexia. Infections die out naturally within six months of leaving the endemic area.

Incubation period

The incubation period is 90 days after infection when eggs will begin to be passed.

Symptoms and signs[163]

Diarrhoea develops towards the end of the incubation period with *abdominal pain*, which is preprandial and relieved by food, resembling a duodenal ulcer. *Anorexia, nausea* and *vomiting* may all be present. *Oedema* of the face, abdominal wall and lower extremities is common and *ascites* may be present. Later *malabsorption* may develop with pale offensive stools and wasting. *Paralytic ileus* is a rare complication. *Eosinophilia* is a common finding.

DIFFERENTIAL DIAGNOSIS

Distinction must be made from peptic ulcer and from other causes of malabsorption, and the nephrotic syndrome, in which there will be marked proteinuria. Other causes of chronic diarrhoea must also be distinguished.

DIAGNOSIS

The diagnosis of *F. buski* is unlikely if the individual has been away from the endemic area for more than six months.

Stool examination

Eggs appear in the stool 90 days after infection and are usually very numerous and easy to find. They are larger than those of *F. hepatica* (which are scanty in the stools) and have to be distinguished from echinostome eggs (Fig. 22.41, p. 509) which are similar in size. Serodiagnosis is of little value.

TREATMENT

The treatment of choice is *praziquantel* which has made all other drugs redundant. A single oral dose of 15 mg/kg at bedtime cured 100% of infections. Flukes evacuated were dead and showed blistering of the integument.[164] Thiabendazole, mebendazole and levamisole are ineffective and the only drug effective other than praziquantel is tetrachlorethylene 0.1 mg/kg on an empty stomach in the morning after a low fat meal the previous evening. However, the use of tetrachlorethylene is associated with severe anaphylactic reactions which can be prevented by prior antihistaminics.[165] Other drugs which have been used are niclosamide and hexyl-resorcinol.

EPIDEMIOLOGY

Human infection is limited to the distribution of the water plants on which the metacercariae encyst and is associated with their cultivation in ponds fertilized by human and pig excreta.

CONTROL

Understanding of the life-cycle from health education has had some success in China. The cycle of transmission could be broken by cooking or drying of the water plants before eating, snail control, storage of night soil for some period and avoidance of pig manure as fertilizer. Mass treatment of the population is now feasible with praziquantel; the average cost for an adult is about £St. 0.60 ($1.00).

Heterophyiasis. 1　*Heterophyes heterophyes*

Two heterophyid flukes can infect man: *Heterophyes heterophyes* and *Metagonimus yokogawai* (see section on *M. yokogawai* below).

GEOGRAPHICAL DISTRIBUTION

Heterophyes is a common human parasite in the Nile Delta and Israel. It is also found in Japan, South Korea, Taiwan, central and south China, the Philippines and western India.

AETIOLOGY

Heterophyes heterophyes is a small fluke which inhabits in large numbers the small intestine of man, rat, fox, dog, cat and other fish-eating mammals, and also the black kite (*Milvus migrans aegyptus*) and a bat (*Rhinolophus divosus acrotis*) in the Yemen. It is a very small grey pyriform fluke measuring 1–1.7 × 0.3–0.7 mm (Figs. 22.39 and II.7, p. 1327) with an oral and ventral sucker. The egg is similar to that of *C. sinensis* measuring 20–30 × 15–17 μm (Plate III.3) but is shorter and broader without an opercular ring. Other species have been recognized, *H. brevicaeca* and *H. taihokui* in Africa and *H. katsuradai* in Japan, the eggs of which are smaller, 25–26 × 14–15 μm.

Life-cycle

The eggs are passed out into water where they hatch, the miracidia entering brackish water snails, *Pirinella conica* (Fig. 22.40A) in the Middle East and *Cerithidia cingulata* and *Tympanotonus micropterus* in the Far East. The cercariae have membranous tails and encyst as metacercariae in the mullet (*Mugil cephalus*) and minnow (*Gambusia affinis*), and in Japan a species of *Acanthogobius* and other freshwater fish (Table 22.2). The adult fluke is short-lived with a life-span of not more than two months.

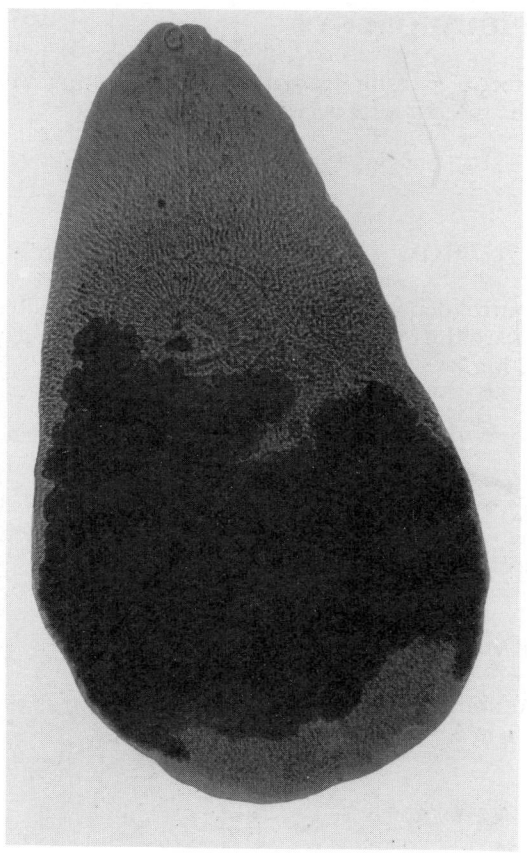

Fig. 22.39 Adult *Heterophyes heterophyes*. Cuticle covered by fine spines and oral sucker less conspicuous than ventral sucker. (Courtesy WTIM.)

TRANSMISSION

Transmission to man is by eating raw, improperly cooked, salted or pickled fish.

PATHOLOGY

Pathology is caused by both adult flukes and eggs. The adult flukes live attached to the mucosa of the small intestine where they cause superficial necrosis. They may invade the mucosa where they and the eggs induce a granulomatous reaction. Sometimes the eggs are carried by the general circulation to ectopic sites where granulomas form in the brain, spinal cord and heart (producing a cardiac syndrome similar to cardiac beriberi).

IMMUNITY

There is little immunity to reinfection and the fluke lives for no more than two years so reinfection is the rule.

CLINICAL FEATURES

Natural history

Most infections are light and asymptomatic. In heavy infections there are abdominal symptoms. The infection dies out naturally within two years of leaving an endemic area.

Symptoms and signs

In heavy infections there is a *chronic diarrhoea* with abdominal discomfort, vomiting, *preprandial pain* (resembling peptic ulcer) and weight loss but there is no evident malabsorption. Eggs in ectopic sites may cause epilepsy and cardiac failure. An eosinophilia may be present.

DIAGNOSIS

The differential diagnosis is from peptic ulcer and other causes of chronic diarrhoea.

Stool

The eggs are easily found in the stool and must

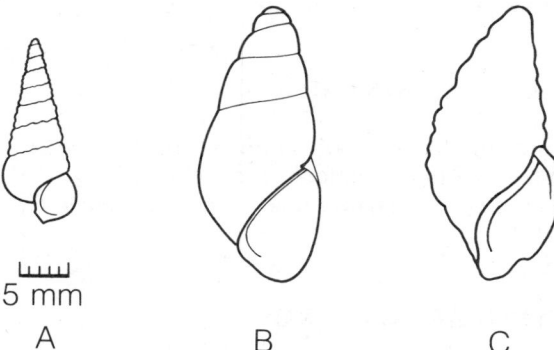

5 mm

A   B   C

Fig. 22.40 A, *Pirinella conica*, molluscan host of *Heterophyes heterophyes*. B, *Semisulcospira libertina* and C, *Thiara granifera*, molluscan hosts of *Metagonimus yokogawai*.

be distinguished from those of *C. sinensis* and opisthorchid eggs which they resemble (Plate III.3). Important points to be noticed are the shape (broader in the centre) and that eggs of *Heterophyes* are not found in the stools over two years after leaving the endemic area, nor in duodenal aspirates of biliary drainage.

TREATMENT

The drug of choice is praziquantel. An oral dose of 20 mg/kg daily for 3 days cured 100% of infections.[135]

EPIDEMIOLOGY

Infections result from the habit of eating raw fish. Infection rates rise with age.

CONTROL

Control depends upon health education directed toward the proper cooking of fish or their correct salting.

Heterophyiasis. 2 *Metagonimus yokogawai*

GEOGRAPHICAL DISTRIBUTION

M. yokogawai is found in China, Japan, Korea, the Philippines, Indonesia, Balkans, Spain, Israel and the USSR. In Korea it is the most important intestinal trematode affecting 1.2% of the whole population.[166] In parts of Japan and the Amur estuary in Siberia prevalence rates of 15–50% have been recorded.

AETIOLOGY

M. yokogawai is the smallest fluke found in man measuring 1.1 × 0.42–0.7 mm and resembles *Heterophyes* (Fig. II.9, p. 1327). The egg (Plate III.6) measures 27 × 16 μm and is more regularly ovoid than that of *C. sinensis*.

Life-cycle

Dogs, cats and rats are the main mammalian hosts as well as man, pig and pelican. The first intermediate hosts are freshwater snails, *Semisulcospira libertina* (Fig. 22.40B) and *Thiara granifera* (Fig. 22.40C) or *Koreanomelania* spp. The second intermediate hosts are the freshwater trout (sweetfish) or ayu (*Plecoglossus altivelus*) which is the most important host and many species of cyprinoid fish and a brackish water fish *Tribolodon taczanouski* in the Far East (Table 22.2). The adult life-span of the fluke seldom exceeds two months.

TRANSMISSION

Human infection is acquired from eating raw fish, especially the freshwater trout or sweetfish, one of which may have more than 10 000 metacercariae in its musculature.[166]

IMMUNITY

No immunity is acquired and reinfection is the rule in endemic areas.

PATHOLOGY

In experimental infections the young flukes live in the crypts of Lieberkühn in the jejunum for 5 days moving to the intervillous spaces when adult where they damage the enterocytes. In moderate infections mucosal damage (villus fusion and shortening, crypt hypertrophy, goblet cell depletion and shortening of the microvilli) occurs but regresses back to normal after four weeks, although the flukes may still be present.

NATURAL HISTORY

Since the life-span of the fluke does not exceed two months infections are self-limiting and unless heavy, asymptomatic. Reinfection is the rule.

CLINICAL FEATURES

The majority of infections are asymptomatic but consumption of a single raw ayu which is heavily infected may cause severe abdominal pain, prostration and watery diarrhoea, which is self-limiting.

EPIDEMIOLOGY

Endemic areas are scattered along rivers where up to 20% of the villagers may be infected.[166] Transmission rates peak in the autumn when the ayu are most edible.

DIAGNOSIS

The shape and size of the egg distinguishes it from *Heterophyes* and *Clonorchis* (Plate III.6).

TREATMENT

Praziquantel is the treatment of choice given as a single oral dose of 20 mg/kg.[135]

Echinostoma

GEOGRAPHICAL DISTRIBUTION

Echinostoma is found in Japan, Philippines, Indonesia, Malaysia, the Celebes, Taiwan, Canton and Assam.

AETIOLOGY

There are several species of *Echinostoma* which can be found in man: *E. lindoensis, E. malayanum* and *Euparyphium ilocanum*. The adult flukes measure 1 cm × 2 mm and have a collarette of spines surrounding the oral sucker. The eggs, which are straw-coloured and operculate (Fig. 22.41), measure 83–116 × 58–69 µm and resemble those of *Fasciolopsis buski* but tend to be smaller.

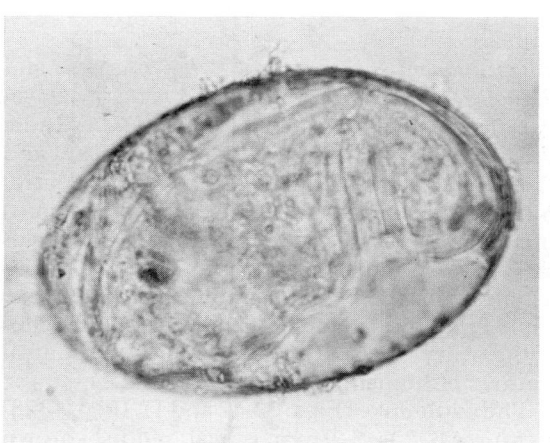

Fig. 22.41 Egg of *Echinostoma malayanum* containing a fully grown miracidium. (Courtesy Dr Lie Kan Joe.)

Life-cycle

The mammalian hosts are man, rat and pig and other mammals. The first intermediate hosts are snails and the second intermediate hosts snails and molluscs (Table 22.2 and Appendix IV).

CLINICAL FEATURES

The echinostomes are attached to the small intestine and most infections are symptomless. Heavy infections are accompanied by abdominal pain, diarrhoea and eosinophilia.[167]

DIAGNOSIS

The eggs, which are found in the stools, resemble those of *F. buski* but their smaller size and geographical area will help to distinguish.

TREATMENT

Praziquantel would appear to be the drug of choice.

EPIDEMIOLOGY

Until recently *E. lindoensis* was common in Lake Lindoe, Celebes but has now died out.

Gastrodiscoides hominis

GEOGRAPHICAL DISTRIBUTION

G. hominis is found in Assam, Bangladesh, Malaya, Thailand, Philippines and Indonesia.

AETIOLOGY

G. hominis is a small, dorsally convex fluke measuring $5-8 \times 3-5$ mm with a large posterior and small anterior sucker. It inhabits the large intestine. The egg is greenish-brown and ovoid with a narrowed anterior end measuring $150-170 \times 60-70\,\mu$m which matures in 16–17 days at 27°C.

Life-cycle (see Fig. II.23, p. 1338)

The adult fluke lives in the caecum and large intestine. The eggs pass into water where they hatch into miracidia which enter a freshwater snail, *Helicorbis coenosus*. The cercariae encyst as metacercariae on freshwater plants which are eaten by the mammalian host.

CLINICAL FEATURES

Light infections are asymptomatic, while heavy infections cause diarrhoea.

DIAGNOSIS

The eggs, which are found in the stool, resemble those of *F. buski* but differ from them in that the anterior third is narrower than the rest.

TREATMENT

Praziquantel would appear to be the treatment of choice.

EPIDEMIOLOGY

Human infection is dependent upon the cultivation of freshwater plants fertilized by pig and human faeces. Pigs are commonly infected in India and Assam but the fluke can occur in the absence of pigs and in Malaya the mouse deer (*Tragulus napu*) is a reservoir host. The incidence is highest in children and in Assam prevalence rates of 40% have been found.

CONTROL

Proper cooking of vegetation before eating will prevent infection.

3 LUNG FLUKES

Paragonimiasis

GEOGRAPHICAL DISTRIBUTION

Many species of *Paragonimus* are widespread throughout the world as infections of fish-eating mammals but only a few can infect man, principally in the Far East.

AETIOLOGY

The most important member of the species is *Paragonimus westermani* which infects man quite commonly in the Far East, China, Japan, Korea, Taiwan and the Philippines, where it is the main cause of human paragonimiasis. Thirteen other species can infect man, in China three species, *P. szechuanensis* (*skrijabani*), *P. huietungensis* and *P. tuanshenensis*;[168] in Thailand and Malaya, *P. heterotremus*; in Japan *P. myazaki*; in India *P. compactus*, in Africa *P. africanus* and *P. uterobilateralis*, and in South and Central America *P. caliensis*, *P. mexicanus* (*peruvianus*) and *P. ecuadorensis*. These less important species can be distinguished by the shape and distribution of the cuticular spines covering the adult fluke, the shape and number of branches of the ovary, the size of the eggs and the clinical features of human infection (Table 22.2).

The adult fluke (Figs. 22.42 and II.10, p. 1328) measures $8-20 \times 5-9$ mm, is oval, reddish-brown and translucent. There is an oral and a larger ventral sucker. The ovary is branched to the

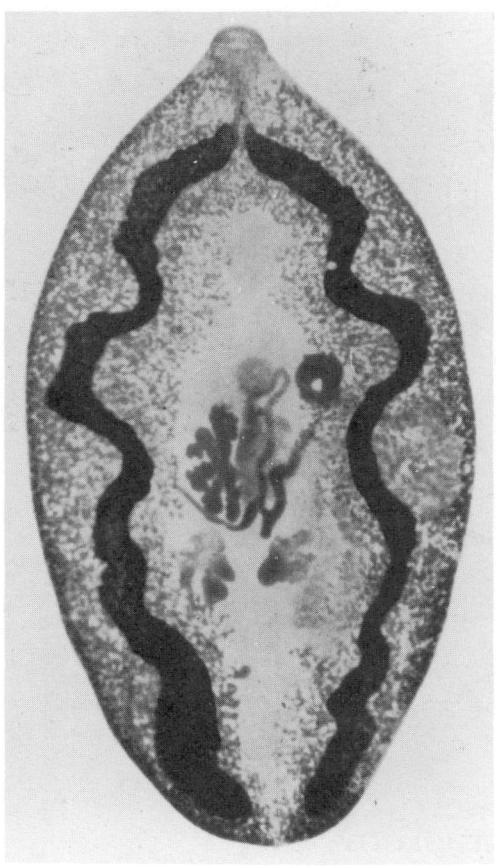

Fig. 22.42 Adult *Paragonimus westermani*. (Courtesy WTIM.)

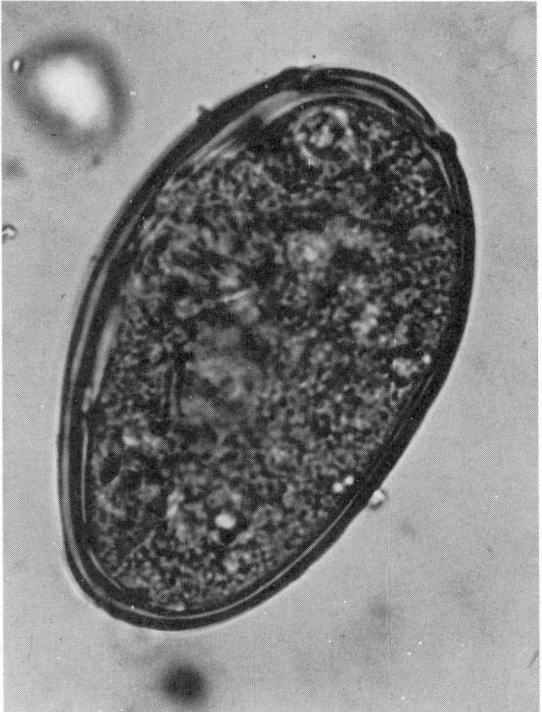

Fig. 22.43 Egg of *Paragonimus westermani*. (Courtesy WTIM.)

left and right of the midline and the uterus is opposite. The cuticle is covered with wedge-shaped spines (cuticular spines) which in association with the numbers of branches of the ovary can be used to distinguish species. The egg, which is brown and operculate, varies in size in the different species (Table 22.2) and shows a thickening at the pole opposite to the operculum (Fig. 22.43 and Plate III.2).

Life-cycle (Fig. 22.44)

The life-cycle involves a vertebrate host (crustacean-eating mammal), a first intermediate host, a snail, and a second intermediate host, a freshwater crab or crayfish. The adult fluke lives in the cystic cavities in the lungs where it can survive for up to 20 years. The eggs which are laid in these cystic cavities in the lung are voided in the sputum or passed via the faeces from swal-lowed sputum into water where they hatch into a ciliated miracidium after 16 days to seven weeks and enter the first intermediate host—a fresh-water snail of various species (Table 22.2)—in which they encyst as metacercariae. The vertebrate hosts are infected by eating raw crabs or crayfish. After passing through the stomach the metacercariae excyst in the jejunum. The young flukes penetrate the intestinal wall to become localized in the peritoneal cavity where there appears to be considerable migration before they arrive in the chest cavity via the diaphragm to enter the lungs. They mature in bronchi after forming cystic cavities in which they mature and lay eggs five to six weeks after infection. In some species the young flukes do not settle in the lungs but wander round the body immature, while others lay eggs in ectopic sites.

TRANSMISSION

Man is infected by eating the flesh or juices of uncooked crabs or crayfish and the raw flesh of a paratenic host such as the wild boar.

Paragonimus westermani

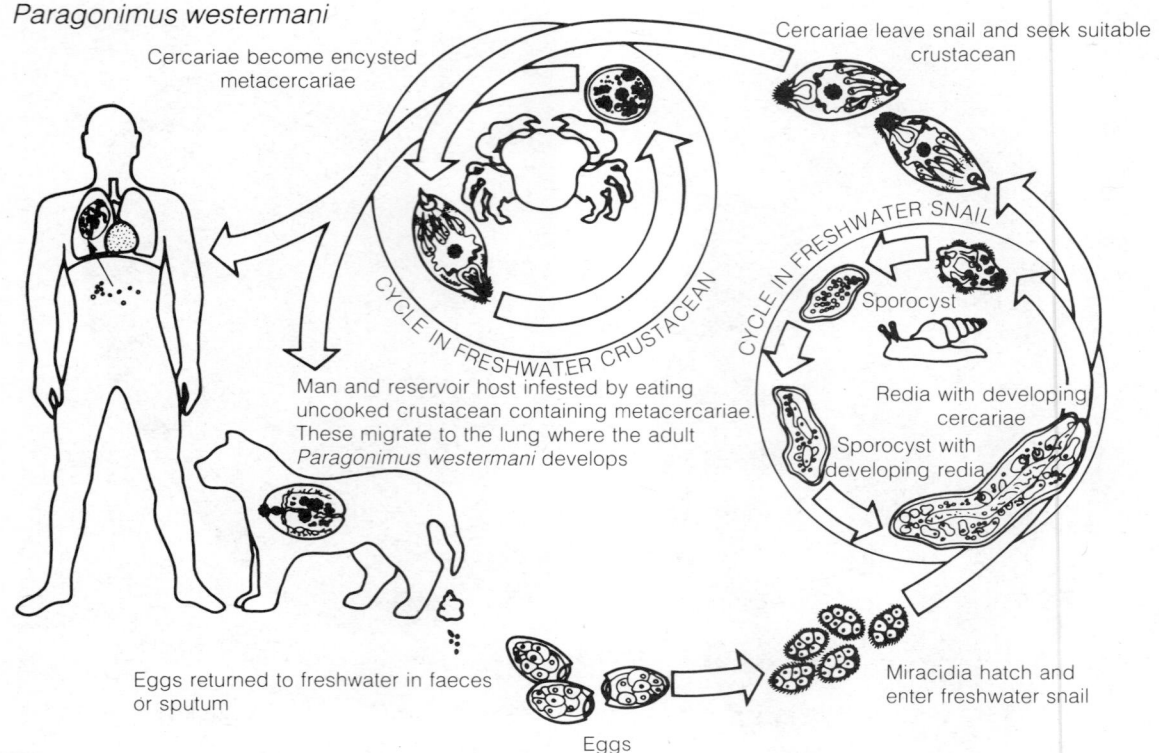

Fig. 22.44   Life-cycle of *Paragonimus westermani*. (Courtesy WTIM.)

Raw crabs and crayfish

In Japan the most important crab host, *Eriocheir japonicus,* is used in the preparation of crab soup. In Korea the crab, *Eriocheir sinensis,* is eaten raw and the raw juice of a crayfish, *Cambaroides similis,* is used as a medicine for diarrhoea. In China the stone crab, *Sinopotamon (Potamon) denticulatus* is eaten alive after being immersed in wine as 'drunken crab'.

Contamination by raw juice

The hands of cooks can become contaminated from the chopping block and knives, and accidental infection occurs from contact with the mouth. The juice of crabs is used in the Philippines to prepare a special dish, 'Kinagang'.

Raw flesh

Wild boar and martens can act as paratenic hosts of *P. myazaki* and infection occurs in Japan after eating the raw flesh containing the immature flukes.[169]

PATHOLOGY

Both adults and eggs cause pathology.

Flukes

In experimental infection the first pathological changes can be detected in the pleural cavity with a haemorrhagic or pleural exudate about 20 days after infection. The diaphragm develops an intense inflammatory reaction after 25 days and mature flukes appear in the lung parenchyma usually in pairs where they induce active pneumonitis and haemorrhage.[170] Adult flukes are found inside the bronchial lumen where they cause 'worm cysts' or 'burrows' (abscess cavities). A leukocytic infiltration initially surrounds the fluke to be followed by the formation of a granuloma and encapsulation in fibrous tissue forming a cyst with an opening into a bronchiole, the columnar epithelium of which is replaced by stratified squamous epithelium. The worm cysts, up to 20–25 in number and 2 cm in diameter, occupy the surface of the lung but to a greater extent the deeper tissues. They can be seen on the pleural surface as deep, red, tumour-like swellings, like a grape or plum. On section the cysts are seen to be distended, greyish-white nodules containing irregular cavities while the lung underneath is seen to contain a number of 'burrows' which are formed of infiltrated lung tissue containing brown material in which the adult flukes may lie (Fig. 22.45) side to side. The septa between the tunnels may break down and a considerable cavity produced to give the appearance of a dilated bronchus. Microscopically the walls of these cavities are composed of fibrous tissue consisting of fibroblasts, mononuclear and plasma cells, and sometimes eosinophils. There is no connection with bronchial carcinoma.

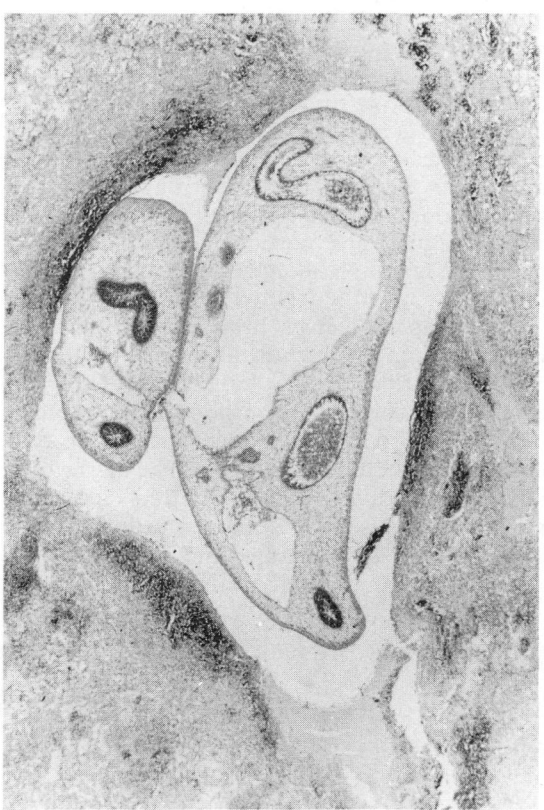

Fig. 22.45 Segments of *Paragonimus westermani* in a cavity in the lung. (Courtesy Dr S. T. Chou.)

Eggs

The eggs incite a granulomatous reaction to form 'egg tubercles' consisting of epithelioid cells, lymphocytes, plasma cells and eosinophils

surrounded by fibroblasts. Both foreign body and Langhan's giant cells may be present. Numerous *Paragonimus* eggs with egg tubercles surround the cavities and the whole histological picture closely resembles tuberculosis (Fig. 22.46).

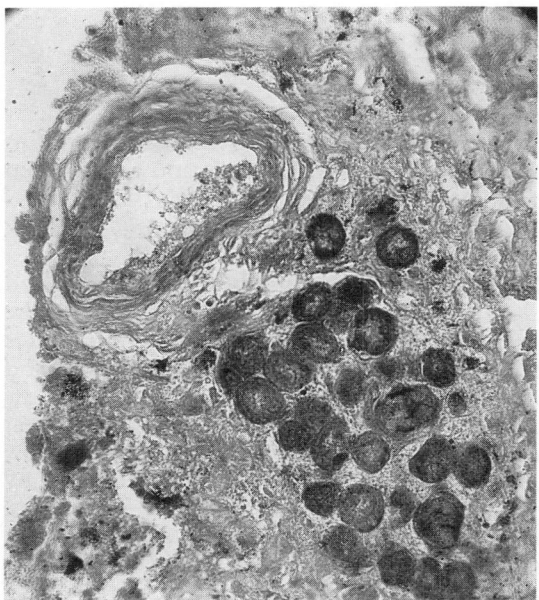

Fig. 22.46 Lung in *Paragonimus westermani* infection. Extensive fibrosis peribronchially and in cyst wall. Nonspecific inflammatory changes and numerous ova present.

Extrapulmonary paragonimiasis

Cerebral and spinal paragonimiasis

Cerebral paragonimiasis is caused by the adult flukes and cannot occur without pulmonary infection. The flukes migrate to the brain along the soft tissues round the neck veins, where they produce eggs, and may return to the lungs. This migration occurs about 10 months after the appearance of the pulmonary lesions.[171] The flukes migrate to the brain either along the internal carotid arteries, through the foramen lacerum, or along the jugular veins, through the jugular foramen.[168] After laying eggs they may return to the lungs.

Cerebral or spinal paragonimiasis accounts for 30– 60% of all cases of extrapulmonary paragonimiasis. In the brain the lesions seen in the temporal or occipital lobes are older and more extensive than newly formed ones elsewhere, and may be either cystic or solid or combined. The solid foci show a central area containing eggs, giant cells and Charcot–Leyden crystals, while in the middle there is a layer of connective tissue and an outer layer of plasma cells and lymphocytes. Similar lesions may be present in the spinal cord causing a transverse myelitis.

Other ectopic lesions

EGGS

Paragonimus eggs may be found in liver, peritoneum, testes, skin and muscle. When found in the skin the eggs may resemble and be mistaken for those of *S. japonicum*.

LARVA MIGRANS

With some species, notably *P. szechuanensis* and *P. hueitungensis* man is not a normal host and the worm cannot develop into an adult but migrates all over the body causing much damage and pathological lesions.[172] The migrating worms cause subcutaneous nodules, mostly in the chest and abdominal wall, which on biopsy show burrows with necrotic centres surrounded by granulation tissue and eosinophilic infiltration with numerous Charcot–Leyden crystals. Older lesions show as an eosinophilic granuloma with foreign body giant cells. Living juvenile worms can be found in these nodules. Similar lesions may be found in the brain forming burrows with eosinophilic infiltration or eosinophilic abscesses. No eggs are laid.

IMMUNITY

Little is known about immunity. A well-marked cell-mediated immunity is shown by the egg granulomas and a humoral immunity by the development of antibodies. Little is known about protective immunity or the mechanism of limiting the number of flukes.

CLINICAL FEATURES

Natural history

Most infections are asymptomatic. In heavier infections recurrent cough and haemoptysis may occur for many years but never threaten life, since the lung disease is not progressive. The development of cerebral lesions is serious. The majority of infections are very chronic but some

may progress on to chronic bronchitis, bronchiectasis, lung abscess, pleural effusions and pulmonary fibrosis.

Incubation period

The incubation period is five to six months after infection until the flukes have matured and started to lay eggs.

Symptoms and signs

No symptoms are caused by the immature flukes while migrating from the intestine to the lungs.

Pulmonary paragonimiasis

The onset of symptoms is insidious with a persistent *cough* and a vague feeling of distress in the chest. A spasmodic cough produces *sputum* containing a large number of *Paragonimus* eggs. The sputum is rusty-brown from blood and eggs. In one series of cases egg counts in the sputum varied from 1000 to 100 000 per day but in over half were under 10 000 per day.[173] *Haemoptysis* is slight, irregular and never profuse. *Clubbing of the fingers* is usual but chest signs are usually absent.

The symptoms may progress to recurrent bronchopneumonia or lung abscess with fibrosis and calcification of the lung. There are few general signs in the uncomplicated pulmonary disease. The *sputum* is characteristic, the red-brown colour being due mostly to the eggs which are thick-walled, operculate (Fig. 22.47), varying in size and shape with a smooth yellow double outer shell: on adding water and replenishing it from time to time ciliated miracidia will hatch

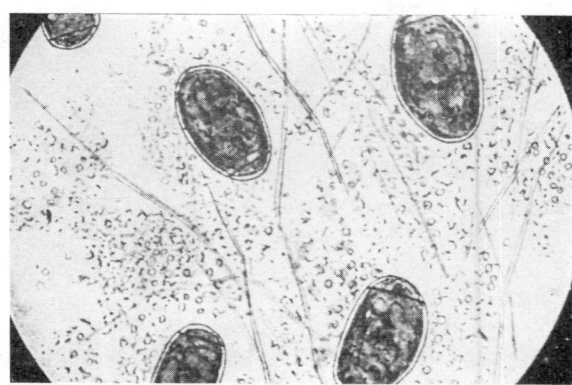

Fig. 22.47 *Paragonimus* ova in sputum.

after four to six weeks. There is usually a mild to moderate eosinophilia, which may be high during the migration phase.

RADIOGRAPHIC APPEARANCES

Radiographic changes in pulmonary paragonimiasis are very similar to those of pulmonary tuberculosis. Tomography is essential for diagnosis (Fig. 22.48). Abnormal shadows are found in the middle, upper and lower parts of the lungs but are rarely seen in the apex, and they are commoner in the right than the left lung. There are three types of shadow which are considered typical: nodular, ring and infiltrative. The nodular shadow is suggestive of a tuberculoma and has a sharply marked rounded or oval contour. The ring shadow is a cystic form with a relatively thin wall and is round, oval or irregular in shape (Fig. 22.48).[174] Radiographic changes at the bases strongly resemble bronchiectasis.

and pneumoencephalography showed the severity of the brain atrophy associated with the infection.[176]

Other ectopic sites

ADULT FLUKES

Worm cysts may develop in the skin and subcutaneous tissues, causing abscesses in the wall of the intestine, with diarrhoea and the passage of eggs in the stool, and in the peritoneum, where they may cause considerable abdominal pain and adhesions.

EGGS

Eggs may enter the circulation and be carried throughout the body causing egg granulomas in the heart, liver, kidneys and brain. In generalized paragonimiasis there is a general lymphadenopathy associated with cutaneous ulcer-

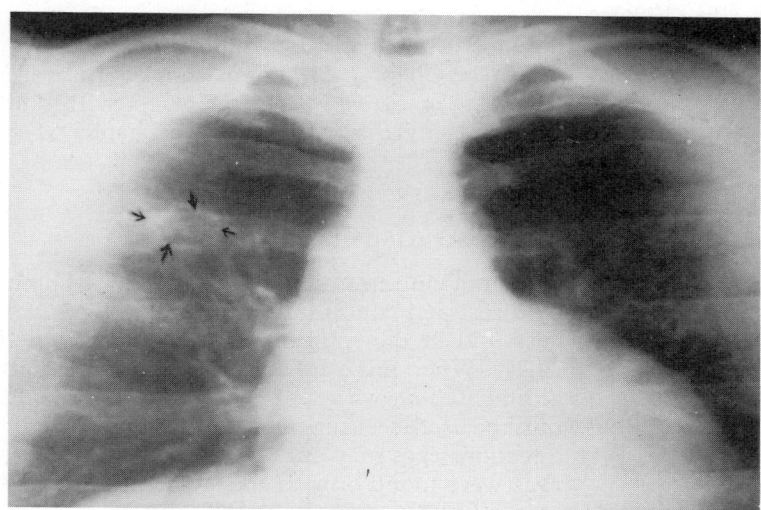

Fig. 22.48 Tomogram showing a cavity (arrowed) in the right upper lobe of the lung in paragonimiasis.

Cerebral paragonimiasis

The clinical symptoms of cerebral paragonimiasis are similar to those of cerebral tumour or embolism—jacksonian epilepsy, ending in hemiplegia, aphasia, visual disturbances, homonymous hemianopia and monoplegias of various degrees. Common eye signs are optic atrophy and papilloedema. Spinal involvement with paraplegia was reported by Oh and Lauyen.[175]

Radiological findings in cerebral paragonimiasis showed calcification in half the cases

ation and abdominal symptoms. Paragonimiasis of the uterus has been described.

LARVA MIGRANS

Lesions caused by migrating immature flukes are responsible for a 'larva migrans' syndrome similar to that of other migrating helminths, migratory subcutaneous nodules associated with deeper visceral lesions and eosinophilia. Three species of *Paragonimus* are responsible: *P. szechuanensis*,[168] *P. hueitungensis*,[177] *P. heterotremus*.[178] Symptoms appear as early as the thirteenth day after infection, usually in children, with a high eosinophilia, fever and general malaise. A number of subcutaneous nodules appear which 'migrate' steadily through the tissues. Although there are some pulmonary symptoms and haemoptysis, eggs can never be demonstrated in the sputum or faeces. In the cases of *P. szechuanensis* and *P. hueitungensis* the young flukes may also migrate through the internal organs causing an 'eosinophilic brain syndrome' (coma, stroke, monoplegia and cranial nerve lesions), pericardium (pericarditis), the eye or abdominal viscera, where they cause abdominal pain and hepatic dysfunction with eosinophilic liver granulomas or abscesses.

African paragonimiasis

Two species are found in West Africa: *P. africanus*[179] in Zaire and *P. uterobilateralis* in Nigeria. The reservoir hosts of *P. africanus* are the mongoose *Crossarchus obscurus* and *Atilax paludinosus*,[179] and the African drill (*Mandrillus leucophaeus*).[180] The host of *P. uterobilateralis* is the African civet cat (*Viverra civetta*)[181] (see Table 22.2). Infections are mild with cough and recurrent small haemoptyses. There are no cerebral symptoms and no radiological signs. There is a good response to treatment with praziquantel.[182]

Neotropical paragonimiasis

In South and Central America only a few cases of paragonimiasis are found. These are caused by *P. caliensis*,[183] *P. mexicanus* (*peruvianus*)[184] and *P. ecuadorensis*.[185] Infections are characterized chiefly by pulmonary symptoms but cerebral lesions have occurred in *P. mexicanus*[186] associated with hepatic lesions.

DIFFERENTIAL DIAGNOSIS

Pulmonary paragonimiasis

The main differential diagnosis is from pulmonary tuberculosis. The absence of general symptoms and wasting and presence of eggs in the sputum will serve to distinguish paragonimiasis. Other lung diseases to be distinguished are bronchiectasis, lung abscess, amoebic lung abscess, hydatid cyst and chronic fungus infections.

Cerebral paragonimiasis

The main differentiation is from other space-occupying lesions: cerebral abscess, cerebral tumour, cerebrovascular disease with stroke, and eosinophilic brain syndromes, *Schistosoma japonicum* (see Chapter 22), toxocariasis (see Chapter 21), *Strongyloides* (see Chapter 21), cerebral gnathostomiasis (see Chapter 24), cysticercosis and *Angiostrongylus cantonensis* (see Chapter 24), all of which may be found in the same geographical area.

Ectopic paragonimiasis

Egg granulomas in ectopic sites may also be found with *Clonorchis sinensis*, and *S. japonicum*, while hepatic eosinophilic granulomas may also be found with *Fasciola hepatica* and *Toxocara canis*. An important point is that eggs of *Paragonimus* are not found in duodenal aspirate whereas those of liver flukes are. Cutaneous larva migrans features are also found in *Fasciola hepatica* (see Chapter 22), animal hookworms (see Chapter 21), *Strongyloides* (see Chapter 21) and cutaneous myiasis (cattle bots, see Chapter 51).

DIAGNOSIS

Demonstration of eggs

The stools and sputum should be examined both by direct and concentration methods. Eggs can be found in the sputum by direct smear (Fig. 22.47). When there are only few eggs centrifuge sedimentation with 1–2% sodium hydroxide must be used (see Appendix IV, p. 1499). In light infections eggs may only be found in the stools; eggs were found only in the stools in 13.2% of cases.[187]

In the stools the eggs can be concentrated by the formol ether concentration method (see Appendix IV, p. 1490). *Paragonimus* eggs can be recovered from gastric juice[188] and on aspiration from the bronchi.[189]

The eggs must be distinguished from *S. japonicum* which are single shell and non-operculated, and from other flukes, *Fasciola hepatica* and *F. buski*, which are larger.

Serodiagnosis

The recovery of eggs from the sputum and stool is often difficult in mild cases, after treatment and in ectopic lesions. The indirect haemagglutination test is highly sensitive but the test of choice is the ELISA which is highly sensitive and specific and differentiates from clonorchiasis, but can give cross reactions at low titre with hydatid cyst, cysticercosis and tuberculosis.[168] These tests become negative within three to four months after successful treatment and are a good test of cure.

TREATMENT

Praziquantel is the drug of choice. Three divided doses orally, each of 25 mg/kg daily for 2 days, cured 100% of cases.[190] Eggs disappeared two to three weeks after treatment with general improvement in signs and symptoms. Radiological lesions in the lungs took a few months to clear. Side-effects were minimal but serious effects may occur in the treatment of cerebral paragonimiasis. *Niclofolan* has also been used with a cure rate of 100% with a single dose of 2 mg/kg but side-effects were more pronounced than with praziquantel.

Other drugs have been used: mebendazole alone was not effective but mebendazole 50 mg/kg three times a day for 28 days plus intramuscular emetime hydrochloride 1 mg/kg/day for 10 days gave a cure rate of 70%.[173]

EPIDEMIOLOGY

Human paragonimiasis is limited in its distribution to where food habits make infection possible, such as Japan, Korea, China, Taiwan, Thailand and the Philippines. Elsewhere, since flukes of the *Paragonimus* genus are found widely distributed in a variety of mammals which eat crabs and crayfish, unusual circumstances can lead to human infection. During the Nigerian Civil War crabs were eaten as the result of food shortages and many cases of paragonimiasis occurred. Sporadic infection may be found among small groups of forest-dwelling aboriginals.

CONTROL

Health education in the handling and preparation of crabs for food can reduce the incidence.

REFERENCES

1 Jordan, P. & Webbe, G. (1982) *Human Schistosomiasis* 2nd edn. London: Heinemann.
2 Sathe, B.D., Mukerji, S., Gaitonde, B.B. et al (1981) *Bull. Haffkine Inst.* **9**, 34–37.
3 Greer, G.J. & Anuar, H. (1984) *S.E. Asian J. trop. Med. publ. Hlth* **15**, 303–312.
4 Attawibol, S., Bunnag, T., Thirachandra, S. et al (1983) *S.E. Asian J. trop. Med. publ. Hlth* **14**, 463–450.
5 Warren, K.S., Mahmoud, A.A.F., Cummings, P. et al (1974) *Am. J. trop. Med. Hyg.* **23**, 902.
6 Goddard, M.J. & Jordan, P. (1980) *Trans. R. Soc. trop. Med. Hyg.* **74**, 185.
7 Fenwick, A. (1969) *Trans. R. Soc. trop. Med. Hyg.* **63**, 557.
8 Theron, A. (1982) Thèse de Docteur d'État, Académie de Montpellier, Université de Perpignan.
9 Wright, C.A. & Ross, G.C. (1982) *Trans. R. Soc. trop. Med. Hyg.* **74**, 326–332.
10 Mao, S. & Shao, B. (1982) *Am. J. trop. Med. Hyg.* **31**, 92–99.
11 Appleton, C.C. & Eriksson, I.M. (1983) *S. Afr. J. Sci.* **79**, 333–334.
12 Webbe, G. & Msangi, A.S. (1958) *Ann. trop. Med. Parasit.* **52**, 302–314.
13 Nduku, W.K. & Harrison, A.D. (1976) *Hydrobiologia* **49**, 143–170.
14 Beadle, L.C. (1974) *The Inland Waters of Tropical Africa*. London: Longman.
15 Giglioli, G. (1964) *Br. med. J.* **i**, 767.
16 Appleton, C.C. (1977) *Int. J. Parasit.* **7**, 335–345.
17 Sturrock, R.F. (1966) *Ann. trop. Med. Parasit.* **60**, 100–105.
18 Appleton, C.C. (1975) *Ann. trop. Med. Parasit.* **69**, 241–245.
19 Smithers, S.R. (1956) *Trans. R. Soc. trop. Med. Hyg.* **50**, 354–365.
20 Webbe, G. (1966) *Ann. trop. Med. Parasit.* **60**, 78–84.
21 Warren, K.S. (1976) *J. Invest. Derm.* **67**, 464.
22 Ashworth, T.G. (1970) *Cent. Afr. J. Med.* **16**, 123.
23 Maldonado, J.F. (1967) *Schistosomiasis in America*. Barcelona: Cientificio-Medica.
24 Gelfand, M. & Hammar, B. (1966) *Trans. R. Soc. trop. Med. Hyg.* **60**, 231.
25 Farid, Z., Miner, W.F., Higashi, G.I. et al (1976) *J. trop. Med. Hyg.* **79**, 164–166.
26 Cheever, A.W. & Andrade, Z.A. (1967) *Trans. R. Soc. trop. Med. Hyg.* **61**, 625.
27 Farid, Z., Bassily, S., Lehman, J.S. et al (1970) *Trans. R. Soc. trop. Med. Hyg.* **64**, 811.
28 Lehman, S.J., Farid, Z. & Bassily, S. (1970) *Gastroenterology* **59**, 433.
29 Malik, M.O.A., Satir, A.A., Veress, B. et al (1975) *E. Afr. med. J.* **52**, 183–195.
30 Owor, R. & Madda, J.P. (1977) *E. Afr. med. J.* **4**, 137–141.
31 Wydell, S.H. (1958) *E. Afr. med. J.* **35**, 413.
32 Pieron, R., Mafart, Y., van den Akker, M. et al (1974) *Med. Afr. Noire* **21**, 255.
33 Cook, J.A. & Jordan, P. (1970) *Trans. R. Soc. trop. Med. Hyg.* **64**, 793.
34 Radstrake, H.N.J., Collenteur, J.C., Hendershee, D. et al (1973) *Trop. Geog. Med.* **25**, 84.
35 Lucas, S.B. (1982) *E. Afr. med. J.* **59**, 345–355.

36 Hicks, R.M., Gough, T.A. & Walters, C.L. (1978) In *Environmental Aspects of N-Nitroso Compounds* (IARC Scientific Publications No. 19 p 465), ed. E.A. Walker et al. Lyon: International Agency for Research on Cancer.

37 Hicks, R.M. (1983) *J. R. Soc. Med.* **76**, 16–22.

38 Bambirra, E.A., Andrade, J. de S., Cesarini, I. et al (1984) *Am. J. trop. Med. Hyg.* **33**, 76–79.

39 Andrade, Z.A., Andrade, S.G. & Sadigursky, M. (1971) *Am. J. trop. Med. Hyg.* **20**, 77.

40 Bassily, S., Farid, Z., Barsoum, R.S. et al (1976) *J. trop. Med. Hyg.* **72**, 256.

41 Sabrour, M.S., Elsaid, W. & Abou-Gabal, I. (1972) *Bull. Wld Hlth Org.* **47**, 549.

42 Barsoum, R.S., Bassily, S., Soliman, M.M. et al (1979) *Trans. R. Soc. trop. Med. Hyg.* **73**, 367.

43 Higazi, A.M., El-Brashy, N., Elsa, A.A. et al (1972) *J. Egyp. med. Ass.* **55**, 439.

44 Edington, G.M., Von Lichtenburg, E., Nwabuebo, I. et al (1970) *Am. J. trop. Med. Hyg.* **19**, 982.

45 Houston, W. (1964) *Br. J. Urol.* **36**, 220.

46 Arean, U.M. (1956) *Am. J. Obst. Gyn.* **72**, 1038–1153.

47 Gelfand, M. (1950) *Schistosomiasis in Central Africa.* Capetown: Juta.

48 Edington, G.M., Nwuabebo, I. & Jnaid, T.A. (1975) *Trans. R. Soc. trop. Med. Hyg.* **69**, 153.

49 Olurin, E.O. & Olurin, O. (1969) *Br. med. J.* **iv**, 534.

50 Rappaport, J., Abukerk, J. & Schneider, I.J. (1973) *Archs Path.* **99**, 227.

51 Wood, M.G., Siolovitz, H. & Schelman, D. (1976) *Archs Derm.* **122**, 690.

52 Macdonald, D.M. & Morrison, J.G.L. (1976) *Br. med. J.* **ii**, 619.

53 Gendrel, D., Richard-Lenoble, D., Kombila, M. et al (1984) *Am. J. trop. Med. Hyg.* **33**, 1166–1169.

54 Bassily, S., Dunn, M.A., Farid, Z. et al (1983) *J. trop. Med. Hyg.* **86**, 67–71.

55 Mahmoud, A.A.F. & Woodruff, A.W. (1972) *Trans. R. Soc. trop. Med. Hyg.* **66**, 75–84.

56 Farid, Z., Bassily, S., Schulert, A.R. et al (1967) *Trans. R. Soc. trop. Med. Hyg.* **61**, 621–625.

57 Jamra, M., Maspes, V. & Meira, D.A. (1964) *Revta Inst. Med trop. São Paulo* **6**, 126–136.

58 Farid, Z., Bassily, S., Schulert, A.R. et al (1968) *Trans. R. Soc. trop. Med. Hyg.* **62**, 496–500.

59 Greenham, R. (1978) *Trans. R. Soc. trop. Med. Hyg.* **72**, 72–75.

60 Forsyth, D.M. (1969) *Bull. Wld Hlth Org.* **40**, 771.

61 Smithers, S.R. & Hockley, D.J. (1968) *Trans. R. Soc. trop. Med. Hyg.* **62**, 466.

62 Smithers, S.R. & Terry, R.J. (1967) *Trans. R. Soc. trop. Med. Hyg.* **61**, 517.

63 Bradley, W.H. & McCullough, F.S. (1973) *Trans. R. Soc. trop. Med. Hyg.* **67**, 491

64 Nelson, G.S. & Saoud, M.F.A. (1968) *J. Helminth.* **42**, 339.

65 Webbe, G., James, C., Lelson, G.S. et al (1979) *Trans. R. Soc. trop. Med. Hyg.* **73**, 42.

66 Amin, M.A. & Nelson, G.S. (1969) *Bull. Wld Hlth Org.* **41**, 225.

67 Madwar, M.A. & Voller, A. (1975) *Br. med. J.* **i**, 435.

68 Mahmoud, A.A.F. (1981) In *Modern Genetic Concepts and Techniques in the Study of Parasites*, Vol. 4, ed. F. Michal, pp. 303–322. Tropical Diseases Research Series. Basel: Schwabe & Coy.

69 Hofstetter, M., Fasano, M.B. & Otteson, E.A. (1983) *J. Immunol.* **130**, 1376–1380.

70 Gazzinelli, G., Katz, N., Rocha, R.S. et al (1983) *Am. J. trop. Med. Hyg.* **32**, 326–333.

71 Butterworth, A.E., Dalton, P.R., Dunne, D.W. et al (1984) *Trans. R. Soc. trop. Med. Hyg.* **78**, 108–123.

72 Clarke, V. de V., Warburton, B. & Blair, D.M. (1970) *Cent. Afr. med. J.* **16**, 123.

73 Gelfand, M., Clarve, V. de V. & Bunbury, H. (1981) *Cent. Afr. med. J.* **27**, 219–221.

74 Webel, O.T., Elmasry, N.A., Castell, D.O. et al (1974) *Gastroenterology* **67**, 939.

75 Mackenjee, M.K.R., Coovadia, H.M. & Chutte, C.H.J. (1984) *Trans. R. Soc. trop. Med. Hyg.* **78**, 13–15.

76 Besson, A., Stahel, E., Anani, P. et al (1982) *Schwietz. med. Woch.* **112**, 454–457.

77 Barsoum, R.S., Bassily, S., Baligh, O.K. et al (1977) *Trans. R. Soc. trop. Med. Hyg.* **72**, 256.

78 Lichtenberg, R. & Vaida, G.A. (1977) *Neurology* **27**, 55.

79 Hamlyn, A.N., McKenna, K. & Douglas, A.P. (1977) *Br. med. J.* **i**, 1258.

80 Lucas, A.O., Adenyi-Jones, C.C., Cockshutt, W.P. et al (1966) *Lancet* **i**, 631.

81 Powell, S.J., Engelbrecht, H.E. & Welchman, J.M. (1968) *Trans. R. Soc. trop. Med. Hyg.* **62**, 231.

82 Buchanan, W.M. & Gelfand, M. (1970) *Trans. R. Soc. trop. Med. Hyg.* **62**, 393.

83 Wright, E.D., Chiphangwi, J. & Hutt, M.S.R. (1982) *Trans. R. Soc. trop. Med. Hyg.* **76**, 822–829.

84 Barlow, C.H. & Meleney, H.E. (1949) *Am. J. trop. Med.* **29**, 79.

85 Pugh, R.N.H. & Gilles, H.M. (1979) *Ann. trop. Med. Parasit.* **73**, 89–90.

86 Wilkins, H.A., Goll, P.H. & Moore, P.J. (1985) *Ann. trop. Med. Parasit.* **79**, 159–161.

87 Van Wijk, H.B. & Elias, E.A. (1975) *Trop. geogr. Med.* **27**, 237.

88 Deschiens, R. & Delas, A.E. (1969) *Trans. R. Soc. trop. Med. Hyg.* **63**, 557.

89 Most, H., Kane, C.A., Lavietas, P.H. et al (1950) *Am. J. trop. Med.* **30**, 239.

90 Robinson, A. & Lewert, R.M. (1983) *Infect. Immun.* **39**, 1477–1480.

91 Cavallo, C., Galvanek, E.G., Ward, P.A. et al (1974) *Am. J. Path.* **433**, 445.

92 Gilles, H.M., Greenwood, B.M., Greenwood, A.M. et al (1983) *Trans. R. Soc. trop. Med. Hyg.* **77**, 24–31.

93 Bell, D.R. (1963) *Bull. Wld Hlth Org.* **29**, 525.

94 Sung, C.K. & Dresden, M.H. (1984) *Am. J. trop. Med. Hyg.* **33**, 1178–1181.

95 Barakat, R.M., El-Gassim, E.E., Awadalla, H.N. et al (1983) *Trans. R. Soc. trop. Med. Hyg.* **77**, 109–111.

96 Deelder, A.M. & Kornelis, D. (1981) *Trop. geogr. Med.* **33**, 36–41.

97 Gold, R., Rosen, F.S. & Weller, T.H. (1969) *Am. J. trop. Med. Hyg.* **18**, 545.

98 Phillips, T.M. & Draper, C.C. (1975) *Br. med. J.* **ii**, 476.

99 McMahon, J.E. & Kolstrup, N. (1979) *Br. med. J.* **ii**, 1396–1399.

100 Katz, N., Rochas, S. & Chabbes, A. (1979) *Bull. Wld Hlth Org.* **57**, 773–779.

101 Santos, A.T., Blass, B.L., Nosenas, J.L. et al (1979) *Bull. Wld Hlth Org.* **57**, 793–799.

102 Feldmeier, H., Zwingenberger, K., Steiner, A. et al (1981) *Tropenmed. Parasit.* **32**, 39–42.

103 Nash, T.E., Hofstetter, M., Cheever, A.W. et al (1982) *Am. J. trop. Med. Hyg.* **31**, 977–982.

104 Kardaman, M.W., Fenwick, A., El Igail, A.B. et al (1985) *J. trop Med. Hyg.* **88**, 105–109.

105 Keittivuti, B., Keitivutti, A., O'Rourke, T. et al (1984) *Trans. R. Soc. trop. Med. Hyg.* **78**, 477–479.

106 Bella, H., Ghaffar, A., Rahima, A. et al (1982) *Am. J. trop. Med. Hyg.* **31**, 775–778.

107 Simpson, T.R. (1965) *Cent. Afr. med. J.* **ii**, 53.

108 Hussein, A.M.T., Medany, S., El-Magd, A.M.A. et al (1983) *Lancet* **i**, 673–674.

109 Kean, B.H. & Goldsmith, E. (1968) *Eighth Int. Congr. trop. Med. Malar. Teheran*, Abstracts 7, Reviews 31.

110 Bousfield, D. (1979) *Nature, Lond.* **279**, 573–574.

111 Appleton, C.C. & Bruton, M.N. (1979) *Ann. trop. Med. Parasit.* **73**, 547–561.

112 Forsyth, D.M. & Macdonald, G. (1966) *Trans. R. Soc. trop. Med. Hyg.* **60**, 568.

113 J.D. Bradley (ed.) (1985) *J. trop. Med. Hyg.* **88**, 45–182.

114 Wilkins, H.A., Goll, P.H., Marshall, T.F. et al (1984) *Trans. R. Soc. trop. Med. Hyg.* **78**, 227–232.

115 Tayo, M.A., Pugh, R.N.H. & Bradley, A.K. (1980) *Ann. trop. Med. Hyg.* **74**, 347–354.

116 Farook, M. & Mallah, M.B. (1966) *Bull. Wld Hlth Org.* **35**, 377.

117 Witenberg, G. & Yofe, J. (1938) *Trans. R. Soc. trop. Med. Hyg.* **31**, 549.

118 Webbe, G. & James, C. (1969) *Trans. R. Soc. trop. Med. Hyg.* **63**, 541.

119 Macdonald, G. (1965) *Trans. R. Soc. trop. Med. Hyg.* **59**, 481.

120 Coutinho, F.A.B., Griffin, M. & Thomas, J.D. (1982) *Parasitology* **82**, 111–120.

121 World Health Organization (1983) SCHISTO/83.72. VBC/83.879.

122 Kloos, H. & McCullough, F.S. (1982) *Planta Med.* **46**, 195–209.

123 Machado, P. (1982) *Am. J. trop. Med. Hyg.* **31**, 76–86.

124 Mobarak, A.B. (1982) *Am. J. trop. Med. Hyg.* **31**, 87–91.

125 Hussein, M.F., Saeed, A.A. & Nelson, G.S. (1970) *Bull. Wld Hlth Org.* **42**, 745.

126 Allen, A.M., Taplin, D., Lagteres, L.J. et al (1974) *Lancet* **i**, 1175.

127 Facey, R.V. & Marsden, P.M. (1960) *Br. med. J.* **ii**, 619.

128 Belding, D.L. (1965) *Textbook of clinical parasitology*, 3rd edn. New York: Appleton Century Crofts.

129 Biggart, J.H. (1937) *J. Path. Bact.* **44**, 488.

130 Neghme, A. & Ossandon, M. (1943) *Am. J. trop. Med.* **23**, 545.

131 Jones, E.A., Kay, J.M., Milligan, H.P. et al (1977) *Am. J. Med.* **63**, 836.

132 Flores, M., Merino-Angulo, J. & Aguirre Erasti, C. (1982) *Eur. J. resp. Dis.* **63**, 231–233.

133 Taillez, R. & Korach, S. (1970) *Ann. Inst. Pasteur* **118**, 330.

134 Pautrizel, P., Baillenger, J., Duret, J. et al (1962) *Rev. Immunol.* **26**, 167.

135 Andrews, P., Thomas, H., Pahlke, R. et al (1985) *Med. Res. Rev.* **3**, 147.

136 Akhtar, B.N. & Abibi, V. (1977) *J. trop. Med. Hyg.* **80**, 179.

137 Attwood, H.D. & Chou, S.T. (1978) *Pathology* **20**, 153.

138 Hsu, H.F. (1939) *Chin. med. J.* **55**, 542.

139 Faust, E.C. & Khaw, O.K. (1927) *Am. J. Hyg., Monogr. Ser.* **8**, 1.

140 Yamagata, S. & Yaegashi, A. (1964) *Prog. med. Parasit.* **1**, 633.

141 Katsurada, F. (1922) *Nisshin Igaku* Suppl., 1.

142 Hou, P.C. (1956) *J. Path. Bact.* **72**, 239.

143 Bhamarapravati, N. & Thamavit, W. (1978) *Lancet* **i**, 205.

144 Yamagata, S. (1962) *S. Nakayama Shoten Tokyo* **1**, 134.

145 Strauss, W.G. (1962) *Am. J. trop. Med. Hyg.* **11**, 625.

146 McFadzean, A.J.S. & Yeung, R.T.T. (1965) *Trans. R. Soc. trop. Med. Hyg.* **59**, 179.

147 Oshima, T., Kagai, N., Kimata, M. et al (1965) *Kise-ichugeka Zasshi* **14**, 195.

148 Flavell, D.J., Flavell, S.U. & Field, G.F. (1983) *Trans. R. Soc. trop. Med. Hyg.* **77**, 538–543.

149 Okuda, K., Enura, T., Morukama, K. et al (1973) *Gastroenterology* **65**, 457.

150 Sadun, E.H., Walton, B., Buck, A.A. et al (1959) *J. Parasit.* **45**, 129.

151 Rim, H.J., Lyu, K.S., Lee, J.S. et al (1981) *Ann. trop. Med. Parasit.* **75**, 27–31.

152 Rim, H.J., Lee, Y.M. & Lee, J.S. (1982) *Korean J. Parasit.* **20**, 1–8.

153 Inatomi, S. & Kimura, M. (1955) *Okayama Igakki Zasshi* **67**, 651.

154 Sadun E.H. (1955) *Am. J. Hyg.* **62**, 81.

155 Rodriguez, M.J.D., Gomez, L.L. & Montalvan, C.J.A. (1949) *Revta ecuad. Hig. Med. Trop.* **6**, 11.

156 Sirisinha, S. (1984) *Arzneimittel Forschung* **34**, 1170–1172.

157 Flavell, D.J. (1981) *Trans. R. Soc. trop. Med. Hyg.* **75**, 814–824.

158 Feldmeier, H. & Horstman, R.D. (1981) *Ann. trop. Med. Parasit.* **75**, 462.

159 Janechaiwat, J., Tharavanu, S., Vajrasthira, S. et al (1980) *J. Med. Ass. Thailand* **63**, 439.

160 Pung Pak, S., Bunnag, D. & Harinasuta, T. (1983) *S.E. Asian J. trop. Med. publ. Hlth* **14**, 363–366.

161 Bhaibulaya, M. & Punthuprasa, P. (1984) *S.E. Asian J. trop. Med. publ. Hlth* **15**, 389–393.

162 Sornmani, S., Schelp, F.P., Vitanaseth, P. et al (1984) *Arzneimittel Forschung* **34**, 1231–1234.

163 Daengsvang, S. & Mangalasmaya, M. (1941) *Ann. trop. Med. Parasit.* **35**, 43.

164 Bunnag, D., Radomyoso, P. & Harinasuta, T. (1983) *S.E. Asian J. trop. Med. publ. Hlth* **14**, 216–219.

165 Rabbani, G.H., Gilman, R.H., Kabiri, T. et al (1985) *Trans. R. Soc. trop. Med. Hyg.* **79**, 513–515.

166 Cho, S.Y., Kang, S.Y & Lee, J.B. (1984) *Arzneimittel Forschung* **34**, 1211–1213.

167 Arizono, N., Uemoto, K., Kondo, K. et al (1976) *Jap. J. Parasit.* **25**, 36.

168 Zhong, H.E.K., Xu, L. & Cao, W. (1981) *Chin. med. J.* **94**, 483–494.

169 Myazaki, I. & Habe, S. (1976) *J. Parasit.* **62**, 646.

170 Choy, W.Y. (1984) *Arzneimittel-Forschung* **34**, 1184–1185.

171 Lei, H.K. & Yen, C.K. (1957) *Chin. med. J.* **75**, 986.

172 Chung H.L., Hasu, C.P., Ho, L.Y. et al (1977) *Chin. med. J.* **3**, 379–394.

173 Benjapong, W., Naeypatimaivond, S., Benjapong, K. et al (1984) *S.E. Asian J. trop. Med. publ. Hlth* **15**, 354–359.

174 Diaconita, C.H. & Goldis, G.H. (1964) *Acta tuberc. scand.* **44**, 51.

175 Oh, S.J. & Lauyen, L. (1964) *J. Korean med. Ass.* **6**, 580.

176 Galatius-Jensen, K. & Uhm, I. (1956) *Br. J. Radiol.* **38**, 494.

177 Chung, H.L., Hasu, C.P., Ho, L.Y. et al (1977) *Chin. med. J.* **3**, 379–394.

178 Myazaki, I. & Harinasuta, T. (1966) *Ann. trop. Med. Parasit.* **60**, 509.

179 Vogel, H. & Crewe, W. (1965) *Z. Tropenmed. Parasit.* **16**, 109.

180 Sachs, R. & Voelker, J. (1975) *Tropenmed. Parasit.* **26**, 205–206.

181 Voelker, J., Sachs, R., Volkman, J.K. et al (1978) *Vet. Med. Rev.* 158–172.

182 Monson, M.H., Koenig, J.W. & Sachs, R. (1983) *Am. J. trop. Med. Hyg.* **32**, 371–375.

183 Little, M.D. (1968) *J. Parasit.* **54**, 738–746.

184 Myazaki, I. & Ishii, Y. (1968) *Jap. J. Parasit.* **17**, 445–453.

185 Voelker, J. & Arzube, M. (1979) *Tropenmed. Parasit.* **30**, 249–263.

186 Madrigal, R.B., Rodrigues-Ortiz, B., Soland, G. et al (1982) *Am. J. trop. Med. Hyg.* **31**, 522–526.

187 Komiya, Y. & Yokogawa, M. (1953) *Jap. J. med. Sci. Biol.* **6**, 207.

188 Okuda J. (1959) *Nichon Eisegaku Zasshi* **13**, 783.

189 Kitamoto, O., Okado, T., Ueno, A. et al (1958) *Kokyuki Shinryo* **13**, 92.

190 Vanijanonta, S., Bunnag, D. & Harinasuta, T. (1984) *Arzneimittel-Forschung* **34**, 1186–1188.

Chapter 23
Tapeworms (Cestodes)

Tapeworms are long flat worms which inhabit the intestine of mammals. They have a head (scolex) on top of a number of segments (proglottides) which absorb nutriment through the cuticle. They are hermaphroditic, the segments containing both testes and ovary. There are two main types, one with a head and rostellum with suckers (Cyclophyllidea) consisting of the tapeworms *Taenia* and *Echinococcus*, and another with slit-like suckers on the head but no rostellum (Pseudophyllidea) consisting of *Diphyllobothrium* species.

The *Taenia* worms have a life-cycle with one intermediate host in which the cysticercus stage is passed while the *Diphyllobothrium* tapeworms have two intermediate hosts in which cysticercoid and plerocercoid stages are passed respectively.

Pathology is caused in man as a definitive host by adult tapeworms, *Taenia saginata*, *T. solium*,

Table 23.1 Adult *Taenia* infections in man.

Adult	Egg	Definitive host	First stage larva	Intermediate host	Clinical features in man	Geographical distribution
Taenia saginata Multibranched uterus No hooks on scolex 4–10 m long	Outer shell and acid fast. Two oncospheric membranes. No hooks on oncosphere 30–40 μm in diameter	Man	Cysticercus bovis. No hooks on scolex 7.5–9 × 5.5 mm	Cattle, also camel and reindeer	Adult infection only. Mild abdominal symptoms	Worldwide in beef-eating countries. Common in Ethiopia, South America and Mexico
Taenia solium Simple branched uterus Hooks on scolex 4–10 m long	Double shelled. No acid-fast staining. Hooks on oncosphere 31–56 μm in diameter	Pig	Cysticercus cellulosae. Hooks on scolex 4.6–7.5 × 10 mm	Man, also macaque monkeys, sheep and dogs	Cysticercosis in man. Subcutaneous nodules. Cerebral cysticercosis with epilepsy and cerebral symptoms	Common among pork-eating peoples. Mexico, Latin America, Manchuria, India, Irian Jaya
Hymenolepis nana 20–45 × 0.5–0.9 mm. Hooks on scolex	40–60 μm diameter	Man	Cysticercoid	Intestinal villi of man. Also haemocoele of larvae of fleas and grain beetles	Asymptomatic. Fever, abdominal symptoms and eosinophilia	Warm countries. Egypt, Sudan, Thailand, India, Japan, southern Europe
Hymenolepis diminuta 20–60 × 3.5 mm. Hooks on scolex	60–80 μm in diameter	Rat	Cysticercoid	Haemocoele of larva of fleas and grain beetles	Asymptomatic. Eosinophilia.	Italy, Zaire, South America and Caribbean
Dipylidium caninum 15–40 cm × 2–3 mm. Hooks on scolex	Egg 30–40 μm in egg packet with 8–13 eggs	Dog	Cysticercoid	Haemocoele of larvae of dog flea, cat flea and human flea	Asymptomatic	Europe

Table 23.2 *Diphyllobothrium* and *Spirometra* worms in man.

Adult	Egg	Definitive host	First larval stage	First intermediate host	Second larval stage	Second intermediate host	Clinical features in man	Geographical distribution
Diphyllobothrium latum (fish tapeworm) 3–10 metres long, groove-like suckers on head	Operculated 70 × 40 μm	Domestic and wild fish-eating mammals and man	Coracidium 22–30 μm long Procercoid 50–60 μm long	*Cyclops. C. strenuus. Diaptomus gracilis. D. graciloides (oregonensis). C. brevispinosus. C. prasenus*	Plerocercoid or sparganum 3–12 × 2.5 mm	Pike, perch, salmon, trout, grayling, wall-eyed pike and turbot	Adult worm infects man, may cause megaloblastic anaemia	Europe, Baltic, Scandinavia, Roumania, Danube Delta, Manchuria and Japan
Diphyllobothrium pacificum								Chile, Peru and Argentina
Diphyllobothrium alascense								North American Eskimos
Spirometra mansoni 20–60 cm long		Domestic and wild canines and felines		*Cyclops*	20–30 cm long	Frogs, snakes, birds and mammals (man)	2nd larval stage infects man. Sparganosis. Migratory subcutaneous nodules	South-East Asia, Japan and China
Spirometra mansonoides 20–60 cm up to 1 metre long		Domestic and wild canines and felines		*Cyclops*		Cat and dog	Sparganosis. Migratory subcutaneous nodules	North America
Spirometra theileri (*pretoriensis*)		Domestic and wild canines and felines		*Cyclops*		?	Sparganosis. Migratory subcutaneous nodules	East and central Africa

Hymenolepis sp., other rarer tapeworms and *Diphyllobothrium latum*. In larval tapeworm infection in man (larval taeniasis) pathology is caused by the cysticercus stages of *T. solium* (cysticercosis), *Echinococcus* (hydatid), *Multiceps* (*Taenia*) *multiceps* and *M*. (*Taenia*) *brauni* (coe-nurus cerebralis) and by the plerocercoid stage of *Diphyllobothrium* species using man as a second intermediate host (sparganosis). The main features of the tapeworms are given in Tables 23.1–23.3).

Table 23.3 Larval tapeworm infections in man.

Adult	Egg	Definitive host	First larval stage	First intermediate host	Geographical distribution	Clinical features in man
Echinococcus granulosus granulosus 3–8.5 × 0.3 mm	Spherical 32–28 × 21–30 μm	Dog	Unilocular hydatid cyst	Man, sheep, buffalo, camel	South Australia, New Zealand, East Africa (Turkana), North and South Africa, Middle East, Mongolia, north China, Vietnam	Unilocular hydatid cyst in liver, lungs and brain
Echinococcus granulosus canadensis	Spherical 32–28 × 21–30 μm	Wolf	Unilocular hydatid cyst	Moose, deer, man	North America	Generally more benign
Echinococcus multilocularis	Spherical 32–28 × 21–30 μm	Arctic fox, wolves and sledge dogs	Multilocular (alveolar) hydatid cyst	Tundra vole, field mice, ground squirrel, shrews	High latitudes of North America, Alaska and USSR	Multilocular hydatid cyst spreading cancerous type of cyst
		Red fox, dog, cat	Multilocular (alveolar) hydatid cyst	Field mouse		
Echinococcus vogeli (*oligarthrus*)	Spherical 32–28 × 21–30 μm	Bush dog	Polycystic hydatid cyst	Paca and spiny rat	Panama, Colombia, Ecuador	Polycystic hydatid cyst. Proliferation externally forming small separate cysts
Smaller, 1.5–4 × 0.15 mm	Spherical 32–28 × 21–30 μm					
Multiceps (*Taenia*) *multiceps* 50 cm long	33 μm in diameter	Dog	Coenurus cerebralis (bladder-worm)	Sheep, cattle, goats, horses	Northern hemisphere and North Africa	Coenurus cerebralis cyst in brain (staggers in sheep)
Multiceps (*Taenia*) *brauni* (tropical tapeworm) 50 cm long	33 μm in diameter	Dog, fox, genet and jackal	Coenurus cerebralis	Swamp rat, porcupine and gerbil	Central and East Africa	Coenurus cerebralis cysts in brain and eye

TAENIA SAGINATA (BEEF TAPEWORM, UNARMED TAPEWORM)

GEOGRAPHICAL DISTRIBUTION

T. saginata has a worldwide distribution where beef is eaten undercooked or raw. It is especially common in Ethiopia and East Africa where the occurrence of 'measly' beef containing cysticerci renders much of the meat unsuitable for export markets.

AETIOLOGY

T. saginata (Fig. 23.1) is a white semitransparent

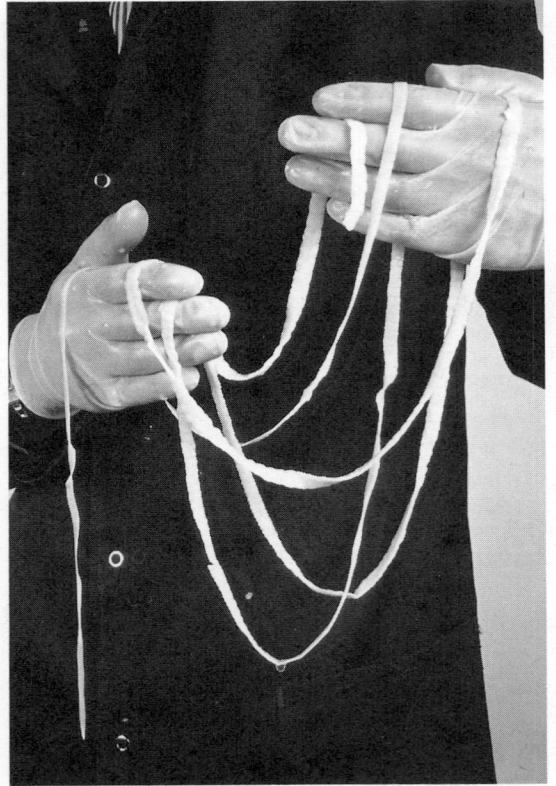

Fig. 23.1 Adult beef tapeworm (*T. saginata*). (Courtesy Professor G. S. Nelson.)

worm measuring 4–10 metres long which when fully adult may contain 2000 segments. The head (scolex) (Figs. 23.2, 23.3D) is 1–2 mm in diameter with four lateral suckers but no rostellum or hooks (unarmed tapeworm). The segments (proglottides) contain a uterus with 20–25 lateral segments which ramify (Fig. 23.4B) but no accessory ovary and 300–400 testes (twice the number found in *T. solium*). (Self-fertilization occurs and eggs are formed containing an *oncosphere* or young cysticercus. The egg is globular, 30–40 × 20–30 μm (Figs. 23.5, 23.6A and Plate III.17) and has an outer shell enclosing the chorionic and two oncospheric membranes (the embryophorous membrane inside the shell is acid fast which distinguishes the egg from that of *T. solium*).[1] Each segment when mature contains about 100 000 eggs and there may be 2000 segments with a total annual output of around 600

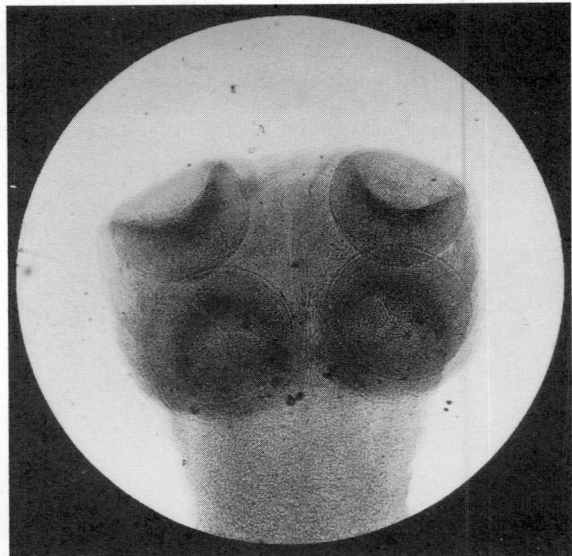

Fig. 23.2 *T. saginata* (unarmed tapeworm) scolex. Suckers without hooklets. (Courtesy WTIM.)

Fig. 23.3 Heads of human cestodes, showing suckers and, when present, the arrangement of the hooklets. A, *Hymenolepis nana.*
B, *Dipylidium caninum.* C, *Taenia solium.* D, *Taenia saginata.*

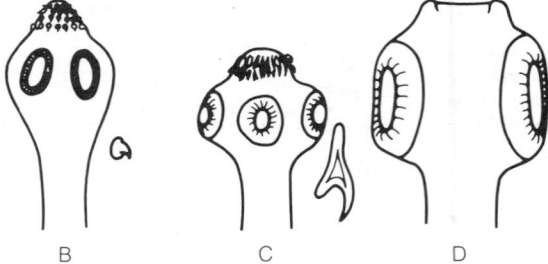

A   B   C   D

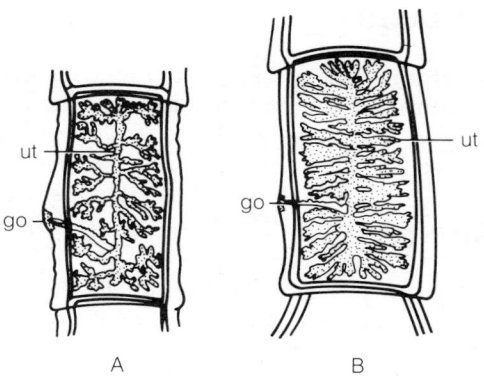

Fig. 23.4 Segments of tapeworms, showing the charac-teristic branching of the uterus as seen in the mature segments. A, *T. solium*. B, *T. saginata*. ut, Uterus; go, genital opening.

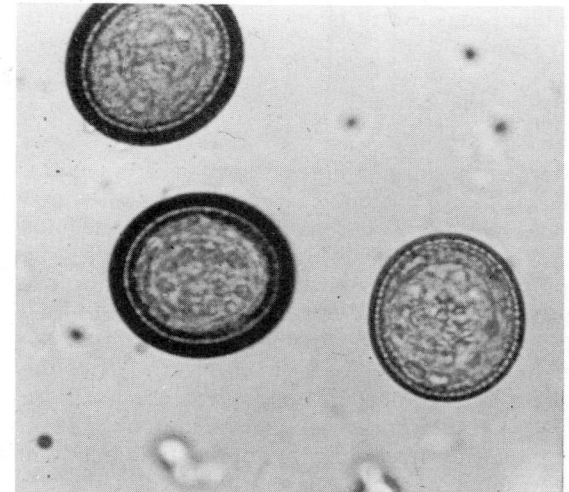

Fig. 23.5 *Taenia* ova. (Courtesy WTIM.)

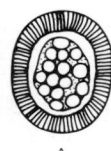

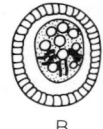

A   B

Fig. 23.6 Eggs of *T. saginata* (A) and *T. solium* (B) showing hooklets.

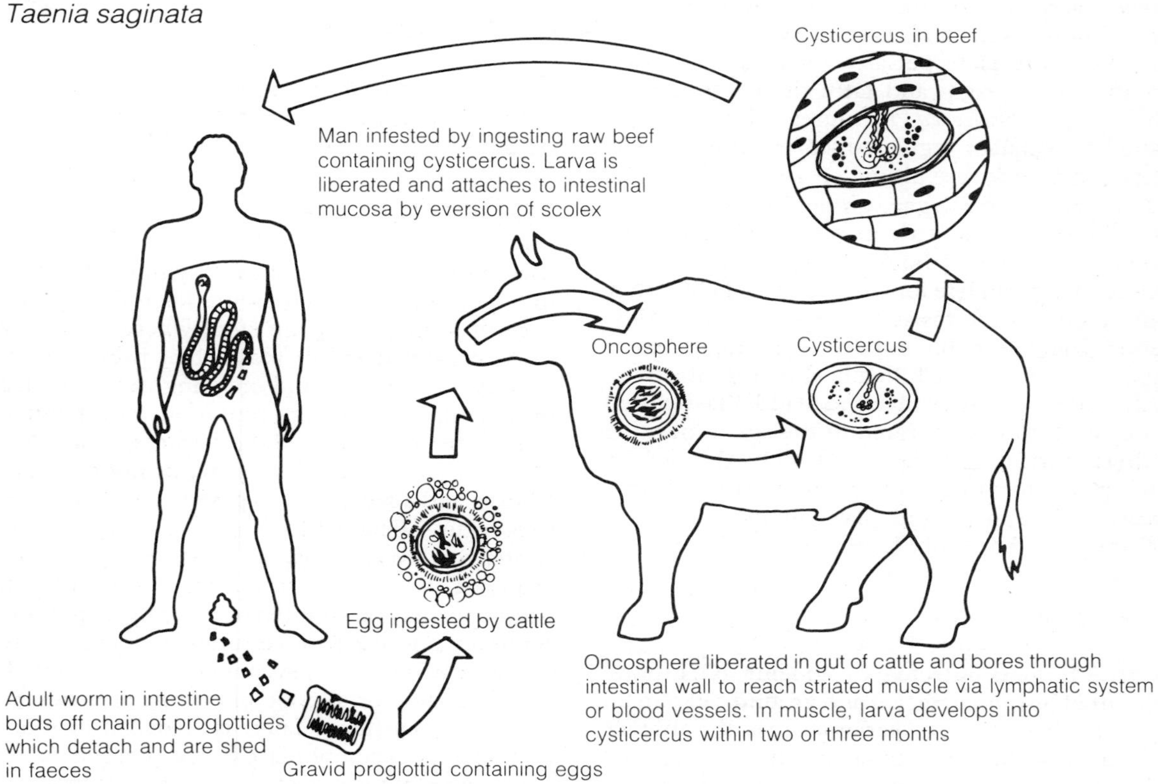

Taenia saginata

Cysticercus in beef

Man infested by ingesting raw beef containing cysticercus. Larva is liberated and attaches to intestinal mucosa by eversion of scolex

Oncosphere

Cysticercus

Egg ingested by cattle

Oncosphere liberated in gut of cattle and bores through intestinal wall to reach striated muscle via lymphatic system or blood vessels. In muscle, larva develops into cysticercus within two or three months

Adult worm in intestine buds off chain of proglottides which detach and are shed in faeces

Gravid proglottid containing eggs

Fig. 23.7 Life-cycle of *T. saginata*. (Courtesy WTIM.)

million eggs. Adult tapeworms can live for up to 25 years.

Life-cycle (Fig. 23.7)

Man is the only *definitive* host of *T. saginata*. The eggs are passed in an intact segment which can move on its own, may crawl out of the anus and move down the leg. When they reach the ground the segments disintegrate releasing the eggs which can live for eight weeks before they are eaten by the intermediate host. Cattle are the main *intermediate* hosts but in North Africa the camel is an important host and in the northern USSR the reindeer.[2] In Africa unhooked (? *T. saginata*) cysticerci can be found sporadically in wild ungulates[3] and there are records from zoo animals[4] and wild goats in Taiwan.[5] A few cases of *T. saginata* cysticercosis in man have been reported but their identification is questionable.

Cysticercal stage (cysticercus bovis)

On ingestion by the intermediate host the *oncosphere* is released in the small intestine, burrows through the wall and is carried by the circulation to the muscles, especially those of the jaws, tongue, diaphragm and fatty tissues round the heart. The *cysticercus* measures $7.5–9 \times 5.5$ mm and has a small unvaginated scolex without hooklets and a neck resembling an adult taenia. The different cestode larvae can be distinguished by variations in these structures especially the presence or absence of hooklets (absent in *T. saginata*). They can live for eight months before they are eaten and can resist temperatures up to $48°C$ and refrigeration, but not deep freezing, for more than three weeks. (Chilled beef is still infective.) After being eaten by man the bladder is digested and the scolex is liberated in the small intestine where it attaches itself to the wall by the suckers and grows to adulthood. (For the distinguishing features of cysticercoid larvae found in man see Table II.6, Appendix II, p. 1343.)

TRANSMISSION

Cattle become infected by grazing on ground polluted by human faeces and ground can remain infected from up to a year or more in the absence of human pollution. Human infection is acquired by eating raw or undercooked 'measly' beef containing the cysticerci.

PATHOLOGY

Apart from slight erosion of the mucous membrane at the site of attachment there is no pathology.

IMMUNITY

There is no protective immunity in the adult stage and multiple infections and reinfections are common. No humoral antibodies develop.

CLINICAL FEATURES

Natural history

Most cases are asymptomatic and the infection is only noticed when segments are seen in the stools. There is no rejection by the host and *T. saginata* can remain in the small intestine causing little or no harm for up to 25 years.

Incubation period

From the time of infection to the passage of segments the incubation period is five to 12 weeks.

Symptoms and signs

Most tapeworm infections are symptomless and the commonest way of presentation is the appearance of segments in the stool where they may cause consternation or make their presence felt by leaving the anus and crawling down the leg producing a tickling sensation. Abdominal symptoms can occur and the commonest are epigastric or umbilical pain, often like hunger pain. Nausea and a feeling of epigastric distension can also occur. Weight loss is rare and can be correlated with a decrease in appetite. Symptoms of peptic ulcer or gallstones may be simulated. Segments may be vomited or enter the appendix, common bile duct or respiratory tract. There may be considerable psychological reaction with severe anxiety or allergic phenomena, urticaria, pruritus and asthma. There is no malabsorption. A moderate eosinophilia may be present in the early stages but is not a feature of the established disease.

DIAGNOSIS

Almost any abdominal condition may be mimicked by a tapeworm. The diagnosis is made by finding eggs or segments in the stool. *Segments* are most commonly found and may not be evident unless the stool is carefully examined with the naked eye (Appendix IV, p. 1492). A purge will often produce segments. Identification from *T. solium* is by the uterine pattern (Fig. 23.4A). The egg (Figs. 23.5 and 23.6A) can be distinguished from that of *T. solium* by the acid-fast shell.

TREATMENT

See section on *T. solium*, below.

PREVENTION

All beef or other meat should be inspected for cysticerci and, if these are present, boiled before consumption. Adequate cooking ensures protection and the critical temperature is 56°C. Insufficiently defrosted hamburgers are a common source of infection and chilled beef is not safe—only deep freezing for three to four weeks is safe.

TAENIA SOLIUM (PORK TAPEWORM, ARMED TAPEWORM)

GEOGRAPHICAL DISTRIBUTION

T. solium has a cosmopolitan distribution and is common wherever pork or ham is eaten raw. It is most common among Slavic peoples and in Mexico, other Latin American countries, Manchuria and India. Recently it has become common in Irian Jaya (West New Guinea) following its introduction to the native pig.[6]

AETIOLOGY

T. solium has a length of 2–3 metres with 800–1000 segments. The head is globular, quad-rangular, 1 mm in diameter with a short pigmented rostellum and a double row of 20–50 hooklets (Figs. 23.3C and 23.8) (armed tapeworm). The mature segments measure 12×6 mm and contain a uterus with seven to 10 stout branches (Fig. 23.4A). Each gravid segment contains 30 000–50 000 eggs. The *egg* (Fig. 23.9 and Plate III.16) measures 31–56 μm, is double-shelled (not acid fast in contrast to *T. saginata*) and contains hooklets. Eggs can be found in the stools since some segments disintegrate in the intestine. The egg contains a hooked *oncosphere* (Fig. 23.9).

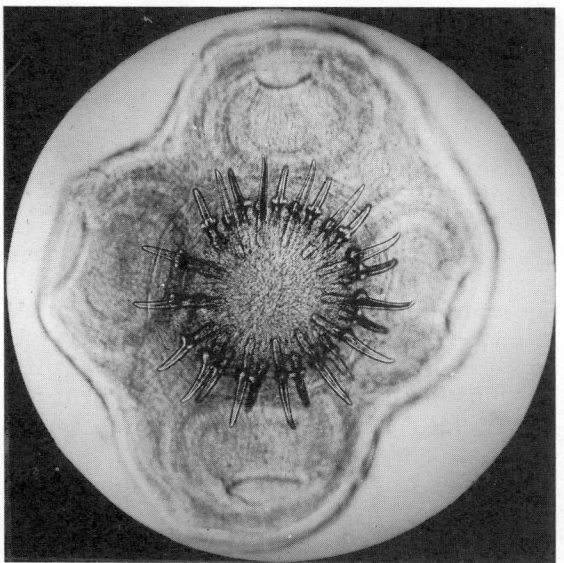

Fig. 23.8 *T. solium* (pig tapeworm) (armed tapeworm). Scolex showing hooklets. (Courtesy WTIM.)

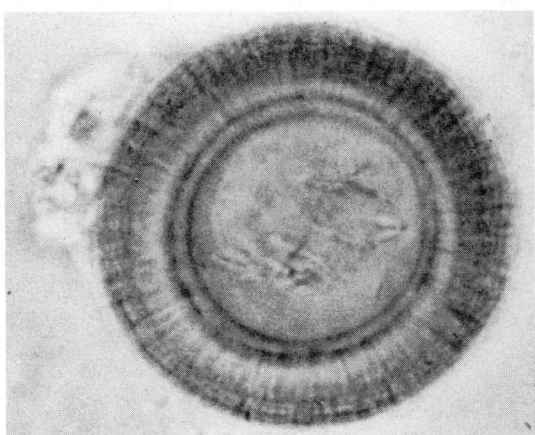

Fig. 23.9 *T. solium*. Ovum showing hooklets in oncosphere.

LIFE-CYCLE (Fig. 23.10)

This is similar to that of *T. saginata*. The eggs are passed out in the faeces and eaten by a pig, the

Taenia solium

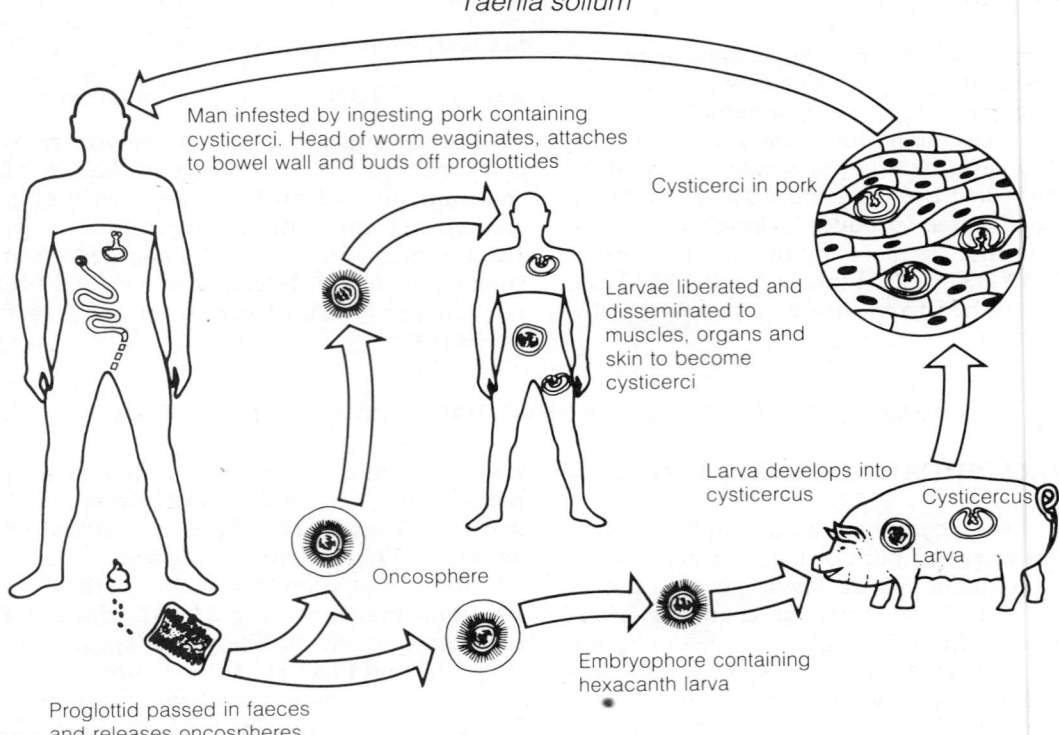

Man infested by ingesting pork containing cysticerci. Head of worm evaginates, attaches to bowel wall and buds off proglottides

Cysticerci in pork

Larvae liberated and disseminated to muscles, organs and skin to become cysticerci

Larva develops into cysticercus

Cysticercus

Larva

Oncosphere

Embryophore containing hexacanth larva

Proglottid passed in faeces and releases oncospheres

Fig. 23.10 Life-cycle of *T. solium*. (Courtesy WTIM.)

usual intermediate host, in which the cysticerci develop as in *T. saginata*, to form cysticercus cellulosae (4–6 × 7.5–10 mm). Infected pork is known as 'measly' pork. Man can also be an intermediate host as can macaque monkeys, sheep and dogs, from autoinfection. After digestion of the shell in the gastric juice the oncosphere penetrates the intestinal wall, enters the bloodstream and settles in the muscles, especially the heart. After eating the measly pork the bladder of the cysticercus is digested in the stomach and the scolex evaginates and attaches itself to the intestinal wall.

TRANSMISSION

Infection with the adult worm is acquired from eating uncooked pork or ham.

PATHOLOGY

The adult *T. solium* causes little pathology in the bowel.

CLINICAL FEATURES

The clinical features are similar to those of *T. saginata*.

DIAGNOSIS

The differentiation between *T. solium* and *T. saginata* is made by examination of the egg, segments and scolex. The embryophorous membrane inside the shell of the egg of *T. solium* is not acid fast and the uterus in the segment has seven to 10 branches in *T. solium* (Fig. 23.4A) as opposed to 20–35 in *T. saginata* (Fig. 23.4B). Examination of the scolex after treatment will show the armed rostellum in the case of *T. solium* (Figs. 23.7 and 23.8).

TREATMENT

The drug of choice is praziquantel, in a single oral dose of 10 mg/kg.[7] Other drugs which have been used are *niclosamide* (Yomesan) taken in tablet form, each of 500 mg, four tablets in two (1 g) doses at an interval of one hour. The tablets should be chewed. *Dichlorophen* has been used, 3–6 g before breakfast. Evidence of previous tapeworm infection was found in 26% of cases of cysticercosis[8] but the cysticercosis probably resulted from autoinfection by contamination of food with faecally contaminated fingers. There is no evidence of internal autoinfection, and this has never been shown to follow treatment with taenicidal drugs.

HYMENOLEPIS NANA (DWARF TAPEWORM)

GEOGRAPHICAL DISTRIBUTION

H. nana is found in warm countries, Egypt, Sudan, Thailand, India, Japan, South America (Brazil, Argentine and especially Cuba) and south Europe (Portugal, Spain and Sicily, where it affects 10% of the children).

AETIOLOGY

H. nana is 25–45 mm long by 0.5–0.9 mm and has 100–200 proglottides (Fig. 23.11). The scolex

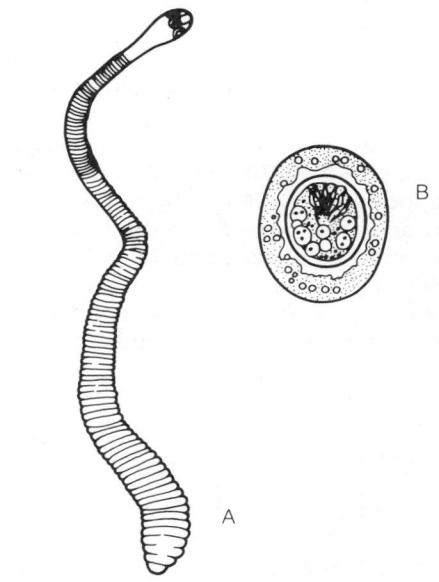

Fig. 23.12 *H. nana* (dwarf tapeworm). Magnified. A, adult. B, egg.

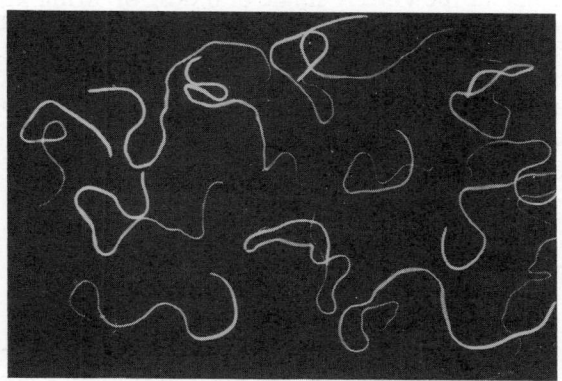

Fig. 23.11 *H. nana* (dwarf tapeworm). (Courtesy WTIM.)

measures 139–480 μm, is subglobular with a well-developed rostellum, a single crown with 20–30 hooklets (14–18 μm) and four globular suckers (80–150 μm) (Fig. 23.3A). The neck is long, the proglottides short anteriorly, but the posterior ones increase in size and are broader than they are long (Fig. 23.12). The genital pores are marginal and placed near the anterior border. There are three testes. The vas deferens widens into the seminal vesicle and the gravid uterus occupies an entire segment.

The egg is oval and globular and there are 80–180 in each segment. It has two membranes, a

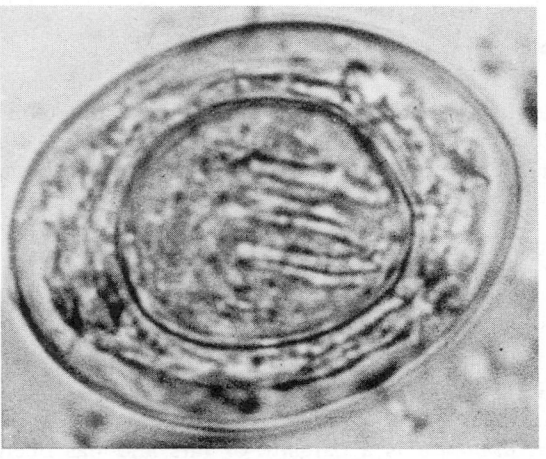

Fig. 23.13 *Hymenolepis nana* (dwarf tapeworm). Ovum. (Courtesy WTIM.)

thin outer vitelline membrane 40–60 μm separated from an inner one, 20–30 μm, by an area
containing radial filaments (Figs. 23.12 and
23.13). There is a conspicuous mamillate projection at each pole enclosing an oncosphere with
three pairs of hooklets.

The segments, when freed, are partially
digested and the eggs, set free in the faeces, are
easily detected.

Life-cycle (Fig. II.32, p. 1345)

Man is the only definitive host and this worm
forms an exception to other members of the
group in that it has no intermediate host; the
larva enters the villus of the intestine to become
a cysticercoid. In 40–70 hours after infection the
scolex appears; in 80–90 hours the rostellum has
hooklets and then passes into the lumen of the
intestine attached to the epithelium of the villus
by a short neck. The rapidity of development
varies greatly. Strobilization is rapid; the proglottides mature in 10–12 days and after 30 days
eggs appear in the faeces.

TRANSMISSION

Humans are the natural reservoir and infection
is direct from human to human by faecal-oral
infection. Transmission by fomites is of less
importance. The larvae of fleas and grain beetles
can become infected and develop cysticercoids
in the haemocoele but insects are of little importance in transmission to humans.

PATHOLOGY

Light infections cause no significant damage but
very heavy infections (over 1000 worms plus) are
not uncommon in children and cause symptoms.

CLINICAL FEATURES

General symptoms, headache, weakness, dizziness and weight loss and abdominal symptoms
of epigastric pain, nausea, diarrhoea with anal
pruritus and urticaria have all been associated
with heavy infections. A moderate eosinophilia
is present.

DIAGNOSIS

Eggs (Fig. 23.13) and not segments are passed
in the stools. Several negative stool results are
necessary to rule out infection.

TREATMENT

Praziquantel is the drug of choice since it acts
against both the adult worms and the cysticercoids in the villi. A single oral dose of 30 mg/kg
cured 27/30 cases while 40 mg/kg cured all.[9]
Niclosamide has been used: adults, 2 g daily for 7
days; children, up to 34 kg, 1 g on the first day
then 0.5 g for 6 days; over 34 kg, 1.5 g on the first
day and then 1 g daily for 6 days.

EPIDEMIOLOGY AND CONTROL

Overcrowding and poor personal and environmental hygiene are responsible for a high incidence of infection. Prevalence rates of 10% are
common. It is a familial and institutional infection. *Control* depends on improved personal and
environmental hygiene allied to mass chemotherapy in institutions.

HYMENOLEPIS DIMINUTA (RAT TAPEWORM)

GEOGRAPHICAL DISTRIBUTION

H. diminuta is a parasite of rats and has been
found in man in Italy, Zaire, South America and
the Caribbean.

AETIOLOGY

The adult worm measures 20–60 × 3.5 mm. The
head is small and cuboidal with a rudimentary
rostellum with four small suckers without hook-

lets (in contrast to *H. nana*). The egg is circular or ovoid and measures 60–80 μm in diameter and a thin, yellowish outer membrane is separated from the inner embryonic envelope by a clear area containing only indistinct radiations (in contrast to *H. nana*) (Fig. 23.14). The gravid segments disintegrate in the bowel and discharge eggs in the faeces.

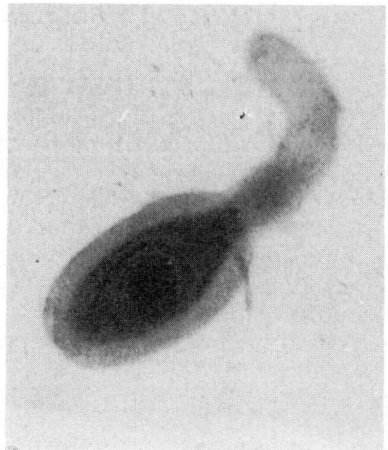

Fig. 23.15 *H. diminuta* (rat tapeworm). Cysticercoid larva from insect intermediate host. (Courtesy Dr H. Zaiman.)

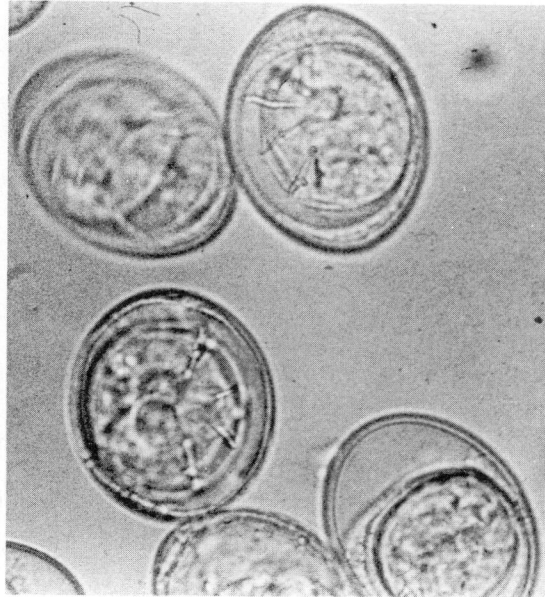

Fig. 23.14 *H. diminuta* (rat tapeworm). Ova. (Courtesy Dr H. Zaiman.)

Life-cycle (Fig. II.33, p. 1346)

The adult worm lives in the small intestine of the rat which is the definitive host. The obligatory intermediate hosts are the larvae of fleas and grain beetles in which the cysticercus develops in the body cavity (haemocoele (Fig. 23.15)). The fleas and beetles are then infective to the rat when eaten. (See also Appendix II, p. 1345.)

TRANSMISSION

Transmission to man is accidental by the consumption of mealworms or grain beetles in dried grains or fruit.

PATHOLOGY

The adult worms are attached to the duodenal or jejunal mucosa and multiple infections are common.

CLINICAL FEATURES

Children are mainly affected. Almost all infections are asymptomatic but mild gastrointestinal symptoms and eosinophilia have been noted.

DIAGNOSIS

The diagnosis is made by finding eggs in the stool which differ from those of *H. nana* in that the space between the outer and inner membranes is only faintly striated.

TREATMENT

The treatment is the same as for *H. nana*: praziquantel in a single oral dose of 30 mg/kg. Niclosamide has also been used.

DIPHYLLOBOTHRIUM LATUM (FISH TAPEWORM)

GEOGRAPHICAL DISTRIBUTION

D. latum is found in Europe in northern Italy, Switzerland, parts of Germany, the Baltic and Scandinavia, from where it has largely disappeared as a result of health education. It is also found in Roumania, the Danube Delta, Israel, Siberia, northern Manchuria (*D. minus*) and Japan. In North America there are foci in the lake region of Minnesota and Michigan and it is common in eastern Canada and among Canadian and Alaskan Eskimos (*D. alascense*). In South America, in Peru, Chile and Argentina a related species, *D. pacificum*, is responsible for the infection. *Diphyllobothrium* has also been found in Australia and possibly East Africa, Botswana, Angola and Papua New Guinea.

AETIOLOGY

The *adult* is a long, fleshy worm up to 3–10 metres in length in the small intestine (Fig. 23.16). The scolex, 3 mm in diameter, has no rostellum or hooklets but two slit longitudinal grooves like suckers (bothria) (Fig. 23.17). There is a thin neck followed by 3000–4000 segments (Fig. 23.18) which become broader as they mature, a single worm discharging as many as 36 000 to one million eggs daily. Infections are often multiple, the number corresponding to the number of individual plerocercoids swallowed. The *egg* (Fig. 23.19) is operculated with a brown shell $70 \times 45\,\mu$m. Eggs are discharged into the faeces in the intestine in large numbers.

Life-cycle (Fig. 23.20)

Diphyllobothrium species differ from *Taenia* in that two intermediate hosts, a crustacean and a freshwater fish, are required for completion of the life history. The egg is passed into water where the operculum is detached and a ciliated

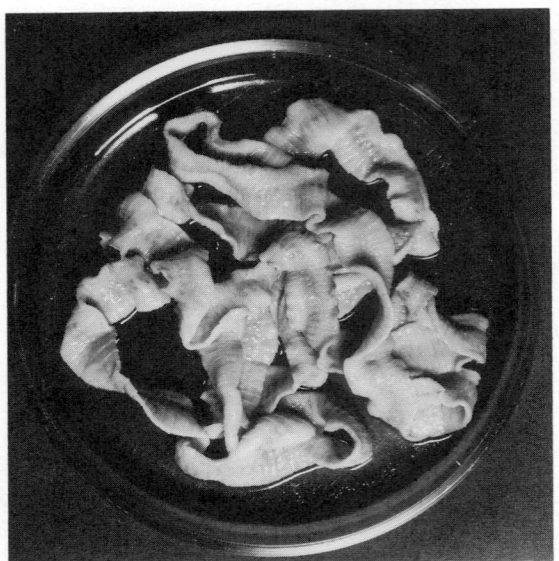

Fig. 23.16 *D. latum* (fish tapeworm). Adult. (Courtesy WTIM.)

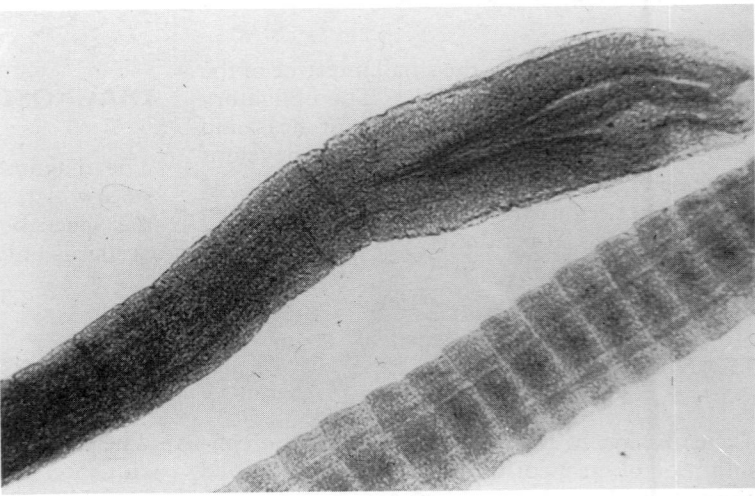

Fig. 23.17 *D. latum* (fish tapeworm). Scolex without suckers or hooks but two grooves (bothria) which attach to the mucosa. (Courtesy WTIM.).

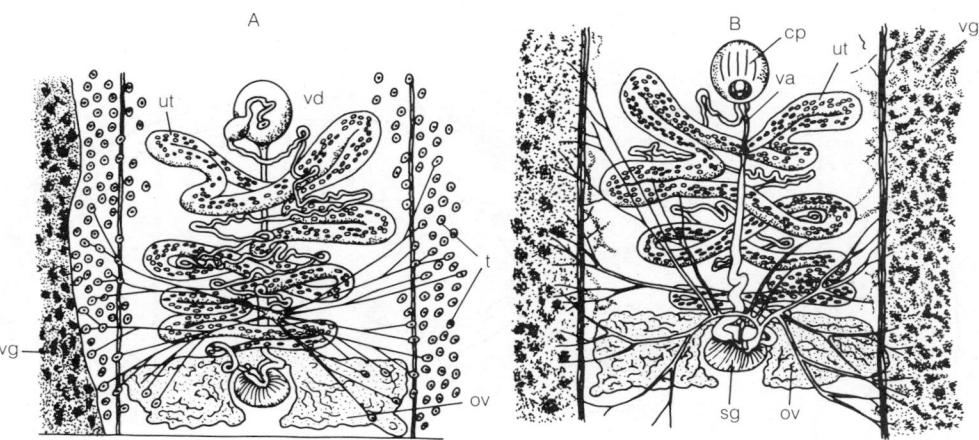

Fig. 23.18 Mature segment of *D. latum*. A, Dorsal or male aspect. B, Ventral or female aspect. t, Testes; vd, vas deferens; vg, vitelline glands; cp, cirrus pouch; ov, ovary; sg, shell gland; ut, uterus; va, vagina.

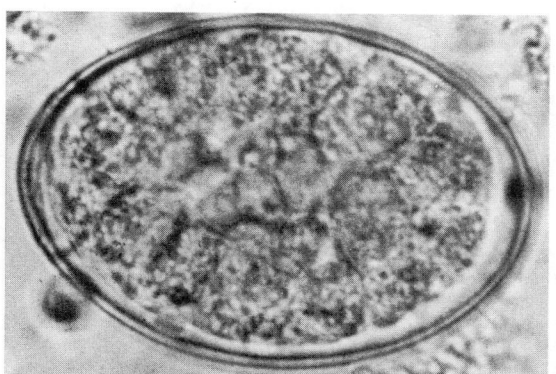

Fig. 23.19 *D. latum* (fish tapeworm). Ovum. (Courtesy Dr D.S. Ridley.)

when ingested by man the plerocercoid develops into an adult diphyllobothrium in five to six weeks. Kippering and ordinary smoking do not destroy the plerocercoids but brine soaking does. Adult worms can live for 29 years but may be discharged spontaneously before this.

TRANSMISSION

Man is infected by eating raw fish or roe and although many fish-eating mammals carry the infection, man is himself responsible for propagation of infection in most endemic areas.

six-hooked *coracidium* 20–30 μm in size emerges and swims by means of its cilia. It dies in 24 hours, unless it is swallowed by freshwater crustacea of certain species (cyclops). In the cyclops the outer layer is digested and the hooks tear a hole in the gut wall passing into the body cavity sometimes killing the cyclops in the process. Lying outside the gut wall it becomes a *procercoid* larva which is ovoid, 50–60 μm long, with a terminal spherical appendage and a terminal appendage at the other end containing six hooklets. Up to two may be found in one cyclops.

The cyclops is swallowed by freshwater fish of certain species (Table 23.2) and reaching the stomach the procercoid penetrates to the body cavity where it encysts as a *plerocercoid* or *sparganum*. Here sucking grooves are developed and

PATHOLOGY

The adult worm lives in the small intestine where it causes little or no trouble in the majority of cases. In some cases it absorbs so much vitamin B_{12} that the host becomes deficient with megaloblastic haemopoiesis and even anaemia. This only occurs in Finland where 9% of carriers had megaloblastic haemopoiesis but only 2% anaemia.[10] Elsewhere in the world there is no anaemia since the strains do not take up vitamin B_{12}. Although all infections show a low serum B_{12} only a few develop anaemia because it is thought that the site of the adult tapeworm, the presence of atrophic gastritis or the presence of blocking antibodies to intrinsic factor are the important factors.

Diphyllobothrium latum

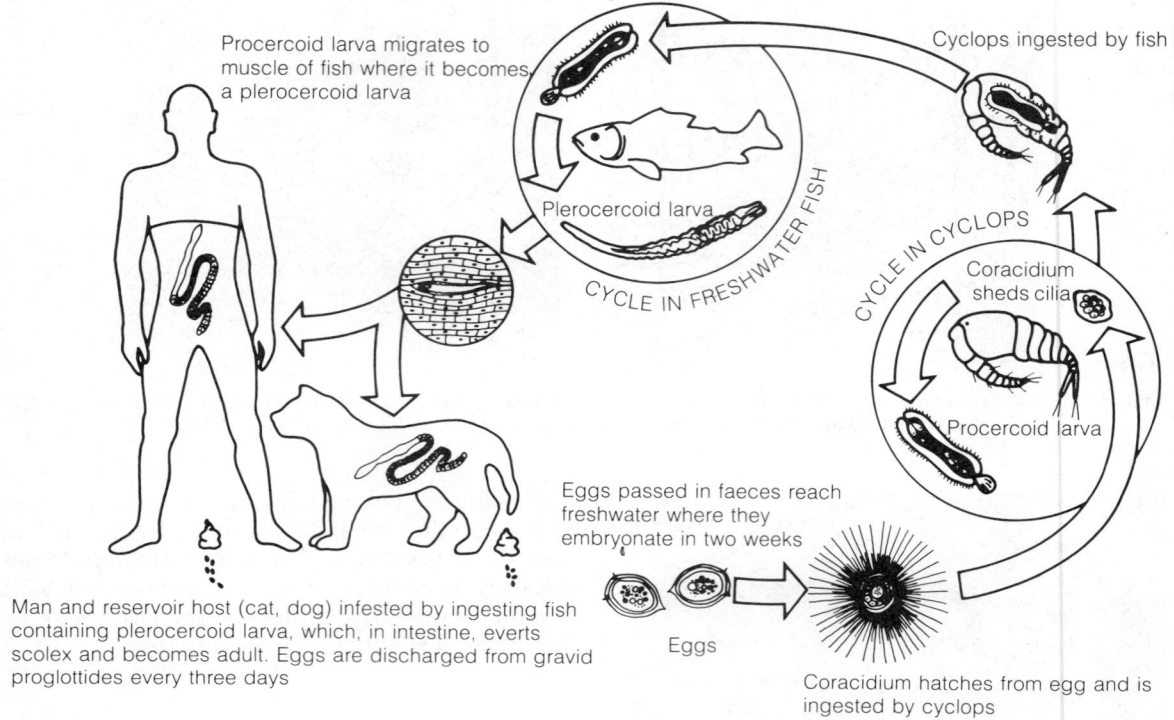

Procercoid larva migrates to muscle of fish where it becomes a plerocercoid larva

Cyclops ingested by fish

Plerocercoid larva

CYCLE IN FRESHWATER FISH

CYCLE IN CYCLOPS

Coracidium sheds cilia

Procercoid larva

Eggs passed in faeces reach freshwater where they embryonate in two weeks

Eggs

Man and reservoir host (cat, dog) infested by ingesting fish containing plerocercoid larva, which, in intestine, everts scolex and becomes adult. Eggs are discharged from gravid proglottides every three days

Coracidium hatches from egg and is ingested by cyclops

Fig. 23.20 Life-cycle of *D. latum*. (Courtesy WTIM.)

CLINICAL FEATURES

In most cases there are no symptoms or signs other than a peripheral eosinophilia. If there are many worms they may obstruct the intestine. Where there is a megaloblastic anaemia cord changes may develop.

DIAGNOSIS

Numerous eggs (Fig. 23.19) are found in the stools.

TREATMENT

Praziquantel is the treatment of choice but 25 mg/kg is necessary for cure.[11] Niclosamide and dichlorophen can also be used.

EPIDEMIOLOGY

Although humans are the main definitive host many fish-eating mammals such as fox, mink, bear, dog, domestic and wild cats, walrus and seal are also hosts. Secondary intermediate hosts are freshwater fish and fish that spawn in fresh water (salmonids). Marine fish may be implicated in South America. While health education has reduced infection in Scandinavia almost to vanishing point, elsewhere spread of the infection has been encouraged by emigration, construction of dams and pollution of lakes with sewage. The habit of tasting raw fish before cooking is responsible for higher rates in women.

CONTROL

Health education regarding eating raw fish and raw roe can control the infection.

DIPYLIDIUM CANINUM (DOG TAPEWORM)

This is a common parasite of the dog, cat and jackal.

GEOGRAPHICAL DISTRIBUTION

D. caninum is found in Europe.

AETIOLOGY

The adult worm measures 15–40 cm × 2–3 mm (Fig. 23.21). The scolex is small and globular,

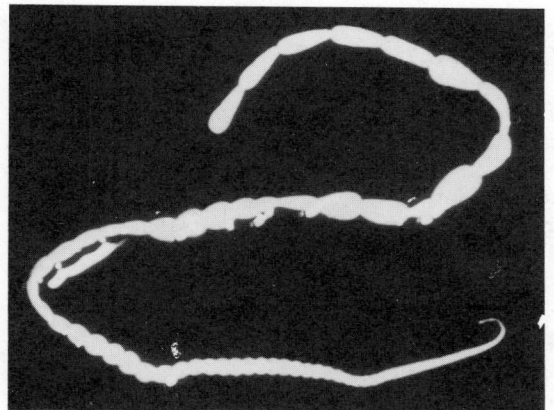

Fig. 23.21 *Dipylidium caninum* (dog tapeworm). Adult. (Courtesy WTIM.)

0.5 mm in diameter with a rostellum retracted into the infundibulum possessing three to four circles of 28–30 hooklets (14–18 μm) in size resembling 'rose thorns' and four elliptical

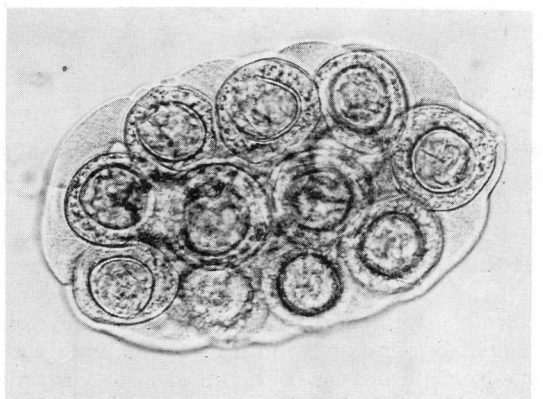

Fig. 23.22 Egg packet of *Dipylidium caninum*. (Courtesy Dr D. S. Ridley.)

suckers (Fig. 23.3D). There are 200 or more segments each measuring 6–7 × 2–3 mm, with two genital pores and containing a number of egg packets containing eight to 15 eggs (Fig. 23.22). The segments leave the intestine intact to discharge eggs on the ground outside the body. The *egg* is round 30–40 μm in diameter (Fig. 23.23).

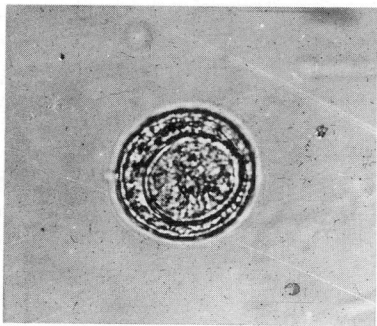

Fig. 23.23 Egg of *Dipylidium caninum*.

Life-cycle

The eggs are ingested by larval lice and fleas: the dog louse (*Trichodectes canis*), the dog flea (*Ctenocephalides canis*), the cat flea (*C. felis*) and the human flea (*Pulex irritans*). The *procercoid* and *cysticercoid* stages are passed in the adipose tissue and muscles of the larvae. The adult fleas are then swallowed by the dog.

TRANSMISSION

Infection of man is accidental due to swallowing adult fleas or the result of a dog licking the face of a child and transferring crushed fleas.

CLINICAL FEATURES

Most cases are asymptomatic but abdominal pain, diarrhoea, irritability and anal pruritus have all been ascribed to infection. Urticaria and eosinophilia are also features.

DIAGNOSIS

Eggs are difficult to find in the stools since segments are passed intact to the outside.

TREATMENT

Praziquantel, as for the other tapeworms, is the treatment of choice.

EPIDEMIOLOGY AND CONTROL

Children are mainly affected due to their close contact with pets. Control may be achieved by keeping pets dewormed and clear of ecto-parasites.

OTHER TAPEWORM INFECTIONS

RAILLIETINA CELEBENSIS AND *R. MADAGASCARIENSIS*

These are tapeworms normally found in birds and, rarely, rats. The intermediate hosts are flies. The adult rostellum is characterized by numerous hooklets of 'coal hammer' shape. Cases of human infection have been found in Celebes, Thailand, Guyana, Mauritius and Taiwan.

BERTIELLA

Infection with tapeworms of the *Bertiella* genus has been reported in man. Normally a parasite of monkeys, *B. mucronata* has been reported from man in Paraguay.[12]

INERMICAPSIFER

These tapeworms closely resemble *Bertiella* but can be distinguished by the absence of hooklets. No fewer than 12 species are parasites of hyraxes and rodents in Africa. Human infection is commoner than supposed, *I. cubensis* being common in Cuba.

LARVAL TAENIASIS

Cysticercosis (Cysticercoid stage of *T. solium*)

GEOGRAPHICAL DISTRIBUTION

Cysticercosis is endemic on all continents except Australia. It is far more prevalent than suspected and the arrival of simple diagnostic tests may show a higher prevalence than has been thought up till now. It is prevalent wherever pigs are extensively raised. In Europe cysticercosis is now uncommon except in countries of the Eastern bloc. In Asia it has a focal distribution, while in Irian Jaya (West New Guinea) there is now a high incidence due to recent infection of the pigs with *T. solium* and the extensive pig culture of the inhabitants. In the American continent it is heavily endemic in Mexico and other South American countries.

AETIOLOGY

Cysticercosis is caused by infection with the larval stage (cysticercus) of *T. solium* (Fig. 23.24).

TRANSMISSION

Man is the only known definitive host and pig and man the only intermediate hosts of *T. solium*. Human infection is acquired from ingestion of *T. solium* eggs which must come from a human source.

Heteroinfection

Person-to-person infection occurs from ingestion of food or water contaminated by another person.

Autoinfection

External autoinfection occurs from transmission of eggs from anus to mouth by inadequate personal hygiene and care of hands after defecation. Internal autoinfection is a theoretical possibility which results when eggs are carried back from the small intestine to the duodenum or stomach

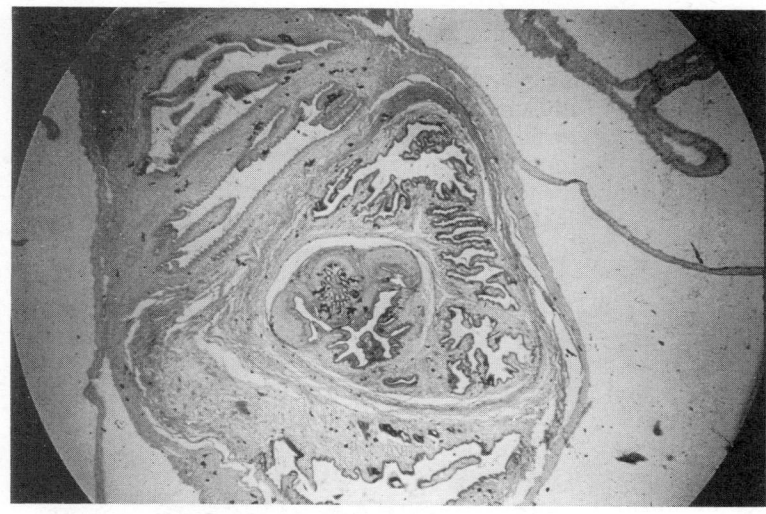

Fig. 23.24 Cysticercus in the brain. (Courtesy WTIM.)

where the oncosphere hatches, migrates to the body tissues and encysts. It has never been proven to occur.

PATHOLOGY

Whether ingested or regurgitated from the small intestine the shells of the ova disintegrate within 24–72 hours and the emergent oncospheres penetrate through the intestinal wall, either by their hooklets or possibly by lytic secretions, into the mesenteric vessels and are carried throughout the body typically filtering out between the muscles where in the course of 60–70 days they change into cysticerci. Cysticerci have been found in nearly every organ and tissue of the body, most commonly in the subcutaneous tissues and muscles of the tongue, neck or ribs, next in the eye and then in the brain, where they may develop in the ventricles or as cyst capsules on the surface of the brain. Less commonly they are found in the heart, liver, lungs and abdominal cavity. Except in the eye viable cysts induce a granulomatous reaction, the cysticercus being surrounded by a fibrous capsule surrounded by neutrophils and eosinophils and later lymphocytes, plasma cells and giant cells. Dying cysts provoke acute inflammation associated with tissue damage. Contrary to previous thinking, live as well as dead cysts, cause pathology.

Recent observations on the timing of the onset of epilepsy after infection suggest that disturbance is caused in the brain by fresh, live cysticerci, which have been recovered in autopsies from such cases.[6] In the brain where the cysts may be parenchymal, meningeal or ventricular, the cysticercus is surrounded by a wall of neuroglia which later undergoes degenerative changes and which is visible as a discoloured ring which is walled off from the normal brain by a ring of neuroglia (Fig. 23.24). After a variable period the parasite dies and becomes calcified, which may not affect the cyst capsule and its contents. However, the cyst wall may collapse and be flattened out by pressure of the surrounding tissues and calcify in a spindle shape. This does not happen in the brain. There is a lapse of three years between death of the cysticerci and calcification in the tissues but in the brain this process takes longer.

IMMUNITY

There is some evidence of protective immunity and immunization has been attempted in cattle against *cysticercus bovis*. There is an antigen present in the activated embryo (oncosphere) which acts against the larval cysts in the tissues.[13]

CLINICAL FEATURES

Natural history

Unless the cysticercus invades the brain infection is usually benign and cysts may be present in large numbers in the body without the patient's knowledge. The cysts may remain viable for many years or calcify when any symptoms present may subside. If the brain is affected (cerebral cysticercosis) then epilepsy and other more serious consequences may result.

Incubation period

Symptoms of cysticercosis may develop 60–70 days after infection.

Symptoms and signs

These depend on the number and site of the cysticerci. The *onset* is usually unnoticed, the invasion of oncospheres giving rise to no general reaction, but the patient may notice the appearance of small subcutaneous nodules or intramuscular swellings.

Cerebral cysticercosis (neurocysticercosis)

Cysticerci may invade the brain but symptoms are only found in half of the affected people.

EPILEPSY
The commonest manifestation of cerebral cysticercosis is epilepsy caused by parenchymatous cysts. Cysticercosis was found to be the main cause of epilepsy in British soldiers in India[14] and is a common cause in South Africa.[15] More recently it has occurred in an epidemic form in Irian Jaya (West New Guinea) where it was brought to light by the extensive burns sustained by falling into fires.[6] Cerebral manifestations appear after an average of four to eight years after infection but may occur after 30 years.[8] The fits may be focal (Jacksonian) or general, varying from petit mal to grand mal. Other features are transient hemiplegia, psychotic states, acute mania and slow mental deterioration of insidious onset. *Meningeal cysts* in the basal meninges excite an intense inflammatory response and may cause obstructive hydrocephalus. *Ventricular cysts* commonly found in the fourth ventricle may float about blocking the aqueduct of Sylvius causing intermittent hydrocephalus with severe headache and vomiting, resembling a cerebral tumour. *Spinal cysts* cause an arachnoiditis with transverse myelitis.

Subcuticular nodules

These may number from one to 30 or more. They

may be the size of a hard pea, a hazel-nut or even a pigeon's egg. Their situation varies widely. They have been found in the lips, masseter muscles, neck, chest, abdominal wall, back and groin. Unless evidence of cysticercosis is systematically sought the diagnosis may be missed, as nodules may be absent at the time of examination only to come out at a later date. Radiological evidence may not appear for some years as calcification does not usually take place for three to five years after infection. Calcified larvae were detected in skeletal muscles in 97% of patients examined radiologically or at necropsy five or more years after the assumed date of infection.[8] Intracranial calcification was found in 36% within 10 years (Fig. 23:25).

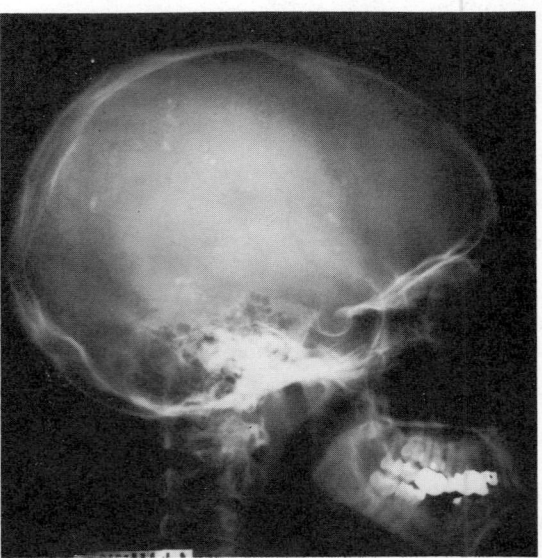

Fig. 23.25   Multiple calcified lesions in the brain in cerebral cysticercosis.

Ocular cysticercosis (see Chapter 70)

The cysticerci remain alive and unencapsulated in the vitreous humour and anterior chamber of the eye where they are constantly changing shape and may cause some discomfort from shadows cast by the larva (Figs. 70.11, p. 1165, and 70.13, p. 1167). Other eye changes which may be caused are uveitis, retinitis, choroidal atrophy and palpebral conjunctivitis.

Other forms

Cysticerci may cause trouble in other sites, such

as the bundle of His, where heart block has been recorded as the result of the presence of a cyst. Numerous cysticerci causing intramuscular swellings may simulate a myopathy.[16].

Course and prognosis

No prophecy can be made of the duration of the epileptic symptoms. Sometimes the fits cease without apparent cause, in others they persist. MacArthur[14] recorded one cysticercus alive after 15 years. The commonest causes of death are status epilepticus and intracranial hypertension.

DIFFERENTIAL DIAGNOSIS

Cerebral cysticercosis may mimic idiopathic epilepsy, multiple space-occupying lesions of the brain, chronic meningitis and increased intracranial pressure. Other conditions causing similar manifestations are tuberculosis, meningitis, coccidioidomycosis, cryptococcosis, neurosyphilis, sarcoidosis and primary and metastatic malignancies.

DIAGNOSIS

Cysticercosis occurs most frequently in the 20–50 year age group whereas idiopathic epilepsy usually starts in childhood. Residence in an endemic area is important but the disease may manifest itself many years (30) after leaving the area. The stools should be examined for ova from adult tapeworms and the patient's body examined carefully for the pea size nodules, which can be excised.

Biopsy

To demonstrate cysticerci a suitable cyst is excised under local anaesthesia and the host capsule is enucleated. The appearance of the translucent membrane with its central 'milk spot' is characteristic. If alive, the parasite may evaginate the head and neck or it may be induced to do so by immersion in hot saline. Distinguishing features of larval cestodes found in human tissues are given in Table II.6 (p. 1343).

Radiography

Radiography is very useful for diagnosis. When partially calcified a good radiograph may show it as a small elongated shadow but the completely calcified cyst gives a characteristic appearance (Fig. 23.26). In the muscles cysticerci are oat-shaped due to pressure, whilst in the brain they are circular (Fig. 23.25). In showing up calcification, 'high penetration' is more effective than slight underexposure. The exposure should be that employed for bone detail. In the early stages the cysts are diaphanous and do not show up so that a negative radiograph of the skull is of no significance. The size of the cysts depends mostly upon their age and situation. Computerized tomography was found to be the most helpful method of diagnosis of cerebral cysticercosis.[17]

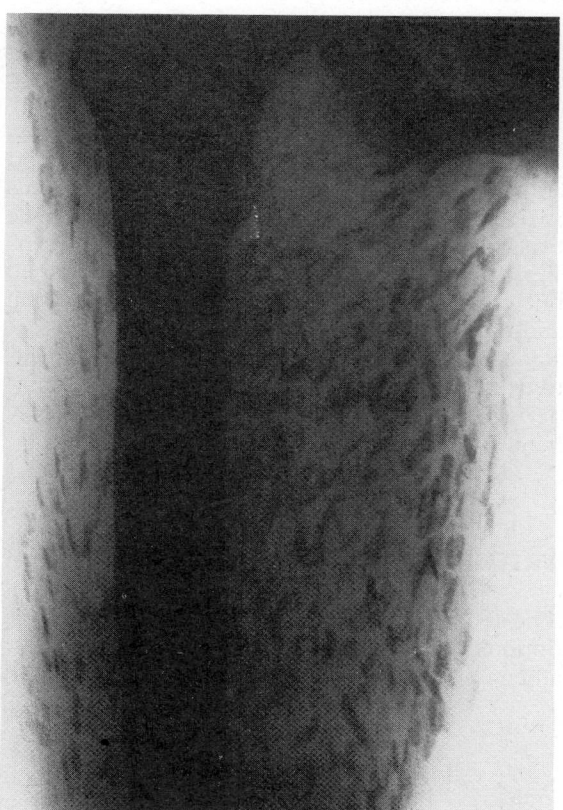

Fig. 23.26 Radiograph of the thigh showing massive invasion of the musculature with cysticercus cellulosae.

Clinical pathology

Eosinophilia affords no aid in diagnosis.

Cerebrospinal fluid

In cysticercosis of the brain changes in the cerebrospinal fluid are variable. Cysticerci are rare. The pressure may be raised and there may be a pleocytosis of five to 500 cells which may be lymphocytes but sometimes eosinophils of 2–42%.[18] Protein changes are non-specific. Among Africans in Durban, cell changes and eosinophilia in the cerebrospinal fluid were found to be inconstant.[15]

Serodiagnosis

The diagnosis relies heavily on immunodiagnosis but this has still not yet reached a reliable stage. Tests used have included complement fixation (CFT), haemagglutination (HA), immuno-electrophoresis (IEP), immunofluorescence (IFA) and enzyme-linked immunosorbent assay (ELISA).[19] Antigens from cysticercus bovis, cysticercus cellulosae (difficult to obtain) and adult tapeworms have all been used. Cysticercus antigen together with adult worm antigen have been used together in an ELISA test and a sensitivity of between 61% and 79% was obtained but cross reactions occurred with schistosomal and echinococcal infections.[20] With indirect HA significant titres are 1/128 and above, but negative tests do not rule out infection.[17] Hybridoma-derived reagents for use with larval cestodes may help in the future.

TREATMENT

The arrival of praziquantel has altered the whole outlook for cerebral cysticercosis, which is now amenable to chemotherapy. Praziquantel should be used in hospital inpatients under expert neurological supervision and additional corticosteroid treatment must be given to prevent the development of intracranial hypertension which may result as a reaction to disintegrating cysts. Epileptic seizures subside in many cases following treatment but may require a second course of treatment given up to six months after the first; 30 mg/kg in three divided doses daily for 6 days caused subcutaneous nodules to disappear after three months, while for cerebral cysticercosis the same dose repeated after one to two months with covering corticosteroids produced great improvement or cure in 17/31 cases.[17] The current situation has been recently reviewed.[21]

EPIDEMIOLOGY

T. solium is present in communities where there is close contact between pigs and man and where standards of sanitation are low. Man is the only source of eggs and transmission depends upon promiscuous defecation in the environment, most commonly round the houses. Flies may also be responsible for spreading the eggs. These conditions are responsible for the high incidence of cysticercosis in West New Guinea. Other cultural practices may cause infection, such as the use of worm segments as medicine or direct and indirect oro-anal sexual contact.

CONTROL

Control of cysticercosis depends upon the control of *T. solium* infections in the community and the prevention of environmental pollution which allows the spread of eggs.

Cysticercus racemosus

Cysticercus racemosus is an aberrant larval stage of *T. solium* or *T. multiceps* species. The oncosphere, instead of invaginating and forming a cyst, buds externally without any scolices forming a multilocular cyst resembling a bunch of grapes. It occurs in the brain where it may form an eosinophilic granuloma (phlegmon) which results in an immunological reaction and the presence of immune complexes. It can be distinguished histologically by the presence of microtriches (hairs) on the surface of the larva, characteristic muscle bands separating cortex from medulla, and a large cavity lined with parenchymal not epithelial cells.[22]

Hydatid disease. 1. Unilocular hydatid

Hydatid disease is caused by the larval stage in man acting as an intermediate host of the canine tapeworm *Echinococcus granulosus*, which normally has its intermediate stage in sheep or other herbivorous animals (unilocular hydatid), and *E. multilocularis*, which has its normal intermediate stage in rodents (see section on multilocular hydatid, below). Other worms rarely seen are *E. oligarthrus* and *E. vogeli* (see section on polycystic hydatid below).

GEOGRAPHICAL DISTRIBUTION

Unilocular hydatid is found extensively in sheep raising countries: South Australia, New Zealand, Tasmania, parts of North and South Africa, East Africa (where in Turkana man himself may be the main intermediate host[23]) and, until recently, Iceland. In the American continent it is common in Argentina and southern Brazil. It is found sporadically in the USA, Britain (Wales), southern and eastern Europe, the Middle East (Iran), Mongolia, Turkestan, north China, southern Japan and North Vietnam.

AETIOLOGY

E. granulosus, which is found in wild and domestic canines, is a very small tapeworm, 3–8.5 mm long, with a pyriform scolex, 0.3 mm in diameter, provided at the apex with a projecting rostellum, four suckers and two circular rows of hooks, varying in size and number (Fig. 23.27). The neck is short and thick; there are usually four proglottides, the last one is the longest (2–3 mm) and only one is sexually mature containing up to 5000 eggs. The genital apertures are marginal, one to each proglottid, in an alternating arrangement. The testes are spherical and numerous. The cirrus pouch is large and pear-shaped. The uterus is tubular and median with short unbranched lateral diverticula. The adult is difficult to remove from the small intestine of the dog without breaking its head. Eggs appear in the dog's faeces. Sometimes the fourth segment also comes away. The egg is spherical, 32–38 × 21–30 μm and is double-shelled, the inner shell being thick. The egg is so similar to those of other tapeworms that it cannot be distinguished from

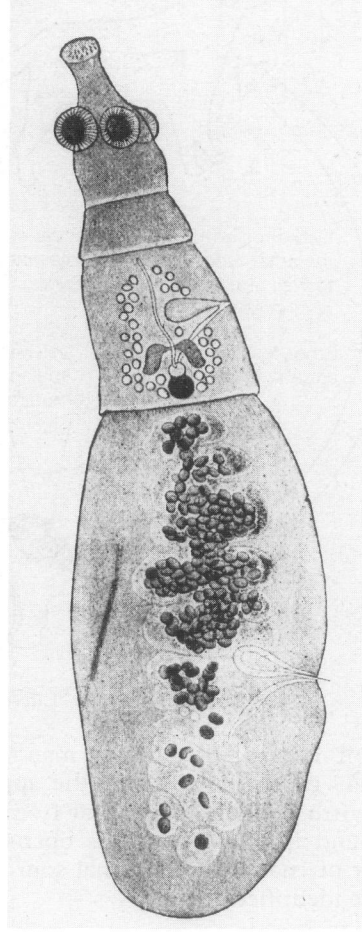

Fig. 23.27 *Echinococcus granulosus*. Adult. (Courtesy WTIM.)

them or from *Multiceps*. The oncosphere contains three pairs of embryonal hooklets.

Life-cycle (Fig. 23.28)

The definitive hosts are wild and domestic canines and the intermediate hosts, sheep and other ruminants.

E. granulosus develops in dogs but generally not in foxes and uses ungulates as intermediate hosts. There are strains which are host adapted and can be differentiated by their isoenzymes. Horse/dog is not infective to man but sheep/dog, buffalo/dog and camel/dog are all infective. A separate strain, (*E. g. canadensis*), deer and

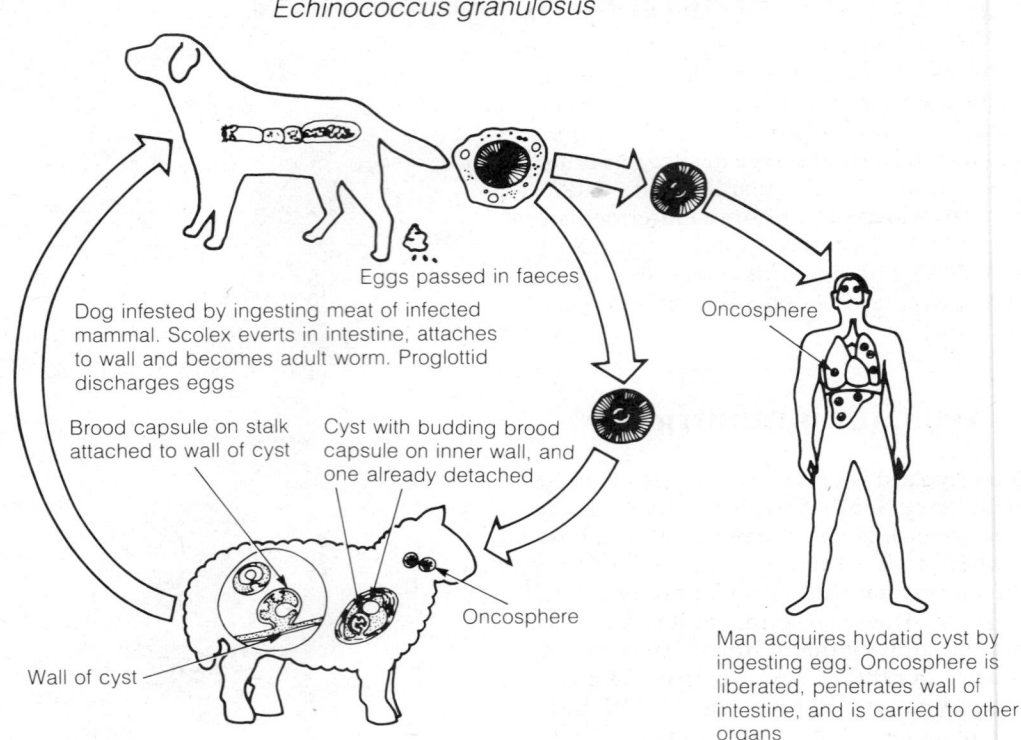

Echinococcus granulosus

Eggs passed in faeces

Dog infested by ingesting meat of infected mammal. Scolex everts in intestine, attaches to wall and becomes adult worm. Proglottid discharges eggs

Oncosphere

Brood capsule on stalk attached to wall of cyst

Cyst with budding brood capsule on inner wall, and one already detached

Wall of cyst

Oncosphere

Man acquires hydatid cyst by ingesting egg. Oncosphere is liberated, penetrates wall of intestine, and is carried to other organs

Fig. 23.28   Life-cycle of *E. granulosus*. (Courtesy WTIM.)

moose/wolf is also infective to man. Further strains may be developing and the application of an in vitro culture of material from human hydatids and isoenzyme studies opens up the possibility of enabling the animal source of the cysts to be identified.[24]

When the egg is swallowed by the intermediate host the shell is digested, the oncosphere emerges and within 8 hours reaches the portal vein and liver which is the first filter, and the lung which is a second filter. The oncosphere develops into a *hydatid* cyst which is made up of an ectocyst,

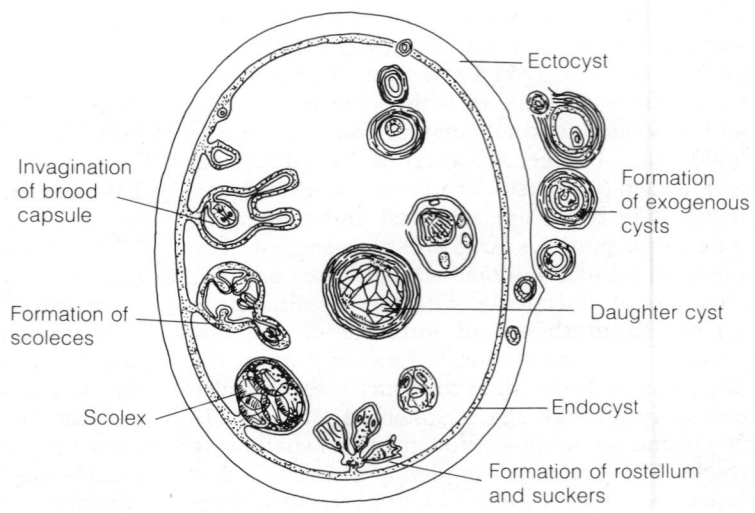

Ectocyst

Invagination of brood capsule

Formation of exogenous cysts

Formation of scoleces

Daughter cyst

Scolex

Endocyst

Formation of rostellum and suckers

Fig. 23.29   Schema of a hydatid cyst.

the fibrous layer of host tissue surrounding the cyst and an endocyst consisting of a striated layer and an inner 'germinal' layer from which *brood capsules* develop, from which larval scolices form, the wall of the brood capsule evaginating to form a protective cup for the growing scolex. Near the head end of the scolex the cuticle thickens and a circle of hooklets develops. The contractile body of the scolex contracts and invaginates the head so that the scolex has the hooklets inside to form a daughter cyst. In endogenous development (unilocular hydatid) the brood capsules grow inwards, the scolices and daughter cysts breaking free into the cyst cavity to form hydatid sand. In exogenous development (multilocular hydatid) the growth is outwards (Fig. 23.29). When the cyst is eaten by the definitive canine host the scolex evaginates and attaches to the intestinal wall where it becomes an adult echinococcus.

TRANSMISSION

Dogs are infected by eating the discarded offal of the intermediate hosts—sheep, buffalo, camel, deer and moose—and convey the infection to man by close contact and fouling of the environment. In Turkana, where dogs are treated as part of the family, the environment in which children crawl is contaminated by dog faeces and the dogs also lick the children to clean them, transferring eggs from their tongue. Elsewhere they contaminate the hands of their masters (shepherds).

PATHOLOGY

Each cyst develops from one oncosphere. The most common site is the liver where the oncosphere arrives within 8 hours after infection. The next filter is the lung. After three weeks it becomes visible as a small vesicle 3 mm in size which elicits a cellular reaction of eosinophils, endothelial and giant cells. The cyst grows in size and in five months measures 1 cm across, eventually forming a large fluid-filled cyst (Fig. 23.30).

There are three types of proliferation: *endogenous* (*E. granulosus*, unilocular hydatid) in which the germinal layer proliferates inwards towards the cavity of the cyst forming brood capsules containing scolices which may become detached and float around (hydatid sand); *exogenous* (*E. multilocularis*, multilocular hydatid) in which the proliferation is outwards into the host tissue invading it like a malignant growth without the development of brood capsules or scolices; or *exogenous* (*E. vogeli*, polycystic hydatid) in which the germinal membrane proliferates outwards to form new cysts, and endogenously to form septa from which brood capsules containing scolices develop. Brood capsules which do not produce scolices are known as *acephalocysts*.

Daughter cysts may be produced by injury or by mechanical interference with the mother cyst, inside which they arise from the detached germinal layer, and also from the brood capsule cells; rarely by vesicular changes from the

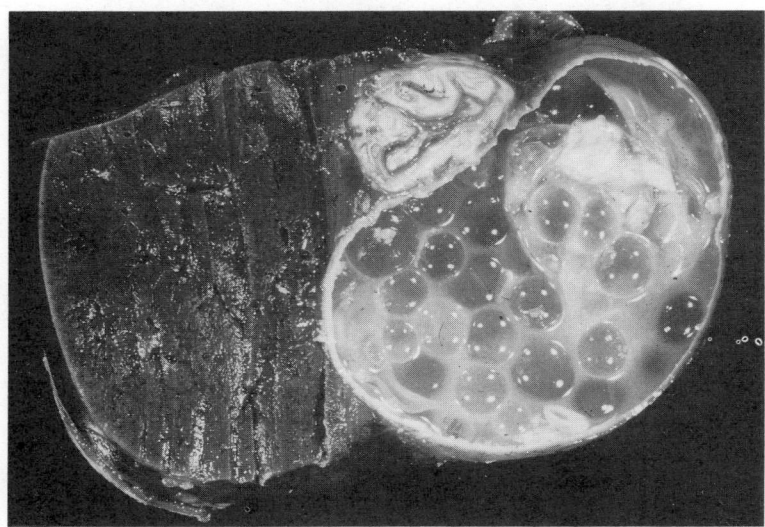

Fig. 23.30 Unilocular hydatid cyst (*E. granulosus*). (Courtesy WTIM.)

detached scolices. In the liver the daughter cysts are bile-stained. Intramuscular injection of scolices causes formation of new cysts and this accounts for the dissemination of hydatid cysts throughout the body which sometimes occurs after operation.

Exogenous daughter cysts in the omentum and bones are secondary, caused by herniation or rupture of both germinal and laminated layers through weakened parts of the adventitia from intracystic pressure. By final exclusion of these herniations new cysts form.

Microscopically the wall of the hydatid cyst consists of the fibrous ectocyst, and the endocyst,

the outer striated layer of which has a brush border consisting of numerous small hairs or *microtriches* and an inner germinal layer containing small nuclear masses which become vacuolated to form brood capsules. This germinal layer contains numerous *calcareous corpuscles*. In microscopical sections of tissue containing parts of old and degenerate cysts, the hydatid nature of the tissue can be identified by the presence of microtriches, calcareous corpuscles and the acid-fast hooklets of the scolices (Fig. 23.31) (see also Table II.6, p. 1343).

Hydatids are slow-growing, sterile, and in man tend to die and calcify. The hydatid fluid

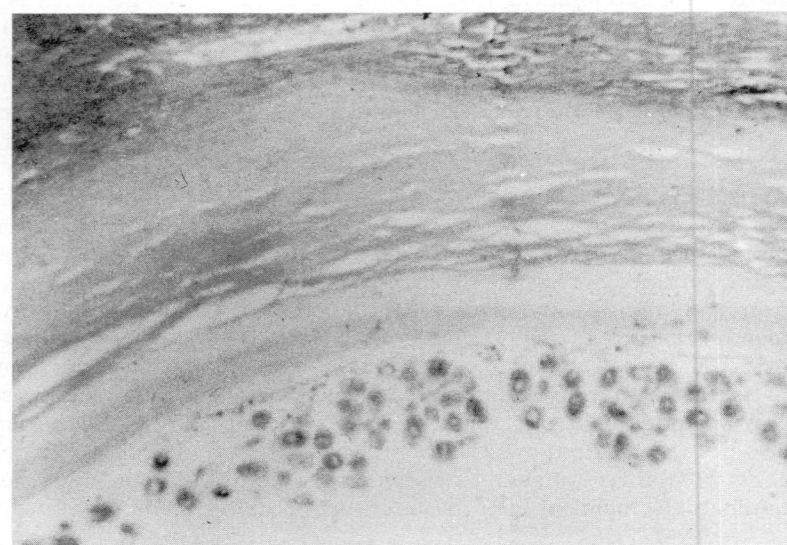

Fig. 23.31 Unilocular hydatid cyst (*E. granulosus*). Section through edge of unilocular hydatid cyst showing the outer cuticular layer and inner germinal layer with numerous thin-walled brood capsules budding off from the germinal layer. The whole cyst is surrounded by a fibrous host tissue reaction. (Courtesy Dr H. Zaiman.)

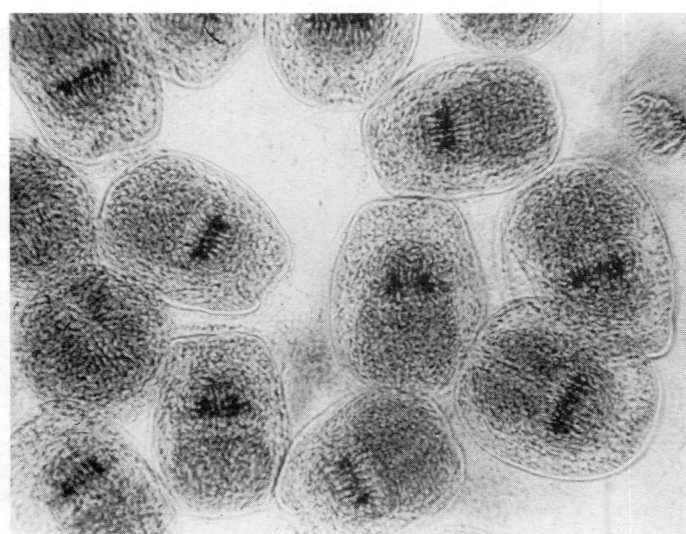

Fig. 23.32 Hydatid sand. Numerous scolices with hooklets. (Courtesy Dr B. H. Kean.)

(protein, salts and a toxin allied to albumin) contains the hydatid sand (Fig. 23.32) and daughter cysts. When released into the abdominal or pleural cavity it may cause anaphylactic shock. The commonest site is the liver (50%) and lung (40%), in 25% of which there are also cysts in the liver. Cysts may also occur in the omentum, mesentery, peritoneum (after rupture), skin, subcutaneous tissues, heart, kidney, spleen, brain, spinal cord, bone (osseous hydatid) and muscles.

The main pathological changes are produced by pressure.

IMMUNITY

Little is known about protective immunity. Cellular immunity does not develop and the wall around the cysts is fibrous tissue without any granulomatous reaction. Antibodies are important in diagnosis, but their protective function is questionable.

CLINICAL FEATURES

Natural history

The course of hydatid disease is very variable. Although infection occurs during childhood the cysts grow slowly and except in the brain do not cause symptoms until middle age. If they do not press on important structures they may give rise to no symptoms. In many cases they develop to a certain size and then die and calcify. Surveys in Turkana in East Africa using ultrasound have shown the presence of symptomless hydatids in a high proportion of the population. In the lung and liver they usually cause no trouble but, in the brain and spinal cord, they lead to raised intracranial pressure and paralysis. They may rupture into body cavities with fatal results.

Incubation period

The incubation period is long, 10–30 years, except in the brain and eye where cysts may present in childhood.

Symptoms and signs

A gradually increasing tumour of the liver may be found in the right subcostal margin. Jaundice is rare.

Lung lesions are often found on routine examination. Other symptoms are caused by pressure on neighbouring structures, collapse of the lung and the mediastinal syndrome. In the pleural cavity a pleural effusion may result.

In the kidney it resembles a hypernephroma and may present as haematuria. In the brain there will be symptoms and signs of a cerebral tumour. In bone (osseous hydatid) there may be spontaneous fracture of long bones and compression fracture of the vertebra.

The cyst may rupture with immediate pyrexia, urticaria and multiple cutaneous eruptions and in the peritoneum general peritonitis may result.

Hydatid cyst of the liver can cause portal hypertension[25] and cysts have been removed from both ventricles of the heart.[26] An extensive myopathy complicating a case of pulmonary hydatid resolved following treatment of the hydatid cyst.[27]

The hydatid cyst, if near the surface, appears as a smooth, round, tense swelling which may give rise to a 'hydatid thrill'. If by any chance the cyst is needled (and this should not be a normal diagnostic procedure) a clear, watery fluid is obtained which contains scolices and hooks. Otherwise the signs are those of a space-occupying lesion in the area involved.

The radiological appearances of a hydatid cyst are characteristic. There is a smooth round outline and in the lung a wavy line crossing the middle of the cyst represents the 'lily' sign which looks like lilies on the surface of a pond in cross-section and is produced by the numerous daughter cysts lying inside the mother cyst. Scanning of the affected organ will show a smooth round cold area. Exploratory puncture should be avoided because of the danger of spread of the daughter cysts. If it occurs then immediate operation and excision of the cyst must be undertaken.

A generalized eosinophilia is present in 20–25% of cases.

DIFFERENTIAL DIAGNOSIS

Unilocular hydatid cysts resemble abscesses or tumours. They may be recognized by their smooth round outline, absence of tenderness and lack of reaction in the surrounding tissues. In the *liver* they must be distinguished from liver abscess and hepatoma, in both of which there is more constitutional disturbance and, in the case of the latter, jaundice. In the *lung* they can be confused with abscess and lung cysts. Aspiration must be avoided at all costs if there is any suspicion of hydatid because of the danger of massive spread of the daughter cysts. In the *brain*, hydatids resemble brain tumours but tend to be more localized. In the *kidney* they resemble hypernephroma and cystic kidneys (usually bilateral).

In histological sections of excised tissue, the features which can identify the presence of a degenerate or destroyed hydatid cyst are the presence of a scolex, the acid-fast hooklets, microtriches and calcareous corpuscles (see section on pathology, above).

DIAGNOSIS

The most important point in diagnosis is the 'index of suspicion'. The patient has come from an endemic area perhaps many years before and in an endemic area every space-occupying lesion must be suspected of being a hydatid cyst. The diagnosis is made by radiology, ultrasound and immunodiagnostic tests. Diagnostic aspiration must be avoided but if a needle has been inserted and what appears to be water is found, then the needle must be left in situ until a surgical team has been assembled to remove the cyst without allowing it to leak.

Radiology

This is best seen in the lung where characteristic appearances are seen (Fig. 23.33).

Ultrasound

This is a very satisfactory technique and can be made available with portable machines in isolated areas; a round, smooth area containing fluid can be demonstrated.

Immunodiagnosis

In general the presence of an active cyst is associated with the production of antibodies and the rupture of a cyst frequently produces a marked rise in antibody levels. Surgical removal as well as suppuration, degeneration and calcification of a cyst results in a marked reduction in antibody levels. High levels of circulating antibody are found with liver cysts but much lower levels with

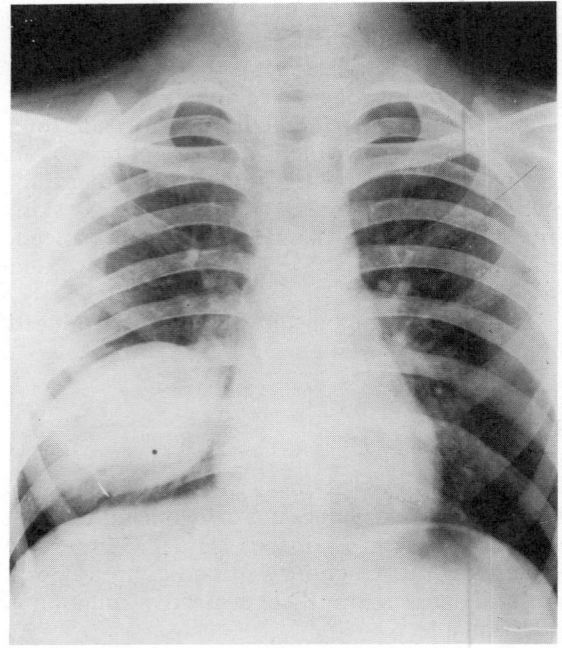

Fig. 23.33   Hydatid cyst of the right lung.

lung cysts; antibodies may be completely absent in lung, intact and hyaline cysts but appear rapidly when they rupture.

IgA and IgG levels are raised but the IgM is highest in active infections. High IgE levels were found in 60% of cases.[28]

An antigen, *Fraction 5*, specific for *E. granulosus*, has been prepared from hydatid fluid and used to measure specific IgE antibodies by IEP; they were present in 30% of active cases.[29] IgG antibodies are measured by the complement fixation, flocculation and fluorescent antibody tests,[30] while IgE antibodies are measured by IEP and can be used to monitor the effectiveness of treatment.

Intradermal test (ID) (Casoni test). The Casoni test is an immediate hypersensitivity reaction produced by the intradermal injection of small amounts of hydatid antigen. The test has a fairly high sensitivity but its low specificity has made the interpretation of results impossible.[31]

Complement fixation test (CFT). Standardized potent antigens and adequate control have improved the accuracy of the CFT;[32] it has proved a valuable diagnostic tool, especially for liver cysts and in the cerebrospinal fluid for brain cysts, as well as a test of cure after surgical removal, when a negative CFT is of better prognostic value than HA or IFA tests.[33] The CFT has a lower sensitivity and cross reactions can occur in patients previously immunized with rabies vaccine.

Haemagglutination (HA) test. This is a more sensitive test than the CFT and a slide test using chromic chloride-treated erythrocytes sensitized by exposure to formalinized hydatid antigen has proved successful.[34]

Latex agglutination (LA) test. The LA test has been found to be easy, fairly specific and sensitive and slide agglutination using latex particles coated with antigen has proved very useful for surveys and screening populations.[35] Confirmation of the diagnosis is made by immunoelectrophoresis.

Indirect fluorescent antibody (IFA) test. Antigen is absorbed on to a glass surface and forms a specific complex with specific antibody which fluoresces.[36] IgG, IgM and IgA antibodies are detectable by this method. The IFA test is sensitive but cross reactivity may occur in patients with hepatic disorders.

Immunoelectrophoresis (IEP). Using specific *E. granulosus* Fraction 5 antigen the precipitation of a band called Arc 5 specific for *E. granulosus* IgE is now considered to be one of the most specific diagnostic tests for the disease,[37] although the antigen is now considered to be genus and not species specific and there are reports of cross reactions with a neoplastic antigen,[38] an important disadvantage.

Enzyme-linked immunosorbent assay (ELISA). ELISA has been applied to the diagnosis of human hydatid using Fraction 5 antigen and is a simple, fairly specific and sensitive diagnostic test.[39]

Radioimmunoassay (RIA) and lymphocyte transformation (LTT) test. These have been used and may be of value in lung cysts when circulating antibodies are often absent.

Circulating antigen in human hydatidosis

As well as the presence of specific antibodies in the serum of some hydatid patients, there is substantial evidence for the presence of specific circulating antigen and immune complexes.[40] Serum antigen has recently been detected using ELISA with purified rabbit antihydatid cyst fluid or human antisera.[40, 41] The circulating antigen appears to be derived from hydatid cyst fluid and also forms circulating immune complexes. Levels of circulating antigen and immune complexes tend to fall more rapidly than specific antibodies following surgical removal of cysts, and their detection may be useful in the diagnosis of antibody-negative cases.[42] Hydatid patients from the hyperendemic focus in Turkana, Kenya were found to have a greater percentage of serum antigen-positive cases with higher levels of antigen, than British hydatid cases and this may be due in part to the generally much larger size of hydatid cysts in the Turkana people.

TREATMENT

Surgical

Solitary cysts in the liver and lung, and in more unusual sites such as the brain, may be removed at operation. The particular risk is the spillage of cyst contents with the immediate complication of anaphylactic shock and the long-term complication of dissemination of secondary cysts. Various techniques have been evolved to prevent spillage, and the injection of a 0.1% cetrimide solution into the cyst prior to attempted removal has minimized the risk of dissemination if spillage should occur.[43] Generally the ectocyst, the outer part of the cyst wall formed by the host, is exposed over the most prominent part of the tumour and walled off with towels. The cyst is then aspirated. A cryogenic cone[44] is used if available but there may be technical difficulties in awkward sites. Cetrimide 0.1% solution is then injected. It will probably kill all cyst material within one minute but is usually left for 5 minutes. Formalin solutions much used in the past are more toxic and less effective. The true cyst wall, thickness 1–5 mm, is then separated from the ectocyst and removed. The inner wall of the ectocyst is swabbed with 0.1% cetrimide, the cavity obliterated with sutures and the incision closed without drainage. Bone cysts cannot be dissected out. The only surgical treatment is amputation.

Medical

Mebendazole in very large and potentially toxic

doses, 10–40 mg/kg, one to three times daily given for prolonged periods (one to three months) often causes regression of the cysts though the death of all cyst material may not be achieved.[27, 45] It may be necessary to continue mebendazole almost indefinitely. Agranulocytosis has been reported with high dose mebendazole.

Albendazole is better absorbed; 10 mg/kg daily for 30 days usually causes regression of cysts and 50 mg/kg daily for 30 days probably kills cysts.[46] The safety of high doses of albendazole is not yet established but such treatment offers the only hope to patients with widespread disease, usually a consequence of spillage at previous surgery.

Praziquantel, while very effective against the adult worms, has no effect on mature cysts. In vitro it is lethal to protoscolices so might reasonably be given over the period of surgery to reduce the risk of dissemination. Albendazole and mebendazole may be used in the same way.

PROGNOSIS

There is little information on the long-term outcome of hydatid cysts without treatment, though it is generally assumed that many deaths occur from anaphylactic shock following spontaneous leakage of cyst material, and also from widespread dissemination of cysts. The prognosis after surgery for a solitary cyst is fair. Prior to the use of cetrimide recurrence of the disease from scolices spilled at operation occurred in up to 50% of cases. Cetrimide has reduced the recurrence rate to less than 10%. The use of mebendazole or albendazole has altered the prognosis of patients with widespread disease.

EPIDEMIOLOGY

Unilocular hydatid may involve wild animals (canids and ungulates) or may enter the domestic cycle involving sheep, camel and dog.

Wild canids and ungulates

In *North America E. g. canadensis*, which involves cervids (deer, moose and wild reindeer or caribou), is found in the high latitudes. Pack dogs eat the viscera of infected moose and provide the source of infection for man.[47] The disease is relatively benign, seldom requiring

surgical treatment. Elsewhere cycles of jackal/deer in Sri Lanka,[48] coyotes/deer in California[49] and wallabies/dingoes in Australia may represent a reservoir of infection for domestic stock.

In *East Africa* in Turkana the incidence of hydatid disease is the highest in the world. There is a high incidence in dogs which have an intimate association with children acting as their 'nurses', cleaning them up after vomiting or defecation.[50] Wild jackals are infected as secondary hosts from eating dead human bodies. Man may also be infected from eating the intestines of wild canids as a delicacy.[23] In this area cysts from cattle, sheep and goats were non-infective and sterile, whereas those from man were very active suggesting that man is playing the part of an active intermediate host.[23] In Masailand, on the other hand, where there is a carnivore (lion etc.)/wildebeest cycle, disease in man is rare.[23]

Domestic dog/sheep, camel cycle

This is the commonest and most widespread form. The dog is the optimum definitive host and in most endemic areas in the world the infection is maintained by dogs which eat the flesh of infected sheep. Sheep, cattle and pigs are the common reservoirs of the larval form of hydatid disease which is found chiefly in sheep-rearing countries. In Iceland in the past 16–33% of the human population were infected with hydatid but in recent years it has disappeared. In southern Australia 40–50% of adult dogs are infected and 2% of the population in certain districts. The camel is an important host in camel-raising areas.

In New Zealand hydatid disease used to be a major health problem with 100 new cases a year.[51] The endemic areas where hydatid is of most concern today are the sheep- and cattle-raising areas of Argentina, Uruguay, southern Brazil and Chile.[52] In Chile the maximum human incidence is in the third decade and in southern Brazil in the second decade.

Most hydatid cysts are acquired in childhood and the unilocular cyst may grow for five to 20 years before it is diagnosed. There is a tendency for hydatid to be more common in members of the same family.[53]

PREVENTION

Infection of dogs can be prevented by controlling

the disposal of raw offal. Dogs should be kept out of abattoirs and no killing of sheep or cattle should be allowed outside authorized places. Dogs may be treated with arecoline hydrobromide in a dosage of 4 mg/50 kg, or with praziquantel (Droncit). Hydatid disappeared from Iceland when a change was made from the production of mutton to lamb which did not allow the hydatids time to develop and so infect the dogs on the island.

2 Multilocular hydatid (alveolar hydatid)

GEOGRAPHICAL DISTRIBUTION

E. multilocularis has a restricted geographical distribution. In the high latitudes of North America the distribution corresponds to that of the arctic fox. There is also a focus in central North America. It is also found in extensive areas of the USSR from the Black Sea, with an extension into Turkey to the Far East and north to Siberia and northern Japan. Definitive records exist in France, Germany, Switzerland, Austria, Belgium and probably England and Sardinia and more recently in Australia and India[54] and in Iraq.

AETIOLOGY

Multilocular hydatid is caused by *E. multilocularis*, which is smaller than *E. granulosus*, 1.4–3.4 mm (as against 3–8.5 mm); the number of testes is 21–29 (as against 45–65). The egg is indistinguishable and is extremely resistant to cold.

Life-cycle (Fig. 23.34)

The definitive hosts are canines and the intermediate hosts rodents. The adult worm lives in

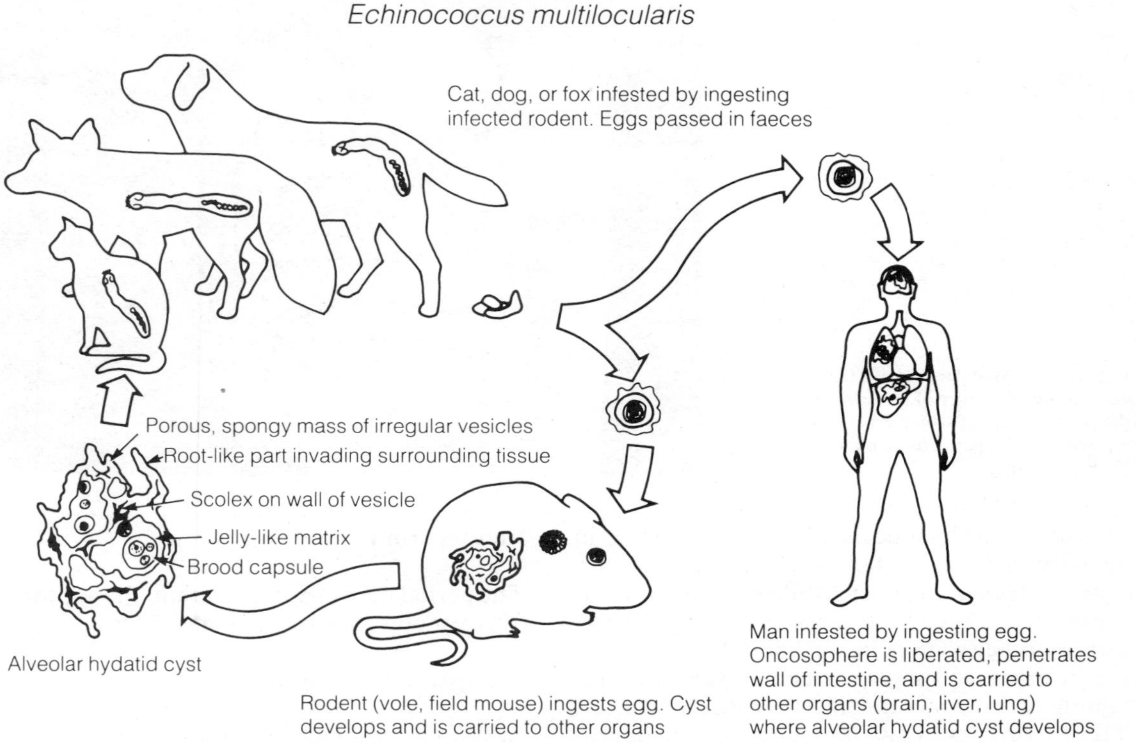

Echinococcus multilocularis

Cat, dog, or fox infested by ingesting infected rodent. Eggs passed in faeces

Porous, spongy mass of irregular vesicles
Root-like part invading surrounding tissue
Scolex on wall of vesicle
Jelly-like matrix
Brood capsule

Alveolar hydatid cyst

Rodent (vole, field mouse) ingests egg. Cyst develops and is carried to other organs

Man infested by ingesting egg. Oncosphere is liberated, penetrates wall of intestine, and is carried to other organs (brain, liver, lung) where alveolar hydatid cyst develops

Fig. 23.34 Life-cycle of *Echinococcus multilocularis*. (Courtesy WTIM.)

the intestines of foxes, wolves and dogs and the egg is ingested by a variety of small rodents in the liver of which the alveolar hydatid cyst develops, to be eaten in turn by a canine.

TRANSMISSION

Man is infected by ingestion of eggs from raw fruit and vegetables contaminated by foxes, sledge dogs and other wild canids.[55] In Europe, strawberries, huckleberries and cranberries contaminated by foxes are the source of infection.[56]

PATHOLOGY

Man is not a normal intermediate host and the cyst grows slowly and aberrantly.

The alveolar cyst (Fig. 23.35) grows by exogenous proliferation, is invasive and frequently metastasizes to other organs. It is solid and not cystic, consisting of many irregular cavi-

by the fine germinative layer. Central necrosis and cavitation are common findings and there is a persistent eosinophilia in the surrounding tissues.

IMMUNITY

Mammals, such as sheep and goats, are resistant to infection and man is partially resistant, so that the cyst grows more slowly than in the natural reservoir, undergoes necrosis and produces few scolices.

CLINICAL FEATURES

Natural history

Alveolar hydatid is a slowly progressive disease which gradually spreads into the surrounding tissues eventually destroying them. It metastasizes to the lung and brain.

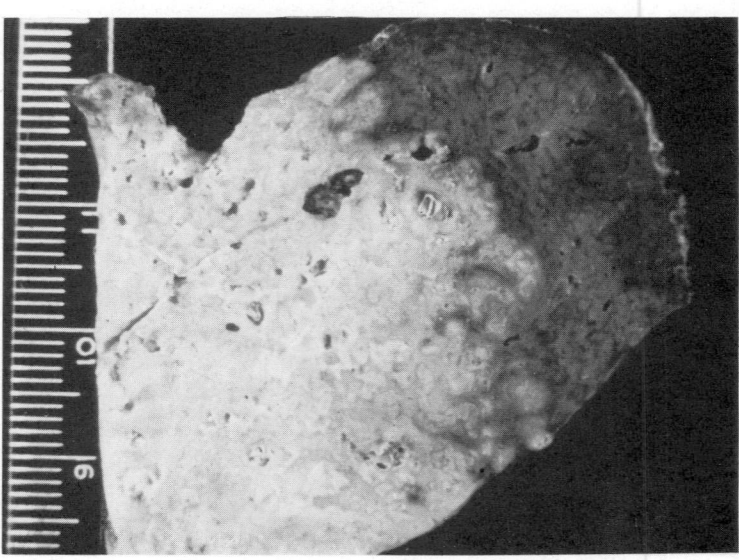

Fig. 23.35 Alveolar hydatid (*E. multilocularis*). Liver of an Eskimo, the parenchyma of which has been replaced by the parasite. (Courtesy Dr R.L. Rausch.)

ties containing hyaline membrane, all enclosed in a relatively avascular fibrous adventitia. Primary lesions occur in the liver, while secondary metastatic lesions have been reported in lung, lymph glands and elsewhere in the body. Embedded in the stroma are minute irregular vesicles containing little or no fluid and very rarely scolices. These vesicles may be recognized microscopically by their upright stratified cuticle lined

Incubation period

The period between infection and the appearance of symptoms may be as long as 30 years.

Symptoms and signs

Symptoms and signs do not develop before the age of 50. The clinical picture is that of intrahepatic portal hypertension. The primary lesion is always in the liver, either the right or left lobe, or both. The presenting symptom is pain in the right upper quadrant of the abdomen along with a palpable liver. Jaundice is common. Growth continues and there may be metastases to the brain and lungs. In the later stages alveolar hydatid resembles a slow-growing carcinoma without fever but with hepatosplenomegaly and ascites.[55]

Radiology and ultrasound will show a diffuse solid space-occupying lesion.

DIAGNOSIS

It is difficult to differentiate from a hepatoma but hydatid grows much more slowly.

Immunodiagnosis

The diagnosis is best made by serology. An indirect HA test using hydatid fluid as antigen is highly successful and an ELISA or gel diffusion test using Factor 5 as antigen is also very useful.

Biopsy

Examination of biopsy material can show the multilaminated cyst wall which is diagnostic; scolices are hardly ever found.

TREATMENT

This is difficult. Surgical removal is usually not possible but partial hepatectomy where feasible can be effective. *Mebendazole* in a daily dose of 40 mg/kg for three years produced some improvement but did not kill the cyst.[57] *Alben-*

dazole used as in unilocular hydatid[46] may be successful in arresting the spread.

EPIDEMIOLOGY

E. multilocularis is an arctic or alpine parasite overwintering as an adult in the intestine of canids and as a cyst in the livers of small rodents. The egg is resistant to cold and lies ready to infect rodents in the spring. In the short summer the cysts grow rapidly in the liver of rodents, scolices developing in a few months in large numbers so that the infected livers produce heavy infections in the canids. Eggs develop after 30–35 days and contamination of the environment is heavy. In the Arctic the numerous sledge dogs, which are heavily infected, contaminate human food which is left out without storage.

In Alaska the definitive hosts are mainly the arctic fox, but also wolves and dogs, and the intermediate host in which the larval forms are found is the tundra vole (*Microtus aeconomus*).[58] In St Lawrence Island in Alaska hosts of *E. m. sibericensis* are field mice (*Clethrionomys rutilis*), ground squirrels (*Citellus undulatus*) and shrews (*Sorex jacksoni*).[59] In North Dakota the host is the deer mouse (*Peromyscus maniculatus*).[60] In southern Germany the larval stages are found in the field mouse (*Microtus arvalis*) and the adult stages in the red fox (*Vulpes vulpes*)[56] and domestic dog and cat.[61]

CONTROL

In villages where there are numerous sledge dogs mass treatment of the dogs with praziquantel has been tried with success. Careful washing of raw fruit and vegetables and the hands before eating is essential.

3 Polycystic hydatid (*E. vogeli, E. oligarthrus*)

GEOGRAPHICAL DISTRIBUTION

Human cases have been recorded from Panama, Colombia and Ecuador but better diagnosis will probably show many more cases and a wider distribution.

AETIOLOGY

E. oligarthrus is a parasite of wild felines with the agouti as an intermediate host. *E. vogeli* is a parasite of the bush dog with the paca and spiny rat as intermediate hosts and is probably the cause of most human cases of polycystic hydatid. *E. vogeli* is half the size of the other echinococci and may be distinguished by the rostellum and two rows of hooklets, the larger ones 38–46 μm in length and the smaller 30–37 μm.

PATHOLOGY

Polycystic hydatid proliferates exogenously but forms small septate cysts. It is a greyish-white polycystic mass containing yellow fluid and gel like a bunch of grapes. The size of the cyst can vary from 10 mm in size to occupying the whole liver.

Microscopically

Multiple vesicles from a few millimetres to centimetres across are divided by septa composed of hyaline laminated membrane which is lined with germinal epithelium containing numerous calcareous corpuscles, and from which the brood capsules containing scolices are formed. Necrotic and dead cysts can be recognized by the hooklets and calcareous corpuscles.

CLINICAL FEATURES

The clinical features are extremely variable depending upon where the cyst is sited. In the liver it presents as a liver tumour, in the stomach and bone as tumours.

DIAGNOSIS

The same serological tests as used for hydatid cyst are very useful.

TREATMENT

Surgical treatment is often possible. Chemotherapy is as yet untried.

Coenurus cerebralis (bladderworm)

GEOGRAPHICAL DISTRIBUTION

Coenurus infection of man is found in North Africa, Zaire, East Africa[62–64] and also in the USA and England.

AETIOLOGY

Coenurus cerebralis is the larval cystic form of *Multiceps* (*Taenia*) *multiceps* where the definitive hosts are dogs and the intermediate hosts sheep, goats, cattle and horses, and *Multiceps* (*Taenia*) *brauni* a tropical tapeworm found in East Africa with definitive hosts dog, fox, genet cat and jackal, and intermediate hosts swamp rat, porcupine and gerbil; *Multiceps* (*Taenia*) *serialis* has as definitive hosts canids, and intermediate hosts rabbit, squirrel and coypu.

The adult *Multiceps* worms are 50 cm long with a scolex and a double row of hooklets. The segments measure 9 × 3–4 mm and the uterus has 22 lateral branches. The eggs are 33 μm in diameter.

Life-cycle

Domestic and wild canids are the definitive hosts and eggs are passed which are ingested by intermediate hosts, herbivorous mammals. The larval or cystic stages have a preference for the brain where they cause 'staggers' in sheep. In the brain the cyst forms a coenurus in which multiple scolices develop endogenously into the cavity from brood capsules on the germinal membrane.

TRANSMISSION

Transmission is by ingestion of raw fruit and vegetables contaminated by dog, cat or genet faeces.

PATHOLOGY

The cysts, which are usually found in the brain, are like bladders and measure from a few millimetres to 2 cm or more in diameter. There are multiple scolices projecting into the bladder cavity from the germinal layer (Fig. 23.36) in which hooklets can be identified (Fig. 23.37). In the brain they obstruct the pathways of circulation of the cerebrospinal fluid and cause raised intracranial pressure. At the base of the

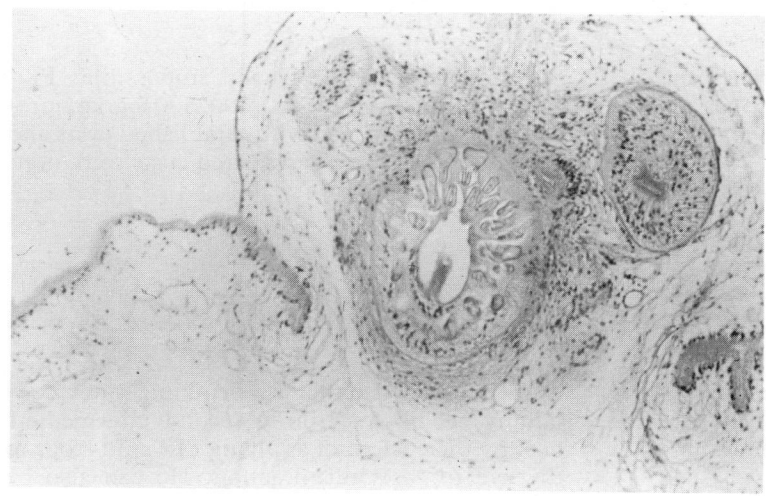

Fig. 23.36 Coenurus cerebralis. *M. multiceps* cyst. Section through membranes and scolex of cyst. (Courtesy Dr G. R. Healy.)

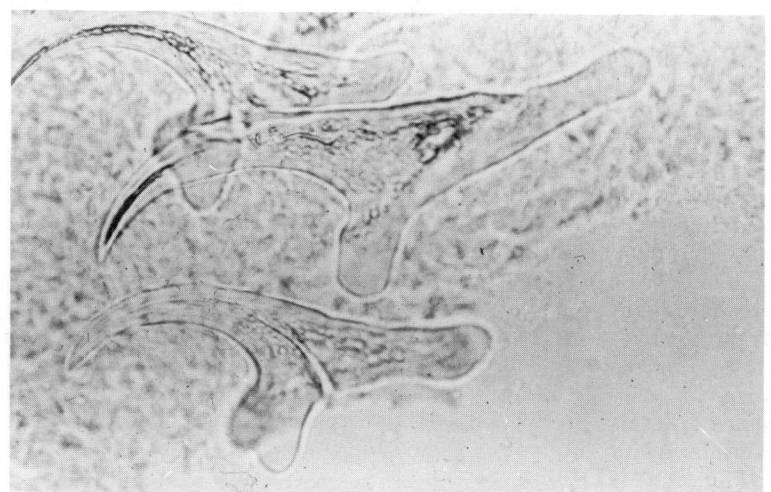

Fig. 23.37 Coenurus cerebralis. *M. multiceps*. High-power view showing hooklets on scolex in brood capsule. (Courtesy Dr G. R. Healy.)

brain they cause a chronic cystic arachnoiditis in which the cyst is embedded. Microscopically the grouping of scolices is linear or in clusters. There is no calcification.

CLINICAL FEATURES

Natural history

Situated in the brain the cysts invariably cause symptoms at an early stage and death occurs from raised intracranial pressure.

Symptoms and signs

Onset is at an early age and the cerebral symptoms are very varied. Intermittent increased intracranial pressure gives rise to transient cerebral episodes of epilepsy and confusion. The tumour is essentially benign and does not infiltrate structures. There may be focal signs, jacksonian epilepsy, hemiplegia, monoplegia and cerebellar ataxia. The spinal cord may be affected with paraplegia. Sometimes there is a toxic psychosis. Cysts may occur beneath the conjunctiva and in the eye[63] (see Chapter 70).

DIAGNOSIS

Brain scan will show dilated ventricles and the presence of a space-occupying lesion. Serological tests are positive, as in the other larval tapeworm diseases.

TREATMENT

Surgical removal is usually impossible. Praziquantel in large doses, 200–500 mg/kg, prevented death in sheep with established cysts and the proscolices from the treated cysts were noninfective.[65]

Sparganosis

GEOGRAPHICAL DISTRIBUTION

Most infections occur in South-East Asia and east central Africa. Cases have also been reported from Japan, China, Australia, Guyana and North America.

AETIOLOGY

Sparganosis is caused by infection with spargana which are the second stage or plerocercoid larvae of *Spirometra* (*Diphyllobothrium*) tapeworms. Many species are probably involved but three have been identified: *Spirometra mansoni*, which is the cause in South-East Asia, Japan, China and scattered cases in America; *Spirometra mansonoides*, which is the cause of sparganum proliferum in the American continent; *Spirometra theileri* (*pretoriensis*), which is a tropical sparganum and is the cause in East Africa (Masailand).[62] Adult spirometra are 20–60 cm long and the segments number 200–300. The egg is pointed, $67 \times 37 \mu m$, with a conical operculum.

Life-cycle

Spirometra differ from other *Diphyllobothrium* worms in that the second intermediate hosts are amphibia, reptiles or mammals (in contrast to fish). The adult stages are found in domestic and wild canines and felines, the eggs are passed into water and the procercoids develop in cyclops. The cyclops are swallowed by tadpoles which develop into frogs in which the plerocercoid develops. The frogs can be eaten by predators, reptiles, snakes, birds and mammals which can act as third intermediate hosts until finally a dog or cat becomes involved. Man acts as a second or third intermediate host.

TRANSMISSION

Man is infected either by drinking water containing cyclops or from a second intermediate host by the custom of applying raw split frogs to the eye to ease inflammation. He can also be infected from eating raw snakes which contain plerocercoids from the frogs which are their usual food.

PATHOLOGY

The plerocercoid burrows through the mucosa of the intestine or eye and enters the tissues and may wander anywhere in the intramuscular fasciae, walls of the alimentary canal, mesentery, kidney, lung, heart and brain. The sparganum resembles the adult tapeworm 3×2.5 cm up to 20–50 cm (Korea) in size with a smooth, glistening coat and undulating movements (Fig. 23.38). The sparganum cyst contains the

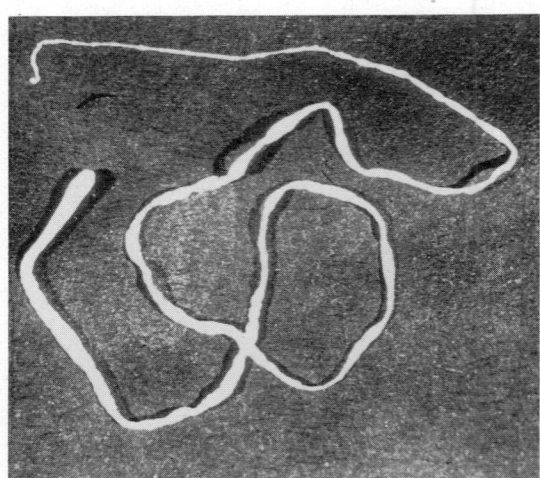

Fig. 23.38   Sparganum mansonoides. Plerocercoid larva. (Courtesy Dr H. Zaiman.)

grooved head of the worm (Fig. 23.39b) and calcareous corpuscles.

In the tissues, as long as they are alive, the spargana cause honeycombing of the tissues and if they get into a lymphatic channel, lymphoedema. When they die they excite an acute inflammatory response which may destroy the eye. Microscopical examination shows a larval tapeworm surrounded by a cellular infiltrate of neutrophils with many eosinophils (Fig. 23.40) (cf. Pentastomids, Chapter 24, p. 562).

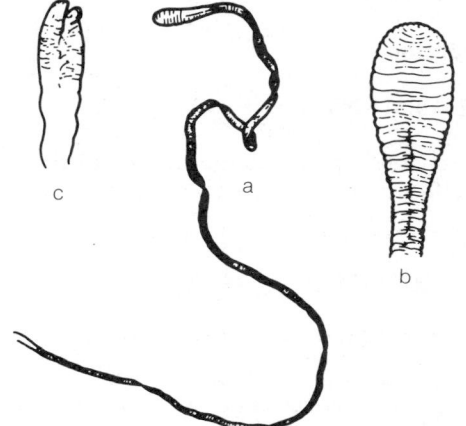

Fig. 23.39 *Spirometra mansoni*. Plerocercoid, extracted from an abscess in a Masai. (a) Natural size; (b) anterior extremity; (c) posterior extremity.

CLINICAL FEATURES

Natural history

Spargana may live up to nine years and few cause symptoms unless they migrate near the surface or damage the eye. If there are many then serious effects can result.

Symptoms and signs

The usual signs are the presence of migratory subcutaneous swellings which may become painful and tender to form abscesses from which the sparganum is discharged. Parts of the body most often affected are the chest wall, breast and legs. The swellings may be very numerous scattered all over the body. In the eye they cause conjunctivitis and periorbital oedema (Fig. 70.20, p. 1175). When they are discharged or removed at operation they appear as glistening, white, opaque worms several centimetres in length resembling tapeworms. Death of the worm excites acute inflammation and, if there are many, severe constitutional disturbance.

DIAGNOSIS

Spargana are mistaken for other helminths which

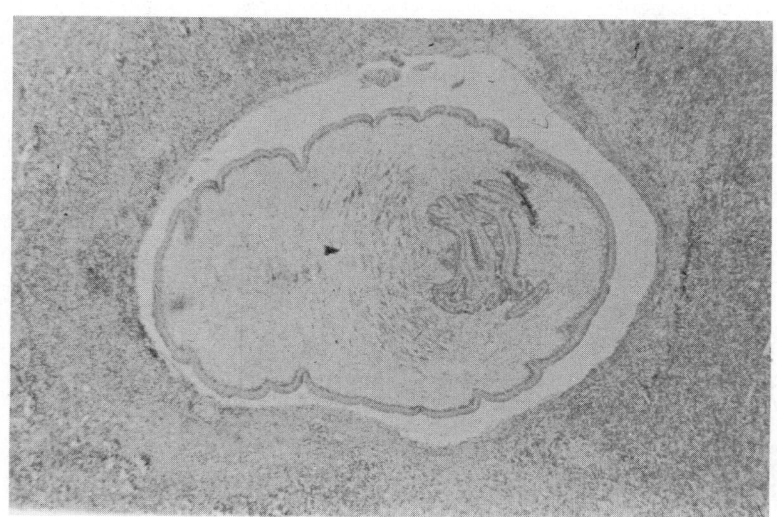

Fig. 23.40 Sparganosis. Cross-section showing typical tapeworm morphology. A dense eosinophilic infiltration is present in the adjacent muscle. (Courtesy Dr H. Zaiman.)

IMMUNITY

Little is known about immunity but multiple infections are found.

are found in the subcutaneous tissues such as guinea-worm, filaria, *Loa loa*, migrating helminths, cutaneous larva migrans, gnathostomiasis, larval flukes and myiasis. A history of the use of raw frogs or drinking infected water may be obtained. The diagnosis is made by biopsy and removal of the swelling, which can be identified as a spirometra by its solid body and deep grooves on the head with absence of suckers and hooklets, distinguishing it from other cestodes. Serological tests appear to be of little use.

Proliferative sparganosis

Proliferative sparganosis is a rare condition in which the worm is pleomorphic and proliferates buds which break off from the parent body and migrate to new locations in the body, where they grow and repeat the process. The condition is seen predominantly in males and runs a chronic course spreading into the viscera.

CLINICAL FEATURES[67]

There are two main types: in one there is a primary tumour in the skin which swells, becomes painful and fluctuant, spreading rapidly to other parts of the body; in the other a small number of asymptomatic or pruritic nodules appear which do not form tumours but propagate to other parts of the body. Once the worms penetrate, haemoptysis, hepatosplenomegaly and cerebral signs develop and the patient becomes weak and emaciated and dies.

DIAGNOSIS

Biopsy shows a well-developed cyst containing one or more worms (Fig. 23.41).

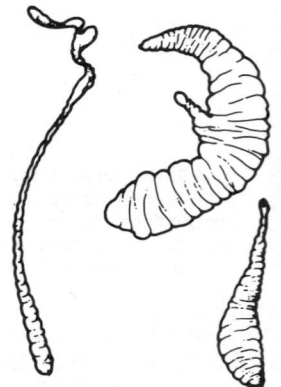

Fig. 23.41   Different forms of sparganum proliferum.

TREATMENT

Praziquantel in large doses of 40 mg/kg in six divided doses failed to affect the course in a case of sparganum proliferum.[66]

PREVENTION

Boiling doubtful water and stopping the use of raw frogs as poultices and raw snakes as food will prevent infection.

TREATMENT

Praziquantel in very large doses failed to have any effect on one case.[66]

REFERENCES

1   Brygoo, E. R. & Randriamalala, J. C. (1959) *Bull. Soc. Path. éxot.* **52**, 26.
2   Abuladze, K. I. (1964) *Principles of Cestology*, Vol. 4. Moscow. Quoted by Dawes, B. (1972) *Adv. Parasit.* **10**, 273.
3   Nelson, G. S., Pester, F. R. N. & Rickman, R. (1965) *Trans. R. Soc. trop. Med. Hyg.* **59**, 507.
4   Dawes, B. (1972) *Adv. Parasit.* **10**, 273.
5   Huang, S. W. (1967) *Bull. Inst. Zool. Acad. Sin.* **6**, 29.
6   Gajdusek, D. C. (1978) *Papua New Guin. med. J.* **21**, 329.
7   Andrews, P., Thomas, H., Pohlke, R. et al (1983) *Med. Res. Rev.* **3**, 147–200.
8   Dixon, H. B. F. & Lipscomb, F. M. (1961) *Spec. Rep. Ser. med. Res. Coun.*, 299.
9   Farid, A., El-Marry, N. A. & Wallace, C. K. (1984) *Trans. R. Soc. trop. Med. Hyg.* **78**, 280.
10   Editorial (1976) *Br. med. J.* **ii**, 1028.
11   Bylund, G., Bang, B. & Wikgren, K. (1977) *J. Helminth.* **51**, 115–119.
12   d'Alessandro, B. A., Beaver, P. C. & Pallares, R. M. (1963) *Am. J. trop. Med. Hyg.* **12**, 193.
13   Gemmel, M. A. (1966) *Immunology* **4**, 325.
14   MacArthur, W. P. (1933) *Trans. R. Soc. trop. Med. Hyg.* **26**, 525.
15   Powell, S. J., Procter, E. M., Wilmot, E. J. et al (1966) *Ann. trop. Med. Parasit.* **60**, 152.
16   McGill, R. G. (1948) *Lancet* **ii**, 728.
17   Botero, D. & Castano, S. (1972) *Am. J. trop. Med. Hyg.* **31**, 811–821.
18   Reinlein, J. M., Trihueros, A., Arjona, E. et al (1951) *Bull. Inst. med. Res. Madrid* **4**, 67.
19   Flisser, A., Willms, K., Laclette, J. P. et al (1982) *Cysticercosis. Present State of Knowledge and Perspectives*. London: Academic Press.
20   Diwan, A. R., Coker-Vann, M., Brown, P. et al (1982) *Am. J. trop. Med. Hyg.* **33**, 364–369.
21   Bell, D. R. (1984) *Br. med. J.* **289**, 857.

22 Ali-Khan, Z., Siboo, R., Meerovitch, E. et al (1981) *Trans. R. Soc. trop. Med. Hyg.* **75**, 774–779.

23 MacPherson, C. N. L. (1983) *Am. J. trop. Med. Hyg.* **32**, 397–404.

24 Smyth, J. D. (1979) *Symp. Br. Soc. Parasit.* **17**, 75.

25 Mansouri, M., Benebadji, R. & Hadjiatan (1970) *Ann. Alger. Chir.* **4**, 7.

26 Calamari, G., Derna, A. M. & Veturini, A. (1974) *Thorax* **4**, 451.

27 Bhattacharya, D. N. & Harries, J. R. (1984) *Trans. R. Soc. trop. Med. Hyg.* **78**, 78–80.

28 Dessaint, J. P., Bout, D., Wattre, P. et al (1975) *Immunology* **29**, 813.

29 Danis, M., Richard-Lenoble, D., Bruckner, G. et al (1977) *Br. med. J.* **ii**, 1356.

30 Kagan, I. G., Maddison, S. E. & Norman, L. (1968) *Am. J. trop. Med. Hyg.* **17**, 79.

31 Capron, A., Vernes, A., Dessaint, J. P. et al (1976) *Rev. fr. Allerg.* **16**, 9.

32 Bradstreet, C. M. (1969) *J. med. Microbiol.* **2**, 419.

33 Matossian, R. M. & Araj, G. F. (1975) *J. Hyg. Camb.* **75**, 333.

34 Matossian, R. M., Mamo, A. J. & Dahrour, R. (1976) *J. clin. Path.* **29**, 39.

35 Varela-Diaz, V. M., Coltorti, V., Ricardes, M. et al (1976) *Am. J. trop. Med. Hyg.* **25**, 617.

36 Matossian, R. M., Kane, G. J., Chantler, S. et al (1972) *Immunology* **22**, 423.

37 Arzabel, L. A., Schantz, D. M. & Lopes-Lemes, M. H. (1975) *Am. J. trop. Med. Hyg.* **24**, 843.

38 Varela-Diaz, V. M., Coltorti, V., Ricardes, M. et al (1978) *Am. J. trop. Med. Hyg.* **27**, 554–557.

39 Farag, H., Bout, D. & Capson, A. (1975) *Biomedicine* **23**, 276.

40 Craig, P. S. & Nelson, G. S. (1984) *Ann. trop. Med. Parasit.* **78**, 219–227.

41 Gottstein, B. (1984) *Am. J. trop. Med. Hyg.* **33**, 1185–1191.

42 Craig, P. S. (1986) *Parasit. Immunol.* **8**, 171–188.

43 Frayha, G. J., Bikhazi, K. J. & Kachachi, T. A. (1981) *Trans. R. Soc. trop. Med. Hyg.* **75**, 447–450.

44 Saidi, F. (1977) *Ann. R. Coll. Surg. Eng.* **59**, 155.

45 Bryceson, A. D. M., Cowie, A. G. A., MacLeod, C. et al (1982) *Trans. R. Soc. trop. Med. Hyg.* **76**, 510–518.

46 Morris, D. L., Dykes, P. W., Dickson, B. et al (1983) *Br. med. J.* **286**, 103–104.

47 Miller, M. J. (1953) *Can. med. Ass. J.* **68**, 423.

48 Paramanthanan, D. C. & Dissanaike, A. S. (1961) *Trans. R. Soc. trop. Med. Hyg.* **55**, 483.

49 Romano, M. N., Brunett, O. A., Schwabe, C. W. et al (1974) *J. Wildlife Dis.* **10**, 225–227.

50 Nelson, G. S. & Rausch, R. L. (1963) *Ann. trop. Med. Parasit.* **57**, 136–149.

51 Forbes, L. (1962) *Trans. R. Soc. trop. Med. Hyg.* **56**, 7.

52 Neghme, R. A., Feigenbaum, A. J., Pilotto, A. et al (1949) *Boln. Sanit. Pan-Am.* **28**, 469.

53 Ferro, A. (1946) *Archos int. Hidatid* **6**, 135.

54 Aikat, B. K., Bhusnurmath, S. R., Cadersa, M. et al (1978) *Trans. R. Soc. trop. Med. Hyg.* **72**, 619.

55 Rausch, R. (1956) *Am. J. trop. Med. Hyg.* **5**, 1086.

56 Vogel, H. (1955) *Dt. med. Wschr.* **80**, 931.

57 Wilson, J. F., Davidson, M. & Rausch, R. L. (1978) *Ann. Rev. Resp. Dis.* **118**, 747.

58 Rausch, R. & Schiller, E. L. (1951) *Science, N.Y.* **113**, 57.

59 Thomas, L. J., Babero, B. B., Gaillichio, V. et al (1954) *Science N.Y.* **120**, 1102.

60 Leiby, P. D. & Kristy, D. C. (1974) *Am. J. trop. Med. Hyg.* **23**, 675.

61 Eckhert, J., Muller, B. & Partridge, A. J. (1974) *Tropenmed. Parasit.* **25**, 334.

62 Fain, A. & Piraux, A. (1960) *Bull. Soc. Path. éxot* **52**, 804.

63 Raper, A. B. & Dockeray, G. (1956) *Ann. trop. Med. Parasit.* **50**, 121.

64 Wilson, V. L. C., Wayte, D. M. & Addae, R. O. (1972) *Trans. R. Soc. trop. Med. Hyg.* **66**, 611.

65 Verster, A. & Tustin, R. C. (1982) *J. S. Afr. Vet. Ass.* **53**, 107–108.

66 Torres, J. R., Noya, O. O., Noya, B. A. et al (1981) *Trans. R. Soc. trop. Med. Hyg.* **75**, 846–847.

67 Moulinier, R., Martinez, E., Torres, J. et al (1982) *Am. J. trop. Med. Hyg.* **31**, 358–363.

Chapter 24
Unusual Parasites

Some parasites, common in nature, may occasionally infect man because of certain practices and habits. These may be the consumption of uncooked tadpoles, frogs or snakes for medicinal purposes or marinated and uncooked snails, slugs and marine fish as food. Insects such as beetles and dragonfly nymphs may be eaten deliberately, accidentally or taken for medicinal purposes, while contaminated soil or water is responsible for other infections. Often the parasite does not develop to maturity in man, who acts as a paratenic host; in other cases it does develop to maturity and eggs are passed. Trematodes, nematodes and free-living amoebae may all be involved.

TREMATODES (T)

A number of trematodes whose life-cycle normally involves mammals, birds and bats have a life-cycle with two intermediate hosts: a snail and a frog. Many land snakes are infected and act as paratenic hosts. In other cases grubs and insect larvae may act as second intermediary hosts.

NEMATODES (N)

Some nematodes have a larval stage in grubs and beetles while others hatch from eggs which are passed on to the soil where they hatch and contaminate food or are accidentally ingested (Table 24.1).

1   TADPOLES, FROGS AND SNAKES

Gnathostomiasis (N)

Gnathostomiasis is caused by a nematode worm, the adult of which lives in tumours in the stomach of dogs and cats which are the definitive hosts. Two intermediate hosts are necessary for complete development: a cyclops as first intermediate host, and fish, frogs or snakes as second intermediate hosts. Dogs and cats are infected from eating the second intermediate hosts. Man is a paratenic host infected from eating raw snakes or amphibians, fish or a paratenic host such as a chicken or duck infected with third stage larvae. Larvae are unable to reach full development in man and wander through the tissues causing human gnathostomiasis.

GEOGRAPHICAL DISTRIBUTION

Gnathostomiasis as a human infection is found mainly in central Thailand where it has become somewhat of a problem. Cases have also occurred in Vietnam, Philippines, Malaysia, Burma, Cambodia, Laos and Indonesia[1] and formerly Japan.

AETIOLOGY

Ten to twelve species of *Gnathostoma* are known of which only two are found in man: *Gnathostoma spinigerum*, which is the commonest, and *Gnathostoma hispidum*, which is rare and causes ocular gnathostomiasis. Both species are morphologically similar. The adult worms live in tumours in the stomach of felines. They are short, reddish coloured nematodes (male 11–25 mm, females 25–54 mm). The anterior half is covered with leaf-like spines which are species specific. The eggs are ovoid, 65–70 × 38–40 μm in size, transparent and superficially pitted with a plug at one end. They are unembryonated when laid (Fig. II.36F, p. 1349).

Life-cycle (Fig. 24.1)

The eggs hatch in water and a motile first stage larva emerges which penetrates one of four species of cyclops as the first intermediate host in which they develop into a second stage larva.

Table 24.1 Unusual parasites.

Method of infection	Parasite	Stage in man	Clinical features	Geographical area
1 Eating raw tadpoles, frogs, snakes, fish, chicken	*Gnathostoma spinigerum* (N)	Paratenic host	Visceral larva migrans and eosinophilic brain syndrome	Thailand and Indo-China
	Fibricola seoulensis (T)	Definitive host	Intestinal infection. Diarrhoea and eosinophilia	Korea
2 Eating raw liver	*Pentastomids Linguatula*	Paratenic host	Halzoun and cysts	Middle East, Sudan and Africa
3 Eating raw snakes	*Armillifer (Porocephalus)*	Paratenic host	Metastatic calcifications Ocular lesions	Africa, Far East and China
4 Eating snails and slugs	*Angiostrongylus* (N) *cantonensis*	Paratenic host	Eosinophilic brain syndrome	Western Pacific, Japan, Indo-China
	costaricensis		Eosinophilic granuloma of bowel	Central and South America
	Hyperoderaeum (T)	Definitive host	Intestinal infection. No symptoms	Thailand
5 Eating raw sea fish	*Anisakis* (N)	Paratenic host	Eosinophilic granuloma of bowel	Japan and north Europe
	Haplorchis (T)	Definitive host	Intestinal infection. No symptoms	Hawaii
6 Eating raw freshwater crabs	*Poikilorchis* (T)	Definitive host	Cysts and abscesses of neck	Nigeria and Zaire
7 Eating insects, nymphs, beetles and grubs	*Prosthodendrium molenkampi* (T) *Phaneropsolus bonnei* (T)	Definitive host	Intestinal infection. No symptoms	Thailand
	Plagiorchis (T)	Definitive host	Intestinal infection. No symptoms	Thailand
	Macracanthorhynchus hirudinaceus (N)	Definitive host	Eosinophilic granuloma of bowel	China
	Physaloptera caucasica (N)	Definitive host	Intestinal infection. No symptoms	Central Africa
	Gonglyonema pulchrum (N)	Definitive host	Abscesses in mouth and oesophagus	Central Africa
8 Soil-transmitted	*Oesophagostomum* (N)	Definitive host	Eosinophilic granuloma of bowel	Africa and South America
	Ternidens deminutus (N)	Definitive host	Intestinal infection. No symptoms	Central Africa
9 Water	Free-living amoebae (P)	Definitive host	Meningoencephalitic disease	Worldwide

T = trematode; N = nematode; P = protozoon.
In a *definitive host* the parasite develops to maturity and eggs are laid.
In a *paratenic host* the parasite does not develop further than a second or third stage larva and eggs are not laid.

The cyclops is then eaten by a second intermediate host (freshwater fish, frog or snake), the important species of fish being in Thailand the catfish (*Charias batrachus*) and snake headed fish (*Ophicephalus striatus*),[1] and in Japan *O. argus* and *O. tadianus*. Snakes (rock python, cobra) and frogs are second intermediate hosts in other areas. A third stage larva develops in the second intermediate host and enters the definitive host, a dog or cat, in which it develops into maturity in the stomach. In man, the third stage larva is incapable of developing further. Other paratenic hosts in which the third stage larva is arrested are crabs, other crustacea, amphibia and rodents.

The third stage larva (Fig. II.36A, p. 1349), which is about 1 cm long with a bulbar head armed with hooklets, is very active.

TRANSMISSION

Man is infected by eating inadequately cooked or processed fish containing third stage larvae or raw snakes, frogs or crustaceans, amphibia or

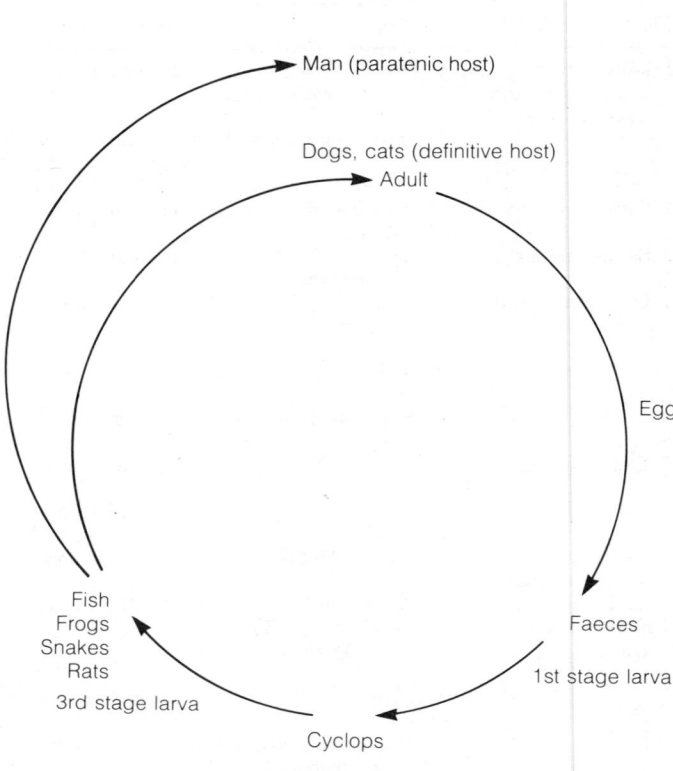

Fig. 24.1　Life-cycle of *Gnathostoma*.

even undercooked chicken. He cannot be infected from swallowing cyclops containing second stage larvae.[2]

PATHOLOGY

Pathology and clinical symptoms and signs may all be caused by one larva. The third stage larva actively migrates from the stomach to the subcutaneous tissues causing subcutaneous tunnels between the germinal layer and corium surrounded by an infiltration of eosinophils and plasma cells causing *larval gnathostomiasis*. If it enters the spinal cord via a nerve root and migrates up to the brain it causes *eosinophilic myeloencephalitis*; blood vessels, especially the subarachnoid, subdural and subventricular vessels, are injured by haemorrhages. Tracks may be visible in the cerebral substance surrounded by an infiltration of eosinophils and lymphocytes. The brain and spinal cord are swollen and congested. Any part of the body or organ may be affected. Granulomatous lesions occur in any organ, especially the liver, and in muscles where they cause abscesses. The eye (*ocular gnathostomiasis*) may be involved with subconjunctival oedema, haemorrhage and retinal damage (Chapter 70). Adult worms and eggs are not found in man.

CLINICAL FEATURES

Natural history

Gnathostomiasis is a prolonged infection, the third stage larva living as long as 10 years. Cerebral gnathostomiasis carries a high mortality.

The *incubation period* may be as short as 24–48 hours after the ingestion of infected material.

Symptoms and signs

Larval gnathostomiasis

This form is characterized by creeping eruption

(larva migrans) and abdominal symptoms. Symptoms start with nausea, vomiting and urticaria with circumscribed oedema of the abdominal wall. These are followed by low-grade fever, right upper quadrant abdominal pain (penetration of liver), pleuritis, and pneumonitis suggesting episodes of acute cholecystitis or pulmonary lesions. Radiographs are suggestive of pulmonary tuberculosis, and there is a hypereosinophilia. These symptoms may be followed by a *creeping eruption* which is characterized by migrating intermittent subcutaneous oedema as the larva moves from one area to another. The episodes of swelling last 7–10 days at intervals of two to six weeks but the larva may persist for as long as 10 years. There is a high peripheral eosinophilia at first which subsides later.

Cerebral gnathostomiasis (eosinophilic myeloencephalitis)

Severe agonizing root pain is followed by paraplegia and sudden loss of sensation often followed by coma or focal cerebral lesions. There is a high fatality rate and many permanent neurological sequelae. The cerebrospinal fluid is bloody, xanthochromic and showing a high eosinophilic pleocytosis.

DIFFERENTIAL DIAGNOSIS

The main differential diagnosis of cerebral gnathostomiasis is from eosinophilic meningitis caused by *Angiostrongylus cantonensis* (p. 564) and other helminths. The diagnostic feature of cerebral gnathostomiasis is the severity of the lesions with coma and paraplegia and bloody xanthochromic cerebrospinal fluid. Larval gnathostomiasis must be distinguished from other causes of creeping eruption, hookworm (see Chapter 21), strongyloidiasis (see Chapter 21), cutaneous myiasis (see Chapter 51), cutaneous paragonimiasis (see Chapter 22) and sparganosis (see Chapter 23). The condition causes oedema resembling calabar swellings (see Chapter 20) rather than truly cutaneous lesions.

DIAGNOSIS

An enzyme-linked immunosorbent assay (ELISA) using a crude water extract of third stage larvae of *G. spinigerum* as antigen has been devised which gave positive results in 100% of parasitologically confirmed cases at a titre of 1/400 or above. The sensitivity (59%) and specificity (84%) were, however, not too satisfactory.[3]

TREATMENT

There is no specific treatment. Quinine sulphate 900 mg daily for four weeks reduced the swelling more quickly than prednisolone and both were more effective than no treatment.[4]

EPIDEMIOLOGY AND CONTROL

The disease occurs in Thailand throughout the year with a variable monthly incidence. Cats and dogs are important reservoirs for human infection. Infection can be prevented by sterilization of fish by boiling or immersion in vinegar for four and a half hours, and chickens should be well cooked rather than lightly toasted.

Pentastomids (tongue worms)
(see also Appendix III)

The pentastomids are neither helminths nor typical arthropods. They form a group of parasites of uncertain origin. The adult body is annular but not segmented, the larvae or nymphs are stumpy and have four legs each with a bifurcated claw. The adults live in the respiratory passages of reptiles, birds and mammals and the females lay eggs which are discharged in the respiratory mucus. After ingestion by another host the first stage larvae migrate to the liver, spleen and lymph glands where they are transformed into nymphs which become encapsulated and calcified. Two genera may infect man as a dead-end infection: *Linguatula*, which normally infects other mammals, and *Armillifer* (*Porocephalus*), which normally infects snakes. *Linguatula* is contracted from mammals while *Armillifer* is contracted from eating raw python meat.

LINGUATULA SERRATA

Geographical distribution

L. serrata is found worldwide.

Morphology

The body of the adult linguatula (Fig. 24.2) is somewhat pear-shaped, flattened and transversely striated with about 90 rings; the mouth is quadrangular with two pairs of simple, retractile

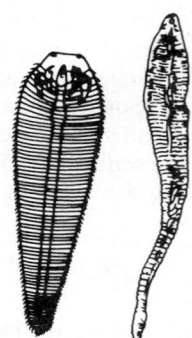

Fig. 24.2　*Linguatula serrata*. Left, nymph, × 6. Right, adult, natural size.

hooks laterally. The female is 80–130 mm in length, grey in colour but with reddish-brown eggs visible through the median line of the body, the body tapering from 8–10 mm anteriorly to 2 mm posteriorly. The male is white, 18–20 mm long and 3 mm broad anteriorly to 0.5 mm posteriorly. The eggs are avoid and 99 μm in length by 70 μm in breadth. They contain mature embryos which hatch into first stage larvae; these are stumpy and have four 'legs' which each bear a bifurcate claw. The nymphs (Fig. 24.2) are worm-like and 4–6 mm in length; they have distinctive spines arranged in transverse rows at the posterior margin of each annulus. These are sufficient to distinguish *Linguatula* spp. in any tissue section.

Life-cycle

The adults live in the nasal passages of mammals, especially dogs, foxes and wolves. These are the definitive hosts. Eggs are passed in the nasal mucus, saliva and faeces and hatch in the gut of the intermediate host, rodents, domestic animals such as sheep and goats. The first stage larva emerges, penetrates the gut wall and migrates to the viscera, where it moults, eventually forming an infective larva or nymph and becomes encysted. The definitive host is infected by ingesting viscera containing the encysted infective stage.

Transmission

Man is infected in two ways.
1　*Ingestion of eggs* from food contaminated by the respiratory mucus of a mammal, in which case the nymphs encyst in various tissues of the body forming *cysts*.
2　*Ingestion of nymphs*. Nymphs are transmitted from raw sheep's or goat's liver or lymph glands to man. The nymphs migrate up from the stomach to attach themselves to the throat and nasopharynx to cause halzoun.[5,6]

Pathology

Encysted larvae are well tolerated and are frequently met with in the mesenteric glands of domestic animals as well as rabbits and hares. They have been found in 4.6% of human livers where they appear to cause no symptoms. Occasionally single cysts in certain locations may obstruct bile ducts or bronchi or cause cerebral compression. When they enter the anterior chamber of the eye they may cause glaucoma (see Chapter 70). In tissue sections the linguatula presents a well-defined body cavity which contains an intestinal tract and distinctive reproductive organs. The muscle fibres are striated and the spines on the cuticle are distinctive. These characteristics will serve to distinguish from sparganum (Fig. 23.40, p. 555).

Clinical features

Cysts

Cysts cause little trouble and are usually asymptomatic being found only when the calcified cysts show up on an X-ray.

Nymphs

Halzoun (parasitic pharyngitis, marrara syndrome in the Sudan). As early as several hours after eating infected tissues there is pain and itching in the throat, paroxysmal coughing and sneezing, and lacrimal and nasal discharge. Often there is hoarseness, dyspnoea, dysphagia and vomiting, less frequently haemoptysis and temporary loss of hearing. There may be enlargement of the submaxillary and cervical lymph glands. The disease is self-limiting, with spontaneous recovery within a week or 10 days. Very occasionally death has been recorded by asphyxiation, possibly caused by a sensitivity reaction. Cases of recurrent epistaxis have occurred as a result of an adult Linguatula in the nose.

Diagnosis

Diagnosis is by biopsy when the characteristic structure can be seen or by the 1 cm opacities on X-ray of muscular tissues.

Treatment

There is no treatment. Halzoun is a self-limiting disease but parasites may have to be removed surgically from the eye.

ARMILLIFER (POROCEPHALUS)

Geographical distribution

Armillifer armillatus infects humans in tropical Africa; *Armillifer moniliformis* causes human infections in Malaysia, Java, Manila, Sumatra and China.

Aetiology

The adult parasite is found in the lungs of pythons and other snakes, the larval and nymphal forms in many mammals, including monkeys and

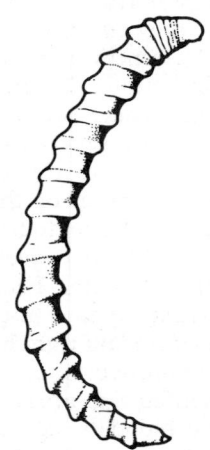

Fig. 24.3 *Armillifer armillatus*, natural size.

man. The parasite is cylindrical, vermiform, yellowish and translucent with conspicuous, opaque annulated rings around the body, 1–2 mm apart (Fig. 24.3). The female of *A. armillatus* is 90–130 mm long and 5–9 mm wide, the male 30–45 mm long and 3–4 mm wide. *A. moniliformis* is more slender and has more rings (26 and above) than *A. armillatus*. The nymphs lie coiled within their cysts, with the ventral surface corresponding to the convexity of the curve. In shape and structure they resemble the adult. A third species of *Armillifer* (*A. grandis*) has been reported from man in central Africa where the nymphs are smaller (9–15 mm long) than those of *A. armillatus* (13–23 mm long).

Life-cycle

The life-cycle of *Armillifer* is similar to that of *Linguatula*, although man can act only as the intermediate host. The ingested eggs hatch in the intestine and the larvae bore through the wall to lodge in any tissue, where they moult over a period of six months to a year to form infective nymphs. Man acquires the infection by eating poorly cooked snake meat or by drinking water contaminated by snakes. In man the infection comes to a dead end and the larvae or nymphs encyst on the surface of the liver, in the intestinal mucosa, peritoneal cavity or lungs. Calcification may take place in the liver and other organs.

Transmission

Man acquires infection by eating raw python meat or other snakes or drinking water contaminated by snakes.

Clinical features

Usually the infection is asymptomatic and infection of man has been found in 33 of 133 postmortems in Zaire and in 45% of Malaysian aborigines. A large number of parasites were found within the lumen of the small intestine and encysted in the lungs as well as the liver. Pathological changes occur around the dead parasites and vary from very little reaction around live parasites to the formation of a necrotic granulomatous reaction followed by fibrosis and calcification round the dead parasites. These may be seen on X-ray pictures as characteristic horseshoe- or crescent-shaped bodies. The parasite has appeared under the bulbar conjunctiva (Fig. 70.16, p. 1172) and caused intestinal obstruction, pneumonitis, meningitis, pericarditis, nephritis and obstructive jaundice. A blood eosinophilia occurs, especially after death of the larva. A highly significant number (*p* < 0.001) of *Armillifer* infections are associated with malignancy.[40]

Treatment

Treatment is usually not necessary. There is no chemotherapy available.

Fibricola seoulensis (T)

This is a trematode worm normally found in Korea in the intestines of rats with a snail as first intermediate host and a frog (*Rana nigromaculata*) and its tadpole as secondary intermediate hosts. Many land snakes which eat frogs are paratenic hosts. Man is infected by eating raw frogs or snakes, the metacercariae developing into adults in the small intestine, and large operculated eggs are passed in the stools. Most infections are asymptomatic but abdominal pain, diarrhoea and eosinophilia may result. Praziquantel is effective in treatment.[7]

2   SNAILS AND SLUGS
Angiostrongyliasis (N)

Angiostrongyliasis is the result of infection of man with a rodent nematode worm of which rodents are the definitive host and slugs and snails intermediate hosts. Two species can infect man as an abnormal definitive host but cannot complete their development. *Angiostrongylus cantonensis* normally occupies the pulmonary artery of rodents but needs a period of migration to the brain first. It causes eosinophilic meningitis in man. *Angiostrongylus costaricensis* normally occupies the mesenteric artery of rodents and needs a preliminary period of development in the lymphatic vessels of the abdominal cavity. It causes abdominal angiostrongyliasis in man.

ANGIOSTRONGYLUS CANTONENSIS (EOSINOPHILIC MENINGITIS)

Geographical distribution

First described from Ponape in the western Pacific[8] *A. cantonensis* was first recovered from the human brain in Hawaii.[9] Human infection is now known to occur in most islands of the western Pacific, New Caledonia, Micronesia, New Hebrides, Cook Islands, Tahiti, Hawaii and, more recently, Papua New Guinea,[10,11] Samoa,[12] Okinawa and southern Japan,[13] Thailand, Vietnam, Cambodia, Sumatra, Philippines and Taiwan.

Aetiology and life-cycle (Fig. 24.4)

The adult worms, male (15.5–22.0 × 0.25–0.35 mm) and female (18.5–33 × 0.28–0.5 mm), are transparent, smooth nematode worms with faint transverse striae. They live in the pulmonary artery of rodents and have a complicated life-cycle involving slugs and the central nervous system of rodents (see Appendix II, p. 1355).

Definitive host (rodent, man)

After ingestion of the slug by the rodent the infective larvae pass from the stomach as far as the ileum where they enter the bloodstream and congregate in the central nervous system some 17 hours after ingestion. The anterior cerebrum is the normal site where the third moult takes place on the sixth and seventh days and a final moult on the eleventh to thirteenth day. The young adult worms emerge on the surface of the brain from the twelfth to fourteenth day and spread out over the next two weeks on the arachnoid surface of the brain. From the twenty-eighth to thirty-first day they migrate to the lung via the venous system and right heart where they inhabit their definitive site, the pulmonary artery. Unsegmented eggs are laid which are discharged into the bloodstream and lodge in the small pulmonary arteries. Here they hatch into first stage larvae which break into the respiratory

Angiostrongylus

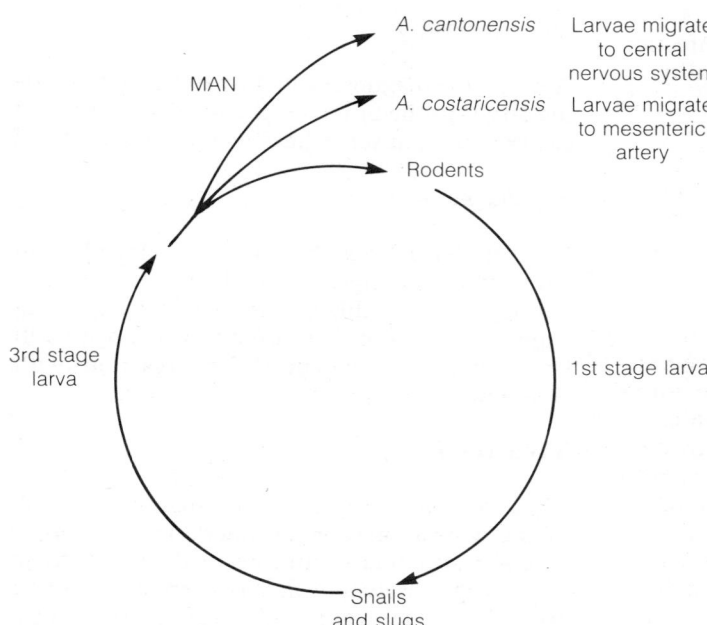

Fig. 24.4 Life-cycle of *Angiostrongylus*.

tract, migrate up the trachea and down the oeso-phagus to pass out into the faeces where they penetrate into, or are ingested by, the inter-mediate host—land snails, slugs and aquatic snails—the normal host being the slug, *Agrio-limax leavis*. The whole cycle and prepatent period in the rodent host is 42–45 days.

Intermediate host (slug, snail)

In the intermediate host two stages of develop-ment occur resulting in a third stage infective larva after 17 days.

Transmission

Man is not a normal host and is infected when he eats third stage infective larvae in the normal intermediate hosts (snails and slugs) or in other crustacea which are not normal but paratenic hosts (crabs, prawns and land planarians) which have not been correctly cooked.

Pathology

Since *A. cantonensis* larvae pass to the brain,

meningitis and meningoencephalitis are the main pathological effects. The pathological changes are caused by dead and degenerating worms. Larvae can be recognized in brain tissue, the subarachnoid space and spinal cord. Numerous tracks and microcavities can be seen[14] sur-rounded by a cellular reaction of lymphocytes, plasma cells and eosinophils with occasional giant cells.[15] Tissue necrosis occurs round the dead worms.[9] In the meninges there is a diffuse eosinophilic infiltration of the meninges with many Charcot–Leyden crystals. Larvae have been recovered from the eye where lesions may cause visual impairment and blindness. In a few cases dead almost adult worms have been found in the pulmonary vessels.

Immunity

There is no immunity to reinfection and second and third attacks have occurred. During infec-tion an immediate hypersensitivity develops which can be demonstrated with skin tests, and humoral antibodies appear. However, there is little specificity with present antigens and cross reactions with other helminths occur.

Clinical features

Natural history

Angiostrongyliasis is a self-limiting infection lasting four to six weeks with a low mortality.

Incubation period

This is short, usually 6–15 days, but in an outbreak recorded in Samoa, was 1–6 days.[12]

Symptoms and signs

The disease is of relatively short duration, four to six weeks, and self-limiting with a case mortality of less than 0.5%. Acute severe intermittent occipital or bitemporal headache is the main and most significant symptom with neck stiffness and paraesthesiae of the limbs in 50% of cases. Fever is uncommon and no neurological findings were present in 58% of cases, while 16% of patients showed visual impairment and 12% an abnormal fundus. Ocular angiostrongyliasis can lead to visual impairment and blindness and iritis, keratitis,[11] vitreous haemorrhages and retinal detachment are serious complications (see Chapter 70). In some there is impairment of the sensorium of a slowly progressive type, and weakness of the limbs without any localization can occur. Involvement of the cranial nerves is found in about one-fifth of the cases, facial nerve and external rectus palsy being the commonest. There is usually a peripheral eosinophilia and the cerebrospinal fluid is characteristically turbid with a cell count of 500/mm^3 with 50–70% eosinophils in the majority of cases.[16] Sequelae are rare but may persist for many years and 3% of patients in Tahiti showed a residual facial palsy.[9]

Differential diagnosis

Any patient in South-East Asia or the Pacific exhibiting a brain syndrome with a peripheral and cerebrospinal eosinophilia should be suspected of angiostrongyliasis. Other helminthic causes are gnathostomiasis, paragonimiasis (see Chapter 22), coenurus cerebralis (see Chapter 23), hydatid of the brain (see Chapter 23), *Schistosoma japonicum* (see Chapter 22), ascariasis, trichinosis and disseminated strongyloidiasis (see Chapter 21). An eosinophilic pleocytosis in the cerebrospinal fluid strongly suggests angiostrongyliasis or gnathostomiasis.

Diagnosis

A definitive diagnosis can only be made by finding larvae in the brain, cerebrospinal fluid or eye (where they can sometimes be seen moving).

Serodiagnosis

An intradermal test has been developed from adult worm antigen and if negative angiostrongyliasis is unlikely.[17] An ELISA test using angiostrongylus antigen gave positive results in 96% of cases in Thailand.[18] Cross reactions with *Gnathostoma* sp. could not be ruled out.

Treatment

Since the pathology is caused mainly by death of the worms there is considerable doubt as to whether attempts should be made to kill them with drugs. *Mebendazole* has been shown to be 100% effective against all stages in rats[19] in a single dose of 20 mg/kg body weight. The headache can be controlled temporarily by removal of 10 ml of cerebrospinal fluid. Marked amelioration of symptoms has been achieved with 30 mg daily of prednisone.[20]

Epidemiology

The rodents known at present as final hosts of *A. cantonensis* in nature are those of the genera, *Rattus*, *Melomys* and *Bandicota*[21] which have been found infected in most islands of the western Pacific, Queensland, South-East Asia, Indo-China and some islands off the East African coast. So far no infected rodents have been found on the African continent. In the western Pacific the infection is associated with the presence of the giant African snail *Achatina fulica* and evidence suggests that angiostrongyliasis is a relatively new infection in the Pacific having been introduced as a result of the spread of *Achatina fulica* to this area.[22]

The method of infection varies in different areas of the Pacific according to the local cultural customs. In Tahiti raw freshwater prawns are consumed at feasts in special sauces from March to June which is the season of maximum incidence, and small epidemics may occur.[17] In New Caledonia the disease is acquired by eating land planaria or small molluscs on raw vegetables and the maximum incidence is during the vegetable season, June to November. Elsewhere the disease is sporadic; in Micronesia infection may have occurred as a result of eating certain species of mangrove crabs.[21] Males and females are affected equally except under the age of 15 when twice as many males as females are affected. Eosinophilic meningitis is prevalent and widely distributed in Thailand. Twice as many males are infected as females. Most have eaten 'pila' (snail) within 30 days and there is a seasonal incidence varying with rainfall.[23]

Prevention and control

Infected slugs and snails may be demonstrated by mincing them with scissors and digesting the material overnight with pepsin at 25–28°C. The larvae recovered from this material are used to inoculate white rats and the faeces are examined for first stage larvae after 40–60 days. Later the rats may be killed and the pulmonary arteries examined for adult worms.

Control methods should include public education into the manner of spread of the infection, proper cooking or freezing of crustaceans (−15°C for 12 hours) and proper washing and inspection of vegetables intended to be eaten raw.[21]

ANGIOSTRONGYLUS COSTARICENSIS (ABDOMINAL ANGIOSTRONGYLIASIS) (N)

Geographical distribution

A. costaricensis has been found in humans from Mexico to Brazil.

Aetiology and life-cycle[24]

A. costaricensis closely resembles *A. cantonensis* in morphology but its life-cycle is different. The adult worm lives in the mesenteric arteries of naturally infected rodents, mainly the cotton rat (*Sigmodon hispidus*) and the black rat (*Rattus rattus*) and further development takes place in a slug (*vaginulus plebeius*).

Definitive host (rodent, man)

The infective third stage larva from an ingested slug enters the intestine at the level of the lower ileum and caecum from where it migrates to the lymphatic vessels of the abdominal cavity. Here two moults take place before the young adult migrates to the mesenteric arteries where it matures. Eggs are laid in the intestinal wall and first stage larvae hatch out to penetrate the wall and pass out into the faeces where they infect slugs either by ingestion or penetration. The prepatent period is 24 days. Man is not a normal host but can act as a definitive host and adults and eggs can be found in human tissues but no infective stage larvae develop.

Intermediate host (slug)

After infection from rodent faeces, complete maturation from first to third stage larva takes from 16 to 19 days. The third stage larvae are then ingested by the definitive host.

Transmission

The slug discharges third stage larvae in its secretions so that contamination of green vegetables which are eaten raw is the cause of human infection.

Pathology

Lesions mostly occur in the ileocaecal region where they cause an eosinophilic granuloma. Ectopic lesions can affect the liver, abdominal lymph glands and testicles. The adult worms may cause thrombosis and necrosis of the intestinal walls but the main lesion is an eosinophilic granuloma. Scattered eggs may be seen in other tissues where they produce a granuloma surrounded by lymphocytes, plasma cells and eosinophils.

Symptoms and signs

The main symptoms are pain in the right iliac fossa and flank. There may be fever, vomiting and anorexia. A mass may be felt in the right iliac fossa. Ectopic sites for the worms and eggs are the liver where lesions resembling visceral larva migrans may be produced[25] and spermatic artery thrombosis with necrosis of the testicle. There is a peripheral leukocytosis of $15–50 \times 10^9$/litre with 10–80% eosinophils.

Differential diagnosis

Other causes of an eosinophilic granuloma of the bowel are *Trichuris* (see Chapter 21), oesophagostoma (see p. 571), schistosomiasis japonicum (see Chapter 22) and visceral larva migrans of toxocariasis (see Chapter 21). Diagnosis from amoeboma, carcinoma, tuberculosis, appendicitis and Crohn's disease should be made by the absence of eosinophilia in these conditions.

Diagnosis

Eggs and larvae do not appear in the stool and an ELISA test is not generally available.

Treatment

Mebendazole in a single dose of 20 mg/kg body weight should be tried.

Epidemiology

Rodent infections have been found from Texas to southern Brazil.[24] The definitive host are five species of rodents: cotton rat (*Sigmodon hispidus*), black rat (*Rattus rattus*), *Zigodontomys microtinus*, *Leomys adspersus* and *Oryzomys fulvescens*.[26] Fresh raw green vegetables should be well washed with disinfectant.

Hyperoderaeum conoideum (T)

H. conoideum is normally a parasite of birds including ducks, geese and fowl. Intermediate hosts include many land snails. Man is infected by eating raw snails. It is a common intestinal infection of man in Thailand, where it causes no symptoms.

3   RAW FISH
Anisakiasis (herring worm) (N)

Anisakiasis is caused by the larval stages of worms, the adult stages of which inhabit the intestinal tract of marine mammals and less commonly fish. Man ingests these larvae as third stage larvae with the flesh of certain salt-water fish and acts as a paratenic host, harbouring only the third stage larvae.

GEOGRAPHICAL DISTRIBUTION

Anisakiasis is found wherever fish are eaten raw, undercooked, salted or pickled, as in Japan,[27] Holland and California.[28]

AETIOLOGY

Adult anisakids (round worms) which are found in the intestinal canal of marine animals and some fish are of three genera: *Anisakis* (Japan and Holland), *Phocanema* (North America) and *Contracaecum* (Appendix II, p. 1350).

Life-cycle

The adults live in the intestinal canal of marine

mammals, seals, porpoises, whales and dolphins. Eggs are passed in the faeces which hatch in water liberating second stage larvae which are ingested by many forms of crustacea (krill) in which third stage larvae develop. When the crustacea are eaten by fish third stage larvae are released but undergo no further development and encyst, invading body cavities and muscles, and are carried passively (transport host) until the fish is eaten by a mammal when the third stage larvae develop into adults in marine mammals, but not in man. One case where an adult was recovered from a human has been reported.[28]

TRANSMISSION

Man is infected by third stage larvae from raw fish ('sushi' and 'sashemi' in Japan) and 'green' herrings in Holland.

PATHOLOGY

Larvae attach to the mucosa of the bowel which

may ulcerate or they may penetrate the bowel wall giving rise to extraintestinal infection. They may invade the mesentery, omentum or pancreas causing lesions from well-developed abscesses to eosinophilic granulomas, when they die.

CLINICAL FEATURES

Natural history

Anisakiasis is a self-limiting infection of a few weeks with a low mortality.

The incubation period is within 12 hours of eating the infected material.

Symptoms and signs

The infection is essentially self-limiting as the larvae die. Nausea, vomiting, epigastric pain and haematemesis may result. Eosinophilic lesions of the bowel and intestinal obstruction are the main features. Peritonitis and death may result.[29] There is a peripheral eosinophilia.

DIFFERENTIAL DIAGNOSIS

Anisakiasis of the bowel resembles Crohn's disease and patients often undergo laparotomy.

Other causes of eosinophilic granuloma of the bowel are *Angiostrongylus costaricensis* (see above), *Ascaris* (see Chapter 21), *Oesophagostomum* (see below) and *Strongyloides* (see Chapter 21).

DIAGNOSIS

Diagnosis is difficult. A definitive diagnosis can be made by identifying larval worms in the vomit or biopsy material. Surgical specimens of bowel showing eosinophilic infiltration should be suspect. Serology is not helpful.

TREATMENT

There is no specific treatment.

EPIDEMIOLOGY AND CONTROL

Wherever raw or undercooked fish is eaten as a result of ethnic eating habits, anisakiasis may occur. Proper cooking or pickling of fish will prevent the disease. Freezing herrings at sea has eliminated the disease in Holland.

Haplorchis yokogawi (T) and *H. taichui* (T)

These are trematode worms which normally parasitize dogs. Man is infected from eating raw mullet containing metacercariae. It causes an intestinal infection. Eggs have been found in the spinal cord and heart.

4 RAW CRABS

POIKILORCHIS CONGOLENSIS (T)

P. congolensis is a fluke which causes postauricular cysts and abscesses in man and has been mistaken for *Paragonimus*. Cases have been recorded from Zaire, Nigeria[30] and Sarawak.[31] The eggs which are found in the discharges resemble those of *Paragonimus* but are smaller (60–68 × 38–41 μm).

5 INSECTS

PROSTHODENDRIUM MOLENKAMPI (T) AND PHANEROPSOLUS BONNEI (T)

The normal hosts of *Prosthodendrium molenkampi* are rats and bats, and of *Phaneropsolus bonnei*, monkeys.

Adult worms live in the intestine. Eggs are passed out in the stools and infect water snails. The cercariae which emerge are captured rectally by dragonfly nymphs (naiads). These nymphs are caught and swallowed raw as a delicacy in the rice fields in Thailand where they are numerous. In man the infection becomes patent. In one sample of 24 people 58% were passing eggs of *Prostodendrium* and 63% of the same sample *Phaneropsolus* in the stools.[32] There were no apparent clinical ill effects.

PLAGIORCHIS JAVANENSIS AND P. PHILIPPINENSIS (T)

Plagiorchis is a trematode, normally a parasite of birds, amphibia and bats. Man is infected by eating grubs containing metacercariae. It causes an intestinal infection.

MACRACANTHORHYNCHUS HIRUDINACEUS (N)

M. hirudinaceus is a nematode worm normally found in the small intestine of pigs, dogs and monkeys in China. Eggs are passed in the stool and taken up by beetles in which an infective stage forms. Man is infected by eating beetles taken as a cure for asthma. In man the adult worms attach themselves to the intestinal mucosa of the small bowel, the eggs are not passed in the stool but penetrate the bowel wall and deposit on the peritoneum. The results may be severe with intestinal perforation, intussusception, peritonitis and abscess formation. There is an eosinophilia. Treatment with tetramisole 3 mg/kg or praziquantel is satisfactory.[33]

PHYSALOPTERA CAUCASICA (N)

Normal hosts are monkeys. In man it has been found in central Africa, Mozambique, Uganda and Malawi. It lives in the oesophagus, stomach, small intestine and occasionally the liver.

The female (2.4–10 cm $\times$ 1.14–2.8 mm) has a posterior end tapering to a sharp point, two ovaries, a single uterine tube and a vulva in the anterior part of the body. The male (1.4–5 cm $\times$ 0.7–1 mm) has two lateral alae on the tail, formed by expansion of the cuticle, four pairs of pedunculated papillae—six pairs sessile—one unpaired postanal papilla and two spicules of unequal length. In both sexes the mouth is guarded by two large lips, armed with two papillae and rows of teeth, which serve to grip the mucous membrane (Fig. II.37, p. 1350).

The egg ($45 \times 35\,\mu$m) has a double contour, smooth, thick, colourless shell.

The life-cycle is unknown; insects possibly act as intermediaries. The clinical symptoms are indeterminate. The worms live with heads embedded in the digestive tract from the oesophagus to the ileum.

GONGLYONEMA PULCHRUM (N)

This is a spirurate nematode of a genus in which there are six species. It is a rare infection in man and pig but ruminants are the optimum hosts.

The worm lives most commonly in the upper portion of the digestive tract where it forms sinuous galleries in the mucosa and submucosa of the oesophagus, buccal cavity and tongue. The male is 62×0.15–0.3 mm and the female much larger, 145×0.2–0.5 mm. The anterior extremity is covered with a variable number of bosses arranged in eight longitudinal series.

The transparent thick-shelled oval eggs are embryonated when laid and are 50–$70\,\mu$m in length by 25–$37\,\mu$m. Development takes place in dung beetles of genera *Apodius* and *Onthophagus*, as well as in a small cockroach. About ten human cases are recorded in tongue, mouth and oesophagus, mostly in the southern USA. One was recorded from the lower lip of a man in Georgia.[34] Treatment is to remove the worm from its tunnel; antiseptic mouthwashes or novocain applied locally help to extrude it.

6 SOIL-TRANSMITTED

Some soil-transmitted nematodes, normally parasites of monkeys, baboons and apes, infect man when he ingests soil contaminated with their eggs. Normal development occurs in man and eggs are passed in the stool.

Oesophagostomum spp.

GEOGRAPHICAL DISTRIBUTION

Oesophagostomum spp. are widely distributed throughout the tropical and neotropical world.

AETIOLOGY

There are two species: *Oesophagostomum apiostomum*, normally parasites of monkeys in Africa, Philippines and China, and *Oesophagostomum stephanostomum*, found in monkeys in Brazil, French Guiana and West Africa.

The adult worms inhabit the caecum and colon of primates where they lie free attached to the lumen or encysted under the mucosa of the bowel. They have a mouth and oesophagus and the male (0.8–1 cm × 0.35 mm) a copulatory bursa and the female (1 cm × 0.325 mm) a vulva (Fig. II.47, p. 1354). The egg, which measures $60 \times 40\,\mu$m, closely resembles that of hookworm but is passed in man in an advanced stage of development which may lead to its recognition.

Life-cycle

The eggs are passed out in the faeces and hatch in the soil into *rhabditiform* larvae. These develop into infective *filariform* larvae which, after being swallowed by a new host, pass through the stomach to the caecum and colon where they invade the mucosa to form submucosal cysts, later to re-enter the lumen of the bowel and attach themselves to the mucosa as adults.

PATHOLOGY AND CLINICAL FEATURES

Transmission is via contaminated water and soil. In man the worms cause *eosinophilic granuloma* of the bowel which may be found in the ileocaecal region.[35] In the colon the submucosal forms may cause polyposis with dysentery or the larvae may penetrate the bowel wall and cause peritonitis. Adult worms cause no symptoms and have been found in 4% of prisoners in jails in the north of Nigeria.

DIAGNOSIS

The egg is difficult to distinguish from that of hookworm but the almost fully formed larva inside the shell should lead to suspicion.

TREATMENT

Albendazole, mebendazole and thiabendazole should prove effective.

Ternidens deminutus (N)

GEOGRAPHICAL DISTRIBUTION

T. deminutus is found in Malawi, Mozambique, Zimbabwe and northern Transvaal.

AETIOLOGY

T. deminutus normally inhabits the small intestine of monkeys and baboons in Africa and Asia. Both male and female resemble female hookworms. The anterior extremity is straight, terminating in a mouth capsule guarded by three serrated teeth. The male (9.5 × 0.73 mm) has a branching copulatory bursa (Fig. II.48, p. 1355) and the female (14–16 × 0.73 mm) a posterior genital opening leading to two uterine tubes. The egg ($84 \times 40\,\mu$m) is transparent and when segmented resembles that of hookworm but is larger.

The *life-cycle* is similar to that of hookworm. The eggs hatch in the soil into rhabditiform larvae and then into infective filariform larvae which are drought resistant, resisting desiccation and reviving with water. These are ingested with soil-contaminated food, or contaminated water to pass into the small intestine where the adults attach themselves to the mucosa.

PATHOLOGY AND CLINICAL FEATURES

Normally it is non-pathogenic and eggs are not uncommonly found in the faeces of man in central Africa. If present in large numbers there may be some abdominal symptoms.

DIAGNOSIS

The egg is difficult to distinguish from that of hookworm, which is slightly smaller ($60 \times 40\,\mu$m).

TREATMENT

Both mebendazole and thiabendazole are effective in treatment. Reports on albendazole are awaited.

7 WATER: INFECTION CAUSED BY FREE-LIVING AMOEBAE (P)

Amoebae living a non-parasitic life in stagnant water may under certain circumstances infect man. These are the free-living amoebae. They are of two groups: *Naegleria* and *Hartmanella* (*Acanthamoeba*).

Naegleria infection[36] (primary amoebic meningoencephalitis)

GEOGRAPHICAL DISTRIBUTION

Since the first published cases in 1965[37] cases have been reported from Australia, New Zealand, the USA, Czechoslovakia, Great Britain, India and Africa.[36]

AETIOLOGY

Most of the human infections, though not all, have been caused by *Naegleria fowleri*, which has been isolated from streams, ponds, lakes and indoor swimming pools where the water is warm.

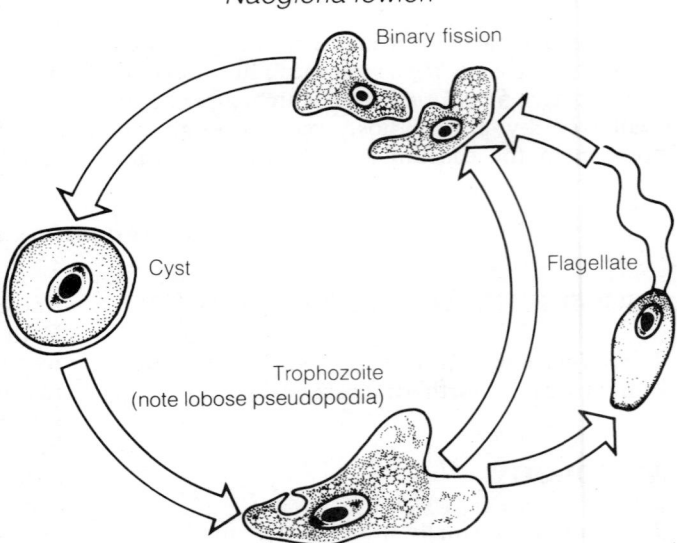

Fig. 24.5 Life-cycle of *Naegleria fowleri*. (Courtesy Dr D. C. Warhurst.)

The related *N. gruberi* is generally thought to be non-pathogenic. *N. fowleri* has an amoeboid and a free-swimming flagellate stage. The *trophozoite* (amoeboid stage) (Fig. 24.5) averages $22 \times 7 \, \mu m$ in size and moves rapidly in wet preparations by means of a wave-like extension of a single anterior pseudopod (slug-like or *Limax* movement). It divides by binary fission to form cysts. On transferring from a wet preparation to distilled water it assumes a *flagellate* (Fig. 24.5) free-swimming form which eventually resumes the amoeboid form. *N. fowleri* can be distinguished from *N. gruberi* on electron microscopy when the mitochondria are dumbbell-shaped rather than oval as in *N. gruberi*. The *cyst* is $9 \, \mu m$ in diameter and does not form large numbers in culture. *N. fowleri* can be distinguished from *Acanthamoeba* by its more rapid movement, a temporary flagellate stage and rounded cysts. *Acanthamoeba* (Fig. 24.6) has acanthapoda, moves much more slowly, there is no flagellate stage and the cysts are not round but are angular and double walled (Fig. 24.6).

have been isolated from air and from nasal swabs taken from children in northern Nigeria during the harmattan (dry, dusty wind).

PATHOLOGY

Infection occurs via the olfactory tract and infection of the brain is direct; haematogenous spread does not occur in man. *Macroscopically* the olfactory mucosa is inflamed and the brain and spinal cord infected and opaque. The main changes are found around the cribriform plate and olfactory bulbs.

Microscopically a thin fibrinopurulent meningitis is found throughout the brain and spinal cord. Amoebae can be identified in the exudate (cysts are not found in the brain) sparsely dispersed in macrophages in the deep perivascular spaces clustered around blood vessels with little inflammatory response. In the brain the amoebae are distributed superficially in the grey matter underlying the meninges where they elicit little

Acanthamoeba (Hartmannella)

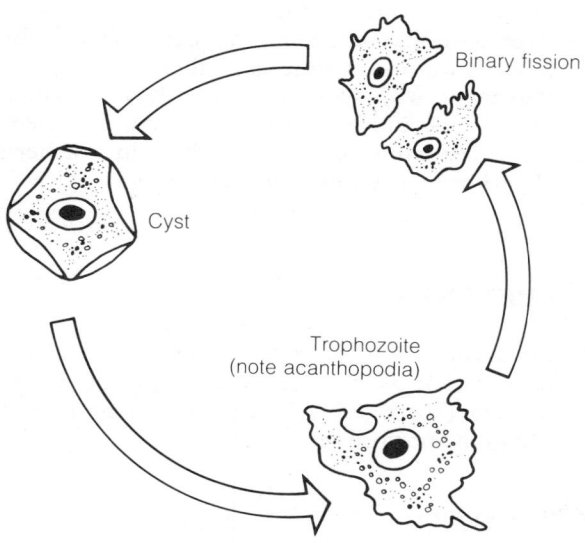

Fig. 24.6 Life-cycle of *Acanthamoeba* (*Hartmannella*). (Courtesy Dr D. C. Warhurst.)

TRANSMISSION

Infection is via the intranasal route. Usually only the trophozoites are infective and only a few amoebae from infected water are required for infection to take place. Inhalation of cysts is possible but improbable although *N. fowleri* cysts

inflammatory response, but in some cases there is purulent and haemorrhagic disruption of the brain.

IMMUNITY

N. fowleri is not opportunist, patients have a

normal immune response and are otherwise healthy. They do not appear to develop any immune response to the amoebae.

CLINICAL FEATURES

Natural history

Naegleria attacks healthy persons causing an acute disease of short duration terminated by death in 5–6 days from a progressive purulent meningoencephalitis.

The *incubation period* is around 3–7 days.

Symptoms and signs

The *onset* is acute in previously healthy young children and adults. A sore throat and rhinitis have been prominent in some cases but not all. This is followed by headache, vomiting and neck rigidity and a condition resembling a fulminating bacterial meningitis with death in 5–6 days.

DIAGNOSIS

The diagnosis is from bacterial meningitis. Suspicion should be aroused when the cerebrospinal fluid is purulent with no bacteria. In such cases a wet drop preparation should be made. The cerebrospinal fluid should be shaken before examination but not centrifuged or refrigerated. The amoebae are easily seen and recognized by their slug-like movement. Confirmation is obtained by the examination of stained specimens when the typical *Limax* nucleus with a large central nucleolus and fine nuclear membrane can be identified (Fig. 24.5). Any amoeboid cell seen in the cerebrospinal fluid should be regarded with suspicion. Immunofluorescent staining is a useful aid to retrospective diagnosis in tissue sections. Amoebae may be cultured in a liquid medium.[38]

TREATMENT

The results of treatment have on the whole been disappointing. The only drug that has shown some promise is *Amphotericin B* in one patient who recovered completely. Amphotericin B was given in high dosage (1 mg/kg/day). Amoebae were still present in the cerebrospinal fluid 5 days later although the drug was given intrathecally and intraventricularly. Amphotericin B and miconazole were given intravenously and intrathecally and rifampicin orally in the successful treatment of a young girl from whose cerebrospinal fluid *N. fowleri* had been cultured.[39] Corticosteroids should not be given.[34] High doses of metronidazole have not yet been tried. As other regimens have been so disappointing it would be reasonable to try huge doses of metronidazole orally or intravenously if necessary; up to 10 g daily have been used in tumour therapy.

EPIDEMIOLOGY

Most, although not all, infections have been associated with bathing in streams, ponds or lakes and indoor swimming baths where the water is warm. In some cases there has been no association with swimming or with water, and a death occurred from primary meningoencephalitis in a young child in northern Nigeria who had not been swimming.

PREVENTION

To ensure the destruction of cysts superchlorination is necessary; 2 p.p.m. of active chlorine (at pH 7.2–7.3) should be used at least 30 minutes before the bath is used.

Acanthamoeba infection

GEOGRAPHICAL DISTRIBUTION

Acanthamoeba infection occurs sporadically worldwide but is much rarer than *Naegleria*.

AETIOLOGY

Two species are responsible: *A. castellani* and *A.* *polyphaga*. Both are opportunist infections. The *trophozoite* has a rough exterior (Fig. 24.6) with several projections (acanthopoda) which move slowly. The cysts are not round and have a wrinkled surface with pores (Fig. 24.6). Dry cysts can survive for several years and can be regularly isolated from dust and the air. There is no free-living stage.

TRANSMISSION

The method of transmission is not known but is not due to contact with water.

PATHOLOGY

In the *brain* the lesions are essentially focal. There 'are multiple areas of granulomatous inflammation with lymphocytes, plasma cells, epithelioid cells and giant cells, mainly in the thalamus, pons or corpus callosum. In *ocular* infections the cornea is ulcerated and destroyed and a purulent exudate appears in the anterior and posterior chambers with uveitis. Amoebic cysts as well as trophozoites are found in the tissues. The trophozoites are indistinguishable from those of *N. fowleri* and identification is made with fluorescent staining.

IMMUNITY

Acanthamoeba infection of the brain is only found in people who have been immunosuppressed with drugs.

CLINICAL FEATURES

Natural history

In immunocompromised people *Acanthamoeba* causes chronic progressive brain disease with focal brain damage and death after weeks or months. In normal people it can cause corneal ulcers and keratitis.

The *incubation period* is more than 7 days.

Symptoms and signs

The usual picture is that of single or multiple brain abscesses. Headache occurs and fever is present, focal epileptiform attacks occur and midbrain lesions are common. The cerebrospinal fluid shows a mononuclear pleocytosis but amoebae are seldom seen.

Ocular lesions occur without any brain involvement. They are usually, but not always, preceded by a history of trauma. A corneal ulcer is found which progresses and eventually destroys the eye.

DIAGNOSIS

Diagnosis is made by culturing on agar plates seeded with *Escherichia coli* or axenically in liquid media.[38]

TREATMENT

There is no treatment for meningoencephalitis. Ocular lesions can be treated with enucleation of the ulcer and corneal transplant.

REFERENCES

1 Daensvang, S. (1981) *S.E. Asian J. trop. Med. publ. Hlth* **12**, 319–332.
2 Myazaki, I. (1966) *Progress in Medical Parasitology in Japan,* Vol. 111: Tokyo: Meguro Parasitological Museum.
3 Suntharasamai, P., Desakorn, V., Migasena, S. et al (1985) *S.E. Asian J. trop. Med. publ. Hlth* **16**, 274–279.
4 Jaroonvesama, M. & Harinasuta, T. (1973) *J. med. Ass. Thailand* **56**, 312.
5 Schacher, J. F., Sabbe, S., Germanos, R. et al (1969) *Trans. R. Soc. trop. Med. Hyg.* **63**, 854.
6 Hopps, H. C., Keegan, H. L., Price, D. L. et al (1971) In *Pathology of Protozoal and Helminthic Diseases,* p. 970. Baltimore: Williams & Wilkins.
7 Hong, S. T., Cho, T. K., Hong, S. J. et al (1984) *Korean J. Parasit.* **22**, 61–65.
8 Bailey, C. A. (1948) *US Navy Med. Res. Inst. Proj.* No. 005007. Rep. No. 7.
9 Rosen, L., Loison, G., Laigret, J. et al (1967) *Am. J. Epidemiol.* **85**, 17.
10 Scrimgeour, E. M., & Welch, J. S. (1984) *Trans. R. Soc. trop. Med. Hyg.* **78**, 774–775.
11 Scrimgeour, E. M., Chambers, B. R. & Kaven, J. (1982) *Trans. R. Soc. trop. Med. Hyg.* **76**, 538–540.
12 Kliks, M. M., Kroenke, K. & Hardman, J. M. (1982) *Am. J. trop. Med. Hyg.* **31**, 1114–1122.
13 Sato, Y. & Otsuru, M. (1983) *S.E. Asian J. trop. Med. publ. Hlth* **14**, 515–524.
14 Tangehai, P., Nye, S. W. & Beaver, P. C. (1967) *Am. J. trop. Med. Hyg.* **16**, 454.
15 Weinstein, P. P., Rosen, L., Laqueur, G. et al (1963) *Am. J. trop. Med. Hyg.* **12**, 358.
16 Punya Gupta, S., Juttijudata, P. & Bunnag, T. (1975) *Am. J. trop. Med. Hyg.* **24**, 921–931.
17 Alicata, J. E. & Brown, R. W. (1962) *Can. J. Zool.* **40**, 119.
18 Jaroonvesama, N., Chardenlarp, K., Buranasin, P. et al (1985) *S.E. Asian J. trop. Med. publ. Hlth* **16**, 110–112.
19 Ambu, S., Kwa, B. H. & Mak, J. W. (1982) *Trans. R. Soc. trop. Med. Hyg.* **76**, 458–462.
20 Cuckler, A. C., Egerton, J. R. & Alicata, J. E. (1965) *J. Parasit.* **51**, 392.
21 Alicata, J. E. (1969) *J. trop. Med. Hyg.* **72**, 53.
22 Alicata, J. E. (1966) *Can. J. Zool.* **44**, 1041.
23 Punya Gupta, S., Bunnag, J., Juttijudata, P. et al (1970) *Am. J. trop. Med. Hyg.* **19**, 950.

24 Morera, P. (1973) *Revta Biol. trop.* **18,** 173.

25 Morera, P., Perez, E., Mora, F. et al (1982) *Am. J. trop. Med. Hyg.* **31,** 67–70.

26 Tesh, R. B., Ackerman, K. J., Dietz, W. H. et al (1973) *Am. J. trop. Med. Hyg.* **22,** 348–356.

27 Yokogawa, W. & Yoshimura, A. (1976) *Am. J. trop. Med. Hyg.* **16,** 723.

28 Kliks, M. M. (1983) *Am. J. trop. Med. Hyg.* **32,** 526–532.

29 Van Thiel, P. H., Kuipers, F. C. & Roskam, T. H., (1960) *Trop. geog. Med.* **12,** 97.

30 Oyedrian, A. B. O. O., Fajemisin, A. A., Abioye, A. A. et al (1975) *Am. J. trop. Med. Hyg.* **24,** 268.

31 Wong Soon Kai & Lie Kan Joe (1965) *Med. J. Malaya* **19,** 229.

32 Manning, G. S., Lerthprasert, R., Watnasirinkit, K. et al (1971) *J. med. Ass. Thailand* **54,** 466.

33 Zhong, H. L., Feng, L. B., Wang, C. X. et al (1983) *Chin med. J.* **96,** 661–668.

34 Dismuke, J. C. Jun. & Routh, C. F. (1963) *Am. J. trop. Med. Hyg.* **12,** 73.

35 Anthony, P. P. & McAdam, U. W. J. (1972) *Gut* **13,** 8.

36 Carter, R. F. (1972) *Trans. R. Soc. trop. Med. Hyg.* **66,** 193.

37 Fowler, M. & Carter, R. F. (1965) *Br. med. J.* **ii,** 740.

38 Diamond, L. S. (1968) *J. Parasit.* **54,** 1047–1056.

39 *Morbidity and Mortality Weekly Report* (1978) **27,** 343.

40 Smith, J., Oladiran, B., Langundoye, S.B. et al (1975) *Ann. trop. Med. Parasit.* **69,** 503–512.

SECTION IV
OTHER BACTERIAL DISEASES

Chapter 25
Tetanus

GEOGRAPHICAL DISTRIBUTION

Although tetanus occurs worldwide it is most frequently seen in Third World countries where neonatal tetanus may account for 10% of neonatal deaths (e.g. Papua New Guinea).

AETIOLOGY

Clostridium tetani is a straight, slender, rod-shaped organism, 2–5×0.4–$0.5\,\mu$m, which forms terminal spores that resemble drumsticks. It is gram-positive and an obligate anaerobe and grows well on ordinary media.

TRANSMISSION

Infection is through an injury to the skin from the entry of a contaminated instrument or an open wound contaminated by dust and earth or dung used to dress the umbilical cord. Vegetative *C. tetani* organisms are present in the faeces of animals and 25% of humans so that faecal contamination of soil is the main source of tetanus.

PATHOLOGY

The pathological features of tetanus are due to the action of tetanus toxin which is produced by the organism. The spores of *C. tetani* that gain entry to the tissues cannot germinate and make toxin unless conditions are anaerobic. Such conditions are most often found in wounds with tissue necrosis, foreign bodies or infection with anaerobic organisms. Spores may persist at the site of inoculation and remain dormant until infection with other organisms provides a suitable environment for growth.

Tetanus toxin made at the site of entry travels to the central nervous system either by absorption at the myoneural junction and migration through the perineural tissue spaces or via the lymphatics and blood to the central nervous system. In the central nervous system the toxin becomes bound to gangliosides in the central nervous system where it suppresses inhibitory influences on the motor neuron, allowing uninhibited stimulation of muscles with sustained muscular contractions.

IMMUNITY

There is no naturally acquired immunity and one attack of clinical tetanus does not confer any immunity. It is difficult to distinguish between relapses and recurrent attacks but, when several months have elapsed, then a second attack is probably responsible. The mortality rate in second attacks is high. Active immunization with tetanus toxoid should be performed in all cases of tetanus after recovery, because a natural attack of tetanus does not produce a significant antibody response.

CLINICAL FEATURES

Once the toxin has reached the central nervous system painful muscular contractions occur on the slightest stimulus or with none at all. The contractions involve any area of the body and in generalized tetanus death occurs from asphyxiation. In local tetanus where there is no asphyxiation spasms may last for months before recovery.

Incubation period

The incubation period is usually 7–21 days but may be extended for two months or even longer in the case of tetanus spores lying dormant in a healed wound. The shorter the incubation period the worse the prognosis and it is unusual for a case with an incubation period of under 7 days to recover.

Generalized tetanus

Signs of tetanus may follow injuries ranging from

a trivial injury which has been forgotten to a severe crush injury. The first sign is the onset of painful trismus (lockjaw) caused by spasm of the masseter muscles. The spasms then spread to involve the muscles of the neck, vertebral column and abdominal wall, following which the generalized spasms typical of tetanus occur. The paroxysms are initiated by some stimulus, such as light, but may be spontaneous. Spasms of the muscles of the jaws give rise to the 'risus sardonicus' (Fig. 25.1) or sardonic smile, and of the muscles of the back to opisthotonos. Spasms of other muscles give rise to flexion and adduction of arms, clenched fists and lower extremities. Involvement of the autonomic nervous system causes widespread fluctuations of blood pressure, tachycardia, sweating, hyperthermia and cardiac arrhythmias. There is often electrolyte imbalance.

Physical examination shows a board-like rigidity best seen in the abdominal muscles, resembling that seen in generalized peritonitis. There is severe respiratory distress due to interference with the respiratory muscles and anoxia. Death may occur quite suddenly from asphyxia due to

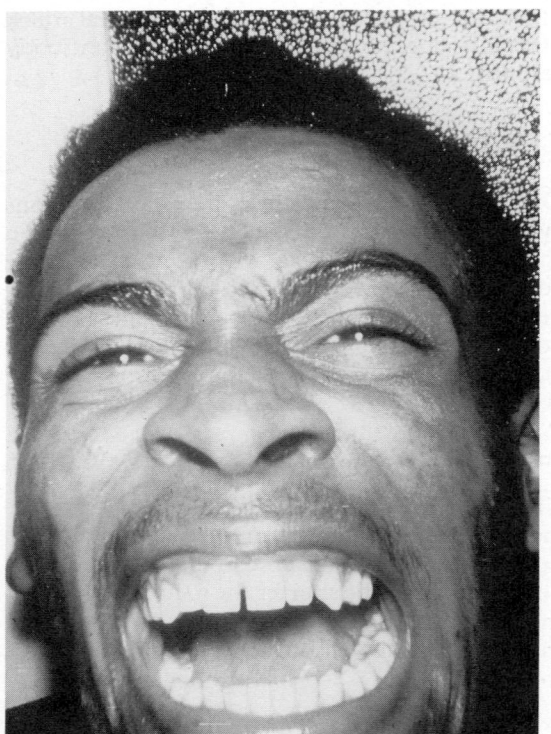

Fig. 25.1 Tetanus. Severe muscular spasm of risus sardonicus (lockjaw). (Courtesy Dr P. D. Marsden.)

laryngeal or respiratory muscle spasms. Other complications are fractures of limbs, pulmonary emboli and coma.

Atypical tetanus

A chronic ambulatory form is not uncommon, lasting for some weeks, with some stiffness of the jaw and muscular rigidity.

Cephalic tetanus

This follows a head wound or otitis media complicated by *C. tetani* infection. The incubation period is 1–2 days and there is severe dysfunction of the cranial nerves, especially the seventh nerve. It may remain localized or progress to generalized tetanus. The prognosis is poor.

Neonatal tetanus

This is a highly lethal form of the disease due to infection of the umbilical stump with spores usually conveyed by the application of a contaminated dressing or instrument. In some parts of the world applications of cow dung are used.

The incubation period is between 3 and 10 days. The onset is gradual and the first symptom is inability to suck the breast, due to trismus. This is followed by constipation and rigidity of the abdominal muscles and then by tetanic spasms which occur at first infrequently but increase in number until they become almost continuous.

DIAGNOSIS

The diagnosis is mainly clinical. The major differential diagnosis is from alveolar abscess (usually unilateral), peritonitis, meningitis, encephalitis, phenothiazine toxicity, rabies, muscular dystonia and in children under two years of age, tetany. In tetanus the level of consciousness is not reduced, the cerebrospinal fluid is normal and there are no convulsions. There is a moderate leukocytosis. *C. tetani* can be recovered from the wound in only one-third of cases.

TREATMENT

Treatment is based upon supportive care to prevent death from asphyxiation until recovery, the injection of human hyperimmune globulin (human tetanus immunoglobulin, HTI), antibiotic therapy and the use of sedatives to control the spasms.

Immunotherapy

HTI, 500–6000 units, must be injected in three equal doses intramuscularly at three different sites. If HTI is not available then heterologous antitoxin (refined horse serum antitoxin) must be injected *subcutaneously* as a single dose of 10 000 units. Complete active immunization with tetanus toxoid must be given after recovery.

Supportive measures

The patient must be nursed in a darkened, quiet ward, by himself. *Meprobamate* and *diazepam* are safe over a wide range of doses and should be given to control spasms: 400 mg meprobamate every 2–4 hours intramuscularly (children 2–5 years: 100–200 mg; infants: 50–100 mg per dose). The body electrolytes should be estimated and corrected. Penicillin G (Crystapen) 1.2–6.0 g daily should be given intravenously or intramuscularly in four divided doses.

Tracheostomy is needed in cases of laryngeal spasm if curarization and artificial ventilation cannot be provided.

Artificial respiration and paralysis can be lifesaving in severe cases but good results are only obtained if a very high standard of medical and nursing care is available. Paralysis is with curare or synthetic paralytic drugs used to achieve muscle relaxation in anaesthesia. In severe cases paralysis may have to be continued for several weeks.

PREVENTION

Immunization

Tetanus toxoid will prevent tetanus and an aluminium salt improves antigenicity. A complete course comprises three doses of alum-adsorbed toxoid with about six weeks between the first and second and six to 12 months between the second and third. The dose is 0.5 ml intramuscularly for all ages. All patients with tetanus treated in hospital should be given the first dose of toxoid while in hospital, to be followed by a second and third after discharge. Neonatal tetanus may be prevented by immunization of pregnant women. Two doses of alum-adsorbed toxoid are given at least one month apart; the first at the first antenatal visit and the second between the seventh and eighth months of pregnancy.[1]

Reactions

Reactions to toxoid are usually regarded as symptoms of delayed type hypersensitivity to antigenic impurities not eliminated by purification. They may be due to precipitating antigen–antibody complexes with tetanus toxoid antigen in excess. Reactions rarely occur in children but the incidence in adults increases with age and correlates with the number of previously administered doses. Local reactions consist of pain, redness and swelling lasting for 3 or 4 days; general reactions consist of urticaria with or without angioneurotic oedema, but serum sickness and peripheral neuropathy have occurred. The reactions, which develop after an interval varying from a few minutes to several days, can be reduced by inoculation into the gluteal region.

Booster doses

Immunity can be maintained by giving booster doses every five to 10 years. Shortening the interval to less than five years increases the risk of hypersensitivity.

Prevention of tetanus in the wounded

Wounded patients who are known to be actively immune do not usually require passive protection but may be given a reinforcing dose of toxoid at the time of treatment.

All wounded patients should be treated surgically. The tetanus proneness of a wound is determined after surgical toilet in the light of factors such as the success of surgery, the extent of remaining contamination, the age of the injury, the presence of wound infection, the possibility of a retained foreign body and the immune state of the patient.

For non-immune patients with a tetanus-prone wound passive protection is required and is best provided by HTI. If human antitoxin is not available heterologous antitoxin should be used.

Treatment with heterologous antitoxin should be preceded by a test dose. Should a hypersensitivity reaction develop, further horse serum should not be given, and a course of intramuscular penicillin administered instead.

When passive protection is given it is accompanied by a first dose of adsorbed toxoid administered in a different limb.

Tetanus toxoid injected for the first time into a non-immune individual at risk from tetanus provides no protection against the risk at this time.

If any antimicrobials are used as prophylactic agents they must be given in adequate doses for an adequate time. Systemic anaerobicidal antimicrobials are advisable before surgical toilet in badly soiled or severe injuries. Metronidazole and benzylpenicillin are the drugs of choice for antimicrobial prophylaxis. For detailed accounts of tetanus prophylaxis see Cotter and Wilson,[2] Furste,[3] and Willis et al.[4]

REFERENCES

1 McLennan, R., Schofield, F. D., Pittman, H. et al (1965) *Bull. Wld Hlth Org.* **32,** 683.
2 Cotter, E. H. J. & Wilson, K. V. (1975) *Jl R. Coll. gen. Pract.* **25,** 812–820.
3 Furste, W. (1974) *Am. J. Surg.* **128,** 616–623.
4 Willis, A. T., Jones, P. H. & Reilly, S. (1981) *Management of Anaerobic Infections. Prevention and Treatment.* Letchworth: Research Studies Press.

Chapter 26
Anthrax

GEOGRAPHICAL DISTRIBUTION

Anthrax is distributed worldwide. In the tropics cutaneous anthrax is the commonest form in cattle-owning countries. It is especially common in Iran;[1] intestinal anthrax is very common in parts of Africa.[2]

AETIOLOGY

Bacillus anthracis is a non-motile, gram-positive, sporing, capsulated bacillus which is both an aerobe and a facultative anaerobe, growing only readily on agar at 35°C. Spores are not produced in tissues, forming at temperatures below 30°C. In culture the colonies produce a typical 'medusa head' or 'curled hair' appearance caused by chains of bacilli growing out from the edge of colonies. The spores are very resistant and will resist dry heat at 140°C for 1–3 hours and 100°C moist heat for 5–10 minutes.

B. *anthracis* possesses three distinct antigen components: a somatic protein, a capsular polypeptide and a somatic polysaccharide. The protein somatic antigen is the anthrax toxin.

TRANSMISSION

Animals are infected via the intestinal tract from food. Man is infected directly by contact with infected hides (cutaneous anthrax or malignant pustule), by the inhalation of spores into the lungs (pulmonary anthrax) or by ingestion from infected meat (intestinal anthrax).

Transmission by insects[3] and house flies[4] has been recorded.

PATHOLOGY

The anthrax toxin acts on the vascular endothelium making it permeable, causing oedema and platelet aggregation leading to thrombosis and gangrene. The essential lesion is a haem-orrhagic area with central necrosis at the site of entry—the malignant pustule. The infection spreads via the circulation to cause septicaemic anthrax with widespread areas of haemorrhagic necrosis and thrombosis in the spleen and other organs. Haemorrhagic meningitis may develop. In pulmonary anthrax the spores are carried to the pulmonary lymph glands and thence to the circulation and spleen. The lungs are filled with serosanguineous fluid. In intestinal anthrax the bacilli enter through the intestinal tract causing severe haemorrhagic inflammation of the ileum and caecum with submucosal abscesses, and often septicaemia.

IMMUNITY

There is some protective immunity which is short-lived and accounts have been given of second attacks one year later. The protein somatic antigen (anthrax toxin) stimulates immunity and can be neutralized by the anthrax antiserum (Sclavo's serum).

CLINICAL FEATURES

Natural history

Anthrax is a very severe disease; it is not known whether there are any subclinical infections although antibodies present in the serum of contacts suggests this is so. Cutaneous anthrax is the mildest form. The pustule develops and in many cases eventually heals but in some the infection becomes generalized. Pulmonary anthrax carries a very high mortality. Intestinal anthrax has a low mortality rate, the majority recovering in a few days.

Cutaneous anthrax

Incubation period

The incubation period is 1–7 days, usually 2–5 days.

Symptoms and signs

A small papule develops at the site of infection, sometimes on the face and neck but more usually on the arm. It becomes a blister within 12–48 hours and then a pustule with a surrounding area of inflammation (malignant pustule). Coagulation necrosis of the centre results in the formation of a large, dark-coloured eschar which is later surrounded by a ring of vesicles containing serous or serosanguineous fluid, and outside this an area of oedema and induration which may become very extensive (Fig. 26.1). There is fever and malaise but further spread to septicaemic anthrax is rare. The typical eschar 7–10 days after onset is fully developed and round, 1–3 cm in diameter; then the edges begin to separate from the crater, the eschar loosens and falls off and heals by granulation leaving a scar. Lesions in the periorbital area may develop extensive oedema that may involve the entire face extending down to the neck and upper chest.

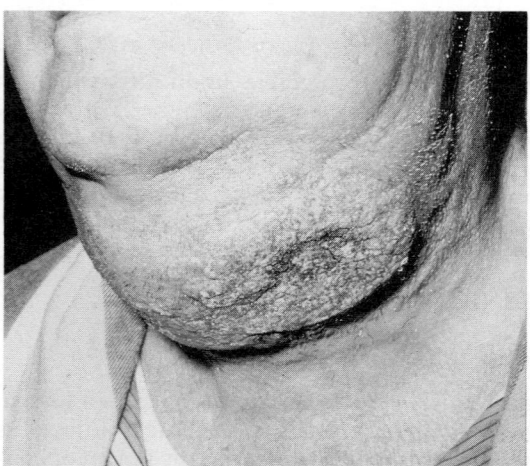

Fig. 26.1   Anthrax pustule on the jaw.

Pulmonary anthrax

Incubation period

The incubation period is 1–5 days.

Symptoms and signs

The clinical pattern is that of a biphasic illness. It starts with malaise, lethargy, mild fever and non-productive cough with signs of bronchitis. Within 2–4 days the symptoms may improve but then the second stage develops with severe respiratory distress, cyanosis, stridor and profuse sweating. Subcutaneous oedema of the chest and neck may develop. The lungs show moist rales and sometimes a pleural effusion. X-ray of the chest shows widening of the mediastinum from enlarged glands. Death usually follows within 24 hours of the onset of this phase.

Intestinal anthrax

Incubation period

The incubation period is 12–18 hours after the infective meal.

Symptoms and signs

The onset is with nausea, vomiting, occasionally haematemesis, and fever with abdominal pain and diarrhoea, which is sometimes bloody. The presentation resembles that of an acute surgical abdominal condition. The majority of cases recover after a few days but some continue on to septicaemic anthrax and death. Ingestion of contaminated meat may cause oropharyngeal anthrax, a syndrome characterized by a mucosal lesion in the oral cavity or oropharynx with subsequent necrosis and cervical adenopathy and oedema.[5]

Meningeal anthrax

Anthrax meningitis may complicate any of the forms of anthrax. The onset is within several days of the primary lesion and a haemorrhagic meningitis develops with death in 1–6 days. Encephalomyelitis and cortical haemorrhages have also been described.

DIFFERENTIAL DIAGNOSIS

Cutaneous anthrax should be considered whenever a painless pruritic papule on an exposed surface proceeds to become pustular and then black, regardless of antibiotic therapy. Other conditions are tularaemia, plague, pox viruses, contagious pustular dermatitis or orf, rickettsialpox and scrub typhus. Pulmonary anthrax must be distinguished from pneumonic plague and severe influenzal pneumonitis, and intestinal anthrax from an acute surgical abdomen.

DIAGNOSIS

The most important requirement is an awareness of the condition from the history and occupation.

Isolation of *B. anthracis*

Cultures must be taken within 24 hours of starting treatment; otherwise the organisms may not be recovered. Anthrax bacilli may be isolated from the anthrax pustule, sputum, blood or stools, depending on the form of anthrax, by culture on ordinary media.

TREATMENT

Patients must be nursed in isolation. Pulmonary anthrax cases require sealed units to prevent aerosol spread. Oral penicillin (ampicillin) is given, 250 mg 6-hourly for 5–7 days, for mild cases. For extensive lesions or systemic disease intramuscular procaine penicillin, 20–25 mg/kg, should be given in two divided doses every 12 hours for 5–7 days. Other antibiotics are also effective including tetracycline 15 mg/kg by mouth in four divided doses daily for 5–7 days.

PROGNOSIS

In cutaneous anthrax the mortality rate in untreated cases is between 10% and 20%; with treatment it falls to 1%. Pulmonary anthrax is invariably fatal. Gastrointestinal anthrax has a variable mortality from 25% to 50% in different epidemics.

EPIDEMIOLOGY

In the tropics cutaneous anthrax is an occupational disease associated with cattle-owning tribes who prepare and sell hides. In The Gambia, on the other hand, it is not an occupational disease but is spread from human to human by the use of communal loofahs, a toilet article. Here it causes widespread morbidity and some subclinical infections. Although the strain of *B. anthracis* is a good toxin producer it is only weakly antigenic, which accounts for the repeated clinical infections.[6] Intestinal anthrax in Africa occurs in explosive epidemics with many people affected by communally eating an animal which has died of anthrax.

PREVENTION

Prevention relies on an awareness of the disease and proper treatment of hides, and the prevention of anthrax in cattle; animals dying of anthrax should be buried in quicklime. Persons exposed should be placed under surveillance for 7 days. If there is a history of consumption of contaminated meat or inoculation of virulent bacilli, oral penicillin should be given daily for 7 days.

Immunization

A cell-free anthrax vaccine is suitable for use in humans and should be given to those exposed to high risk.

REFERENCES

1 Amidi, S., Dutz, W., Kohout, E. et al (1974) *Z. Tropenmed. Parasit.* **25,** 96.
2 Fendall, N. R. E. & Grounds, J. G. (1965) *J. trop. Med. Hyg.* **68,** 77.
3 McKendrick, D. R. A. (1980) *Cent. Afr. J. Med.* **26,** 126.
4 Turner, M. (1980) *Cent. Afr. J. Med.* **26,** 160.
5 Sirisanthana, T., Nauachareon, N., Tharavichitkul, P. et al (1984) *Am. J. trop. Med. Hyg.* **33,** 144–150.
6 Heyworth, B., Ropp, M. E., Meunel, H. et al (1975) *Br. med. J.* **ii,** 79.

Chapter 27
Plague and Melioidosis

PLAGUE

Plague, which is endemic in many parts of the world, has been an extremely important infection in the past, during which it has caused three world pandemics: the first in the sixth century (the Justinian plague), the second in the fourteenth century (the Black Death) which wiped out half the population of Europe, and the third which started in China in 1860 and reached the rest of the world in the early years of the twentieth century. Since then the spread has been halted and only 191 cases were reported to the World Health Organization in 1981. However, it is still an important infection and will always remain a threat, since enzootic wild rodent foci exist in many parts of the world.

GEOGRAPHICAL DISTRIBUTION

Plague exists all over the world in Asia, Africa and the Americas (Fig. 27.1) as an enzootic in wild rodents. Recently it has appeared in epidemic form in Vietnam, Burma, Brazil and Kenya. In the USA it occurs sporadically.[1]

AETIOLOGY

The specific cause of plague is the bacillus which was discovered by Yersin and Kitasato in 1894. It occurs in great profusion in the characteristic buboes, generally in pure culture, and is also present in great abundance in the spleen, intestines, lungs, kidneys, liver and other viscera and, though in smaller numbers, the blood; in the pneumonic type it is found in profusion in the sputum. It may also be found in the urine and faeces. Towards the termination of rapidly fatal cases it occurs in great numbers in the blood.

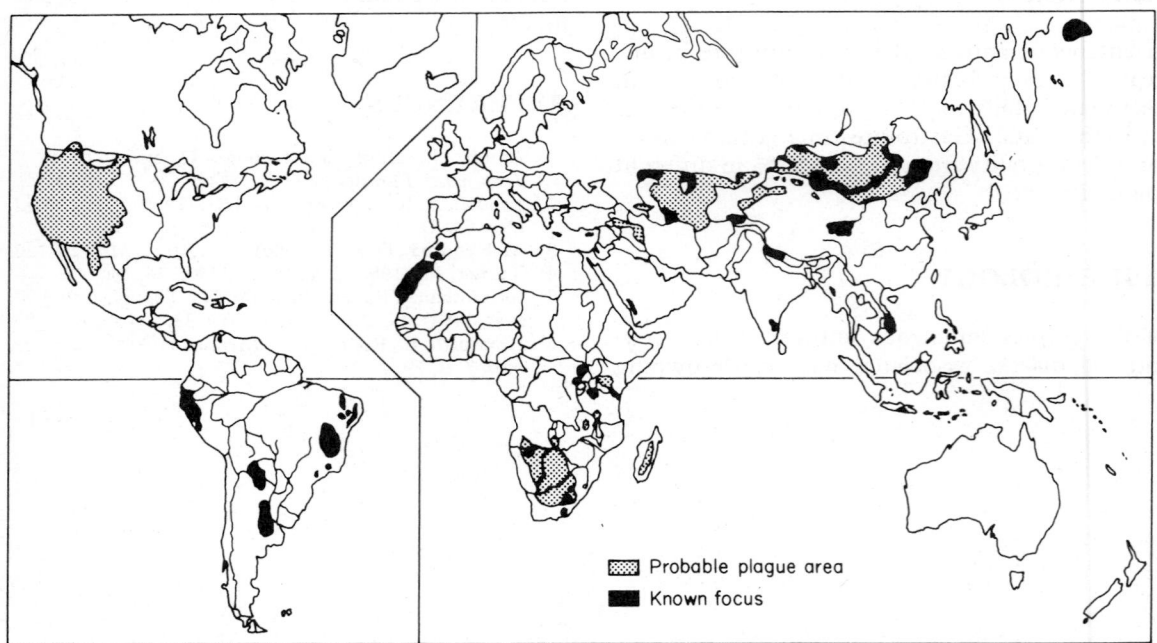

Probable plague area
Known focus

Fig. 27.1 Foci of transmission of plague (*Yersinia pestis*) to humans.

Yersinia pestis (now called *Yersinia pseudo-tuberculosis* ssp. *pestis*) as seen in the blood film or in preparations from any of the other tissues, is a short, thick coccobacillus ($1.5–2 \times 0.5–0.7 \mu m$) with rounded ends, very like the bacillus of chicken cholera. A capsule, or the appearance of one, can generally be made out, especially in bacilli in the blood. The organism is readily stained by aniline dyes, especially by Romanowsky stains, the extremities taking on a deeper colour than the interpolar part, giving a bipolar appearance. Virulent strains of *Y. pestis* can be recognized by the abundance of the envelope substance.

It is non-motile, gram-negative, indole-positive and gives a nitrite reaction with sulphanilic acid and α-naphthylamine.

Cultural characters

When sown on blood serum and kept at body temperature, in 24–48 hours an abundant moist, yellowish-grey growth is formed without liquefaction of the culture medium. On agar, but better on glycerin agar, the growths have a greyish-white appearance. On agar plate cultures they show a bluish translucence, the individual colonies being circular, with slightly irregular contours and a moist surface; on mannite neutral red bile salt agar the colonies are bright red, but are colourless on a similar medium in which lactose is substituted for mannite. Litmus milk and glucose broth are rendered slightly acid; lactose broth is unchanged. Young colonies are glass-like, but older ones are thick at the centre and more opaque; they are singularly coherent and may be removed en bloc with a platinum needle. Stab-cultures show after 1–2 days a fine dust-like line of growth. Cultivated on broth in which clarified butter or coconut oil is floated, *Y. pestis* usually presents characteristic stalactite growths which gradually fall off, forming a granular deposit. Examined with the microscope, these various cultures show chains of a short bacillus, presenting large bulbous swellings here and there. In gelatin the bacilli sometimes form fine threads, sometimes thick bundles made up of many laterally agglomerated bacteria, and involution forms are common. The bacillus does not produce spores.

The most favourable temperature for culture is 28°C. When *Y. pestis* is cultivated on human serum, growth is enhanced by the addition of iron.[2]

Three varieties of *Y. pestis* are recognized.[3] They can be distinguished by their ability to acidify glycerol and reduce nitrites.

	Glycerol-acidifying	Nitrite-reducing
Y. pestis var. *orientalis* or *oceanica* (adapted to rats)	−	+
Y. pestis var. *antiqua*	+	+
Y. pestis var. *mediaevalis* (adapted to *Meriones*)	+	−

There is a fourth subgroup of a mixed nature.

A distinction between the varieties of *Y. pestis* can be epidemiologically important, since if the *Y. orientalis* variety is found in both wild and domestic rodents, the original source of infection for both was the same, plague was imported into the area and passed from domestic to wild rodents. If, however, as in Kenya, two varieties have been found coexisting, this would indicate two separate sources of infection, one ancient and the other more recent and imported.

The plague bacillus can be modified by artificial methods and it is well known that some process of this kind takes place in nature, for as a plague epidemic decreases so the case mortality falls. There is difficulty in producing virulent mutants from an avirulent strain.

TRANSMISSION

The commonest method of transmission between rodents and to man is by *fleas*. Other less common methods are droplet spread from man to man in pneumonic plague, direct contact from handling infected animals (skinning) and laboratory infections. Soil can be infected and plague bacilli can remain dormant in the soil of rodent burrows for a long time. Aerosol transmission of plague is one of the suggested forms of biological warfare.

Transmission by fleas

Plague is readily communicated from rat to rat by fleas, principally by *Xenopsylla cheopis* (see Appendix III, p. 1483, and Fig. III.84, p. 1484), the rat flea of the tropics, *Ceratophyllus fasciatus*, the rat flea of temperate climates, and *Ctenocephalus canis* and *C. felis*, which bite man, dogs and cats indifferently. *Pulex irritans*, the human flea, though important in the Middle Ages, does not often act as carrier now, although in Manchuria it may convey the bacillus directly from one patient to another without the intervention of the rat. Wild rodent fleas transmit infection in a similar manner in wild rodent plague. The Indian Plague Commission showed that if fleas were excluded, healthy rats would not contract the infection from diseased rats and young rats suckled by infected mothers remained healthy in the absence of fleas. The transfer of fleas to a healthy animal or placing them in jumping range of fleas (about 4 cm above the floor) permitted infection. The capacity of a flea's stomach is about $0.5\,mm^3$ and in most cases of bubonic plague there are not sufficient bacilli in the peripheral blood to infect fleas except in the terminal stages of fatal cases. After the ingestion of infected blood *Y. pestis* multiplies in the flea's stomach and is then passed out in the faeces so that the flea serves as a multiplier of the bacillus. The life-span of an infected flea is about 3.2 days and a proportion become 'blocked', a condition in which the stomach and oesophagus become obstructed with a pure culture of *Y. pestis*. Blocked fleas die rapidly in a warm dry atmosphere. When such a flea feeds the culture is regurgitated and communicates infection. The flea transmits infection either by fouled mandibles, regurgitation in the act of feeding, or by provoking scratching and the inoculation of infection via the faeces.

Species of flea

Fleas are the main method of transmission of plague between rodents but not all species can transmit. Wild rodent plague is maintained in nature by a large number of different species of flea in many parts of the world (see Table 27.1). Domestic rat plague depends on three main species of rat flea: *Xenopsylla cheopis*, *X. braziliensis* and *X. astia*. Since *X. cheopis* is a much more efficient transmitter of plague than *X. astia*, where *X. cheopis* is the predominant rat flea, then plague is more likely. The situation is measured by the 'cheopis index' (number of fleas per rat) which, if in excess of five, is an indication of a likely outbreak of plague. (For diagnostic characters see Figs. III.84, and III.85, p. 1484.)

Bionomics of the rat flea (see also Appendix III, p. 1482, and Fig. III.83, p. 1483)

The rat flea ordinarily completes its developmental cycle in 14–21 days but in warm damp weather this may be shortened to 10 days. The average life of a flea separated from its host is about 10 days but it is capable of remaining alive without food for two months at low temperatures. In temperate climates fleas are most numerous during the warmer months and summer and autumn are the plague seasons. In warm climates plague is likely to become epidemic at temperatures between 10°C and 30°C but over 30°C is unfavourable. *X. cheopis* can flourish in northern countries in super-heated houses and factories even during the winter months.

Persistence of infection in the absence of fleas

The Indian Plague Commission has shown that floors of cow dung contaminated with *Y. pestis* do not remain infective for more than 48 hours and that mud floors ('chunam') cease to be infective in 24 hours, but plague bacilli can remain dormant in the soil of wild rodent burrows for a long time in the absence of any fleas.

PATHOLOGY

The toxin of *Y. pestis* causes vascular damage and leakage of fluid into the tissues, with haemoconcentration and shock.

Experimental plague

In the guinea-pig within a few hours of the introduction of the bacillus a considerable amount of oedema appears around the puncture and the adjacent gland is peceptibly swollen. At the end of 24 hours the animal is very ill; its coat is rough and staring; it refuses food. Presently it becomes convulsed and usually dies on the third or fourth day. If the body is opened immediately after death a sanguineous oedema is found at the point of inoculation, with haemorrhagic inflammatory effusions around the nearest lymphatic gland, which is much swollen and full of bacilli. The intestines are hyperaemic; the adrenals, kidneys and liver are red and swollen. The much enlarged spleen frequently presents an eruption of small whitish granulations resembling miliary tubercles. All the organs, and even any serous fluid that my be present in peritoneum or pleura, contain plague bacilli. In the blood, besides those free in the liquor sanguinis, bacilli are found in the mononuclear, though not, it is said, in the polymorphonuclear leukocytes.

Table 27.1 Established wild rodent plague foci, showing main reservoir hosts and fleas found naturally infected.

Plague focus	Main reservoir	Also found infected	Wild rodent fleas
USA North-western	Sciuridae (*Citellus*) (ground squirrels) *Citellus beecheyi* *Citellus* sp. (other ground squirrels)	Dipodomyinae (pocket mice) *Microtus, Peromyscus* (wood mice) Geomyidae (gophers) *Glaucomys* (flying squirrels) *Tamiasciurus* (chickadee chipmunks) Leporidae (jack rabbit, cottontail rabbit) *Neotoma* (wood rats)	*Anomiopsyllus nudatas* *Catallagia decipiens* *Diamanus montanus* *Echidnophaga gallinacea* *Euhoplopsyllus glacialis affinis* *Hoplopsyllus anomalus* *Hystrichopsylla dippei* *Hystrichopsylla linsdalei* *Malaraeus sinensis* *Malaraeus telchinus* *Megabothris abantis* *Megabothris clantoni clantoni* *Meringis shannoni* *Monopsyllus eumolpi* *Monopsyllus wagneri* *Neopsylla inopina* *Opisocrostis bruneri* *Opisocrostis hirsutus* *Opisocrostis labis* *Opisocrostis tuberculatus* (ssp.) *Opisodasys keeni nesiotus* *Oropsylla idahoensis* *Oropsylla rupestris* *Stenistomera alpina* *Thrassis acamantis* (ssp.) *Thrassis arizonensis* *Thrassis bacchi* (ssp.) *Thrassis fotus* *Thrassis francisi* (ssp.) *Thrassis pandorae* (ssp.) *Thrassis petiolatus* *Thrassis stanfordi*
South-western	Sciuridae (*Cynomys*) (prairie dogs) *Cynomys mexicanus*	*Marmota* (marmots) Bats	*Anomiopsyllus hiemalis* *Dactylopsylla* (*Foxiella*) *ignota* *Monopsyllus exilis* *Polygenis gwyni* *Stenistomera macrodactyla*
South America Peru/Ecuador	Sciuridae (*Sciurus*)	Cavidae (guinea-pigs) Leporidae (hares) Cricetinae Bats *Orizomys* (rice rat) *Sigmodon hispidus* (cotton rat)	*Adoratopsylla intermedia copha* *Cediopsylla spillmani* *Euhoplopsyllus andensis* *Euhoplopsyllus manconis* *Hectopsylla eskeyi* *Hectopsylla suarezi* *Neotyphloceras rosenbergi* *Pleochaetis dolens quitanus* *Pleochaetis equatoris* *Plocopsylla hector* *Polygenis brachinus* *Polygenis liturgus* *Tiamastus cavicola*
Argentina/Venezuela	Cavidae (guinea-pigs) *Microcavia australis* *Microcavia galea* *Grammomys griseoflavus* *Holochilus balnearum* Heteromyinae *Heteromys anomalus* Cricetinae *Sigmodon hispidus* (cotton rat)	Chinchillidae (chinchillas) Leporidae (hares) *Lagotomus maximus* (vizcacha or Peruvian hare) *Orizomys* (rice rat)	*Craneopsylla minerva* *Delostichus talis* *Polygenis platensis cisandinus* *Rhopalopsyllus* sp. indet.
European Russia South-eastern and northern (steppe)	Sciuridae (*Citellus*) (ground squirrel) *Citellus pygmaeus* (suslik)	Dipodidae (jerboas) Microtinae (voles) *Lagurus* (lemmings)	*Amphypsylla rossica* *Ctenophthalmus breviatus* *Ctenophthalmus congener secundus*

Table 27.1 (*continued*)

Plague focus	Main reservoir	Also found infected	Wild rodent fleas
South-eastern and southern (sandy stretches)	Gerbillinae (Meriones) *Meriones meridianus* (midday gerbil) *Meriones tamariscinus* (tamarisk gerbil) (gerbils and jirds)		*Frontopsylla semura* *Neopsylla setosa* *Nosopsyllus consimilis* *Nosopsyllus laeviceps* *Nosopsyllus mokrzeckyi* *Ophthalmopsylla volgensis* *Oropsylla ilovaiskii* *Rhadinopsylla cedestis* *Rhadinopsylla ucrainica* *Stenoponia tripectinata*
Asiatic Russia			
Desert	*Rhombomys opimus* (great gerbil) *Meriones lybicus erythrourus*	Leporidae (hares)	*Amphypsylla primaris mitis* *Citellophilus lebedewi*
Mountains	Sciuridae (marmots) *Marmota barbacina* *Marmota caudata* (long-tailed marmot)		*Citellophilus tesquorum* *Echidnophaga oschanini* *Neopsylla bidentatiformis* *Nosopsyllus aralis* *Nosopsyllus tersus* *Nosopsyllus turkmenicus* *Ophthalmopsylla volgensis* (ssp.) *Oropsylla silantiewi* *Paradoxopsyllus curvispinus* *Paradoxopsyllus teretifrons* *Rhadinopsylla liventricosa* *Stenoponia conspecta* *Stenoponia vlasovi*
Transbaikalia *Manchuria*	*Marmota babak* (Tarabagan)	Dipodidae (jerboas) Microtinae (voles)	*Oropsylla silantiewi*
Mongolia			
Central	*Marmota barbacina* *Marmota sibirica*		*Amphipsylla primaris mitis* *Echidnophaga oschanini*
Southern	*Meriones meridianus* *Meriones unguiculatus* (Mongolian jird) *Rhombomys opimus. Citellus pallicauda* (white tailed ground squirrel) *Citellus dauricus* (ground squirrel)		*Neopsylla bidentatiformis* *Neopsylla mana* *Oropsylla silantiewi* *Paradoxophilus dashidorzhü*
Central Asia			
Iran/Kurdestan	*Meriones persicus* (Persian jird) *Meriones lybicus* *Meriones vinogradoui*	Dipodidae (jerboas) Mictrotinae (voles)	*Coptopsylla bairamaliensis* *Coptopsylla lamellifer* *Mesopsylla apscherionisa* *Mesopsylla tuschkan* *Nosopsylla iranus iranus* *Xenopsylla conformis*
Africa			
North Africa/Mauretania	*Gerbillus gerbillus*	*Jaculus* (jerboa) *Psammomys obesus* (fat mouse)	*Synosternus cleopatrae* *Xenopsylla nubica* *Xenopsylla ramesis*
Egypt	*Acomys* (spiny mouse) *Arvicanthis niloticus* (Nile rat)		
West Africa	*Cricetomys gambianus* (giant rat)	*Arvicanthis* (grass rat) *Xerus erythropus* (striped ground squirrel) *Cryptomys* (mole rat)	*Synosternus pallidus*
Madagascar East Africa	Rodents and insectivores *Arvicanthis* (grass rat) Rats, mice. *Acomys* spp. *Praeomys* (*Mastomys*) *natalensis* (multimammate rat) *Otomys angionensis* (swamp rat) *Aethiops kaiseri* *Tatera* spp.	*Laeniscomys* (grass mouse) *Mus* (pygmy mouse)	*Sinopsyllus fonquerniei* *Ctenophthalmus cabirus* *Ctenophthalmus phyris* *Dinopsyllus lypusus* *Leptopsylla aethiopica* *Xiphopsylla lippi*

Table 27.1 (*continued*)

Plague focus	Main reservoir	Also found infected	Wild rodent fleas
South Africa	*Tatera brantsi* (Brant's gerbil) *Praeomys* (*Mastomys*) *natalensis* (multimammate rat) *Desmodillus* (Namaqua gerbil)	Cricetinae Dendromyinae Leporidae (hares) (Cape, zulu, karoo hare) Muridae Otomyinae Pedetidae (spring hares) Sciuridae (ground squirrels) *Xerus*	*Chiastopsylla rossi* *Dinopsyllus ellobius* *Listropsylla dorippae* *Xenopsylla hirsuta* *Xenopsylla philoxera* *Xenopsylla phyllommae* *Xenopsylla piriei* *Xenopsylla versuta*
India	*Tatera indica* (Indian gerbil or antelope rat)	*Millandia* (metad or field rat)	*Nosopsyllus nilgeriensis*
Java	*Rattus exulans* (Polynesian rat)	*Bandicota* (bandicoot rat)	*Neopsylla sondaica* *Stivalius cognatus* *Stivalius ahalae*

After Smith[18] and Pollitzer.[3]

Human plague

After death from plague the surface of the body very frequently presents numerous ecchymotic spots or patches. Buboes are characteristic; they are enlarged, congested lymphatic glands with haemorrhagic points and late necrosis in which plague bacilli are numerous. The glands are hard and can be moved under the skin. Occasionally there are also furuncles, pustules and abscesses.

The characteristic appearance of plague in a necropsy is that of engorgement and haemorrhage, nearly every organ of the body participating more or less. There is also parenchymatous degeneration in most of the organs. The brain, spinal cord and their meninges are markedly congested and there may be an increase of subarachnoid and ventricular fluid.

Ecchymoses are common in all serous surfaces; the contents of the different serous cavities may be sanguineous. Extensive haemorrhages are occasionally found in the peritoneum, mediastinum, trachea, bowel, stomach, pelvis of kidney, ureter, bladder or in the pleural cavities. The lung frequently shows evidence of bronchitis and hypostatic pneumonia; sometimes haemorrhagic infarcts and abscesses are found. The right side of the heart and the great veins are usually distended with feebly coagulated or fluid blood. In pneumonic plague the superficial lymphatic glands are not enlarged; the pleural cavities contain bloodstained fluid; the infected lungs are deeply congested and oedematous and, at a later stage, pneumonic consolidation is found. The bronchi contain bloodstained mucus and the bronchial glands are swollen and haemorrhagic.

The liver is congested and swollen, its cells are degenerated and may be the seat of miliary plague abscesses. The spleen is enlarged to two or three times its normal size. The kidneys are in a similar condition.

The lymphatic system is always involved; around the glands there is much exudation and haemorrhagic effusion, with hyperplasia of the gland cells and enormous multiplication of plague bacilli.

IMMUNITY

There is no known natural immunity to plague. Acquired immunity is short-lived and there is no protection against second attacks. This is borne out by the short-lived protection provided by vaccination.

Y. pestis has a complicated antigenic structure. The antigens so far defined are fraction I (envelope substance), which is stable, initiates a strong antibody response and provides the main protective effect against wild strains of plague bacilli, fraction II (murine toxin), fractions V, W, L, PF, antigen 4, Ph6 and the specific polysaccharide.[4] Three of these antigens are held in common with *Y. pseudotuberculosis*: the PF antigen, which has been shown to protect guinea-pigs against plague, and the V and W antigens, which enable organisms to survive and multiply within monocytes (i.e. determine virulence).

The main mechanism of immunity to plague is the formation of antibodies which neutralize the antiphagocytic properties of the fractions I, V and W antigens.[5] Protective immunity does not depend upon antitoxins to murine toxin (fraction II).

Toxins

Y. pestis has potent endo- and exotoxins. The endotoxin produces fever, disseminated intravascular coagulation and complement activation. Exotoxins include a protein murine toxin which is cardiotoxic but its action in man is not known.

Complement-fixing and haemagglutinating antibodies are found in both man and rodents and appreciable antibody levels against fraction I can be found for months in the sera of persons recovered from plague. The passive haemagglutination test (HA),[6] which is widely used for epidemiological studies on plague, is especially useful for detecting plague foci in rodent populations. Antitoxin is found in the sera of patients with pneumonic plague and of convalescent patients but does not persist for long; vaccinated individuals who contracted plague showed both antibodies and antitoxins for months or years.[3]

When purified, fraction I is used as antigen for the complement fixation (CF) and HA tests, which are sensitive and specific. The HA test is useful in rodents and the CF test will demonstrate antibodies in immunized or infected hosts. The presence of fraction I can be detected in animal tissues by immunofluorescence and microtechniques, which can be used to determine the presence of *Y. pestis* in small amounts of tissue.[7] The serological identification of *Y. pestis* is best made by immunofluorescence when the organism can be identified within 2 to 3 hours.[8]

CLINICAL FEATURES

Natural history

Plague can be a very virulent infection with a high mortality as history can relate, but this is not so in the majority of infections. Subclinical cases are probably not uncommon and bubonic plague, which forms the vast majority of infections, can be mild or moderate and only in a small minority of cases severe, leading to septicaemic plague and death.

Incubation period

Symptoms of plague begin to show themselves after an incubation period of from 2 to 8, rarely 15 days.

Symptoms and signs

The average case of plague: prodromal stage

In a certain but small proportion of cases there is a prodromal stage characterized by physical and mental depression, anorexia, aching of the limbs, feelings of chilliness, giddiness, palpitations and sometimes dull pains in the groin at the seat of the future bubo.

Pestis minor ambulatory stage

Abortive or ambulatory cases of bubonic plague have been reported in connection with almost every true outbreak of the disease and in some constitute a high proportion. Clinically these cases present mild, general febrile symptoms with a bubo; when that suppurates the temperature falls and the patient recovers. The diagnosis may be difficult because the plague bacilli may be scanty in the pus. The differential diagnosis has to be made from climatic bubo (lymphogranuloma venereum).

Marshall et al[9] have isolated *Y. pestis* from throat swabs of patients with plague, as well as from healthy contacts. This suggests that healthy carriers of plague can be found. Treatment with streptomycin did not hasten clearing of the carrier state.

Bubonic plague (zootic plague)

This is the most common form and constitutes about three-quarters of the total number. The incubation period is usually very short; a small vesicular primary lesion has been described at the site of the infective flea bite. The characteristic bubo or buboes (Fig. 27.2) develop within 24 hours. It is possible to distinguish three

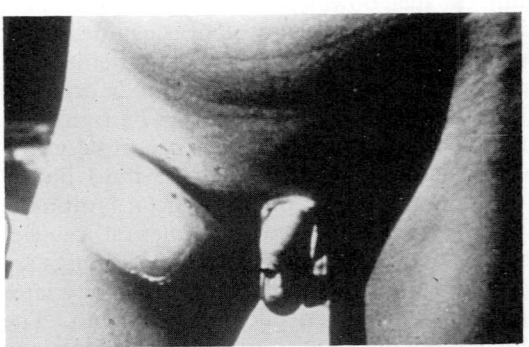

Fig. 27.2 A plague bubo in the groin.

varieties of bubonic plague: (a) well-marked bubonic infection not leading to secondary septicaemia; (b) bubonic affection followed by secondary septicaemia; (c) serious general septicaemia combined with slight affection of lymph glands. Generally (in 70%) the bubo appears in the groin (Fig. 27.2), especially on the right side and affecting one or more of the femoral glands; less frequently (20%) the axillary; more rarely still (10%, especially seen in children) the submaxillary lymphatic gland may be the seat of the bubo. In rare cases the tonsil may be the primary focus of infection. Buboes are usually single but in about one-eighth of the cases they form simultaneously on both sides of the body. Very rarely buboes form in the popliteal, epitrochlear or clavicular glands. Occasionally they develop simultaneously in different parts of the body. A curious point, noted in north-west America, is that axillary buboes are more common in plague conveyed by squirrels than in plague conveyed by rats. Plague buboes vary very much in size. Sometimes they are not as large as a walnut; in others again they may be as large as a goose's egg. Pain may be very severe, but sometimes it is hardly felt. Besides the enlargement of the gland there is, in most instances, considerable pericellular infiltration and oedema.

Stage of fever

The stage of invasion may last for a day or two without serious pyrexia but usually it is much shorter or it may be altogether absent. The disease usually develops abruptly without a definite rigor or other warning, the thermometer rising rapidly to 39.4°C or 40°C, or even to 41.7°C, with corresponding acceleration of temperature and pulse. Sordes form on the teeth and about the lips and nostrils. Thirst is intense, prostration extreme and from utter debility the voice is reduced to a whisper. Sometimes there is wild delirium or it may be of the low muttering type.

Coma, convulsions, sometimes tetanic retention of urine, subsultus tendinum and other nervous phenomena ensue. Vomiting is in certain cases very frequent. Some patients are constipated but in others there is diarrhoea. The spleen and liver are usually enlarged. Urine is scanty, but rarely contains more than a trace of albumin. The pulse at first is full and bounding; in the majority it rapidly loses tone, becoming small, frequent, fluttering, dicrotic and intermittent. There is usually a polymorphonuclear leukocytosis.

Stage of recovery

In favourable cases, sooner or later, after or without the appearance of the bubo, the constitutional symptoms abate with the onset of profuse perspiration. The tongue begins to moisten, the pulse rate and temperature to fall and the delirium to abate. The bubo, however, continues to enlarge and to soften. After a few days, if not incised, it bursts, discharges pus, sometimes very ill-smelling, and sloughs. Owing to the contracture and fibrosis of lymphatic tissue, oedema of the leg on the affected side usually supervenes.

Skin affections

In a very small proportion of cases, what are usually described as carbuncles, in reality small patches of moist gangrenous skin that may gradually involve a large area, develop on different parts of the integument. These occur either in the early stage or late. Sometimes they slough and lead to extensive gangrene.

A generalized papular rash on the hands, feet and pectoral region has been described. Should life be continued sufficiently long, the vesicles become converted into pustules resembling smallpox. These observations confirm in a remarkable manner the old writers who described manifestations in the Plague of London of 1665 as 'blains'.

Complications

Occasionally a pyaemic condition with boils, abscesses, cellulitis, parotitis or secondary adenitis, succeeds the primary fever. During convalescence fatal sudden cardiac failure is not uncommon. Secondary pneumonic plague with bloodstained sputum may supervene, but the patient may recover.

Septicaemic plague (pestis siderans)

In this type there is no special enlargement of the lymphatic glands during life, although after death they are somewhat enlarged and congested throughout the body. The high degree of virulence and the rapid course of the disease depend on the entry of large numbers of the bacilli into the blood, where they can be readily found during life. The patient is prostrated from the outset; he is pale and apathetic; there is generally little febrile reaction (37.8°C). Great weakness, delirium, picking of the bed-clothes, stupor and coma end in death on the first, second or third day or it may be later. Frequently in these cases there are haemorrhages.

Subclinical plague

Subclinical cases are probably not uncommon in the human population in areas of wild rodent plague. Using the HA survey technique it has been shown that 4.7% of human sera showed antibodies when the disease was quiescent, whereas 46.8% did so when it was active[10] and that these antibodies were still detectable four years later.[11]

Pneumonic plague (demic plague)

This occurs frequently in epidemic form among the marmot trappers of northern China, who live under very insanitary conditions, but may occur spontaneously wherever the bubonic form is found. It is especially dangerous to the patient's attendants and visitors because of the multitude of bacilli which are scattered about in the patient's expectoration, because the clinical symptoms are unlike those of typical plague and are apt to be mistaken for some ordinary form of lung disease. The illness commences with rigor, malaise, intense headache, vomiting, general pains, fever and intense prostration. In the early stages there may be little to suggest pneumonic plague, except the marked discrepancy between the almost negligible physical signs and the gravity of the patient's condition. Cough and dyspnoea set in, accompanied by a profuse, watery, blood-tinged sputum. The sputum is not viscid and rusty, as in lobar pneumonia. From the outset clouding of consciousness is very marked. Moist rales are audible at the bases of the lungs; the breathing becomes hurried; other symptoms rapidly become worse, delirium sets in and the patient usually dies on the fourth or fifth day. This is the most fatal as well as the most directly infectious form of plague. Epidemics of 50 000 and more cases have occurred in Manchuria, where the plague bacillus exists as an intestinal infection in the marmot, which acts as a reservoir. Pneumonic plague has been recorded from Nigeria, Ghana, Ecuador, New Orleans and elsewhere. In these countries haemorrhage into the intestinal canal occurs in about 8% of plague-infected rats and the organism is passed out in the faeces; in this manner the plague bacillus can be disseminated in dust and inspired by man directly into the lungs.

It has been pointed out that whereas in rat-borne plague pneumonia is rare, in wild rodent plague it is common.

Meningeal plague

Primary plague meningitis has been found in Dakar, Zaire, East Africa,[12] Chuanchow, south China,[13] southern California and South America. In most cases meningeal involvement was a complication of the bubonic form from the ninth to the seventeenth day. In clinical features it rather resembles cerebrospinal meningitis with headaches, stiff neck and Kernig's sign. Special symptoms are meningeal irritation, convulsions, vestibulocerebellar symptoms and coma. The cerebrospinal fluid is under pressure and yellow in colour, closely resembling that of acute suppurative meningitis; *Y. pestis* may be obtained by lumbar puncture. The initial infection is probably due to droplet spread. The brain shows congestion and flattening of sulci and is covered with a thick fibrinopurulent exudate.

MORTALITY

The mortality is usually greatest at the beginning and height of the epidemic. The death rate may be anything from 60% to 95% of those attacked. Much appears to depend on the social condition of the patient and the attention and nursing available. Thus, in a Hong Kong epidemic while the case mortality among the indifferently fed, overcrowded, poor Chinese amounted to 93.4%, it was only 77% among the Indians, 60% among the Japanese and 18.2% among the Europeans— a gradation in general correspondence with the social and hygienic conditions of the different races. Modern treatment has greatly reduced the mortality.

DIFFERENTIAL DIAGNOSIS

Bubonic plague has sometimes to be distinguished from other affections associated with enlarged glands, such as streptococcal infections, lymphogranuloma venereum, filarial adenitis and occasionally anthrax pustule.

In filarial and streptococcal infections lymphangitis tracks are usually visible but in bubonic plague there is usually no visible sign of the primary infection. In glandular fever the cervical glands are as a rule primarily affected and there is an excess of heterophil antibodies in the serum (Paul–Bunnell test).

Generalized pustular plague has to be differentiated from chickenpox or smallpox; carbuncular plague may be confused with typhus. In the USA, north Europe and Russia, tularaemia may resemble plague.

Pneumonic plague differs from other forms of pneumonia in three main characteristics.

1 The patient is extremely prostrated, although his critical state can hardly be accounted for by such physical signs as are present in the chest; but by the time definite involvement of the lung can be demonstrated, he generally dies.

2 The sputum is watery, never thick, and soon becomes very bloodstained.

3 Pleural effusion is usually present in pneumonic plague.

DIAGNOSIS

Fever and adenitis during a plague epidemic must invariably be viewed with suspicion. Blood culture has been recommended by inoculating blood into broth containing 1% of sodium citrate, and in Java splenic puncture is valuable in establishing a diagnosis and was not opposed by the local population. In western America the differentiation of mild cases of plague from tularaemia is important (see Chapter 7), but the discovery of the bacillus in the glands, blood, sputum or discharges is the only thoroughly reliable test. Should a coccobacillus with the characteristic bipolar staining be found it should be cultivated by Haffkine's method in broth on which clarified butter (ghee) or coconut oil is floated. In case of doubt, animal inoculation should be used; infective material from the patient or a culture is rubbed into a shaven area (2.5 × 2.5 mm) on the abdomen of a white rat or a guinea-pig. *Y. pestis* inoculated in this way kills the guinea-pig in 7 days, the rat sooner and white mice in 48 hours. The latter may be inoculated at the root of the tail.

Before rats suspected of being plague infected are handled, they should be immersed in insecticide to destroy ectoparasites.

The lymphatic glands should be first exposed. If the rat is infected, subcutaneous injection around the glands is generally recognizable. If the glands are inflamed this is almost diagnostic of plague; the liver will be yellow, sprinkled with innumerable pinky-white granules. The spleen is enlarged, congested and occasionally granular. The serous membranes are of dull lustre with petechial or diffuse haemorrhages. Serous or bloodstained serous effusions are present in 72% of such rats; if, on microscopical examination of scrapings from glands or spleen, bipolar-staining bacilli are detected, the case is probably plague.

Y. pestis, *Y. pseudotuberculosis rodentium*, *Y. suiseptica* and *Y. aviseptica* closely resemble each other and are scarcely distinguishable by the usual cultural methods, but the last two have no 'envelope substance', though they have a common antigen with *Y. pestis*. A textbook of bacteriology should be consulted for cultural details of these differences.

In cases of doubt some assistance is afforded by the fact that *Y. pseudotuberculosis* has not been found in central Africa, China, Indo-China and Madagascar.

The most satisfactory means of differentiation is animal inoculation. Rabbits, guinea-pigs and white mice are susceptible to *Y. pseudotuberculosis*, but white rats are not. The Indian Plague Commission laid stress on the latter point as white rats are quickly killed by *Y. pestis*. Some strains of *Y. pestis* from Brazil, however, do not affect guinea-pigs; they depend on asparagine, and guinea-pigs possess circulating asparaginase.[14]

Y. pestis can be identified by serological methods, most satisfactorily by immunofluorescence (see section on immunity; above).

In the investigation of rodent plague the inoculation into animals of pooled fleas is important. Cyanide gas is the best method of collecting fleas from rodents. The long bones of rodents and finger bones from human cadavers may be sent to the laboratory for culture of marrow.

TREATMENT

Cases must be treated in a rat- and flea-free environment. Pneumonic plague cases must be isolated with strict precautions against aerial spread, the attendants must wear masks and be protected (see section on personal prophylaxis, below).

Streptomycin

Streptomycin is the most effective drug against plague; 30 mg/kg in two divided doses daily for 10 days, but severe intoxication can occur because its highly bactericidal effect causes massive destruction of plague bacilli.

Tetracycline

Tetracycline is more usually preferred; 2–4 g daily in four divided doses for 10 days.

Chloramphenicol

Chloramphenicol is used in meningitis since it crosses the blood–brain barrier. It is given intramuscularly at first in a loading dose of 25 mg/kg followed by 60 mg/kg daily in four divided doses, and when the condition permits, orally for 10 days.

Results

Most cases of bubonic plague recover with treatment without any permanent disability, and most cases of pneumonic plague treated early recover. Some are left, however, with a permanently diminished vital capacity due to destruction of lung tissue.

EPIDEMIOLOGY

Plague is a disease of 'natural foci'[15] and a typical

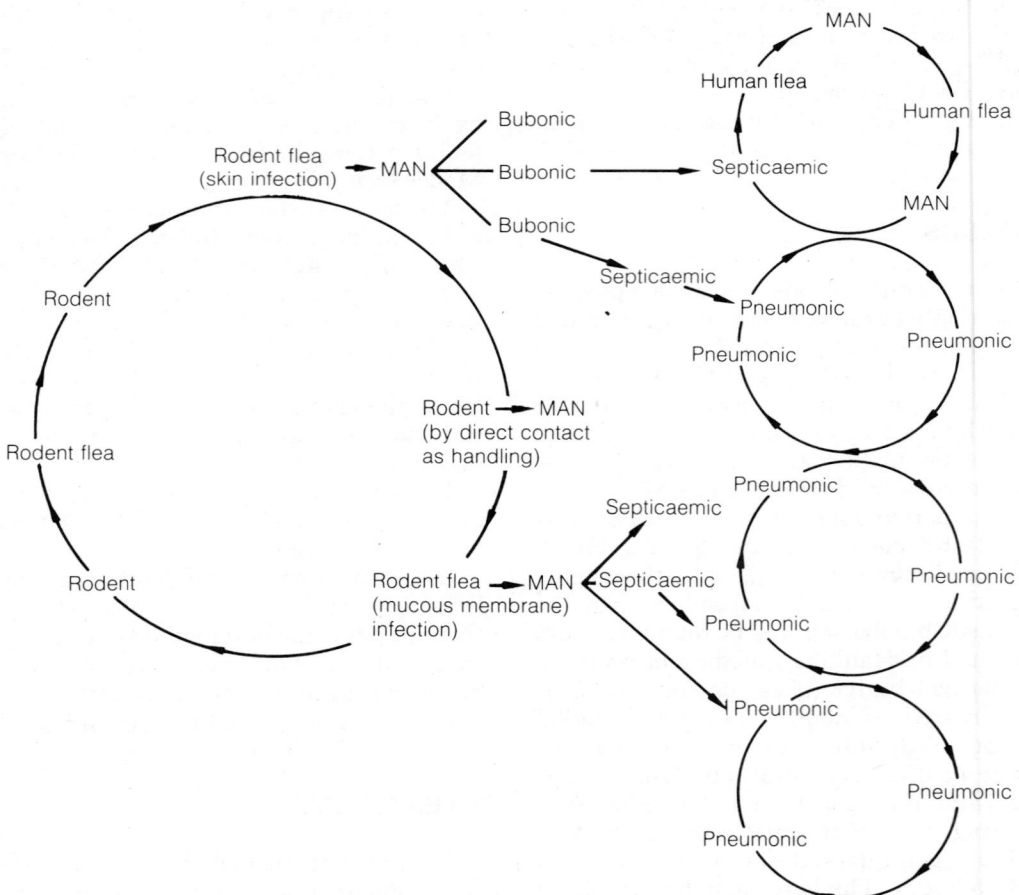

Fig. 27.3 Transmission cycles of plague. On the left, the enzootic cycle; on the right the potential epidemic cycles in man. (After Faust and Russell.[16])

zoonosis (Fig. 27.3).[16] It exists in two forms: sylvatic or wild rodent plague, existing in nature independent of human populations and their activities, and domestic plague, intimately associated with man and rodents living with man (commensal rodents).

Wild rodent plague

Plague exists all over the world in wild rodents. In all some 200 or more species of rodents representing all the major families throughout the world can harbour plague naturally.[17] It occurs among the marmots (tarabagan) of Siberia and Manchuria, the susliks, mice and jerboas of the desert region of south-east Russia, the gerbils and Muridae of the African veld and high regions, the chipmunks and ground squirrels of California and the prairie dogs of the south-west USA, and in the cavies ('cuis', wild guinea-pigs) and other rodents of the pampas of South America. In these areas the infection is maintained permanently by hosts which are relatively resistant, termed 'permanent reservoir hosts' (Table 27.1).[3,18] They pass the infection to less resistant animal hosts and cause epizootics (murine plague) which affect rodents dependent on man for their food—commensal rodents—and thus cause outbreaks of plague in man. In tropical areas the spread of infection from natural foci to domestic rats and then to man is influenced by rainfall characteristics and agricultural practices as well as human behavioural patterns.[17] Certain wild rodents, such as *Arvicanthis* and *Otomys* in Africa, are relatively resistant and form permanent foci of plague. Rodents which are highly susceptible to plague during the active period of their lives become less so as hibernation approaches and may be quite refractory whilst in hibernation,[19] and thus serve as a source of permanent infection in a natural focus. Epizootics, which usually begin in northern regions after hibernation, attack rodent colonies and wipe out the susceptible population. The infection then dies out, only to return when a susceptible population builds up again.

Cyclic plague outbreaks in central Asia involve the interaction of two gerbil (*Meriones*) species, one resistant and the other susceptible. The susceptible species spreads the infection when the population is high, but following the rapid fall in numbers, infection persists in the resistant species until the susceptible population recovers.[17] It has been shown that in Iran plague

bacilli can survive in the soil of burrows in the absence of rodents and fleas for a long time and thus maintain a permanent focus of plague in the rodents of that region.[20] Serological testing with the haemagglutination test has shown the persistence of rodent plague in the foothills of Kenya.[21] Rodent fleas play the main part in transmission and proventricular blocking with plague bacilli occurs in the gerbil fleas, *Citellophilus tesquorum* and *Nosopsyllus laeviceps*, *Neopsylla setosa*, which infests susliks, and *Oropsylla silantiewi*, which sticks in the fur and is found in pelts of the tarabagan (*Marmota bobak*). A large number of wild rodent fleas have been found naturally infected with *Y. pestis* (Table 27.1).

Infection is also transmitted by the intestinal tract and carnivores, such as mongoose, are susceptible to plague from feeding on dead and dying rodents. In South Africa the discovery of gerbil remains in the faeces of the suricate and yellow mongoose is a valuable indication of the existence of rodent plague, as these animals do not normally eat them unless they are sick. When epizootics occur in the wild rodents the infection is passed on to rats commensal with man and outbreaks of human plague occur. Man can acquire plague directly by inhalation from wild rodent skins, such as the tarabagan (*Marmota bobak*) in Manchuria and Siberia, or indirectly via commensal rodents, as in parts of Africa. Foci of wild rodent plague may be very ancient, as in Iran and Africa, or recent following the introduction of plague by the brown rat, as occurred in California after the San Francisco outbreak in 1903.

Commensal rodents

Commensal rodents are those dependent on man for their food supplies. The rodents implicated are *Rattus norvegicus*, *Rattus rattus* (and its races, see Table 27.2) and less commonly *Mus musculus*. In India wild and commensal rodents live close together and interbreed.

The brown or sewer rat (*Rattus norvegicus*) is the prime originator and main means of spread of bubonic plague. Originally the infection is picked up from susceptible secondary reservoirs of plague (murine plague), the commensal semi-domestic rodents which come into contact with permanent reservoirs which initiate the epizootic in the commensal rodents. The brown rat is a great traveller but does not come into direct contact with man. It frequents cities, sewers and docks and when it dies the fleas leave the dead rat and in some circumstances infect the black rat (*Rattus rattus*, domestic rat) which lives in close contact with man in his houses. Rat plague is seasonal and spreads during the period when fleas are most numerous. The first sign of plague is the appearance of dead rats, and dead sewer rats first appear in the region of docks and grain stores. When the black rat becomes infected dead rats appear in houses and the phenomenon of 'rat fall' occurs when rats fall from the rafters and die on the floor. This is a sign of the imminent outbreak of epidemic bubonic plague in man. The sewer rat also lives on ships, spreading the infection from one port to another, and was responsible for the spread of plague around the world during the great pandemics. Rats also accompany certain trade goods, such as wool and cotton, which in older times spread plague along the trade routes.[22]

Rattus rattus, Linn, the black rat (Fig. 27.4). Principal features: build slender; muzzle sharp; ears large, translucent, cover eyes when folded down; tail usually long, never much shorter than head and body; coarse hair on rump; hind foot (heel) to tip of longest toe, without claw) 35–40 mm; weight of adults rarely more than 225 g.

Indigenous, wild, more or less arboreal in Indo-Burmese countries. In the tropics it is generally the dominant domestic rat in houses and ships. The chief domestic races are distinguished as shown in Table 27.2.

The forms *R. frugivorus*, *R. alexandrinus* and *R. rattus* have now acquired an almost worldwide distribution; *R. frugivorus* is the least and *R. rattus* the most modified race. These are climbing rats, common on ships, frequent in dwellings in warm countries and not shunning man; they are of especial importance as plague-carriers. They attain sexual maturity early (minimum weight sexually mature, 70 g), breed throughout the year; gestation about 21 days, but with concurrent lactation about 31 days; litter of from four to 11; average litter five or six.

Rattus norvegicus, Berkenhout (= *decumanus*), *the brown, grey or sewer rat* (Fig. 27.5). Principal features: robust; muzzle blunt; ears small, opaque; tail noticeably shorter than head and body; fine hairs on rump; hind foot 40–45 mm; weight of adults commonly 460 g, often much more; colour brown or grey above, silvery below. A melanic form (often confused with *R. rattus*) is quite common.

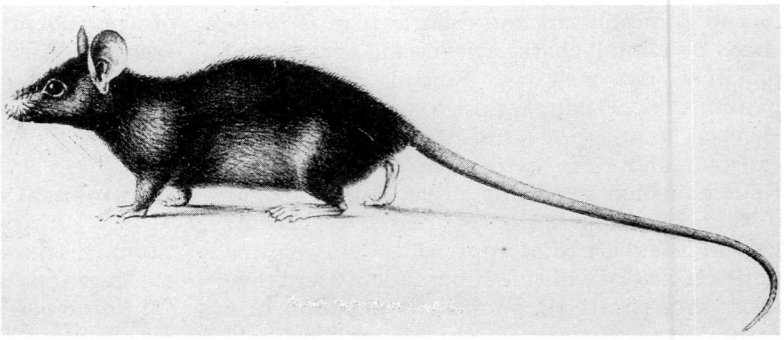

Fig. 27.4   The black rat, *Rattus rattus*. (Courtesy London School of Hygiene and Tropical Medicine.)

Table 27.2   Domestic races of *Rattus rattus*.

Colour	Race
Back reddish or greyish-brown	
Underparts white or pale lemon	*R. r. frugivorus* Raf. (= *tectorum*), common in the Mediterranean region or *R. r. kijabius* in Uganda
Underparts darkened	
Ventral hairs with rusty tips	*R. r. rufescens* Gray, the common rat of Indian houses
Ventral hairs without rusty tips	*R. r. alexandrinus* Geoff
Back black; underparts dusky or slate grey	*R. r. rattus*, a domestic form evolved in cold temperate countries

N.B. The black rat tends to be brown in the tropics.

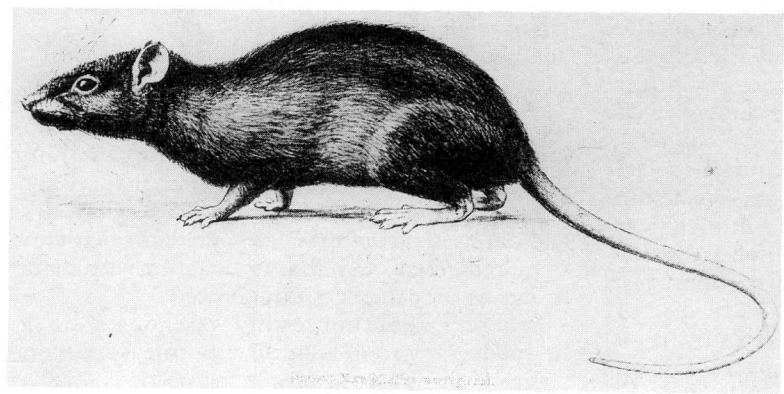

Fig. 27.5 The common sewer rat, *Rattus norvegicus*. (Courtesy London School of Hygiene and Tropical Medicine.)

Human plague

Man can become infected directly from wild rodents by handling them during skinning or trapping. Under these conditions plague is sporadic and only a few cases occur every year. Under some circumstances commensal rodents which have become infected may introduce the infection to rural houses or villages and cause small outbreaks. This occurs in Kenya and India, in the mountain foothills, but not on the plains below.

In Mongolia and Siberia outbreaks of pneumonic plague occur when trappers, who have become infected from tarabagans, in which there is an intestinal infection, spread the infection directly by inhalation in crowded tents and huts during the Siberian winter.

Plague was once common in eastern Europe, occurring as great epidemics such as the Black Death in the fourteenth century and the Plague of London in the seventeenth century. These ceased shortly after and the reason is thought to be that the brown rat (*R. norvegicus*) ousted *R. rattus* from Europe. As *R. norvegicus* is a sewer or stable rat, contact with man was greatly reduced.

During the last great pandemic, which started in 1896, plague spread from Hong Kong to Bombay and then rapidly to other parts of India, as well as to Mauritius, whence it was introduced to East Africa causing outbreaks in Mombasa, Zanzibar, Delagoa Bay, Cape Town, Port Elizabeth and Durban. Alexandria and the Nile Delta were invaded from the same source, as was Australia, with outbreaks in Sydney and Brisbane. In 1903 plague appeared in the New World in San Francisco and spread later to Brazil and Argentina. Plague appeared in Colombo, Sri Lanka in 1914 and in Java in 1910 where for the next 40 years there were some 3000 to 4000 cases each year.

Sometimes human plague spreads rapidly from point to point but more generally it creeps slowly from one village to another, from one street or house to another. Sometimes it skips a house or a village.

PREVENTION

Surveillance

In any focus of plague, surveillance[23] of human cases, vertebrate reservoirs and vectors should be undertaken on a permanent basis and should be a feature of the health programme, so that the circulation of *Y. pestis* in populations of rodents and their flea parasites can be monitored in known permanent foci and in peridomestic and commensal rodents. The methods used are the identification of human cases and the collection of data on mammalian hosts and vectors. Animals are inspected for signs of plague; a sample of blood is taken for the HA test and fleas are removed and identified and pools inoculated into test animals. A flea index should be established and monitored. The total flea index is the average number of fleas of all species per host, the specific flea index the average number of fleas of each species per host and the burrow and nest flea index the average number of each species of flea per burrow or nest. By monitoring the changes in the flea indices an outbreak of plague can be foreseen.

General prevention

Quarantine

Modern systems of land or sea quarantine

directed against plague take cognizance of the facts that the incubation period of the disease may extend to 10 days and that plague may affect certain of the lower animals (e.g. rats) as well as man.

Eradication of rats from ships requires special measures. At present Cyanogas (calcium cyanide, Ca(CN)$_2$), is employed as a fumigant. It is a fine greyish-white powder which is dusted or pumped into rat burrows and harbourages, where it liberates hydrocyanic acid. In disc or granular form it is used in the treatment of rooms, ships' holds and enclosed spaces. For rat holes on land a sturdy and powerful pump or blower should be available, usually with a cut-out device which renders it possible to blow in air after the required amount of dust has been delivered. The pump is adjusted so as to clear a known amount of dust with a given number of strokes (e.g. 28 g with 30 strokes), the exact delivery being ascertained beforehand. Before or during pumping all openings of burrows, except one, should be blocked and care must be taken that no unblocked holes lead into rooms in houses; 28 g suffice for average burrows but under Indian conditions 450 g suffice for 60 burrows.

For fumigation the ship is divided into sections, each of which is measured by volume. Water bottles and cabin water tanks are emptied, moist food removed and mattresses turned on edge. All apertures are sealed. Danger boards are prominently displayed. Ships may be fumigated loaded or unloaded. A plague-infected ship should be treated before unloading.

In an outbreak in a town it must be borne in mind that plague, once established in human beings, is communicable to others and to rats by expectoration and by discharges from the buboes or glandular swellings, and that plague in rats usually precedes plague in human beings. The main efforts should be directed towards destruction of rats by methods detailed below.

After death the rat is treated with insecticide or soaked in lysol. Smears are made from lymph glands, liver and spleen, and stained by Leishman. Broquet's medium (calcium carbonate 2; glycerin 20; distilled water 80 parts) is a good preservative for fleas and permits isolation of *Y. pestis* after 6 days.

In India the compulsory inspection of all dead bodies before burial has been found a valuable measure.

Destruction of vermin and other measures in anticipation of the introduction of plague bacilli

The campaign against rats is usually carried on by rat-traps and rat-catchers and the cautious laying down of poisons. The pumping of sulphur dioxide gas under pressure is useful for warehouses. So long as the sulphurous acid gas is dry, and not used on damp articles, no damage is done to merchandise. Care has to be taken with damp things as they may get discoloured.

Where possible houses and warehouses should be made rat-proof—not an easy measure, considering the burrowing and climbing habits of the rat. *R. norvegicus* can penetrate ordinary lime-mortar or soft brick but is stopped by cement and concrete. Its burrows may attain a depth of 46 cm but *R. rattus* is not so active in this respect.

Walls should be at least 15 cm thick when made of hard brick or concrete and they should extend to not less than 46 cm below the level of the ground floor; the latter should be paved with concrete 8 cm thick, covered with 1.24 cm of cement. All ventilators should be protected with iron gratings and all openings around wires and pipes cemented. In New Orleans some warehouses are elevated, leaving a clear open space beneath: in others an impervious wall is built around the ground floor, penetrating 60 cm into the ground. In a third, and a most effective type, the ground floor is laid out in concrete with a protective wall round the edges sinking 60 cm into the ground. The mooring cables of ships should be shielded in such a way as to prevent egress or ingess of rats and all gangways should be taken up at night or when not in use. Village food stores are sometimes set out on poles and can be protected from rat invasion by suitable wooden discs.

Control of fleas (Appendix III, p. 1485)

Some resistance of the classic vector *X. cheopis* to organochlorine insecticides such as DDT has been demonstrated but fleas can normally be destroyed by this substance. Flea control measures have been well described.[24]

Rodenticides (Table 27.3)

All rodenticides should be handled with great care; they can affect man.

Warfarin is an anticoagulant derived from cou-

Table 27.3 Rodenticides.

Rodenticide	Recommended strength by weight	Relative safety	Relative effectiveness
Warfarin	0.025%	2	2
Red squill*	5–10%	1	7
ANTU (1-naphthylthiourea)	2–3%	3	6
Zinc phosphide	1%	4	5
Arsenic trioxide	3%	5	4
Thallium sulphate	0.5%	6	3
Sodium fluoroacetate (1080)	—	7	1

* The Cruel Poisons Act prohibits the use of red squill in Great Britain.

marin; it easily takes first place for combined safety and effectiveness. Water-soluble warfarin can be used in addition to the solid bait. War-farin-treated oats are prepared with warfarin 0.025%, white mineral oil 11%, *p*-nitrophenol 0.25% and rolled oats 88.73%.

Sorexa warfarin (3(2-acetyl-1-phenylethyl)-4-hydroxy-coumarin) has fewer disadvantages than other poisons. It acts slowly and creates no suspicion in rats; it kills without pain. Sorexa (1% warfarin in fine oatmeal) kills rats by drastically reducing the clotting power of the blood and by causing leaks in the small capillary vessels. This leads to extensive internal haemorrhages which are rapidly fatal. It inhibits the formation of prothrombin which is produced in the liver.

Initial clearance is readily achieved by making available to rats sufficient bait to satisfy the appetites of the whole population. Reinfestation can be controlled by the use of permanent baiting points which attract the migratory rats. Perimeter defence of premises is by use of permanent or semipermanent bait containers. Some populations of *Rattus norvegicus* and *R. rattus* are resistant to anticoagulant rodenticides in Europe and America. New rodenticides available include norbormide effective against *Rattus norvegicus* and *R. rattus*. A combination of calciferol and warfarin kills rats and house mice otherwise resistant.[25]

Bait

Any bait that causes rats to feel ill is immediately suspect and the entire colony is warned against the bait. No prebaiting is necessary with Sorexa. Ground cereals are used as a basis for bait. In the UK it is medium oatmeal; in the USA yellow corn meal and in South Africa maize meal. Palatability is increased by the addition of 2–10%

fine sugar or 1–2% refined vegetable oil. Good results are obtained if Sorexa is dusted on to soft egg shells. When conditions are dry and warm and foodstuffs available with low moisture content, increased bait-take can be achieved if water is placed near the dry bait.

RULES OF BAIT REPLACEMENT
1   Lay many baits (116–168 g) wherever rats are known to run.
2   Inspect baiting points and replenish where bait is being taken.
3   Replenish bait as long as there are signs of feeding (7–14 days).
4   Maintain permanent baiting points to destroy any rats which may come into the cleared area.

The quickest clearance of rats is obtained where enough attractive bait is laid in the correct places. Mix 1 part Sorexa to 10 parts of bait base.

SITING OF THE BAIT
Rats are particular where they feed and while preferring quiet corners they do not like feeling hemmed in. Rats like a quick and easy 'get-away' but seldom feed in a draught or open space. It is generally accepted that for every rat seen there are at least 10 living in the area and enough bait must be laid for the whole colony. Rats will not eat food which is mildly rancid or made unpalatable.

Control of wild rodent reservoirs of plague

Wild rodent reservoirs of plague have been successfully controlled and eradicated in some areas in the USSR, California and South Africa. There are three main methods of control.
1   Complete clearing principle. Rodent extermination is carried out over a number of years. No antiflea measures are necessary.

2 Current prophylaxis. This is more of an emergency method and is undertaken when an epizootic of plague is occurring in the rodents. Rodent destruction must be accompanied by disinfestation of the burrows.

3 Long-term prophylaxis.

Methods of rodent destruction

The chief methods are gassing with chloropicrin and black cyanide, and poison bait of oats impregnated with 10–20% zinc phosphide.

How to deal with an epidemic

The principles of dealing with an epidemic are breaking the rat–man contact and protection of the population and health workers at risk.

Breaking rat–man contact

This can be done by destruction of rats and their fleas. Rats can be destroyed by burning dwellings if these are temporary and made of wood and grass. Rats must be prevented from leaving the area by killing them as they try to escape. In more permanent buildings a crash programme of rodenticides is practical. Fleas can be destroyed by spraying the infected buildings with insecticide (DDT) (Appendix III, p. 1485).

Protection of population and health workers

This can be done by chemoprophylaxis and vaccination.

VACCINATION AGAINST PLAGUE

Although both live and inactivated vaccines are available their effectiveness is not well established. The use of vaccines may reduce the morbidity and mortality in bubonic but not in pneumonic plague.[6] The immunity conferred is of short duration, not longer than six months, so that revaccination is necessary to maintain immunity and must be spread over a period and reinforced by booster injections.[26] Mass vaccination cannot be recommended for general plague control but under highly endemic conditions or for high risk groups vaccination may be given for individual protection.

To be effective against plague a vaccine must contain an adequate amount of fraction I antigen or, in the case of live vaccines, they must produce sufficient fraction I in vivo. Two types of vaccine are available: inactivated highly virulent cultures of *Y. pestis*, originally prepared by Haffkine, and live avirulent cultures of the EV strain, available from the Pasteur Institute, Paris.

Inactivated vaccine. Meyer's modification of Haffkine's vaccine consists of *Y. pestis* grown for 3 days at 37°C and killed by formaldehyde. The adult dose is 0.5 ml (containing 1500 million organisms) subcutaneously followed by 1 ml 10–28 days later and then 0.5 ml every six months to persons at risk.

Live vaccine. The EV strain of *Y. pestis* which is kept as the original strain[6] gives a better immunity in experimental animals than that obtained with dead cultures. This immunity is long-lasting, of high degree and protects against any form of plague[26] and was used in Java in 1935–1939 and more recently in Madagascar with great success. Lozenge vaccine containing the EV strain is stable at 4°C and taken orally enhances the antibody response, but a local pharyngeal and tonsillar reaction occurred in 45% of persons.[27] Anyone wishing to work with plague or enter a plague area should have at least two doses of killed plague vaccine which should be followed up by a dose of EV vaccine or a third dose of killed vaccine, since a single dose does not give much protection.[28]

CHEMOPROPHYLAXIS

Chemoprophylaxis is recommended for persons in contact with plague and for individuals contaminated in laboratory accidents. In selected populations it may also be used as a short-term measure in small explosive outbreaks until other measures can be instituted. Tetracycline should be used wherever possible in a dose of 250 mg every 6 hours for one week or, failing this, sulphonamides 6 g daily for 3 days or 3 g daily for one week.

PERSONAL PROPHYLAXIS

The attendants on pneumonic cases should provide themselves with masks of muslin, three- or fourfold, changed when at all damp, and also with goggles to protect the eyes. In Mukden a mask of absorbent cotton-wool (16×12 cm) enclosed in muslin and retained in position by a many-tailed gauze bandage, together with goggles, rubber gloves and cotton uniform, proved thoroughly effective.

MELIOIDOSIS

Melioidosis (Stanton's disease, pneumoenteritis, pseudocholera) is a rare glanders-like disease endemic in South-East Asia, mainly in Burma, Malaysia, Vietnam and Sri Lanka.

GEOGRAPHICAL DISTRIBUTION

The infection was first recognized by Whitmore in Rangoon in 1911,[29] Malaysia in 1921,[30] Vietnam in 1925,[31] in Sri Lanka in 1927, in Singapore in 1931 and in Indonesia in 1932.

Melioidosis occurred during the Second World War in Burma, Malaysia and Thailand and is no longer a rare infection in northern Queensland.[32]

Melioidosis has also been described in patients who have never visited a known endemic area or had contact with a case. Three cases have been reported from the USA, two from Panama, one from Ecuador, one from central India and one from Turkey.[33]

AETIOLOGY

Pseudomonas pseudomallei (*Loefflerella whitmori*, *Pfeifferella whitmori*), resembles *Pseudomonas mallei*, the cause of glanders in horses. It is a small bacillus about the same size and shape as *P. mallei* and occurs in very large numbers in all acute lesions of the disease. It is a saprophyte and can be isolated from soil, stagnant water and rice fields in endemic areas. In films stained with Leishman bipolar staining is common. On culture it resembles the glanders bacillus closely but is more actively motile and liquefies gelatin more rapidly. It grows luxuriantly upon peptone agar, forming a dense wrinkled culture especially when the medium contains glycerin. A peculiar aromatic odour reminiscent of truffles is given off, though on repeated subcultures this feature is lost. On broth cultures a pellicle is formed. *P. pseudomallei* can be distinguished from *P. mallei* by its behaviour on a peptonized medium containing 1% sodium fumarate. The organism is pathogenic for most laboratory animals and, for guinea-pigs at any rate, the infection is more rapidly fatal than glanders, but in each case acute orchitis is produced by intraperitoneal injection (Strauss reaction). There may be difficulty in distinguishing *P. pseudomallei* from *P. pyocy-*

anea. Susceptible animals can be infected by scarification, by feeding or by simple application of cultures to the nasal mucosa. A characteristic feature in infected laboratory animals is discharge from the nose and eyes and the organism is excreted in the urine and faeces.

TRANSMISSION

The route of infection is uncertain. It has been considered that the bacillus enters through open skin lesions, a view supported by the fact that patients had scars and lacerations received during outdoor activities, and in addition two patients showed some evidence of an associated leptospiral infection which is water-borne and enters through the skin and mucous membranes. Pulmonary lesions which preceded septicaemia were present in eight cases[33] which suggested that inhalation was a likely source of infection.

Source of infection

Several cases of natural infection have been observed in rats, cats and dogs and for many years it was thought that this disease was spread by rats, but extensive surveys have shown only a few infected rats. After the Second World War the disease appeared in sheep, horses, pigs, cattle and goats in Queensland. Soil and surface water is the natural habitat of *P. pseudomallei* in Vietnam,[34] Malaysia,[35] Singapore[36] and northern Australia[37] and infection is from direct contact with water, since the bacillus is most prevalent in rice-growing areas and surface water from a housing development contained *P. pseudomallei*.

Serological surveys among healthy people have shown that subclinical infections may be commoner than is realized.[35]

PATHOLOGY

The lesions vary very considerably. Numerous small pulmonary abscesses, roughly resembling those of miliary tuberculosis, are produced. Nodules which coalesce and break down into abscesses are found in the spleen and liver; they somewhat resemble those of portal pyaemia and have to be distinguished from amoebic abscesses. The organisms have been recovered from the blood, urine, sputum and fluid from cutaneous vesicles of patients dying from the disease. In laboratory animals, artificially infected, small nodules form in the internal organs.

IMMUNITY

Natural immunity is high and the majority of infections are subclinical.[32] Clinical infections occur in people whose resistance has been reduced, such as alcoholics and diabetics. Immunity is mediated by both humoral and cell-mediated systems. Antibodies are formed and are used in diagnosis.

CLINICAL FEATURES

Natural history

Melioidosis is mainly a subclinical infection but when resistance has been reduced by diabetes or chronic alcoholism or malnutrition it may appear in a clinical form. In the chronic and subacute forms recovery can occur but in the septicaemic form the mortality is very high.

The *incubation period* is unknown but in an accidental infection was as little as 3 days.

Signs and symptoms

The clinical features are very variable and are well described by Thin et al.[33] Cases can be divided into acute, subacute and chronic[38] and a fourth group who have experienced subclinical infections. The first three types are rare but the fourth is probably not uncommon. It is possible that the acute form develops only in debilitated persons and that previously healthy people develop the subacute and chronic disease.

Acute septicaemic form

The acute septicaemic form usually occurs only in persons debilitated from alcoholism or diabetes or who are extremely obese.[33] The onset is gradual and the intestinal and pulmonary systems are usually involved. Fever is high, remittent and often irregular. There is commonly a generalized pustular rash and *P. pseudomallei* can be isolated from the pustules. Vomiting and diarrhoea, which may be so severe as to cause collapse and resemble cholera, are common. Pneumonia is usual with other signs of

septicaemia and *P. pseudomallei* can be isolated from the sputum. Often there is a synovitis with effusion into a large joint from which the organism can be cultured. The spleen is soft and enlarged. The cerebral system may be involved and death invariably occurs after a few days or weeks with delirium or mania.

Subacute form (pulmonary)

The subacute form starts as an intestinal infection with diarrhoea, and pulmonary signs develop with consolidation of one lung and rapid cavitation, closely resembling tuberculosis. The sputum is profuse and often bloodstained and *P. pseudomallei* can be isolated from it. Fever is usual and there are widespread abscesses in the subcutaneous tissues, liver (Fig. 27.6) and spleen. Recovery can occur in this form after antibiotic treatment.

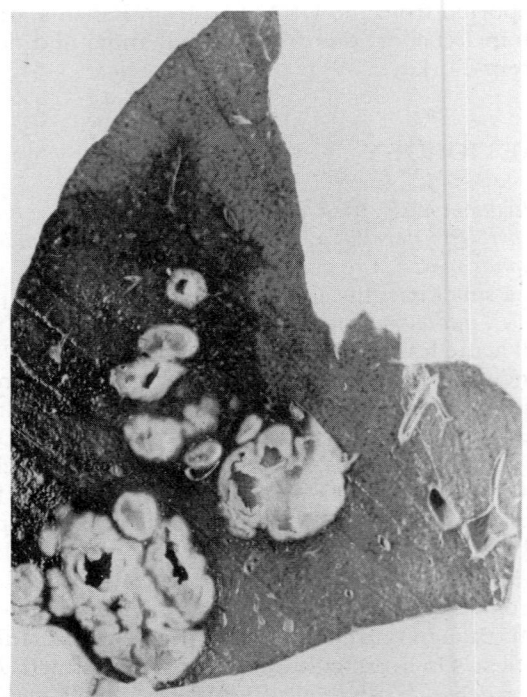

Fig. 27.6 The characteristic appearance of liver abscesses due to melioidosis. (Courtesy Sir A. T. Stanton.)

Chronic form (local suppurative)

This is very variable. Lesions occur in the skin and subcutaneous tissues leading to subcutaneous abscesses and collections of pus in the liver, lungs and spleen. The initial signs may be those of acute parotitis. In one case[39] there was a latent period of three years between possible infection and the development of parotid swelling, abscesses, osteomyelitis of the frontal bone, perispinal abscesses and bronchopneumonia. An afebrile case with cervical adenitis and recovery was reported in an Indian.[40] Ten cases of all three types have been reported from Malaysia.[33] Localized cutaneous melioidosis has been described. Few cases have been described in women in whom the bladder and kidneys are chiefly involved.

Subclinical infections

Subclinical infection is the commonest manifestation of infection and significant antibody titres have been found in the general population in endemic areas in northern Queensland[32] with a rate of 5.7% in the general population, 29% in Vietnamese refugees and 15% in alcoholics.

Relapse

Relapses may occur after many years triggered off by some factor which reduces immunity, such as chronic illness or immunosuppressive drugs and treatment.

DIFFERENTIAL DIAGNOSIS

The pulmonary form must be distinguished from pulmonary tuberculosis, chronic lung abscess and fungal infections; the septicaemic form from chronic disseminated tuberculosis, systemic fungal infections and chronic pyogenic infections; the local suppurative form from tuberculosis of bone, chronic osteomyelitis and fungal infections.

DIAGNOSIS

The essential in diagnosis is to be aware of the possibility of melioidosis in any patient from an endemic area who presents with multiple abscesses or pyrexia of unknown origin or doubtful aetiology since melioidosis is a rare infection. The diagnosis is made by isolation of the organism from pustules in the skin, blood or urine. Although it may be found in the stool, isolation is difficult. *P. pseudomallei* may also be isolated from the cerebrospinal fluid and synovial fluid. *P. pseudomallei* grows on most media when characteristic wrinkled colonies can be seen after 48–72 hours. The definitive diagnosis is made by biochemical tests.

Serological tests

Indirect haemagglutination is the most widely used test. IgM titres must be measured and an IgM titre of 1/40 or over is highly suggestive of active infection.[41]

TREATMENT

P. pseudomallei is resistant to most antibiotics and treatment varies with the form of disease. The chronic and subacute non-septicaemic forms should be treated daily with tetracycline (2–3 g) orally, chloramphenicol (3 g) orally or co-trimoxazole (four tablets) orally for 60–150 days.[42] The septicaemic form demands much more treatment and combinations of drugs should be used: tetracycline and chloramphenicol, or co-trimoxazole and kanamycin—all by the parenteral route.

EPIDEMIOLOGY

Soil and water are the natural habitat of *P. pseudomallei* in Vietnam,[34] Malaysia,[35] Singapore[36] and northern Queensland.[37] It can infect animals including rats, sheep, goats and horses but these are not the source of human infection, which takes place from stagnant water and infected soil, perhaps through abrasions in the skin or mucous membranes. Subclinical infections are common in endemic areas of the disease.[35]

CONTROL

There is little that can be done to control the spread but protective clothing in rice fields and other marshy areas should be used.

REFERENCES

1 Akiev, A. K. (1982) *Bull. Wld Hlth Org.* **60**, 165–169.
2 Jackson, S. & Morris, B. C. (1961) *Br. J. exp. Path.* **42**, 363.

3   Pollitzer, R. (1960) *Bull. Wld Hlth Org.* **23,** 313.
4   Chen, T. H. (1965) *Acta trop.* **22,** 97.
5   Pollitzer, R. (1954) *Monograph Ser. Wld Hlth Org.*, 22.

6   World Health Organization (1970) *Wld Hlth Org. tech. Rep. Ser.* **447.**
7   Chen, T. H. & Meyer, K. F. (1966) *Bull. Wld Hlth Org.* **34,** 911.
8   Cherry, W. B. (1960) *Fluorescent Antibody Technique in the Diagnosis of Transmissible Disease*, PHS publication No 729. Washington, DC: US Government Printing Office.
9   Marshall, J. D. Jr, Quy, D. V. & Gibson, F. L. (1967) *Am. J. trop. Med. Hyg.* **16,** 175.
10 Isaacson, M. & Hallett, A. F. (1975) *S. Afr. med. J.* **29,** 1165.
11 Isaacson, M., Qhobula, Q. M., Davis, D. H. S. et al (1976) *S. Afr. med. J.* **50,** 929.
12 Williams, A. W. (1934) *E. Afr. med. J.* **ii,** 229.
13 Landsborough, D. & Tunnell, N. (1947) *Br. med. J.* **i,** 4.
14 Burrows, T. W. & Gillett, W. A. (1971) *Nature, Lond.* **229,** 51.
15 Pavlovsky, E. N. (1966) *Natural Nidality of Transmissible Diseases with Special Reference to the Landscape Epidemiology of Zooanthoponoses*. Urbana: University of Illinois Press.
16 Faust, E. C. & Russell, P. F. (1964) *Craig and Faust's Clinical Parasitology*, 7th edn. Philadelphia: Lea 2 Febiger.
17 Baltazard, M. (1963) *Bull. Soc. Path. éxot.* **56,** 1230.
18 Smith, K. G. V. (1973) *Insects and other Arthropods of Medical Importance*. London: British Museum (Natural History).
19 Zhigilev, D. S. & Otdelskaya, A. A. (1956) *Coll. Pap. Anti-plague Inst.* Rostov. Quoted by Pollitzer (1960) *Bull. Wld Hlth Org.* **23,** 313.
20 Baltazard, M., Bahmanyar, M., Chamsa, M. et al (1963) *Bull. Soc. Path. éxot.* **56,** 1108.

21 Davis, D. H. S., Heisch, R. B., McNeill, D. et al (1968) *Trans. R. Soc. trop. Med. Hyg.* **62,** 838.
22 Hirst, I. & Fabian, M. D. (1953) *The Conquest of Plague. A Study of the Evolution of Epidemiology*. Oxford: Clarendon Press.
23 World Health Organization (1974) *WHO Chron.* **28,** 71.
24 World Health Organization (1970) *Wld Hlth Org. tech. Rep. Ser.* **553,** 4.
25 World Health Organization (1970) *Wld Hlth Org. tech. Rep. Ser.* **443,** 7.
26 Ehrenkrantz, N. J. & Meyer, K. F. (1955) *J. infect. Dis.* **96,** 138.
27 Vorbiev, A. A. et al (1973) *Zh. Mikrobiol. Epidem. Immunobiol.* **10,** 77.
28 Meyer, K. F. (1972) *Suppl. Proc. Symp. Live influenza and bacterial vaccine*. Yugoslav. Acad. Sci. & Inst. Immunolski. Zagreb.
29 Whitmore, A. (1913) *J. Hyg., Camb.* **13,** 1.
30 Stanton, A. J. & Fletcher, W. (1921) *Studies from the Institute of Medical Research*. Kuala Lumpur: FMH Government Printing Office.
31 Pons, R. & Advier, M. (1927) *J. Hyg., Camb.* **26,** 28.
32 Ashdown, L. R. & Guard, R. W. (1984) *Am. J. trop. Med. Hyg.* **33,** 474–478.
33 Thin, R. N. T., Brown, M., Stewart, J. B. et al (1970) *Q. Jl Med.* **39,** 115.
34 Chambon, L. (1965) *Ann. Inst. Pasteur* **89,** 299.
35 Strauss, J. M., Groves, M. G., Mariappan, M. et al (1969) *Am. J. trop. Med. Hyg.* **18,** 698.
36 Thin, R. N. T., Groves, M. G., Radmund, G. et al (1971) *Singapore med. J.* **12,** 181.
37 Laws, L. & Hall, W. K. T. (1964) *Aust. vet. J.* **40,** 309.
38 Alain, M. St., Etienne, J. & Reynes, V. (1949) *Med. trop.* **9,** 119.
39 Grant, A. & Barwell, C. (1943) *Lancet* **i,** 119.
40 Green, R. & Mankikar, D. S. (1949) *Br. med. J.* **i,** 308.
41 Ashdown, L. R. (1981) *J. clin. Microbiol.* **14,** 361–364.
42 Guard, R. W., Kwafagi, F. A., Brigden, M. C. et al (1984) *Am. J. trop. Med. Hyg.* **33,** 467–473.

Chapter 28
Rhinoscleroma

GEOGRAPHICAL DISTRIBUTION

Rhinoscleroma is spread over widely distributed regions in special nests or foci and occurs all over the world. According to Kouwenaar[1] between 3000 and 4000 cases have been recorded. Small foci exist in Switzerland and Italy. The most extensive area of infection is in eastern Europe, Hungary, Poland, Galicia, the Ukraine and the northern shores of the Black Sea and Caspian Sea. Other foci have been noted in Tomsk in Siberia, Turkestan, Bengal, Java, Sumatra, central and southern France, Morocco, Egypt, New England, Argentina, Cuba, Mexico, Panama, Colombia, Brazil, Peru, Chile, El Salvador and Costa Rica.

AETIOLOGY

The cause of rhinoscleroma is *Klebsiella rhinoscleromatis* which is a gram-negative organism closely related to *Klebsiella pneumoniae* or Friedländer's bacillus, from which it can be distinguished by its growth as well as by its reactions in media containing bile. It is easily cultivated and forms knob-like colonies on gelatin or agar, greyish on the whole and less conspicuous than *K. pneumoniae*. In sections it is found in hard fibrotic swellings in the nose, scattered throughout the mucosa and submucosa. It exhibits a very low order of pathogenicity for laboratory animals with the exception of mice and has to be differentiated from other capsulated pneumococcus-like organisms in the nose. Other klebsiellae (*K. ozaenae*, *K. pneumoniae*) have been found to be causative agents in a minority of cases.[2]

TRANSMISSION

Little is known about transmission but its existence in small restricted foci and the absence of any animal host suggests direct transmission from man to man, the portal of exit and entry being the nasal passages.

PATHOLOGY

Rhinoscleroma is characterized by a peculiar form of plasma-cell infiltration of great density and by gaps or 'foam cells' which consist of swollen cells with foamy cytoplasm ('foam cells' or 'Mikulicz cells') (Fig. 28.1). Very frequently there are also hyaline drops or gram-positive Russell's bodies which occur in all kinds of degenerative tissue and are probably derived from the plasma cells. The rhinoscleroma nodule is known as a plasmoma. It never breaks down but becomes progressively sclerosed. The scleromatous process may spread and via the paranasal sinuses may grow into the upper lip and infiltrate the alveolar process of the maxilla, involve the pharynx by direct extension from the nose and may affect the lacrimal duct. In rare cases it may spread through the cribriform plate and invade the brain, giving rise to a tumour affecting the base of the brain. The nasal septum and the alveolar border of the maxilla may show local destruction. The cervical glands are often enlarged.

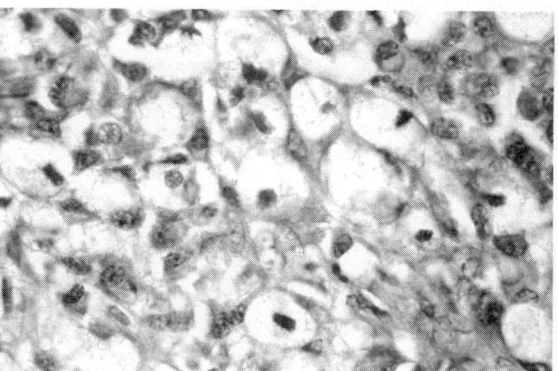

Fig. 28.1 Photomicrograph of tissue from a case of rhinoscleroma showing Mikulicz cells and general histological picture. (Courtesy Professor M. S. R. Hutt.)

IMMUNITY

Little is known about immunity. *K. rhinoscleromatis* has both somatic and capsular antigens, the capsular inducing specific antibodies which are used in serological diagnosis.

CLINICAL FEATURES

Natural history

Rhinoscleroma causes a very chronic, slowly progressive, inflammatory growth in the nose and respiratory passages anywhere from the nostrils to the hilum of the lung, which leads to great disfigurement and eventual death.

The *incubation period* is not known.

Symptoms and signs

The disease starts as a painless, chronic, inflammatory swelling causing nasal or respiratory tract obstruction which gradually increases in size to produce gross deformity of the nose and distortion of the respiratory tract. The typical splayed out nasal organ is known as the 'hebra nose' (Fig. 28.2) and is most commonly found in Sumatra but is rare elsewhere. Sometimes there is perforation of the nasal septum with total destruction of the uvula. The process extends along the respiratory passages with little change in the surrounding tissues. On the whole it tends to form metastases with enlargement of the neighbouring lymphatic glands but, in spite of this, the general health and condition remain unaffected.

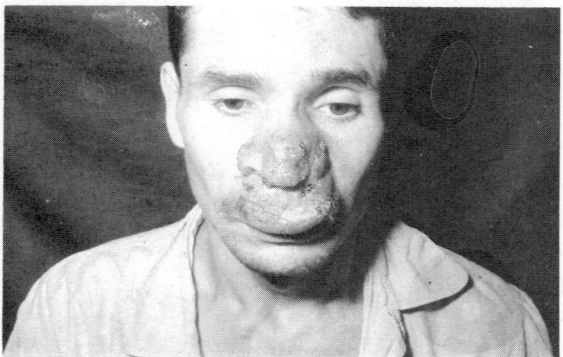

Fig. 28.2   Hebra nose in a patient with rhinoscleroma. (Courtesy Dr F. Kerdel-Vegas.)

DIFFERENTIAL DIAGNOSIS

Similar appearances of the nose are seen in espundia, rhinosporidiosis, leprosy and late syphilis and yaws.

DIAGNOSIS

A portion of tissue is teased out and a smear is made and stained by Pappenheim's method when the characteristic foam cells can be demonstrated in 30 minutes.

Serology

Capsular antibodies can be detected by complement fixation and haemagglutination tests. The Middlebrook–Dubos haemagglutination test is both specific and sensitive.[3]

TREATMENT

The treatment is mainly surgical by plastic operation to remove the unsightly growths. Intramuscular streptomycin is effective in some cases in doses of 1 g daily intramuscularly for a month. More extended courses may be necessary.[1]

EPIDEMIOLOGY

Rhinoscleroma occurs in small discrete foci in widely distributed areas with direct transmission. Little is known about the reasons for this distribution or where the reservoir of organisms is found. The disease is associated with poor and crowded living conditions.

REFERENCES

1 Kouwenaar, W. (1956) *Documenta Geogr. trop.* **8,** 13.
2 Rees, T. A. & Gregory, M. M. (1977) *Lancet* **i,** 650.
3 Hencner, Z. & Tuskiewicz, M. (1958) *Ann. Univ. Marie Curie-Sklódowska* **13,** 128. (Quoted by *Trop. Dis. Bull.* (1960) **57,** 73.)

Chapter 29
Diphtheria

GEOGRAPHICAL DISTRIBUTION

Diphtheria has a worldwide distribution but is not uncommon in hot tropical countries where it is becoming more obvious since improving standards of hygiene have reduced the incidence of immunization from cutaneous diphtheria.

AETIOLOGY

Corynebacterium diphtheriae is a pleomorphic non-motile, non-spore bearing, gram-positive organism. It grows aerobically on Loeffler's and tellurite media and can be differentiated into three types: *C. d. mitis, C. d. gravis* and *C. d. intermedius.*

TRANSMISSION

Man is the only known host and infection is transmitted by droplet, dust or, more rarely, fomites direct from man to man from carriers and cases. Transfer to the throat from abraded skin infections is common and these are major sources of infection.

Carriers

Healthy carriers of the organism in the throat or on the skin are common and a throat carrier rate of 7% was found in Ugandan children.[1]

PATHOLOGY

Exotoxin

Most bacilli produce a protein exotoxin which is responsible for the clinical illness but non-toxic *C. diphtheriae* can also cause infections.

The infection occurs in the upper respiratory tract where invasion of the epithelial cells of the pharynx causes an adherent membrane formed of bacteria, necrotic tissue and fibrin. The infection may spread to the laryngeal and nasal mucosa, the skin, genitalia and the umbilical cord of infants, especially in the tropics.

The exotoxin circulates in the blood causing toxic manifestations, especially in the heart (myocarditis) and the peripheral nerves (peripheral neuropathy).

IMMUNITY

Infection induces a well-marked immunity to reinfection and second attacks are rare. The immunity is mediated by humoral antibodies especially antitoxins which neutralize the diphtheria toxin and kill the bacteria. These antibodies cross the placenta and protect infants for up to six months. Protective immunity may be acquired by inapparent infection of the throat or skin.

CLINICAL FEATURES

Natural history

Most infections are asymptomatic, especially skin infections. These immunize those infected, many of whom become carriers. A varying proportion develop mild pharyngeal (mitis) or severe (gravis) infection. These may heal spontaneously but many develop cardiac and nerve complications with heart block and paralysis.

Incubation period

The incubation period is 1–7 days.

Symptoms and signs

Pharyngeal diphtheria

The onset may be gradual or sudden with sore throat and malaise. Other symptoms may be nausea, vomiting, and painful dysphagia. The throat may appear inflamed just like a streptococcal throat but usually a membrane forms which is grey-green in colour and adherent to the underlying tissues which when removed leaves a bleeding surface. The cervical glands become enlarged causing a 'bull neck' appearance.

Laryngeal diphtheria

Infection may spread to the larynx and can occur without any pharyngeal infection. Laryngeal diphtheria causes laryngeal obstruction with cough and laryngeal stridor (croup). Croup has a typical presentation with a weak cough and evidence of palatal paralysis with inspiratory stridor, best heard by holding the ear close to the patient's mouth.

Nasal diphtheria

Rarely infection is restricted to the nose with unilateral serosanguineous or purulent nasal discharge.

Cutaneous diphtheria

See Chapter 39.

Complications

Myocarditis

The exotoxin causes cardiac arrhythmias and heart failure. It becomes apparent during the first week of illness when electrocardiographic changes will be seen (AV block and left bundle branch block). At this stage sudden death may occur from complete heart block. Myocarditis can be detected by the rapid weak pulse, dyspnoea and increased jugular venous pressure. Myocarditis is completely reversible with treatment and there are no permanent effects.

Neuropathy

The exotoxin affects the peripheral nerves especially of the lower limbs and the cranial nerves with paralysis of the soft palate (nasal voice and return of food and water through the nose on swallowing), blurred vision and loss of accommodation. The neuropathy appears up to four weeks after onset and completely recovers with treatment.

DIAGNOSIS

Laryngeal and faucial diphtheria must be dis-

tinguished from other bacterial causes of acute pharyngitis, especially streptococcal pharyngitis. The membrane is adherent and leaves a bleeding surface when removed in contrast to the other causes. Acute viral pharyngitis and infectious mononucleosis with cervical adenitis must all be distinguished.

The organisms can be seen on direct smear from the throat and cultured on Loeffler's medium.

TREATMENT

Laryngeal and pharyngeal diphtheria is a medical emergency and treatment must be instituted on suspicion before laboratory confirmation. All patients should be nursed in bed and isolated and not discharged until two throat cultures are negative. All contacts should be tested for the carrier state and treated with penicillin or erythromycin.

Antitoxin

All patients must be first tested for sensitivity. Mild cases require 10 000–20 000 units intramuscularly or intravenously. Nasopharyngeal cases require 50 000–100 000 units half intramuscularly and the rest intravenously by drip in 200 ml saline.

Antibiotics

Procaine penicillin 300 mg intramuscularly 12-hourly or erythromycin 250 mg 6-hourly should be given for 10 days.

Carriers will respond to penicillin or erythromycin.

EPIDEMIOLOGY AND CONTROL

Laryngeal and pharyngeal diphtheria used to be uncommon in the tropics where the high incidence of cutaneous infection immunized the population. Improving standards of hygiene and residence in towns have reduced the incidence of cutaneous infection so that now, as with paralytic poliomyelitis, laryngeal and pharyngeal diphtheria have become more common. Non-immunized expatriates are at risk.

CONTROL

Contacts of cases of diphtheria must be examined for the carrier state and susceptible contacts treated with penicillin.

IMMUNIZATION

The *Schick test* is used to determine the susceptibility of individuals to infection; 0.1 ml of diphtheria toxin is injected intradermally and the site examined after 48 hours. A positive reaction is shown by an area of erythema. This means the person has no immunity since there is no antitoxin in the system to neutralize the toxin. A negative reaction denotes immunity.

Immunization with diphtheria toxoid prevents the disease. Infants should be immunized in the first year of life with DPT (diphtheria, pertussis, tetanus) vaccine—first dose at two or three months then the second and third doses at four to six week intervals. Booster doses should be given at one and five years of age. Children over six years and adults should be given the first dose and then the second after six weeks and the third after six months. Booster doses should be given to expatriates moving to developing countries.

REFERENCES

1   Bezjak, V. & Farsey, S. J. (1970) *Bull. Wld Hlth Org.* **43**, 543.

Chapter 30
Acute Bacterial Meningitis

Acute bacterial meningitis is a common cause of illness in tropical countries where it is a significant cause of mortality in children under five years of age. Three organisms are responsible.

Streptococcus pneumoniae (pneumococcal meningitis)

Haemophilus influenzae (influenzal meningitis)

Neisseria meningitidis (meningococcal meningitis)

The commonest causes of bacterial meningitis throughout both the wet and dry tropics are *S. pneumoniae* and *H. influenzae*. Meningococcal infection is most common in the northern savannah belt of tropical Africa (meningitis belt, see Fig. 30.1) where major epidemics occur. A major epidemic has recently occurred in Brazil.

All three organisms have capsular polysaccharide antigens which are specific, dividing them into a number of different groups and exciting a powerful antibody response. *H. influenzae* and *N. meningitidis* in addition possess a powerful endotoxin.

TRANSMISSION

Transmission is by droplet spread from person to person from asymptomatic infections in the nasopharynx although pneumococci may spread from a focus in the lung.

PATHOLOGY

Pathogenesis

From a rhinopharyngitis the organisms reach the bloodstream from which they reach the meninges. *H. influenzae* and *N. meningitidis* both possess a powerful *endotoxin* which is responsible for the pathological manifestations of acute infection and the meningitis. *Endotoxin* activates both the complement and clotting pathways causing circulatory collapse and disseminated intravascular coagulation. Some pneumococcal infections lacking endotoxin may activate the alternative pathway. Local endotoxin production contributes to the polymorphonuclear infiltration of the meninges. Other manifestations of infection are caused by immunopathological effects. Antigen–antibody immune complexes form and are responsible for arthritis, cutaneous vasculitis, episcleritis, iritis and pericarditis which may develop several days after the onset of illness, appearing at a time when the patient is improving. These lesions are sterile and are characterized by a vasculitis in which antigen–antibody and complement can be demonstrated by immunofluorescence suggesting that immune complexes are deposited locally around organisms which have reached there. These lesions occur most frequently when antigen disappears from the circulation and antibody appears.[1] These immunopathological effects are most commonly seen in meningococcal infections.

Morbid anatomy

The surface of the brain is flattened and the ventricles distended. The pia arachnoid is covered with a purulent exudate, white to greenish (in the case of pneumococcal infection), situated between the pia and arachnoid. The exudate is composed of neutrophils, red cells and organisms. Subarachnoid block occurs on the roof of the fourth ventricle. Throughout the brain there are perivascular foci of pus cells, red cells and organisms (pneumococci penetrate deeper and cause an encephalitis). Metastatic infection may cause pleurisy, pericarditis, pneumonia, ophthalmitis, peritonitis (especially pneumococci). Adrenal haemorrhage is caused by endotoxin.

IMMUNITY

There is a well-marked immunity against further infection in all three infections. Protection against pneumococcal, meningococcal and *H. influenzae* infection is mediated by antibody. Little is known about cell-mediated immunity. The capsular polysaccharide antigens stimulate a protective immunity against the organisms and both the asymptomatic carrier state and clinical infection can immunize. Cross protection can be achieved by related organisms containing common antigens which are harmless commensals. As a result most adults possess bactericidal antibodies against meningococci, *H. influenzae* and some pneumococcal strains, and are immune. Susceptible individuals have no antibodies and are not immune.

CLINICAL FEATURES

Natural history

Infection in the majority of cases is completely symptomless apart from a mild pharyngitis in the carrier state. In susceptible persons infection with meningococci may cause acute meningococcaemia (see p. 616) with rapid death. In all infections a small proportion develop acute meningitis.

The *incubation period* is 2–5 days.

Symptoms and signs

The onset is usually sudden, the presenting symptoms being headache, fever and malaise. There may also be photophobia, vomiting and convulsions, especially in young children. On examination, there will be signs of meningitis. The neck is stiff and the head retracted. In pneumococcal infections there is a greater degree of impairment of consciousness than in the other infections. In infants there may be bulging of the anterior fontanelle. Cranial nerve palsies (III, VI, VII and VIII) may all occur. In meningococcal infection a petechial rash may be present and signs of myocardial involvement with electrocardiographic changes and arrhythmias. In pneumococcal infection there may be signs of infection elsewhere—pneumonia, sinusitis and otitis media.

Laboratory findings

The blood shows a polymorphonuclear leukocytosis and thrombocytopenia. Blood culture is most likely to be possible in *H. influenzae*. Capsular polysaccharide antigen can be detected in the serum of some patients.

Cerebrospinal fluid (CSF)

The CSF is usually turbid and under pressure.

The cell count shows a high leukocyte count with high protein and a low glucose, lower than the blood glucose (cf. tuberculous meningitis). Organisms may be difficult to demonstrate especially if antibiotics have been given but polysaccharide capsular antigen can be demonstrated and is a useful diagnostic tool.

Complications

Complications may occur in the nervous system: extradural collections of fluid or empyema, cerebral thrombosis and encephalopathy (common in pneumococcal infection). Raised intracranial pressure may cause coning and there may be disseminated pyogenic lesions in the eyes and joints. Herpes simplex eruption around the mouth is not uncommon when the patient is in hospital.

DIFFERENTIAL DIAGNOSIS

Meningitis can be easily missed in its early stages when there may be no fever. It must be thought of in any child with febrile convulsions and in older patients who suddenly become confused. Other causes of fever and meningism are many: falciparum malaria, typhus, relapsing fever and other conditions causing meningism. Viral and tuberculous meningitis may be excluded by examination of the cerebrospinal fluid. A rash favours meningococcal pneumonia and otitis media, pneumococcal meningitis.

DIAGNOSIS

A turbid CSF confirms the diagnosis of meningitis but clear fluid can show a white cell count of $200/mm^3$ or more. The CSF should be centrifuged and a fresh portion examined for amoebae (see Chapter 24). The rest must be stained to determine the type of cellular exudate and the presence of organisms. Lymphocytes are found in viral meningitis and both polymorphs and lymphocytes in tuberculous meningitis. Often the CSF findings have been obscured by previous antibiotic treatment.

Immunodiagnosis

The two main methods of immunodiagnosis are detection of specific polysaccharide and detection of endotoxin.

Meningococcal and pneumococcal meningitis can be diagnosed rapidly and typed by direct countercurrent immunoelectrophoresis (CIE) of the CSF against specific antisera.[2] Antibody-coated latex particles have also been used to detect polysaccharide antigens in the CSF.[2] This is a simple and easy method of diagnosis in rural hospitals needing a minimum of equipment. Latex particles precoated with antibody to the appropriate organisms can be stored ready for use. On adding the particles to serum or CSF they will agglutinate when the homologous organism is present.

Endotoxin may be detected by the limulus test[3] which can be used as a side room investigation, but only distinguishes gram-negative from gram-positive meningitis. Antigen levels in the CSF are of value in prognosis since patients with severe brain damage and late sequelae have a higher concentration in the CSF than those who recover without any sequelae.[4] Antigen usually disappears from the CSF 24–48 hours from the start of treatment; longer persistence is ominous and antigen in the serum, especially if present in high titre or for more than 2 or 3 days, is another bad sign.

TREATMENT

Antibiotic therapy

The choice of antibiotic depends upon the causative organism which may not always be easy to identify, especially after previous antibiotic therapy.

Where the organism cannot be identified

Chloramphenicol is the antibiotic of choice in the treatment of acute bacterial meningitis where the organism cannot be isolated. It crosses the brain barrier and is effective against most isolates of pneumococci, meningococci and *H. influenzae*. Chloramphenicol 500 mg (children 25 mg/kg) by parenteral and then oral administration 6-hourly should be given for 14 days. A single injection of 3 g of long-acting chloramphenicol (Tifomycine) has proved an effective method of treatment suitable for the management of epidemics in areas with limited resources.[5]

Meningococcal meningitis

Crystalline penicillin 1.2 g (children 600 mg) should be given intramuscularly or intravenously 6-hourly for 5–7 days. Chloramphenicol is an effective alternative to penicillin if this cannot be given.

Pneumococcal meningitis

Crystalline penicillin 2.4 g (children 600 mg to 1.2 g) should be given 6-hourly for 14 days. If there is any evidence of resistance, change must be made to another penicillin (ampicillin), chloramphenicol or another antibiotic.

H. influenzae

Chloramphenicol 500 mg (children 25 mg/kg) should be given at first parenterally and then orally 6-hourly for 10 days.

General measures

The patient should be treated in hospital and if unconscious nursed in a position which maintains the airway open. Regular turning to prevent bedsores is important as is rehydration in hot countries where fever and coma prevent drinking.

Response to treatment

The temperature and degree of consciousness should be monitored and failure to improve within 48 hours should lead to suspicion of an intra- or extradural collection of pus or lead to a change of antibiotic.

Deterioration of the neurological condition of the patient should lead to search for pus by exploratory burr holes. Relapse with a rise in temperature after improvement should lead to a definite suspicion of intracerebral pus. Pneumococcal meningitis may relapse two weeks after a full course of antibiotics and the CSF should be examined 2–3 days after termination of treatment in all cases. Most patients with meningococcal and influenzal meningitis recover but the prognosis in pneumococcal meningitis is much worse.

PREVENTION

Chemoprophylaxis of pneumococcal and *H. influenzae* infection

Sustained prophylaxis with penicillin has been used to protect high risk individuals such as splenectomized people and cases of sickle cell disease.

Vaccines

Pneumococcal polysaccharide vaccines are now available. They work poorly, however, in young people, do not confer a lasting immunity and are only group specific. Their use in the tropics is confined to special groups, such as patients with sickle cell disease or the nephrotic syndrome.

Meningococcal infection

GEOGRAPHICAL DISTRIBUTION

Meningococcal infection is cosmopolitan in distribution, endemic in large towns but breaking out in epidemics in villages. In Africa these epidemics occur in the 'meningitis belt' spreading from west to east between 10° and 12° north (Fig. 30.1).

lapse and the inflammatory changes in the meninges in meningitis.

There are a number of antigenic groups of which three are important: A, B and C, each with its own specific polysaccharide capsular antigen, the chemical structure of which is known, and diseases due to meningococci of groups A and C can be controlled by vaccination with material

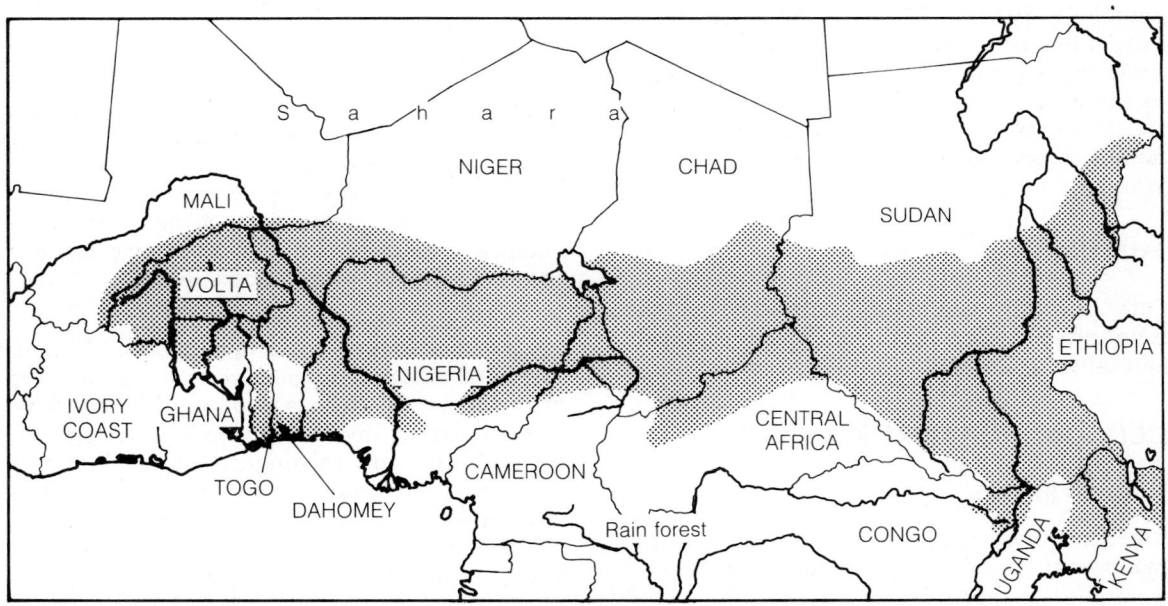

Fig. 30.1 Cerebrospinal meningitis. The African meningitis belt.

AETIOLOGY

The meningococcus (*Neisseria meningitidis*) is a gram-negative coccus $0.8 \times 0.6\,\mu m$ occurring in pairs or tetrads in the nasopharynx of man in neutrophil leukocytes or free. It grows well aerobically on blood or serum enriched media at 37°C, ferments glucose and maltose but not sucrose with acid formation. Meningococci produce a large amount of endotoxin which is responsible for the peripheral circulatory col-

containing their group specific polysaccharide. Since the chemical nature of the polysaccharides is known those of groups Y and W 135 have been incorporated with groups A and C antigen in a quadrivalent vaccine. Large scale epidemics are usually due to group A but group C meningococci caused a large outbreak in Brazil[6] and this group is increasing in prevalence in Africa.[7] Meningococci are delicate organisms, sensitive to heat, not surviving for more than half an hour at 40°C. They are sensitive to sunlight and changes in temperature.

TRANSMISSION

Transmission is from person to person by droplet spread from asymptomatic carriers.

PATHOLOGY

Meningococci produce large amounts of endotoxin, which is important in causing the peripheral circulatory collapse characteristic of acute meningococcaemia. A patient who has died from acute meningococcaemia may show few abnormalities. Extensive haemorrhage may be present in the adrenals. Factors other than acute adrenal insufficiency may, however, be responsible for the shock. Spread from the nasopharynx to the cerebrospinal fluid causes meningitis with involvement of the pia arachnoid (see section on pathology, p. 612). Arthritis, cutaneous vasculitis, episcleritis and pericarditis, which develop some days after the start of the illness, are caused by immune complexes in these tissues which are sterile. These complexes can be shown by immunofluorescence to be situated around small blood vessels.[8]

IMMUNITY

One infection confers an antibody-mediated immunity against both the organism responsible and other strains and second attacks are rare.

CLINICAL FEATURES

Natural history

Most meningococcal infections are asymptomatic with a mild pharyngitis conferring an immunity against further attacks. These mild infections are carriers who may consist of 30% of the population at times and who are responsible for transmitting the infection. Some susceptible individuals may develop meningitis while a small proportion develop a severe meningococcaemia leading to peripheral circulatory collapse and death.

The *incubation period* is 2–5 days.

Acute meningococcaemia (spotted fever)

Symptoms and signs

The onset is sudden, the patient being well one morning and possibly dead by evening. Fever, headache, general malaise and sometimes diarrhoea are the main symptoms. At first there is nothing to find except fever and tachycardia and even fever may not be present in a severely ill patient. Later petechiae appear in the skin and conjunctiva which rapidly progress to ecchymoses. The blood pressure falls dramatically, the electrocardiogram suggests myocardial involvement and the patient goes into shock.

Laboratory investigations

There is a marked polymorphonuclear leukocytosis (except in very ill patients), blood culture is positive and meningococci may be seen in a peripheral thick blood smear.

Complications

Disseminated intravascular coagulation occurs early with haemorrhage; pulmonary oedema and renal failure result from myocardial complications. Later, if the patient lives, immune complex complications occur: arthritis, cutaneous vasculitis leading even to gangrene of the extremities and skin ulceration.

Arthritis. Patients with meningococcal meningitis or acute meningococcaemia may develop arthritis during the stage of septicaemia from direct bacterial invasion of the joint with purulent effusion and meningococci, or they may develop it later during recovery about 6 days after onset when one joint, usually the knee, is affected. There is a secondary rise in temperature and a serous effusion into the joint. The arthritis resolves gradually over a period of days or weeks and no permanent effects are noted. It may be accompanied by other immune complex-related complications.

Chronic meningococcaemia

This is a rare condition characterized by recurrent fever, rash, arthritis and splenomegaly. The rash is most frequently maculopapular, although petechial, nodular and ecchymotic lesions are also seen. The condition is accompanied by many of the immune complex complications.

DIAGNOSIS

Acute meningococcaemia is very easy to miss. The patient may at first sight not appear to be ill and may even be afebrile. The early petechial rash may not be discovered. Other septicaemias with endotoxic shock (*Escherichia coli*) must be distinguished. Typhus fever, plague, viral haemorrhagic fevers all produce fever, a haemorrhagic rash and shock. The diagnosis is made by demonstrating the meningococcus in blood or CSF, by culture or smear.

Demonstration of organisms

Meningococci are delicate organisms. They are sensitive to heat, not surviving more than one and a half hours at 40°C, which is quite usual in the epidemic season. They are very sensitive to sunlight and to changes in temperature; although they survive freezing, they suffer badly at the usual temperature found in a refrigerator.[9] Specimens of cerebrospinal fluid or throat swabs should therefore not be kept in a refrigerator or in sunlight, but should be taken at body temperature at once to the laboratory and inoculated on to culture medium as soon as possible.

Nasopharyngeal carriers can be detected by taking swabs but the technique needs care. Metal rods (for instance bicycle spokes) are better than wooden sticks since wood releases harmful substances. The toxicity of cotton-wool swabs can be reduced by rolling them in finely powdered vegetable charcoal before sterilization. The swabs can be dipped in 0.1 M phosphate buffer solution at pH 7.4, boiled in this for 10 minutes and then dried and sterilized.[9] Meningococci can be isolated in Thayer–Martin medium but this is a task for the specialist.

Biopsy of the skin rash may show meningococci.

Serology

Detection of polysaccharide capsular antigen in the serum or CSF is a rapid way of making a diagnosis. The latex test (see section on immunodiagnosis, p. 613) can be used in rural hospitals.

TREATMENT

Acute meningococcaemia is a very serious illness and should be managed if possible in intensive care. The principles of treatment are to maintain the blood pressure, treat the shock, treat the infection with penicillin and, in some cases, corticosteroid therapy.

Treatment of shock

Infusion of plasma or dextran should be started but care must be taken to avoid pulmonary oedema. The peripheral vascular resistance can be controlled by noradrenaline by intravenous infusion and careful combination of both these methods should be used to keep the systolic blood pressure at 100 mmHg. Phentolamine 20–80 μg/minute by intravenous drip will to a certain extent counteract the noradrenaline but may be added if the condition of the patient requires it.

Antibiotic treatment

Penicillin must be given by intravenous drip, 2.4 g 6-hourly for an adult, and later intramuscularly and continued for 7 days.

Corticosteroids

The use of corticosteroids is controversial. In some patients with a low plasma cortisol who are hypotensive, hydrocortisone and prednisone should be given in high dosage; heparin therapy is ineffective.

EPIDEMIOLOGY

Meningococci are spread from one person to another via the nasopharynx and the nasal and buccal discharges. In general the epidemiology is that of a respiratory infection in which the numbers of patients who become ill are very much less than the numbers of healthy carriers in the general population. In closed communities, such as military units living in barracks, the proportion of carriers may reach 50% within the first three months of barrack life, but only a small proportion are ill. In these conditions the proportion of carriers is influenced by the inflow of new recruits, most of whom are not infected before arrival.

The proportion of carriers to the numbers diseased is inverted. Those who get meningitis do so early in their exposure when the numbers of carriers are increasing; when the carriers are at their peak the numbers of clinical cases fall off.

The disease often tends chiefly to affect children. In Delhi, India, an epidemic in 1966 did so with a case mortality rate of 37% below the age of one year. In other outbreaks the incidence may be highest at age 15–19. Like other epidemics, the Delhi outbreak was most severe in congested areas.

Special conditions exist in Africa which favour the occurrence of epidemic waves. In a wide belt of country between the Sahara to the north and the equatorial forest to the south, stretching from the Sudan westwards through Chad, northern Nigeria, Benin, Ghana and Upper Volta, there are some 10 000 cases of meningitis each year with an average case mortality of around 12%[9] and the incidence is seasonal. The feature of this area which probably determines the epidemic waves is that between January and March the weather is dry and the nights are very cold (Fig. 30.2). The people therefore sleep inside their houses at this time, though at other seasons they tend to sleep outside or on the roofs. In this dry weather the mucous membranes of the nasopharynx tend to be dry, ceasing to act as an efficient barrier to infection. Conditions for transmission from carriers are favourable and cases of meningitis occur. This cycle tends to end in about three months when a degree of immunity has been established.

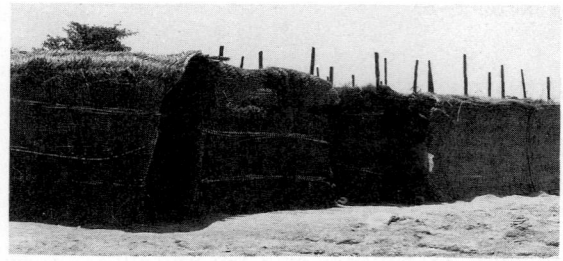

Fig. 30.2 Cerebrospinal meningitis isolation camp outside a large village 12 miles north of Zaria, northern Nigeria. The graves of the dead can be seen on the lower flats below the camp. In the wet season these flats, just outside the village, become a large pond from which the inhabitants draw their drinking water. (Courtesy Dr A. J. Duggan.)

At other times of the year in this area carriers maintain the infection at a low rate and actual disease is sporadic. There seems to be no evidence that disease is provoked solely by organisms of increased virulence, but lack of immunity in individuals is probably a factor. Subclinical infections may provide some immunity. The seasonal incidence in West Africa may be due to changes in the ratio of clinical to subclinical infection while the frequency of transmission remains the same. The reason for these changes remains obscure.[10]

PROPHYLAXIS

Prevention of overcrowding in schools and villages in the cold dry season helps to prevent spread but there are two further measures which can be very effective.

Chemoprophylaxis

Sulphonamides protect against clinical disease and remove meningococci from the nasopharynx of carriers. A single dose of the drug can give protection for several weeks. Many meningococci are, however, now resistant to sulphonamides.

Sulphadiazine

Dose: 1 g twice daily for adults for 2 days; children one to 12 years 500 mg twice daily and infants under one year 500 mg once a day.

Other antibiotics

Rifampicin has been used successfully but is expensive and resistance develops rapidly. *Dose*: adults 600 mg twice daily for 2 days; children one to 12 years 10 mg/kg, infants under one year 5 mg/kg.

Vaccination

Group A and C meningococcal polysaccharide capsular vaccines are now available in a quadrivalent vaccine and are effective, and serious epidemics of meninogcoccal disease have been brought under control in Brazil. Whereas vaccines protect against disease it is not known whether they stop the spread of infection by carriers. They do not work well in young children and booster doses do not always enhance the antibody response. Epidemiological studies suggest that protection lasts for three years and three immunizations are necessary during the first five years of life.

Control of infection

A combination of chemotherapy and vaccination is necessary. Where the organism is sensitive to sulphonamides then vaccination plus sulphonamide chemoprophylaxis should be given to household contacts and the occupants of the crowded accommodation where the outbreak has occurred. Where the organism is insensitive then rifampicin plus vaccination should be given to household contacts and the rest of the population vaccinated. Mass vaccination of the population can bring an epidemic of group A or C meningococcal infection to a halt, but it may only be necessary to vaccinate the two to 20 year age group.

REFERENCES

1 Greenwood, B. M., Whittle, H. C. & Bryceson, A. D. M. (1973) *Br. med. J.* **i,** 797.
2 Whittle, H. C., Tugwell, P., Egler, L. J. et al (1974) *Lancet* **ii,** 619.
3 Ross, S., Rodriguez, W., Contoni, G. et al (1975) *J. Am. med. Ass.* **233,** 1366.
4 Whittle, H. C., Greenwood, B. M., Davidson, N. McD. et al (1975) *Am. J. Med.* **58,** 283.
5 Wali, S. S., MacFarlane, T., Weir, W. R. C. (1979) *Trans. R. Soc. trop. Med. Hyg.* **73,** 698.
6 Morais, J. S., Munford, R. S., Risi, J. P. et al (1974) *J. inf. Dis.* **129,** 568–571.
7 Rey, J. L., Adamov, E. J. & Picq, J. J. (1983) *Med. trop.* **43,** 60.
8 Whittle, H. C., Abdullahi, M. T., Fakunle, F. A. et al (1973) *Br. med. J.* **i,** 733.
9 World Health Organization (1970) *WHO Chron.* **23,** 54.
10 Greenwood, B. M., Bradley, A. K., Blakeborough, I. S. et al (1984) *Lancet* **i,** 1339–1342.

SECTION V
DISEASES CAUSED BY SPIROCHAETES

Chapter 31
Endemic Treponematoses

The treponematoses include:
Venereal syphilis (*Treponema pallidum*)
Non-venereal syphilis (endemic syphilis, bejel, njovera) (*T. pallidum*), treponarid
Yaws (buba, pian, framboesia) (*T. pertenue*)
Pinta (carate, mal del pinto) (*T. carateum, T. herrejoni*)

GEOGRAPHICAL DISTRIBUTION

The geographical distribution of the treponematoses is shown in Fig. 31.1. Since 1900 there has been a great diminution in the incidence of yaws and treponarid in all the areas shown, but in only one (treponarid in Bosnia) has eradication been accomplished.

AETIOLOGY

Two opinions are held about the origin of the treponematoses. Hackett[1] considers that the progenitor of the group was pinta, which probably arose from an animal infection about 15 000 BC, spreading throughout the world but later becoming isolated in the Americas. Yaws arose from mutants of the pinta treponeme and by about 10 000 BC had spread throughout much of the world but did not reach the Americas, which were then isolated by the flooding of the Bering Strait as a result of the melting of the polar ice caps. Treponarid arose from yaws about 7000 BC when arid climates followed the retreat of the last glaciation, favouring the selection of suitable treponemes. Venereal syphilis appeared from

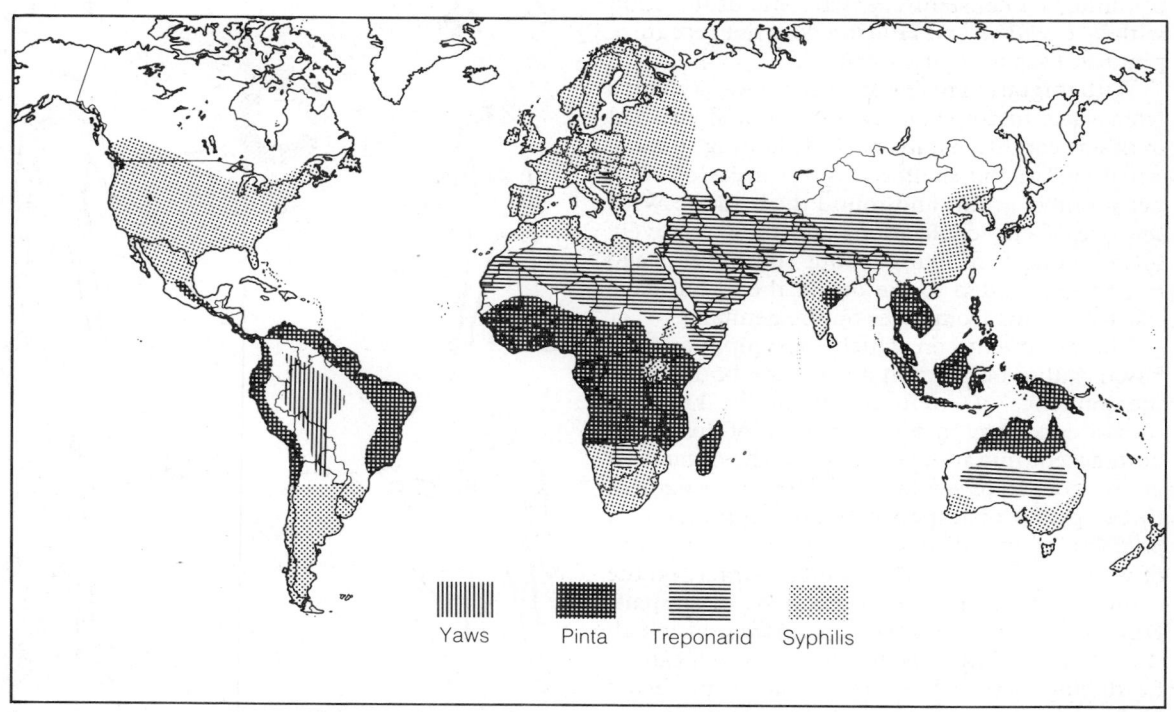

Yaws   Pinta   Treponarid   Syphilis

Fig. 31.1   Geographical distribution of human treponematoses about AD 1900. (Courtesy Dr C. J. Hackett.)

treponarid about 3000 BC, when big cities developed in south-west Asia, favouring the selection of suitable mutants. Venereal syphilis spread through Europe after the first century AD as a mild disease, until a mutation to the present form took place towards the end of the fifteenth century. It was carried throughout the world with the European expansion which has taken place since then.

Hudson,[2] however, thinks that the group of diseases probably originated in Africa, possibly from spirochaetes living on decaying vegetable matter, which in the course of time became parasitic in man. The infection was then non-venereal (like yaws) and existed, again like yaws, in conditions of heat, humidity and naked human skin. About 100 000 years ago people migrated from Africa to as far as Australia and Oceania and may have taken yaws with them—it could even have reached the Americas. Pinta probably developed from yaws as a result of some environmental factor; although there are more cases of pinta in Central and South America than anywhere else, Hudson holds that 'pinta' cases can be found constantly, but in varying degree, in association with yaws and syphilis all over the world. Disturbance of pigmentation, the prominent feature of pinta, is a constant characteristic of infection with *T. pallidum* and Hudson does not recognize pinta as a separate disease.

With migration to dry areas there was a change from yaws to treponarid which now flourished in desert conditions, the parasite finding suitable situations in the sheltered moist areas of skin, neck, limbs, groins and round the orifices. With the rise of city civilizations and their relatively high standards of living, about 10 000 years ago treponarid tended to die out in them, but gave rise to syphilis from sores on the genitalia.

The arguments on which these opinions are based cannot be given in detail here; both accept the influence of environment on the kinds of disease encountered in various parts of the world; both accept mutational change in the organisms in the course of evolution. Hackett recognizes three species of treponemes infecting man—*T. pallidum* of syphilis and treponarid, *T. pertenue* of yaws and *T. carateum* of pinta—largely on the evidence of experimental infections in animals. Hudson recognized only *T. pallidum*, of which the others are intraspecific strains, which cannot be distinguished. The nomenclature preferred by Hackett is used for convenience in this book.

Whatever the truth of these interpretations, the fact remains that clinically and epidemiologically there are differences between the various diseases and that although treatment is the same for all, prevention is not.

T. pallidum, *T. pertenue* and *T. carateum* are all highly motile organisms. They are morphologically identical and serological tests fail to differentiate them. They have not been cultivated in artificial media.

TRANSMISSION (Fig. 31.2)[3]

Each treponematosis has a different method of transmission: yaws direct from person to person

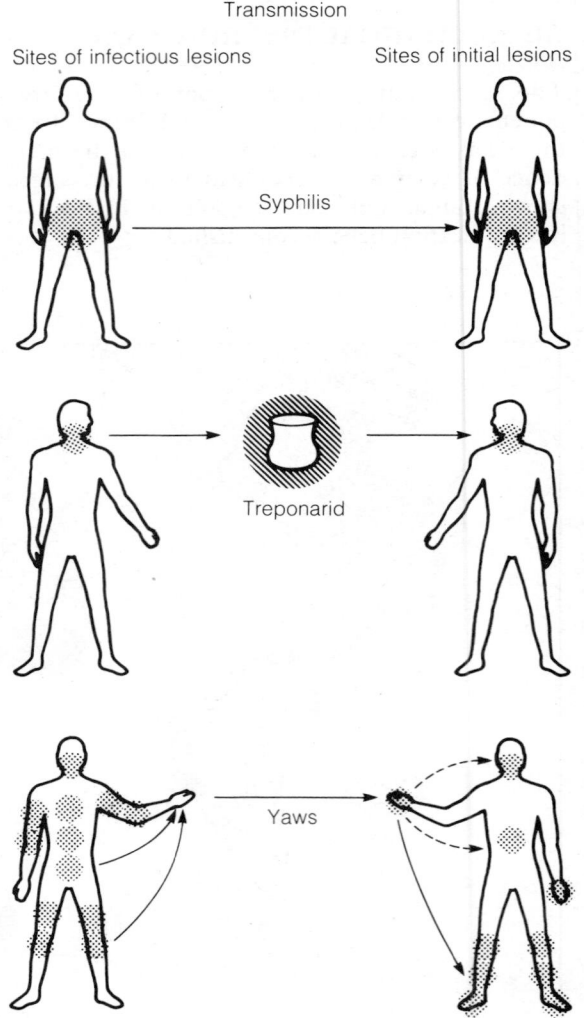

Transmission

Sites of infectious lesions   Sites of initial lesions

Syphilis

Treponarid

Yaws

Fig. 31.2 Transmission of syphilis, treponarid and yaws. (After Hackett.[3])

via the fingers, treponarid via shared utensils and syphilis by sexual contact. Other methods of transmission are of course possible but not so common. Congenital transmission is only found in syphilis.

PATHOLOGY

Pathogenesis

On infection the treponeme attaches to the mammalian cell by specific receptor sites[4] and, although they are more usually seen in the cellular spaces, they can be found in cells[5] where they evade the host's immune responses and persist in latent periods. The lesions (initial, early and late) are characterized by acute inflammatory reactions and since there is no treponemal toxin it is probable that the damage to the tissue is caused by the host response to persistent treponemes.

Pathological features

The basic tissue reactions in the treponematoses are:[6]
1 an exudate with infiltration of lymphocytes, plasma cells and macrophages;
2 proliferation of fibroblasts;
3 endarteritis.

In initial (local) and early (blood-borne) lesions exudation is prominent with little or no fibrosis; these lesions can resolve with little or no permanent trace. Treponemes are present in most of them, especially in the primary and early secondary stages. The initial lesion may be associated with enlargement of the lymph nodes draining the area; this constitutes the initial complex.

In the late stage the notable feature is tissue loss of two main types.[6]
1 Chronic degeneration and atrophy with replacement of the specialized cells of the affected part by fibrous tissue. These changes are permanent. Treponemes are scanty in these lesions except in the brain in general paresis.
2 Gummas, which are localized necrotic processes surrounded by fibroblasts, capillaries, cellular infiltrations and occasional giant cells. Healing is by fibrosis. Treponemes are seldom seen.

All the treponemes of these diseases almost certainly become blood-borne early in the infec-

tion and therefore reach all tissues of the body, but they exhibit affinities for certain tissues.

In pinta the early lesions remain active and contain treponemes for many years before they become inactive and depigmented. They are therefore infective for long periods (which is unique among the treponematoses). Palmar and plantar lesions do not occur and there are no bone lesions or late destructive lesions.

In the early stages of treponarid and yaws, skin, palmar, plantar and bone lesions occur; later there are destructive skin and bone lesions.

In the early stages of syphilis there are skin lesions and not infrequently bone lesions. In the late stages there are destructive lesions of skin, bone and other tissues and lesions of the heart and brain.[1]

In the early stages of syphilis and yaws the lesions may be of two kinds.[6]

1 *Minor*. These are more or less symmetrical generalized eruptions, profuse or sparse. They are either macules or tiny papules, often grouped, and they seldom increase in size; they are short-lived and benign and never ulcerate. Treponemes are very scanty or cannot be demonstrated.

2 *Major*. The major lesions in yaws and pinta often resemble the initial lesions and treponemes are present in large numbers.

IMMUNITY

Resistance to symptomatic infection has been recognized in syphilis for many years and this has been proved experimentally.[7] Immunity also develops in yaws and treponarid, but not in pinta.[8] In experimental infection with yaws treponemes in rabbits, resistance to infection develops by the third month and continues as long as infection is present. In the field there is considerable protection against adult syphilis from childhood yaws. The mechanisms of this immunity are not yet well understood. Both humoral and cellular mechanisms play a part. Antibody contributes by bactericidal action in the initial infection and also by complement-mediated mechanisms. Cellular immunity also is active, T lymphocytes and macrophages leading to healing of the lesions.[9]

There is some reciprocal immunity between all common pathogenic treponemes owing to common antigenic components.[10] Most strains of syphilis give some cross immunity in rabbits and the same in yaws, and although there is no general cross immunity between syphilis and yaws, it is often quite good.

Although a few cross infections of yaws with syphilis in man have been reported (especially when only a month or two separated the infections) most field workers agree that there is considerable protection against syphilis from yaws in childhood. There is no cross immunity between non-pathogenic treponemes and pathological ones except with *T. cuniculi* of the rabbit. Tre-

ponemal antigens are under study but no vaccine has yet been developed.

CLINICAL FEATURES

The treponematoses vary in their clinical characteristics, the main features of which are shown in Table 31.1.

EPIDEMIOLOGY

The treponematoses vary greatly in their epidemiology (Table 31.2).

Table 31.1 Some clinical characters of the treponematosis (after Hackett[1]).

Character	Pinta	Yaws	Treponarid	Syphilis
Usual source of treponemes	Skin anywhere	Skin anywhere	Buccal mucosa	Genital and mucosal lesions
Size of infectious area	Large	Large	Small	Small
Duration of:				
Infectiousness of individual lesions	Many years	A few months	A few months	A few months
Infectiousness of patients, including infectious relapses	Many years	3–5 years	3–5 years	3–5 years
Latency	Absent	Characteristic	Characteristic	Characteristic
Lesions:				
Initial, site	Exposed skin	Skin of legs	Mouth?	Genital
Initial, occurrence	Infrequent	Frequent	Unusual	Frequent
Generalized skin, extent	Extensive	Extensive	Limited	Moderate
Genital, occurrence	Unusual	Scanty	Scanty	Frequent
Buccal mucosal, occurrence	Absent	Scanty or absent	Moderate	Scanty
Palmar and plantar hyperkeratoses occurrence	Absent	Frequent	Scanty	Scanty
Bone, occurrence	Absent	Moderate	Moderate	Scanty
Juxta-articular nodules, occurrence	Absent	Frequent	Scanty	Scanty
Heart, brain and other viscera occurrence	Absent	Absent	Scanty and mild or absent	Moderate
Congenital transmission	Absent	Absent	Absent	Present
Age group of most infections	Children	Children	Children	Adults

Table 31.2 Epidemiological features of the treponematoses.

	Syphilis	Treponarid	Yaws	Pinta
Environment	Urban cosmopolitan	Rural dry Africa	Rural moist	Rural arid, South and Central America
Peak incidence (years)	20–30	2–10	4–15	18–30
Transmission				
congenital	Frequent	Very rare	Never	Never
sexual contact	Usual	Rare	Never	Never
direct fingers	Only occasionally	Common	The usual method	Probable
fomites (utensils)	Rare	Usual	Possible	Never

YAWS

GEOGRAPHICAL DISTRIBUTION
(Fig. 31.1)

Yaws is restricted to tropical countries with a coastal distribution in South America because of its limitation to populations of African descent and a limited distribution in India in certain previously isolated aboriginal tribes. Formerly more prevalent in Africa, it still persists at a low level and in a latent state, and there has recently been a considerable recrudescence; in Ghana there was a 12-fold increase between 1968 and 1981[11] and it has returned to Benin, Ivory Coast, Togo and central Africa where it is found especially among the Pygmies; outbreaks have also occurred in New Guinea.[12]

AETIOLOGY

The cause of yaws is *Treponema pertenue*, which is a slender, delicate spirochaete 8–16 μm long × 0.2 μm wide with some eight to 16 regular spirals of about 1 μm. It cannot be distinguished morphologically from the other treponema, its relationship to which is discussed on p. 623.

TRANSMISSION (Fig. 31.2)

Yaws is essentially a disease of primitive rural people living in moist, humid climates.

Congenital transmission does not occur and healthy babies are born of mothers with early yaws. The infection is transmitted by direct contact of the fingers with a infective lesion in the skin of another person. The treponemes probably enter through a breach in the epidermis.

The treponemes are present in the skin wherever there are early lesions, which remain infective for a few months. There are latent periods after the initial and early lesions but relapses tend to occur when infective lesions may appear. Transmission occurs from child to child.

Early cases are much more common in children than in adults, possibly because adults tend to be immune through previous infection, or because they do not have such close physical contact with infective persons and such a propensity to minor skin injuries.

Transmission is particularly likely in hot and humid conditions where little clothing is worn, the skin is constantly moist (and therefore the lesions tend to be open) and bodily cleanliness is not generally stressed.

Transmission by non-biting flies (especially *Hippelates pallipes*) which are attracted to raw surfaces has been suggested but not satisfactorily proved. If it does occur it is probably of minor importance.

It is to be noted that as rural yaws dies out men from rural villages who visit cities, for instance to attend fairs, are likely to acquire venereal syphilis, to return to their villages with secondary syphilitic sores and from them to infect children non-venereally. The result is syphilis, not yaws, in the children, though the infection is by the skin.

PATHOLOGY

Initial lesion

The initial lesion is a granular papilloma, raised above the skin and usually covered with a scab. There is oedema of the epidermis and infiltration with polymorphs, plasma cells and lymphocytes; there may be an irregular fungating mass of granulation tissue. Sometimes the initial lesion takes the form of an ulcer with a granulating base which is rarely indurated. Healing takes place by scab formation and epithelialization from the periphery.[6,13]

Treponemes are most numerous in the tips of the dermal papillae and in the foci of polymorphs.

Early lesions

The early lesions[6,13,14] resemble the primary lesions in degree rather than in character. They are often very prominent, coming in a general eruption.

The histological picture of the papilloma shows acanthosis and fusion of some of the rete pegs giving an appearance of islands of dermal papillae. There is hyperkeratinization and thickening of the epidermis, infiltration with polymorphs and focal necrosis (microabscesses), oedema and reduction of melanin but without ulceration. The papules are granular but there is no true granulation tissue; they consist of greatly proliferated epithelium and there is little scarring. Small papules often occur in groups.

Infiltration with plasma cells and lymphocytes occurs; there is some swelling of the capillary endothelium but there is little change in the larger vessels.

Macular lesions show increased keratinization but only slight thickening of the epidermis; there is little cellular infiltration; treponemes are relatively scanty. There are other lesions intermediate between papillomas and macules.

Other early lesions include pigmented macules and localized serpiginous areas of fine desquamation. Enlargement of lymph glands is common.

Late lesions

Late skin lesions[6,14] include gummas in which the centre consists of hyalinized fibrous tissue which may go on to necrosis. Capillaries may be blocked by epithelioid cells but there is no destruction of the vessel walls. Healing takes place by replacement of the necrotic mass by scar tissues. Ulcers occur with fibrous tissue in the depths.

Hyperkeratosis of the palms and soles is seen mostly in the later stages but can occur in all but the very earliest stage. The stratum corneum may be five to ten times its normal thickness. Bone lesions consist of periosteal thickening with small foci of lymphocytes and plasma cells, vascular sclerosis, decalcification, osteoclasis with increase in fibrous tissue and plasma cell infiltration in the medullary spaces. Fluid may form in the knee joints.

Gangosa is an ulcerating gummatous lesion of the nose (see Fig. 31.17).

Juxta-articular nodes are composed of subcutaneous fibrous tissue which is loose on the outside and more dense in the middle, with hyaline material going on to softening. They are freely movable and rubbery, painless and multiple, occurring in several sites—over the ankle, head of the fibula, olecranon, greater trochanter and sacrum. They are usually found in adults and may be related to trauma which provides a nidus for treponemes. Though usually thought of as late lesions they may perhaps originate earlier.

IMMUNITY

It has always been recognized that there is a well-marked immunity in yaws. It was a common observation in the Pacific that when yaws was prevalent there was no syphilis and now that yaws has been greatly reduced there syphilis may take its place (see section on immunity, p. 625).

Cure, with gradual loss of acquired immunity, may occur at any stage during a latent phase and during the early stage reinfection may then occur, though the lesions may be modified as a result of residual immunity. The same is true of the late stages.

Immunity to yaws probably carries cross immunity to syphilis and vice versa, though in some areas of the world the two diseases apparently coexist, and primary chancres have developed in subjects with old latent yaws who were subsequently inoculated with *T. pallidum*.

Serological tests for syphilis (STS) become positive three or four weeks after appearance of the primary lesion of yaws and rapidly increase in titre; they are strongly positive in the secondary stage, continuing into the tertiary stage. The same is true of pinta, except that positive reactions are less common in the primary stage. Tests with treponemes (*Treponema pallidum* immobilization (TPI) etc.) and fluorescent antibody tests are difficult to carry out in field conditions but are positive in yaws, as in syphilis.[15]

How far the antibodies detected in these serological tests reflect resistance or immunity is problematical, since complement-fixing and flocculating antibodies are not necessarily protective. Susceptibility to infection, however, does seem to increase in a community as the proportion of seroreactors falls and we assume that a seronegative person is susceptible to infection. Little is known of reinfection of people who have been treated in the course of mass campaigns. This is of little importance at present but may become so in the future.

CLINICAL FEATURES

Natural history (Fig. 31.3)

Yaws should be regarded as a latent infection with periodic relapses of active disease and it is this which can give rise to outbreaks of yaws after mass treatment campaigns when surveillance has been inadequate. The course of yaws may be divided into an early infectious and late stages

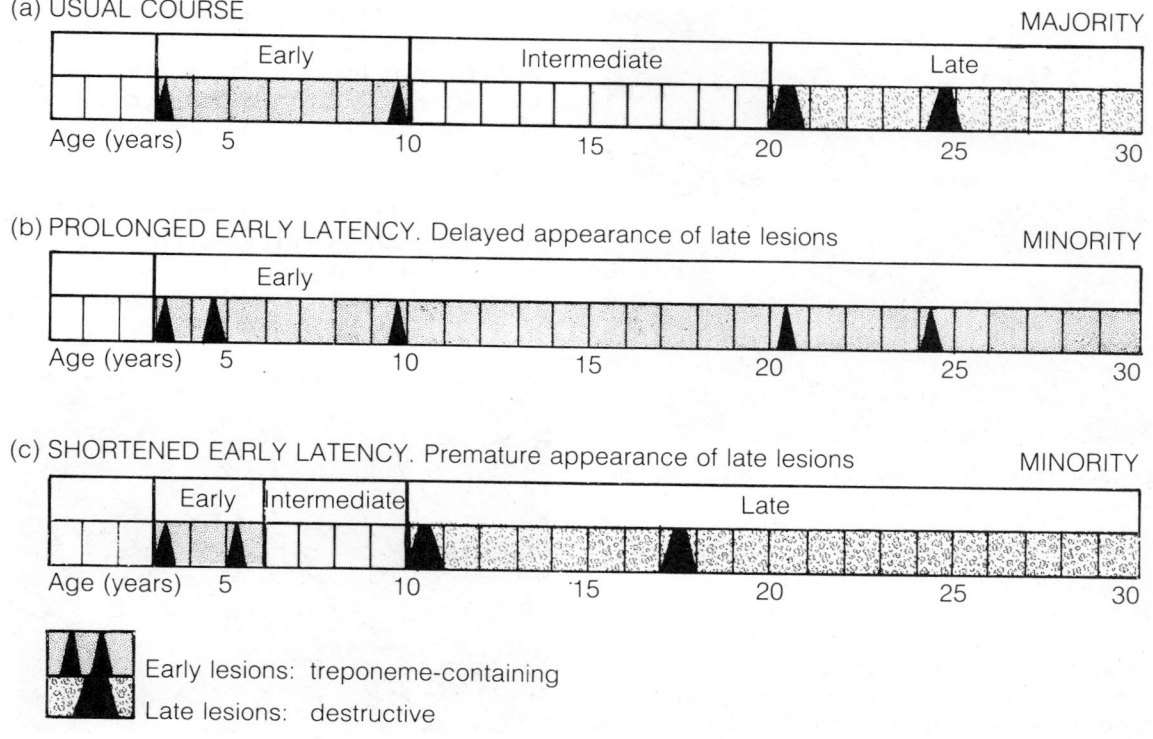

Fig. 31.3 The natural history of yaws. (Courtesy Dr C. J. Hackett.)

with latent periods in between. Infection gives rise to an initial lesion or to early lesions without the initial lesion, to be followed by a period of latency with positive serology and spontaneous cure, or extremely painful and crippling late lesions of skin and bone.

In the *usual course* (Fig. 31.3a) the early and late stages are separated by an *intermediate interval* of 10 or more years in which hyperkeratoses of the palms and soles may develop. Some of these may resemble those seen in the early stages and others those of the late stages. When no clinical symptoms are present serological tests are positive, as in syphilis, and the infection is latent. For each person with active yaws there will be five or more with latent infections.

In a minority the course follows a *prolonged early latency course*. Relapses of infectious lesions may appear in young adults many years after their usual appearance (Fig. 31.3b). In a further minority of cases, *shortened early latency*, the infectious lesions soon cease and late destructive lesions may appear in children (Fig. 31.3c).

Incubation period

The incubation period varies from three to five weeks.

Symptoms and signs

Initial lesion

An initial lesion develops at the site of inoculation after an incubation period of three to five weeks or longer and was found in 80% of persons who developed generalized yaws.[16] The initial lesion, which is round or oval and 2–5 cm in diameter, resembles a large papilloma. It develops most often on an exposed area of the body particularly the lower third of the leg and the wrist (Fig. 31.4). It is uncommon on the soles of the feet but may occur on the edges or outer edges or between the toes. The papilloma persists, usually for six to nine months, resolving spontaneously, often leaving no scar.

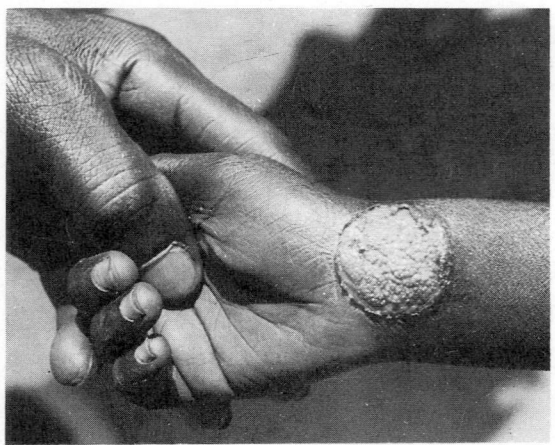

Fig. 31.4 Yaws: initial lesion. (Courtesy Dr C. J. Hackett.)

Early lesions

GENERAL[3,6]

Early lesions usually erupt six to 16 weeks after the appearance of the initial lesion but may do so at any time from three weeks to two years; the two stages may therefore overlap and early lesions may develop years after the initial lesion has healed. The early lesions may be ushered in with pains in the joints, loins and head and fever. Early lesions of the skin are usually multiple, disseminated and proliferative containing many treponemes and heal without permanent trace, or they may persist for a long period (prolonged early lesions).

The early eruptions are due to treponemes carried in the blood from the initial lesion or to local spread by lymphatics. These lesions are usually exudative but may be dry. The serum exuding from them contains treponemes and even non-exudative lesions, especially papules, contain them. Early lesions are therefore infectious. There is no definite evidence of involvement of the eyes, cardiovascular system or central nervous system in spite of the fact that treponemes at this stage are blood-borne. At this stage generalized enlargement of the lymph glands may be notable.

SKIN LESIONS (CUTANEOUS EARLY YAWS)

These may be divided into two groups, major and minor. The major lesions are large raised papillomas and papules with raised convex granular surfaces which have been compared to that of a pickled cauliflower. They are red-yellow in colour, exude a dark yellowish highly infec-

tious serum containing many treponemes which dries to form a yellow-brown scab which may be shed or remain for some time and become black (Figs. 31.5–31.7). They are discoid, annular, crescentic or irregular in shape and occur on any part of the body—limbs, face, body and anogenital region (which should always be examined in children). The anal condylomas are often large and bilaterally contiguous. In debilitated patients shallow ulcers may form and become covered by crusts resembling oyster shells (rupia).

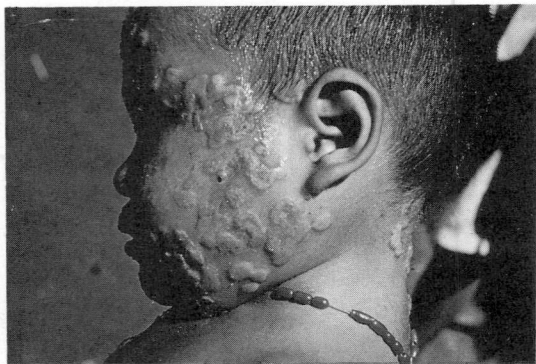

Fig. 31.5 Cutaneous early yaws: papillomas. (Courtesy Dr C. J. Hackett.)

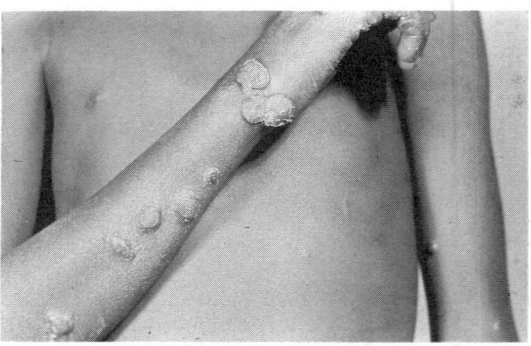

Fig. 31.6 Cutaneous early yaws: papilloma. (Courtesy Dr C. J. Hackett.)

The papular form consists of much smaller lesions about the size of a small grain of rice. They may be very numerous, simulating the rash of chickenpox or smallpox and they may be umbilicate.

The minor lesions are less obvious and are easily missed. They are small and dry. They may occur as small papules or collections of small pale buff-coloured lesions, slightly raised, with flat

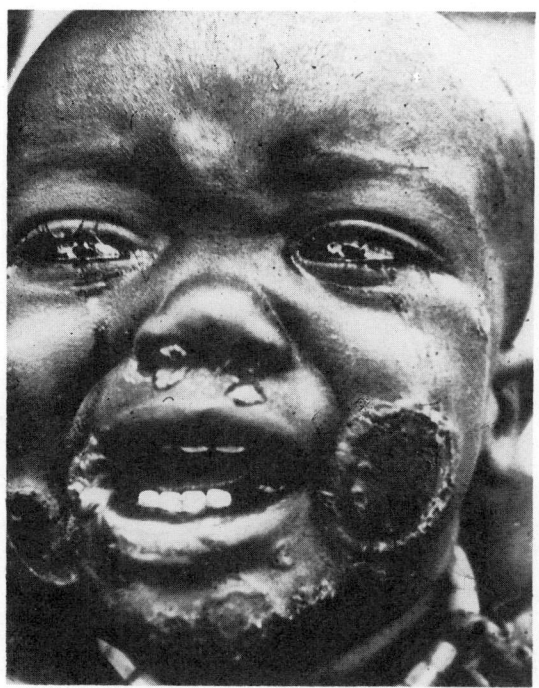

Fig. 31.7 Cutaneous early yaws. Papillomas. (Courtesy Dr C. J. Hackett.)

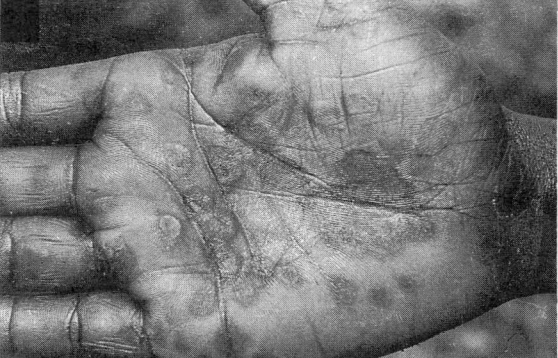

Fig. 31.8 Indeterminate yaws: palmar hyperkeratosis.

tops. They are scattered over the trunk and may itch.

Macular lesions are 12.5–25 mm in diameter and are sometimes confluent. The edges may be pigmented. Erythematous macules are rare and the erythema is transient. Early lesions of the buccal mucous membrane and vagina have been reported. The early generalized eruption heals after a few months with little or no scarring.

PLANTAR LESIONS

Plantar lesions are common and often painful and the sole is the commonest site of infectious recurrences.

In communities accustomed to walking barefoot, the foot is constantly subject to trauma and hyperkeratosis is the response. There may also be cracks, pittings and erosions. The plantar and palmar skin may develop diffuse, non-ulcerative dermatitis with permanent sequelae (Fig. 31.8). Plantar papillomas are quite common as part of a general eruption but they are most important as the commonest infectious lesions to reappear later, possibly appearing up to 20 years after the main eruption. They take longer to erupt than elsewhere on the skin and are extremely painful

(crab yaws) (Fig. 31.9), patients walking painfully with a sideways crab-like gait. They are constantly disturbed by trauma and scabs are rare. Papillomas of long duration tend to develop a firm, dry centre but with a gap between the hard core and the margin. On healing there is a flat-bottomed crater in which the skin appears to be normal.

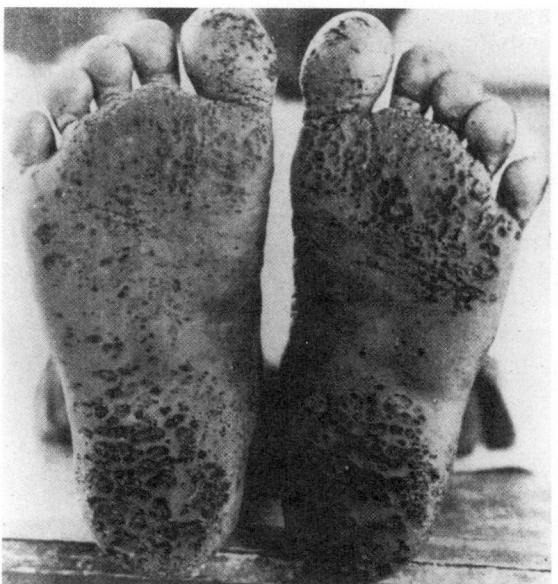

Fig. 31.9 Indeterminate yaws: plantar hyperkeratosis (crab yaws).

Lesions which could appear as macules on the skin elsewhere may occur on the soles; they have a papular element.

Squamous macular lesions are flat or slightly raised areas, firmer and paler than the unaffected parts. They are dry and measure 6–30 mm across but may be confluent. They eventually desquamate, leaving erythematous patches in the soft soles of young people.

Hyperkeratotic lesions are similar to macules but are exaggerated because of the abnormally thick skin of the soles; they are rare in young people but commoner in older patients. They crack and become fissured and often involve the sides of the feet and clefts between the toes. They may be painful. Spontaneous healing occurs but treatment helps.

BONE LESIONS[3]

Bones are commonly affected in yaws; 15–20% of patients voluntarily attending clinics may have obvious lesions. Bone pain is a common complaint; it is a deep-seated ache, worse at night and aggravated by damp conditions. It may be present in the absence of radiographic changes but is commonly associated with such changes. Bone lesions are common in the early stages. The changes consist fundamentally of osteoperiostitis with cortical rarefaction and periosteal deposits going on to bony expansion. Spontaneous healing occurs within a few months without ulceration. The bones involved in order of frequency are the ulna, the hand bones, tibia, fibula, the foot bones and the radius. Polydactylitis is not uncommon in children (Fig. 31.10). Chronic, painless effusions into synovial lined spaces causing ganglion in the wrist and painless effusions into the wrist and knee joints are not uncommon (Fig. 31.11). In the early stages the tibiae are commonly bowed

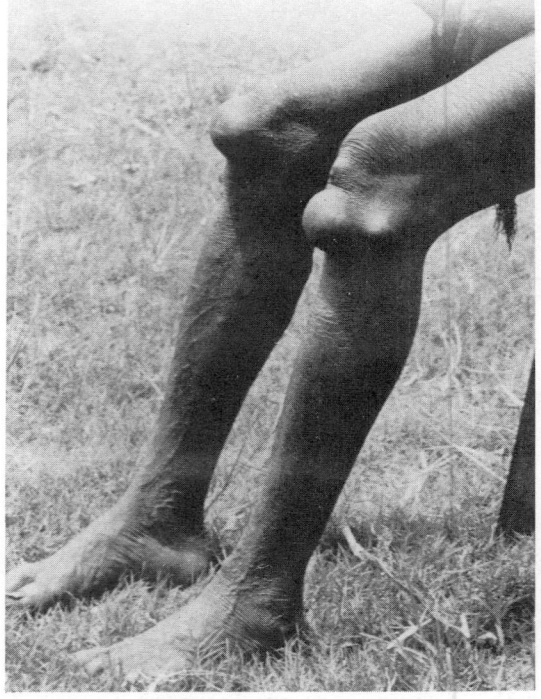

Fig. 31.11 Early yaws: chronic bilateral prepatellar bursitis.

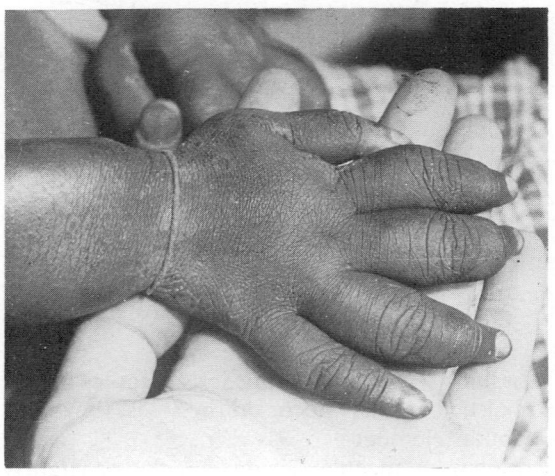

Fig. 31.10 Early yaws: polydactylitis.

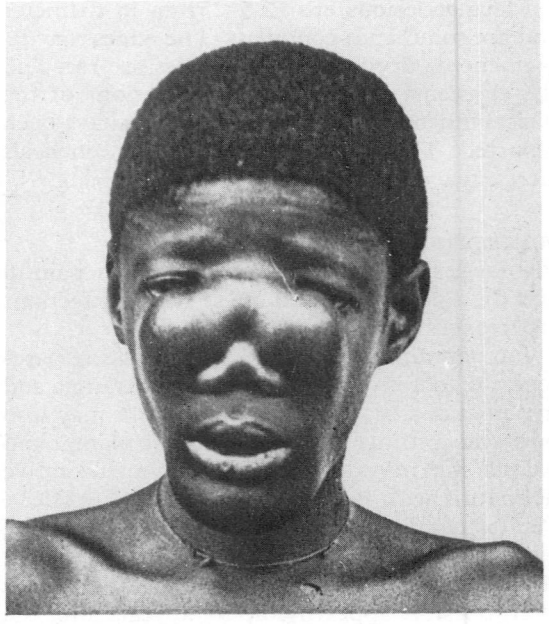

Fig. 31.12 Early yaws: goundou. (Courtesy Dr C. J. Hackett.)

with thickening and expansion of the cortex and periosteal deposits.

Goundou, involving the nasal processes of the maxillae bilaterally, is one form of yaws osteitis. It is not found in some areas (such as the Far East) where yaws is endemic and doubt has been expressed as to its aetiology. It is an early lesion usually beginning in childhood though adults may be attacked. There is a discharge from the nostrils and the formation of small bony swellings on either side of the nose, not involving the cartilages. The swellings persist and can grow to a large size tending to obstruct the nostrils, and sometimes involving the hard palate[17] (Fig. 31.12). In the early stages goundou may respond to medical treatment but in the later stages bone may have to be removed surgically.

COURSE OF THE EARLY STAGES

During the first five years of infection (the duration of the early stage) several relapses of early stage lesions may occur. With each relapse there are fewer lesions and the palms and soles may be involved in painful papillomas and crab yaws.

When most infectious relapses cease there is a symptomless latent period usually of at least three years before late lesions appear; lesions of the two stages do not appear at the same time.

Three courses may be recognized (see section on natural history, above and Fig. 31.3).

1 In childhood the infection passes into the early stage and with the appearance of the early lesions latency persists through an intermediate period when the main yaws lesions are hyperkeratoses of the palms and soles which last about 10–15 years.

2 In infections with a prolonged early stage, early infectious lesions may relapse in adults and this is of epidemiological importance, as was demonstrated in an outbreak of yaws in deep South African mines.[18]

3 In the third course the early latent stage is shortened and late lesions appear in children. It may be possible to distinguish the relapse of early lesions by the absence of an initial lesion whereas the first eruption of papillomas may appear while the initial lesion is present.

Late lesions

These are characteristically destructive, leaving scars and depigmentation. They are solitary and most frequent in older adolescents and adults. In a yaws-endemic population fewer patients have late-yaws ulcers and bone lesions than early lesions but palmar and plantar hyperkeratoses are often the most frequent lesions.

Late lesions are often of two types: hyperkeratotic lesions characteristic at the start and end of the intermediate period, and destructive lesions (gummas) of skin and bone.

SKIN LESIONS[6]

These are gummas which pass through four stages: nodule, central necrosis and abscess formation, rupture and ulceration and healing with scarring. The gummatous process may be superficial or may involve the subcutaneous tissues as well as the skin.

The localized gumma (Fig. 31.13) begins as a

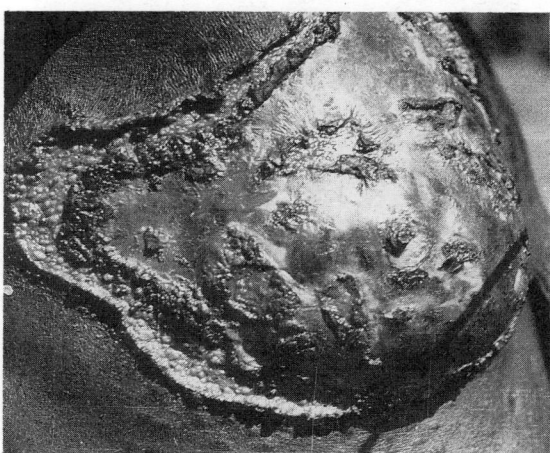

Fig. 31.13 Late yaws: gumma of the right breast. (Courtesy Dr C. J. Hackett.)

small painless nodule enlarging to about 2.5 cm across. There are no signs of acute inflammation though softening is present. The skin above this abscess ultimately gives way and the contents are discharged, leaving an ulcer with a yellowish slough, later showing irregular granulations becoming indurated. The gummas are often grouped and may coalesce; they can persist for years. Secondary infection may involve deeper structures, tendons and joints. When they ultimately heal they leave thin depigmented scars.

A localized swelling may arise secondary to underlying osteitis, particularly on the skull, face, sternum and superficial bones of the extremities.

Serpiginous (spreading) gummas start as small

nodules which coalesce and break down, resulting in an area of affected skin which spreads centrifugally and may be enormous. The centre of the area tends to heal while the edge is still spreading. Keloid formation is common. Scars from these processes may produce contractures of joints, crippling or disfigurement, so as to interfere with the economic contribution to the community.

PLANTAR AND PALMAR LESIONS[3,6]

Late stage palmar lesions are much less common than plantar lesions. Late stage lesions tend to be diffuse, the margins are often ill-defined and the pathological processes affect deeper tissues.

They may appear within a few years of first infection.

The outstanding feature of late lesions is hyperkeratosis. The lesions are probably due to a diffuse chronic inflammatory process which tends to affect all layers of the skin. These lesions may persist for months or years but eventually spontaneous arrest occurs leaving permanent changes due to fibrosis. The skin is thin but stiff and smooth, there may be contractures of the fingers, depigmentation (leukoderma) is common especially of the hands and feet (pintoid yaws) and STS are positive.

BONE LESIONS[6,19]

The bone lesions of this stage are due to periostitis, gummatous osteitis or a combination of the two. Gummas may become necrotic and involve overlying tissues, going on to ulceration.

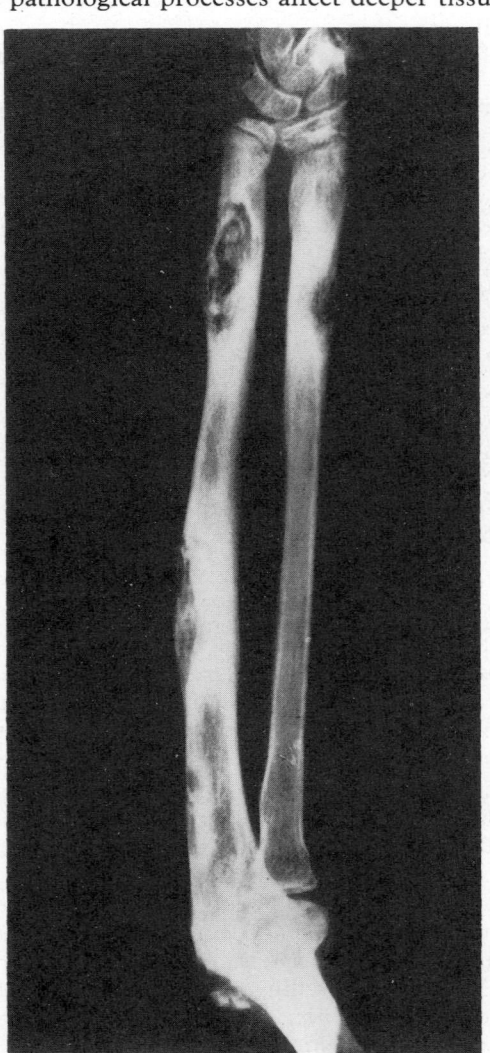

Fig. 31.14 Late yaws: gummatous osteitis of radius and ulna. (Courtesy Dr C. J. Hackett.)

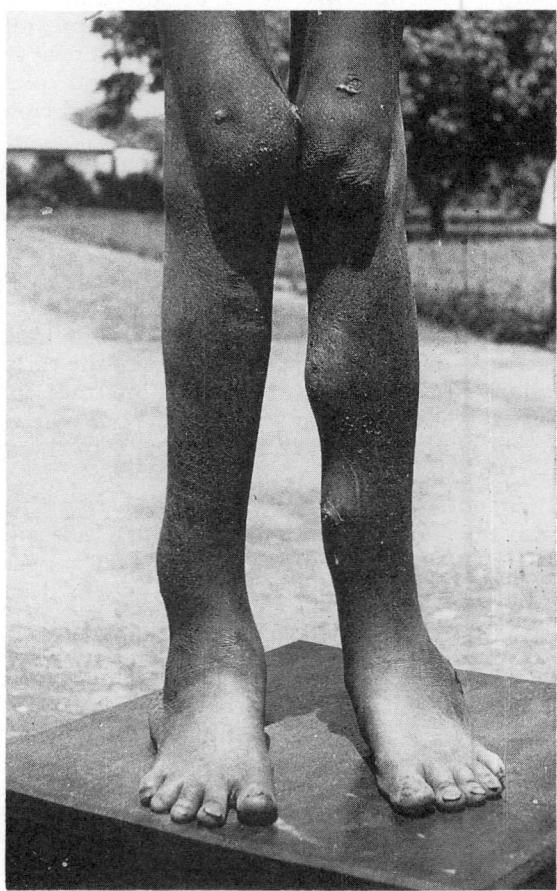

Fig. 31.15 Late yaws: bone lesions. Cortical thickening and deformity of the lower legs (bowed tibia, sabre tibia, boomerang leg). (Courtesy Dr C. J. Hackett.)

These changes cause well-defined rarefied areas in the cortex, either large or small (Fig. 31.14). Pathological fractures are uncommon.

Painless firm fibrous nodes over bony prominences (juxta-articular nodes), prepatellar bursal enlargement (Fig. 31.11) and ganglion of tendon sheaths may occur in both stages of the disease, usually resolving spontaneously. Bone pain is common.

The main change is cortical thickening with multiple rarefied foci, especially in the tibia but also in all bones of the leg and arm. A characteristic result of cortical thickening due to organizing periosteal deposits is the condition known as sabre tibia and, in Australia, boomerang leg[20] (Fig. 31.15).

Lesions of the hand have minor thickening and expansion of the metacarpals and phalanges or destructive focal rarefactions with periosteal deposits which sometimes result in shortening of the bones, or even complete destruction of a diaphysis with resulting deformity (Fig 31.16). Bone lesions of the foot resemble those of the hand but damage is less common, although pain and swelling are constant. The metatarsals may also be involved (Fig. 31.16).

In the skull there are localized thickenings of the calvarium. These nodes are rounded swellings 40 mm or more in diameter and raised. The centre is usually fluctuant with an indurated rim attached to the bone. They may resolve or ulcerate. The bone may be rarefied in the area.

Gangosa, with collapse of the nose and perforating ulceration of the palate, is sometimes seen (Fig. 31.17). It usually starts as a painful ulcer on the palate or nasal septum spreading to perforation and destruction of the turbinates, and to the pharynx causing dysphagia. A foul nasal discharge may be due to gangosa of parts inaccessible to direct examination in the field, and a voice suggesting cleft palate may have a much more serious cause. Gangosa, however, often responds to penicillin.

Apropos the bone lesions of yaws and syphilis,

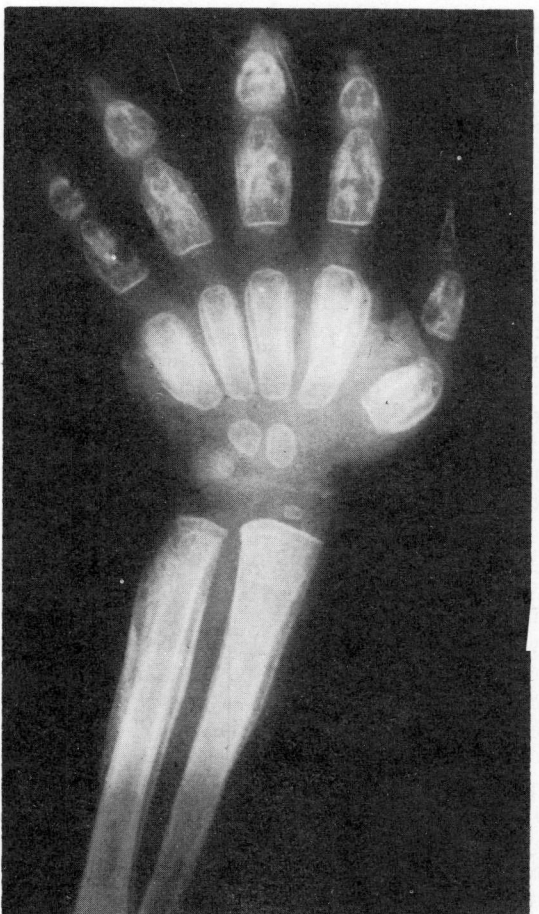

Fig. 31.16 Late yaws: osteoperiostitis with rarefaction of the bones of the hand.

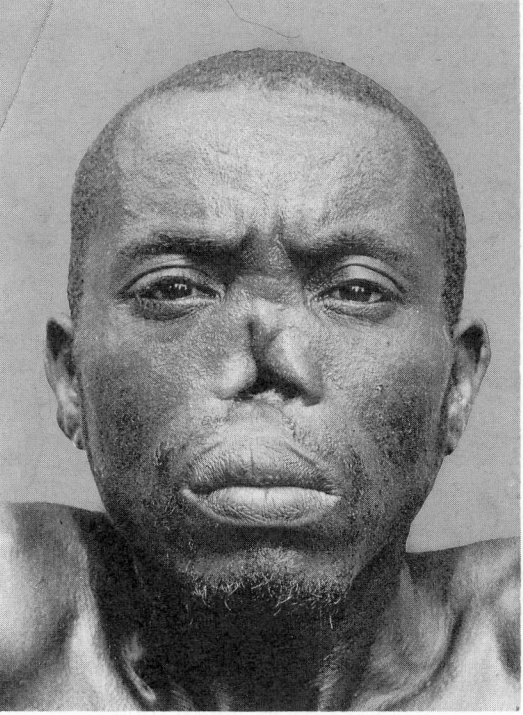

Fig. 31.17 Late yaws: gangosa. (Courtesy Dr C. J. Hackett.)

apart from the absence of osteochondritis in yaws there are probably no bone lesions that occur in one disease that may not be observed in the other.[19]

COURSE OF LATE YAWS

Late yaws lesions relapse as do early ones, but less frequently and at longer intervals. The last lesions to appear are those of the palms and soles. With increasing age the active disease becomes less frequent and ceases. Spontaneous cure with seroreversal probably can occur at any stage of the infection although this is probably rare.

Attenuated yaws[21]

Receding yaws in the community has led to the appearance of attenuated yaws characterized by scanty (usually only one) small dry papillomas of short duration (a few weeks), long dominant latent period and low reagin levels. Attenuated yaws is important since it can so easily be missed during surveys, seldom appears at clinics and can revert to classical yaws with a high rate of transmission.

Several other lesions have been attributed to yaws among which are flexor contractures of the fingers resembling Dupytren's contractures (in the absence of palmar skin changes) and depigmentation of areas other than the hands and feet. General agreement about these is lacking.

DIFFERENTIAL DIAGNOSIS

In mass treatment of yaws, accuracy of diagnosis is needed especially towards the end of the campaign to indicate the number of active cases of yaws remaining, upon which the immediate operations must depend. Accuracy is less essential, though desirable at the start, when all persons are treated. Initial prevalence figures early in yaws campaigns are often exaggerated. This may arise from attributing to yaws certain conditions resembling it, e.g. impetigo, tropical ulcer, ecthyma, tungiasis, occupational hyperkeratoses, the effects of vitamin deficiencies, mycoses, certain palmar and plantar lesions that are not due to yaws and also by counting 'yaws scars' and 'history positive' as active yaws.

A tropical ulcer commences as an inflammatory oedema and vesicle, which soon gives way to an extensive necrosis; on separating, this leaves a chronic granulating ulcer. It responds to penicillin therapy. Impetigo results in scabs covering inflammatory areas. Ecthyma may accompany impetigo or be present alone. On removing the scab a depressed loss of dermis is seen that is very different from the raised, more granular yaws papillomas. Tungiasis (chiggers) is likely to be confused with plantar papillomas. It occurs frequently on parts of the sole not in direct contact with the ground. The posterior extremity of the parasite should be sought extruding ova or red-brown pellets of faeces. *Tunga penetrans* may parasitize the buttocks. Certain vitamin deficiencies may result in papular lesions, especially at the angles of the lips, which may resemble early yaws lesions; other signs of the deficiencies may be present. Mycoses of the soles have less induration than yaws lesions.

Macular leprosy lesions may resemble early yaws macules or maculopapules. Other manifestations of leprosy, especially loss of sensation, and acid-fast bacilli should be sought. Perforating ulcers may be mistaken for plantar papillomas, but they are always painless. Gangosa has been confused with leprosy or syphilitic lesions and also with mucosal leishmaniasis and blastomycosis. Bone lesions of sickle cell anaemia and the dactylitis of tuberculosis also may need to be differentiated from early yaws bone lesions. Pyogenic osteomyelitis and periostitis are usually more painful and of more rapid development than yaws bone lesions. Pyogenic osteomyelitis may occasionally complicate ulcerated late yaws bone lesions when its recognition may be difficult without radiography. In many rural populations in tropical countries pyogenic osteomyelitis may be infrequent.

There are a number of palmar and plantar lesions not well understood and of which the causes are not known. They are characterized by thickening and fissuring of the epithelium and by pitting of the surface. They are usually worse in the wet season. These and other conditions to be differentiated from yaws lesions have been dealt with in a WHO monograph.[18]

Pigmentary changes in the skin may occur in any of the treponematoses, but in patients with pinta there also might be areas of earlier changes in which treponemes should be sought in expressed serum. Depigmentation alone should not be attributed to yaws.

The differentiation of yaws from syphilitic lesions, especially late lesions in adults, may be very difficult. Often the only help is the rural or urban childhood origin of the patient (Table 31.2).

Corns and callosities caused by ill-fitting shoes, warts, and even lesions resulting from rats gnawing the thickened soles while the victim sleeps; all may be mistaken for yaws plantar lesions.

DIAGNOSIS

In early lesions *T. pertenue* may be demonstrated by dark-field microscopic examination of the exudate from a suspected lesion but cannot be differentiated from syphilis or treponarid. In the field diagnosis is essentially clinical.

Serology

STS all become positive three to four weeks after the appearance of the initial lesion, rapidly increasing in titre. These tests (fluorescent treponemal antibody absorption—FTA–ABS) are strongly positive in the early stages continuing through the latent period up to the late stages. They revert to negative after treatment but only after a prolonged period. In an adult, apparently healthy, with a positive STS it may be difficult to say whether this is syphilis or yaws, a question which must be decided on geographical and epidemiological criteria.

TREATMENT

T. pertenue is very susceptible to penicillin; a single injection of 1.2 g of long-acting penicillin (procaine penicillin G) is given to adults. *Benzathine penicillin* has largely replaced PAM (penicillin aluminium monostearate) because of its greater stability in the tropics and its availability in multiphial doses. The present recommended dose of benzathine penicillin is 300 mg (1 ml) to all under 10 years of age, and 1.2 g (4 ml) to all over that age.

Drug resistance

Penicillin has been used for many years for the treatment of yaws without the emergence of penicillin-resistant strains. However, this could change quite quickly and a strain of *T. pallidum* resistant to penicillin has been found.[22] The tetracyclines (1–2 g daily for 5 days) and chloramphenicol are effective in the treatment of yaws[23,24] and erythromycin and the cephalosporins are effective in syphilis.

Mass treatment campaigns

For mass campaigns when the prevalence of clinically active cases in a community is over 10% total mass treatment (TMT) should be given, i.e. all patients with clinically active yaws should be given the full dose, and the remainder of the population should be given half doses. In areas of lower incidence of active disease (5–10%), in addition to the actual patients (at full doses) all children under the age of puberty are treated with half doses (juvenile mass treatment, JMT).

If the incidence of yaws is under 5%, selective mass treatment (SMT) may be given. In this only those with active disease (full doses) and their contacts (half doses) are treated. In many mass campaigns, because of the low cost of the drug, TMT is practised whatever the prevalence of active yaws.

Results of treatment

The response to these small doses of drug is excellent. Early lesions become non-infectious within a few days and are healed in 7–10 days. Subsequent relapses of infectious lesions also heal, but a little more slowly. A 10% prevalence of active lesions at the first survey will probably be less than 2% at a resurvey a year later; a second single injection to patients with active lesions and to latent infections is followed by a further fall in prevalence figures the following year.

Probably many of the patients with *active yaws seen at resurveys* were among those *not seen at the initial treatment survey*.

Individual treatment of early lesions may result in seroreversal, but for late lesions this change is slower and less frequent. Following mass treatment with single injections seroreversal is less rapid and less frequent. The almost complete suppression of infectious relapses is of great value to the health of the community.

Early treatment rapidly heals all early lesions, thus stopping transmission, and limits the destruction of the late ones. Early slight goundou lesions become smaller and may disappear with treatment but large lesions may need surgical removal.

Surveillance

In all mass campaigns annual resurveys with at least 80% attendance are important. These treatment policies have been widely adopted with great success but they depend on careful organization and supervision to detect cases, assess conditions and ensure acceptable response on the part of the people.

Penicillin, as is well known, may give rise to reactions, sometimes fatal. The fatalities have been estimated at slightly more than 1 per million injections;[25] non-fatal anaphylactic reactions probably number 10 times as many.

For the treatment of these reactions immediate and repeated injections of adrenaline are essential and prolonged administration of antihistamine drugs. An emergency kit of suitable antishock drugs, portable oxygen should be available for immediate use.[25] The procedure recommended is:

1 immediately on the appearance of signs of reaction the patient should be made to lie down (head down, feet up);
2 0.5–1.0 ml of adrenaline (1 in 1000) should be injected subcutaneously into the upper arm;
3 in angioneurotic oedema, urticaria or conjunctivitis, antihistamines should be given intramuscularly or intravenously.

EPIDEMIOLOGY

Yaws is a rural disease of warm humid climates and under naturally endemic conditions the infection is usually contracted from about the age of two or three years. By the age of 15, most of the population has been infected. Susceptible children are infected by contact with infected children from other households rather than from their older siblings whose infections are latent. In some countries the prevalence is not uniform throughout the yaws-endemic area. In some African countries active yaws has been reported more prevalent during the wet than during the dry, warmer season.[26]

The delayed relapses of the prolonged early latency may be responsible for some of the 'last cases' of yaws following a mass treatment campaign. This may start a recrudescence of early yaws. Such relapses of early yaws lesions may occur mainly in patients who have not received an injection of long-acting penicillin in the treatment phase of the campaign. Early and late lesions are never present together. The end of the early stage and the beginning of the late stage can only be recognized by the appearance of the first late lesion.

Yaws transmission does not occur in cities or towns. It is not transmitted by sexual contact nor to the unborn child probably because of infection long before sexual maturity, so that the patient is no longer infectious.

ERADICATION AND CONTROL

The maintenance of yaws eradication depends on the continued improvement of standards of living, including adequate water supplies for domestic use, adequate nutrition, and road communications, all of which depend upon economic development. The factors favouring the transmission of yaws are so insecure that they appear to be rather readily displaced by such simple measures as the use of good body soap and water. Recession of the infection has been happening everywhere since the 1920s. What formerly required a generation to accomplish now can be done in two to three years if the mass treatment is carried out thoroughly.

When after some five years of resurveys at which 80% of the population is seen, and all active cases are given the full dose and direct contacts half doses and less than 0.5% of infectious patients are found, the mass treatment phase ceases and the campaign then passes into the consolidation phase when careful surveillance is maintained to recognize and treat any cases without delay. The activity should be carried out from basic health centres suitably sited in the yaws area.

It is essential for yaws eradication, and for economic reasons, that this should be combined with measures against other diseases, especially those that need only a brief single annual contact with each individual.

This was done with considerable success in Indonesia, where the campaign was carried out from over 3000 well-established rural dispensaries. This extension of activities can be introduced with the early resurveys.

The claim has been made that in the eradication of yaws the prophylactic treatment of contacts is important. This seems to overlook the greater part played by latency in transmission.

It must be stressed again that the proper use of long-acting penicillin preparations in mass treatment of yaws depends upon taking into account the *high prevalence of latent infections.* Treatment of these will take care of contacts, which are impossible to recognize until the initial lesion appears.[27] Eradication is defined by the World Health Organization[28] as being achieved when no indigenous active case of yaws has appeared in the population for three years and no seroreactors are found among persons under five years of age. This may take five years.

In the Nigerian national mass treatment campaigns, a team of 10 trained auxiliary persons with an experienced field supervisor (and under medical direction) examined and treated 1500 people daily as long as those numbers were available.[29] After a few days two or three members of the staff remained while the others moved to the next community where preparations already had to be made. Examinations of over 80% of the population by surveys at intervals of not more than one year are important for success. In the Haiti campaign the surveys were made by house-to-house visits because of the scattered population; this has not been used so successfully elsewhere.[30] In Indonesia the campaign has been carried out by careful surveys and frequent resurveys, with TMT.

The long-established village health administration in Java made this successful, but it may not be so successful in other countries lacking this important service.[31,32]

In national yaws eradication campaigns assisted by the World Health Organization and UNICEF up to 1963, more than 350 million persons had been examined in all surveys and resurveys, and 50 million had received penicillin. The prevalence of active yaws in most of these populations is now well below 0.5%.[33]

There still may be some millions of infected persons with a low prevalence of active yaws. For this reason governments may not regard the problem as justifying very active measures while there are so many more urgent calls on limited national finances, but some reliable system of surveillance should be maintained. The success of yaws eradication campaigns by mass treatment surveys has depended upon the recognition of the latency of yaws, the efficacy and proper use of long-acting penicillin, and the rising standards of living. It should not be forgotten that yaws was a grave infliction in many populations only a few decades ago.

In the early days of mass treatment campaigns against yaws it was recognized that a growing population freed from childhood yaws infection would become susceptible to venereal syphilis unless, following the campaign, adequate steps were taken to prevent this. In some countries where yaws has been greatly reduced venereal syphilis recently has been reported to have been carried from towns to some such rural populations.

TREPONARID (ENDEMIC SYPHILIS)

GEOGRAPHICAL DISTRIBUTION

Treponarid is found in Africa extending across the Sahara to the Middle East, Arabia (bejel)[34] and central Asia and in central Australia.[35] Foci occur in Zimbabwe (njovera), Botswana (dichuchwa) and Gambia (siti). Formerly present in Bosnia (skerlievo), it has now been eradicated (Fig. 31.1).

AETIOLOGY

T. pallidum identical to the spirochaete causing syphilis is the cause.

TRANSMISSION

It is transmitted from person to person by con-

tagion from infectious lesions on the skin and mucous membranes by the use of common feeding utensils and pipes (Fig. 31.2).

PATHOLOGY

The pathology is the same as syphilis. The viscera are involved but there is much less involvement of the central nervous system and cardiovascular system where lesions are rare.

IMMUNITY

There is the same tendency to latency as in the other treponematoses.

CLINICAL FEATURES

Natural history

The classical form of treponarid is a small insignificant initial lesion usually on the mouth, followed by the appearance of early lesions, infectious patches in the mouth and a general eruption. Late stages (gummas and bone lesions) may occur following a period of latency. The classical form has now been replaced within a generation by a milder form with less severe lesions of shorter duration.[36]

The *incubation period* is not known.

Symptoms and signs

Initial. Initial lesions are rarely seen but have been found on the mouth and lips, the nipples of women and the genitalia, but in Bosnia less than 1% of early cases showed a primary lesion.

Early. Characteristic early lesions[2] (which are usually the first manifestations) include mucous patches on the lips and tongue and papules or macules favouring the warm and moist areas (e.g. the flexures), especially round the genitalia and anus, neck, axilla, elbows and knees, though the eruption may be generally distributed over the whole body (Figs. 31.18 and 31.19). The eruption is florid and luxuriant and the picture is clinically unmistakable.[2] The lips, tongue, palate, tonsils, nasal septum or larynx may be involved, going on to dysphagia and dysphonia.

Adenitis of the groin and cervical, axillary and epitrochlear lymph nodes is marked but the nodes do not break down; they remain discrete, elastic and not tender. Periostitis, usually of the tibia, but also of the humerus, radius and bones of the hand, can occur at this stage.

Late. In the late stage[2] lesions include occasional erosions and ulcers of the mouth, the nasal structures (gangosa) (Fig. 31.20) and larynx. On the skin gummatous ulcers are characteristic and may persist for years. Hyperkeratosis of the soles of the feet occurs, causing great thickening of the skin, with fissures, and disability. Juxta-articular nodules are also seen. Depigmentation of the skin can be extensive but is not common (Fig. 31.21).

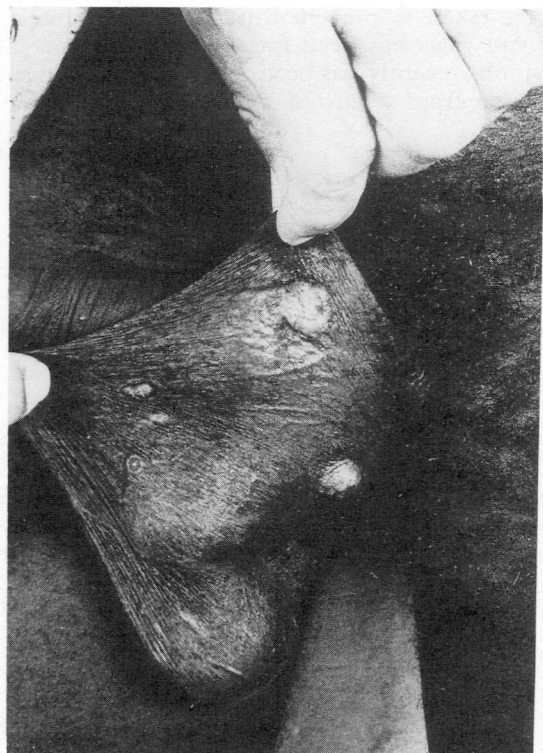 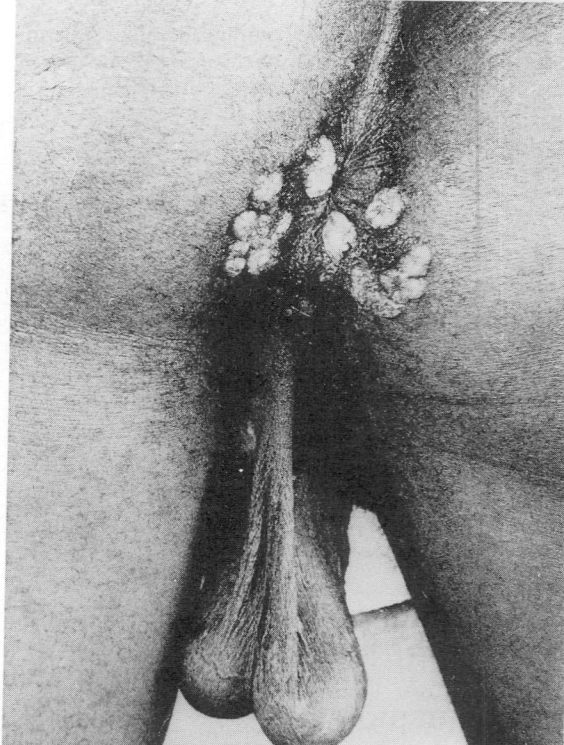

Fig. 31.18   Early treponarid: moist papules involving anus and scrotum. (Courtesy Dr P. D. Marsden.)

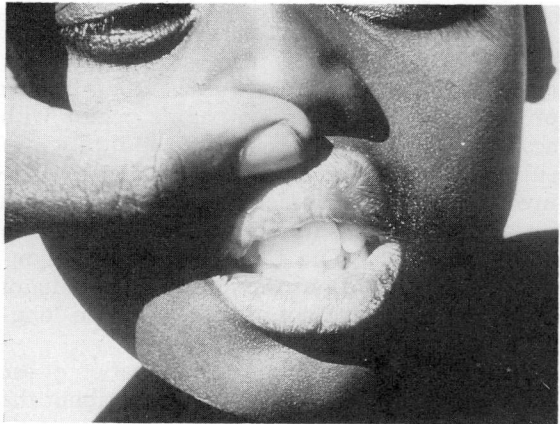

Fig. 31.19   Early treponarid: mucous papules on the buccal surface of the upper lip.

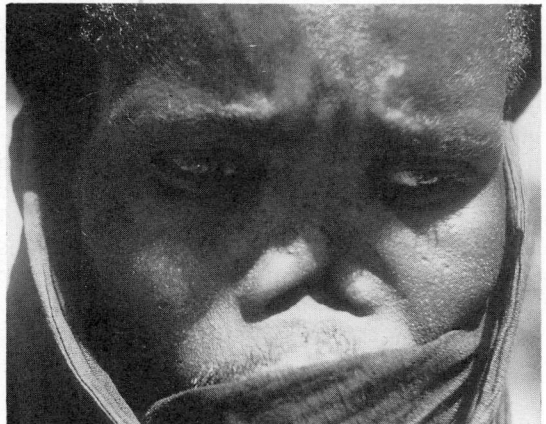

Fig. 31.20   Late treponarid: gangosa in a female adult.

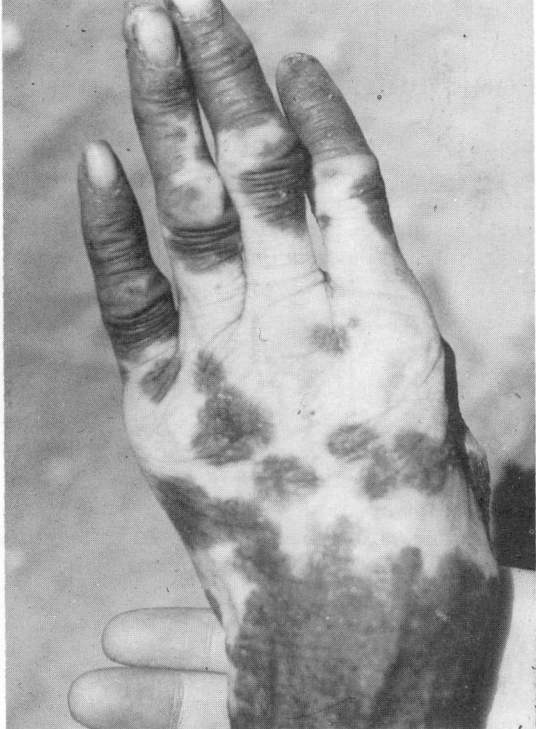

Fig. 31.21   Late treponarid: depigmentation of hand.

Periostitis, with bone pain, gummas of various bones, and even osteomyelitis, have been reported. Sabre tibia indistinguishable from the same condition in yaws is reported by Hudson.[2]

It is noticeable that in treponarid, as in yaws, the cardiovascular and central nervous systems escape damage, except in very rare cases.

DIAGNOSIS

The differential diagnosis from other treponematoses is given in Table 31.2. Serological tests for syphilis (STS) are positive.

TREATMENT

Treatment with repository penicillin is as effect-ive as in other treponematoses. Mass treatment campaigns have been carried out in the same way as yaws.

EPIDEMIOLOGY

Treponarid is confined to nomadic and semi-nomadic communities living in the more remote rural areas in dry, semi-arid climates where the standard of hygiene is low and access to static health services limited. Children are the chief reservoir of infection, the age of peak incidence being two to 10 years. Existing disease of the mucous membrane, such as the stomatitis associated with vitamin B_2 deficiency, predisposes to infection by affording suitable sites for the treponemas to enter. This vitamin deficiency is common in these rural communities. The change of seasons may be associated with an increase in infectious lesions.

CONTROL

Improved environmental hygiene, the availability of water and penicillin treatment have greatly reduced the infection.

PINTA (CARATE, MAL DEL PINTO)

GEOGRAPHICAL DISTRIBUTION

Pinta is found only in the Americas. Formerly it extended from Mexico and Cuba, through Central America, down to the upper Amazon basin. Presently it is much reduced in incidence although it still persists in Colombia and southern Mexico.[35]

AETIOLOGY

The cause is *T. carateum* which cannot be differentiated from *T. pallidum* or *T. pertenue* and like them has not been cultivated in artificial media but has successfully been inoculated into chimpanzees, although not small laboratory animals.

TRANSMISSION

Congenital transmission does not occur. *T. carateum* is present in the skin lesions, especially early lesions. The lesions tend to be dry and scaly, rather than exudative, but the papules are itchy and scratching can cause excoriation of the skin, releasing serum to the surface; in this serum the treponemes are abundant and may find the way to the skin of another person, especially if abraded. Treponemes can be found with dark-ground microscopy in fluid expressed from the lesions. They have also been found in abrasions of the skin of infected persons and by puncture of lymph nodes.

Direct contact is therefore the route of transmission, but venereal transmission via the genitalia is not a feature since lesions of the genitalia are unusual.

PATHOLOGY

In pinta the lesions are confined to the skin; no other structures are affected. The treponemes are located chiefly in the malpighian cells, especially in small areas of acanthosis in the epidermis. They are present in primary lesions and in fluid from such lesions.

The initial lesions in pinta are never moist or eroded and the epithelium is intact unless broken or excoriated. The earliest papule begins with acanthosis and diffuse round cell infiltration of subepithelial tissues and the rete malpighii. The involvement of the epidermis never proceeds to intradermal abscess formation such as is seen in secondary yaws. The blood vessels and lymphatics are dilated but the intima and media of the vessel walls are not affected, even in longstanding lesions.

In the secondary pintid the localization of the infiltration (often rich in plasma cells) about the vessels of the cutis is characteristic. The elastic tissue is rarefied and stretched.

In later pintids a hyperkeratosis may develop which, together with existing local oedema of the cutis, leads to progressive atrophy and flattening of the rete malpighii. There is diffuse infiltration of the corium and perivascular nodulation of the deeper cutis. In the later lesions the inflammatory changes recede, pigment is reduced or atrophied and may collect and clump in the deep cutis. In this stage depigmented leukodermic areas coexist with blue, red or copper coloured lesions. Eventually there may be accumulations of epithelioid cells but no changes occur in the walls of the blood vessels.[37]

IMMUNITY

Léon y Blanco[38] successfully inoculated *T. carateum* into persons with advanced syphilis and a patient with pinta may develop an unmodified syphilitic chancre. Yaws can develop in a pinta subject and pinta can develop in persons who have had yaws. There seems, therefore, to be no protection in pinta against the other treponematoses, though sera from pinta patients react to the same antigens as sera from subjects with yaws, venereal and non-venereal syphilis. The tests reveal no differences between the treponemes causing these conditions.

In pinta the total prevalence of clinically active disease approaches that of the seroreactors, which might be as high as 80%, because latency apparently does not occur and active lesions are usually present. Yet one attack of pinta does not protect against reinfection.

CLINICAL FEATURES

Natural history

Eighty per cent of persons infected with pinta have lesions and infective lesions may be present for many years. There is no latent non-infectious stage, such as occurs in the other treponematoses. The course of the disease is an initial lesion followed by an early and a late stage.

Incubation period

The initial lesion appears 30–50 days after infection.

Symptoms and signs

Initial. Initial lesions are almost always found on uncovered parts of the body—leg or dorsum of the foot (common), thigh, buttock, forearm or dorsum of the hand (common), arm, face, neck. The lesion appears as an itchy erythematous papule becoming in 30–50 days an erythematous raised squamous patch, round which other papules may develop and spread.

Early. In the early stage there are skin rashes or multiplication of papules described as pintids and seen five to 12 months after the initial lesions, which themselves continue to develop. These lesions are widespread. Pigmented patches may appear in the mouth. Generalized lymphadenitis is fairly common.

Late. In the late stage pigment changes occur with coloured or blanched spots, keratoderma or superficial atrophy (Fig. 31.22). The lesions may be grey with bluish tones or almost black, red or copper coloured. They are round, oval or irregular, not elevated, but always visible.

Hyperkeratosis has been said to occur on the palms and soles in the late stages but Hackett[1] does not accept the diagnosis, considering that they may have been confused with hyperkeratosis due to yaws. There are no lesions of bone, heart, brain or other viscera.

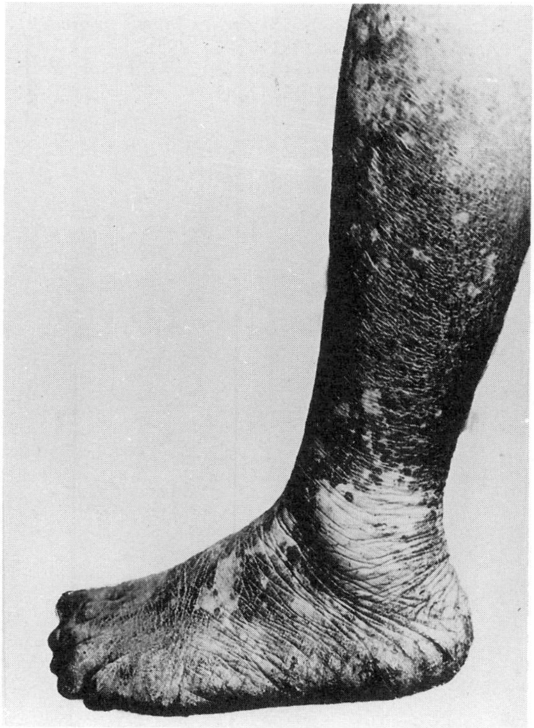

Fig. 31.22 Late pinta: depigmentation of foot and lower leg. (Courtesy Dr L. A. Leon.)

DIAGNOSIS

Treponemes can be found in fluid expressed from the early lesions especially but even from those of all stages and examined under darkground illumination. Fungi from the surface of the skin have often been seen and wrongly considered to be the cause of the condition. They should be ignored. The appearance of the patient with developed pinta is striking.

The characteristic colour or depigmentation of the skin gives the clue to diagnosis in endemic areas but depigmented patches of skin are occasionally found in late yaws, and may resemble those of pinta. Pinta is also to be differentiated from leprosy, vitiligo and other skin conditions.

Serological tests of the reagin type become positive two to four months after onset, and are usually positive at high titre thereafter.

TREATMENT

Treatment rests on penicillin in the same dosages as for yaws.

REFERENCES

1   Hackett, C. J. (1963) *Bull. Wld Hlth Org.* **29,** 7.
2   Hudson, E. H. (1958) *Non-venereal Syphilis. A Sociological and Medical Study of Bejel.* Edinburgh: Livingstone.
3   Hackett, C. J. (1957) *An International Nomenclature on Yaws. WHO Monogr. Ser.,* 36.
4   Fitzgerald, T. J., Johnson, R. C., Miller, J. N. et al (1977) *Infect. Immunol.* **18,** 467–478.
5   Sykes, J. A., Miller, J. N. & Kalan, N. J. (1974) *Br. J. vener. Dis.* **50,** 40–44.
6   Turner, L. H. (1959) *Notes on the Treponematoses with an Illustrated Account of Yaws.* Kuala Lumpur: Institute for Medical Research.
7   Magnuson, H. J., Thomas, E. W., Olansky, S. et al (1956) *Medicine* **35,** 33–38.
8   Turner, L. H. (1936) *Am. J. Hyg.* **23,** 431–448.
9   Lukehart, S. A. (1985) *Rev. infect. Dis.* **7,** S304–313.
10 Turner, T. B. & Hollander, D. H. (1957) *Biology of the Treponematoses. WHO Monogr.,* 35.
11 Agadzi, V. K., Aboagye-Atta, Y., Nelson, J. W. et al (1983) *Lancet* **ii,** 389–390.
12 Reid, M. S. (1985) *Rev. infect. Dis.* **7,** S254–259.
13 Hill, K. R., Kodijat, R. & Sardadi, M. (1951) *Monogr. Ser. WHO* 5.
14 Hackett, C. J. (1946) *Trans. R. Soc. trop. Med. Hyg.* **40,** 206.
15 Hackett, C. J. (1967) *Trans. R. Soc. trop. Med. Hyg.* **61,** 148.
16 Powell, A. R. (1923) *Proc. R. Soc. trop. Med. Hyg.* **42,** 16. *Sect. trop. Med. Parasit.* 15.
17 Botreau-Rousell, P. (1925) *Osteitis pianques à goundou.* Paris: Masson.
18 Hackett, C. J. & Lowenthal, L. J. A. (1984) *Differential Diagnosis of Yaws. WHO Monogr. Ser.,* 45.
19 Hackett, C. J. (1951) *Bone Lesions of Yaws in Uganda.* Oxford: Blackwell Scientific.
20 Hackett, C. J. (1936) *Boomerang Leg and Yaws in Australian Aborigines.* Monograph 1. Royal Society of Tropical Medicine and Hygiene, London.
21 Vorst, F. A. (1985) *Rev. infect. Dis.* **7,** S327–331.
22 Norgard, M. U. & Miller, J. N. (1981) *Science* **215,** 553–555.
23 Loughlin, E. H., Joseph, A. & Schaeffer, K. (1951) *Am. J. trop. Med. Hyg.* **31,** 20–25.
24 Payne, E. H., Bellerive, A. & Jean, L. (1951) *Antibiot. Chemother.* **1,** 88–91.
25 World Health Organization (1960) *Wld Hlth Org. Tech. Rep. Ser.* 5.
26 Harding, R. D. (1949) *Trans. R. Soc. trop. Med. Hyg.* **47,** 347–366.
27 Hackett, C. J. & Guthe, T. (1956) *Bull. Wld Hlth Org.* **15,** 869.
28 Hackett, C. J. & Guthe, T. (1956) *Bull. Wld Hlth Org.* **15,** 869.
29 Zahra, A. (1956) *Bull. Wld Hlth Org.* **15,** 911–935.
30 Petrus, F., Leutans, S., Paolielloa et al (1953) *Bull. Wld Hlth Org.* **8,** 271.
31 Soetopo, M. & Wasito. R. (1953) *Bull. Wld Hlth Org.* **8,** 273–291.
32 Soetopo, M., Wasito, R., Soedarsono, H. et al (1956) *Bull. Wld Hlth Org.* **15,** 937–958.
33 World Health Organization (1964) *WHO Chron.* **18,** 403–417.
34 Pace, J. L. (1983) *Saudi med. J.* **4,** 211–220.
35 World Health Organization (1982) *Wld Hlth Org. tech Rep. Ser.* **674,** 16–19.
36 Csonka, G. & Pace, J. L. (1985) *Rev. infect. Dis.* **7,** S260–265.
37 Hasselmann, C. M. (1955) *Arch. klin. exp. Derm.* **201,** 1 (*Abstr. Trop. Dis. Bull.* (1957) **54,** 295).
38 Léon, Y., Blanco, F. (1940) *Revta Med. trop. Parasit. Habana* **6,** 13, 21, 39, 43, 47, 49.

Chapter 32
Other Spirochaetal Diseases

RELAPSING FEVER

Relapsing fever is also known as recurrent fever, spirillum fever, tick fever and tick bite fever.

AETIOLOGY

The spirochaetes which cause relapsing fever are of two morphologically indistinct species: *Borrelia recurrentis* and *Borrelia duttoni*.

The spirochaetes are actively motile spiral organisms 6–10 μm long × 0.4 μm wide with five to 10 fairly regular but loose waves (Fig. 32.1). They multiply by transverse fission. They have tapering ends but no flagella and under electron microscopy each consists of a bundle of 12 filaments twisted round the spirochaete body, external to the cell wall, with a thin covering layer of viscid material. They have a rapid corkscrew movement and may be seen in blood films between the red cells, staining pink with Giemsa or Leishman and appearing sometimes beaded

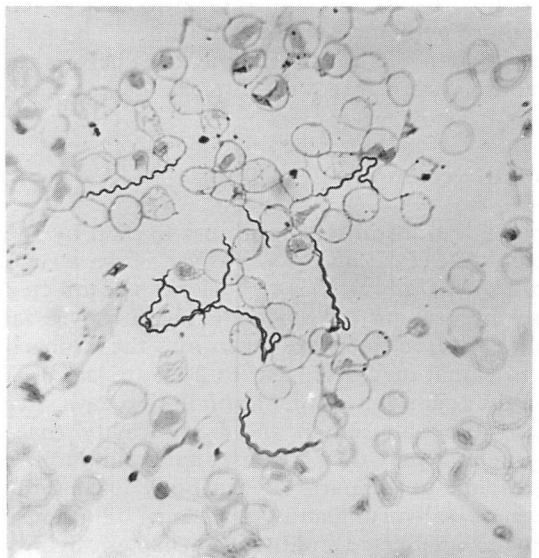

Fig. 32.1 *Borrelia recurrentis* in a blood film.

or granular. They may assume irregular shapes and appear tangled together towards the end of a pyrexial attack. They can be seen by dark-ground illumination, can be grown only with difficulty in enriched media in the allantoic fluid of fertile hen's eggs, but can be demonstrated best by animal inoculation.[1] Susceptible animals include newborn rabbits, monkeys, mice, rats and ground squirrels. Normally guinea-pigs are not susceptible.

Species differentiation

B. recurrentis infects lice but not ticks, and guinea-pigs are resistant except in East Africa. Sudanese strains are not infective to monkeys. *B. duttoni* infects soft ticks and can infect lice and most rodents.

PATHOLOGY

Cycle in man

During pyrexial attacks the spirochaetes occur in the blood where they may be seen in leukocytes but disappear during the crisis and can only be detected by animal inoculation. Some resistant spirochaetes persist in the brain and other tissues until a fresh immunologically distinct strain increases in number and reaches the blood.

Pathogenesis

Borreliae enter the skin and subcutaneous tissues without causing a primary lesion and enter the systemic and lymphatic circulation. They multiply in the blood and are phagocytosed by the reticuloendothelial system. They do not multiply in extravascular sites. There is sequestration of platelets in the marrow with thrombocytopenia which is responsible for petechial rashes in the skin and haemorrhages. In the liver there is intrahepatic obstruction of the flow of bile and hepatocellular disturbance causing jaundice.

The fever is caused by the large number of borreliae which do not produce toxins but are pyrogenic, since the outer envelope of the borrelia, which is heat-stable, stimulates mononuclear cells to produce pyrogens. A Jarisch–Herxheimer reaction may occur spontaneously or after treatment following phagocytosis of the large number of borreliae and disseminated intravascular coagulation may also occur.

Pathology

The general features found at post-mortem are jaundice, congestion of the organs and petechial haemorrhages in the pleura, lungs, heart, brain, kidneys, stomach and intestines.

In the liver borreliae accumulate and multiply causing focal necrosis of the parenchyma cells, which they invade. The fixed phagocytes do not respond to live borreliae but do ingest dead ones. Shortly before the crisis the borreliae roll up and are taken in by the endothelial cells of the liver, spleen and bone marrow. Surviving borreliae remain in these organs and in the brain until the next relapse.[2]

In the spleen the borreliae accumulate and multiply in the sinuses causing cellular infiltration; they may enter the endothelial cells and cause infarcts and necrosis; they can be demonstrated in the infarcts. The spleen is large, soft and red and perisplenitis is common. Borreliae may also be found in the kidneys.

In the blood vessels the damage to the endothelium tends to cause haemorrhage which may show as petechiae on the skin.

The bone marrow is hyperaemic. There is polymorphonuclear leukocytosis and borreliae may sometimes be seen within the polymorphs. Lymph glands may be involved.

The heart shows cloudy swelling. Bronchopneumonia is common.

The borreliae are distinctly neurotropic affecting the meninges and central nervous system. In infected animals they may be found in the brain and cerebellum as much as a year after infection. In the brain they are found in capillaries. There are no changes in the nerve cells but there is intense microglial reaction in the cortex. Meningitis is sometimes found.

IMMUNITY

Immunologically borreliae behave like African trypanosomes. Antigenic variation overcomes the specific humoral antibodies formed to give rise to a series of relapses. When the spirochaetes first appear in the blood IgM antibodies (agglutinins, immobilizing antibodies, spirochaeticidins, lysins and leukostatic antibodies which promote phagocytosis) specific to the antigenic type of borrelia overcome the blood forms but do not eradicate the organisms from the tissues. The remaining borreliae which are antigenically unstable develop fresh antigens, only to be removed by fresh IgM antibodies specific to that type. This process leads to waves of IgM antibodies succeeding one another, to be followed by the formation of IgG antibodies which are more permanent and not specific.[3] The lytic activity depends on complement.[4] There is no immunity to subsequent attacks of relapsing fever.

Louse-borne relapsing fever (epidemic cosmopolitan type)

GEOGRAPHICAL DISTRIBUTION

The main endemic area is now the highlands of Ethiopia and Burundi but it can appear anywhere in areas of low endemicity in Peru and Bolivia, north-west and East Africa, India, Asia and China whenever environmental conditions are suitable and in times of social unrest and war (Fig. 32.2).

TRANSMISSION

Louse transmission

Man is the only known mammalian host and the disease is transmitted from man to man by the body louse (*Pediculus humanus* var. *corporis*) and head louse (*P. h.* var. *capitis*). Lice can be infected only by feeding on blood during the pyrexial attack. Spirochaetes are taken into the stomach from which they disappear in 24 hours at 28°C, and they cannot be found again until 6 days later when they appear in the body cavity (haemocoele), where they increase rapidly in number spreading to all parts of the body except the ovaries, salivary glands and gut. The louse remains unaffected and the spirochaetes can only escape from the louse by injury to the body or limbs. Lice are not infective until 6 days after

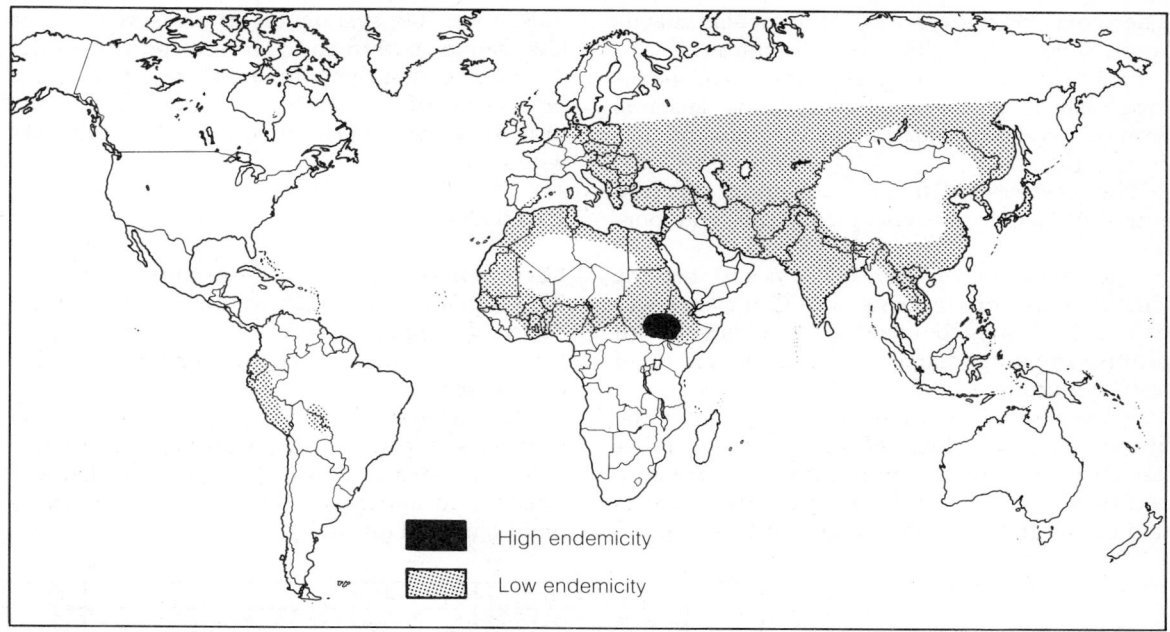

Fig. 32.2 Geographical distribution of louse-borne relapsing fever (*Borrelia recurrentis*). (Courtesy Department of Entomology, London School of Hygiene and Tropical Medicine.)

taking a feed and man can only become infected by crushing lice on the skin and not by bite. There is no transovarial transmission.

Other methods of transmission

Congenital. Transplacental transmission and abortion are not uncommon.

Blood transfusion. Transmission by blood transfusion has been recorded.[5]

CLINICAL FEATURES

Natural history

Louse-borne relapsing fever can be a severe disease. It is a febrile illness characterized by a primary attack of fever followed by not more than four relapses. There is a great variation in the degree of severity, varying from an asymptomatic parasitaemia to a severe febrile illness with death from hepatic or cardiac failure. In some epidemics mortality rates are high reaching 70%.

Incubation period

The incubation period is 2–10, usually 4–8 days.

Symptoms and signs[6]

The onset is sudden with chills and fever rising rapidly to 40.5°C or even higher when the patient may become delirious. He sits or lies on the bed or on the ground, silent, with a glazed expression, apathetic manner, and mentally dull or confused. There is dizziness, severe headache and pain in the back, chest, abdomen and legs (especially the calves) and joints. Nausea, vomiting and dysphagia are common. *Dyspnoea*, which is characteristic, is common; it is loud and hissing and can be heard for some distance away from the patient so that it is possible to diagnose a cause of relapsing fever from a distance. *Cough* is common and the sputum may contain borreliae. The spleen becomes enlarged, often to such a degree as to lead to spontaneous rupture. The liver is enlarged and *jaundice* is common. *Bleeding* often occurs into the skin (petechial rash), over the flanks and shoulders and into the mucous membranes; epistaxis is common. An erythematous *rash* over the upper part of the body may appear during the first attack resembling the rash of typhoid. The conjunctival vessels are congested and may bleed (clumps of adherent borreliae become impacted in capillaries, enmesh red cells, causing rupture of the capillaries and bleeding).

There may be widespread intravascular coagulation. There is usually heavy albuminuria.

Liver function tests show extensive hepatocellular damage. The blood shows anaemia with a *polymorphonuclear leukocytosis* of 15–30 × 10⁹/litre.

The *cerebrospinal fluid* may be under pressure and show a lymphocytic pleocytosis and borreliae.

The attack of fever lasts 5–7 days and then the temperature drops by crisis to 36°C or even lower (when there may be a state of collapse) with profuse sweating, diarrhoea, weakness and relief from symptoms.

Relapse occurs 5–9 days (Fig. 32.3) after the first attack in two-thirds of the patients, is rather less severe and there is no rash. A second relapse occurs in one-quarter of the patients and it is said there are never more than four relapses.

pulse over 100, systolic blood pressure of 90 or less, gallop rhythm and reversed splitting of the second sound in the pulmonary area. There may be a phase of critically low cardiac output due to myocardial damage which mostly disappears with treatment.

PROGNOSIS

Case mortality rates vary—usually around 2–9%—but are occasionally as high as 12%. Death occurs during the first febrile attack due to prothrombin deficiency, hepatic coma, myocarditis or disseminated intravascular coagulation. During the first crisis death may be due to hyperpyrexia with convulsions, heart failure, shock or cerebral oedema. Death is usually sudden and unexpected and may occur shortly after treatment has been given.

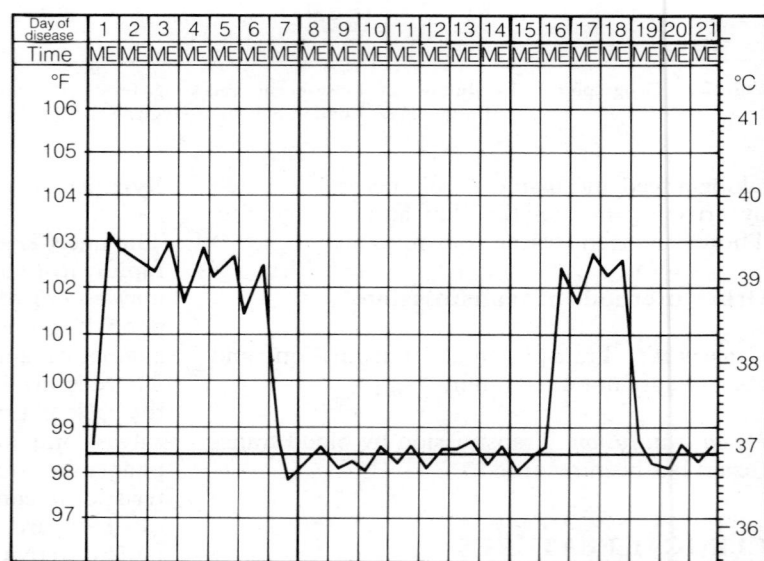

Fig. 32.3 Temperature chart in louse-borne relapsing fever. There is usually one relapse but not more than four.

COMPLICATIONS

Complications include pneumonia (pneumonic type) which may be a leading feature of the presentation, nephritis, parotitis, diarrhoea, arthritis, neuropathy, acute ophthalmitis and iritis, meningoencephalitis, meningitis and meningism.

Cardiac complications

Myocardial damage is not uncommon on the day of crisis with prolonged QTc, altered T waves,

DIFFERENTIAL DIAGNOSIS

In parts of East Africa, epidemics of a febrile illness in which jaundice is a noted feature are usually louse-borne relapsing fever. During the first attack other causes of febrile jaundice can present in a similar manner: yellow fever (does not usually present with jaundice as a marked feature), viral hepatitis, leptospirosis, severe falciparum malaria, typhoid, louse-borne typhus fever (with which it often coexists in the same patient), trench fever and cerebrospinal meningitis (a cerebrospinal fluid (CSF) specimen has been known to show meningococci and borreliae in the same microscopical field). After the first attack and during relapses other conditions may be relapsing typhoid, relapsing malaria (benign tertion), pyelonephritis, gallstones and kala-azar.

DIAGNOSIS

Borreliae are usually found in thick blood films taken during a febrile attack. They may be isolated at any time by inoculation of blood or CSF into young rats or white mice in which the blood will become positive in 2–3 days. Guinea-pigs, adult rabbits and dogs are refractory.

Serological tests

These are not very reliable. Serological tests for syphilis may be positive. A complement fixation test (CFT) has been devised[7] and an *immobilization* test has proved sensitive while a fluorescent antibody test using borrelia antigen is not quite so sensitive but cross reacts with *T. pallidum*.

TREATMENT

The treatment of choice is *tetracycline* alone or combined with *penicillin*. Procaine penicillin 300 mg units with tetracycline 500 mg 6-hourly for 7 days was effective and safe.[8] In Ethiopia a single oral dose of 500 mg tetracycline or erythromycin was effective[9] and this is the best dosage. Intravenous tetracycline 250 mg is effective if oral therapy cannot be given. A Jarisch–Herxheimer reaction quite commonly occurs after the administration of tetracycline or penicillin, especially if given intravenously. The patient is restless and there is a rigor lasting 10–30 minutes with a quick rise of temperature, pulse rate, breathing and blood pressure and intense shivering. This is followed by a phase of flushing and profuse sweating and the blood pressure falls. The patient becomes more comfortable and falls asleep, the temperature being normal next day. Borreliae disappear from the blood about the time of the peak of this reaction.[6] Few patients die. Steroids are not effective in relief but 300–500 mg of meptazinol (an opioid antagonist with agonist properties) intravenously reduces the severity of the reaction.[10] Intravenous fluid support is necessary since dehydration is an important cause of collapse.

EPIDEMIOLOGY

Louse-borne relapsing fever behaves in a similar manner to louse-borne typhus with which it usually coexists. It is a disease of great antiquity and epidemics have occurred in times of war. Refugees and great migrations with human overcrowding and poor hygiene all favour epidemics.

Between 1910 and 1945 it is estimated that there were 15 million cases in sub-Saharan Africa, Sudan, Ethiopia, eastern Europe and Russia with over five million deaths and mortality rates up to 75%. It is a disease of overcrowding and cold with poor hygiene, conditions which lead to heavy louse infestation (although it is seen in the tropics at high altitudes where head lice may be important).

CONTROL

With modern methods of delousing with insecticides, epidemics can be brought to a halt immediately. Insecticide powder is blown into the clothes of the population at risk to eliminate lice and heat sterilization of the clothing kills the eggs. Personal prevention may be achieved by careful delousing without crushing the lice and avoiding scratching. Lice cannot transmit the infection by bite or faeces (see also Appendix III, p. 1470).

Tick-borne relapsing fever

GEOGRAPHICAL DISTRIBUTION

Tick-borne relapsing fever has a wide distribution in both the Old and New Worlds in five main areas (three in the Old World and two in the New World), each with a specific borrelia tick vector complex (Fig. 32.4).

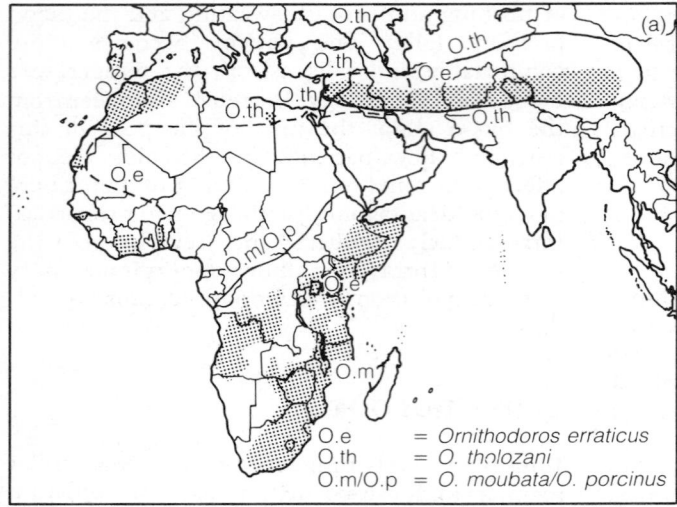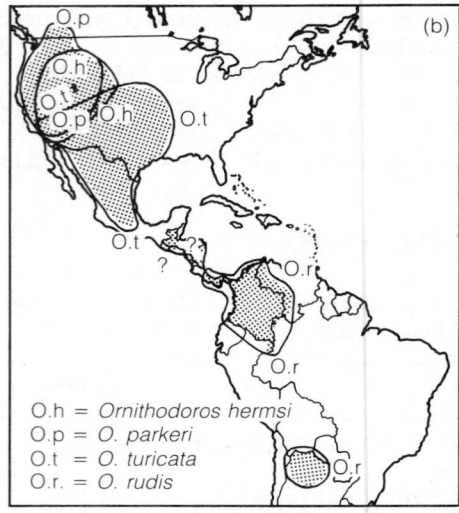

Fig. 32.4 Geographical distribution of tick-borne (endemic) relapsing fever in the Old World (a) and New World (b). (Courtesy Department of Entomology, London School of Hygiene and Tropical Medicine.)

AETIOLOGY

There are seven species of *Borrelia* involved (Table 32.1).

Table 32.1 *Borrelia* species involved in tick-borne relapsing fevers (see also Table III.2, p. 1389).

Species	Vector	Geographical area
B. duttoni	*O. moubata* (*O.m. porcinus* and *O. savignyi*)	East, central and South Africa
B. hispanica	*O. erraticus*	Mediterranean region (part), North and West Africa, Portugal and Spain
B. persica	*O. tholozani* (=*papillipes*) including var. *crossi*	Mediterranean region (part), Tobruk, Cyprus, Israel, through Iran to Kashmir and Sinkiang province of western China
B. parkeri	*O. parkeri*	Central and western USA, Mexico
B. turicata	*O. turicata*	Central and western USA, Mexico
B. hermsi	*O. hermsi*	Central and western USA, Mexico
B. venezuelensis	*O. rudis* (=*venezuelensis*)	Northern, South and Central America southwards to northern Argentina

TRANSMISSION

Ticks

The main method of transmission is by soft ticks of the genus *Ornithodoros* (Appendix III, p. 1387, and Figs. III.10, III.11 and III.12A, p. 1388.

Cycle in the tick

Both nymphs and adults transmit the infection by the salivary glands and bite and by the coxal fluid. The borreliae penetrate the gut wall after being ingested at a blood meal and invade the haemocoele and other organs, including salivary glands, coxal glands and ovary, where they multiply. They are not found in tick faeces. Infection of a susceptible animal can take place through the bite of an infected tick, which is a relatively large puncture into which infective saliva is pumped or which may be the portal of entry for coxal fluid secreted while the tick is feeding. Nymphs of *O. moubata* transmit both by salivary and coxal fluid while *O. turicata*, *O. parkeri*, *O. hermsi* and *O. tholozani* do not produce coxal fluid while feeding. Transmission can take place in less than a minute after attachment of the tick.

Transovarial transmission is usual. A tick remains infected for many years and transmits the infection to its offspring. The organisms perpetuate themselves enzootically in ticks without need for other hosts to the extent of at least five generations.

Other methods of transmission

Borreliae can enter through intact mucous membrane and skin. Accidental infection via the conjunctiva can occur and transfusion, transplacental transmission and infection by intravenous drug administration can all occur. Borreliae can survive in lice and bed bugs but do not develop further.

Hosts

Man is the only source of infection for *O. moubata* while for other soft ticks the main sources of infection are rodents which live in open country, caves and burrows and do not infest human dwellings. Infection is transmitted to man only as an incidental infection. Animal hosts also include monkeys, squirrels, chipmunks, rats, hedgehogs and possibly bats and other cave dwelling mammals.

IMMUNITY

Tick-borne relapsing fever is more serious in expatriates than among indigenous people who have had previous experience of the disease, and neurological complications are much commoner in visitors.

CLINICAL FEATURES

Natural history

Tick-borne relapsing fever is a milder disease than the louse-borne form. A primary attack of fever is followed by a number of relapses not exceeding 11 before the infection dies out. Mortality is low but neurological complications are a feature. However, recovery is usually complete and there are no sequelae.

Incubation period

This may be quite short; 1–2 days has been reported in the Spanish form, but is usually longer, up to 14 days.

Symptoms and signs

Onset

The primary attack begins abruptly with severe headache and fever up to 40°C. Rarely the attack may be fulminating leading to coma and death but, on the other hand, it may take the form of a chronic low fever. During this attack the spleen (45%) enlarges and may develop infarcts and haemorrhage. The liver also enlarges (11%) but jaundice is not so common or so intense as in the louse-borne form. There may be diarrhoea, bronchitis and pneumonia. Massive haematuria with nephritis has been recorded in Israel.[11]

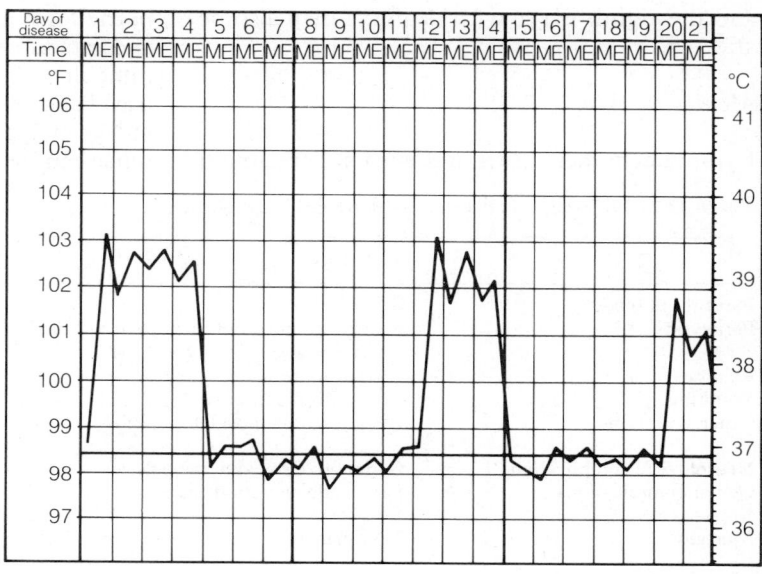

Fig. 32.5 Temperature chart in tick-borne relapsing fever. There are usually three to six relapses but may be as many as eleven.

Blood changes

Borreliae are not so numerous in the blood as in the louse-borne form. There is a poly-morphonuclear leukocytosis. The primary attack may last 4–5 days (less in the African form) ending in crisis which can lead to collapse.

Relapses

Relapses are characteristic of the tick-borne form. They may occur at intervals of a day or two or as long as three weeks. There are usually three to six relapses but may be as many as 11 in the African form (Fig. 32.5).

COMPLICATIONS

Neurological

The borreliae of tick-borne relapsing fever are neurotropic and have a distinct affinity for the nervous system. They may be present in the CSF detected by microscopical examination or by animal inoculation. Various neurological syndromes may result appearing at the end of the initial fever or during relapses.

Cranial nerve involvement

This is the commonest neurological complication. The seventh nerve is the most affected (22% in one series in North Africa) but the third, fourth, fifth and sixth with ophthalmoplegia and the eighth nerve with deafness may also be affected.

Meningitic form

Lymphocyte meningitis and even subarachnoid haemorrhage may occur. The CSF is under pressure with a pleocytosis. This form is not uncommon in expatriates in the Dakar area.

Other cerebral syndromes

Hemiplegia, aphasia, encephalitis, optic atrophy, iritis and iridocyclitis are not uncommon. The spinal nerves may be involved especially with *O. moubata* and *O. tholozani* transmitted infections. There may be facial nerve involvement and sciatic neuralgia with anaesthesia. Most cerebral complications recover without leaving any permanent effects.

Other complications

Bronchitis, hepatic failure and arthritis may all occur.

DIFFERENTIAL DIAGNOSIS

Other fevers must be distinguished as with louse-borne relapsing fever from other relapsing fevers (rat bite fevers), while the differences between the tick-borne and louse-borne form are given in Table 32.2.[12]

DIAGNOSIS

In the febrile period borreliae can be seen in the peripheral blood but are fewer than in the louse-borne form and may need inoculation into mice and rats to demonstrate them. Diagnosis can be difficult in the afebrile period but a history of travel and residence in a known infected camp or village helps and in a subsequent relapse borreliae can be demonstrated at the onset and peak

Table 32.2　Differences between tick-borne and louse-borne relapsing fevers (after Coghill[12]).

	Tick-borne	Louse-borne
Parasites in blood	Scanty	Numerous
Paroxysms	Relatively short, not more than 5–7 days. Often chronic, irregular fever	Relatively long, up to 10 days
Relapses	Two or more	Two or less, often none
Vomiting	Only with meningitis	At any stage
Other symptoms	Lethargy, loss of weight, debility	Diarrhoea, jaundice, coma, severe haemorrhage
Neurological complications	Common. Cranial nerve palsies	Infrequent
Ocular complications	Papilloedema with meningitis	Infrequent
Illness	Less severe	More severe
Mortality	Less than 10%	May be high, up to 50%

of the fever. Serological tests may be used in the same way as in louse-borne relapsing fever.

TREATMENT

The treatment is the same as for louse-borne relapsing fever using tetracycline in one 500 mg dose or procaine penicillin 300 mg. The Jarisch–Herxheimer reaction is not a complication of treatment.

EPIDEMIOLOGY

Tick-borne relapsing fever is an endemic disease found in certain places (it is a place disease). In central, East and South Africa, where man is the only reservoir, it is found in human habitations and wherever man collects together; certain types of house, staging camps for migrant workers and old camping sites. In East Africa *O. moubata* is of two types, one preferring to feed on chickens living in hot humid conditions and not important in transmission, and the other preferring to feed on man and found in cooler, wetter conditions (highlands) where it is an important vector.[13]

O. moubata porcinus, which is widely distributed in African dwellings at all altitudes in East Africa, feeds on man and is favoured by higher rainfall and a high relative humidity. It is a better vector than *O. moubata*.[14]

O. savignyi prefers a hot, dry climate and infests market places and cattle byres around wells where it comes into contact with man.

In North Africa, the eastern Mediterranean, central Asia and North and South America rodents are the main reservoir and the infection is only transmitted to man incidentally. The ticks live in animal burrows and caves, and in North America in holiday homes where chipmunks live in the roof.

CONTROL

Control of infection where dwellings are the source of infection is effected by building concrete floors and better walls so that ticks do not have access. Ticks can be killed by insecticides: they are relatively unaffected by DDT but can be killed by BHC at 20 mg/900 cm^2 used to dust on the floor. Travellers must never sleep on the floor. Old camping sites and mud houses must be avoided.

Lyme disease caused by a spirochaete *Borrelia burgdorferi* in the eastern USA is described in Appendix III, p. 1391.

RAT BITE FEVERS

Two forms of fever have been ascribed to infection through the bites of rats: Sodoku (sokosha), named by Japanese workers and caused by *Spirillum minus* (*S. morsus-muris*), and Haverhill fever (infectious erythema), named by American workers and caused by *Actinobacillus muris* (formerly known as *Streptobacillus moniliformis* and other names).

These are not strictly tropical diseases but are included here because they are relapsing diseases which may be confused with other similar infections.

Sodoku

GEOGRAPHICAL DISTRIBUTION

Most cases have occurred in Japan but it has also been reported from Australia, Africa, the Americas and Europe.

AETIOLOGY

Spirillum minus is a short spiral organism (2–4 µm long), rather thick, with regular rigid spirals and pointed ends continued into one or more flagella. It moves rapidly, like a vibrio. It is easily stained by methylene blue or Giemsa.

S. minus can be cultivated but subcultivation has been unsuccessful.[1] It can be grown by intraperitoneal inoculation into guinea-pigs, mice and rats.

TRANSMISSION

S. minus is a parasite of rats which are healthy

carriers. Transmission is from rat to man although it can also be caused by the bite of cats, ferrets and bandicoots. It may also be transmitted by rat urine contaminating food.

PATHOLOGY

The organism enters at the site of the bite, which develops local inflammation and even necrosis. It travels to the regional lymph glands. In fatal cases neuronal degeneration has been seen in the brain and degenerative changes in liver and kidneys.

CLINICAL FEATURES

Natural history

Sodoku is a relapsing fever which may subside spontaneously or go on for months. It is a relatively mild disease and the death rate has been about 10%.

Incubation period

The incubation period varies from 5 to 30 days, the average being 5–10 days.

Symptoms and signs

There is usually a history of a bite which heals but may later break down to form an ulcer (Fig. 32.6) and then the scar itself and sometimes the surrounding tissues becomes inflamed with the formation of blebs and even necrosis. The lymphatics draining the area are implicated and the glands themselves become swollen and tender. The onset of fever is characterized by rigors and malaise; the temperature gradually rises in 3 days to a maximum of 39.4–40°C and after a further period of 3 days ends in crisis with profuse sweating.

After the primary attack a quiescent interval of 5–10 days ensues. One or more relapses associated with the same symptoms and a characteristic purple papular exanthem, or urticaria, on the chest and arms, have been noted. The eruption is sometimes nodular. With each bout of fever the cicatrix at the site of the original bite becomes inflamed.

In most cases the reflexes are increased; there may be pains in the muscles and joints, hyperaesthesia and oedema of various parts of the

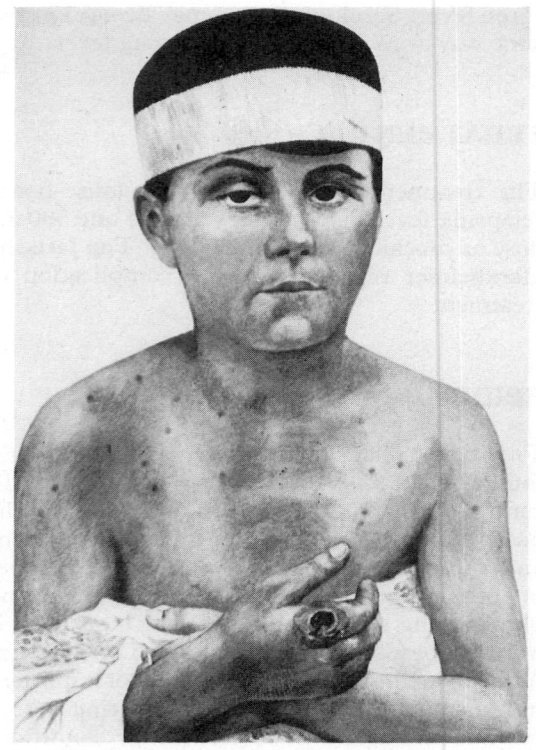

Fig. 32.6 Rat bite fever produces an initial lesion at the site of the bite, followed by relapsing fever and rash. (Courtesy WTIM.)

body. In some cases arthritis has been reported. The death rate is about 10%. In fatal cases the end is ushered in by delirium, often lapsing into coma. Some cases subside spontaneously, others go on for months.

As in relapsing fever, the organism can be demonstrated in the blood during the fever only, disappearing during the apyrexial intervals. There is an eosinophilia during the paroxysm and a moderate leukocytosis of about 15×10^9/litre and an increase in CSF pressure.

DIFFERENTIAL DIAGNOSIS

Differential diagnosis has to be made from the different forms of relapsing and trench fevers with which the temperature chart (Fig. 32.7) has much in common. In tropical countries the possibility of a coexistent malaria has to be taken in to account. The puffiness of the face accompanying the urticarial eruption may simulate acute nephritis.

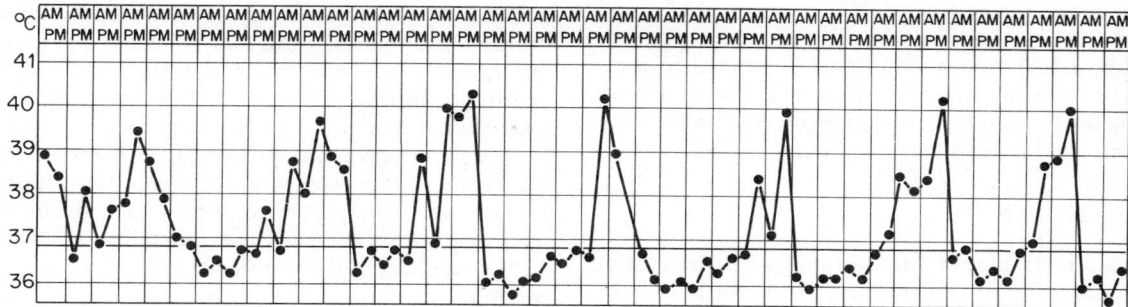

Fig. 32.7 Temperature chart in rat bite fever showing the periodic relapses.

The reaction occurring around the site of the scar is apt to be confused with erysipelas or cellulitis.

DIAGNOSIS

In many cases the diagnosis of rat bite fever can be fully established from the history, the infiltration at the seat of the bite, the typical temperature chart, the rash, and the effects of the administration of penicillin. This diagnosis can be confirmed either by dark-ground illumination when spirilla may be seen in the exudate obtained from the site of the bite, or in the serous fluid from the papule, or by Giemsa-stained smears. It is seldom possible to demonstrate spirilla in a thick blood film. If a number of relapses have occurred, probably the best examination to make is for the presence of lytic antibodies. Absolute proof of the clinical diagnosis may be obtained by inoculating the patient's blood, lymph gland, or a piece of excised wound into guinea-pigs and mice.

S. minus is not easily found in the blood though it does invade the blood after a few days but it can be found in the exudate near the bite and in juice from the local lymph nodes. Inoculation of infected material into mice and rats produces blood infection and in guinea-pigs a febrile disease. Dogs can be infected but remain symptomless. Monkeys and rabbits are also susceptible. The spirilla appear to be present in the muscles of the rat tongue and rats, mice and guinea-pigs may be healthy carriers.

Serology

The serum gives weak treponemal serological reactions and a positive Weil–Felix to the proteus OXK strain.

TREATMENT

The infection responds rapidly to penicillin; one injection of 300 mg of a repository penicillin is adequate. Streptomycin and tetracycline are also effective.

EPIDEMIOLOGY

Single sporadic cases occur following a rat bite but small epidemics are found when contaminated raw milk is the vehicle of infection.[15]

Haverhill fever

GEOGRAPHICAL DISTRIBUTION

Haverhill fever is found in the USA, Europe and elsewhere.

AETIOLOGY

Actinobacillus muris (*Actinobacillus moniliformis,* *Streptobacillus moniliformis*) is a natural parasite of the nasopharynx of rats. It is a pleomorphic organism which forms slender, branching filaments 1–3 × 0.3–0.4 μm which break up to form chains of bacilli or coccoid bodies. It is a commoner cause of rat bite fever than *Spirillum minus*.

TRANSMISSION

Although infection can often be traced to a rat bite, transmission can occur via raw milk that has been contaminated by rat urine, which has been the cause in many epidemics.[15]

PATHOLOGY

Little is known of the pathology but ulcerative endocarditis and subacute myocarditis have been reported and the liver is enlarged.

CLINICAL FEATURES

Natural history

Haverhill fever consists of fever, an erythematous rash most prominent on hands and feet, arthralgia and the subsequent development of a sore throat. The fever may relapse and continue for months without treatment.

Incubation period

The incubation period is 3–10 days during which there may be gastrointestinal upset.

Symptoms and signs

If there is a bite the local wound heals to be followed by fever, extreme prostration, severe generalized muscular pain and tenderness, head-ache and a widespread morbilliform rash, most marked on the hands and feet. There is a general enlargement of the lymph glands. A non-suppurative shifting arthritis is characteristic. In untreated cases the disease may subside spontaneously after 9–10 days but can continue with a relapsing fever which is prolonged with night sweats, and can recur for weeks or months at irregular intervals.[16,17] Case mortality is about 10% from bacterial endocarditis and abscess formation.

DIAGNOSIS (Table 32.3)

Differential diagnoses include Coxsackie viral illness, meningococcal septicaemia and erythema multiforme. The organism can be isolated from the blood on an aerobic culture and subcultured on blood agar in a carbon dioxide atmosphere after 48 hours.

Serology

Actinobacillus muris can be agglutinated by serum and a fluorescent antibody titre (IgM) of 1/400 was given against an antigen consisting of *Actinobacillus* organisms.[15]

TREATMENT

Tetracycline is the drug of choice, 250 mg 6-hourly for two weeks. Some of the coccobacillary variants are resistant to penicillin.

Table 32.3 Differentiation of sodoku and Haverhill fever.

	Sodoku	Haverhill fever
Transmission	Bite of rat	Bite of rat or other animal. Possibly contaminated food
Incubation period	5–30 days	3–10 days, average 5
Wound from bite	Apparent healing, followed by chancre-like ulceration	Heals promptly
Lymph glands	Regional lymphadenitis	Not involved
Systemic manifestations	Regularly relapsing type of fever	Intermittent, but not regularly relapsing type of fever
	Generalized maculopapular rash	Macular, pustular and petechial eruption
	Varying degrees of prostration and debility	Varying degrees of prostration
	Arthritis very rare	Metastatic arthritis fairly common
Laboratory findings	Polymorphonuclear leukocytosis	Same
	Secondary anaemia	Same
	Kahn test, usually +	Negative
	Isolation of *Spirillum* by animal inoculation of blood or infected gland	Isolation of *A. muris* by blood culture and from pustules on veal infusion broth enriched with rabbit serum
	Agglutination test negative	Agglutination test with *A. muris* positive. Serum agglutinates a polyvalent antigen of the bacillus

LEPTOSPIROSIS

Sheena A. Waitkins

Leptospirosis is a zoonotic disease caused by the spirochaetal organisms *Leptospira*.[18–20] It has been known by many different names such as mud fever, swamp fever, sugar cane fever (Table 32.4). This disease is found worldwide and is caused by many different serologically related serovars of the genus *Leptospira*.

Table 32.4 Synonyms used for leptospirosis.

Weil's disease	Japanese autumnal fever
Seven-day fever	Swamp fever
Queensland fever	Canicola fever
Cane cutters' fever	Infectious jaundice
Fort Bragg fever	Rice-field workers' disease
Harvest fever	Red water fever
Mud fever	

AETIOLOGY

Leptospires were first observed and described by Stimson in 1907.[21] They are fine spiral-shaped bacteria with characteristic morphology seen by dark-field, phase-contrast, fluorescence and electron microscopy (Fig. 32.8). The organism appears straight with both ends characteristically hooked. Their diameter is about 0.1 μm and their length varies from 6 μm to 20 μm (Fig. 32.8).

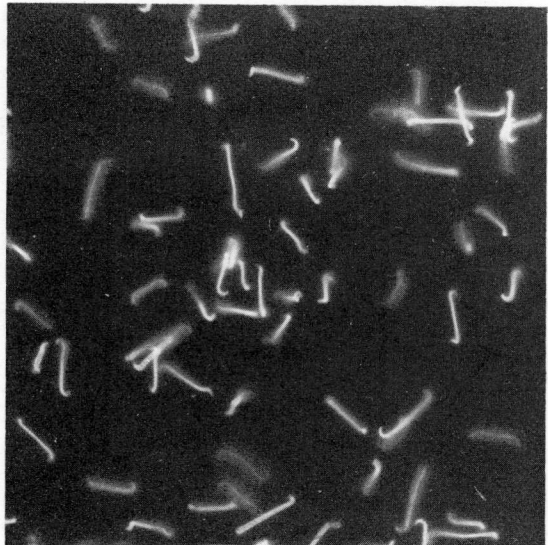

Fig. 32.8 Leptospires under dark-ground illumination—characteristically hooked at both ends.

The genus *Leptospira* was created by Noguchi in 1918[22] and belongs to the family Spirochaetaceae. It is currently divided into two species: *Leptospira biflexa* (saprophytic and free-living strain) and *Leptospira interrogans* (parasitic and potentially pathogenic strain). Within each strain are serologically related serogroups which are arranged according to their antigenic interrelationships demonstrated by the micro-agglutination test (MAT) and cross-absorption reactions with high titre rabbit homologous antisera.[20] Currently there are 188 serovars antigenically arranged into 26 major serogroups within the strain *L. interrogans*. *L. biflexa* contains 36 serogroups with corresponding 65 serovars.[20] The genus specific antigen is found in the *L. biflexa* serogroup semaranga serovar patoc (Table 32.5).

Table 32.5 Recognized serogroups of *Leptospira*.

L. interrogans	
Australis	Icterohaemorrhagiae
Autumnalis	Javanica
Ballum	Kenya
Bataviae	Louisiana
Bufonis	Manhao
Butembo	Mini
Canicola	Panama
Celledoni	Pomona
Cynopteri	Pyrogenes
Djasiman	Ranarum
Grippotyphosa	Sejroe
Hebdomadis	Shermani
Huanuco	Tarassovi

L. biflexa	
Abaete	Maritza
Ancona	Muggia
Andamana	Nazara
Aurisina	Nomentano
Basrich	Ondina
Basovizza	Orvenco
Bessemans	Parapatan
Cadore	Percedol
Camtachia	Poona
Cau	Pulpudeva
Codice	Semaranga
Dindio	Sidonia
Doberdo	Sorbradinoho
Garcia	Tevere
Holland	Tharcia
Khoshamian	Tororo
Lazio	Udine
Malomievo	Vinzent

The two species can be separated on biological and serological criteria. Table 32.6 illustrates the common tests used to differentiate both species. They are used routinely by reference laboratories to identify unknown strains or newly isolated leptospires. Pathogenic leptospires are parasites and do not usually multiply in great numbers outside the body of their maintenance host while saprophytic biflexa strains are often found in muddy soils, freshwater rivers and canals and humid environments. It is generally thought that the presence of biflexa in river waters indicates that the environmental conditions are satisfactory for the survival of pathogenic leptospires excreted from their maintenance host.

survive in environmental elements such as fresh water (sea water contains sodium chloride which kills leptospires). However, they are destroyed by the gastric juices, bile, human and cow's milk and killed by 1 p.p.m. of chlorine.[23]

CLASSIFICATION

Classification of *L. interrogans* serogroup is based mainly on serological criteria involving a two-way cross absorption–agglutination reaction between the strain under test and known serovars. Two strains are considered to be the same, if after cross agglutination–absorption with adequate amounts of high titre homologous

Table 32.6 Differentiation of saprophytic and pathogenic leptospires.

Strain	Growth at 13°C	Growth in 8-azaguanine (200 µg/ml)	Hamster challenge experiments
Pathogenic: *L. interrogans*	No growth	No growth	Death/clinical symptoms
Saprophytic: *L. biflexa*	Growth	Growth	No symptoms

Leptospira interrogans is an obligate aerobe requiring demanding growth factors for multiplication; optimal pH range is 7.2–7.6, temperature 28–30°C, generation times vary between 7 and 16 hours depending on media used. Essential vitamins such as B_1 and B_{12} are required for their growth and their major source of energy are long chained fatty acids. Leptospires do not catabolize amino acids but use ammonium salts as their source of nitrogen.[23,24]

Media for the cultivation of leptospires incorporate the above ingredients and are usually enriched with fresh rabbit serum and/or bovine serum albumin, such media as Fletcher's,[25] Korthof's[26] or modifications of it[27,28] and Stuart's medium.[29] All these have been successful in the past but the need to obtain fresh animal products presents difficulties and in 1965 Ellinghausen and McCullough[30] prepared a semisynthetic media containing bovine serum albumin and Tween 80 which was further modified by Johnson and Harris[31] and can be commercially obtained from Difco Laboratories (EMJH).

Despite the fastidious growth requirements the leptospires have a remarkable ability to

serum, less than 10% of the homologous antibody titre remains in both test and known criteria. This classification procedure was originally described by Wolff and Broom[32] and further modified by Kmety et al.[33] Alternatively a shortened but equally successful classification procedure based on Kmety's factor serum analysis was described by him in 1966.[34] Although the leptospires are identified by their 'major antigenic factors' the method works well with some groups such as sejroe but less efficiently with others such as tarassovi. Because of the variation in results obtained Kmety's shortened method is not recognized officially.

The methods described above rely on standard high titre antisera for all known leptospiral serovars; this is difficult because standard inoculum, rabbit's age and variety and the exact method of absorption are still not fully standardized within the *Leptospira* reference laboratories. Furthermore, they are also tedious, labour intensive and technically difficult and are therefore, not easily undertaken by all national reference laboratories. Alternative methods of taxonomy are being developed and applied. Monoclonal antibodies are such a method. Developed to recognize 'major antigens' these have proved to be useful in recognition of certain groups such as hebdomadis, pomona and icterohaemorrhagiae.[35,36] However, the successful hybridization of clones is a very 'hit and miss' procedure and depends on checkerboard titrations similar to Kmety's factor analysis scheme. Despite these limitations monoclonals do have the advantage that 'libraries' of clones can be set up and good standardization of techniques can be assessed. When monoclonals are available for a serogroup they work very well.

Another method which is now being widely applied to leptospiral taxonomy is the bacterial restriction endonuclease DNA analysis (BRENDA). These were first used by Robinson and his colleagues in 1982.[37] These workers used the ability of endonucleases to digest and split the DNA of *Leptospira interrogans* serovars hardjo, balcanica and tarassovi; the lengths of DNA were then run on agarose gels and produced a characteristic pattern of 'bands of DNA'. These patterns were then visually compared with each other and identification achieved. Understandably, this method relies on the subjective analysis of like band patterns with like bands. This can be tedious and 'errors' can occur if patterns are similar. Hookey and his colleagues[38] examined the DNA patterns obtained in the australis serogroup and quantified these results by means of a computer assisted analysis scheme whereby percentage similarities and disimilarities could be detected. It is now possible to grow an unknown leptospiral organism, digest the DNA by means of recognized DNA endonucleases and then run the resulting DNA patterns in a microcomputer enabling the match of similar organisms to be quantifiably recognized. This is a considerable saving in time and energy over the classical taxonomic methods and is reproducible in any country or laboratory where it is attempted. The use of such modern analysis will lead to more accurate and reproducible classification and a more precise epidemiological understanding of the relationship between strains and their hosts.

TRANSMISSION

Infected animals carry the leptospires in the tubules of their kidneys and shed the organisms in their urine. Man and other susceptible animals become infected through contact either directly with urine or indirectly through contact with fresh water, soil, mud and foodstuffs contaminated with pathogenic leptospires. Water is one of the most important agents in the transmission of leptospires. Stagnant water and slow-moving water is particularly dangerous in temperate climates in late summer. However, in tropical countries rapidly flowing water in the jungle is also an important danger.

Pathogenic leptospires require moist, warm (about 25°C) environmental conditions and a pH value of soil, mud and surface water to be about 7.0 for optimum conditions of survival. These are often found throughout the year in tropical countries but are limited to summer and early autumn in temperate climates. If the optimal conditions are present, then leptospires can survive for months in warm muddy waters.

Leptospires enter via fresh cuts and abrasions in the skin and through mucosal surfaces of nose, throat and conjunctiva. Fresh wounds should always be covered if handling suspected materials such as animal foodstuffs or before coming in contact with potentially infected fresh water.

CLINICAL PRESENTATION AND PATHOLOGY

Leptospirosis is *not synonymous* with Weil's disease for milder, febrile illnesses are also associated with leptospiral infections. These are often mistaken for malaria, yellow fever, viral hepatitis and bacterial fevers in the tropics. In temperate climates, leptospirosis may often be diagnosed as influenza, viral hepatitis or meningitis. The severity of the disease varies from the classical presentation of Weil's syndrome, namely hepatorenal failure and meningitis and occasionally, in severe cases, haemoptysis, erythema nodosum and acute pancreatitis to a milder flu-like illness with severe headache which may persist for several months. It must be remembered that there is considerable overlap in the clinical presentation.

Two distinct phases of leptospirosis are noted. The first is essentially a leptospiraemia while the second is predominantly a leptospiruria. The bacteraemic phase corresponds to the incubation period and varies between 2 and 20 days (average 7–12 days) with subsequent spread to tissues and organs. This accounts for the various presenting symptoms during the first week of illness. Onset is often sudden with fever, malaise and myalgia. The fever lasts for about 7 days and blood cultures taken during this period may give positive growth of *Leptospira*. During the second phase of illness the leptospires have been removed from the blood and tissues by phagocytes and increasing concentrations of antibodies. In most tissues they are eradicated and the tissues return to their normal function. The kidney is the only organ which retains leptospires, which migrate to the convoluted tubules of the cortex where they may multiply producing renal failure. Corza[39] demonstrated that even in relatively mild cases of human leptospirosis in which glomerular filtration remains unaffected, tubular function is reduced markedly; therefore impaired renal blood flow constitutes the major leptospiral nephropathy. Because the kidney is involved the leptospires may be excreted via the urine and can persist for several months, even after clinical cure has been achieved.[18] It is unlikely that the numbers of leptospires excreted in the urine ($<10^4$ organisms/ml) represent a hazard of man-to-man transmission. During the second week increasing amounts of antibodies may be detected and by the tenth day of illness sufficient IgM has normally been produced to confirm the original clinical diagnosis. When meningitis is a clinical feature, leptospires may be isolated from the CSF and antibodies demonstrated; lymphocytes are present and the condition may be mistaken for a 'viral meningitis'. There may be a macular or maculopapular rash and enlarged lymph nodes and clinical signs of pneumonitis may be present. There may be haemorrhaging in the muscles, skin, kidneys, lungs and alimentary canal. Conjunctivitis is pathognomonic. By the third week extreme icterus is often accompanied by severe glomerulo-interstitial nephritis. The mortality rate for leptospirosis with severe jaundice may be as high as 20%.

The milder forms of leptospirosis lack the severity of classical cases. The illness usually presents with flu-like symptoms including fever, severe headache and often mental confusion. Recovery is prolonged, usually eight to 10 weeks and lethargy is common. In a small minority of cases the symptoms proceed to meningitis and renal failure but rarely death. Leptospirosis is commonly misdiagnosed.

So, if a successful diagnosis is to be achieved an overall knowledge of the clinical features and the epidemiological likelihood of the disease should be first sought from the clinician before laboratory tests are undertaken. A useful 'check list' of epidemiological data such as: date of onset, any animal contact, which ones, contact with fresh water courses, which kind of contact, e.g. total immersion, contact with fresh wounds. All this information should be available from the clinician.

Clinical features

The course of the disease may be divided into three stages: the septicaemic, the leptospiruric and finally the convalescent phase.

The septicaemic stage

This stage is one of sudden onset with flu-like illness and myalgia. It proceeds to involve the central nervous system and is characterized by meningism. As mentioned above, hepatorenal failure occurs and the urine shows albuminuria and bile pigment. Biochemical parameters are usually helpful in a differential diagnosis of leptospirosis from other hepatic diseases.[40] The CSF shows increased protein levels and a predominant leukocytosis; if jaundice is present there is xanthochromia, as the infection increases the permeability of the meninges to bile pigment.

SERUM
Liver function tests. Alkaline phosphatase and transaminase are slightly raised while the serum bilirubin is usually significantly increased. Alkaline phosphatase, 140–150 IU/litre (120–130 IU/litre), AST, 40–45 IU/litre (<38 IU/litre), ALT, 40–45 IU/litre (<36 IU/litre), bilirubin total $>50\,\mu$mol/litre ($17\,\mu$mol/litre) (normal values in brackets).

BLOOD
The organism is present in the blood during the first 10 days and therefore cultural investigations should be undertaken during this period before antibiotics are given (see below).

Antibodies may develop in the first week of illness but these are usually IgM and therefore acute-phase serological antibodies may be measured and used for subsequent rising antibody titres.

The leptospiruraemic phase

This phase represents the stage of deepening

jaundice and increasing renal and myocardial involvement, particularly with serogroup ictero-haemorrhagiae. This is classical Weil's syndrome, while in milder forms the second phase of the illness may proceed only to meningeal involvement. Death may occur at this stage. Leptospires may be found in the urine, provided the patient's urine has been alkalinized, in vivo, with for example potassium citrate; otherwise recovery is very unpredictable. Antibodies may be demonstrated in the serum.

Convalescent stage

Clinical improvement occurs, with increased mental awareness, fading jaundice and renal improvement. The usual convalescent phase involves no permanent renal or hepatic damage.

DIFFERENTIAL DIAGNOSIS

Leptospirosis like other spirochaetes 'mimics' most bacterial and viral diseases. It should always be considered in patients suffering from pyrexia of unknown origin and especially, flu-like illness. Aseptic or viral meningitis, particularly if the patients also complain of conjunctivitis, needs to be investigated for leptospirosis. Risk related occupations such as rice-workers, miners, sewermen etc., must always be considered in the differential diagnosis of jaundice especially in tropical countries. Finally, because leptospirosis is primarily a zoonotic disease, farmers and those in contact with wildlife and domestic animals must always be suspected of leptospirosis.

DIAGNOSIS

Since leptospirosis may be confused with other diseases, clinical diagnosis is difficult. A definite diagnosis can only reliably be performed in the laboratory where both clinical features and laboratory tests are supportive of one another.

Microbiological diagnosis

The extreme variability in clinical symptoms in most cases of leptospirosis makes laboratory confirmation an absolute requirement for definitive diagnosis.

Serology

The serological diagnosis of leptospirosis is often difficult, particularly the interpretation of results. These may be masked either by the 'prozoning' effect of the test sera or the anti-complementary activity of the antigen used. Despite the complex nature of the antigen components of *Leptospira*, detection of leptospirosis by serodiagnostic methods is still the easiest way to confirm leptospirosis.

There are three established serological methods used: the microscopic agglutination test (MAT), which is serogroup specific and a confirmatory test; the complement fixation test (CFT) which is a genus specific test and can be routinely used to screen sera and the enzyme-linked immunosorbent assay (ELISA) which is also a genus specific test and can be used to detect early IgM. Others include a macroscopic slide test, a sensitized erythrocyte lysis and an indirect immunofluorescence test; all are genus specific.[41]

Whenever leptospirosis is suspected serum should be taken as early in the illness as possible. Usually antibodies can be detected within the first 5 to 6 days depending on the system used to detect them. Therefore, an early acute serum sample may be negative but could be a vital comparison for later samples. IgM may be detected at high titres using the ELISA method 3 to 4 days after the onset of illness.

The MAT may be performed using either live or formalized leptospires as antigens and is serogroup specific. Live antigens comprise 4- to 10-day-old cultures incubated at 30°C. Alternatively, formalized cultures of leptospires may be used; the cultures are grown as for live antigen and killed with 0.2% v/v neutralized formaldehyde. In both cases the test is performed using a battery of leptospiral antigens representing all known pathogenic serogroups as shown in Table 32.5. The patient's serum is tested in doubling dilutions ranging from 1:40 to 1:10 400. One drop of patient's diluted serum is mixed with one drop of each antigen incubated at either 30°C for 2 hours if live antigen is used or overnight at room temperature if formalized. The resulting agglutination is read by means of a dark-ground microscope with ×40 objective and ×10 ocular lenses. In positive results, agglutination of the leptospires are seen. Agglutination may be incomplete in high titre serum at low dilutions because of the 'prozoning effect'. Microscopic agglutinations may be detected as early as day 6 of the illness but more commonly after day 10. Both IgG and IgM are detected by MAT.

The CFT is a useful screening method which is genus specific and involves a heated/acid extracted antigen of serogroups australis, canicola, hebdomadis and patoc. The ELISA is also a genus specific test utilizing only one serogroup. The test is easy to perform and may use a variety of antihuman conjugates for detecting antibody. IgM is generally detected very early, 3 to 4 days after onset of illness and is therefore an ideal laboratory method. The ELISA is specific, does not require sophisticated equipment if 5-aminosalicylic acid is used as substrate, which may be read by eye.[42]

A more detailed description of serological methods may be found in Turner[41] and Waitkins.[24]

Culture methods

The success and reliability of laboratory investigations depends largely on specimens of good quality and adequate amounts which are obtained at the right time in the course of infection. Samples from both man and animals for culture include urine from the leptospiruric phase (after 10 days) and blood in the acute phase (first 10 days). Cerebrospinal fluid may be of value in the leptospiruric phase for culture. It must be remembered that the human urine is acidic and therefore if culture of urine is to be successful, in vivo alkalinization is required.

Small volumes of biological fluid serially diluted in large volumes of media (see below) are necessary to dilute the inhibitory substances such as lysozyme, antibodies and other bacteria. The most commonly used media is EMJH with and without the selective agent 5-fluorouracil.[43] 5-fluorouracil (5-FU) was found to be lethal to most microorganisms but surprisingly not to leptospires at concentrations of 200–400 μg/ml. The addition of agar at 0.1–0.2% enhances the isolation rate as does increased rabbit serum of 2%.[44]

Direct microscopy of the biological fluid by dark-ground microscopy may be difficult and will certainly lead to false-positive results due to proteinaceous artefacts of red blood cell membranes that can easily be mistaken for true leptospirosis. Culture and serological diagnosis must be attempted.

Animal inoculation

Inoculation of suspect biological fluids may be undertaken. Young hamsters and guinea-pigs may be inoculated intraperitoneally and observed for clinical symptoms of infection. Blood and kidneys are then inoculated as described above.[20] This method of diagnosis should only be attempted by experienced laboratory workers; many reported cases of leptospirosis have found their way into medical publications because inexperienced operators have mistaken pseudoleptospires for the true organisms.

TREATMENT

The primary aim in clinical management of leptospirosis is to prevent the organisms from invading the tissues, particularly the kidneys. The principles of treatment are the same irrespective of the infecting serogroup, namely early administration of antibiotics, maintenance of water and electrolyte balance and supporting renal and cardiac function.

In man, the place of antibiotic treatment for classical Weil's syndrome caused by the serogroup icterohaemorrhagiae is still contentious. High doses of penicillin at least 6–7.2 g per day should be given within 4 days from the start of the fever; if the patient is seriously ill then higher doses of 10 g per day have been recommended.[18] On the other hand studies by Hall and his colleagues in 1951 and Fairbain and Semple 1956, showed that there was no benefit gained from using penicillin treatment.[45,46] Despite the uncertainty and until there is definite medical evidence against treatment, clinicians should be recommended to start parenteral penicillin as soon as possible. Alternatively, if the patient is hypersensitive to penicillin then tetracycline at an initial dose of 500 mg followed by 250 mg 8-hourly intravenously for 24 hours and then 500 mg, 6-hourly for 10 days may be used or erythromycin 500 mg initially and followed by 250 mg 6-hourly for 10 days.

Pre-exposure prophylaxis of doxycycline (200 mg on a weekly basis) may be given to soldiers and others on short-term jungle exposure.[47] It must be emphasized that although doxycycline is an excellent *pre-exposure* treatment, patients suspected of leptospirosis *post-exposure* should always be treated as a case of leptospirosis and full antibiotic therapy undertaken.

EPIDEMIOLOGY

The natural reservoir of *Leptospira* is wild animals, particularly the rodent family. Domestic animals such as farm livestock and dogs may also become infected, either indirectly by contact with infected urine from maintenance host reservoirs, or directly with leptospiral serogroups specific for their own species; for example, sejroe serovar hardjo affects cows and var. canicola, dogs (Fig. 32.9).

Occupations at special risk are people working in moist environments such as sewermen, abattoir workers, farmers, rice-field workers, sugar-cane planters and cutters, miners, water and ditch workers. Any environment which is moist and is rat infested is a special risk area. Control of leptospirosis depends on control of the rodent population. Other occupations such as those workers in the veterinary or farming industry with livestock such as cattle, pigs, sheep and others, e.g. dogs, are also at risk. In Great Britain the epidemiology of leptospirosis has changed from the predominating serogroup of ictero-haemorrhagiae to the cattle-associated form known as hardjo. Knowledge of the changing epidemiological patterns must remain a priority in the control of leptospirosis.

In tropical countries the prevalence of leptospirosis is closely associated with contact with wildlife. The predominant infecting serogroups found in the wildlife population reflects the type

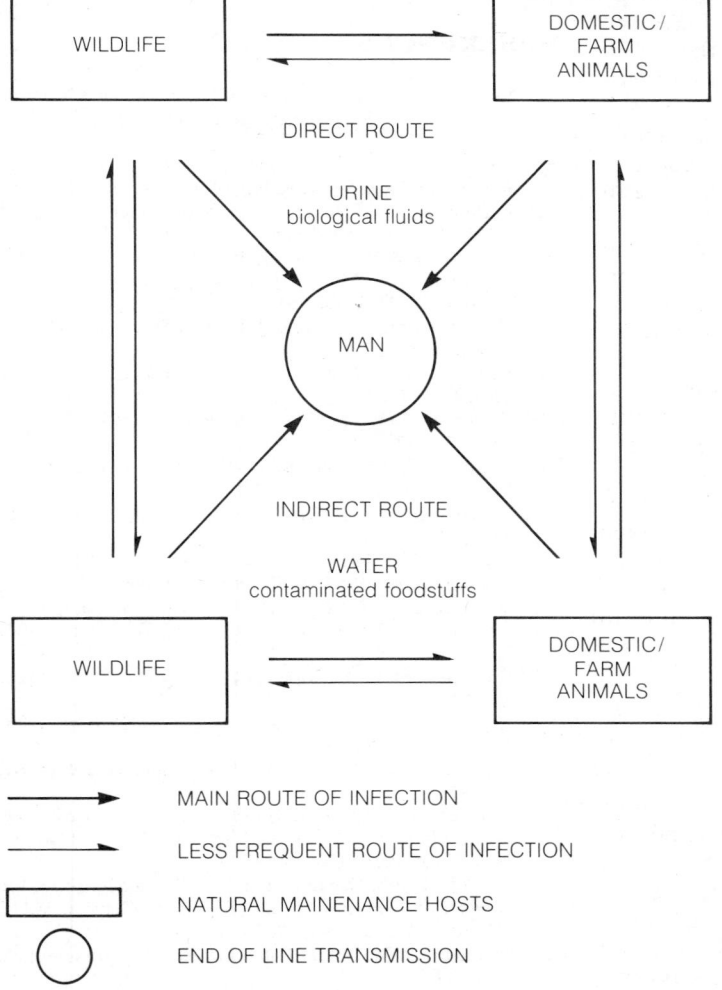

Fig. 32.9 Natural reservoirs of leptospires and their transmission routes to man.

of leptospirosis seen in the human population. This in turn determines the severity of the human clinical presentation.

ECONOMIC ASPECTS

It is probable that leptospirosis is the most widespread zoonosis in the world.[48] It is geographically widespread throughout the world producing a wide range of clinical manifestations of varying severity which is undoubtedly underdiagnosed. In countries such as Australia, where extensive studies have been undertaken, it is estimated that one in every four meat inspectors is likely to acquire leptospirosis in a working life of 30 years.[49] In 1980, Little and his colleagues estimated that about 10% of bovine abortions in the south-west of England were due to leptospirosis,[50] whereas in 1954, in the USA the government estimated that more than 100 million dollars was lost annually because of leptospirosis.[51] These estimates are based on the developed temperate countries: the economic problem facing the emerging tropical countries must be much worse. In 1959 the World Health Organization noted that bovine leptospirosis was a major disease rivalling brucellosis in certain countries.[52] Today both human and animal leptospirosis is still a worldwide problem and the incidence and prevalence of leptospirosis in tropical countries is still high, Everard and his colleagues have shown that leptospirosis is one of the major infectious diseases found in the south-eastern Caribbean and is still underdiagnosed.[53]

Zoonotic diseases have direct consequences for national economic development. Leptospirosis reduces the available supply of much needed protein due to death of livestock and additional expenses incurred in both veterinary care of the animal and medical costs and loss of earnings in the human.

PREVENTION

Leptospirosis is a notifiable disease in most developed countries and adequate guidelines for its control have been drawn up by the World Health Organization.[20] In man prophylactic measures against leptospirosis include general awareness of the risks involved, particularly to those working in high risk occupations and environmental conditions, personal hygiene and proper rodent control.

Chemical treatment of domestic water supplies with, for example, chlorine or filtration should be an adequate measure. Environmental conditions are more difficult to control and the source of leptospirosis, the wildlife and farm livestock, should be controlled. Vaccination of domestic animals has been long recommended and is successful[20] but human vaccination is less successful and more contentious.

Since leptospirosis is a classical zoonosis, educational programmes must involve veterinary, medical, public health and wildlife control programme personnel. Farmers, water workers and those with direct contact with animals or infected water have to be warned of the potential dangers of contracting leptospirosis.

REFERENCES

1   Wilson, G. S. & Miles, A. A. (1964) *Topley and Wilson's Principles of Bacteriology and Immunity.* London: Arnold.
2   Felsenfeld, O. (1965) *Bact. Rev.* **29,** 46.
3   Felsenfeld, O. & Wolf, R. H. (1969) *Acta trop.* **26,** 156.
4   Felsenfeld, O., Decker, W. J., Wohlhieter, J. A. et al (1965) *J. Immunol.* **94,** 805.
5   Chen, J. H. & Wu, Y. K. (1946) *Chin. med. J.* **64,** 309.
6   Bryceson, A. D. M., Parry, E. H. O., Perine, P. L. et al (1970) *Q. Jl Med.* **39,** 129.
7   Wolstenholme, B. & Gear, J. H. S. (1948) *Trans. R. Soc. trop. Med. Hyg.* **41,** 513.
8   Salih, S. Y. & Mustafa, D. (1977) *Trans. R. Soc. trop. Med. Hyg.* **71,** 49.
9   Butler, T., Jones, P. K. & Wallace, C. K. (1978) *J. infect. Dis.* **137,** 573.
10 Teklu, B., Habt-Michael, A., Warrell, D. A. et al (1983). *Lancet* i, 835–839.
11 Eisenberg, S., Gunders, A. E. & Cohen, A. M. (1968) *Trans. R. Soc. trop. Med. Hyg.* **62,** 679.
12 Coghill, N. F. (1949) *J. R. Army med. Corps.* **93,** 2.
13 Walton, G. A. (1957) *Bull. ent. Res.* **42,** 669.
14 Walton, G. A. (1961) *Symp. zool. Soc. Lond.* **6,** 83.
15 Shanson, D. G., Midgley, J., Gazzard, B. C. et al (1983) *Lancet* ii, 92–94.
16 Sprecher, M. H. & Copeland, J. R. (1947) *J. Am. med. Ass.* **134,** 1014.
17 Brown, T. M. & Nunemaker, J. C. (1942) *Bull. Johns Hopkins Hosp.* **70,** 201.
18 Turner, L. H. (1967) *Trans. R. Soc. trop. Med. Hyg.* **61,** 842–855.
19 Turner, L. H. (1968) In *Some Diseases of Animals Communicable to Man in Britain,* pp. 231–245. Oxford and New York: Pergamon Press.
20 World Health Organization (1982) *Guidelines for the Control of Leptospirosis,* ed. S. Faine. Geneva, WHO Offset publication No. 67, 1–169.
21 Stimson, A. M. (1907) *Pub. Hlth Rep. (Washington)* **22,** 541–549.

22 Noguchi, H. (1918) *J. exp. Med.* **27**, 575–592.
23 Waitkins, S. A. (1983) *Lab. Technol.* **17**, 178–184.
24 Waitkins, S. A. (1985) In *Isolation and Identification of Micro-organisms of Medical and Veterinary Importance*, ed. C. H. Collins & H. G. Grange, pp. 251–274. Society for Applied Bacteriology.
25 Fletcher, W. (1928) *Trans. R. Soc. trop. Med. Hyg.* **21**, 265–287.
26 Korthof, G. (1932) *Zentralbl. Bakteriol. Parasitol. Abt. 1. Orig.* **125**, 429–434.
27 Alston, J. M. & Broom, J. C. (1958) *Leptospirosis in Man animals.* London: Livingstone.
28 Babudieri, B. (1961) Laboratory diagnosis of leptospirosis. *Bull. Wld Hlth Org.* **24**, 45–58.
29 Stuart, R. D. (1946) *J. Path. Bact.* **58**, 343–349.
30 Ellinghausen, H. C. & McCullough, W. G. (1965) *Am. J. Vet. Res.* **26**, 45–51.
31 Johnson, R. C. & Harris, V. G. (1967) *J. Bacteriol.* **94**, 27–31.
32 Wolff, J. W. & Broom, J. C. (1954) *Doc. Med. Geogr. Trop.* **6**, 78–84.
33 Kmety, E., Galton, M. M. & Sulzer, C. R. (1970) Further standardization of the agglutinin absorption test in the serology of leptospires. *Bull. Wld Hlth Org.* **42**, 733–745.
34 Kmety, E. (1970) *Ann. Soc. Belg. Med. Trop.* **46**, 103–108.
35 Ono, E., Naiki, M. & Yanagawa, R. (1982) *Zentralbl. Bakteriol. Mikrobiol. Hyg.* **252**, 414–424.
36 Terpstra, W. J., Korver, H., van Leeuwem, J. et al (1985) *Zentralbl. Bakteriol. Mikrobiol. Hyg.* **259**, 498–506.
37 Robinson, A. J., Ramadass, P., Alison, L. et al (1982) *J. med. Microbiol.* **15**, 331–338.
38 Hookey, J. V., Waitkins, S. A. & Jackman, P. J. H. (1985) Numerical analysis of *Leptospira* DNA-restriction endonuclease patterns. *FEMS Microbiol. Lett.* **29**, 185–188.
39 Corza, D. (1956) *Clin. Med.* **37**, 1295–1297.
40 Sherlock, S. (1981) *Disease of the Liver and Biliary System*, 6th edn. Oxford: Blackwell Scientific Publications.
41 Turner, L. H. (1968) *Trans. R. Soc. trop. Med. Hyg.* **62**, 880–899.
42 Terpstra, W. J., Lighart, G. S. & Schoone, G. J. (1980) *Zentralbl. Bakteriol. Mikrobiol. Hyg.* **A247**, 400–405.
43 Johnson, R. C. & Rogers, R. (1964) *J. Bacteriol.* **87**, 422–426.
44 Turner, L. H. (1970) *Trans. R. Soc. trop. Med. Hyg.* **64**, 623–646.
45 Hall, H. E., Hightower, J. A., Rivera, D. et al (1951) Evaluation of antibiotic therapy in human leptospirosis. *Annals of Internal Medicine* **35**, 981–988.
46 Fairburn, A. C. & Semple, S. J. G. (1956) *Lancet* **1**, 13–16.
47 Takafuji, E. G., Kirkpatrick, J. W., Miller, R. N. et al (1984) *New Engl. J. Med.* **310**, 497–500.
48 Van der Hoeden, J. (1964) In *Zoonoses*, pp. 241–274. Amsterdam: Elsevier.
49 Faine, S. (1983) *Med. J. Austral.* **1**, 445–446.
50 Little, T. W. A., Richards, M. S., Hussaini, S. M. et al (1980) *Vet. Rec.* **106**, 221–224.
51 United States Department of Agriculture (USDA) (1954) *Losses in Agriculture*, Agriculture Research Services, Washington.
52 World Health Organization (1959) *WHO tech. Rep. ser.* **169**.
53 Everard, C. D. R., Fraser-Champong, G. M., Bhagwardin, L. J. et al (1979) *Trans. R. Soc. trop. Med. Hyg.* **73**, 303–305.

SECTION VI
DISEASES CAUSED BY FUNGI

Chapter 33
Superficial Mycoses
John H. S. Pettit

INTRODUCTION

Tinea in the tropics

There are many thousand different fungi living in the world ranging from moulds to mushrooms but less than 100 are known to cause disease in man.[1] The spores of these fungi not infrequently get on to the epidermis and establish themselves there, particularly if they belong to the limited group which can exist on keratin.[2] Other fungi, not keratinophilic or keratolytic, can grow in the dermis, usually as a result of a penetrating wound, and a few others exist in the deeper parts of the body (see Chapters 34 and 35).[3,4]

People living in the warmer and moister parts of the world are more prone to superficial epidermal infections because the increased humidity combined with increased perspiration softens the keratin and thereby renders it more susceptible to invasion.

Causes

The epidermal mycoses can be divided into three subsections (Table 33.1), the largest of which, dermatophyte infections, produce lesions usually called 'tinea' or 'ringworm'. Other subsections compose a few yeast-like infections (*Candida* and *Pityrosporon*) and some other fungi and pseudo-fungi whose classification is often somewhat uncertain which produce abnormalities such as trichomycosis and piedra.

Dermatophytes are a subgroup of the Ascomycetes and produce a wide range of clinical appearances according to the part which is infected. Most dermatophytes belong to the genus *Trichophyton*: they affect the skin and nails in both of which they exist predominantly in their hyphal state but, when they invade hair, they produce spores either inside the hair-shaft (endothrix infection) or clustered around the outside (ectothrix infection).

Other dermatophytes from the genus *Microsporum* usually affect hair and can be recognized by the presence of small-spored ectothrix.

Lastly, there is a single member of the genus *Epidermophyton* which has never been known to affect hairs.

Recognition of a fungus

Although the various forms of tinea can often be suspected clinically the diagnosis should always be confirmed microscopically. The spreading edge of a ringworm lesion should be moistened by a drop of 10% potassium hydroxide, the skin is then scraped with a small curette or a blunt scalpel and the epidermal debris mounted in a further drop of potassium hydroxide and covered

Table 33.1 Organisms causing chronic superficial mycoses.

	Species	Site of infection
Dermatophytes		
	Trichophyton	May affect skin, hair or nails
	Microsporum	Usually hairs, rarely skin or nails
	Epidermophyton	Always on skin, never affects nails
Yeast infections		
	Candida albicans	Skin, nails, mucosae (not hairs)
	Pityrosporon orbiculare (also known as *P. ovale*)	Limited to the skin
Other fungi or pseudofungi		
	Corynebacterium tenuis	Axillary hairs, sometimes pubic hairs
	Piedraia hortai	Scalp hairs
	Trichosporon beigelii	Usually the beard
	Exophiala werneckii	Usually the palm or sole

with a coverslip. In a few minutes the keratin of the epidermal cells will be clear and examination under the high dry (× 40) objective of a microscope will permit recognition of the fungal elements. Inexperienced workers sometimes confuse the intercellular spaces with hyphae but, as a fungus grows directly *through* the epidermal cells and not round them, only a little experience is necessary to be able to recognize the presence of an active infection. Some mycologists prefer to add 1% methylene blue or a drop of ink such as Parker's 'Quink' to the potassium hydroxide solution making the hyphae more easily visible (Appendix IV, p. 1499).

If it is suspected that hairs are involved they can be removed manually and mounted in the potassium hydroxide solution.

The combination of clinical and microscopic findings is usually enough to confirm the presence of ringworm infection but sometimes Wood's light (an ultraviolet light filtered through cobalt-nickel glass) may clarify the diagnosis as some affected hairs fluoresce a green or yellow colour. It must be remembered that a negative finding does not disprove the presence of a fungal infection and also that not all fluorescent dermatoses are caused by fungi.

Principles of treatment

The ointment originally developed by Whitfield consists of 6% benzoic acid and 3% salicylic acid in unguentum emulsificans and this is still of great value, particularly for clinicians working in less affluent communities. If applied twice daily until two weeks after the clinical clearance of the infection this ointment will cure most cases. For moister lesions, e.g. those in the groin or between the toes, Castellani's paint (Magenta Paint *BPC*, Carbol-Fuchsin *USP*) can be used twice a day until the lesion has dried up and then Whitfield's ointment can be used to complete the cure.

The many proprietary fungicides on the market, particularly imidazoles such as clotrimazole, miconazole, econazole and tioconazole,[5] can all be used effectively provided the treatment is not stopped too soon. None of these is markedly superior to the others.

The development of griseofulvin completely revolutionized the treatment of ringworm. Clean, not too expensive and relatively free from side-effects, if given by mouth it is absorbed from the gut and selectively concentrated into keratin and, as the stratum corneum and the hair grow outwards, infections are in effect pushed off the surface of the patient. Dosage (see Table 33.2) has to be modified according to the age/weight of the patient—it is almost never necessary to give griseofulvin to children under three years of age.

Table 33.2 Dosage schedule for fine particle griseofulvin.

Under five years	125 mg daily
5–10 years	250 mg daily
10–15 years	375 mg daily
Over 15 years	500 mg daily

Never less than 4 weeks' therapy
Six months for fingernails
One year for toenails

DERMATOPHYTE INFECTIONS

Tinea capitis

This condition is almost entirely limited to children. It is often called ringworm of the scalp but in actual fact most cases of tinea capitis affect the hair more than the scalp. Spores, either airborne or acquired by sharing infected head-gear, penetrate hairs at scalp level; the hyphae grow along the hair in both directions producing spores either inside or outside the shaft. These spores spread to the neighbouring hairs and extending bald patches develop in which the hairs, having become deformed and lustreless, break off some 5 mm above the scalp. As the patches extend the hairless areas are seen to be slightly erythematous and scaly (Plate VI.5).

Twenty or thirty years ago tinea capitis was usually caused by a microsporum infection, either *M. canis* acquired from infected animals or *M. audouini* which spread from child to child. More recently *Trichophyton mentagrophytes* and *T. rubrum* seem to have become major causes of tinea capitis in several parts of the world, these fungi producing a rather more angry looking bald patch while other trichophyton infections, *T. violaceum*[6,7] and *T. tonsurans*,[8] produce large-spored endothrix which distend the hairs to such an extent that they break off at scalp level and the only part of the shaft that shows is seen to fill the mouth of the hair follicle. This is called 'black-dot' ringworm.

All these infections have a tendency to spontaneous improvement at puberty but it is unwise to postpone therapy in the expectation of a natural cure, as not infrequently the picture is complicated by an unpleasant condition known as kerion (Plate VI.6), in which a secondary infection is established at the roots of the affected hairs causing a warm boggy swelling which completely destroys the infected follicles to leave permanent patches of scarred alopecia.

The differential diagnosis should be simple although the uninitiated may be confused by the exclamation-mark hairs found in the actively spreading edge of alopecia areata patches, but these never contain spores or hyphae. In other forms of alopecia the diagnosis is simple. Telogen effluvium is diffuse and shows no broken hairs, and conditions like lupus erythematosus, lichen planopilaris and secondary syphilis occur in a later age group and with their own diagnostic signs.

Examination of affected hairs may suggest which dermatophyte is involved but, if further investigations are required, these fungi can easily be cultured on Sabouraud's glucose agar to produce diagnostic coloured colonies showing subtle differences of micro- and macroconidia which delight the mycologist but rarely assist the clinician.

TREATMENT

All ringworm of the scalp responds to treatment. It should not be treated with antifungal ointments nor, since the advent of griseofulvin, is it any longer necessary to use X-irradiation or poisons such as thallium acetate to produce a therapeutic epilation of the scalp. Griseofulvin is the recommended therapy. It is necessary at the same time to ensure that the scalp is shaved as otherwise viable spores remain in the longer hairs and if griseofulvin is stopped after only one months' treatment such spores from the terminal parts of the hairs will soon reinfect the scalp. The treatment routine is:

day 1:   shave head and start griseofulvin;
day 25:   shave head again;
day 31:   stop griseofulvin.

If possible the head should be examined under Wood's light at day 42 (after the hairs have reappeared on the scalp) and if the patient has been infected by a form of fungus which fluoresces it will be possible in a suitably darkened room to see if any infected hairs remain. If found they can be removed manually.

SPECIAL CASE—FAVUS

A fungus known as *T. schoenleinii* breaks many of the rules that have been outlined above. It occurs particularly frequently in the Middle East and along the Mediterranean littoral. Not only are the hairs and scalp equally infected but it is also the one form of ringworm of the scalp which does not resolve spontaneously at puberty. This disease is known as 'favus' and the affected hairs fluoresce a dull greyish-green colour under Wood's light; patients are often found with fluorescent hairs 15, 20 or more centimetres long which are full of fungus but have not broken. The infection spreads back down the hair root which is consequently destroyed and as the years go by an extensive cicatricial alopecia develops. If the patient remains untreated saucer-shaped yellow crusts containing a profuse growth of fungus can be seen adhering to the scalp—they are known as scutula (Fig. 33.1).

Microscopically, and again unusually, not only are there chains of large-spored endothrix but they are interspersed with numerous air bubbles in the shaft. These gaps are diagnostic of favus.

If the routine treatment for tinea capitis is carried out in detail patients can be cured with one month's treatment. It must be remembered that untreated the condition carries on into adult life.

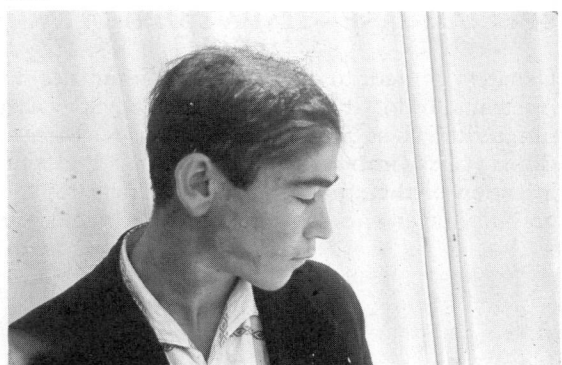

Fig. 33.1 Favus. Extensive hair loss and scaliness on the vertex of the scalp. Hair loss will be permanent.

Tinea corporis (tinea circinata)

When spores of the dermatophytes penetrate the skin of the trunk or limbs the hyphae grow in all directions; those which penetrate through the granular layer cause a vesicular or inflammatory reaction but those growing less deeply will spread centrifugally to produce a clinical picture which, starting with a small itching papule, enlarges peripherally and clears in the centre to produce an annular lesion with a rather scaly centre and an advancing edge of vesicles and papules (Plate VII.1). Often such lesions coalesce to produce serpiginous plaques.

It is usually easy to suspect the diagnosis as other vesicular conditions (discoid eczema, dermatitis herpetiformis or palmoplantar pustulosis) do not have vesicles limited to the periphery. If a microsporum has infected the skin any hairs in the patch will be fluorescent but with trichophyton infections hairs are not usually affected. The diagnosis can be confirmed by finding fungus in the skin scrapings from the peripheral vesicles and by growing it on Sabouraud's medium.

TREATMENT

Small lesions can be satisfactorily treated with Whitfield's ointment or Castellani's paint or by an imidazole cream but patients in warmer climates do not appreciate the use of ointments in large areas, and it is recommended that such cases should be treated with griseofulvin for 28 days.

SPECIAL CASE—TINEA IMBRICATA

Usually limited to aborigine communities in Australia, Indo-China, Indonesia and Malaysia a fungus known as *T. concentricum* causes a disease called tinea imbricata. This very superficial infection of the epidermis rarely penetrates the granular layer and consequently the lesions are not vesicular. They start as small papules which extend centrifugally to produce rosettes of concentric scaly rings which, coalescing, cover large areas of skin that slowly becomes somewhat hypochromic (Fig. 33.2). These lesions may affect the face, the palms and the soles but do not penetrate on to the scalp or into the hair.

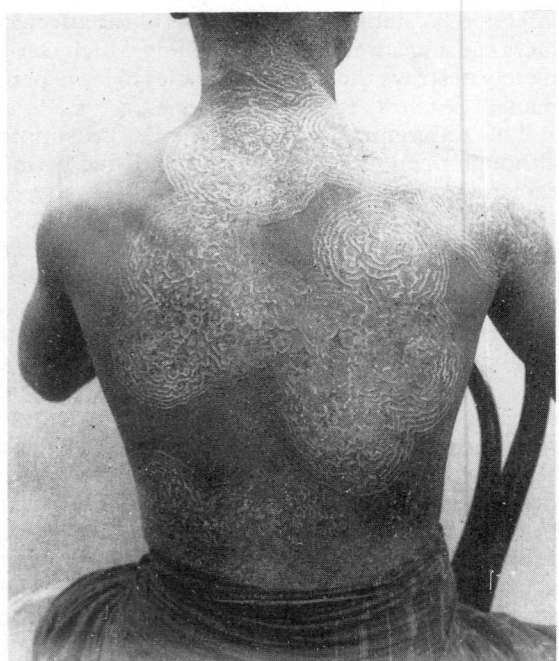

Fig. 33.2   Tinea imbricata. Concentric rings of superficial scaliness in a Malay aborigine.

The treatment recommended for other forms of tinea corporis will be rapidly effective but, unfortunately, the condition often relapses equally quickly; persistence, however, pays off and the condition is much less common than it used to be before griseofulvin was used. The aborigines in Malaysia think that a paint based on Whitfield's formula (5% salicylic acid and 5% benzoic acid in methylated spirits) is equally effective.

Tinea cruris

It seems to have become traditional to discuss ringworm of the groin separately from tinea of the body but this is only necessary because tinea cruris looks somewhat different from the annular lesions of tinea corporis. The vesicular edged lesion will spread outwards down and across the thigh but the same patch extending in the opposite direction seems to falter and die off when it reaches the pubic hair or the genitalia and produces an arciform rather than an annular lesion (Plate VII.2). The condition should not be confused with seborrhoeic dermatitis of the groin, which has a diffuse ill-defined margin and is usually associated with other signs on the scalp, the eyebrows and nasolabial folds. *Candida* of the groin looks quite different as its lesions classically have a peripherally attached collarette of scaling.

The most common causes of tinea cruris are *Epidermophyton floccosum*, *T. mentagrophytes* and *T. rubrum*. Perspiration, diabetes and friction from 'jockey'-type nylon underwear are all said to be predisposing factors but most probably the commonest way for a fungus to affect the groin is for it to be spread with a towel by a patient who also has athlete's foot.

The diagnosis can be easily confirmed by the demonstration of hyphae in suitable skin scra-pings and the treatment is the same as that for tinea corporis.

SPECIAL CASE—ERYTHRASMA

Another condition which affects the groins is this mild, scaly, reddish-brown discoloration which is neither vesicular nor does it have the well-demarcated extending edge typical of tinea. Originally believed to be due to a fungus infec-tion the causative organism has now been recog-nized as *Corynebacterium minutissimum*.

The affected areas fluoresce pink under Wood's light and respond well to oral erythro-mycin 250 mg four times a day for two weeks. The erythromycin lotion recently marketed for acne vulgaris is often quicker and cheaper than systemic treatment, while if both of these prove to be too expensive other antibiotic creams such as tetracycline or nitrofurazone can be tried.

Tinea pedis

Fungi affect the feet rather more often than they affect the hands producing different lesions depending on the site of infection: the dorsum of the foot, the sole or the interdigital spaces. Infection of the dorsum of the foot looks like any other form of tinea corporis being more or less annular spreading peripherally. If the infection is on the sole the considerable thickness of the stratum corneum will modify the presentation and pruritic vesicles or pustules will be embed-ded in the keratin layer. In such cases skin scra-pings are often unsuccessful and, if the organisms also fail to grow in Sabouraud's medium, it may be necessary to treat suspected cases with gri-seofulvin for a few weeks in a therapeutic trial.

The differential diagnosis is often a problem—persistent palmoplantar pustulosis, pustular pso-riasis or podopompholyx may present diagnostic challenges but these patients often have a longer history and bilateral lesions.

SPECIAL CASE—ATHLETE'S FOOT

Large numbers of the world's population have chronic fissured and scaly lesions of the toe-webs. Miners, soldiers and sportsmen are particularly prone to this condition, all complaining of itching soggy skin between the fourth and fifth toes (Fig. 33.3). Although sometimes called tinea interdigitale, athlete's foot is not due to a single infection; often scrapings and cultures show the presence of dermatophytes coexisting with *Candida* while erythrasma organisms are often present. It is best to consider these symptoms

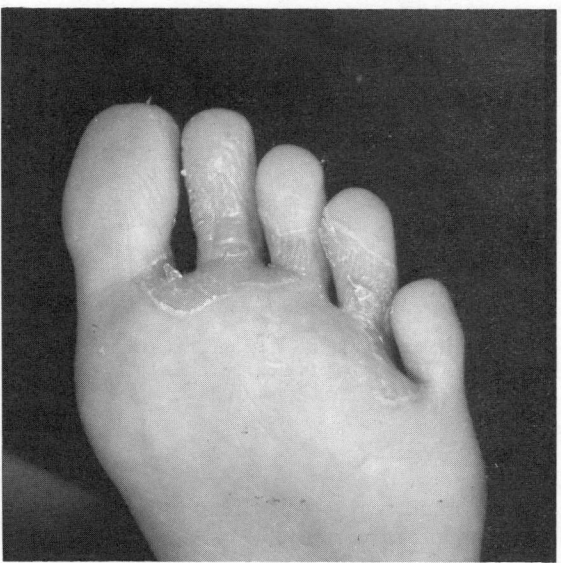

Fig. 33.3 Athlete's foot. Pruritic scaling and fissuring between the toes.

to be due to multiple infections and although griseofulvin may be administered in the usual dose for the usual period it is often not particularly successful. Recently ketoconazole has been more useful but it is now considered the side-effects are too dangerous to justify the use of this drug in such a mild disease.

More effective than systemic treatment is

Whitfield's ointment rubbed between the toes every day for several weeks, the toes being separated with large pledgets of cotton wool. If the condition is acute and moist twice daily applications of Castellani's paint to the whole of the forefoot will be effective. The proprietary antimycotics do not help to rid the toes of *Candida* or erythrasma organisms.

Tinea unguium

Spores not infrequently penetrate the nails on fingers or toes; the infection usually starting under the free edge of the nails growing in the subungual debris and later invading the undersurface of the nail plate. It slowly grows down towards the nail matrix and up through the plate producing first a yellow discoloration under the nail edge and finally a rough, ragged, distorted and broken nail (Fig. 33.4). Clinically, this is almost indistinguishable from subungual psoriasis but clippings or scrapings from the undersurface of the nail may contain hyphae. The commonest organisms that affect the nails are *E. floccosum, T. rubrum* and *T. mentagrophytes* and even the favus organism can sometimes be found. Attempts to culture these organisms from nail clippings are often disappointing.

at least six months' oral therapy with griseofulvin and toenails from 12 to 15 months. In an attempt to reduce the cost and duration of this treatment some dermatologists recommend avulsion of affected nails after a few weeks' systemic treatment but most patients reject this suggestion. If avulsion is permitted griseofulvin need only be given for a further three months if at the same time the nail bed is treated with an imidazole ointment or lotion.

A new technique for the chemical removal of psoriatic nails has recently been adapted for tinea unguium.[9] The following ointment:

urea	40%
anhydrous lanoline	20%
white wax	5%
white petrolatum	35%

is applied to the affected nails, carefully avoiding the surrounding skin; after two weeks the softened nail is painlessly scraped away and miconazole cream or lotion is applied to the nail bed.

SPECIAL CASE—SUPERFICIAL NAIL INFECTION

Sometimes a dermatophyte manages to establish

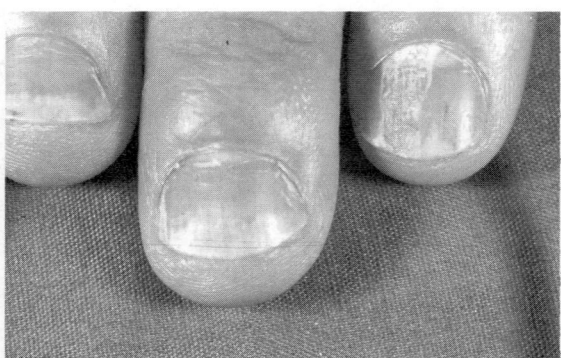

Fig. 33.4   Tinea unguium. The infection is under the nails giving a yellow discoloration easily confused with subungual psoriasis.

TREATMENT

There is no reason to believe that treatment of ringworm of the nail will be rapidly successful. The slow growth of the fingernails and even slower growth of the toenails means that effective treatment will be prolonged; fingernails will need

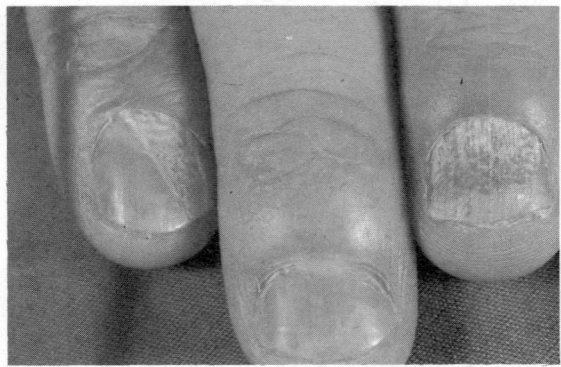

Fig. 33.5   Tinea unguium. Superficial damage to the surface of the nails due to fungal infection of the nail matrix.

itself either in the cuticle or under a paronychial fold in which case it will ultimately involve the dorsal surface of the nail. As it grows out a roughened surface extends distally; lateral spread proves that the infection is slowly spreading along the nail base (Fig. 33.5).

Systemic therapy is not needed: an alcoholic solution of an imidazole should be applied twice daily under the nail fold and to the dorsum of the nail.

YEAST INFECTIONS OF THE SKIN

Yeasts are a group of microorganisms which are neither well-defined nor homogeneous.[10] Several of these (including *Cryptococcus* and *Torulopsis*) are known to grow on the skin but the only two forms to be considered here are the *Candida* species and that organism which has been given various names in the past but is now usually called *Pityrosporon orbiculare*.

Candidal infections

C. albicans is an opportunistic organism growing only when local conditions are favourable; it not infrequently affects patients in temperate climates but is even more widely recognized in the tropics. Most commonly it invades the skin and the nails but it also affects the mucosae (particularly the mouth and the vulva) and may even become established in the alimentary tract and the lungs. *Candida* organisms grow extremely rapidly on Sabouraud's glucose agar producing small moist-looking creamy-white colonies containing spherical vegetative cells which may be budding and among which numbers of germ tubes are found. Sometimes these are produced in such amounts they produce pseudomycelia. Many candidal species have been named (*C. tropicalis*, *C. parapsilosis*, etc.) and there is considerable debate as to whether these actually produce the skin lesions in which they are occasionally found, but it is not believed that they play any great part in the pathogenesis of superficial infections of the skin.

C. albicans is usually considered to be a normal resident of the alimentary tract and will grow profusely from swabs taken from the mouth, stool or vagina. In the tropics the organism may be detected in superficial infections of the skin (infected eczema, infected scabies, etc.) but in such cases it is not considered to be a pathogen. It may be difficult to determine whether these organisms have caused the dermatosis in which they are living and sometimes it is necessary to carry out a therapeutic trial to see if anti-candidal therapy alleviates the signs and symptoms.

There are, however, a number of lesions with a classical appearance in which *Candida* is not only to be found but also to be blamed as the causative agent. These lesions are usually in flexures, particularly the groins and interdigital spaces. They classically present as a moist erythematous intertrigo with superficial erosions surrounded by a delicate, peripherally attached, bluish-white scale; if the initial lesions are on the trunk or the groin they are often surrounded by small erythematous satellite pustules.

CANDIDA IN CHILDREN

The most common infection in children is probably the form of mucosal candidiasis known as 'thrush'—well-defined, soft, milky-looking patches may grow on any part of the mouth (tongue, tonsil, palate etc.). These patches rarely ulcerate and can often be scraped off with a wooden spatula. While thrush is common and relatively unimportant in infants, if it affects older children or adults it may be a warning that the patient has some form of immunological incompetence.

The organisms produce little or no sign of trouble when they live in the gastrointestinal tract but, particularly if the child is on oral antibiotics, *Candida* may spread from the anus to the perineum from whence it can invade or even cause a napkin rash (Fig. 33.6).[11]

In those less sophisticated parts of the world in which sweetened condensed milk plays an unfortunately large role in nutrition, many infants develop obesity with deep folds in the skin which are not related to flexures. If *Candida* organisms invade these folds they produce sore

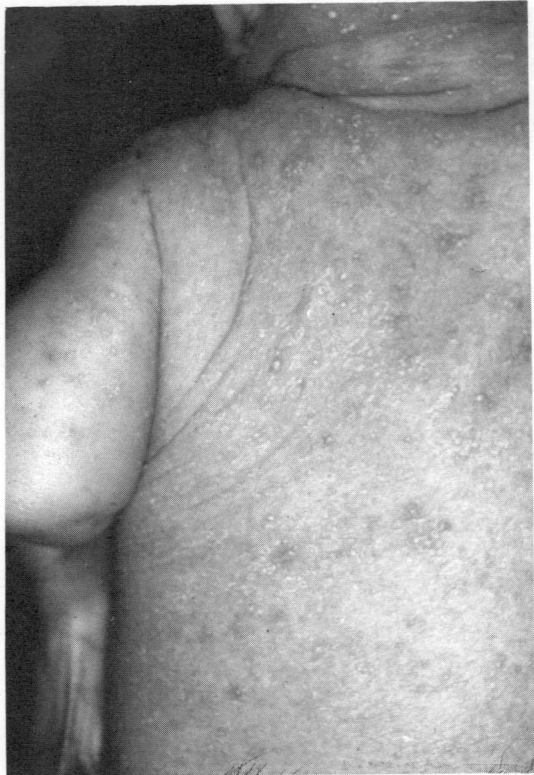

Fig. 33.6   Candidiasis. Extensive candidiasis (mainly folliculitis) in a baby.

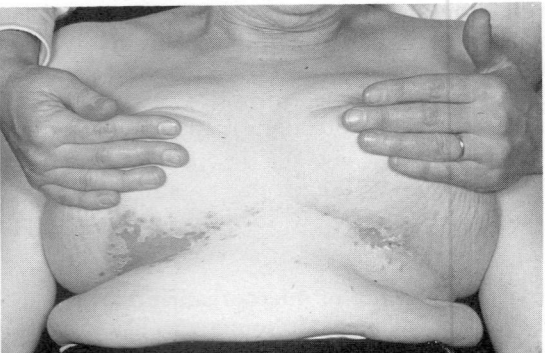

Fig. 33.7   Candidiasis. Erythematous sub-mammary erosions with a peripheral collarette of scaling.

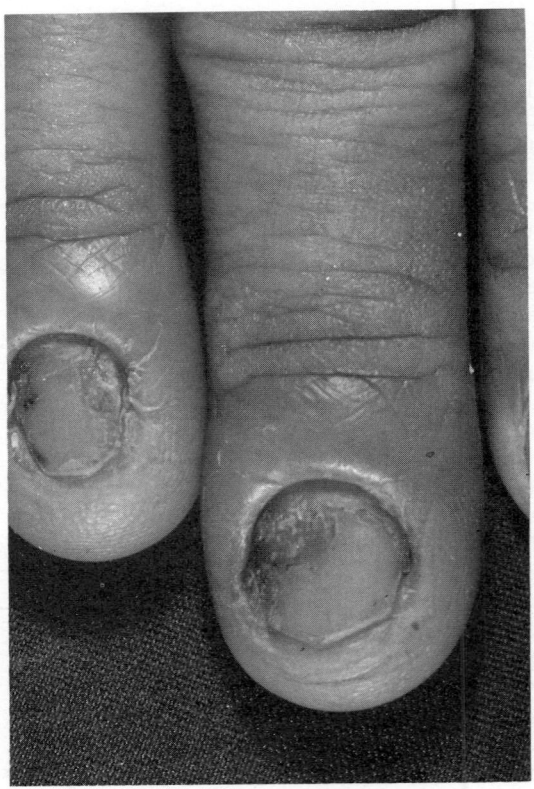

Fig. 33.8   Candidiasis. Extensive swollen paronychial infection has deformed nail growth.

red intertriginous areas with erosions showing the peripheral collarettes of scale; elsewhere the skin may be studded with pustules and vesicles.

CANDIDA IN ADULTS

In adults *Candida* usually affects the more obese and sweaty individuals (Fig. 33.7). In the warmer parts of the world, particularly in males, the inguinal region is often troubled by a sore moist erythema, not infrequently aggravated by the use of close-fitting nylon underwear. Women may develop a candidal vulvovaginitis while in uncircumcized males a candidal balanoposthitis may develop either spontaneously or as a conjugal infection.

More frequently seen in women is that form of swollen red bolstering which surrounds nail folds to give a paronychia (Fig. 33.8); it particularly affects mothers whose recent pregnancy has led to a considerable increase in wet work, laundry and child-bathing. The infection penetrates deeply under the nail folds and although gram-negative anaerobes are not infrequently also present it is usually held that *C. albicans* plays an important aetiological role in these infections. Affected mothers not infrequently transmit infection to their children.

TREATMENT

Candidal infections of the skin have for many years been treated with nystatin cream which is the drug of choice. Equally satisfactory is Castellani's paint, diluted for children to half or even quarter strength, although some people find its colour unacceptable. (Certain workers nowadays urge the use of a paint made with Castellani's formula but excluding the carbol-fuchsin; opinions vary as to its therapeutic value.) Local application of various imidazoles, particularly clotrimazole and miconazole, may also be used. Patients using any form of local treatment should be advised to apply it widely, at least 3 cm beyond the visible infection, to forestall the development of potential satellite lesions.

Nystatin lozenges can be sucked by patients whose infection is limited to the mouth and pharynx but as nystatin is not absorbed into the bloodstream oral medication will have no success in treating other than local infections of the gut. Infections of the rectum or of the female genitalia can be handled by nystatin pessaries nightly for two to four weeks. Recently imidazole pessaries have been shown to be rapidly effective; isoconazole or clotrimazole pessaries need be used for not more than 3 days.

Other anti-candidal drugs include amphotericin B, which is not absorbed from the gut but can be used locally for skin infections or intravenously for systemic manifestations, and flucytosine, a synthetic antifungal drug only active against yeasts, which can be used for systemic candidiasis as well as *Cryptococcus* and *Torulopsis* infections. It can be given by mouth as it is well absorbed from the gut (100–200 mg/kg daily in four divided doses).

Candidal paronychia needs a special routine. An orange stick that has been pared to a flat blade (*not* a point) can be used to insert Castellani's paint or miconazole lotion under the affected nail folds. This must be done twice daily for three to four weeks while the infected pockets slowly heal up from the bottom.

SPECIAL CASE—MUCOCUTANEOUS CANDIDIASIS

Both children and adults may suffer from immunological defects which permit a chronic candidiasis to be established both superficially and systemically.[12] Extensive candidal granulomas occur in the skin, mouth and the nails. Patients show signs of endocrine deficiency, immunological abnormalities, iron deficiency or other forms of severe ill-health and the combination of severe infection and immunological defect not infrequently leads to a fatal conclusion.

Active anti-candidal measures must be taken supplemented by oral iron therapy; flucytosine, amphotericin B and even ketoconazole should be used in severe cases. Individuals with a primary immune deficiency may need to be immunologically reconstituted.

Pityriasis versicolor

This condition is caused by a yeast-like organism which is not a dermatophyte and therefore the frequently used name 'tinea' versicolor is inappropriate and mentioned here only to be condemned. In the past the causative organism was often called *Malassezia furfur* but it is increasingly accepted that it is better known as *Pityrosporon orbiculare*.[13,14]

Superficial scaly patches are found most frequently on the trunk, the face and the proximal portions of both upper and lower limbs. They vary in size from 1–2 mm to many centimetres in diameter. In the initial stages of infection most patches are somewhat darkish in colour but later (especially in the more pigmented races) these areas become hypopigmented and it is often this change in colour that causes patients to seek treatment (Plate VII.3). Not infrequently these lesions are mildly pruritic but only rarely is this a presenting symptom. Dyschromic patches are not always scaly when the patient is first seen but if the skin is slightly stretched the scale becomes more visible.

The disease is often associated with hyperhidrosis and in Europe it has been said that patients on systemic corticosteroids or immunosuppressives tend to be more frequently affected, but most patients in the tropics do not have a detectable predisposing abnormality.

If a Wood's light is available it will cause the affected scales to fluoresce a yellowish-green in a darkened room; the use of this light is particularly valuable as fluorescence will often be seen in sites which are not visibly affected and this demonstration that the condition was more widespread than has been suspected will encourage a patient to agree to treating the whole body and not just the visible lesions. Wood's light is particularly useful in showing if an infection of the face has spread into the scalp.

Often Wood's light is not available but the Sellotape test can be carried out in even the most primitive conditions (Fig. 33.9); a 5 cm length of Sellotape (sometimes called Scotch tape) is applied over two or three small active lesions and rubbed firmly with the back of a fingernail. When it is removed superficial scales from the lesions will be found to have adhered to the tape in a pattern that exactly reproduces the clinical appearance. This precision of replication is not seen in tinea imbricata, ichthyosis, pityriasis alba or any other superficial scaly dermatosis and is of itself positive evidence of *P. orbiculare* infection. The diagnosis can be further confirmed if the scales are stained with a drop of 1% gentian violet for 1–2 minutes, then blotted and mounted on a microscope slide. Spores and hyphae are easily seen; in recent infections hyphae are predominant but if the condition has been present for many months there will be more grape-like clusters of spores and relatively few hyphae.

The differential diagnosis should present no difficulties; superficial psoriasis, pityriasis alba or an early vitiligo may be suspected but in these conditions both Wood's light and the Sellotape test will be negative.

TREATMENT

In the past decade therapy has become much easier. It used to be recommended that a 10% solution of sodium thiosulphate should be scrubbed with a toothbrush on to all visible lesions twice a day for several weeks. If carried out conscientiously this was successful but most patients simply got tired and gave up, so leading to the suspicion that *P. orbiculare* infection was less a disease than a symbiosis and that treatment was unlikely to be curative.

Nowadays selenium disulphide shampoo is recommended by most dermatologists although they disagree as to the frequency and the duration of treatment. Some workers think that the

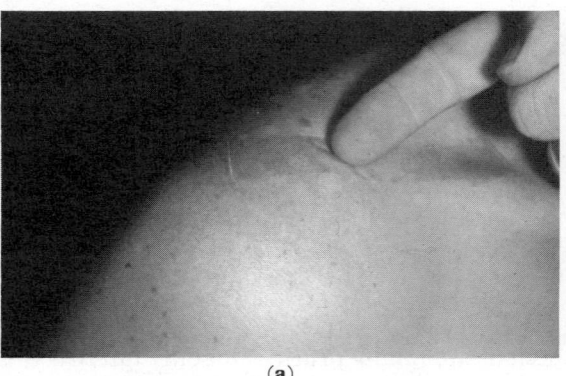

(a)

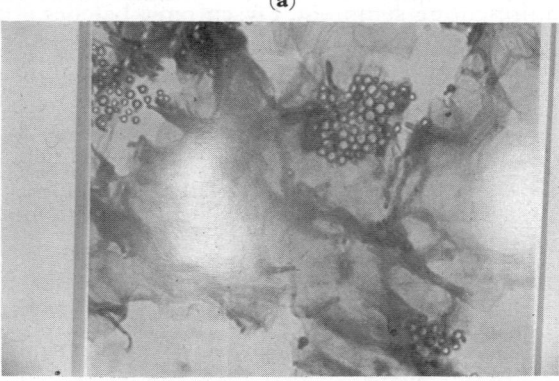

(c)

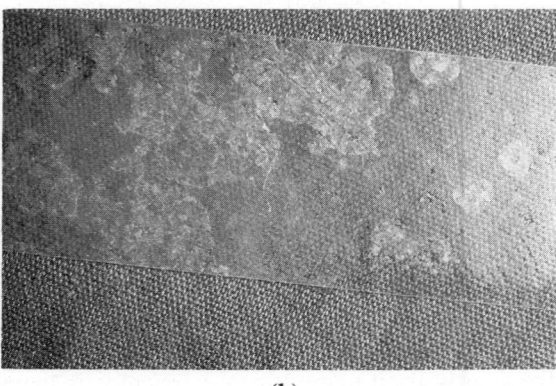

(b)

Fig. 33.9 Sellotape test. (a) Sellotape applied and stroked firmly with fingernail. (b) Diagnostic replication of scales on strip. (c) Staining with 1% gentian violet shows clusters of spores and some germ tubes.

shampoo should be applied all over the body (except around the eyes and mouth) for half an hour every day for up to two weeks while others have found that application of the shampoo for an 8–12 hour period and repeated in 3 days will usually clear the infection; this latter routine may irritate the groins and the genitalia but it has the advantage of using less medication and so being less expensive. Swedish doctors prefer zinc pyrithione shampoo as it is cosmetically elegant and lacks the unpleasant odour of selenium disulphide.

In areas where neither selenium disulphide nor zinc pyrithione shampoos are available it is suggested that a 50% solution of propylene glycol in water will be equally useful if applied every night for 10–14 days.

Griseofulvin is of no use either locally or systemically but even small doses of ketoconazole (a single dose of 400 mg) have been dramatically successful. The recent recognition of ketoconazole-induced liver damage[15] has made this drug contraindicated in the less serious dermatomycoses.[16]

Many individuals with darker skins will not be satisfied with the simple removal of the scales but will want the hypochromic macules to be returned to normal colour before they feel they have been properly treated. They must be reassured that repigmentation will take place in due time and that this period can be shortened if they do not expose themselves excessively to sunlight.

SPECIAL CASE—*PITYROSPORON* FOLLICULITIS

It has recently been recognized[17] that patients may develop small dome-shaped follicular papules, markedly pruritic and often indistinguishable from those erythematous papules called 'prickly heat'. Usually found in adults with greasy or sweaty skins these lesions contain spores and hyphae which grow in a lipid-enriched medium.[18] It is believed that *P. orbiculare* is the aetiologic agent.

Treatment with selenium disulphide $2\frac{1}{2}\%$ or 50% propylene glycol usually takes several weeks. Some doctors use ketoconazole systemically for this condition but others are more wary.

OTHER FORMS OF SUPERFICIAL FUNGUS INFECTION

Nodular trichomycoses

In various parts of the world hair, of the scalp or body, can become infected by a variety of organisms (*Trichosporon*, *Piedraia* or corynebacteria) which produce coloured concretions along the hair shaft. Usually they have a nodular or beaded appearance but sometimes considerable lengths of hair are so sheathed with disease that patients have believed their hair has changed colour.

Trichomycosis axillaris, as the name suggests, occurs mainly on axillary hair but may occasionally be seen also in pubic hair. Different varieties of *Corynebacterium tenuis*[19] produce hard, coloured accretions along the hairs. Most frequently they are yellow but in other cases red, white or black nodules are found. They are made of tightly packed bacteria which invade the outer cells of the hair cuticle but do not penetrate to the cortex. They do not affect surrounding skin but sometimes nearby clothing is stained the colour of the nodules.

Black piedra is most commonly found in South America and South-East Asia; it is caused by *Piedraia hortai* which affects the scalp hair. Hard, black nodules, just visible to the naked eye, spread along the hair shafts which consequently feel gritty to the touch. If a large area of scalp is involved, combing the hair can produce a whistling sound.

White piedra is entirely different from black piedra, being caused by *Trichosporon beigelii*[20] which particularly affects the beard and has been recognized in South America and many parts of Europe and Asia. The light-coloured concretions are occasionally beaded but more often produce a sheath around the hair.

It is not known how any of these forms of trichomycosis are spread so there is no known method of prevention. Treatment is simple: all that is necessary is to shave the affected part. This is usually acceptable to patients with trichomycosis axillaris or white piedra but patients with black piedra are often unwilling to be shaved and may prefer to apply Whitfield's lotion twice daily (5% benzoic and 5% salicylic acid in methylated spirits).

Tinea nigra

This is a misnomer as it is not caused by a dermatophyte but, as no one seems to have suggested an acceptable alternative, this name has become well established.

The condition is caused by *Exophiala werneckii* (previously called *Cladosporium werneckii*) and appears as a very superficial spreading discoloration, most frequently on the palms, which looks as if it has been caused by black ink. It is much rarer in temperate zones but has been reported on the neck and elsewhere in European and North American patients, in which case the patches are rarely black but more frequently a golden brown. The incubation period may vary from several weeks to many years.

The only dermatosis that it resembles is a junctional naevus but this may easily be differentiated by scraping the affected skin and recognizing the presence of pigmented hyphae and cells in a 10% potassium hydroxide preparation.

Persistent use of any local antimycotic preparation will be successful especially if it is prepared in an alcohol or dimethylsulphoxide base.

REFERENCES

1 Wilson, J. W. & Plunkett, O. A. (1965) *Fungus Diseases of Man*. Berkeley, California: University of California Press.
2 Rebell, G. & Taplin, D. (1970) *Dermatophytes*, revised edn. Coral Gables, Florida: University of Miami Press.
3 Beneke, E. S. (1974) *Scope Monograph on Human Mycoses*, 5th edn. Kalamazoo, Michigan: The Upjohn Company.
4 Vanbreuseghem, R. (1966) *Guide Pratique de Mycologie*. Paris: Masson et Cie.
5 Clayton, Y., Hay, R. J., McGibbon, D. H. et al (1982) *Clin. exp. Derm.* 7, 273.
6 Barth, J. H. & Billington, H. (1984) *Clin. exp. Derm.* 9, 625.
7 Bhakhtaviziam, C., Shafi, M., Mehta, M. C. et al (1984) *Clin. exp. Derm.* 9, 84.
8 Gaisin, A., Holzwanger, J. & Leydon, J. J. (1977) *Int. J. Dermatol.* 16, 188.
9 White, M. I. & Clayton, Y. (1982) *Clin. exp. Derm.* 7, 273.
10 Lodder & Kreger van R. (1952) *The Yeasts*. Quoted by Vanbreuseghem (1966) *op. cit.* p. 9.
11 Dixon, E. N., Warin, R. B. & English, M. (1969) *Br. med. J.* 25.
12 Mackie, R. N., Parrott, D. & Jenkins, W. H. H. (1978) *Br. J. Derm.* 98, 343.
13 Faergemann, J. & Fredriksson, T. (1982) *Int. J. Dermatol.* 21, 8.
14 Fredriksson, T. & Faergemann, J. (1984) *Int. J. Dermatol.* 23, 110.
15 Lewis, J. H., Zimmermann, J. H., Benson, C. D. et al (1984) *Gastroenterology,* 86, 503.
16 Hay, R. J., Clayton, Y., Griffiths, W. A. D. et al (1985) *Br. J. Derm.* 112, 691.
17 Back, O., Faergemann, J. & Hornquist, R. (1985) *J. Am. Acad. Derm.* 12, 56.
18 Roberts, S. O. B. (1969) *Br. J. Dermatol.* 81, 264.
19 Crissey, J. T., Rebell, G. C. & Laskas, J. J. (1952). *J. invest. Derm.* 19, 189.
20 Benson, T. N., Lapins, M. A. & Odom, R. B. (1983) *Archs Derm.* 119, 602.

Subcutaneous mycoses are caused by fungi which normally inhabit soil or vegetation and infect man by inoculation into the skin. They include mycetoma, chromomycosis and phaeo-hyphomycosis, caused by several species of fungi, and zygomycoses caused by single species, sporotrichosis and rhinosporidiosis.

MYCETOMA

Mycetoma (madura foot, maduromycosis) is a clinical syndrome caused by any one of many species of fungi. It may affect any part of the body exposed to trauma and occurs most frequently in the foot or hand. It can also affect the skull. Madura foot is the term applied to the disease as it affects the foot.

GEOGRAPHICAL DISTRIBUTION

Mycetoma occurs round the world in tropical and temperate regions. In India where mycetoma was first described it is an important disease and is endemic in widely scattered districts, although whole provinces, such as Lower Bengal, enjoy an almost complete freedom.

Africa is the chief home of mycetoma, extending from the east across the southern Sudan and equatorial Africa to the west coast and down through Nigeria to Zaire. Cases are commonly seen in Mexico, Central America and adjacent areas and have been described from Italy and South Vietnam.

AETIOLOGY

Mycetoma is caused by two main groups of organisms, true fungi (*Madurella*, etc.) and acti-nomycetes. *Eumycetoma* is the term used for infections caused by fungi and *actinomycetoma* for those caused by actinomycetes (*Nocardia* and *Streptomyces*, etc.) (Table 34.1).[1,2]

The dominant species vary in different parts of the world. In the Sudan the commonest agents are Eumycetes, *Madurella mycetomatis* (70%) and actinomycetes (30%) with *Streptomyces somaliensis* (20%) and *Actinomadura* (*Streptomyces*) *madurae* and *A.* (*S.*) *pelletieri* (10%). In Mexico most of the mycetomas are caused by *Nocardia brasiliensis*. The causative micro-organism of mycetoma is seen in the lesion as a small compact colony or 'grain' of various sizes and colours according to the species.

The mycelium in the grain is arranged in radial formation and in the case of some fungi the peripheral part is formed of large thick-walled cells usually known as chlamydospores. Surrounding the grain in many species is a layer of hyaline eosinophil material often drawn out into club-like bodies forming a kind of corona on the grain which is more or less characteristic of the species of microorganism. These hyaline formations, which are common also in most other species of fungi, notably *Sporotrichum* and *Aspergillus*, represent a reaction by the host which is probably defensive. The maduromycoses which are caused by true fungi possess grains composed of coarse septate mycelium (Fig. 34.1), whereas the grains of the actinomycoses show only very slender non-septate hyphae, usually not exceeding $1 \mu m$ in diameter, which respresents the characteristic bacillus-like thallus of the actinomyces.

Carter's black mycetoma (*M. mycetomatis*)

This is found mainly in tropical Africa, India, other Asiatic countries and also in parts of North and South America. There and perhaps also in

Table 34.1   Eumycetes and actinomycetes capable of causing mycetoma.

		Grain size (mm)	World distribution	Rainfall (cm/year)
Eumycetoma (infections caused by true fungi):				
Dark grain eumycetoma	*Madurella mycetomatis*	1.0	Africa, South America, India, Madagascar, Indonesia	25–50
	Madurella grisea	1.0	Mainly North and South America	
	Exophiala jeanselmi	1.0	Senegal and Chad	
	Pyrenochaeta romeroi			
	Leptosphaeria senegalensis			
	Curvularia lunata			
Pale grain eumycetoma	*Petriellidium boydii*		Europe, America, Africa	100–200
	Acremonium spp. (*A. kiliense, A. recifei*)		South America, Africa, Europe, India	
	Fusarium spp. (*F. solani, F. oxysporum*)			
	Neotestudina rosati			
	Aspergillus nidulans, A. flavus			
	Dermatophytes (*Microsporum ferrugineum*; *M. audouinii*)			
Actinomycetoma (infections caused by actinomycetes):				
Pale grain actinomycetoma	*Actinomadura madurae*	>2.0	Africa, North and South America	5–25
	Streptomyces somaliensis	1.0	Africa, North and South America, Israel	
Red grain actinomycetoma	*A. pelletieri*	0.5	Africa, South America	25–100
Small microscopic actinomycetoma	*Nocardia* spp. (*N. brasiliensis*); *N. asteroides*; *N. caviae*)	<0.5	Cosmopolitan	100–200

After Hay and Mackenzie.[2]

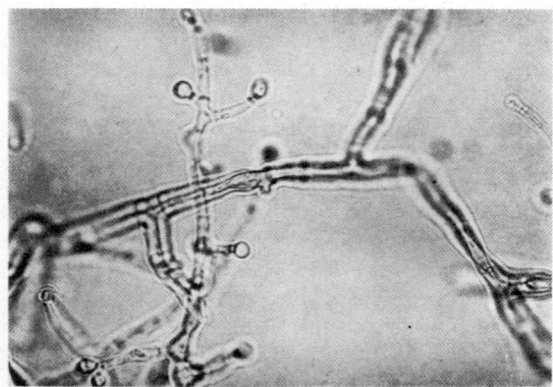

Fig. 34.1   Aleurospores of *Mycetoma mycetomatis*.

India the geographical distribution of *M. myce-tomatis* and *M. grisea* may overlap.

The parasitic grains of *M. mycetomatis* consist of a radially spreading septate and branching mycelium, measuring 1–5 μm in diameter with chlamydospores up to 25 μm. The actual grains are dark brown or black and measure 1–2 mm in diameter. They are also hard and brittle. This fungus grows readily on Sabouraud's medium. It has been shown that the grains remain viable for three months or longer.[3] In culture *M. myce-tomatis* can utilize glucose, maltose and galactose, but not sucrose, as sources of carbon; as sources of nitrogen it makes use of potassium nitrate, ammonium sulphate, asparagine and urea.

M. grisea may be the predominant form in the geographical range of mycetoma in South America. The parasitic grains of this species differ from those of *M. mycetomatis* in the unpigmented central part surrounded by a blackish, cortical zone. In this marginal zone the mycelium is embedded in a brown cement. On culture *M. grisea* is unable to utilize sucrose, in addition to other sugars already mentioned.

The colonies on glucose agar are hard, creased and folded, almost black in colour, and covered with greyish-white pulvesence. In Czapek's medium puff-ball colonies are formed with dark centres. Hyphae are either cylindrical, measuring 2–3 μm in diameter, or moniliform and thicker, 3–4 μm. They are branched and septate and give rise to more slender, almost colourless hyphae.

Madura foot—Vincent's white mycetoma (*Actinomadura madurae*)

The organism is *Actinomadura madurae* (formerly *Streptomyces madurae*) (Vincent 1894). It has been found in Algeria, Ethiopia, Somalia, Cyprus, India, Argentina, Cuba and Brazil.[4] The species is monomorphic and constant. The grains may reach a size larger than that of any other species. They are whitish-yellow, sometimes with a pink tinge. The central part of the grain may be hollow and contain scant, loosely and irregularly packed filaments which radiate. Clubs are usually observed. They are elongated, up to 25 μm, tape-like and sometimes branched. The ends may be pointed and they usually stain pink with eosin. (*A. madurae* is synonymous with *Actinomyces brumpti* and *Discomyces bahiensis*.)

Yellow-grained mycetoma (*Streptomyces somaliensis*)

The fungus is *Streptomyces somaliensis* Brumpt 1906, and has been extensively studied in the Sudan.[3] It occurs also in Ethiopia, Egypt, commonly in the Sudan and Somalia, West Africa and São Paulo. (The fungus appears to be identical with *Indiella somaliensis* of Brumpt and at one time the disease was called Bouffard's white mycetoma.) On Krainsky's medium it forms a thin, smooth pellicle and a short, light, ochreous aerial mycelium. On glucose peptone agar, cream coloured pellicles are produced and the culture may become brownish or blackish.

The mycelium is non-segmented with some chlamydospores about 1 μm in diameter. The aerial conidia are 1.25 μm, typical of the genus *Streptomyces*.

Peptone and asparagine are assimilated but ammonium sulphate, potassium nitrate and urea are not. The grains are yellowish, 1.25 mm in diameter, round, oval and compact. They are composed of a matrix of amorphous material showing slits and embedded on this the filaments of actinomyces are easily observed. Inoculations of mice and guinea-pigs have proved unsuccessful.

Red-grained mycetoma (*Actinomadura pelletieri*)

This form has been shown by Abbott to be widespread in the Sudan. In its gross pathology it is similar to the others, but it is of greater virulence.

The organism is *Actinomadura pelletieri* (*Streptomyces pelletieri*) (Laveran 1906). It is found in the Sudan, Senegal, Nigeria, India, Arabia and other countries. It produces (according to Mackinnon) slow growth in all media. On Krainsky's medium it forms hard, red, purple, adherent colonies. There is a poor growth on Czapek's medium.

Non-segmented branched vegetative mycelium is produced with some swellings up to 1 μm in diameter. No conidia are observed. The organism is not acid-fast and stains well by Gram's method. On basal medium with asparagine only glucose favours growth. Peptone and asparagine are utilized; urea and potassium nitrate are not.

The parasitic grains are deep red in colour, rather small, and rarely reach 1 mm in diameter. They are very irregular in shape and have smooth or denticulate edges. Some are seen to be enveloped by a refringent hard pellicle.

Nocardia brasiliensis

The general term *Nocardia* is reserved for the semi-acid-fast species. This species is found in Mexico, Brazil and Venezuela.

It is a rapid growing actinomycete and on Krainsky's medium forms heaped-up colonies with membranous consistency and marked furrows. The colour varies from pale ochre to orange or red ochre. Scarce aerial mycelium is formed on Krainsky and more abundantly on Czapek's media. The cultures produce an earthy odour.

A non-pigmented mycelium prevails. All strains are semi-acid-fast and stain well by Gram's method.

On basal medium with asparagine, glucose and galactose are utilized, but maltose, sucrose and lactose are not.

The parasitic grains are irregular, of moderate size, built up by lobules without clubs. Mice inoculated in the peritoneum developed abscesses, 1–3 mm in diameter, in pancreas, omentum and in between the liver and diaphragm.

Nocardia asteroides

This species was isolated by Fonseca in Rio de Janeiro and in Montevideo. On Krainsky's medium it produces a soft, inconsistent, creamy growth which acquires some orange and rose colour. On liquid media an inconsistent veil is formed.

The cultures are similar to those of *N. brasiliensis*. The mycelium may be segmented.

This fungus has no proteolytic activities and does not hydrolyse starch and can utilize all the nitrogenous compounds.

When inoculated into mice it produces small abscesses similar to those described above.

Leptosphaeria senegalensis

This organism was found in maduromycosis in Senegal and Mauritania and isolated in pure culture.[5]

Cultures can be made, as in actinomycosis, under aerobic and anaerobic conditions on glucose or glycerol agar plates, in shake cultures or in Löffler's serum, as well as on Krainsky's and Czapek's media. Some workers recommend keeping cultures in an atmosphere of carbon dioxide. The medium should be inoculated directly with colonies from the pus but, owing to slow growth of the actinomyces, pure cultures are somewhat difficult to obtain unless the pus is free from contamination with other organisms.

Petriellidium (Allescheria) boydii

Petriellidium (Allescheria) boydii is widely distributed and causes a mycetoma with yellowish-white grains in Zaire.[6] It grows well on Sabouraud's medium.

Acremonium (Cephalosporium) falciforme has been isolated from cases of mycetoma in Puerto Rico and *A. acremonium, A. recifei* and *A. granulomatis* have been isolated from human and animal cases of mycetoma.[7]

Corynespora cassiicola has been isolated from mycetoma in the Sudan.[8]

TRANSMISSION

Mycetoma is not contagious. Transmission is probably by puncture of the skin by infected thorns. Thorns were found embedded in the tissues at operation in seven subjects of yellow and two of black mycetoma.[3]

PATHOLOGY

On cutting into a mycetomatous foot or hand the knife passes readily through the mass, exposing a section with an oily, greasy surface in which the anatomical elements in many places are unrecognizable, being as it were fused together, forming a pale, greyish-yellow mass. The bones have in parts entirely disappeared; where their remains can still be made out, the cancellous structure is very friable, thinned, opened out and infiltrated with oleaginous material. Of all the structures the tendons and fasciae seem to be the most resistant.

The most remarkable feature revealed by section is a network of sinuses and communicating cyst-like cavities of various dimensions from a mere speck to a cavity 2.5 cm or more in diameter. Sinuses and cysts are occupied by a material unlike anything else in human morbid anatomy. In the black varieties this material consists of a black-brown, firm, friable substance which, in many places, fills the sinuses and cysts; manifestly it is from this that the black particles in the discharge are derived. In the white varieties the sinuses and cysts are also more or less filled with a white or yellowish roe-like substance, evidently an aggregation of particles identical with those escaping in the corresponding discharge. In the very rare red variety the colour of the accretions is red or pink.

Under the microscope the mycotic elements can be readily recognized in the concretions. In microscopic sections of the tissues, evidence of extensive degenerative changes, the result of a chronic inflammatory process, can be made out. Numerous microabscesses are present and there is a difference on microscopy in the character of the granules in the various types of mycetoma. *Streptomyces somaliensis* (actinomycetoma) shows a structureless pink homogeneous centre whereas *M. mycetoma* (eumycetoma) shows a structured centre containing fungal elements. The main differences are shown in Tables 34.2 and 34.3.[9]

Black mycetoma shows a marked tendency to spread along tissue planes and through fibrous tissue in the foot where numerous fibrous septa pass between the muscles and tendons. In the earlier stages of this deeper growth it may be possible to remove the tumour and it will be found enclosed in a capsule of fibrous tissue and may be dissected out.

Muscle tissue is resistant to invasion. A black mycetoma in a sheet of muscle on the back or

Table 34.2 Characters of grains of mycetoma.

Organism	Naked eye			Microscopically	
	Colour	Diameter (mm)	Intrinsic colour	Diameter of filaments (μm)	Staining affinities
M. mycetomatis *M. grisea* *L. senegalensis* *P. romeroi*	Black	*ca* 1	Brown	>2.0	None in particular
P. boydii *Acremonium* species	White or yellow	*ca* 1	None	>2.0	PAS positive[a]
Nocardia species	White or yellow	<0.5	None	<1.0	Acid-fast[b]
S. somaliensis	Yellow	*ca* 1	None	<1.0	Eosinophilic[c] Not acid-fast
Actinomadura pelletieri	Red	<0.5	Not pronounced	<1.0	Stain deeply and uniformly with haematoxylin[c] Not acid-fast
Actinomadura madurae	Yellow	>1.0	None	<1.0	Margin stains deeply with haematoxylin[c] Not acid-fast

Modified from Murray.[9]
[a] Periodic acid–Schiff stain.
[b] Decolorize with 1% sulphuric acid.
[c] Standard haematoxylin and eosin stain for tissues.

Table 34.3 Histological features of non-pigmented eumycetoma grains.

	P. boydii	*Acremonium* spp.	*Fusarium* spp.	*Neotestudini rosatii*
Diameter (mean μm)[a]	480 × 350 (80–940)	490 × 366 (130–890)	560 × 483 (100 × 1100)	380 × 320 (30–720)
Eosinophilic fringe	5–15 nm (7)	5–10 nm (2)	—	—
Shape	Variable	Variable	Variable	Variable
Central invasion by neutrophils	Frequent	Infrequent	Infrequent	Infrequent
Vesicles present	Usual	Sometimes	Rare	Yes
Nucleoli visible (HE)	No	Uncommon (1)	Yes	Yes

[a] Mean diameter is expressed as the mean of the maximal diameters of each grain measured at right angles in nm. The range is the minimum and maximum diameters measured. All measurements were made using tissue sections.
After Hay and Mackenzie.[2]

buttock will grow for years without penetrating the muscle fibres. Nerves and tendons are also resistant.

Neurological complications and trophic changes are conspicuously absent in eumycetoma. Yellow mycetoma caused by *S. somaliensis* shows an insidious growth. The edges blend imperceptibly with surrounding tissues. From the first these tumours infiltrate the underlying muscles. Yellow mycetoma is harder than the black. The fibrous stroma is more compact and in it the yellow grains may be embedded. Red mycetoma due to *A. pelletieri* is similar in gross pathology to the yellow. The sinuses are more numerous and active. Systemic spread occurs occasionally with actinomycetoma, but not in eumycetoma.

IMMUNITY

Humoral immunity

Both precipitating and complement-fixing antibodies develop in mycetoma infection; they rise with activity and fall with recovery, disappearing with cure. Precipitating antibodies are used in diagnosis and monitoring treatment. They are measured by immunodiffusion and counterimmunoelectrophoresis, both of which are sensitive and specific.[10,11] Complement-fixing antibodies are less specific.[12]

Cellular immunity

Mycetoma patients seem to be deficient in their cell-mediated immunity as measured by the tuberculin test, dinitrochlorobenzene reaction and lymphocyte transformation test[13] but type 4 skin reactions are produced to purified protein antigens in actinomycetoma and in some cases of eumycetoma with *Madurella* antigens.[14]

CLINICAL FEATURES

Natural history

The course of the infection is slowly progressive, spreading through the tissues and destroying cartilage and bone. Dissemination does not occur with eumycetoma but can with actinomycetoma.

Incubation period

The concept of an incubation period can hardly be applied. The fungus probably starts to develop as soon as it is implanted but a period of 10 years may elapse before the patient seeks treatment.

Symptoms and signs

Whatever the colour of the grains of species of fungus, the clinical course remains remarkably uniform. The first sign noticed is a painless swelling, usually but by no means invariably, on the sole of the foot, which in yellow mycetoma is ill defined and in black mycetoma takes the form of a clearly defined, painless nodule in the subcutaneous tissues.[3]

The growth continues slowly and inexorably. It may be a very long time before the deeper tissues are invaded but the granuloma spreads inwards, invading the bones. Nodules, at first paler than the surrounding skin, form on the surface, revealing the mouths of the sinuses (Fig. 34.2). From there a purulent fluid is discharged containing the characteristic coloured grains of the fungus. With all this the relative lack of pain is most remarkable and it is only when the foot or leg has been rendered quite useless that the patient suffers appreciably. No fever or other systemic effects accompany mycetoma, however long-standing, large or

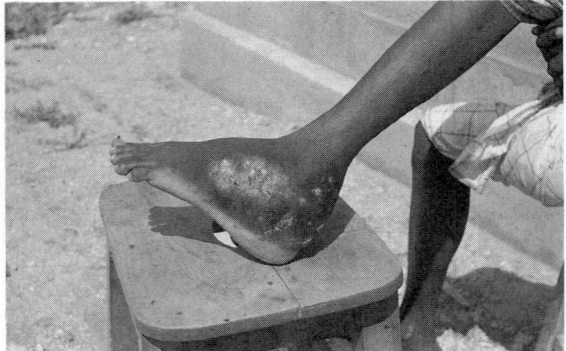

Fig. 34.2   Madura foot.

destructive the lesion may be, unless secondary bacterial infections supervene.

The regional lymph glands are involved in 1% of cases with local sinus formation from which the fungus can be isolated. The visible lesions are situated in less disabling sites. Back, buttocks, or thigh may remain well nourished and in good condition. In the majority of cases it is the effects of inactivity and economic loss which lower the patient's vitality.

An important feature is that the sinuses that are diagnostic may be late in appearing. The interval may be as long as six years. As the foot enlarges, the leg commences to atrophy from disuse, so that in advanced disease an enormously enlarged and misshapen foot, flexed or extended, is attached to an attenuated leg consisting of little more than skin and bone. X-rays show destruction and fusion of the bones of the foot (Fig. 34.3).

The intraosseous mycetoma is primarily a fungous tumour occurring in the metaphysis of a long bone, usually the upper end of the tibia. All the cases of this variety have been in boys under 13 and all were caused by *M. mycetomatis*.

The patient usually complains of dull, aching pains in the affected part. Examination reveals widening of the bone at the site of infection without involvement of the skin. It is probable that in these cases the infection is blood-borne. Periosteal tumours appear in all varieties. When a periosteal tumour forms on a long bone it presents itself as a hard, painless, smooth swelling without sinuses. It is probable that this type is due to direct inoculation of the organism into the periosteum of the tibia.

Cranial maduromycosis (Fig. 34.4) caused by *Streptomyces somaliensis*[15] is not very uncommon

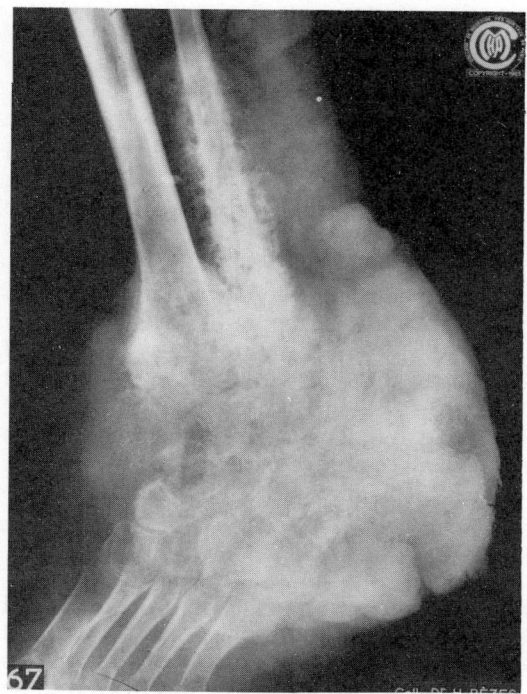

Fig. 34.3 Radiograph of a madura foot.

and causes enlargement and distortion of the skull with loss of vision, proptosis and headache. The X-ray appearances are characteristic; there is expansion of the bone, periosteal new bone formation and punctate areas of osteoporosis without sequestrum formation. The picture may be confused with that of a neoplasm. The radiological appearances can be used to differentiate the causative organisms, since in some bone resorption is dominant, in others osteoblastic activity occurs towards the periphery. In a third type incomplete regeneration of bone results in spicule formation. Differentiation can be made radiologically between mycetomas caused by large (2–4 mm) and small (under 2 mm) grains.[16]

Paranasal Aspergillus granuloma[17] is caused by invasion of the maxillary sinus by *Aspergillus flavus*. Formation of a granuloma causing a painless proptosis or swelling on the medial side of the eye which ultimately invades the brain and kills has been described in farmers from the northern Sudan. Treatment is by surgical excision and radiotherapy.

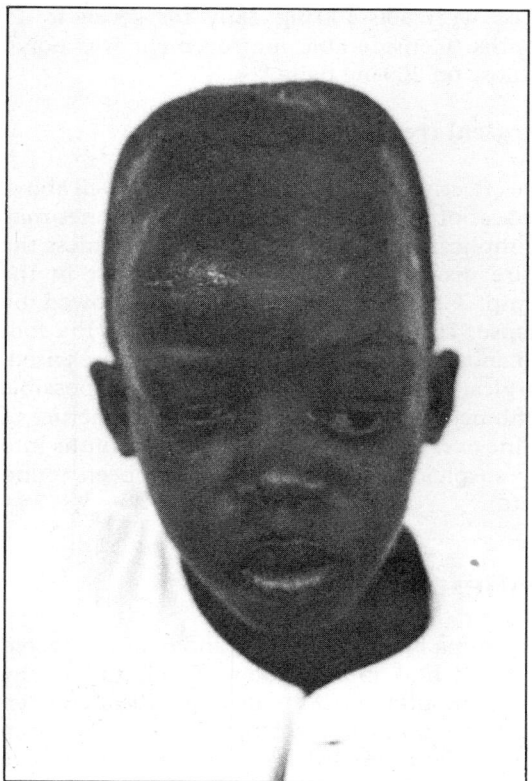

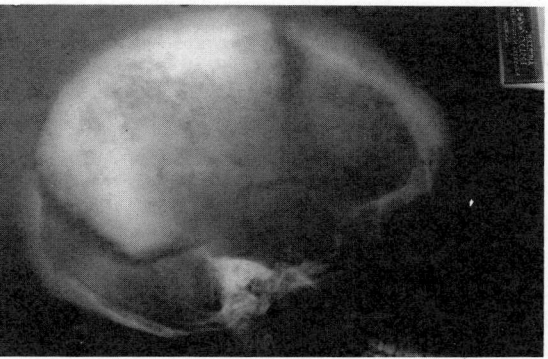

Fig. 34.4 Cranial maduromycosis. Note the periosteal new bone formation and punctate areas of osteoporosis without sequestrum formation.

Unusual lesions caused by Petriellidium (Allescheria) boydii

An asymptomatic coin lesion of the lung,[17] paranasal granuloma and disseminated infections in immunosuppressed people and a fungal arthritis resembling juvenile rheumatoid arthritis have been described.[18]

DIAGNOSIS

Direct examination of pus reveals the presence of the granules which are diagnostic. With knowledge of the usual mycetomas of the area the fungus can be identified by the size, shape, colour and consistency of the granules (Table 34.2). Direct examination is made by placing the granules in a drop of 10% sodium hydroxide and crushing under a coverslip to examine the hyphae. The granules should be crushed in the pus in which they have been obtained for staining (Gram's stain).

Direct culture from a biopsy of deep tissues should be performed on Sabouraud's modified agar (2% glucose, 1% neopeptone, pH 6.5–7.0) at room temperature and at 35–37°C. If granules are to be cultured they must first be washed in saline to remove contamination.

Serological diagnosis

Immunodiffusion and counterimmuno-electrophoresis with the appropriate antigens can define the causative organism with reasonable accuracy. There are cross reactions within the actinomycetoma group but not with the fungus group so that the serological reactions are very valuable in that they can indicate whether treatment will be effective or not. Using titre levels the progress of the disease can be checked since falling titres will indicate response to treatment. An enzyme-linked immunosorbent assay (ELISA) has been developed.

TREATMENT

Actinomycetoma responds readily to chemotherapy and more recently eumycetoma has been found responsive.

Actinomycetoma

Combinations of dapsone (DDS), co-trimoxazole, streptomycin, sulfadoxine–pyrimethamine and rifampicin have all been used successfully. Streptomycin 1 g daily for one month and then on alternate days plus either DDS 100 mg twice daily or co-trimoxazole two tablets twice daily is the cheapest regimen and should be used as a start. Streptomycin plus sulfadoxine–pyrimethamine or streptomycin plus rifampicin may also be used. Successful treatment usually requires six to nine months of therapy and relapse is uncommon. Careful haematological monitoring is essential because of the danger of bone marrow depression.[19] Chemotherapy is much less successful in *Streptomyces somaliensis* cases, in which surgery is often necessary.

Eumycetoma

Previously eumycetoma due to *Madurella* did not respond to any form of chemotherapy and treatment by surgical excision or amputation was the only remedy. *Ketoconazole* has proved to be active and five of 13 patients were completely cured with 300–400 mg daily for seven to 15 months. Considerable improvement was noted in those on 200 mg daily.[20]

Surgical treatment

The effective treatment is amputation well above the seat of the disease since the long bones may be implicated as well as the small and unless the entire disease is removed it will recur in the stump. Complete removal is not followed by relapse. If a toe or a small portion of the foot or hand alone is involved this may be excised. Surgical removal of as much tissue as possible combined with injection of 1–2 ml of tincture of iodine every 10 days for at least two months into any suspicious area remaining has been found useful.

EPIDEMIOLOGY

Mycetoma is not contagious and man is infected by accidental implantation of the fungus by thorns or splinters. Although sporadic cases can occur in temperate countries the disease is seen between latitudes 15° south and 30° north. The grains of mycetoma can withstand drought for prolonged periods and remain dormant but viable until the rainy season moistens the ground. Mycetoma occurs where there is a short rainy season and a daily temperature of 30–37°C with savannah scrub and thorn trees and bushes. There is a clear correlation between incidence and rainfall. Many cases of fungal infection with mycetoma-causing fungi must occur since serological evidence was obtained using the ELISA test of infection in apparently healthy individuals in the Sudan.

CONTROL

The greatest contribution towards control of the disease would be the general use of adequate footwear. Sandals are not sufficient.

CHROMOMYCOSIS

GEOGRAPHICAL DISTRIBUTION

Chromomycosis has a worldwide distribution but is mainly found in tropical rural areas with a particularly high prevalence in Costa Rica and Madagascar.

AETIOLOGY

Chromomycosis is caused by several fungi. The most common and widespread are *Phialophora verrucosa*, *Fonsecaea pedrosoi*, *Fonsecaea compacta*, *Cladosporium carrionii*. *P. dermatidis* is restricted to the Far East and *C. trichoides* is uncommon. In tissues they appear as single or clustered thick-walled dark brown bodies and in culture the first three species produces spores of two diverse types, the proportion of which varies with the species. *P. Verrucosa* produces mainly phialospores (cup-shaped) and rarely arborescent spore heads typical of abbreviated *Cladosporium* sporulation. *F. pedrosoi* and *F. compacta* sporulate predominantly by lateral production of conidia and terminal arborescent spore heads, but rarely produce phialospores. *Cladosporium carrionii* sporulates only by branching chains of spores. The organisms are commonly found in wood and soil as saprophytes.

TRANSMISSION

Infection is acquired through the skin from abrasions contaminated by soil or by thorns.

PATHOLOGY

Lesions of chromomycosis show pseudo-epitheliomatous hyperplasia associated with keratolytic microabscesses in the hyperplastic epidermis and must be distinguished from epithelioma. The deeper dermis contains confluent granulomatous nodules composed of pale, irregularly distributed epithelioid cells bordered by lymphocytes, plasma cells and other inflammatory cells. The centres may contain large foreign body giant cells. When ulceration ensues there is accompanying acute or chronic pyogenic infection. Brown hyphae may occasionally be demonstrated in the superficial crusts, but the characteristic findings are in the dermis where the yeast form is seen as round thick-walled *brown* septate fungus cells 5–12 μm in diameter. Owing to the brown colour special stains are of little use. Six or seven fungus bodies may be found crowded in a giant cell, resembling peas in a pod.

IMMUNITY

Both humoral and cellular mechanisms are involved. Precipitating antibodies were produced against an antigen prepared by ultrasonic destruction of fungal cells of *F. pedrosoi* which showed cross reactions with *F. compacta* but none with a wide range of other fungi including *Cladosporium*.[21] Precipitating, agglutinating and fluorescent antibody tests have been used to separate the various organisms which cause chromomycosis[22,23] but are not much used in practice. Cellular immune mechanisms are responsible for the granulomas seen in pathology.

CLINICAL FEATURES

The *incubation period* is very long. A minor wound may precede by months or years the fully developed lesion.

Symptoms and signs

The primary lesion is minimal, persisting for months as a papule or pustule which finally ulcerates. The ulcer spreads slowly laterally and is replaced by a chronic dry crusted or verrucous violaceous lesion with a raised border (Fig. 34.5). It may remain flat or extend 1–3 cm above the normal skin surface. After many years the lesion becomes pedunculated with a stalk producing a cauliflower-like tumour.

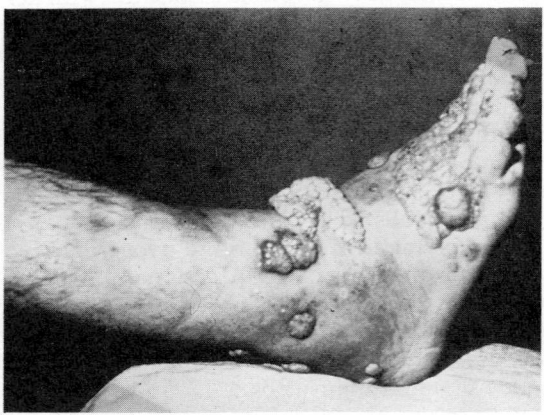

Fig. 34.5   Chromomycosis of the leg.

The lesions may heal at the centre while spreading marginally but spontaneous cure does not occur. There is little pain but considerable irritation. There may be spread by the lymphatic channels to remote areas and a few cases have been recorded of brain abscesses from which *F. pedrosoi* has been isolated. Secondary infection may cause considerable lymph stasis with lymphoedema.

Cladosporium trichoides has caused cerebral lesions[24] and cutaneous infection.[25]

DIFFERENTIAL DIAGNOSIS

Chromomycosis may resemble blastomycosis as well as lymphatic siderosilicosis (see Chapter 44), filarial elephantiasis (see Chapter 20), diffuse cutaneous leishmaniasis (see Chapter 37), cutaneous tuberculosis, syphilis and yaws (see Chapter 31).

DIAGNOSIS

Superficial crusts removed from the lesion contain long brown branching hyphae 2–5 μm wide which can be seen after digestion in sodium hydroxide. On biopsy brown rounded bodies are found within giant cells or extracellularly among the polymorphs in the suppurative areas. Culture of material should be on media containing chloramphenicol or other antibiotics and incubated at 30°C.

TREATMENT

Chemotherapy

Although the organisms which cause chromomycosis are sensitive to *amphotericin B* in vitro, the concentration is too high to be used in vivo. Local infiltration with excision and thermocoagulation of the skin followed by grafting has been helpful but relapses occur.[26] *5-Fluorocytosine* by mouth and by local infiltration has given good results,[27] but resistance occurs. 5-Fluorocytosine 500 mg 6-hourly to a total of 400 g combined with *amphotericin B* 50 mg intravenously on alternate days to a total of 1.5 g produced a cure after two months with no remission after six months.[28] *Ketoconazole* has shown some activity.[29] *Thiabendazole* was given, 3.0 g daily in three divided doses for 10 weeks, after which the dose was reduced to 2.0 g daily. After eight months only scars and thickening of the skin were noticeable.[30]

Heat therapy

Since the maximum temperature of growth of these fungi lies between 35°C and 39°C heat has been used and cases caused by *P. verrucosa* have been cured with infrared heat.

EPIDEMIOLOGY

Chromomycosis is seen more often in males than females and in rural than urban workers and in those people who are exposed to thorn and puncture wounds while working without shoes.

It is suspected that *Phialophora* are saprophytes in soil or timber and *P. verrucosa* has been isolated in a few instances from the soil and is responsible for the blue discoloration of wood pulp. *F. pedrosoi* has been isolated from saprophytic sources only rarely but probably occurs commonly in decaying vegetation in the soil. In Madagascar infections with *C. carrionii* occurred in areas of low rainfall (50–60 cm annually) whereas infections caused by *F. pedrosoi* were found in areas of high rainfall (220–300 cm annually).

Spores of *Cladosporium* can be identified in surveys of airborne spores and perhaps sometimes cause allergic respiratory disease.

SPOROTRICHOSIS

Sporotrichosis is a chronic, subcutaneous, lymphatic mycosis which may remain localized for months but may become generalized involving bones, joints and other organs. Lesions may be granulomatous or may suppurate, ulcerate and drain.

GEOGRAPHICAL DISTRIBUTION

Sporotrichosis occurs worldwide but is commonest in warm, tropical and subtropical countries.

AETIOLOGY

Sporotrichosis is caused by *Sporothrix schenckii*, also known as *S. beurmanni*. *S. schenckii* is dimorphic. In tissues the yeast form appears as spherical budding cells which may reach a diameter of $10\,\mu m$ or as cigar-shaped budding cells 1×3–$10\,\mu m$. This form grows well on a high glucose medium at 37°C. In culture at room temperature (24°C) *S. schenckii* forms branching septate hyphae not exceeding 1–$2\,\mu m$ in diameter. Conidiophores bearing elliptical conidia 2–3×3–$6\,\mu m$ arise from the hyphae. At room temperature *S. schenckii* forms a moist colony with a wrinkled surface and newly isolated strains produce pigment, at first yellow, later becoming black.

Intraperitoneal inoculation into a male mouse causes orchitis within a week to 10 days.

TRANSMISSION

The infection is transmitted by direct inoculation into the skin or a pre-existing abrasion or cut from an infected source.

IMMUNITY

Skin sensitivity tests are of use in diagnosis of the common lymphatic variety and in the rare cases of disseminated disease complement fixation and agglutination tests may be of great value.

Skin test (sporotrichin test)

The specific capsule polysaccharide antigen of *S. schenckii* is most specific and a positive sporotrichin test is almost invariably a sign of infection with *S. schenckii*, either past or present, since positive reactions have been obtained in 6–24% of subjects in an endemic area compared with one of 55 in a non-endemic area,[31] and in 11–30% of healthy individuals the highest percentage being found in nursery gardeners.[32] The sporotrichin skin test is especially useful in the differential diagnosis from cutaneous leishmaniasis.

Complement fixation and agglutination tests

The most specific antigens used in serological tests are prepared from yeast phase cells by autoclaving or grinding acetone treated cells. The precipitin test appeared most useful[33] and has been used in the diagnosis of the disseminated disease.

Fluorescent antibody tests

These tests have proved useful in detecting *S. schenckii* in exudate from lesions and homologous *S. schenckii* fluorescein-labelled sera stained both yeast and mycelial phase cultures of eight different strains and showed no cross reactivity with heterologous species.[34]

PATHOLOGY

The infection starts as a primary lesion at the site of inoculation and extends along a superficial lymphatic vessel causing an ascending mycotic lymphangitis with development of secondary gummas along the course of the thickened vessel. These secondary gummas tend to break down and ulcerate but except for secondary bacterial infection there is generally an absence of secondary lymphadenopathy.

Histopathology

The basic histopathological lesion is a combination of a pyogenic and granulomatous reaction also seen in blastomycosis, coccidioidomycosis and chromomycosis. Typically there are small nodules composed of histiocytes, some of which are epithelioid cells; in these small granulomas there is a central focus of neutrophils bordered by a rim of epithelioid cells. Langhans' giant cells may be present. *S. schenckii* is difficult to demonstrate in skin lesions and those which are characterized by pseudoepitheliomatous hyperplasia and a mixed pyogenic epithelioid cell granulomatous reaction in which neither fungi nor bacteria can be demonstrated should be suspected as sporotrichosis. In secondary and disseminated lesions the histological picture is the same.

The asteroid body consists of a central rounded or oval yeast-like somewhat basophilic structure 3–5 μm in diameter which is bordered by a radiate eosinophilic substance which forms a covering of approximately 10 μm thickness. The central yeast-like body reacts positively to fungus stains. Although asteroid bodies can be found in coccidioidomycosis and aspergillosis, if they are present in skin and secondary lesions they are presumptive evidence of sporotrichosis. *S. schenckii* may be more easily identified in lesions of susceptible animals and in visceral sporotrichosis by special fungus stains as oval, cigar-shaped or rounded bodies.

CLINICAL FEATURES

Localized lymphatic sporotrichosis

The commonest type of sporotrichosis follows the subcutaneous implantation of spores in a penetrating wound caused by a thorn or splinter. The incubation period is from 7 to 14 days but can be as long as one month and very rarely six months.

The primary lesion is a cutaneous gumma or chancre, firm, elastic, painless and movable on the deeper tissues, measuring on the average about 1.5–2 cm. As the gumma enlarges its centre becomes necrotic and breaks down, becoming fluctuant, and the surface becomes dull red or violaceous in colour. A shallow ulcer with a little sinus may form at the apex and become crusted but eventually the sinus enlarges, the summit breaks down and the contents of mucoid pus in which the fungus can be found by culture are discharged, leaving an indolent ulcer with overhanging violaceous walls and a non-sloughing granulomatous base from which a serosanguineous fluid exudes and forms a crust (Fig. 34.6).

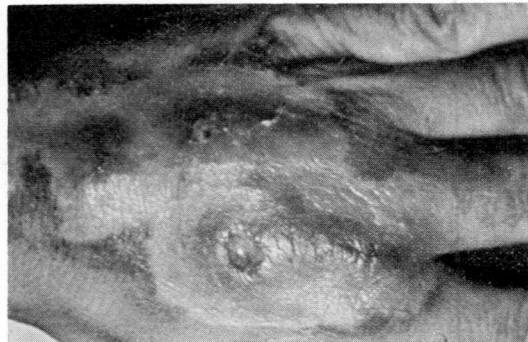

Fig. 34.6   Spirotrichosis.

Lymphatic spread occurs along the lymphatics draining the area, which become indurated and cord-like; the lymph glands become swollen and eventually suppurate. The lesions may persist for years.

Primary pulmonary sporotrichosis caused by inhalation of spores has been described.[35]

Disseminated sporotrichosis

Rarely there may be haematogenous spread from the primary lesion or from suppurating lymph glands. In some cases it seems possible that the infection could have had a respiratory origin.

Dissemination to the skin is manifested by numerous widespread skin lesions starting as nodules and developing into papules, pustules, ulcers and confluent areas of folliculitis. Occasionally there are lesions of the oral and nasal mucosa.

Dissemination to the visceral organs is rarely observed and is accompanied by fever. Pyelo-nephritis, orchitis, mastitis and pulmonary disease may all occur. Lesions of the bones are characterized by periostitis and osteomyelitis and of the joints by synovitis and destruction of cartilage. Granulomatous synovitis and osteitis caused by *S. schenckii* have been described;[36] in one case there was a lesion on the wrist, and the ulnar bone and synovial covering were involved, and in the other there was a chronic synovitis of the knee.

DIFFERENTIAL DIAGNOSIS

Sporotrichosis must be distinguished from a wide range of cutaneous skin lesions, such as tularaemia, cutaneous leishmaniasis (*L. L. major*), anthrax, tuberculosis and some pyogenic bacteria, as well as from other mycoses.

DIAGNOSIS

The diagnosis by culture is made by sowing material from a gumma on glucose agar slants or Sabouraud's medium and incubating at room temperature (24°C). After 5–12 days the young colonies of characteristic appearance will be found.

TREATMENT

Potassium iodide is specific in this disease, commencing with 600 mg to 1 g by mouth in 100 ml of milk or water thrice daily after food and increasing by about 300 mg/dose/day until a maximum of 3–3.3 g/dose is reached. This dosage should be maintained until clinical cure is achieved and continued in a diminishing scale for a further four weeks to insure against recurrence. In simple cases the treatment takes about six to eight weeks but the response will depend on the state of the disease and the individual patient.

EPIDEMIOLOGY

S. schenckii is a saprophyte which grows in man's environment and causes disease after accidental inoculation. It occurs naturally on berberis, rose, poinsettia, sphagnum and salt marsh green. It can grow on wood and causes 'bud rot' when inoculated into carnations. Infection is often related to minor punctures by rose or barbary thorns, splinters or even metal particles such as steel wool, which may have been contaminated by soil containing spores.

Sporotrichosis has been found in wild rats, dogs and horses and mules, in which it resembles epizootic lymphangitis, but the disease in lower animals does not constitute a reservoir of infection for man.

Sporotrichosis occurs sporadically or in groups in many parts of the world and is particularly common in florists, horticulturists and people who handle raw packing material. From 1941 to 1944 an epidemic of sporotrichosis involving 2825 cases occurred in two mine shafts on the Witwatersrand where conditions of temperature (26.1–28°C) and humidity (96–100%) were very favourable for the growth of *S. schenckii* on the sound but unpreserved mine timbers. The infection was associated with contamination of cutaneous abrasions common in the mine workers. In Uruguay it was found that the infection rate was related to seasonal conditions of temperature and rainfall comparable to the temperature and humidity recorded in the Transvaal mines.[37]

PHYCOMYCOSIS (MUCORMYCOSIS) (ENTEROPHTHOROMYCOSIS)

AETIOLOGY

Infection by one of two general phycomycetes belonging to the order Entomophthorales results in one of two clinical conditions, neither of which is opportunist. One type of disease is caused by the genus *Basiodobolus*, *B. meristosporus*, *B. haptosporus*[38] and is known as subcutaneous phycomycosis, creeping granuloma or eosinophilic granuloma. The other type is caused by *Coniodobolus coronatus* and less often by *Basiodobolus* species and involves the nasal cavities. It is known as zygomycosis or rhinoentomophthoromycosis.

Most of the pathogenic phycomycetes grow rapidly on neopeptone agar and other media at 27–37°C. On Sabouraud's medium they appear as broad irregularly branched non-septate hyphae up to 15 μm in diameter which stain deeply with haemotoxylin. They have a tendency to penetrate blood vessels with resultant thrombosis and disseminated lesions. In immunosuppressed people and diabetics the organisms enter through superficial lesions of the nose, nasal sinuses or bronchi causing a systemic infection with infarcts, suppuration and necrosis.

Subcutaneous phycomycosis (*Basiodobolus* spp.)

The fungi which cause subcutaneous phycomycosis in man are numerous in the environment on the dung of herbivorous animals and decaying vegetation and fruit. *Basiodobolus meristoporus* (*B. ranarum*) is present as a saprophyte in the intestinal canal of beetles, frogs, toads and lizards.

Subcutaneous phycomycosis has been described from Indonesia,[39] Nigeria and Uganda[40] which is the main area of infection. Males are attacked more frequently than females and it is predominantly a disease of childhood and adolescence.

Basiodobolus species cause a granuloma with a chronic inflammatory reaction in the centre of which are found large degenerated poorly stained hyphae. Necrotizing eosinophilic debris surrounds the hyphae and the cellular reaction contains many eosinophils, neutrophils, fibroblasts and thick-walled capillaries. Foreign body giant cells are common.

The infection begins as one spot of hard, woody, subcutaneous infiltration which spreads rapidly to involve extensive areas over the neck, arms and upper chest (Fig. 34.7). The process involves subcutaneous tissue and muscle fascia. The infection usually heals spontaneously but deeper structures may be involved and visceral involvement has been reported.[41] Sometimes some cheesy material may be squeezed out of the

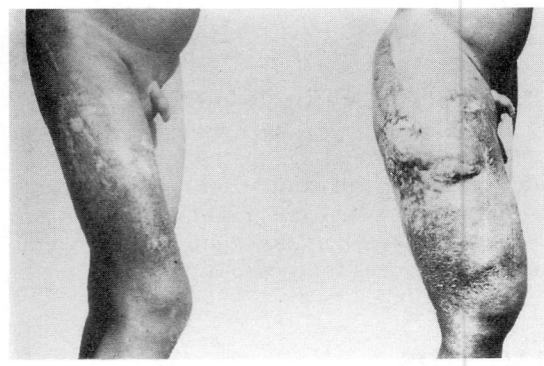

Fig. 34.7 Subcutaneous phycomycosis before (right) and after (left) treatment.

indurated areas. The buttocks are the usual site but rhinopharyngeal, orbital and orocutaneous phycomycosis has been reported. In Senegal *B. meristoporus* (*B. ranarum*) can cause, rarely, massive oedema of the lower limbs resembling filarial lymphoedema, but subcutaneous nodules can be palpated and granulomas with fungal elements seen on biopsy.[42]

Potassium iodide has been used successfully in treatment. The drug should be administered commencing with 600 mg to 1 g by mouth in 100 ml milk or water thrice daily and increasing by about 300 mg/dose until a maximum of 3–3.3 g/dose is reached.

Rhinoentomophthoromycosis (*Coniodobolus*)

Coniodobolus coronatus (*Entomophthora coronata*) occurs in soil and decaying vegetation and causes disease in insects. The disease occurs in adult males in the third and fourth decades of life living in lowland regions of tropical rain forest in Nigeria, India, Colombia and Brazil. Transmission is probably by the inhalation of spores.

The primary site of infection is in the nasal mucosa and cases present with a nasal obstruction which eventually involves the paranasal sinuses, pharynx and subcutaneous muscles of the face in a chronic granulomatous swelling. The disease is discussed by Clark.[44]

PHAEOHYPHOMYCOSIS

This is a group of dark-pigmented fungi distinct from chromomycosis and mycetoma which includes cladosporidiosis, phaeosporotrichosis and cystic chromomycosis. They are very uncommon but may also occur in immuno-compromised individuals.

Entry is assumed to be via the skin from a puncture from a contaminated object.

PATHOLOGY

There is an intense suppurative and granulomatous response in the dermis with micro-abscesses and spherical or filamentous brown pigmented hyphae.

CLINICAL FEATURES

Lesions start as a single small papule becoming verrucous increasing gradually in size over a number of years, which extends into the deeper tissues invading the chest and other cavities. A case caused by *Exophiala spinifera* has been described.[43]

Rarely brain abscesses may be caused in immunocompromised people.

DIAGNOSIS

Diagnosis is made by the presence of pigmented (brown) hyphae in the lesion.

TREATMENT

There is no specific treatment.

CERCOSPORAMYCOSIS

Cercosporamycosis caused by *Cercospora apii* has been described in a single case from Indonesia.[45] The patient was a boy with extensive indurated verrucous and ulcerated cutaneous and sub-cutaneous lesions of the face which later extended to other areas. The patient later died.

The disease had started in early infancy. The fungus was easily seen in biopsy specimens as brown septate hyphae and was also cultured. Experimental infection of tomato plants gave rise to 'leaf spot disease'.

PROTOTHECOSIS

Geographical distribution

Protothecosis is a very rare infection first described from Sierra Leone[46] since when isolated cases have occurred in South Africa, China, Vietnam, New Zealand, Panama and the USA.

AETIOLOGY

Prototheca has a life-cycle similar to green algae. It consists of an ovoid or spherical hyaline cell (mother cell) or *sporangium* 3–20 μm which grows and ruptures to release sixteen or more *sporangiophores* each of which grows into a sporangium. There are two species, *P. wickerhamii* and *P. zopfi* (*segbwema*). They stain well with

PAS or Gomori methenamine silver stains and occur naturally in vegetable matter, sludge, stagnant water or acid lakes causing natural infections of animals.

TRANSMISSION

Infection is contracted through the skin from a subcutaneous penetrating wound.

IMMUNITY

Protothecosis occurs mainly in immuno-compromised persons.

PATHOLOGY

The infection is usually limited to skin and sub-cutaneous tissue causing a localized dermatitis or granulomatous nodule. There is hyperkeratosis and acanthosis with a cellular infiltrate of lymphocytes, plasma cells and many eosinophils with central caseation and Langhans' giant cells. Lymphatic spread to the local glands is rare and haematogenous spread very rare.

DIAGNOSIS

Prototheca can be demonstrated with PAS in caseous material and cultured on Sabouraud's medium.

TREATMENT

Local excision is the only form of treatment.

EPIDEMIOLOGY

Infection is contracted in an aquatic environment of rice fields, stagnant ponds and acid lakes.

RHINOSPORIDIOSIS

A disease due to a yeast-like organism, *Rhinosporidium seeberi*, infects the mucous membrane of the nose, producing nasal polyps and tumours on the cheek, conjunctiva, lacrimal sac, uvula, ear, glans penis and skin.

GEOGRAPHICAL DISTRIBUTION

Rhinosporidiosis is found most often in India and Sri Lanka but has also been reported from Indonesia, Malaysia, Philippines, Iran, South Africa, England, Scotland, southern United States, Mexico, Cuba, Argentina, Brazil, Paraguay and Ecuador.

AETIOLOGY

Rhinosporidium seeberi is a spherical or oval non-motile organism which occurs in polypoid growths, usually lying between the connective tissue cells. The earliest stages are about 6 μm in diameter with a chitinous envelope, vacuolated cytoplasm and vesicular nucleus containing a karyosome. When fully grown, the cyst, or sporangium, may measure 0.25–3 mm in diameter. In early stages the nucleus commences to divide by binary fission, until thousands are produced, of which the majority become daughter spores, though a considerable proportion remain unchanged. The fully formed sporangium finally bursts and discharges the spores, which are enclosed in chitinous envelopes; they then spread into the connective tissues via the lymph channels and on reaching suitable spots the trophic stage at once begins and the cycle is repeated.

Attempts at cultivation proved partially successful in Ashworth's hands, and multiplication of the spores took place, but slowly, on Sabouraud's medium.

PATHOLOGY

The most striking feature is the presence in the stroma of polyps of numerous sharply defined globular cysts varying in size from 10 to 200 μm in diameter. There is a chronic inflammatory reaction and occasionally microabscesses occur. Eosinophils are inconspicuous.

CLINICAL FEATURES

Friable, highly vascular, sessile and pedunculated polyps may appear on almost any mucosal surface, but only rarely on the skin. Extension can occur beyond the mucocutaneous border. The nose, nasopharynx and soft palate are most commonly affected, but the eye, lacrimal sac and to a less extent the larynx, penis and vagina may also be involved.[47]

Multiple pedunculated tumours on the nose and face (Fig. 34.8) generally with secondary tumours on both feet, which ultimately became distributed over the whole body, have been described.[47] Haematogenous dissemination with

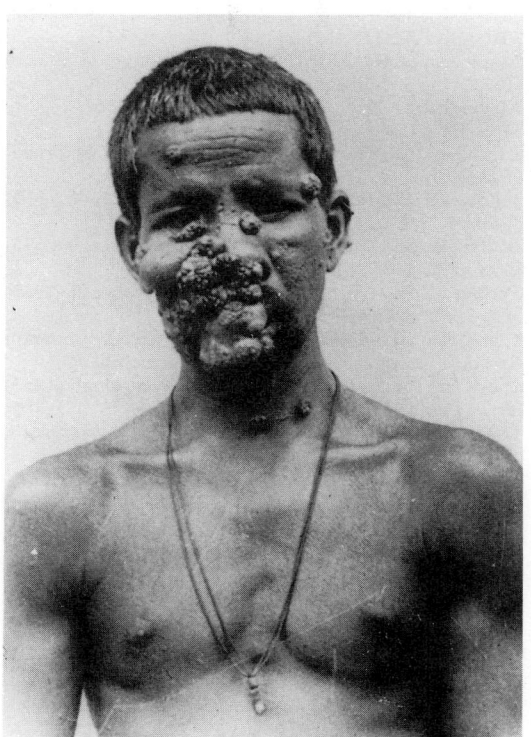

Fig. 34.8 Rhinosporidiosis involving the face.

rhinosporidial cells in the urine, peripheral blood and ascitic fluid has been described[48] and nodules on the palate and lower eyelid with visceral involvement of the lungs, liver, spleen and skin.[49]

DIFFERENTIAL DIAGNOSIS

Rhinosporidiosis must be differentiated from nasal polyps, and genital and anal lesions from warts, condylomata and haemorrhoids.

DIAGNOSIS

The diagnosis is made by demonstrating the sporangia up to 350 μm in diameter in sections of excised tissue. Culture and animal inoculation are unsuccessful.

TREATMENT

Treatment is essentially surgical and consists in removing the polyps from the nares by a wire snare. Pentavalent antimony compounds, as used by Allen and Dave[47], proved not always to be effective.

EPIDEMIOLOGY

Rhinosporidiosis is most often seen in children and young adults and in men more than women, but can also occur at any age. There are no racial differences in susceptibility. Infection is most often seen in labourers who are frequently exposed to water in streams and pools, and cases have occurred in groups of men diving to recover sand. This suggests that *R. seeberi* has a natural habitat in water, growing either as a saprophyte or as a parasite of fish or water insects. A closely related form, *R. equi*, has been found in the nasal cavities of horses and cattle and an organism closely resembling *R. seeberi* has been found in nasal polyps of two waterfowl in Zaire.[50]

REFERENCES

1 Mahgoub, E. S. & Murray, U. G. (1973) *Mycetoma*, London: Heinemann Medical.
2 Hay, R. J. & Mackenzie, D. W. R. (1982) *Trans. R. Soc. trop. Med. Hyg.* **77**, 49–50.
3 Abbott, P. (1956) *Trans. R. Soc. trop. Med. Hyg.* **50**, 11.
4 Renato, C. & Melo, I. S. (1975) *Revta Patol. Trop.* **4**, 49.
5 Baylet, J., Camain, R. & Segretain, G. (1959) *Bull. Soc. Path. éxot.* **52**, 448.
6 Courtois, G., de Loof, C., Thys, A. et al (1954) *Ann. Soc. belge Med. trop.* **34**, 371.
7 Baylet, J., Camain, R., Bezes, H. et al (1961) *Bull. Soc. Path. éxot.* **54**, 902.
8 Mahgoub, E. (1969) *J. trop. Med. Hyg.* **72**, 218.
9 Murray, I. G. (1966) *Trans. R. Soc. trop. Med. Hyg.* **60**, 554.
10 Mahgoub, E. S. (1975) *Pan. Am. Hlth Org. Sci. Pub.* 304.
11 Gumaa, S. A. & Mahgoub, E. S. (1975) *Sabouraudia* **13**, 309.
12 Gumaa, S. A. & Mahgoub, E. S. (1973) *J. trop. Med. Hyg.* **76**, 140.
13 Mahgoub, E. S. (1977) *Trans. R. Soc. trop. Med. Hyg.* **71**, 184.
14 Murray, I. G. & El Moghraby, I. (1964) *Trans. R. Soc. trop. Med. Hyg.* **58**, 557.
15 Hickey, B. B. (1956) *Trans. R. Soc. trop. Med. Hyg.* **50**, 393.
16 Peyron, J. P., Herouin, P., Lesquere, C. et al (1979) *Med. trop.* **39**, 27.
17 Woodward, B. H. (1982) *Southern med. J.* **75**, 229–230.
18 Kaapasari, J., Essen, R. V., Kahandaa, A. et al (1982) *Br. Med. J.* **285**, 923–924.
19 Mahgoub, E. S. (1976) *Bull. Wld Hlth Org.* **54**, 303.
20 Mahgoub, E. S. & Gumaa, S. A. (1984) *Trans. R. Soc. trop. Med. Hyg.* **78**, 376–379.

21 Buckley, H. R. & Murray, I. G. (1966) *Sabouraudia* **5,** 78.

22 Seeliger, H. P. R., Lacaz, C. da S. & Ulson, C. M. (1959) *VIth Int. Cong. trop. Med. Malar.* **4,** 636.

23 Gordon, M. A. & Al-Doory, Y. (1965) *Fonsecaea J. Bact.* **89,** 551.

24 Desai, C. S., Bhantikar, M. L. & Nehta, R. S. (1966) *Neurology, Bombay* **14,** 6.

25 Gugnani, H. C., Susehan, A. V., Nwokolo, C. et al (1977) *J. trop. Med. Hyg.* **80,** 177.

26 Whiting, D. A. & Cloete, G. N. P. (1968) *S. Afr. med. J.* **42,** 883.

27 Lopes, C. F., Alvarenga, R. J., Cisalpino, E. O. et al (1969) *Hospital, Rio de J.* **75,** 1335.

28 Bopp, C. (1974) *Dermatologia Mexico* **18,** 109.

29 Cuce, L. C., Wroclawski, E. L. & Samdaio, S. A. (1980) *Int. J. Derm.* **19,** 405–408.

30 Olle-Goig, J. E. & Domingo, J. (1983) *Trans. R. Soc. trop. Med. Hyg.* **77,** 773–774.

31 Wernsdorfer, R., Pereira, A. M., Goncalves, A. P. et al (1963) *Rev. Inst. Med. trop. São Paulo* **5,** 217.

32 Schneidau, J. D., Lamar, L. M. & Hauston, M. A. (1964) *J. Am. med. Ass.* **188,** 371.

33 Norden, A. (1951) *Acta path. microbiol. scand.*, Supplement 89.

34 Kaplan, W. & Ivens, M. S. (1960) *J. invest. Derm.* **35,** 51.

35 Jay, S. J., Platt, M. R. & Reynolds, C. R. (1977) *Am. Rev. resp. Dis.* **115,** 1051.

36 Marrocco, G. R., Thien, W. S., Goodnough, C. P. et al (1975) *Am. J. clin. Path.* **64,** 345.

37 Mackinnon, J. E. (1948) *Mycopathologia* **4,** 367.

38 Dreschler, C. (1956) *Mycologia* **48,** 655.

39 Lie-Kian-Joe, Eng, N. I. T., Rohan, A. et al (1956) *Archs Derm.* **74,** 378.

40 Jelliffe, D. B., Burkitt, D. P., O'Connor, G. T. et al (1961) *J. Pediat.* **59,** 124.

41 Ridley, D. S. & Wise, M. (1965) *J. Path. Bact.* **90,** 675.

42 Cornic, J. (1975) *Med. Trop.* **35,** 248.

43 Padhye, A. A., Ajello, L., Chandler, F. W. et al (1983) *Am. J. trop. Med. Hyg.* **32,** 799–803.

44 Clark, B. M. (1968) *Systemic Mycoses.* Ciba Foundation Symposium, pp. 179–197. London: Churchill.

45 Lie-Kian-Joe, Eng, N. I. T. & Sartona Kertopati (1957) *Archs Derm.* **75,** 864.

46 Davies, R. R. & Wilkinson, J. L. (1967) *Ann. trop. Med. Parasit.* **61,** 112.

47 Allen, F. R. W. K. & Dave, M. (1936) *Indian med. Gaz.* **71,** 276.

48 Rajam, J. V. (1955) *Indian J. Surg.* **17,** 269.

49 Agarwal, S., Sharma, K. D. & Shrivastan, J. B. (1959) *Archs Derm.* **80,** 22.

50 Fain, A. & Herrin, V. (1957) *Mycopath. Mycol. appl.* **8,** 54.

Chapter 35
Systemic Mycoses

The systemic mycoses are primarily contracted via the respiratory tract. They comprise histoplasmosis, coccidioidomycosis, paracoccidioidomycosis, blastomycosis and cryptococcosis.

Finally, there are fungi which are opportunistic and cause systemic infection in immunocompromised persons, systemic candidiasis.

HISTOPLASMOSIS

Histoplasmosis comprises two mycosal diseases: classic or small form histoplasmosis and large form or African histoplasmosis.

Classic or small form histoplasmosis

Classic histoplasmosis is an intracellular mycosis of the reticuloendothelial system involving lymphatic tissues, lung, liver, spleen, adrenals, kidneys, skin, central nervous system and other organs of the body. It may be asymptomatic, a benign acute or chronic pulmonary disease or widely disseminated and fatal.

GEOGRAPHICAL DISTRIBUTION

Histoplasmosis has been reported from 30 countries of the world and occurs in both temperate and tropical zones. It is chiefly a disease of the New World, particularly the USA. Sporadic cases and small groups of infection have been identified in the Old World—Australia, Austria, Belgium, Bulgaria, Great Britain, France, Germany, Holland, Spain, Turkey, India, Indonesia, Philippines, East Africa, South Africa and Portugal.

AETIOLOGY

Histoplasma capsulatum is a dimorphic fungus which grows within cells of the reticuloendothelial system (rarely in giant and polymorphonuclear cells) in the form of budding oval cells $2-3 \times 3-4 \mu$m. It grows readily on Sabouraud's medium at room temperature as a white to brown mould which reproduces by spherical smooth to spiny conidia $2-5 \mu$m in diameter and by spherical macroconidia $8-14 \mu$m in diameter. A yeast-like phase can be obtained by sowing the mycelial form on to blood agar and by incubating at 37°C. The mycelial phase only occurs below 34°C.

TRANSMISSION

Infection from human and animal cases does not occur. *Histoplasma capsulatum* is found in soil and man is usually infected by inhalation of spores from the soil. *Histoplasma* may be isolated from soil by culture or by exposing animals in cages in suspected caves or by the intraperitoneal injection of soil into mice.

PATHOLOGY

A primary lesion, the histoplasmoma ('coin lesion'), occurs at the site of infection and is followed in the majority of cases by healing without any signs, causing a subclinical infection. Healing may occur with calcification, which may appear in later life on X-ray examination of the chest. If the infection is heavy the development of delayed hypersensitivity is accompanied by pulmonary signs (benign pulmonary histoplasmosis) or more rarely the infection disseminates with lesions spread throughout the reticuloendothelial system.

The characteristic and diagnostic feature is the appearance of histoplasma cells. These are histiocytes containing the yeast form of the organism which appear as small spherical bodies measuring 1–5 μm in diameter averaging approximately 3 μm. In haematoxylin and eosin (H&E) sections they appear to have a rigid wall from which the protoplasm has been retracted by the fixative, giving the appearance of an unstained capsule (Fig. 35.1). Under low magnification the appearances closely resemble *Leishmania* and more superficially *Toxoplasma*, but they can be differentiated by periodic acid–Schiff stain (PAS) stain. They also have to be differentiated from other PAS-positive fungi: *Coccidioides immitis*, *Cryptococcus neoformans*, and *Blastomyces dermatitidis*. The characteristic cellular reaction is an epithelioid granuloma with or without Langhans' giant cells.

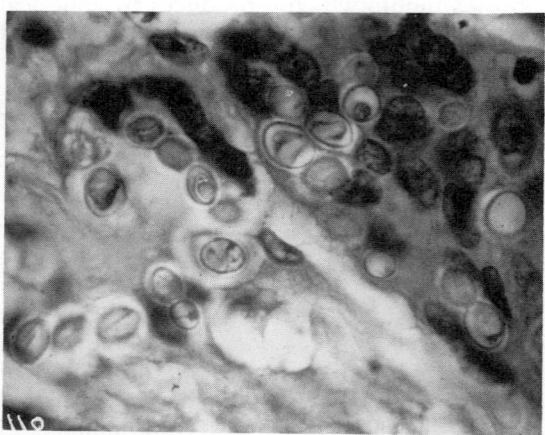

Fig. 35.1 *Histoplasma duboisii* in a skin section.

The solitary pulmonary nodule or histoplasmoma of primary histoplasmosis is situated just beneath the pleura and there is fibrous thickening on the pleural surface and the centre is caseous. Healing occurs by fibrosis and later calcification. All the demonstrable histoplasma cells are usually within the caseous part.

In fatal disseminated histoplasmosis the reticuloendothelial system is invaded by *Histoplasma* and histoplasma cells multiply in great numbers eroding and replacing the normal tissue. Lesions

may occur in any part of the body but chiefly the liver (Fig. 35.2), spleen, adrenals, lymph glands, mucous membrane of the mouth, gastrointestinal tract and bone marrow. Caseous necrosis develops especially in the adrenals but abscesses may occur anywhere in the body including the brain. Oropharyngeal lesions are not uncommon.

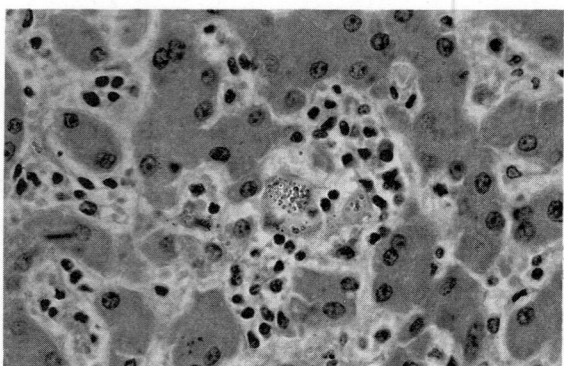

Fig. 35.2 *Histoplasma capsulatum* in the liver. (Courtesy Professor W. St C. Symmers.)

IMMUNITY

Most primary infections with *Histoplasma* are asymptomatic or benign with rapid recovery and a lasting immunity to reinfection. Immunity is both cellular and humoral. Cellular immunity develops along with delayed hypersensitivity and humoral immunity is shown by the presence of serum antibodies. 'Benign pulmonary histoplasmosis' is the result of a delayed hypersensitivity reaction.

Where the immune process breaks down or fails to develop, widely disseminated lesions result. Histoplasmosis is a common 'opportunist' infection.

Histoplasmin is a standardized preparation of a filtered culture autolysate of the mycelial form of *H. capsulatum* grown for several weeks in a chemically defined synthetic liquid medium at room temperature. The usual dilution is 1/1000. Both immediate (type 1) and delayed (type 4) reactions occur. Histoplasmin 0.1 ml is injected intradermally and the reaction read at 12, 48 and 72 hours. The minimum positive reaction is an area of induration 5 mm in diameter. The skin test with histoplasmin is capable of producing serum antibodies, and cross reactions with North

American blastomycosis are very strong. Serial skin tests which show a change from negative to positive during an illness may be diagnostic but a positive skin test merely means past infection. Serological tests in regular diagnostic use are the intradermal, complement fixation and precipitin tests.

Intradermal test

The first test to become positive is the intradermal reaction to histoplasmin which becomes positive within 2 to 20 days.

Complement fixation test

The antigens used are prepared in different ways either from the mycelial (histoplasmin) or yeast form. Tests should be performed with both types of antigen because some sera react with histoplasmin or with yeast cell antigen. Complement-fixing antibodies are found in moderately severe and severe cases about the end of the acute stage during the first one to three months. The antibody titre rises sharply and falls as steeply although a low titre may persist for a time and is proportional to the degree of infection; antibodies may never appear, may appear only transiently or may persist for months. Transient cross reactions occur with tuberculosis. A complement-fixing titre of 1 in 8 with either histoplasmin or yeast phase antigen is generally considered as presumptive evidence of histoplasmosis although not necessarily an active or present infection.[1]

Precipitin test

Precipitin tests in agar gel using concentrated histoplasmin have been reported.[2] Both specific (H) and non-specific (M) bands occur. M bands may be induced by histoplasmin skin testing but in the absence of a recent skin test the M band may be an early indication of disease.[3]

Latex agglutination test[4]

A commercial antigen has been used to coat latex particles and a titre of 1 in 32 or greater is significant and there were few false-positives. The antibodies appear earlier but do not persist so long as complement-fixing antibodies.

Fluorescent antibody test

Fluorescent antibody methods have been used to differentiate between *H. capsulatum* and *H. duboisii* and fluorescent antibody inhibition tests have proved to be simple and effective in detecting yeast antibody and in differentiating from other serologically related mycotic infections.[5]

Fluorescent antibody tests on sera in combination with agar gel precipitation tests allow early recognition of the true-positives among *H. capsulatum* reactive sera.

The serological response to *H. duboisii* is relatively weak in African histoplasmosis. The histoplasmin skin test may be negative even in proved cases.

CLINICAL FEATURES

Histoplasmosis is a universal infection in endemic areas, the majority of cases being asymptomatic. Acute histoplasmosis occurs in individuals exposed to heavy concentrations of airborne fungal spores (as in 'cave' disease).

Primary infection occurs in people visiting an endemic area for the first time. The incubation period is 10–18 days, there is a moderate to severe illness and scattered soft patchy pneumonic infiltrates which eventually calcify.

Reinfection acute histoplasmosis occurs in persons previously exposed. There is a shorter incubation period (3–7 days) and disseminated granulomas in the lungs resembling miliary tuberculosis.

Pulmonary histoplasmosis

Chronic pulmonary histoplasmosis is superimposed on pulmonary centrilobular or bullous emphysema.[6] In some instances a primary histoplasmosis may develop mediastinal granulomas characterized by confluence and encapsulation of the mediastinal lymph nodes with marked fibrinogenesis. The type of infection is thus determined by the resistance of the host, the previous experience of the infection and size of dose to which the host is exposed.

Benign pulmonary histoplasmosis resembles primary tuberculosis, is the form most commonly associated with 'epidemic' histoplasmosis ('cave' disease) and develops as a result of delayed hypersensitivity. The incubation period is 9–14 days and in the acute stage the symptoms are those of a moderately severe pneumonitis with lassitude, headache, fever, pains in the limbs and joints, backache, coryza and non-productive cough. There may be high fever with rigors and a persistent dyspnoea. There may be patchy dullness suggesting virus pneumonia and X-ray of the lungs shows widespread miliary nodules or localized groups of pea-sized nodules and a general increase in the bronchovascular shadows and enlarged hilar glands.

This acute stage lasts one to three weeks and is usually followed by complete recovery. All cases develop specific cutaneous hypersensitivity to histoplasmin in four to eight weeks after the onset of symptoms, which persists, and complement-fixing antibodies appear in the blood. Other forms of pulmonary histoplasmosis are a chronic infection with the development of fibrotic disease resembling phthisis, a mediastinal form resembling lymphoma and a diffuse interstitial form resembling miliary tuberculosis.

X-ray appearances show widespread diffuse 'fluffy' miliary mottling in the early stages, associated with hilar adenopathy and many large areas of consolidation, either widely disseminated miliary lesions or a lung lesion with mediastinal glandular enlargement. Healing occurs with either miliary calcification or a calcified focus with calcified hilar glands.

Disseminated histoplasmosis

Disseminated histoplasmosis is invariably associated with deficiency of some of the host's immune defence mechanisms.

This is a rare form and appears only sporadically. Symptoms include continued fever, sweating, malaise, weakness and loss of weight. A syndrome may result, closely resembling kala-azar, with fever, leukopenia and anaemia often of a severe form with involvement of the blood-forming organs and haemorrhage. The adrenals may be involved with symptoms of Addison's disease. In infants the blood picture resembles that of an 'aleukaemic leukaemia'.

Mucous membrane lesions are common and ulcerative lesions of the tongue, mouth and oropharynx may be the presenting signs of the infection.

Skin lesions may occur, sometimes papular and sometimes ulcerative.

A chronic meningitis lasting many years with H. capsulatum first isolated from the cerebrospinal fluid in 1959 has been described.[7]

Repeated courses of amphotericin B failed to control the infection. This form of the infection in the absence of underlying disseminated infection can be a chronic disease with few sequelae.

DIFFERENTIAL DIAGNOSIS

Histoplasmosis resembles a wide variety of infections. In its pulmonary form it can easily be mistaken for pulmonary tuberculosis; in its disseminated form for visceral leishmaniasis, disseminated tuberculosis, other disseminated granulomatous infections, other fungal infections such as coccidioidomycosis and paracoccidioidomycosis and Addison's disease. Any granulomatous tumour or focus anywhere in the body could be due to Histoplasma.

DIAGNOSIS

In the benign form diagnosis is by serology. Serological diagnosis is discussed in the section on immunity, above.

In the disseminated form examination of sputum, urine, excised lymph glands, ulcer base, bone marrow or peripheral blood may show Histoplasma. Smears and culture may be made from bone marrow aspirate and liver biopsy, while culture may be made from splenic aspirate.

Smears may be stained with Giemsa or Wright's stain. The fungus appears intracellularly within the macrophages or lying as an oval cell $2–3 \times 3–4\ \mu m$ with a large vacuole and a cup-shaped mass of red-stained protoplasm at the large end of the cell. The fungus may be isolated by culture on Emmons' modification of Sabouraud's medium (1% neopeptone, 2% glucose, 2% agar, pH 6.5–7); cultures should be incubated at or below 34°C.

Material may be mixed with penicillin and streptomycin and inoculated intraperitoneally into a mouse which should be killed two to four weeks after inoculation and cultures made from the liver and spleen.

TREATMENT

Ketoconazole is the drug of choice. It should be given in a daily dose of 200 mg after meals for as long as is necessary to effect a cure, however, it can be hepatotoxic (p. 1215).

Amphotericin B is a second line drug. It should

be started in a low daily dosage of 0.25 mg/kg body weight increasing to a maximum daily dose of 1 mg/kg body weight. Total dosage need not be more than 2 g. When the adrenals are involved supporting treatment with cortisone is necessary. In histoplasmosis caused by *H. capsulatum* a favourable response has been observed in some patients but relapses are frequent. In 29 cases of active histoplasmosis treatment with amphotericin B the total dosage varied between 600 mg and 2.1 g and lasted from three to six weeks to three to five months.

Of patients with severe histoplasmosis treated with amphotericin B 12 showed apparent recovery, 33 some improvement, nine relapsed, seven showed no change and two died.[8]

Trimethoprim–sulphamethoxazole (Septrin) and rifampicin are valuable adjuncts.[9] Septrin, two tablets three times a day for four weeks, is the usual course and a very satisfactory response was obtained[10] in *Histoplasma duboisii*.

Test of cure should include negative cultures and smears for *Histoplasma*, falling titres of complement-fixing antibodies and arrest or remission of lesions.

EPIDEMIOLOGY

Reservoirs of infection

Soil. Histoplasma has been isolated from the soil of chicken houses, caves, hollow trees and barnyard soil. Growth of the fungus is most frequently associated with the decayed or composted manure of chickens, birds or bats.

Animals. In the USA *H. capsulatum* has been found to cause natural infection in the dog, cat, brown rat, mouse, spotted skunk and opossum. Chickens cannot maintain the infection, although they may harbour it for a few weeks. Fourteen species of bats have been found naturally infected in America. The infections are systemic and bats are active reservoirs passing the organism in the faeces causing infected bat guano to be found in caves.[11] In Africa natural infection has been found in the baboon[12] and in Brazil *Histoplasma* was isolated by the inoculation of tissues from four rodents, *Proechimys guyanensis*, and a sloth, *Choloepus didactylus*, into hamsters.[13]

Endemicity

All age groups are affected with a maximum incidence in the second decade. Males are affected more than females.

Histoplasmosis is endemic in an enormous area in the Mississippi–Missouri–Ohio river valleys in a relatively mild and usually subclinical form. Histoplasmin skin testing has shown significant reactor rates in areas where histoplasmosis had not been expected. Histoplasmosis has a predominantly rural or village distribution and its occurrence is related to exposure to soils enriched by the faecal material of chickens, other birds and bats. Important urban sources of exposure have been shown by the isolation of *Histoplasma* from soil collected under trees used by starlings as roosting areas in cities.

Epidemics

Small epidemics of the benign pulmonary form of the disease occur in groups of persons infected through cleaning of chicken coops, pigeon lofts or disused silos. Others have been infected on visits to cellars or bat infested caves (cave disease). Outbreaks of histoplasmosis or cave disease have been reported in Venezuela, the Transvaal,[14] Zimbabwe[15] and Tanzania[16] where the benign pulmonary form has attacked caving expeditions.

CONTROL

Care should be taken not to expose oneself to infected caves, chicken houses and bird roosts. Protective immunization is not available.

African histoplasmosis (large cell histoplasmosis)

GEOGRAPHICAL DISTRIBUTION

Histoplasma duboisii[17] is confined mainly to the rain forest zone of West Africa extending to Uganda but has been found in Madagascar.[18]

AETIOLOGY

H. duboisii[17] can be distinguished from the classical form by the large size of the intracellular form which measures three or four times the size of

H. capsulatum (Fig. 35.1). The oval cells are 6–12 μm in length and are readily cultivated at 26°C on glucose agar and maltose agar producing white cottony colonies.

PATHOLOGY

The localized form of the disease may present as a solitary skin nodule or an isolated bone lesion but at the other extreme the disseminated form may involve the skin, subcutaneous tissues, lymph glands, bones, joints, lungs and abdominal viscera. A detailed classical description has been given.[19]

Skin and subcutaneous tissues

The skin granulomas may present as nodular, ulcerative, circinate, eczematous or psoriasiform lesions with a well-defined hyperpigmented halo surrounding them. In the disseminated form in the tissues these skin lesions are multiple and are continuously evolving.

Subcutaneous abscesses may arise from lesions in the underlying bone or independently. The abscesses present as firm, tender, hot swellings and the pus contains numerous yeast cells of *H. duboisii*.

Bone

The occurrence of bone lesions (Fig. 35.3) is an important feature. The bone lesions may be isolated or widespread in disseminated cases and are often asymptomatic and discovered only in the course of a radiological survey of the skeleton. When the abscess ruptures through the skin the resultant mass of granulation tissue may simulate a malignant neoplasm. Spontaneous fractures occasionally occur.[20]

Other lesions

Neurological complications may arise from compression of the spinal cord by lesions in the vertebrae. Lymphadenopathy is usually confined to the area of a local lesion but is generalized in the

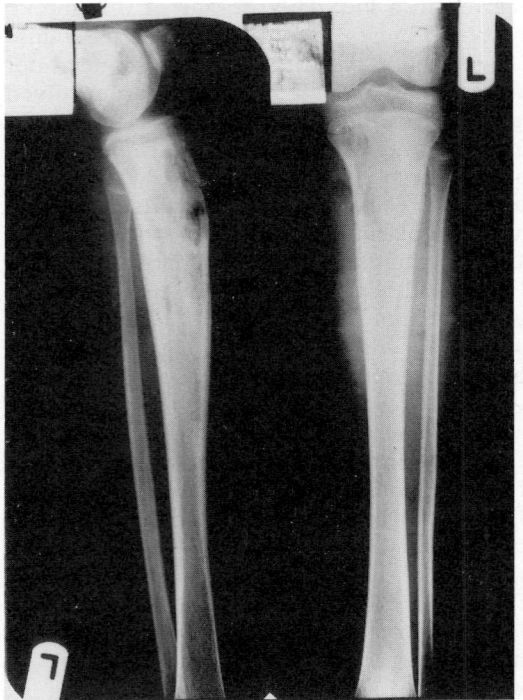

Fig. 35.3 Bone lesions of *Histoplasma duboisii* infection.

disseminated form. Abdominal visceral lesions may be found in the liver, spleen, bladder and large bowel. The manifestations have included abdominal pain with jaundice.[21] Systemic reaction with fever and rigors is often present in patients who have the disseminated form of the disease. Lungs are involved only rarely but cases have been recorded[22] and miliary lesions have been found in the lungs in the disseminated disease.

TREATMENT

Ketoconazole is the drug of choice. An oral dose of 200 mg daily for six weeks completely cured a case of African histoplasmosis with skin and bone involvement.[23] African histoplasmosis also responds quickly and well to amphotericin B.[19]

COCCIDIOIDOMYCOSIS

Coccidioidomycosis (Posada's disease, coccidioidal granuloma, valley fever, desert rheumatism) is an inapparent and benign or severe and fatal mycosis. It is respiratory in origin and in benign forms limited to the lung. In disseminated cases the infection spreads to other visceral organs and to the skin and subcutaneous tissues.[24]

GEOGRAPHICAL DISTRIBUTION

Coccidioidomycosis is limited to the western hemisphere where the area of highest endemicity is in Arizona and the San Joaquin valley of southern California. Other areas include New Mexico, south Texas, Nevada, Utah and northern Mexico. In Central America there are small areas in Guatemala and Honduras, and rare cases in El Salvador, in South America, Venezuela and the Chaco regions of Paraguay and Argentina. A few cases have been found in Bolivia and Colombia.

AETIOLOGY

Coccidioidomycosis is caused by *Coccidioides immitis* (Fig. 35.4), which is a dimorphic organism. The parasitic form is a spherical cell 30–60 μm in diameter (spherule) which does not bud but divides internally forming numerous endospores (2–5 μm in diameter) creating a multinucleate cell. The endospores are freed by rupture of the cell walls.

The mycelial form, which grows rapidly in culture on Sabouraud's and other media, grows

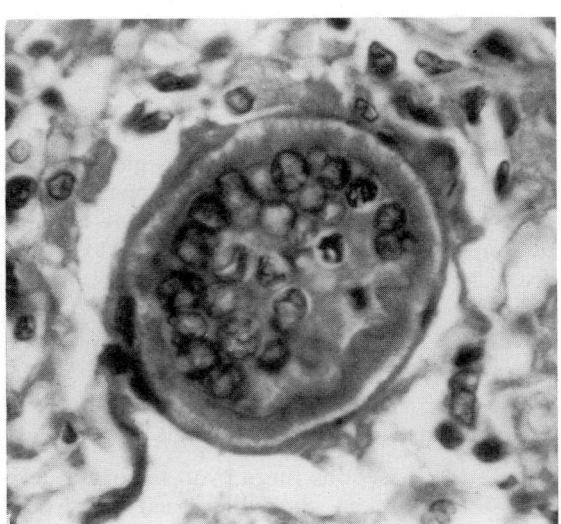

Fig. 35.4 Sporangium of *Coccidioides immitis*.

readily in soil, producing great numbers of arthrospores which are easily disseminated by air currents.

TRANSMISSION

Coccidioidomycosis is not contagious and infection is from exogenous sources. Man is infected via the respiratory route by the inhalation of arthrospores from the soil disseminated by air currents in endemic areas. Laboratory infections are common.

PATHOLOGY

Primary coccidioidomycosis is a benign self-limiting respiratory disease in the majority of cases. Progressive coccidioidomycosis is a relatively malignant disseminated infection involving cutaneous, subcutaneous, visceral and osseous tissues.

Primary lesion

The early lesions of coccidioidomycosis are indistinguishable from focal pulmonary pyogenic pneumonitis of bacterial origin except that spherules with endospores may be obtained in the lesions. The pyogenic reaction may be attributed to the released endospores, while the delayed hypersensitivity cellular response to the spherules is a granulomatous exudate with giant cells. Small developing spherules are seen intracellularly in histiocytes and giant cells; small released endospores are smaller than neutrophils and are difficult to identify with H & E stains. Both forms are readily seen with PAS.

Coccidioidal granuloma (coccidioidoma) is a solitary circumscribed pulmonary granuloma which closely resembles the solitary lesions found in tuberculosis and histoplasmosis. Calcification is not so pronounced and the diagnosis can only be made by identification of the causal agent.

Disseminated coccidioidomycosis

At autopsy lesions are widespread, involving lymph glands, spleen, skin, subcutaneous tissue, liver, kidney, bones, joints and meninges. The lesions may be miliary or extensive and the histological picture is a combination of suppuration and granulomatous cellular reaction in which many spherules may be demonstrated.

Central nervous system

The characteristic lesion is that of a diffuse granulomatous meningitis which encases the brain and may cause obstruction to the flow of cerebrospinal fluid. Small granulomatous lesions occur within the brain substance. In rapidly progressive cases the meningeal exudate is more suppurative in character. In some cases a fatal meningitis has been found in persons without any evidence of a pulmonary lesion.

IMMUNITY

Coccidioidomycosis is in the main an asymptomatic infection in which there is a primary infection followed by delayed hypersensitivity and recovery with permanent immunity. The recovered persons show hypersensitivity to coccidiodin. In white females allergic-type lesions of erythema nodosum and erythema multiforme may develop but these are rare in dark-skinned males. In a very small percentage of cases no resistance develops and there is disseminated spread.

Delayed hypersensitivity is measured by a skin reaction and circulating antibodies by complement fixation, immunodiffusion and fluorescent antibody tests. The most valuable tests are the skin test, complement fixation and precipitin tests. Coccidioidin is prepared from a pool of cultures of *C. immitis* grown under carefully standardized conditions[25] and is used as antigen for both skin hypersensitivity tests and circulating antibody.

Skin hypersensitivity is a delayed type (type 4) reaction and a positive reaction is manifested by an area of induration 5 mm or more at the site of intradermal injection of 0.1 ml coccidioidin. Reactivity develops 2 to 21 days (80% within a week) after the appearance of symptoms and persists for at least 20 years in persons who have left the endemic zones. The test is relatively specific, although a few patients react mildly to histoplasmin, blastomycin and paracoccidioidin. The degree of hypersensitivity is very great in patients with erythema nodosum. Reactivity to coccidioidin may decrease or disappear at the time of dissemination of the infection only to reappear with recovery. The coccidioidin skin test is of great diagnostic value and positive serological tests were not obtained in patients with primary coccidioidomycosis or with impending dissemination in the absence of a positive skin test.[26]

Spherulin derived from the spherule phase is more sensitive than coccidioidin and will detect approximately one-third more skin sensitive persons than coccidioidin.

Complement-fixing antibodies[26] are of the IgG type and appear late in the infection, not until three months after symptoms, and may never be detectable in asymptomatic and mild cases. When present they disappear in six to eight months. They are best used to detect disseminated disease in which they persist until death or after recovery, and a high and rising titre of complement-fixing antibodies indicates a poor prognosis.

Positive titres of 1 in 2 or 1 in 4 can be significant but have occasionally been obtained in patients not known to have coccidioidomycosis. Negative serological tests do not exclude the disease.

Precipitins are of the IgM type and appear in 50% within the first week and 90% by the third week. They disappear from 12 to 16 weeks after infection, even in disseminated disease. An immunodiffusion test has been perfected and gives a 95% accuracy.[27]

With a combination of complement fixation and immunodiffusion tests 90% of primary cases with clinical symptoms can be confirmed.[26]

Fluorescent antibody inhibition tests can be used for the rapid detection of antibodies to *C. immitis*.[28]

Immunization

A vaccine prepared from washed killed whole *Coccidioides immitis* spherules was given to volunteers and seroconversion and positive skin tests were obtained. Three injections—the first two one week apart, with a booster dose after six to seven weeks—were given with complete safety.[29]

CLINICAL INFECTIONS

Inapparent infections

In 60% of infections there is no history of anything which can be diagnosed as coccidioidomycosis. In these persons the diagnosis of past infection is based upon a positive skin reaction to coccidioidin. The remaining 40% develop a mild upper respiratory infection, primary pulmonary coccidioidomycosis and less than 0.5% disseminated infection.

Primary pulmonary coccidioidomycosis

This form is discussed by Richardson et al.[30] The incubation period is between 7 and 28 days. The onset is with fever, varying from a few hours (valley fever) to months in duration, which may be remittent, when eventual dissemination is more probable. The fever exhibits diurnal variation and sweats are common.

Pulmonary symptoms are frequent with pleuritic pains which may be severe, dyspnoea and cough, which may be productive with white purulent or bloodstained sputum. There may be no cough, however, even in the presence of pulmonary disease. The lungs may show pneumonic spread or pleural effusion with rales, signs of consolidation or pleural friction rub. There may be associated pericarditis. Later pulmonary cavitation may occur.

X-ray appearances are not specific but show patches of consolidation as nodular lesions 2–3 cm in diameter and widening of the hilar shadows although there is no peripheral lymphadenopathy. Calcified lesions may be found later after recovery.

Dermal lesions

Dermal lesions are caused by hypersensitivity. An early generalized macular erythematous rash in 10% of cases may precede the onset of sensitization.

Erythema nodosum and erythema multiforme (desert rheumatism) occur in about 20% of symptomatic cases, are observed most frequently in adult white females and denote a good prognosis. Erythema nodosum occurs as crops of bright red nodules on the anterior surface of the tibia and lasts a few days. Erythema multiforme on the thighs may be associated with joint pains. They are both accompanied by a pronounced eosinophilia.

Healed or residual coccidioidomycosis

Chronic pulmonary cavitation occurs in 2–8% of symptomatic infections, the chronic cavity is solitary, has a thin wall with little surrounding reaction and may contain fluid. It may be almost symptomless or associated with chest pain, cough and haemoptysis, and may persist for many years without dissemination. Coccidioidoma (coccidioma) is a benign residual granulomatous lesion in the lungs, varying in size, usually discovered by accident as a 'coin lesion', and is difficult to diagnose from carcinoma.

Cutaneous coccidioidomycosis

The skin lesions which have been described may be determined by local trauma but are almost certainly of primary pulmonary origin. The lesions ulcerate, exuding pus in which the organisms can be found, and after a few weeks become papillomatous. A scrofulodermic type of lesion is associated with the superficial cervical glands. Progressive coccidioidomycosis of the skin (Fig. 35.5) is found in the disseminated form of the disease.

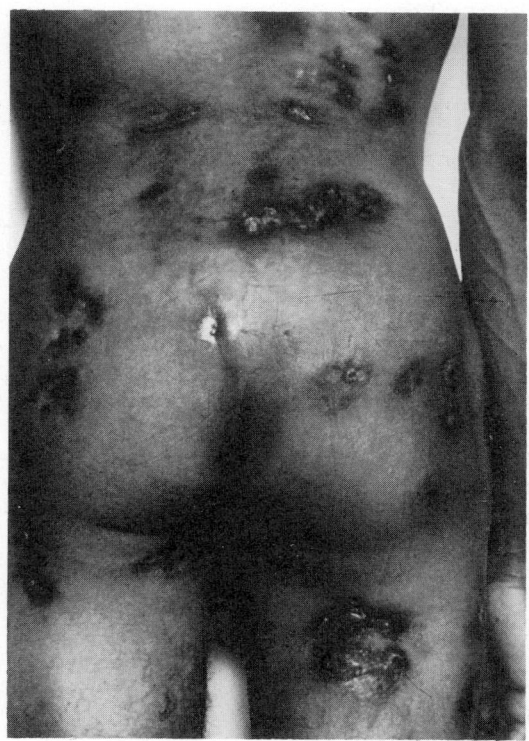

Fig. 35.5 Disseminated lesions of coccidioidomycosis on the back and buttocks.

Disseminated coccidioidomycosis

Massive dissemination following immediately after the primary infection occurs most often in Negroes and Filipinos. In other groups the dissemination is preceded by primary disease characterized by pneumonia, pleural effusion and high eosinophilia. There may be a remission but this is followed after a few days or weeks by recurrence of fever and a rise in titre of complement-fixing antibodies. Disseminated lesions may be found in skin, subcutaneous lesions, bones, joints and all visceral organs. The course of the disease is marked by remission and exacerbations with recovery or a slow or rapid progression. Acute miliary dissemination and meningitis are always fatal.

DIAGNOSIS

Direct examination of exudates may show the sporangia of *C. immitis* in sputum or pus prepared with sodium hydroxide and examined both with and without ink under the low-power microscope. Heat fixed stained films are of no value.

Culture of the organism may be made on Sabouraud's medium incubated at 25–30°C and kept for one or two weeks.

Animal inoculation of material into mice may be useful.

TREATMENT

Treatment is indicated in the disseminated disease. Amphotericin B is active against *C. immitis* when given by the intravenous route,[31] but relapses occur frequently. Surgical resection may be necessary for chronic residual pulmonary lesions. Miconazole is a potentially useful drug in the treatment of coccidioidomycosis. Up to 3.6 g daily can be given by intravenous infusion. Complete remission was obtained in three of 10 patients with coccidioidal

meningitis with systemic treatment combined with the direct injection of 20 mg into the cerebrospinal fluid where the drug persisted for at least 24 hours.[32]

Ketoconazole 400 mg daily has been successful in cases of disseminated lung and bone lesions, but not so successful in meningitis.

EPIDEMIOLOGY

Coccidioidomycosis is endemic in the Lower Sonoran life zone in the USA including areas of southern California, Arizona, New Mexico, south Texas and northern Mexico, which is characterized by a short but intense rainy season, high summer temperature and a characteristic association of certain plants, cacti and creosote bushes, with certain species of rodents, *Perognathus*, *Dipodimys* and *Citellus*. Similar areas also occur in the Chaco of northern Argentina and Paraguay.

Cases in other areas can be explained on the basis of fomites brought in from an endemic area. Many of the rodents have pulmonary lesions caused by *C. immitis* and play an important part in the maintenance of endemic infection and *C. immitis* can be isolated from both the soil and rodents.[33]

The greatest endemic focus is in the San Joaquin valley where skin tests have shown that 75–97% of children react positively to coccidioidin. No age group is immune and the condition is a mild disease of early childhood, most apparent in the adult migrant population. There is no evidence of sex or racial differences in susceptibility to infection but there is a marked difference in the occurrence of progressive and disseminated disease. About 1 in 400 adult white males develop granulomatous disease. In white females the rate is one-fifth of this and in male Negroes the rate is 10–15 times greater than in white males.

PARACOCCIDIOIDOMYCOSIS (SOUTH AMERICAN BLASTOMYCOSIS)

Paracoccidioidomycosis is also known as Brazilian blastomycosis, Lutz–Splendore–de Almeida disease and paracoccidioidal granuloma. It is a chronic mycosis characterized by ulcerative

granulomas of the buccal and nasal mucosa with extension to the skin by regional and generalized lymphadenopathy and by metastases to the lungs, spleen and other viscera.

GEOGRAPHICAL DISTRIBUTION

Paracoccidioidomycosis is an uncommon infection confined to the New World. Most of the reported cases have occurred from the state of São Paulo in Brazil but cases have been found in southern Mexico, Central and South America.

AETIOLOGY

Paracoccidioidomycosis is caused by a dimorphic fungus *Paracoccidioides brasiliensis* which grows in tissue cells (and often in giant cells) in the yeast form of spherical or oval cells which reach diameters of 30 μm and reproduce by budding (Fig. 35.6); the distinctive feature is the cell which bears buds (gemmules) 1–5 μm in diameter over the external surface (ectosporulation). This budding type of growth can be maintained *in vitro* by incubation at 37°C on blood agar. In culture at room temperature the mycelial form grows slowly on Sabouraud's medium.

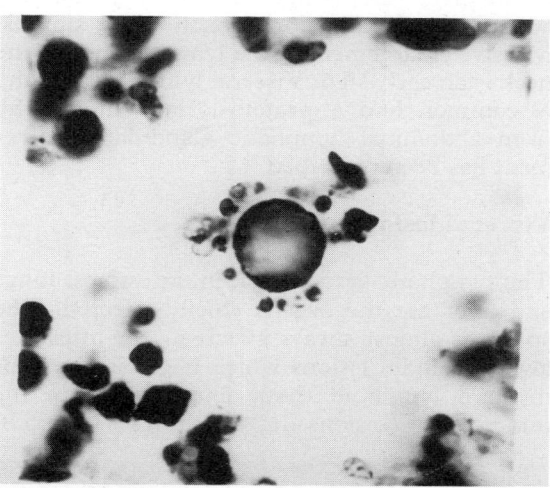

Fig. 35.6 Yeast forms of *Paracoccidioides brasiliensis* in the sputum.

TRANSMISSION

Clinical records and epidemiological studies suggest that this mycosis is not transmitted from person to person. The organism has been isolated from soil and primary lesions are usually on the buccal mucosa, suggesting the introduction of the fungus to these tissues by fragments of wood used in cleaning the teeth. It is also possible that primary infection of the lung occurs through inhalation.

PATHOLOGY

A characteristic feature is a tendency to involve lymphoid tissue, first in the lymph glands draining the lesions in the skin or mucous membranes and later by widespread involvement of lymphatic tissues including the spleen. Lesions of the intestinal tract are common. In the disseminated form of the disease granulomas are found in most organs, including the liver, heart, pancreas and kidney. Occasionally the caseous necrosis of the suprarenal glands resembles histoplasmosis. Osteomyelitis may occur. The central nervous system is rarely involved; there is a granulomatous basal meningitis with large numbers of giant cells containing *P. brasiliensis*.

IMMUNITY

Although benign cases of the disease are not known, patients who develop some resistance after a primary infection show delayed hypersensitivity, but disseminated cases are anergic and there is immunodepression in severe infections with a correlation between severity and immunodepression.[34]

Skin tests of delayed hypersensitivity (type 4) have been developed using a wide variety of culture filtrates and cellular antigens which have produced confusing results. A polysaccharide antigen[35] gave positive results in 87% of patients with confirmed disease. A positive result produced a small granuloma of foreign body type beneath the epithelium after 10–15 days.[36] Positive tests may be expected in clinically well people living in endemic areas and the test can distinguish between paracoccidioidomycosis, cutaneous leishmaniasis and sporotrichosis.

Complement-fixing antibodies (IgG) using the polysaccharide antigen are present in the highest titre in disseminated disease and in low titre or negative in localized disease.[35] A combination of complement fixation and precipitin tests demonstrated antibodies in 98.4% of patients. Complement-fixing antibodies persist for a long time but decrease in titre in cured patients. Cross reactions occur with histoplasmosis but higher titres are found with the homologous antigen.

Precipitating antibodies (IgM) demonstrated

by agar gel precipitation using a concentrated culture filtrate of the yeast phase as antigen are the first antibodies to appear and disappear.[37] No cross reactions occur with North American blastomycosis, histoplasmosis, coccidioidomycosis, sporotrichosis, tuberculosis or healthy individuals.

CLINICAL FEATURES

The incubation period is usually very prolonged, between five and nine years.[38] There are four main clinical types.

Mucosal lesions

The primary lesion is usually in the nasal or oral mucosa (gums) but may be in the conjunctiva or the anorectal mucosa. A severe ulcerative painful stomatitis develops which may extend to the tonsils. Mucosal lesions of the oronasal junction resemble espundia (Fig. 35.7). Laryngeal lesions

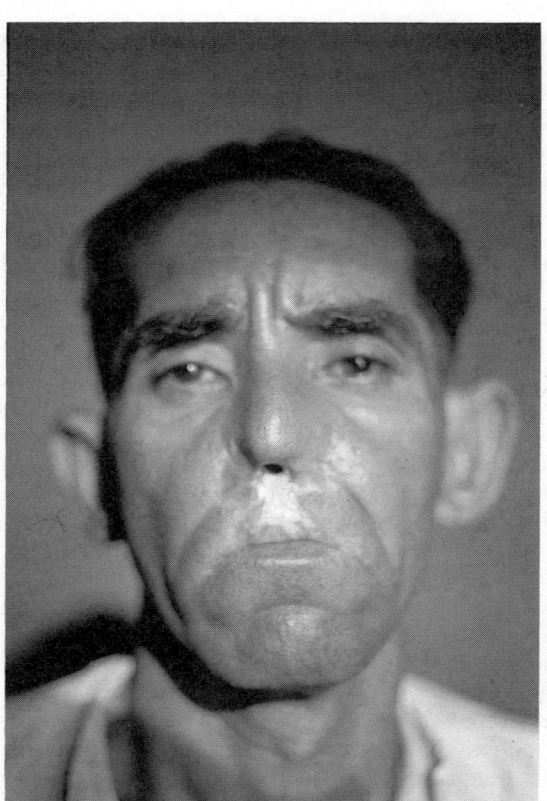

Fig. 35.7 Mucosal lesions (healing) of paracoccidioidomycosis.

are usually secondary to the pulmonary lesions and may cause great diagnostic difficulty because of the close resemblance to tuberculosis. The appearance is that of hyperaemia, oedema, ulceration and granulations on the epiglottis and vocal cords. Gingival lesions are accompanied by ulceration and spontaneous loss of teeth, and lesions may develop on the tongue.

Cutaneous lesions

The typical lesions are an ulcerative and crusted granuloma of the skin arising by direct extension from the mucosal lesions or by autoinoculation. Spread to the skin may also take place via the blood and lymph channels. Occasionally a solitary pustular lesion may represent a primary implantation of the fungus.

Lymphatic lesions

The lymphatics draining the primary lesion are invariably involved. The cervical lymph glands are involved early. They are painlessly enlarged, adherent and may suppurate, forming sinuses. Massive enlargement of the lymph glands of the neck is an early sign. Visceral lymphadenopathy is common and a protein-losing enteropathy from abdominal lymphatic glandular involvement has been described.[39]

Visceral lesions

The lymphatic system, spleen, intestines, lungs and liver are the organs chiefly affected. The spleen is almost always affected. The intestines always contain lesions which begin in the submucosal lymphoid tissue and erode into the lumen. The lesions in the lungs (Fig. 35.8)

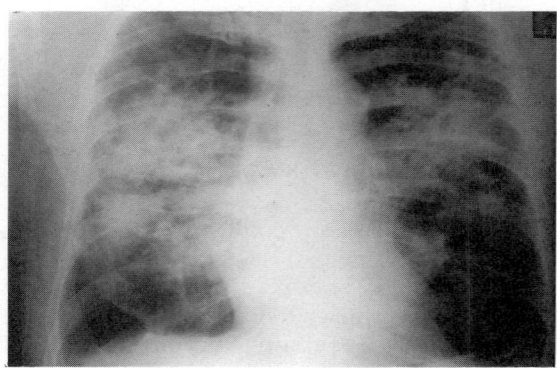

Fig. 35.8 Pulmonary lesions of paracoccidioidomycosis.

resemble those of pulmonary tuberculosis and involve chiefly the apex. Diffuse hilar lesions also occur.

X-ray appearances are those of nodular lesions, patchy infiltration, fibrosis and emphysema. Ventilatory studies show an obstructive form of respiratory insufficiency.

The adrenals may be affected. Osteolytic lesions of the bones may be found and lesions of the central nervous system may predominate with a high protein content in the cerebrospinal fluid caused by basal meningitis. Anal, rectal and penile lesions also occur.

DIAGNOSIS

Paracoccidioidomycosis differs from blastomycosis in its predilection for the mucosal tissues, in the frequency of gingival lesions, in a tendency to central healing and in regional and generalized lymphadenopathy. It must also be differentiated from tuberculous adenitis, cutaneous tuberculosis, syphilis, yaws, sporotrichosis and leishmaniasis, which it closely resembles but in which the lungs remain free. The diagnosis is made by examination of fresh sputum and other discharges for the typical spherical or oval cells with external buds.

The fungus may be cultured on blood agar incubated at 37°C or as the mycelial form on Sabouraud's medium.

Serodiagnosis

The skin test is of little use. The complement fixation test is satisfactory (see section on Immunity, p. 701).

Although a benign form of the disease is suspected, clinical cases of the disease as actually known are fatal unless effective treatment is given.

TREATMENT

Ketoconazole

Ketoconazole is the treatment of choice; 400 mg daily for ·90 days followed by maintenance therapy of 200 mg three times daily for 10 months was curative[40] (but see p. 1215).

Other drugs

Most clinical forms of the disease except lymphoidal and central nervous system disease may be kept in remission by maintaining a serum level of 5 mg/100 ml of sulphonamide. This is achieved by the use of long-acting sulphonamides. However, relapse follows cessation of therapy.

Sulfadoxine (Fanasil) 1 g daily for 10 days followed by 2 g weekly gave the best results[41] and should be continued for one to two years. Resistance to sulphonamide therapy may develop.

Trimethoprim has been used in conjunction with sulphonamides as Septrin, especially in the treatment of sulphonamide-resistant cases.[42]

Amphotericin B gives good results and should be used in all severe forms of the disease especially where the central nervous system is involved. It is given in the usual way to a total dosage of 2 g (see p. 745).

Miconazole has been used very successfully in the treatment of both localized and disseminated paracoccidioidomycosis intravenously in a dose of 0.6 or 1.2 g daily for 25–44 days. It may be feasible to give the drug orally for longer periods.[32]

Complications

Complications of treatment can occur from sensitivity to the organism developing during treatment of pulmonary disease with asthma which may necessitate the use of steroids to control it.

The results of treatment are followed by observations on the presence of the fungus in sputum and tissue, radiological appearances of the lungs and the titre of complement-fixing antibodies.

EPIDEMIOLOGY

No animal reservoir is known and the organism probably lives saprophytically in the soil. Paracoccidioidomycosis is confined to South America. Most of the reported cases have been from the state of São Paulo, Brazil, but it occurs not uncommonly elsewhere in Brazil and has been reported from all South American countries. It occurs at all ages but with the highest incidence between 30 and 50 years of age. Skin test surveys show that in endemic areas a substantial proportion of the population have positive tests suggesting that subclinical infections are common.

KELOIDAL BLASTOMYCOSIS (LOBO'S DISEASE)

Keloidal blastomycosis is a localized cutaneous benign process observed primarily in the Amazon and Orinoco river areas,[43] but also in Surinam and Costa Rica. About 69 cases have been observed to date. Clinically it is a mycosis characterized by keloidal skin lesions without lymphangitis or visceral dissemination. The disease is probably distinct and a clinical variant and the fungus is called *Loboa loboi*.

BLASTOMYCOSIS (NORTH AMERICAN BLASTOMYCOSIS)

Blastomycosis (Gilchrist's disease) is a chronic granulomatous and suppurative disease which originates as a respiratory infection and disseminates usually with pulmonary, osseous and cutaneous involvement predominating.

GEOGRAPHICAL DISTRIBUTION

This mycosis is almost entirely American in distribution extending southwards from North America to Mexico and Central America, with a few cases in South America, but recently verified cases have been reported from the Middle East, Zaire, South Africa, Tunisia and Uganda[44] and it is an important cause of deep systemic mycoses in Mashonaland in Zimbabwe.[45]

AETIOLOGY

The cause of blastomycosis is *Blastomyces dermatitidis*, a dimorphic fungus which grows in mammalian tissues as budding cells 8–15 μm in diameter (rarely reaching 30 μm) and in culture as a dry white mould, bearing spherical or ovoid conidia 2–10 μm in diameter or short slender conidiophores. The parasite grows *in vitro* by incubation at 37°C on blood agar. Budding is usually single and *Blastomyces* differs from *Histoplasma* and *Cryptococcus* by its multinucleate condition.

TRANSMISSION

The exact form of transmission is unknown. There is no evidence of transmission to patient contacts. Occasional cases have been attributed to fomites.

PATHOLOGY

There are two main types of blastomycosis, systemic and cutaneous. The primary lesions occur in the lungs. The characteristic response to *Blastomyces dermatitidis* is a combination of suppuration and epithelioid cell granulomatous reaction with giant cells. The reaction closely resembles tuberculosis or histoplasmosis with extensive caseous necrosis. The fungus can be demonstrated as a rounded intracellular body 8–15 μm in diameter with the protoplasm shrunk away from the cell wall leaving a clear space. Budding is difficult to demonstrate.

IMMUNITY

There is a well-marked cellular immune response with delayed hypersensitivity which is responsible for the pathology and a humoral response of antibodies used for diagnosis. Four basic antigens have been used: culture filtrates of a broth supporting the mycelial phase (blastomycin), extracts of mycelium, suspension of yeast phase cells and extract of yeast phase cells. There is considerable antigenic overlap with *Histoplasma capsulatum* and *Coccidioides immitis*. From the diagnostic point of view serological results have proved disappointing owing to the large percentage of negative reactions and the incidence of cross reactions. Blastomycin has been used in skin tests but is frequently associated with histoplasmin reactivity and has been regarded as useless. Using a heat-killed yeast phase antigen, positive reactions were obtained in 84% of active cases.[46]

The complement fixation test is unsatisfactory, confirmed diagnosis being obtained in only 46% of tests with blastomycin.[47] An antigen from yeast phase cells gave a positive result in 71% of affected patients but cross reacted with *H. capsulatum*.

Precipitins against blastomycin were present in the sera of 14 of 22 patients with blastomycosis and could be distinguished from the cross reactions occurring with coccidioidomycosis and histoplasmosis.[48]

CLINICAL FEATURES

Pulmonary blastomycosis

Primary pulmonary blastomycosis begins as a mild respiratory infection which progresses with dry cough, hoarseness and low grade fever. The symptoms and signs closely resemble those of pulmonary tuberculosis with increasing blood-stained sputum, dyspnoea, loss of weight, fever and night sweats. Features of the adult respiratory distress syndrome with diffuse pulmonary infiltration, pulmonary oedema, poor lung compliance and refractory hypoxaemia have been ascribed to *B. dermatitidis*.[49]

X-ray examination of the chest shows widespread miliary lesions, homogeneous consolidation, solitary or multiple nodular shadows or abscesses or fibrotic lesions. Cavitation is rare.[50]

Systemic blastomycosis

In the systemic infection there is involvement of the skin, subcutaneous tissues, respiratory organs, bones, urogenital canal and central nervous system. The gastrointestinal tract is rarely involved. Dissemination to the skin is common.

Cutaneous blastomycosis

The presenting complaint of many patients is in the skin. The infection may start as a papule or pustule which ulcerates and develops into an ulcerated or warty granuloma. Characteristic organisms can be demonstrated in the pus. The lesions spread slowly over a period of months or years leaving their atrophic scars in the centre. Cutaneous lesions associated with bone lesions are sinuses.

Course of the disease

Cutaneous blastomycosis is very chronic and indolent and the lesions may clear up with antifungal treatment without cure of the deep mycosis.

In the widely disseminated disease the prognosis is poor in spite of treatment.

DIAGNOSIS

Blastomycosis must be differentiated from squamous cell carcinoma, mucosal leishmaniasis and paracoccidioidomycosis. Laryngeal blastomycosis is very like laryngeal epidermoid carcinoma. The diagnosis may be made by biopsy and the characteristic pathology and by culturing the fungus from sputum, pus and biopsy material. Tissue may be stained with PAS to show up the fungi. Skin and serological tests are of little use.

TREATMENT

Ketoconazole has been used successfully in a dose of 400 mg daily in treatment of the cutaneous lesions.

Hydroxystilbamidine isethionate has been used successfully in some cases in intravenous doses of 150–200 mg daily for 30 days at a time. Courses may be repeated. Many cases relapse.

Amphotericin B is preferable and should be given in standard doses (see p. 745) up to a total of 2 g. A smaller percentage of patients relapse.

Experimentally, 81 cases were treated with diamidines and 30 with amphotericin B; 15 were treated with both drugs; 54 (67%) were arrested by diamidines and five (6%) died; 27 (90%) were arrested by amphotericin B and two (7%) died. Using both drugs 12 of 15 were arrested and two died.[8]

EPIDEMIOLOGY

The occurrence of benign respiratory forms of North American blastomycosis has not yet been proved. Cases of the established disease are sporadic in incidence and when groups of cases have occurred these have been small. Natural infection has been recorded in dogs and the infection is probably saprophytic from the soil, yet the fungus has never been isolated from soil. Blastomycosis occurs at all ages with a slightly higher incidence in the third and fourth decades; males are affected nine times as frequently as females.

CRYPTOCOCCOSIS

Cryptococcosis (torulosis, European blasto-mycosis, Busse–Buschke disease) is an acute, subacute or chronic pulmonary, systemic or meningeal mycosis caused by *Cryptococcus neo-formans*.

GEOGRAPHICAL DISTRIBUTION

C. neoformans occurs in both temperate and trop-ical countries especially throughout South America, Africa, India and the Far East. Most human cases have been recorded from North America.

AETIOLOGY

C. neoformans is seen as a thick-walled spherical cell surrounded by a wide capsular structure of mucoid character which is less refractile than the cell.

Mounted in a suspension of China ink or nigrosin the cell is seen to measure 5–15 μm in diameter, occasionally up to 20–30 μm, and the entire parasite with its capsule 15–45 μm in diam-eter. The young cryptococci are easily stained by Gram's stain but the best differentiating stain is mucicarmine with haematoxylin, which colours the cell wall an intense red and the contents and capsule a faint pink. The parasite multiplies by gemmation, does not produce endospores or mycelium and can be cultivated in glucose broth or Sabouraud's medium at 37°C. The colonies are honey-coloured and semifluid.

C. neoformans has been divided into a number of serotypes;[51] the capsular polysaccharides are antigenic and cross reactions are found with *Candida albicans* and other fungi as well as types 2 and 14 pneumococci.

TRANSMISSION

Cryptococcosis is not contagious and *C. neo-formans* cannot be isolated easily from the skin, mucous surfaces or faeces of man. *C. neoformans* grows frequently in accumulations of pigeon droppings, and inhalation of cells of cryptococci and infection of the respiratory tract from this source is probably the usual method of infection.

PATHOLOGY

The portal of entry is most likely the lung with haematogenous spread to the skin, bones, abdominal viscera and especially the central nervous system.

Benign pulmonary cryptococcosis

A few sporadic cases of a pneumonic form of cryptococcosis have been reported. Benign pul-monary cryptococcosis may be found only at autopsy by finding a small encapsulated healed granuloma.

Pulmonary cryptococcosis

The histological reaction in the lung may be a marked cellular reaction indistinguishable from those of other granulomatous diseases. Where the cellular reaction is slight the cryptococci are numerous and there is a mucoid quality of the lesion suggesting a myxomatous condition.

The 'primary' pulmonary lesion, a solitary cryptococcal granuloma, may be seen as a nodule 1–7 cm in diameter near the pleural surface. It is sharply circumscribed but does not have a thick or calcified wall.

Cryptococcus lesions present histologically as pure histiocytic granulomas with large mono- or multinucleate histiocytes supported by a delicate vascular stroma containing spherical or oval bodies without visible internal structure but a clear halo 3–5 μm in thickness separating the fungus wall from the cytoplasm of the histiocyte. In actively growing lesions budding cells are found. In progressive infection there are miliary granulomas, small abscesses or large solid or mucoid lesions varying from granulomatous to pure mucoid reaction involving one or more lobes of the lung.

Central nervous system

Gross changes are usually minimal. The arach-noid space contains adherent mucoid exudate. A coronal section shows numerous gelatinous or myxoid foci predominantly located in the grey matter. Tumour-like granulomas may be found. Microscopically the lesions contain great numbers of thickly capsulated cryptococci and the almost total absence of any inflammatory reaction.

Cryptococci reach the brain through the bloodstream or from the subarachnoid space along the perivascular lymph channels or the cortical branches of the pial vessels. The cryptococci multiply in these channels within endothelial and multinucleate cells and also extracellularly and form a gelatinous nodule around the little vessels. These nodules usually multiply and increase in size and coalesce, causing pressure atrophy of the surrounding and intervening brain tissue.

IMMUNITY

Although there is some evidence that man can be resistant to infection there is no evidence that an initial benign exposure immunizes man against subsequent exposure. Most mammals have a high degree of innate resistance to infection and there is a relatively high incidence of cryptococcosis in people with disorders of the reticuloendothelial system, which suggests that a humoral mechanism is involved in this resistance, and cryptococcosis is an 'opportunist' infection occurring with immunosuppression whether from therapy or from Hodgkin's disease and other immunosuppressive conditions.

CLINICAL FEATURES

Natural history

Subclinical cryptococcosis is quite frequent and skin tests have shown 48% of the healthy population may be sensitized.[52] Progressive disease seldom follows inhalation of the organism and a subacute pulmonary form may resolve without chemotherapy but overt cryptococcosis carries a high fatality rate.

The *incubation period* is unknown.

Symptoms and signs

Three main forms of infection present: pulmonary, central nervous system and dermal cryptococcosis. Cryptococcosis most frequently presents as a meningitis.

Pulmonary cryptococcosis

A subacute form which resolves naturally does

occur, with fever, cough and lung shadows seen on radiography which later resolve.

PRIMARY FOCUS
A primary lung focus forms which may resolve spontaneously or form a well-circumscribed granuloma or cryptococcoma which may be detected on a routine chest X-ray.

DIFFUSE PULMONARY CRYPTOCOCCOSIS
The disease spreads and is accompanied by cough and scanty blood-tinged sputum. Low grade fever, malaise and loss of weight may occur. There may be signs of bronchitis, consolidation or pleural effusion, all closely resembling pulmonary tuberculosis. X-ray appearances are not diagnostic. Spherical or oval tumour-like masses may resemble a neoplasm. There is no hilar gland enlargement, caseation or calcification but these changes may be obscured by surrounding cavitation.[53]

Extrapulmonary infections follow dissemination from the lungs, meningitis, dermal lesions and visceral spread.

Central nervous system cryptococcis

This closely resembles tuberculous meningitis. The onset is usually insidious and the course chronic. The first symptom is intermittent headaches increasing in frequency and severity without any previous pulmonary symptoms, associated with the development of granulomatous lesions of the meninges. More rarely there is a sudden severe onset indicating the presence of rapidly spreading cerebral lesions. The signs are those of chronic meningitis with low grade fever and neck stiffness. There are general

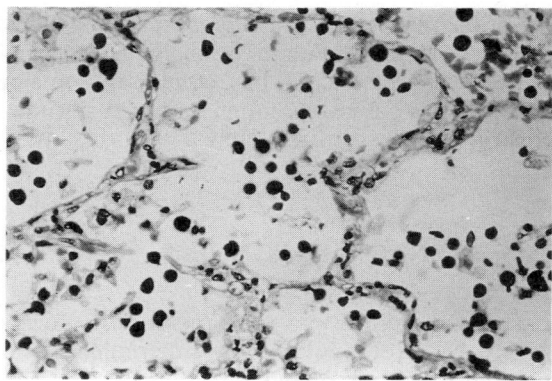

Fig. 35.9 Cryptococci stained by silver impregnation.

signs of meningitis with changes in personality and local signs which may include papilloedema, amblyopia, oculomotor paresis and optic atrophy. The duration varies from a few months to 15 or 20 years. The cerebrospinal fluid shows a raised protein content with reduced glucose and chlorides. There is a lymphocytosis as in tuberculous meningitis. The cryptococci may be present in abundance but may only be demonstrated by washing the deposit in saline and mounting in China ink to show up the particles (Fig. 35.9). In periods of remission cryptococci may be present in the cerebrospinal fluid although cultures may remain negative.

Dermal cryptococcosis

This is usually associated with a systemic infection but cases have been diagnosed without previous pulmonary infection. The skin lesions may be papules, pustules or subcutaneous abscesses which ulcerate. The ulcers may be solitary or multiple and may resemble carcinoma. Similar lesions may occur on the oral or nasal mucosa.

Involvement of bones

Bone involvement occurs in 10% of reported cases. They are associated with pain and swelling of many months' duration and are osteolytic, often spreading to the skin. The cryptococci can be demonstrated only with difficulty in the glairy pus. Biopsy material can be mistaken for Hodgkin's disease unless special stains are used to demonstrate the cryptococci.

Visceral spread

Infection may spread to any part of the body where the granulomatous lesions bear a resemblance to carcinoma. Cryptococcal granuloma of the breasts is a rare phenomenon in man. Endocarditis is a rare manifestation.

DIFFERENTIAL DIAGNOSIS

Both the pulmonary and meningitic forms closely resemble pulmonary tuberculosis and meningitis. Other fungal infections are benign pulmonary histoplasmosis and blastomycosis.

DIAGNOSIS

The organism is best seen using a capsular stain, the China ink or silver impregnation method (Fig. 35.9). Cryptococci can be so numerous in the cerebrospinal fluid deposit that they can be mistaken for dust particles contaminating the slide. The organism can be cultured on glucose agar or Sabouraud's medium at 37°C to distinguish it from non-pathogenic fungi. Identification can be obtained by mouse inoculation.

Serological diagnosis

The most helpful test is the latex test for cryptococcal polysaccharide antigen in the serum or cerebrospinal fluid. It is positive in 96% of cases and is useful in prognosis as well as diagnosis since a fall in antigen titre in the cerebrospinal fluid is a good prognostic sign.[54]

Fluorescent antibody techniques have been used to detect the presence of cryptococcal polysaccharide lining the bronchial epithelium and in alveolar exudate and macrophages in a granulomatous reaction.[55]

Fluorescent antibodies have been demonstrated in the sera of seven of eight proved cases of cryptococcosis but false-positive reactions were obtained with *C. albicans* sera[56] and positive reactions were reported in 18 of 23 patients with proved cryptococcosis.[3]

Skin tests of delayed hypersensitivity type have not yet proved of any use in the diagnosis of infection.

TREATMENT

Combined amphotericin B and flucytosine is the treatment of choice.

Amphotericin B is given as a total dose of 2 g over an extended period (see Section 17).

Flucytosine (Fluorocytosine) is given in a dose of 2–4 g orally daily for seven to 40 weeks.

Miconazole has been used successfully in meningitis in a dose of 0.6–1.2 g intravenously daily for 25–44 days.[57]

Ketoconazole has shown promise in mice[58] but experience has been patchy and not all cases, especially meningitis, respond.

It is very difficult to assess cure since cryptococci may disappear from the cerebrospinal fluid for long periods, up to one year, only to reappear at a later date.

EPIDEMIOLOGY

Cryptococcosis is worldwide in distribution and all ages, sexes, races and occupations may be affected.

Reservoirs of infection

Soil reservoir

Emmons[59] found a frequent saprophytic association of *C. neoformans* with pigeon manure; it has been isolated frequently from old nests and excreta under roosting sites of pigeons in the upper floors of buildings in cities and in stables in rural areas. Accumulations of pigeon droppings are the most important source of the fungus.

Animal reservoir

Cryptococcosis has been described in the horse, rat, mouse, dog, cat, tiger, cheetah, marmoset, monkey, cow, koala and domestic pigeon. Extensive outbreaks of cryptococcal mastitis have been reported in dairy herds in the USA.[60] The infection was transmitted through the suction cups of milking machines and the disease was generally confined to the udder. Nevertheless, there is no evidence that the disease in lower animals is a source of direct infection of man.

CANDIDIASIS

Candidiasis is also known as moniliasis, thrush, *Candida* perionychia, *Candida* endocarditis, bronchomycosis and mycotic vulvovaginitis. It is an acute, chronic, superficial or disseminated mycosis caused by species of *Candida*.

GEOGRAPHICAL DISTRIBUTION

Candidiasis is a worldwide infection.

AETIOLOGY

Candida albicans is the most frequent cause of any of the clinical types of the mycosis but *C. parapsilosis*, *C. krusei*, *C. tropicalis* and *C. stellatoidea* may also be responsible.

C. albicans grows on corn meal as spherical macroconidia (chlamydospores), $8-12\,\mu m$ in diameter, and characteristic spherical clusters of blastospores or yeasts. Fermentative reactions are useful in differentiating species of *Candida*.

TRANSMISSION

C. albicans is a frequent commensal in the alimentary canal and transmission is by direct inoculation on to the mucous surfaces of the mouth, vulva or intestines, from which systemic spread may occur rarely.

PATHOLOGY

In autopsy material *Candida* may be seen in superficial ulcers of the mucous membrane of the alimentary tract developing in the last stages of a terminal illness.

Systemic candidiasis

In this form the lesions caused are widespread, occurring as microabscesses in lungs, heart, kidney, brain and other organs. In candidiasis endocarditis the exuberant vegetations contain large numbers of hyphae and blastospores. Meningitis and intracranial candidiasis have been described.[61] The histological picture of terminal candidiasis is that of focal suppuration with the formation of small abscesses in which neutrophils abound.

Granulomatous form

Chronic granulomatous lesions occur in the mouth, skin and nails, causing leukoplakia-like lesions with ulceration and deforming scars. It starts in infancy or early childhood and is associated with debilitating conditions and nutritional deficiencies. It lasts until early adult life when death occurs from intercurrent disease.

Pulmonary candidiasis

This is a frequent terminal infection in pulmonary tuberculosis as an extension from the mouth and has not been recognized as a primary disease. Complete casts of the bronchial tree have been recorded in pulmonary candidiasis.

Alimentary candidiasis

Alimentary infection occurs as a local or general invasion of the alimentary mucosa followed by a *Candida* septicaemia as a terminal event in diabetics and others suffering from chronic cachexial conditions. Alimentary candidiasis provoked by antibiotic therapy may lead to systemic infection of various organs and sometimes embolism and infarction. The pathogenicity of these fungi in the deeper tissues is not great, so that if the alimentary infection is treated with nystatin, spontaneous cure will occur.[62]

IMMUNITY

Man is normally resistant to infection with *Candida* which usually causes a local infection of the skin, nails and mucous membranes, but where the immune response has been altered by the presence of lymphoma or leukaemia or suppressed by immunosuppressive drugs or steroids and where long courses of broad-spectrum antibiotic treatment have been given, systemic candidiasis occurs. *Candida* endocarditis is well recognized following cardiac catheterization and open-heart surgery. The antibody response depends on the depth and site of infection and is of little use in diagnosis.

CLINICAL FEATURES

Oral candidiasis (oral thrush)

The tongue, soft palate, buccal mucosa and other oral surfaces are characteristically covered with discrete or confluent patches of a creamy-white to grey pseudomembrane composed of hyphae and yeasts of *C. albicans*, which may be deep and extensive enough to interfere with swallowing or breathing. Oral lesions may be associated with hypertrophy of the papillae of the tongue (black hairy tongue) and *C. albicans* grows freely in this environment although it is not the cause. When oral candidiasis extends to the angles of the mouth it may be a fortuitous invasion of the lesions of perlèche.

Cutaneous candidiasis (see also Chapter 33)

This is of particular importance in warm climates where the humid state of the skin especially in the intertriginous areas greatly conduces to the disease.

These cutaneous lesions generally resolve spontaneously with the removal to a cool climate or with the onset of the cool season, but recur with return to warm humid conditions. The forms of cutaneous candidiasis are intertriginous, generalized, paronychia, onychia, perianal and anogenital perlèche.

The intertriginous form occurs in the inguinal, genital, crural, gluteal, perianal, inframammary, axillary and interdigitial clefts of the hands and feet.

The genitocrural infection is manifested at first by little papules or vesicles 1–2 mm in diameter, isolated or in groups. The papule is slightly raised, of a dull red colour with a scaly surface and surrounded by a narrow inflammatory zone. These initial lesions increase in size and coalesce to form large raised plaques and as these increase in size the central part becomes less scaly, is erythematous or violaceous in hue and still shows the crusts of dried vesicles and some excoriations. The marginal zone is active and covered with a thick layer of whitish sodden epithelium in which vesicles are common and ends abruptly in a prominent raised border surrounded by a zone of inflammation. Satellite lesions are common and in consequence the border often presents as a festooned outline. Although the appearance may be slightly modified by the chafing of opposed surfaces the general character is very typical of candidiasis, being unlike the picture of tinea cruris.

The interdigital type presents the same basic character and on the foot may be mistaken for tinea pedis.

The generalized form is found chiefly in infants associated with oral candidiasis or infection of the napkin area. It spreads to the main flexures and eventually may involve the entire skin in an erythematosquamous vesicular and pustular eruption.

Among United States personnel in Japan, intertriginous candidiasis occurred more or less severely every summer owing to unsuitable uniform, although the local civilian population were free.[63]

Paronychia (perionychia), onychia

This occurs in persons exposed occupationally to water, such as housewives and fruit packers. There is swelling, redness and pain at the base of the paronychia containing very little pus covered with an intact skin showing little scaling. The nail is brownish and sometimes shows striation.

Vulvovaginal candidiasis

Vulvovaginal infection consists of eczematoid lesions with slight erythema or with severe pustules, excoriations or even ulcers covered with a grey membrane composed of hyphae and yeasts of *C. albicans*.

Bronchocandidiasis

This is described as a chronic bronchitis characterized by cough, varying amounts of sputum, medium and coarse rales at the lung bases and X-ray appearances of peribronchial thickening or hazy linear fibrosis. It is difficult to evaluate the importance of *C. albicans* as the cause of this syndrome since it may be present in any chronic condition of the respiratory tract.

Pulmonary candidiasis

Pulmonary symptoms are characterized by low grade fever, cough with mucoid and sometimes bloodstained sputum, pleurisy and effusion. There may be patchy bronchopneumonia.

Candida endocarditis

Candida endocarditis follows heart surgery or in drug addiction. Large vegetations are produced on the mitral or aortic valves and cause emboli.

Other visceral forms

With intravenous catheters *Candida* may occur in the blood but cause no lesions. Other organs that can be involved are the kidneys, liver, muscle, skin, brain and retina.

DIAGNOSIS

Diagnosis is made by demonstration of the fungus. Direct examination of sputum, pus or scrapings is made in a drop of sodium hydroxide warmed gently and examined for the egg-shaped budding cells and hyphae of *Candida*. The yeast is gram-positive in stained films. Culture is made on Sabouraud's modified agar with chloramphenicol and incubated at 30°C or room temperature.

Skin tests

Both immediate (type 1) and delayed (type 4) hypersensitivity reactions are found in 10–15% of the adult population and are probably related to early repeated contacts.[64] They are of little diagnostic significance.

Serum antibodies

High titres are found in *Candida* endocarditis.

Precipitin tests

These have been made especially with mannan A and positive results have been obtained in healthy subjects as well as 72% of asthmatics with pulmonary infiltrations and eosinophilia.[65] Quantitative precipitin and agar gel diffusion tests using group specific cell wall polysaccharides have been used to separate groups A and B of *C. albicans*.

TREATMENT

Nystatin is specific in the treatment of all forms of candidiasis. It can be administered orally in the treatment of deep forms of the infection or it can be given in conjunction with broad-spectrum antibiotics to counteract their effect.

Amphotericin B intravenously has also been used successfully in the treatment of severe forms of the infection.

Cutaneous candidiasis

A nystatin lotion or powder gives immediate relief and eventual cure in many cases. Nystatin lotion is prepared by suspending the antibiotic powder in 60 ml of a basic lotion of talc 6 g, zinc oxide 6 g, glycerin 6 ml, bentonite magna 12 ml and water to 60 ml, to give a concentration of 35 000 units of nystatin per ml. The lotion is applied thrice daily. It does not keep and should therefore be dispensed in small quantities and stored in the cold.

EPIDEMIOLOGY

Reservoir of infection

C. albicans causes candidiasis in monkeys, fowls, turkeys and pigeons and occurs as a commensal in the cat, dog, goat, hedgehog, rabbit and rat. It can survive in contaminated soil but is not known to have a natural habitat in inanimate nature.

The other species of *Candida* have a common saprophytic existence apart from the animal host.

Human infection

Oral candidiasis (thrush) is seen in the newborn and aged and in debilitated patients and is also associated with long continued therapy with broad-spectrum antibiotics. Intertriginous candidiasis and paronychia are seen in diabetic and obese persons and in those whose hands are frequently immersed in water for prolonged periods.

Vulvovaginitis occurs during pregnancy. Bronchopulmonary candidiasis is secondary to another disease and endocarditis is associated with indwelling cardiac catheters.

Systemic candidiasis is an 'opportunist' infection associated with prolonged use of immunosuppressive drugs or the presence of lymphoma and leukaemic disorders.

Oral and intestinal candidiasis have been found as terminal infections in sprue in the tropics and at one time were thought to be the cause of the disease.

REFERENCES

1 Schubert, J. H. & Wiggins, G. L. (1963) *Am. J. Hyg.* **77**, 240.
2 Heiner, D. C. (1958) *Pediatrics, Springfield* **22**, 616.
3 Kaufman, L. (1966) *Pub. Hlth Rep. Wash.* **81**, 177.
4 Hill, G. B. & Campbell, C. C. (1962) *Mycopathologia* **18**, 169.
5 Kaufman, L. & Kaplan, W. (1963) *J. Bact.* **85**, 986.
6 Goodwin, R. A., Jr & Des Prez, R. M. (1978) *Am. Rev. resp. Dis.* **117**, 929.
7 Gelfand, J. A. & Bennett, J. E. (1975) *J. Am. med. Ass.* **233**, 1294.
8 Furcolow, M. D. (1963) *Med. Clins N. Am.* **47**, 1119.
9 Seribi, O., Alderele, W. I., Johnson, A. et al (1975) *J. trop. Med. Hyg.* **78**, 248.
10 Brown, K. G. E., Molesworth, B. D., Boerrighter, F. G. G. et al (1974) *E. Afr. med. J.* **51**, 584.
11 Ajello, L., Hosty, T. S. & Palmer, J. (1967) *Am. J. trop. Med. Hyg.* **16**, 329.
12 Walker, J. & Spooner, E. T. C. (1960) *J. Path. Bact.* **80**, 346.
13 Lainson, R. J. & Shaw, J. J. (1975) *Trans. R. Soc. trop. Med. Hyg.* **69**, 505.
14 Murray, J. F., Lurie, H. I., Kaye, J. et al (1957) *S. Afr. med. J.* **31**, 245.
15 Dean, G. (1957) *Cent. Afr. J. Med.* **3**, 79.
16 Ajello, L., Manson-Bahr, P. E. C. & Moore, J. C. (1959) *Am. J. trop. Med. Hyg.* **9**, 623.
17 Van Breuseghem, R. (1952) *Bull. Acad. r. Méd. Belg.* **23**, 686.
18 Coulanges, P., Raveloarison, G. & Rauisse, P. (1983) *Bull. Path. éxot. Fil.* **75**, 400–403.
19 Cockshott, W. P. & Lucas, A. O. (1964) *Q. J. Med.* **33**, 233.
20 Cockshott, W. P. & Lucas, A. O. (1964) *Br. J. Radiol.* **37**, 653.
21 Cole, A. C., Ridley, D. S. & Wolfe, H. R. (1965) *J. trop. Med. Hyg.* **68**, 92.
22 Clark, B. M. & Greenwood, B. M. (1968) *J. trop. Med. Hyg.* **71**, 4.
23 Mabey, D. C. W., Ajdukiewicz, A. B. & Hay, R. J. (1983) *Trans. R. Soc. trop. Med. Hyg.* **77**, 219–220.
24 Fiese, M. J. (1962) *Coccidiomycosis*, p. 99. Springfield, Ill: Charles C. Thomas.
25 Smith, C. E., Whiting, E. G., Baker, E. E. et al (1948) *Am. Rev. Tuberc.* **57**, 330.
26 Smith, C. E., Saito, M. T. & Simons, S. A. (1956) *J. Am. med. Ass.* **160**, 546.
27 Bailey, J. W., Huppert, M. & Chitjian, P. (1965) *Bact. Proc.* **11**, 19.
28 Kaplan, W. & Clifford, M. K. (1964) *Am. Rev. resp. Dis.* **89**, 651.
29 Williams, P. L., Sable, D. L., Sorgen, S. P. et al (1984) *Am. J. Epidemiol.* **119**, 591–602.
30 Richardson, H. V., Jr, Anderson, J. A. & McKay, R. M. (1967) *J. Pediat.* **70**, 376.
31 Baker, K. C. & Kemberling, S. R. (1960) *Archs Derm.* **81**, 373.
32 Stevens, D. A., Restrepo, M. A., Cortés, A. et al (1978) *Am. J. trop. Med. Hyg.* **27**, 801.
33 Emmons, C. W. (1942) *Pub. Hlth Rep. Wash.* **57**, 109.
34 Mota, N. G. S., Rezkallah-Iwasso, M. T., Peracoli, M. T. et al (1983) XIX Cong. Brazilian Society tropical Medicine, Rio de Janeiro. Annals, p. 126.
35 Fava Netto, C. (1965) *Mycopathologia* **26**, 349.
36 De Brito, T. Raphael, A., Fava Netto, C. et al (1961) *J. invest. Derm.* **37**, 29.
37 Restrepo, M. A. (1966) *Sabouraudia* **4**, 223.
38 Scarpa, C., Nini, G. & Geraldi, G. (1965) *Minerva derm.* **40**, 413.
39 Laudanna, A. A., Bettarello, A., van Bellen, B. et al (1975) *Arq. Gasteroenterol.* **12**, 195.
40 Cuce, L. C., Wroclawski, E. L. & Sampaio, S. A. (1981) *Rev. Inst. Med. trop. São Paulo* **23**, 82–85.
41 Lopes, C. F., Furtado, T. A., Cisalpino, F. et al (1966) *Hospital, Rio de J.* **70**, 285.
42 Lopes, C. F. & Armand, S. (1968) *Hospital, Rio de J.* **73**, 1245.
43 Dias, L. B., Sempaio, M. M. & Silva, D. (1970) *Rev. Inst. Med. trop. São Paulo* **12**, 8.
44 Ajello, L. (1967) *Systemic Mycoses*, Ciba Foundation Symposium, p. 132. London: Churchill.
45 Ross, M. D. & Gelfand, M. (1978) *Cent. Afr. J. Med.* **24**, 262.

46 Balows, A. (1963) *VII Int. Cong. Microbiol.*
47 Busey, J. F. (1964) *Am. Rev. resp. Dis.* **89,** 659.
48 Abernethy, R. S. & Heiner, D. C. (1961) *J. Lab. Clin. Med.* **57,** 604.
49 Evans, M. E., Haynes, J. B., Atkinson, J. B. et al (1983) *Ann. Rev. resp. Dis.* **126,** 1099–1102.
50 Boswell, W. L. (1959) *Am. J. Roentg.* **81,** 224.
51 Evans, E. E. (1950) *J. Immunol.* **64,** 432.
52 Bennett, J. E., Hasenclever, H. F. & Baum, G. L. (1965) *Am. Rev. resp. Dis.* **91,** 616.
53 Donnan, M. G. F. (1959) *J. Fac. Radiol.* **10,** 17.
54 Snow, R. M. & Dismukes, W. E. (1975) *Archs int. Med.,* **136,** 1155.
55 Kase, A. & Marshall, J. D. (1960) *Am. J. clin. Path.* **34,** 52.
56 Vogel, R. A., Sellers, T. F. & Woodward, P. (1961) *J. Am. med. Ass.* **178,** 921.

57 Graybill, J. R. & Levine, H. B. (1977) *Archs int. Med.* **138,** 814–816.
58 Craven, P. C., Graybill, J. R. & Jorgensen, J. H. (1982) *Am. Rev. resp. Dis.* **125,** 696–700.
59 Emmons, C. S. (1955) *Am. J. Hyg.* **62,** 227.
60 Pounden, W. D. (1952) *Am. J. vet. Res.* **13,** 121.
61 Miale, J. B. (1943) *Archs Path.* **35,** 427.
62 Mackinnon, J. E. & Artagaveytia-Allende, R. C. (1956) *Trans. R. Soc. trop. Med. Hyg.* **50,** 31.
63 Higdon, R. S. (1956) *Archs Derm.* **74,** 620.
64 Holti, G. (1966) In *Symposium on Candida Infections,* ed. H. I. Winner & R. Hueley, p. 73. Edinburgh: Livingstone.
65 Pepys, J., Faux, J. A., Longbottom, J. L. et al (1967) In *Clinical Aspects of Immunology,* ed. P. G. M. Gell & R. R. A. Coombes, 2nd edn, p. 108. Oxford: Blackwell Scientific Publications.

SECTION VII
DISEASES COMMONLY PRESENTING AS ULCERS

Chronic ulceration of the skin is an important cause of disability in the tropics. There are many causes and when a cutaneous ulcer presents the following conditions must be thought of:

Tropical ulcer (Chapter 36)
Cutaneous leishmaniasis (Chapter 37)
Tuberculosis (Chapter 59)

Buruli ulcer (Chapter 38)
Cutaneous diphtheria (Chapter 39)
Systemic mycosis (Chapter 35)
Leprosy (Chapter 40)
Yaws (Chapter 31)
Tertiary syphilis (Chapter 68)
Chronic ulceration of the lower leg may occur in sickle cell disease (Chapter 58)
Cancer of the skin (Chapter 67)

Chapter 36
Tropical Ulcer

GEOGRAPHICAL DISTRIBUTION

Tropical ulcer is common in Africa, India (Naga sore) and tropical America (Fig. 36.1).

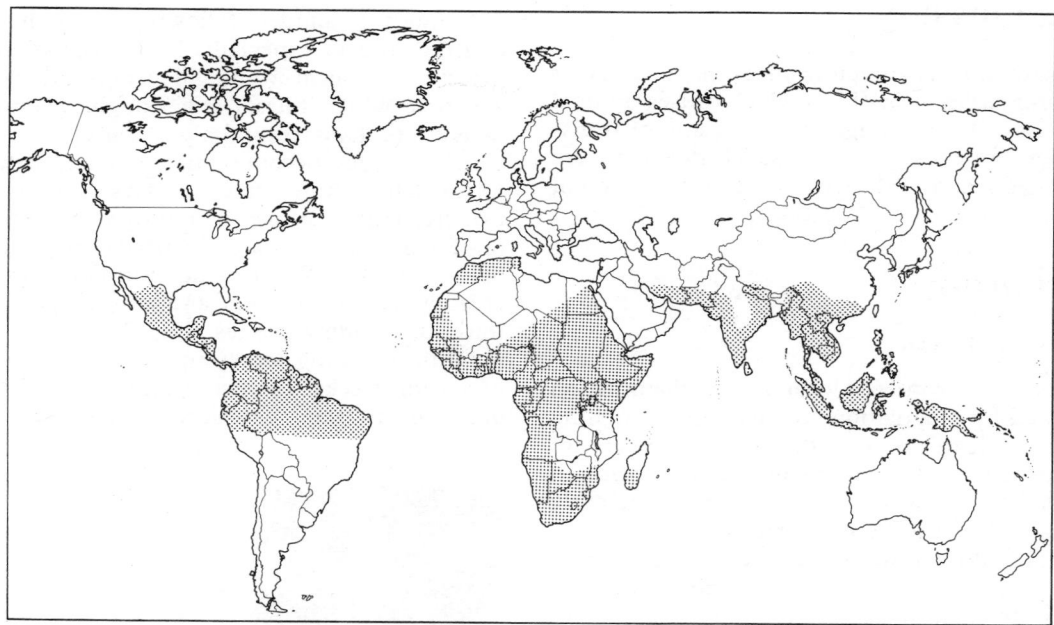

Fig. 36.1   Geographical distribution of tropical ulcer.

can be readily cultured anaerobically at 37°C on serum agar or broth. It is found in large numbers in acute but not chronic ulcers. *Borrelia vincenti* is a delicate spirochaete, 7–18 μm long, with three

AETIOLOGY

The aetiology is still not clear but three factors are involved: infection, possibly nutritional deficiency, and trauma.

Infection

Two organisms, *Fusobacterium fusiforme* and *Borrelia vincenti,* are so closely connected with tropical ulcer that they are almost certainly concerned directly in its cause. *Fusobacterium fusiforme* is a straight or curved rod-like bacillus, 5–14 μm long, thickened in the middle with pointed ends. It is non-motile and gram-positive and

to eight coils. It is an actively motile gram-negative organism and can be cultured on the same media as *F. fusiforme*. Other organisms are also found: *Proteus, Pseudomonas* and diphtheroids, but these are probably contaminants.[1]

Nutritional deficiency

Nutritional deficiency has been suggested as an important predisposing factor since malnutrition and tropical ulcers are frequently found together and tropical ulcers are common in famine conditions. In Zambia, however, a significant minority of the ulcer patients were well nourished and their diet contained plenty of fish.[2] These observations suggest that nutritional deficiency is not a major cause.

Trauma

Although ulcers have been produced experimentally in healthy volunteers by contact with ulcer pus,[3] the high incidence of ulcers on the anterior and lateral aspects of the lower leg in people who go around with bare feet and legs suggests that trauma plays an important role.

TRANSMISSION

Transmission is direct from cases to cases or contamination of an object which causes trauma. Flies have been thought to be agents of transmission but those cases on which flies fed were not infective[2] and flies are not thought to be of importance in rural conditions.

PATHOLOGY

The early lesion

At first there is intense local, acute inflammation followed by coagulation, necrosis and sloughing of the whole thickness of the skin and sometimes deeper tissues. Granulomatous tissue forms in the base of the ulcer and scrapings in the early stages will reveal the fusiform bacilli and spirochaetes. Fibrin thrombi are seen in the smaller vessels with infiltration with polymorphonuclear leukocytes, histiocytes, eosinophils, lymphocytes and plasma cells. At the growing edge the epithelium is raised and thickened and deep papillary processes project into the corium. Microabscesses underlie the edge. Deeper tissues are involved rarely.

The chronic lesion

The edges thicken with epithelial hyperplasia, inflammatory infiltration and oedema. The ulcer may remain stationary for many years. Extensive fibrosis occurs under the ulcer and there may be epithelialization and scarring.

CLINICAL FEATURES

Natural history

Tropical ulcer runs a varied course, some developing acutely and healing spontaneously, others persisting for many years. Some slowly extend, destroying muscle tendons and bone, leading eventually to loss of a leg from secondary infection or epithelioma.

Incubation period

The incubation period is 2 days to four weeks.

Symptoms and signs

The onset is sudden following a minor penetrating injury, especially from vegetation, or insect bite. A local swelling develops followed by a vesicle which bursts and sloughs leading to ulceration. Less commonly a papule develops which enlarges, becomes pustular and discharges foul-smelling fluid after 6–7 days. The ulcer is usually single but may be multiple and situated on the anterior and lateral surfaces of the lower half of the leg. When it has formed it spreads rapidly, has a raised edge and inflamed, oedematous surrounding tissues (Fig. 36.2). It is very painful, spreading deeply and widely for a period of several weeks. In severe ulcers there is gangrene of muscle, exposure of tendons, pen-

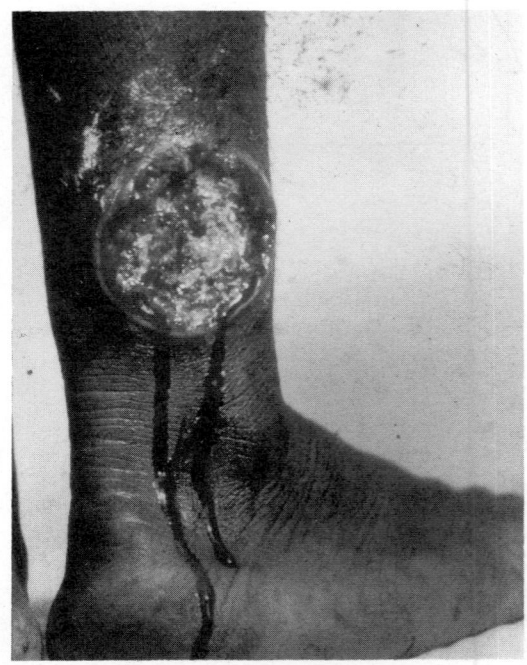

Fig. 36.2   Tropical ulcer. (Courtesy Dr J. Saave.)

etration to bone causing periostitis, local necrosis and even osteomyelitis. The regional lymph glands may be enlarged. There is general malaise and fever in some cases but most patients experience no constitutional upset. After the acute stage a more chronic phase supervenes. The ulcer develops firm, sclerotic edges and a base of unhealthy pinkish granulation tissue. The surrounding skin is thin, atrophic and depigmented with fibrosis in and around the ulcer. If healing takes place a scar is left which is fixed to deeper structures but healing may never occur without treatment.

Malignant change

In a small proportion of cases a well-differentiated squamous cell carcinoma forms at the edge which is locally invasive and may metastasize to local lymph glands, but haematogenous spread is rare (Fig. 67.3, p. 1092).

DIAGNOSIS

In the acute stage the ulcer has a typical appearance which is usually diagnostic and the fusiform bacilli and Vincent's spirochaetes can usually be found. In the chronic stage these organisms may not be present.

Tropical ulcer has to be distinguished from cutaneous leishmaniasis in which ulcers are usually painless and do not heal with the measures used for tropical ulcer. Tropical ulcer must also be distinguished from veld sore and Buruli ulcer. Varicose ulcers may be contaminated by Vincent's spirochaetes and fusiform bacilli; varicose veins are always present. Malignant melanoma may cause confusion but, when cleaned, the true nature of the pigmentation becomes apparent and can be confirmed by biopsy. Squamous cell carcinoma may develop producing a rolled, everted edge with destruction of the underlying bone demonstrable by radiography and possibly accompanied by enlarged lymph nodes. A biopsy should give the diagnosis. Late yaws also causes chronic ulcers in which case serological tests for syphilis are always positive.

Tetanus and gas gangrene are rare but possible complications requiring appropriate treatment. Chronic lymphoedema may result from constriction of lymphatics by scar tissue and from chronic lymphangitis and lymphadenitis.

TREATMENT

Antibiotics

Penicillin should be given in the acute stage; 900 mg of procaine penicillin daily for 5 days, rapidly abolishing pain and all signs of acute inflammation. Metronidazole 200 mg orally three times daily for 7 days also quickly reduces inflammation and initiates healing.[4]

Local treatment

In the early stages the patient should if possible be admitted to hospital for complete rest to the affected limb. There are two phases:
1 Antiseptic soaks to clean the ulcer. Suitable wet dressings are: eusol (sodium hypochlorite solution), hydrogen peroxide (1 vol%) and physiological saline. These should be used initially with the aim of cleaning the ulcer and encouraging the formation of healthy granulation tissue. Plain gauze is soaked in the chosen solution, applied to the ulcer and *occluded by a sheet of impermeable plastic* to prevent the dressing from drying out. The dressing should be reviewed daily until the floor of the ulcer is completely clean and free of pus and slough.
2 Non-adherent dressings to allow undisturbed healing. This stage of the treatment is designed to protect the ulcer from trauma and contamination and allow unhindered growth of new epithelium from the skin margins over the ulcer floor. Several materials are satisfactory:
  paraffin gauze (tulle gras)
  gauze soaked in a locally available oil, such as coconut or groundnut (after heat sterilization) or petroleum jelly (Vaseline). Newer synthetic gel or plastic wound dressings are effective but expensive.

Once covered with a non-adherent dressing the ulcer should be left undisturbed for 7–14 days. When the dressing is taken down action should be governed by what is found.
1 The ulcer is clean: reapply another non-adherent dressing.
2 The ulcer shows signs of infection (pus or slough is present): reapply wet *antiseptic* dressings as already described. Renew them daily until the ulcer is clean again. Then resume non-adherent dressings and review once a week as before.

Dressings which are allowed to dry out in contact with the ulcer will adhere to new epithelium and will cause loss of this delicate tissue when the dressing is changed. Drying dressings of this sort must *never* be applied to tropical ulcers, or any other sort of ulcer. Sadly, this simple rule is ignored in countless dispensaries, clinics and hospitals throughout the world every day. Enormous, entirely avoidable, suffering is the consequence of this ignorant practice.

EPIDEMIOLOGY AND CONTROL

Tropical ulcer is a disease of rural farmers, plantation labourers and inhabitants of large camps for prisoners of war or famine victims. The highest incidence is in the second decade of life, children under five years of age being rarely affected. Where both sexes work in the fields the incidence is equal in both sexes. Incidence is high in the rainy season and occasionally there is an outbreak amounting to a small epidemic, the cause of which is unknown.[5] Prevention of tropical ulcer chiefly depends upon the prompt treatment of minor injuries with topical antiseptic application and occlusive dressings and the liberal use of penicillin to treat any developing ulcer.

CANCRUM ORIS

Cancrum oris is a rapidly developing necrotic ulceration of the face occurring predominantly in malnourished children due to infection with *Fusobacterium fusiforme* and *Borrelia vincenti*. It is not uncommon in kala-azar (see Chapter 4) but also occurs in measles and other systemic infections. The ulceration, which is painful, is unilateral and involves the mouth causing large defects (Fig. 36.3). Diagnosis is made by exclusion of other infections such as mycetoma

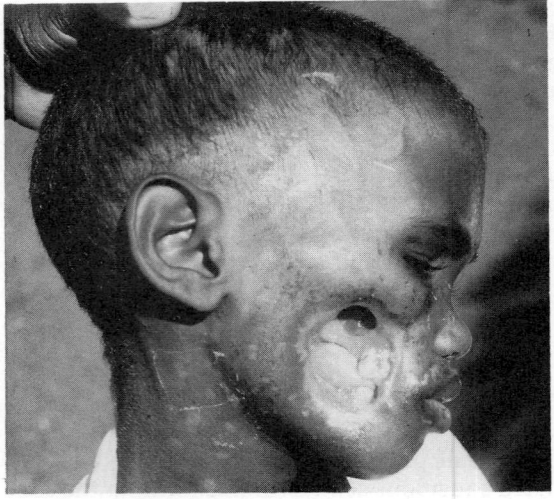

Fig. 36.3   Cancrum oris.

(see Chapter 34) and discovering the primary cause.

Treatment

The primary cause must be treated and parenteral penicillin should be given in generous doses without delay. Restoration of good nutrition is essential. Reconstructive surgery may be needed to repair defects resulting from loss of tissue.

REFERENCES

1   Ngu, V.A. (1967) *Br. med. J.* **i**, 283.
2   Robinson, D.C. & Hay, R.J. (1986) *Trans. R. Soc. trop. Med. Hyg.* **80**, 132–137.
3   McAdam, I. (1966) *J. R. Coll. Surgs Ed.* **II**, 196–205.
4   Lindner, R. & Adenyi-Jones, C. (1968) *Trans. R. Soc. trop. Med. Hyg.* **62**, 712.
5   Kuberski, T. & Koteka, G. (1980) *Am. J. trop. Med. Hyg.* **29**, 291–297.

Chapter 37
Cutaneous Leishmaniasis

This is an important disease presenting as skin ulceration. There are two forms, Old World cutaneous leishmaniasis and New World (neotropical or American) cutaneous leishmaniasis.

AETIOLOGY

The parasites which cause cutaneous leishmaniasis are leishmaniae of various species which have an amastigote form in mammals and a promastigote form in the sandfly invertebrate host as described in Chapter 4.

Life-cycle

This is essentially the same as described for *L. (L.) donovani* in Chapter 4. The amastigote form is ingested from a skin ulcer by a female sandfly and undergoes development in the sandfly gut, in the anterior part in the cases of *L. (L.) tropica*, *L. (L.) major* and *L. (L.) mexicana* complexes (suprapylarian development), and in the midgut in the case of *L. (V.) braziliensis* complex (peripylarian development). The infection is then transmitted by sandfly bite at the second blood meal.

OLD WORLD CUTANEOUS LEISHMANIASIS
(oriental sore; Biskra button; Delhi boil)

GEOGRAPHICAL DISTRIBUTION

Old World cutaneous leishmaniasis is widely distributed in central Asia, the Middle East, Mediterranean, Africa both north and south of the Sahara, and India (Figs. 37.1 and 37.2).

AETIOLOGY

There are three species which cause Old World cutaneous leishmaniasis: *L. (L.) tropica*, *L. (L.) major* and *L. (L.) aethiopica*. All are identical morphologically but can be distinguished from each other by their enzyme structure (zymodemes) and by the serological reactions of the excreted factor (EF).[1] The three species differ clinically and epidemiologically.

L. (L.) tropica causes anthroponotic cutaneous leishmaniasis (ACL), which is a complex of different strains (zymodemes) throughout its distribution (Fig. 37.1). In the western Medi-

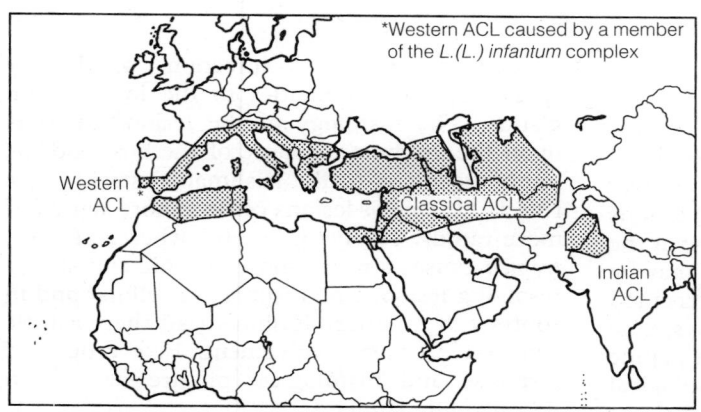

Fig. 37.1 Geographical distribution of cutaneous leishmaniasis caused by the *L. (L.) tropica* complex (ACL). (Courtesy Department of Entomology, London School of Hygiene and Tropical Medicine.)

729

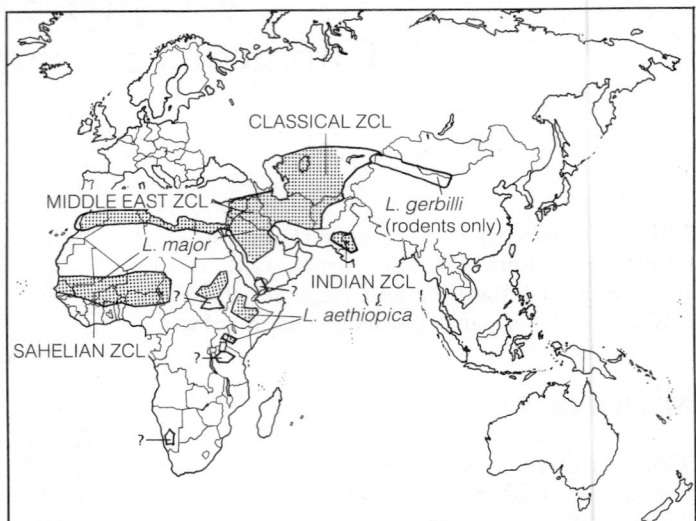

Fig. 37.2   Geographical distribution of cutaneous leishmaniasis caused by the *L. (L.) major* complex and *L. (L.) aethiopica* (ZCL). (Courtesy Department of Entomology, London School of Hygiene and Tropical Medicine.)

terranean (western ACL) a strain of *L. (L.) infantum* is responsible.[2] *L. (L.) major* causes zoonotic cutaneous leishmaniasis (ZCL) which is a remarkably uniform parasite throughout its distribution (Fig. 37.2).[3]

L. (L.) aethiopica causes cutaneous leishmaniasis in eastern Africa with a high incidence of diffuse cutaneous leishmaniasis (DCL) (Fig. 37.2). In the southern part of this area the causative parasite has not yet been clearly identified.

TRANSMISSION (Appendix IV, p. 1401, and Table III.3, p. 1400)

Transmission is by sandfly bite but can also be achieved by inoculation of amastigote parasites or promastigote cultures into or under the skin, deliberately or accidentally.

PATHOLOGY

Old World cutaneous leishmaniasis is a localized infection confined to the skin. There is no permanent visceral or mucosal spread. The lesions are single or multiple, localized to the skin at the site of the sandfly bite. Multiple lesions may be due to multiple infective bites, from interrupted feeding or possibly from transient systemic spread. The cutaneous lesion starts as a papule which may ulcerate (Fig. 37.3). The pathological process is confined to the skin except in the case

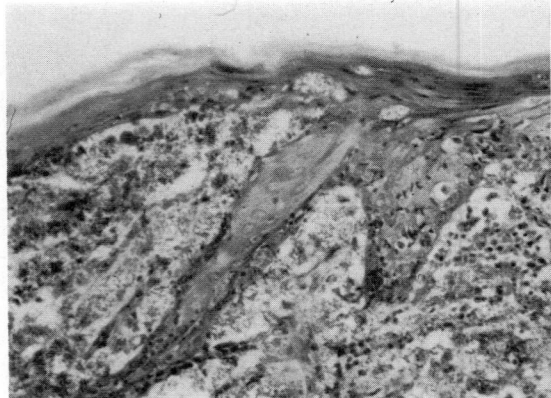

Fig. 37.3   *L. (L.) tropica* ulcer from which the epidermis has disappeared. Adjacent epidermis thinned with destruction of tissue and inflammation of the subepithelial tissue. (Courtesy Dr H. Zaiman.)

of some *L. (L.) major* infections which may spread up the lymphatics to the local lymph glands. The histology of the lesions depends upon the immune response of the host and the immunogenicity of the leishmanial strain. As a rule *L. (L.) major* lesions cause a more acute but more rapidly resolving lesions, whereas *L. (L.) tropica* causes a much more chronic and slowly resolving lesion. The response is cellular and in contrast to American leishmaniasis there is little connective tissue involvement. Five groups of response and histological picture have been described by Ridley:[4]

Group 1. Undifferentiated parasite-laden macrophages throughout the lesion with little or no cellular response. No ulceration, an anergic response as in diffuse cutaneous leishmaniasis (DCL).

Group 2. Focal macrophage granuloma formation containing parasites. Some central necrosis. Some macrophage destruction with extracellular parasites on the periphery of the necrotic area. The granulomas are surrounded by a dense zone of plasma cells and lymphocytes.

Group 3. Heavy cellular infiltration. No granulomas, scanty parasites.

Group 4. Abundant lymphocytes, a few Langhans' giant cells. Scanty parasites; small epithelioid cell granulomas (tuberculoid).

Group 5. Well-developed epithelial cell granulomas with Langhans' giant cells. No necrosis. Heavy fibrosis. Hypersensitive reaction as in leishmaniasis recidiva.

IMMUNITY

The majority of infections with *L. (L.) tropica* and *L. (L.) major* subside spontaneously and are usually followed by a solid immunity to reinfection but reinfections have been recorded.[5] A well-marked cellular immunity develops accompanied by delayed hypersensitivity. Immunity is to reinfection with the homologous strain: *L. (L.) major* protects against *L. (L.) tropica*, but the reverse is not true. The immunity is accompanied by delayed hypersensitivity which is measured by the *leishmanin* skin test (see p. 89). Elimination of parasites is dealt with by the mechanism outlined in Chapter 4 (p. 89). There is a spectrum of immune responses for the anergic (DCL) forms at one end to the hypersensitive delayed healing (recidiva) at the other with self-healing forms in the middle.

CLINICAL FEATURES

Natural history

Both *L. (L.) tropica* and *L. (L.) major* lesions are usually self-limiting, *L. (L.) tropica* usually being single, growing and healing slowly over a period of a year or more, whereas *L. (L.) major* typically causes multiple lesions which grow and heal more rapidly over a period of six months. In both cases there is a permanent immunity to reinfection with the homologous strain and, in the case of *L. (L.) major*, with *L. (L.) tropica*. In a small number of cases of *L. (L.) tropica* the infection is chronic and non-healing (leishmaniasis recidivans) and a proportion of *L. (L.) aethiopica* cases show anergy, allowing the parasite to spread throughout the skin (diffuse cutaneous leishmaniasis).

Incubation period

The incubation period varies from a few days to several months. Senekji and Beattie[6] in studying the development of experimentally produced oriental sores in man found that the incubation period after infection with three million promastigotes of *L. (L.) tropica* ranged from two to eight weeks. Wenyon inoculated himself with oriental sore in Aleppo but it was not until six and a half months later that a lesion developed. In some cases the incubation period appears to be as long as three years.[7]

Symptoms and signs of *L. (L.) tropica* infection (ACL)

The local lesion commences as a minute itching papule which expands as a shotty congested infiltration of the dermis. Later the surface becomes covered with fine white scales which then become darker and thicker, falling off to reveal an ulcer. A crust forms and the ulcer continues to spread under the edge which is firm and raised. The centre of the crust may contain a horny spicule (Montpellier sign). Satellite

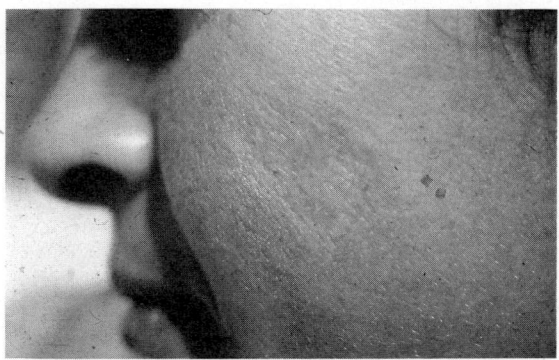

Fig. 37.4 Healed *L. (L.) tropica* lesion. Characteristic scar on face.

lesions appear and may merge to form a larger lesion. Depending on the host reaction the lesion heals spontaneously after six to 12 months, seldom longer. A depressed scar follows. The characteristic scar on the face can be recognized in most of the adult inhabitants of endemic areas (Fig. 37.4). The lesions may be multiple, either as a result of interrupted feeding by the sandfly or blood spread, since as many as 150 lesions have been counted on the same individual accompanied by a bout of fever. According to the immune response, lesions may be papular, ulcerative or warty and when multiple appear at the same stage of development, growing and fading together. Lesions occur mostly on the uncovered parts of the body, hands, feet, arms and legs and especially the face. Lesions are rare on the trunk and are never seen on the palms, soles or hairy scalp. When near the nasolabial folds lesions may cause a destructive lesion resembling espundia but never involve the bone.

The infection usually resolves spontaneously and many inapparent infections occur since most adults in endemic areas show a positive leishmanin reaction without the presence of any characteristic scars.

Leishmaniasis recidiva

This is a chronic relapsing form of L. (L.) tropica infection with much scarring (Fig. 37.5), most common on the face. The appearance is often much like lupus vulgaris. Amastigotes are difficult or impossible to find but the leishmanin test is strongly positive. Lesions may persist for up to 50 years.

Symptoms and signs of L. (L.) major infection

Lesions are more florid than those of L. (L.) tropica and are more likely to be multiple with satellite lesions (Figs. 37.6 and 37.7). Infection may spread in nodular fashion along the lymphatics and involve the glands (Fig. 37.8), and so resemble sporotrichosis. L. (L.) major infection does not develop into chronic recidiva lesions.

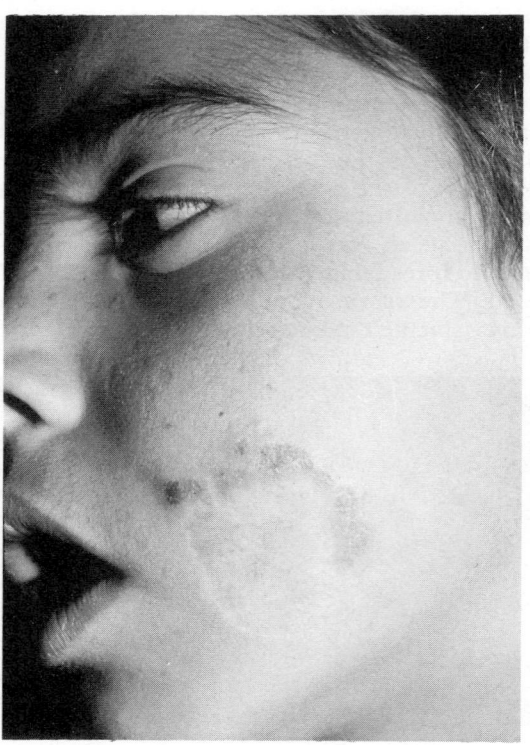

Fig. 37.5   Leishmaniasis recidiva. Scarring and active lesion present together.

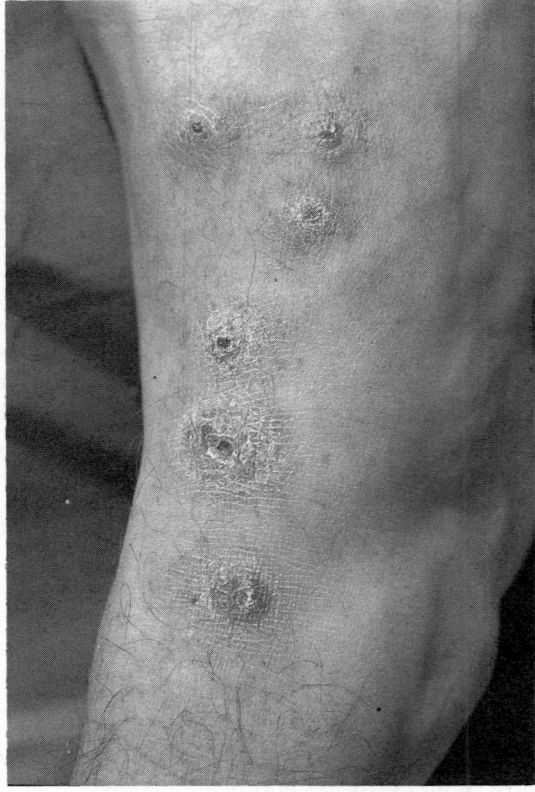

Fig. 37.6   Multiple lesions caused by L. (L.) major.

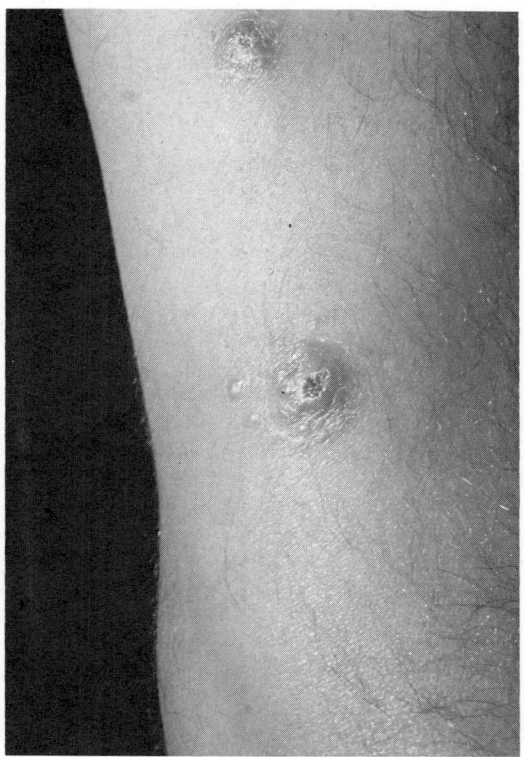

Fig. 37.7 Lesion caused by *L. (L.) major* with satellite lesions.

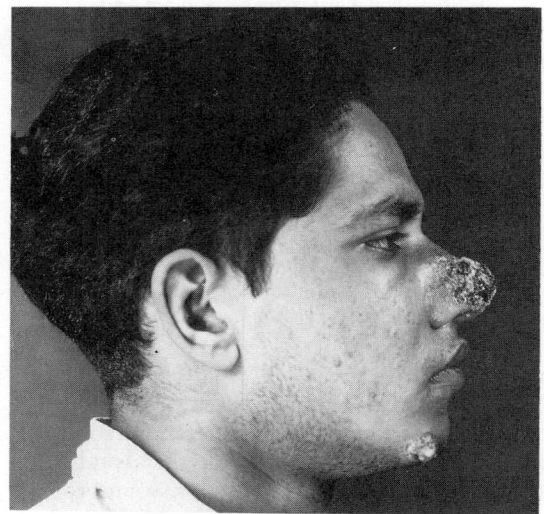

Fig. 37.8 Lesion on nose caused by *L. (L.) major* showing lymphatic spread (Medical Department of the Navy).

Symptoms and signs of *L. (L.) aethiopica* infection

The lesions caused by *L. (L.) aethiopica* are in the majority of cases similar to those caused by *L. (L.) tropica* but there is a high incidence of diffuse cutaneous leishmaniasis, an attribute which this species shares with *L. (L.) mexicana* species in north-eastern South America.

Diffuse cutaneous leishmaniasis (DCL, leishmaniasis diffusa, leproid or cheloid leishmaniasis)

DCL was first described from Ethiopia[8] and from Venezuela.[9]

The species of *Leishmania* which can cause DCL are *L. (L.) aethiopica* in Africa (Ethiopia, Kenya, Namibia), *L. (L.) amazonensis*, *L. (L.) pifanoi* in north-eastern South America and *L. (L.) mexicana* species in the Dominican Republic. In these areas, although most cases of infection are simple single cutaneous lesions, a varying proportion of the cases exhibit DCL. In the cases of *L. (L.) amazonensis* and *L. (L.) pifanoi*, although human infection is rare, the incidence of DCL is high (30%) and in the Dominican Republic only DCL exists,[10] although inapparent infections outnumber the cases of DCL.

DCL is a very chronic disease and may persist for 20 years. It starts as a single non-ulcerating lesion, usually on the face, and spreads slowly over the entire body, affecting mainly the face, limbs and buttocks which become covered with lepromatous-type nodules (Fig.37.9). There is

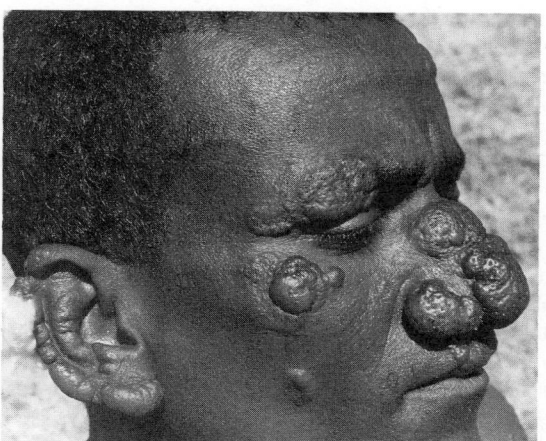

Fig. 37.9 Diffuse cutaneous leishmaniasis. (Courtesy Dr A.F. Bryceson.)

never any ulceration but the nose may become affected and cause obstructive symptoms. There is little or no tissue reaction and the leishmanin test remains negative unless recovery occurs. Histologically the dermis is full of leishmania-filled macrophages and free leishmania with little cellular reaction, group 1.[4] There is no visceral disease but leishmaniae have been recovered from the marrow and blood by cultural and sub-inoculation techniques. The cause of DCL is a combination of the failure of the cell-mediated immune response on the part of certain individuals and the toxigenicity of certain strains of *Leishmania.*

Differential diagnosis includes lepromatous leprosy but skin smears and biopsy will show many leishmaniae and no acid-fast bacilli. Lepromatous leprosy and DCL may coexist in the same patient but this may be due to the fact that many DCL patients were kept for long periods in leprosaria where they contracted leprosy. There is no evidence that the immunological defects found in each disease are the same.

Treatment of DCL

Treatment is difficult. Pentavalent antimony in the usual dosage has no effect or the case will relapse after an initial response. Pentostam (sodium stibogluconate) intravenously in doses of 20 mg Sb[v]/kg twice daily for 30 days was successful in three cases in Kenya.[11] Pentamidine also is useful but must be given for a long time intravenously—4 mg/kg three times a week—for as long as it takes to eliminate parasites and for three months longer. Some, but not all, cases will respond and the appearance of leishmanin sensitivity indicates a good prognosis.[12] The topical application of 2% chlorpromazine in Vaseline ointment was of help.[13]

DIAGNOSIS

Cutaneous leishmaniasis in its varied clinical forms from a simple single or multiple nodule to ulcers and large warty growths has to be distinguished from a number of conditions found in the tropics: desert or veld sore (see Chapter 39), tropical ulcer, tertiary syphilis and yaws (see Chapter 31), lupus vulgaris and fungal infections, blastomycosis and paracoccidioidomycosis (see Chapter 35), rodent ulcer and epithelioma.

The distribution of the lesions on the exposed surfaces of the body and the geographical history are important but demonstration of the parasite and serological tests are critical.

Demonstration of the parasite

Parasites may be demonstrated by direct examination, culture or subinoculation of material into hamsters.

Touch preparations

These are best. A small full thickness biopsy is taken from the lesion's edge and touch preparations made on a number of slides which can be stained with Giemsa and examined (Fig. 37.10, Appendix IV, p. 1497). The biopsy is divided into two; one portion is placed in culture (Schneider's insect medium, see Appendix I) and the other into Carnoy's fixative for histology.

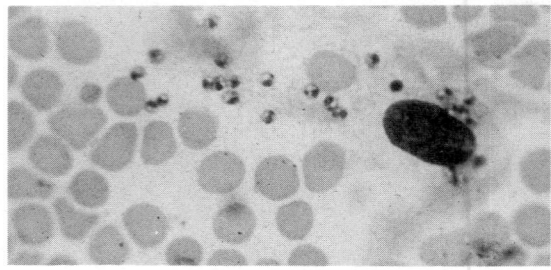

Fig. 37.10 Touch preparation from cutaneous leishmaniasis showing amastigotes and red cells.

Needle preparations

Material can be aspirated from beneath the edge of the ulcer and tissue sampling with a dendritic broach (used in dentistry) can be accomplished by rotating the broach around under the edge; this can be repeated many times without trouble (Appendix IV).

Biopsy

The histological picture will vary with the degree of host resistance. Parasites when present can be seen enclosed in macrophages often surrounded by granulomatous tissue. There is usually an unorganized granulomatous response with round cells, plasma cells and occasional giant cells (but no tubercles). There may be areas of tissue necrosis.

Serology

The leishmanin skin test becomes positive within three months of the appearance of the lesion, remaining positive for life. It is of little use in areas of high endemicity.

Immunofluorescence

Immunofluorescence is of little help in diagnosis since no antibodies are found in *L.* (*L.*) *tropica* infections and only in some *L.* (*L.*) *major* infections, especially those from Iraq and Arabia where titres similar to those found in kala-azar may be found.[14]

In leishmaniasis recidiva the differential diagnosis is from skin tuberculides, lupus vulgaris and Bazin's disease and from tuberculosis leprosy and syphilis. There is no sensory loss. The leishmanin test is always strongly positive and a negative test should bring the diagnosis under suspicion. Since parasites are so rarely found culture must always be undertaken and the biopsy examined for the typical 'tuberculoid histology'. Unlike in leprosy the nerves are unaffected.

TREATMENT

The majority of lesions caused by *L.* (*L.*) *major* and *L.* (*L.*) *tropica* heal spontaneously (*L.* (*L.*) *major* three to five months, *L.* (*L.*) *tropica* longer—up to 12 months) and do not necessarily require treatment. However, when they become large and threaten neighbouring structures (such as the eye, see Chapter 70, p. 1168) then some form of treatment is necessary.

Pentavalent antimony

Pentostam intravenously 20 mg Sb/kg/day for 10 days is usually successful. Other drugs which have been used with varying success are metronidazole, levamisole and dehydroemetine. Rifampicin has a varying effect but has been useful in difficult cases.[15,16]

Outpatient procedures

The following treatments are suitable for outpatient use.

Intra-lesional injection

For many years intra-lesional injection, using at first 5% mepacrine (no longer available) but more lately, pentavalent antimony and dehydroemetine have been used. Injections are given into one or more nodules at 3–5 day intervals for one to three occasions.

Cryosurgery

Many dermatologists have used cryosurgery and in one series[17] healing was complete with a good cosmetic result in all of 30 cases in four to five weeks.

Curettage

Simple curettage alone cured 73/78 cases within four weeks with little scarring and requires only one attendance.[18]

Local heat treatment

Leishmaniae do not grow above 33°C, so raising the intra-lesional temperature to 37–43°C for 12 hours at a time has been very successful.

Treatment of leishmaniasis recidiva

Since this form of leishmaniasis is so chronic, treatment is very difficult. Pentavalent antimony is of little use. Rifampicin has been used successfully[16] and intra-lesional injection of emetine hydrochloride 0.1–0.2 ml once a week into each nodule for two months successfully cured a chronic lesion after 42 years.[19] Heat treatment has also been successful.

EPIDEMIOLOGY (see also Appendix I, p. 1308)

The epidemiology of Old World cutaneous leishmaniasis depends upon the habits and ecology of the rodent hosts and sandfly vectors (Table III.3, p. 1400). There are three main types: zoonotic cutaneous leishmaniasis (ZCL) caused by *Leishmania* (*L.*) *major*; anthroponotic cutaneous leishmaniasis (ACL) caused by *Leishmania* (*L.*) *tropica* and cutaneous leishmaniasis caused by *Leishmania* (*L.*) *aethiopica*.

Zoonotic cutaneous leishmaniasis (ZCL) (rural leishmaniasis)

There are four types of ZCL: classical ZCL with major host the great gerbil; Middle Eastern ACL with major host the fat sand rat; Indian ZCL (major host the jird) and Sahelian ZCL (major host the Nile grass rat) (Fig. 37.2).

ZCL major host the great gerbil (*Rhombomys opimus*) (*classical ZCL*)

The great gerbil is distributed throughout large areas of Soviet Asia, northern Iran and northern Afghanistan where it lives in burrows in large colonies on the steppes and is highly susceptible to *L. (L.) major*. Persisting leishmanial lesions form on the ears which last over the winter season. In many areas 100% of the gerbils are infected. Their burrows are an ideal habitat for sandflies which live and breed in intimate contact with the gerbils and maintain the infection, among them *P. papatasi*, *P. caucasicus*, *P. antrejevi* and *P. mongolensis*. *P. papatasi* transmits the infection to man; *P. ansarii* (Iran) may also be a vector.[20]

Man is involved when he settles on the steppe and develops agriculture, building villages close to the gerbil colonies where up to 100% of inhabitants may show scars, and the infection is mainly in children. Man may intrude as fisherman, hunter or soldier in uninhabited areas. The gerbil does not adapt to intensive agriculture and the burrows can be destroyed by deep ploughing.

Other rodents *M. persicus*, *M. meridianus*, suslik (*Spermophilopsis leptodactylus*), jerboa (*Allactaga servtzovi*) and mouse (*Mus musculus*) are of minor importance although sometimes infected. Mustelids such as the weasel (*Mustela* sp.), marbled polecat (*Vormela peregusna*) and badger (*Meles meles*) may contract the infection by predation although cutaneous lesions do occur.

ZCL major host the fat sand rat (*Psammomys obesus*) (*Middle East ZCL*)

The fat sand rat is found throughout North Africa in Algeria, Morocco, Libya,[21] the Dead Sea area of Israel and Jordan,[22] southern Iran, Iraq and Saudi Arabia,[23] Kuwait[24] and the Yemen.[25] It lives in burrows under bushes in the semidesert and increasingly comes into contact with man with agricultural development (Fig III.16A, p. 1396). The vector in the western Mediterranean is *P. papatasi*, with possibly *P. chabaudi* in Algeria and Tunisia. *P. dubosqui* and *P. bergeroti* may be vectors in the Arabian peninsula.

Jirds (*Meriones* sp.) which live in the same burrows are secondary hosts in most areas but where the great gerbil does not occur, the red-tailed jird (*Meriones erythrourus*) can act as a major host. *M. shawi* in North Africa and *M. libycus* (Libya) can also act in this manner. Susliks are infected but are of little epidemiological importance.

Indian ZCL

In north-west India on the irrigation canals of Rajasthan the jird *Meriones hurrianae* is the only host and *P. salehi* is the vector.[26]

Sub-Saharan Africa (*Sahelian ZCL*)

ZCL is found in a wide zone between 10° and 13° north, from Thies in Senegal almost on the Atlantic coast to the central Sudan (Darfur) and a focus north of Khartoum.[27] In Senegal the main host is the Nile grass rat (*Arvicanthis niloticus*) in which infections have been visceral.[28] The multimammate rat (*Mastomys erythroleucus*) and a gerbil (*Tatera gambiana*) are secondary hosts.[29] The main sandfly vector is *P. dubosqui*. *P. bergeroti* is a suspected vector.[28]

L. (L.) major has also been isolated from rodents in the Rift Valley of Kenya where *L. (L.) major* isolated from cryptic infections of *Tatera robusta*, *Arvicanthis niloticus*, *Taterillus emini*, *Mastomys natalensis* and *Aethiomys kaiseri* were found to be identical to *L. (L.) major* from Israel and one of the *L. (L.) major* strains from West Africa. The other West African strain of *L. (L.) major* corresponds to other West African strains.[30] *P. dubosqui*, the major vector in West Africa, is also present in the Rift Valley[31] showing the extensive range of this sandfly from Senegal to East Africa and the Arabian peninsula. The absence of ZCL from East Africa must be due to the purely zoophilic habits of *P. dubosqui* but a focus of *L. (L.) major* has now been demonstrated here and a human case reported.[32]

Cutaneous leishmaniasis caused by *L. (L.) aethiopica*

Cutaneous leishmaniasis caused by *L. (L.) aethiopica* occurs in cool, high-altitude zones (1500–

2000 m) on the Ethiopian plateau[33] and in Kenya on Mount Elgon and Meningai crater. The main hosts are the rock hyrax (*Procavia habessinica*) and tree hyrax (*Heterohyrax brucei*).[21] The vectors are *P. longipes* and *P. pedifer* in Ethiopia and *P. pedifer* in Kenya. The disease is similar to that caused by *L. (L.) tropica* but a proportion of cases of disseminated cutaneous leishmaniasis (DCL) are found. The infection passes from hyrax to man in small villages and collections of houses near the rocky outcrops and trees where the hyrax live. A similar condition occurs in south-west Africa in the warm semi-arid plateau uplands of Namibia (1000–2000 m)[34] and in the Orange river area of Cape province.[35] Leishmaniae but not *L. (L.) aethiopica* have been isolated from man and a sandfly, *P. rossi*, but differ from leishmaniae isolated from the rock hyrax (*Procavia capensis*) in the area.

Anthroponotic cutaneous leishmaniasis (ACL) (*L. (L.) tropica*)—urban leishmaniasis

ACL is a natural infection of the dog and man although transmission occurs in the absence of dogs which may be secondarily infected only. It is an urban infection and is found in cities and towns. Up until recent years when there has been a steep decline in incidence caused by residual spraying of insecticides for malaria control, almost every adult long-term resident in these cities bore the scars of the disease on their faces, and it was a disease of children. There are three main epidemiological areas (Fig. 37.1).

Classical ACL

Classical ACL is or was found as an urban infection in all the major cities of the Middle East, Tashkent, Teheran, Baghdad, Aleppo and Damascus. It is transmitted by *P. sergenti*. Other possible vectors are *P. caucasicus* (Iran), *P. bergeroti*, *P. dubosqui* (Arabia), *P. mongolensis* (Iran, southern USSR) and *P. alexandri* (Iraq, Turkey, Yemen). As yet there has been no resurgence in the infection.

Western ACL

Western ACL is or was found throughout the western Mediterranean including central Italy, Sicily, Greek islands and North Africa, transmitted by *P. papatasi*. Another possible vector is

P. perfiliewi (Italy, Sardinia, Sicily). Although many scars can still be found in older people, few new cases occur. It is now thought that western ACL is caused by a zymodemne of *L. (L.) infantum*.[2]

Indian ACL

Indian ACL occurs in north-west India and the cities of Afghanistan, especially Kabul where there has been a great increase in incidence; 11.6% of the population show signs of the disease and there are many recent scars. Infected dogs are common and *P. sergenti* is the vector. Other possible vectors are *P. caucasicus* and *P. alexandri* (Afghanistan). Any alteration in sanitary conditions which follow natural or man-made disasters can cause a great upsurge in the sandfly population and an outbreak of ACL happened in the Quetta earthquake in Pakistan in the early years of the twentieth century.

Infection rates can be calculated on the percentage of active lesions in a population and incidence by counting scars of past infection and leishmanin sensitivity on an age-related basis. If the disease has become epidemic recently then the leishmanin rates will be approximately equal in all age groups. If the infection has been endemic for a long time then there will be a steady increase in leishmanin positivity with age. Interruption of transmission in the past can be shown in a similar manner by a sudden drop in leishmanin positivity under a certain age.

PROPHYLAXIS AND CONTROL

Reduction and control of cutaneous leishmaniasis in the population requires a knowledge of the epidemiology, sandfly vectors and animal hosts in the area. Clinical surveys for active cases and scars with a leishmanin survey will reveal the past and present extent of the infection. Surveys for infected dogs and rodents can be helped by serology and satisfactory indirect immunofluorescence (IFAT) titres were obtained in rodents infected with *L. (L.) major*.[36]

Sandfly control (Appendix III, p. 1403)

If the sandfly is peridomestic, general sanitary measures including removal of refuse and rubble and provision of good housing will reduce infection. Residual spraying for malaria eradication had eliminated *L. (L.) tropica* from most urban areas but since cessation of the spraying both the sandflies and the disease have returned.

Control of the animal reservoir

In central Asia colonies of the great gerbil (*Rhombomys opimus*) have been removed from the environs of villages and irrigation schemes by ploughing up the communal burrows which are in soft, sandy soil and creating conditions in which the gerbils cannot survive.[37] In many countries the identification and removal of infected dogs has proved very useful.

Immunization

Prophylactic inoculation with live cultures (pro-

mastigotes) of *L. (L.) major* has been practised for many years in Russia, Israel and Jordan. Freshly isolated virulent strains are necessary and these rapidly lose virulence on subculture. A frozen promastigote vaccine used after 11 months in storage given by intradermal jet in a dose of 4 million organisms gave a 100% take[38] with a high ulceration rate which is necessary to produce a good immunity. Frozen vaccines lose their immunity after prolonged storage. The formation of nodules alone may not produce such a good immunity. The ulcers must be allowed to run their natural course and heal spontaneously. Since they are on covered regions of the body and the scarring is usually minimal this is an effective procedure. Difficulties can arise in certain individuals who may develop recidiva-like lesions.

NEW WORLD (NEOTROPICAL) CUTANEOUS LEISHMANIASIS (AMERICAN LEISHMANIASIS)

GEOGRAPHICAL DISTRIBUTION
(Figs. 37.11 and 37.12)

Cutaneous leishmaniasis of the New World is found from southern Texas south through Central America to South America and Brazil as far south as northern Argentina and on the western slopes of the Andes in Peru and northern Argentina.

AETIOLOGY

A number of leishmanial species and subspecies are the cause of American leishmaniasis. These *Leishmania* are normally found in small forest rodents and other larger mammals, existing as inapparent infections or small cutaneous lesions. They are transmitted in a forest environment on the ground or in the trees by ground dwelling or

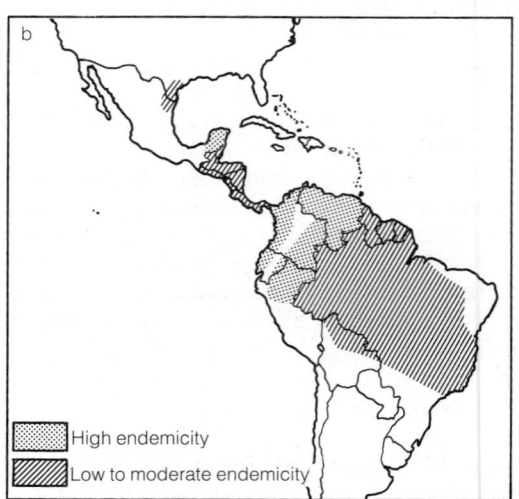

Fig. 37.11 Geographical distribution and endemicity of cutaneous leishmaniasis caused by the *L. (L.) mexicana* complex. (Courtesy Department of Entomology, London School of Hygiene and Tropical Medicine.)

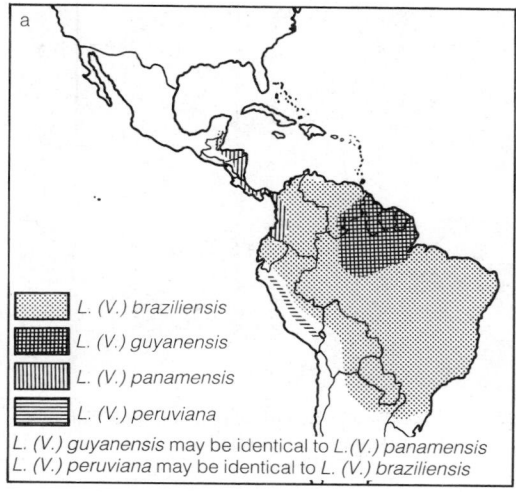 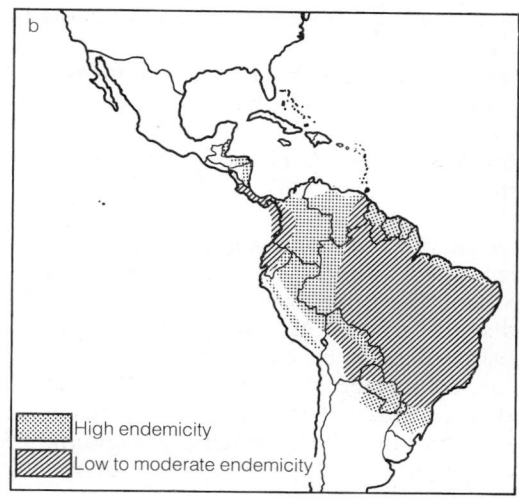

Fig. 37.12 Geographical distribution and endemicity of cutaneous and mucosal leishmaniasis caused by the *L. (V.) braziliensis* complex. (Courtesy Department of Entomology, London School of Hygiene and Tropical Medicine.)

arboreal sandflies of the *Lutzomyia* and *Psychodopogus* genera which live in this environment.

In the main there are two main complexes: *L. (L.) mexicana* and *L. (V.) braziliensis* complex, each with a number of strains which can be distinguished clinically, epidemiologically and biochemically. The *Leishmania* which cause American leishmaniasis are:

L. (L.) mexicana complex	*Clinical condition*
L. (L.) mexicana	Chiclero's ulcer
L. (L.) amazonensis (*L. (L.) garnhami*)	Enzootic rodent leishmaniasis
L. (L.) pifanoi	Enzootic rodent leishmaniasis
L. (L.) mexicana (from the Dominican Republic)	DCL[10]
L. (V.) braziliensis complex	
L. (V.) guyanensis	Pian bois. Bush Yaws
L. (V.) panamensis	Panamanian leishmaniasis
L. (V.) braziliensis	Espundia. Mucosal leishmaniasis
L. (V.) peruviana	Uta

These *Leishmania* can be identified by cultural methods, study of their enzymes and by serology of the excreted factor (EF) (see Section on diagnosis, p. 743, and Appendix I).

L. (L.) mexicana develops in the sandfly in the same way as other *Leishmania* causing visceral and Old World cutaneous leishmaniasis in the anterior position in the gut (suprapylarian development), whereas *L. (V.) braziliensis* develops behind in the midgut (peripylarian development) (see Appendix III, Fig III.19, p. 1402, and Appendix I, p. 1295).

TRANSMISSION

Transmission is by sandfly bites of the genus *Lutzomyia or Psychodopogus* which inoculate promastigotes into the skin (Table III.3, p. 1400). Direct transmission by contact has been reported.[39]

PATHOLOGY

The ability to distinguish between *L. (L.) mexicana* and *L. (V.) braziliensis* has been of great help in the understanding of the pathogenesis and pathology of the lesions. In *L. (L.) mexicana*-type lesions the pathological features are similar to those seen in *L. (L.) major* infection. The anergic DCL seen in a proportion of infections caused by *L. (L.) amazonensis, L. (L.) pifanoi* and the Dominican Republic *Leishmania* has a similar pathology to DCL caused by *L. (L.) aethiopica* (see p. 733). In lesions of the ear (Chiclero's ulcer) the cartilage is involved in the granulomatous process and there is necrosis of the cartilage.

In the lesions caused by *L. (V.) braziliensis* the pathology is somewhat different.

Cutaneous lesions *L. (V.) braziliensis* complex

The strain of *Leishmania* is important; the more virulent the leishmaniae the less they are tolerated and the greater the connective tissue and vascular disturbance on release of the antigens suggesting damage by extracellular parasites or immune complexes. Scarring is the hallmark of this disease, macrophages are few and parasites seldom seen but, where present, 'garlanding' of the amastigotes round the periphery of vacuolated histiocytes is a feature.

Histologically, there is a spectrum of change varying from little to intense cellular infiltrate, granuloma formation or necrosis. Parasites are scanty and show 'garlanding' in histiocytes. In some cases there is fibrinoid necrosis and vasculitis in the dermis or small scattered foci of less severe fibrinoid change. Where there are granulomatous changes there is a well-developed epithelioid cell granuloma (tuberculoid) with necrosis (Fig. 37.13) or with large Langhans'

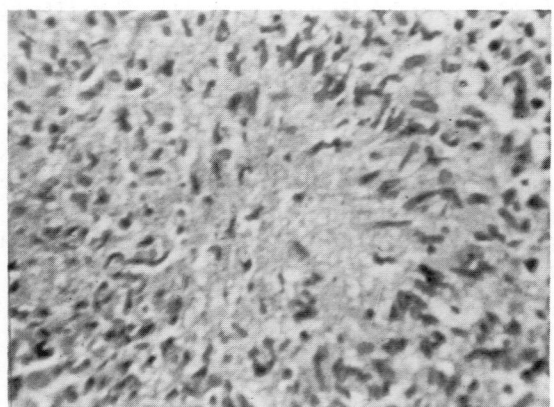

Fig. 37.13 *Espundia.* Tuberculoid reaction with central necrosis but no parasites. (Courtesy Dr B.H. Kean.)

giant cells and scanty lymphocytes (Fig. 37.14). There may be epidermal hyperplasia with pseudoepitheliomatous down-growths which can progress to a basal cell carcinoma. Necrosis leading to ulceration is a favourable prognostic sign.

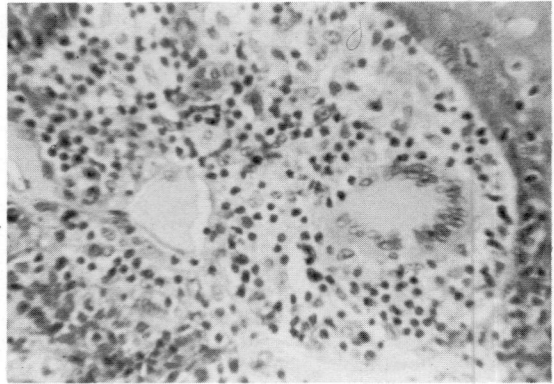

Fig. 37.14 *Espundia.* Tuberculoid reaction with Langhans' giant cells and invasion of nasal cartilage. (Courtesy Dr H. Zaiman.)

Mucosal leishmaniasis (espundia)

An important feature is the development of mucosal lesions around the nose and mouth. The cutaneous lesion starts as a papule usually on the lower part of the leg which ulcerates and may involve the local lymphatic glands (in *L. (V.) guyanensis* this is a major feature). The ulcer heals and after a period of time, usually up to two years or more, mucosal lesions (espundia) appear in the nose.

What pathological processes cause these lesions to appear, often after many years, is still not clear. An immunological process is possible and the intense destruction of nasal cartilage in the absence of any parasites suggests an autoimmune process.

The nose and nasal septum are the main areas involved (in contrast to the oropharyngeal mucosal lesions seen in kala-azar—see Chapter 4). The oropharynx and larynx may become involved with nodules and granulomas spreading down even to involve the trachea and oesophagus, causing obstruction. The disease starts at the junction of the nose and mouth spreading to the nasal septum (Fig. 37.14) which can be entirely destroyed and eventually the whole of the front of the face may be transformed into a hideous open sore.

Lupoid form

This is a chronic non-healing form found in patients with mucosal involvement which is very resistant to treatment.

Histological changes in the lesions

Ridley et al[4] have classified the changes into five groups.

Group 1. Mild changes, inflammatory cells, scanty or absent; no granulomas (non-reactive).

Group 2. Necrosis and vasculitis with light infiltrate of polymorphs and chronic inflammatory cells (reactive).

Group 3. Heavy cellular infiltrate; no granuloma (infiltrative).

Group 4. Abundance of lymphocytes; a few Langhans' giant cells; small epithelioid cell granulomas (tuberculoid).

Group 5. Well-developed epithelioid cell granuloma with Langhans' giant cells; no necrosis; fibrosis heavy (hypersensitive).

This classification has prognostic value. Groups 1 and 5 are mostly mucosal and respond poorly to treatment. Groups 2 and 4 are all cutaneous responding relatively well to treatment. Group 3 response to treatment is variable with a tendency to relapse and a small number develop mucosal disease.

IMMUNITY

There is no natural immunity and all ages, races and both sexes can be attacked. In endemic areas where there is a raised positive leishmanin rate in the population, presumably from inapparent infection, a positive leishmanin reaction gives protection against the homologous strain. Recovery from *L. (L.) mexicana* and *L. (V.) panamensis* and *L. (V.) guyanensis* will provide protection against infection by the homologous strain but in some cases of *L. (L.) mexicana* and *L. (V.) guyanensis* there is a spectrum of cell-mediated immune response, so that *L. (L.) amazonensis* commonly causes diffuse cutaneous leishmaniasis, and in *L. (V.) guyanensis* there may be relapses and reinfection.[40]

CLINICAL FEATURES

Natural history

American leishmaniasis is basically an infection of small rodents. Man is not a normal host and is only infected accidentally when he intrudes on rodent habitats.

There is a wide spectrum of response to infection. With *L. (L.) mexicana* strains a single skin lesion develops which heals spontaneously in six months in the great majority of cases and there is immunity to reinfection with the homologous strain. In chiclero's ulcer (*L. (L.) mexicana*) the lesion on the ear is very chronic because of localization in the relatively poorly blood-supplied cartilage. At the other end of the spectrum is the anergic response to *L. (L.) amazonensis* strains with the development of DCL, a very chronic and progressive infection. With *L. (V.) braziliensis* strains the original lesion may heal and, in many cases, not progress any further; in others *L. (V.) braziliensis* may heal only to be followed from two or more years later by the development of hypersensitivity and appearance of espundia, a very destructive lesion of the mucosa of the nose and mouth. Once this stage has been reached there is usually no spontaneous cure and eventually death results from secondary infection.

In another strain *L. (V.) guyanensis* the original lesion may spread to the rest of the skin causing multiple lesions or may extend up the lymphatics to the regional lymph glands, with resolution after a long period.

In many cases both of mexicana and braziliensis types there are many inapparent infections and leishmanin surveys in endemic areas have shown a proportion of the population with positive leishmanin skin tests who have never shown signs of disease.

Incubation period

The incubation period is similar to that of *L. (L.) tropica* and *L. (L.) major* lesions, a few days or weeks after the original sandfly bite.

Symptoms and signs

L. (L.) mexicana (chiclero's ulcer)

L. (L.) mexicana causes a single benign self-limiting lesion except where it occurs on the ear where the infection is very chronic. The incubation period is a few weeks to several months. A small erythematous, often pruritic papule develops at the site of inoculation. This becomes scaly and ulcerates with a raised indurated margin which heals after six months. When situated on the ear the pinna becomes swollen and inflamed and the cartilage is invaded. A very chronic lesion results with slow destruction of the auricle over a period of as long as 20 years (chiclero's ulcer, oreja de chicleros—Fig. 37.15).

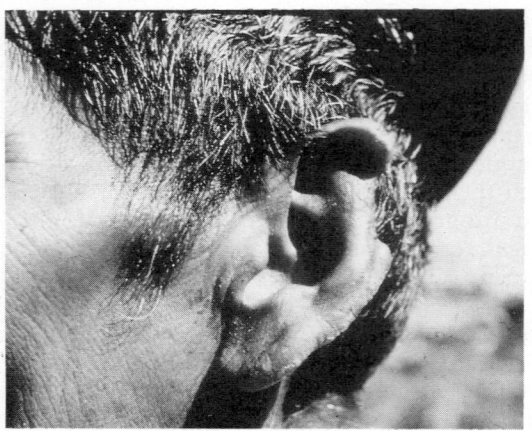

Fig. 37.15 *L. (L.) mexicana* infection of the pinna of the ear (chiclero's ulcer—oreja de chicleros): early and late stages.

L. (L.) amazonensis

L. (L.) amazonensis causes a similar benign lesion but with no predilection for the face or ear, which heals in six months. However, in a proportion of cases (as much as 30%) the infection disseminates and is of the DCL type (see p. 733) so that although rare in man, the results of *L. (L.) amazonensis* infection can be severe.

L. (L.) pifanoi is similar in its clinical effects to *L. (L.) amazonensis* and, although it rarely infects man, causes a high proportion of DCL cases. *L. (L.) mexicana* from the Dominican Republic causes, as seen so far, only DCL cases.

L. (V.) braziliensis (espundia)

PRIMARY LESION
The incubation period can be as short as 15 days. The initial lesion begins as a small painless nodule which may itch intensely and then ulcerates within one to two months forming a round shallow ulcer with prominent raised borders. The most frequent presentation is a large ulcer on the lower third of the leg.[41] In about a third of cases the lesions are multiple and other sites include the foot, forearm, head, hip, elbow and nasal mucosa. Multiple lesions tend to develop mucosal lesions to a greater extent than single lesions.

MUCOSAL LESIONS (ESPUNDIA)
Mucosal lesions are found most commonly in *L. (V.) braziliensis* infection but may also occur in *L. (V.) panamensis* but not in *L. (V.) guyanensis*. The further south the higher the percentage of mucosal involvement from 2% in Panama to 80% in Brazil (60%[42]). The process starts at the junction of the nose and upper lip (Fig. 37.16) and in some cases destruction of the whole of the front of the face occurs. This process may occur rapidly or may take many years, often appearing to remain static. Very rarely, self-healing has been noted. In the nose crusting of the anterior septum, polyp formation, ulceration and perforation of the septum with scarring and sinking of the external nose 'tapir nose' (Fig. 37.17) may destroy the whole of the septum so that it is

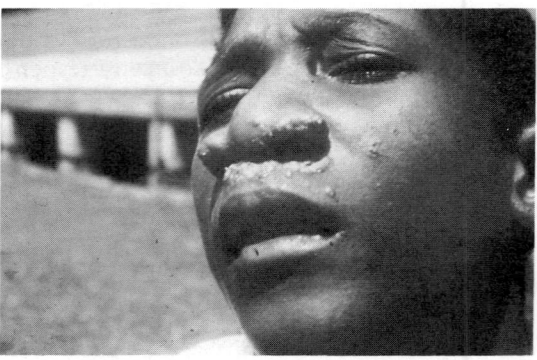

Fig. 37.16 Mucosal leishmaniasis (espundia) caused by *L. (V.) braziliensis*. Early stage involving junction of nose and upper lip.

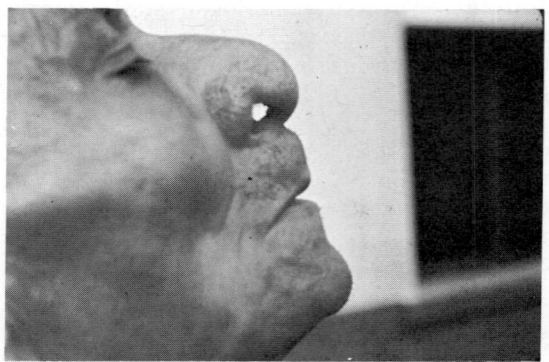

Fig. 37.17 Mucosal leishmaniasis (espundia) caused by *L. (V.) braziliensis*. Destruction of nasal septum (tapir nose). (Courtesy Dr D.A. Leon.)

possible to look right down to the larynx from the nose. Mucosal lesions may be single involving the nose alone or more rarely the larynx, or may be multiple (Fig. 37.18), involving the pharynx, palate, larynx and upper lip. Death eventually results from aspiration pneumonia from destruction of the pharynx.

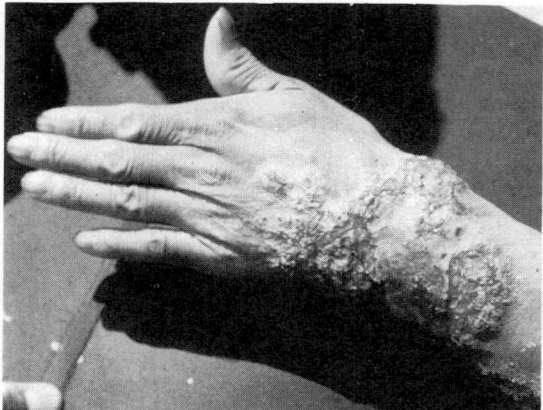

Fig. 37.19 Pian bois. Cutaneous leishmaniasis caused by *L. (V.) guyanensis*. Ulceration of the hand and forearm of the 'pian bois' type. (Courtesy Dr R. Lainson.)

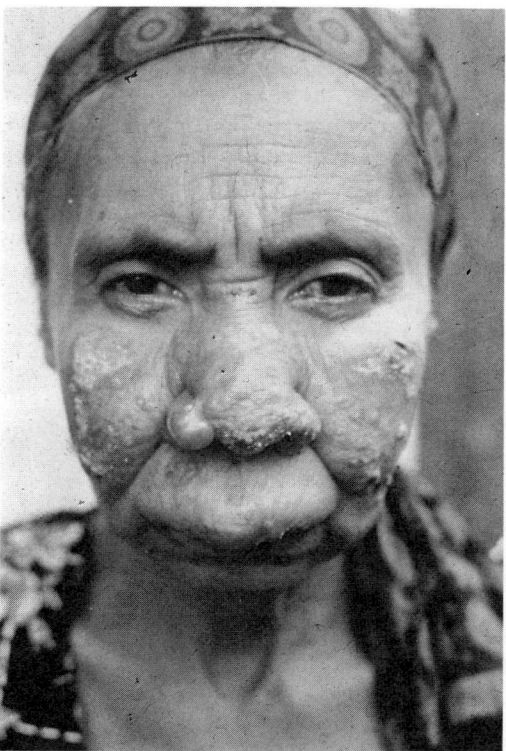

Fig. 37.18 Mucosal leishmaniasis (espundia) caused by *L. (V.) braziliensis*. Late stage involving nose and pharynx. (Courtesy Dr P.D. Marsden.)

L. (V.) guyanensis (pian bois, bush yaws)

A few weeks after exposure a small itchy papule appears which enlarges to form a firm nodule which ulcerates to form a shallow ulcer. The lesions are usually multiple (64%[43]) and spread widely over the upper body and on the dorsum of the hands (Fig. 37.19). Facial lesions may be accompanied by oedema. A special feature is the involvement of the lymphatics with discrete rubbery nodules which may ulcerate and spread to the local lymph glands which become grossly enlarged so that the whole picture resembles that of sporotrichosis. There is no mucosal spread. Relapses and reinfections have been described.[40]

Leishmanids

A leishmanid is a cutaneous eruption found in both Old and New World cutaneous leishmaniasis. It may appear from a few months to many years after the initial lesion has disappeared. Transient hypopigmented lesions appear to be followed by papular or lichenoid lesions which may spread up the lymphatics. The histology is tuberculoid (RIDLEY group V[4]) but no parasites can be identified and the leishmanin reaction is strongly positive. The eruption often appears after the ingestion of alcohol, exposure to the sun, or during the puerperium, suggesting that some form of immunosuppression is responsible[44]. Leishmanids are to be differentiated from Diffuse cutaneous leishmaniasis in which numerous parasites can be seen (p. 733) and post kala azar dermal leishmanoid in which the leishmanin test is negative and some parasites can be demonstrated (p. 105). The condition responds to pentavalent antimony treatment.

DIAGNOSIS

It is important in all American leishmaniasis lesions to determine as soon as possible whether the parasite responsible is *L. (L.) mexicana* or *L. (V.) braziliensis*. Methods of distinguishing them (behaviour in culture, enzyme structure, excreted factor type) are discussed in Appendix I (p. 1321), and development in the sandfly in Appendix III (p. 1401) and Fig. 111.19 (p. 1402). From the point of view of clinical diagnosis, behaviour in culture is most important and cultures should be obtained as soon as possible. If the parasite grows well and rapidly in the usual media, then it is *L. (L.) mexicana*; if it grows slowly or not at all, then it is *L. (V.) braziliensis*.

L.(L.)mexicana infections

Parasites are usually numerous and can be demonstrated by the same methods used for *L. (L.) major* (see p. 734); touch preparations, dendritic broach, biopsy and culture.

Serology

The IFAT is negative throughout and is an important sign that the infection if leishmanial is with *L. (L.) mexicana*. The leishmanin test becomes positive six to eight weeks after the start and remains positive for life and is an important diagnostic test. If the test remains negative and parasites are present, then the case is of the diffusa type and needs treating accordingly.

L. (L.) braziliensis infections

L. (L.) guyanensis (pian bois) must be distinguished from sporotrichosis which it closely resembles and other mycotic infections. Parasites are scanty (one-third only show parasites) and the leishmanin test becomes positive. Biopsy will show a characteristic picture[45] and the IFAT is positive in all cases from a titre of 1/8 to 1/512.[43]

Mucosal lesions (espundia)

Mucosal lesions must be distinguished from yaws (gangosa), syphilis, lupus vulgaris, leprosy, mycotic infections and epithelioma. Parasites are very scanty in smears and every effort must be made to obtain a culture, especially from the primary lesion.

Serology

The IFAT is positive in nearly all cases and has proved very useful in diagnosis, prognosis and monitoring the effect of treatment.[45,46] The use of an amastigote antigen avoids cross reactions with Chagas' disease and titres ranging from 1/16 to 1/1024 were found in 89% of cases.[47] Following successful treatment there is a twofold drop in titre but antibodies never disappear completely and their persistence does not apparently prophesy a recurrence but a subsequent rise does.

ENZYME-LINKED IMMUNOSORBENT ASSAY (ELISA)

The ELISA was more sensitive than any other test[48] and a micro-ELISA has been devised[49] suggesting that this test may replace the IFAT.

LEISHMANIN TEST

The leishmanin test is very useful in the diagnosis of espundia from other conditions. It becomes positive shortly after infection and positive tests were found in 94.6% of cases.[50] As opposed to *L. (L.) mexicana* the leishmanin test may not remain positive for life in *L. (V.) braziliensis* infection and in 52/100 cases treated with Glucantime the test reverted to negative in from 19 days to seven years after treatment.[51] An important point noted was that in mucosal lesions the leishmanin test intensified with reactivation of the disease.

TREATMENT

L. (L.) mexicana complex

Since most mexicana lesions are self-limiting, healing naturally within six months, no treatment is needed. If the lesions are multiple and when the ear is involved (*L. (L.) mexicana*) then treatment is necessary to prevent destruction of the pinna and a very chronic lesion. Glucantime 20 mg/kg daily for 10–12 days will heal the lesion and prevent further destruction.

Most *L. (L.) amazonensis* lesions are self-healing but a proportion will develop DCL. If the biopsy shows many parasites and little cellular response Cat 5 (ref. 4) then treatment must be given. Pentamidine is the drug of choice, 4 mg/kg twice daily for as long as it may take to produce response[52] (see section on diffuse cutaneous leishmaniasis, p. 734). DCL caused by *L. (L.) amazonensis* has been treated successfully by a combination of rifampicin, isoniazid and para-aminosalicylic acid (PAS) but relapsed when the isoniazid was withdrawn.[53] Experimental *L. (L.) amazonensis* has been successfully treated with liposome trapped Pentostam.[54]

L. (V.) braziliensis complex

Once the diagnosis of braziliensis infection has been made by cultural means then treatment must be given.

L. (V.) braziliensis (espundia)

The primary lesion of *L. (V.) braziliensis* must be treated to prevent later mucosal spread and also when mucosal spread is present then a full course of Glucantime must be given. Glucantime 20 mg/kg intravenously is given daily for 30 days or as long as it is necessary to obtain healing. Twice daily doses of 10–20 mg/kg may be employed in resistant cases. When combined with heat treatment, healing occurs quickly. Cases of resistance do occur and are especially common in Peru.[55] Treatment must be monitored by serology especially where only the primary lesion has been treated since mucocutaneous spread can occur as long as the IFAT remains positive and shows no fall.

Pentamidine can be used as a second drug as in pian bois.

Amphotericin B. This is a very toxic and very much a last resort drug but may be used in resistant cases. If dosage, initially 0.15–0.2 mg/kg by drip infusion, is tolerated then the dose may be raised to a maximum of 50 mg dose by drip infusion over 6–8 hours, two to four doses a week for a period of six to 17 weeks with a total dosage of 400–2000 mg.

L. (V.) guyanensis (pian bois)

Most cases of *L. (V.) guyanensis* need treatment in view of the lymphatic spread. The drug of choice is pentamidine methane sulphonate (Lomidine). Lomidine given intravenously in a 120 mg dose every other day for seven injections produced an initial response in all of 30 patients;[43] 19/30 relapsed and needed a second course and one required a third course. Biopsy findings were useful in assessing possible responses (see p. 741).

L. (V.) peruviana (uta)

Lesions of uta are usually self-healing and need no treatment.

Other drugs

Other drugs have been used successfully mostly with mexicana and non-metastasizing infections.

Rifampicin

Rifampicin used in cases with multiple lesions in doses of 1200 mg (adults) and 600 mg (children) at 12-hourly intervals for three to 15 weeks produced total cicatrization in 40/55, partial in 11/55 and complete failure in 4/55.[56]

Heat treatment

Heat treatment as applied in Old World cutaneous leishmaniasis has proved effective in neotropical cutaneous leishmaniasis.

COMPLICATIONS

The complications are due to mucosal disease; secondary infection of the lungs from the destructive laryngeal and palatal lesions and epithelioma which may develop in chronic lesions. Once the parasites have been removed by treatment and the lesion rendered inactive then reconstructive surgery can restore the nose and palate.

EPIDEMIOLOGY AND CONTROL (see also Appendix I, p. 1310)

American leishmaniasis is a rural disease which although it is found in primeval climax forest becomes especially important to man when he clears the forest and establishes secondary growth or plantations. It is an infection which attacks forest workers, hunters and settlers on cleared forest land in new territory. It is a zoonosis, the main cycle of infection being transmitted between small forest rodents and larger forest mammals by arboreal and ground dwelling sandflies.

L. (L.) mexicana complex[57]

Parasites of the mexicana complex have a wide distribution throughout the Americas (Fig. 37.11) and can be expected to be found in any type, primary forest or degraded woodland, in which sandflies of the *Lutzomyia flaviscutellata* group are known to exist in the presence of small terrestrial animals (forest rodents, marsupials and foxes) which share the same habitat.

L. (L.) mexicana (chiclero's ulcer)

L. (L.) mexicana which causes chiclero's ulcer in

man is confined to the low-lying forest areas of the Yucatan in Mexico and the Peten in Guatemala and Belize (the country of the Mayan Indians) (Fig. 37.11). The major host is a cricetid rodent, the big-eared climbing rat (*Ototylomys phyllotis*) with minor hosts, the vesper rat (*Nycromys semichrasti*), the cotton rat (*Sigmodon hispidus*), the spiny pocket mouse (*Heteromys desmaresteanus*). The sandfly vector is *Lutzomyia olmeca* which bites man mainly on the ear so that forest workers, mainly gum collectors (chicleros) are affected. *L. (L.) mexicana* has recently been reported as far north as southern Texas where further reports are of a case of DCL (see p. 734) not previously recorded in *L. (L.) mexicana*[58] and two further cases,[59] one of which resembled espundia but in an immunocompromised host.[60] Two further cases have been reported from Coahuila state in northern Mexico[61] where other sandflies may be involved in transmission.

L. (L.) amazonensis (enzootic rodent leishmaniasis)

Enzootic rodent leishmaniasis has long been known to occur in man in eastern Panama, Amazonian Brazil and Venezuela (Fig. 37.11) but until recent developments have enabled it to be separated from *L. (V.) braziliensis* it has not been possible to clarify the situation. There is a widespread range of hosts. Thirteen species of rodents, marsupials and foxes have been found infected[57] in whom infection is confined to the skin (while *L. (V.) braziliensis* is found in the skin and viscera.[62] The primary host in Panama is the spiny rat (*Proechimys guyanensis*) in which the infection rate is high (25% or more) with the parasite restricted to the skin as an inapparent infection. *Lutzomyia flaviscutellata* is the vector which abounds in secondary growth and plantations of non-indigenous trees in a narrow zone near the ground where it feeds on a wide variety of rodents, especially *Proechimys* or *Oryzomys* which have invaded these new habitats. Few bite man in whom the infection can be severe with a 30% rate of DCL.[63]

A focus of rodent leishmaniasis has been found in Trinidad[64] where 3% of rice rats (*Oryzomys capito*) were found infected but no human cases. In other areas other rodents may be of greater importance, the rice rat (*Oryzomys capito*) and spiny rat (*Proechimys guyanensis*) in Brazil[65] and in north Pará State in Brazil three species of opossums, *Didelphis marsupialis*, *Philander*

opossum and the brown four-eyed opossum *Metachirus nudicaudatus*.[62]

L. (L.) pifanoi

A separate existence for *L. (L.) pifanoi* is still open to doubt but cases of DCL caused by this organism have been described from Venezuela (Fig. 37.11) where the pocket spiny mouse (*Heteromys anomalus*), spiny rat (*Proechimys guyanensis*) and cane mouse (*Zygodontomys microtinus*) are hosts, and *Lutzomyia flaviscutellata* is the vector.

L. (L.) garnhami (*Venezuelan Andean cutaneous leishmaniasis*)

Cases of cutaneous leishmaniasis have been found in the Venezuelan Andes at a height of 800–1000 metres (higher than *L. (L.) amazonensis*) (Fig. 37.11) from which some differences have been noted.[66] *Lutzomyia townsendi* has been named as the vector and a single opossum (*Didelphis marsupialis*) has been found infected. Some observations on *L. (L.) garnhami* have cast doubts on its identity, some isolates being of the mexicana and others of the braziliensis type.

Cutaneous leishmaniasis in the Dominican Republic (Fig. 37.11)

A leishmanial parasite has been found in the Dominican Republic where all the human cases so far discovered have been of the DCL type but where leishmanin surveys have revealed a number of inapparent infections. It differs from *L. (L.) amazonensis* in zymodeme and excreted factor type. It has been found in the small amount of indigenous forest left and only two species of sandfly are present, one of which (*Lutzomyia christophei*) feeds on man.[10]

L. (V.) braziliensis complex

The *L. (V.) braziliensis* complex contains two well-defined subspecies, *L. (V.) panamensis* and *L. (V.) guyanensis*, as well as minor subspecies, *L. (V.) peruviana* and other as yet unknown subspecies.

L. (V.) panamensis (*Panamanian leishmaniasis*)

L. (V.) panamensis is found in Central America,

Panama and north-western South America (Fig. 37.12). *L. (V.) panamensis* causes cutaneous but rarely nasopharyngeal lesions in man. It was identified in Panama and Costa Rica.[69] Sloths are important hosts and the two-toed sloth (*Choloepus hoffmani*) is the main reservoir host, in which the infection is inapparent involving the skin and viscera. The vectors are *Lutzomyia yphiletor* in Costa Rica[67] and *Lutzomyia trapidoi* in Columbia.[68] Other animals may be secondary or accidental hosts, the three-toed sloth (*Bradypus infuscatus*), the night monkey (*Aotus trivirgatus*), Geoffroy's tamarin (*Sanguineus geoffroyi*), olingo (*Bassaricyon gabbi*), coati (*Nasua nasua*) and kinkajou (*Potos flavus*). Dogs also may be hosts and are of importance, since hunting dogs bring infection into the villages.[69] The epidemiology and environment in which *L. (V.) panamensis* is acquired is similar to that of *L. (V.) guyanensis.*

L. (V.) guyanensis (bush yaws, pian bois)[57]

This form is found in Amazonian Brazil, Guyana, Surinam and French Guyana (Fig. 37.12). In primary forest the main hosts are sloths and edentates, the two-toed sloth (*Choloepus didactylus*) and the ant-eater (*Tamandua tetradactyla*) in which the infections are inapparent and visceral.[72] The vector, *Lutzomyia umbratilis*, spends most of the year in the forest canopy but descends to the forest floor to lay eggs for about two weeks at the start of the rainy season[73] where, when disturbed from tree trunks at ground level, it may attack and infect secondary hosts including man. Transmission to man occurs principally during the early part of the day when the sandflies are concentrated on the tree trunks (important for personal prophylaxis).

Where the primary forest has been disturbed for development the primary hosts withdraw and opossums take over so that the opossum (*Didelphis marsupialis*) becomes the primary host and outbreaks of pian bois occur in the suburbs of new towns cut out of the primary forest.

L. (V.) braziliensis (espundia, mucosal leishmaniasis)

L. (V.) braziliensis consists of a number of as yet unidentified subspecies of *Leishmania* recognized by their 'peripylarian' type of development in the sandfly (see Appendix I, p. 1401, and Fig. III.19, p. 1402). *L. (V.) braziliensis* is distributed throughout the forested or wooded regions of most of Latin America (Fig. 37.12). The animal hosts are almost unknown and the primary host has not yet been identified, but three species of rodent have been found infected with braziliensis-type parasites (*Oryzomys capito, O. nigripes, Akodon arviculoides*) and an opossum (*Didelphis marsupialis*). A major vector *Lutzomyia (Psychodopygus) wellcomei*[79] is the predominantly man-biting sandfly by day and night in northern Brazil. *Lutzomyia pessoai* and *Lutzomyia intermedia* have been implicated in southern Brazil.

L. (V.) braziliensis is a major public health problem in Brazil, especially during road operations in Amazonia. It occurs focally in small areas often widely separated. It is of great importance in newly settled areas and in eastern Bolivia this importance has been emphasized where there was a prevalence rate of 16% among 7599 inhabitants with an incidence of 80% in first year settlers one year after arrival, falling to 2–3% in subsequent years; 125 cases of the mutilating espundia were found. In endemic areas there is an equal incidence in both sexes and a decrease in incidence with age.

L. (V.) peruviana (uta)[73]

This *Leishmania* is now known to belong to the braziliensis group by reason of its 'peripylarian' development in sandflies and enzyme structure and may be, in fact, *L. (V.) braziliensis*. It is found in the dry scrubland valleys of the western Andes in Peru and Argentina (Fig. 37.12). Originally it occurred as a peridomestic infection with the dog as the major host and *Lutzomyia verrucarum* as vector.[74] This sandfly frequented houses and animal sheds. In some villages 94% of the children carried scars of infection.

Following the destruction of peridomestic sandflies for the control of bartonellosis, uta completely disappeared. Recently in the Santa Eulalia valley[75] there has been a resurgence and a strong possibility exists that there is a wild animal host with a less domestic sandfly than *Lutzomyia verrucarum* as vector and the pattern of infection is now reverting from semidomestic to its ancient sylvatic state.

CONTROL

Since American leishmaniasis is always a zoonosis, little can be done to control the source of infection. Peridomestic sandflies can be controlled by house spraying with residual insecticide and this eradicated uta in Peru in the 1950s. However, there is little hope of controlling forest sandflies so that two other methods must be considered.

Breaking man–fly contact

Where enough is known of the biology of the vector then sandfly bites can be avoided. In the Guyanas where pian bois *L. (V.) guyanensis* is transmitted by *Lutzomyia umbratilis*, avoiding action can be taken. The sandfly lives in the forest canopy and descends to the floor to lay eggs especially at the start of the rainy season. It becomes active round the bases of the trees in the early morning so that disturbance of these areas must be avoided until later in the day. In other areas the primary hosts will be driven back some kilometres from new settlements so a cleared zone of a few kilometres around new villages will break the man–host contact. However, new more adaptable hosts will take up a peridomestic habitat (opossums) and so new sources of infection may arise.

Immunization

No method of immunization is yet available. This would involve a live vaccine made from a benign strain to protect against espundia (*L. (V.) braziliensis*). Experiments with monkeys[76] and observations in French Guyana[77] suggest that while *L. (V.) braziliensis* can protect against *L. (L.) mexicana*, but *L. (L.) mexicana* cannot protect against *L. (V.) braziliensis* strains.

REFERENCES

1 Schnur, L.F. & Zuckerman, A. (1977) *Ann. trop. Med. Parasit.* **71**, 273.
2 Rioux, J.A., Lanotte, G., Pratlong, F. et al (1985) *Méd. malad. Inf.* **11**, 650–656.
3 Le Blancq, S.M., Schnur, L.F. & Peters, W. (1986) *Trans. R. Soc. trop. Med. Hyg.* **80**, 99–112.
4 Ridley, D.S. (1980) *Trans. R. Soc. trop. Med. Hyg.* **74**, 515.
5 Guirges, S.Y. (1971) *Ann. trop. Med. Parasit.* **65**, 197.
6 Senekji, H.A. & Beattie, C.P. (1941) *Trans. R. Soc. trop. Med. Hyg.* **23**, 523.
7 Smith, P.A.J. (1955) *Br. med. J.* **ii**, 1143.
8 Price, E.W. & Fitzherbert, M. (1965) *Ethiop. med. J.* **3**, 57.
9 Convit, J.A. & Kerdel Vegas, F.T. (1965) *Archs Derm.* **91**, 439.
10 Schnur, L.F., Watton, B.C. & Bogaert Diaz, H. (1983) *Trans. R. Soc. trop. Med. Hyg.* **77**, 756–762.
11 Chulay, J.D., Anzeze, E.M., Koech, D.K. et al (1983) *Trans. R. Soc. trop. Med. Hyg.* **77**, 717–721.
12 Bryceson, A.D.M. (1969) *Trans. R. Soc. trop. Med. Hyg.* **63**, 708.
13 Henricksen, T.H. & Lende, S. (1983). *Lancet* **i**, 126.
14 Latif, B.M.A., Al Shenawi, F.A. & Al Alousi, T.I. (1979) *Ann. trop. med. Parasit.* **73**, 31.
15 Sande, M.A. (1983) *Rev. infect. Dis.* **5**, suppl. 3.
16 Even-Paz, Z., Weinrauch, L., Livshin, R. et al (1982) *Int. J. Derm.* **21**, 110–112.
17 Bassiouny, A., El-Meshad, M., Talaat, M. et al (1982) *Br. J. Derm.* **107**, 467–474.
18 Currie, M.A. (1983) *Br. med. J.* **287**, 1105.
19 Cohen, H.A. & Wahaba, A. (1979) *Acta Derm. Venerol.* **59**, 549–552.
20 Bray, R.S. (1982) *Biol. Dis.* **4**, 257–267.
21 Ashford, R.W., Schnur, L., Chance, M.L. et al (1977) *Ann. trop. med. Parasit.* **71**, 265–271.
22 Egoz, N. & Michaeli, D. (1978) *Rev. Int. Servs. Sante Armees* **51**, 151–157.
23 Bienzle, V., Ebert, F. & Dietrich, M. (1978) *Tropenmed. Parasit.* **29**, 188–193.
24 Al-Taqi, M. & Behbehan, K. (1980) *Ann. trop. Med. Parasit.* **74**, 495–501.
25 Shmakov, V.V. & Lavrik, A.V. (1979) *Medskit. Parazit. Bol.* **48**, 9–11.
26 Sharma, M.I., Suri, J.C., Kalra, N.L. et al (1973) *J. comm. Dis.* 149–53.
27 Abdalla, R.E. & Sherif, H. (1978) *Ann. trop Med. Parasit.* **72**, 349–352.
28 Ranque, P., Quilici, M. & Camerlynck, P. (1974) *Bull. Soc. Path. éxot.* **67**, 167–175.
29 Dedet, J.P., Hubert, B., Desjeux, V. et al (1981) *Bull. Soc. Path. éxot.* **74**, 71–77.
30 Githure, J.I., Beach, R.F. & Lightner, L.K. (1984) *Trans. R. Soc. trop. Med. Hyg.* **78**, 283.
31 Beach, R., Young, D.G. & Mutinga, M.J. (1982) *Trans. R. Soc. trop. Med. Hyg.* **76**, 707–708.
32 Beach, R., Kiilu, G., Hendricks, L. et al (1984) *Trans. R. Soc. trop. Med. Hyg.* **78**, 747–751.
33 Ashford, R.W., Bray, M.A., Hutchinson, M.P. (1973) *Trans. R. Soc. trop. Med. Hyg.* **67**, 568.
34 Grove, S.S. (1978) *S. Afr. med. J.* **53**, 712–715.
35 Rutherfoord, G. & Uys, C.J. (1978) *S. Afr. med. J.* **53**, 716–718.
36 Zovein, A., Edrissian, Gh. H. & Nadim, A. (1984) *Trans. R. Soc. trop. Med. Hyg.* **78**, 73–77.
37 Dergashova, T.I. & Zherikhina, I.I. (1980) *Med. Parasitol. Parasit. Bol.* **49**, 40–45.
38 Green, M.S., Kark, J.D., Witztum, E. et al (1983) *Trans. R. Soc. trop. Med. Hyg.* **77**, 152–159.
39 Marsden, P.D., Almeida, E.A., Llanos-Cuentas, E.A. et al (1985) *Br. med. J.* **290**, 433–443.
40 Barbier, D., Goyot, P. & Dedet, J.P. (1985) *Trans. R. Soc. trop. Med. Hyg.* **79**, 47–50.
41 Llanos-Cuentas, E.A., Cuba, C.C., Barreto, A.C. et al (1984) *Trans. R. Soc. trop, Med. Hyg.* **78**, 845–846.
42 Sampaio, R.N.R., Rocha, Ara, A., Marsden, P.D. et al (1980) *Anais Brasil. Derm.* **55**, 69–76.
43 Low-a-Chee, R.M., Rose, P. & Ridley, D.S. (1983) *Ann. trop. Med. Parasit.* **77**, 255–260.
44 Rotberg, A. (1960) *Rev. Ass. Med. Argentina* **74**, 190.
45 Ridley, D.S., Marsden, P.D., Cuba, C.C. et al (1980) *Trans. R. Soc. trop. Med. Hyg.* **74**, 508.

46 Walton, B.C., Brooks, W.H. & Arjona, I. (1972) *Am. J. trop. Med. Hyg.* **21**, 296.

47 Shaw, J.J. & Lainson, R. (1975) *Trans. R. Soc. trop. Med. Hyg.* **69**, 323.

48 Luzzio, A.J., McRoberts, A. M.J. & Euliss, N.H. (1979) *J. infect. Dis.* **140**, 370–371.

49 Anthony, R.C., Christensen, H. & Johnson, C.M. (1980) *Am. J. trop. Med. Hyg.* **29**, 190–194.

50 Cuba Cuba, C.A., Marsden, P.D., Barreto, A.C.R. et al (1980) *Bol. Of. Sanit. Panam.* **89**, 195–208.

51 Mayrink, W., Melo, M. N., C. A. da et al (1976) *Rev. Inst. Med. trop. São Paulo* **18**, 182–185.

52 World Health Organization (1979) *Document TRR/ Leish* (MCL 79).

53 Peters, W., Lainson, R., Shaw, J.J. et al (1981) *Lancet* **i**, 1122–1124.

54 New, R.R.C., Chance, M.L. & Heath, S. (1981) *Parasitology* **83**, 519–527.

55 Mayer, P.J.J. (1974) *B. Münch. Med. Wscher.* **116**, 1539–1546.

56 Dourado, H.V., Birborema, C.T., Alecrim, W. et al (1975) *Revta Bras. clin. Terapeut.* **4**, 1–5.

57 Lainson, R. (1983) *Trans. R. Soc. trop. Med. Hyg.* **77**, 569–596.

58 Simpson, M.H., Mullins, J.F. & Stone, A.J. (1968) *Arch. Derm. Syph.* **51**, 124–128.

59 Shaw, P.K., Quigg, L.T., Allain, D.S. et al (1976) *Am. J. trop. Med. Hyg.* **25**, 788–796.

60 Walton, B.C., Shaw, J.J. & Lainson, R. (1977) *J. Parasitol.* **63**, 1118–1119.

61 Ramos-Aguirre, C. (1970) *Derm. Res. Mex.* **14**, 39–45.

62 Lainson, R., Miles, M.A. & Shaw, J.J. (1981) *Ann. trop. Med. Parasit.* **75**, 251–253.

63 Lainson, R. (1982) In *Parasitic zoonoses,* ed. J.H. Steele, Vol. 1, pp. 41–103. Boca Paton: CRC Press.

64 Tihasingh, E.S. (1974) *Bull. Pan-Am Hlth Org.* **8**, 232–242.

65 Shaw, J.J., Lainson, R. & Ward, R.D. (1972) *Trans. R. Soc. trop. Med. Hyg.* **66**, 718–723.

66 Scorza, J.V., de Valera, M., Scorza, C. et al (1979) *Trans. R. Soc. trop. Med. Hyg.* **73**, 293.

67 Zeledon, R., Ponce, C. & de Ponce, E. (1975). *Am. J. trop. Med. Hyg.* **4**, 706–707.

68 Morales, A., Corredor, A., Cacares, E. et al (1981) *Biomedica* **1**, 198–207.

69 Herrer, A. & Christensen, H.A. (1976) *Am. J. trop. Med. Hyg.* **25**, 59.

70 Christensen, H.A., Arias, J.R., de Vasquez, A.M. et al (1982) *Am. J. trop. Med. Hyg.* **31**, 239–242.

71 Pajot, F.X., Le Pont, F., Gentile, B. et al (1982) *Trans. R. Soc. trop. Med. Hyg.* **76**, 112–113.

72 Lainson, R., Shaw, J.J., Ward, R.D. et al (1973) *Trans. R. Soc. trop. Med. Hyg.* **67**, 184.

73 Lainson, R. & Shaw, J.J. (1979) In *Biology of the Kinetoplastida,* ed. W.H.R. Lumsden-Evans, Vol. 2, pp. 1–116. London: Academic Press.

74 Herrer, A. (1951) *Rev. Med. exp., Lima* **8**, 87–117.

75 Herrer, A., Hidalgo, V. & Meneses, O. (1980) *Rev. Inst. Med. trop. São Paulo* **22**, 203–206.

76 Lainson, R. & Shaw, J.J. (1977) *J. trop. Med. Hyg.* **80**, 29.

77 Pradinaud, R., Grossman, E. & Roche, J.C. (1976) *Bull. Soc. Path. éxot.* **67**, 167–175.

Chapter 38
Buruli Ulcer

GEOGRAPHICAL DISTRIBUTION

Buruli ulcer, named after the part of Uganda where it has been studied, has been found in localized foci in Uganda, Nigeria, Zaire, India, Malaysia, Sumatra, New Guinea, Queensland and South Australia, Mexico and a focus in north-east America. The major foci of infection are Uganda and New Guinea.

AETIOLOGY

Buruli ulcer is caused by *Mycobacterium ulcerans* which is an acid-fast bacillus 3–6 μm long, 0.2–0.35 μm wide, first described in Australia.[1] It occurs singly or in groups, mainly in the centre of the lesion but best cultured from the bases and edges of the ulcer. It grows in three to four weeks in tubercle bacillus media at 30–35°C.[2] Rats, mice and cattle are susceptible but not guinea-pigs.

TRANSMISSION

The probable method of transmission is through the skin by an abrasion or insect bite. *M. ulcerans* has not been recovered from soil, water or insects but saprophytic mycobacteria closely resembling it have been isolated from grass, and the distribution of Buruli ulcer in Uganda is similar to that of the grass *Echinocloa pyramidalis*.[3,4]

PATHOLOGY

The lesion begins as a small subcutaneous nodule attached to the skin and the pathological process is a spreading non-caseous necrosis of the subcutaneous tissue. The epidermis is not at first affected.[5] Microscopically it starts as a small opaque area of subcutaneous necrotic fat with little inflammatory response in which organisms may be seen. It spreads with a necrotizing vasculitis at the periphery extending laterally with necrosis underneath the dermis and epidermis

for up to 15 cm. Healing takes place with granulation tissue and non-caseating epithelioid granuloma. Granulations in the ulcer bed tend to have a gelatinous appearance and calcification may occur.[6]

IMMUNITY

There is no immunity to reinfection but tuberculin negative individuals are more susceptible.

CLINICAL FEATURES

Buruli ulcer is a chronic ulcerating condition of the skin which heals naturally after months or years leaving severe scarring. Subclinical infections occur so that there is a spectrum of disease in the endemic foci.

Incubation period

The incubation period has been estimated retrospectively as six to 12 weeks.

Symptoms and signs

The onset is gradual with a small indurated subcutaneous swelling attached to the skin but not the deep fascia. Usually single and commonest on a limb near the joint, the lesion may occur on any part of the body except the palms and soles and may itch. Slight fever is often present. It extends slowly during several months though it can be fulminating in two to three weeks; there is no tenderness or adenopathy. The overlying skin becomes hyperpigmented and then breaks down to form an ulcer with undermined edges which may become very large (Fig. 38.1). Secondary infection causes a foul smelling sloughing ulcer. In fulminating cases the limb is not hot or tender but becomes tense and shiny owing to massive oedema which must be differentiated from cellulitis (in which there is inflammation and fever). Satellite ulcers or nodules may

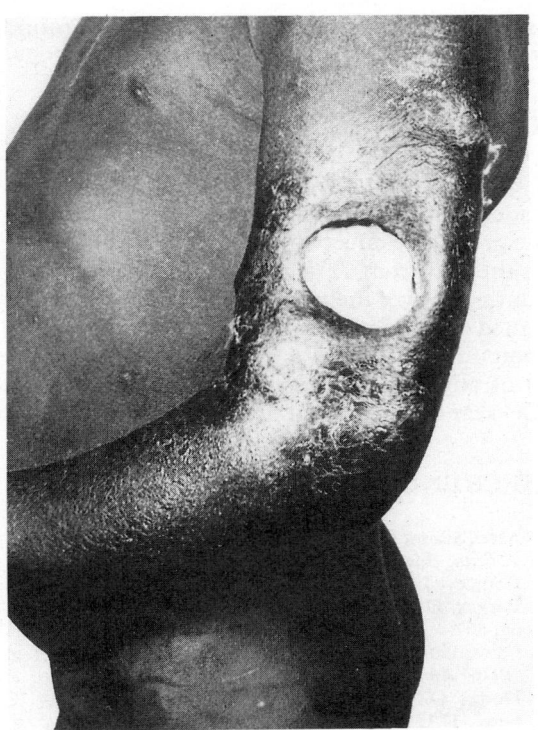

Fig. 38.1 Buruli ulcer before preparation for grafting. (Courtesy Dr H.F. Lunn.)

appear. Metastatic spread is uncommon but may involve the bone and cartilage. The ulcer tends towards natural healing after many months or even years and heals with scarring. Local recurrence may occur in 7% of cases but may be due to ineffective treatment.

DIFFERENTIAL DIAGNOSIS

The lesion must be distinguished from foreign body granulomas (history of trauma), fibroma or low grade fibrosarcoma, phycomycosis (biopsy) (see Chapter 34), injection abscess, cellulitis and panniculitis and sebaceous cysts.[7]

DIAGNOSIS

Biopsy will show numerous bacilli in necrotic areas and material should be cultured from the ulcer edge in tuberculin media at 33°C.

Burulin is a skin test antigen prepared from *M. ulcerans* which is highly specific in the reactive stage but most patients who react to burulin also give positive reactions to tuberculin.[8]

TREATMENT

The small preulcerative lesions can be excised completely under local anaesthesia in an outpatient department and the wound usually heals by first intention. Somewhat larger lesions can often be excised and grafted (Fig. 38.2) but they are usually more extensive than preoperation examination suggests.[7]

In very large lesions the object is to excise nonviable skin and skin bridges and to cut flaps to gain access to diseased fascia; it is usually not possible to remove all the diseased tissue initially and repeated operations may be needed, but the diseased tissue should be removed completely as soon as possible (Fig. 38.2). If healthy granu-

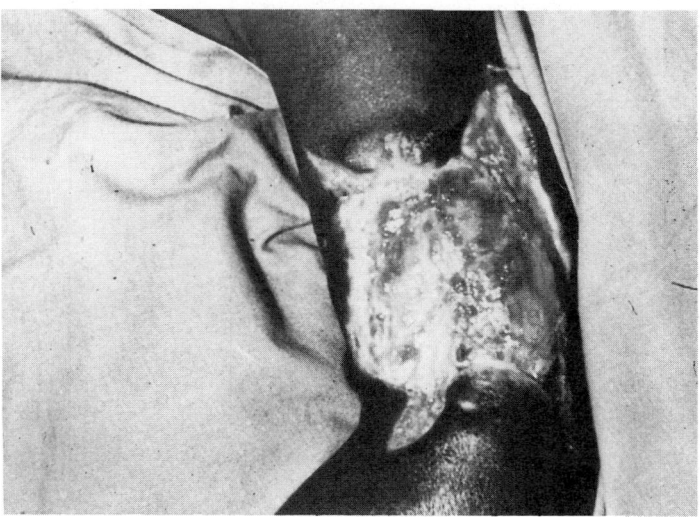

Fig. 38.2 Buruli ulcer on the upper arm after removal of irreparably damaged skin and fat. The granulated area is awaiting grafting. (Courtesy Dr H.F. Lunn.)

lations do not appear and skin flaps do not stick down in one or two weeks after operation the disease is still present and if further operation is delayed the discharge and organization of necrotic material take months, leaving considerable fibrosis which limits the final result.

In one series of cases[6] wet dressings of 0.25 or 0.5 silver nitrate were applied to the ulcers, repeatedly, after they had been surgically cleaned up. This arrested and cleaned them so that pinch grafts could be applied in due course. If the lesions are large before treatment, fibrosis tends to be extensive and may affect joint movement, for instance by contracture near the knee.

Treatment by drugs is disappointing though clofazimine (Lamprene, B 663) and rifampicin have been suggested because of their actions in leprosy, and the important treatment is surgical.

Because the growth of *M. ulcerans* is inhibited at 37°C, heat was applied to the ulcers by means of hot water circulating through a water jacket which kept the temperature at the base of the ulcer at 40°C. Considerable improvement was reported with healing or inactivity after an average of 41 days.[9]

EPIDEMIOLOGY

The highest incidence is in children and in Uganda in women more than men. In Uganda the annual incidence was more than 10/1000 per year for a few years but fluctuates widely. The disease is found in relatively small foci round swamps and river banks.

CONTROL

BCG seems to give some protection: 18% in high incidence areas and 74% in low incidence areas.[10] The protective effect of BCG has been confirmed but this fell from 72% in the first six months to about 50% over the two years of the trial.[11] BCG seemed to be of value only in those whose initial tuberculin reaction was less than 4 mm; it was not of any value in patients who had an initial BCG scar or evidence of previous ulcer infection.

REFERENCES

1 MacCallum, P., Tolhurst, J.C., Buckle, G. et al (1948) *J. Path. Bact.* **60**, 93, 102, 110, 116.
2 Clancey, J.K. (1964) *J. Path. Bact.* **88**, 175.
3 Barker, D.J.P. (1977) *Trans. R. Soc. trop. Med. Hyg.* **66**, 867.
4 Oluwasanmi, J.O., Solante, T.F., Olurn, E.O. et al (1976) *Am. J. trop. Med. Hyg.* **25**, 122.
5 Dodge, O.G. (1964) *J. Path. Bact.* **88**, 167.
6 Gray, H.H., Kingma, S., Kok, S.H. (1967) *Trans. R. Soc. trop. Med. Hyg.* **61**, 712.
7 Uganda Buruli Group (1970) *Br. med. J.* **ii**, 390.
8 Stanford, J.L., Revill, D.W.L., Gunthorpe, W.J. et al (1975) *J. Hyg., Camb.* **74**, 7.
9 Meyers, W.M., Shelley, W.M., Connor, D.H. et al (1974) *Am. J. trop. Med. Hyg.* **23**, 919.
10 Uganda Buruli Group (1969) *Lancet* **i**, 111.
11 Smith, P.G., Revill, D.W.L., Lukwago, E. et al (1976) *Trans. R. Soc. trop. Med. Hyg.* **70**, 449.

Chapter 39
Cutaneous Diphtheria (Veld Sore)

GEOGRAPHICAL DISTRIBUTION

Diphtheritic infection of the skin is common in many areas of the hot, humid tropics as well as in hot, dry desert areas where veld sore is found.

AETIOLOGY

Corynebacterium diphtheriae mitis has been isolated from unabraded skin on the Pacific coast of Colombia where it was surprisingly common and has been isolated from veld sores on a number of occasions.[1]

TRANSMISSION

Infection may arise from the patient's throat or skin or from a contact. Transfer of *C. diphtheriae* to the skin is easy and infection of a scratch or abrasion may occur from organisms already present on the skin. The sore can be aggravated by sand, and serum oozing from it contaminated by *C. diphtheriae* from the patient's skin, throat or from a contact.[2] The organism can be isolated from acute but not chronic sores.

PATHOLOGY

The organism multiplies in the ulcer and produces a toxin which can cause the same neurological and cardiac complications as in faucial diphtheria.

CLINICAL FEATURES

The sore (usually single but may be multiple) shows first as a vesicle full of straw-coloured fluid and is very painful. On bursting this leaves a shallow ulcer with a thin grey pellicle or chamois-leather slough, which may spread; the raw surface is exquisitely tender. After two to three weeks the ulcer becomes chronic. It is punched-

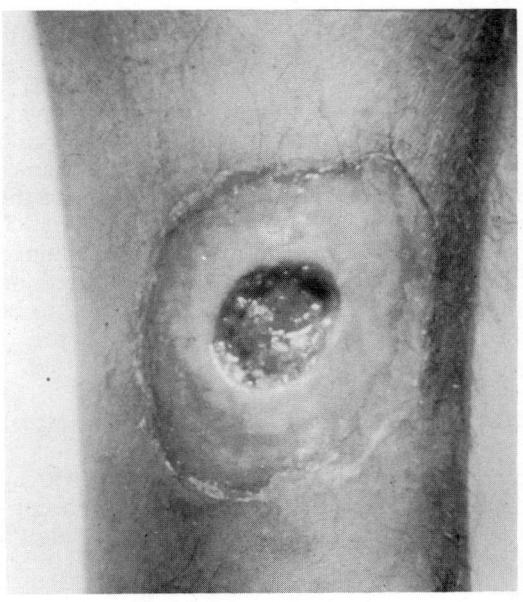

Fig. 39.1 Diphtheria ulceration of the leg (veld sore).

out, circular, with undermined edges and thick margins (Fig. 39.1). The base is covered with grey and scaly debris, beneath which there may be an adherent membrane. The edges become indurated and the thickened tissue has a cyanotic appearance. The ulcer may persist for many months. If healing takes place a thin, paper-like scar is left.

The nervous system is likely to become involved, the first symptom being blurring of vision, numbness and coldness of the extremities. Paralysis of accommodation and of the pharynx, wrist drop and ankle drop may follow and there may be ataxia, loss of knee jerks, anaesthesia and incoordination. The initial local paresis is related to the site of the sore which possibly indicates direct passage of toxin along the nerves to the central nervous system. General pareses usually appear in the second week; polyneuritis is usually delayed for three weeks or more.

Sudden death from cardiac involvement may occur as in faucial diphtheria.

IMMUNITY

C. diphtheriae infection produces a long-lasting immunity and the common presence of *C. diphtheriae* on the skin of people in the hot, humid tropics is responsible for the rarity of faucial diphtheria in these areas.

DIAGNOSIS

Veld sore must be differentiated from tropical ulcer, varicose ulcer, mycotic ulcer, yaws and cutaneous leishmaniasis. Veld sore has a characteristic undermined edge, is very painful and the base of the ulcer has a peculiar grey colour. *C. diphtheriae* can be seen in direct smears stained with Gram's and Neisser's stain, cultured on Löffler's and tellurite medium and proved to be pathogenic in 24 hours and typed in 48 hours.

TREATMENT

Penicillin, 600 mg daily, or erythromycin 250 mg with the first dose of antitoxin and then continued by mouth for 4 or 5 days, three times a day, will control the infection.

Antitoxin

Diphtheria antitoxin (at least 20 000 units) should be injected subcutaneously or intra-muscularly (with usual precautions against sensitivity) near the sores which should also be dressed with antitoxin.

EPIDEMIOLOGY

Diphtheria infection of the skin is common in the hot, humid tropics but diphtheria ulceration or veld sore is found in hot, dry desert conditions and was common in South Africa and North Africa during war when it was noted to be commonly associated with work with horses and camels, as well as being common in soldiers in North Africa in the Second World War.

PREVENTION

Active immunization of all Schick positive individuals who are susceptible to infection should be carried out. The Schick test consists of the intradermal injection of diphtheria toxin, a positive result being shown by an area of erythema denoting susceptibility. Immunization with aluminium precipitated toxoid (APT) is protective for life. Care of abrasions in the desert is important.

REFERENCES

1 Prior, A. (1970) *Lancet* **i**, 1395.
2 Walton, H.C.M. (1970) *Lancet* **i**, 1395.

SECTION VIII
LEPROSY

Chapter 40
Leprosy

GEOGRAPHICAL DISTRIBUTION

Leprosy probably affects 12–15 million people throughout the world but is most common in the tropics and subtropics. Tropical Africa has the highest disease rates, ranging from 1 to 43 per 1000 of the population in some parts of Uganda, and even more in parts of West Africa, where surveys have been made. In surveys in East Africa Ross Innes found prevalences of 12–33 per 1000, about 20% of which were lepromatous.

It is also common throughout the Far East (5.8 per 1000 in Burma, 10 in Nepal, 3.6 in Singapore) and the Pacific islands, and in South America (1.34 per 1000 in Brazil, 4.25 in Surinam). It was formerly endemic in Europe, though in Biblical times and the Middle Ages the name leprosy was given to some conditions which were probably not true leprosy. Nevertheless, true leprosy did exist as an endemic disease, for instance in Norway and Spain, until recent times. In the last decade there has been an increase in the number of registered cases, now around five million, but no significant change in prevalance, now estimated to be 10.6 million.[1]

For some of the countries in Europe the numbers of cases of leprosy registered in 1975 were: UK 122, France 1800, Italy 517 and The Netherlands 600. Numbers in Spain and Portugal were high, 3725 and 2540 cases respectively, and Greece notified 3000 cases. The USA (including Puerto Rico) had 1965 cases on the register in 1973.[2] In Britain and other countries of western Europe the disease is now confined to immigrants and persons who have lived abroad.

Figures quoted from many parts of the world may be unduly low because people are reluctant to report leprosy for fear of local ostracism or a restraint on their movements or from natural reticence. These reactions tend to be intensified if there is any suggestion of compulsory segregation, an idea now almost universally rejected.

AETIOLOGY

Mycobacterium leprae is the accepted cause of leprosy. It is a strongly acid-fast rod-shaped organism with parallel sides and rounded ends. In size and shape it closely resembles the tubercle bacillus. It occurs in large numbers in the lesions, chiefly in masses within the lepra cells, often grouped together like bundles of cigars or arranged in a palisade. Chains are never seen. Most striking are the intracellular and extracellular masses, known as globi, which consist of clumps of bacilli in capsular material.

Under the electron microscope the bacillus appears to have a great variety of forms. The commonest is a slightly curved filament 3–10 μm in length containing irregular arrangements of dense material sometimes in the shape of rods. Short rod-shaped structures can also be seen (identical with the rod-shaped inclusions within the filaments) and also dense spherical forms. Some of the groups of bacilli can be seen to have a limiting membrane.

It is now generally accepted that only leprosy bacilli which stain with carbol-fuchsin as solid acid-fast rods are viable and that bacilli which stain irregularly are probably dead and degenerating. This is not to say that all solid bacilli are viable; there must be stages at which they are dead but not yet disintegrated. The differences are very apparent in preparations examined under the electron microscope, but can be appreciated under the light microscope. These differences are valuable pointers in biopsy specimens to the effects of treatment. In patients receiving standard treatment with DDS (dapsone) a very high proportion of bacilli are killed within three months, which suggests that many of the manifestations of leprosy, including reactions of the erythema nodosum type, which follow initial treatment, must be due in part to dead rather than living bacilli. We therefore need drugs which will help the body to dispose of dead but still intact leprosy bacilli.

Two indices[3] which depend on observation of *M. leprae* in smears from skin or nasal smears are important in assessing the amount of infection, and the viability of the organisms and also the progress of the patient under treatment. They are the morphological index and the bacteriological index.

1 *The morphological index (MI).* This is calculated by counting the numbers of solid-staining acid-fast rods in a smear made by nicking the skin with a sharp scalpel and scraping it; the fluid and tissue obtained are spread fairly thickly on a slide and stained by the Ziehl–Neelsen method and decolorized (but not completely) which 1% acid alcohol. Only the solid-staining bacilli are viable. It is not unusual for solid-staining *M. leprae* to reappear for short periods in patients being successfully treated with drugs.

2 *The bacteriological index (BI).* This is an expression of the weight of infection. It is calculated by counting six to eight stained smears under the 100 × oil immersion lens. The results are expressed on a logarithmic scale.

1+   At least 1 bacillus in every 100 fields.
2+   At least 1 bacillus in every 10 fields.
3+   At least 1 bacillus in every field.
4+   At least 10 bacilli in every field.
5+   At least 100 bacilli in every field.
6+   At least 1000 bacilli in every field.

The bacteriological index is valuable because it is simple and is representative of many lesions but is affected by the depth of the skin incision, the thoroughness of the scrape and the thickness of the film.

A more accurate and reliable index of the bacillary content of a lesion is given by the logarithmic index of biopsies (LIB). This is mainly used in research and the details should be sought in the original paper.[3] These indices help to assess the state of patients at the beginning of treatment and to assess progress.

A review of methods of study of leprosy by laboratory techniques was published by Rees.[4]

Ultrastructure and chemical composition

The ultrastructure and composition of the DNA can lead to rapid identification and chemical composition of the organism to test for viability and drug sensitivity within a few days. The ultrastructure of *M. leprae* shows no special features except that it can be distinguished from *M. lepraemurium* by the absence of a fibrillar capsule.[5] The biochemical study has revealed two extracellular lipids, one of which, a glycoprotein, appears to be a species specific antigen.[6] Biochemical study of the organism has advanced so that viability and sensitivity to drugs could be estimated within a few days[7] and the DNA differs from that of other mycobacteria.[8]

Culture in vitro

Claims of successful culture have been made in the past but none have been substantiated and *M. leprae* has not yet been successfully cultured in vitro. There have been many reports of cultivation in *artificial* media of acid-fast bacilli from the skin or other tissues of leprosy patients and many authors have claimed such bacilli to be true leprosy bacilli, but no satisfactory evidence of this has been produced. Most of the organisms isolated in culture from lepromatous tissues appear to be mycobacteria related to *M. scrofulaceum*.

Culture in vivo

Normal mice

The Shepard mouse foot-pad system is still the mainstay of bacteriology. Inoculation of 10^4 bacilli into the hind foot-pads yields 10^6 bacilli after five to six months although no clinical disease develops. During the logarithmic phase the mean generation time is 10–20 days which is consistent with the natural history of disease in man and is responsible for the chronicity of the foot-pad test.[9] No subsequent local increase in bacterial numbers takes place and the bacilli slowly degenerate but the infection may spread via the bloodstream and, after two years or more years, give rise to granulomas and neural damage at the site of inoculation and the nose, ears and tail skin. The histological features of human leprosy in the borderline range are reproduced.[10] Similar results have been found in the ear and foot-pad of hamsters and the foot-pad of rats.

Immunologically deficient mice

Experimental lepromatous leprosy was obtained by inoculating thymectomized irradiated (TR) mice.[11] The generation time remained unchanged but the bacilli continued to multiply until 10^8–10^9 bacilli per foot-pad were obtained after nine to 12 months. The histological picture is that of lepromatous leprosy and numerous bacilli can be found in the liver and spleen although the main spread is to the nose, tail, front paws and ears. The TR mouse has been used to detect small numbers of variable organisms (three to ten viable out of an inoculum of 10^5) and is used to detect 'persisters' after 12 months.

The mouse foot-pad has been used to test the minimum concentration of drugs necessary and the sensitivity of the bacilli to drugs in different strains of *M. leprae*.

The nine-banded armadillo (*Dasypus novemcinctus*)

An important development has been the discovery that the nine-banded armadillo can be infected with leprosy[12] and now this animal is the main source of *M. leprae* for biochemical research and the supply of antigen for immunological research and the development of a vaccine. The armadillo has a primitive immunological system and a lower body temperature. Intravenous inoculation produces widespread disseminated disease with yields from the liver and spleen reaching 10^{12} organisms per gram of tissue.

Monkeys

The white-handed gibbon develops lepromatous leprosy after an interval of 15 years[13] and the sooty mangabey after two years.[14]

TRANSMISSION

Transmission is direct from a case of leprosy to an uninfected person.

Infectivity of *M. leprae*

It is generally believed that tuberculoid leprosy is not infective and that tuberculoid (TT) and borderline tuberculoid (BT) patients present no danger. Lepromatous leprosy in which large numbers of viable bacilli are excreted is the source of infection. Previously it has been thought that prolonged intimate contact was necessary but there is now strong evidence that this is not necessary and that the susceptibility of the individual is more important.

A comparison of the response to exposure to *M. leprae* using the lymphocyte transformation test (LTT) showed that newly arrived volunteers had a much lower rate of transformation than those who had worked for some years with leprosy patients,[15] suggesting that leprosy, like tuberculosis, has a high infective rate but a low attack rate with clinical disease.

Route of transmission

Formerly it was believed that leprosy was contracted through the skin but it is now clear that the upper respiratory tract is more important. Few *M. leprae* are shed from the intact skin[16] whereas large numbers are shed from the upper respiratory tract of lepromatous patients.[17] The epidemiology of leprosy has been compared to that of tuberculosis,[18] suggesting droplet infection from the upper respiratory tract. Immunologically suppressed mice have been infected by an aerosol spray containing *M. leprae*[19] and *M. leprae* can remain viable in dried nasal secretions for up to 7 days.

Other methods of transmission

Other methods of transmission which are of little importance are *arthropods* in which bacilli are able to persist for several days in the gut, mouth parts and legs, mosquitoes[20] and flies[21] and bed bugs. *Maternal* and *transplacental* infection has been suggested. *M. leprae* has been found in the breast milk of lepromatous mothers[22] and transplacental infection of babies of untreated or relapsing lepromatous (LL) and borderline lepromatous (BL) mothers has been found.[23]

CLASSIFICATION OF LEPROSY

Leprosy may be classified by the pathological reaction of the tissues and the number of bacilli contained in them. When leprosy bacilli gain access to the tissues they may quickly be destroyed by the protective phagocytes of the host; phagocytes with engulfed bacilli can sometimes be found in skin biopsies of normal contacts who do not develop overt leprosy. Genetic characters are no doubt factors in this process.

If the bacilli do obtain a foothold the defence mechanisms of the host (varying from effective to poor) create a reaction which at first is named indeterminate because the lesion is too immature to be classifiable. This may persist for months or years or go on to complete healing, or to one of the fairly clearcut forms of clinical leprosy but the indeterminate form shows no signs of the form which will emerge.

The recognizable forms of leprosy show a continuous spectrum of severity according to the immune status of the host from the tuberculoid form, in which resistance is high, to the lepromatous form at the other pole in which resistance is low. Between these extremes there is a borderline (sometimes known as dimorphous) form which may show some characters of tuberculoid tendency, or some of lepromatous tendency.

This differentiation into three forms has been widely accepted and is adequate for many purposes but the general spectrum of the disease may be more usefully divided, histologically and clinically, into five grades.[24] This classification is shown in Tables 40.1 and 40.2. Leprosy may also be classified according to the bacillary load and this is extensively used in deciding treatment and in prognosis.

Multibacillary leprosy (MBL) contains all LL, BL and BB patients and also those BT patients where the bacillary index (BI) is 2+ at one or more sites.

Paucibacillary leprosy (PBL) contains TT and BT patients who are smear negative or if positive show no BI greater than 1+ at any one site.

Tuberculoid leprosy tends towards healing though neural damage may be permanent.

The polar forms, tuberculoid (TT) and lepromatous (LL) are relatively stable but the borderline form is unstable. Without treatment it tends to deteriorate to lepromatous. After treatment it sometimes reverts. Lepromatous leprosy which may develop directly from indeterminate or from borderline leprosy is less likely to revert to borderline after treatment.

A subdivision of the lepromatous (LL) group

Table 40.1 Histological classification of leprosy.

Histological feature	TT	BT	BB	BL	LL
Granuloma	Epithelioid cells with or without giant cells, in foci	Like TT	Epithelioid cells but no giant cells	a. Histiocytes evolving to epithelioid cells; scanty foamy change. Lymphocytes scanty b. Histiocytes sometimes foamy; no large globi. Many lymphocytes	*Active*: Macrophages round or spindle-shaped, with very many bacilli *Regressive*: Histiocytes with fatty change; foam cells or globi often large; multinucleate
Lymphocytes	Dense zone of infiltration round foci of granuloma	Like TT	Usually scanty. If present they are diffusely spread through granuloma	a. Scanty b. Numerous occupying whole segments of granuloma, or forming perineural cuffs	Scanty, diffuse
Nerves	Those in granuloma usually destroyed beyond recognition. Occasional caseation	Greatly swollen by Schwann cell proliferation. Perineural sheath intact	Moderate Schwann cell proliferation. Sheath intact	No cell proliferation in nerve bundle, which is often structureless. May be infiltration of histiocytes in perineurium	May show structural damage but not infiltration or cuffing
Subepidermal zone	Granuloma extends to basal layer of epidermis. No clear zone	Clear subepidermal zone, usually narrow	Clear subepidermal zone, broad or narrow	Like BB	Like BB
Bacilli in granuloma	None seen	0–3+	3–5+	5 or 6+	5 or 6+

After Ridley and Jopling.[24]
TT = tuberculoid; BT = borderline tuberculoid; BB = borderline; BL = borderline lepromatous; LL = lepromatous.

Table 40.2 Clinical classification of leprosy.

TT	BT	BB	BL	LL
Lesions consist of a few macules and/or plaques. Plaques tend to be large, have a rough dry hairless surface and well-defined edges from which there is a gradual slope to a flattened centre Distribution of lesions asymmetrical	May be confused clinically with TT but differentiated by: (*a*) Lesions more numerous, surface less dry and rough, edges less well defined, and hair growth may be slight; and (*b*) Annular lesions common, the peripheral band of tissue being raised and having well-defined outer and inner edges	Macules and plaques are intermediate in number and size between TT and LL. 'Punched-out' lesions are characteristic. Annular lesions occur as in BT Distribution of lesions asymmetrical	May be confused clinically with LL but differentiated by: (*a*) Macules and plaques not consistently small, edges less vague, and less tendency to bilateral symmetry. Some may have 'punched-out' appearance. (*b*) Papules and nodules unusual and few. Nodules may be dimpled. (*c*) Rare and less marked are iritis and keratitis, nasal ulceration, madarosis, thickened ear lobes, testicular damage and bone changes	Macules, papules, nodules and plaques may all be present. Lesions small, multiple, distributed bilaterally and symmetrically with smooth shiny surface. Macules and plaques have vague edges and no hair loss. May be nasal ulceration, iritis and keratitis, madarosis, leonine facies, thickened ear lobes, testicular damage, oedema of legs, and bone changes in limbs and skull
Lesions markedly anaesthetic	Lesions moderately anaesthetic	Lesions show mild anaesthesia	Some lesions may show slight patchy anaesthesia	Lesions not anaesthetic
Nerve thickening early, often single. First manifestations may be neural	Nerve thickening early, more numerous than in TT. First manifestations may be neural	Nerve thickening early, more numerous than in BT. First manifestations may be neural	Nerve thickening early, more numerous than in BB. First manifestations may be neural	Nerve thickening (and damage) late and tends to be bilateral and symmetrical (e.g. glove and stocking anaesthesia). First manifestations never neural
Lepromin test strongly positive	Lepromin test moderately or weakly positive	Lepromin test negative	Lepromin test negative	Lepromin test negative

After Ridley and Jopling.[24]
TT = tuberculoid; BT = borderline tuberculoid; BB = borderline; BL = borderline lepromatous; LL = lepromatous.

is now accepted into LLp (polar lepromatous) and LLs (subpolar lepromatous). Clinically a patient with LLs will have typical early lepromatous lesions and also some typical lesions of borderline type with one or more thickened nerve trunks with or without evidence of nerve dysfunction.[25] Whereas LLp is immunologically stable, LLs is not, for LLs patients may regain lost cell-mediated immunity. During chemotherapy LLs may become bacteriologically negative sooner than LLp. The two types can be differentiated histologically.[26] It is probable that a similar division of tuberculoid leprosy into polar and subpolar groups will come to be made.

PATHOLOGY

Portal of entry

Although the chief method of spread of *M. leprae* is via the upper respiratory tract the site of entry is not known. Some people believe that the portal of entry is via the upper or lower respiratory tract while others believe it is through the skin.[7]

Pathological changes

In very early infection (and in skin biopsies of some presumably healthy contacts) the fixed cells of the dermis near the acid-fast bacilli proliferate and monocytes from the blood migrate towards the bacilli engulfing and disintegrating them. Leprosy bacilli may also enter nerves causing focal damage related to the blood vessels near their site of entry into the nerves. They spread along the fine fibres of cutaneous nerve twigs and are carried centripetally, multiplying and bursting into the endoneural spaces where they are phagocytosed by histiocytes. In this way an incipient infection may be eradicated, though this is less likely once the bacilli have gained a foothold in nerves. If a skin lesion develops a biopsy specimen at this stage shows foci of inflammatory cellular exudate, mainly round the finest nerve fibres in plexuses in the dermis. The exudate is determined by the ability of the host to react immunologically and it consists of lymphocytes, histiocytes and other cells; clinically it is marked on the skin by wheal-like papules or pink or pale macules. This is the *indeterminate* stage of infection which usually occurs in children in whom resistance has not been determined and which may last for months or resolve or progress to *tuberculoid*, *dimorphous (borderline)* or *lepromatous* leprosy, depending on the immunological response of the body.

In lepromin-negative persons (whose resistance is poor) the histiocytes gradually change into lepra cells which in more severe cases become foamy; the ingested bacilli are not destroyed. In lepromin-positive persons (whose resistance is good) the histiocytes change into epithelioid cells after ingesting the bacilli, which they destroy.

But although the manner of evolution of these cells' containing *M. leprae* is important the mediators of immunity are the lymphocytes and although the lymphocytes in skin lesions are not all immunologically active the numbers present in tuberculoid and borderline lesions are significant indications of the degree of resistance to the infections.

Tuberculoid leprosy

The change from indeterminate to tuberculoid leprosy involves the appearance of groups of epithelioid cells (derived from histiocytes) inside fine nerve twigs and the formation of sharply circumscribed foci of these cells in the dermis, often surrounded by a zone of lymphocytes, which are fairly numerous. The epithelioid cells often coalesce to form giant cells. The epidermis

is thinner than normal and there are foci of inflammatory cells reaching the epidermis without a clear space. In the dermis the granulomatous cords follow the lines of neurovascular bundles (Fig. 40.7). The nerve bundles in the skin are swollen by proliferation of Schwann cells which develop into epithelioid cells. The nerves become difficult to recognize; they occasionally undergo caseation which does not occur in leprosy except in nerves (Fig. 40.1).

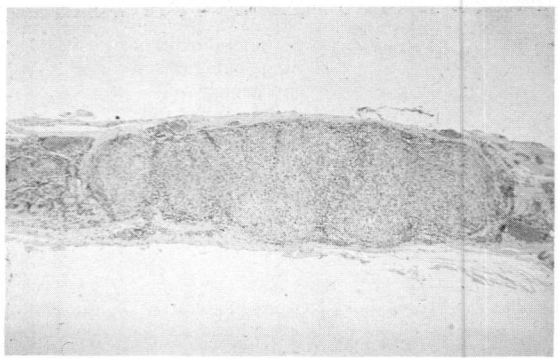

Fig. 40.1   Nerve lesions (low power) in tuberculoid leprosy. (Courtesy Dr S. G. Browne.)

Acid-fast bacilli are very rare in the cells of the inflammatory exudate in tuberculoid leprosy except in reaction phases but bacilli may be found in the active extending margin of a tuberculoid macule.

The most consistent feature of tuberculoid leprosy is the early involvement of peripheral nerves and ganglions, both somatic and sympathetic. In the upper extremity this often goes on to weakness and paralysis of the intrinsic muscles of the hand (main-en-griffe) and in the leg to drop foot. Damage to the sympathetic nerves leads to slow atrophy and absorption (osteoporosis) of the small bones of the hands and feet through interference with vasodilatation.

Borderline leprosy

Indeterminate leprosy often goes on to the borderline form in which large hypopigmented patches appear, often on the limbs, usually with loss of sensations of touch and temperature. Satellite macules with varying degrees of sharpness in the edges also appear; they are usually small. Acid-fast bacilli can always be found in these lesions by concentration techniques or even by routine methods. The lepromin reaction is variable but is usually weakly positive.

The histological picture shows features intermediate between those of lepromatous and tuberculoid lesions. There is an inflammatory reaction with cellular exudate in the superficial layers of the dermis; it consists of small round cells, histiocytes and clumps of epithelioid cells but no giant cells. Nerves may show large numbers of bacilli and round cells or epithelioid cells with few bacilli, i.e. they may resemble nerves in lepromatous or tuberculoid disease (Figs. 40.1 and 40.2). This dimorphous leprosy is unstable and tends to progress to the lepromatous form if not treated.

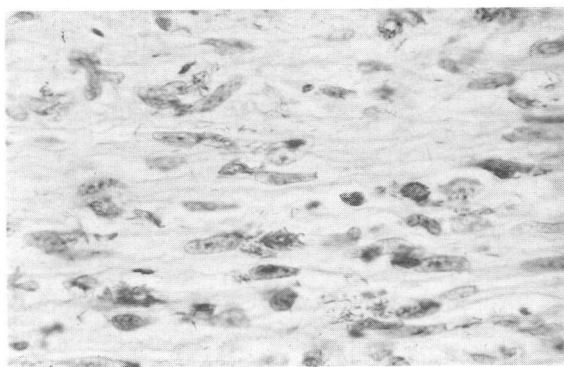

Fig. 40.2 Nerve lesions (high power) of lepromatous leprosy. (Courtesy Dr S. G. Browne.)

Lepromatous leprosy

In the skin lesions in fully developed lepromatous disease large areas of the dermis are connected into continuous sheets of chronic inflammatory tissue containing enormous numbers of bacilli in slabs of lepra (Virchow) cells (derived from histiocytes) (Fig. 40.3), interspersed with groups of mononuclear and plasma cells. Lymphocytes are scanty. The subepidermal zone of the dermis is clear of infiltrate. The disease is now systemic, the bacilli being transported by blood or lymph to distant parts of the body, for instance, the testes, though most of them are trapped by lymph nodes, liver, spleen and bone marrow, where miliary lepromas and even large lepromas may be found and subcutaneous veins may be involved.

The mucous membrane of the upper respiratory tract from the nose to the larynx, including the root of the tongue and the peritonsillar tissues, is heavily infiltrated in advanced lepromatous leprosy. It is oedematous, thickened and ulcerated and the nasal cartilages may be perforated. If the disease regresses, however, either spontaneously or as a result of treatment, the skin lesions heal in a remarkable manner.

IMMUNITY

Leprosy bacilli are not killed or eliminated by humoral antibodies but by cellular immune mechanisms similar to those which eliminate tubercle bacilli. Although not killed by humoral antibodies leprosy bacilli stimulate the production of humoral antibodies against various constituent antigens. The type of leprosy produced depends on the ability to produce and develop cell-mediated immunity (CMI). CMI (mediated by lymphocytes) is strong in tuberculoid leprosy but weak or absent in lepromatous leprosy.[27] However, antibodies are produced plentifully in lepromatous leprosy but are immunologically useless. Tuberculoid leprosy patients give a positive lepromin test showing allergy to *M. leprae*. The histological picture shows numerous lymphocytes and epithelioid cells whereas lepromatous patients show little cellular reaction (Fig. 40.3).

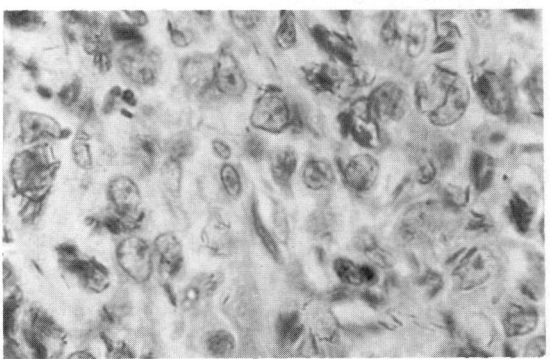

Fig. 40.3 Skin lesions of lepromatous leprosy (high power) showing the lepra cellular tissue. (Courtesy Dr S. G. Browne.)

Leprosy patients can resist other infections so that the anergy is specific. Reactions associated with an increase in immunity move the pathological and clinical response towards the tuberculoid pole, while reactions associated with a decrease in immunity move towards the lepromatous pole. The causes of these variations in response to *M. leprae* are complicated and various.

Genetic factors

It has been thought that a small proportion of communities are genetically incapable of mounting an effective CMI response to *M. leprae* but studies have failed to confirm this although some have shown that HLA types do play a small part in the process.[28, 29]

Lymphocyte depletion

Using the lymphocyte transformation test (LTT) and *M. leprae* as antigen the cellular defect in leprosy is due to a specific lack of *M. leprae* reacting lymphocytes.[15]

Variation in T cells

Studies on T lymphocyte subpopulations have shown that the distribution of T helper and T suppressor cells varies in the different types of leprosy and that the distribution of helper and suppressor cells in tuberculoid leprosy resembles that found in sarcoidosis.[30]

Macrophage function

Whereas macrophage function in lepromatous leprosy is satisfactory there is a deficiency in lymphokines.[31]

Other factors

The route of infection may be important in deciding the type of disease. While the intradermal route of immunization with *M. leprae* is best,[32] should the bacilli reach a nerve before being recognized they become shut off in the nervous system, the antigens reach the liver and spleen before the lymph glands, leading to a suppression of CMI and an increase in antibody production.

Humoral immunity

M. leprae possesses comparatively few antigens but some are specific[33] but a wide variation in antibody concentration has given inconstant results with immunological tests.

CMI in tuberculoid leprosy

CMI is intact in tuberculoid leprosy but the appearance of lesions may appear after treatment for some reason with antileprosy drugs or BCG vaccination, suggesting that tuberculoid leprosy may result from delayed recognition of *M. leprae* or as a reaction to dead but not live bacilli.

Bacillaemia

Bacillaemia occurs in leprosy. Of 240 biopsy specimens from leprosy patients in India, 21% of those with tuberculoid disease and 62% of those with lepromatous disease showed leprous granulomas in the liver;[34] BT, BB and BL patients gave intermediate results. This indicates that bacillaemia occurs even in the 'immune' group. Acid-fast bacilli were also seen in the liver in BT, BB, BL and LL groups, even when treatment had produced negative bacterial indices in the skin.

Lepromin

The lepromin test is used widely in leprosy. Lepromin is a substance derived from nodular lepromatous tissue from which epidermis and fat are removed and which contains masses of leprosy bacilli, or from infected lymph nodes rich in bacilli; it is autoclaved and either ground up in saline and then filtered and phenolized or prepared by some other convenient method, and it represents a suspension of the bacilli together with much cellular matter from the host tissues. Lepromin is injected intradermally in a dose of 0.1 ml. Standard Mitsuda lepromin contains 160 million leprosy bacilli per millilitre.

Reactions to lepromin are of two kinds.

1 The early (Fernandez) reaction which becomes positive in 48 hours and shows erythema and infiltration 10–15 mm in diameter (+ reaction), 15–20 mm (+ +) or over 20 mm (+ + +).

2 The late (Mitsuda) reaction read at four to five weeks, positive results giving + reaction (3–5 mm), + + (6–10 mm) or + + + (over 10 mm or a reaction of any size which ulcerates).

It is generally understood that the early (Fernandez) reaction in which desiccated *M. leprae* from lepromatous tissue were originally suspended in oil, and injected intradermally in a dose of 0.1 ml, is an allergic reaction similar to the tuberculin reaction. It is positive in all forms of leprosy (unlike the Mitsuda reaction), but most strongly positive in the tuberculoid form. It is a reflection of the sensitivity of the tissues to the protein of the leprosy bacilli. The late (Mitsuda) reaction, however, which is elicited only by whole leprosy bacilli—not by separate fractions—does not reflect the allergic state but is an index of resistance. Dharmendra lepromin, much used in India, is a purified suspension of *M. leprae* extracted with chloroform–ether. The early (Fernandez) reaction is best seen when this lepromin is used.

The Mitsuda reaction is strongly positive in tuberculoid leprosy, usually negative or weakly positive in borderline leprosy and almost invariably negative in lepromatous leprosy. It is sometimes positive in persons who have never been in contact with the leprosy bacillus and the test is therefore of no diagnostic value. A positive result indicates resistance to leprosy bacilli; a negative result in a patient with the disease is a sign of poor resistance.

In lepromatous leprosy the Mitsuda reaction is negative, partly, it is thought, owing to a subnormal response of leukocytes to physical stimuli and to antigens totally unrelated to *M. leprae*. These responses are suppressed by factors in lepromatous serum. Some severe lepromatous leprosy cases are associated with the delayed allergic response to skin test antigens or delayed rejection of skin grafts.[35]

Reversal of a negative to a positive Mitsuda test in a leprosy patient is taken as a sign of increased resistance and therefore of improved prognosis; in fact this test is used to assess progress. Over-use of the test, however, is said to produce a temporary allergic sensitization to lepromin, which may have no relation to resistance and could therefore confuse the issue.

Injections of BCG in leprosy patients negative to lepromin have some effect in converting the Mitsuda reaction to positive; in patients with a positive Mitsuda reaction, BCG may increase the intensity of that reaction. How far this is related to true resistance is still a matter for conjecture.

CLINICAL FEATURES

Natural history

The natural history of leprosy is very variable. The majority of people who come into contact with infectious lepromatous patients develop no symptoms or signs of infection although the lymphocyte transformation test shows that a majority will have experienced infection which they overcome. The majority of those who experience clinical effects mount a strong CMI response to the initial primary lesion, develop tuberculoid leprosy and eventually eradicate the infection. A minority who mount a weak CMI response or none at all develop lepromatous leprosy, a chronic progressive disseminated infection leading to deformity and death after many years. A proportion of cases mount varying degrees of CMI response and develop borderline or indeterminate leprosy and may then swing one way or the other on the pendulum, downgrading or upgrading, depending on outside circumstances and changes in the immunological response.

Incubation period

This is undoubtedly very variable and the chief difficulty of establishing the incubation period in any given case is the fact that early symptoms and signs of the disease may be overlooked or ignored for years. Another difficulty is that patients often attempt to hide the true facts about leprosy. Although short incubation periods of a few months have been recorded in infants born of leprous parents, the average is about three and a half years. Longer incubation periods are not unusual, especially in those who fail to observe early signs of the disease and the late Sir Philip Manson-Bahr in London diagnosed as leprosy a case which had been regarded as seborrhoea of the face and ears in which the incubation period appeared to be as long as 31 years.

Symptoms and signs

The mode of onset is very variable. A *primary* lesion may be found, an indeterminate depigmented patch with some anaesthesia. The initial manifestation in children is especially hypopigmentation with anaesthesia; no other disease produces this. Bacilli may be hard to find. In Uzuakoli 13 patients with confluent macular lepromatous leprosy were described[36] in whom for some time a generalized hypopigmentation was the only sign of the disease until other manifestations of lepromatous leprosy appeared. The hypopigmentation grew from the confluence of macular areas, but spared the inguinal region, the axillae and part of the lumbar region; these areas of apparently normal skin usually contained *M. leprae* and globi. In all the patients .the confluent hypopigmentary condition had been unnoticed.

Spontaneous healing may take place after the early lesions of childhood but, though this is quite common in some communities, it obviously cannot be taken for granted; a definite diagnosis is an indication for treatment.

As compared with tuberculosis one of the chief characteristics of leprosy is the absence of toxicity; enormous numbers of bacilli may be present in the body with few signs. The local inflammatory reactions to lepra bacilli vary within wide limits. Thus, in one patient the disease is so localized that it affects one small skin area or its main nerve supply. There may be acute inflammatory swelling, local pain and trophic, sensory and other disturbances. Bacilli can be demonstrated with great difficulty. In contrast, a second case may show involvement of almost the whole body, so that a preparation taken from any part of the skin may reveal numerous bacilli, though the patient is not acutely ill and is able to go about and do his work. The nerves are not noticeably thickened and superficially the skin appears normal. At any stage during invasion sudden exanthematous reactions may appear, accompanied by fever and general symptoms.

The *chronic onset* is so gradual and insidious that the disease has advanced to a considerable extent before any abnormality is evident. There may be tenderness, tingling or thickening of a nerve, an area of anaesthesia, perhaps with some change in the appearance of the skin, insensitiveness to burning, formication, tingling or numbness of extremities. Discoloured skin patches may be mistaken for eczema or ringworm; these may at first be small, gradually increasing in size.

In the *acute onset* there are occasionally multiple lesions with less diffused margins, which tend to spread rapidly and which contain very numerous bacilli. The first noticeable sign may be an evanescent rash. The onset may be determined by some other acute disease, such as malaria or typhoid, which lowers resistance. It may also be the sequel to chronic infection, such as syphilis, ancylostomiasis or chronic disease of the gastrointestinal tract. The period of life may also have some bearing, e.g. extra strain imposed on the body during puberty, parturition and the menopause.

Lepromatous leprosy

This is the type seen in persons with a negligible resistance; leprosy bacilli are widely disseminated throughout the skin, nerves and reticuloendothelial system. In addition, there may be bacillary invasion of eyes, testes, bones and mucous membranes of mouth, nose, pharynx, larynx and trachea; one of the earliest signs in children is swelling and tenderness of the tip of the nose, oedema and infiltration of the alar cartilages.

Skin lesions

These are multiple, small and symmetrically distributed; they take the form of macules, infiltrations (plaques), papules and nodules (Fig. 40.4), all of which may be present in the same patient at the same time once the disease has become well established. The pure diffuse type is an exception and will be described later. The earliest skin lesions are macules; these are

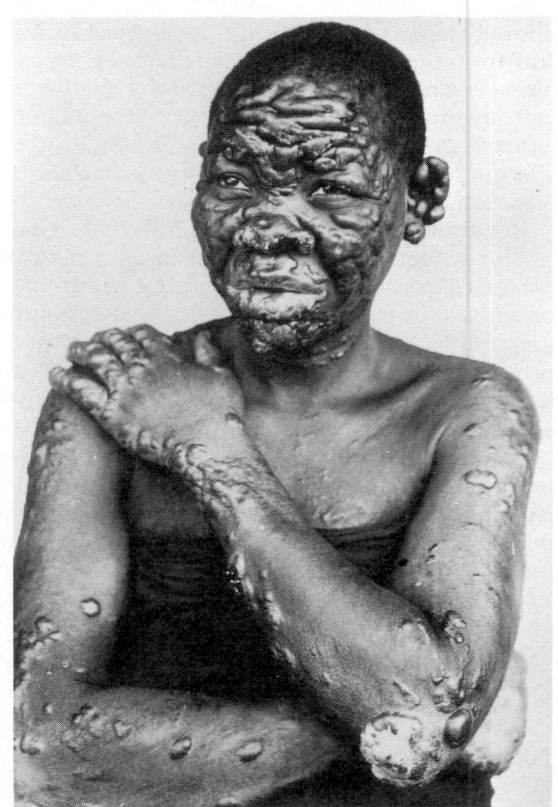

Fig. 40.4 Nodular skin lesions of lepromatous leprosy. (Courtesy Dr S. G. Browne.)

level with the skin and therefore cannot be palpated. They are small, circular or elliptical; they are erythematous in light skins, sometimes with a coppery or purple hue, and coppery in dark skins, sometimes with a faintly hypopigmented background. They have a smooth and shiny surface, their edges are indistinct and they are not anaesthetic or anhidrotic. Owing to the fact that these macules are often difficult to see and are not associated with itching or anaesthesia, they may be ignored by the patient. They may be situated on any part of the body, but are unusual in the axillae, groins, perineum, on the external genitalia or on the scalp. They are most commonly found on the face, buttocks and extremities; on the limbs the flexor surfaces may be involved as well as the extensor, and the palms and soles as well as the backs of hands and feet.

Infiltrated lesions are raised above the level of the skin and give a sensation of thickening when gripped between finger and thumb. Their distribution and colouring are the same as those of lepromatous macules, except that they do not appear on palms and soles owing to the thickness and tightness of the skin. They are raised in the centre and slope away peripherally to merge imperceptibly with the surrounding skin, have a smooth and shiny surface, and do not exhibit sensory loss, unless situated in a region of skin which is already anaesthetic as a result of peripheral nerve damage. Papules and nodules make their appearance as the disease advances and particularly favour the face, ears and buttocks. Ears should always be carefully examined, for the lobes are more constantly affected than any other part and appear thickened quite early in the course of the disease, such thickening being readily confirmed by palpation with finger and thumb. Advanced infiltration and nodulation of the face give rise to leontiasis or 'leonine facies', in which the normal wrinkles on the forehead and cheeks have become deep furrows. Nodules and infiltrations may undergo superficial necrosis and ulceration and large ulcers may form on the lower legs when leprous infiltration of the skin is associated with chronic bilateral lymphoedema, secondary to massive bacillary invasion of the lymphatics. Thinning of the eyebrows is common, commencing in the lateral half and sometimes progressing to complete loss of eyebrows and eyelashes (superciliary and ciliary madarosis). Alopecia may occur but is uncommon. Jopling[25] has seen eight cases of vitiligo among 114 patients with lepromatous leprosy

attending his clinic in London; the condition developed after several years of treatment.

One particular variety of skin infiltration requires separate mention, namely the pure diffuse type described by Lucio and Alvarado in Mexico in 1852 and later by Latapi in 1938. The skin of the whole body becomes diffusely infiltrated (no macular stage being observed) rendering it stiff and smooth as in scleroderma. There is no obvious disfigurement apart from loss of eyebrows and eyelashes which always occurs, but there may be widespread small telangiectases; nasal destruction may develop and sometimes there is alopecia and loss of body hair. Laryngeal ulceration has been recorded but cutaneous nodules and ocular involvement are absent. Mexican physicians have described, in these patients, a unique form of lepra reaction known as 'Lucio's phenomenon' in which painful, purpuric, ulcerating patches appear on the skin, becoming crusted and leaving scars.[25] This may be differentiated from erythema nodosum leprosum (ENL) reaction by the absence of fever and leukocytosis, absence of tender lesions, and a good response to antileprosy drugs, but not to thalidomide. It may also be distinguished histologically.[37, 38]

Nerve involvement

Nerve involvement, in the absence of skin involvement, has not been described in lepromatous leprosy, but combined dermal and neural changes are a usual finding. Nerves do not show signs of damage as early as in the other types of leprosy, but nerve thickening and associated sensory or motor dysfunction can usually be demonstrated as the disease advances. As sensory loss is often more pronounced than muscular wasting, patients continue to use the affected limbs and the skin suffers much damage from repeated trauma owing to insensitivity to pain. Thus the hands become scarred from injuries and burns and trophic ulcers develop on the soles of the feet. Nerve thickening, like skin involvement, tends to be bilateral and symmetrical but there may be a difference in degree on the two sides. It is found in those peripheral nerves which are superficial in some part of their course, the thickening being localized to the superficial portion, e.g. the great auricular nerves in the neck (Fig. 40.5), the supraclavicular nerves as they cross the clavicles, the ulnar nerves just above the elbows, the antebrachial cutaneous

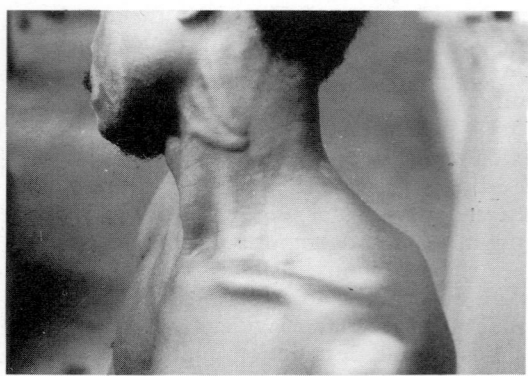

Fig. 40.5 Gross enlargement of the auricular nerve in tuberculoid leprosy. (Courtesy Dr S. G. Browne.)

nerves in the forearms, the radial and median nerves at the wrists, the femoral cutaneous nerves, the common peroneals as they wind round the necks of the fibulae, the superficial peroneals in front of the ankles and the posterior tibial nerves immediately below the internal malleoli. The earliest sensory disturbances may take the form of paraesthesia, hyperaesthesiae and hyperalgesia, to be followed later by impairment of light touch, temperature or pain sensation. All three modalities should be tested when examining a patient, as sometimes only one is affected (dissociated anaesthesia); in such a case it is usually the ability to differentiate between hot and cold which is lost first. Loss of position sense, vibration sense and tendon reflexes may occur, but not commonly. Muscle wasting may produce deformities such as claw hand (ulnar nerve), main-en-griffe (combined ulnar and median nerves), drop foot (common peroneal nerve) and facial palsy (facial nerve), but careful examination of muscles will show evidence of weakness long before paralysis occurs.

Involvement of autonomic nerves manifests itself in the early stages by slight oedema of the hands or feet; more marked vasomotor disturbance develops later causing the skin of hands and feet to be puffy and cyanosed.

Other tissues involved in lepromatous leprosy

Nails of fingers and toes. These are affected when trophic changes take place in digits, and appear dry, lustreless, narrowed and longitudinally ridged.

Mucous membranes. The patient may complain of nasal discharge, possibly bloodstained, and of blocking of the airway; examination reveals hyperaemia and swelling of the mucosa together with nodules or ulcers on the nasal septum. Ulceration leads to septal perforation and later to cartilage destruction and consequent 'saddle-nose' deformity. Nodules may also form on the lips, tongue, palate and larynx, leading to ulceration. Laryngeal involvement gives rise to hoarse cough, husky voice and stridor. Oedema of the glottis, occurring as part of a reactional state, used to be a dreaded complication in the pre-cortisone era, calling for immediate tracheotomy. Perforation of the palate may occur in the absence of syphilis or yaws. Jopling[25] stresses the importance of nasal symptoms (stuffiness, crust formation, bloodstained discharge) and of bilateral oedema of the legs as early signs which may point to a diagnosis of lepromatous leprosy long before the appearance of the classical skin lesions.

Eye. For the effects of leprosy on the eye, see Chapter 70.

Bones. Changes in bones in lepromatous leprosy are confined to the skull and limbs. In the limbs the changes are almost solely concentrated in the hands and feet and are due to a combination of factors which include: (a) deposition of bacilli; (b) neurotrophic atrophy; (c) repeated trauma resulting from analgesia; (d) disuse owing to paralysis and contractures; (e) secondary infection from trophic ulceration; (f) generalized osteoporosis of hormonal origin. Deposition of bacilli in the medullary cavities, the periosteum and the nutrient vessels gives rise to bone cysts, enlarged nutrient foramina, aseptic necrosis and spindle-shaped leprous dactylitis closely simulating that of tuberculosis or syphilis. Leprous periostitis of the tibia, fibula and ulna has been described. Neurotrophic atrophy affecting the hands is localized to the phalanges. Metacarpals and carpal bones are spared. In the feet the atrophic changes are localized to the metatarsals and phalanges, commencing in the proximal phalanges or in the heads of the metatarsals. In the proximal phalanges the diaphyses become gradually thinned by rarefying osteitis, known as 'concentric bone atrophy', so that eventually there is but a fine needle of bone left. This may be followed by disappearance of the affected bones and the shortened toes are connected to the foot by soft tissue only.

In the metatarsals absorption begins at the distal ends which become thinned and pointed—the 'sucked candy stick' appearance. The tarsal bones are spared.

Sensory loss results in repeated trauma, both major and minor, and this is an important contributory factor to the production of bone atrophy and absorption. Brand[39] states: 'By far the greatest proportion of finger absorption is secondary to burns and trauma which follow anaesthesia.' In addition, sensory loss can lead to the development of Charcot joints in the fingers, toes, wrists or ankles.

Muscle paralysis can lead to disuse and, in neglected cases, to fibrous or bony ankylosis of the interphalangeal, metacarpophalangeal and metatarsophalangeal joints. Disuse also results in osteoporosis owing to decreased osteoblastic activity.

Secondary infection commonly follows neglected trophic ulceration of feet or hand and can result in pyogenic osteomyelitis.

Generalized osteoporosis may follow defective production of testosterone as a result of testicular damage.

Changes in the skull in lepromatous leprosy consist of atrophy of the anterior nasal spine and the maxillary alveolar process, probably caused by a combination of aseptic necrosis, due to leprous endarteritis, and pyogenic osteomyelitis, due to gross ulceration in the nose.

Reticuloendothelial system. Lymph glands may be enlarged and painless with the consistency of soft rubber, particularly the femoral, inguinal and epitrochlear glands but occasionally one or more glands become very swollen and tender as part of a reactional state. The reticuloendothelial elements of the abdominal viscera are invaded by bacilli, especially in the spleen and liver, and the red marrow is similarly invaded. Lymphoedema of the lower legs may occur, giving rise to elephantiasis in neglected cases.

Testes. Testicular atrophy may occur, resulting in sterility and gynaecomastia.

Kidneys. Glomerulonephritis, interstitial nephritis and pyelonephritis may occur. Renal amyloidosis is a prevalent complication in some geographical areas but is uncommon in others; it appears to be related to the severity and frequency of type 2 lepra reactions (ENL).

Serological tests for syphilis are usually positive in lepromatous leprosy but the *Treponema pallidum* immobilization (TPI) test remains negative in the absence of syphilis.

Tuberculoid leprosy

This is the type seen in persons with a good resistance and may be purely neural or combined neural and dermal. The infection is never widespread but is localized to one area or to a few areas asymmetrically. Affected nerves are thickened, sometimes irregularly, and there are associated sensory or motor changes depending on the type of nerve involved. Sensory disturbance occurs as described under lepromatous leprosy except for the fact that it occurs earlier in the course of the disease and can be noted before the onset of skin lesions. If the patient complains of sensory disturbance such as paraesthesiae or anaesthesia, a search must be made for palpable thickening of the nerve responsible for the sensation of that area, e.g. face (trigeminal nerve); neck (great auricular nerve) (Fig. 40.5); forearm (antebrachial cutaneous nerve); fifth finger (ulnar nerve); hand (median nerve at the wrist); thigh (femoral cutaneous nerve); lower leg (common peroneal nerve at the neck of the fibula); dorsum of foot (superficial peroneal nerve); and sole of foot (posterior tibial nerve just below the internal malleolus).

Loss of position sense, vibration sense and tendon reflexes occur rarely. Motor changes are shown by muscle weakness or wasting and must be sought in the face, the intrinsic muscles of the hand and the dorsiflexors of the foot. It is extremely rare for the dorsiflexors of the wrist to be affected, owing to the fact that the radial nerve in the arm and forearm follows a deep course among the muscles and is therefore rarely involved. It is interesting to note that the same nerve, when it becomes superficial at the end of its course, often becomes thickened and can be palpated as a firm mobile cord as it lies against the lower end of the radius.

Abscesses in the course of affected nerves are not uncommon in tuberculoid leprosy.

Skin lesions take the form of macules or infiltrations (plaques) (Fig. 40.6). A tuberculoid macule is erythematous on fair skins and hypopigmented (not depigmented) on dark ones, has a dry and rather rough surface, its edges are well defined, and it is anaesthetic (except on the face) and anhidrotic. Infiltrated lesions are erythematous, whether on fair or dark skins, some-

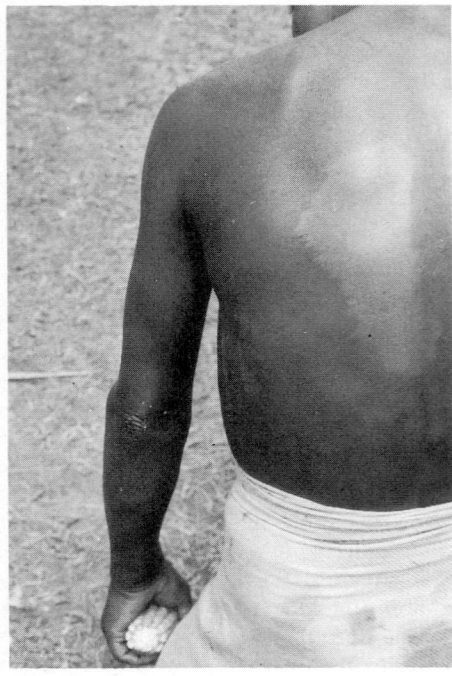 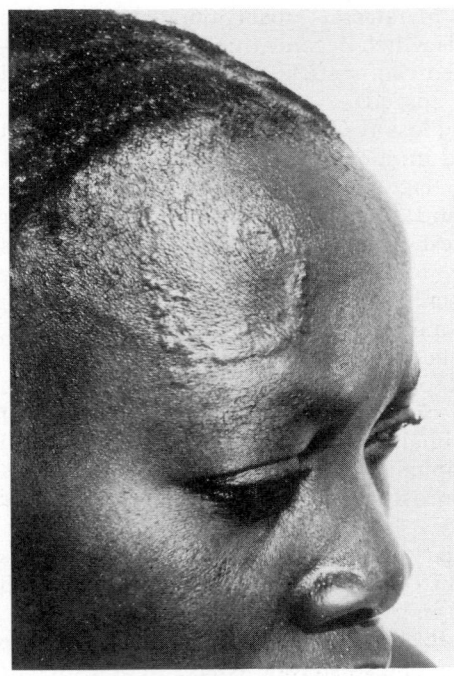

Fig. 40.6   Skin lesions of tuberculoid leprosy. Left, macular. Right, infiltrated. (Courtesy Dr S. G. Browne.)

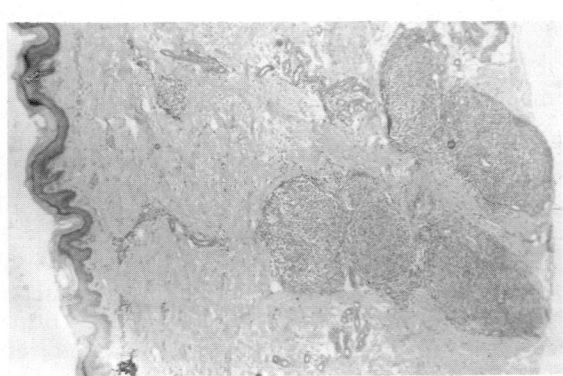

Fig. 40.7   Skin lesions in tuberculoid leprosy (high power).
(Courtesy Dr S. G. Browne.)

For descriptive purposes these infiltrated lesions are divided into minor and major tuberculoids (leprides), the major ones being larger, more grossly infiltrated and more deeply coloured.

Lesions of tuberculoid leprosy are usually few, large and asymmetrically situated; they favour the face, extensor surfaces of limbs, back and buttocks, while tending to avoid the chest, abdomen, scalp and flexor aspects of limbs. If palms or soles are involved the lesions are not raised owing to the thickness and tightness of the skin. Sometimes one or two small 'satellite' lesions are seen in the vicinity of a large plaque and may look like nodules, but the fact that they are less elevated in the centre than at the edges can be confirmed by palpation. Thickened cutaneous nerves may be palpated in the vicinity of the lesions, but tissues other than skin and nerves are not involved directly. The eye may suffer indirectly from corneal ulceration when there is damage to the facial nerve (exposure keratitis) and also when there is damage to the trigeminal nerve (neuropathic keratitis) (Plate V.6). Loss of eyebrows does not occur unless there is an infiltrated lesion traversing the eyebrow, and then the loss of hair is confined to that portion of the eyebrow, which is actually covered by the lesion.

times with a coppery, brownish or purple hue, have a dry and rather rough surface which may be irregular or pebbled, are sometimes scaly, have well-marked sensory loss and have edges which are raised and clearcut while the centres show variable flattening. In dark skins the colouring of the lesions obscures the underlying hypopigmentation. Central healing and peripheral extension give rise to annular lesions in which the *outer* edges are raised and well defined and the *inner* ones are flattened and indistinct.

Bone changes in hands or feet are less common than in the lepromatous type as leprosy bacilli are not deposited in the bones or their nutrient arteries; also, the early development of muscle wasting and paralysis results in disuse and therefore reduced risk of repeated trauma. However, neuropathic atrophy may occur in the phalanges of fingers or in the metatarsals and phalanges of feet but, unlike the changes in lepromatous leprosy, they are never bilateral and symmetrical. Bone changes secondary to disuse, to loss of sensation and to trophic ulceration may occur as described under lepromatous leprosy. Indolent ulcers of the feet are common (Fig. 40.8).

skins. They may appear on trunk or limbs but have a predilection for the back; in number and character they are intermediate between the macules of the two polar types. Careful testing will reveal impairment of sensation in some if not all of the macules.

Infiltrated lesions have their own distinctive features in which the characteristics of the two polar types are merged. They are moderate in number, asymmetrical in distribution, their erythema has an admixture of purple or brown, their surface is smooth and often shiny and they slope away peripherally from raised centres. The edges are well defined in places and indefinite in others.

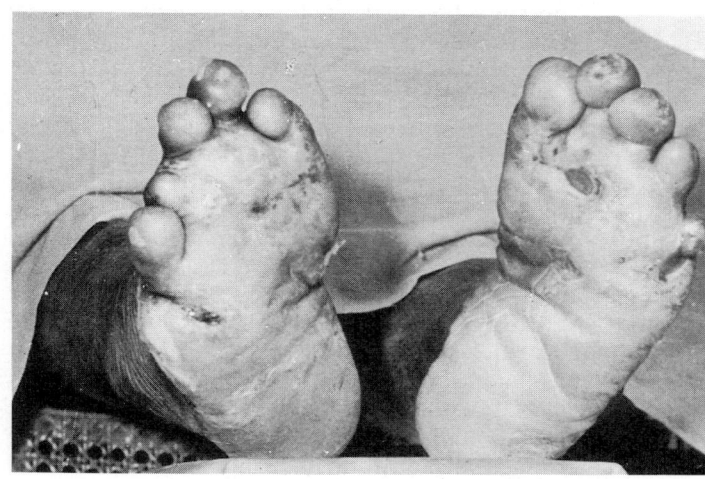

Fig. 40.8 Trophic ulceration and deformity of the feet. (Courtesy Dr S. G. Browne.)

Borderline (dimorphous) leprosy

This is the type seen in persons with a limited or variable resistance and usually presents with skin and nerve involvement. At the Sixth International Congress of Leprosy in Madrid (1953)[40] the existence of a pure neural form was not accepted but careful observation since then has proved that a polyneuritic form does exist.

The infection is neither as strictly localized as in tuberculoid leprosy nor as widespread as in the lepromatous type but is somewhere between the two. Some patients remain dimorphous throughout but others progress to one or other of the two polar types, depending on immunological factors not yet understood.

Skin lesions are macular, infiltrated or both, the earliest lesions being macules which are erythematous in fair skins or hypopigmented (sometimes with an erythematous periphery) in dark

Some of these infiltrations may take the form of bands, annular lesions and small nodules. Annular lesions have a characteristic form in which an oval area of normal looking but anaesthetic skin is surrounded by a band of infiltrated tissue of varying width, the *inner* edge being raised and clearcut (giving the oval area a punched out appearance), the *outer* merging imperceptibly with the surrounding skin. These should not be mistaken for annular tuberculoid lesions for in the latter the outside edges are raised and clearcut while the inner edges are indistinct. Sometimes there is an oval band of infiltrated tissue, even in width, and more raised in the central part of the band which has well-defined outer and inner edges. Infiltrated lesions are invariably anaesthetic and may be found on any part of the body, with the exception of axillae, groins, perineum and scalp but favour the limbs and buttocks (Fig. 40.9).

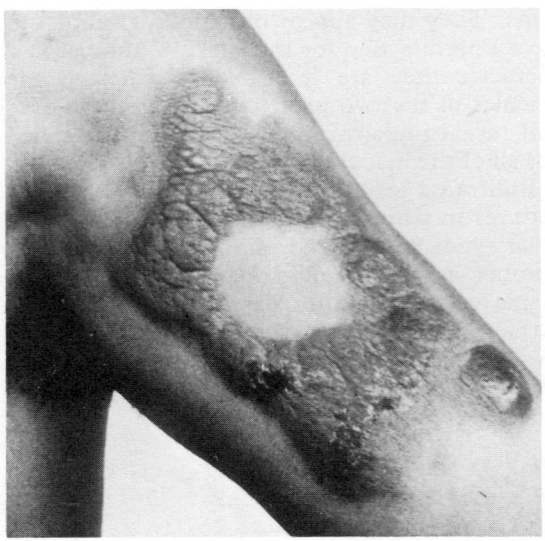

Fig. 40.9   Borderline leprosy. (Courtesy Dr S. G. Browne.)

Nerve involvement can always be demonstrated in borderline leprosy and neurological symptoms such as paraesthesiae and hyperalgesia often precede the onset of skin manifestations. Nerves are involved asymmetrically and show palpable thickening and impaired function (sensory, motor or both). Other tissues are not affected directly but only indirectly as in the tuberculoid type.

Indeterminate leprosy

This is an early phase in the natural history of leprosy. At this stage the disease has not yet determined into which type it is going to evolve. Manifestations may be neural or macular (or both), macules being nondescript with uncharacteristic histology and absence of bacilli.

DIFFERENTIAL DIAGNOSIS

The characteristic marks of leprosy are sufficiently distinctive, but they have to be differentiated from psoriasis, seborrhoeic dermatitis, various forms of tinea, eczema, lichen planus, pellagra and filarial disease. Blastomycosis produces skin lesions reminiscent of leprosy. From syphilis and yaws, diagnosis may not always be so easy. Syphilitic and yaws skin lesions may often closely resemble the maculae of leprosy but the absence of sensory changes and

reaction to treatment are sufficiently distinctive. The VDRL reaction alone cannot always be depended upon in differential diagnosis as syphilis and leprosy may coexist; also a false-positive reaction is not uncommon in lepromatous leprosy. Leprophilia is the name given for a hysterical condition with false anaesthesia developed by a peculiar kind of psychoneurotic who craves for sympathy.

The thickened skin of crab yaws on the feet may roughly resemble leprotic hyperkeratosis and may give a semblance of anaesthesia. Gangosa of yaws may be mistaken for nasal leprosy.

The early lesions of mycosis fungoides might possibly be mistaken for early nodular leprosy and leukoderma is not infrequently associated with leprosy in the popular mind. It is extremely common, especially in India and in Negro races, and unfortunate sufferers are sometimes to be found in leprosy institutions. Depigmentation in leukoderma, however, is more complete and sensory changes are absent. Lupus vulgaris and other tuberculides are very likely to be mistaken for leprides and in both diseases acid-fast bacilli are difficult to demonstrate. Lupus evinces a greater tendency to scar formation and there are no sensory changes.

Cutaneous leishmaniasis and in South America espundia may be mistaken for leprosy. The lesions on the skin of the face tend to concentrate round the mouth and nose and form a more raised margin than those in leprosy. Demonstration of the Leishman–Donovan body will always settle the matter but leishmanial lupus-like lesions on the ears may cause difficulty. Burns and other injuries may leave behind anaesthetic scars. Eunuchism has been mistaken for leprosy on account of the absence of eyebrows and the smooth, shiny appearance of the skin.

Polyneuritic leprosy affecting the hands has to be differentiated from syringomyelia in which analgesia and loss of heat sense are accompanied by retention of sense of touch and normal sweat function. The absence of nerve swelling and tenderness is important. The nerve injuries caused by trauma of the ulnar nerve or by cervical rib may possibly be called into question, but can be settled by X-ray examination. Meralgia paraesthetica (Bernhardt's syndrome) may cause anaesthesia of the anterolateral region of the thigh and Raynaud's disease can cause trophic changes in the extremities. Familial hypertrophic interstitial neuritis (Déjérine–Sottas disease) may cause confusion because of the characteristic thickening of peripheral nerves, together with sensory and motor changes in the limbs. Anaesthesia of the feet, leading to trophic ulceration and mutilation, can occur in diabetes, tabes, familial sensory radicular neuropathy and primary amyloidosis involving peripheral nerves. Von Recklinghausen's disease (neurofibromas) may sometimes resemble leprosy. Scarring and anaesthesia caused by extensive herpes zoster on the chest may give rise to difficulty. Scleroderma, localized or diffuse, may be confused with lepromatous leprosy but madarosis is not present, nerves are not thickened, acid-fast bacilli are absent from smear and skin biopsy is diagnostic. The absence of fever and the presence of neural signs should differentiate tuberculoid leprosy in reaction from erysipelas. Erythema nodosum leprosum may be mistaken for other forms of erythema nodosum or for the Weber–Christian syndrome (a relapsing, febrile, non-suppurative, nodular panniculitis). Sarcoidosis can resemble tuberculoid leprosy but there is no sensory loss and no nerve thickening. Although a peripheral neuropathy has been reported complicating sarcoidosis, there is no nerve thickening. Granuloma annulare may simulate tuberculoid leprosy but there is no sensory loss or nerve thickening and the histological appearances are different. Granuloma multiforme may resemble tuberculoid leprosy; it appears to be localized to Nigeria. There is no sensory loss or nerve thickening and the histological appearances are different.

DIAGNOSIS

The diagnosis of leprosy rests upon three cardinal signs and an awareness of the disease:
1 palpable thickened nerves,
2 demonstration of anaesthesia,
3 demonstration of *M. leprae* in skin, nasal mucous membrane or nerve biopsy.

Leprosy should be considered in any untypical or unfamiliar skin disorder in a patient from an endemic area and in any obscure neurological disorder.

Thickened nerves may be felt on palpation and tenderness elicited by striking an area sharply with the finger or patellar hammer. The ulnar nerve is commonly affected above the elbow; the common peroneal at the head of the fibula behind the knee; the superficial peroneal in front of the ankle; the terminal branch of the radial as it passes over the lower end of the radius; the posterior tibial below the inner malleolus; the great auricular as it runs parallel to the external jugular vein; and the branches of any particular nerve supplying a tuberculoid lesion.

To test sensation the patient should be stripped and blindfolded. For testing anaesthesia to light touch a feather should be used; analgesia is tested by pinprick, using an area of normal skin as control. The two-pin test is often positive when the feather test is negative. Loss of thermal sensation is important and can be elicited by using a test-tube containing hot water and another containing iced water. Hyperaesthesia and paraesthesia may precede anaesthesia to light touch. *The possibility of leprosy should be considered in any patient presenting with a painless burn, injury or ulcer of one limb.*

Bacteriological examination

This is essential in order to establish proof of the disease and to assist in correct classification; it consists in carrying out a series of smears from the lesions. The scrape-incision method is recommended and is carried out as follows. The lesion is cleaned with ether and a fold is firmly held between thumb and forefinger of the left hand (to render it avascular); with a small bladed scalpel an incision is made about 5 mm long and 3 mm deep, pressure of the fingers being maintained; the blade is then turned at right angles to the cut and the wound is scraped several times so that tissue fluid and pulp collect on one side of the blade; this is *gently* smeared on a glass slide. Smears are fixed by heat and are then stained by Ziehl–Neelsen technique (Appendix IV, p. 1500). By this method acid-fast bacilli will always be found in lepromatous leprosy and frequently in the borderline form, but will usually be absent in the tuberculoid type (except in reaction) and in the indeterminate group. Nasal scrapings have been advocated in the past but experience has shown that skin smears are far more valuable in diagnosis; not only are bacilli always readily demonstrated in the skin when they are present in the nasal mucosa, but often they are present in the skin when absent from the nose. For example, in borderline leprosy, nasal scrapings may be negative when the skin smears contain large numbers of bacilli and bacilli may disappear from the nasal mucosa long before they disappear from the skin. Nasal scrapings are helpful in deciding whether a patient is infectious. In untreated lepromatous leprosy they are always positive but bacilli disappear from the nose more quickly after chemotherapy than they do from the skin. Nasal scrapings are always negative in BB, BT and TT leprosy and negative in most BL cases.

In lepromatous leprosy the skin of the fingers is rich in bacilli and this site should be included in the assessment of new cases and in follow-up examinations. Jopling[41] suggests that for these purposes no more than four smears are necessary, one from each ear lobe and one from the terminal phalanx of each middle finger.

Skin biopsy

Biopsy of the skin is essential for correct classification as it enables the histological changes in the skin to be studied. In addition several biopsies carried out at regular intervals provide a valuable method of assessing prognosis and treatment. In carrying out a biopsy the most active part of the lesion must be chosen; this will be at the edge of the lesion in tuberculoid leprosy and in the centre in the lepromatous type. After ensuring local anaesthesia with 2% procaine a portion of skin is removed with a scalpel or by a skin biopsy punch possessing a circular cutting edge, 5–7 mm in diameter. It is essential that the incision should reach the subcutaneous fat, otherwise the deeper layers of the dermis may not be included in the biopsy material. Paraffin sections are stained with haematoxylin and eosin to show the histological changes and, with a modification of the Ziehl–Neelsen method, using pinene to demonstrate acid-fast bacilli. A nerve biopsy will be necessary in a purely neural case or where a skin biopsy has not given sufficient information; a thickened sensory nerve is chosen, such as the great auricular in the neck, the antebrachial cutaneous in the forearm, the radial at the lateral aspect of the wrist, the femoral cutaneous in the thigh or the superficial peroneal on the dorsum of the foot.

In lepromatous leprosy bacilli can often be found in the sternal marrow but this is not a practical method of diagnosis as bacilli are always readily demonstrable in the skin if present in the marrow.

Subsidiary signs

Anhidrosis, often preceded by hyperhidrosis, is characteristic of chronic cases and is usually present in tuberculoid macules. In doubtful cases pilocarpine 0.2 ml of 1 in 1000 solution is injected intradermally in a suspected patch and a similar amount in adjacent healthy skin. Both areas are then painted with tincture of iodine and, when dry, powdered with starch. The control area sweats, turning the starch blue. Absence of sweat at the point of injection indicates leprosy.

A useful diagnostic aid is the intradermal mecholyl test for anhidrosis. The action of mecholyl chloride (almost identical with acetylcholine) is similar to that of pilocarpine. Denervation of sweat glands by leprous neuritis is the cause of anhidrosis, usually affecting the most distal portions of the post-ganglionic nerve fibres. In carrying out the test, equal areas of leprous and healthy skin are painted with a solution of castor oil, iodine and absolute alcohol. Then 0.05–0.1 ml aqueous solution of mecholyl chloride is injected intradermally at the border of the lesion so as to produce a wheal. The whole area is lightly dusted with powdered starch. Within a few minutes sweat droplets appear on the functionally intact skin, which becomes blue from the iodine and starch combination. The response is negative when no sweat drops appear within the area tested.

The histamine test of Rodriguez is somewhat similar in slight or early cases. A drop of 1 in 1000 solution of histamine is placed within the margin of the suspected area and a second outside. A prick is made with a needle through the drops. A red flare appears in normal skin. This test can be of great value in a purely neural case with sensory loss in one or more limbs, for it will exclude hysteria and organic disease of the central nervous system, such as syringomyelia. In all those conditions a red flare develops in the anaesthetic skin but no flare appears if the anaesthesia is due to leprosy or other forms of peripheral neuritis.

REACTION

The reactional state in leprosy has been described and interpreted many times and the subject has been much disputed with confusing results. The following description is taken from Ridley[42] and essentially relates the reactional state to the immune status of the patient. It is important to remember that simple extension or regression of lesions does not constitute the true leprosy reaction. An agreed terminology has still to be generally accepted. For the types of reaction described below some leprologists use the term 'lepra reaction' for the reaction associated with borderline leprosy. Others use the term 'type 1 reaction' to refer to this. The reaction almost exclusively occurring in lepromatous leprosy is termed 'ENL reaction' by some and 'type 2 lepra reaction' by others. Some prefer to use the term 'upgrading reaction' in place of 'reversal reaction'. See Jopling[25] for a discussion of this subject.

The reactions in leprosy are all acute episodes associated with alterations in the immunological balance between the bacilli and the host and they have an allergic basis. The reactions take place in borderline (BT, BB, BL) and lepromatous leprosy and are described by Ridley[42] as follows:

Borderline	Downgrading	Both associated with changes in cell-mediated immunity
	Reversal	
Lepromatous	Exacerbation nodules	
	Erythema nodosum leprosum (associated with humoral mechanisms)	

Reactions in borderline patients

Downgrading

This is unfavourable, associated with movement towards lepromatous leprosy and occurs only in untreated, near tuberculoid patients.
1 Decline of immunity.
2 Increase in bacilli.
3 Extension of infection.

Histological features include:
1 increase in bacilli;
2 dispersion of lymphocytes encompassing the lesions;
3 infiltration through the dermis of large giant cells of foreign-body type;
4 loss of the usual compact focalization of the granuloma;
5 spread of the granuloma;
6 oedema, intracellular and extracellular;
7 dermal reaction, as in reversal reaction (below), replaced by granuloma; no heavy fibrosis.

Reversal

This is favourable and occurs in near-lepromatous and borderline patients when the bacterial load is diminished by treatment.
1 Increase of immunity.
2 Decrease in bacilli.

Clinical features are similar in both downgrading and reversal reactions. They may appear rapidly and violently. There may be fever (in severe reaction) to 37.7–40.0°C, possibly lasting several months. Erythema and swelling of skin lesions occurs and possibly ulceration. Hands and feet may be swollen and acutely tender. Nerve involvement is common; lesions are very tender. Gross paralysis may develop in a few days. New lesions (towards the tuberculoid type in reversal reactions) may occur. The nasal passages may be blocked by swollen mucosa. The patient may be in a miserable state.

Histological features may be seen in marked reversal cases (in mild cases there is little histological sign):
1 decrease in bacilli;
2 influx of lymphocytes usually; transient;
3 change of host cells towards the epithelioid form;
4 giant cell formation (foreign body type at first, later Langans' type);
5 necrosis in severe reactions;
6 oedema in and around the granuloma which enlarges;
7 dermal reaction; influx of undifferentiated cells and fibrocytes in parts of the skin not affected by granuloma;
8 fibrosis later.

The most severe reactions tend to occur in patients who are in the middle of the classification spectrum—a considerable shift, from BL to BT, would be associated with a heavier reaction than would a slight shift.

Reactions in lepromatous patients

Exacerbation nodules

These are not of great practical importance since they do not produce systemic upset. They occur in exceptionally large lesions with excessive bacilli.

Clinical features include:
1 large nodules, possibly erythematous;

2   no systemic upset.

Histological features are:

1   heavy polymorph infiltration;
2   cellular disintegration (see ENL, below);
3   related to histoid lesions which are histologically similar to hyperactive lepromatous nodules.

Erythema nodosum leprosum (ENL)

This may be precipitated by treatment especially by dapsone or by intercurrent infection etc. This is not an indication of shift in immunological status. It occurs usually when patients have been under treatment for about one year and the bacterial load has fallen, the bacilli are disintegrating and releasing antigenic material and are relatively numerous in the circulating blood. It is probably associated with humoral mechanisms and represents a manifestation of the Arthus phenomenon.

Clinical features include:

1   fever;
2   transient crops of small painful red nodules lasting a few days;
3   large painful red plaques if severe, with necrosis and ulceration;
4   enlargement of lymph nodes, liver and spleen;
5   iridocyclitis (allergic), orchitis and painful enlargement of nerves (neuralgia);
6   swollen joints occasionally;
7   nephritis (allergic) occasionally;
8   polymorphonuclear leukocytosis.

These manifestations are found mostly where bacilli are common except the lesions in joints, kidneys and possibly the eyes, which may be allergic. Changes in the kidneys, apparently due to deposition of protein complexes (probably antigen–antibody complexes) within the nephrons, tend to occur in patients subject to severe reactional states. The nephrons may be destroyed. The condition seems to resemble the nephrosis sometimes seen in quartan malaria.

Histological features of mild ENL. Reaction is not in the major skin lesions but in small, clinically inapparent lesions with few bacilli. The centre is never in normal skin. Polymorphs are present and predominant in the early stage. Cellular disintegration is marked. Lymphocytes appear later. Vasculitis is seen in about half the lesions.

Severe ENL. This occurs in advanced lepromatous leprosy with heavy bacillary load. There are large necrotizing lesions which may be wedge-shaped like infarcts. Oedema is intense. Cellular infiltration is intense often affecting the whole dermis except the fat. Lymph node and nerve involvement with polymorphs occurs and there is heavy infiltration of bacilli into walls of large vessels and necrosis of small vessels. Dermal reaction (as in reversal reaction) can be intense. (A similar reaction sometimes occurs in the dermis in very mild ENL.)

TREATMENT

Treatment should not be started until a definite diagnosis has been made and the case classified as multibacillary (LL, BL or BB) or paucibacillary (BT, TT or indeterminate). Although multidrug therapy is now standard the management and prognosis of the case depends on the original classification.

It is probably unwise to begin treatment in very anaemic patients and this should be delayed until the haemoglobin has been increased to 5 g/dl. Once the diagnosis is established most patients can be treated by medical auxiliaries at mobile or static clinics but patients who are undergoing reaction or who are sensitive to drugs are better treated in hospital. Lepromatous patients should be kept isolated until they are not discharging any viable bacilli, which with rifampicin treatment is four to five weeks. Tuberculoid patients are not infectious. Modern drug therapy has led to the establishment of country-wide rural outpatient schemes for the treatment of leprosy, like those for tuberculosis.

Drug treatment

Five drugs are available for treatment (Table 40.3) and two or more are given concurrently as standard treatment.

Dapsone (DDS; 4,4'-diaminodiphenylsulphone)

Dapsone is slowly bactericidal. The dose is 6–10 mg/kg weekly, i.e. a dose of 100 mg daily for adults and suitably reduced for children. A lepra reaction may be precipitated by dapsone but type 2 reactions are not dose dependent and the drug may be given to lepromatous patients in full dosage from the start of treatment. There is a risk of type 1 reaction in borderline cases with a

Table 40.3. Bactericidal drugs available for the chemotherapy of leprosy.

Drug	Dose (mg)	Minimal inhibitory concentration (ng/ml)	Ratio of peak serum concentration to MIC	Bactericidal activity
Dapsone	100	3	500	Low
Rifampicin	600	300	30	High
Clofazimine	50–100	?	?	Low
Ethionamide	375	50	60	Intermediate
Prothionamide	375	50	40	Intermediate

From Waters.[7]

reversal reaction leading to nerve damage and in certain cases where this would lead to extensive nerve damage (facial nerve) then smaller doses should be given to start with.

Dapsone may be given by injection. For this it is suspended (20–25%) in various oils (chaulmoogra, arachis) and is intended for intramuscular injection in initial (adult) doses of 0.2 ml (50 mg dapsone in 25% suspension) once each week, rising to a maximum of 0.8 ml.

Another preparation for injection consists of 5 g dapsone dissolved in 40 ml absolute alcohol to which 55 ml propylene glycol is added, and 5 ml benzyl alcohol is incorporated to reduce discomfort on intramuscular injection.[43]

Other injectable preparations of dapsone are also available. No advantage is apparent for the injectable preparations except perhaps that the doses are known to be given, whereas a patient given a supply of tablets to be taken at intervals for a week or more by mouth may fail to take them regularly.

Side-effects of dapsone are uncommon but include haemolytic anaemia, methaemoglobinaemia, hepatitis, skin conditions including fixed eruptions (blackish macules or diffuse hypermelanosis) in dark skins, together with systemic symptoms, slight or severe. Subjects with a deficiency of glucose-6-phosphate dehydrogenase (G-6-PD) are more susceptible to haemolysis than are normal subjects. Agranulocytosis has been reported in patients taking dapsone for other conditions in much larger doses than are usually given in leprosy. Psychotic symptoms, including disorders of speech and thought, and delusions may occur on large doses although other factors may be concerned.

Dapsone is now no longer so effective as it once was and this is due to two factors: poor compliance with treatment and the development of dapsone resistance.

COMPLIANCE

Failure to take the drug regularly developed out of the practice of stopping administration of the drug from time to time for fear of reaction and the patients not noticing any deterioration in their condition. Studies on compliance using the detection of dapsone in the urine[44] revealed a loss of half the patients, both lepromatous and tuberculoid, over four years. This has led to the establishment of shorter courses using multidrug therapy.

DAPSONE RESISTANCE

Proof of bacterial resistance to dapsone depends either on the results of inoculation of the bacilli into mouse foot-pads or on the response, judged by skin smear examinations, to supervised treatment over a period of three months in hospital. The possibility of drug resistance should be considered if there is no obvious clinical improvement after treatment for six months.

Resistance developing during the course of treatment (secondary resistance) may be recognized by the appearance of new skin lesions, erythematous papulonodules, accompanied by the presence of morphologically normal leprosy bacilli in skin smears and sections from the lesions and in nasal mucus. These lesions should not be mistaken for those of ENL which are often tender, fade under pressure and disappear in a few days. Bacteriological reactivation usually precedes clinical signs of relapse and regular examination of skin smears every six to 12 months should prevent the occurrence of clinical relapse. A disquieting development has been the development of primary resistance to dapsone, i.e. infection by dapsone-resistant bacilli. To avoid the emergence of resistant organisms, patients with multibacillary leprosy should not be given dapsone alone.

Prevalence of dapsone resistance. Secondary

dapsone resistance has been detected wherever it has been looked for—the highest so far being 40% in central Burma.[45] For this reason treatment with only one drug is no longer possible.

Persistence of M. leprae. It has been found that a small number of dapsone-sensitive bacilli may persist in the body for many years leading to relapse up to 20 years later.[7]

DADDS (acedapsone, 4,4'-diacetyldiamino- diphenyl sulphone)

DADDS is a repository sulphone suspended in a mixture of benzyl benzoate and castor oil which releases dapsone slowly. In intramuscular doses of 225 mg every 75–77 days it is as active as dapsone in patients with lepromatous leprosy. Some patients have experienced ENL in some degree.[46] DADDS is an excellent prophylactic drug to treat contacts in some communities (see section on Control, below).

Rifampicin

This antibiotic, an addition to leprosy therapy in 1970, has proved its value. It is bactericidal to the tubercle bacillus whereas other antileprosy drugs are bacteriostatic to that organism. An early report[47] showed that it rapidly reduced the morphological index (MI) of bacilli in skin to zero in five weeks, compared with five months in control patients with lepromatous leprosy receiving dapsone. It is no more effective than dapsone in eradicating a lepromatous infection. Rifampicin is rapidly effective in relieving nasal symptoms in lepromatous leprosy and in healing leg ulceration resulting from the breaking down of nodules.[25] Rifampicin is effective given monthly[25] in a dose of 1200 mg or 600 mg on 2 consecutive days every four weeks on an empty stomach (this is important).

SIDE EFFECTS

Rifampicin may produce a reddish-brown colour in urine, sputum and sweat. Other side-effects include nausea, abdominal discomfort and, rarely, toxic effects on the liver but these are more likely when the drug is given twice weekly. Care should be taken in borderline leprosy because there is a risk that a type 1 reaction might be precipitated.

It should be noted that the effects of steroids are reduced by rifampicin (see below, in section on treatment of reactional states) and the drug also impairs the effectiveness of oral contraceptives.[48]

Leprosy may be worsened during pregnancy and the puerperium and the disease may show its first signs at these times. There is also a high risk to the infant. Jopling[25] recommends that for a pregnant woman with lepromatous leprosy rifampicin, together with dapsone, should be given for at least three months before the birth of the child. This will make it unnecessary to separate the infant from the mother at birth. (It is not yet known how long the course of rifampicin must be to ensure that the breast milk does not contain viable leprosy bacilli.)

The first two cases of rifampicin resistance were reported in 1976.[49]

Clofazimine (Lamprene; B 663 (Geigy); G 30320)

This is a rimino compound derived from phenazine dye. It appears to have a remarkable action on ENL and on the course of lepromatous leprosy itself. It is indicated:

1   in lepromatous leprosy, particularly if the patient is liable to severe and prolonged exacerbation;

2   in lepromatous leprosy with long-standing ENL severe enough to necessitate continuous corticosteroids;

3   in patients harbouring dapsone-resistant M. leprae;

4   in patients responding only slowly to dapsone or who are intolerant of or hypersensitive to dapsone.

Clofazimine has been given by mouth in doses of 100–300 mg daily for long periods to patients in reaction, formerly dependent on corticosteroids, and the steroids have been reduced gradually and eventually abandoned completely, with good clinical and bacteriological results. Once reaction is controlled the dose can be reduced.[50] If reaction does break through the dose should not be reduced but should be increased. Clofazimine has now been found effective in previously untreated lepromatous leprosy in doses of 100 mg two or three times each week; this treatment is as effective as the standard dapsone regimen. Monthly administration has been used in lepromatous leprosy with success after a loading dose. In reactional states larger doses are needed.

Clofazimine is slowly eliminated from the body. The main adverse reaction is deep and persistent redness followed by pigmentation of the skin which is resented by patients with light skins but not by others who appreciate its therapeutic value. It not only controls ENL but also improves the clinical condition, the bacillary index and the morphological index. It may rarely cause abdominal pain and diarrhoea.

Information on clofazimine has been published by members of the medical department of Ciba-Geigy, makers of Lamprene.[51] Because of occasional reports of serious adverse effects in patients who have received this drug in high dosage over long periods, it is recommended that a dosage of more than 100 mg daily should be given for as short a period as possible (less than three months) and only under supervision. A few cases of fatal diarrhoea have been reported[52] when dosage has been continued for many months or years. One case of resistance has been reported.[53]

Clofazimine is now available in capsules of 50 mg, an ideal daily dose for many patients.

Ethionamide and prothionamide

Ethionamide and prothionamide (better tolerated) are given in a dosage of 250–500 mg daily, larger doses cause gastrointestinal upsets and jaundice. The usual dose is 375 mg daily after the main meal. They kill *M. leprae* faster than dapsone but more slowly than rifampicin. Resistance can develop after years of single drug treatment.[54] The indication for ethionamide or prothionamide is as an alternative to clofazimine in triple drug therapy where skin coloration is unacceptable.

Treatment regimens

Antileprosy drugs are no longer given alone and multidrug regimens are necessary to overcome dapsone resistance, prevent rifampicin resistance in cases with a significant bacterial load and to encourage compliance. Two standard regimens are recommended:[55]

Multibacillary
leprosy

For adults: Rifampicin 600 mg once a month supervised.
Dapsone 100 mg daily unsupervised.
Clofazimine 50 mg daily self-administered, plus 300 mg once a month supervised.

For others: Dapsone 1.2 mg/kg daily.
Rifampicin 450 mg < 35 kg.
300 mg < 20 kg.
150 mg < 12 kg.

As an alternative to 50 mg daily of clofazimine, 100 mg may be given every other day.

An alternative to clofazimine, if it is unacceptable, is ethionamide or prothionamide 250–375 mg daily unsupervised after the main meal. (Jaundice may be a problem in some areas.)

This triple drug regimen must be given for a minimum of two years or until the smears have become negative. The duration of treatment should be: LL five to 11 years; BL three to six years and BB two to three years. Relapsed smear positive patients should be given a minimum of two years and treated until they become smear negative.

Paucibacillary leprosy

Rifampicin 600 mg supervised once a month for six doses.

Dapsone 100 mg daily unsupervised for six months.

If the patient is on steroids for a reaction then the dapsone must be continued until the steroids have been stopped. As well as drug therapy patients with anaesthetic hands or feet will require long-term care to prevent ulceration (see section on surgical treatment, below).

Treatment of reactional states

The main therapeutic weapons in the treatment of reactional states are steroids, clofazimine and, where not contraindicated, thalidomide.

ENL (type 2 reactions)

Antileprosy drugs must be continued in full dosage throughout treatment.

Steroids. These may be used in repeated short courses[45] but in chronic ENL steroids plus clofazimine or thalidomide must be given.

For pain and swelling in the motor nerve, with weakness or paralysis, an injection of 1 500 units of hyaluronidase in 1 ml of 2% procaine solution, mixed with 1 ml hydrocortisone suspension (25 mg/ml) may be given slowly into or around the nerve through a size 14 needle—for instance, just above the elbow for the ulnar nerve and the neck of the fibula for the common peroneal nerve. The solution should be freshly made each time. Nerve stripping is not now in vogue. If surgery is necessary it suffices to incise the epineurium and decompress nerves where they pass through tunnels, such as the median nerve in the carpal tunnel and the ulnar nerve in the epitrochlear tunnel. For severe reactions treatment with corticotrophin or corticosteroids is indicated if other measures fail. It is important to give only the smallest dose which will control the condition. For corticotrophin a gel preparation can be given intramuscularly in daily doses of 40 units, gradually increasing the intervals to one injection every second day, or twice each week, and then reducing the dose; for cortisone a 5-day course by mouth (in divided dosage) as follows: 100 mg the first day, decreasing each day to 75 mg, 50 mg, 25 mg and 12.5 mg. With these courses the patient should reduce dietary salt and take a daily dose of a potassium salt equivalent to 3–5 g of potassium chloride. Prednisone and prednisolone are suitable alternatives, but their doses are much smaller (20 or 30 mg daily in divided doses). Prednisone is important for acute epididymo-orchitis; it causes less electrolyte disturbance than cortisone.

One advantage of corticosteroids is that antileprosy treatment can be continued; but the steroids should be withdrawn as soon as possible. The danger that the patient may become accustomed to bed rest and habituated to corticosteroids is real and must be avoided. Graded physical exercises, passive at first, are valuable in this connection.

One point about treatment with corticosteroids is that when such patients complain of abdominal pain or diarrhoea, trophozoites of *Entamoeba histolytica* can often be found in their stools. These exacerbations of amoebic colitis respond to standard antiamoebic treatment and do not indicate cessation of steroid treatment.[56] The development of the hyperinfection syndrome of strongyloidiasis *does* demand immediate withdrawal of corticosteroids, however, and pre-emptive treatment of strongyloidiasis is a wise precaution in endemic areas (see Chapter 21). The effects of steroids are reduced by rifampicin and if this drug is being given for leprosy a poor response to steroid therapy may be expected. This can be offset by increasing the dose by about 50% over the normal level.

Clofazimine. In addition to its antileprosy effect, clofazimine has an anti-inflammatory action which is useful in controlling both type 1 and type 2 lepra reaction but the dosage must be large, 300–600 mg daily.[25] It is slower in its effect than steroids.

Thalidomide. This has proved useful in type 2 lepra reaction (ENL) but is of no value in type 1 reaction. It is given in a dosage of 300–400 mg daily in divided doses, the dose then being reduced as the reaction subsides to 100 mg daily or on alternate days. Both thalidomide and clofazimine are helpful in reducing dependence on steroids but Jopling[25] stresses that it is important that the steroid (prednisone) is not stopped but continued in slowly reducing dosage; otherwise the thalidomide, which appears to require the presence of steroid, or of a functioning adrenal cortex, lacks effect. Because of its teratogenic effect thalidomide must not be given to women of childbearing age.

Type 1 reactions
Treatment in type 1 reactions may be urgent because of the possibility of permanent nerve damage.

In tuberculoid and dimorphous leprosy the reactionary state is less severe but the lesions may become painful or ulcerate and a peripheral nerve may be involved with pain and weakness. Dapsone, or other antileprosy drug, should be continued in full dosage. Analgesics will be required for the pain associated with the neuritis characteristic of the type 1 lepra reaction. Steroids and thalidomide are effective in relieving nerve pain in leprosy but thalidomide is of use only in type 2 reaction (ENL).

If a motor nerve is involved weakened muscles should be splinted and steroid treatment should be started in doses higher than for ENL. Intraneural injection may be called for. If a nerve abscess develops it should be aspirated or incised. Lesions which ulcerate require appropriate dressings.

Immunotherapy

Immunotherapy, with a view to increasing cell-mediated immunity in lepromatous leprosy, is under investigation. Transfer factor, prepared from lymphocytes from healthy donors with strongly positive lepromin tests, has been tried, but with varying results. For example, it has been shown that clinical reversal reactions developed in patients with lepromatous leprosy who had received transfer factor for 12 weeks with evidence of effective cell-mediated immunity; but no suggestion was found that transfer factor given for 20 weeks was of value. BCG vaccine given every two weeks combined with chemotherapy has shown promising results when continued for a year or longer.

Eye conditions

For the treatment of eye conditions associated with leprosy and with the reactional state, see Chapter 70.

Surgical treatment

The results of nerve involvement in leprosy lead to ulceration, paralysis and deformity of the limbs so often that the prevention or correction of the deformities involves a multitude of special techniques up to full orthopaedic surgery. A discussion of these complicated treatments is outside the scope of this book and surgeons who wish to study the subject are referred to books on surgery in leprosy by Carayon et al,[57] Fritschi[58] and McDowell and Enna,[59] and to the book on foot problems by Brand.[39]

Primary deformity is due to the activity of the disease, for instance to erosion of the phalanges due to lepromatous granulomas. Secondary deformity is due to damage which the patient inflicts on himself as a consequence of anaesthesia or paralysis.

It is important to keep the hands under constant examination for swelling, sensation and function and to ensure as far as possible that the hands are protected from trauma during the period when decalcification of the bones may be taking place. Examination by X-ray is essential for complete assessment. The same is true of the feet, but in the feet deep plantar damage may occur before anaesthesia is complete and nerve damage must therefore be recognized when loss of localization of light touch occurs on the sole. In England, lepromatous leprosy is far more important than tuberculoid or borderline leprosy as a cause of plantar ulceration. Plantar damage and ulceration can be prevented, partly by provision of footwear with rigid wooden soles and soft insoles and by the use of Plastazote insoles placed inside orthopaedic shoes.[60] It is important regularly to scrape away the callus which forms over a healed ulcer. Dry cracked skin can be treated by soaking in water for several hours each day and then covering with soft paraffin. Ulcers can be treated by rest, dressings and antibiotics; a plaster cast may obviate the need for more than a few days' bed rest.

Foot drop and other signs of damage to nerves need special apparatus or surgical measures such as tendon transplantation.

In all cases the need for physiotherapy must be borne in mind; it can do much to help the patient. The same is true of occupational therapy, which should satisfy the patient's need to be a useful member of the community in which he can do productive work, mental or physical. Occupational therapy is limited because many manual skills involve the risk of damage to the hands, for instance, carpentry. But some form of satisfactory occupation should be sought; the mental effect of enforced idleness can be disastrous to the personality of the patient.

PROGNOSIS

Leprosy in its milder forms is a self-healing disease; it is also curable. Of those who become infected, only a small proportion develop overt signs. Its old terrible reputation is justifiable only in extreme cases.

In *macular tuberculoid leprosy* the prognosis after treatment is excellent, though with severe hypopigmentation the pigment may not return to completely healed lesions, and if anaesthesia is extensive, sensation may not be restored completely, even after complete cure.

In *infiltrated tuberculoid leprosy* also the prognosis is excellent after treatment but if nerves have been grossly enlarged there may be some permanent anaesthesia and the patient should be warned not to damage hands and feet because of the risk of permanent ulceration or deformity.

In *lepromatous leprosy* the prognosis, though now much better than ever before, must be guarded. The earlier the treatment is instituted, the better the prognosis, but cure must not be promised lightly. If the patient suffers from acute ENL, especially if this goes on to progressive reaction, the prognosis becomes more grave. No estimate of prognosis can be given until the patient has been treated for at least two years, possibly five years or even longer. In advanced lepromatous leprosy permanent sequelae—deformity, paralysis or paresis from nerve injury, damage to the eyes—may occur, though modern treatment can do much to prevent these.

In *infiltrated borderline leprosy* the prognosis should be guarded at first; there is a tendency to severe deformity after reactional borderline lesions; careful physiotherapy is needed, with avoidance of trauma, such as accidental burns. Moreover, this form may go on to lepromatous leprosy. This borderline group is particularly prone to lead to serious deformities and to relapse; the patients need careful attention.

With modern treatment, including drug treatment, surgery and physiotherapy, much deformity can be avoided or relieved, but treatment must be continued for a long time.

Relapse may occur, especially when full courses of treatment are not observed. Even after five years of treatment 11 of 98 lepromatous patients relapsed[61] and in Nigeria 6% of relapses were found in treated patients,[62] mostly with lepromatous or borderline disease. The commonest cause of relapse appeared to be insufficient treatment in conditions prone to relapse. High relapse rates were reported in patients who had received treatment regularly for periods considered in 1974 to be adequate: for example, a relapse rate of about 15% in those with BT leprosy who had been treated for at least five years, and one-third of the patients who had been treated for BL/LL leprosy for at least 10 years after inactivity relapsed.

Clinically, a relapse shows itself by the appearance of new skin lesions, erythematous papulonodules, and these are accompanied by the presence of morphologically normal leprosy bacilli in skin smears and sections from the lesions and in nasal mucus. These lesions should not be mistaken for those of ENL which are often tender and disappear in a few days. Only small numbers of granular bacilli are found in an ENL lesion. The subject of relapse in leprosy has been reviewed in the *British Medical Journal*.[63]

EPIDEMIOLOGY

The classical view is that leprosy is an infectious disease but that for infection to spread from one person to another there must be close and prolonged contact or challenge by large numbers of bacilli at one time, such as occurs within families or among close associates. On the other hand, many cases have been reported in which contact was apparently neither prolonged nor very intimate but in which repeated contact was a factor. Sexual contact has been suggested as the source of infection, not presumably via the sex organs but through the close physical contact involved. Cases have also been reported in which leprosy was transmitted apparently by blood transfusion and in the process of tattooing and possibly that of variolation.

The mycobacteria are present in large numbers in the nasal mucosa and skin of lepromatous patients and are presumably spread in discharges from open lesions; they may be airborne. Whether there is a hereditary factor, a genetically controlled susceptibility, as postulated in Uganda, is a subject of research with methods of genetic study now becoming available. The study of marriage patterns may help in this. This question of genetic constitution in relation to susceptibility is difficult; it is discussed at length in Spickett[64] and the view taken that of the various environmental factors thought to influence susceptibility, climate is not important and nor are hygiene, the standard of living or diet. Variation in the probability of contact with infectious patients does not provide a sufficient explanation for the distribution within populations or families. The evidence suggests that there must be some other factor and that this factor must be genetic. It would be strange if this were not so.

The attack rate for household contacts of lepromatous patients is six to eight times as high as for non-contacts, but the rate for contacts of tuberculoid patients is less than twice as high as for non-contacts. Nevertheless, it is probably true that most patients, whatever the form of leprosy they have, are infectious at some time or another to susceptible persons.

The lymphocyte transformation test was performed on household contacts of patients with leprosy and on medical attendants who had been working with leprosy patients in various parts of the world. It was found that more than 50% of contacts in both groups showed immunological evidence of exposure to leprosy and it concluded that a subclinical infection commonly follows exposure to *M. leprae*. A relatively low response in contacts of patients with active lepromatous leprosy suggested that 'super exposure' to *M. leprae* could result in a decrease in host resistance.[65]

A high rate of conjugal leprosy (106 spouses in 1830 couples, one of whom had leprosy—58 per 1000) has been reported[66] and somewhat higher rates have been reported elsewhere, but these may suggest an exaggerated estimate of true conjugal transmission, in that in some cases the infection was probably contracted before marriage. Nevertheless, conjugal infection has been substantiated, as in the case reported by the late Sir Philip Manson-Bahr, of leprosy in the wife of a patient who died of leprosy. She had never been out of England, but developed the disease after an incubation period of seven years.

Age is probably a factor and it has usually been considered that infants and children are more susceptible than adults. It was concluded from a study at Uzuakoli in eastern Nigeria,[36] that incidence of new infections increases with age for the first four decades. Nevertheless, there have been many reports indicating that adults are susceptible and that age is much less important than contact and the intimacy of contact. Children are likely to have more intimate contact with parents and other children than older persons have among themselves. Children have been known to infect their parents.

It has often been said that males are rather more susceptible than females but it seems to be more likely that the difference in incidence is due rather to the fact that males have more opportunities for contact than females in many communities. Where opportunities are equal, incidence is equal. But lepromatous leprosy does seem to be more common in males than in females (1.6 : 1).

Great variations have been recorded in the proportions of lepromatous and tuberculoid leprosy in different countries. Skinsnes[67] quotes 60.7% lepromatous in Brazil, 63.5% in Japan, 69.8% in the USSR, against only 21.2% in Papua New Guinea, 12% in India and 7% in Angola; these reports were made on several thousands of observed cases in each instance. Conversely, the tuberculoid or non-lepromatous percentages were high: 78.7% in Papua New Guinea, 88% in India and 47% (tuberculoid) and 46% (indeterminate) in Angola. Similarly, low or moderate rates were found in Brazil, Japan and the USSR.

These findings suggest a racial factor in resistance to leprosy but this may be the result of a long experience of the disease in the countries with low lepromatous rates and vice versa; that is, a matter of natural selection. The figures had not changed significantly 10 years later.[2]

Skinsnes distinguishes between the epidemic patterns of leprosy in fresh populations and in endemic foci (Table 40.4).

Table 40.4 Epidemic patterns of leprosy.

Fresh populations	Endemic foci
Rapid spread	Slow spread
In most houses of a village	In foci and families
Endemic of tuberculoid, few macules	More lepromatous (20–25%)
Adults and children almost equally susceptible	Mostly in young adults and children
Mostly no contact with lepromatous leprosy. Not prolonged intimate contact	Most patients have contact with lepromatous leprosy, often prolonged and intimate

A sense of proportion is necessary. Thousands of doctors and nurses have attended leprosy patients without becoming infected, though there have been some tragedies. Whatever the relative importance of constitution on the one hand and opportunity for infection on the other, it is true to say that leprosy flourishes most where life is lived in primitive conditions and where overcrowding exists—not necessarily in cities, but wherever people live and sleep in close intimate contact, as in village life. Poverty and diet may be factors but in spite of much speculation no clear evidence has been adduced that diet has any direct bearing on susceptibility to leprosy. It is interesting to note that in spite of the occasional introduction of leprosy patients into such countries as Britain and the USA, there is no indication that the disease has spread to the communities to which they entered. This is not to say that they do not infect close physical contacts.

CONTROL

For prevention Cochrane and Davey[61] suggest certain factors.
1 A well-informed and educated public opinion (including medical and paramedical personnel).
2 Reasonable measures for controlling infective persons to prevent infection of healthy persons.
3 Successful treatment.
4 A rise in the standard of living, resulting in reduction of overcrowding.

They make the points that the public should realize that leprosy is an infection not a hereditary disease to be controlled on that basis, and that control of infective persons must depend upon their willingness to accept restrictions, which should not be excessive—otherwise, as so often in schemes of compulsory segregation, the disease will be concealed. Case finding, which should include the regular examination of household contacts and of schoolchildren, is very important.

Persons suffering from bacilliferous leprosy should avoid skin-to-skin contact with others, particularly children, since pus from ulcerating succulent lesions or from skin, which is the seat of chronic diffuse lepra reaction, contains large numbers of bacilli.[68]

Treatment has not yet become available to most persons suffering from leprosy in remote areas and has not yet made a great impact on the prevalence of the disease, but with more extensive organization and more money it can become much more widespread. Prevention therefore depends upon knowledge of prevalence and this in turn depends upon deliberate surveys of whole populations, such as have been done in Africa and elsewhere. The layout and amenities of settlements for isolation of patients must obviously be attractive.

Where children are in close contact with infective parents or siblings the one obvious preventive measure is to treat the infective persons, but this is slow. The question whether to give healthy children prophylactic half doses of sulphones has been raised; this can be successful, as in an investigation in India. Prophylactic DDS is allowable if there is proper supervision. It has shown remarkable prophylactic effects in a long trial in a small, highly infected community in Micronesia[69] but is probably not suitable for this in the widely scattered African and Asian regions where infection is not so intense. The dose is 225 mg (in suspension) every 75 days. In a prophylactic campaign in Micronesia, after an initial cessation of new cases during the three-year campaign (1967–1970) there was a slow rise at a rate of two cases per 1000 population per year. A secondary wave of cases occurred since 1973 among children born after 1968, probably owing to relapsing multibacillary cases. A long-term control programme was suggested with DDS prophylaxis limited to contacts of multibacillary cases.[70] If dapsone is used as the prophylactic, the dosage ranges from 25 mg/week for children up to the age of four years, to 200 mg/week for contacts aged over 15 years. Regular doses of this sort, given to child contacts

of patients with leprosy, give a high degree of protection.

Immunization

Major field trials using BCG against leprosy have been carried out in Burma, Uganda, Papua New Guinea and India with contradictory results. Except for Uganda the results were disappointing for reasons probably connected with the number of lepromatous patients in each area.[71]

Leprosy vaccine

BCG plus killed armadillo derived *M. leprae* has been used for immunotherapy. With repeated vaccination every two to three months using BCG and *M. leprae* as a vaccine, histopathological reversion of LL to BL, BB and BT was obtained in 80% of BL and LL patients.[70] Organisms similar to *M. leprae* (*M. vaccae*) have also been used.

REFERENCES

1 Sansarricq, H. (1981) *Lepr. Rev.* Special Issue 15S–31S.
2 World Health Organization (1979) *Wkly epidem. Rep.* **3**, 17.
3 Ridley, D.S. (1967) *Trans. R. Soc. trop. Med. Hyg.* **61**, 596.
4 Rees, R.J.W. (1969) *Bull. Wld Hlth Org.* **40**, 785.
5 Draper, P. (1982) In *The Biology of the Mycobacteriae*, ed. C. Ratledge & J.L. Stanford, pp. 39–47. London: Academic Press.
6 Hunter, S.W. & Brennan, P.J. (1981) *Bacteriology* **147**, 728–735.
7 Waters, M.F.R. (1984) In *Recent Advances in Tropical Medicine*, ed. H.M. Gilles. Edinburgh: Churchill Livingstone.
8 Imaeda, T., Kirchheimer, W.F. & Barksdale, L. (1982) *J. Bact.* **150**, 414–417.
9 Rees, R.J.W. (1967) *Trans. R. Soc. trop. Med. Hyg.* **61**, 581.
10 Rees, R.J.W., Weddell, A.G., Palmer, A.G.M. et al (1969) *Br. med. J.* **iii**, 216.
11 Rees, R.J.W., Waters, M.F.R., Weddell, A.G.M. et al (1967) *Nature, Lond.* **215**, 599–602.
12 Kirchheimer, W.F., Storrs, E.E. & Binford, C.H. (1972) *Int. J. Lepr.* **40**, 229.
13 Waters, M.F.R., Bakri Bin, H.J., Isa, M.D. et al (1978) *Br. J. exp. Path.* **59**, 551.
14 Maugh, T.H. (1982) *Science, Washington* **215**, 1083–1086.
15 Godal, T., Lofgren, M. & Negassi, K. (1972) *Int. J. Lepr.* **40**, 243–250.
16 Pedley, J.C. (1973) *Lepr. Rev.* **44**, 33–35.
17 Davey, T.F. & Rees, R.J.W. (1974) *Lepr. Rev.* **45**, 121.
18 Rees, R.J.W. & Meade, T.W. (1974) *Lancet* **i**, 47–49.

19 Rees, R.J.W. & McDougall, A.C. (1976) *Int. J. Lepr.* **44**, 99.

20 Narayanan, E., Sreevatsa Raj, A.D., Kirchheimer, W.F. et al (1978) *Lepr. India* **50**, 26.

21 Geater, J.G. (1975) *Lepr. Rev.* **46**, 279.

22 Pedley, J.C. (1967) *Lepr. Rev.* **38**, 239–242.

23 Duncan, M.E., Melsom, R., Pearson, J.M.H. et al (1983) *Int. J. Lepr.* **51**, 7–17.

24 Ridley, D.S. & Jopling, W.H. (1966) *Int. J. Lepr.* **34**, 255.

25 Jopling, W.H. (1978) *Handbook of Leprosy*, 2nd edn. London: Heinemann.

26 Ridley, D.S. (1974) *Bull. Wld Hlth Org.* **51**, 451.

27 Turk, J.L. (1969) *Immunology in Clinical Practice.* London: Heinemann.

28 Eden, W., Van Vries, R.R.P., de Mehra, N.K. et al (1980) *J. inf. Dis.* **141**, 693–701.

29 Eden, W., Van Vries, R.R.P., de Marao, J.D. et al (1982) *Hum. Immun.* **4**, 343–350.

30 Narayanan, R.B., Bhutani, L.K., Sharma, A.K. et al (1983) *Clin. Exp. Immunol.* **51**, 421–430.

31 Haregewoin, A., Godal, R., Mustafa, A.S. et al (1983) *Nature, Lond.* **303**, 542–544.

32 Shepard, C.C., Walker, L.L., Landingham, R.M. van et al (1982) *Infect. Immun.* **38**, 673–680.

33 Harboe, M. (1982) *Int. J. Lepr.* **50**, 342–350.

34 Karat, A.B.A., Job, C.K. & Rao, P.S.S. (1971) *Br. med. J.* **i**, 307.

35 Turk, J.L. & Waters, M.F.R. (1968) *Lancet* **ii**, 436.

36 Browne, S.G. (1965) *Lepr. Rev.* **36**, 157.

37 Rea, T.H. & Levan, N.E. (1978) *Archs Derm.* **114**, 1023.

38 Rea, T.H. & Ridley, D.S. (1979) *Int. J. Lepr.* **47**, 161.

39 Brand, P. (1966) *Insensitive Feet: A Practical Handbook on Foot Problems in Leprosy.* The Leprosy Mission, London.

40 International Congress of Leprosy (1953) *Int. J. Lepr.* **21**, 484.

41 Jopling, W.H. (1979) *Lepr. Rev.* **50**, 271.

42 Ridley, D.S. (1969) *Lepr. Rev.* **40**, 77.

43 French, T.M. (1968) *Lepr. Rev.* **39**, 171.

44 Ellard, G.A., Gammon, P.T., Helmy, H.S. et al (1974) *Am. J. trop. Med. Hyg.* **23**, 464.

45 Pearson, J.M.H. (1981) *Int. J. Lepr.* **49**, 417–420.

46 Shepard, C.C., Tolentino, J.G. & McRae, W.H. (1968) *Am. J. trop. Med. Hyg.* **17**, 192.

47 Rees, R.J.W., Pearson, J.M.H. & Waters, M.F.R. (1970) *Br. med. J.* **i**, 89.

48 Joplin, W.H. & Pettit, J.H.S. (1979) *Int. J. Lepr.* **40**, 229.

49 Jacobson, R.R. & Hastings, R.C. (1976) *Lancet* **ii**, 1304.

50 Browne, S.G. (1966) *Lepr. Rev.* **37**, 141.

51 Yawalkar, S.J. & Vischer, W. (1979) *Lepr. Rev.* **50**, 135.

52 Jopling, W.H. (1976) *Lepr. Rev.* **47**, 1–3.

53 Warndorff-Van Diepen, J. (1982) *Int. J. Leprosy* **50**, 139–142.

54 Pattyn, S.R., Rollier, M.-T., Rollier, R. et al (1975) *Int. J. Lepr.* **43**, 356–363.

55 World Health Organization (1982) *Wld Hlth Org. tech. Rep. Ser.*, 675.

56 Goodwin, C.S. (1969) *Br. med. J.* **iii**, 174.

57 Carayan, A., Bourrel, P. & Languillon, J. (1964) *Surgery in Leprosy.* Paris: Masson.

58 Fritschi, E.P. (1971) *Reconstructive Surgery in Leprosy.* Bristol: John Wright.

59 McDowell, F. & Enna, C. (1974) *Surgical Rehabilitation in Leprosy and Other Peripheral Nerve Disorders.* Baltimore: Williams & Wilkins.

60 Jopling, W.H. (1969) *Lepr. Rev.* **40**, 175.

61 Cochrane, R.G. & Davey, T.F. (1964) *Leprosy in Theory and Practice.* Bristol: John Wright.

62 Browne, S.G. (1965) *Int. J. Lepr.* **33**, 267–273.

63 Leading article (1977) *British Medical Journal* **ii**, 914.

64 Spickett, O. K. (1964) In *Leprosy in Theory and Practice*, eds. R.C. Cochrane & T.F. Davey. Bristol: John Wright.

65 Godal, T. & Negassi, K. (1973) *Br. med. J.* **ii**, 557.

66 Mohamed Ali, P. (1965) *Int. J. Lepr.* **33**, 223.

67 Skinsnes, S. G. (1964) In *Leprosy in Theory and Practice*, eds. R.C. Cochrane & T.F. Davey. Bristol: John Wright.

68 Browne, S.G. (1967) *Trans. R. Soc. trop. Med. Hyg.* **61**, 265.

69 Sloan, N.R., Worth, R.M., Jano, B. et al (1971) *Lancet* **ii**, 525.

70 Russell, D.A., Worth, R.M., Jano, B. et al (1979) *Am. J. trop. Med. Hyg.* **28**, 559.

71 Nordeen, S.K. & Sansarricq, H. (1984) *Bull. Wld Hlth Org.* **62**, 1–6.

72 Convit, J., Aranzuzu, N., Ulrich, M. et al (1982) *Int. J. Lepr.* **50**, 415–424.

SECTION IX
POCK DISEASES

Chapter 41
Pock Diseases

ORTHOPOX VIRUSES

The orthopox viruses are DNA double strand viruses, brick- or ovoid-shaped, 200–250 nm in size, which are all antigenically related and contain the following members: camelpox, cowpox, ectromelia (mice), monkeypox, Turkmenia rodent pox, vaccinia, and variola. The only ones that infect man are variola (smallpox), vaccinia, monkeypox and cowpox. Tanapox is not an orthopox virus, but is a fairly close relation.

It now seems that the most important virus in this group, the variola virus which causes smallpox, has been eradicated[1] by the World Health Organization global vaccination programme. But the possibility of its resurgence remains, because virus may, under certain conditions, survive for many years outside the body. As the pool of susceptible people increases year by year, vaccination programmes now having been abandoned, some old blanket chest containing infective material may one day unleash this ancient scourge again. And there is always the possibility that laboratory-maintained variola might be used as an agent of germ warfare.

But these are hypothetical scenarios, and the world at present seems free of smallpox. For this reason, we shall not deal with the disease in this edition. But its close relative monkeypox, a disease of tropical Africa easily mistaken for smallpox, does deserve a place.

MONKEYPOX

GEOGRAPHICAL DISTRIBUTION (Fig. 41.1)

The disease is confined to Africa. Although monkeypox virus has been known since 1958 in captive monkeys, the first human case was recognized in 1970 in Zaire, since when there have been more than 200 reported cases, mainly in Zaire, but also in Liberia, Nigeria, Ivory Coast, Cameroon and Sierra Leone. It has seldom been reported outside the areas of tropical rain forest.

AETIOLOGY

Monkeypox is a brick-shaped orthopox virus 200–250 nm in size which forms cytoplasmic inclusions and is morphologically indistinguishable from variola. It can readily be distinguished in culture since the pocks on chick chorioallantoic membrane are slightly larger and more haemorrhagic than those of variola. Unlike variola, monkeypox virus is pathological to rabbits and has a higher temperature ceiling for growth. It grows readily on green monkey and

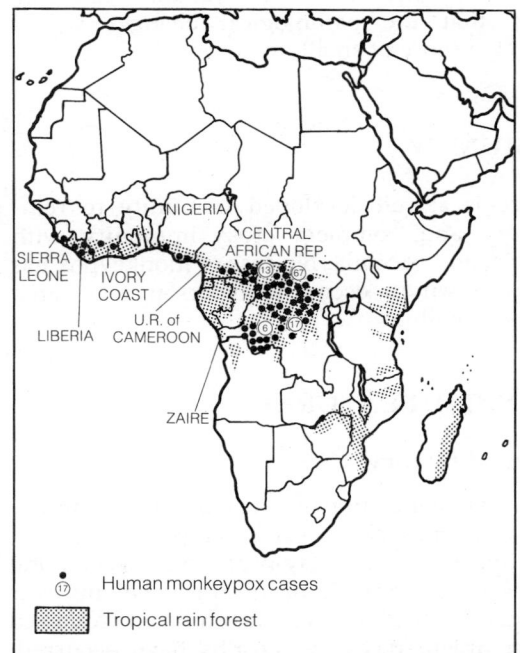

Fig. 41.1 Geographical distribution of human monkeypox showing number of cases reported from 1970 to 1 March 1984. (Courtesy World Health Organization.)

789

rodent cell cultures. Four strains of pox virus have been isolated from monkey kidney cells and rodents, which differ from monkeypox but are closely related to variola, from which they can only be distinguished by DNA analysis. These are known as 'white pox' viruses and their relation to human infection is unknown.

TRANSMISSION

The usual method of transmission from monkey to man is unknown, but infection is sometimes direct from handling dead monkeys for eating, or by droplet via the respiratory tract. Transmission by chimpanzee bite has recently been recorded.[2] The disease is not readily transmitted from man to man, but secondary cases have occurred. Little tertiary spread occurs and epidemic spread is not a feature.

PATHOLOGY

Few persons are known to have died from monkeypox and no post-mortems have been performed, so no information is available. It seems likely that the pathological changes would resemble those of smallpox.

IMMUNITY

There is a well-developed immunity to reinfection, and complete cross immunity with variola, and vaccinia. No case of monkeypox has been known to occur in a person vaccinated against smallpox.

CLINICAL FEATURES[3]

Natural history

Monkeypox infection of man is a dead-end infection which manifests itself as a typical smallpox-like illness with a 2-day prodromal period, and appearance of a smallpox-like rash evolving over 2–4 days. The illness is usually mild and followed by complete recovery. Deaths have occurred, mainly in children.

The *incubation period* is 5–17 days. In the cases described by Mutombo et al[2] it was 6 days.

Symptoms and signs

The onset is abrupt with fever and a prodromal period of illness of 2–3 days. On the third day a rash appears, a single crop of discrete papules more abundant on the face and extremities than on the trunk. The soles of the feet and palms of the hands are involved. The papules form pustules which become umbilicated and covered with crusts which separate after about 10 days, leaving small scars. Marked lymphadenopathy may occur (Fig. 41.2). Mild atypical cases occur in which there may be fewer than 10 lesions, separation of the crusts occurring by the fifth day. There appear to be no complications.

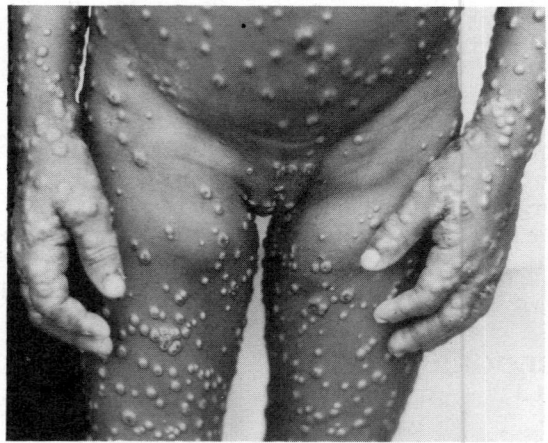

Fig. 41.2 Monkeypox showing characteristic inguinal and femoral adenopathy. (From Breman et al[3] with permission.)

DIAGNOSIS

The differential diagnosis from smallpox is based on the epidemiology and a history of contact with monkeys. Lymphadenopathy is an important distinguishing feature. Isolation of the virus and its cultural characteristics and antigenic structure[4] provide definitive diagnosis.

TREATMENT

Treatment is symptomatic and supportive.

EPIDEMIOLOGY

It is not known whether the primary maintenance hosts are chimpanzees, other primates or smaller mammals. Most patients give a clear account of contact with monkeys which they have caught and eaten. Most cases occur during the dry season. Children are affected more than adults. The attack rate is 10% in susceptibles in close contact with the primary case, in contrast to smallpox where it is 20%. Secondary spread among families occurs but tertiary spread is rare and epidemics are not a feature. When the level of vaccination in the community falls, monkeypox in man may become much commoner.

TANAPOX

GEOGRAPHICAL DISTRIBUTION

Tanapox was first described by Downie et al[5] who reported epidemics in 1957 and 1962 from the lower Tana river in Kenya.

Human infections have since been found in the forest area of Zaire. A closely related virus has been isolated from outbreaks in primate colonies in the USA and in contact cases in man. Serological surveys have shown continuing transmission along the lower Tana river.[6,7]

AETIOLOGY

Tanapox virus is not an orthopox virus, but with the yaba pox virus of monkeys forms a distinct subgroup of pox viruses. It does not grow on chick chorioallantoic membrane, but grows well on green monkey kidney cell and Vero cell cultures.

TRANSMISSION

Epidemiological features suggest that the virus is transmitted from monkeys to man by mosquitoes, since outbreaks in man have occurred in low lying country near the Tana river after floods had isolated wild animals, people and their domestic animals on islands in the flood water, on which *Mansonia uniformis* and *M. africanus* had proliferated in immense numbers. There is no evidence of direct spread from person to person.

PATHOLOGY[5]

Pathology is limited to the epidermis where the pock forms. There are few or no destructive changes. Hypertrophied epidermal cells containing acidophilic inclusion bodies are predominant. Cellular infiltration is slight and the dermis escapes.

IMMUNITY

Nothing is known about second attacks. Antibodies which develop in infected persons and monkeys persist for some years. There is no cross immunity with vaccinia and recently vaccinated people can develop the disease.

NATURAL HISTORY

The infection is usually mild: fever heralds the appearance of one or two pock-like lesions followed by complete recovery.

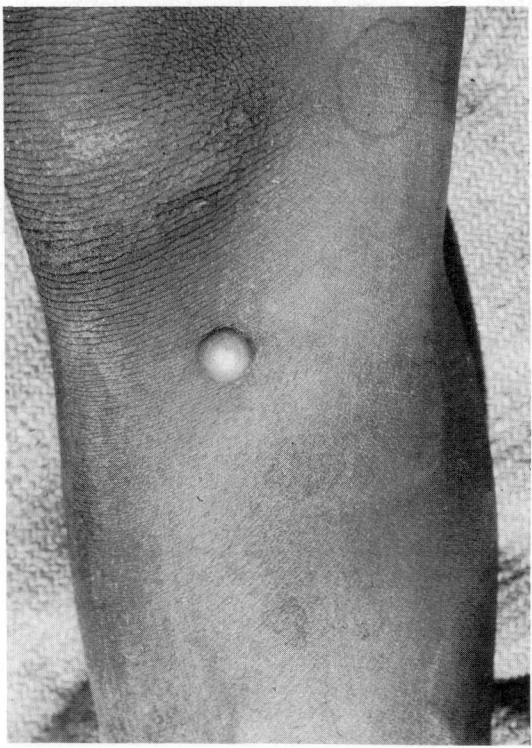

Fig. 41.3 Tanapox. Solid pock containing firm cheesy material.

SYMPTOMS AND SIGNS

The incubation period is unknown. The onset is abrupt with fever lasting 3–4 days and in some cases severe headache and prostration (the severity is open to doubt since histories were taken retrospectively a long time after the event in the major study published (Downie et al[5]). During the fever one or two (but never more) pock-like lesions appear on the skin resembling those of smallpox. Lesions become umbilicated but never proceed to pustule formation, forming firm cheesy contents instead (Fig. 41.3). The pocks occur mainly on the exposed surfaces of the body, the upper arms, face, neck and trunk, but never on the hands, legs or feet. Recovery follows rapidly, no scars are left and there are no complications.

DIAGNOSIS

Tanapox has to be distinguished from modified smallpox in a vaccinated person. The character of the pock which at first looks like smallpox differs in its larger size, firm, solid nature and absence of pustulation. Electron microscopic appearances are similar to those of smallpox. Virus can be isolated by culture in green monkey kidney cells or Vero cell cultures, and clearly distinguished by antigenic structure from orthopox viruses. Serum antibodies develop only slowly but complement fixation and neutralizing tests on both human and monkey sera show antibody at low titre which persist for some years, and so can be used for retrospective diagnosis.

TREATMENT

No treatment is necessary.

EPIDEMIOLOGY

The epidemiology is not well known. The primary maintenance hosts are unknown, but many monkeys especially vervet (*Cercopithecus aethiops*) are susceptible and are common in the endemic area. Small outbreaks occur after flooding but transmission was still continuing along the lower Tana river as shown by serological surveys[6,7] in 1971 and 1976, showing infection had persisted since 1962. Antibodies were found in 9.2% of the population and in children between the ages of two and 12. There is no evidence of any direct person-to-person transmission.

REFERENCES

1 Henderson, D.A. (1975) *J. clin. Path.* **28**, 843.
2 Mutombo, M.W., Arita, I. & Jezek, Z. (1983) *Lancet* **ii**, 735–737.
3 Breman, J.G., Kalisa-Ruti, Steniowski, M.V. et al (1980) *Bull. Wld Hlth Org.* **58**, 849–868.
4 Gispen, R. (1975) *Trans. R. Soc. trop. Med. Hyg.* **69**, 299.
5 Downie, A.W., Taylor-Robinson, C.H., Caunt, A.E. et al (1971) *Br. med. J.* **i**, 363.
6 Manson-Bahr, P.E.C. & Downie, A.W. (1973) *Br. med. J.* **ii**, 151.
7 Axford, J.S. & Downie, A.W. (1979) *J. Hyg., Camb;* **83**, 273.

SECTION X
RABIES AND SLOW VIRUSES

Chapter 42
Rabies and Slow Viruses

RABIES

GEOGRAPHICAL DISTRIBUTION

Rabies is enzootic in most areas of the world. Rabies-free areas include the UK, Scandinavia (except Denmark), west Malaysia, Taiwan, Japan, Australasia and the Pacific Islands. Animal rabies is distributed much more widely than human disease. Rabies is a true zoonosis. It cannot be maintained in a human population without help from other animals.

AETIOLOGY

Rabies is an RNA virus of the rhabdovirus group, one of the genus of antigenically related lyssaviruses. The virus is bullet-shaped (Fig. 42.1), 180×75 nm in size, consisting of a helical single-stranded protein nucleocapsid, surrounded by a protein matrix and an envelope bearing single spikes of glycoprotein. It is readily inactivated by sunlight, ultraviolet radiation, drying and heating, especially at a pH outside the range 5–10, by lipid solvents and by a variety of antiseptics. It is relatively resistant to phenol. Virus isolated from naturally infected animals is known as 'street virus' or 'field virus'. Repeated intracerebral passage in rabbits produces 'fixed virus' which has a relatively constant incubation period, shortened from 9–15 to 5–6 days, and with reduced pathogenicity for many non-human species. Many antigenically distinct strains of rabies virus have been identified, using monoclonal antibodies raised against nucleocapsid and glycoprotein antigens. Rabies virus can be cultivated in embryonated bird eggs and on human diploid cell cultures.

Rabies-related viruses[1,2]

Six rabies-related viruses have been isolated in Africa, all serologically related to, but distinguishable from, classical rabies virus, only two

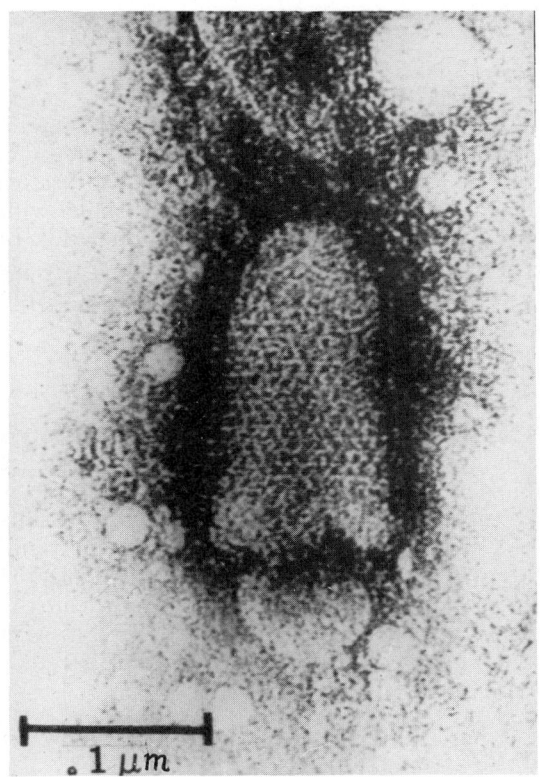

Fig. 42.1 The rabies virus shown on an electron micrograph.

of which have been associated with human infection.

Lagos bat virus: isolated from fruit-eating bats in Nigeria, the Central African Republic and Natal (South Africa).

Nigerian horse virus: isolated from a horse in Nigeria which died of 'staggers'.

Obodhiang virus: isolated from *Mansonia uniformis* mosquitoes in the Sudan.

Kotonkan virus: isolated from *Culicoides* midges in Nigeria.

Mokola virus: isolated from shrews in Nigeria and Cameroon, and from two children in

795

Nigeria with encephalomyelitis and aseptic meningitis.

Duvenhage virus: isolated from a man with a rabies-like illness following a bite from an insectivorous bat in South Africa.

Strains of rodent variants of rabies virus have been isolated in Europe from *Apodemus flavicollis, Clethrionomys glareolus* and *Microtus arvalis* but there is no evidence to link these isolations with rabies in foxes, the principal reservoir of rabies in Europe.

TRANSMISSION

Rabies virus can penetrate broken skin and intact mucosa. Routes of transmission may be saliva inoculated by a bite, the contact of saliva with a pre-existing wound or scratch, inhalation of aerosol, inoculation of the conjunctiva, or via tissue transplant from an infected cadaver as in corneal transplantation.

Animal bite

By far the commonest method of transmission is by the inoculation of virus-laden saliva from the bite of a rabid animal. Most human rabies is transmitted by the domestic dog, but in Trinidad, Central and South America, the main transmitter is the vampire bat *Desmodus rotundus*; the bats are not diseased and virus persists in the saliva for long periods. Insectivorous bats can also be infected and have been found in Yugoslavia, Germany and Turkey.

Aerosol

Inhalation of rabies virus may be an important method of transmission among cave-dwelling bats which excrete virus in the urine. Visitors to the caves and laboratory workers exposed to airborne infection from infected animals may acquire infection in this way.

Ingestion

Animals can become infected from eating infected meat but there is no well-documented case of man being infected in this way.

Transplacental

Transplacental transmission of rabies has been reported in natural infections of dogs, bats and a cow but infants appear to survive rabid mothers and a rabid mother gave birth at 38 weeks to an infant who remained well thereafter.[3]

Person-to-person

Although, theoretically, nursing staff and medical attendants could be infected from rabies-infected saliva, respiratory excretions and the urine of rabies patients, no such cases have been documented. Nevertheless, it is prudent to nurse rabies patients with barrier precautions, including the use of goggles, and to have all attendants vaccinated against rabies when possible.

Tissue grafts

Human-to-human transmission has occurred via corneal grafts from donors who have died from undiagnosed neurological disease[4,5] and this danger must be recognized in endemic areas.

PATHOLOGY

Virus multiplies locally at the site of inoculation, and after a period of days or weeks enters the peripheral nerves and travels up the axons to the dorsal root ganglia where further multiplication takes place. From here it spreads into the central nervous system, where it escapes the humoral defences of the host if these exist. In the central nervous system virus multiplies in neurons and glial cells and is transmitted from cell to cell. The virus then spreads outwards via the axons of the peripheral nerves to many tissues including skeletal and cardiac muscle, adrenal medulla, kidney, cornea and nerves in hair follicles. Most important to transmission is the spread of virus to the salivary glands, where it escapes from the acini by a process of budding,[6] the lacrimal glands, taste buds and the respiratory tract. Virus may also be shed in milk and urine. Viraemia is not significant.

Changes on microscopy

Changes are most marked in the midbrain and medulla in 'furious' rabies, and in the spinal cord in paralytic rabies. The presence of Negri bodies is characteristic of rabies. Negri bodies are intracytoplasmic inclusion bodies 24–27 μm in diameter, composed of an acidophilic matrix within which are smaller basophilic inner bodies 0.2 to 0.5 µm in size arranged in rosette fashion (Fig. 42.2). They are found mainly in Ammon's horn and in the cerebellar Purkinje cells. They can be demonstrated best by Seller's or Mann's stains, or by direct fluorescence microscopy using a fluorescein-conjugated antirabies serum. Negri bodies contain altered virus particles.

lies between 20 and 90 days. It tends to be shorter after proximal bites, after severe bites, and after bites from wild animals.

There are prodromal symptoms of fever and headache in most cases, followed by signs of encephalitis or paralysis which progress inexorably to a fatal conclusion. Recovery has been claimed after heroic attempts at life support[7] but even in the most sophisticated centres, death is

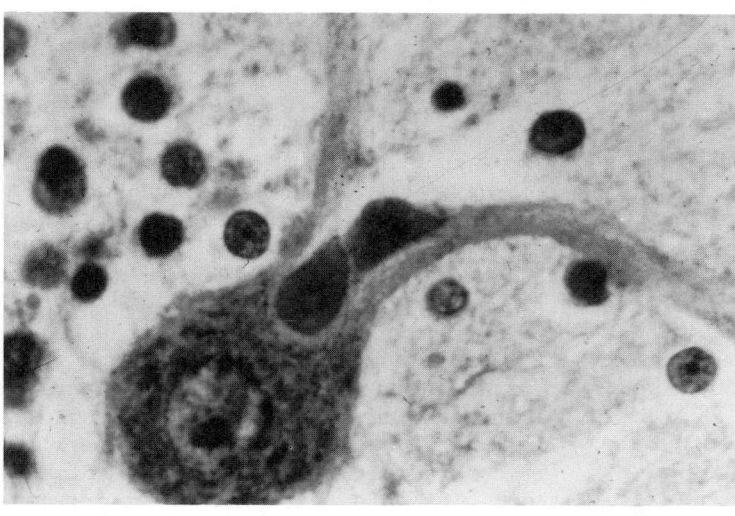

Fig. 42.2 Rabies. Typical appearance of Negri bodies in a neuron. (Courtesy WTIM.)

Neuronolysis is seen in foci of degenerate neurons associated with leukocytic infiltration and gliosis forming distinctive patterns known as 'Babès' nodes'. Other organs are infected and there is focal degeneration in the salivary gland, pancreas, adrenal medulla and lymph glands. An interstitial myocarditis with round cell infiltration is found in about one-quarter of the cases.

IMMUNITY

No immune response can be detected until after symptoms develop. Neutralizing and fluorescent antibodies can be detected in the blood after 7 days of illness, and a little later in the cerebrospinal fluid. Interferon production has been detected.

CLINICAL FEATURES

The incubation period varies in man from 4 days to two years or more, but in over 90% of cases

virtually invariable once the first symptom has appeared.

There are two main types of clinical picture, 'furious' and 'dumb'. In furious rabies symptoms are those of overaction of the central nervous system and in dumb rabies inhibition or paralysis is the outstanding feature.

Symptoms and signs

The first symptoms are fever, anxiety, malaise, headaches, photophobia, and myalgia. The mood changes towards irritability and depression and there is often marked anxiety. A characteristic symptom in paraesthesiae or pain at the site of the original bite.

Rabies is usually of the 'furious' type in man. The most characteristic symptom is spasm of the muscles of deglutition often precipitated by an attempt to swallow, from which the disease gets its name 'hydrophobia'. Spasmodic contractions of the muscles may spread to the respiratory and other muscles leading to attacks of apnoea.

Hydrophobia

Spasms of the muscles of deglutition are accompanied by obvious pain and extreme distress, and the anticipation of swallowing, such as when the patient is offered food or drink, often precipitates a reaction of terror. Spasms may also be stimulated by air playing on the face which gives rise to the expression 'aerophobia'. Almost any other tactile, visual or auditory sensation may in extreme cases precipitate spasms, as may even the mention of water or drinking. Spasms often spread to involve the respiratory muscles, and spasms of the neck and back muscles resemble a momentary convulsion. These responses are believed to be due to destruction of the brain stem inhibitory systems.[8]

Death usually occurs 5–10 days after the onset of symptoms, and is often preceded by paralysis of varying extent. Symptoms of autonomic dysfunction include excessive lacrimation (the saliva is copious and often ropy, and the patient spits), excessive sweating, derangement of temperature control, and the development of diabetes insipidus. Cranial nerves III, VI, VII, IX, X, XI and XII may be involved. Systems outside the central nervous system are seldom clinically involved, although myocarditis has been reported.[9]

Paralytic rabies

In man this form is less common than furious rabies, and occurs normally in only about 20% of cases; it is the usual form in bat rabies. After the usual prodromal symptoms the patient develops an acute progressive ascending myelitis, symmetrical or asymmetrical, with flaccid paralysis, root pain, and fasciculation in the affected muscles with mild sensory disturbance. A complete paraplegia develops eventually with fatal paralysis of the respiratory and pharyngeal muscles. Death may be delayed for up to four weeks after the onset of symptoms, and in the absence of spasms the diagnosis is often only made at post-mortem examination.

Haematemesis from stress ulcers has been reported in rabies.

DIAGNOSIS

In most endemic areas specific diagnosis cannot be made before death, and diagnosis has to be clinical. Specific diagnosis can be made in a proportion (perhaps 20% of cases) before death by the identification of virus in corneal impression smears using the fluorescent antibody technique.[1] The differential diagnosis in furious rabies includes tetanus and hysterical reactions in people who are afraid of rabies. In the paralytic form of rabies, virus encephalitis of various sorts, poliomyelitis, the Guillain–Barré syndrome may be difficult to distinguish.

Serodiagnosis is not of much practical help, because antibodies often fail to appear before death. Antibodies can be detected in blood and cerebrospinal fluid from the eighth day of illness, and high titres of antibody in the cerebrospinal fluid suggest a diagnosis of rabies rather than post-vaccinal encephalitis when an illness develops in the post-exposure period in a patient who is being vaccinated. The specificity of the antibodies is doubtful in areas where rabies-related virus infections occur.

Post-mortem diagnosis is made by the finding of Negri bodies and the typical encephalomyelitis, although gross changes may be minimal. The most rapid and sensitive diagnostic method is the fluorescent antibody test, in which tissue is examined under the fluorescence microscope after treatment with fluorescein-conjugated antirabies serum, but this is only possible if fresh, unfixed tissue is available. Diagnosis can be confirmed in properly equipped laboratories by animal inoculation.

TREATMENT

The clinician will have to decide for himself whether active treatment is justifiable, or whether relief of symptoms only should be the aim. In endemic areas the alternatives do not usually present, because the high technology demands of prolonged intensive life support are insuperable in most developing countries. Only three reasonably well-documented cases of recovery following rabies attack are reported in the world literature[7] and there have been many reports of failure despite heroic attempts at life support. Further, severe changes in the central nervous system after prolonged life support have been reported, making it difficult to believe that recovery in such cases could have occurred, no matter what was done.

If symptomatic treatment alone is to be carried out, the aim should be relief of spasms and suffering by continuous narcosis. A combination of chlorpromazine, diamorphine and barbiturate is invariably effective in producing narcosis and analgesia.

Despite the fact that person-to-person transmission of rabies has not been reported, patients should be barrier nursed and staff should in addition to protective clothing and gloves, be provided with goggles, as patients may spit.

Post-exposure treatment

This is treatment given after exposure to infection, but before symptoms have developed. It should be given as soon as possible after exposure. The objective of this form of treatment is firstly to inactive virus at the site of inoculation by proper wound toilet, and secondly to produce effective antirabies antibody levels as quickly as possible.

Suspect animals should if possible be kept under observation. If an animal is alive 10 days after attack, then it is believed that it could not have been excreting rabies virus at the time of the attack. Most cases of prolonged excretion of rabies virus by asymptomatic dogs have been shown to involve a virus of reduced pathogenicity, only capable of producing rabies if directly inoculated intracerebrally.

Suspect animals should not normally be killed, but if natural death occurs during the 10 days of observation, the animal's brain should be examined for rabies virus, preferably using the fluorescent antibody test. If this is not possible fixed brain can be examined for Negri bodies in the usual way.

Local treatment

The wound should be thoroughly washed with soap and water or a quaternary ammonium compound such as benzalkonium. The two agents should not be used together as they inactivate each other.

After cleansing the wound can be treated with tincture of iodine or iodine solution. If suturing is necessary it should be delayed. Experiments have shown that local treatment alone is capable of preventing many cases of rabies after inoculation of virus, even if immunotherapy is not given.

Hyperimmune serum

This is given if there is a delay between exposure to rabies and vaccination, or if there is reason to believe that the incubation period will be unusually short. The dose is 40 units/kg for immune serum of animal origin, or 20 units/kg if human immune rabies serum is used. If there is a gross wound it is usual to infiltrate the wound with half the dose, and give the remainder by deep intramuscular injection. If there is no obvious site for infiltration, the whole dose is given intramuscularly. Simultaneous administration of vaccine and immune serum does *not* neutralize the active immunizing effect *provided* they are injected into different limbs.

Rabies vaccine: post-exposure regimens

The most effective vaccine is human diploid cell vaccine (HDCV). It is apparently free of the risk of producing central nervous system complications. The manufacturer's recommendation is to give 1 ml reconstituted freeze-dried vaccine subcutaneously or intramuscularly on days 0, 3, 7, 14, 30 and 90. It has, however, recently been shown in Thailand that, doses of 0.1 ml intradermally produce equally satisfactory protection. A total of four doses (0, 3, 7, 14) appears to be completely effective and reconstituted vaccine was stored for up to 7 days in the refrigerator without apparent loss of potency.[10] A single session at which 0.2 ml is injected intradermally into one site or 0.1 ml into two sites on each limb may prove to be just as effective.

The main disadvantage of HDCV is its cost, currently about £18 sterling per 1 ml dose. Its use as recommended by the makers is totally impracticable in most developing countries on grounds of cost. The use of the 0.1 ml × 4 regimen reduces the cost to less than £10, surely a low price for a human life.

Reactions with HDCV are extremely rare, and usually confined to slight swelling, redness and itching at the site of inoculation. If the intradermal route is used, increased effectiveness of the vaccine depends on its delivery to the local lymph glands via the lymphatics; hence the extreme importance of making sure that the injection is given strictly intradermally and not subcutaneously. In pale-skinned people the accuracy of the intradermal injection can be checked by the pink coloration of the skin, as the vaccine contains an indicator dye.

In Third World countries where expense is a major consideration, Semple vaccine is still used in a dose of 2 ml daily for 14 days with two booster doses after a further 10 and 20 days.

Pre-exposure immunization

The arrival of HDCV means that pre-exposure immunization is possible, and is appropriate for adults and children who will live in high risk areas and those who visit these areas where post-exposure treatment is not possible. The intradermal route is quite satisfactory; 0.1 ml is given intradermally on days 0, 7, and 28. Failures of this regimen may be associated with the concomitant administration of chloroquine.

EPIDEMIOLOGY

Although the main transmitter of rabies to man is the domestic dog, in many parts of the world the infection is maintained as an epizootic in wild life. In the USA and Canada foxes, skunks and rodents; in the Caribbean bats; and in Europe the fox is the main vector and reservoir of the virus, which since the Second World War has spread from Austria to the English Channel.

CONTROL

Quarantine of all imported animals for six months on arriving in a rabies-free country is mandatory. Dogs must be immunized annually. Attempts are being made with some success to immunize foxes with oral vaccine on bait.

SLOW VIRUS INFECTION

Subacute and chronic progressive degenerative diseases of the central nervous system in man and animals caused by viruses fall into two groups. The first group is caused by conventional viruses but with long incubation periods and includes subacute sclerosing panencephalitis (measles, see Chapter 6), chronic focal virus encephalitis and progressive multifocal leukoencephalopathy (polyoma virus). The second group, the spongiform encephalopathies are caused by atypical viruses, which include two diseases of man, Kuru and Creutzfeldt–Jakob disease (a form of presenile dementia), and two diseases of animals, scrapie and mink encephalopathy. All the diseases in this second group have incubation periods extending to years and, unlike the first group, produce no detectable immunological response.[11]

Kuru

GEOGRAPHICAL DISTRIBUTION

Kuru is found only in the Fore tribe in a small area of the eastern highlands of Papua New Guinea.

AETIOLOGY

It is now well established that kuru is transmissible to a variety of animals including subhuman primates.[11] The agent responsible has not been identified but it does not behave like a conventional virus and is resistant to many procedures which destroy common viruses. It is closely associated with the plasma membrane of brain cells and is inactivated by membrane disrupting procedures.[12]

TRANSMISSION

Transmission is direct and was related to the practice of cannibalism formerly widespread in the Fore region but which has now died out. It seems that kuru is acquired from the consumption of the brains of persons who have died from the disease.[13]

PATHOLOGY[14]

The cerebellum is primarily involved. Degenerative changes occur in the vermis and its connections where there is marked degeneration of the neurons and loss of Purkinje cells, the axons becoming ballooned (torpedo cells). The cytoplasm of cells becomes basophilic and vacuolated and the Nissl substance is reduced. The areas where the cells have disappeared are occupied by astroglial and microglial cells but neuronophagia is minimal. A distinctive feature is the development of amyloid plaques (kuru plaques). Perivascular cuffing is occasionally present. The changes are found in the cerebellar cortex, dentate nucleus, thalamus, corpus striatum, globus pallidus and focal areas in the cerebral cortex, giving rise to the spongiform appearance. The spinocerebellar and lateral corticospinal tracts are also affected. Electron microscopy studies show changes in the plasma membrane of cells leading to proliferation and the formation of intracytoplasmic vacuoles.[12]

CLINICAL FEATURES

Natural history

The disease has an insidious onset and there is gradual progression involving the cerebellum and adjacent structures. Death after three months to two years is inevitable (average six to nine months).

The *incubation period* is 10–20 years. The youngest known patient with kuru was five years old.

Symptoms and signs

The onset is insidious, usually with ataxia. As the ataxia progresses a fine tremor appears involving the head, trunk and limbs which is exaggerated by fatigue but subsides during sleep. Choreiform and athetoid movements occur when the patient tries to stand up. There are pronounced emotional changes and easily provoked inordinate laughter. Later there is a progressive convergent strabismus, a flexed posture and Parkinsonism. The course of the disease is inexorably progressive with death in three months to two years. In the terminal stages patients are mute and doubly incontinent and die from inanition or intercurrent infection. The rest of the nervous system is unaffected, the pyramidal tract is not involved and the cerebrospinal fluid is unchanged.

TREATMENT

There is no effective treatment.

EPIDEMIOLOGY

Kuru is principally a disease of the Fore-speaking peoples and occurs in a strictly limited area south of Mount Michael in the eastern highlands of Papua New Guinea.[15] Although confined mainly to the Fore people about 20% of kuru deaths each year occurred in people of other linguistic groups[16] and the disease has occurred in a few women who entered the area from outside. When first described the disease affected children of either sex and young adult females and adult males were only rarely affected. But there has been a progressive rise in adult male deaths each year since 1957. Since 1957 there has been a rapid decline in the disease until now there are hardly any cases to be found.

Cannibalism, formerly practised in the area, in which the brains of dead people were eaten, was abandoned in the 1950s. If kuru was transmitted by cannibalism then the generation born since its cessation would not be affected and this has come about. Although kuru was confined to the Fore tribe, cannibalism was widely practised in other tribes who escaped the horrid consequences of kuru. But perhaps we all owe our existence to a kuru-like disease that extinguished our Neanderthal competitors, whose 'skull nests' suggest a taste for brains.

CONTROL

Cessation of the cultural habit of consuming the brains of the dead has resulted in complete elimination of the disease.

Motor neuron disease

Chronic degenerative neurological diseases have been found in various parts of the world in well-defined foci connected with isolated homogeneous population groups. These diseases are amyotrophic lateral sclerosis (ALS), Parkinsonian dementia (PD) and hereditary cerebellar ataxia which probably bears no relation to ALS or PD.

GEOGRAPHICAL DISTRIBUTION

Foci of ALS and PD have been identified[17] among:

1 the Chamorro people of Guam, Rota and Tinian in the Marianas in Micronesia;
2 Japanese in two villages on the Kii peninsula on Honshu;
3 New Guineans of the Auyu and Jakai cultural groups in southern West New Guinea.

Other similar conditions have been found in Australian Aborigines in Arnhem Land, Filippino immigrants to Hawaii and the Yakut people in Siberia.

AETIOLOGY

Several causes have been suggested, toxic and infective.

Toxic

Originally it was suggested that in the Chamorros on Guam, ALS and PD were caused by intoxication with *cycasin,* a cyanogenic glucoside present in food prepared from the cycad nut. Another suggestion was poisoning from heavy metals found in the central nervous system, but this was probably secondary.

Infective

Infection with a slow virus is strongly suggested by epidemiological studies[17] and a transmissible agent has been identified in the Yakut people of Siberia, but studies over a long period have failed to show in ALS and PD an agent which can be transmitted to primates.[18]

TRANSMISSION

The method of transmission is unknown.

PATHOLOGY

The pathology of ALS is similar to that found elsewhere with loss of anterior horn cells and loss of voluntary muscle tissue over the whole body. In the PD syndrome there is cortical and pallidal atrophy and depigmentation of the substantia nigra with widespread ganglion cell degeneration without inflammatory changes. These changes are widespread throughout the frontal and temporal lobes and tegmenta of the brain stem.

CLINICAL FEATURES

In ALS there is rapid wasting of all the muscles with fibrillation and eventual paralysis leading to dysphagia and respiratory failure with death from secondary infection. In the PD syndrome the mean age of onset is 50 and death occurs after three to five years. The onset is rapid with Parkinsonism and dementia.

EPIDEMIOLOGY

Extensive studies have been undertaken to find whether genetic or environmental factors were the most important. In the Marianas where there has been a considerable movement of populations it was found that the incidence of ALS and PD varied in the various groups and that environment or the 'place' where they lived was most important.[19] If Guam males outnumber females 4 to 1 and nearly 10% of the Chamorro population is affected by ALS and 7% die from PD.

REFERENCES

1 World Health Organization (1973) Expert committee on rabies. *Wld Hlth Org. tech. Rep. Ser.,* 523.
2 Crick, J. & Brown, F. (1976) *Trans. R. Soc. trop. Med. Hyg.* **70**, 196.
3 Caffrey, K. (1983) *Postgrad. Doc. Africa* **5**, 230.
4 Shouff, S.A., Burton, R.C., Wilson, R.W. et al (1979) *New Engl. J. Med.* **300**, 603–604,
5 Anon (1980) *Morbid. Mortal. Weekly Rep.* **29**, 25–26.
6 Macrae, A.D. (1969) *Lancet* **ii**, 1415.
7 Hattwick, M.A.W., Weis, T.T., Stechschulte, C.J. et al (1972) *Ann. intern. Med.* **76**, 931.
8 Warrell, D.A. (1976) *Trans. R. Soc. trop. Med. Hyg.* **70**, 188.
9 Cheetham, H.D., Hart, J., Coghill, N.F. et al (1970) *Lancet* **i**, 921.
10 Warrell, M.J., Warrell, D.A., Suntharasmai, P. et al (1983) *Lancet* **ii**, 301–304.
11 Gajdusek, D.C. (1977) *Science* **197**, 943–960.
12 Beck, E., Daniel, P.M., Davey, A.J. et al (1982) *Brain* **105**, 755–786.
13 Mathews, J.D., Glasse, R.M. & Lindebaum, S. (1968) *Lancet* **ii**, 448.
14 Beck, E., Bak, I.J., Christ, J.F. et al (1975) *Brain* **98**, 595–612.
15 Zigas, V. & Gajdusek, D.C. (1957) *Med. J. Aust.* **2**, 21.

16 Hornabrook, R.W. & Moir, D.J. (1970) *Lancet* **ii**, 1175.

17 Gajdusek, D.C. (1982) In *Human Motor Neuron Disease,* ed. L.P. Rowland, pp. 363–392. New York: Raven Press.

18 Gibbs, J.G. & Gajdusek, D.C. (1982) In *Human Motor Neuron Disease,* ed. L.P. Rowland, pp. 343–353. New York: Raven Press.

19 Yanagihara, R.T., Garruto, R. M. & Gajdusek, D. C. et al (1983) *Ann. Neurol.* **13**, 79–86.

SECTION XI
DISEASES OF THE ENVIRONMENT

Chapter 43
Disorders Due to Heat

We make no apology for the fact that this chapter differs little from that in the last edition. The reason is simple: nobody has made any significant discovery in this area since 1972.

Body temperature fluctuates only slightly in healthy people so long as they are reasonably protected against extremes of environmental heat or cold and consume suitable amounts of food and water. Body temperature depends upon the following factors.

1 Heat created by the metabolic processes of the body acting upon food and fluid ingested.

2 Physical activity which can quickly raise the metabolic rate, and therefore body temperature, but only moderately in health.

3 Heat absorbed by the body from the environment, which may be:

(a) radiant heat from hot objects (e.g. in engine rooms),

(b) convected heat from the air (e.g. in deserts). Conducted heat from actual contact with hot objects is rarely significant.

4 Heat lost from the body via:

(a) the lungs;

(b) the skin, partly by dissipation due to vasodilatation in the skin, which entails vasoconstriction of the splanchnic vessels, and partly (more important) through evaporation of sweat from the skin surface.

Evaporation of sweat is the main defence against heat stress and sweat is apparently produced solely to provide water for evaporative cooling.

Sweat can be absorbed by the keratinaceous layers of the skin, which may swell and block the sweat ducts, reducing the amount of sweat and causing the condition of miliaria.

The control of heat exchange is governed by complex physiological mechanisms, ultimately from a centre situated in the hypothalamus, which also controls water balance and vasomotor and humoral activities aimed at maintaining the temperature level. The heat-regulating centre comprises two distinct subcentres, one for dissipation of heat (cutaneous vasodilatation and sweating) and one for heat conservation (cutaneous vasoconstriction and shivering). The mechanisms activating these centres are not precisely known.[1]

In hot conditions the heat lost by evaporation of moisture from the lungs and from the surface of the body (as insensible perspiration or actual sweat) is greater than in cool conditions, but evaporation depends not only on external heat, but also on humidity. Skin exposed to hot dry wind remains dry because of the intense evaporation, though the actual production of sweat is very great; body temperature is therefore reduced in proportion. Skin covered from such wind remains wet because sweat is continually produced and evaporation is prevented. Skin exposed to even moderate heat in conditions of high humidity remains wet because evaporation is slow; body temperature is therefore less effectively reduced.

In all cases fluid is lost in sweat much more quickly in hot conditions than in cool, and therefore the secretion of urine is reduced unless the intake of fluid is increased. Fluid balance is therefore a primary factor in heat regulation. With fluid loss in sweat there is loss of salt, and salt depletion is another important factor in heat balance.

The hormone system is involved, and in dehydration through excessive sweating, an antidiuretic hormone is released from the pituitary. This hormone acts by reducing the output of urine through reabsorption of water in the renal tubules and thus conserving body fluid. The production of aldosterone and possibly other adrenocortical substances is also increased, resulting in reduction of salt loss in sweat.

Acclimatization

There is definite evidence that people can become to some degree acclimatized to heat, so that body temperatures and pulse rates do not rise as high in experienced persons, whose sweating mechanism becomes more efficient,[2] as in people unaccustomed to heat. There is also evidence that, especially in older subjects, heavy work in the heat produces fatigue of the sweat glands during the work session, with consequent rise in body temperature and increased strain on the cardiovascular system.

For young healthy adults, for example men in the armed forces, acclimatization, either natural or artificial, has been shown to reduce greatly the incidence of heat illness. In the gold mines in South Africa, acclimatization chambers in which graded work is performed at raised temperatures have proved very effective in achieving the same effect.

HEAT STRESS AND HEAT STRAIN

Heat stress is defined as the total load of heat which must be dissipated if the body is to remain in heat balance. There are five components of four main features.

1 The metabolic rate of the subject, which varies with physical activity, body build and constitution.
2 Air temperature:
   (*a*) dry bulb;
   (*b*) wet bulb.
3 Air movement.
4 Radiant temperature (black globe reading).

Various indices based upon these factors have been devised, of which the corrected effective temperature scale is perhaps the most well known. The details of these should be studied by doctors working in ships, mines and other places where heat stress is great; descriptions and references are available in the works of Leithead,[3] Leithead and Lind[1] and Edholm.[2]

Heat strain is defined as the physiological or pathological displacement resulting from heat stress; it includes sweating, raised heart rate and body temperature, dehydration, syncope, and other disorders discussed below.[3] The important factors are sweat loss, heart rate, deep body temperature, acclimatization, age, body build, physical fitness and clothing. Increasing age (because of the cardiovascular strain) and obesity are detrimental. Some of these factors can easily be measured—the heart rate, for instance, indicates the demands imposed by work and heat load on the circulatory system.[4] A continuously rising rectal temperature can easily be measured and is a serious danger signal. Intercurrent infectious disease adds to this risk. Sweating can be assessed clinically. A dry skin, indicating absence of sweating (except where sweat is evaporated at once in hot dry air), is easily noted and is a sign of serious heat effect in a person with a high pulse rate and rectal temperature. A sweat rate of 1 litre/hour in a desert environment may achieve thermal equilibrium even with heavy work, without rise in body temperature or cardiovascular strain, but in a humid climate it could be accompanied by great strain if only 0.5 litre/hour evaporated and the rest was deposited on clothing, or dripped off the body.

The normal adult intake of water in food and drink, in a moderate climate, is about 2.5 litres daily; the loss of water is about 1.5 litres in urine and 1 litre in sweat, faeces and expired air. Similarly, the normal intake of sodium chloride is about 10 g, most of which is excreted in urine and a small amount in sweat. When a man is suddenly exposed to severe heat the salt content of sweat is initially high, up to 4 g/litre. But if severe sweating continues, maximal reabsorption of sodium and chloride from the renal tubules may be enough to maintain balance, and the salt content of the sweat may fall to as little as 1 g/litre. The speed at which this mechanism of salt conservation develops is important, and salt-depletion heat exhaustion is mostly observed in newcomers to heat.

When sweating is heavy—over 5 litres in 8 hours of work—however, the intake of salt, as well as that of water, should be increased. Excess salt can be harmful and the use of salt tablets is not recommended unless salt loss is exceptionally high.

HEAT DISORDERS

The pathological conditions resulting from failure to maintain heat balance are of three types.[1]

1 Disorders resulting from the processes of heat regulation:

   (*a*) Circulatory instability:
      Heat syncope
   (*b*) Water and electrolyte imbalance:
      Heat oedema
      Water-depletion heat exhaustion
      Salt-depletion heat exhaustion
      Heat cramps
   (*c*) Skin changes:
      Prickly heat
      Anhidrotic heat exhaustion

2 Disorders resulting from failure of heat regulation:

  (*a*) Heatstroke
  (*b*) Heat hyperpyrexia

3 Disorders resulting from apathy, fatigue etc.:

  (*a*) Chronic tropical fatigue
  (*b*) Acute heat fatigue

The conditions in group 3 are discussed by Pepler in Leithead and Lind[1] under the heading of psychological effects of heat, and may not be attributable solely to heat. The various factors are shown in Fig. 43.1.

down. The patient may recover quickly or may be shaken by the experience and need a period of rest and quiet before complete recovery.

Other causes of loss of consciousness must be excluded; such an attack may be the prelude to more serious disorders due to heat. The patient should be taken to lie down in cool surroundings are given drinks if necessary.

Heat oedema

This affects the feet and usually occurs within 10 days of first experience of hot climates; it disappears with acclimatization. The patho-

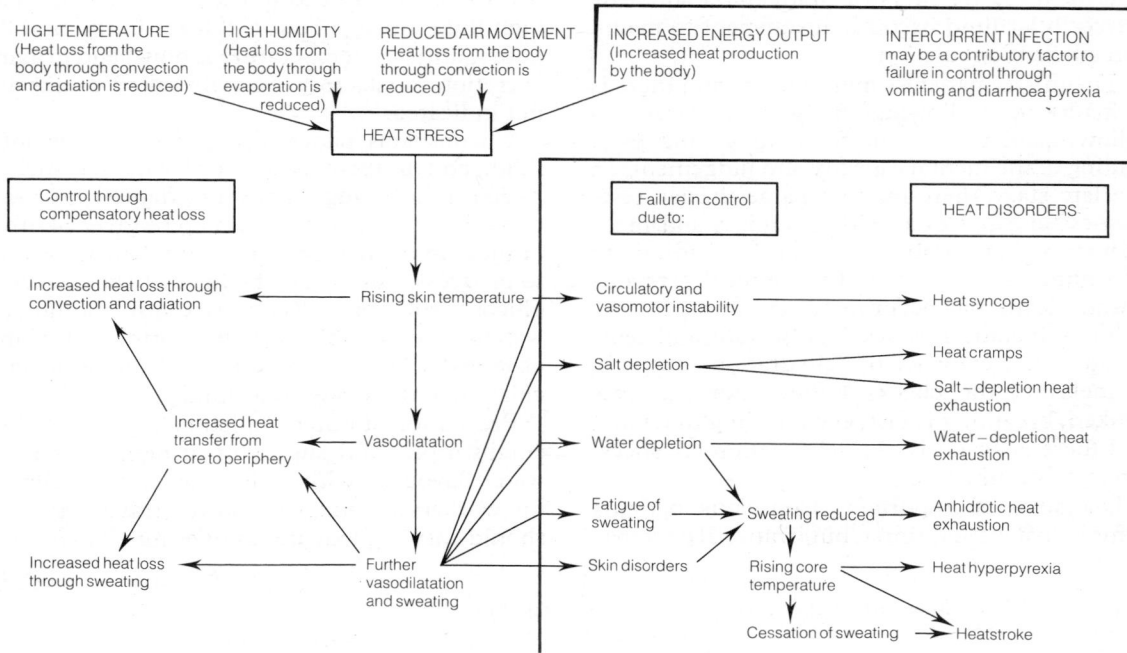

Fig. 43.1 Heat stress and heat disorders.

Heat syncope

This is a fainting attack due to collapse in vasomotor tone leading to cerebral anoxia, in the absence of water depletion or salt depletion. It is more common in hot humid conditions than in hot dry conditions.

The patient becomes pale, with slow pulse and slow, sighing breathing; consciousness is usually lost for a few minutes, but returns as the cerebral circulation is restored when the patient lies

genesis is uncertain. The swelling is usually slight and is partially relieved by a night's rest. A short period of rest is usually enough to end the condition.

Water-depletion heat exhaustion

This is due to loss of fluid by sweating and insufficient intake of fluid to replace it; an accessory factor may be loss of fluid by vomiting or diarrhoea. The commonest factor is an inadequate supply of water to labourers or troops. It should be remembered that a man doing heavy work in severe heat (say 43°C) can lose more than 1 litre of sweat/hour, and if working in the sun or in a boiler room, or if marching, for 8 hours a day, can lose up to 10 litres of sweat.

The patient becomes thirsty and the secretion of urine is much reduced. The extracellular fluid is reduced and water moves from the cells themselves into the extracellular fluid. If this process is severe, reabsorption of sodium from the renal tubules is increased, although the plasma sodium is already high and this further induces water to move from the intracellular fluid to the extracellular fluid, including the plasma. Potassium excretion, however, continues. Eventually, in spite of these transfers of fluid, the amount of extracellular fluid becomes insufficient to maintain efficient circulation.

The thirsty patient's mouth is dry and there is difficulty in swallowing. Fatigue and weakness follow, with a sense of foreboding, and even dulling of the mental capacity and judgement. In the late stage there may be paraesthesiae restlessness and hysteria, with giddiness and incoordination of limb movements, leading to delirium, coma and death. In extreme desert conditions death may occur in 12–48 hours.

Signs include increased pulse rate and temperature and evidence of dehydration—the skin is inelastic, the cheeks hollow and the eyes sunken; breathing is fast, even leading to tetany, and there is cyanosis. As dehydration advances, sweating diminishes.

Diagnosis is important. Conscious patients complain of intense thirst, but irrational or comatose patients cannot do so. There is little urine and its specific gravity is high; unlike the urine in salt-depletion heat exhaustion, it contains measurable quantities of sodium chloride. The patient may be anuric.

It is obviously important to decide whether the heat exhaustion is due mainly to water depletion or to salt depletion (see p. 811) and the sodium content of plasma is significant in this respect. Sweat being hypotonic, more water is lost than salt, but if the patient has drunk some water without salt, more salt may have been lost than water. The distinguishing features of the two conditions are set out in Table 43.1 (from Leithead and Lind).[1]

Treatment of water-depletion heat exhaustion consists of rest in bed in cool surroundings and high fluid intake, about 6–8 litres in the first 24 hours, until the temperature is down and urinary excretion satisfactory. Heavily salted drinks are not indicated.

Unconscious patients may need intravenous fluid, and if there is a doubt whether such a patient is suffering from water depletion or salt depletion, isotonic saline should be given, 4 litres or more in the first 24 hours, and then according to progress. Otherwise the fluid of choice is 5% glucose solution. Plasma sodium should be watched if possible and the output of urine observed. There is a risk of overloading the circulation with intravenous fluid.

Prevention of water-depletion heat exhaustion entails a plentiful supply of drinking water, or water flavoured with fruit juice, easily available for workers in the heat and for travellers, who should ensure adequate supplies for all journeys.

Table 43.1 Differential diagnosis of heat exhaustion.

	Predominant salt depletion	Predominant water depletion
Duration of symptoms	3–5 days	Often much shorter
Thirst	Not prominent	Prominent
Fatigue	Prominent	Less prominent
Giddiness	Prominent	Less prominent
Muscle cramps	In most cases	Absent
Vomiting	In most cases	Usually absent
Thermal sweating	Probably unchanged	Diminished
Haemoconcentration	Early and marked	Slight until late
Urine chloride	Negligible amounts	Normal amounts
Urine concentration	Moderate	Pronounced
Plasma sodium	Below average	Above average
Mode of death	Oligaemic shock	High osmotic pressure; oligaemic shock; heatstroke

Salt-depletion heat exhaustion

The average daily diet of Europeans contains about 10 g of salt and about as much is excreted daily, but in hot conditions sweating increases the loss of salt, even though sweat is hypotonic. This applies especially to newcomers.

The deficit of sodium is more important than the deficit in chloride. The extracellular fluid contains most of the sodium; when sodium is lost in sweat the osmolarity of the extracellular fluid is reduced and some of that fluid passes into the cells. Less water than usual is reabsorbed from the renal tubules and there is therefore an increase in urine, with secondary depletion of water, and further reduction of extracellular fluid. In cases with marked symptoms plasma sodium and chloride are clearly reduced, and both are virtually absent from urine and sweat.

Plasma volume is reduced and haemoconcentration therefore occurs, with high blood urea; this may be a factor in the tendency to nausea and vomiting.

The clinical features are fatigue, giddiness, anorexia, nausea, vomiting and muscle cramps. Fatigue is very marked; the patient is too desperately weary to give an account of his condition. Anorexia, diarrhoea and vomiting reduce the already inadequate intake of salt, establishing a vicious circle. Muscle cramps are common and very painful. Thirst is not a feature, but becomes prominent in progressive water depletion. The body temperature is usually normal and the condition does not predispose to heat stroke.

The sodium chloride content of urine is negligible and this, together with the other symptoms, helps in diagnosis. In the absence of laboratory facilities for estimating sodium and chloride the Fantus test on urine is simple and useful.

Fantus test for chlorides in urine.[1] To 10 drops of clear centrifuged urine in a clean test-tube add one drop of 20% potassium chromate solution as an indicator. Then add 2.9% silver nitrate solution drop by drop, shaking well after each drop, until the colour changes from yellow to the brick red of silver chromate. This is the point at which the silver has combined with all the chloride and is therefore available to combine with the chromate. The number of drops of the silver nitrate solution required to produce the endpoint colour-change is the concentration of chloride in the urine, expressed as grams of sodium chloride per litre. If the colour change occurs with the first drop of silver nitrate it means that for practical purposes there is no chloride in the urine. The silver nitrate should be kept in a coloured bottle in the dark and each reagent should be tested from time to time against distilled water. The normal sodium chloride value is 9 (3–15) g/litre of urine and in the presence of the appropriate history and clinical features a level of 1–3 g/litre warrants a diagnosis of salt-depletion heat exhaustion.

Treatment involves rest in bed in cool conditions and plenty of salt in the form of salted drinks. One teaspoonful of salt should be added to 0.5 litre of cool fruit drink (7 g/litre) and salty foods such as soup, beef tea and tomato juice should be encouraged, salt being added liberally to all appropriate food. The daily intake of salt in predisposing surroundings should be 20 g and this should be weighed out each day; discipline is needed to ensure adequate intake.

For comatose patients isotonic saline may be given intravenously in doses of 2–4 litres during 12–24 hours. Pulse rates and blood pressures should be watched and the volume, chloride content and specific gravity of the urine measured and recorded. The neck veins and lung bases must be examined for signs of overloading of the circulation and cardiac failure.

Prevention entails the provision of salt for fluids and food, especially for people working in severe heat such as in engine rooms, and especially for people not acclimatized.

Heat cramps

These painful cramps are probably due to water intoxication or salt depletion and occur in people who are sweating heavily and are at the same time drinking large amounts of unsalted fluids.[1] The cramps may be mild or quite severe, with the affected muscles contracted into stony hard lumps. They usually last less than one minute, occasionally for 2 or 3, but they may recur every few minutes for several hours.

For severe cramps intravenous normal saline (0.5–1 litre) can be given, or even a small quantity of 5% (hypertonic) saline. This should be followed by liberal salt taken by mouth until the urine contains 2–3 g of chloride/litre.

Prevention entails the provision of salted drinks at the place of work; men differ in their need for extra salt.

Skin changes

Prickly heat (miliaria rubra)

This common condition is due to prolonged wetting of the skin by sweat, and is found in those parts of the skin in which evaporation is poor, for instance where the skin is covered and chafed by clothing and there is friction. A high concentration of salt in sweat, possibly due to adrenocortical hypofunction or fatigue, may be a factor; bathing in sea water is thought to aggravate the condition.[5]

The essential lesion is obstruction of the sweat ducts by plugs of keratin debris, and distension of the ducts by retained sweat. There is round cell infiltration round the ducts. In skin persistently wet with sweat the epidermis tends to become oedematous and liable to infection; injury may also play a part.

The rash consists of many small red papules, going on to vesicles, on a mildly erythematous skin, chiefly in the bends of the elbows and knees, over the sternum, round the waist and in the axillae. In severe cases most of the trunk is involved, but not the palms or soles. The rash is accompanied by a prickling or tingling sensation which comes on in waves and which may be so irritating as to interfere seriously with sleep and therefore with general health. The rash may go on to pustule formation or eczema.

The best treatment is to remove the patient to a cooler climate. Otherwise the condition may be relieved by avoiding sweating, by wearing light, airy, loose clothing or remaining as naked as possible and by careful drying of the skin when wet by water or sweat.

Mildly astringent lotions, such as mercuric chloride (1 in 2000 in 95% alcohol), are useful. Another lotion[6] is:

Arachis oil	5.0%
Adeps lanae	2.2%
Lanette wax	6.7%
Salicylic acid	2.0%
Glycerin	6.7%
Tragacanth mucilage	25.0%
Water to	100.0%

Mercuric chloride or hexachlorophane can be added to this. Hexachlorophane soap, or a lotion or cream containing neomycin, helps to avoid infection.

Prickling can be relieved by a cool shower, thorough drying of the skin and the application of calamine lotion or zinc oxide powder. Oral promethazine (Phenergan) relieves it.

For prevention, measures to avoid sweating are obviously desirable and excessive use of soap (especially alkaline soap) is to be avoided. Hindson[7] advises ascorbic acid, 15 mg/kg daily, for children subject to prickly heat.

Anhidrotic heat exhaustion

This affects people exposed for several months to heat and is characterized by numerous discrete vesicles (miliaria profunda, mammillaria) in the skin, mainly of the trunk and proximal parts of the limbs, and by diminished or absent sweating (anhidrosis) in the area of the rash.[1] It was described in troops in the Second World War, but not much since then.

The skin is relatively dry because there is obstruction to the delivery of sweat to the surface, caused by keratin plugs deep in the epidermis. The condition may evolve from prickly heat. The pathogenesis is disputed; there may be a factor of unexplained failure of the renal tubules to respond to antidiuretic hormone and a defect in the secretion of aldosterone.

The patient is unduly fatigued, with headache and a feeling of uncomfortable warmth at first in the heat of the day, but later throughout the day but worst during exercise. The skin is dry, hot and tense (except the palms, which may sweat) and there is dizziness, nausea, tachycardia and hyperpnoea. Some patients pass more urine than usual because loss of fluid by sweating is reduced. The rectal temperature may be raised to 38.9°C.

The miliaria rash consists of discrete pale elevations like those of gooseflesh and is present everywhere except on the palms and soles, perineum, groins and axillae.

Treatment involves cool surroundings, 10% salicyclic acid in 70% alcohol may be applied to the anhidrotic area, followed after desquamation by inunction of lanolin cream.

Heatstroke and heat hyperpyrexia

In heatstroke the patient is usually unconscious, with or without convulsions, there is no sweating and the body temperature is very high. In heat hyperpyrexia the patient is conscious and may be sweating; the body temperature is not so high as in heatstroke.

The factors are heat, humidity, physical activity and lack of acclimatization. Except in industry these conditions are most common in infancy and in old age, when degenerative cardiovascular disease is a factor. In desert climates the failure of mothers to provide for their infants adequate fluid to compensate the great losses due to sweat is very important. In older people excessive food or alcohol is probably deleterious. Administration of atropine, for instance as a prelude to operation, can be dangerous by inhibiting sweating. Infections such as malaria and other fevers increase the risk of heatstroke.

The sweat mechanism may become fatigued, and anhidrotic heat exhaustion and severe water depletion (with some reduction of sweat) predispose to heatstroke, as does that rare condition in which sweat glands are defective or absent. Clothing is also a factor.

Pathology

The basic change is widespread cellular damage of vital organs, as a result of high body temperature.[8]

At post-mortem there may be cyanosis and ecchymoses. The meninges and brain are oedematous, with petechial haemorrhages (except in the cerebral cortex and hypothalamus). Haemorrhages are also common in serous cavities, heart, kidneys, adrenals, liver and gastrointestinal mucosa. The blood coagulation mechanism is affected, prothrombin and fibrinogen levels fall and platelet counts are below normal, with raised urinary Fibrin degredation products indicating DIC. The organs are congested. The kidneys are damaged, with hyperaemia and petechial haemorrhages, and the urine is scanty and turbid, with protein and abundant casts. Intravascular clotting may lead to renal insufficiency.[9] There may be acute renal failure. Liver damage is one of the most prominent features, with raised serum bilirubin, iron and SGOT, SGPT, lactic dehydrogenase (LDH) and creatine phosphokinase, and reduction in prothrombin and fibrinogen already mentioned. SGOT, SGPT and LDH are not raised in acute infections without heatstroke.

Polymorphonuclear leukocytosis (10 000–30 000) is usual in severe cases.

Clinical findings

The onset of heatstroke may be acute, relatively acute or insidious.

The acute onset is the most common, occurring without warning. The relatively acute onset if preceded by prodromal symptoms lasting minutes or hours. The insidious form is preceded by prodromal symptoms lasting several days, but this is not common.

The prodromal symptoms may include headache, confusion, disorientation, stupor, emotional outbursts, faintness, dizziness, anorexia, locomotor disturbances, excessive thirst and polyuria.[8]

Typically, the patient is in coma, with a temperature of 40.6°C or more, and there may be involuntary movements closely resembling epilepsy, with tonic and clonic convulsions and incontinence of urine and faeces. It has often been said that the skin is hot and dry and this may be so, but if the patient has been engaged in strenuous physical exercise in the heat, he may be sweating freely though suffering from heatstroke. This indicates that the thermoregulatory mechanism has been overloaded, rather than that it has broken down.[8]

The eyes are fixed and the pupils do not react to light; the conjunctiva is injected and the corneal reflex is lost. The face is cyanosed or blotched and there may be petechiae on the head, neck and arms. Watery diarrhoea and vomiting (both with blood) are common and tend to a state of dehydration. Hyperpnoea is also common and may lead to tetany. The pulse is fast and in severe cases the blood pressure is low (systolic below 90) indicating a state of shock, which is a bad sign; peripheral circulatory failure sometimes occurs. The myocardium may be damaged.

The patient may die before or during treatment or the response to cooling may be only temporary, or may be complete. Delay of more than 4 hours in beginning active cooling, or ineffective cooling, may mean that the patient fails to respond; if he does recover, he may have a residual neurological disability such as paresis of a limb. Shock, jaundice, oliguria, pulmonary oedema and myocardial infarction are sometimes present and there may be acute adrenal insufficiency.

In differential diagnosis the most important disease is *Plasmodium falciparum* malaria, for which appropriate treatment is urgently needed. Other fevers, such as meningitis and arbovirus infections, and nervous affections, such as tetanus and cerebral (pontine) haemorrhage, can lead to difficulty. It is important to examine the skull and surrounding parts for signs of injury;

patients may have been aggressive or have injured themselves during convulsions or at the onset of coma.

Treatment

Heatstroke is a medical emergency requiring prompt treatment. Rapid cooling is paramount. In the field the patient should be placed in the shade, all clothing removed and the skin kept wet and fanned. In the hospital the patient must be cooled efficiently and immediately by a combination of convection and evaporation. He is placed on a slatted bed which exposes as much of his skin as possible to the air and he is subjected to a fine spray of cold water in good air movement, by an electric fan if possible. The room should preferably be air-cooled or at least made as cool as possible by other means. Alternatively, the patient can be placed in a bath of water and ice, or cold water alone, and his body and limbs should be massaged vigorously to promote good circulation. However, these measures may cause vasoconstriction of the blood vessels of the skin, impeding heat loss, and the patient may struggle. Evaporative cooling is preferable. The patient should be suspended over a cooling bath and sprayed with atomized tap water;[10] warm dry air should be blown over the body at the same time. This avoids severe skin vasoconstriction.

These measures can reduce body temperature to 38.9°C within 20–60 minutes and it is extremely important to stop cooling at this temperature, otherwise it may fall to subnormal levels and shock may occur.

These facilities (ice and electric fans) should be available in hospitals where heatstroke is to be expected. If not available, the patient can be cooled by sponging in cold water or by wrapping him in a wet sheet and fanning him. The room should not only be cool but should be large so that it does not become humid.

Cooling is effective but drugs may be useful; for instance, chlorpromazine as a sedative. For shock oxygen is valuable if there is cyanosis or pulmonary oedema; intravenous 5% dextrose in saline is used for water or salt depletion or prolonged coma, though with care to avoid overloading the circulation. Disseminated intravascular coagulation (DIC) has been successfully treated with heparin,[11] but fresh plasma provides a safer alternative.

Pressor agents such as noradrenaline or meta-raminol (Aramine) can be at least temporarily beneficial in hypotensive patients. These should not be given until the patient has been cooled, because they produce vasoconstriction which could interfere with heat loss.

The most serious complication arising during treatment is bleeding. Low molecular weight dextran 500 ml should be given in the first 3 hours to prevent sludging of platelets.[12] Death from aspiration pneumonia may be avoided by keeping the airway clear and nursing in the semi-lateral position.[12]

If treatment is not given, heatstroke is fatal and even in treated patients mortality is high (20–50%). In heat hyperpyrexia (in which the patient is conscious) treatment reduces mortality to about 5%.

Sequelae include persistent headache, difficulty in concentrating, personality changes and neurological damage of various kinds.

Epidemiology

Heatstroke occurs particularly during heat waves in temperate countries when the elderly, those with heart disease and alcoholics are equally susceptible;[13] also during the Mecca pilgrimage during the summer months[14] and in unacclimatized young men taking part in athletic pursuits or unaccustomed physical work.[15]

Prevention

Prevention of the ill-effects of heat entails, for doctors working in mines, ships and other places where the risk occurs, knowledge of the techniques for measuring the various environmental factors—heat, humidity and air movement to assess the corrected effective temperature—and the factors relating to people at work or rest in those conditions. These techniques require more information than can be given here, and the reader is referred to Leithead and Lind,[1] World Health Organization[4] and other standard works on the physiology of people under heat stress. An essential is to have a prepared centre where effective cooling treatment can be given at once, without delay, to any patient in need.

In three valuable papers Ellis[16] reviews the epidemiology and pathogenesis of heat illness and discusses acclimatization.

REFERENCES

1 Leithead, C.S. & Lind, A.R. (1964) *Heat Stress and Heat Disorders*. London: Cassell.
2 Edholm, O.G. (1969) *J.R. Coll. Physns London* **4**, 27.
3 Leithead, C.S. (1967) *Trans. R. Soc. trop. Med. Hyg.* **61**, 739.
4 World Health Organization (1969) *Wld Hlth Org. tech. Rep. Ser.*, 412.
5 *British Medical Journal* (1964) **ii**, 772,
6 Wardle, E.N. (1966) *Br. med. J.* **ii**, 221.
7 Hindson, T.C. (1968) *Lancet* **i**, 1347.
8 *Lancet* (1968) **ii**, 31.
9 Haanen, C. (1968) *Lancet* **ii**, 400.
10 Weiner, J.S. & Khogali, M. (1979) *Lancet* **i**, 1135.
11 Weber, M.B. & Blakely, J.A. (1969) *Lancet* **i**, 1190.
12 Khogali, M., Mustafa, M.K.E. & Gumaa, K. (1982) *Lancet* **ii**, 1225.
13 Kilbourne, M.E., Choi, K., Jones, S. et al (1982) *J. Am. med. Ass.* **247**, 3332–3336.
14 Khogali, M. & Weiner, J.S. (1980) *Lancet* **ii**, 276–278.
15 Sutton, J.R. (1979) *Med. J. Aust.* **ii**, 463–464.
16 Ellis, F.P. (1976) *Trans. R. Soc. trop. Med. Hyg.* **70**, 402, 412, 419.

Chapter 44
Lymphatic Siderosilicosis (Endemic Non-filarial Elephantiasis)

GEOGRAPHICAL DISTRIBUTION

Lymphatic siderosilicosis is found in widely separated areas: Kenya and Ethiopia,[1] Ruanda, Uganda,[2] West Africa,[3] Ecuador and India.

AETIOLOGY

Careful epidemiological and pathological studies have shown that the cause is an obstructive lymphopathy of the peripheral lymphatics resulting from aluminosilicate and silicon absorbed through the skin of the feet in areas where the rocks are rich in colloidal iron, alumina and silicon, and is a 'geochemical disease'.[4]

TRANSMISSION

The condition is contracted through the skin of the feet by walking in these areas without shoes.

PATHOLOGY

The main changes[5] are found in the femoral nodes, the skin of the feet and the connecting lymph channels. In the lymph nodes groups of macrophages are found in the mid-zone containing small spherical or rod-shaped birefringent particles in a disorganized PAS-positive cytoplasm and in the early cases granulomas. Changes in the lymph vessels are most marked distally and below the knees. The vessels are dilated, with failure of the valve mechanisms, and contain a reflux of lymphocytes. Later, hypertrophy and multiplication of the endothelial cells fill the lumen and a progressive fibrosis replaces the vessel with a fibrous strand. The site of lymph blockage is in the peripheral lymphatics. The skin of the foot shows lymphatic cuffing of the sweat ducts with small granulomas, birefringent particles and positive iron-staining ferric crystals.

CLINICAL FEATURES

The disease begins commonly in youth and starts at the toes proceeding proximally. Progress is insidious or episodic with acute episodes of swelling. It very rarely extends beyond the knee. It starts unilaterally but spreads to the other leg after a varying period of time so that it is asymmetrical. The femoral lymph nodes are enlarged and often tender. A variety of clinical forms are found, varying between two extremes: the soft 'water bag' type where the swelling is largely fluid and easily reduced by compression, and the hard type characterized by a massive fibrotic thickening of the skin, not responding to compression. In the latter type the hyperkeratoses and verrucosities limited to the slipper area has led to a mistaken diagnosis of 'mossy foot' or mycetoma (Fig. 44.1).

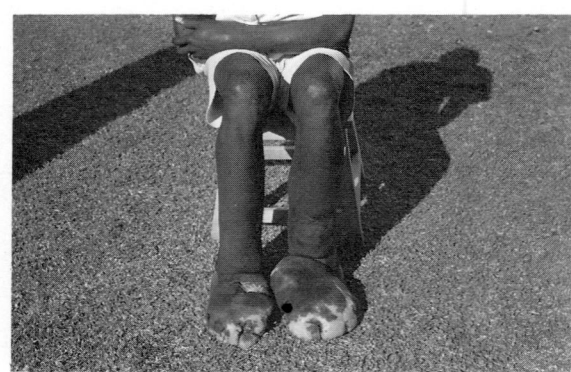

Fig. 44.1 Lymphatic siderosilicosis (endemic non-filarial elephantiasis).

DIAGNOSIS

The main differential diagnosis is from filarial lymphoedema. Filariasis occurs in low-lying areas in contrast to lymphatic siderosilicosis which is most often found in highland areas where filariasis does not occur. In filariasis there are other signs of filariasis—oedema of the scrotum and hydrocele—which are not found in lymphatic siderosilicosis. Lymphangiography shows marked hypoplasia of the lymphatic channels below the knees in contrast to the dilated channels, with back-flow characteristic of filariasis. In mycetoma chronic fungal infections may discharge through sinuses and the bones may be affected.

TREATMENT

Treatment is disappointing, but reduction of the swelling can be obtained with intermittent positive pressure using FLOWTRON apparatus as in elephantiasis (Chapter 20, p. 366); however, permanent support must be maintained.

EPIDEMIOLOGY

The distribution is related to the distribution of red soil derived from volcanic rocks, particularly basalt,[4] usually in highland areas but also in river delta systems which drain such areas. The condition occurs during the second decade of life in both sexes in people who do not wear shoes.

PREVENTION

The wearing of shoes from childhood will prevent the condition.

REFERENCES

1 Cohen, L.L. (1961) *E. Afr. med. J.* **37**, 53.
2 Loewenthal, L.J.A. (1934) *Ann. trop. Med. Parasit.* **28**, 47.
3 Manuwa, S.L.A. (1935) *Trans. R. Soc. trop. Med. Hyg.* **62**, 715.
4 Price, E.W. (1976) *Trans. R. Soc. trop. Med. Hyg.* **70**, 288.
5 Price, E.W. (1975) *Trans. R. Soc. trop. Med. Hyg.* **69**, 177.

SECTION XII
NUTRITIONAL DISEASES

Chapter 45
Nutritional Deficiency Syndromes

NUTRITIONAL REQUIREMENTS IN THE TROPICS

The energy requirement for an adult man of 25 years working an 8 hour day is estimated at 3200 calories (13 000 kJ) per 24 hours in the temperate countries. The effect of a hot climate on these requirements is not more than a 10–20% decrease at the most.

It has been estimated that some villagers consume only 2,040 calories (8,500 kJ) per day and are permanently hungry.

Pregnancy and breastfeeding increase the energy requirement and a baby during the first six months at the breast will require an extra 600 calories (2500 kJ) each day in the mother's food intake. Growing children require extra, so that pregnant women and nursing mothers, as well as growing children, are the most vulnerable to food deficiencies. This is shown by the average lower weight of children from underdeveloped countries as compared with well-fed children from the temperate countries. Diets in the tropics are unbalanced as well as being deficient in calories. In the UK, of the 3200 calories (13 000 kJ) daily intake, 88 g are protein of which 54 g are animal protein. In India of the 2040 calories (8500 kJ) daily intake 53 g are protein of which only 6 g are animal protein.

In addition to the energy-deficient unbalanced diet available to tropical people there is the added effect of the bacterial and parasitic infections which are so prevalent. Social and cultural customs and the breakdown of society from the impact of towns and industrial development have all played a major part in producing the nutritional deficiencies which are so common in many tropical areas.

NUTRITION AND INFECTION

The relationship between infection and nutrition is reviewed in detail by Scrimshaw et al.[1] Infection may have an effect on the nutritional status or the nutritional status may affect the resistance to infection of the individual.

Infection has its most serious effect in protein nutrition on the nitrogen balance. Intestinal infections may cause some decrease in absorption of nitrogen from the gastrointestinal tract but the most important effect is from increased excretion of urinary nitrogen and diminished intake from anorexia.[1] An outstanding feature of kwashiorkor is the frequency with which it is precipitated by an attack of acute diarrhoeal disease. The increased excretion of nitrogen and decreased intake of food associated with active tuberculosis is of considerable importance in regions where protein malnutrition is common. All virus diseases exert a detectable adverse effect on nitrogen balance and measles of all the communicable diseases imposes an unusually severe nutritional stress. Morley[2] believes that measles precipitates kwashiorkor in West Africa more frequently than any other infectious disease. Measles is an important contributory cause of kwashiorkor in many tropical areas and there is a strong association between failure to thrive, diarrhoeal disease and bacterial colonization of the upper bowel.[3] Heavy *Ascaris* infection especially many divert protein from the host, since an adult worm contains a lot of protein. Any unusually heavy infection with an intestinal helminth can probably induce protein malnutrition in persons whose diet is otherwise adequate and many observers believe that infection with helminths may precipitate kwashiorkor. The consequence of moderate and light helminthic infections is more debatable and adequate epidemiological studies to determine their effect are not available.

Infection may have an effect on vitamin deficiencies. There is some evidence[4] that blindness caused by onchocerciasis is less common in areas where red palm oil, which is high in vitamin A content, is used.

Infectious diseases can precipitate clinical beriberi in persons on a diet deficient in vitamin B_1.

Systemic infections are able to induce anaemia

when folic acid is deficient and fish tapeworm may cause anaemia because of its high requirement of vitamin B_{12}.

Hookworm disease is responsible for iron-deficiency anaemia, due to iron loss from blood passing through the worms' intestinal canal. Chronic infections of bacterial or viral origin produce an 'anaemia of infection' by interfering with iron binding capacity and red cell life span.

Heavy infections with *Giardia* or *Strongyloides* may interfere with fat absorption but unless the infection is heavy, intestinal helminths as a rule do not interfere with fat absorption.

Immunocompetence in malnutrition

It is now well recognized that immunocompetence is severely affected in malnutrition. Both T cell and B cell dependent immune systems are depressed but this is reversible with nutritional repletion.[5] Defects in cellular immunity were found in 75% of children with protein–energy malnutrition[6] and malnourished children show thymic atrophy and depressed cell-mediated immunity, possibly, it has been suggested, the result of zinc deficiency.[7] The effect on humoral immunity is not so clear. Low IgG, albumin and secretory IgA levels were found in malnutrition,[8] but the production of antibodies was found not to be inhibited[9] and it is probable that it is the quality of antibody formed which is important, which limits the ability to remove antigen. Immunosuppression from infections such as malaria play an important part in susceptibility to infections in malnutrition.

Malnutrition and resistance to infection

When malnutrition weakens resistance to infection the effect is termed synergic; when malnutrition affects the infectious agent more than the host then it is termed antagonistic. Many observations have shown that tuberculosis is commoner in malnourished persons and that diarrhoeal diseases and upper respiratory illnesses occur more frequently and last longer in malnourished than among well-nourished children. There is some evidence, especially in Africa, that amoebic dysentery is more severe in persons who are on a deficient diet. Synergism is usual and antagonism is rare. From experimental studies on animals synergism is the characteristic reaction with bacteria, rickettsiae, intestinal protozoa and helminths. On the other hand antagonism is relatively common with viruses.

The results of studies support a general view that moderate to severe nutritional deficiencies increase the seriousness of infection in man.

MALNUTRITION

Malnutrition is extremely common throughout the Third World. Estimates of incidence are:

	Africa	Asia	South America
Severe malnutrition	3 million	6 million	1 million
Moderate malnutrition	16 million	64 million	10 million

In the world 10 million children are at risk of death and one-third will die even if treated. Certain well-defined syndromes occur:
　　protein–energy malnutrition (kwashiorkor, marasmus);
　　vitamin deficiencies;
　　nutritional neuropathies.

Protein–energy malnutrition (kwashiorkor) (PEM)

Kwashiorkor has very many other names including: Mehlnährschaden (Germany), obwosi (Uganda), diboba, m'buaki (Zaire), culebulla (Mexico), bouffisure d'Annam (Indo-China), depigmentation oedema syndrome, pellagroide beri-berico (Cuba). The disease is similar to Mehlnährschaden, a starch or flour dystrophy described by Czerny and Keller in Vienna in 1906. The first clinical description in the tropics was given in Kenya.[10,11] In Ghana Cicely Williams first gave it its distinctive name, kwashiorkor or 'deprived child' and described its pathology.[12]

GEOGRAPHICAL DISTRIBUTION

PEM is found in Africa, India, New Guinea,

Indonesia, China, Japan, Malaya, Mexico and many South American countries. Cases have been found in Hungary, Italy and in Puerto Rican families living in New York.

AETIOLOGY

The cause of PEM is multifactorial though dietary intake is the most important, but infection and psychosocial factors are also important.

Diet

The primary cause of PEM is a diet low in protein but containing some calories derived from carbohydrate in infancy when protein needs are much greater than in adult life. For the first six months the breastfed infant gains weight and is protected from infections by the transfer across the placenta of antibodies. In the second six months the breast milk decreases and supplementary foods are insufficient and mainly carbohydrate and, at the same time, the passive immunity wears off. In the second year of life breastfeeding may cease or if it continues is insufficient and supplementary foods are mainly carbohydrate. At this time the non-immune child is exposed to infection with nutritional consequences. The child's weight remains constant or it may decline and PEM develops (Fig. 45.1).

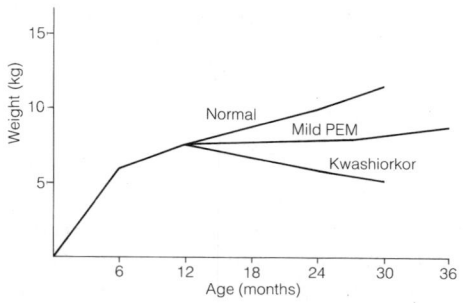

Fig. 45.1 Weight gain in mild malnutrition and kwashiorkor.

In the third and fourth year weight gain will resume its upward trend but at a lower level than would be regarded as normal. The diet is then deficient in protein and the calorie intake may

also be reduced due to the low quality of staple food. In addition, there may be deficiencies of minerals and vitamins. Cultural habits, ignorance and poverty all contribute to this poor diet.

Infections

Infection is an important cause of kwashiorkor (Fig. 45.2). The body's defence against invading organisms is to produce free radicals (lipid peroxides and toxic carbonyls) to kill them. There are a number of protective pathways against these free radicals which require micronutrients (zinc, selenium) for their efficient function. A recent hypothesis states that a deficiency of any of these micronutrients will lead to a loss of protection, resulting in cellular damage giving rise to the oedema, fatty liver, pigmentary changes, diarrhoea, immunoincompetence and mental changes typical of kwashiorkor.[52]

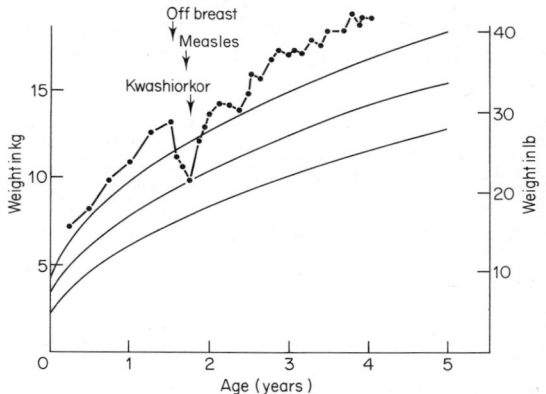

Fig. 45.2 The effect of measles on weight gain. Recovery occurs after a stay in hospital. (After Morley.[31])

Psychosocial factors

Weaning and the arrival of another child cause feelings of deprivation which result in anorexia and decrease in food intake.

Toxins

Aflatoxin has been blamed as a factor in the cause of kwashiorkor[13] but as a major factor it is probably not to blame.[14] The finding of high levels of aflatoxin in kwashiorkor could well be due to the inability of the fatty liver to eliminate the toxin.

PATHOLOGY

Protein deficiency has a severe effect on nutrition

by interfering with carbohydrate, fat and protein metabolism. Changes occur in the enzyme-secreting organs but all tissues are affected. The bones become osteoporotic and the skeletal muscles flabby.

Liver

The liver is fatty and greasy. Fat first appears in the periphery of the lobules and moves towards the centre as small droplets which coalesce to form large fat globules filling practically the whole cell (Fig. 45.3). There is a fibrous stellate pattern round each portal tract and, although there is an increase in lymphocytes and plasma cells in the sinusoids during recovery, there is no evidence that cirrhosis is a late result.[15] With adequate treatment the fat disappears in the reverse order and the fatty changes are totally reversible. Liver function is well preserved and, when in advanced cases the serum bilirubin and transaminases are raised, the prognosis is bad and sudden death may occur probably from liver failure.

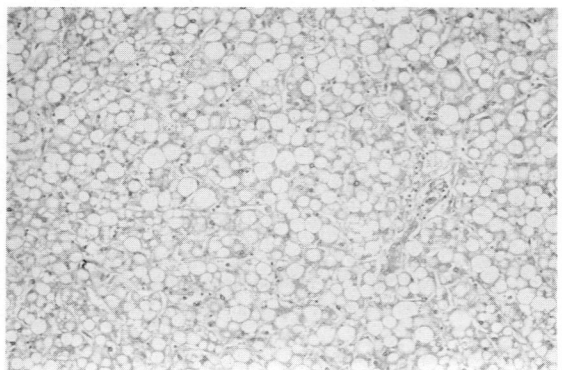

Fig. 45.3   The liver of a patient with kwashiorkor showing severe fatty vacuolation of the hepatocytes.

Pancreas

The pancreas is pale and atrophic. Microscopically there is atrophy, vacuolation and loss of zymogen granules from the acinar cells with dilatation of ducts and interstitial fibrosis. Calcification can occur and there is some evidence connecting PEM with the juvenile tropical pancreatitis syndrome leading to pancreatic calcification in adults (see Chapter 60). The salivary glands show marked atrophy with loss of acinar cells.

Gastrointestinal tract

The enzyme-secreting cells of the mucosa are atrophied and there is atrophy and broadening of the villi with an increase of cells in the lamina propria. This leads to loss of disaccharidases and monosaccharidases with lactose and glucose intolerance seen in PEM on recovery when lactose and glucose cause diarrhoea. Bacterial contamination of the upper bowel causes malabsorption and protein loss; diarrhoeal diseases and measles further worsen the position.

Heart

The heart is small and atrophied with histological and biochemical evidence of myocardial dysfunction. A rise in cardiac enzymes and return to normal with recovery suggests dead or dying myocardial cells.[16] The cardiac output is reduced one-half to one-third of normal with a great danger of circulatory overload during treatment.

Thymus

The thymus is atrophied which is related to the immunodepression evident in PEM.

Brain and central nervous system

The true weight of the brain is decreased. Atrophy, vacuolation, chromatolysis with neurofibrillary disorganization is seen in the central nervous system in experimental animals. The anterior horn cells in the spinal cord show similar changes. There are degenerative and atrophic changes in the central ganglia and a reduction in size of the cortical neurons.

Skin

The skin shows hyperpigmentation with subsequent exfoliation, atrophy, hypopigmentation and a mixture of ulcers, fissures and hyperkeratosis. The nails are thin and soft. Microscopically the horny layer is thickened with basophilia and atrophy of the cells of the granular layer, and vacuolation and atrophy of the cells of the Malpighian layer. The dermis is congested and oedematous and the collagen bundles swollen and fragmented. The hair bulbs are atrophic with loss of pigment from the shafts.

Kidneys

Hyalinization of the glomeruli and fatty degeneration of the convoluted tubules have been observed. Albuminuria indicates reduced glomerular flow and tubular activity which with a reduced cardiac output leads to electrolyte and water imbalance.

Hormone changes

Hormone changes are an adaptation to nutritional stress. The plasma cortisol levels are raised with an increase in growth hormone (sometimes they are reduced and lead to nutritional dwarfism) and the level of insulin is reduced. With recovery the growth hormone and cortisol levels return to normal but the insulin level remains low with a reduced ability to handle glucose.[16]

Anaemia (see also Chapter 58)

Some degree of anaemia is always found in children with PEM. There is usually a moderate but occasionally severe normocytic normochromic anaemia.

B_{12} and folate

Macrocytosis and megaloblastic marrow changes have been described in some patients[17,18] and giant metamyelocytes have been reported in the marrow.[19] However, there is no demonstratable deficiency of vitamin B_{12} or folate in the serum and the defect may be due to a failure to convert folic acid.[20]

Iron

Iron deficiency is not a consistent feature of the anaemia of PEM although on refeeding the iron stores become depleted and an iron deficiency anaemia may appear.

Erythropoietin

An adequate erythropoietin response for the degree of anaemia has been demonstrated.[21]

The anaemia of PEM usually responds to refeeding and treatment of infections, and with the restoration of marrow function iron deficiency limits haematological recovery, but because of the possibility of a flare up in malaria and other infections on recovery iron therapy should be postponed until after refeeding.[22]

Oedema

Oedema is a constant feature of PEM. Its causation is a matter of controversy. The classical view is that it is due to hypoalbuminaemia but other factors can also contribute. The cardiac output is reduced and there are decreases in renal blood flow, glomerular infiltration and an inability to concentrate urine and handle sodium.[23] There are also electrolyte deficiencies, potassium depletion which can cause oedema as well as magnesium and phosphorus depletion.[24] All these factors may operate but a low serum albumin is probably the key factor.[25]

Carbohydrate metabolism

Hypoglycaemia is frequently observed and may be due to liver failure; it is one cause of death. Glucose absorption and the handling of intravenous glucose and galactose loads is abnormal.[26] Enzymatic abnormalities of glucose oxidation have been described.[24]

Lipid metabolism

An intestinal mucosal defect is responsible for marked reduction in the absorption of different fat fractions[26] which persists for many weeks after clinical recovery. Intolerance to milk fats has been described.[27] Abnormalities in lipid transport are probably related to a deficiency of protein carriers.

Protein and amino acid metabolism

There is a severe disturbance of protein metabolism in kwashiorkor. The serum proteins are invariably reduced. The serum albumin is low owing to decreased albumin synthesis.[28] The α_1 and α_2 globulins are relatively increased and the β globulin frequently decreased. The γ globulin is also high and the albumin/globulin (A/G) ratio inverted. As a result of impaired hepatic circulation and altered serum proteins the flocculation and turbidity liver function tests are abnormal and there is a high bromsulphthalein retention in kwashiorkor. Nitrogen balance studies have shown that there is retention of a larger proportion of dietary protein than in normal children and there is increased recycling of body amino acids.[28]

Blood urea and urinary excretion of urea are low. Urinary creatinine is reduced but amino acid nitrogen, purine derivatives and protein and amino acid metabolites are high.

The serum activity of various enzymes, amylase, pseudocholinesterase and alkaline phosphatase, is constantly reduced but the levels of other enzymes associated with destruction of parenchymatous organs are raised.

IMMUNITY

Immunocompetence is severely affected in PEM; both T cell and B cell dependent systems are depressed but recover with nutritional repletion (see section on immunocompetence and malnutrition, above). Infections such as measles and malaria further depress immunity and secondary infections are common. Tuberculosis is very common and bronchitis and bronchopneumonia frequently cause death.

CLINICAL FEATURES

The main clinical features of kwashiorkor are failure to grow, oedema, skin and hair changes, diarrhoea and mental changes. The *onset* during the second year of life is often quite abrupt and is triggered off by an attack of diarrhoea, measles or removal from the mother (displacement by a new infant). Kwashiorkor has been seen in breastfed infants who are fed an excess of sugar and starch in addition to small amounts of breast milk,[29] and who are called 'sugar babies' in the Caribbean.[30]

Failure to grow

Of all the measurements made which can foretell PEM, weight records are the most valuable,[31] and the effect of removal of a child from the mother or an attack of measles are well shown in Fig. 45.2. In prolonged PEM the growth becomes stunted and ossification of bone is delayed.

Oedema

Pitting oedema is of variable degree, from a slight pitting of the legs to a generalized oedema in which the child is blown up, with massive swelling of the eyelids which block the eyes (Fig. 45.4). The oedema may be deceptive and the child looks fat and plump so that when recovery begins and the oedema is lost he changes into a wizened little creature with sunken cheeks, pot-belly and spindly legs. In 'sugar babies' who receive adequate calories but an excess of carbohydrate the body tissues under the oedema are not wasted.

Skin lesions

Skin lesions, which may be slight or absent, are very characteristic of kwashiorkor (Fig. 45.5). The skin always shows some degree of atrophy but the typical dermatosis is seen with varying frequency. It starts as large areas of erythema resembling second degree burns which become progressively dry, hyperkeratotic and hyperpigmented. In other cases the lesions start as small areas of hyperkeratosis and hyperpigmentation which grow and become confluent. The epidermis peels off, leaving a depigmented, often tender and reddish oozing surface known

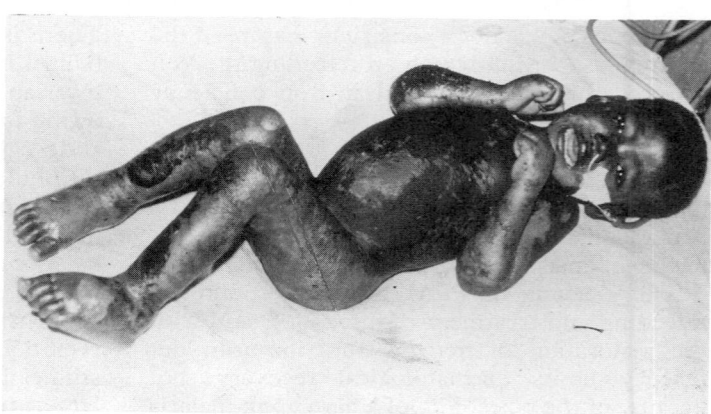

Fig. 45.4 Oedema and dermatosis in kwashiorkor. (Courtesy Dr Jelliffe and Dr Barber.)

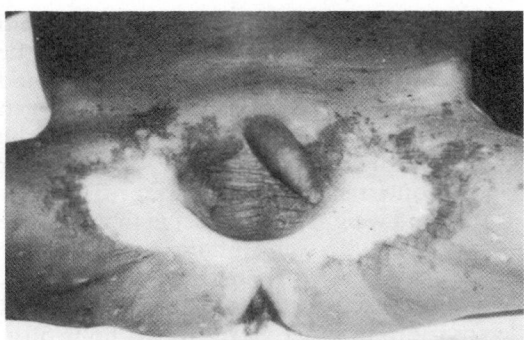

Fig. 45.5 Kwashiorkor in a Fijian male child aged two, showing characteristic dermatosis, depigmentation and hyperpigmentation.

as 'crazy pavement', 'alligator' or 'mosaic' skin. The dermatosis affects mainly the pressure areas and is not, like the dermatosis of pellagra, limited to areas exposed to sunlight. It first appears in the napkin areas or lower legs, spreading to the thighs, elbows and flexures of the knee and groin. Linear flexural fissures extending into the subcutaneous tissues may be seen around the pinna of the ear and back of the knee. In severer cases the dermatosis is well marked over the legs and in milder cases over the lumbar region. There is a tendency for the skin to break down, giving rise to deep necrotic ulcers of the skin, and gangrene of the limbs may ensue.

Hair changes (achromotrichia)

Hair changes are almost a constant feature, but are variable. The hair becomes dry and thin, loses its normal sheen and can easily be pulled out. Hair grown during periods of malnutrition loses its colour; black hair becomes brown or reddish yellow or even white and periods of depigmented growth alternating with periods of more pigmented growth are responsible for the 'flag sign' (signale la bandera).[32] Similar but less marked changes may be seen in the eyelashes and nails.

Diarrhoea

A recent history of diarrhoea is almost always present. The diarrhoea is non-specific with undigested food in the faeces. A large stool volume indicates malabsorption. Vomiting is common, especially if the child is made to eat more than he is accustomed to. Dehydration and electrolyte imbalance resulting from diarrhoea allows hypovolaemia to coexist with oedema.

Mental changes

The kwashiorkor child is dull, apathetic and miserable. He rarely screams or cries but gives rise to a low and miserable whimper and resists examination. He never fights or screams. There is a great falling off in expression and comprehension.[33] A syndrome resembling encephalitis has been described with coarse tremors, postural abnormalities, exaggerated tendon reflexes and myoclonus, which are transient features and disappear with treatment.[34] Transient electroencephalogram (EEG) abnormalities have been reported.[35] Brain weights of children dying of malnutrition are significantly lower than in control non-malnourished children.[36] EEG and histological evidence of brain damage has been found in protein-deficient animals[37] but there is as yet no evidence that these findings are applicable to the progress of children recovering from protein–energy malnutrition.

Cardiovascular changes

Since the heart is small and atrophied pathologically, some disturbance of cardiovascular function is to be expected and anaemia and fluid retention are important causes of heart failure. The heart is small on X-ray and there is a low cardiac output. The extremities are frequently cold and cyanotic and the blood pressure is low with a small pulse pressure. The low serum potassium and magnesium affect the myocardial excitability and the heart is extremely sensitive to digitalis. During recovery there may be marked cardiovascular changes with an increase in heart diameter with gallop rhythm, and cardiac failure may occur after blood or plasma infusions.[38]

The electrocardiogram shows non-specific changes, dwarfing of all complexes and abnormally short or long P-R interval and flat or inverted T waves over the left precordium. During recovery bizarre S-T and T patterns have been noted, often with asymmetrical peaking of the T wave.[38]

Associated nutritional deficiencies

Associated vitamin deficiencies are frequently seen but are not constant and vary from one region to another. Vitamin A deficiency is favoured since its absorption, transport and utilization are impaired in kwashiorkor[39] and there is a high frequency of severe ocular lesions due to vitamin A deficiency in children with protein-energy malnutrition in areas where vitamin A deficiency is endemic[40] (see p. 835).

Trace metals

Deficiency of trace metals, particularly copper and zinc, may be important. Zinc deficiency is now assuming a more important role (see p. 823).

Associated infections

Associated infections are common. Bronchitis and pneumonia may occur in a patient with kwashiorkor who may die quite suddenly of respiratory failure due to bronchopneumonia without having shown any fever or dyspnoea. Paradoxically, during recovery malaria may flare up due to the improved nutritional status of the patient and other infections may relapse.

TREATMENT

Treatment is based fundamentally upon the administration of a diet high in protein of good biological value and containing sufficient energy. Dehydration and electrolyte imbalance must be corrected and since there is usually a severe potassium deficiency potassium must be given. Since the cardiac reserve is diminished intravenous fluids must be given cautiously. The basis of treatment is skim milk powder (50 g) which can be used with calcium caseinate (50 g), sugar (20 g) and cottonseed oil (30 g) in water to 1 litre. The milk powder is made to a paste with cold water, hot water is added and brought to the boil and the whole is blended and made up to 1 litre.[41] A total intake of 3–5 g/kg body weight of protein of high biological value should be maintained and the total energy intake should be about 120–140 calories (500–600 kJ)/kg body weight/day. Small frequent feeds are necessary from the start. Specific supplements are needed only if there is a particular deficiency, such as vitamin A, which should be given intramuscularly. Potassium chloride 1 g daily is also recommended and rapid improvement in the electrocardiogram and in the child is achieved by adding magnesium. Blood transfusion may be needed; iron should be given in the case of iron-deficiency anaemia and folic acid for megaloblastic anaemia. The weight curve and consistency of the stools form important guides and weight may be lost at first because of loss of oedema. In some infants diarrhoea may develop owing to carbohydrate intolerance, especially of lactose.[42] Lactose-free material made from groundnuts 150 g, wheat flour 50 g, maize flour 100 g, cottonseed oil 25 g and sugar 75 g, made into biscuit, has been used successfully.

Recovery takes place in two stages.[43] During the first stage the oedema disappears and the major biochemical and physiological alterations return to normal values. This stage lasts two or three weeks and weight is lost. During the second stage the child recovers the weight lost and reaches the normal weight for his height. This takes two to three months.

PREVENTION

Prevention depends on educating the mothers to avoid artificial feeding in the absence of the correct knowledge of how to handle it and on adopting satisfactory weaning habits using local products containing available protein.

Incaparina prepared by the Institute of Central America and Panama is an economic, easily cooked mixture of ground maize, whole ground sorghum, cottonseed flour, yeast and calcium carbonate, enriched with vitamin A, and is a protein supplement widely used in Central America to prevent the development of protein–energy malnutrition.

MILD TO MODERATE PEM

This is manifested by inadequate physical growth. The child is smaller and less active. Bone maturation is retarded and mental development slowed but whether this is irreversible or not is debatable (see section on mental changes, above).

Marasmus

The commonest form of marasmus in the tropics is of primary origin and is the result of starvation in small children.

Children are fed a diet which is adequate qualitatively but is grossly deficient in energy to fill the requirements of the rapidly growing child. Energy is the limiting factor and the child lives on its own tissues. The picture develops in infants fed on mother's milk, which is deficient in amount in malnourished mothers, or fed by prolonged breastfeeding, with inadequate supplementation or inadequate artificial feeding with over-diluted cow's milk or starchy gruels. Social changes and urbanization are forcing mothers to wean early and the adoption of artificial feeding brings infective diarrhoea. An important cause of marasmus is malabsorption caused by bacterial colonization of the upper bowel brought about by the constant intake of infected water and food from an insanitary environment.

There is marked atrophy of all the organs and tissues. There is no anaemia unless a superimposed cause is present. Intestinal absorptive mechanisms are adequate.[44] The duodenal enzymes are normal in marasmus, in contrast to kwashiorkor.[45]

Serum proteins are normal and serum enzymes like amylase and pseudocholinesterase are not affected.[46]

Marasmus is more frequent in infants than older children because they are growing more rapidly and are more likely to be subject to the marasmus-producing type of diet. With restriction of food intake growth almost ceases and the infant utilizes the subcutaneous fat and then the muscles. The infant is hungry and cries continuously. There may be constipation because of the diminished food intake. Infectious diseases act as precipitating and aggravating factors. The child is extremely emaciated; the muscles are atrophic. The skin is thin, flaccid and wrinkled. The hair is not altered. The mind is alert, but the typical face of the marasmic child looks like that of a very little old man. Often there is added dehydration from infective vomiting and diarrhoea.

Practically all cases will recover with adequate dietary treatment unless severe complications, such as dehydration, electrolyte imbalance or infection, are present. The diet should be complete and balanced and be adequate for the apparent biological age and higher in energy than would be required for a normal child, 200 calories (850 kJ)/kg body weight daily are needed.[47] Progress must be followed by regular weighing.

ENDEMIC GOITRE

This is a slowly developing enlargement of the thyroid gland caused by a deficiency of iodine in the diet or the influence of goitrogens.

GEOGRAPHICAL DISTRIBUTION

Endemic goitre is distributed worldwide in certain restricted localities, away from the sea, at the head of rivers, and isolated valleys with poor soil and high rainfall. In the tropics it is found in Africa, Central and South America and in Asia.

In *Africa* it is found in the Atlas mountains, the Nile valley, highland areas of Kenya, Tanzania, Ruanda, Burundi, Cameroon, Gambia, Congo basin and Nigeria.

It is found in large areas of *Central* and *South America*.

In *Asia* it is found in the Himalayas from the Pamirs to Kashmir, Nepal, Burma and China (Yunnan) and also in Thailand, Vietnam and Malaysia.

AETIOLOGY

The cause of endemic goitre is failure of the thyroid gland to obtain a sufficient supply of iodine to maintain its normal structure and function.[48] This failure may be brought about by a deficiency of iodine in the diet which is caused by a deficiency in the environment, accounting for the geographical distribution of endemic goitre. It may also be caused by goitrogens, which are substances which impose an abnormal demand on the thyroid or interfere metabolically with the utilization of iodine by the thyroid.[49] Goitrogens include cyanide compounds (cassava) and fluoride, which interfere with the ability of the gland to trap iodine from the circulation and antimony and cobalt, which interfere with the production of thyroid hormone. Goitrogens are also found in vegetables of the *Brassica* (cabbage) family.

PATHOLOGY

The thyroid enlarges in response to secretion of TSH by the pituitary. In the early stages hyperplasia of the follicles occurs and colloid is reduced. In the later chronic stages when the iodine stores have been exhausted the gland becomes soft and enlarged with large amounts of colloid in the follicles. Nodular formation takes place and haemorrhage and calcification may occur. The gland does not become toxic and there is no evidence that malignancy ensues.

Severe iodine depletion may interfere with corneal neuronal dendrites and is a factor in the pathogenesis of endemic cretinism.

CLINICAL FEATURES

Large goitres are easy to recognize. Moderate degrees of thyroid enlargement are diagnosed on goitre surveys and are graded by inspection, palpation and neck measurement. The presence of thyroid enlargement in a significant number of persons living in an area is sufficiently strong evidence for the diagnosis of endemic goitre. Pressure on the trachea may produce symptoms and interference with the recurrent laryngeal nerve hoarseness. The patient is almost always euthyroid.

DIAGNOSIS

The urinary excretion of iodine can be as low as $10 \mu g$ a day. The uptake of radioactive I^{131} is increased. Thyroid hormones are normal. Rarely, the hormone levels are depressed and the patient is hypothyroid.

TREATMENT

If treated early the goitre may disappear completely with the administration of iodine as 30 mg potassium iodide made up to 20 ml distilled water and administered as four to six drops daily in a glass of water. Results will be observed in four to six weeks and then the patient should be maintained on a daily regimen. Advanced goitres have to be treated surgically if they are causing symptoms.

EPIDEMIOLOGY

Areas of iodine deficiency may be plotted by the presence of isolated areas of poor soil where rainfall has leached the soil far away from the sea and so there is no natural supply of iodine. Areas of endemicity can be found by surveys and measurement of thyroid glands in the population. Protein bound iodine levels in the serum are low and the uptake of ^{131}I low in these areas.

PREVENTION

Goitre can be prevented by the use of iodized salt and $100 \mu g$ of iodine added to the daily diet are sufficient. It is more practical to give a deep intramuscular injection of 5 ml of iodized oil containing about 400 mg I_2 per ml, which is effective for several years.[50]

ENDEMIC CRETINISM

Endemic cretinism[51] is the most serious effect of endemic goitre and is found where the urinary iodine excretion is less than $20 \mu g$/day. In Papua New Guinea the prevalence of cretinism approaches 15%. There are two forms, the 'neurological', which predominates and is characterized by mental retardation, deaf mutism, spastic diplegia and strabismus, and the 'myxoedematous', with signs of congenital hypothyroidism which predominates in central Africa where dietary goitrogens may play a part.

Cretinism can be prevented by iodine supplements which must be given before conception since iodine deficiency causes neurological damage in early fetal development, and by iodized oil prophylaxis of the general population.

FAMINE OEDEMA

True famine oedema is due to a deficiency of protein in adults. It occurs during war and other social disturbances and was common in central Europe during the First World War. Famine oedema was common in Japanese prison camps during the Second World War and was confused with beriberi. The 'hungeroedem' of the Dutch was synonymous with the wet beriberi of the British medical staff.

The condition is due to a lack of fat and protein in the diet. The primary effect is a reduction in the serum protein below 4–5 g/100 ml. A generalized oedema develops without albuminuria or evidence of heart failure or peripheral neuritis. The serum albumin is greatly reduced. Recovery takes place when the patients are placed on a diet containing sufficient protein of high biological value. Many of the cases of so-called adult kwashiorkor are in reality famine oedema. Epidemic dropsy caused by the consumption of contaminated cottonseed or mustard oil can also produce a similar picture.

REFERENCES

1 Scrimshaw, N.S., Taylor, C.E. & Gordon, J.E. (1968) *Wld Hlth Org. Monograph,* 57.
2 Morley, D.C. (1962) *Am. J. Dis. Childh.* **103**, 230.
3 Rowland, M.G.M. & McCollum, J.P.K. (1977) *Trans. R. Soc. trop. Med. Hyg.* **71**, 199.
4 Rodger, F.C. (1957) *Trans. ophthal. Soc. UK.* 77, 267.
5 Law, D.K., Dudrick, S.J. & Abdou, N.I. (1973) *Ann. intern. Med.* **79**, 545.
6 Suskind, R.M., Olson, R.C. & Olson, R.C. (1973) *Pediatrics, Springfield* **51**, 25.
7 Golden, H.N. & Golden, B.E. (1978) *Lancet* i, 1226.
8 Sirinha, S., Suskind, R., Edelman, R. et al (1975) *Pediatrics, Springfield* **55**, 166.
9 Rosen, E.G., Geefhuysen, J. & Ipp, T. (1971) *S. Afr. med. J.* **45**, 990.
10 Procter, R.A.W. (1927) *Kenya med. J.* 3, 284.
11 Gillan, R.W. (1934) *E. Afr. med. J.* **11**, 88.
12 Williams, C.D. (1933) *Archs Dis. Childh.* 8, 423.
13 Hendrickse, R.G. (1984) *Trans. R. Soc. trop. Med. Hyg.* **78**, 427–435.
14 *Lancet* (1984) **ii**, 1133–1134.
15 Umana, C.R. & Tejada, V.C. (1961) *Revta clin. Méd. Guatemala*
16 Wharton, B. (1973) *J.R. Coll. Phys. Lond.* 7, 259.
17 Walt, F., Holman, S. & Hendrickse, R.G. (1956) *Br. med. J.* i, 1199–1203.
18 Fondu, P., Kabeya-Mudiay, S., De Maertelaere-Laurent, E. et al (1973) *Biomedicine* **18**, 51–58.
19 Spector, I. & Metz, J. (1966) *Br. J. Haem.* **12**, 737–746.
20 Wickramasinghe, S.N., Akinyanju, O.O., Grange, A. et al (1983) *Br. J. Haem.* **53**, 135–143.
21 Wickramasinghe, S.N., Cotes, P.M., Gill, D.S. et al (1985) *Br. J. Haem.* **60**, 515–524.
22 Murray, M.J., Murray, A.B., Murray, N.J. et al (1978) *Br. med. J.* **ii**, 1113–1115.
23 Klahr, S. & Alleyne, G.A.O. (1973) *Kidney Int.* 3, 129–141.
24 Metcoff, J., Frenk, S., Antonowicz, I. et al (1960) *Pediatrics, Springfield* **26**, 960.
25 Waterlow, J.C. (1984) *Trans. R. Soc. trop. Med. Hyg.* 78, 436–441.
26 Viteri, F.E., Arroyave, C. & Behar, M. (1966) *7th Int. Congr. Nutr.* **12**, 170, 46.
27 Dean, R.F.A. & Swanne, J. (1963) *J. trop. Pediat.* 8, 97.
28 Picou, D. & Waterlow, J.C. (1962) *Clin. Sci.* **22**, 459.
29 Davies, J.N.P. (1955) *E. Afr. med. J.* **32**, 283.
30 Jelliffe, D.B., Bras, G. & Stuart, K.L. (1954) *W. Indian med. J.* 3, 43.
31 Morley, D.C. (1968) *Trans. R. Soc. trop. Med. Hyg.* **62**, 200.
32 Pena Chavarria, A., Saenz Herrera, C. & Cordero, C.E. (1948) *Revta med. Costa Rica* **6**, 170.
33 Geber, M. & Dean, R.F.A. (1956) *Courrier* **6**, 3.
34 Kahn, E. & Falcke, H.C. (1956) *J. Pediat.* **49**, 37.
35 Nelson, G.K. & Dean, R.F.A. (1959) *Bull. Wld Hlth Org.* **21**, 779.
36 Brown, R.E. (1965) *E. Afr. med. J.* **42**, 584.
37 Platt, B.S., Heard, C.R.C. & Stewart, R.J.C. (1964) Experimental protein deficiency. In *Mammalian Protein Metabolism,* ed. H.N. Munro & J.B. Allison. New York: Academic Press.
38 Smythe, P.M., Swanepoel, A. & Campbell, J.A.H. (1962) *Br. med. J.* **i**, 67.
39 Arroyave, G., Viteri, F., Behar, M. et al (1959) *Am. J. clin. Nutr.* **9**, 186.
40 Oomen, H.A.P.C. (1954) *Br. J. Nutr.* **8**, 307.
41 Dean, R.F.A. & Skinner, M. (1957) *J. trop. Pediat.* **8**, 97.
42 Dean, R.F.A. (1956) *Bull. Wld Hlth Org.* **14**, 798.
43 Brock, J.F., Hansen, J.D.L., Howe, E.E. et al (1955) *Lancet* **ii**, 355.
44 Thomson, M.D. & Trowell, H.C. (1952) *Lancet* **i**, 1031.
45 Vegelhyi, P. (1948) *Acta chir. belge* 2, 347.
46 Waterlow, J.C. (1959) *Fedn Proc. Fedn Am. Socs exp. Biol.* **18**, 113.
47 Jelliffe, D.B. (1970) *Diseases of Children in the Tropics and Subtropics,* 2nd edn. London: Arnold.
48 Stanbury, J.B. & Ramalingaswami, V. (1964) *Nutrition* **i**, 373.
49 Scrimshaw, N.S. (1958) *Fedn Proc. Fedn Am. Socs exp. Biol.* **17**, 57.
50 Buttfield, I. & Hetzel, B.S. (1967) *Bull. Wld Hlth Org.* **36**, 243.
51 *Lancet* (1979) **ii**, 1165.
52 Golden, M.H.N. & Ramdath, D. (1987) *Proc. Nutr. Soc.* **46**, 53–68.

Chapter 46
Vitamin Deficiency

SCURVY

GEOGRAPHICAL DISTRIBUTION

Scurvy is found worldwide especially in hot, dry desert areas where fresh vegetables and fruit are lacking.

AETIOLOGY

Scurvy is due to a lack of vitamin C (ascorbic acid) which catalyses oxidation by the introduction of hydroxyl groups and is essential for the formation of collagen.

PATHOLOGY

Inadequate formation of collagen leads to extravasation of blood, loosening of the teeth and easily fractured bones with haemorrhages under the periosteum. Autopsy shows extensive haemorrhage in the internal organs.

CLINICAL FEATURES

Scurvy may occur in adults or infants.

Adult scurvy

The onset is insidious with loss of weight, progressive weakness and, characteristically, stiffness in the leg muscles and any other muscle groups that are in extensive use. Haematomas in the calf muscles may be the first sign. The acute symptoms are brought on by physical exertion. The gums soon become affected with swelling and sponginess of the alveolar margin and fungating masses projecting beyond the teeth which loosen and fall out. Subcutaneous petechiae form on the limbs and trunk producing scorbutic purpura, and wounds fail to heal. The anaemia is characteristically microcytic and hypochromic and responds only to ascorbic acid.

Infantile scurvy

The majority of cases present in the second half of the first year especially in premature and artificially fed infants. There is a triad of irritability, tenderness of the legs and failure to use them (pseudoparalysis). Bleeding manifestations are confined to the site of erupting teeth. The infant lies in a characteristic position with legs flexed at the knees and hips partially flexed and internally rotated due to pain from subperiosteal haemorrhages, which may be felt at the distal end of the femur and proximal end of the tibia. Costochondal beading (scorbutic rosary) is usually palpable. Anaemia is microcytic and hypochromic but may be megaloblastic due to accompanying folate deficiency from lack of folate coenzymes associated with vitamin C.

X-ray of the bones shows characteristic epiphyseal changes with a line of rarefaction at the line of epiphyseal growth with a ground glass appearance of the shafts of the bones.

DIAGNOSIS

The main differential diagnosis is from rickets which may coexist as 'scurvy rickets'. In rickets there is a dense line at the epiphyseal junctions. The capillary permeability test of Hess is performed using a sphygmomanometer to occlude the venous return of the arm when petechiae will appear in scorbutic cases. The vitamin C saturation test which is performed by saturating the body with ascorbic acid and measuring excretion in the urine; if any ascorbic acid is retained then there is a deficiency of vitamin C.

TREATMENT

Ascorbic acid 50 mg four times daily should be given for one week in infantile scurvy followed by 50 mg twice daily for one month. Vitamin C may also be given as 100–200 ml fresh orange juice per day. Adult scurvy should be treated with 250 mg four times daily until all signs have disappeared.

EPIDEMIOLOGY

Scurvy is not common in tropical areas since vitamin C is abundant. Cases can occur in infants who are fed on dried cereal and boiled milk and soldiers, prisoners and refugees in camps in dry desert areas who are not given fresh fruit and vegetables.

PREVENTION

Vitamin C is destroyed by heat, especially prolonged cooking, and the presence of alkalis. Foods which are steamed and cooked rapidly retain much of their vitamin C content. The recommended allowance of vitamin C is 30 mg daily for infants, 40–45 mg daily for children and 70 mg daily for adults. Scurvy may be prevented in camps and bodies of men living on dry rations by giving 100 mg of ascorbic acid daily in tablet form. Artificially fed infants should receive supplements in the form of fresh orange juice daily or an ascorbic acid supplement.

RICKETS AND OSTEOMALACIA

GEOGRAPHICAL DISTRIBUTION

Rickets is now rare in temperate countries but still occurs sporadically in many parts of the world where custom deprives the infant or woman of sunlight by confining them because of social or religious custom.

AETIOLOGY

Rickets and osteomalacia are caused by a deficiency of vitamin D. Vitamin D is a sterol; vitamin D_1 (calciferol) results from the action of ultraviolet light on ergosterols in plants, and vitamin D_2 (cholecalciferol) from the action of sunlight on 7-dehydrocholesterol in the skin of mammals. Vitamin D has a direct effect on the calcification of bone where it increases the rate of secretion and resorption of minerals. A high phytate content of the diet may upset the absorption of calcium and phosphorus.

PATHOLOGY

Defective calcification of developing long bones results in the slowing down of the precipitation of calcium and phosphorus in the newly formed matrix, resulting in the formation of a mass of osteoid tissue which fails to calcify causing enlargement at the growing ends of the bone in rickets (rickety rosary) along the costochondral junction, and a softening of all the bones in rickets and osteomalacia.

CLINICAL FEATURES

Rickets

The onset during the first two years of life is later than scurvy. The child becomes ill, pale, flabby and irritable, prone to tetany and laryngeal stridor. There is general physical and mental retardation and deformity in ribs, spine, pelvis and limbs (Fig. 46.1). The skull shows bossing

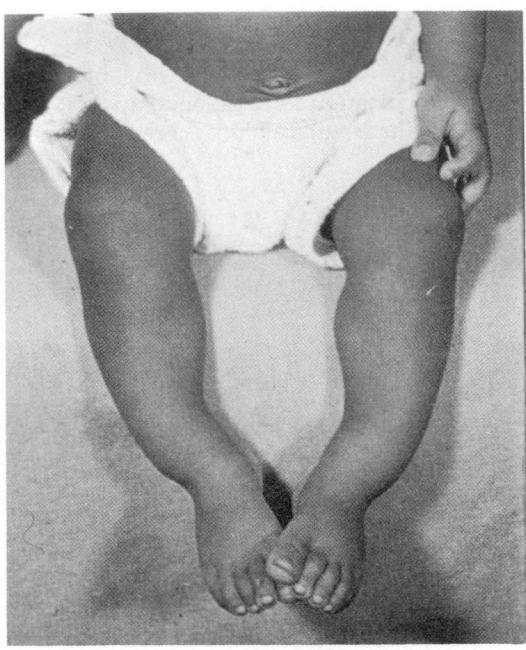

Fig. 46.1 Curvature of the legs caused by rickets.

(craniotabes). The liver and spleen may be palpable. As the child grows older the skeletal changes heal but marked deformities may remain, such as pigeon-chest, spinal curvature, knock-knees and bow-legs.

Osteomalacia

Osteomalacia occurs only in women of child-bearing years, usually in the first pregnancy. The bones, especially those of the pelvic girdle, ribs and femora become soft, painful and deformed. The gait is characteristic, the patient swaying the leg outward before putting the foot to the ground. Tetany is common. Anaemia is present and spontaneous fractures may occur. The bones of the fetus show no signs of rickets.

DIFFERENTIAL DIAGNOSIS

The differential diagnosis of rickets from infantile scurvy may be difficult but rickets occurs in older infants and there are no subperiosteal haemorrhages; other conditions are congenital syphilis, achondroplasia and osteogenesis imperfecta. Renal rickets in chronic renal disease does not respond to vitamin D.

DIAGNOSIS

X-ray of the wrist may show characteristic changes in the epiphyses. The line of osteochondral calcification is broadened and rarefied (Fig. 46.2). The serum calcium is low (6–7 mg/dl) but clinical rickets can occur with normal calcium and phosphorus levels.

TREATMENT

Treatment is based on providing an adequate intake of calcium and vitamin D. Vitamin D should be given, 2000–5000 international units (IU) daily and calcium as milk 500 ml daily.

EPIDEMIOLOGY

Rickets

In the tropics rickets may occur where sunlight is cut off by high rise buildings in Asia[1] where it is a disease of cities. The San Blas Indians of Panama protect their children from the sun because of the high incidence of albinism.[2] In Guatemala some cases have been found in sunny rural areas where the toddlers are kept in houses because the mothers have to go out to work. It has been suggested that rural rickets in Iran[3] and Kashmir might be due not to a high phytate content but to an 'anti-calcifying' factor present in high extraction flour (chupatty).[4]

Osteomalacia

In India osteomalacia is widespread in women whose diets are inadequate in calcium and vitamin D and who are kept in 'purdah' which prevents the sunlight acting on the skin and in northern China a similar cause in osteomalacia

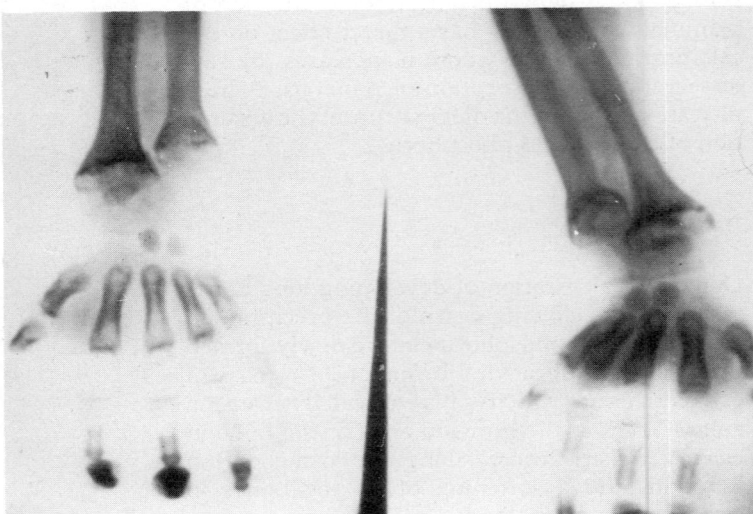

Fig. 46.2 Radiograph of the hands in rickets, with a normal radiograph on the left for comparison.

as for rickets has been suggested, namely, an 'anti-calcifying' factor in chupatty flour, and biochemical healing has been obtained with a chupatty-free diet.[5]

PREVENTION

An adequate intake of milk, clearance of slums and action against atmospheric pollution should be undertaken, as well as health education for children and women to obtain adequate sunlight and daily intake of 400 IU of vitamin D as cod-liver oil or bread fortified with calcium and vegetable fats with calciferol.

VITAMIN A DEFICIENCY (NIGHT BLINDNESS, XEROPHTHALMIA, KERATOMALACIA)

GEOGRAPHICAL DISTRIBUTION

Vitamin A deficiency is common in parts of south and South-East Asia, the Middle East, Africa and Latin America where it usually accompanies protein–energy malnutrition (PEM) (see p. 828).

AETIOLOGY

Vitamin A (retinol) is used by epithelial cells throughout the body which undergo squamous metaplasia, the cells becoming flattened and heaped upon each other. The sweat glands become blocked with secretion and sweat diminishes. The lack of tears and the change in the conjunctiva leads to *xerophthalmia* and, on the cornea, *keratomalacia*, and the diminished supply to the rod cells of the retina to failure of dark adaptation and *night blindness*. Similar changes in the skin of the body lead to *follicular keratosis*.

The pathology, clinical features, treatment and prevention of these conditions is dealt with in Chapter 70.

VITAMIN B₁ DEFICIENCY (BERIBERI)

GEOGRAPHICAL DISTRIBUTION

Until recently beriberi was common in tropical and subtropical areas and was formerly the scourge of mines and plantations in Malaysia, China, Indonesia and other parts of the Far East, wherever rice was the staple diet, and was the cause of an enormous mortality and morbidity. It was common among workers in the tropics on such major engineering projects as the Panama Canal and Congo (Zaire) Railway. Outbreaks have occurred in institutions such as mental homes in Ireland, the USA and France and in fishermen in Newfoundland, the North American coast and Iceland. Beriberi was formerly a major problem in the Japanese Navy and was almost universal in prisoner-of-war and internment camps in the Far East in the Second World War. Beriberi was formerly prevalent in the crews of ships on the high seas. From 1894 to 1920 the disease was common in the crews of Swedish and Norwegian ships and yet was comparatively rare in British ships. The explanation was that during these years bread baked from white flour or a mixture of wheat and rye was used in the Scandinavian ships so that the crew's diet was inadequate in vitamins.

AETIOLOGY

Vitamin B₁ deficiency or beriberi is due to a deficiency of vitamin B₁ or thiamine. Vitamin B₁ is found in the tissues in the phosphorylated form as diphosphothiamine which acts as a coenzyme for the metabolism of carbohydrate in the Krebs citric acid cycle and plays a part in the oxidative breakdown of pyruvic acid. Since the brain and all nervous tissue and heart muscle use glucose in large amounts as a primary source of energy, carbohydrate metabolism is especially deranged in these tissues in vitamin B₁ deficiency. Pyruvic acid accumulates in the blood and central nervous system and is excreted in excess in the urine. Vitamin B_1 is also involved in the synthesis of acetylcholine and in nerve transmission. Another factor resulting from breakdown in the Krebs cycle is the metabolic acidosis resulting from the accumulation of lactic acid in the blood, which is important in alcoholic beriberi.[6]

Vitamin B_1 is widely distributed in raw foodstuffs, the richest sources being whole cereals and especially rice, in which it is found in the pericarp in the aleurone layer and in the embryo of the grain. The rice grain in its natural condition is enclosed in a husk. In 'husking' the husk is removed but the pericarp is retained; this is unpolished rice. In milling and 'polishing' both the embryo and pericarp are removed and the grains are polished by rubbing with talc between sheepskins. This is known as polished or white rice. Vitamin B_1 is also found in yeast which is an exceptionally potent source and can be used as a dietary supplement. Vitamin B_1 is a colourless, water-soluble, crystalline substance melting at 248–250°C and in dry conditions is stable at 100°C for 24 hours. The rate of destruction is increased by the presence of water and alkali but ordinary cooking in the absence of soda does not destroy the vitamin; it is, however, destroyed by pressure cooking and autoclaving when yeast and liver are subjected to heat and pressure. The larger part of vitamin B_1 is stored in the liver, kidneys and muscles and it is abundant in the normal heart. Vitamin B_1 is excreted in the urine in which the kidney concentrates it from the plasma, but only a small part of the vitamin given by the mouth is excreted, the rest being destroyed in the body. It is also excreted in the milk but not in the faeces. An excretion of less than 12.1 IU/day in the urine is evidence of vitamin B_1 deficiency. The international unit is the antineuritic activity of $3\,\mu g$ of pure vitamin B_1. The minimum daily requirement of an adult of 70 kg on 3000 calories (12 600 kJ)/day would be 300 IU or 1 mg, but 500–700 IU (1.75–2.3 mg) is desirable. A larger amount is required where metabolic rates are increased in pregnancy, lactation, infancy and childhood and there is a high incidence of beriberi among pregnant women and mothers. Hard physical work also increases the requirements; thus beriberi is more prevalent among stokers than sailors. Since the metabolic rate rises during fever there is an association of beriberi with malaria and other pyrexias.

Secondary (alcoholic) beriberi

Alcoholic cardiomyopathy causes a low output type of heart failure, has a complicated aetiology and is not due to beriberi.[7]

True alcoholic beriberi is a form of oedematous heart disease with high output failure occurring in certain severe alcoholics, which responds rapidly to vitamin B_1. It is not common in the West but has been described as 'palm-wine tapper's heart' in Gambia[8] which develops in palm tappers whose work is arduous and involves the climbing of many palm trees and the consumption of the fermenting sap.

Drug-induced beriberi has been reported from East Africa from the use of nitrofurazone in the treatment of trypanosomiasis which interferes with pyruvate metabolism.

PATHOLOGY

As a result of the breakdown of carbohydrate metabolism those systems of the body which utilize glucose most rapidly are affected. These are the central nervous system, peripheral nerves and cardiac muscle. Degenerative nerve changes may be detected in the neurons in the anterior and posterior horn cells and sympathetic ganglia. The vagus is involved with degenerative changes in its nucleus in the floor of the fourth ventricle. Microscopically the nerve trunks show changes from a slight medullary degeneration to complete destruction of the nerve (Wallerian degeneration). Regenerative processes can occur side by side with the degenerative. Some fibres of the vagus and sympathetic nerves escape and the bronchial and oesophageal twigs are usually unaffected. In Wernicke's encephalopathy foci of congestion and haemorrhage are scattered symmetrically in the grey matter of the brain stem and hypothalamic regions. The mamillary bodies are nearly always affected. The lesions show specific selectivity for the vegetative centres, being most severe in the lateral horns and Clarke's nuclei at the thoracic level. There are also numerous perivascular haemorrhages and widespread degenerative changes throughout the brain. In the heart the primary lesion is a loss of contractibility of the heart muscle due to water retention. Microscopic examination of the heart muscle shows intracellular oedema, sarcolysis and hydropic degeneration probably due primarily to an excess of lactic acid brought about by defective oxygenation.[9] These changes cause 'beriberi heart', the essential feaures of which are a hyperkinetic circulation, peripheral vasodilatation, enlargement of the right side of the heart and dilatation of the pulmonary artery with an increased circulation time, causing a high output failure.[10]

The cause of the hyperkinetic circulation is a low peripheral arterial resistance from vasodilatation, in spite of increased plasma catecholamines, due to a loss of control of muscular arteriole tone.[11] It may be a compensatory mechanism which is brought into play to counteract tissue anoxia, which is simulated by a failure of carbohydrate metabolism, or the vasodilatation in the muscles may be responsible by causing an arteriovenous shunt.

The post-mortem appearances are those of severe right heart failure. The right side of the heart is dilated, especially the right atrium, the walls of which may be paper thin. There is gross congestion of the venous return and right atrium and ventricle. There are serous effusions into the pleural and peritoneal cavities and cellular tissues. There is oedema of the lungs and severe central congestion of the liver with 'nutmegging'.

CLINICAL FEATURES

Beriberi assumes varying clinical forms according to the extent and degree of cardiac involvement. There are two main forms of the disease; neurological or 'dry' beriberi and oedematous or 'wet' beriberi. In all its forms beriberi is the same disease and a mixture of the two forms is usual.

The period of development of beriberi in man after being placed on a vitamin B_1-deficient diet has been determined as between 80 and 90 days. The onset is usually insidious but may occasionally be ushered in by acute symptoms, ending fatally within a few hours without any symptoms referable to the central nervous system.

Paraplegic or dry beriberi

The signs and symptoms are those of a peripheral neuropathy of a mixed motor and sensory type. There is a gradual onset of weakness of the lower limbs followed by ataxia; there may be paraesthesiae with burning and tingling in the limbs.

Motor signs. A flaccid weakness with wasting develops at first in the muscles of the lower limbs.

The extensors of the foot and toes are involved with foot and toe drop and the gastrocnemii become weak and wasted. This weakness gradually spreads up to involve the extensors of the legs and later the extensors and flexors of the thigh. At this stage the patient is not able to rise from the squatting position with his hands held above his head. This is the 'jongck' or 'squatting test'. The upper limbs are eventually affected with weakness and wasting of the thenar, hypothenar, plantar and arm muscles, which may show fibrillary twitchings. There may be marked wrist drop. There is a loss of the deep reflexes. The knee jerks, ankle jerks and arm reflexes are all lost. The fibres of the affected muscles show myoedema and contract painfully when struck by the patella hammer. Electrical reactions show the reaction of degeneration.

Sensory changes. Sensory changes are marked. There is a sensory neuropathy of the peripheral type with glove and stocking anaesthesia spreading up from the feet over the tibiae to the thighs.

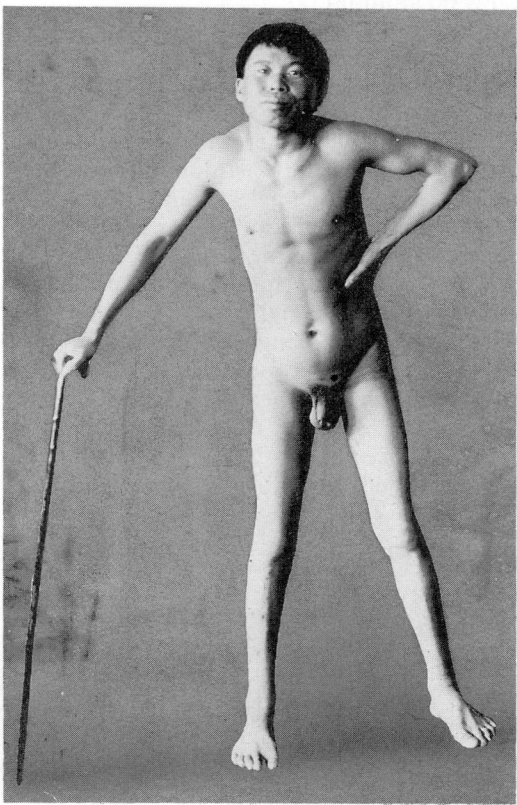

Fig. 46.3 Ataxic or paraplegic beriberi, showing the characteristic attitude.

A similar loss of sensation spreads up from the tips of the fingers. There is loss of sensation to pain, light touch and heat and cold, and deep sensibility elicited by compression of the Achilles tendon is lost.

A severe ataxia develops owing to the marked loss of postural sensation and the patient is unable to button his jacket or pick up a pin. The gait becomes ataxic and he walks with a high-stepping gait on a broad base, requiring the use of a stick (Fig. 46.3). The cranial nerves are not involved and there are no tremors. The bladder and rectal sphincters are not involved until the terminal stages.

Cardiac or wet beriberi (see also Chapter 61)

Cardiac beriberi is a high output right heart failure in which the circulation time is increased.

Oedema. There is generalized oedema of the arms, legs, hands and trunk and the face is puffy. The urine is scanty, of high specific gravity and contains no albumin.

Circulatory changes. In the early stages the extremities are warm and the pulse rapid. The blood pressure is low with a high pulse pressure. In the later stages when heart failure appears the hands may become cold. 'Pistol shot' sounds may be heard over the larger arteries and occasionally heart block may occur. The jugular venous pressure is greatly raised with a marked venous pulse in the neck due to tricuspid incompetence. The heart is enlarged to the right and the heart sounds are evenly spread, causing a tic-tac rhythm with reduplication of the second heart sound. A loud pansystolic murmur is heard over the whole of the precordium including the tricuspid area. Paralysis of the recurrent laryngeal nerve by a grossly distended atrium has been recorded. The liver is enlarged and tender and may pulsate. There is usually a single or double hydrothorax and ascites.

Radiography of the heart shows a typical globular enlargement affecting the right and left ventricles (Fig. 61.4, p. 1015). Pericardial effusion is rare at this stage. The electro-cardiogram shows distinct changes of low voltage, inverted or flattened T waves in all leads, a decreased P-R interval and a prolongation of the Q-T interval. Changes of right ventricular strain are also found.

Progress

Most patients die from paralysis and right heart failure complicated and aggravated by oedema of the lungs, diaphragmatic paralysis, hydrothorax or hydropericardium. Sudden cardiac failure is common (Shoshin of the Japanese).

Infantile beriberi

Infantile beriberi occurs in breastfed infants of vitamin B_1-deficient mothers, especially if they are taking a high carbohydrate diet. It can also occur in artificially fed infants if the feed is deficient in vitamin B_1 or the carbohydrate level is too high.

It is probable that vitamin B_1 deficiency is not the only cause of infantile beriberi[12] and that some of the features are caused by certain toxic products in the breast milk. It is considered that breakdown products from the incomplete metabolism of carbohydrate, especially methyl glyoxal,[13] are toxic to the infant.

Characteristically the onset is during the second and third months of life especially the ninth, tenth and eleventh weeks.[14] The baby is rather fat and flabby. The onset is with restlessness, attacks of crying, oliguria and a little

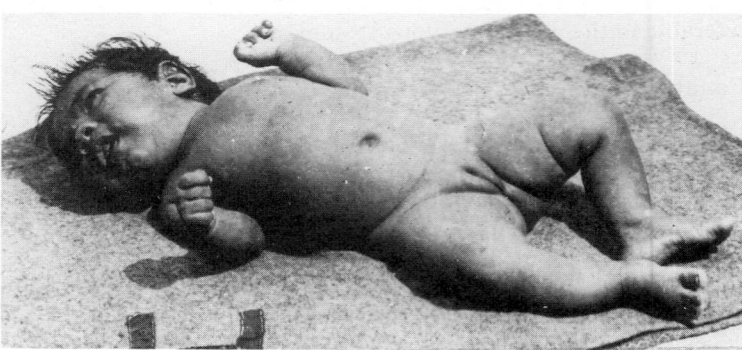

Fig. 46.4 A child in the convulsions of infantile beriberi. Note the generalized anasarca.

puffiness of the body. This may be followed by vomiting of the milk (Fig. 46.4).

The cardiorespiratory phase is the most dramatic and rapidly fatal form of the disease. There is a fairly sudden onset of peripheral and central circulatory failure. The lungs become moist, the heart enlarges with a tic-tac rhythm and the pulse becomes rapid and thready. There is venous engorgement of the neck veins with tender enlargement of the liver. Oedema collects and the child may die in 36–48 hours from cardiorespiratory failure.

A chronic phase occurs in slightly older infants. There is anorexia, loss of weight and constipation. Dysphonia and aphonia, ascribed to a paralysis of the left recurrent laryngeal nerve from pressure of the left auricle, are common and give rise to a characteristic cry. There is oedema and oliguria. Paralysis of muscles and loss of tendon reflexes are found (polyneuritic phase).

The thiamine concentration in the milk can be estimated.[15] The critical level may be about 6–7 μg/100 ml.

Wernicke's encephalopathy

The combination of ataxia, clouding of consciousness and ophthalmoplegia was described by Wernicke in 1881. Subsequently this syndrome was associated with chronic alcoholism. From 1933 onwards its connection with vitamin B_1 deficiency was suspected and a similar condition was described in a nutritional disease of silver foxes in America. Outbreaks of this disease occurred in prisoner-of-war camps in the Far East in the Second World War.[16,17] Diagnosis was established at autopsy by demonstration of haemorrhages in the mamillary bodies (see section on pathology, above). The cause of the syndrome was established as vitamin B_1 deficiency by the rapidity with which it responded to injections of vitamin B_1. Predisposing causes were dysentery, diarrhoea, failure to adapt to a rice diet and febrile conditions such as sepsis and malaria.

In 90% of cases of the B_1 deficiency type other forms of beriberi are associated. There are signs of severe disturbance of the midbrain with oculomotor signs and cranial nerve lesions with general clouding of the consciousness. The first symptom is persisting anorexia followed by cranial nerve lesions.

General signs include clouding of consciousness, insomnia, disorientation and semi-coma.

Oculomotor signs and symptoms include wavering of the visual fields on looking to the side, diplopia and photophobia. Horizontal nystagmus is the earliest sign. In a quarter of the cases there is an external rectus palsy, sometimes with complete disconjugate wandering of the eyes. There are loss of visual acuity, ptosis and retinal haemorrhages.

Other cranial nerve lesions occur in the trigeminal, facial, auditory and glossopharyngeal nerves.

The symptoms and signs are relieved promptly by injections of vitamin B_1, 50–100 mg daily.

DIFFERENTIAL DIAGNOSIS

Dry beriberi must be distinguished from alcoholic peripheral neuropathy in which there are associated tremors and mental changes including Korsakoff's psychosis; from tabes dorsalis in which there are Argyll Robertson pupils and posterior column changes; from arsenical neuritis in which there are pigmentation of the skin and hyperkeratosis of the palms and soles of the feet: from chronic lead poisoning in which there is a blue line on the gums and the neuropathy is purely motor; from lathyrism, in which there is a pyramidal lesion with spasticity of the legs, increased tendon reflexes and extensor plantar responses; from triorthocresyl phosphate (ginger or jake) paralysis in which there is a pure motor flaccid paralysis; from other nutritional neuropathies such as burning feet and combined degeneration of the cord when both posterior columns and the pyramidal tracts are involved. In the rapidly ascending paralysis of the Guillain–Barré syndrome the cerebrospinal fluid shows a raised protein content. Wet beriberi must be distinguished from other causes of right heart failure with a high cardiac output: anaemic heart failure, hookworm disease and also chronic nephritis. In famine oedema and epidemic dropsy signs of peripheral neuropathy are absent.

DIAGNOSIS

Laboratory tests. The pyruvic acid level of the blood is raised and is of diagnostic value. In acute beriberi the level of pyruvic acid is about 2 mg/dl and in untreated chronic beriberi about

1.5 ml/dl. After aneurine injection the level falls to about 0.5 mg/dl.

Red blood cell transketolase (RBCTK) levels are reduced and blood lactic acid levels raised.[18]

Meyer's test. There is an increase in the audible sounds in the antecubital fossa after the subcutaneous injection of adrenaline.

Volhard's diuresis test. In a normal fasting person after drinking one litre of water all the fluid is excreted in 4 hours. In beriberi there is water retention which disappears after treatment with aneurine.

Acute cardiac beriberi will respond dramatically within a few hours to the intravenous injection of 50–100 mg of vitamin B_1.

SEQUELAE: WET BERIBERI

It has been thought that there were no sequelae to wet beriberi but a case of gradually progressive congestive cardiomyopathy following severe wet beriberi in a Far Eastern prisoner-of-war camp proved fatal 30 years later.[19]

TREATMENT

Wet beriberi

The specific treatment of beriberi is with thiamine. Dramatic effects are observed in acute cardiac cases when large doses are given intravenously.[20] Immediate intravenous injections of 50 mg of thiamine should be repeated two or three times in the 24 hours until serial X-rays show that the heart has been reduced to a normal size. In moribund patients the injection has been made straight into the jugular vein. In severe cases venesection taking 250–300 ml of blood from the arm is of great value. In the ordinary case the patient should be confined to bed and given a high protein diet with restriction of salt and fluids and the addition of aneurine to the diet in the form of tablets or by intramuscular injection.

Dry beriberi

The treatment with injections of thiamine will relieve the pain and subjective dysthesiae. The signs of peripheral neuropathy take some time to disappear but results are disappointing in some parts of the world where the patients will inevitably relapse when they return home and resume a diet of polished rice.

Infantile beriberi

After an injection of thiamine improvement will be noted in a few hours; sometimes it is dramatic. In acutely ill children 25 mg of thiamine should be injected intravenously and a further 25 mg given intramuscularly once or twice a day until the symptoms have subsided, when an oral dose of 10 mg should be given daily for several weeks. The child should be removed from the breast and given artificial feeds for 24 hours while the mother is given thiamine. The breast milk must be drawn off and discarded so that after 24 hours she is ready to feed her baby again.

PREVENTION

Beriberi can be eradicated by the prohibition of the use of polished rice. This has been attempted in some countries but to legislate against the use of white rice in countries where rice is the staple food leads to the appearance of a black market in polished rice. Unpolished (red) rice and parboiled rice, in which the vitamin is retained, are good foods. Beriberi can also be prevented by using mixed diets containing other sources of thiamine, such as pulses, groundnuts, whole wheat, vegetables, fruit and milk.

Health education and the development of methods of milling rice in which the germ is not removed have led to the disappearance of beriberi from most eastern communities.

PELLAGRA

GEOGRAPHICAL DISTRIBUTION

Pellagra has been reported from most parts of the world where maize is consumed as a staple diet. Since the Second World War pellagra has vanished from most of its former range and is now found in parts of Kenya, Malawi, Lesotho and South Africa. It follows social disturbances and the establishment of large camps for internment or for refugees.

AETIOLOGY

Pellagra is a syndrome caused by a deficiency of a variety of specific factors with nicotinic acid (nicotinamide, niacin) as the most important. The amino acid tryptophan is a precursor of nicotinic acid in man, so that a diet with a high tryptophan but low nicotinic acid content is not pellagrogenic.

The richest sources of nicotinic acid are liver, kidney and yeast; important sources are wholemeal flour and green vegetables. Of staple foods maize contains the least available nicotinic acid, possibly because a large proportion of the nicotinic acid is in a bound form which can be liberated by alkaline hydrolysis and is achieved by the treatment of maize with lime practised in Central America. The daily need of nicotinic acid is about 10–15 mg but can be replaced by excess dietary tryptophan. Nicotinic acid is found in the tissues as a neucleotide, diphosphopyridine nucleotide (DPN) usually called coenzyme I, formed by the combination of adenine ribose phosphate and nicotinamide. There is also a corresponding coenzyme II, triphosphopyridine nucleotide.

Coenzymes I and II are the coenzymes responsible for the oxidative enzyme dehydrogenases and act as intermediate carriers for the hydrogen released from various substrates by the dehydrogenase enzymes. The enzymes containing nicotinamide are concerned with many of the important energy producing reactions of metabolism. Nicotinic acid deficiency leads to metabolic disturbances in many tissues and the nervous system is seriously involved. There is also an impairment of pyruvic acid metabolism in pellagra which is more marked in pellagrins with neurological manifestations than in those without. After the administration of nicotinic acid alone for 15 days the pyruvic acid levels returned to normal in a group of pellagrins, suggesting that nicotinic acid deficiency was the cause of the deranged pyruvate metabolism and there was a significant improvement in neurological status after nicotinic acid therapy alone.[21]

Pellagra appeared soon after the introduction of maize to Europe and advanced with the extension of maize cultivation. Epidemics of pellagra occur among maize (or sorghum) eaters. Pellagra is also found in non-maize-eating countries, such as India, Cuba and Brazil. In Central America where maize is the staple, pellagra is rare. This may be due to the treatment of the maize with lime which releases more tryptophan or to the consumption of coffee, which is rich in niacin. The cause of pellagra is more complicated than a simple deficiency and is due to the disturbance of a delicate chemical balance between certain toxins present in relatively large amounts in maize and some essential dietary factors, of which nicotinic acid and tryptophan are the most important. Leucine, for instance, which is plentiful in sorghum, affects the metabolism of tryptophan and nicotinic acid in man. Analogues of nicotinic acid can produce pellagra-like effects in animals but it is not certain whether these are the poisonous substances present in maize. The problem of pellagra is one of biochemical imbalances.

Secondary pellagra is due to non-absorption of the necessary vitamins by a non-functioning intestinal mucosa. It also occurs after prolonged treatment with large doses of isoniazid which replaces the nicotinic acid in the oxidative reduction coenzyme DPN.

PATHOLOGY

There is an increased excretion of coproporphyrin in the urine in pellagra which has been regarded either as indicating faulty metabolism or abnormal absorption. It occurs especially in alcoholic pellagra but Beckh et al[22] have shown that the amount of coproporphyrin in the urine is inversely proportional to the nicotinic acid intake. Since the oral gastrointestinal and neurological manifestations of pellagra can be evoked by exposure to sunlight it has been suggested that there is an abnormal porphyrin metabolism in pellagra. There is great emaciation of the body. The viscera show fatty degeneration and a characteristic deep pigmentation. The intestinal walls and villi, the liver and the spleen are atrophied. The suprarenal capsules may be atrophied and the cortex black; the medulla may be the seat of haemorrhages. The heart shows brown atrophy.

Central nervous system

The central nervous system manifestations were discussed by Spillane.[17] In the brain the main alterations are found in the Betz cells of the motor cortex and to a less extent in the Purkinje cells, the periventricular cell groups and the nuclei of cranial motor nerves. Chromatolysis, poor staining of nuclei and nucleoli and an increase of intracellular pigment are the most constant findings. The frontal lobes are most affected but the basal ganglia may show some degree of change. There is some endothelial thickening and hyaline degeneration of the walls of capillary blood vessels. In advanced cases there may be some gliosis.

The spinal cord shows a more or less symmetrical degeneration of the dorsal columns in the form of scattered demyelinization. The spinocerebellar and pyramidal tracts are involved to a lesser extent. The cells of Clarke's column show chromatolysis and pigmentary degeneration, the column of Goll being most affected. Myelin degeneration of the peripheral nerves of some degree is common. The myelin sheaths become irregular from swelling and atrophy and may present a honeycombed appearance.

CLINICAL FEATURES

The cardinal signs of pellagra constitute the well-known diagnostic triad: 'diarrhoea, dermatitis and dementia'.

Prepellagrous state

The initial symptoms are composed of vague psychological digestive disturbances which recur with repeated exacerbations and periods of quiescence for years without the appearance of skin eruptions. The patient appears pale, has a peculiar lifeless staring look with dilated pupils and complains of non-specific symptoms, giddiness and vague but often severe pains in the back and joints. The complexion is muddy with bluish leaden-coloured sclerae. The character changes, becoming irritable and at the same time stupid and morose. Since the earliest signs are difficult to define a great many people who suffer from chronic ill-health in an endemic pellagra area may really be in the prepellagrous state.

Other early vitamin B deficiencies may be associated with the prepellagrous state: angular stomatitis, an atrophic condition of the lips (per-lèche) and cheilosis (see p. 846) are associated with ariboflavinosis.

The disease may not advance beyond this point but may progress to the fully developed syndrome.

Gastrointestinal symptoms and signs

The gums become swollen and bleed easily (alpine scurvy). The tongue may be scarlet, raw and fissured and the lingual papillae atrophied. A characteristic symptom is pyrosis or a burning sensation in the oesophagus causing dysphagia. The appetite is variable. There is tenderness in the epigastrium and over the lower abdomen. There may be constipation but diarrhoea is common and the stools are often pale and fermenting, resembling those of sprue.

Skin lesions

The skin lesions appear on sites exposed to the sun and pressure. At first an erythema not unlike a severe sunburn is observed on the parts of the body which are as a rule unclothed and exposed to the sun. The eruption is symmetrical and characteristic. It appears suddenly first on the back of the hands and feet, then on the forearms, legs, chest, neck, face and sometimes on the scrotum and female genitalia, anus and other regions subject to mechanical pressure and irritation. The patches of erythema are irregular in outline and intensity. Very characteristic is a symmetrical eruption behind the mastoid process or a ring and collar round the neck (Casal's necklace) (Fig. 46.5). The affected area is swollen and tense and is the seat of burning or itching sensations, which become acute on exposure to the sun.

The congestion disappears completely but temporarily on pressure. Petechiae are common on the affected parts; blebs with clear opaque or bloodstained contents of feebly alkaline reaction may form. The eruption usually lasts about a fortnight and is followed by hyperkeratosis and desquamation, which leaves the skin rough, thickened and prolongedly stained a light sepia. This is specially marked on the backs of the hands and on the elbows, thus constituting recognizable evidence of pellagra. There may be malar or supraorbital pigmentation. Hyperkeratosis may follow and involve the whole body. Linear haemorrhagic strips of purpura may occur after exposure to the sun and after trauma, caused by increased permeability of the blood vessels[23] and was observed in prisoners in Indonesia.

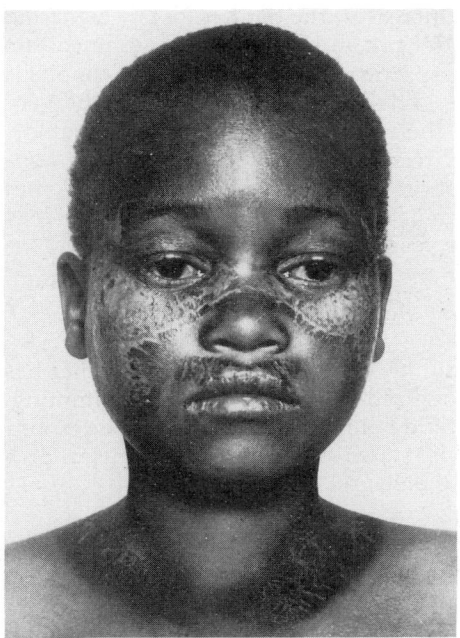

Fig. 46.5 Butterfly skin lesions and Casal's necklace in pellagra.

Pellagra differs in coloured races and erythema becomes a blackish or purplish patch on black skin. In olive-skinned races these appear sepia.

After the eruption has subsided atrophic patches of skin remain in the interdigital clefts and these, combined with wasting, produce the appearance of 'washer-woman's fingers'. The hands become aged and the nails atrophic and brittle.

Nervous system

The brain, cord and peripheral nervous system may all be involved.

Central nervous system

The time of appearance of mental symptoms is subject to the widest variations. They may be present from the start or occur during convalescence. The patient suffers from obstinate insomnia but occasionally from sleepiness. In general there is anxiety neurosis with depressive features and depression is common. Psycho-sensory disturbances are common with intolerance of bright light, colours and noises and the patient becomes fidgety, quarrelsome and irritable. General deterioration of mental and physical health may antedate continued manifestations of disease or acute mania and confusion may herald the end.

Encephalopathy and nicotinic acid deficiency

Acute encephalopathic states associated with a deficiency of nicotinic acid are accompanied by an acute metabolic disturbance of a reversible nature.[17] Certain stuporose and psychotic states in malnourished individuals have been found to respond in a significant manner to nicotinic acid. A certain clinical picture has been described of clouding of consciousness, cogwheel rigidity of the extremities and uncontrollable gasping and sucking reflexes. This syndrome has been observed in association with pellagra, alcoholism, polyneuritis, Wernicke's encephalopathy and scurvy. No response was obtained with thiamine, but after 1000 mg of nicotinic acid daily in divided doses parenterally, recovery occurred between the third and fifth days of treatment.[24] Stupor, delirium and acute psychotic symptoms are sometimes seen in association with a mild pellagrous rash and may respond dramatically to intravenous nicotinic acid.

Psychosis and pellagra

Pellagra may not only cause insanity but may result from it. It has been estimated that 4–10% of patients with pellagra become permanently insane and in the USA pellagrins used to be numerous in the lunatic asylums. Not only may pellagra lead to insanity but those insane from other causes used to be very liable to pellagra. It was found[25] that in certain mental institutions in the USA the number of mentally insane developing pellagra was a constant proportion of the total. In a review of pellagra in asylums in England it was found that at the time of onset pellagrins had been resident from six months to several years. The type of psychosis is a most profound melancholia with suicidal tendencies preceded by restlessness and insomnia; it may closely resemble general paralysis of the insane. The mental aberration may be characterized by profound dementia, hallucinations and catatonia.

Spinal cord and peripheral nerve disturbances

Disturbance of the spinal cord or peripheral nerves may precede, accompany or follow the cutaneous, oral and alimentary lesions of pellagra. In the early stages of pellagra the neurological manifestations are commonly those of a psychoneurotic kind but later peripheral neuropathy or paraplegia of the ataxic or spastic type or a combination of both may develop. Cord changes are commoner than those of a neuropathy. Tremors and rigidity, possibly of extrapyramidal origin, may occur. Burning, tingling and aching feet suggest neuropathy; exaggerated knee jerks and extensor plantar responses suggest a pyramidal lesion and ataxic paraplegia is not uncommon in the late stages of pellagra. The cranial nerves may be involved and eighth nerve deafness, retrobulbar neuritis and central scotomas have all been recorded.

The variable incidence of these neurological complications in different pellagrous communities and the fact that they sometimes appear after recovery from pellagra and are resistant to treatment with nicotinic acid suggest that they are caused by associated vitamin B deficiencies and are not features of pure pellagra. They are considered more fully in nutritional neuropathies (see Chapter 47).

Associated vitamin B deficiencies

Ariboflavinosis with angular stomatitis and cheilosis may occur in the early stages of pellagra. Burning feet is a common symptom in pellagra and is probably associated with pantothenic acid deficiency.

Ocular changes

The eyes may be affected with oedema of the conjunctiva, corneal dystrophy and lens opacities of three types—powder-like, multiple, irregular and tongue-like opacities—extending from the peripheral zone towards the centre of the lens.

Progress

The symptoms may abate two or three months after onset and although the affected skin areas remain dark and rough the disease appears to be arrested. Next spring, however, if the diet is the same, it recurs in a more severe form. The eruption assumes a darker colour and the depression of spirits deepens into melancholia which may have maniacal interludes with a peculiar tendency to suicide. The general feeling of weakness increases, the patient loses weight and is unable to work and his gait becomes uncertain and of the spastic paraplegic type. The tongue is tremulous. The pains in the back become very acute and there may be lightning pains, cramps, twitching, tremors and even epileptiform convulsions of the cortical type. Diarrhoea becomes troublesome. The symptoms of pellagra may persist for years unless the diet is improved.

Secondary pellagra

Pellagra due to voluntary restriction of diet has been recognized for several years; slimming, ketogenic and faddist diets have all been responsible. It is stated that hyperthyroidism predisposes to pellagra.

Surgical pellagra

Pellagra may follow upon surgical operations on the gastrointestinal tract, such as partial colectomy or total or partial gastrectomy. It may also be associated with some organic lesion in the gastrointestinal tract, such as oesophageal stricture, carcinoma of the stomach, pyloric ulcer, pyloric stenosis, carcinoma of the ileum, stricture of the rectum, rectal polyposis, Crohn's disease, chronic intestinal amoebiasis and malabsorption syndromes such as coeliac disease and sprue. Failure of biosynthesis of vitamins is a possible cause in these cases.

Alcoholic pellagra

Alcoholic pellagra occurs especially in America in those who drink methyl alcohol; it is possible that chronic gastritis interferes with the production of intrinsic factor and the absorption of nicotinic acid.

Drug-induced pellagra

Isoniazid, which is used in the treatment of tuberculosis, may cause pellagra when administered in doses of more than 300 mg daily by displacing nicotinic acid in the oxidative reduction coenzyme DPN. In these cases extra nicotinic acid must be given along with the isoniazid. Sulphonamides are also capable of interfering with the action of nicotinic acid and may cause pellagrous rashes.

DIAGNOSIS

In acute pellagra the blood nicotinic acid has been found to be below 0.31 mg/dl and to rise on treatment to above 0.55 mg/dl. A combination of localized erythema of seasonal recurrence with neurological, particularly mental, disturbance in a person coming from an endemic pellagrous area is not likely to be confused with any other disease.

The rash may be mistaken for acrodynia, erythema multiforme, dermatitis venenata, lupus erythematosus or eczema solare. The combination of mental and neurological signs must be distinguished from hysteria, cerebrovascular syphilis, general paresis of the insane, ergotism, lathyrism and other nutritional neuropathies. 'Pink disease' in children may also be mistaken for pellagra as the distribution of the skin lesions is similar.

TREATMENT

The most important part of the treatment of pellagra is to provide an ample and balanced diet and most pellagrins will improve as rapidly on a good hospital diet as on any other treatment. There is evidence that rapidly increasing the intake of one vitamin may precipitate imbalance and produce deficiency in another. A high energy diet is necessary—3000–4000 calories (12 600–16 800 kJ) with good supplies of fresh meat, liver, milk, eggs and in addition a source of the vitamin B complex, such as yeast 25–50 g daily.

Nicotinic acid

Nicotinic acid should be given in doses of 50 mg three times a day for 10–14 days and double this quantity in severe cases. There is usually a pharmacological reaction with tingling and warmth over the malar regions and neck, caused by vasodilatation. Overdosage may cause tingling and numbness of the tongue and lower jaw.

In acute mania or encephalopathy associated with pellagra intravenous nicotinic acid in large doses (1000 mg daily in divided doses) may cause a dramatic recovery. The spinal symptoms of pellagra are largely resistant to treatment and nicotinic acid has not been of much use in chronic psychotic pellagrins.[26]

Maize and sorghum, both associated with pellagra, contain large amounts of leucine, which affects the metabolism of tryptophan and nicotinic acid. Isoleucine counteracts this metabolic effect and Krishnaswarmy and Gopalan[27] have treated pellagrous patients (sorghum eaters) with 5 g of isoleucine daily, curing them in about 15 days. Controls kept on the sorghum diet without isoleucine did not improve.

Riboflavine

Since ariboflavinosis frequently accompanies pellagra, treatment should be reinforced with riboflavine 1–3 mg daily.

Parentrovite

Parentrovite is a multivitamin preparation which is of great use in the treatment of pellagra.

EPIDEMIOLOGY

Seasonal incidence

In Europe pellagra used to appear during the spring and autumn quarters, being most severe in the spring. In Egypt the incidence was similar. In Malawi, south of the equator, pellagra was prevalent during August, September and October, the southern spring. In the northern USA the disease exhibited the usual double incidence, the spring outbreak occurring during May and June and the autumnal in September and October. In the Deep South the disease used to appear as early as January. This definite seasonal periodicity indicates that climatic factors have an important though indirect effect and it is likely that exposure to sunlight, which exacerbates all the manifestations of pellagra, is responsible.

Sex

Both sexes are liable to the disease but in different places the disease exhibits a different predilection for one or other sex in accordance with the occupation and habits of the people. In the USA it was more prevalent in women of childbearing age because of the debilitating effects of menstruation, pregnancy and lactation. Old people living alone are especially liable, owing to their monotonous diet.

Age

Pellagra is a disease of middle age, the majority of cases occurring between 20 and 50. 'The so-called 'Infantile pellagra' is now known to be due to protein–energy malnutrition and is not a pellagrous condition.

Occupation

Pellagra is most prevalent amongst field labourers doing hard manual work. It is very prevalent among the prison population. Epidemics of pellagra commonly occur when an apparently healthy prison or camp population is suddenly exposed to hard physical labour to which they are unaccustomed, such as building an airfield or road.

Diet

The dietary factor is all-important. In the southern USA pellagra was common when the main diet was molasses and corn (maize). With improved social and economic conditions and the development of supermarkets, pellagra preventing foods such as milk and eggs became more freely available and pellagra has vanished from the community. Pellagra is a disease of poverty, backwardness and subsistence agriculture, in large populations of plantation labour.

PREVENTION

Pellagra may be prevented by a change in the economic and social conditions that cause it. In institutions and prisons the diet must not be confined to maize meal but must include fresh fruit and vegetables and foods containing vitamin B. Hard physical work must be avoided when the diet is not of a good mixed nature.

ARIBOFLAVINOSIS

GEOGRAPHICAL DISTRIBUTION

Ariboflavinosis is found worldwide associated with other deficiency syndromes such as pellagra and PEM and was common in prisoner-of-war camps in the Far East in the Second World War.

AETIOLOGY

Ariboflavinosis is due to deficiency of riboflavine (vitamin B_2). Riboflavine (vitamin B_2) is found in tissues as a dinucleotide, flavinadenine dinucleotide (FADN) or flavine, which occupies a key position in reactions leading to the oxidation of hydrogen to water. The main sources are meat, legumes, milk and wholemeal flour. Riboflavine is destroyed on exposure to light and signs of riboflavine deficiency occur when the daily intake is below 0.2–0.3 mg/1000 calories (4200 kJ). A daily intake of 0.35–0.5 mg/1000 calories (4200 kJ) is adequate but a daily intake of 2 mg of riboflavine is considered ideal for an adult.

PATHOLOGY

Lack of tone in small blood vessels is believed to be the cause of the lesions at the junction of skin mucous membranes and epithelial surfaces.

CLINICAL FEATURES

Sore red lips (cheilosis), a marked increase in the vertical fissuring of the lips (perlèche), a sodden fissured condition at the angles of the mouth (angular stomatitis) and a purplish raw tongue covered with granular enlarged papillae are among the most constant signs of ariboflavinosis.[28] Other signs are facial lesions consisting of seborrhoeic excrescences (dyssebacea), varying in length up to 1 mm and sparsely scattered over the face. The mouths of the sebaceous glands are plugged with inspissated sebum giving the skin a roughened appearance which, when it occurs on the shoulders, arms and legs, is known as follicular hyperkeratosis, phrynoderma or toad's skin. This may, however, be a manifestation of vitamin A deficiency and not caused by ariboflavinosis. Scrotal dermatitis, an eczematous condition of the scrotum, is due to ariboflavinosis. Ariboflavinosis frequently complicates other deficiency syndromes such as pellagra and PEM and was frequently associated with the deficiency syndromes occurring in prisoner-of-war camps in the Far East in the Second World War.

TREATMENT

Ariboflavinosis is quickly cured by the administration of 2–5 mg of riboflavine daily. Measures designed to improve the diet in a general manner and an increased diet of legumes, roots and animal proteins will prevent any deficiency.

REFERENCES

1   Jelliffe, D.B. (1955) *Monogr. Ser. WHO*, 29.
2   Jelliffe, D.B. & Jelliffe, E.F.P. (1961) *J. pediat.* **59,** 271.
3   Dunnigan, M.G., Childs, W.C., Smith, C.M. et al (1975) *Scott. med. J.* **20,** 217.
4   Dunnigan, M.G., McIntosh, W.B. & Ford, J.A. (1976) *Lancet* **i,** 1346.
5   Ford, J.A., Colhoun, E.M., McIntosh, W.B. et al (1972) *Br. med. J.* **ii,** 446.
6   Campbell, C.H. (1984) *Lancet* **ii,** 446–449.
7   Brigden, R.W. & Robinson, J. (1964) *Br. med. J.* **ii,** 1238.
8   Walters, J.H. & Smith, D.A. (1952) *W. Afr. med. J.* **1,** 21.
9   Wenckebach, K.A. (1928) *Lancet* **ii,** 265.
10 Weiss, S. & Wilkins, R.W. (1937) *Ann. intern. Med.* **2,** 104.
11 Blacker, R.E. & Palmer, A.J. (1960) *Br. Heart J.* **22,** 485–501.
12 Fehily, L. (1944) *Br. med. J.* **ii,** 591.
13 Sato, A. (1964) *Tukuku J. exp. Med.* **83,** 103.
14 Bray, G.W. (1928) *Trans. R. Soc. trop. Med. Hyg.* **22,** 9.
15 Simpson, I.A. & Chow, A.J. (1956) *J. trop. Pediat.* **2,** 3.
16 De Wardener, H.E. & Lennox, B. (1947) *Lancet* **i,** 11.
17 Spillane, J.D. (1947) *Nutritional Disorders of the Nervous System.* Edinburgh: Livingstone.
18 Sauberlich, H.E. (1967) *Am. J. clin. Nutr.* **20,** 529.
19 Gill, G.V., Hendre, L. & Reid, H.A. (1980) *Br. J. Nutr.* **44,** 273–274.
20 Hawes, R.B. (1937) *Trans. R. Soc. trop. Med. Hyg.* **31,** 474.
21 Bedi, H.K., Bombe, B.S., Agarwal, M.P. et al (1977) *Trans. R. Soc. trop. Med. Hyg.* **71,** 28.
22 Beckh, W., Ellinger, P. & Speis, T.D. (1937) *Lister Inst. prev. Med. coll. Pap.* **33,** 4.
23 Simons, R.D.G.P. (1946) *Ned. Tijdschr. Geneesk.* **90,** 351.
24 Jolliffe, N., Wortis, H. & Fein, H.D. (1941) *Archs Neurol. Psychiat.* **46,** 569.
25 Goldberger, J. & Wheeler, G.A. (1920) *Archs intern. Med.* **25,** 451.
26 Sydenstricker, V.P., Schmidt, H.L., Fulton, M.C. et al (1938) *Sth med. J., Nashville* **31,** 1155.
27 Krishnaswamy, K. & Gopalan, C. (1971) *Lancet* **ii,** 1167.
28 Bicknell, F. & Prescott, T. (1953) *The Vitamins in Medicine,* 3rd edn. London: Heinemann.

Chapter 47
Nutritional and Toxic Neuropathy

The peripheral nerves and spinal cord are susceptible to damage from nutritional and toxic factors and the result is the occurrence of a diverse group of disorders, the tropical ataxic neuropathies.

The syndrome of ataxic neuropathy, posterior cord and pyramidal lesions together with retrobulbar neuropathy and eighth nerve disturbances has been described from Africa (Central;[1] West;[2] East[3]) and from the Caribbean.[4,5] Similar syndromes have been described from the Far East in prisoners of war.

AETIOLOGY

An intact nervous system depends upon a series of intricate biochemical reactions. A variety of factors operating at different levels can produce selective damage to the most susceptible tissues. Those parts of the nervous system which carry the heaviest metabolic load are the upper motor neuron, first sensory neuron for proprioception and the optic and auditory nerves. The aetiological agent varies and may be a vitamin deficiency, a toxin or a combination of the two. Some of the toxins responsible are organic complexes in which cyanide is bound.

NUTRITIONAL NEUROPATHY

GEOGRAPHICAL DISTRIBUTION

In peace-time nutritional ataxic neuropathy, as distinct from dry beriberi, is or was common in Malaya,[6] Somalia,[7] India[8] and Jamaica.[5] During the Second World War it was almost universal among prisoners of war in the Far East and was common in German prisoners of war in the Middle East.[9]

AETIOLOGY

The exact nutritional deficiencies are not yet clear but two vitamins are known to cause similar conditions: pyridoxine and pantothenic acid.

Pyridoxine deficiency

Pyridoxine and its derivatives and their phosphates (the vitamin B_6 group) act as coenzymes for many of the metabolic reactions of amino acids including the transamination reactions. Pyridoxine deficiency may occur in patients undergoing treatment with isoniazid for tuberculosis. The symptoms of pyridoxine deficiency under these circumstances are pains in the soles of the feet which can be cured by adding 10 mg pyridoxine daily to the dose of isoniazid.

Pantothenic acid deficiency

Pantothenic acid occurs in nearly all foodstuffs, being especially abundant in liver, kidneys and yeast. The bran of cereals is a good source. It is concerned as a dinucleotide referred to as coenzyme A with reactions involving the active form of organic acids. Volunteers in whom pantothenic acid deficiency was induced by an antagonist, omega-methyl pantothenic acid, developed burning pains in the feet which rapidly improved on the addition of pantothenic acid to the diet.[5]

PATHOLOGY

The main lesion is central distal axonopathy[10] in which degeneration of the axons starts at the periphery and spreads towards the centre affecting those axons which terminate in the posterior columns. The optic and eighth nerves show similar degenerative changes.

CLINICAL FEATURES

This disorder is also known as chachaleh[7] (Somalia); barasheh; kalerichal; Gopalan syndrome;[8] dysaesthetic phenomenon;[9] pyralgia; melalgia; and happy feet. 'Burning feet' have been the only or outstanding complaint.

The symptoms commence slowly, taking some months to develop, with a deep aching in the soles of the feet spreading to the toes and instep, until eventually the whole of both feet is involved with the most acute 'pins and needles'. The pain is worse at night so that the legs are kept outside the blankets. The condition progresses with excruciating pain shooting up and down the feet and calves. The palms of the hands are only rarely involved. There is no erythromelalgia. Signs of peripheral neuropathy are minimal with some analgesia to pinprick and light touch, of stocking distribution, and diminution of the knee and ankle jerks. Most of the advanced cases exhibit signs of associated deficiencies with retrobulbar neuritis, eighth nerve palsy and ariboflavinosis.

DIAGNOSIS

Nutritional neuropathy differs from dry beriberi in that there is no history of oedema and the posterior columns are chiefly affected with evidence of a pyramidal lesion not found in beriberi.

TREATMENT

The condition responds well to the administration of yeast and other products rich in vitamin B as well as to pantothenic acid and pyridoxine.

SEQUELAE

Although many cases recover completely permanent sequelae have been noted in Far Eastern prisoners of war over 30 years after they were released. Persistent peripheral neuropathy, amblyopia and deafness with 'burning feet' were the main manifestations.[11]

TOXIC ATAXIC NEUROPATHY

The cause of toxic ataxic neuropathy is now known to be connected with a high concentration of cyanides in the diet.

CHRONIC CYANIDE INTOXICATION

The staple diet in many endemic areas such as East and West Africa and the West Indies is a root (cassava) or other vegetable rich in cyanogenic glucosides. Thiocyanate has been found in high concentration in the serum of patients with ataxic neuropathy and, although the total level of serum vitamin B_{12} is high in these patients, the proportion of free hydroxocobalamin and cyanocobalamin has been upset resulting in an inability to detoxify cyanide.[12]

PATHOLOGY

There are widespread patches of demyelination with a peripheral distribution affecting chiefly the posterior and lateral columns. There is perivascular inflammation involving the vessels of the pia arachnoid and spreading into the cord via the penetrating vessels.

CLINICAL FEATURES

The presenting features of these syndromes vary in different areas. Severe posterior column damage, retrobulbar neuropathy and eighth nerve deafness are the commonest presenting features. Pyramidal tract damage is rare and the burning feet syndrome is intermediate in occurrence.

The patients have a loss of joint position leading to a sensory ataxia. There is a relatively slight loss of superficial sensation or impairment of lower motor neurons and it is uncommon for there to be much impairment of upper motor neurons. The condition involves especially the lower limbs and is slowly progressive. Bilateral nerve deafness, often preceded by tinnitus, and bilateral visual deterioration, leading to optic atrophy are common.

In any one case it may not be possible to find out whether a toxic substance (cyanide) or a vitamin deficiency is the major factor. The diet should be a good mixed one and possible cyanide-containing staples must be avoided. Large doses of vitamin B_{12} (0.1 mg daily for 12–14 days), vitamin B_1, pantothenic acid and pyridoxine should all be administered. Response to treatment is poor and not much improvement can be expected in advanced cases.

EPIDEMIC ATAXIA[13]

Epidemic ataxia has been described from Nigeria[14] and Mozambique.[15] The cause is cyanogenic glycosides derived from cassava which under drought conditions formed 80% of the staple food and contained 85 mg/kg hydrocyanic acid (HCN). Owing to the drought the cassava was not stored and thus the breakdown of the HCN did not occur and the poor nutritional state of the people did not allow biochemical detoxification of cyanide in the body.

There are two variations in the clinical picture; in one, after a meal, there is acute onset of vomiting with coarse tremors of a parkinsonian nature and various extrapyramidal symptoms[14] with sometimes impaired consciousness and coma. In the other form the clinical picture is of an acute spastic paraplegia with sometimes optic and auditory nerve involvement and mild sensory disturbance.

TREATMENT

Improvement occurs with food and nutritional supplements and removal of the unstored cassava, but many patients are left with severe residual disability. The benefits of vitamin B_{12} injections are uncertain.

LATHYRISM

In this neurological disease changes take place in the lateral columns of the spinal cord, characterized by ataxic spastic paraplegia and caused by nitrile neurotoxins found in the hardy pea, *Lathyrus sativus*.

The disease occurs in Ethiopia, Algeria and India in the districts in which vetches, 'khashari', *Lathyrus sativus* and allied species are the staple food. There are two varieties of vetch, one larger called 'lakh' or 'teova', the other smaller called 'takhori' or 'teovi'. Cyanide-containing compounds have been isolated from the lathyrus family. *Lathyrus sativus* is more drought resistant and as the percentage of *Lathyrus* consumed rises during droughts, so the incidence of paraplegia increases, especially among active young males.

The lateral columns of the spinal cord are chiefly affected by a demyelinating process although associated posterior column changes have been described.[16]

The disease is very chronic. There is gradual onset of a spastic paraplegia which causes a typical 'scissors gait' (Fig. 47.1). Incontinence of urine and impotence are common and early symptoms. Ataxia due to posterior column changes is less marked but is found in advanced cases.

It is claimed that cases rapidly improve on dietetic and vitamin treatment.

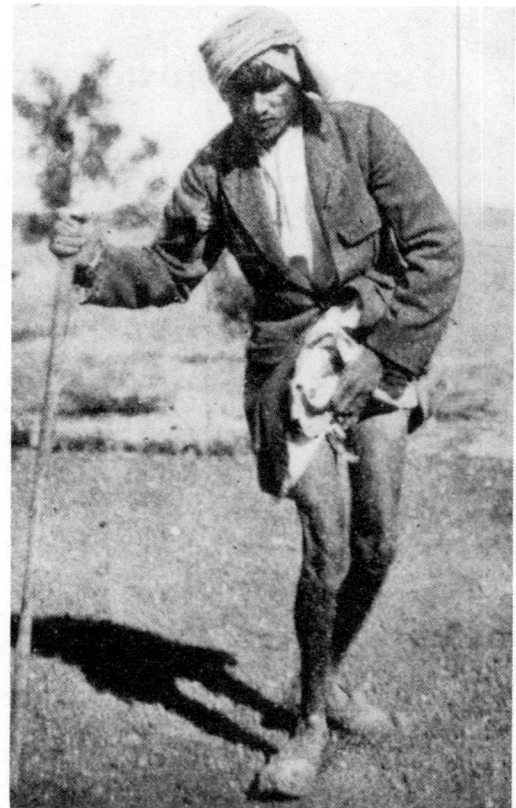

Fig. 47.1 Scissors gait due to adductor spasm in lathyrism.

REFERENCES

1 Stannus, H.S. (1936) *Trop. Dis. Bull.* **33**, 729.
2 Monekosso, G.L. (1968) *Abbottempo* **3**, 6.
3 Makene, W.J. & Wilson, J. (1972) *J. Neurol. Neurosurg. Psychiat.* **35**, 31.
4 Scott, H.H.(1918) *Ann. trop. Med. Parasit.* **12**, 109.
5 Cruickshank, E.K. (1969) In *Neurological Disorders in the Tropics*, ed. D. Williams. London: Butterworths.
6 Dugdale, J.N. (1928) *Malay med. J.* **3**, 74.
7 Buchanan, J.C.R. (1932) *Trans. R. Soc. trop. Med. Hyg.* **25**, 383.
8 Gopalan, C. (1946) *Indian med. Gaz.* **81**, 22.
9 Spillane, J.D. (1947) *Nutritional Disorders of the Nervous System.*Edinburgh: Livingstone.
10 *British Medical Journal* (1983) **286**, 917–918.
11 Gill, G.V. & Bell, D.R. (1982) *J. Neurol. Neurosurg. Psychiat.* **45**, 861–865.
12 Osuntokun, B.O., Monekosso, G.L. & Wilson, J. (1969) *Br. med. J.* **i**, 547.
13 *Lancet* (1984) **ii**, 904–905.
14 Osuntokun, B.O. (1972) *Br. med. J.* **ii**, 589.
15 World Health Organization (1984) *Bull. Wld Hlth Org.* **62**, 477–484.
16 Buzzard, E.F. & Greenfield, J.G. (1921) *Pathology of the Nervous System.* London: Constable.

SECTION XIII
VENOMS AND POISONS

Chapter 48
Animal Poisons
D. A. Warrell

VENOMOUS BITES AND STINGS

INTRODUCTION

Venoms are toxic, irritant or allergenic substances elaborated by some groups of animals to be injected into their prey or squirted at their enemies. Possession of venom by an easily recognizable and often highly coloured animal may confer protection on its species and the harmless species which mimic its appearance or behaviour. The venoms secreted on to the skin of some amphibians may protect their moist integument against infection as well as being distasteful, poisonous and therefore deterrent to predators.

Animals have evolved various methods of injecting venom into their prey or aggressors. Snakes, lizards, spiders, centipedes, ticks and octopuses inject their venoms by biting; fish, coelenterates, echinoderms, insects and scorpions do so by stinging. Poisoning which results from the ingestion of the flesh and viscera of aquatic animals is discussed in the second part of this chapter (see p. 893). Allergic reactions to injected venoms and ingested poisons are in some cases far more dangerous than their direct toxic effects. This is a large subject in its own right; here it will be referred to only briefly.

VENOMOUS SNAKES

TAXONOMY, IDENTIFICATION AND DISTRIBUTION

Of the more than 2700 species of snakes, about 500 belong to the four families of venomous snakes, Atractaspididae, Elapidae, Hydrophiidae and Viperidae. Only about 200 species have caused death or permanent disability by biting húmans. More than 40 species of another family, Colubridae, once considered non-venomous, have produced signs of envenoming in man[1] and three species have caused fatal bites. Among non-venomous snakes, only the giant constrictors (family Boidae) are potentially dangerous to man. There have been a number of fatal attacks by these snakes reported from Africa, South-East Asia (especially Indonesia) and South America. Some of the victims, even adults, were swallowed.

Snakes are classified on morphological grounds, from the arrangement of their scales (lepidosis), dentition, osteology, myology, sensory organs and hemipenis, and more recently by immunological studies of their venoms and serum proteins.[2]

Most legless lizards, such as slow worms and glass lizards (Anguidae), and legless skinks, may easily be distinguished from snakes by their closable eyes, friable tails or lack of enlarged ventral scales. Amphisbaenids have worm-like annular grooves along the length of their bodies and caecilians (legless amphibians) lack obvious eyes and scales.

All medically important species of snakes have one or more pairs of enlarged teeth, the fangs, in the upper jaw, by which venom is introduced through the skin of a human victim. Very rarely, bites by species with venomous oral secretions but no fangs have resulted in local envenoming (e.g. *Cyclagras-Hydrodynastes-gigas*). Approximately 400 species of Colubridae have short, immobile fangs at the posterior end of the maxilla (Fig. 48.1). The African burrowing asps (Atractaspididae), also known as burrowing or mole vipers or adders, false vipers, side-stabbing or stiletto snakes, have very long front fangs on

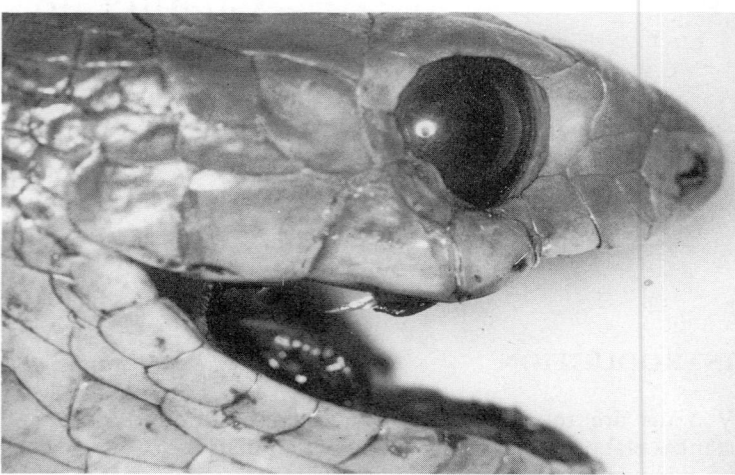

Fig. 48.1 Rear fangs of the boomslang (*Dispholidus typus*), a dangerous African colubrid.

which they impale their victims by a side-striking motion, the fang protruding from the corner of the partially closed mouth (Fig. 48.2).[3] The Elapidae (cobras, kraits, mambas, shield-nosed snakes, coral snakes and laticaudine sea snakes or sea kraits) have relatively short, fixed front fangs (Fig. 48.3). The Hydrophiidae, true sea snakes (Fig. 48.4) and terrestrial venomous Australasian snakes (formerly Elapidae), have short, fixed fangs like elapids. The Viperidae

(vipers, adders, rattlesnakes and pit vipers) have highly developed long, hinged front fangs containing a closed venom channel, giving them a structure like a hypodermic needle (Fig. 48.5). The subfamily Crotalinae (pit vipers) includes

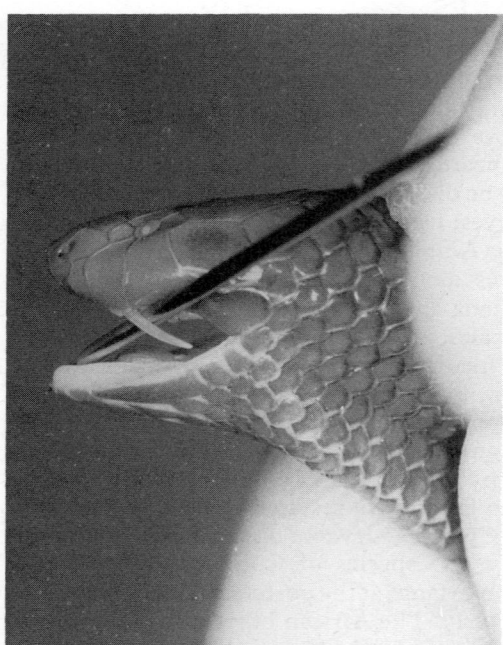

Fig. 48.2 Very long fang of a West African burrowing asp (*Atractaspis aterrima*: family Atractaspididae).

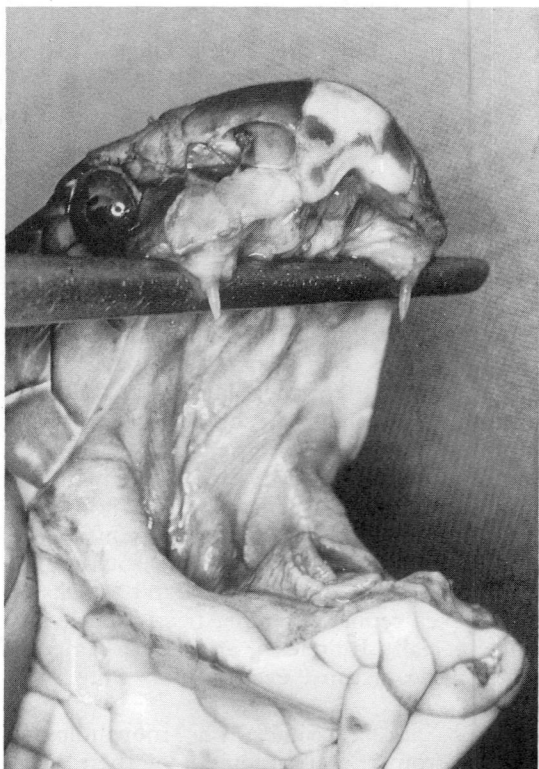

Fig. 48.3 Short front fangs of the monocellate Thai cobra (*Naja kaouthia*: family Elapidae).

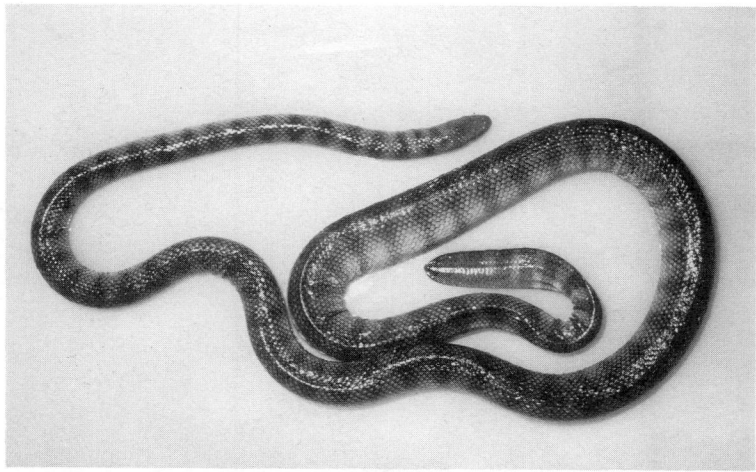

Fig. 48.4 A common sea snake of South-East Asia (*Hydrophis cyanocinctus*: family Hydrophiidae). Note flattened tail. Specimen 1.5 metres long, from the Gulf of Siam.

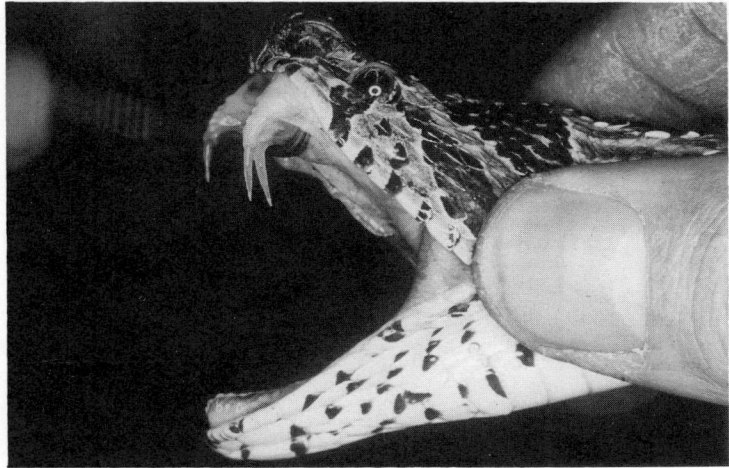

Fig. 48.5 Long hinged front fangs, with reserve fang on the left side, enclosed in dental sheath, in a Thai Russell's viper (*Vipera russelli siamensis*: family Viperidae; subfamily Viperinae).

the rattlesnakes (genera *Crotalus* and *Sistrurus*), moccasins (*Agkistrodon*) and lance-headed vipers (genera *Bothrops* and *Lachesis*) of the Americas and the Asian pit vipers (genera *Agkistrodon*, *Deinagkistrodon*, *Calloselasma*, *Trimeresurus* etc.). The pit of crotaline snakes is a heat-sensitive organ, situated between the eye and nostril, which detects warm-blooded prey (Fig. 48.6). Snakes of the subfamily Viperinae, the Old World vipers and adders, have no pit organ. The English words viper and adder have not been strictly applied to distinguish those species which produce live young (ovoviviparous) and those which lay eggs.

None of the care and skill lavished on the identification of parasites and their vectors is devoted by medical staff to the identification of venomous snakes. In some cases, however, a

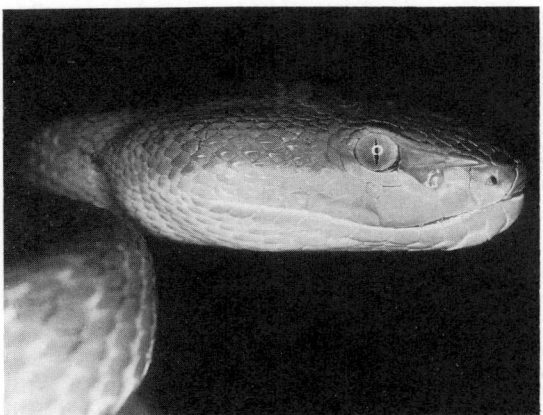

Fig. 48.6 Heat-sensitive pit organ of a common South-East Asian green pit viper (*Trimeresurus albolabris*: family Viperidae; subfamily Crotalinae).

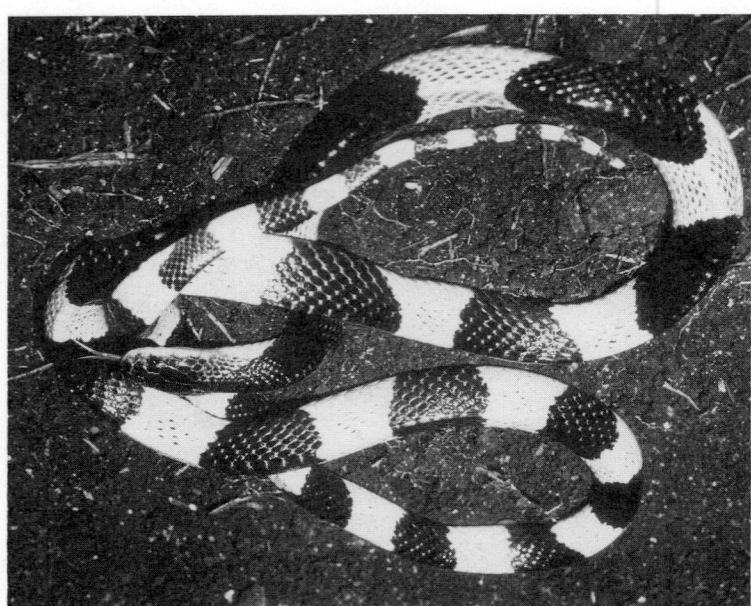

Fig. 48.7 Malayan krait (*Bungarus candidus*: family Elapidae). Specimen one metre long from southern Thailand.

precise diagnosis can be life-saving. For example, the two common South-East Asian kraits, *Bungarus fasciatus* and *B. candidus* (Fig. 48.7), are superficially similar in appearance, but monospecific *B. fasciatus* antivenom is ineffective in patients envenomed by *B. candidus*.[4] There is no simple and reliable method of distinguishing venomous from non-venomous snakes. The mouth can be examined for the presence of fangs but these may be very small in the case of elapids, and folded back inside a sheath in vipers. However, the most dangerous species are usually well known in the areas where they occur. The characteristic hood of cobras and some other elapids is evident only when the snake is rearing up in a defensive attitude (Fig. 48.8). Vipers are often identifiable by their repeated and sometimes colourful dorsal pattern (Fig. 48.9). Russell's viper (*Vipera russelli*) makes a very loud hissing sound by expelling air through its large nostrils, the saw-scaled or carpet viper (*Echis carinatus*) produces a characteristic rasping sound by rubbing its coils together (Fig. 48.10) and rattlesnakes produce an unmistakable sound. Some harmless species are readily confused with the venomous ones which they mimic: for example *Telescopus* and *Dasypeltis* species in Africa and *Boiga trigonata* in Sri Lanka with *Echis carinatus*; *Boiga multimaculata* with *Vipera russelli* in Thailand; various species of *Dryocalamus*, *Lycodon*, *Rhinophis* and *Cercaspis* with *Bungaris candidus*, *B. caerulus* and *B. ceylon-*

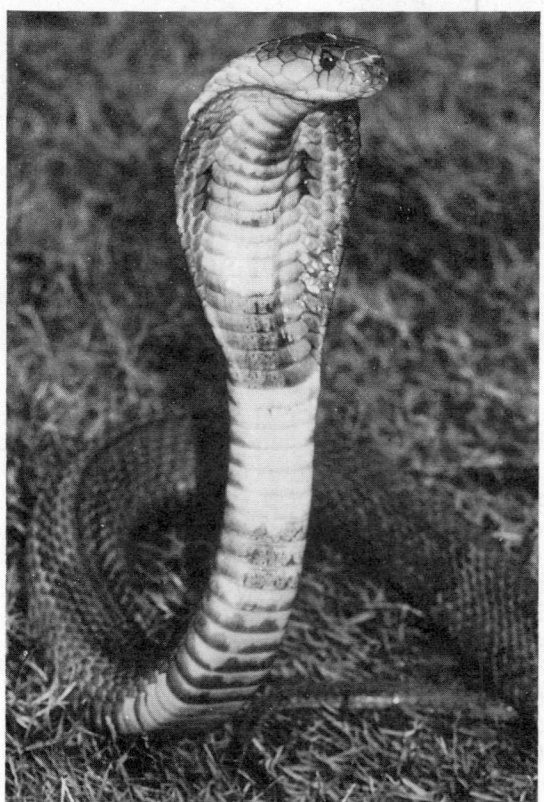

Fig. 48.8 Thai spitting cobra, brown phase (*Naja naja sputatrix*: family Elapidae) showing spread hood in threatening/defensive attitude. Specimen 1.3 metres long from central Thailand.

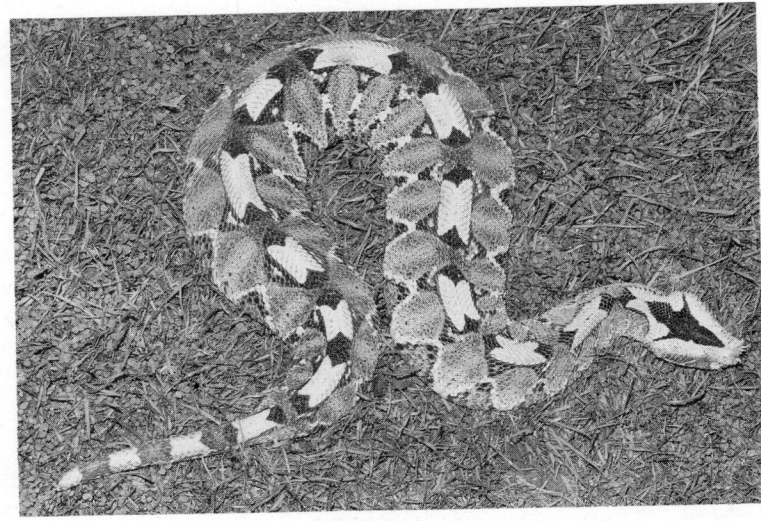

Fig. 48.9 Rhinoceros or nose-horned viper of the African rain forest (*Bitis nasicornis*) showing distinctive repeated dorsal pattern. Specimen 90 cm long from Cameroon. (Photographed by courtesy of Cotswold Wildlife Park.)

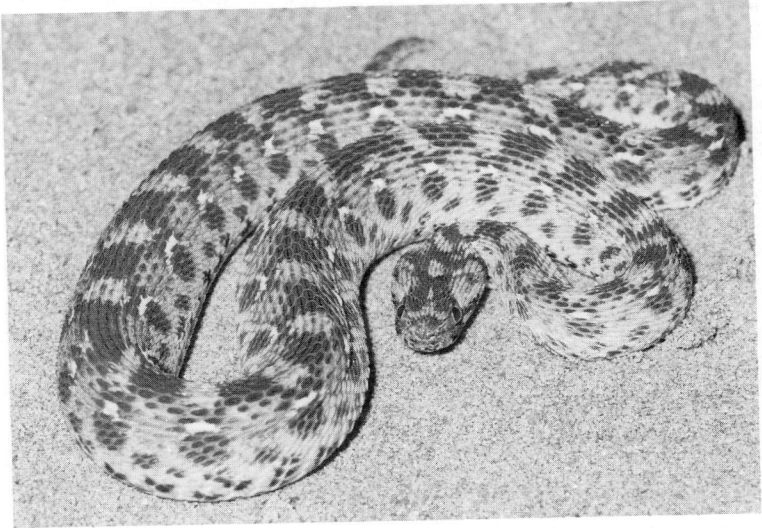

Fig. 48.10 Saw-scaled or carpet viper (*Echis carinatus ocellatus*). This species probably causes more bites and deaths than any other, worldwide. Specimen 55 cm long from north-eastern Nigeria. (Photographed by courtesy of London Zoo.)

icus. Table 48.1 lists the species which, in each continent, are responsible for most snake bite deaths and severe morbidity. Some species, although notorious for the potency of their venom (e.g. many species of sea snakes and Australian snakes), or their great size (e.g. king cobra, *Ophiophagus hannah*; gaboon viper *Bitis gabonica*; bushmaster *Lachesis muta*), have not been included because they rarely bite humans. The African night adders (genus *Causus*) and Asian green pit vipers (genus *Trimeresurus*) (Fig. 48.6) bite many people but rarely cause severe envenoming. Illustrated books, papers and keys have been published for the identification of venomous snakes in most parts of the world, but most are out of print and available only in librar-ies or through antiquarian booksellers.

Venomous snakes are widely distributed, up to altitudes of 4000 metres, especially in tropical countries. One species (*Vipera berus*) occurs within the Arctic Circle. There are no venomous species in the Antarctic, in most of the islands of the western Mediterranean, Atlantic and Caribbean (except in Martinique, Santa Lucia, Margarita, Trinidad, Tobago and Aruba), in Madagascar, Chile, New Caledonia, New Zealand, Hawaii and some other Pacific Islands, Ireland and Iceland. Sea snakes exist in the Indian and Pacific Oceans as far north as Siberia (*Pelamis platurus*), and in some freshwater lakes (e.g. *Hydrophis semperi* in Lake Taal, Philippines).

Table 48.1 Snakes responsible for most deaths and morbidity.

Area	Scientific name	English name
North America	*Crotalus adamanteus*	Eastern diamondback rattlesnake
	Crotalus atrox	Western diamondback rattlesnake
	Crotalus viridis subspecies	Western rattlesnakes
Central America	*Crotalus durissus durissus*	Central American rattlesnake
	Bothrops atrox asper	Terciopelo, caissaca
South America	*Bothrops atrox atrox*	Fer-de-lance, barba amarilla
	Bothrops jararaca	Jararaca
	Crotalus durissus terrificus	South American rattlesnake
Europe	*Vipera berus*	Viper, adder
	Vipera ammodytes	Long-nosed viper
Africa	*Echis carinatus*	Saw-scaled or carpet viper
	Bitis arietans	Puff adder
	Naja nigricollis	Black-necked spitting cobra
	Naja haje	Egyptian cobra
	Dendroaspis species	Mambas
Asia, Middle East	*Echis carinatus*	Saw-scaled or carpet viper
	Vipera lebetina	Levantine viper
	Vipera palaestinae	Palestine viper
Indian subcontinent and South-East Asia	*Naja naja, N. kaouthia*	Asian cobras
	Bungarus caeruleus	Indian krait
	Vipera russelli	Russell's viper
	Calloselasma (Agkistrodon) rhodostoma	Malayan pit viper
	Trimeresurus	Green pit vipers
	Echis carinatus	Saw-scaled or carpet viper
Far East	*Naja naja*	Asian cobra
	Trimeresurus flavoviridis	Habu
	Trimeresurus mucrosquamatus	Chinese habu
Australasia	*Acanthophis antarcticus*	Death adder
	Notechis scutatus	Tiger snake
	Pseudonaja textilis	Eastern brown snake

EPIDEMIOLOGY

The incidence of snake bite and its related morbidity and mortality has been determined most precisely in industrialized countries such as the USA[5] and Australia.[6] In the tropical countries where snake bite is a serious problem, reliable data are elusive. In many areas, traditional herbal remedies remain more popular than western style treatment for snake bite. Until recently, the majority of snake bitten patients in Sri Lanka were treated by ayurvedic doctors. Most patients treated at rural hospitals in Nigeria, Thailand and Burma had already taken 'native' remedies. Except in countries such as Sri Lanka, where ayurvedic and western medicine are accorded equal status, records of patients treated by these traditional methods are lost to the official statistics. Hospital records, the sole source of most snake bite reporting, are likely to over-represent the more seriously envenomed patients, and depend on the enthusiasm and workload of the hospital superintendent. Population surveys[7] and seroepidemiological methods may give a more accurate picture of the incidence of snake bite. Certain hunter gatherer tribes are at greatest risk from snake bite. Snakes were responsible for 2% of adult deaths in the Yanomamo of Venezuela and 5% in the Waorani of Ecuador. Gajdusek[8] found that snake bite was the most important cause of death in some villages in the kuru-endemic area of the Papua New Guinea highlands. The Phi Tong Luang of the Thailand–Laos border, the Hadza of Tanzania and the Aborigines of central Australia have also suffered a high mortality from snake bite. An estimated 15 000–20 000 people die each year from snake bite in India. In the 1930s the annual snake bite mortality reported in Burma exceeded 2000 (15.4 per 100 000 population).[9] Thirty years later it was still estimated to exceed 1000 (3.3 per 100 000) per year and has been as high as the fifth most important cause of all deaths. In 1984, about 900 snake bite deaths were recorded in Sri Lanka, an incidence of 6 per 100 000 per year. In the Benue valley of north-eastern Nigeria the incidence of snake bites was found to be 497 per 100 000 population per year with a mortality of 12.2%. Snake bite is also common in Latin America. There are an estimated 2000 deaths each year in Brazil and more than 10 000 bites a year with 200–300 reported deaths. In the USA there are 7000 venomous snake bites each year with nine to 14 deaths, and in Australia more than 200 bites per year with an average of 4.5 deaths per year during the 30 years up to 1977.[6] In Britain, there are more than 100 adder bites (*Vipera berus*) each year but there have been only 14 deaths during the last hundred years. There were 44 deaths caused by this species in Sweden between 1911 and 1978, and in Finland 21 deaths in 25 years with an annual incidence of almost 200 bites.

In tropical countries, snake bite is an occupational disease of farmers, herders and hunters. Rice farmers in Burma, Sri Lanka and central Thailand tread on Russell's vipers or inadvertently pick them up in a handful of paddy during the harvest[10] (Fig. 48.11). In the savannah of West Africa farmers are bitten by *Echis carinatus* as they dig the fields at the start of the rainy

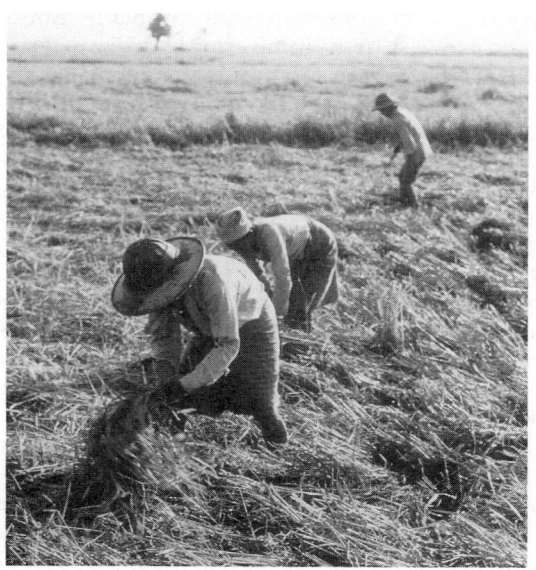

Fig. 48.11 Burmese rice farmers harvesting the paddy, an occupation with a high risk of Russell's viper bite.

season.[11] Rubber tappers in South-East Asia tread on Malayan pit vipers in the dark and are bitten as they make their early morning rounds of the rubber trees.

Sea snake bites have been an occupational hazard of fishermen in those parts of South-East Asia where hand nets are used. Records of 144 sea snake bites were collected by Reid and Lim[97] in north-west Malaya in 1955–1956. Mechanization of fishing methods in this region has resulted in a dramatic decrease in sea snake bites. The beaked sea snake (*Disteira-Enhydrina-schistosa*) has caused most bites and deaths. Other common and medically important species are *Hydrophis cyanocinctus*, *H. spiralis* and *Lapemis hardwickii*).

In the more industrialized countries, however, venomous snakes are increasingly popular as pets. Most bites are inflicted on the hands when the snakes are picked up and in the USA 25% of bites resulted from snakes being attacked or handled. Stories of unprovoked attacks by such species as mambas and king cobras can be discounted, but snakes will bite if they are cornered or feel threatened. Some species, notably *Bungarus caeruleus* in India and Sri Lanka, *Bungarus candidus* in South-East Asia and *Naja nigricollis* in West Africa, enter human dwellings at night in pursuit of their prey (rodents, lizards, toads) and may strike at a sleeping person if startled. Epidemics of snake bite have resulted from a sudden increase in snake population, for example after flooding in Colombia, Pakistan, India and Bangladesh, but in the case of *Echis carinatus* in Togo in the 1950s a dramatic increase in snakes and bites was unexplained.[11] Invasion of the snake's habitat by a large number of people may also be followed by an increased incidence of snake bite. This has happened during the building of new roads through jungles in South America and moving farmers to newly irrigated areas in the former dry zone of Sri Lanka.

VENOM APPARATUS[12]

Colubridae

The most primitive method for injecting venom is found in the back-fanged Colubridae. The posterior part of the superior labial gland (Duvernoy's gland) drains into a periodontal fold of buccal mucosa. The venom tracks down grooves in the anterior surfaces of the several enlarged posteriorly situated fangs (Fig. 48.1).

This arrangement is effective for envenoming the natural prey, for example a chameleon, which is held in the snake's mouth until it is dead. Human envenoming is a very rare accident. The snake must seize and chew at the finger of its victim, usually a herpetologist.

Atractaspididae

The venom apparatus of Atractaspididae differs from all other venomous snakes in many respects and the homology of the venom glands is uncertain.[12] In *Atractaspis engaddensis* and *A. microlepidota*, as in some species of Elapidae (*Maticora*) and Viperidae (*Causus*) the venom glands are very long—perhaps one-sixth of the snake's total length. The fangs and method of striking are also distinctive (see page 856).

Elapidae, Hydrophiidae and Viperidae

In these families, the venom glands lie behind the eye. Compressor muscles, principally the adductor superficialis in Elapidae and Hydrophiidae, and the compressor glandulae in Viperidae, squeeze venom out of the gland through the venom duct to the base of the fang. Venom is transmitted to the tip of the fang through a partially closed groove in its anterior surface or through a closed canal in the case of the Viperidae (Solenoglypha). In six species of elapid, the African spitting cobras *Naja nigricollis*, *N. katiensis*, *N. pallida* and *N. mossambica*, the South African ringhals or rinkals (*Hemachatus haemachatus*) and Asian spitting cobras (*Naja naja sputatrix*), the fang is modified to allow the snake to eject a spray of venom into the eyes of an aggressor. Instead of opening downwards at the tip of the fang, the venom channel is angled forward at its point of exit in the anterior surface of the fang, a few millimetres above its tip.[13]

The performance of the venom apparatus has been studied in very few species. The Palestine viper (*Vipera palaestinae*) can inject doses of venom lethal to its natural prey at each of 10 or more consecutive strikes. When snakes have bitten two or more humans in rapid succession the second or third victims were sometimes more severely envenomed than the first. However, Russell's viper appears to inject most of its available venom at the first strike. A high proportion of people bitten by some venomous species (e.g. Malayan pit viper) show little or no venoming. This suggests that snakes might be capable of biting defensively without injecting venom. There is little evidence that snakes can control their injection of venom or vary the amount according to the size of the prey. The snake's venom apparatus has been evolved to deliver a mechanically effective bite with injection of a supralethal dose of venom into the snake's natural prey. When the snake strikes at a human foot or ankle, it is far less likely, for purely anatomical reasons, that an adequate injection of venom will be achieved.

VENOM COMPOSITION[13a]

The most complex of all poisons, snake venoms may contain 20 or more components. More than 90% of the dry weight is protein, comprising a rich variety of enzymes, non-enzymatic polypeptide toxins and non-toxic proteins. Non-protein ingredients of venom include carbohydrate and metals (often in the form of glycoprotein and metalloprotein enzymes), lipids, free amino acids, nucleotides and biogenic amines. The precise role of most venom enzymes in the process of natural envenoming and digestion of the snake's prey is unknown. Enzyme function and pathophysiological disturbances are most clearly related in case of venom coagulants or procoagulants. For example, Russell's viper venom contains at least two proteases which activate the mammalian blood clotting cascade. RVV-X, a glycoprotein (but probably not a serine protease or arginine ester hydrolase), activates factor X by a calcium dependent reaction and also acts on factor IX and protein C. RVV-V, an arginine ester hydrolase, activates factor V. *Echis carinatus* venom contains a zinc metalloprotein, 'Ecarin', which activates prothrombin. Malayan pit viper venom contains a glycoprotein serine protease, ancrod (Arvin), which cleaves fibrinopeptide A from the fibrinogen molecule. Phospholipase A_2 is the most widespread and extensively studied of all venom enzymes. Under experimental conditions it damages mitochondria, red blood cells, leukocytes, platelets, skeletal muscle, vascular endothelium and other membranes, produces presynaptic neurotoxic activity, opiate-like sedative effects and the autopharmacological release of histamine. Few, if any, of these properties can be linked with certainty to pathophysiological disturbances in man. The acetylcholinesterase found in most elapid venoms is no longer thought to contribute to their neurotoxicity. Hyaluronidase may serve to promote the spread of venom through tissues, proteolytic enzymes (hydrolases) may be responsible for local changes in vascular permeability leading to oedema, blistering and bruising, and to necrosis. L-amino acid oxidase, which gives yellow viper venoms their colour, may have a digestive function.

The polypeptide toxins, often called neurotoxins, are low molecular weight, non-enzymatic proteins found almost exclusively in elapid and hydrophiid venoms. Postsynaptic (alpha-) neurotoxins such as alpha-bungarotoxin and cobrotoxin, contain about 60–70 amino acid residues and bind to acetylcholine receptors on the motor end-plate. Presynaptic (beta-) neurotoxins such as beta-bungarotoxin, crotoxin and taipoxin, contain about 120–140 amino acid residues and a phospholipase A subunit and prevent release of acetylcholine at the neuromuscular junction. Biogenic amines such as histamine and 5-hydroxytryptamine, found particularly in viper venoms, may contribute to the local pain and permeability changes at the site of a snake bite.

Clearly, snake venom cannot be regarded as a single toxin. The variation of venom composition from species to species explains the clinical diversity of snake bite. There is also considerable variation in the relative proportions of different venom constituents within a single species throughout its geographical distribution, at different seasons of the year, and as a result of ageing.

PATHOPHYSIOLOGY

Relevance of animal models

Studies of the effects of venom fractions in vitro and in experimental animals have contributed most of the available knowledge about the mechanism of envenoming. Many of the results of such studies are irrelevant to the interpretation of human envenoming. Unlike most experimental models, the human snake bite victim receives, usually by subcutaneous or intramuscular injection, a dose of the whole venom which is small in relation to body weight. Species differences in the response to venoms may also contribute to the different effects of venoms in animals and men. Thus, rodents, the natural prey of most vipers, die of massive intracardiac and intravascular coagulation within minutes of being struck by the snake and receiving a deep, often intraperitoneal, injection of venom, whereas humans die of haemorrhage, shock or renal failure days after the bite. The venom of the African spitting cobra, *Naja nigricollis*, contains neurotoxins which kill small animals by paralysing their respiratory muscles, but in humans the venom causes local necrosis.[14] Venoms of true sea snakes and Australasian terrestrial snakes (Hydrophiidae) also contain neurotoxins and produce paralysis in small animals, whereas in humans the most prominent clinical effect is generalized skeletal muscle breakdown.

Absorption, distribution and elimination of venom

Absorption of venom from the site of the bite depends on where the venom is injected, on the tissue binding affinities of the various venom components and their molecular sizes, and on local effects of the venom on tissue permeability and blood supply. Four hours after subcutaneous injection of *N. naja atra* venom, 70% of the neurotoxin, but only 33% of the cardiotoxin (which is basic and has high affinity for tissues) had been absorbed.[15] Intravenous injection of viper venoms may explain rare cases in which severe systemic envenoming develops rapidly with minimal local changes. At the site of injection, Russell's viper venom stimulates mast cells to release heparin which partly neutralizes the effects of the venom.[16] Viper bite wounds in humans show the histological changes of acute inflammation, haemorrhage, fat necrosis, and fibrinoid or hyaline degeneration of dermal and subcutaneous tissues. Krait (*Bungarus multicinctus*) bite wounds showed oedema with little inflammation whereas the necrotic wounds produced by cobras (*N. naja atra*) showed purulent inflammation and coagulation necrosis.[17] High local concentrations of viper venom coagulants may cause thrombosis of small blood vessels leading to ischaemic necrosis and, on rare occasions, the occlusion of a major artery. Venom hyaluronidase may promote the spread of other venom components through the tissues and contribute to tissue destruction. The toxic polypeptides of elapid and hydrophiid venoms are relatively small molecules which are absorbed rapidly into the bloodstream, whereas the much larger molecular weight toxic enzymes of vipers are taken up more slowly through lymphatics. The distribution and elimination of several isotopically labelled snake venoms has been studied in animals.[18] Most of the work was done using crude whole venom and it is uncertain which components were labelled. Most venoms appear to be concentrated and bound in the kidney and some components, but not Arvin,[19] are eliminated in the urine. Venom of the cottonmouth moccasin (*Agkistrodon piscivorus*) is selectively bound in the lungs, a number of crotaline venoms are concentrated in the liver and excreted in the bile, while neurotoxins such as alpha-bungarotoxin, are tightly bound at neuromuscular junctions. Most venoms and their components do not cross the blood–brain and blood–cerebrospinal fluid barriers, but some have been shown to increase their permeabilities. Some elapid venoms, notably those of the spitting cobras, can be absorbed through the intact cornea, causing systemic envenoming and even death in animals, and damage to the cornea, anterior chamber and uveal tract in man. Envenoming after ingestion of snake venom has not been reported in humans. In patients bitten by snakes, the symptoms and signs are explained by fear, the direct action of the various venom components on tissues, indirect effects such as complement activation and autopharmacological release of endogenous vasoactive substances, effects of treatment and complications such as secondary infections.

Local swelling

In the bitten limb, increased vascular permeability leads to swelling and bruising. The factors responsible include proteases, phospholipases, membrane damaging polypeptide toxins, hyaluronidase and endogenous autacoids released by the venom, such as histamine, 5-hydroxytryptamine and kinins. Venoms of some Viperidae, such as *V. russelli*, *V. berus* and *Crotalus* species, can produce a diffuse increase in vascular permeability resulting in pulmonary oedema, serous effusions, conjunctival and facial oedema and haemoconcentration.

Local tissue necrosis results from the direct action of myotoxic and cytolytic factors, possibly polypeptide toxins, and ischaemia caused by thrombosis, external compression by a tight tourniquet, or compression of arteries by swollen muscle within a tight fascial compartment.

Hypotension and shock

Profound hypotension is part of the autopharmacological syndrome which may occur within minutes of bites by *Vipera palaestinae*, *V. berus*, *V. russelli* and *Atractaspis engaddensis*. Presumably, this is caused by release of vasodilating autacoids. Leakage of plasma or blood into the bitten limb and elsewhere or massive gastrointestinal haemorrhage may cause hypovolaemia after viper bites. Vasodilatation, especially of splanchnic vessels, and a direct myocardial action may contribute to hypotension after viper and rattlesnake bites.

Bleeding and clotting disturbances

These are seen after bites by many vipers and pit vipers, some of the terrestrial Australasian snakes and the few dangerously venomous colubrids. Snake venoms can cause haemostatic defects in a number of different ways: venom coagulants can activate intravascular coagulation or, at lower doses, produce consumption coagulopathy leading to incoagulable blood. For example, procoagulants in the venom of Colubridae, *Echis carinatus* and *Notechis scutatus* activate prothrombin, *Vipera russelli* venom has procoagulants activating factors V and X, and many Crotalinae venoms have a direct thrombin-like action on fibrinogen. Some venoms, such as those of the rattlesnakes *Crotalus atrox*[20] and *C. adamanteus*,[21] cause defibrinogenation by activating the endogenous fibrinolytic system. Anticoagulant activity, sometimes identifiable with phospholipase, does not seem to be clinically significant. Thrombocytopenia is a common accompaniment of systemic envenoming and many venoms affect platelet function in vitro. Few studies of platelet function in envenomed humans have been attempted. In patients bitten by Malayan pit vipers and green pit vipers (*Trimeresurus albolabris*) there was initially inhibition of platelet agglutination followed by activation and the appearance of circulating clumps of platelets.[22] In the absence of trauma, defibrination induced by venom coagulants such as arvin is a relatively benign state. Spontaneous systemic bleeding is attributable to distinct venom components, haemorrhagins, which damage vascular endothelium. Some venoms, such as those of *Vipera palaestinae* and Saudi Arabian *Echis carinatus*, exhibit haemorrhagic activity without causing incoagulable blood.[23] The combination of defibrination, thrombocytopenia and vessel wall damage will result in massive bleeding, a common cause of deaths from viper bites. This group of venom activities is often referred to, inappropriately, as 'vasculotoxic', 'haematotoxic' or even 'haemolytic'.

Intravascular haemolysis

Although most snake venoms are haemolytic in vitro, this effect is rarely of clinical significance. However, envenoming by the South American rattlesnake (*Crotalus durissus terrificus*), some *Bothrops* species, Russell's viper (in India and Sri Lanka) and members of the colubrid genera *Dispholidus*, *Thelotornis* and *Rhabdophis* may be associated with massive intravascular haemolysis contributing to renal failure. Evidence of mild microangiopathic haemolysis is sometimes found in patients with severe bleeding and clotting disturbances.

Complement activation

Elapid and some colubrid venoms activate complement via the alternative pathway (e.g. 'cobra venom factor' may be the cobra's C_3b), whereas some viperid venoms activate the classical pathway. The role of complement activation in the pathogenesis of envenoming is unknown, but there are many possible interactions with the clotting system and other humoral mediators.[14]

Renal failure

Renal failure is a rare complication of severe envenoming by almost any species of snake, even those which usually cause only mild envenoming such as *Trimeresurus albolabris*, the hump-nosed viper (*Hypnale hypnale*) and *Vipera berus*. However, it is a common event following bites by Russell's viper and the tropical rattlesnake (*Crotalus durissus terrificus*); in these cases it is the major cause of death. Possible mechanisms of acute tubular necrosis are prolonged hypotension, disseminated intravascular coagulation, a direct toxic effect of the venom on the renal tubule, haemoglobinuria, myoglobinuria and hyperkalaemia. Russell's viper venom produces hypotension, disseminated intravascular coagulation, direct nephrotoxicity and, in Sri Lanka and possibly India, intense intravascular haemolysis. The mechanism in victims of *C. d. terrificus* is most likely to be intravascular

haemolysis combined with hypotension in some cases. Generalized rhabdomyolysis (see below), following bites by some Hydrophiidae (sea snakes and Australasian terrestrial snakes) causes renal failure through the production of myoglobinuria and hyperkalaemia. A large variety of renal histological changes have been described after snake bite.[26] Pre-existing chronic renal disease and the effects of antivenom (serum sickness) may confuse interpretation.

Neurotoxicity

The neurotoxic polypeptides and phospholipases of snake venoms cause paralysis by blocking transmission at the neuromuscular junction. Paralytic symptoms are characteristic of most elapids, such as kraits, coral snakes, mambas and cobras, but not of the African spitting cobras (*Naja nigricollis* and *N. mossambica*). Venoms of terrestrial Australasian snakes, sea snakes and a few species of Viperidae, notably *C. d. terrificus*, Pallas' pit viper (*Agkistrodon halys*), Sri Lankan and possibly South Indian *V. russelli* and berg adder (*Bitis atropos*) are also neurotoxic to man. Patients with paralysis of the bulbar muscles may die of upper airway obstruction or aspiration, but the commonest mode of death after neurotoxic envenoming is respiratory paralysis. Anticholinesterases, by prolonging the life of the neurotransmitter, may lead to a dramatic improvement in paralytic symptoms in patients bitten by snakes whose neurotoxins are predominantly postsynaptic in their action (e.g. Asian cobras). Some patients bitten by elapids or vipers are unphysiologically drowsy in the absence of respiratory or circulatory failure. This is unlikely to be an effect of neurotoxic polypeptides as these do not cross the blood brain barrier. An intriguing possibility is the release of endogenous opiates by a venom component or binding to an opiate receptor. For example, intracerebral injection of β-RTX (receptor-active protein) from *V. russelli* venom produced sedation in rats.[25]

Rhabdomyolysis

Generalized rhabdomyolysis with release of myoglobin, muscle enzymes and potassium is the principal effect in man of presynaptic neurotoxins of most species of true sea snakes and many of the terrestrial Australasian snakes (Hydrophiidae) such as taipan (*Oxyuranus scu-*

tellatus), tiger snake (*Notechis scutatus*), mulga snake (*Pseudechis australis*) and small-eyed snake (*Cryptophis nigrescens*). Patients may die of bulbar and respiratory muscle weakness, from acute hyperkalaemia or later renal failure.

Venom ophthalmia

Venoms of the spitting cobras and ringhals are intensely irritant and even destructive on contact with mucous membranes such as the conjunctivae and nasal cavity. Corneal erosions, anterior uveitis and secondary infections may result.

CLINICAL FEATURES

The symptoms and signs of snake bite victims result from fear and treatment as well as from the venom. Many patients anticipate a rapidly fatal outcome and the clinical picture may be dominated by physiological manifestations of anxiety or even frank hysteria. Thus, non-envenomed patients may complain of feeling flushed, dizzy and breathless, may feel constriction of the chest, palpitations and tingling and spasm of the extremities resulting from hyperventilation. Fashionable first aid and traditional remedies may produce harmful effects: congested and ischaemic limbs from the use of tight tourniquets, profuse bleeding and sensory loss from local incisions, vomiting and diarrhoea from herbal medicine, ruptured ear drums, and aspiration pneumonia or even respiratory arrest caused by the forceful insufflation of oil through a nasal tube, a popular ayurvedic treatment used in Sri Lanka. Patients may be physiologically drowsy, especially children who are reacting to an exhausting rush to hospital and parental anxiety.

The earliest symptoms directly attributable to the snake bite are local pain and bleeding from the fang punctures, followed by pain, tenderness and swelling extending up the limb and, later, by pain in regional lymph nodes. Early syncope, vomiting, colic, diarrhoea, angioneurotic oedema and wheezing may occur after bites by some vipers.[23] Nausea and vomiting are common early features of severe envenoming by many species of snake. There follows a description of the main clinical features following bites by the main taxonomic groups of venomous snakes.

Colubridae (back-fanged snakes)

Severe or fatal envenoming is reliably reported in patients bitten by five species of back-fanged colubrid snake: boomslang (*Dispholidus typus*) (Fig. 48.1),[26] vine, twig or bird snake (*Thelotornis kirtlandi* and *T. capensis*)[27] of central and southern Africa, yamakagashi (*Rhabdophis tigrinus*)[28] of Japan and the red-necked keelback (*R. subminiatus*)[29] of South-East Asia. Snakes of this family claimed the lives of two outstanding herpetologists; K. P. Schmidt (*Dispholidus typus*) and R. Mertens (*Thelotornis kirtlandi*). Severe envenoming is possible only if the snake is able to retain its grip and chew for 15 seconds or longer. All five species give rise to similar symptoms. Nausea with repeated vomiting, colicky abdominal pain and headache develop hours after the bite. There is bleeding from old and recent wounds such as venepunctures, and spontaneous gingival bleeding, epistaxis, haematemesis, melaena, subarachnoid haemorrhage, haematuria and extensive ecchymoses. Intravascular haemolysis and microangiopathic haemolysis have been described. Most of the fatal cases died of renal failure from acute tubular necrosis many days after the bite. Local effects of the venom are usually trivial but several patients showed some local swelling and one bitten by *Dispholidus typus* had massive swelling with blood-filled bullae. Investigations reveal incoagulable blood, defibrination, elevated fibrin degradation products (FDPs), severe thrombocytopenia and anaemia. These clinical features are explained by disseminated intravascular coagulation triggered by a venom procoagulant which activates prothrombin.

Atractaspididae (burrowing asps)

Thirteen species of the genus *Atractaspis* have been described in Africa and the Middle East. All are venomous, but fatal or near fatal envenoming has been described in only three species: *A. microleptidota*, *A. irregularis* and *A. engaddensis*.[30] Local effects include pain, swelling, blistering, necrosis, tender enlargement of local lymph nodes and in some cases local numbness or paraesthesiae in areas conforming to the distribution of a cutaneous nerve. The commonest systemic symptom is fever. Most of the fatal cases died within 45 minutes of the bite after vomiting, producing profuse saliva and lapsing into coma. Severe envenoming by *A. engaddensis* may produce violent autonomic symptoms (nausea, vomiting and diarrhoea) within minutes of the bite. One patient developed severe dyspnoea with acute respiratory failure and two showed abnormal electrocardiograms (ST-T changes and prolonged PR interval). Rarely, mild abnormalities of blood coagulation and liver function have also been described. *Atractaspis* venom has very high lethal toxicity. Recently, the venom of *A. engaddensis* was shown to contain a cardiotoxin which causes coronary vasoconstriction. The venom also contains haemorrhagic and necrotic factors.[31]

Elapidae (cobras, kraits, mambas and coral snakes)

Elapid venoms are best known for their neurotoxic effects. In the case of kraits, mambas, coral snakes and some of the cobras (e.g. Egyptian cobra, *Naja haje*; Cape cobra, *Naja nivea*), local effects are minimal. However, patients bitten by African spitting cobras (*N. nigricollis*, *N. pallida* and *N. mossambica*) and Asian cobras (*N. naja*, *N. kaouthia*, etc.) commonly develop tender local swelling which may be extensive (Fig. 48.12) and

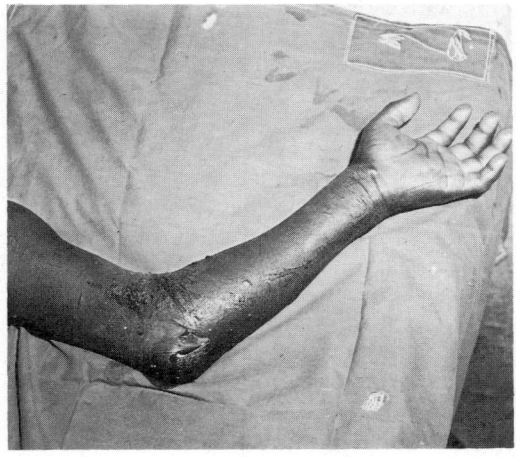

Fig. 48.12 Massive swelling of arm and trunk in a Nigerian boy 3 days after being bitten on the elbow by a black-necked spitting cobra (*Naja nigricollis*). Early necrosis is visible at the site of the bite.

regional lymphadenopathy. Blistering may appear within 24 hours, often at the edge of a demarcated pale or blackened anaesthetic area of skin (Fig. 48.13). The lesion smells putrid and eventually breaks down with loss of skin and subcutaneous tissue which may be extensive

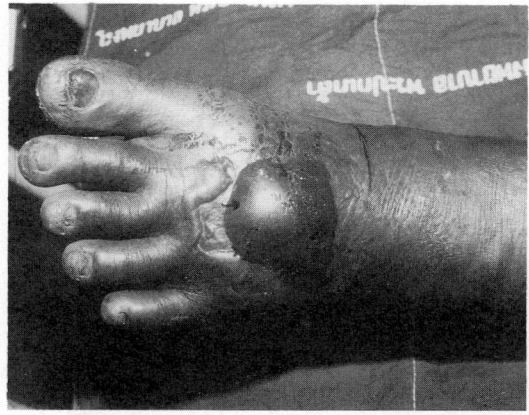

Fig. 48.13 Blistering which appeared 36 hours after a bite by a monocellate Thai cobra (*Naja kaouthia*). Necrosis is an inevitable consequence of blistering caused by cobra bites.

(Fig. 48.14). Prolonged morbidity may result and some patients may lose the affected limb if there is secondary infection. Severe envenoming by the king cobra (*Ophiophagus hannah*) resulted in swelling of the whole limb and formation of bullae at the site of the bite but there was minimal local necrosis.[98] However, rapidly developing

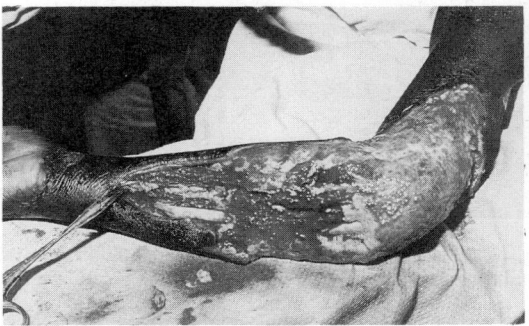

Fig. 48.14 Extensive loss of skin and ulnar compartment muscles in a patient bitten by a black-necked or spitting cobra (*Naja nigricollis*).

neurotoxicity is the dominant clinical feature of patients envenomed by this species. Neurotoxic effects[32] are also seen in patients envenomed by Asian cobras and other elapids, but have yet to be documented adequately in victims of African spitting cobras. The earliest symptom of systemic envenoming is repeated vomiting, but the use of emetic herbal medicines may confuse the interpretation of this symptom. Other early preparalytic symptoms include contraction of the frontalis (before there is demonstrable ptosis), blurred vision, paraesthesiae especially around the mouth, hyperacusis, headache, dizziness, vertigo and signs of autonomic nervous stimulation such as hypersalivation, congested conjunctivae and 'gooseflesh'. Paralysis is first detectable as ptosis and external opthalmoplegia, as these muscles are most sensitive to neuromuscular blockade (Fig. 48.15). These signs may

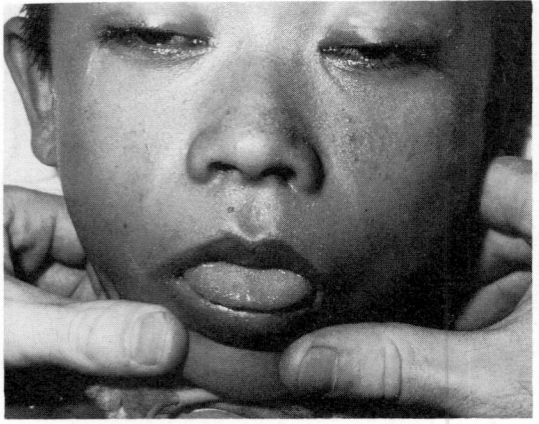

Fig. 48.16 Ptosis and inability to open the mouth or protrude the tongue in a Thai patient bitten by a Malayan krait (*Bungarus candidus*).

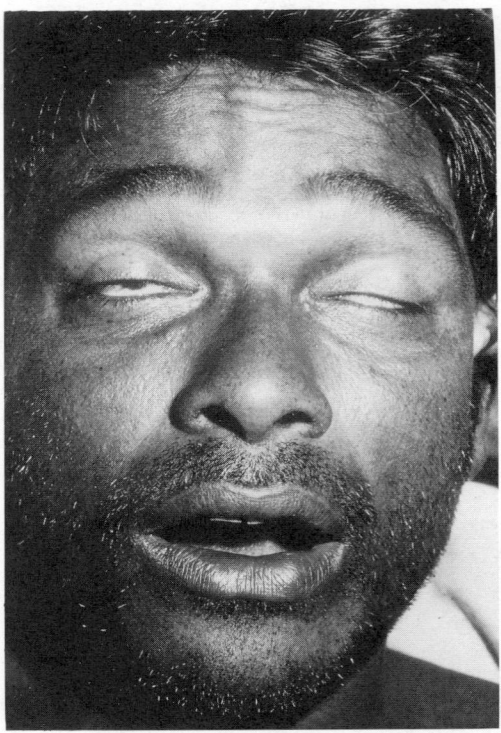

Fig. 48.15 Severe ptosis, external ophthalmoplegia and inability to open the mouth, protrude the tongue or swallow in a Sri Lankan patient bitten by a common Indian krait (*Bungarus caeruleus*).

appear as early as 15 minutes after the bite (cobras or mambas) but may be delayed for 10 hours or more following krait bites. Later, the palate, jaws, tongue, vocal cords, neck muscles and muscles of deglutition may become paralysed (Fig. 48.16). At this stage respiratory arrest may be precipitated by obstruction of the upper airway by the paralysed tongue or inhaled vomitus. Intercostal muscles are affected before the limbs, diaphragm and superficial muscles and, even in patients with generalized flaccid paralysis, slight movements of the digits may be possible. Loss of consciousness and generalized convulsions are usually ex-

plained by hypoxaemia in patients who have respiratory paralysis. However, drowsiness, before the development of significant paralysis, has often been described but remains unexplained. In patients whose eyelids are drooping as a result of physiological tiredness, ptosis may be inferred incorrectly, unless the extent of lid retraction with upward gaze is formally assessed. Patients with systemic envenoming suffer from headache, malaise, and generalized myalgia. Intractable hypotension can occur in patients envenomed by Asian cobras, despite adequate respiratory support. Neurotoxic effects are completely reversible either acutely in response to antivenom or (for example in Asian cobra bites) anticholinesterases,[33] or they may slowly wear off spontaneously. In the absence of specific antivenom, patients supported by mechanical ventilators recover sufficient diaphragmatic movement to breathe adequately in 1–4 days. Ocular muscles recover in 2–4 days and there is usually full recovery of motor function in 3–7 days.

Snake venom ophthalmia (see also Chapter 70, p. 1179)

Venom ophthalmia may result when venom of the spitting elapids (see above) enters the eye. There is intense local pain, blepharospasm, palpebral oedema and leukorrhoea (Fig. 48.17). Slit lamp or fluorescein examination reveals corneal erosions in more than half the patients spat at by *N. nigricollis*.[34] Secondary infection of the corneal lesions may result in permanent opacities causing blindness or panophthalmitis with loss

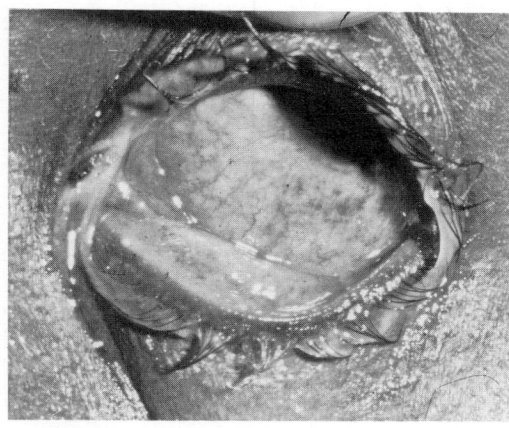

Fig. 48.17 Intense conjunctivitis with leukorrheoa (and corneal erosions) in a patient 'spat' at 3 hours previously by a West African black-necked or spitting cobra (*Naja nigricollis*).

of the eye. Rarely venom is absorbed into the anterior chamber causing hypopyon and anterior uveitis.

Hydrophiidae (true sea snakes and terrestrial Australasian snakes)

Bites by terrestrial Australasian snakes

Venoms of these snakes formerly classified as Elapidae result in three main groups of symptoms: neurotoxicity similar to that seen with elapid bites, generalized rhabdomyolysis and haemostatic disturbances. Local signs are usually mild, but extensive local swelling and bruising with localized necrosis has been reported, especially after bites by the king brown or mulga snake (*Pseudechis australis*). Painful and tender local lymph nodes are a common feature in patients developing systemic envenoming. Early symptoms include vomiting, headache and syncopal attacks similar to those experienced after some viper bites (see below).

Persistent bleeding from wounds and spontaneous systemic bleeding from gums and gastrointestinal tract is found in association with incoagulable blood following bites by many Australasian species. Venoms of 15 out of 19 species exhibited procoagulant activity in vitro.[35] Haemostatic abnormalities are particularly frequent and serious in patients bitten by tiger snakes (*Notechis* species), taipans (*Oxyuranus* species), and brown snakes (*Pseudonaja* species), but never with bites by death adders (*Acan-*

thophis species) and rarely, if ever, with bites by black snakes (*Pseudechis* species).

In the past, there has been some confusion between haemoglobinuria and myoglobinuria in patients passing dark urine. It is now clear, however, that haemoglobinaemia and haemoglobinuria occur as a result of intravascular haemolysis (e.g. with envenoming by *Pseudechis australis*) but that myoglobinuria caused by generalized rhabdomyolysis (see below) is also a feature of envenoming by some species (e.g. *Notechis*, *Oxyuranus* and *Pseudechis australis*). Renal failure may result from haemoglobinuria or myoglobinuria.

Neurotoxicity is an important feature of bites by terrestrial Australasian hydrophiids. Clinical features are identical to those produced by elapid venoms (see above) and develop 1–10 (mean $5\frac{1}{2}$) hours after the bite.[32]

Bites by true sea snakes[36]

Generalized rhabdomyolysis is the dominant feature of envenoming by these snakes and also occurs after bites by some of the terrestrial Australasian snakes such as the taipan (*Oxyuranus scutellatus*), tiger snake (*Notechis scutatus*), mulga snake (*Pseudechis australis*) and small-eyed snake (*Cryptophis nigrescens*). Early symptoms of sea snake bite poisoning include headache, a thick feeling of the tongue, thirst, sweating and vomiting. Generalized aching, stiffness and tenderness of the muscles becomes noticeable between 30 minutes and $3\frac{1}{2}$ hours after the bite. Trismus is a common feature. Passive stretching of the muscles is resisted. Later, there is generalized flaccid paralysis but the patient remains conscious until the respiratory muscles are sufficiently affected to cause respiratory failure. Myoglobinaemia and myoglobinuria develop 3–8 hours after the bite. These are suspected when the serum/plasma appears brownish and the urine dark reddish brown. 'Stix' tests will appear positive for haemoglobin/blood in urine containing myoglobin. Myoglobin and potassium released from damaged skeletal muscles may cause renal failure, while hyperkalaemia may lead to cardiac arrest.

Viperidae (Old World pitless vipers and adders, New World rattlesnakes, moccasins and lance-headed vipers, Asian pit vipers)

In general, venoms of vipers and pit vipers

produce more local effects than other snake venoms. Swelling may appear within 15 minutes, but rarely is delayed for several hours. It spreads rapidly, sometimes involving the whole limb and adjacent trunk. There is associated pain, tenderness and enlargement of regional lymph nodes. Bruising, especially along the path of superficial lymphatics and over regional lymph nodes is commonly seen and there may be persistent bleeding from the fang marks. Swollen limbs can accommodate many litres of extravasated blood leading to hypovolaemic shock. Blistering may appear at the bite site as early as 12 hours after the bite. Blisters may be filled with clear or bloodstained fluid and, in cases of severe envenoming, extend up the bitten limb (Fig. 48.18). Necrosis of skin, subcutaneous tissue and muscle (Fig. 48.19) may develop in up to 10% of

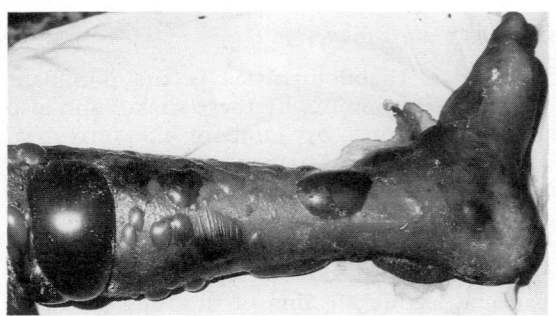

Fig. 48.18 Massive swelling and bulla formation in a Thai patient 36 hours after being bitten by a Malayan pit viper (*Calloselasma rhodostoma*).

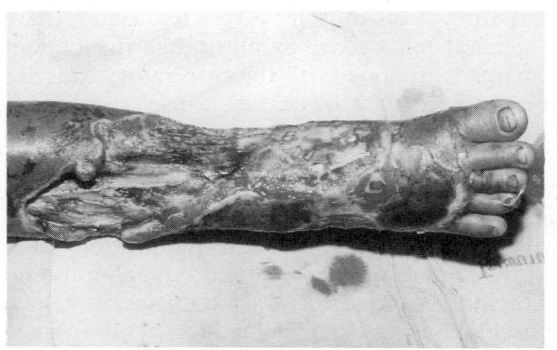

Fig. 48.19 Extensive necrosis of skin and muscle in a 5-year-old child 10 days after being bitten by a Malayan pit viper (*Calloselasma rhodostoma*).

hospitalized cases, especially following bites by rattlesnakes (e.g. *Crotalus adamanteus*, *C. atrox*, *C. horridus* and *C. viridis*), South American lance-headed vipers (genus *Bothrops*) and the

bushmaster (*Lachesis muta*) and Asian pit vipers (e.g. *Calloselasma rhodostoma*, *Deinagkistrodon acutus* and *Trimeresurus flavoviridis*), African giant vipers (genus *Bitis*), saw-scaled viper (*Echis carinatus*) and Palestine viper (*V. palaestinae*). Bites on the digits and in areas draining into the tight fascial compartments, such as the anterior tibial compartment (Fig. 48.20), are particularly likely to cause necrosis.

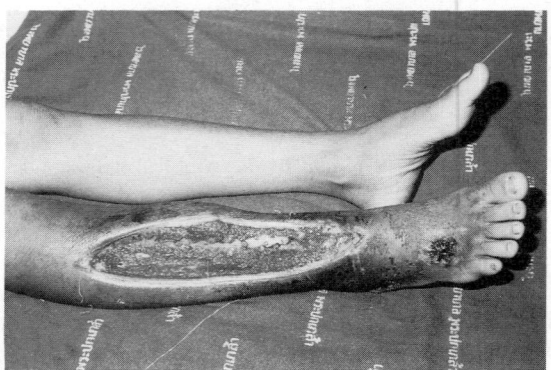

Fig. 48.20 Necrosis of muscles of the anterior tibial compartment in a Thai woman bitten on the dorsum of the foot by a Malayan pit viper (*Calloselasma rhodostoma*). There is healing with granulation tissue after surgical débridement.

In these cases high intracompartmental pressure may add ischaemic necrosis to the direct necrotic effects of the venom. Very severe pain associated with tense swelling, subcutaneous anaesthesia, and pain on stretching the intracompartmental muscles (e.g. dorsiflexion of the foot in the case of the anterior tibial compartment) should raise the possibility of raised intracompartmental pressure.[37] Sudden severe pain, absence of arterial pulses and a demarcated cold segment of limb suggests thrombosis of a major artery. The absence of detectable local swelling 2 hours after a viper bite usually means that no venom was injected. However, there are important exceptions to this rule: fatal systemic envenoming by the tropical rattlesnake (*Crotalus durissus terrificus*), Mojave rattlesnake (*Crotalus scutellatus*) and Burmese Russell's viper (*V. r. siamensis*) may occur in the absence of local signs. In fact, patients bitten by *C. d. terrificus* rarely show any local swelling.

Haemostatic abnormalities are characteristic of envenoming by Viperidae, but are usually completely absent in patients bitten by the smaller European vipers (*V. berus*, *V. aspis*, *V. ammodytes*, etc.) and some species of rattlesnakes. Persistent bleeding from the fang puncture wounds and from new injuries such as venepuncture sites and from old partially healed wounds may be the first clinical evidence of a bleeding diathesis. Spontaneous systemic haemorrhage is most often detected in the gingival sulci (Fig. 48.21). Saliva and sputum may contain

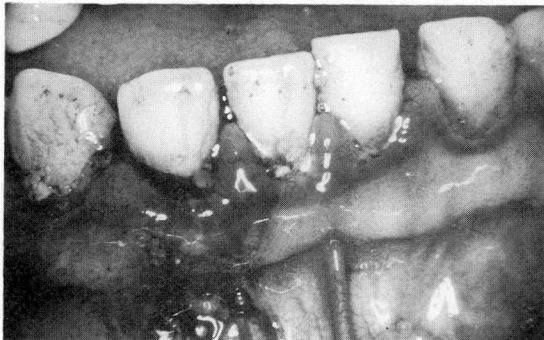

Fig. 48.21 Bleeding from gingival sulci in a Nigerian patient bitten by a saw-scaled or carpet viper (*Echis carinatus ocellatus*).

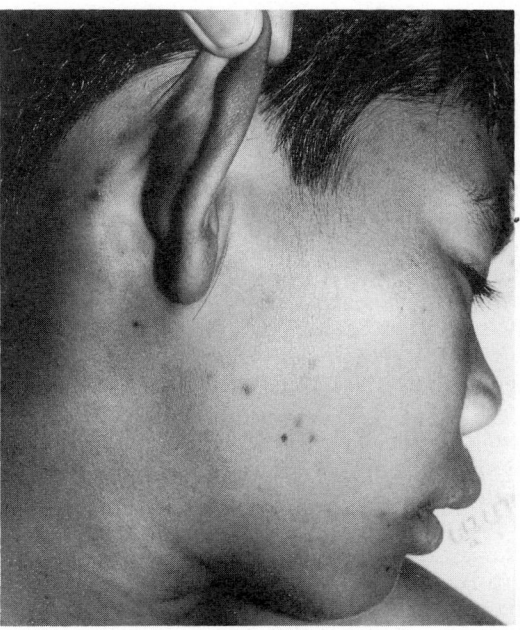

Fig. 48.22 Discoid haemorrhages in a Thai boy 6 hours after being bitten by a Malayan pit viper (*Calloselasma rhodostoma*).

blood which usually derives from bleeding gums or epistaxis. True haemoptysis is rare. Haematuria may be detected a few hours after the bite. Ecchymoses, intracranial and subconjunctival haemorrhages, bleeding into the floor of the mouth, tympanic membrane, gastrointestinal and genitourinary tracts also occur. Discoid ecchymoses, especially of the face and trunk, are seen in patients bitten by *Calloselasma rhodostoma* (Fig. 48.22). Bleeding into the anterior pituitary (resembling Sheehan's syndrome) has been described in patients bitten by Burmese and Indian Russell's vipers and by *Bothrops jararacussu* (Fig. 48.23). Menorrhagia and ante and postpartum haemorrhage have been described in women envenomed by vipers. Severe headache and meningism suggests subarachnoid haemorrhage, evidence of a developing central nervous system lesion (e.g. hemiplegia), irritability, loss of consciousness and convulsions suggests (in the absence of cardiorespiratory failure) an intracranial haemorrhage. Abdominal distension, tenderness and peritonism with signs of haemorrhagic shock but no external blood loss(haematemesis or melaena) suggests retroperitoneal or intraperitoneal haemorrhage. Incoagulable blood resulting from defibrination is a common and important finding in patients systemically envenomed by members

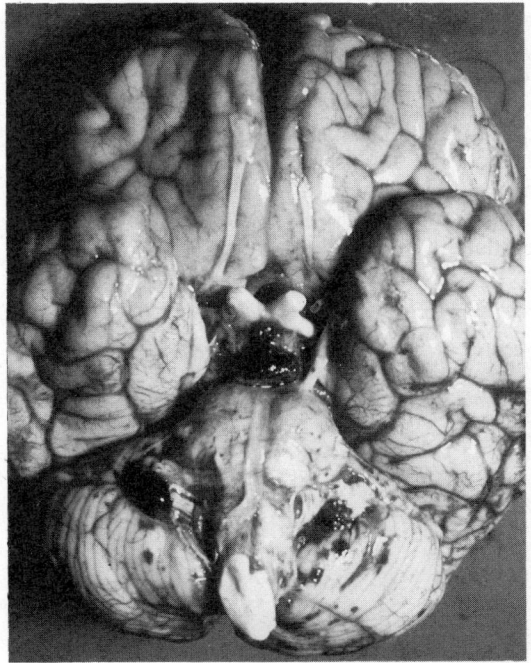

Fig. 48.23 Pituitary haemorrhage in a Burmese patient who died in shock 5 days after being bitten by a Russell's viper (*Vipera russelli siamensis*). (Courtesy Dr U Hla Mon, Rangoon.)

of the following genera: *Atheris, Vipera, Echis, Lachesis, Agkistrodon, Bothrops, Calloselasma, Crotalus, Deinagkistrodon,* and *Trimeresurus.*

Intravascular haemolysis, causing haemoglobinaemia (pinkish plasma) and black or greyish urine (haemoglobinuria or methaemoglobinuria), has been convincingly described in patients bitten by tropical rattlesnakes (*Crotalus durissus terrificus*), Sri Lankan Russell's viper (*Vipera russelli pulchella*), South American *Bothrops* species and the three genera of medically important colubrids (*Dispholidus, Thelotornis* and *Rhabdophis*). Progressive severe anaemia and renal failure may result.

Circulatory shock (hypotensive) syndromes. A fall in blood pressure is a common and serious event in patients bitten by vipers, especially in the case of some of the North American rattlesnakes (e.g. *Crotalus adamanteus, C. atrox* and *C. scutellatus*), South American Crotalinae (e.g. *Lachesis muta*) and Old World Viperinae (e.g. *V. russelli, V. palaestinae, V. berus, Bitis arietans* and *B. gabonica*). The pulse rate will be rapid if the patient is compensating for hypovolaemia resulting from external haemorrhage, blood loss into the tissues or local or generalized increase in capillary permeability. Patients envenomed by Burmese Russell's viper (*Vipera russelli siamensis*) show evidence of increased vascular permeability. They may have conjunctival oedema (Fig. 48.24), serous effusions (Fig. 48.25), pulmonary oedema (Fig. 48.26), haemoconcentration and a fall in serum albumin concentration.[10] The pulse rate may be slow or irregular if the venom is affecting the heart directly or reflexly (e.g. *Vipera berus, Bitis arietans, Calloselasma rhodostoma*). Vasovagal

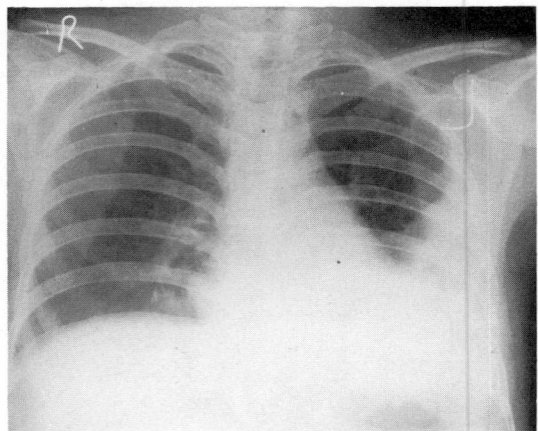

Fig. 48.25 Chest radiograph showing a pleural effusion in a Burmese woman bitten by a Russell's viper (*Vipera russelli siamensis*).

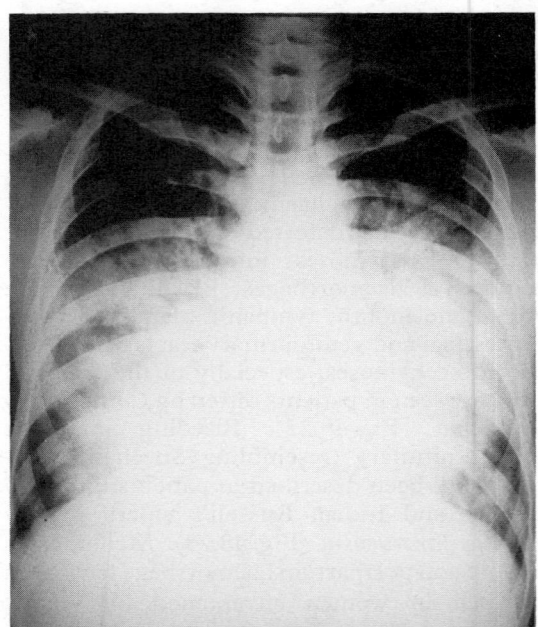

Fig. 48.26 Chest radiograph of a Burmese man who developed pulmonary oedema after being bitten by a Russell's viper (*Vipera russelli siamensis*).

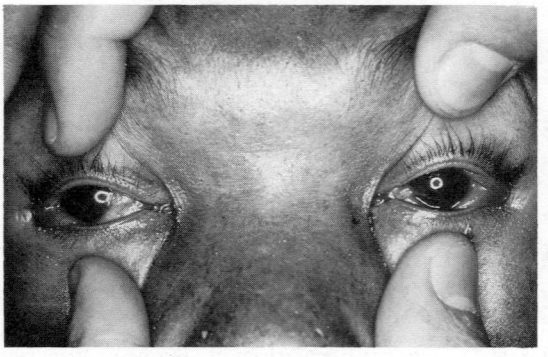

Fig. 48.24 Bilateral conjunctival oedema in a Burmese patient envenomed by Russell's viper (*Vipera russelli siamensis*).

syncope may be precipitated by anxiety in certain individuals. Early repeated and usually transient syncopal attacks associated with features of an autopharmacological or anaphylactoid reaction are seen in patients bitten by some members of the genus *Vipera* (e.g. *V. palaestinae, V. berus, V. aspis* and *V. russelli*). Vomiting, sweating, colic, diarrhoea (with incontinence), shock and angioneurotic oedema of the face, lips, gums, tongue and throat may appear as early as 5 minutes or as late as many hours after the bite. These symptoms may resolve spontaneously or recur and persist leading to death. Hypotension is also an important feature of the systemic anaphylaxis which may complicate antivenom therapy (see below). *Renal failure* is a rare complication of severe envenoming by any species of snake, but it is a regular occurrence and the most frequent cause of death in victims of Russell's viper throughout its range, tropical rattlesnake (*Crotalus durissus terrificus*), some species of *Bothrops*, and the bushmaster (*Lachesis muta*). Patients bitten by Russell's viper may become oliguric within a few hours of the bite. Loin pain and tenderness may be experienced within the first 24 hours and, in 3 or 4 days, the patient may become irritable, comatose or convulsing, with hypertension and evidence of metabolic acidosis. Neurotoxicity, possibly attributable to venom phospholipase, is a feature of envenoming by a few species of *Viperidae* (e.g. *Crotalus durissus*

terrificus, *Bitis atropos* and Sri Lankan *Vipera russelli pulchella*). The clinical features are the same as with elapid envenoming (Fig. 48.27) but progression to respiratory or generalized paralysis rarely if ever occurs. Associated myalgia suggests the possibility of rhabdomyolysis.

CLINICAL COURSE AND PROGNOSIS

Local swelling is usually evident within 2–4 hours of bites by vipers and cytotoxic cobras and may develop even more rapidly following bites by some rattlesnakes. Swelling is maximal and most extensive on the second or third day after the bite. Resolution of swelling and restoration of normal function in the bitten limb may be delayed for months especially in the older age group (e.g. after bites by the European adder *Vipera berus*). The earliest systemic symptoms such as vomiting and syncope may develop within minutes of the bite, but even in the case of elapid venoms which are thought to be the most rapidly absorbed, deaths are most unusual in less than an hour after the bite. Patients may become totally defibrinated within one or two hours of the bite (e.g. saw-scaled or carpet viper *Echis carinatus*) and neurotoxic signs may progress to a state of generalized flaccid paralysis and respiratory arrest within a few hours. If the venom is not neutralized by antivenom, these effects may be prolonged. Defibrination can persist for weeks (*E. carinatus* and Malayan pit viper *Calloselasma rhodostoma*). Patients with neurotoxic envenoming have recovered after being artificially ventilated for up to ten weeks. Tissue necrosis usually declares itself within a week of the bite. Sloughing of necrotic tissue and secondary infections including osteomyelitis may occur during subsequent weeks or months. Early deaths from neurotoxic envenoming are caused by airways obstruction or respiratory paralysis, whereas later deaths may result from technical complications of mechanical ventilation or intractable hypotension. Late deaths, more than 5 days after the bite, are usually the result of renal failure. Delayed shock with recurrent spontaneous haemorrhage has been described in Burmese victims of Russell's viper: pituitary and other intracranial haemorrhages have been found at autopsy.

Even when the fangs of a venomous snake have pierced the skin, envenoming is not inevitable.

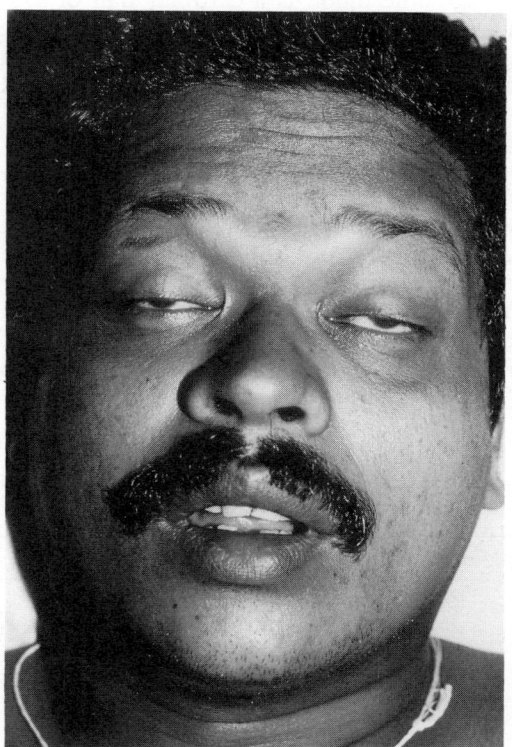

Fig. 48.27 Sri Lankan patient envenomed by Russell's viper (*Vipera russelli pulchella*). There is ptosis, ophthalmoplegia and inability to open the mouth or protrude the tongue.

About 20% of patients bitten by North American rattlesnakes, Central American lance-headed vipers (mainly *Bothrops*), *Calloselasma rhodostoma* and *Vipera russelli* show absolutely no evidence of envenoming, and as many as 80% of those bitten by sea snakes and 50% by *C. rhodostoma* or *V. russelli* have trivial or no envenoming. Untreated snake bite mortality is hard to assess, for hospital admissions include a disproportionate number of severe cases, and data for untreated snake bite are available only from the pre-antivenom era or from occasions when antivenom supply is limited, an antivenom of low potency is used[11] or when antivenom is withheld by doctors who doubt its efficacy. The untreated mortality of *C. d. terrificus* is said to have been 74%, but has been reduced to 12% by antivenom, while the mortality of *E. carinatus* bites has been reduced from about 20% to 3% with antivenom. Prognosis appears to be worst in infants and in the elderly, but there is no convincing evidence that children have a worse prognosis than young adults, despite the larger dose of venom relative to their body weight.

Interval between bite and death

Death after snake bite may occur as rapidly as 'a few minutes' (reputedly after a bite by the king cobra *Ophiophagus hannah*) or as long as 41 days after a bite by the saw-scaled or carpet viper (*Echis carinatus*). However, the rapidity of death after snake bite has generally been exaggerated. Most elapid deaths occur several hours after the bite, most sea snake bites between 12 and 24 hours after the bite, and viper bites within days of the bite (Table 48.2).

LABORATORY INVESTIGATIONS

Systemic envenoming by most species excites a neutrophil leukocytosis: counts above 20 000 cells/μl indicate severe envenoming. Haematocrit may be high initially because of haemoconcentration when there is generalized increase in capillary permeability (e.g. *Crotalus* species, Burmese *V. russelli*). A subsequent fall in haematocrit is usual: the causes include bleeding into the bitten limb and elsewhere and, uncommonly, from intravascular haemolysis, especially from microangiopathic haemolysis in patients with disseminated intravascular coagulation. In these cases, the blood film will show fragmented erythrocytes (schistocytes or helmet cells). Thrombocytopenia is commonly associated with snake venom coagulopathies (e.g. *V. russelli*, *Calloselasma rhodostoma* and *Crotalus viridis helleri*) and is also a feature of bites by the puff adder (*Bitis arietans*) although there are no other disturbances of haemostasis in humans bitten by this species.

Incoagulable blood is a cardinal sign of systemic envenoming by the majority of Viperidae, many of the terrestrial Australasian snakes and the medically important Colubridae. For clinical purposes, a simple all-or-nothing test of blood coagulability is adequate. A few millilitres of blood taken by venepuncture is placed in a clean, dry glass test-tube, left undisturbed at room temperature for 20 minutes, then tipped to see if there is clotting or not. The test interval can be reduced to 5 minutes by adding approximately 20 units of thrombin per 2 ml of blood (as in the commercially available tubes for collection of FDP samples (Wellcome FDP assay kits). More

Table 48.2 Interval between snake bites and death.

Species	Number of cases	Range	Mean	Source
Bungarus caeruleus	18	3 h–63 h	18.0 h	Reid[38]
Naja naja	27	$\frac{1}{4}$ h–60 h	8.4 h	Reid[38]
Naja kaouthia	3	1 h– 3 h		Viravan et al[39]
Hydrophiidae	48	$2\frac{1}{2}$ h–12 days		Reid[40]
Vipera berus		6 h–60 h	34 h	Reid[41]
Vipera russelli	7	$\frac{1}{4}$ h–9 days	41.3 h	Reid[38]
Vipera russelli (Burma)	10	15 h–7 days		Myint-Lwin et al[10]
Echis carinatus	33	25 h–41 days	5 days (median)	Warrell and Arnett[11]
Calloselasma rhodostoma	23	5 h–240 h	64.6 h (median 32 h)	Reid[38]
Crotalus species	8	2 h–26 h	15.9 h	Russell[42]

sensitive tests which are reasonably simple to perform are whole blood or plasma prothrombin times for the detection of an unequivocally elevated FDP concentration (e.g. $80\,\mu g/ml$) by agglutination of sensitized latex particles (Thrombo-Wellcotest). Serum concentrations of creatine phosphokinase and aspartate aminotransferase, and blood urea are commonly raised in patients with severe envenoming, probably because of muscle damage. In patients with generalized rhabdomyolysis caused by venoms of sea snakes and Australasian snakes there is a steep rise in creatine phosphokinase, myoglobin and potassium concentrations. Plasma usually appears brownish in the presence of myoglobinaemia, but is stained pink when there is intravascular haemolysis. Heparinized blood should be allowed to sediment spontaneously (without centrifugation) for detection of haemoglobinaemia. The urine of patients with intravascular haemolysis is black (as in 'blackwater fever') but brownish, pinkish or reddish in those with haematuria or myoglobinuria. Blood urea and serum creatinine and potassium concentrations should be measured in patients who become oliguric, especially in cases with a high risk of renal failure (e.g. *V. russelli*, *C. d. terrificus*, *Bothrops* species, terrestrial Australasian snakes and Colubridae). Severely sick, hypotensive and shocked patients will develop lactic acidosis (increased anion gap), those with renal failure will also develop a metabolic acidosis (decreased plasma pH and bicarbonate concentration, reduced arterial P_{CO_2}), and patients with respiratory paralysis will develop respiratory acidosis (low pH, high arterial P_{CO_2}, decreased P_{O_2}) or respiratory alkalosis if they are over-ventilated.

All snake-bitten patients should be encouraged to empty their bladder on admission. Urine should be examined for blood/haemoglobin and protein ('stix' test) and for microscopic haematuria and red cell casts.

Electrocardiographic abnormalities are unusual but important. Sinus bradycardia, ST-T changes, various degrees of atrioventricular block and evidence of hyperkalaemia have been described, especially in patients envenomed by Viperidae and Atractaspididae.

Chest radiographs are useful for detecting pulmonary oedema (e.g. European *Vipera* and *V. russelli*) (Fig. 48.26), intrapulmonary haemorrhages and pleural effusions (*V. russelli*) (Fig. 48.25).

Immunodiagnosis

The immunological detection of venom antigens and antibodies in body fluids of snake bite victims promises greatly to improve diagnosis, understanding of pathophysiological mechanisms, assessment of first aid methods[43] and control of antivenom treatment. Enzyme-linked immunosorbent assay (ELISA) has been the most widely used[44, 45] but immunodiagnostic test kits are generally available only in Australia (from the Commonwealth Serum Laboratories). The prevalence of venom antibody in a community could be used to assess the incidence of snake bite. These tests are highly sensitive but their specificity may be inadequate to distinguish between different species and false-positive reactions are common especially in the sera of rural populations in the tropics. Relatively high venom antigen concentrations (e.g. from wound swabs or aspirates) can be detected within 15–30 minutes, which is just fast enough to allow the selection of the appropriate monospecific antivenom. For retrospective diagnosis, including forensic cases, tissue around the fang punctures, wound and blister aspirate, serum and urine should be stored for ELISA immunodiagnosis.

MANAGEMENT OF SNAKE BITE

First aid

First aid can only be carried out by the person who is bitten or people nearby, using materials which are readily available at that site.

1 Reassure the victim who will almost certainly be terrified.
2 Do not tamper with the bite wound in any way, but immobilize the bitten limb using a splint or sling. If available, firm binding of the splint with a crepe bandage is an effective form of immobilization.
3 Take the patient as quickly as possible to the nearest health clinic, dispensary or hospital where medical treatment can be given. Muscular contraction in the bitten limb will promote spread of venom, so this should be avoided as far as possible. Ideally, the patient should be transported by motor vehicle, stretcher or (as a passenger) by bicycle.
4 Avoid harmful and time-wasting treatments (see below).
5 Since species diagnosis is critically important, the snake should be taken along to hospital

if it has been killed. However, if the snake is still at large, do not risk further bites and waste time by searching for it. Even snakes which appear to be dead should not be touched with the bare hands but carried in a bag or dangling across a stick. Some species (e.g. *Hemachatus haemachatus*) sham death, and even a severed head can inject venom!

Rejected or controversial first aid methods

Procedures which inflict further trauma or pressure to the bite site are potentially harmful and should not be used. These include cauterization, incision or excision, amputation of the bitten digit, suction by mouth, vacuum pumps or 'venom-ex' apparatus, instillation of chemical compounds such as potassium permanganate and cooling with ice (cryotherapy). Incisions will lead to uncontrolled bleeding in patients with incoagulable blood, may damage nerves, blood vessels or tendons and may introduce infection. Suction, chemicals and cryotherapy may cause necrosis of tissues. None of these methods aimed at removing venom from the site of the bite has received consistent support from the results of animal experiments. No clinical studies have been attempted. The use of tourniquets, compression pads and bandages in an attempt to impede the systemic uptake of venom, remains controversial. In animals, tight (arterial) tourniquets have been shown to prevent the absorption of venom and to prolong survival after the injection of venoms of elapids, Australasian terrestrial snakes and vipers. The splinting and crepe bandaging method advocated by Sutherland[46] also proved effective in limiting the absorption of venom in restrained monkeys. In the original experiments, crepe bandaging was thought to exert a pressure of about 55 mmHg, that of a venous tourniquet. The splint and crepe bandage is certainly an effective way of immobilizing the bitten limb, and is a less painful way of applying an obstructive pressure than is the arterial tourniquet. However, in practice, it is difficult to judge how tightly to apply the crepe bandage. Dangers of tourniquets and other occlusive methods include ischaemia and gangrene, if they are applied for long periods, damage to peripheral nerves (especially the lateral popliteal nerve), increased fibrinolytic activity, and congestion, swelling, increased bleeding and increased local effects of venom. Few convincing clinical data are available, but in Thai patients bitten by *Calloselasma rhodostoma*, and Burmese patients bitten by *V. russelli*, systemic venom antigen concentrations did not increase after tight tourniquets were released.[43, 47] However, if a patient is bitten by a dangerous elapid, terrestrial Australasian snake or sea snake, and medical attention is likely to be delayed for 1–2 hours, there is a risk that he might develop respiratory paralysis en route. In these cases alone it seems reasonable to apply a tight tourniquet (upper arm or thigh) or a firm crepe bandage and splint, in the hope that it will delay the onset of life-threatening neurotoxicity until the patients reach a place where they can be resuscitated.

Treatment of early symptoms

Distressing or even dangerous manifestations of envenoming may appear before the patient reaches hospital.

Local pain may be intense. Oral paracetamol is preferable to aspirin which commonly causes gastric erosions and could lead to persistent gastric bleeding in patients with incoagulable blood.

Severe pain can be treated with pethidine or pentazocine.

Vomiting is a common early symptom of systemic envenoming. Patients should lie on their side with their head down to avoid aspiration. Persistent vomiting can be treated with intravenous chlorpromazine (25–50 mg in adults, 1 mg/kg in children).*

Syncopal attacks and anaphylactic shock

Patients may collapse within minutes of the bite and show features either of a vasovagal attack or of an autopharmacological reaction with angioneurotic oedema, sweating, abdominal colic and diarrhoea. An antihistamine such as chlorpheniramine maleate (10 mg in adults, 0.2 mg/kg in children) can be given by intravenous or intramuscular* injection. Hypotension or bronchoconstriction can be treated with adrenaline 0.1% (1 in 1000) (0.5 ml in adults, 0.01 ml/kg in children) by *subcutaneous injection*.

---

* In patients with incoagulable blood, intramuscular and subcutaneous injections can lead to haematoma formation. Pressure dressings should be applied to venepuncture sites to prevent oozing.

Respiratory distress

This may result from upper airway obstruction if the jaw and tongue are paralysed or from paralysis of the respiratory muscles. Patients should be laid on their side, the airway cleared, if possible using a suction pump, an oral airway inserted and the jaw elevated. If the patient is cyanosed, or respiratory movements are very weak, oxygen should be given by any available means. If clearing the airway does not produce immediate relief, artificial ventilation must be given. In the absence of any equipment, mouth-to-mouth or mouth-to-nose ventilation can be life-saving. Manual ventilation by Ambu bag and anaesthetic mask is rarely effective. Ideally, the patient should have a cuffed endotracheal tube inserted using a laryngoscope, or a cuffed tracheostomy tube inserted. The patient can then be ventilated by Ambu bag. If no femoral or carotid pulse can be felt, external cardiac massage should be instituted.

Treatment at health clinic, dispensary or hospital by medically trained staff

Clinical assessment

Snake bite is a medical emergency. The history, symptoms and signs must be rapidly assessed so that appropriate treatment can be started without delay. The three most important preliminary questions are: Where (in which part of your body) were you bitten? How long ago were you bitten? Have you brought the snake, or if not, did you see what kind of snake it was? If the snake has been killed but not brought, one of the accompanying friends or relatives should be despatched to collect it posthaste. If the snake can be diagnosed confidently as non-venomous, the patient can be discharged immediately after receiving a booster dose of tetanus toxoid. Patients should be asked whether they have taken any herbal or other treatment, whether they have vomited, fainted, or have noticed any bleeding or other ill-effects of the bite. Physical signs should be assessed before any tourniquet is removed. Fang marks are sometimes invisible and rarely help the diagnosis. Local swelling, tenderness and lymph node involvement are early signs of envenoming. The gingival sulci should be examined carefully as this is usually the first site of spontaneous bleeding. Bleeding from recent wounds and skin lesions suggests that the blood is incoagulable. If the patient is shocked (collapsed, sweating, cold, cyanosed extremities, low blood pressure, tachycardia) the foot of the bed should be raised, and an intravenous infusion of a plasma expander such as fresh frozen plasma, dextran, Haemaccel or fresh blood started immediately. The jugular venous pressure or, preferably, the central venous pressure should be observed. The earliest symptom of neurotoxicity after elapid bites is often blurred vision, a feeling of heaviness in the eyelids and drowsiness. The earliest sign is contraction of the frontalis muscle (raised eyebrows and puckered forehead) even before true ptosis can be demonstrated. Signs of respiratory muscle paralysis (dypsnoea, exaggerated abdominal respiration and contraction of intercostal muscles and cyanosis) must be detected and the blood pressure measured. Patients with generalized rhabdomyolysis have trismus and stiff and tender muscles which resist passive stretching. Urine output may dwindle very early in the course of Russell's viper bite. Dark urine suggests myoglobinuria or haemoglobinuria.

It may be obvious from this preliminary assessment that antivenom should be given, but even if there is no evidence of significant envenoming the patient should be admitted to a ward where they can be observed closely for at least 24 hours. Every hour, ptosis should be looked for and symptoms, level of consciousness, pulse rate and rhythm, blood pressure, respiratory rate, extent of local swelling and other new signs should be recorded. If there is any evidence of neurotoxicity, the ventilatory capacity or expiratory pressure should also be recorded every hour. Useful investigations include the simple whole blood clotting test (or more sensitive tests of haemostasis, FDP estimation etc. if available), peripheral leukocyte count, haematocrit, urine microscopy and 'stix' testing and electrocardiogram.

ANTIVENOM (ANTIVENIN, ANTIVENENE, ANTI-SNAKE BITE SERUM)

Antivenom is the whole serum or partially purified immunoglobulin of animals, usually horses, which have been immunized with venom. It is the only specific treatment available and has proved effective against many of the lethal and damaging effects of venoms. In the management of snake bite, the most important clinical decision is whether or not to give antivenom, for only a minority of snake-bitten patients need it, it may produce severe reactions, and it is expensive and often in short supply.

Indications for antivenom

Systemic envenoming

1 Haemostatic abnormalities: spontaneous systemic bleeding, incoagulable blood or prolonged clotting time, elevated FDP, thrombocytopenia.
2 Cardiovascular abnormalities: hypotension, shock, abnormal electrocardiogram, cardiac arrhythmia, cardiac failure, pulmonary oedema.
3 Neurotoxicity.
4 Generalized rhabdomyolysis.
5 Impaired consciousness.
6 In patients with definite signs of local envenoming, the following indicate significant systemic envenoming: neutrophil leukocytosis, elevated serum enzymes such as creatine phosphokinase and aminotransferases, haemoconcentration, uraemia, hypercreatininaemia, oliguria, hypoxaemia, acidosis, and vomiting in the absence of a history of ingesting emetic agents.

Severe local envenoming

The development at any stage of local swelling involving more than half the bitten limb or extensive blistering or bruising, especially in patients showing the abnormalities listed above under **6**, and in patients bitten by species known to cause local necrosis (e.g. Viperidae, Asian cobras, African spitting cobras, *Naja nigricollis*, *N. pallida* and *N. mossambica*).

Some wealthy countries can afford a wider range of indications for the use of antivenom. The following *additional* indications have been suggested.

United States and Canada. Following bites by the most dangerous rattlesnakes (*Crotalus atrox*, *C. adamanteus*, *C. viridis*, *C. horridus* and *C. scutellatus*) antivenom therapy has been recommended if there is rapid spread of local swelling, even without evidence of systemic envenoming,[42] and after bites by coral snakes (*Micruroides euryxanthus* and *Micrurus fulvius*) if there is immediate pain or any other symptom or sign of envenoming.

Australia. Antivenom is recommended in any proved or suspected case of snake bite if there is any evidence of systemic spread of venom including tender regional lymph nodes, and if there has been an effective bite by any identified highly venomous species.[6]

Europe. To improve the rate of recovery of local swelling after bites by *Vipera berus*, antivenom has been recommended in adults with swelling extending up the forearm or leg within 2 hours of the bite.[41]

Contraindications

Atopic patients and those who have had reactions to equine antiserum on previous occasions have an increased risk of developing severe antivenom reactions. In such cases antivenom should not be given unless there are definite signs of severe (potentially life-threatening) systemic envenoming. Reactions may be ameliorated by pretreatment with adrenaline, antihistamine and corticosteroid (doses given below). Rapid desensitization is not recommended.

Prediction of antivenom reactions

Hypersensitivity testing by intradermal or subcutaneous injection or intraconjunctival instillation of diluted antivenom has been widely practised in the past. However, these tests delay the start of antivenom treatment, are not without risk, and have recently been proved to have no predictive value for early (anaphylactoid) or late (serum sickness type) antivenom reactions.[48]

Administration of antivenom

The range of venoms neutralized by an antivenom should be stated in the package insert. If the biting species is known or can reliably be deduced, the appropriate monospecific antivenom should be used. In parts of the world where several species produce identical signs, patients who fail to bring the dead snake must be treated with polyspecific antivenom which will contain a lower concentration of specific antibody to each species than the monospecific antivenom.

Manufacturers' expiry dates are often extremely conservative. Liquid and lyophilized antivenoms stored at below 8°C usually retain most of their activity for five years or more.

Opaque solutions should not be given as precipitation of protein indicates loss of activity and increased risk of reactions. Antivenom should be given as soon as it is indicated, but it is almost never too late to give it as long as signs of systemic envenoming persist (e.g. up to 2 days after a sea snake bite and many days or even weeks for prolonged defibrination following bites by Viperidae). In contrast, local effects of venoms are probably not reversible by antivenom delayed more than 1–2 hours after the bite. The intravenous route is the most effective. An infusion over 30–60 minutes of antivenom diluted in isotonic fluid may be easier to control than an intravenous 'push' injection of reconstituted but undiluted antivenom given over 10–20 minutes. There is no difference in the incidence of severity of antivenom reactions in patients treated by these two methods.[48] In the rural tropics, the intravenous push method has the advantage that it involves less expensive equipment, is quicker to initiate and compels someone to remain with the patient at least while the injection is being given.

In the absence of someone capable of giving an intravenous injection, antivenom may be given by deep intramuscular injection (e.g. into the lateral thigh) followed by massage to promote absorption. However, the volumes of antivenom normally required would make this route impracticable as would the risk of haematoma formation in patients with incoagulable blood. Local injection of antivenom, for example into the fang marks, seems rational but is difficult, painful and hazardous (especially when the bite is on a digit or other tight compartment) and has not proved effective in animal studies.

Table 48.3 Guide to initial dosage of some important antivenoms.

Species		Manufacturer, antivenom	Approximate initial dose
Latin name	English name		
Acanthophis antarcticus	Death adder	CSL,[a] monospecific	3000–6000 units
Bitis arietans	Puff adder	Behringwerke, SAIMR,[b] polyspecific	80 ml
Bothrops atrox *Bothrops jararaca*	Lance-headed vipers	South American Institutes, *Bothrops* polyspecific	40 ml
Bungarus caeruleus	Indian krait	Haffkine polyspecific	100 ml
Calloselasma (Agkistrodon) rhodostoma	Malayan pit viper	Thai Red Cross (Saovabha), Bangkok, monospecific	100 ml
		Thai Government Pharmaceutical Organization, monospecific	50 ml
		Twyford Pharmaceuticals	10 ml
Crotalus adamanteus	Eastern diamondback rattlesnakes		
Crotalus atrox	Western diamondback rattlesnakes	Wyeth, (Crotalidae) polyspecific	30–100 ml
Crotalus viridis subspecies	Western rattlesnakes		
Echis carinatus	Saw-scaled or carpet viper	SAIMR, *Echis*, monospecific	20 ml
		Behringwerke, *Bitis–Echis–Naja*, polyspecific	100 ml
Hydrophiidae	Sea snakes	CSL, *Enhydrina schistosa*	1000 units
Naja kaouthia	Monocellate Thai cobra	Thai Red Cross, monospecific	100 ml
Naja naja	Indian cobra	Haffkine, Kasauli, polyspecific	100 ml
Notechis scutatus *Pseudonaja textilis*	Tiger snake Eastern brown snake	CSL, monospecific	3000–6000 units
Trimeresurus albolabris	Green pit viper	Thai Red Cross, monospecific	100 ml
Vipera berus	European adder	Imunoloski Zavod-Zagreb Vipera polyspecific	10 ml
Vipera palaestinae	Palestine viper	Rogoff Medical Research Institute, Tel Aviv, Palestine viper monospecific	50–80 ml
Vipera russelli	Russell's viper	Burma Pharmaceutical Industry, monospecific	40 ml
		Haffkine, polyspecific	100 ml

[a] Commonwealth Serum Laboratories, Australia.
[b] South African Institute for Medical Research.

The average initial dose of antivenom required should be based on results of clinical studies, but these are rarely available. Most manufacturers base their recommendations on the mouse assay which may not correlate with clinical findings.[49] Initial doses of some important antivenoms are given in Table 48.3. The apparent serum half-lives of antivenoms in envenomed patients range from 26 to 95 hours depending on how they are prepared.[50,51] Systemic envenoming may recur several days after an initial good response to antivenom.[43] This is probably the result of continuing absorption of venom from the injection site after antivenom has been largely cleared from the circulation. The implication is that an initial dose of antivenom, however large, may not prevent late or recurrent envenoming. Children must be given the same or larger doses of antivenom than adults. The response to antivenom will determine whether further doses should be given. Neurotoxic signs may improve within 30 minutes of antivenom treatment[32] but usually take several hours. Hypotension, sinus bradycardia and spontaneous systemic bleeding may respond within 10–20 minutes and blood coagulability is usually restored between one and 6 hours provided sufficient antivenom has been given. A second dose of antivenom should be given if severe cardiorespiratory symptoms persist more than 30 minutes, and incoagulable blood persists for more than 6 hours, after the start of the first dose. Enormous doses of antivenom may be required to treat patients bitten by species capable of injecting very large amounts of venom or extremely potent venom. Thus a patient bitten by the king cobra (*Ophiophagus hannah*) required 1150 ml of specific antivenom and prolonged artificial ventilation.[98] Other exceptionally large species include bushmaster (*Lachesis muta*),[99] gaboon viper (*Bitis gabonica*)[100] and black mamba (*Dendroaspis polylepis*).

Antivenom reactions

Antivenom treatment may be complicated by three types of reaction: early (anaphylactoid), pyrogenic and late (serum sickness type).

Early antivenom reactions are not type I IgE-mediated hypersensitivity reactions to equine serum proteins for they are not predicted by hypersensitivity tests.[48] Antivenoms activate complement in vitro[52] while the clinically similar reactions to homologous serum are associated with complement activation and immune complex formation in vivo. The complement system is probably activated by aggregates of IgG. Reactions usually develop within 10 to 180 minutes of starting antivenom. There is itching, urticaria, fever, tachycardia, palpitations, cough, nausea and vomiting. The reported incidence, which varies from 3 to 54%, appears to increase with the dose and to decrease when refined antivenom is used and administration is by intramuscular rather than intravenous injection. Unless patients are watched carefully for 3 hours after treatment, mild reactions may be missed and deaths may be misattributed to the envenoming itself. Up to 40% of patients with early reactions show features of severe systemic anaphylaxis: bronchospasm, hypotension or angioneurotic oedema, but deaths are rare. Early reactions respond readily to adrenaline given by a subcutaneous injection of between 0.5 and 1.0 ml of 0.1% (1 : 1000, 1 mg/ml) in adults (children 0.01 ml/kg) at the first sign of trouble. Antihistamines such as chlorpheniramine maleate (adult dose 10 mg, children 0.2 mg/kg) should be given by intravenous injection to combat the effects of histamine released during the reaction.

Pyrogenic reactions result from contamination of the antivenom by endotoxin-like compounds. High fever develops 1–2 hours after treatment and is associated with rigors, followed by vasodilatation and fall in blood pressure. Febrile convulsions may be precipitated in children. Patients should be cooled and given antipyretic drugs such as pyrazolones (e.g. Dipyrone 1 g in 2 ml intramuscularly for adults) or paracetamol, powdered and washed down a nasogastric tube (15 mg/kg) or in the form of a suppository.

Late (serum sickness-type) reactions develop 5–24 (mean 7) days after treatment. The higher the dose of antivenom the higher the incidence of these reactions and the speed of their development. Symptoms include fever, itching, urticaria, arthralgia including the temporomandibular joint, lymphadenopathy, periarticular swellings, mononeuritis multiplex, albuminuria and rarely encephalopathy. This is an immune complex disease which responds to corticosteroid (prednisolone 5 mg four times a day for 5 days in adults, 0.7 mg/kg per day in divided doses for 5 days for children) and an antihistamine such as chlorpheniramine (adults 2 mg four times a day, children 0.25 mg/kg per day in divided doses).

Supportive treatment (assuming that adequate doses of antivenom have been given)

Artificial ventilation was first suggested for neurotoxic envenoming more than one hundred years ago but patients continue to die for lack of this simple procedure. Neurotoxic effects are fully reversible with time: a patient bitten by *Bungarus multicinctus* in Canton recovered completely after being ventilated manually for 30 days, and a patient probably envenomed by *Tropidechis carinatus* recovered after 10 weeks' mechanical ventilation in Queensland, Australia. Endotracheal intubation or tracheostomy, using cuffed tubes, is needed. The patient can be ventilated manually with an anaesthetic or Ambu bag or, preferably, with a mechanical ventilator.

Anticholinesterase drugs may produce a rapid useful improvement in neuromuscular transmission in some patients envenomed by Asian and African cobras, mambas and kraits.[4, 33] It is worth trying the Tensilon test in all cases of severe neurotoxic envenoming as with suspected myasthenia gravis. Atropine sulphate (adults 0.6 mg, children 50 µg/kg) is given first by intravenous injection to block unpleasant muscarinic effects of acetylcholine (increased secretions, abdominal colic). Edrophonium chloride ('Tensilon') is then given intravenously in an adult dose of 10 mg, or 0.25 mg/kg for children. Patients who respond convincingly can be maintained on neostigmine methylsulphate, 50–100 µg/kg and atropine 4-hourly or by continuous infusion.

Hypotension and shock. These usually result from hypovolaemia and should be treated by infusing a plasma expander, preferably fresh whole blood or, failing that, fresh frozen plasma. Central venous pressure or pulmonary arterial catheter monitoring is the safest way to control volume replacement. Hypotensive patients envenomed by Burmese Russell's viper responded to dopamine 2.5–5 µg/kg per minute by intravenous infusion; but methylprednisolone 30 mg/kg and naloxone were not effective.[10]

Renal failure. If urine output drops below 400 ml/24 hours, urethral and central venous catheters should be inserted. If urine flow fails to increase after cautious rehydration, diuretics (e.g. frusemide up to 1000 mg intravenously) and dopamine (2.5 µg/kg per minute) should be given, and the patient should be placed on strict fluid balance. Peritoneal or haemodialysis will be required in most patients with established renal failure.

Local infection. Infection at the site of the bite should be prevented with penicillin or erythromycin and a booster dose of tetanus toxoid should be given. An aminoglycoside such as gentamicin should be added if the wound has been tampered with or there is evidence of local necrosis. Bullae are best left alone. Snake-bitten limbs should be nursed in the most comfortable position. *Necrotic tissue* should be excised as soon as possible and the denuded area covered with split skin grafts.

Intracompartmental syndromes. Swelling of muscles within tight fascial compartments may raise the tissue pressure to such an extent that perfusion is impaired and ischaemic damage is added to the effects of the venom. The signs of intracompartmental syndrome include excessive pain, weakness of the compartmental muscles and pain when they are passively stretched, hypoaesthesia of areas of skin supplied by nerves running through the compartment and obvious tenseness of the compartment.[37] Palpation of peripheral pulses or their detection by Doppler ultrasound does not exclude intracompartmental ischaemia. An intracompartmental pressure of more than 45 mmHg indicates a high risk of ischaemic necrosis.[37] In these circumstances, fasciotomy may be justified to relieve the pressure in the compartment, but this treatment did not prove effective in saving envenomed muscle in animal experiments.[53] Necrosis occurs most frequently after digital bites. Fasciotomy must not be performed before blood coagulability has been restored by antivenom, accelerated if possible by the transfusion of fresh whole blood or clotting factors.

Corticosteroids, heparin, antifibrinolytic agents such as Trasylol and epsilon aminocaproic acid, antihistamine, trypsin and a variety of traditional herbal remedies have been used and advocated for snake bite. Most are potentially harmful and none has been proved to be effective.

Snake venom ophthalmia

The 'spat' venom should be washed from the eye or mucous membrane as soon as possible using large volumes of water or other bland fluid. Unless a corneal abrasion can be definitely excluded by fluorescein staining or slit lamp examination, treatment should be the same as for any corneal abrasion—a topical antimicrobial agent such as tetracycline or chloramphenicol and closure of the eye with a dressing pad.[34]

PREVENTION

The incidence of snake bite can be greatly reduced by taking simple precautions. Unfortunately, these methods are impracticable for those, such as farmers, who have to do hard physical work in hot snake-infested areas. Snakes should never unnecessarily be disturbed, attacked or handled even if they are thought to be harmless species or appear to be dead. Venomous species should never be kept as pets or as performing animals. Protective clothing—boots, socks, long trousers—should be worn when walking in undergrowth or deep sand and a light should always be carried at night. Particular care should be taken while collecting firewood, moving logs, boulders, boxes or debris likely to conceal a snake and climbing rocks and trees covered with dense foliage or swimming in overgrown lakes and rivers. Wading in the sea, especially in sand or near coral reefs, is a dangerous pastime (see below fish stings) and should be avoided if possible. Shuffling is safer than a high stepping gait. Divers should keep clear of sea snakes. Fishermen who catch sea snakes in nets or on lines should return them to their element without touching them.

Prophylactic immunization against snake venoms

Venom toxoids (venoids) have been used to immunize farmers at high risk of habu bite (*Trimeresurus flavoviridis*) in the Ryukyu and Amami Islands in Japan.[54] Elsewhere, there has been some progress with producing venoids to protect against Russell's viper bite. In this case, the rapid development of renal damage, irreversible by antivenom, is a strong argument for pre-exposure prophylaxis.[10] The production and modification of venom antigens by genetic engineering is an exciting new development which could lead to the production of snake venom vaccines.[55, 56]

VENOMOUS LIZARDS[57]

Two species of venomous lizard (genus *Heloderma*) are capable of envenoming man. The venom glands are in the lower jaw. The Gila monster (*H. suspectum*) is striped with a short, thick tail and grows up to 60 cm in length. It occurs in the south-western USA and adjacent areas of Mexico. The Mexican beaded lizard or escorpión (*H. horridum*) is spotted with a relatively long, thin tail and reaches 80 cm in length. It is found in western Mexico and Central America. Bites are rare. The lizard hangs on with its powerful jaws and is difficult to disengage. The application of a flame to the underside of the animal's jaw is said to be the most effective and least inhumane method of loosening its grip. There is immediate severe local pain with tender swelling and regional lymphadenopathy. Symptoms include weakness, dizziness, hypotension, syncope, sweating, rigors, tinnitus, nausea and vomiting. There may be leukocytosis and electrocardiographic changes. No fatal cases have reliably been reported. Specific antivenom is not generally available. A powerful analgesic may be required. Hypotension should be treated with plasma expanders and perhaps adrenaline or a pressor agent such as dopamine.

VENOMOUS FISH[58]

TAXONOMY

More than 100 species of fish, inhabiting temperate and tropical seas, possess a defensive venom-injecting apparatus which can inflict dangerous stings. Fatal stings from members of the groups have been reported: order Chondrichthyes (cartilagenous fish); order Squaliformes (sharks and dogfish); order Rajiformes (stingrays and mantas); order Osteichthyes (bony fish); suborder Siluroidei (catfish); family Trachinidae (weever fish); family Scorpaenidae (scorpion fish, stonefish) and family Uranoscopidae (stargazers or stonelifters).

VENOM APPARATUS

Venom is secreted around spines or barbs in front of the dorsal, anal or pectoral fins and tail and opercular spines in the gill covers. The venom gland in stingrays lies in a groove beneath a membrane covering the barbed precaudal spine up to 30 cm long. The most advanced venom apparatus is found in the genus *Synanceja* (stonefish): bulky venom glands drain through paired ducts to the tips of the short, thick spines.

VENOM COMPOSITION[58]

Fish venoms are unstable at normal ambient temperatures and so have been difficult to study. Venoms of the North American round stingray (*Urolophus halleri*) and weever fish (*Trachinus*) were found to contain peptides, protein, enzymes and a variety of vasoactive compounds (kinins, 5-hydroxytryptamine, histamine, adrenaline and noradrenaline). Pharmacological effects include local necrosis, direct actions on cardiac, skeletal and smooth muscle causing electrocardiographic changes, hypotension and paralysis, and central nervous system depression.

INCIDENCE AND EPIDEMIOLOGY OF FISH STINGS

There are hundreds of weever fish stings around the British coast each year especially in Cornwall. The peak incidence is in August and September. Fifty-eight cases were seen at a hospital in Pula on the Adriatic over 13 years. In the USA, 1500 stings by rays and 300 stings by scorpion fish are thought to occur each year. Eighty-one cases of stonefish sting were seen over a 4-year period at a hospital in Pulau Bukom, an island near Singapore. Ornate but highly venomous and aggressive members of the genera *Pterois* and *Dendrochirus* (zebra, lion, tiger, turkey or red fire fish or coral or fire cod) are popular aquarium pets. Fatal fish stings are very rarely reported. Stings usually occur when people wading near the shore tread on fish which are lying in the sand in shallow water. Most victims are stung on the sole of the foot, but stingrays lash their tails and usually impale the ankle. Fishermen, scuba divers and aquarium enthusiasts are often stung on the fingers while carelessly handling or attempting to touch the fish.

SYMPTOMS OF ENVENOMING

Immediate, sharp, agonizing pain is the dominant symptom. Even stoical adults may collapse screaming with pain and are thought to be hysterical. Bleeding may be seen from single or multiple puncture sites. Hot, erythematous swelling extends rapidly up the stung limb.

Stingrays[60]

These fish are widely distributed. The large barbed spine may cause severe lacerating injuries, usually to the lower part of the legs but occasionally penetrating the body cavities, heart and viscera when the swimmer falls or lies on the fish. Deaths from this mechanical trauma have been reported from Mexico and New Zealand. The spine and fragments of its integument may remain in the wound. The venom produces local swelling and sometimes necrosis with a high risk of secondary infection unless the broken spine and other foreign material is removed from the wound. Systemic effects include hypotension, cardiac arrhythmias, muscle spasms, generalized convulsions, vomiting, diarrhoea, sweating and hypersalivation.

Weevers[61]

Stings by Trachinidae produce intense local pain with slight swelling. Systemic symptoms are rare, but some patients develop severe chest pain simulating myocardial ischaemia, cardiac arrhythmias and hypotension.

Scorpion fish and stonefish

The family Scorpaenidae comprises more than 350 species which are widely distributed in some temperate and all tropical seas and are especially abundant around the coral reefs of the Indo-Pacific region. The stonefish (genus *Synanceja*) are the most dangerous of venomous fish. They occur from East Africa, across the Indian Ocean, to the Pacific. Stings are excruciatingly painful, as are all fish stings, but symptoms may persist for 2 days or more. There is local swelling, discoloration, sweating and paraesthesia and sometimes local lymphadenopathy. Systemic symptoms are more common than with other fish stings. They include nausea, vomiting, hypotension, cardiac arrhythmias, respiratory distress, neurological signs, convulsions and evidence of autonomic nervous system stimulation. People have died within an hour of being stung by *S. verrucosa.*

TREATMENT

The most effective treatment for pain is to immerse the stung limb in water that is uncomfortably hot but not scalding (i.e. just under 50°C). Temperature can be assessed with the unstung limb. It is not necessary to add magnesium sulphate to the water. Injection of local anaesthetic such as 1% lignocaine, for example as a ring block in the case of stung digits, is less effective. The spine, membrane and other foreign material must be removed from the wound. Prophylactic antibiotics and tetanus toxoid should be given to patients stung by rays or scorpionfish because of the size of wound and risk of necrosis, but these measures are not justified for weever fish stings. Local injection of potassium permanganate solution or acidifying solutions such as emetine hydrochloride were said to cure local pain, but they may promote local necrosis and are less effective than immersion in hot water. In patients with severe systemic envenoming, an adequate airway should be established and cardiorespiratory resuscitation instituted when necessary. Severe hypotension can be treated with adrenaline and bradycardia with atropine. The only antivenom now available commercially is manufactured by the Commonwealth Serum Laboratories in Australia. It neutralizes the venoms of *S. trachynis*, *S. verrucosa* and *S. horrida* and has paraspecific activity against venoms of the North American scorpion fish (*Scorpaena guttata*) and other members of the Scorpaenidae family. Two millilitres (2000 units), one ampoule, is given intravenously for each two puncture marks found at the site of the sting. The dose is increased in patients with severe symptoms.[6]

PREVENTION (see p. 882)

PREVENTION (see p. 882)

Bathers and waders should adopt a shuffling gait to reduce the risk of stepping on a venomous fish skulking in sand or mud. Footwear protects against most species except stingrays.

VENOMOUS MARINE INVERTEBRATES[58]

Coelenterates (hydroids, stinging corals, medusae, Portuguese men-of-war or bluebottles, jellyfish, blubbers, box-jellies, stinging algae, sea anemones and sea pansies)

The venom apparatus of the coelenterates is the stinging capsule or nematocyst which, when triggered by physical contact or chemicals, everts a thread-like tubule with sharpened tip which can penetrate the skin and inject toxin. The tentacles of coelenterates are armed with myriads of these nematocysts which produce lines of painful irritant wheals on the skin of swimmers unlucky enough to make contact with them. Coelenterate venoms contain peptides together with vasoactive compounds such as 5-hydroxytryptamine, histamine, prostaglandins and kinins which cause immediate severe pain, inflammation and urticaria.

EPIDEMIOLOGY

The most dangerous coelenterate to man, the box-jellyfish (*Chironex fleckeri*) has been found along the northern coast of Australia from Darwin to Port Curtis and has been responsible for more than 70 deaths since 1900.[6] Most stings occur in December and January. Fatal jellyfish stings have also been reported from Bougainville Island in the east to the west coast of India and north to the Philippines where a similar species *Chironex quadrigatus* is common. During a three-and-a-half year period, 116 cases of marine stings were seen in Cairns, north Queensland.[62] Forty per cent of the patients had clinical features of 'Irukandji sting' caused by *Carukia barnesi*. Prodigious swarms of the Scyphomedusa *Pelagia noctiluca* appeared along the northern Adriatic coast during the summers of 1977–1979. In 1978 it was estimated that 250 000 swimmers had been stung.[63] At Pula on the Adriatic coast, 55 patients stung by a sea anemone (*Anemonia sulcata*) were seen from 1965 to 1980. This coelenterate is widely distributed in the eastern Atlantic and Mediterranean. Coelenterate stings are common in most parts of the world but few reliable statistics are available.

CLINICAL FEATURES

The imprint of nematocyst stings on the skin may have a diagnostic pattern. *Chironex fleckeri* produces immediate brownish or purplish wheals 8–10 mm wide with cross striations. More extensive swelling, erythema and vesiculation develops with areas of necrosis and eventual healing with scar formation. *Carukia barnesi* produces an oval erythematous area about 7 cm in diameter and then transient papules with surrounding hyperhidrosis. Portuguese man-of-war stings (*Physalia*) produce chains of oval wheals surrounded by erythema. These lesions persist for only about 24 hours. Histological sections of the skin lesions may reveal identifiable nematocysts, allowing differentiation between stings by different genera.[64]

The dominant symptom of coelenterate sting is immediate severe pain coming in waves and sometimes becoming incapacitating in its intensity. Systemic symptoms are most severe following stings by cubomedusae (box-jellyfish), genera *Chironex* and *Chiropsalmus*. The victim, usually a child swimming in shallow water, suddenly screams with pain and within minutes becomes cyanosed, suffers generalized convulsions and is found to be pulseless. The whole jellyfish or length of tentacles may still be adherent to the patient's skin. Autopsies reveal pulmonary oedema. Patients envenomed by *Carukia barnesi* develop severe systemic effects minutes to hours after the sting but with little or no local effect. Systemic effects of coelenterate stings include cough, nausea, vomiting, abdominal colic, diarrhoea, rigors, severe musculoskeletal pains, syncope and signs of autonomic nervous system stimulation such as profuse sweating. The Portuguese man-of-war (*Physalia*) occasionally causes systemic symptoms and has been known to produce intravascular haemolysis leading to haemoglobinuria and renal failure. No deaths have reliably been attributed to *Physalia*. The sea anemone *Anemonia sulcata* produces painful local papules, erythema, oedema and vesiculation. Systemic symptoms such as sleepiness, dizziness, nausea, vomiting, myalgia and periorbital oedema are occasionally produced.[65]

TREATMENT

First aid is all important as patients may die within minutes of the sting. Lifeguards and others working on coelenterate infested beaches should be trained how to deal with jellyfish stings. The patient must be taken out of the water. The nematocysts in fragments of tentacles stuck to the skin must be inactivated to prevent further discharge and envenoming. For *Chironex* and *Physalia*, commercial vinegar or 3–10% aqueous acetic acid is effective;[65] but for *Chrysaora*, a widely distributed Atlantic genus, baking soda and water (50% w/v) proved effective. Alcoholic solutions (methylated spirits, suntan lotion, aftershave, etc.) were advocated until recently when it was shown that they cause massive discharge of nematocysts. Tourniquets and pressure immobilization are not recommended because the stings are usually extensive and the value of these first aid methods has not been investigated. Mouth-to-mouth artificial ventilation has proved life-saving in several patients who developed severe respiratory depression with cyanosis, coma and pulselessness.[67] If no pulse can be detected, external cardiac massage should be started. Experimentally, the venom of *Chironex* affects the heart directly and the central nervous system. Clinically, respiratory depression appears to be more important than cardiotoxicity but recent work suggests that verapamil might reverse this effect.

A specific 'sea wasp' antivenom is manufactured by the Commonwealth Serum Laboratories in Australia for *Chironex fleckeri* stings. The antivenom should be administered intravenously (or in the absence of a medically qualified person intramuscularly) if symptoms of systemic envenoming persist after first aid treatment.

Prevention

People, and especially children, should keep out of the sea at times of the year when dangerous coelenterates are most prevalent and especially when they have been sighted and warning notices have been displayed. Wet suits and other clothing will protect against the stings.

Echinoderms (starfish and sea urchins)[58, 68]

Echinoderms have hard protective exoskeletons. Starfish (Asteroidea) sprout numerous sharp spines which can penetrate human skin releasing a violet coloured liquid. *Acanthaster planci* of the

Red Sea, Indian and Pacific Oceans, is up to 60 cm in diameter and possesses venomous spines 6 cm long. The venom causes severe pain, redness, swelling, muscle weakness, hyper/hypoaesthesia, facial oedema, cardiac arrhythmias, vomiting and paralysis. Sea urchins (Echinoidea), especially of the tropical families Diadematidae and Echinothuridae, have brittle, articulated spines (30 cm long in *Diadema*) and grapples (globiferous pedicellariae). Both contain venom which is released when they are embedded in the skin. Severe pain, syncope, numbness, generalized paralysis, aphonia, respiratory distress and even death may result. The fragments of spines embedded in the skin may cause secondary infection, and granuloma formation several months later. Penetration of bones and joints may cause destructive changes.

Treatment

Spines and pedicellariae must be removed as soon as possible as they may continue to inject venom and give rise to later complications. The sites of penetration are usually on the soles of the feet. The superficial layer of thickened epidermis should be pared down and 2% salicylic acid ointment applied for 24–48 hours to soften the skin. Most spines can then be extruded, but deeply embedded ones may require surgical removal under local anaesthetic.[58, 68]

Molluscs (cone shells and octopuses)

Cone shells (family Conidae), up to 20 cm in length, are found in the Pacific and Indian Oceans. They kill their prey of small fish and other marine animals by implanting a detachable venom-filled radular tooth or dart. In humans, the venom produces local paraesthesiae and numbness and paralysis which progressed to fatal respiratory paralysis in eight out of 30 reported cases. The venom of *Conus geographus* was found to contain several neurotoxic peptides including one that produced irreversible inhibition of the release of transmitter at neuromuscular junctions by preventing calcium entry. No specific treatment is available. If respiratory paralysis develops mouth-to-mouth respiration may be needed, followed by prolonged mechanical ventilation. An arterial tourniquet or crepe bandage and splint might delay absorption of the venom until the patient had reached hospital.

Cephalopods (cuttlefish, squids and octopuses) secrete toxic saliva which is inoculated by the sharp and powerful beak. The venom contains tetrodotoxin-like activity (see p. 895), other toxins, vasoactive amines and hyaluronidase. Cephalopod bites are usually painful and produce bleeding, swelling, redness, heat and irritation. Systemic symptoms include numbness of the mouth and tongue, blurring of vision, dysphonia, dysphagia, and paralysis of the legs and arms. A number of severe cases including two fatalities have been reported from Australia; they were caused by small (20 cm long) octopuses, the common blue-ringed or banded octopus (*Octopus maculosus*, also known as *Hapalochlaena maculosa*) and the blue-ringed octopus (*O. lunulatus*). *O. maculosus* is abundant around the coast of Australia, especially in the south and frequents shallow water and rock pools. The two patients who died had handled octopuses while they were out of the water. They vomited soon after the bite, then developed respiratory paralysis and died 90 and 120 minutes later.

There is no specific treatment for octopus bites; the effects resemble rapidly developing tetrodotoxin poisoning. Mouth-to-mouth respiration combined with external cardiac massage (if the patient is pulseless) may be life-saving. An arterial tourniquet or crepe bandage and splint should be applied to delay absorption of the venom until the patient has reached hospital. Mechanical ventilation and other intensive care may be needed. It would be worth testing the response to anticholinesterase (see Tensilon test, p. 881) and treating bradycardia with atropine.

INSECT STINGS

Hymenoptera stings (bees, wasps, yellow jackets, hornets)

In most temperate countries, anaphylactic reactions to *Hymenoptera* stings are a commoner cause of death than direct effects of envenoming by any animal.

For example, between 1959 and 1972 there were 61 deaths from insect stings in England and Wales but only one death from adder bite. In the USA, there are between 40 and 50 deaths a year from *Hymenoptera* stings. Deaths from *Hymenoptera* sting anaphylaxis are probably under-reported because a sting is not suspected in patients found dead and assumed to have had myocardial infarctions or cerebrovascular accidents. *Hymenoptera* venoms also have direct toxic effects but these are not seen in man unless there have been many, usually hundreds of, stings.

The commonest, and most severe *Hymenoptera* stings are caused by members of the family Apidae (e.g. *Apis mellifera*, the honey-bee) and Vespidae (e.g. wasps such as *Paravespula*—formerly *Vespa vulgaris*, American yellow jackets genus *Dolichovespula* and hornets genus *Vespa* (Fig. 48.28), including the enormous East Asian *V. mandarinia* which can reach a length of almost 4 cm and a weight of 3 g).

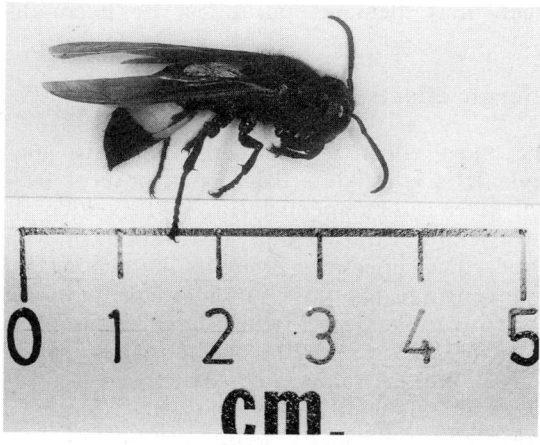

Fig. 48.28 Asian hornet (*Vespa* sp). Specimen from Sri Lanka.

VENOM APPARATUS AND COMPOSITION[68a,68b]

Venoms are injected through a barbed sting. Bees inject approximately 50 μg of venom, the total capacity of the venom sac, and leave the stings embedded in the skin, but wasps and hornets can sting repeatedly. The venoms contain biogenic amines (histamine, 5-hydroxytryptamine and acetylcholine), enzymes such as phospholipase A and hyaluronidase and toxic peptides; kinins in the case of Vespidae, apamin, melittin and anti-inflammatory compounds such as mast cell degranulating peptide ('401') in Apidae.

CLINICAL FEATURES

Toxic effects

In people who are not allergic to the venom, stings usually produce only local effects attributable to the injected biogenic amines, particularly 5-hydroxytryptamine. Pain, redness, swelling, whealing and heat develop rapidly but rarely last more than a few hours (Fig. 48.29). Local effects are dangerous only if the airway is obstructed, for example following stings on the tongue.

Fatal systemic toxicity can result from as few as 30 stings in children. Adults have survived more than 2000 stings by *Apis mellifera*. The clinical effects of massive envenoming resemble histamine overdose: vasodilatation, hypotension,

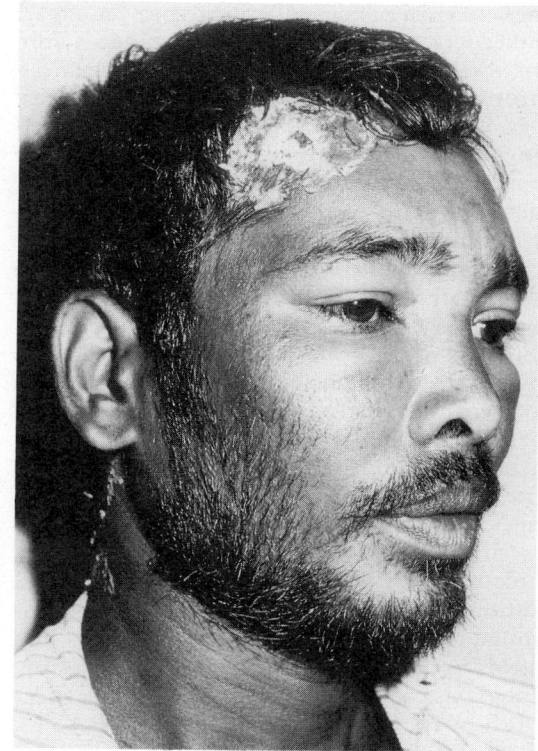

Fig. 48.29 Sri Lankan patient with facial swelling after multiple stings on the head by hornets. Herbal medicine has been applied to the stings.

vomiting, diarrhoea, throbbing headache and coma. Rhabdomyolysis followed by myoglobinuria and renal failure can occur after multiple hornet stings (*Vespa affinis*). Intravascular haemolysis with haemoglobinuria (*Vespa orientalis*), thrombocytopenic purpura, myasthenia gravis (*Polistes* sp.) and various renal lesions including nephrotic syndrome have also been described. A child who suffered about 1000 bee stings in northern Nigeria developed epidermal necrolysis and severe anaemia, presumably haemolytic.[69]

Allergic effects[70, 71]

These are seen in the 0.5% of the population who have become hypersensitized to *Hymenoptera* venoms. Clinical suspicion of venom hypersensitivity arises when reactions to successive stings are increasingly severe, or when systemic symptoms follow a sting. In England, sensitization to bee venom appears to require more stings (average 81 on 23 occasions) than sensitization to wasp venom (average four stings).[70] Most patients allergic to bee venom are bee-keepers or their relatives. Systemic symptoms include tingling scalp, flushing, dizziness, syncope, wheezing, abdominal colic and diarrhoea, tachycardia and visual disturbances developing within a few minutes of the sting. Over the next 15–20 minutes urticaria, angioneurotic oedema, oedema of the glottis, profound hypotension and coma may develop. Patients may die within minutes of the sting. In a few cases, serum sickness develops a week or more after the sting. Atopy does not predispose to sting allergy but asthmatics who are allergic to venom are likely to suffer severe reactions. The diagnosis of venom hypersensitivity can be confirmed by intradermal skin testing with dialysed specific venoms in concentrations of 0.01 to 1 μg/ml. The test may be negative if years have elapsed since the last sting. Specific IgE antibodies can be measured in serum by radioimmunoassay (RAST test). Whole body extracts (WBE) of bees and wasps, traditionally used for skin testing, do not discriminate between hypersensitive patients and controls. A post-mortem diagnosis of insect sting anaphylaxis can be supported by detecting specific IgE by the radioallergosorbent test (RAST). Pathological findings in cases of fatal systemic anaphylaxis include acute pulmonary hyperinflation, laryngeal oedema, pulmonary oedema and intra-alveolar haemorrhage.[72, 73]

TREATMENT

The embedded bee sting should be removed without squeezing, which will inject more venom. It can be scraped out with a blade or fingernail. Domestic meat tenderizer (papain) diluted roughly 1 in 5 with tap water is said to produce immediate relief of pain. Aspirin is an effective analgesic favoured from long experience by bee-keepers. Local antiseptics are acceptable, but topical antihistamines should not be used as they promote sensitization.

Toxic effects

In cases of severe systemic envenoming, life-threatening effects of biogenic amines can be treated with adrenaline (adults 0.5 ml of 0.1% solution subcutaneously) and systemic antihistamine (adults chlorpheniramine maleate 10 mg intravenously). No specific antivenoms are available. Renal failure complicating myoglobinuria, haemoglobinuria or a direct nephrotoxic effect, may demand peritoneal or haemodialysis.

Allergic effects

The most effective treatment for sting anaphylaxis is adrenaline 0.1% in a dose of 0.5–1 ml given subcutaneously or, if the patient is unconscious or pulseless, by intravenous or even intracardiac injection. Patients known to be hypersensitive should wear an identifying tag (such as provided by Medic-Alert in Britain) as they may be discovered unconscious after a sting. They should be trained to give themselves adrenaline subcutaneously and should always carry a preloaded syringe of adrenaline for this purpose. Adrenaline delivered by a pressurized inhaler ('Medihaler-epi' delivering 200 μg of adrenaline acid tartrate per puff) will relieve bronchospasm, but insufficient is absorbed to combat other effects of anaphylaxis. Injection of an antihistamine (e.g. chlorpheniramine maleate 10 mg intravenously or intramuscularly) will alleviate the mild urticarial symptoms, and antihistamine should be given for the next 24–48 hours to combat the effects of histamine released during the reaction. Severe reactions may require cardiorespiratory resuscitation. Salbutamol is an effective bronchodilator and large doses of hydrocortisone may help the resolution of massive oedema. Respiratory tract obstruction is the main cause of death. Stings in the mouth may cause serious airway obstruction even in people who are not hypersensitive to venom.

Prevention of *Hymenoptera* sting anaphylaxis

Desensitization with WBE was practised for many years and was believed by many experienced allergists to be effective. However, it had not been subjected to controlled trials, lacked a sound theoretical basis and could produce early (anaphylactic) or late (serum sickness) reactions. In 1978, a controlled trial proved that hyposensitization using pure venom was effective in protecting allergic patients against anaphylactic reactions to sting challenge.[74] A mild protective effect observed in the group treated with WBE was no greater than in untreated controls and probably reflected spontaneous loss of sensitivity rather than any effect of WBE immunization. However, immunotherapy is probably only necessary in a few patients with histories of severe reactions and an unusual risk of being stung. Most people are stung when they inadvertently crush the bee or wasp or interfere with their nests (i.e. bee-keepers). Wasps congregate where sweet things are manufactured or consumed and in orchards and wine plantations. Vespidae are attracted by brightly coloured floral patterns and perfumes.[75] Some of the largest hornets (*V. velutina* and *V. mandarinia*) are so aggressive that their territory cannot be cultivated until the nests have been destroyed.

SCORPION STINGS

Scorpions (order Scorpionida) capable of inflicting fatal stings in humans are all members of the family Buthidae.[76] Examples of the most deadly species are: *Androctonus australis* (North Africa and Middle East) (Fig. 48.30), *A. crassicauda* (Turkey, Middle East and North Africa), *Buthus occitanus* (countries bordering the Mediterranean and Middle East), *Leiurus quinquestriatus* (North Africa and Middle East) (Fig. 48.31), *Parabuthus* (South Africa), *Tityus trinitatis* (Trinidad and Venezuela), *T. serrulatus* and *T. bahiensis* (Brazil, Argentina), *Centruroides sculpturatus* (California, New Mexico, Arizona and Baha California), *C. limpidus* and *C. suffusus* (Mexico) and *Buthotus* (formerly *Buthus*) *tamulus* (India).

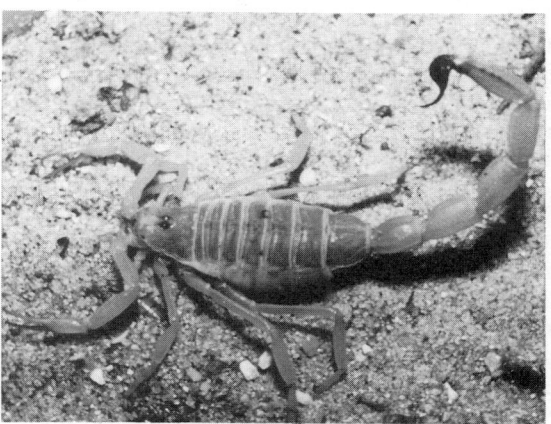

Fig. 48.31 One of the most dangerous scorpions of North Africa and the Middle East (*Leiurus quinquestriatus*). Specimen from the Sudan.

EPIDEMIOLOGY

Painful scorpion stings are common throughout the tropics; however, fatal envenoming is frequent only in Mexico, Brazil, Trinidad, parts of North Africa and the Middle East and in India. In southern Libya there were 900 stings with seven deaths per 100 000 population in 1979. There has been no death from scorpion sting in the USA since 1968, but in Mexico there are between one and two thousand deaths each year, with an incidence of 84 deaths per 100 000 per

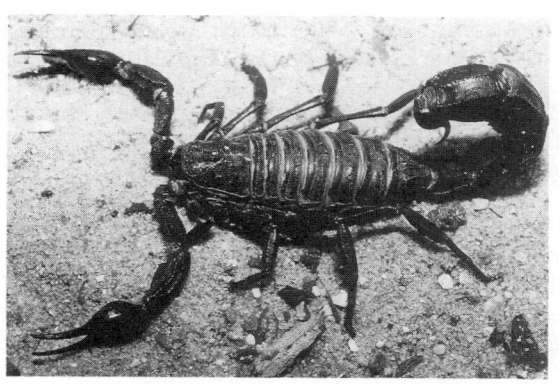

Fig. 48.30 One of the large species of lethal North African scorpion (genus *Androctonus*).

year in Colima state and a mere three deaths per 100 000 per year in the infamous Durango state. Case mortality is about 50% in children up to four years old. In Trinidad, *Tityus trinitatis* is a scourge of canefields and cocoa plantations: there were 33 deaths in a group of 698 cases. Mortality was 25% amongst the children under five years compared with 0.25% in adults.[77] In Brazil, mortality increases from around 1% in adults to 15–25% in children less than six years old. In Algeria there were an average of 1260 stings and 24 deaths per year. In India there are many cases of scorpion stings with fatalities in adults and children.

CLINICAL FEATURES

Rapidly developing, very intense local pain is the commonest symptom. Local signs such as swelling, redness, heat and regional lymph node involvement are never extensive. Local necrosis is most unusual. Systemic symptoms may develop within minutes, but may be delayed for as much as 24 hours. Features of autonomic nervous system excitation include dilated pupils, hypersalivation, profuse sweating, hyperthermia, vomiting, diarrhoea, abdominal distension, loss of sphincter control, and priapism. Release of catecholamines, as in phaeochromocytoma, produces hypertension and toxic myocarditis with arrhythmias (most commonly sinus bradycardia), cardiac failure and pulmonary oedema.[78] These cardiovascular effects are particularly prominent following stings by *Leiurus quinquestriatus* and *Buthotus tamulus*. Neurotoxic effects such as fasciculation, spasms and respiratory paralysis are a particular feature of stings by *Centruroides sculpturatus*.

Hemiplegia and other neurological lesions have been attributed to fibrin deposition resulting from disseminated intravascular coagulation. Hypercatecholaminaemia could explain hyperglycaemia and glycosuria in patients stung by scorpions, but in the case of stings by the black scorpion on Trinidad (*Tityus trinitatis*), acute pancreatitis may be the mechanism. Fifteen to 120 minutes after the initial searing pain of the sting, patients stung by this scorpion begin to salivate, feel nauseated and vomit persistently producing coffee grounds or frank haematemesis. Hyperglycaemia, glycosuria and sometimes albuminuria, can be detected a few hours after the sting. There is abdominal pain with distension and rigidity. Electrocardiogram abnormalities (T wave inversion, QRS segment abnormalities and QTC prolongation) are common and may last for 3–6 days.[79] Other features include pyrexia, sweating, bradycardia, cardiac arrhythmias, hypotension and neuromuscular irritability. Acute oedematous or haemorrhagic pancreatitis with development of pancreatic pseudocysts has been demonstrated at autopsy or laparotomy.[77] This may be explained by the venom stimulating pancreatic exocrine secretion and causing contraction of the sphincter of Oddi.[80]

TREATMENT

Pain may respond to local infiltration or ring block with local anaesthetic. Local injection of emetine is said to relieve the pain but may cause necrosis. Parenteral opiate analgesics such as pethidine and morphine may be required but are alleged to be dangerous in victims of *Centruroides sculpturatus*.

The treatment of choice for systemic envenoming is specific antivenom which should be given by intravenous injection (as described above for snake bite). Antivenom is manufactured in the USA, Britain, Germany, Mexico, Brazil, Turkey, Algeria, South Africa, Egypt and Iran.

Many accessory treatments have been suggested. There is some clinical evidence to support the use of the following treatments:

1 For patients with the hypercatecholaminaemia syndrome (hypertension, bradycardia and early pulmonary oedema) rapid digitalization, potent loop diuretics and alpha-blocking vasodilators. Beta-blockers may be dangerous once cardiac failure has developed.

2 Atropine for patients with signs of parasympathetic nervous system stimulation such as bradycardia.

3 Anticonvulsants such as phenobarbitone for neurotoxic symptoms (*Centruroides sculpturatus*).

No antivenom is commercially available for the treatment of *Buthotus tamulus* stings in India. In this case, patients who develop priapism, dilated pupils, sweating and bradycardia are at high risk of progressing to pulmonary oedema. Early energetic treatment of cardiac failure may prevent this.

Prophylactic immunization with scorpion venom toxoid is under trial in Mexico.

SPIDER BITES[81]

The spiders (Araneae) are an enormous group containing more than 30 000 known species. A single family, containing less than 1% of these species, is non-venomous. Only 12 species of spider are known to cause dangerous envenoming in humans while another 24 are suspected of doing so. Spiders bite with a pair of fangs, the chelicerae, to which the venom glands are connected. A central venom duct opens near the tip of the fang.

CLINICAL FEATURES

Two main clinical syndromes, 'necrotic' and 'neurotoxic', are caused by spider bite.

Necrotic araneism

Skin lesions, varying in severity from mild localized erythema and blistering to quite extensive tissue necrosis, have been attributed to a variety of species of spiders. The members of the genus *Loxosceles* are the most important causes of the syndrome. Many of these spiders are extending their geographical ranges. *L. laeta* is widely distributed in Central and South America, especially in Chile. *L. reclusa*, the brown recluse spider, has caused at least 200 bites with six deaths in the USA this century. More than 60 cases were reported in Texas between 1959 and 1962. *L. rufescens* occurs in the Mediterranean region, North Africa, Israel and elsewhere.

Eighty per cent of patients are bitten indoors, usually in their bedrooms while asleep or dressing and in the USA a number of men were bitten on their genitals while they sat on outdoor lavatories in which the spiders had spun their webs. There is burning pain at the site of the bite, oedema and development of a violaceous plaque which, over the course of a few days, becomes a black eschar which sloughs in a few weeks, sometimes leaving a necrotic ulcer. Rarely, the necrotic area may cover an entire limb. In 12% of cases there are systemic effects including haemoglobinuria and jaundice resulting from haemolytic anaemia, fever, respiratory distress and collapse. The average mortality among all reported cases is 6% and about 30% in those with systemic envenoming.

Neurotoxic araneism

Members of the genus *Latrodectus* (widow, hourglass, button or red-back spiders) are the most widespread and numerous of all venomous animals dangerous to man. *L. mactans mactans* (black widow spider) (Fig. 48.32) occurs in the Americas. Sixty-three deaths were attributed to this species in the USA from 1950 to 1959.

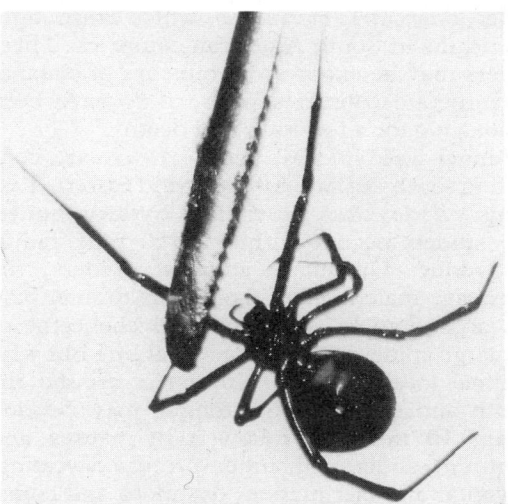

Fig. 48.32 'Black widow' spider (*Latrodectus mactans*). Note 'hourglass' pattern on undersurface of abdomen.

L. mactans tredecimguttatus, widely but incorrectly known as 'tarantula' lives in fields in the Mediterranean countries where it has been responsible for epidemics of bites. Nine hundred and forty-six cases were reported in Italy between 1946 and 1951.

L. mactans hasselti, the Australian and New Zealand 'red-back spider' or 'katipo' causes up to 340 reported bites each year in Australia. Twenty deaths are known to have occurred.

L. mactans and a related species *L. geometricus* also causes some bites in South and eastern Africa.

L. m. hasselti bites produce local heat, swelling and redness which is rarely extensive. Intense local pain develops in about 5 minutes and after 30 minutes there is pain in local lymph nodes and after about an hour headache, nausea, vomiting and sweating. Tachycardia and hypertension may follow and there are muscle tremors and spasms which may be severe enough to demand artificial ventilation.

L. m. mactans bites produce minimal local changes. Local dull aching or numbness may develop after 30–40 minutes. Painful muscle spasms and lymphadenopathy spread and increase in intensity during the next few hours until the trunk, abdomen and limbs are involved and respiration may be embarrassed. Other features include tachycardia, hypertension, irritability, psychosis, vomiting and priapism. Similar effects are produced by the banana spider, *Phoneutria nigriventer*, which causes bites and deaths in South American countries. These spiders may be exported in bunches of bananas to temperate countries where they have been responsible for a few bites and deaths.

Funnel-web spiders, genus *Atrax*, are confined to south-eastern Australia and eastern Tasmania.[6] *A. robustus*, the famous Sydney funnel-web spider, occurs within a 160 mile radius of Sydney. Unusually amongst spiders, the aggressive male is more dangerous to man than the larger female. The powerful chelicerae of this large spider produce a painful bite but with minimal local changes. Numbness around the mouth and spasm of the tongue may develop within 10 minutes, followed by nausea and vomiting, abdominal colic, profuse sweating, salivation and lacrimation, dyspnoea and coma. There are local or generalized muscle fasciculations and spasms, hypertension and in some of the fatal cases, pulmonary oedema, thought to be neurogenic in origin. Thirteen deaths, occurring between 15 minutes and 6 days after the bite, were reported between 1927 and 1980.

TREATMENT

First aid treatment

In the case of bites by spiders with rapidly active potent venom such as *A. robustus*, firm crepe bandaging and splinting of the bitten limb or a tight tourniquet may delay venom spread until the patient reaches hospital.

Specific treatment

Antivenom for *Latrodectus* bite is made in Australia, USA, USSR, Italy, Yugoslavia, South Africa and South America; for *Atrax* bite in Australia; for *Loxosceles* in Peru, Brazil and Argentina and for *Phoneutria* and *Lycosa* in Brazil. Neurotoxic araneism seems more responsive to antivenom than does the necrotic type. Oral dapsone (100 mg twice a day) is said to reduce the extent of necrotic lesions.

Supportive treatment

Calcium gluconate (10 ml of a 10% solution given by slow intravenous injection) relieves the pain of muscle spasms caused by *Latrodectus* venom rapidly and more effectively than muscle relaxants such as diazepam or methocarbamol. Antihistamines, corticosteroids, beta-blockers and atropine have also been advocated.

TICK BITE PARALYSIS[82, 83]

TAXONOMY AND EPIDEMIOLOGY

Ticks, with mites, form a subgroup of the class Arachnida. Adult females of about 30 species of hard tick (family Ixodidae) and immature specimens of six species of soft ticks (family Argasidae) have been implicated in human tick paralysis. The tick's saliva contains a neurotoxin which causes presynaptic neuromuscular block and decreased nerve conduction velocity. The tick embeds itself in the skin with its barbed hypostome introducing the salivary toxin while it engorges with blood.

Although tick paralysis has been reported from all continents, most cases occur in western North America (*Dermacentor andersoni*), eastern USA (*D. variabilis*), and eastern Australia from north Queensland to Victoria (*Ixodes holocyclus* known as the bush, scrub, paralysis or dog tick). In British Columbia there were 305 cases with 10% mortality between 1900 and 1968. About 120 cases have been reported in the USA, and in New South Wales there were at least 20 deaths between 1900 and 1945.

CLINICAL FEATURES

Ticks are picked up in the countryside or from domestic animals, particularly dogs, in the home.

A majority of patients and almost all fatal cases are children. After the tick has been attached for about 5 or 6 days a progressive ascending, lower motor neuron paralysis develops with paraesthesiae. Often a child, who may have been irritable for the previous 24 hours, falls on getting out of bed first thing in the morning, and is found to be weak or ataxic. Paralysis increases over the next few days: death results from bulbar and respiratory paralysis and aspiration of stomach contents. Vomiting is a feature of the more acute course of *Ixodes holocyclus* envenoming.

This clinical picture is often misinterpreted as poliomyelitis, although in North America the peak incidence of tick paralysis is earlier in the year than the epidemic season for poliomyelitis. Other neurological conditions including Guillain–Barré syndrome, paralytic rabies, Eaton–Lambert syndrome, myasthenia gravis, or botulism may also be suspected. Diagnosis depends on finding the tick, which is likely to be concealed in a crevice, orifice, or hairy area of the body. The scalp is the commonest place. Fatal tick paralysis has been caused by a tick attached to the tympanic membrane.

TREATMENT

The tick must be detached without being squeezed. It can be painted with ether, chloroform, paraffin, petrol or turpentine, or prised out between the partially separated tips of a pair of small curved forceps. Following removal of the tick there is usually rapid and complete recovery; but in Australia, patients have died after the tick has been detached. An antivenom, raised in dogs, is available in Australia and, recently, rabbits have been used to produce an antitoxin against *I. holocyclus* saliva.[84] This is recommended for severely affected or very young patients; 20–30 ml are given intravenously.

CENTIPEDE AND MILLIPEDE BITES

CENTIPEDES

Many species of centipede (Chilopoda) can inflict painful bites producing local pain, swelling, inflammation, and lymphangitis. Systemic effects such as vomiting, headache, cardiac arrhythmias, and convulsions are extremely rare and the risk of mortality was probably greatly exaggerated in the older literature. The most important genus is *Scolopendra* which is distributed throughout tropical countries. Local treatment is the same as for scorpion stings. No antivenom is available.

MILLIPEDES (DIPLOPODA)

Most species possess glands in each of their body segments which secrete, and in some cases squirt out, irritant liquids for defensive purposes. These contain hydrogen cyanide and a variety of aldehydes, esters, phenols, and quinonoids. Members of at least eight genera of millipedes have proved injurious to man. Important genera are *Rhinocricus* (Caribbean), *Spirobolus* (Tanzania), *Spirostreptus* and *Iulus* (Indonesia), and *Polyceroconas* (Papua New Guinea). Children are particularly at risk when they handle or try to eat these large arthropods. When venom is squirted into the eye, intense conjunctivitis results and there may be corneal ulceration and even blindness. Skin lesions are initially stained brown or purple, blister after a few days, and then peel. First aid is generous irrigation with water. Eye injuries should be treated as for snake venom ophthalmia (see p. 881).

POISONING BY INGESTION OF MARINE ANIMALS

A variety of illnesses, usually categorized as 'food poisoning', are caused by eating seafood. The commonest are attributable to bacterial or viral infections. These include *Vibrio parahaemolyticus* (after eating crustaceans, especially shrimps), *V. cholerae* (crabs and molluscs), non-01 *V. cholerae* (shellfish), *Salmonella typhi* (molluscs), *Campylobacter jejuni* (clams), Hepatitis A virus (molluscs, especially clams and oysters), Norwalk agent (oysters and other molluscs)[85] and 'small round viruses' (cockles and other molluscs). Botulism has been reported in people eating smoked fish. Since 1953, approximately 100 000 Japanese are thought to have been affected by methyl-mercury poisoning ('Minamata disease') after eating fish and molluscs contaminated with methyl-mercury derived from industrial waste dumped in Minamata Bay and at the mouth of the Agano river in Japan. The victims developed severe central nervous system damage with a mortality of 33% in the initial outbreak. Pregnant women exposed to the methyl-mercury gave birth to infants who were mentally retarded and had cerebral palsy and convulsions.[58]

A number of clinical syndromes have been recognized which are related to the presence in the ingested flesh or viscera of marine animals of toxins either derived ultimately from dinoflagellates (e.g. ciguatera, tetrodotoxic or paralytic shell fish poisoning) or resulting from the decomposition of fish during storage (scombrotoxic fish poisoning).[86, 87]

GASTROINTESTINAL AND NEUROTOXIC SYNDROMES

Nausea, vomiting, abdominal colic, tenesmus and watery diarrhoea may precede the development of neurotoxic symptoms. Paraesthesiae of the lips, buccal cavity and extremities are early symptoms. Other neurotoxic manifestations include a peculiar distortion of temperature perception so that cold objects feel hot (like dry ice) and vice versa, dizziness, myalgia, weakness starting with muscles of phonation and deglutition and progressing to respiratory paralysis and flaccid quadriplegia in some cases, ataxia, involuntary movements, convulsions, visual disturbances, hallucinations and psychoses, cranial nerve lesions and pupillary abnormalities. Cardiovascular abnormalities include hypotension and bradycardia and some patients develop florid cutaneous lesions.

Distinguishable within this general pattern of symptoms are a number of conditions related to the ingestion of a particular taxonomic group of animals. Some of the more important syndromes are described below.

Ciguatera fish poisoning

The word ciguatera seems to derive from the Cuban word 'cigua' for a poisonous marine snail (*Livona pica*, the west Indian top shell) which was coined by early Spanish settlers.[58] Ciguatera is now applied to an illness resulting from the ingestion of more than 400 species of warm-water, shore or reef fish. The highest incidence of ciguatera seems to be in the Pacific region. Three thousand and nine cases with 0.1% mortality were reported during a 14-year period from New Caledonia, where it is known as 'la gratte' ('the itch'),[88] and more than 400 cases a year occur in Vanuatu. In Guadeloupe (Antilles) there were an average of 30 cases of ciguatera poisoning per 10 000 inhabitants each year. The fish most often associated with ciguatera are from the families Serranidae (groupers), Lutjanidae (snappers), Scaridae (parrot fish) and Scombridae (mackerel). Other important groups are moray eels (Muraenidae), barracudas (Sphyraenidae) and jacks (Carangidae).[88, 89]

It is now known that the toxins responsible for ciguatera fish poisoning originate from benthic dinoflagellates. *Gambierdiscus toxicus* has been implicated.[90] It settles on algae such as *Spysidia filamentosa* in the neighbourhood of tropical reefs and is ingested by herbivorous fish. These in turn are the prey of the carnivorous fish which, when eaten by humans, may give rise to severe gastrointestinal, neurotoxic and cardiovascular symptoms. Ciguatoxins are concentrated in the intestine, gonads and viscera. The acquisition of toxin by fish cannot be predicted, there is no seasonal variation in its prevalence but the risk of poisoning is greater with some species, e.g. Moray eels, and definitely increases as the fish gets larger.

Three toxins, ciguatoxin, maitotoxin and scaritoxin (from the parrot fish *Scarus sordidus*) have been identified but their molecular structures are not yet known. Until recently there was no better method of deciding whether a fish contained toxin than by feeding part of it to an animal and waiting for clinical symptoms to develop. One recent method is to measure the LD_{50} of fish extract injected intrathoracically in *Aedes aegypti* mosquitoes[91] but an even more promising method consists of piercing the suspect fish with a bamboo stick and detecting ciguatoxin using a monoclonal antibody ELISA method.[92]

The effect of ciguatoxin was thought to resemble anticholinesterase, but more recent work suggests a direct effect on excitable membranes by competing with calcium ions. In animals the venom produces respiratory failure followed by hypotension, bradycardia and cardiac arrhythmias.

Clinical features

Exceptionally, symptoms first appear as early as minutes or as long as 30 hours after eating the poisoned fish. However, the usual interval is 1–6 hours. The earliest symptom is numbness or tingling of the lips, tongue, throat and extremities, a metallic taste and a dry mouth or hypersalivation. Reversed perception of heat and cold is a distinctive symptom. In many cases, especially with milder poisoning, the earliest symptoms are gastrointestinal: sudden abdominal colic, nausea, vomiting and watery diarrhoea. Myalgia, ataxia, vertigo, visual disturbances and pruritic skin eruptions develop later. In severely neurotoxic cases flaccid paralysis and respiratory arrest may develop. Gastrointestinal symptoms resolve within a few hours but paraesthesiae may persist for a week or longer.

Ciguatera poisoning from eating moray eels (*Gymnothorax* species) is particularly rapid and severe because of the high concentration of toxin in these animals.

Chelonitoxication results from the ingestion of marine turtles (Chelonia). Its clinical features resemble ciguatera poisoning.[93] Most outbreaks have been in the Indo-Pacific area. The species usually implicated are green hawksbill and leathery turtles. The mortality rate among reported cases is 28%.[58]

Tetrodotoxic (puffer fish) poisoning

More than 50 species of tropical scaleless fish of the order Tetraodontiformes have proved poisonous. They include porcupine fish (*Chilomycterus*), molas or sunfish (*Mola*) and puffer fish or toadfish (Tetraodontidae—genera *Arothron*, *Fugu*, *Lagocephalus*, etc.). The flesh of the puffer fish (Japanese fugu) is particularly relished in Japan where, despite the stringent regulations and skilful fugu cooks, there are 250 cases of tetrodotoxin poisoning reported each year with a 60% mortality. The peak mortality was probably 470 in 1947. Cases have been reported in Thailand and many other Indo-Pacific countries. Tetrodotoxin is an aminoperhydroquinazoline which has been synthesized. It is one of the most potent non-protein toxins known. It is found mainly in the ovaries, viscera and skin. There is a definite seasonal variation in the toxin concentration which reaches a peak during the spawning season (May to June in Japan). Tetrodotoxin impairs nervous conduction by blocking the sodium ion flux without affecting potassium, producing neurotoxic and cardiotoxic effects. The origin of this toxin is unknown. It may, like ciguatoxin, be acquired through the food chain. An identical toxin has been found in the skin of newts (genus *Taricha*), and frogs (genus *Atelopus*) and the saliva of octopuses (genus *Octopus* or *Hapalochlaena*) (see p. 886).

Clinical features

Paraesthesia, dizziness, and ataxia become noticeable within 10 to 45 minutes of eating the fish. Generalized numbness, hypersalivation, sweating, and hypotension may develop. Some patients remain aware of their surroundings despite appearing comatose. Gastrointestinal symptoms may be completely absent. Death from respiratory paralysis usually occurs within the first 6 hours and is unusual more than 2 hours after eating the fish. Erythema, petechiae, blistering, and desquamation may appear.

Paralytic shellfish and crustacean poisoning

Bivalve molluscs such as mussels, clams (*Saxidomus*), oysters, cockles, and scallops, xanthid crabs, coconut crabs (*Birgus*),[94] and the eggs of horseshoe crabs (*Carcinoscorpius*),[95] may acquire neurotoxins such as saxitoxin from the dinoflagellates *Gonyaulax catenella*, *G. tamarensis*, and *G. excavata* which occur between latitudes 30° north and south. The dinoflagellates may be sufficiently abundant during the warmer months of May to October to produce a 'red tide'. The dangerous season is announced by the discovery of unusual numbers of dead fish and sea birds. Symptoms develop within 30 minutes of ingestion. They include perioral paraesthesia, gastrointestinal symptoms, ataxia, visual disturbances and pareses progressing to respiratory paralysis within 12 hours) in 8% of cases. Milder gastrointestinal and neurotoxic symptoms without paralysis have been associated with ingestion of molluscs contaminated by neurotoxins from *Ptychodiscus brevis*, which also causes a 'red tide'.

Histamine syndrome (Scombrotoxic poisoning)[95a]

The red flesh of scombroid fish such as tuna, mackerel, bonito, and skipjack, and of canned non-scombroid fish like sardines and pilchards may be decomposed by the action of bacteria such as *Proteus morgani*, converting muscle histidine into saurine, histamine, and unidentified toxins. Toxic fish may produce a tingling or smarting sensation in the mouth when eaten. Between minutes and a few hours after ingestion, flushing, burning, urticaria and pruritus of the skin, headache, abdominal colic, nausea, vomiting, diarrhoea, and bronchial asthma may develop. Identical symptoms have been described in Sri Lankan patients who ate a histamine-rich fish the skipjack while taking isoniazid, a histaminase inhibitor, for tuberculosis.[96]

Poisoning by ingestion of carp's gall bladder

In parts of the Far East, the raw bile and gall bladder of various species of freshwater carp (e.g. the grass carp *Ctenopharyngodon idellus*, 'plaa yeesok' *Probarbus jullienii*) are believed to have medicinal properties. Patients in China, Taiwan, Hong Kong, Thailand and elsewhere have developed acute abdominal pain, vomiting and watery diarrhoea 2–18 hours after drinking the raw bile or eating raw gall bladder of these fish. One patient developed flushing and dizziness. Hepatic and renal damage may develop progressing to oliguric or non-oliguric acute renal failure (acute tubular necrosis).[101] The hepatonephrotoxin has not been identified, but is heat stable and may be derived from the carp's diet.[102]

TREATMENT

The differential diagnosis includes bacterial and viral food poisoning and allergic reactions. No specific treatments or antidotes are available. Gastrointestinal contents should be eliminated by emetics and purges. Activated charcoal absorbs saxitoxin and other shellfish toxins. Atropine is said to improve gastrointestinal symptoms and sinus bradycardia in patients with gastrointestinal and neurotoxic poisoning. Oximes, such as pralidoxime and 2-pyridine aldoxime, have been claimed to benefit the anticholinesterase features of ciguatera poisoning but the evidence is not convincing. Calcium gluconate may relieve mild neuromuscular symptoms. In scombroid poisoning, antihistamines and bronchodilators should be used. In cases of respiratory paralysis, endotracheal intubation and mechanical ventilation have proved life-saving. Cardiac resuscitation may also be required.

PREVENTION

Ciguatera, tetrodotoxin, and the other toxins responsible are heat-stable, so cooking does not prevent poisoning. In tropical areas the flesh of fish should be separated, as soon as possible, from the head, skin, intestines, gonads, and other viscera which may have high concentrations of toxin. All scaleless fish should be regarded as potentially tetrodotoxic, while very large fish carry an increased risk of being ciguateratoxic. Moray eels should never be eaten. Some toxins are fairly water-soluble and may be leeched out, so water in which fish are cooked should be thrown away. Scombroid poisoning can be prevented by prompt freezing or by eating the fish fresh. Shellfish should not be eaten during the dangerous seasons and when there are red tides.

REFERENCES

1   Gans, C. (1978) Reptilian venoms: some evolutionary considerations. In *Biology of the Reptilia*, ed. C. Gans & K.A. Gans, vol. 8, pp. 1–42. London: Academic Press.
2   Dessauer, H.C. (1974) Biochemical and immunological evidence of relationships in amphibia and reptilia. In *Biochemical and Immunological Taxonomy of Animals*, ed. C.A. Wright, pp. 177–242. London: Academic Press.
3   Kochva, E. & Wollberg, Z. (1987). A cardiotoxic venom in the burrowing asps genus *Atractaspis*, a tropical group of venomous snakes. *Proceedings XI International Congress for Tropical Medicine and Malaria, Calgary, Canada.* September 16–22, 1984. Bocaraton: CRC Press. (In press.)
4   Warrell, D.A., Looareesuwan, S., White, N.J. et al (1983) *Br. med. J.* **286**, 678–680.
5   Parrish, H.M. (1980) *Poisonous Snakebites in the United States.* New York: Vantage Press.
6   Sutherland, S.K. (1983) *Australian animal toxins. The Creatures, their Toxins and Care of the Poisoned Patient.* Melbourne: Oxford University Press.
7   Pugh, R.N.H., Theakston, R.D.G., Reid, H.A. et al (1980) *Ann. trop. Med. Parasit.* **74**, 523–530.
8   Gajdusek, D.C. (1977) London Ciba Foundation Symposium. In *Symposium on Health and Diseases in Tribal Societies.* New series No. 49. New York: Elsevier.

9 Swaroop, S. & Grab, B. (1954) Snakebite mortality in the world. *Bull. Wld Hlth Org.* **10**, 35–76.

10 Myint-Lwin, Warrell, D.A., Phillips, R.E. et al (1985) *Lancet* **ii**, 1259–1264.

11 Warrell, D.A. & Arnett, C. (1976) *Acta Tropica (Basel)* **33**, 307–341.

12 Kochva, E. (1978) Oral glands of the reptilia. In *Biology of the Reptilia*, ed. C. Gans & K.A. Gans, vol. 8: pp. 43–161. London: Academic Press.

13 Bogert, C.M. (1943) *Bull. Am. Mus. Nat. Hist.* **81**, Art III, 285–360.

13a Mebs, D. (1985) *List of Biologically Active Components from Snake Venoms*. Frankfurt: Zentrum der Rechtsmedizin, University of Frankfurt.

14 Warrell, D.A., Greenwood, B.M., Davidson, N.McD. et al (1976) *Q. J. Med. N.S.* **45**, 1–22.

15 Tseng, L.F., Chiu, T.H. & Lee, C.Y. (1968) *Toxicol. appl. Pharmacol.* **12**, 526–535.

16 Higginbotham, R.D. (1965) *J. Immunol.* **95**, 867–875.

17 Kuo, T.P. & Wu, C.S. (1972) *J. Form. Med. Ass.* **71**, 447–466.

18 Mebs, L.D. (1978) Pharmacology of reptilian venoms. In *Biology of Reptilia*, ed. C. Gans & K.A. Gans, vol. 8, pp. 437–560. London: Academic Press.

19 Regoeczi, E. & Bell, W.R. (1969) *Br. J. Haematol.* **16**, 573–587.

20 Budzynski, A.Z., Pandya, B.V., Rubin, R.N. et al (1984) *Blood* **63**, 1–14.

21 Kitchens, C.S. & Van Mierop, L.H.S. (1983) *Am. J. Hematol.* **14**, 345–353.

22 Hutton, R.A., Warrell, D.A., Looareesuwan, S. et al. Unpublished.

23 Efrati, P. & Reif, L. (1953) *Am. J. trop. Med. Hyg.* **2**, 1085–1108.

24 Sitprija, V. & Boonpucknavig, V. (1979) Snake venoms and nephrotoxicity. In *Snake Venoms. Handbook of Experimental Pharmacology*, ed. C.Y. Lee, vol. 52, pp. 997–1018. Berlin: Springer-Verlag.

25 Bevan, P. & Hiestand, P. (1983) *J. biol. Chem.* **258**, 5319–5326.

26 Lakier, B. & Fritz, V.U. (1969) *S. Afr. med. J.* **43**, 1052–1055.

27 Beiran, D. & Currie, G. (1967) *Cent. Afr. J. Med.* **13**, 137–139.

28 Mittleman, M.B. & Goris, R.C. (1978) *J. Herpetol.* **12**, 109–111.

29 Cable, D., McGehee, W., Wingert, W.A. et al (1984) *J. Am. med. Ass.* **251**, 925–926.

30 Warrell, D.A., Ormerod, L.D. & Davidson, N. McD. (1976) *Am. J. trop. Med. Hyg.* **25**, 517–524.

31 Weiser, E., Wollberg, Z., Kochva, E. et al (1984) *Toxicon* **22**, 767–774.

32 Campbell, C.H. (1979) Symptomatology, pathology and treatment of the bites of elapid snakes. In *Snake Venoms. Handbook of Experimental Pharmacology*, ed. C.Y. Lee, vol. 52, pp. 898–921. Berlin: Springer-Verlag.

33 Watt, G., Theakston, R.D.G., Hayes, C.G. et al (1986) *N. Engl. J. Med.* **315**, 1444–1448.

34 Warrell, D.A. & Ormerod, L.D. (1976) *Am. J. trop. Med. Hyg.* **25**, 525–529.

35 Marshall, L. R. & Herrmann, R.P. (1983) *Thromb. Haemostat (Stuttgart)* **50**, 707–711.

36 Reid, H.A. (1979) Symptomatology, pathology and treatment of the bites of sea snakes. In *Snake Venoms. Handbook of Experimental Pharmacology*, ed. C.Y. Lee, vol. 52, pp. 922–955. Berlin: Springer-Verlag.

37 Matsen, F.A. (1980) *Compartmental Syndromes*, p. 162. New York: Grune & Stratton.

38 Reid, H.A. (1968) Symptomatology, pathology, and treatment of land snake bite in India and Southeast Asia. In *Venomous Animals and their Venom*, vol. I, Chap. 20, pp. 611–642. New York: Academic Press.

39 Viravan, C., Veeravat, U., Warrell, M.J. et al (1986) *Am. J. trop. Med. Hyg.* **35**, 173–181.

40 Reid, H.A. (1961) *Lancet* **ii**, 399–402.

41 Reid, H.A. (1976) *Br. med. J.* **ii**, 153–156.

42 Russell, F.E. (1980) *Snake Venom Poisoning*. Philadelphia: Lippincott.

43 Ho, M., Warrell, D.A., Looareesuwan, S. et al (1986) *Am. J. trop. Med. Hyg.* **35**, 579–587.

44 Theakston, R.D.G. (1983) *Toxicon* **21**, 341–352.

45 Ho, M., Warrell, M.J., Warrell, D.A. et al (1986) *Toxicon* **24**, 211–221.

46 Sutherland, S.K., Coulter, A.R. & Harris, R.D. (1979) *Lancet* **i**, 183–186.

47 Tun-Pe, Tin-Nu-Swe, Myint-Lwin et al (1987) *Trans. R. Soc. Trop. Med. Hyg.* (in press).

48 Malasit, P., Warrell, D.A., Chanthavanich, P., et al (1986). *Br. med. J.* **292**, 17–20.

49 Warrell, D.A., Warrell, M.J., Edgar, W. et al (1980) *Br. med. J.* **280**, 607–609.

50 Thein-Than, Kyi-Thein & Mg-Mg-Thwin (1985) *Trans. R. Soc. trop. Med. Hyg.* **79**, 262–263.

51 Ho, M., Karbwang, J., Warrell, D.A. et al. Unpublished.

52 Sutherland, S.K. (1977) *Med. J. Austral.* April 23, 613–615.

53 Garfin, S.R., Castilonia, R.R., Mubarak, S.J. et al (1984) *Toxicon* **22**, 177–182.

54 Sawai, Y. (1979) Vaccination against snakebite poisoning. In *Snake Venoms. Handbook of Experimental Pharmacology*, ed. C.Y. Lee, pp. 881–897. Berlin: Springer-Verlag.

55 Vandenplas, M.L., Vandenplas, S., Brebner, K. et al (1985) *Toxicon* **23**, 289–305.

56 Tamiya, T., Lamouroux, A., Julien, J.F. et al (1985) *Biochimie* **67**, 185–189.

57 Russell, F.E. & Bogert, C.M. (1981) *Toxicon* **19**, 341–359.

58 Halstead, B.W. (1978) *Poisonous and Venomous Marine Animals of the World*, revised edn. Princeton, New Jersey: Darwin Press.

59 Russell, F.E. (1965) *Marine Toxins and Venomous and Poisonous Marine Animals*. Academic Press, 1965, T.F.H. Publications, 1971.

60 Russell, F.E., Panos, T.C., Kang, L.W. et al (1958) *Am. J. med. Sci.* **235**, 566–584.

61 Maretic, Z. (1973) Some epidemiological, clinical and therapeutic aspects of envenomation by weeverfish sting. In *Toxic of Animal and Plant Origin*, ed. A. de Vries & E. Kochva, pp. 1055–1065. New York: Gordon and Breach.

62 Barnes, J.H. (1960) *Med. J. Austral.* **2**, 993–999.

63 Maretic, Z., Russell, F.E. & Ladavac, J. (1980) Epidemic of stings by the jelly fish *Pelagia noctiluca* in the Adriatic. In *Natural Toxins*, ed. D. Eaker & T. Wadstrom. Oxford: Pergamon Press.

64 Kingston, C.W. & Southcott, R.V. (1960) *Trans. Roy. Soc. trop. Med. Hyg.* **54**, 373–384.

65 Maretic, Z. & Russell, F.E. (1983) *Am. J. trop. Med. Hyg.* **32**, 891–896.

66 Hartwick, R., Callanan, U. & Williamson, J. (1980) *Med. J. Austral.* **1**, 15–20.

67 Williamson, J., Callanan, V.I. & Hartwick, R.F. (1980) *Med. J. Austral.* **1**, 13–15.

68 Alender, C.B. & Russell, F.E. (1966) Pharmacology. In *Physiology of Echinodermata*, ed. R.A. Boolootian, pp. 529–543. New York: Interscience Publisher.

68a Schmidt, J.O., Blum, M.S. & Overal, W.L. (1986) *Toxicon* **24**, 907–921.

68b Schmidt, J.O., Yamane, S., Matsura, M. et al (1986) *Toxicon* **24**, 950–954.

69 Bryceson, A.D.M. Personal communication.

70 Ewan, P.W. (1984) *J. Roy. Soc. Med.* **78**, 234–239.

71 Golden, D.B.K. & Valentine, M.D. (1984) Insect sting allergy. *Anim. Allergy* **53**, 444–451.

72 Delage, C. & Irey, N.S. (1972) *J. forens. Sci.* **17**, 525–540.

73 Hoffman, D.R., Wood, C.L. & Hudson, P. (1983) *J. Allerg. Clin. Immunol.* **72**, 193–196.

74 Hunt, K.J., Valentine, M.D., Sobotka, A.K. et al (1978) *New Engl. J. Med.* **299**, 157–161.

75 Edery, H., Ishay, J., Gitter, S. et al (1978). Venoms of Vespidae. In *Arthropod Venoms, Handbook of Experimental Pharmacology*, ed. S. Bettini, vol. 48, pp. 691–771. Berlin: Springer-Verlag.

76 Keegan, H.L. (1980) *Scorpions of Medical Importance*. Jackson, Missouri: University Press of Mississippi.

77 Waterman, J.A. (1938) *Trans. Roy. Soc. trop. Med. Hyg.* **31**, 607–624.

78 Bawaskar, H.S. (1982) *Lancet* **i**, 552–554.

79 Poon-King, T. (1963) *Br. med. J.* **i**, 374–377.

80 Bartholomew, C., McGeeney, K.F., Murphy, J.J. et al (1976) *Br. J. Surg.* **63**, 807–810.

81 Maretic, Z. & Lebez, D. (1979) *Araneism*. Pula, Yugoslavia: Novit.

82 Pearn, J. (1977) *Med. J. Austral.* **2**, 313.

83 Murnaghan, M.F. & O'Rourke, F.J. (1978) Tick paralysis. In *Arthropod Venoms. Handbook of Experimental Pharmacology*, ed. S. Bettini, vol. 48, pp. 419–464. Berlin: Springer-Verlag.

84 Stone, B.F. (1987) Toxicoses induced by ticks and reptiles in domestic animals. In *Natural Toxins: Animal, Plant, and Microbial*, ed. J.B. Harris. Oxford: Oxford University Press.

85 Morse, D.L., Guzewich, J.J., Hanrahan, J.P. et al (1986) Widespread outbreaks of clam- and oyster-associated gastroenteritis. Role of Norwalk virus. *New Engl. J. Med.* **314**, 678–681.

86 Hughes, J.M. & Merson, M.H. (1976) *New Engl. J. Med.* **295**, 1117–1120.

87 World Health Organization (1984) Aquatic (marine and freshwater) biotoxins. *Environmental Health Criteria* 37, WHO, Geneva.

88 Bagnis, R., Kuberski, T. & Laugier, S. (1979) *Am. J. Trop. Med. Hyg.* **28**, 1067–1073.

89 Bagnis, R.A. (1979) *Rev. Epidem. et Santé publ.* **27**, 17–29.

90 Bagnis, R., Chanteau, S., Chungue, E. et al (1980) *Toxicon* **18**, 199–208.

91 Pompon, A., Chungue, E., Chazelet, I. et al (1984) *Bull. Wld Hlth Org.* **62**, 639–645.

92 Scheuer, P.J. (1986) Recent developments in ciguatera research. In *Natural Toxins: Animal, Plant, and Microbial*, ed. J.B. Harris. Oxford: Oxford University Press.

93 Pillai, V.K., Nair, M.B., Ravindranathan, K. et al (1962) *J. Assoc. Phys. India* **10**, 181–187.

94 Hashimoto, Y. & Konosu, S. (1978) Venoms of Crustacea and Merostomata. In *Arthropod Venoms. Handbook of Experimental Pharmacology*, ed. S. Bettini, pp. 13–39. Berlin: Springer-Verlag.

95 Trishnananda, M., Tuchinda, C., Yipinsoi, T. et al (1966) *J. trop. Med. Hyg.* **69**, 194–196.

95a Russell, F.E. & Maretić, Z. (1986) *Toxicon* **24**, 967–973.

96 Uragoda, C.G. & Kottegoda, S.R. (1977) *Tubercle* **58**, 83–89.

97 Reid, H.A. & Lim, K.J. (1957) *Br. Med. J.* **ii**, 1266–1272.

98 Ganthavorn, S. (1971) *Toxicon* **9**, 293–294.

99 Bolañòs, R. (1984) *Serpientes Venenos y Ofidismo en Centroamérica*. Editoriale, Universidad de Costa Rica.

100 Marsh, N.A. & Whaler, B.C. (1984) *Toxicon* **22**, 669–694.

101 Chan, D.W.S., Yeung, C.K. & Chan, M.K. (1985) *Brit. Med. J.* **290**, 897.

102 Yip, L.L. (1981) *Toxicon* **19**, 567–569.

Chapter 49
Plant Poisons

L. G. Goodwin

People in tropical countries, especially those living in rural areas, rely heavily for medical advice and treatment on local traditional herbalists and do-it-yourself medicines. A small survey in the Transkei in 1982 showed that half of the children admitted to hospital had had previous treatment with herbs, enemas or 'coloured medicine' (remedies made and sold by the coloured population). A third of children attending the outpatient clinic, but not sufficiently ill to need admission, had also received traditional remedies.

The herbs and preparations, although they may have been used for generations, are not necessarily safe. Many are known to contain toxic substances and pharmacological studies on preserved specimens are unlikely to reveal the activity of potent but labile constituents present in the fresh herb and extracts made from it at the place where it is administered. Even if a traditional medicine shows no immediate toxic effects it may have a slow or cumulative hepatotoxic, carcinogenic or mutagenic action. Very few herbal remedies have been submitted to the rigorous scrutiny now demanded by licensing authorities in developed countries for the registration of new synthetic drugs.

It is a paradox that, along with increasingly strict requirements for new drugs, traditional herbal medicines, because of their reputed therapeutic or aphrodisiac virtues, are at present enjoying an increasing popularity in the developed world. Ginseng, for example, is 'a modern Western craze' and it is not surprising that the toxic effects of herbal remedies are on the increase in Europe and North America.

Contact with certain plants or their irritant constituents may cause dermatitis and in addition to their use as medicines plant poisons are also employed for their psychotropic effects and for criminal purposes. Although illegal in many countries 'trial by ordeal' is still carried out, a person suspected of crime or witchcraft being given a toxic dose of a plant poison – vomiting and survival denoting innocence.

Food plants, if carelessly used or processed or contaminated with toxic weeds or fungi, may also result in poisoning.

Plant poisoning may therefore present as:
dermatitis (allergic or toxic);
effects of products used as medicines;
criminal poisoning;
effects of plants used for their psychotropic action;
effects of toxic or contaminated foods.

ALLERGIC AND TOXIC DERMATITIS

Poison ivy dermatitis (dermatitis venenata)

Many tropical plants cause dermatitis which may assume an erythematous, vesicular or urticarial form. Intimate contact with the plant or its leaves is necessary. Poison ivy (*Rhus toxicodendron* and *R. juglandifolia*), poison sumac (*R. vernix*), poison wood (*Metopium toxiferum*) in northeastern and southern USA cause intense dermatitis. Repeated attacks do not produce immunity. The venom is toxicodendrol. Treatment consists of washing the skin with soap and water; alcoholic or oily solutions must be avoided. Clothes must be decontaminated by immersion in 1% calcium hypochlorite for 20 minutes.

Pyrethrum dermatitis

Pyrethrum dermatitis has been noted in Kenya and is caused by the leaves and flowers of *Chrysanthemum cinerariaefolium* which grows at altitudes of 150–2100 m and flowers throughout the year. Absorption is facilitated by constant sweating, and exposure to sunlight greatly exacerbates the lesions. Some persons on contact exhibit merely a local dermatitis; others show a widespread allergy. Itching commences at the corner of the eyes and is followed by lacrimation, an irritating vesicular rash, peeling of the skin and formation of painful fissures.

Manchineel poisoning

The manchineel or manchineale, *Hippomane mancinella* (Euphorbiaceae), is a tree 9–15 m high and of a circumference of 1.5–3 m distributed along the coastline of North, South and Central America and the West Indies. It is particularly common in Barbados, Grenadine Islands and the Archipelago of Les Saintes in French West Indies. Two varieties are recognized, one with 'holly' and the other with 'laurel' leaves; both are equally toxic. The first, which resembles a crab-apple, has a pleasant odour.

The latex contains a greenish resin which is the active toxic principle. Like the upas tree the manchineel has been said to bring death to those who sleep under its shade. All parts of the tree are toxic but the amount of latex in any portion varies with the season; even the dry wood and sawdust are endowed with irritant properties. Hypersensitive people who pick manchineel apples (or fruit) may suffer from a skin eruption with erythema, bullae and vesiculation. Toxic dermatitis is especially likely to affect the genitalia and the anus causing a vesiculopustular eruption which may be confined to the corona penis. Conjunctivitis with pain, photophobia and blepharospasm may result from the introduction of the latex into the conjunctival sac. Severe dermatitis brought about by handling dried wood powder is thought to be allergic.

If the fruit is eaten, as it may be by ignorant visitors, children or insane people, vesiculation of the buccal mucous membrane wih diarrhoea and blood and mucus in the stools may ensue. Fatal poisoning may result.

Manchineel juice on the skin should be washed off with sea water. Blisters should be kept aseptic and, if extensive, treated like a second-degree burn. When the fruit has been eaten emesis should be induced.

Atriplicism

A combination of cutaneous and nervous symptoms in China is caused by eating leaves of the spinach *Atriplex littoralis* (Chenopodiaceae). The earliest symptoms consist of itching of the hands followed by oedema and often by bullae;

the fingertips may become gangrenous, cutaneous haemorrhages may occur and the face and eyelids become cyanotic and oedematous. In many aspects it resembles Raynaud's disease and erythromelalgia. A similar syndrome occurs after the leaves of *Atriplex serrata* or *Chenopodium hybridium* have been eaten and it is thought that the skin lesions can be ascribed to light-sensitive dermatosis.

Other forms of dermatitis

Several other plants and flowers may cause severe allergic dermatitis, such as *Cypripedium* (lady's slippers), *Euphorbia*, primroses, lilies and vanilla beans; sometimes also mangoes and, in Japan, lacquer made from *Rhus vernicifera*.

The juice of some species of the Umbelliferae contains photosensitizing furanocoumarin derivatives which on contact with the skin cause erythema and vesication on exposure to light.

Seaweed dermatitis has been reported from Hawaii and appears to be due to contact with a blue-green filamentous alga tentatively identified as *Lyngbya majuscula*, which produces an erythematous and vesicular rash in persons bathing in the sea off windward beaches. The condition is a reaction to a toxin and is not allergic in origin. It subsides quickly on local treatment.

Idiosyncrasy to wood dust is not uncommon. Iroko is a trade name for *Chlorophora excelsa*, a tree of East and West tropical Africa known as African teak. The dust produces the usual signs of allergy with skin irritation, oedema of face, blepharospasm, acute coryza and pharyngitis. Other woods, such as satin wood, teak and mahogany, also produce allergy in susceptible persons. Obeche or wa-wa (*Triplochiton sclerox-ylon*), a soft wood, produces similar symptoms.

HERBAL MEDICINES

Poisoning from herbal medicines occurs because the herb itself contains toxic substances, because it has been adulterated accidentally or deliberately with other plants or because, as in the Asian 'Kushtays' used as tonics or aphrodisiacs, it has been mixed with appreciable amounts of the oxides of arsenic, mercury, tin, zinc or lead.

Self-medication with herbal medicines sometimes causes problems because they interfere with the effects of treatment with orthodox drugs. The main interactions are listed by Penn.[1]

Bush teas (veno-occlusive disease)

The commonest herbal remedies are bush teas—extracts made from fresh or dried flowers, fruits, leaves, bark or roots by steeping in hot or cold water. Some of them are undoubtedly toxic.

Veno-occlusive disease is an acute, subacute or chronic condition affecting primarily the central and sublobular hepatic veins. It has been reported mainly from the West Indies but also from North and South Africa and India.

It is now generally accepted that the consumption of 'bush tea' containing the alkaloids of *Crotalaria fulva*, which produces a similar condition in rats, is the cause in the West Indies.[2] The pyrrolizidine alkaloids of this group of plants, *Crotalaria*, *Senecio* and *Heliotropium*, have produced liver injury in all animals in which they have been tested, and *Senecio* poisoning occurs naturally in animals in many parts of the world. In South Africa *C. dura* is responsible for hepatic and pulmonary lesions in horses. Outbreaks in people in India have been associated with the contamination of cereals with seeds of *Crotalaria*[3] and *Heliotropium*.[4] An outbreak of a liver disease resembling veno-occlusive disease was attributed to aflatoxins in the food by Krishnamachari et al.[5]

The primary pathological change involves the central and sublobular hepatic veins. There is subendothelial oedema followed by intimal overgrowth of connective tissue and narrowing and occlusion of the lumina. Centrizonal congestion, atrophy or necrosis of liver cells with consequent fibrosis leads to gross changes similar to those described in cardiac cirrhosis.[6] In the West Indies cirrhosis due to veno-occlusive disease accounts for about one-third of all types of cirrhosis.[7] The symptoms and signs are due to portal hypertension with its associated complications. There is no evidence of any association with hepatitis B antigen.

The condition presents as acute hepatomegaly and ascites in children. About half of those affected recover and 20% die in the acute state. The remainder pass into a subacute and chronic stage with the development of portal hypertension.[8]

Ginseng

The roots of *Panax ginseng* (Araliaceae) have been used in China and Korea for centuries in the belief that they counter fatigue and stress and confer health, virility and longevity. Although the pharmacological basis for its reputation is slender, ginseng is at present enjoying a vogue worldwide. Several species of *Panax* are extensively cultivated but the drug is expensive and is frequently found adulterated with *Eleutherococcus* (Russian ginseng), *Mandragora*, *Rauwolfia* and other roots. Ginseng extract contains a complex mixture of sugars, steroids and saponin glycosides. Side-effects include central nervous excitation, nervousness, tremor, oestrogen-like effects and perhaps hypertension.

Cotton root bark

The bark of *Gossypium* (Malvaceae) contains gossypol, which depresses spermatogenesis and has been used as a male contraceptive. Side-effects have been few but increased loss of potassium through the kidney occurs and cases of hypokalaemic paralysis have been reported.

Karela

The fruit of *Momordica charantia* (Cucurbitaceae) is a traditional Indian remedy for diabetes. It has a hypoglycaemic effect that may interfere with the control of diabetes in patients receiving orthodox treatment.

Maklua

The fruit of *Diospyros mollis* (Ebenaceae) is used in Thailand for the expulsion of intestinal worms. The active principle is a hydroxynaphthalene derivative, diospyrol, which has been reported to cause optic neuritis, especially in young children.

Cows' urine poisoning

Cows' urine mixture (CUM) is a well-established tradition among the Yoruba people in Nigeria. It is employed as a prophylactic and treatment for fits and convulsions in children and adults from epilepsy or eclampsia. The ingredients—cows' urine (sometimes human) and green tobacco leaves—are given by mouth or rubbed on the skin[9] and have been shown to cause toxic effects in animals similar to those in humans. They contain nicotine, rock salt, juice of *Citrus medica* and leaves of *Occinium viridae*.[10]

The clinical picture of CUM poisoning is an acute excitation of the central nervous system accompanied by vomiting, diarrhoea and dehydration, later proceeding to depression of the central nervous system with coma which may last for days, causing death or permanent neurological derangement. Hypoglycaemia is a feature.

Immediate control of convulsions is required with intravenous injection of 25% or 50% glucose. The poison must be removed by gastric lavage or cleansing of skin, and fluid and electrolytes corrected. Blood glucose should be monitored.

For a fuller account of the hazards of unorthodox medicine, see Penn.[1]

CRIMINAL POISONING

The plants used for criminal purposes, for trial by ordeal and for arrow poisons are many and varied. Some of their most active constituents—the tropane alkaloids, strychnine, eserine, strophanthin and tubocurarine—are familiar in Western medicine for their useful pharmacological effects. Others are frank poisons. Plant products are not infrequently supplemented with inorganic poisons, usually arsenic introduced into seeds, flour or sweets, for criminal purposes.

In India a large number of vegetable poisons is in use. In the Madras and Bombay states an extract is obtained from the roots of *Nerium odorum* (Apocynaceae), the white oleander, which contains glycosides exerting a specific action on the heart. Similar substances, urechitin and urechitoxin, from *Urechites suberecta* of the West Indies, exert a cumulative action and sudden death may therefore be produced without arousing suspicion of poisoning.

Several other species of the Apocynaceae, such as *Cerbera odollam* and *Thevetia neriifolia*, the sap and seeds of which contain a glycoside, thevetin, are very deadly, death from cardiac failure taking place in 12–15 hours.

The juice of *Asclepias* (milkweed) is used in India as an infanticide; the symptoms are vomiting, salivation and cramps. The roots of various species of aconite (*Aconitum ferox*, etc) are used for the same purpose; death takes place rapidly, in 3–6 hours as a rule.

In southern India, Burma, Sri Lanka and Africa a decoction of tubers of *Gloriosa superba* (Liliaceae) allied to squill, is employed for criminal and suicidal purposes. The active principles,

superbine and colchicine, cause gastrointestinal irritation and cardiac failure within 4 hours.

The commonest poison in India and Sri Lanka is *Datura* (Solanaceae) of which there are several species. The seeds, mixed with food or drink, produce a state of extreme mental exaltation followed by coma; the active principles are atropine, hyoscyamine and scopolamine. The seeds of *Datura fastuosa* were used by Thugs in India. The seeds have a slight taste and are consequently easily introduced into food. *D. stramonium* is found in many parts of the world and accidental poisoning may occur.[11] *D. sanguinea* is used in Peru and Colombia, *D. ferox* and *D. arborea* in Brazil. The characteristic seeds are found in the faeces and, in fatal cases, in the small intestine. The leaves of *Hyoscyamus fahezlez*, also containing hyoscyamine and scopolamine, are used by Tuareg of the Sahara.

In Indonesia a poison extracted from the roots of *Milletia sericea*, a leguminous plant allied to *Wisteria*, is used for poisoning fish and produces debility, headache, diarrhoea, collapse and death.

In the Pacific Islands a fish poison containing saponins is derived from the fruit of *Barringtonia speciosa* (Myrtaceae).

In China, opium is the suicidal poison most frequently used, especially by women.

Curare, the potent arrow poison of South American Indians, was known to Sir Walter Raleigh in 1595. The material was obtained from the giant vines of the Amazon and Orinoco, called 'bushropes' by explorers, which include *Chondodendron tomentosum* which is the main source of curare. Curare poisons by causing paralysis of the muscles as shown by Claude Bernard in 1857. It blocks neuromuscular transmission and relaxation of the muscle is produced. It has now revolutionized anaesthesia; the active principle is D-tubocurarine chloride. Synthetic substitutes for curare have been discovered and are being widely used.

In Zaire almost all the poisons used on arrowheads contain cardiotoxic glycosides derived from species of *Strophanthus*, particularly strophanthin-K and ouabain; many also contain haemolytic saponins.

In Brazil, common poisons are derived from *Paullinia pinnata* which contains an alkaloid, timboin, and from the fruit of *Thevetia ahonai*, the active principle of which is thevetosin; both of these cause vomiting and respiratory failure.

In West Africa one of the commonest plant poisons used for criminal purposes is 'red water' or 'sassy' bark, the bark of the leguminous tree *Erythrophleum guineense*. It contains the alkaloid erythrophleine that causes vomiting, difficulty in respiration, convulsions and an action on the circulatory system resembling that of digitalis. It also has a local anaesthetic action. *Erythrophleum*, like the well-known 'ordeal bean' *Physostigma venenosum* is used for trial by ordeal.

The common African hedge cactus (*Euphorbia* spp.) contains an escharotic and cathartic latex that is used as an ingredient of arrow poison and for criminal purposes.

The seeds of the castor oil plant *Ricinus*, another member of the Euphorbiaceae, contain ricin, a phytotoxic protein that is one of the most poisonous substances known. A single castor oil bean contains enough ricin to kill a child. It has been used for criminal purposes, one of the more recent being the implantation of a 1.5 mm sphere containing ricin into the thigh of the victim by the assassin's umbrella.

PSYCHOTROPIC DRUGS

Alcohol poisoning

This occurs in varying degrees among nearly all tropical races and in symptoms and course does not differ materially from alcoholism in other parts of the world. Rum (65–72% alcohol), obtained from the fermentation of molasses, is used in the West Indies and South America; arrack (50–60% alcohol) is manufactured in India, China and Java from fermented rice or from palm sap; while a slightly fermented drink, toddy, is obtained from sweet sap of various palms and is drunk in India, Sri Lanka and West Africa. In South America a potent alcoholic drink is made from the fermented juice of *Agave americana* and is known as 'pulque'.

Opium poisoning

The opium habit, either eating or smoking—the symptoms of which are too well-known to require description—is common throughout the tropics. Opium poisoning is also a favourite form of suicide, especially among women.

Cannabis indica

Indian hemp, or hasheesh, grows in India, Iran and Arabia and is a variety of the common hemp, *Cannabis sativa*. The leaves are powdered and either chewed or smoked in a preparation known as bhang; an extract of the flowers is known as ganja. Both these preparations cause great nervous excitement and, if persistently used, often lead to permanent insanity, the main features of which are hallucinations and illusions. Hasheesh, in various preparations, often with the addition of extracts of various Solanaceae, such as datura and nux vomica, is habitually taken daily by millions of the inhabitants of Africa and Asia. The most stringent government regulations have been framed in an attempt to suppress trade in this drug, which has become a serious problem also in Europe and North America.

Kava or yangona

The powdered root of *Piper methysticum*, prepared to form a beverage, is drunk on festive occasions throughout Polynesia. Formerly the root was masticated by specially selected girls in the preparation of the drink, a practice which was then a prolific source of tuberculosis. Over-indulgence in kava induces a state of hyper-excitement, with loss of power in the legs. Chronic intoxication produces debility, with coarse roughened skin.

Betel

Chewing betel, the leaves of *Piper betel*, together with lime and areca nut (*Areca catechu*), is a common practice in India and Sri Lanka and generally throughout the East. The mouth, lips and teeth are stained a bright red colour. It produces a flushing of the face and has mild stimulant and possibly anthelmintic properties. In central and West Africa the nuts of the kola tree (*Cola acuminata* and *C. nitida*) are chewed habitually and act as a sialogogue and stimulant without, it is said, producing any detrimental effects but may cause sqamous cell carcinoma of the mouth (Chapter 67).

Cocaine

Erythroxylon coca is widely used in India and in parts of South America as a stimulant and intoxicant. The leaves, first dried in the sun, are chewed with lime, or, as in India, with betel. This drug produces a loss of sensation in tongue and lips, the pulse is accelerated and there ensues a period of hilarity and exaltation. The drug addict soon becomes emaciated and cachectic.

Khat

Khat (miraa, muiragi, cafta) is derived from a tree, *Catha edulis*, about 6 m in height, indigenous to North Africa. The leaves or twigs may be chewed or infused or may even be smoked when they induce a happy mellow sense of friendliness. Cases of mental disturbance in addicts have been described. The leaves contain cathinone, a phenylalkylamine with an effect similar to that of amphetamine.

TOXIC AND CONTAMINATED FOODS

Accidental poisoning, especially of children, occurs as a result of gathering and eating toxic fruits from the bush. More serious outbreaks of poisoning occur from foodstuffs that have been contaminated with the seeds of toxic weeds, adulterated with cheap but dangerous substitutes or carelessly prepared and stored so that they contain poisonous residues or have grown toxic moulds.

Ackee poisoning (vomiting sickness of Jamaica)

An acute and fatal condition, locally termed 'the vomiting sickness', has been known for many years in Jamaica. It is found principally in rural districts in circumscribed epidemics. The causation and nature were neither apprehended nor understood, although several Commissions had attempted to elucidate them. To Sir Harold Scott belongs the merit of clearing up this mystery and of indicating simple and practical methods of prevention which have saved the lives of many children. It is estimated that since 1886 over 5000 lives have been lost in Jamaica from this cause.

Scott showed that vomiting sickness is the result of poisoning by ackee, the fruit of *Blighia sapida*, a native of West Africa where it is known as ishin. When mature and in good condition this fruit is wholesome enough; if gathered before it is quite ripe and before it has opened while on the tree, or if gathered from an injured branch or opened after falling to the ground, it is poisonous.

Vomiting sickness is confined to the West Indian islands, practically to Jamaica, and occurs principally in the cooler months, from November to April.

A previously healthy child suddenly complains of abdominal discomfort, vomits several times, recovers and perhaps falls asleep. Three or four hours later, vomiting—now of a cerebral type—returns. Within a few minutes convulsions and coma supervene and death follows on an average about 12 hours from the initial vomiting, though it may take place in one and a half hours. The case mortality amounts to 80–90%. In those who recover convalescence is complete in 24 hours.

During the attack the temperature is normal or subnormal, rarely rising to 38.3°C; the pulse rate is 90–100; the respirations are 26–30, sometimes, as death approaches of Cheyne–Stokes type. The pupils are slightly dilated and, until near the end, react to light. Except during the convulsive seizures there is no muscular rigidity. Post-mortem examination reveals hyperaemia of viscera with a tendency to minute intestinal haemorrhages together with marked fatty changes, especially in the liver and kidneys and sometimes in the pancreas and heart muscles.

Extreme hypoglycaemia (blood sugar levels as low as 22 mg/dl) was found in children with this illness by Stuart et al (1955).[12] They laid the foundations for its logical treatment by prompt and large doses of glucose. Biopsy and necropsy showed fatty changes in the liver with almost complete absence of glycogen. The course of the disease suggested a temporary enzyme block, inhibiting gluconeogenesis for which the name of *acute toxic hypoglycaemia* is proposed. The ackee contains two polypeptides, hypoglycin A and B, which produces fatal hypoglycaemia in laboratory animals.[13]

An emetic, and washing out the stomach with an alcoholic fluid during the primary vomiting are indicated. This must be followed by intravenous glucose. Glycin in large doses may be of value.[14]

Coral plant

Coral plant poisoning has been reported from Tanzania, the symptoms being colic, cramps and thirst, with subnormal temperature. Two species, *Jatropha curcas* and *J. glandulifera* (Euphorbiaceae) are common in the West Indies. *J. glandulifera*, since it grows rapidly, is used in Jamaica for fencing enclosures. The nuts taste like sweet almonds and the plants are known as 'physic nuts'; a third species, *J. multifida*, is known as the 'French physic nut'. *J. gossypifolia*, which occurs in the West Indies, is known as the wild cassava or 'belly-ache bush' and its seeds contain an intestinal irritant like croton oil. A fifth species, *J. urens*, from the same area, bears leaves provided with stinging hairs, which cause itching, smarting, flushing of the face, swelling of the lips and faintness.

Manioc (cassava) and nami (yams)

Manihot aipi (sweet cassava) and *manihot utilissima* (bitter cassava) (Euphorbiaceae) are ground roots extensively used in the tropics. From the latter are produced starch, tapioca and cassava cakes. Poisoning arises from failure to remove the contained glycoside and enzyme. In the presence of water these release free hydrocyanic acid so that nausea, vomiting, distension of the abdomen and impeded respiration result. How far these widely used foods are responsible for poisoning is problematical. Cassava may contain an antithyroid agent and may cause goitre.[15] A predominantly cassava diet is also reported to cause parotid hypertrophy, ataxic neuropathy (see Chapter 47), chronic pancreatitis and diabetes (see Chapter 66).

Yams are the tubers of *Dioscorea* spp. (Dioscoreaceae). Sweet, edible and bitter, toxic forms are common. The bitter varieties contain the alkaloid dioscorine. In West Africa they are sometimes planted at the edges of fields of sweet yams in order to discourage theft; they have been responsible for deaths in times of food shortage. In areas in which the root stocks of cycads (*Cycas* or *Zamia*) are used to produce flour, poisoning may occur unless the product is washed free from the glycoside cycasin which can cause lesions of the central nervous system and liver cancer.

Epidemic dropsy (argemone oil poisoning)

Epidemic dropsy somewhat resembles beriberi. Clinically, it is characterized by dropsy associated with cardiac symptoms but without paralysis or anaesthesia.

This condition was first noted in Calcutta in 1877; it has since occurred there sporadically but vanishes in the hot season. In Mauritius in 1879 it affected one-tenth of the coolies, of whom a large number died. An epidemic broke out in Fiji in 1926 and was limited to Asians; no native Fijians were affected. In Purulia (Nagpur, India) there have been epidemics at intervals since 1913, the worst being in 1934 when over 2000 were attacked. An outbreak in coloured labourers has been described in the north-west Cape district of South Africa.[16]

In spite of the apparently wide distribution of this disease most of the information comes from India where this form of poisoning is especially seen in the Hindus, particularly in females. Children before puberty are less susceptible than adults; sucklings are seldom affected. The weak and the robust are equally susceptible. It has been remarked that very few are of the poorer class, nearly all coming from the middle and upper classes.

The outbreak in Fiji in 1926 was attributed to mustard oil used in the preparation of curries and later Banerji and Ghosh in Bengal came to the same conclusion. The Mexican poppy, *Argemone mexicana*, is a common weed in India as well as in Australia where it has been mixed with wheat and fed to fowls. In them it produces changes in the comb, paralysis of legs and oedema of wattles and subcutaneous tissues reminiscent of epidemic dropsy in man. Bhattacharjee was the first to bring forward evidence that oil from the seeds of this poppy was responsible for toxic manifestations in man. Later, Pasricha showed that the toxicity of contaminated mustard oil could be eliminated by heating to 240°C for 15 minutes. Lal and his colleagues found that the seeds of *A. mexicana* (sialkanta, in Hindu) are present in many stocks of mustard seed in India, used in the preparation of katakar oil for cooking. Sanguinarine is the toxic principle of argemone oil. It is absorbed by the skin and contaminated oil used for massage has been reported to cause dropsy.[17] In animal experiments it has been found to cause capillary dilatation and interferes with oxidation of pyruvic acid.

The aetiology now appears clear. Argemone oil, under experimental conditions, produces symptoms indistinguishable from those of 'epidemic dropsy'. It can be detected by a paper chromatography test;[18] 10 ml of suspect oil is mixed with an equal volume of 50% methanolic hydrochloric acid in a boiling tube and heated for 15 minutes in a water bath. The tube is cooled and the lower acid layer is carefully removed and dried in a Petri dish at 100°C. The dry residue is taken up in a few drops of chloroform containing 1% acetic acid and spotted for paper chromatography on Whatman paper No. 1. The chromatogram is developed with the organic phase separated out of a mixture of citric acid 6 g completely dissolved in *n*-butanol 64 ml and then shaken up with distilled water 36 ml using descending flow. Sanguinarine is detected under filtered ultraviolet light as a brilliant yellow-orange spot with an *RF* value of 0.45–0.47. Its specificity is further confirmed by changing the orange colour to blue by placing a drop of alkali on the spot. A drop of acid can restore the orange colour.

Extensive vascular dilatation in the deeper layers of the skin is characteristic. The heart muscle shows no degenerative changes but there is thinning of the muscle walls and muscle fibres are separated by dilated capillaries. There is capillary dilatation wherever the vessels are least supported and this is most obvious in fatty tissues, whether subcutaneous, subpericardial or subperitoneal. Similar changes are seen in the lungs, in the cervix uteri, in the ovaries and in the intestines. Liver biopsies in 45 patients showed vascular changes involving the dilatation of hepatic vein radicles and centrilobular sinusoids with mild parenchymal injury including cytoplasmic swelling and the presence of occasional intracytoplasmic granular hyaline inclusions with focal necrosis. Similar changes have been noted in epidemics of veno-occlusive disease in India.[3]

For effects on the eye, see Chapter 70.

In an average case the total erythrocyte count is about 3.8 millions while the haemoglobin is reduced to 11 g/dl. The lymphocyte percentage is raised and there is usually considerable eosinophilia. The reticulocytes are not increased as a rule.

Dropsy is almost invariably present. It usually appears first in the legs and in some instances is confined to them; in others it involves the entire body. Occasionally it is very persistent, recurring during convalescence. Fever also is very constant; sometimes it precedes, sometimes it accompanies, sometimes it follows the dropsy. It is rarely high, ranging usually from 37.2°C to 38.9°C. Diarrhoea and vomiting generally ushered in the disease in the Mauritius epidemic. In Calcutta these symptoms were not so frequent although by no means rare, occurring at both earlier and later stages. The total duration is about six weeks. An outbreak in the employees of the East Indian railway was reported in 1945. There were 476 cases. The largest proportion were oedematous and a considerable number had diarrhoea and pyrexia. Oedema of feet and legs lasted for two weeks. There was patchy pigmentation over nose, malar bones and shins. Tachycardia was common and mortality 4.4%.

Peripheral neuritis is absent and the knee jerk is not abolished but distressing aching of muscles, bones and joints is usually prominent. An exanthem, erythematous on the face, rubeolar on the trunk and limbs, was frequently seen in Mauritius, less so in Calcutta. It appeared about a week after the oedema and lasted from 10 to 12 days. On the skin, vascular naevi often appear and may bleed profusely, while telangiectases are common. The eruptions have been described as nodular, resembling sarcoids in some epidemics, while lesions on the mucous membranes have been noted. They do not inconvenience the patient but may bleed uncontrollably. Ecchymotic patches consist, not of haemorrhage, but of telangiectases. Three to six weeks after the first symptoms nodular excrescences are seen; there may be 100 or more; they may be sessile or pedunculated, varying in size from a pea to a lemon, and they bleed readily.

Disturbances of the heart and circulation are prominent in nearly all the cases. The pulse is weak, rapid and irregular, the blood pressure low; cardiac murmurs are often noted. Breathlessness on exertion occurred in all cases, severe orthopnoea in many. Signs of pleural and pericardial effusion, of oedema of the lungs, of pneumonia, and of cardiac dilatation are common. The lung signs are characteristic and resemble a bronchial spasm with defective aeration. No liver dysfunction can be noted clinically but there is a non-tender hepatic enlargement. Anaemia is usually marked and so are wasting and prostration. The urine is not albuminous but of low specific gravity and greatly increased in amount. Concurrent primary glaucoma is not uncommon (see Chapter 70).

It may be necessary to differentiate epidemic dropsy from the oedema observed in central Europe and Egypt during the First and Second World Wars and more recent famines in Africa. It occurs in populations undergoing severe dietetic restriction and is characterized by great emaciation and a high degree of anaemia. From oedematous beriberi, epidemic dropsy is differentiated by pyrexia, the peculiar erythematous rash and persistence of the deep reflexes. A history of family outbreaks following the use of mustard oil suggests epidemic dropsy.

Treatment is based upon the facts that:
the adulterant argemone oil is the primary cause;

it is a cumulative poison;

it causes capillary dilatation and permeability;

the serum albumin and calcium are reduced and serum globulin is increased;

carbohydrate metabolism is checked at the pyruvic acid stage;

myocardial damage is set up.

Antihistaminic drugs, such as promethazine, are of benefit, though no rise in blood histamine has been demonstrated. Restoration of damaged capillaries by vitamins C and E and by hesperidin, rutin or extracts of citrus fruits, protection of the liver by a diet rich in protein and fat with glucose and insulin (10 units twice daily) is indicated. The calcium deficiency is restored by 10% Calcium-Sandoz intravenously.

Beans

The family Leguminoseae provides much of the world's food but contains many poisonous species, the fruits of which may be eaten by accident, by mistake or through hunger in times of famine. Several of these are mentioned above; others include the jequirity bean (*Abrus*), bright and attractive to children, which contains a lectin that can cause serious gastroenteritis. The toxin is destroyed by heat and the cooked beans are eaten in Egypt.

Jenghol (djenkol) poisoning occurs in Java and Malaysia from eating a bean, *Pithecolobium*. Blockage of the renal tract with crystals of djenkolic acid causes pain in the renal region, dysuria and often anuria. The urine contains blood casts and djenkolic acid crystals. Treatment consists of the removal of the crystals by mechanical means or making the urine alkaline to a pH of 8. With an output of 1 litre a day this may be achieved by 400 mmol/day of sodium bicarbonate (250 ml of 3.5% sodium bicarbonate four times a day for a 70 kg patient). The condition may be prevented by boiling the beans in sodium bicarbonate or carbonate which removes the djenkolic acid.[19]

Favism is caused by consumption, or exposure to the pollen of the broad bean, *Vicia fava*, which causes haemolysis in people with glucose-6-phosphate dehydrogenase deficiency (see Chapter 58).

Fungi

Poisoning may result from eating toxic mushrooms in the belief that they are harmless or from the mycotoxins[20] in stored foods contaminated with moulds and other fungi. Poisonous mushrooms have been used for criminal purposes (*Amanita phalloides*) and for their psychotropic effects (*A. muscaria, Conocybe, Psilocybe*).

Ergot (*Claviceps purpurea*) is the best known example of fungal poisoning in food. The sclerotia, containing ergotoxine and other alkaloids that stimulate smooth muscle, grow in the ears of rye and less frequently other grasses. They are harvested and ground with the grain and contaminate the flour. The result—uterine contraction, thrombosis, arterial occlusion and painful gangrene—was known as St Anthony's fire in the Middle Ages. Although not difficult to prevent, epidemic ergot poisoning still occurs. Vasodilator drugs help to relieve ischaemic pain and prevent gangrene.

Wheat contaminated with the grass *Lolium temulentum* also causes poisoning. The *Lolium* seed carries a fungus (*Endoconidium*?) which is probably the source of the toxin.

Brinton[21] has described recurrent epidemics of food poisoning in the local population of Aden due to Ethiopian wheat containing *Lolium*, known in local Arabic as miscara ('tipsy'). Within a quarter of an hour the patient becomes dizzy with headache, slurred speech and generalized tremors and staggering gait. Sometimes there is diarrhoea, nausea and abdominal pain. Stupor and coma supervene and last for about 10 hours. This state is known as 'lolism' and is common in Ethiopia.

Mouldy grains infected with *Fusarium* or *Stachybotrys* contain toxic tricothecenes that cause alimentary toxic aleukia (ATA). Some strains of *Aspergillus* produce aflatoxins that are toxic to the liver and are associated with liver cancer, or ochratoxins that cause chronic renal disease.

Inhalation of fungal spores may cause respiratory disease due to direct invasion (histoplasmosis, actinomycosis), the effect of toxic metabolites (stachybotryotoxicosis) or allergy.

'Ginger paralysis' (jake paralysis, triorthocresyl phosphate poisoning)

This is a flaccid paralysis of the distal muscles of the limbs without involvement of sensory nerves. The arms are affected later. The deep reflexes, especially the knee jerks, are exaggerated. Deaths have been recorded from respiratory paralysis in South Carolina and Tennessee from eating

Jamaica ginger adulterated with triorthocresyl phosphate.

An extensive epidemic of orthocresyl phosphate poisoning occurred in Morocco when lubricating oil containing 3% mixed cresyl phosphates was added to cooking oil and sold on a large scale. A great number of affected people developed paralyses, particularly flaccid paralysis involving all the muscles below the knee, and muscles of the hand; some patients developed spastic conditions two years later.

REFERENCES

1 Penn, R.G. (1985) In *Iatrogenic Diseases*, ed. P.F. D'Arcy & J.P. Griffin, 3rd edn. Oxford: Oxford University Press.

2 Hill, K.R., Stephenson, C.F. & Filshie, I. (1958) *Lancet* **i**, 623.

3 Tandon, R.K., Tandon H.D., Nayak, N.C. et al (1976) *Indian J. med. Res.* **64**, 1064.

4 Mohalbat, O., Srivastana, R.N., Younis, M.S. et al (1976) *Lancet* **ii**, 269.

5 Krishnamachari, K.A.U.R., Bhat, R.V., Nagarajan, V. et al (1975) *Lancet* **i**, 1061.

6 Edington, G.M. & Gilles, H.M. (1969) *Pathology in the Tropics*. London: Edward Arnold.

7 Bras, G., Brookes, S.E.M. & Walter, D.C. (1961) *J. Path. Bact.* **82**, 503.

8 Stuart, K.L. & Bras, G. (1957) *Q. J. Med.* **26**, 291.

9 Hendrickse, R.G. (1976) *J. trop. Med. Hyg.* **79**, 237.

10 Elegbe, R.A. & Oyebola, D.D.O. (1977) *Trans. R. Soc. trop. Med. Hyg.* **71**, 127.

11 Taha, S.A. & Mahdi, A.H. (1984) *Trans. R. Soc. trop. Med. Hyg.* **78**, 134.

12 Stuart, K.L., Jelliffe, D.B. & Hill, K.R. (1955) *J. trop. Pediat.* **i**, 69.

13 Hassall, C.H. & Reyle, K. (1955) *W. Indian med. J.* **4**, 83.

14 Sherratt, H.S.A. & Al-Bassam, S.S. (1976) *Lancet* **i**, 1243.

15 Ekpechi, O.L. (1967) *Br. J. Nutr.* **21**, 537.

16 Meaker, R.E. (1950) *S. Afr. med. J.* **24**, 331.

17 Sood, N.N., Sachdev, M.S., Mohan, M. et al (1985) *Trans. R. Soc. trop. Med. Hyg.* **79**, 510.

18 Hakim, S.A.E. (1970) *Maharashtra Med. J.* **16**, 10.

19 West, C.E., Peirin, D.D., Shaw, D.C. et al (1973) *S.E. Asian J. trop. Med. pub Hlth* **4**, 564.

20 World Health Organization (1979) *World Health Organization Environmental Health Criteria* 11, Mycotoxins. WHO, Geneva.

21 Brinton, D. (1946) *Proc. R. Soc. Med.* **39**, 173.

FURTHER READING

Kingsbury, J.M. (1964) *Poisonous Plants of the United States and Canada*. Cornell, N.J.: Prentiss Hall.

North, P. (1963) *Poisonous Plants and Fungi*. London: Blandford.

Watt, J.M. & Breyer-Brandwijk, M.G. (1962) *Medicinal and Poisonous Plants of Southern and Eastern Africa*. Edinburgh: Livingstone.

SECTION XIV
ECTOPARASITES AND MYIASIS

Chapter 50
Leeches and Leech Infestation

GEOGRAPHICAL DISTRIBUTION

Land leeches are common in South-East Asia, the Pacific Islands, the Indian subcontinent and South America. Aquatic leeches have a worldwide distribution.

AETIOLOGY

Leeches which attack man have the following position in the animal kingdom:

Phylum	Annelida
Class	Hirudinea
Order	Gnathobdellida
Family	Hirudinidae

Gnathobdellid leeches are invertebrates, having a smooth cuticle, a mouth lacking a proboscis but with three jaws, two suckers (one surrounding the mouth, the other at the posterior end) and powerful muscles, circular and longitudinal. They attach themselves by the posterior sucker, the anterior end moving about freely. When unfed they are usually about 2.5 cm long and 5 mm thick; some are bigger. When full of blood they are dark, bloated objects.

The muscular jaws are covered with chitin and produce a characteristic triradiate wound in the skin of the victim. The mouth leads to a pharynx, with salivary glands which secrete the anticoagulant hirudin, a crop in which ingested blood can be stored, a stomach, intestine, rectum and anal pore near the posterior sucker. The excretory system consists of 17 pairs of nephridia. There is a vascular system and a nervous system.

Leeches are hermaphrodites, each one possessing testes and ovaries, the spermatozoa of one individual being deposited during copulation on the cuticle (to migrate through the tissues to reach the ovary) or into the vagina, of the other member of the copulating pair. Some leeches deposit egg masses on objects submerged in water, others form a cocoon to be deposited in water or mud, from which the young hatch and attach themselves to water plants. Others carry their young until they are able to suck.

Leeches which attack man may be divided into two classes: *land leeches*, which have powerful jaws which can penetrate the skin so that they can attach anywhere on the external surface of the body, and *aquatic leeches*, which have weak jaws and require soft tissues to feed on. They gain entrance to orifices such as the pharynx and vagina.

LAND LEECHES

Land leeches live in the vegetation of tropical rain forests and tend to breed near springs, streams and wells frequented by cattle, horses and other vertebrates. The species noted for attacks on man include *Haemadipsa zelanica, H. sylvestris,* and *H. picta*. Land leeches attach themselves to the skin and feed; when fed they fall off on to the ground having remained attached for a comparatively short time.

Clinical features

The punctures made in the skin by land leeches are painless and remain open and bleeding after the leech has gone; healing is slow. Leeches take much more blood than they need and if they remain attached, or are numerous, they can take so much that the patient becomes seriously anaemic and may die from loss of blood.

Treatment

Leeches which attach themselves to the skin must be induced to detach, but they must not be simply pulled off because they may then leave behind their jaws, which could become the starting point of destructive ulceration. Drops of strong salt solution, alcohol or strong vinegar applied round the mouth, or heat from a lighted match or cigarette applied to the body will cause the leech to release its hold. The wound can then be treated with a styptic and an antiseptic.

Prevention

People in countries where land leeches are common should, when travelling in infested country, wear boots and trousers thick enough to prevent access by the leeches to the skin. Additional protection is afforded if the garments or the skin are treated with repellents such as dimethyl or dibutyl phthalate, Rutgers 612 or indalone. Dibutyl phthalate lasts longer on clothing than dimethyl phthalate and, if applied about once every two weeks at the rate of 28 ml per set of garments, or about 4 ml/30 cm², is a good repellent. On the skin, repellents are effective for only 3–5 hours, less if sweating is excessive. Dimethyl phthalate should not be used on rayon garments.

AQUATIC LEECHES

Aquatic leeches live exclusively in fresh water. Species feeding on man include *Limnatis nilotica*, which is large and haunts quiet water and ponds, and *L. maculosa*. *Phytobdella catenifera*, *Dinobdella ferox* and *Myxobdella africana* occur in sub-Saharan Africa.[1] Aquatic leeches deposit their eggs on water plants and the young may be seen in the water. They do not all require a mammalian host, and can exist on amphibians. Young leeches enter orifices such as the nose and pharynx where they attach themselves for prolonged periods until they become adult, when they drop off into the water. They are more dangerous than land leeches, because they are more likely to cause severe anaemia.

Clinical features

Aquatic leech infestation is less common than land leech infestation, but may be much more harmful. Aquatic leeches can enter the mouth or nostrils during drinking or washing and can also attack the conjunctiva, the vulva, vagina and urethra in persons bathing in infested water.

Having entered the mouth or nostrils the leech can quickly pass to the nasopharynx, epiglottis or oesophagus, and even to the trachea and bronchi. When attached to the mucous membrane the leech secretes anticoagulant and engorges. The result is bleeding, according to the site of attachment—epistaxis, haemoptysis or haematemesis—which may lead to severe anaemia. A leech in the nares may also give prolonged headache; if in the larynx there is a cough with bloody discharge, hoarseness, dyspnoea, pain and even suffocation. Leeches in the pharynx or oesophagus may cause difficulty in swallowing.

Treatment

In treating leech infestation of the upper respiratory passages an attempt should be made to see the leech. If it is in the posterior pharynx, larynx, trachea or bronchi, the patient should be positioned so that the leech cannot fall back and block the lower passages. If it is in the nares or upper pharynx it can be paralysed with cocaine and extracted directly. If lower down, a pair of long hooked forceps can be introduced through a laryngoscope and the leech pulled out gently, but tracheostomy may be necessary. If in the oesophagus the leech should be visualized through an oesophagoscope and treated with cocaine; it will then fall into the stomach where the gastric juice will kill it. For a leech in the genitourinary tract, irrigation with strong salt solution may make it release its hold.

Prevention

To avoid attack by aquatic leeches, it is necessary to wear appropriate clothing and apply repellents, and to drink only water which has been filtered, strained through fine gauze or boiled.

Although they suck blood, leeches have not been incriminated in transmitting infection.

REFERENCE

1   Cundall, D.B., Whitehead, S.M. & Hechtel, F.O.P. (1986). *Trans. R. Soc. trop. Med. Hyg.* **80**, 940–944.

Chapter 51
Myiasis

Myiasis is the condition when dipterous fly maggots invade living tissue or when they are harboured in the intestines or bladder.

Clinically, maggots causing myiasis may attack three parts of the body:

1 *Cutaneous tissue.* Some species of maggots cause furuncles (subcutaneous myiasis), invade sores and wounds (wound myiasis), burrow under the skin (dermal myiasis, a cause of creeping eruption) or suck blood.

2 *Body cavities.* Other species invade the nasal passages (nasal myiasis), mouth, ears and accessory passages, enter the orbit of the eye (ocular myiasis) or penetrate the anus or vagina.

3 *Organs of the body.* Accidental myiasis-producing flies produce eggs or larvae which are ingested, pass out intact through the bowel to emerge in the stool (intestinal myiasis).

Parasitologically, myiasis-producing flies can be divided into three categories (see also Appendix III, p. 1462).

1 *Obligatory myiasis producers.* Here it is essential for the larvae to develop in living tissue because they are unable to develop elsewhere. These obligate parasites are highly specialized insects, the larvae of which have developed highly sophisticated mechanisms to avoid the host's immune system.

2 *Facultative myiasis producers.* These larvae usually develop on carrion but may invade wounds. They may be primary invaders which initiate myiasis; secondary invaders, entering tissue only when the animal has become infested; or tertiary, which only become involved later when decomposition is advanced.

3 *Accidental myiasis producers.* Here eggs or larvae are accidentally ingested and are not killed in the intestine.

1 CUTANEOUS TISSUE MYIASIS

(A) BLOOD SUCKERS (CONGO FLOOR MAGGOT) (see also p. 1466)

Geographical distribution

The adult fly *Auchmeromyia luteola* (Fig. III.66, p. 1466) is widely distributed throughout tropical Africa from 18° north to 26° south, from northern Nigeria and the southern Sudan to Natal, from sea level to 2250 m in both dry and wet climates.

Aetiology

The Congo floor maggot is the larval stage of *Auchmeromyia luteola* (Fig. III.60A, p. 1463), an orange-buff coloured fly covered with numerous small hairs which give it a smoky look. It has a stoutly built body 10–12 mm long.

Life-cycle

The adult fly sits motionless among the thatch, beams and cobwebs of the roof of huts where it is protected by its colour and is difficult to see. Human faeces is its most important source of food. It lays its eggs in the crevices of mud floors, favouring those contaminated by urine, three weeks after its emergence from the pupa. The larva which emerges from the egg is dirty white, semitransparent, 15 mm in length and composed of 11 segments. This stage is known as the Congo floor maggot (Fig. III.60A, p. 1463). The larva which is mobile and emerges from its hiding place to take its blood meal from the host, which must be hairless and immobile, such as a sleeping human. It also feeds on the aardvark and nestling birds. It feeds by scraping with its mouth hooks until it reaches a blood vessel. The first segment is then retracted and its sucker apparatus is then applied. After feeding it becomes conspicuously red as it is filled with blood and retreats into the crack in the floor from which it emerged. Larvae are frequently found under the mats on which people sleep and in the earth to a depth of 7.6 cm.

They feed mainly at night and drop off at once if disturbed. They can be recognized by the characteristic shape of the spiracles (Fig. III.60A). When ready to pupate the larva selects a suitable place and lies dormant. The pupa is dark reddish-brown with an oblong body 9–10 × 4.5 mm and this stage lasts two to three weeks.

Clinical features

The bite is painless. Blood loss has never been found sufficient to cause anaemia. No infections are known to be transmitted by its bite.

Prevention

Sleeping on a bed raised above the floor is sufficient to prevent attack.

(B) SUBCUTANEOUS MYIASIS

The maggot penetrates the skin; no previous lesion is necessary. Two species of fly are the cause; both are obligatory myiasis producers: *Cordylobia anthropophaga* (tumbu fly, putsi fly) in Africa and *Dermatobia hominis* (ver macaque, macaw worm, tropical warble fly) in South America.

CORDYLOBIA   ANTHROPOPHAGA (tumbu fly, putsi fly, ver du cayor) (see also p. 1462)

Geographical distribution

The tumbu fly is widely distributed in sub-Saharan Africa and has been recorded from southern Spain.

Aetiology

Cordylobia anthropophaga (Fig. III.59, p. 1463) is a large robust yellow-brown fly, 7–12 mm long resembling the adult of the Congo floor maggot (*Auchmeromyia luteola*) and it is difficult to distinguish the adults of either from numerous other species of the family. *C. anthropophaga* is an obligate parasite. Adults are active in the early morning and late afternoon laying eggs on sandy ground or contaminated clothing. The eggs hatch and the larvae which emerge invade the subcutaneous tissue and undergo three moults or instars (Fig. III.60B, p. 1463); complete development in the subcutaneous tissues takes 8–12 days. The larvae emerge and fall to the ground where they pupate in 24 hours. The pupa has a characteristic shape with a truncated end. The adult hatches in 10–20 days according to temperature. Rodents and dogs are the usual larval hosts and man is infected only accidentally.

Transmission

The female fly lays its eggs in two batches on sandy ground, preferably contaminated with urine or faeces but can also lay on clothing if also contaminated (although such clothing may appear clean). Clothing laid on the ground to dry is affected but not clothing hanging in bright sunlight since the eggs are only laid in shaded areas. The eggs are not laid directly on the skin.

On hatching, the small first stage larvae hold themselves erect and can remain alive without food for about 9 days. The larvae, which are sensitive to both heat and vibration, become attached to a host and immediately begin to penetrate the unbroken skin taking about one minute. Penetration, which is painless, may involve any part of the body but most commonly occurs on the back, head and neck in man. Larvae are acquired from lying on the ground or from clothing, and infection is more common in children. Dogs are an important reservoir.

Immunity

There is a localized degree of immunity which has been experimentally produced in guinea pigs. There are no antibodies and no general immunity. Larvae penetrating the immune area die in 40 hours and grafted skin retains its immunity.

Clinical features

Initially the lesion starts as a small papule containing the larva which may be itchy or pricking at intervals. As the papule increases in size the symptoms recur and may keep the patient awake at night. Serous fluid may be exuded and local lymphadenopathy occur. There may be fever and general malaise. The lesion, which resembles a boil, grows over a period of 6 days, the larva being noticed by the time the third stage has been reached. During the period of time the larva is in the host (8–12 days) the larva has its posterior segment bearing the respiratory spiracles protruding from the aperture which can be withdrawn when touched. There may be numerous lesions resembling boils situated on the arms, scrotum and other parts of the body coinciding with areas of contact with contaminated clothing. Close inspection of the lesions will reveal that instead of a pustular head the lesions terminate in a 1–3 mm dark line, the site of the respiratory spiracles of the larva (Fig. 51.1).

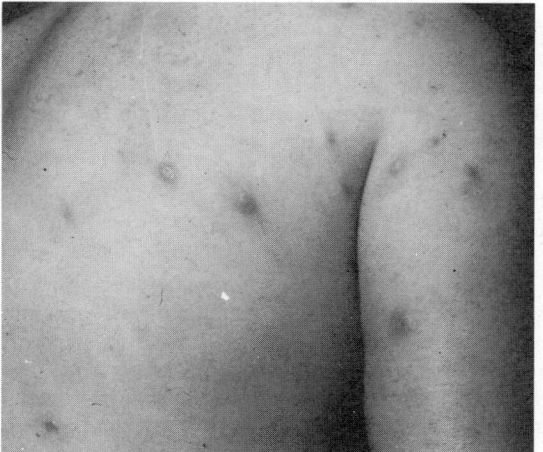

Fig. 51.1 Lesions of tumbu fly (*Cordylobia anthropophaga*).

Diagnosis

There is usually less pain than with an ordinary boil, and the appearance of the spiracles is diagnostic. In case of doubt, the surface of the lesion should be covered with Vaseline, glycerin or oil. The appearance of bubbles clinches the diagnosis.

Treatment

The larvae can be removed by manual expression, and this is assisted by first covering the spiracle with a layer of paraffin oil to stop the oxygen supply. Mature larvae will then wriggle partly out, and can be finally removed by exerting firm digital pressure on each side. Early lesions are best left to develop for a few days, as immature larvae are reluctant to emerge. Rupture of the larvae by injudicious attempts at extraction may cause a severe inflammatory response.

Prevention

All clothing and towels should be ironed on *both* sides, and drip-dry clothes should be hung indoors with the windows closed[1] to prevent contact with the flies.

DERMATOBIA HOMINIS
(VER MACAQUE, BERNE, EL TORSALO, BEEFWORM, HUMAN BOT FLY) (see also p. 1465)

Geographical distribution

Dermatobia hominis is widely distributed throughout Central and South America from Mexico to Argentina and Chile. It is especially common on the forested eastern slopes of the Andes in Colombia. It attacks a wide range of hosts and is a devastating pest of livestock in some areas.

Aetiology

The adult fly is a large bluish-grey fly 1.5 cm long (Fig. III.61, p. 1464) with a strong flight, found primarily on the edge of tropical forests particularly hilly areas of secondary forest between 160 and 3000 m. The adult *D. hominis*, on attaining maturity, lays its eggs directly on other insects or foliage, but especially on day-flying mosquitoes such as *Psorophora* (Fig. III.62, p. 1464), flies (*Sarcophaga, Musca* and *Stomoxys*) and a tick *Amblyoma*.

The packets of eggs, which are enclosed in cement, adhere to the insect's thorax (Fig. III.62, p. 1464) and are thus conveyed to the new host (cattle, dogs and man). This characteristic is called phoresis or 'hitch-hiking'.

The larva remains in the egg until it senses warmth, whereupon it rapidly 'hatches' and penetrates the host's skin in 5–10 minutes remaining at the site of penetration. Each larva penetrates individually and a small nodule develops around it with a central pore through which the larva breathes. The second stage larva has a characteristic shape (Fig. III.63, p. 1464) which makes it difficult to remove. The duration of larval development is uncertain but probably lasts from six to twelve weeks in man during which it grows slowly feeding on tissue exudate. It then emerges and drops to the ground and pupates (Fig. III.64, p. 1465).

Clinical features

Cutaneous swellings harbouring the larva usually occur on exposed areas although the flies can penetrate clothing. They are usually single, being found most commonly on the head but also elsewhere on the body. In the orbit the larva

can cause serious pathology and is a cause of
ophthalmomyiasis (Chapter 70). Lesions can be
multiple and 12 have been reported on one individual. The lesion is an inflamed swelling 2–3 cm
in diameter at the apex of which the small black
spiracles can be seen from which exudes a seropurulent fluid containing the dark faeces of the
larva. The lesions are very painful and itchy but
do not suppurate since the bacteriostatic activity
of the gut of the larva prevents undesirable overgrowth of pyogenic bacteria.

Diagnosis

Diagnosis is made by examining the lesion for
the characteristic spiracles and the faecal-stained
serous exudate.

Complications

Loss of the eye can occur in opthalmomyiasis. A
fatal cerebral myiasis can occur in children but
is rare.

Treatment

Occasionally the first stage larva can be removed
as in *Cordylobia* but more often surgical removal
is necessary with second and third stage larvae.
The larvae are best removed by a cruciate
incision and care must be taken not to go through
the central hole and damage the larva, portions
of which must not be left in the wound.

Control

In Brazil the fly has been controlled with insecticides including DDT, BHC and Toxaphene.
In Curaçao males sterilized by radiation have
been released to render the females sterile after
mating (since females mate only once). After two
years of the sterile male release programme the
fly was exterminated in a similar manner to *Callitroga hominivorax*.

(C) DERMAL MYIASIS OR CREEPING ERUPTION

Dermal myiasis is caused by the maggots of horse
and cattle bot flies which are obligatory myiasis
producers, but in man the maggots cannot
develop further, producing tunnels in the epidermis in which they may wander for some time.

Aetiology

Gasterophilus sp. (horse bots, warble flies) (see also
Appendix III, p. 1465)

These are common parasites of horses, and sometimes of man, especially people who look after
horses. The eggs are laid on the hair of the host
or on grasses. On contact with skin, the larvae
promptly penetrate, but do not develop beyond
the first instar causing a swelling and a wandering
tunnel in the lower epidermis in which they may
wander for a long time.

Hypoderma sp. (cattle bots) (see also Appendix
III, p. 1465)

Hypoderma ovis and *H. lineatum* are parasites of
cattle and cause creeping eruption in persons
connected with cattle. The eggs are deposited on
the hair of cattle and hatch within a week. The
larvae penetrate more deeply into the subcutaneous tissues than those of *Gasterophilus* sp.
and have been reported to have invaded the
nervous system.

Clinical features

The tunnels caused by *Gasterophilus* sp. maggots
resemble the lesions caused by *Ancylostoma braziliense* (cutaneous larva migrans). They itch but
do not discharge unless infected. Lesions caused
by *Hypoderma* sp. are deeper, producing a swelling resembling a boil. The maggots migrate
slowly for considerable distances. *H. ovis* has
been reported to invade the central nervous
system.

Differential diagnosis

Other causes of a creeping eruption are cutaneous
larva migrans (Chapter 21) caused by *Ancylostoma* sp. *Strongyloides* (Chapter 21), *Gnathostoma* (Chapter 24), and *Fasciola hepatica*
(Chapter 22). But *Strongyloides* is transient and
very fast-moving (hence 'larva currens'), and
Gnathostoma and *Fasciola* larvae do not usually
tarry in the skin for long before moving deeper.

Diagnosis

Gasterophilus larvae can be identified if a small
amount of clear mineral oil is smeared over the
lesion. The larva can then be seen and identified

by the black transverse bands of spines on its body.

Treatment

Gasterophilus larvae when identified can be removed with a needle. *Hypoderma* larvae can be removed through a cruciform incision.

2 BODY CAVITY MYIASIS

NASAL MYIASIS

Geographical distribution

Nasal myiasis occurs most commonly in Asia, less commonly in Africa.

Aetiology

Chrysomyia bezziana (Old World screw fly) is the commonest cause, but *Oestrus ovis* (sheep nasal bot fly), *Rhinoestrus purpureus* (Russian gadfly), *Callitroga hominivorax, C. americana* (New World screw fly) are other causes (Appendix III, p. 1465).

Pathology

The flies are obligatory myiasis producers. The female flies lay eggs in the nasal cavity especially where there is a chronic nasal discharge. The larvae require living tissue in which to develop. After the eggs hatch the larvae burrow into the tissue, even to the nasal bone, within a few hours.

Clinical features

The initial symptoms are tickling, sneezing, pain and nasal obstruction. Epistaxis is common, but the discharge soon becomes purulent and fetid. Destruction and erosion of the nose or mouth may facilitate larval migration to the brain with meningitis and death. A mortality of 8% has been recorded in cases of *Callitroga hominivorax* infection.

Diagnosis

The maggots can be seen with a nasal speculum and extracted for examination. They should be preserved in 70% alcohol and sent to a laboratory to be identified by their spiracles (Fig. III.65, p. 1466), or kept alive and hatched to permit identification. Precise identification is academic unless control measures are intended and is of no practical importance to the patients (Appendix III, p. 1468).

Treatment

A few drops of 15% chloroform in light vegetable oil applied to the nasal passages will cause the larvae to appear when they can be removed with forceps. In advanced cases the nasal sinuses may have to be opened surgically.

Control

Callitroga hominivorax has been eradicated from some areas by the large-scale release of male flies sterilized by gamma radiation (see p. 916).

MYIASIS OF THE EAR

The same species may invade the ear causing pain and discomfort accompanied by deafness and tinnitus and the drum can be perforated.

OCULAR MYIASIS (OPHTHALMOMYIASIS) (see also Chapter 70, p. 1171)

External ophthalmomyiasis, where conjunctivitis only results, is caused by *Oestrus* spp. (sheep bots) or *Wohlfahrtia* spp.

Internal ophthalmomyiasis can be caused by *Dermatobium hominis, Oestrus ovis* (sheep bot), *Gasterophilus* spp., *Rhinoestrus* spp. (horse bots) and *Hypoderma* spp. (cattle bots). However, *Oestrus ovis* mainly attacks the conjunctivae (external ophthalmomyiasis). The female fly strikes the eye depositing eggs almost instantaneously while on the wing. Larvae are deposited on the conjunctiva at the inner canthus of the eye, the nasal openings or the lips. The larvae, which do not survive for more than 10 days developing no further, are actively motile possessing characteristic hooks which cause conjunctival irritation. They can be removed under direct vision after applying topical anaesthetic drugs (Fig.III.67, p. 1467).

Internal ophthalmomyiasis involving the orbit and eye can be very destructive leading to the loss of the eye (Chapter 70, p. 1171).

MYIASIS OF THE ANUS AND VAGINA

Wohlfahrtia spp. (flesh fly) (Appendix III, p. 1465) can lay their eggs in large numbers round the anus and vagina of adults and children in poor hygienic circumstances where there are soiling and sores in the anogenital region. Large numbers of maggots can develop within a few hours.

3 WOUND MYIASIS

Aetiology

This includes myiasis produced by both obligatory and facultative myiasis producers. Larvae of several groups of flies usually associated with carrion have been found in wounds and gangrenous tissues where they act as facultative parasites feeding on necrotic tissue although occasionally they may attack living tissues.

Larvae of the facultative parasites *Calliphora, Lucilia, Phormia, Musca* and *Fannia* spp. (Fig. III.65, p. 1466) are found living in moist folds of the skin and enter sores and wounds. At one time it was practice to use the larvae of carefully cultivated *Lucilia* to cleanse wounds by removal of infected tissue, but this practice has now been abandoned.

In some areas of the world the species of fly varies. In southern Europe, Russia, the Middle East and Africa *Wohlfahrtia magnifica* (Old World flesh fly or sheep maggot) (Appendix III, p. 1465) is the common species, and *Wohlfahrtia vigil* (New World flesh fly) in the New World (Appendix III, p. 1466); in India, the Far East and sub-Saharan Africa *Chrysomyia bezziana* (Appendix III, p. 1467) and in the New World *Callitroga hominivorax* (New World screw worm) (Appendix III, p. 1465). These flies are obligatory myiasis producers relying on living tissue for their survival.

4 INTESTINAL MYIASIS

Eggs, and sometimes larvae, of many species of flies are deposited on foodstuffs, and sometimes survive the journey down the intestinal tract. They may then develop in the folds of mucous membrane, even causing some irritation (pain, vomiting, diarrhoea) or even ulceration before being evacuated. If deposited around the anus, such larvae may crawl into the rectum to complete their feeding inside the body. This kind of infestation may persist for months, producing severe nervous symptoms (because of anxiety) as well as internal irritation. The larvae can be recognized in the faeces, sometimes in vomit.

The flies usually implicated include species of *Musca, Fannia, Chrysomyia, Calliphora* and others. Prevention entails the careful covering of food. Treatment with purgatives will aid elimination, and metriphonate, on theoretical grounds, would be worth a trial.

5 URINARY MYIASIS

A mistaken diagnosis of urinary myiasis due to a larva from a contaminated vessel in which urine has been collected, or which has been introduced into the urine after it was passed, is not uncommon. But there have been genuine cases in which larvae have been passed via the urethra from the bladder. If the vulva or vaginal area in women is infested, there are obvious opportunities for larvae to enter the bladder. The flies concerned are usually of the genera *Psychoda, Musca, Calliphora* and *Sarcophaga*.

REFERENCE

1   Radcliffe, W. (1972) *Br. med. J.* **ii**, 164.

Chapter 52
Jiggers (Jigger Flea)

GEOGRAPHICAL DISTRIBUTION

Originally found in Central and South America the jigger has now spread to West and East Africa and parts of the Indian subcontinent.

AETIOLOGY (Appendix III, p. 1485)

Tunga penetrans (the sand flea, jigger flea, chigoe, chique) is the cause, the female being adapted for an intracutaneous permanent attachment to the host (man, pig, poultry and other animals). As with other fleas, the larvae are free-living, dusty or sandy soil being best for *T. penetrans*. Adults are also free-living at first, when copu-

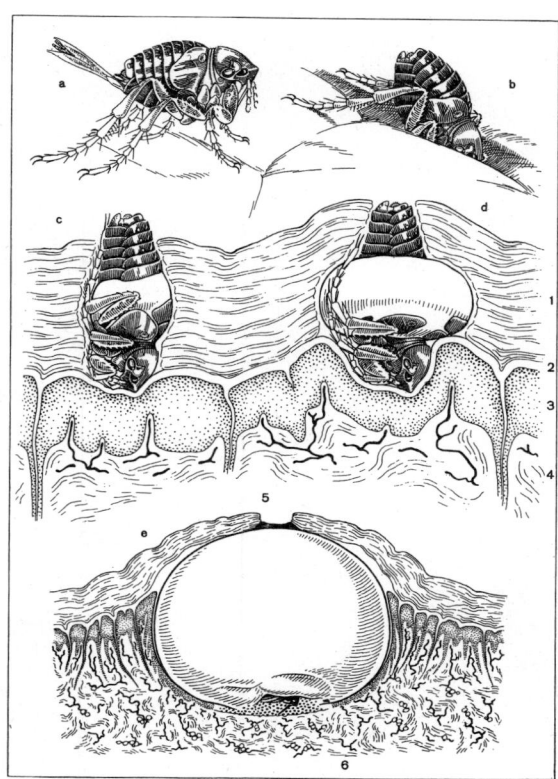

Fig. 52.1 The sand flea or jigger.

lation occurs. The fertilized female then finds a suitable host and tries to penetrate crevices in the skin, such as cracks in the soles of the feet (Fig. 52.1), between the toes and especially around the toenails. Any part of the human anatomy can be affected. By means of the mouthparts, the female *Tunga* becomes firmly attached and soon swells to the size and shape of a small white pea. Somehow the host skin envelops the jigger, which lies below the stratum corneum but above the stratum granulosum, leaving only the posterior spiracles exposed to the air. Only when the jigger is almost mature and distended, after 8–12 days, does the infection begin to irritate. Severe inflammation and ulceration ensues, so that scratching helps to expel large numbers of white eggs from the jigger. (See also Appendix III, p. 1485.)

CLINICAL FEATURES

The jigger seldom attacks the leg above the dorsum of the foot, but no part of the body escapes. The soles (Fig. 52.2), the skin between the toes and that at the roots of the nails are favourite situations. Usually only one or two jiggers are found at a time, but occasionally they are present in hundreds, the little pits left after extraction or expulsion being sometimes so closely set that parts of the surface may look like a honeycomb. During her gestation the jigger causes a considerable amount of irritation. Pus may form around her distended abdomen which now raises the integument into a pea-like elevation. After the eggs are laid the skin ulcerates and the jigger is expelled, leaving a small sore which may become seriously infected or lead to tetanus. Ulceration is common and may follow removal of the jigger or natural extrusion of the egg sac. The ulcer commences as a tiny pit and as it extends the sloping edge may develop into a septic ulcer. It remains more or less circular in outline, except under the nail or nail margin, where the outline is more irregular and a pocket of pus forms beneath it.

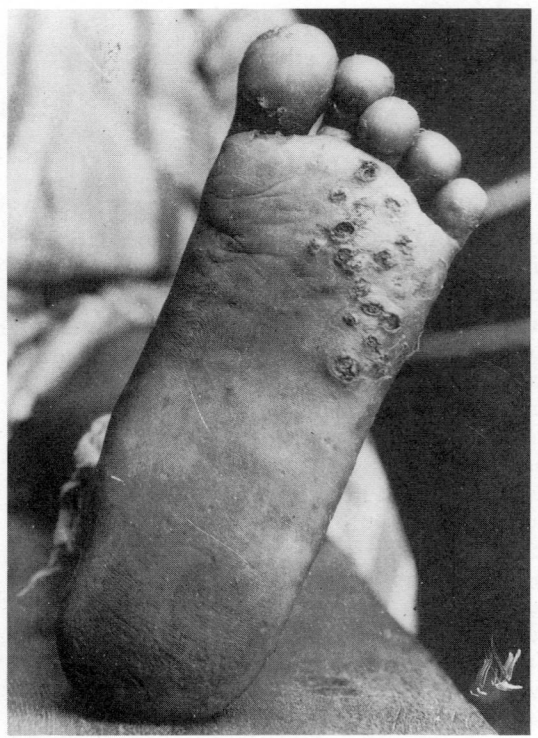

Fig. 52.2 Jiggers in the sole of the foot.

TREATMENT

The mature female jigger should be removed carefully using a sterile needle, so as to pick out the jigger without bursting it. Inexpert attempts at removal may lead to severe secondary infection.

PREVENTION (Appendix III, p. 1486)

Affected areas of soil may be burnt off in an effort to kill the fleas, or residual insecticide applied to infested areas. Since female jiggers are not good jumpers, human infestation is normally confined to the feet. Daily inspection of the interdigital clefts, roots of nails and soles of feet should cause freshly burrowing female jiggers to be detected and removed before they have grown much. To prevent attack, foot-enveloping shoes (not 'flip-flops' or sandals) are effective, and a more sensible solution than repellents.

Chapter 53
Scabies

GEOGRAPHICAL DISTRIBUTION

Scabies is a worldwide infection most common in poor countries irrespective of climate.

AETIOLOGY

Sarcoptes scabiei the itch or scabies mite causes human scabies. A morphologically similar species causes sarcoptic mange in animals and scabies mites of dogs and horses which differ physiologically can establish themselves briefly on humans causing lesions similar to scabies which are milder and cure spontaneously.

The female *S. scabiei* (0.3–0.4 mm) is twice the size of the male (0.2 mm) (Fig. III.1A and B, p. 1381). The gravid female lays her oval eggs (15 × 100 μm) in a burrow in the skin (Fig. III.2, p. 1382). The eggs give rise to adults 10–14 days later after passing through the larval and one or two nymphal stages. The nymphs moult, become sexually mature and pair off on the surface of the skin. The adults live for four to five weeks.

TRANSMISSION

Transmission is from person to person by direct skin contact and through bedding and clothing. Scabies is often transmitted sexually. The newly fertilized female is the infective agent.

PATHOLOGY

Both males and females make short burrows but it is only the fertilized female which makes a permanent burrow in the horny layers of the skin with the female at the end (Fig. III.2, p. 1382). Pathology is the result of sensitization of the host to the mites and their excretions.

A vesicle is present at the point of entry of the tunnel in which eggs and faeces are deposited. The larvae hatch out after 3–4 days when they leave the burrows for the skin surface for food and shelter in the hair follicles. After 4–5 days the adults mate and the female burrows into the cuticle of the skin to complete the cycle.

The population of mites builds up over two to four months and a fully developed case of scabies may have no more than 20 adult mites, often less. When sensitization of the host occurs a generalized rash develops. Infiltration with eosinophils is found round the burrows and foci of lymphocytes and histiocytes can be found deep in the corium after cure.

IMMUNITY

In immunosuppressed persons the mites escape control and multiply considerably leading to encrustation of the skin, when the condition is known as crusted or Norwegian scabies. Steroid therapy to control undiagnosed itching may change ordinary into crusted scabies.

CLINICAL FEATURES (Chapter 65) p. 1061)

Incubation period

There is an incubation period of six to eight weeks before symptoms appear.

Symptoms and signs

The first stage is a small (1–3 mm) slightly raised itchy papule which develops at the site of each mite. Scratching may destroy the mite and convert the papule into a pustule. Local sensitization is followed by the appearance of a rash.

Rash

The generalized rash of scabies is an itching erythematous rash the distribution of which does not correspond to the site of the mites. It is a hypersensitivity phenomenon in which it may be impossible to demonstrate mites. The eruption occurs most commonly in the axillae around the waist, inner aspect of the thighs and back of the legs from which it may spread all over the body. It commonly occurs in reinfection and the number of mites present may be small.

Norwegian or crusted scabies

This is a severe type of scabies accompanied by profuse crusting and hyperkeratotic plaques (Fig. 53.1). It is common in the tropics and used to be common in leprosy. Burrows are not formed and a large number of scabies mites may be present on the surface of the skin.

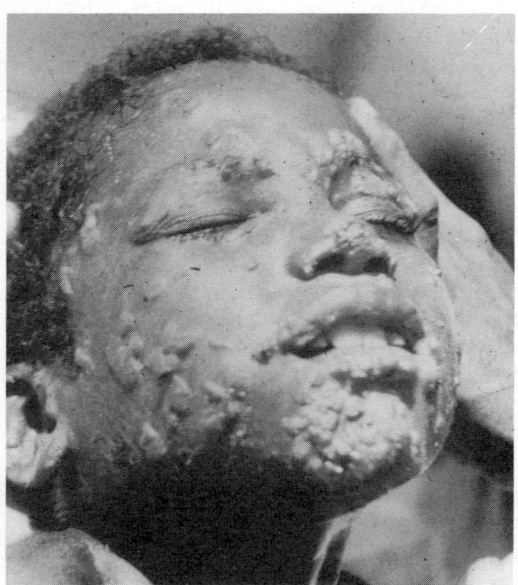

Fig. 53.1 Crusted scabies. (Courtesy Dr P. Rotmil.)

Scabies in children

Scabies in children is atypical. During the first year of life the lesions are general and resemble pemphigus, the buttocks and perineum being most often severely infected. Burrows are often impossible to find and secondarily infected excoriations and scattered pustules are the most characteristic lesion (Fig. 53.1, Plate VIII.3).

Sarcoptic mange (animal scabies)

This is sometimes contracted by man by contact with dogs, cats and cattle infested with zoonotic races of *Sarcoptes*. They may be distinguished from human scabies by the distribution of papules and vesicles on the arms, shoulders, trunks and thighs and by the absence of burrows on the hands. Sarcoptic mange responds rapidly to treatment with sulphur.

Important complication: nephritis

Secondary infection of scabies lesions is very common, especially in children. Scabies infected with nephritogenic strains of β-haemolytic streptococci is an important cause of glomerulonephritis, and in some parts of the world may be a more frequent cause of nephritis than streptococcal throat infection. Secondarily infected scabies should always be treated with a course of penicillin at the same time as antiscabetic treatment.

DIFFERENTIAL DIAGNOSIS

Scabies in the tropics is atypical in appearance especially in children in whom crusted scabies may be very difficult to distinguish from eczema and pyoderma. Itching is severe in scabies in which it may be possible to identify burrows. In adults onchocerciasis, also intensely pruritic, and lepromatous leprosy with which scabies may coexist must be thought of.

DIAGNOSIS

The burrows may be seen between the fingers with a magnifying glass. After opening a burrow the mite at the end can be extracted with a needle and examined under mineral oil. Scrapings from ulcers may reveal mites or eggs.

TREATMENT (see also p. 1061)

All members of the family in contact with the patient should be treated at the same time. It is important to treat the whole body from the neck down. Mites are only found above the neck in infants.

Benzyl benzoate 20% emulsion must be applied from the neck down after a bath and allowed to dry when the clothes may be put on again. After 24 hours a second bath should be taken and the clothes and bedclothes washed in the meantime. A second treatment should be given one week later. Crusted lesions should first be removed with a mixture of sulphur and salicylic acid. Secondary infection is treated with a 5-day course of penicillin.

NBIN emulsion concentrate consists of 68% benzyl benzoate, 6% DDT, 12% benzocaine and 14% polysorbate 80. This requires a dilution of 1 : 15 in water before use.

Tetmosol (tetraethylthiuram monosulphide) in a 5% solution can be used as benzyl benzoate. In soap form it is of little value.

Crotamiton (*Eurax*) is applied daily for 5 days and is suitable for infants. It is more expensive but has powerful antipruritic properties.

An application of 5% γ-benzene hexachloride (BHC) in vanishing cream is rubbed all over the body. Lotions of 0.5% malathion or 1% BHC are also effective, and sting less than benzyl benzoate.

EPIDEMIOLOGY

Human scabies waxes and wanes in incidence in 15–20 years cycles probably due to changing immunity patterns. Scabies is widespread in the tropics especially among children where infection levels are highest in the poorer communities. Infection is associated with poor hygiene, the result of an inadequate water supply.

CONTROL

Good personal hygiene and the search for and treatment of infected families is the best form of control.

Prevention can be obtained by avoidance of skin contact with infected persons and clothing. People able to wash themselves frequently do not suffer much from scabies.

Chapter 54
Louse Infestation

Three species of louse are parasitic on man:

   Pediculus humanus (body louse);
   Pediculus capitis (head louse);
   Phthirus pubis (crab louse).

   Pediculus humanus and *P. capitis* are morphologically similar but have different habits. Although experimental interbreeding is possible this does not happen in nature. The majority of lice are host specific, and although lice from domestic animals may be found on man they do not persist. Most lice do not survive for long when removed from the host.

PEDICULUS HUMANUS (BODY LOUSE) (see also Appendix III, p. 1468)

Aetiology

P. humanus (Fig. III. 69A, p. 1469) is larger (0.4 mm) than *P. capitis* (0.3 mm) (Fig. III.69B, p. 1469) and there are minor morphological differences. The female *P. humanus* sometimes attaches her eggs to body hair, but more often cements them to cloth fibres usually along seams and folds in garments. The female lice produce an average of four to five eggs per day during their life of up to one month. The nymphs hatch in 8 days, becoming adult after three moults in 18 days. Both nymphs and adults take blood meals two to five times a day throughout life.

Transmission

Pediculus infestation is usually acquired through close contact with lousy persons, shared clothes and bedding. Lice tend to leave patients with fever and sweating thus promoting the spread of disease. They leave a corpse as it becomes cold. They avoid light.

Clinical features

Body lice cause generalized itching and a generalized itchy, red maculopapular rash. Scratching may cause secondary infection and impetigo may result. *P. humanus* is the sole transmitter of louse-borne typhus (*Rickettsia prowazeki*), Trench fever (*Rickettsia quintana*) (Chapter 10) and louse-borne relapsing fever (*Borrelia recurrentis*) (Chapter 32).

Diagnosis

Eggs (nits) should be searched for on body hair and the adults may be recovered. Eggs should be looked for in the seams and folds of clothing.

Treatment

See section on control of lice and treatment of lousy patients, below.

PEDICULUS CAPITIS (HEAD LOUSE)

P. capitis females cement their eggs to the base of head hairs and growth of the hair eventually brings the empty egg cases into view after the eggs have hatched (nits). They are confined to the scalp.

Transmission

This is by close contact as for *P. humanus*.

Clinical features

Usually there are no signs or symptoms, and infestation is principally a hygienic and aesthetic nuisance. In heavy infections some dermatitis of the scalp can result from scratching. *P. capitis* is not known to be a vector of any disease.

Diagnosis

Diagnosis is by searching for the presence of 'nits' in the hair or observing the lice themselves.

PHTHIRUS PUBIS (CRAB LOUSE)

Crab lice occur worldwide, and are found exclusively in man.

924

Aetiology

Phthirus is shorter and broader than *Pediculus* and has massive claws on the second and third legs by which it clings to hair (Fig. III.70, p. 1409). It is most commonly found in the genital and inguinal regions but may be found on any of the body hair except the scalp, including the beard, chest hair and eyelashes. They cannot survive off the host for more than 24 hours.

Transmission

This is by sexual and close personal contact.

Clinical features

Infection is normally noticed following irritation caused by the bite. Sometimes a characteristic small 'bluespot' (2–3 mm across) may result from the bite, different from the red spot caused by pediculid lice. *P. pubis* is not known to be the vector of any disease.

CONTROL OF LICE AND TREATMENT OF LOUSY PATIENTS (Appendix III, p. 1470)

Pediculus

Destruction of the lice and eggs on clothes is efficiently achieved by heating to 70°C for 30 minutes. Particular attention should be paid to folds and pleats and the application of a hot iron to these is useful. Head lice may be treated by rubbing an insecticidal preparation into the scalp (such as 1% malathion) and leaving it in contact for at least an hour. Insecticidal shampoos are, because of their short contact time, relatively ineffective. Nits can be removed with a fine-tooth comb. Cropping of the hair is not necessary with modern treatment.

Phthirus

Chemical methods, as outlined above, are normally used for this species. Resistance to insecticides is not widespread.

BODY LICE AND INSECTICIDE RESISTANCE

Mass control of louse infestation was successfully achieved after the Second World War by the use of DDT dusting powder, applied by puffer applicators inside the clothing of lousy people. But DDT resistance is now so common that malathion should normally be used, and a watch should be kept for the development of malathion resistance.

Phthirus pubis is still usually sensitive to DDT and its relations, and is always sensitive to organophosphorus compounds. The application of an insecticide lotion—so as to ensure contact for at least an hour—is usually effective after one application.

Chapter 55
Arthropod Dermatoses, Stings, Bites, Allergies and Neuroses

Kenneth G. V. Smith

ACARINE DERMATOSIS

Intense irritation and dermatitis, somewhat resembling that produced by scabies, can result from various mites (Acari) living as temporary ectoparasites on the skin of man. The commonest occurrence of such infestation is among workers associated with stored food products in which the mites occur as pests. The more familiar of these are grocer's itch caused by *Glycyphagus domesticus*, baker's itch (*Acarus siro*) and copra itch (*Tyrophagus putrescentiae*). *Pyemotes tritici* (=*ventricosus*), the grain or straw itch mite (Fig. 55.1) causes an urticarial and papular eruption of exposed parts of the body in those who handle grain, cottonseeds, beans and especially straw. These mites give rise to a severe pruritus, especially on the trunk. A lotion of warm water and vinegar or a saturated solution of picric acid in 90% alcohol will relieve the irritation. An application of 5% betanaphthol ointment is a preventative treatment and a dilute phenol solution will kill the mites. *Dermatophagoides* mites have been recorded as causing an unusually severe dermatitis in man. In one case infestation of the scalp persisted for seven years. Among the constituents of house-dust it has been found that *Dermatophagoides* produced the most potent allergen. Bites of trombiculid mites, or chiggers,

cause a parasitic dermatitis known as trombidiosis or scrub-itch. This condition is an allergic reaction to the saliva of the mite and can be caused by about 15 species, mostly belonging to the genera *Eutrombicula*, *Schoengastia* and *Neoschoengastia*. Trombiculid bites can be prevented by mite repellents such as diethyltoluamide (see also Appendix III, p. 1382).

TICKS

Extensive subcutaneous haemorrhages can be caused by the anticoagulant inoculated with the saliva of ticks.

BUTTERFLY AND MOTH DERMATOSES

Various moth and butterfly caterpillars, usually of the families Arctiidae, Lymantriidae, Saturniidae, Megalopygidae, Notodontidae and Nymphalidae, possess urticating hairs which can cause dermatitis. These hairs penetrate the skin and poison may be injected through them from attached glands. The poisons include histamine and cause irritation which can be severe if mucous membranes are affected, for example

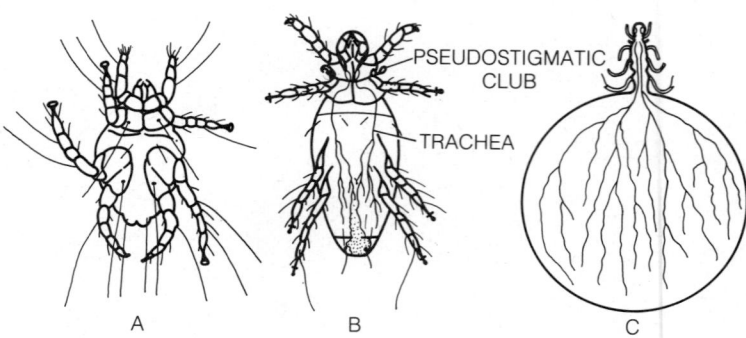

Fig. 55.1 *Pyemotes tritici*. A, male. B, adult female. C, pregnant female with brood sac. × 80.

when detached hairs enter the eye and give rise to nodular conjunctivitis.[1] Both larvae and adults can be involved.

In Papua New Guinea and northern Australia the moth *Ochrogaster lunifer* has caused epidemics of urticaria among troops. In Brazil flannel moths (Megalopygidae) are well known urticators. In the Panama Canal Zone the urticating caterpillars of *Megalopyge lanata* produce rapidly developing eosinophilia (8–22%), numbness and vesication. The 'puss caterpillar', *Megalopyge opercularis*, causes thousands of cases of dermatitis in children in Texas, necessitating the closure of schools. In Japan, some 300 000 people were affected by the moth *Euproctis flava*. In Israel *Thaumetopoea pinivora* causes trouble every year in February and May and caterpillar dermatitis is also common in northern Kenya (Fig. 55.2).

In Africa and Asia some adult moths of the families Pyralidae, Geometridae and Noctuidae feed upon the eye discharges of various mammals, including man. Although their probosces cannot penetrate live tissue, they may well be vectors of mammalian epidemic keratoconjunctivitis and other eye diseases. In Malaya one noctuid fruit-piercing moth *Calyptra eustrigata* can penetrate mammalian skin and suck blood and must therefore be considered a potential vector of disease or producer of allergic reaction.[3]

BEETLE DERMATITIS

Beetle larvae of the family Dermestidae have urticating hairs which produce a dermatitis. Since these beetles are pests of stored products,

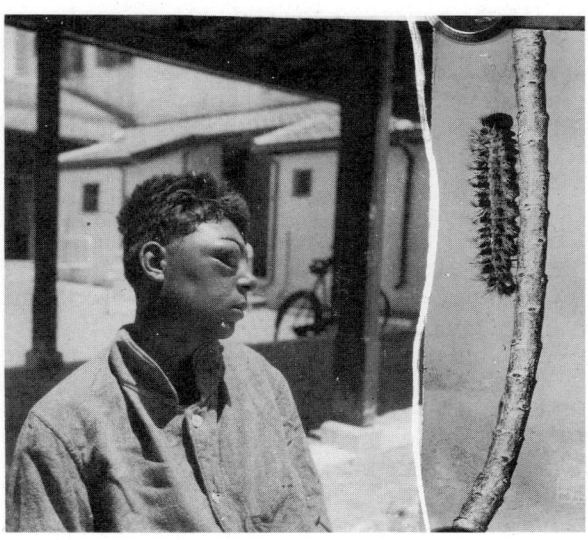

Fig. 55.2 Urticating dermatitis caused by contact with a processionary caterpillar of the moth *Thaumetopoea wilkinsoni*.

Urticating hairs may become detached from the caterpillar and the cocoon spun by the caterpillar before pupation. Such detached hairs may retain their urticating properties for a long time. If inhaled these hairs may cause dyspnoea and if ingested may give rise to stomatitis. In Africa *Anaphe renata* (Notodontidae) and related moths have both imago and larva clothed with detachable irritating hairs.

Caterpillars of the Venezuelan saturniid moth *Lonomia achelous* inject, through their hairs, a powerful anticoagulant if handled or even brushed against and long-lasting fibrinolytic bleeding results.[2]

dockers unloading ships' cargoes have developed dyspnoea and erucic stomatitis from the inhalation and ingestion of detached hairs.

The family Meloidae contains some species known as blister beetles because their body fluids contain cantharidin, a cytotoxic principle which causes vesicular dermatitis when applied to the skin. The best known species is the so-called Spanish fly, *Lytta vesicatoria*, and in India *Mylabris cichorii* and *Epicauta hirticornis* are troublesome. In the Gilbert Islands severe blistering is caused by the coconut beetles *Sessinia collaris* and *Ananca decolor* of the family Oedemeridae. The bushmen of South Africa use body fluids from the larvae of the chrysomelid beetle *Diamphidia nigroornata* as a lethal arrow poison which causes death from a general paralysis. Staphylinid beetles of the genus *Paederus* cause urticaria and blistering and minute species of the genera *Atheta* and *Oxytelus* fly in numbers and may enter the eye, causing a burning sensation.

OTHER INSECTS

Other insects causing dermatitis are ceratopogonid flies (biting midges) of the genus *Culicoides*. In Brazil *C. paraensis* is a public health problem in this way and in El Salvador an increase in biting *Culicoides* was correlated with decreasing standards of sanitation and the cessation of a control campaign against the breeding sites of the mosquito *Aedes aegypti*. In Japan there are records of eczema following the bites of *C. erairai* and long-lasting sores (three to four months) following bites by *C. obsoletus*. Mosquito bites in persons sensitized to their saliva can cause troublesome chronic ulcers which will respond dramatically to topical steroids. Sandflies and black flies can similarly cause quite severe reactions in sensitized persons which will respond quite readily to steroid ointment such as betamethasone valerate. An irritant vesicular rash, superficially resembling scabies, can be caused by Thysanoptera (see also Table III.7, p. 1425).

BEE AND WASP STINGS

The stings of bees, wasps and hornets may produce a mild reaction easily soothed with an ice-pack, diluted vinegar or antihistamine ointment. They may be very serious in the case of multiple stinging or of stings in the mouth. Some people react violently to bee stings and may become increasingly hypersensitive with each successive sting. In such cases anaphylaxis may result which can be fatal. Massive anaphylaxis causes muscular paralysis and suggests a curare-like action on synapses of muscle end-plates. The antidote is an injection of adrenaline.

People extremely sensitive to bee stings should always have access to a pressurized bronchodilator spray and use two puffs when breathing in and this procedure can be repeated in 15 minutes. Such patients, however, may quickly become faint and lose consciousness and should be immediately taken into medical care.[4,5]

Bee and wasp venoms contain histamine, acetylcholine and enzymes (phospholipase A and hyaluronidase); the more superficial aspects of a sting are due to the histamine. The African honey-bee *Apis mellifica adansonii* is abundant in equatorial and warm temperate southern Africa and is a fairly aggressive species. In 1956 this species was introduced into South America and hybridization with local bees has produced an extremely aggressive race of Brazilian honey-bees. The spread of these bees has been very rapid throughout South America and a number of fatalities have resulted from the abundance and special behavioural characteristics of the bee. The slightest disturbance near the hive can cause hundreds of bees to become airborne which then sting any animal or human within 100 m of the apiary and may pursue fleeing victims for over a kilometre.[6] Taylor[7] considers the past and possible future spread of these bees, which have now reached the southern USA.

In the honey-bee the sting is torn out by the act of stinging but the poison gland, which is attached to the sting, continues to inject venom into the wound. For this reason the sting should be carefully removed as soon as possible and the remaining venom expressed from the gland with forceps.

Sometimes stingless social bees (*Melipona* etc.) are prone to aggressive mass biting and some neotropical species squirt caustic fluid, but these insects are rarely more than a nuisance. Some tiny stingless sweat-bees (*Trigona*) can be annoying in the African savannah regions and, because of their numbers and persistence, are sometimes mistaken for *Simulium* (black flies).

Wasps (*Vespula*) and hornets (*Vespa*) can sting repeatedly because, unlike the honey-bee, the sting is not torn out by the action of stinging. Wasp venom contains a higher proportion of histamine and 5-hydroxytryptamine (serotonin) which is distinctly more active than that of the honey-bee. *Scleroderma nipponensis* (Bethylidae), in one incident in Japan, attacked 340 people, who were left with reddish swellings and injuries leading to suppuration and lymphangitis. Some parasitic wasps of the family Ichneumonidae such as *Ophion*, *Netelia* and *Ichneumon* can inflict painful stings. Sensitive patients may be ill for some weeks following these stings.

Paper-wasps of the genus *Polistes* also cause many fatalities in the New World. These wasps build their nests under the eaves of houses or in ornamental shrubs and trees where people are likely to be exposed to their stings.

Arthropod venoms are dealt with in Chapter 48 and by Beard[8] and Bucheri and Buckley.[9]

POISONOUS HONEY

Occasionally the honey produced by hive-bees, wild honey-bees, bumble-bees and stingless bees may be toxic if particular plants are foraged or if polluted liquid resources are used in the absence of clean drinking water (which should be provided in the case of honey-bees).

ANTS

Ants can bite, sting and squirt formic acid. Mostly the attacks of ants produce only mild effects, but, as in wasps, the stinging apparatus is a modified ovipositor which can be extracted after each sting and used repeatedly; multiple stinging may induce an anaphylactic response. Some ants may also be mechanical transmitters of disease; for example, Pharaoh's ants (*Monomorium pharaonis*) have been found to carry *Salmonella*, *Pseudomonas*, *Staphylococcus*, *Streptococcus* and *Clostridium* spp. in hospitals.[10]

The venom of ants is largely proteinaceous but in the south-eastern USA *Solenopsis richteri* is a dangerous fire-ant in which the venom is non-proteinaceous and exhibits necrotic activity resembling the bites of *Loxosceles* spiders. When a colony is disturbed the ants erupt in thousands and 3000–5000 stings may be administered in a matter of seconds. Allergic reactions to such stings, and anaphylactic shock, may sometimes result in death of sensitive individuals. The subject is reviewed by Gurney.[11]

OTHER BITES AND ALLERGIES

Skin reactions of both immediate and delayed hypersensitivity type were common following the bite of *Triatoma infestans* and *T. maxima* in Brazil where the former was the major man-biting triatomid (Hemiptera). The reactions were severe enough to prevent the use of these bugs for xenodiagnosis.[12]

Other orders containing insects capable of inflicting bites or stings include other Hemiptera (plant bugs) and some Orthoptera. Chicken bugs in Mexico (*Haematosiphon inodorus*) and Brazil (*Ornithocoris toledo*) attack poultry but may incidentally bite man and may produce a polymorphous dermatitis with pustules, scabs and linear scars. The bite of the giant water-bugs (Belostomatidae) may be nearly as severe as a bee sting. Many other bugs will bite if incautiously handled. The larger coreid and pentatomid bugs can squirt a jet of irritant fluid from the metathoracic glands into the eye of the beholder which can cause a very painful reaction for a day or two.

The bites of several insects not mentioned above may also produce allergic reactions. Recorded cases involve adult flies of the rhagionid genus *Symphoromyia* and larvae of Therevidae Smith[13] and Tabanidae[14] (Diptera) and the possibility of such reactions following the bite of almost any insect must be considered; if possible suspected specimens should be collected and identified by a specialist.

In addition to bites, other allergic reactions are not uncommon. Inhalant allergens may be acquired from acarine sources in house dust (especially from *Dermatophagoides pteronyssinus*) or among stored products from the grain weevil *Sitophilus granarius* or the Mexican bean weevil *Zabrotes subfasciatus*.

Some aquatic insects such as Ephemeroptera and Trichoptera emerge in vast numbers and their cast exuviae are fragmented and windborne and become inhalant allergens. Chironomidae ('green nimitti') have also been associated with asthma and other allergic symptoms along the Nile.[15] Terrestrial counterparts causing similar allergies are the prolific aphids.

Allergic reactions to the bites and stings of insects and other arthropods are treated by Frazier[16] and Frazier and Brown[17]. Tu[18] surveys the whole field of arthropod poisons, allergens and venoms.

For the identification of arthropods of medical importance Smith[19] should be consulted.

NEUROSES

Many people have a morbid fear of insects and the extreme manifestation of this is in delusory parasitosis (Ekbom's syndrome), also loosely referred to as parasitophobia, acarophobia or entomophobia. In these cases patients suffering from dermatitis artefacta, usually of emotional origin, believe that they are infested with insects or other parasites which cause the itching. They then scratch the affected parts until the skin breaks down. Further skin damage may be caused by the overuse of disinfectants or insecticides. Such cases are difficult, and best treated by a psychiatrist, but every effort should be made to establish that there are in fact no minute biting insects such as *Culicoides* or allergen-producing mites or insects, particularly of the type bearing or shedding urticating hairs. The possibility of inanimate allergens such as paint should also be carefully investigated. Cases of delusory parasitosis may follow an actual infestation by fleas or other arthropods, by seeing or reading about ectoparasites in the popular media,[20,21] or by emotional disturbances.[22] Some success in treating this difficult condition has recently been claimed from use of the drug pimozide. A common feature of these cases is that the persistence of the sufferer often results in a second member of the household presenting similar symptoms, which adds credence to their claims.

Sometimes there are group outbreaks of imagined biting insects, a phenomenon which has only recently received attention.[22] In these cases 'phantom biters' may persist for two or three years in offices or small factories where several people work together. The causative agent may be carpet fibres, fragments of glass fibre lampshades or the coverings of wires on telephone switchboards. Spraying *during working hours* (even with water) has sometimes proved effective in these cases. Here again extreme care should be taken that an actual infestation of mites or minute insects is not the cause.

REFERENCES

1 Watson, P.G. & Sevel, D. (1966) *Br. J. Ophthal.* **50,** 209–217.
2 Arocha-Pinango, C.L. & Layrisse, M. (1969) *Lancet* **i,** 810–812.
3 Bänziger, H. (1980) *Mitt. schweiz. ent. Ges.* **53,** 127–142.
4 Frankland, A.W. (1976) Bee sting allergy. *Bee Wld* **57,** 145–150.
5 Hoffman, D.R. (1977) *Cutis* **19,** 763–767.
6 Michener, C.D. (1975) The Brazilian bee problem. *A. Rev. Ent.* **20,** 399–416.
7 Taylor, O.R. (1977) *Bee Wld* **58,** 19–30.
8 Beard, R.L. (1963) *A. Rev. Ent.* **8,** 1–18.
9 Bucherl, W. & Buckley, E.E. (1971) *Venomous Animals and Their Venoms, III. Venomous Invertebrates.* New York and London: Chapman and Hall.
10 Beatson, S.H. (1972) *Lancet* **i,** 425–427.
11 Gurney, A.B. (1975) Some stinging ants. *Insect World Digest* Sept/Oct, 1975, 19–25.
12 Costa, C.H.N., Costa, M.T., Weber, J.N. et al (1981) *Trans. R. Soc. trop. Med. Hyg.* **75,** 405–408.
13 Smith, K.G.V. (1979) *Lancet* **(i) 8112,** 391–392.
14 Otsuru, M. & Ogawa, S. (1959) *Acta Med. Biol.* **7,** 37–50.
15 Cranston, P.S., Gad-El-Rab, M. & Kay, A.B. (1981) *Trans. R. Soc. trop. Med. Hyg.* **75,** 1–4.
16 Frazier, C.A. (1969) *Insect Allergy. Allergic and toxic reactions to insects and other Arthropods.* St Louis: W.H. Green.
17 Frazier, C.A. & Brown, F.K. (1980) *Insects and Allergy.* Norman: University of Oklahoma Press.
18 Tu, A.T. (ed.) (1984) *Handbook of Natural Toxins,* vol. 2. *Insect Poisons, Allergens and Other Invertebrate Venoms.* New York: Dekker.
19 Smith, K.G.V. (ed.) (1973) *Insects and Other Arthropods of Medical Importance.* London: British Museum (Natural History).
20 Busvine, J.R. (1980) *Insects and Hygiene,* 3rd edn. London: Chapman and Hall.
21 Mester, H. (1977) Das Syndrom des wahnhaften Ungeziefer-befalls. *Angew. Parasit.* **18,** 70–84.
22 Lyell, A. (1983) . *Br. J. Dermatol.* **108,** 485–499.

SECTION XV
CLINICAL PROBLEMS IN THE TROPICS

Chapter 56
Fever

Fever is the cardinal symptom of many tropical infections, and the diagnosis of the cause of fever is one of the commonest problems confronting the clinician in the tropics. This short chapter is intended to refresh the memory, and provide a few useful lists.

THE MECHANISM OF FEVER

Fever is usually caused by exogenous pyrogens, mainly of bacterial origin, which stimulate the release of endogenous pyrogens from a variety of phagocytic cells. These include monocytes, histiocytes, Kupffer cells, alveolar macrophages and splenic sinusoidal cells. Endogenous pyrogen is not realeased in significant quantities by lymphocytes or polymorphonuclear leukocytes.

Endogenous pyrogens cause the release of prostaglandins in the hypothalamus, which reset the thermoregulatory centre. Antipyretic drugs reduce temperature by interfering with prostaglandin synthesis and as they are only effective if prostaglandin synthesis is excessive, they do not reduce the temperature in the absence of fever. On the other hand, corticosteroids reduce fever by inhibiting the release of endogenous pyrogen.

THE PATTERN OF FEVER

Old textbooks used to attach a great deal of importance to the pattern of fever as a diagnostic aid, and there is a danger that modern scepticism has allowed the pendulum to swing too far the other way. There really *are* some diagnostically useful patterns of fever, and for this reason, the 4-hourly temperature chart is still a useful aid to diagnosis in many cases.

1 Mode of onset

An abrupt onset of fever, often accompanied by rigors, is a frequent feature of malaria and many pyogenic and viral infections. On the other hand, a gradual onset is typical of subacute and chronic infections such as typhoid, brucellosis and tuberculosis.

2 Regularly periodic intermittent fever

Fever that occurs at intervals of 48 to 72 hours strongly suggests tertian or quartan malaria respectively. One must remember that it often takes a week or two for schizogony to become synchronized, and so in the early stages of malaria infection the characteristic periodicity is often absent. Many patients with falciparum malaria never develop a regular pattern of fever.

3 Relapsing fevers

This pattern of fever is not only typical of the borrelioses which are named 'relapsing fever', but also of a number of other infections including:

malaria;
African trypanosomiasis;
brucellosis;
subacute bacterial endocarditis.

4 Remittent fevers

These are fevers in which the temperature is always elevated above normal, although the swings may be large. They are typical of typhoid and other septicaemic states.

5 Intermittent fevers

These are fevers in which the temperature fluctuates widely between febrile and afebrile levels.

They are typical of severe pyogenic infections, including ascending cholangitis.

6 Biphasic fever

An initial fever which lasts a few days is followed by an afebrile period lasting a day or two, followed by a return of fever. This 'double hump' pattern is typical of a variety of viral infections, of which dengue is perhaps the best example. The first hump corresponds to viraemia, the second hump occurs when antibody is destroying virus—and sometimes destroying host cells containing virus, too.

DIAGNOSIS OF FEVER

Once the obvious causes of fever in an individual patient have been eliminated, it may be very difficult to find the cause of the fever. This difficulty is even greater in areas where laboratory facilities are very limited.

ACUTE OR CHRONIC FEVER?

A start can be made by calling fevers of more than two weeks' duration chronic fevers. There are far fewer cases of chronic fever than there are of acute fever. Simple laboratory tests combined with experience will enable most fevers to be identified, and a correct decision taken about treatment. Even the rather imprecise diagnosis of 'viral fever' is worth something to the patient. When uncomplicated it predicts a favourable outcome and that there is no need for antibiotic treatment. The white blood-cell (WBC) is often very helpful in identifying the likely cause of a fever.

Routine investigations in all fevers are:
1 thick blood film for malaria parasites;
2 total and differential WBC.

In holoendemic malaria areas, positive blood films are so common it is often very difficult to decide whether the malaria parasites are related to the fever or not. If in doubt, one treats the malaria, and waits to see what happens. When malaria is causing the fever, the WBC is usually normal or reduced and the platelet count is often low.

If the WBC shows a polymorphonuclear leukocytosis (PNL), even if the blood film is positive for malaria, it is likely there is another cause for the fever.

Malaria is the most important cause of fever in the world. It may cause acute, chronic or relapsing patterns.

Acute fevers

Acute fevers with a negative malarial blood film

The WBC divides this group into two as shown.

Polymorphonuclear leukocytosis?	
Yes	*No*
Pyogenic infection	Viral infections*
Leptospiral infection	Rickettsial infections
Relapsing fevers	Typhoid
Amoebic liver abscess	
Acute collagenosis	

*But PNL often develops after the onset of severe viral infections such as Lassa fever.

Acute fevers with PNL and localizing symptoms

Organ-specific symptoms or signs often localize the site of infection:
1 severe sore throat:
   (a) streptococcal tonsillitis;
   (b) diphtheria;
2 cough, pleuritic pain, rusty sputum: pneumonia;
3 severe pain and swelling in a joint: pyogenic arthritis;
4 frequency, dysuria and loin pain: pyelonephritis;
5 severe pain in the head and back of the neck with stiffness: meningitis;
6 severe pain in a bone: osteomyelitis;
7 severe lower abdominal pain: pelvic sepsis;
8 bloody diarrhoea: bacillary dysentery, campylobacter infection;
9 marked localized lymphadenopathy: local sepsis, plague;
10 sharply defined cutaneous inflammation: erysipelas;
11 Ill-defined subcutaneous inflammation: cellulitis.

A delay in seeking medical aid, so common in tropical countries, greatly increases the chances of the patient presenting with a useful localizing sign or symptom.

Acute fevers with PNL and no obvious localizing features

The most important are:
1 septicaemias of all kinds: most commonly staphylococcal, streptococcal and meningococcal, including acute bacterial indocarditis;
2 infections with *Leptospira* and *Borrelia* spp. (Chapter 32):

(a) leptospirosis (there is often jaundice and renal involvement);

(b) tick-borne relapsing fever;

(c) louse-borne relapsing fever;

3 acute non-typhoid *Salmonella* septicaemia (Chapter 15). Gastrointestinal symptoms may be few. Rose spots and splenomegaly may develop.

Acute fevers without PNL and with a negative blood film

The most important are viral and rickettsial infections and typhoid fevers. Most viral fevers are never diagnosed precisely, because of their relatively non-specific features, unless the physician is helped by a good virology laboratory. Features suggesting a viral aetiology are:

1 the double-humped fever pattern already mentioned;

2 many other cases seen in the same space/time envelope.

In some of the rickettsial infections, localized adenopathy may draw attention to a previously unrecognized eschar. In typhoid, persistent complaints of abdominal discomfort or pain draw attention to an abdominal location of infection.

Important non-localizing accompaniments of fever

These include:

1 rash;

2 generalized or multiple adenopathy;

3 splenomegaly;

4 anaemia;

5 jaundice;

6 polyarthritis.

Some patients have localizing features and non-localizing features in addition to fever. These features are just as important in long-term as in short-term fevers. Sometimes the diagnosis unfolds itself as time passes.

Acute fever with a haemorrhagic rash

There are two main causes:

1 viral haemorrhagic fevers (such as dengue, chikungunya, Rift Valley fever) (Chapter 5);

2 acute meningococcal septicaemia (Chapter 30).

Correct diagnosis is vital, because death may follow within a few hours of petechiae appearing in meningococcal infection. Material aspirated from the spots contains meningococci in more than 80% of cases when examined by a simple

stained smear. Other pyogenic septicaemias cause purpura only rarely.

Non-haemorrhagic rashes accompany a great number of acute fevers. One of the few general infections in which a rash never occurs is malaria unless the rash is caused by a drug used to treat it.

Acute fever with anaemia

The main causes are:

1 malaria (Chapter 1);

2 babesiosis (Chapter 1);

3 bartonellosis (Chapter 11);

4 infection in a patient with a pre-existing anaemia such as sickle cell disease or thalassaemia, or with glucose-6-phosphate dehydrogenase (G-6-PD) deficiency (Chapter 58).

Causes 1 and 4 are much the commonest. Polyarthralgia is usual in sickling crises, which are often precipitated by infections. Jaundice often accompanies pneumonia in patients with G-6-PD deficiency, and is partly haemolytic and partly hepatic in origin.

Prolonged fever

By this I mean fever of more than two weeks' duration. There is some overlap with the acute fevers, because sometimes infection with the same organism causes fever for a week, sometimes for a few weeks. Typhoid fever in some individuals causes a mild fever of only a few days' duration, in others a continuous fever for several weeks. Also, infection with *Borrelia* may cause only one bout of fever or several bouts.

The following list contains the commonest causes of prolonged fever, simply subdivided according to the most usual WBC picture.

1 Chronic fever with PNL:

(a) deep sepsis (amoebic liver abscess) ⎫

(b) ALA ⎬ typically a sustained fever

(c) erythema nodosum leprosum ⎭

(d) cholangitis ⎫ typically a relapsing

(e) relapsing fever ⎭ pattern

2 Chronic fever with eosinophilia:

(a) invasive ('toxaemic') *Schistosoma mansoni* and *S. japonicum* infections (Chapter 22);

(b) invasive *Fasciola hepatica* infection (Chapter 22);

(c) acute lymphangitic exacerbations of

Wuchereria bancrofti and *Brugia malayi* infections (Chapter 20);
(d) gross visceral larva migrans due to *Toxocara canis* (Chapter 21).
3 Chronic fever with neutropenia:
  (a) malaria (Chapter 1);
  (b) disseminated tuberculosis;
  (c) visceral leishmaniasis (Chapter 4);
  (d) brucellosis (Chapter 7).
4 Chronic fever with normal WBC:
  (a) localized tuberculosis;
  (b) brucellosis (Chapter 7);
  (c) secondary syphilis;
  (d) trypanosomiasis (Chapter 2);
  (e) toxoplasmosis (Chapter 9);
  (f) subacute bacterial endocarditis (SBE);
  (g) systemic lupus erythematosus (SLE);
5 Chronic fever with a variable WBC picture:
  (a) tumours;
  (b) reticuloses;
  (c) drug reactions;
  (d) deep mycoses (Chapter 35).

I have missed out those conditions where the localizing signs are so obvious that they could not really be overlooked, such as pyogenic arthritis.

Chronic fevers with a relapsing pattern

In these, a period of fever is typically followed by an afebrile period, after which the fever recurs. Some of the above infections may show this feature but the following often do:
1 malaria (Chapter 1);
2 visceral leishmaniasis (Chapter 4);
3 trypanosomiasis (Chapter 2);
4 relapsing fever (Chapter 32);
5 brucellosis (Chapter 7);
6 filariasis (Chapter 20);
7 cholangitis.

Pyrexia of undetermined origin (PUO) in the tropics

A difficult problem at any time, it is even more difficult in the tropics because there is usually a lack of sophisticated techniques for investigation. One often has to rely on very simple investigations combined with clinical acumen.
  Ideally, the following investigations should be carried out:

1 full blood count, including repeated films for malaria;
2 chest X-ray;
3 urine examination;
4 repeated blood cultures;
5 liver biopsy, including cultures for tuberculosis;
6 marrow, including cultures and animal inoculation;
7 intravenous pyelography;
8 Mantoux test to 1, 10 and 100 tuberculin units;
9 *Brucella* cultures and antibody titres;
10 *Toxoplasma* dye test;
11 rickettsial and viral antibodies;
12 blood for LE cells, and antinuclear factor.

  The commonest cause of PUO in the tropics is cryptogenic tuberculosis, and by this I mean disseminated tuberculosis without evidence of its origin. The presence of a negative Mantoux supports the diagnosis, as in many tropical areas it is unusual to find an adult who is not Mantoux positive, and disseminated disease is accompanied by a generalized suppression of cell-mediated immunity. Once the overwhelming infection is overcome, the test becomes positive, often very strongly.

Prolonged fever with a normal WBC and erythrocyte sedimentation rate (ESR)

There are two main causes of this, one is spurious (the patient is simulating fever) and the other is toxoplasmosis.

Prolonged fever with ascites

The commonest cause is tuberculous peritonitis. Decompensated cirrhosis and pneumococcal peritonitis can give similar pictures.

TROPICAL FEVERS: CONCLUSIONS

Most prolonged fevers in the tropics can be diagnosed by fairly simple tests. When all tests fail, one may have to resort to therapeutic trial. There is nothing to be ashamed of about this, for one should never let a patient die of a treatable condition from insisting too rigidly on firm diagnostic criteria.

Chapter 57
Diarrhoea

This chapter is meant to bring together some of the many entries on diarrhoea in other chapters, and to help with problems of differential diagnosis. It deals with conditions whose *primary* feature is diarrhoea, but one remembers that there are many infections in which diarrhoea may be a secondary feature.

CATEGORIES OF DIARRHOEA

I shall use a system that I have used elsewhere,[1] not because it is perfect, but because I find it useful in clinical practice. It is based on the duration of the diarrhoea, the presence or absence of blood in the stool, and the presence or absence of fever. The system divides diarrhoea into these categories:

    with fever and blood,
    with fever but no blood,
    without fever, with blood,
    without fever, without blood.

The same four categories can also be used to categorize chronic diarrhoea. I find it useful to have a third 'temporal' category of 'persistent diarrhoea', which I shall explain later.

ACUTE DIARRHOEA

Acute diarrhoea with fever and blood

The main causes are:

    shigella dysentery,
    campylobacter infection,
    entero-invasive *Escherichia coli* infection,
    salmonella enterocolitis.

Shigella dysentery (Chapter 14)

The more severe clinical picture of shigellosis commonly seen in tropical countries is because of the high prevalence of *Shigella dysenteriae* infections. Although attacks are usually self-limiting and of short duration, the mortality can be high in the absence of good supportive treatment, especially in children and the mal-nourished. Complications include the haemolytic–uraemic syndrome, and convulsions are common in children. A reactive arthritis may follow shigellosis, mostly in people of HLA type B27. Stool culture results, even if available, are of no use in deciding management, for the important decisions have to be taken before culture results are available.

Two decisions that must be taken are: (i) is rehydration needed, and if so, by what route? (ii) should an antibiotic be given, and if so, which one?

The aid that can be given by the laboratory is not of much help. The stool will contain an inflammatory exudate of polymorphonuclear leukocytes, there may be fairly numerous macrophages (an inexperienced microscopist might mistake these for amoebae), and there are usually fairly scanty non-motile bacilli.

Clinical judgement will decide the need for rehydration. The diarrhoea of shigellosis is partly inflammatory and partly secretory in type, and suitable replacement solutions include Ringer lactate solution (Chapter 12), BP or the WHO intravenous diarrhoea treatment solution for parenteral treatment, and the WHO formula oral rehydration solution (ORS) (Chapter 12). Mild cases will be managed quite adequately with the simpler glucose or sucrose/salt solutions.

If an *effective* antibiotic is given to a patient with shigellosis it will shorten the duration of the illness, and will not encourage (cf. salmonellosis) the development of the carrier state. The difficulty is in finding an antibiotic to which the organisms are sensitive. The widespread resistance of shigellae to the commonly used antibiotics is a result of the indiscriminate use of antibiotics and the fact that resistance is spread from one organism to another by the exchange of resistance-encoding plasmids. It is very useful to know the usual resistance pattern in the area in which you are working, so that you can make a rational choice of antibiotic. In general, the antibiotics to which the organisms are most likely to be sensitive are those which have been used the least.

They would usually include nalidixic acid and gentamicin, for example.

Campylobacter infections (Chapter 14)

In tropical countries these infections are mainly seen in children, adults presumably being immune. The organism is widespread in animals, from whom the infection is almost invariably acquired. The contamination of the environment with animal faeces is one source of infection, and milk-borne outbreaks are also common.

The organism causes an enterocolitis, so a feature which distinguishes it from shigellosis is the frequent appearance of upper abdominal pain, and abdominal pain is sometimes severe enough to bring the patient to surgery. Another difference from shigellosis is the duration of the illness: fever and diarrhoea may continue for 10 days or more.

Although campylobacters are usually beyond the resources of the small hospital in the tropics to culture—they require a special medium and a microaerophilic environment to grow—they can usually be recognized by direct microscopy. The small, vibrio-like organisms have a very characteristic 'shunting-engine-like' to and fro movement, best seen with the dark-field condenser, but almost as well recognizable by using the normal condenser well stopped down. When the organisms are present in large numbers, as in patients with frank enterocolitis, they can be recognized in about 90% of cases, whose cultures subsequently prove positive.

Although campylobacters respond to erythromycin, the drug does not seem to alter the course of the illness unless given early.

Enteroinvasive Escherichia coli (Chapter 14)

These organisms can cause an illness clinically indistinguishable from shigellosis. They can only be identified in specialized centres, but the failure to do so is of little clinical importance, as management is the same as for shigella dysentery.

Salmonella enterocolitis (Chapter 15)

The organisms of salmonella food poisoning usually cause enteritis, but sometimes colitis may be sufficiently marked for frank blood to appear in the stool. In the absence of septicaemia, management is supportive only.

Acute diarrhoea with fever but no blood

The main causes are:
    salmonella food poisoning;
    parenteral infections in children;
    enterotoxigenic *E. coli* infection (fever may be absent).

Of course, mild cases of shigellosis and campylobacter infection can also cause this syndrome, when inflammation has not proceeded as far as ulceration. Oddly enough, enterovirus infections do not usually cause diarrhoea (poliovirus is a good example) but rotavirus infections, mainly seen in children, and other viruses such as the Norwalk agent, may produce a very transient fever, lasting a few hours at the onset if present at all.

Salmonella food poisoning (Chapter 15)

All the many animal salmonellae are responsible for human food poisoning at times, numerically the most common being *S. typhimurium* and *S. enteritidis*. Because the infecting dose is high—about 10^8 organisms in contrast to the 10^2 or so organisms needed to transmit bacillary dysentery—the organisms usually need to multiply in food before reaching levels capable of infecting man. So direct human-to-human transmission, although it does occur, is far less common than transmission via food which has acted as a culture medium.

The main clue to the diagnosis of salmonella food poisoning is the presence of many cases occurring all at the same time. When there is a clear history of everyone affected having attended the same wedding party, a common source outbreak is obvious. It is less obvious when the outbreak is due to contaminated food being sold to people coming from a wide area, and here a painstaking investigation may be needed to track down the source of the infection.

The diagnosis of salmonella food poisoning is initially made clinically, and confirmed later by culture if the facilities are available.

THE NATURAL HISTORY OF SALMONELLA FOOD POISONING

The onset is often with fever, followed by vomiting and diarrhoea. Fever and vomiting usually settle within 48 hours, diarrhoea often continues for a week or a little longer. The disease is, therefore, self-limiting, and the mortality is usually very low.

But *some* patients will continue to have fever far more than 48 hours, and go on to develop signs of septicaemia, such as a swinging fever, splenomegaly and a 'rose spot' rash similar to that of typhoid. These patients, if untreated, may die.

THE MANAGEMENT OF SALMONELLA FOOD POISONING

Normal management is supportive only, i.e. oral or parenteral rehydration as required.

Antibiotics should *not* routinely be used because:

1 antibiotics do not shorten the duration of diarrhoea;

2 antibiotics tend to make the patients become carriers.

The indications for antibiotic treatment are:

1 fever lasting more than 48 hours in an adult,

2 signs of septicaemia;

3 a clinical judgement in a small child that septicaemia is likely, mainly based on the degree of toxaemia—in small children it is not safe to wait;

4 the victim has sickle cell disease or sickle cell/haemoglobin C disease: an antibiotic is given to protect against salmonella osteomyelitis.

If it is decided to give an antibiotic for any of the reasons given, it must be continued for 10–14 days as in the case of typhoid, to prevent relapse.

Recurrent or relapsing salmonella septicaemia may complicate *Schistosoma mansoni* infection.

Parenteral infection in children

In very small children, almost any infection can cause diarrhoea. The *localized* infections that can do this include:

otitis media;
acute tonsillitis,
pneumonia,
urinary tract infection.

When confronted with a child with a history of fever and diarrhoea, especially when there is no blood in the stool, the throat, ear, lungs and urine must be examined *and a blood film examined for malaria parasites.*

Malaria is quite a common cause of diarrhoea, especially *Plasmodium falciparum*, but the diarrhoea is usually not bloody.

Acute diarrhoea without fever, with blood

The main causes are:

amoebic dysentery (Chapter 17),
balantidial dysentery (Chapter 17).

Both of these soon become chronic, as the natural history is for the infections to persist for longer than two weeks. In both cases diagnosis is established by the examination of *freshly passed* stools for the presence of the characteristic, motile trophozoites.

Three other important causes of bloody diarrhoea which becomes persistent are infection with:

Schistosoma mansoni (Chapter 22);
Schistosoma japonicum (Chapter 22);
Trichuris trichiura (Chapter 21).

In all these cases, the diagnosis is made by finding the relevant eggs in the stool. In all three cases, bloody diarrhoea only occurs in very heavy infections, and in all three cases, eosinophilia is usual. In the case of *Trichuris* infections heavy enough to cause a bloody diarrhoea—usually only encountered in small children or the mentally defective—the diagnosis is best made by proctoscopy, when worms will be seen embedded in the rectal mucosa (Fig. 21.11).

Acute diarrhoea without fever and without blood

When this occurs in outbreaks, one must think of:

cholera (Chapter 13),
preformed toxin food poisoning,
(severe abdominal pain should make one suspect *Clostridium perfringens* type C) (Chapter 14).

Cholera is suspected whenever a prostrated patient is seen who passes a watery stool without apparently noticing it, whenever an outbreak of diarrhoea is associated with very severe dehydration, and whenever diarrhoea is associated with muscle cramps. This severe, secretory diarrhoea is sometimes almost matched in severity by some attacks of enterotoxigenic *Escherichia coli* (ETEC) infection.

Isolated cases of acute diarrhoea without blood or fever may be due to food toxicants, ETEC infection and various viruses including the rotavirus (Chapter 16).

The problem of persistent diarrhoea

This is diarrhoea which continues, although at lesser severity, following an attack of acute diarrhoea. The main causes are:

giardiasis (Chapter 17),

amoebiasis (Chapter 17),
secondary lactase deficiency (Chapter 19).

In visitors to the tropics, an acute bowel infection of one sort or another commonly seems to initiate non-specific inflammatory bowel disease.

CHRONIC DIARRHOEA

The 'categories' here are not quite so helpful.

Chronic diarrhoea with fever

The main causes are:
    tuberculous enteritis (there is often marked wasting; the sputum smear may be positive);
    visceral leishmaniasis (the diarrhoea may be due to direct involvement of the mucosa or to a variety of secondary infections) (Chapter 4);
    schistosomiasis (fever in the early stages only; eosinophilia provides a clue) (Chapter 22);
    yersiniosis (Chapter 14);
    Acquired immunodeficiency syndrome (AIDS) (Chapter 68).

Chronic diarrhoea with blood, without fever

The main causes are:
    amoebiasis (Chapter 17);
    balantidiasis (Chapter 17);
    schistosomiasis (due to *S. mansoni* or *S. japonicum*) (Chapter 22);
    trichuriasis (Chapter 21).
In each case, the diagnosis is made by stool microscopy.

Chronic diarrhoea without fever or blood

Fatty diarrhoea is common in this category, and the causes include the following.
1   Giardiasis (diarrhoea resolves spontaneously in a few months) (Chapter 17).
2   Coeliac disease (gluten enteropathy: an accompanying iron deficiency is common).
3   Tropical sprue (Chapter 19) (an accompanying megaloblastic anaemia is common). Serum folate levels are low, and B_{12} levels are low also when the condition has been present for some months.
4   Strongyloidiasis (Chapter 21) (upper abdominal pain and eosinophilia are useful clues; the abdominal symptoms usually subside in a

few weeks, when the condition becomes a chronic 'commensal' infection).
5   *Capillaria philippinensis* (Chapter 18) infection (the picture resembles severe strongyloidiasis, and will often not resolve spontaneously. It may cause severe malabsorption which eventually leads to the patient's death).
6   Lymphoma of the small bowel. This usually causes a diffuse infiltration of the bowel wall which renders it thickened and rigid. It is important to make the diagnosis accurately, as this tumour usually responds well to chemotherapy (Chapter 67).
7   Although chronic pancreatitis or mucoviscidosis can cause steatorrhoea—and a calcified pancreas with or without pancreatic lithiasis is common in some parts of the tropics (Chapter 60)—the steatorrhoea is more commonly biochemical than clinical. This means that although fat excretion may be significantly increased, it is often not increased enough to give the patient diarrhoea.
8   Cryptosporidiosis (Chapter 17). This infection causes chronic diarrhoea which is normally self-limiting, seldom lasting for more than a few weeks. But it can be fatal in immunosuppressed patients, and is an important component of the 'slim disease' presentation of AIDS in Africa. Diagnosis is by direct microscopy using a special stain. There is no satisfactory treatment. Isosporiasis (see Chapter 17) also causes diarrhoea in AIDS, but in many AIDS patients no cause for the diarrhoea can be found.

Cosmopolitan causes of diarrhoea

Non-specific inflammatory bowel disease is less common in many parts of the tropics than it is in Western Europe or North America. The reasons are obscure, but it does seem that these diseases may be becoming more common in those parts of the world, such as the West Indies, where the traditional diet is being replaced by more 'westernized' dietary habits.

Carcinoma of the colon is also relatively uncommon in parts of the tropics where a 'traditional' diet is followed, and protagonists of the high fibre diet have suggested that the fibre protects the mucosa from the local action of carcinogens on the mucosa. If this is so, one must expect an increase in this form of carcinoma in people abandoning their traditional fibre-rich diets. But a high fibre intake may itself be causally related to other bowel diseases, such as volvulus of the colon, which occurs relatively frequently in people where dietary fibre intake is traditionally high.

REFERENCE

1 Bell, D. (1985) *Lecture Notes on Tropical Medicine*, 2nd edn. Oxford: Blackwell Scientific Publications.

Chapter 58
Haematological Problems
S. H. Abdalla and *D. J. Weatherall*

ANAEMIA IN THE TROPICS

Anaemia is a common and important cause of morbidity in the tropics. A variety of environmental, nutritional and genetic factors lead to the more common occurrence of certain anaemias. The aim of this chapter is to draw attention to these common factors which lead to anaemia and often in a situation where minimal facilities are available for diagnosis and treatment. This chapter is not intended to be comprehensive, and for a more detailed description a standard haematological textbook should be consulted.

NORMAL VALUES IN THE TROPICS

Anaemia is defined as a condition in which the haemoglobin concentration in the blood is lower than normal. It is important in defining normal levels to recognize that these vary with age, sex, physiological status and altitude.[1]

The normal values for haemoglobin accepted by the World Health Organization are:

children aged six months to six years	11 g/dl
children aged six to 14 years	12 g/dl
adult males	13 g/dl
adult females, non-pregnant	12 g/dl
adult females, pregnant	11 g/dl

A reference range of values has to be defined for any particular population using standardized methods, and should be defined for sex and age groups.

In defining a reference range for a population it is essential to exclude all the common causes of anaemia in the selected healthy subjects. Where this has been done the difference in normal values between indigenous populations in the tropics and in populations in the developed world has not been great. In everyday clinical practice in the tropics it is more important

to recognize and treat anaemia that is life-threatening or that is clinically significant than to define whether any one patient's haematological parameters lie within the normal range. For further discussion of this subject the reader is referred to a review by Gilles.[2]

In recent years it has become recognized that black Africans and Americans of African origin have a lower mean neutrophil count than non-blacks. This neutropenia is thought to be genetically determined as it is also seen in blacks who have lived outside the tropics. The normal range for neutrophils in blacks is $1.1–6.0 \times 10^9$/litre and in non-blacks $1.5–6.5 \times 10^9$/litre.

DIAGNOSIS OF THE CAUSE OF ANAEMIA

In addition to the determination of haemoglobin concentration in the blood other parameters are essential for the diagnosis of the cause of anaemia. If the packed cell volume (PCV) and red cell count (RCC) can be determined then the 'absolute' values (the mean cell volume, mean corpuscular haemoglobin and mean corpuscular haemoglobin concentration) can be calculated.

Mean cell volume (MCV). In most laboratories the MCV is measured directly, electronically. It can also be calculated if the PCV and RCC are known as follows:

$$MCV = \frac{PCV \text{ (ratio)}}{RCC} \times 1000 \quad \text{(result in femtolitres (fl))}$$

The normal range for the MCV is 82–96 fl in adults but may be as low as 70 fl in normal children below 2 years of age. The MCV is raised in megaloblastic and macrocytic anaemias and decreased in iron deficiency, secondary anaemias, thalassaemias, haemoglobin C and E both disease and trait.

Mean cell haemoglobin (MCH). This value is calculated as follows:

$$MCH = \frac{Hb\ (g/l)}{Red\ cell\ count\ per\ litre} \quad \text{(result in picograms (pg))}$$

The MCH is raised in macrocytosis due to any cause and is low in any of the conditions that lead to a low MCV (normal range 27–33 pg).

Mean cell haemoglobin concentration (MCHC). This is calculated as follows:

$$MCHC = \frac{Hb\ (g/dl)}{PCV\ (ratio)} \quad \text{(result expressed as a percentage)}$$

The MCHC is increased in spherocytosis. It is decreased in iron deficiency and to a lesser extent in secondary anaemias. It is, however, usually normal in the thalassaemias and haemoglobinopathies and is useful in discriminating these conditions from mild iron deficiency (normal range 31.7–34.1).

The most important single investigation in the diagnosis of the cause of anaemia is examination of a blood film. Although this requires training and expertise and a good microscope, it is not beyond the capabilities of many hospitals and institutes.

The examination of the blood film will reveal, in most cases of severe anaemia, whether the red cells are normocytic, normochromic, microcytic, hypochromic or macrocytic (Table 58.1).

Normocytic anaemia. This is commonly due to acute blood loss, haemolysis, anaemias associated with splenomegaly, secondary anaemias or marrow infiltration. The blood film shows red cells of normal size although some variation in size (anisocytosis) and shape (poikilocytosis) is usually seen. Rouleaux may also be seen especially in secondary anaemia, myeloma and kala-azar.

Hypochromic microcytic anaemia. This is commonly due to iron deficiency but may also be due to thalassaemia and sometimes secondary anaemia. The red cells show an increase in central pallor (Fig. 58.1B) and there is a marked anisocytosis with many small red cells (microcytes). Poikilocytosis is often marked. 'Pencil cells' which are poikilocytes with parallel sides, are often characteristically seen in iron deficiency (Fig. 58.1A).

Macrocytic anaemias. A proportion of the red cells are often enlarged in macrocytic anaemias. The diameter of a normal red cell is slightly less than that of a nucleus of a lymphocyte. This is a useful inbuilt scale especially in cases where mild macrocytosis is suspected. Macrocytes may be round or oval. Oval macrocytosis, especially when associated with hypersegmented neutrophils, is almost exclusively seen with megaloblastic anaemias (Fig. 58.1C and D). Other conditions associated with round macrocytosis include liver disease, hypothyroidism and alcohol abuse when not complicated by dietary deficiencies.

Bone marrow examination

Even in the absence of an experienced haematologist a physician may be able to obtain useful information by examination of bone marrow smears. The following is a brief description of some of the features that are easy to recognize.

Cellularity. This is best assessed by examination of the particles. These should have a variable amount of fat spaces constituting 30–60% of the fragments. Increased marrow cellularity is seen in iron deficiency, megaloblastic anaemias, haemolysis, hypersplenism and infiltration of bone marrow as in leukaemias and in lymphomas and carcinomas with bone marrow secondaries. A hypocellular bone marrow is a characteristic finding in aplastic anaemia. It must be remembered that bone marrow cellularity may vary widely from different sites and a single hypocellular aspirate may not be sufficient to diagnose aplasia. The marrow is hypocellular in elderly subjects and more so if a sample is taken from the posterior superior iliac spine. Bone marrow is also generally more cellular in young children.

Morphology. Megaloblastic changes can be easily recognized with little practice. Erythroblasts are large and show a granular chromatin pattern and there is a delay in maturation of the nucleus in relation to haemoglobinization of the cytoplasm (Fig. 58.2B).

Micronormoblastic changes occur in iron

Table 58.1 Morphological classification of anaemia.

Type of anaemia	Causes	Comments
1 Microcytic hypochromic	Iron deficiency	Dietary, chronic blood loss from gastrointestinal tract (hookworm etc.), gynaecological causes. Commonest cause of anaemia worldwide
	Anaemia of chronic disease	Common worldwide: may also be normocytic but MCV may be as low as 65 fl
	Thalassaemias	Common in the Mediterranean, South-East Asia, isolated parts of Africa
	HbE	Very common in South-East Asia mild to moderate anaemias
	HbC	Common in West Africa but anaemia if present is usually mild. May also have normal MCV or microcytosis, mild
	Sideroblastic anaemia	Rare
2 Macrocytic anaemias	*Megaloblastic:* Folate deficiency	Dietary, malabsorption syndromes, increased demand, haemolysis, pregnancy, antifolate drugs etc.
	B_{12} deficiency	Pernicious anaemia (may occur at a young age group in blacks), malabsorption, Crohn's, TB etc.
	Non-megaloblastic: Other causes	Drug induced Liver disease Myelodysplastic syndrome Hypothyroidism
	Accelerated erythropoiesis	Chronic haemolytic anaemia without secondary megaloblastosis
3 Normocytic normochronic	Malaria	Common cause in areas of high endemicity especially in children up to 5 years, pregnant women and non-immune adults
	Acute haemorrhage	Gastrointestinal blood loss, trauma, childbirth etc.
	Haemolysis: Sickle cell disease	Commonest haemoglobinopathy in blacks
	HbC disease	Anaemia usually mild (may also be microcytic)
	G-6-PD deficiency	Usually associated with drugs or infections
	Other enzyme deficiencies	
	Associated with an enlarged spleen:	Usually accompanied by thrombocytopenia and leukopenia
	tropical splenomegaly syndrome, kala-azar, trypanosomiasis etc.	
	Marrow infiltration: leukaemias lymphoma myeloma carcinoma	Abnormal cells in peripheral blood or bone marrow
	Marrow failure: aplastic anaemia	Hypocellular bone marrow
	dyserythropoiesis	Hypercellular bone marrow with reticulocytopenia
	anaemia of chronic disorders	Normocellular bone marrow

deficiency anaemia and there is often fragmentation of the cytoplasm.

Iron stain. Presence of storage iron in the fragments rules out iron deficiency as a cause for anaemia. However, it must be remembered that

if iron stores are low, treatment of severe anaemia due to other causes such as megaloblastosis, may lead to limitation of a full response to treatment. Iron stores are generally increased in pernicious anaemia as there is no associated iron malabsorption, in thalassaemias and sickle cell disease,

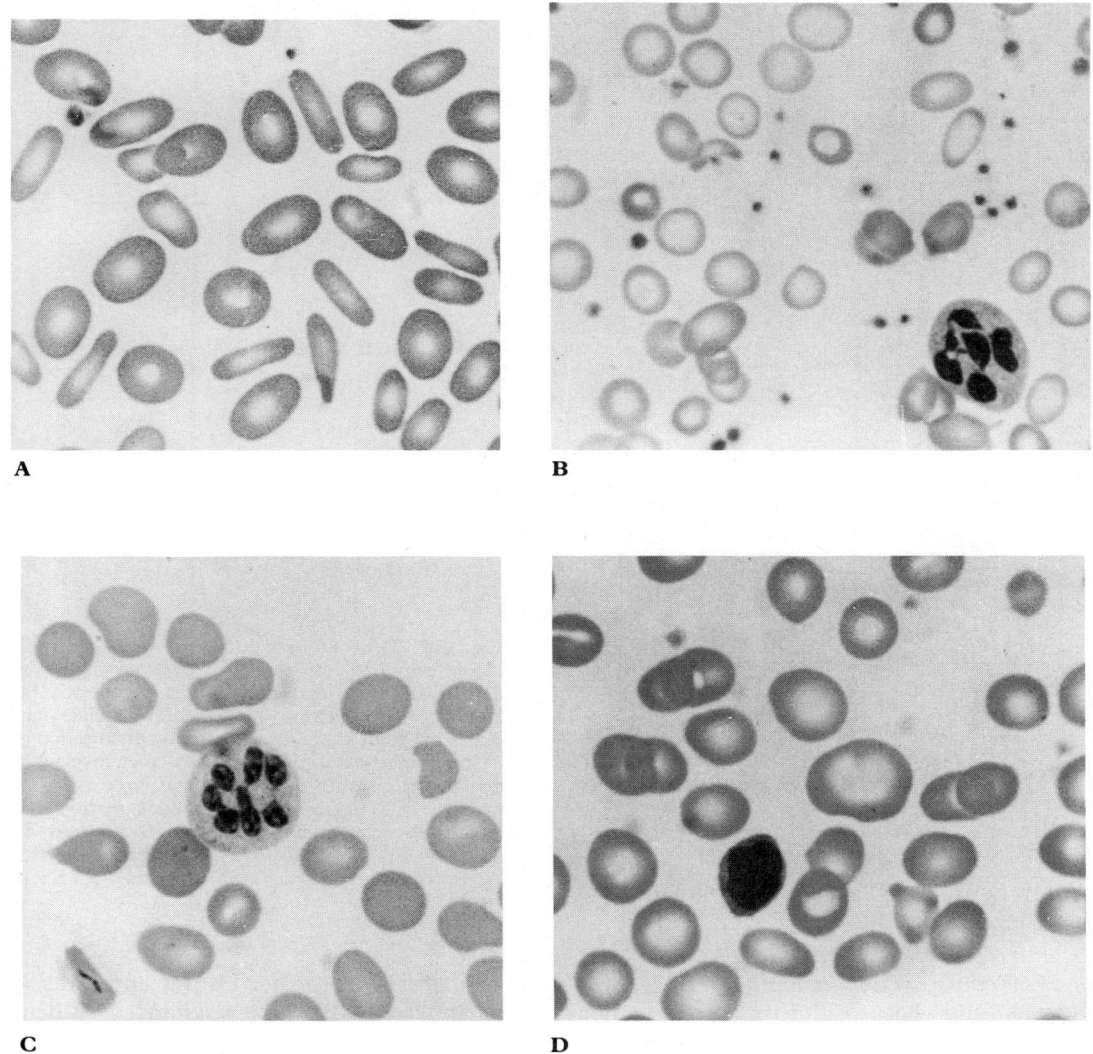

Fig. 58.1 Peripheral blood. A, Elliptocytosis: most of the red cells are elliptical. Most subjects with elliptocytosis do not suffer from anaemia. A minority of cases may have a compensated haemolysis or even a haemolytic anaemia. B, Iron deficiency anaemia: there is an increase in area of central pallor (hypochromia). Some cells are small in size (microcytosis). There is also a hypersegmented neutrophil. This is sometimes seen in uncomplicated iron deficiency. C, Hypersegmented neutrophil from a blood film of a patient with dietary B_{12} deficiency. D, Macrocytosis: most of the cells are larger than normal and some are oval (from a patient with megaloblastic anaemia due to dietary B_{12} deficiency). NB. All photomicrographs in Figs. 58.1–58.4 are at the same magnification.

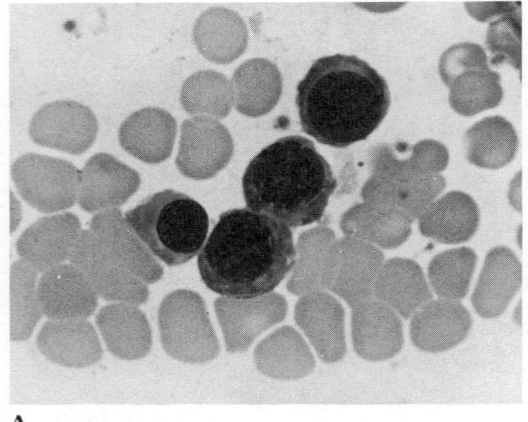

A

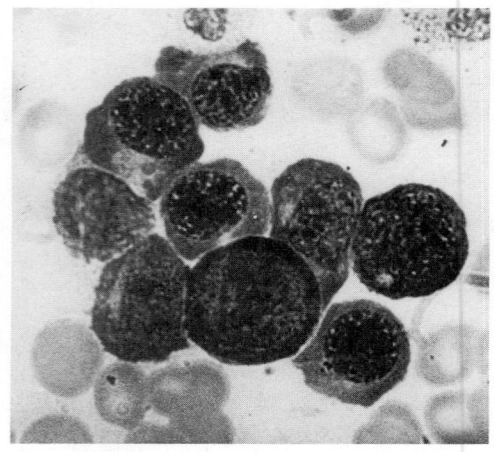

B

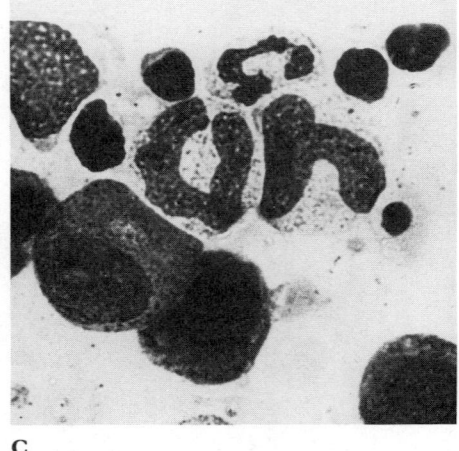

C

Fig. 58.2 Bone marrow. A, Normoblastic erythroid hyperplasia from a patient with haemolytic anaemia to show the normal stages of maturation of erythroblasts. B, Megaloblastic bone marrow: the erythroblasts are large. The nuclear pattern is grainy and there is dissociation of nucleocytoplasmic maturation. C, Giant metamyelocytes: these are characteristically at least twice as large as normal metamyelocytes. They are found in bone marrows in megaloblastic anaemias and less frequently in iron deficiency anaemia. They may also occur in other dyserythropoietic states without evidence of haematinic deficiency (i.e. malaria).

in dyserythropoietic anaemias, sideroblastic anaemias and haemosiderosis. In secondary anaemias there is a characteristic iron distribution (see p. 953). Absence of iron stores indicates iron deficiency.

PATHOPHYSIOLOGY AND CLINICAL FEATURES OF ANAEMIA

A reduction of oxygen carrying capacity by the blood is the main consequence of anaemia. Several compensatory mechanisms occur in order to make the best use of available oxygen and these depend on the speed of onset of the anaemia. In anaemia of gradual onset there is an increase in cardiac output and a decrease in peripheral vascular resistance. When haemoglobin falls below 9 g/dl there is an increase in heart rate, stroke volume and a shortening of the circulation time. There is a shift of the oxygen dissociation curve to the right. This is mainly due to the increase in production of 2,3-diphosphoglycerate (2,3-DPG). There is an increase in plasma volume to compensate the loss of red cells.

The clinical features of anaemia depend upon its severity and rapidity of onset.

The common symptoms are easy fatiguability and muscular weakness and a lower threshold for exercise or work tolerance. Pallor is an easy though not necessarily reliable clinical way of diagnosis of anaemia and is assessed by inspection of the conjunctival and oral mucous membranes. It must be remembered that conjunctivitis and stomatitis may interfere with this assessment and so will shock and peripheral vascular collapse.

Cardiovascular signs and symptoms include tachycardia, palpitations, dyspnoea on exertion and a mid-systolic (haemic) murmur. In severe cases especially where there is underlying heart or circulatory disease more severe ischaemic events such as claudication, angina, myocardial infarction and congestive cardiac failure may occur (Fig. 61.3, p. 1015). In younger subjects and especially in children in whom anaemia occurs gradually there is a much greater tolerance to anaemia especially if it is of gradual onset.

Nutritional Anaemias

IRON

Iron deficiency is the commonest cause of anaemia on a worldwide basis. Iron itself is a very common element and there is no mechanism in the human body for iron excretion. Control of the amount of iron in the body is achieved by a tight control on iron absorption from food.

Iron in the body (total approximately 5 g) is found mainly in haemoglobin (2–3 g) and reticuloendothelial storage iron (0.5–1.5 g). Other iron-containing compounds are myoglobin, iron-containing enzymes and transferrin and ferritin. Transferrin, a beta globulin glycoprotein mol. wt 76 000 is essential for iron transport. It is synthesized mainly in the liver and with a plasma half-life of about 10 days. There are two main transferrin variants which are separated by electrophoretic mobility. Ferritin is a water-soluble protein iron complex. The protein part, apoferritin is made by most cells in the body, the stimulus for synthesis being the presence of iron. The iron content of ferritin is variable but may be up to 20%.

Iron absorption

Several factors affect absorption of iron from the intestinal mucosa. Thus a higher percentage of iron from meat is absorbed than from vegetable or cereal sources. Iron absorption is also enhanced by the presence of low molecular weight chelators in food, such as ascorbate, and also by acid pH, and is inhibited by the presence of high molecular weight chelators, such as phytates, and and by alkaline pH. Iron absorption takes place mainly in the duodenum with lesser amounts being absorbed in the jejunum. This is due to the low pH in the duodenum which favours absorption. Neutralization of gastric juice by pancreatic secretion takes place in the jejunum and this diminishes iron absorption considerably.

Daily requirement

Physiological loss of iron from desquamation of epithelial cells in the body is estimated at between 0.5 mg per day in infants and younger children to about 1 mg in adults. In older children and adolescents there is an added requirement of between 0.5 and 0.9 mg per day according to age. In menstruating women the amount lost in menses leads to a further average requirement of 1–2 mg per day. Pregnancy requirements are 3–4 mg per day. Thus the total daily requirement of iron varies from 1 mg daily in infants and non-menstruating adults to about 2 mg for adolescent males and 2.5–3 mg in menstruating females.

The amount of iron absorbed from food varies from 20–30% in meat and liver to 5% or less from cereals, spinach and eggs. Iron deficiency increases the percentage of iron absorbed.

The normal western diet is said to provide a total of 15–20 mg of iron a day which is barely sufficient for maintenance of iron balance in a menstruating female as only 10% of this is absorbed on average. It is therefore essential to realize that in the tropics, where meat consumption may be low, iron deficiency can easily occur in groups at risk such as pregnant or menstruating women and during adolescence. This can occur even without the added burden of extra blood loss due to intestinal infestation such as hookworm or schistosomiasis (see Table 58.2 for common causes of iron deficiency).

Diagnosis

When iron loss from the body exceeds absorption, iron deficiency ensues; a depletion of storage iron occurs before the onset of anaemia.

Table 58.2   Commonest causes of iron deficiency.

Physiological:	Infancy (aggravated by prematurity) Adolescence Pregnancy	
Chronic blood loss:	Uterine:	Menorrhagia Fibroids Obstetric causes
	Gastrointestinal:	Oesophageal varices Hookworm Carcinoma of gastrointestinal tract Aspirin Peptic ulcers Haemorrhoids etc.
	Other causes:	Haematuria Haemoptysis Haemorrhagic disorders
Insufficient intake:	Dietary	
Malabsorption:	Ileocaecal tuberculosis Coeliac disease Gastrointestinal surgery	

This is followed by a fall in the haemoglobin level with a drop in MCV and MCH. With more severe deficiency the red cell count drops as does the MCHC. The typical blood picture shows hypochromia and microcytosis. Elliptocytosis ('pencil' cells) and occasional target cells may be seen. Hypersegmented neutrophils are sometimes seen in severe iron deficiency not complicated by B_{12} or folate deficiency. The platelet count is sometimes raised especially when there is chronic haemorrhage. Iron deficiency is often easy to diagnose from the examination of a well-prepared, well-stained blood film. However, occasionally other conditions which may cause microcytosis or hypochromia may cause confusion. Hypochromia and microcytosis are characteristic of thalassaemia. The anaemia of chronic disorders is also sometimes hypochromic and microcytic, and hypochromic red cells are seen in sideroblastic anaemia. Other tests are necessary to confirm the presence of iron deficiency in doubtful cases, especially where a full response to iron therapy has not been obtained. The serum iron level is low in iron deficiency and the total iron binding capacity (TIBC) is raised. This is in contrast to the anaemia of chronic disorders where both the serum iron and TIBC are low. Serum ferritin is a sensitive index of iron status (normal range 15–250 μg/litre). However it is raised in some conditions, irrespective of iron status. These include hepatitis, malaria and acute inflammatory conditions.

The definitive method of diagnosing iron deficiency with confidence is the examination of a bone marrow smear stained with Perls' ferrocyanide method. It is important to make a diagnosis of the cause of the iron deficiency especially when this occurs in adult males who do not have the risk factors that females in the childbearing age suffer from (Table 58.2).

Treatment

The most effective treatment of iron deficiency is also the cheapest. Ferrous sulphate tablets 200 mg given two to three times daily will produce a very quick response in most cases. This should be continued until the haemoglobin level is back to normal, then reduced to one tablet daily. It is necessary to continue with treatment for four to six months in order to build up reserve storage iron. If intolerance to iron occurs it is best to either reduce the dosage to once daily or to change the preparation to ferrous gluconate or ferrous fumarate. These preparations contain less iron per tablet and therefore are less irritant. Enteric coated iron tablets, 'spansules', and other such expensive preparations should not be used as they are released beyond the duodenum and are not well absorbed. It is important to realize that iron given before meals is most efficiently absorbed but may cause gastrointestinal irritation in some people. It is therefore usually recommended that iron tablets should be given during or after a meal to minimize these side-effects.

Parenteral iron therapy has limited indications

such as the presence of a constant blood loss which cannot be stopped, i.e. hiatus hernia, ulcerative colitis, hereditary telangiectasia, or when a patient cannot return for follow-up or be relied on to take the tablets. In the latter case a total dose infusion of an iron dextran complex will ensure that the patient has had sufficient iron to bring back haemoglobin level to normal and for storage iron to be replenished.

Iron dextran (Imferon) contains 50 mg of iron per ml the total dose needed whether given intramuscularly daily in divided doses (maximum 2 ml per injection) or as an intravenous total dose infusion can be calculated as follows:

total dose (in ml) $= 0.0476 \times W$ $(14.8 - \text{Hb})$
where W = weight in kg and Hb = haemoglobin in g/dl.

This is sufficient to bring the Hb back to normal levels. An additional 6 ml should be added to the infusion if the patient is female and 14 ml if the patient is male in order to restore body stores. No additional amount is required in children under 15 years. A total dose infusion must be given slowly for the first 30 minutes and must be given in a minimum volume of 500 ml of diluent (either 5% glucose or 0.9% sodium chloride). Not more than 25 ml should be diluted in 500 ml.

Intramuscular iron must be given by deep injection to avoid skin discoloration.

It must be remembered that parenteral iron therapy does not lead to a quicker rise in haemoglobin. Intramuscular iron is painful. Intravenous total dose infusion carries a significant risk of an anaphylactic type reaction which can be fatal. This form of therapy should therefore only be undertaken in a unit where supervision of the patient is possible and where facilities for resuscitation are immediately available.

Failure of response to iron therapy

The causes for this are failure of compliance, prescription of iron preparations that are not easily absorbed, the existence of malabsorption, continuous haemorrhage, usually from the gastrointestinal tract, or that a wrong diagnosis was made.

MEGALOBLASTIC ANAEMIAS

These are a group of anaemias distinguished by characteristic abnormal morphology of erythroblasts in the bone marrow (Fig. 58.2). The common causes are B_{12} or folate deficiencies or abnormal metabolism of these vitamins. Other rare causes include abnormalities of DNA synthesis such as occurs in erythroleukaemia, sideroblastic anaemia and secondary to cytotoxic agents which interfere with DNA synthesis (Table 58.3).

Table 58.3   Causes of B_{12} and folate deficiency.

B_{12} deficiency	
Nutritional:	Vegans
Malabsorption:	Pernicious anaemia
	Gastrectomy
	Stagnant loop syndrome
	Tropical sprue
	Crohn's disease
	Fish tapeworm
Folate deficiency	
Dietary:	Usually associated with general poor nutrition, i.e. poverty, old age, alcoholism and PEM
Malabsorption:	Coeliac disease
	Tropical sprue
	Crohn's disease
	Ileocaecal tuberculosis
Excess utilization:	Pregnancy
	Prematurity
	Chronic haemolytic anaemia
Antifolate drugs:	Cytotoxics
	Anticonvulsants
	Pyrimethamine co-trimoxazole
	(These are important in severely ill patients and those who have borderline nutrition)

Clinical and haematological features

The clinical features are those of anaemia described above. The basic lesion in megaloblastic anaemia is the impairment of DNA synthesis because of the reduced supply of deoxyuribonucleoside triphosphates which are the precursors of DNA. Deficiency therefore affects rapidly dividing cells such as those of the bone marrow and gastrointestinal mucosa. Folate acts as a coenzyme in the synthesis of thymidylate. The coenzyme is oxidized in this reaction and requires another enzyme, dihydrofolate reductase (DHFR), to return folate to its active state. Several drugs inhibit DHFR such as methotrexate and pyrimethamine and to a lesser extent trimethoprim. Vitamin B_{12} is an essential coenzyme in the conversion of methyltetrahydrofolate to the active intracellular folate coenzymes.

The main clinical features of megaloblastic anaemia, apart from those of anaemia (see above), are pigmentation, anorexia, weight loss and diarrhoea, angular stomatitis and atrophic glossitis. A mild splenomegaly is sometimes seen in severe cases. An additional feature which occurs only in B_{12} and not in folate deficiency is peripheral neuropathy. Patients usually present with paraesthesiae and muscle weakness. More severe deficiency may lead to subacute combined degeneration of the cord and paraplegia or quadriplegia.

Pernicious anaemia in blacks has been observed to present in a different manner to that in non-blacks. The age of presentation is often much younger, many patients presenting at the second or third decade of life. The presentation is usually with severe anaemia and neurological complications are common. The incidence seems higher in women. It must also be remembered that macrocytosis, whether judged by electronic measurement of MCV or by inspection of a blood film, may be masked in areas of the world where α thalassaemia is common (reviewed by Abdalla et al[3]).

Haematological changes

In megaloblastic anaemias there is usually anisocytosis and poikilocytosis and oval macrocytosis in the blood film (Fig. 58.1D). The MCV rises. This is usually proportional to the severity of the deficiency until the haemoglobin falls to levels below 8 g/dl. The MCV may then fall but rarely back to normal levels. This is due to the formation of very small red cells in advanced deficiency. The red cell count also falls proportionately.

Neutropenia is usual and may predispose to the increased incidence of infection. Thrombocytopenia in advanced deficiency may be sufficiently severe to lead to haemorrhagic manifestations.

The bone marrow in megaloblastic anaemia is extremely hypercellular and characteristic megaloblastic features are seen in the maturing erythroblasts. Giant metamyelocytes and hypersegmented neutrophils are seen (Figs. 58.1C and 58.2C). Despite the marrow hypercellularity there is reticulocytopenia because of ineffective erythropoiesis as most of the precursors die in the bone marrow. Other biochemical features of ineffective erythropoiesis include a rise in serum lactate dehydrogenase and a mildly raised serum bilirubin.

Dietary sources and absorption of vitamin B_{12} and folates

Vitamin B_{12} is made by bacteria in the gut of higher animals. It is only absorbed from the foregut of herbivores who have a specially adapted gastrointestinal system. Carnivores including man obtain their supply of B_{12} from meat and other animal products, or by faecal contamination of food. Folate is found in large quantities in fresh green vegetables and also in liver and meat and yeast extracts. Folate in food is heat labile and is particularly susceptible to prolonged boiling in a large volume of water. The daily requirement of vitamin B_{12} is 1–3 μg and of folate, about 100 μg. The body stores of B_{12} are about 2–3 mg and can last up to about three years. Folate stores are 10 mg and are only sufficient to last about four months.

Most of the vitamin B_{12} is absorbed by an active process in the ileum. The vitamin has to be coupled to intrinsic factor before it is absorbed. Intrinsic factor is produced by the gastric parietal cells and is a glycoprotein. Folate absorption takes place mainly in the upper small intestine and lesser amounts are absorbed in the jejunum and ileum.

Causes of deficiency (Table 58.3)

Vitamin B_{12}

The two main causes of vitamin B_{12} deficiency

are defective nutrition and malabsorption. Nutritional B_{12} deficiency is common amongst strict vegans who, for religious or other reasons, do not take any animal products. The largest group of vegans are Hindus and subnormal levels of vitamin B_{12} are common in these communities. However, true megaloblastic anaemia is less frequent. Severe deficiency may also occur in cases of extreme poverty. Purely dietary B_{12} deficiency is rare apart from the above exceptions.

Malabsorption of vitamin B_{12} occurs in pernicious anaemia, tropical sprue, terminal ileal disease and a variety of other conditions where chronic intestinal malabsorption occurs. The causes vary in importance in different geographical areas. Pernicious anaemia is the commonest cause of B_{12} malabsorption in the industrialized countries of the world.[4] However, the true incidence of pernicious anaemia in Asians and black Africans is not known. A review by Baker indicates that the disease is rare in Asians.[5] However, other reports indicate that where specific diagnostic procedures are applied pernicious anaemia is found more frequently than previously described, amongst American blacks, South Africans and others.[3]

Folate deficiency

This is much more common than B_{12} deficiency. The main causes are dietary deficiency, malabsorption and increased utilization. Dietary folate deficiency is commonly found in the elderly or in young children and is associated with poverty and general malnutrition. Malabsorption of folate occurs in patients with coeliac disease and tropical sprue. Numerous conditions are also said to be associated with transient malabsorption of folate such as alcoholism and congestive cardiac failure and systemic infections such as tuberculosis. Increased utilization of folate occurs as a result of pregnancy and lactation and folate supplementation during pregnancy is now standard practice in many parts of the world. Excessive utilization also occurs in chronic haemolytic anaemias such as sickle cell disease, in conditions where excessive ineffective erythropoiesis occurs (myelosclerosis), inflammatory disease (tuberculosis, Crohn's disease) and neoplastic disease.

Antifolate drugs may also lead to a tissue deficiency of folate. This is most likely to occur in patients who have borderline folate stores. Common offenders are the antimalarial drug, pyrimethamine and the antibiotic, trimethoprim.

Diagnosis of B_{12} and folate deficiency

After establishing that the anaemia is megaloblastic, the following procedures help to elucidate which of the vitamins is deficient and the likely cause of the deficiency.

1 *Dietary history*. A careful dietary history should be taken in all cases. The presence of gastrointestinal symptoms may point to the presence of chronic malabsorption.

2 *Measurement of vitamin B_{12} in the serum and of folate in the serum and red cells*. Subnormal levels of B_{12} (normal range 160–925 ng/litre) are not necessarily indicative of tissue deficiency of B_{12}, especially in dietary B_{12} deficiency. Lower levels of below 50 μg/litre usually reflect severe deficiency.

Serum folate measurement is not a good measure of tissue stores as it reflects recent folate intake. The red cell folate is a more accurate level of tissue stores of folic acid (normal range serum folate 3–15 μg/litre, red blood cell (RBC) folate 160–640 μg/litre.

3 *Therapeutic trial*. This can be done when patients are not severely ill. The advantages are that it does not require any special assays. For suspected B_{12} deficiency a small physiological dose of vitamin B_{12}—1 μg intramuscularly is given daily. Haematological response should then occur with a reticulocytosis starting after 3 days with a peak at 7–10 days and a rise in haemoglobin of about 1 g/dl per week. Folic acid deficiency may be identified in the same way by giving folic acid, 100 μg daily.

4 *Deoxyuridine suppression test*. Deoxyuridine monophosphate is converted to thymidine monophosphate in normal cells in the presence of active folate coenzymes. The test utilizes the suppression of uptake of tritiated thymidine into normal marrow cells which have been preincubated with deoxyuridine. In B_{12} or folate deficiency this suppression is less efficient and is a sensitive index of B_{12} or folate status in the marrow cells.[6]

5 *B_{12} absorption tests*. The commonest test used is the Schilling test; 1 μg of cyanocobalamin labelled with ^{57}Co or ^{58}Co is administered orally to a patient who has previously fasted overnight. This is followed by an intramuscular flushing dose of non-radioactive B_{12} of 1000 μg/litre. A 24-hour urine collection is then used to estimate the percentage excretion of the dose given orally. If the test is abnormal, it is repeated with the addition of intrinsic factor (IF) orally to test whether the B_{12} malabsorption is corrected by IF as occurs in pernicious anaemia.

6 *Other tests.* If pernicious anaemia is suspected other tests are used to confirm its presence. These include testing for antibodies to gastric parietal cells and to intrinsic factor in the serum, the presence of gastric atrophy and pentagastrin-fast achlorhydria.[4] The finding of neuropathy in a patient with severe anaemia must alert the clinician to the possibility of pernicious anaemia or severe B_{12} deficiency due to other causes.

Treatment

B_{12} deficiency

If B_{12} malabsorption is demonstrated parenteral B_{12} therapy must be instituted for life unless there is an obvious treatable cause such as tropical sprue or fish tapeworm. In severely anaemic patients body stores should be replenished by injection of 1000 μg of vitamin B_{12} every other day for six doses. Hydroxocobalamin is then given in doses of 1000 μg every two to three months as maintenance.

In dietary B_{12} deficiency the vitamin may be given orally or parenterally and needs to be given less frequently than in malabsorption states.

Folate

Folate in daily doses of 5–15 mg orally is absorbed efficiently even in the presence of malabsorption. For full repletion of stores treatment should continue for about three to four months where a treatable cause is found. Where deficiency of B_{12} cannot be excluded vitamin B_{12} should be administered before folate therapy as folate may precipitate neurological damage in patients who are B_{12} deficient.

Long-term therapy with folic acid is required for patients with chronic haemolysis such as sickle cell anaemia. The dose is usually 5 mg daily.

PROTEIN–ENERGY MALNUTRITION (PEM) (Chapter 45)

In this type of malnutrition, which affects mainly preschool children, there are multiple deficiencies of protein, calories and a variety of vitamins and minerals. In addition complications such as bronchopneumonia, tuberculosis and malaria are common. The anaemia of PEM is therefore very complex in its pathogenesis.

Anaemia of PEM

There is usually a moderate or occasionally severe normocytic and normochromic anaemia. Macrocytosis and megaloblastic marrow changes have been described in some patients.[7-9] Other workers have also reported the presence of giant metamyelocytes (GMM) in the marrow.[10] In view of these findings it has been suggested that B_{12} and/or folate deficiency may play an important part in the anaemia of PEM, and some investigators have found low levels of serum folate in children with PEM in Egypt and the Sudan.[11,12] A recent study in Nigeria showed that some children with PEM had GMM and megaloblasts in their bone marrow with abnormal deoxyuridine suppression values. However, there was no demonstrable deficiency of B_{12} or folate as judged by the assay of these vitamins in the serum and red cells respectively and by the lack of the expected correction in the deoxyuridine suppressed values by pteroylglutamic acid.[13] Further studies suggested that the biochemical defect may be due to the impairment of conversion of folic acid to 5,10-methylenetetrahydrofolate or an impairment of the activity of the enzyme thymidylate synthetase. There was no evidence of a deficiency in the enzyme dihydrofolate reductase or of the amino acids homocysteine or methionine.[14]

Whatever the mechanism of impairment in bone marrow function in PEM, an adequate erythropoietin response for the degree of anaemia has been demonstrated.[15]

The anaemia of PEM despite its complex pathology usually responds to refeeding and treatment of infection, if present. Iron deficiency is not a consistent feature of the anaemia of PEM at presentation. However, following treatment of malnutrition and restoration of marrow function iron deficiency may occur and limit haematological recovery. Because of the possibility of a flare up of malaria and infections on administration of iron it has been suggested that iron therapy should be postponed until after refeeding.[16]

Secondary Anaemias

THE ANAEMIA OF CHRONIC DISORDERS

A moderate anaemia usually accompanies chronic inflammatory diseases (rheumatoid arthritis and other autoimmune diseases), infections (tuberculosis, chronic suppurative disease, fungal infections) and malignancies (carcinoma, lymphoma or Hodgkin's disease). This is termed the anaemia of chronic disorders.[17]

The haematological features are a mild to moderate anaemia, the haemoglobin rarely falling below 8 g/dl. The red cells may be mildly microcytic or normocytic. The MCV is usually between 70 and 85 fl but may be even lower in children. A lower MCV may suggest the coexistence of iron deficiency. There may be neutrophilia and the platelet count is often raised. There is an increased erythrocyte sedimentation rate and the blood film shows increased rouleaux formation.

The bone marrow appearances are often unremarkable. Erythropoiesis is often normoblastic with some minor dyserythropoietic features. There may be an increase in plasma cells and this is seen more frequently in inflammatory and in autoimmune disease. The characteristic feature of the bone marrow is a marked reduction or total absence of siderotic granules in erythroblasts when marrow smears are stained with Perls' haemosiderin stain, despite the presence of a normal or increased amount of reticuloendothelial iron. There is also a reduction of both the serum iron level and the total iron binding capacity which contrasts with iron deficiency where the latter is raised.

The serum ferritin may be raised in inflammatory conditions. As a rough rule in uncomplicated suspected iron deficiency a serum ferritin below 12 μg/litre confirms iron deficiency, whereas in the presence of other diseases a value of up to 25 μg/litre also indicates absence of iron stores in patients with anaemia of chronic disorders.

Aetiology

Early work suggested a decrease in red cell lifespan but this has not been confirmed in recent studies. The current opinion is that haemolysis, if it exists, is a minor factor in the pathogenesis of the anaemia and that the impairment of the ability of the bone marrow to respond to the anaemia is the main lesion. The mechanisms of this impairment are not clear and there are many studies producing conflicting results for the role of decreased erythropoietin production, reduced bio-availability of iron to erythroblasts, ineffective erythropoiesis and abnormal development of erythroid progenitors (see Samson[18]). It seems that the mechanisms for the production of anaemia are complex and one or more of these factors may play a part in the pathogenesis of the anaemia.

Treatment

There is no known treatment of anaemia of chronic disease although improvement is achieved by treatment of the underlying cause. Iron therapy is of no benefit despite the presence of hypochromia unless there is also coexistent iron deficiency.

ANAEMIA DUE TO MALARIA

Falciparum malaria has been recognized to be a common cause of anaemia in susceptible groups of the population in areas of high endemicity. The pathogenesis of this anaemia has not been fully worked out but some recent work has helped in the elucidation of some of the mechanisms involved.

Haemolysis of parasitized red cell occurs as the parasite matures into schizonts which then burst and lead to release of a fresh crop of merozoites (see Chapter 1). This mechanism is important in high parasitaemias where 10% or more of red cells may be destroyed in each cycle. However, haemolysis of parasitized cells is not the only factor leading to anaemia as it has been noticed that anaemia persists longer than expected after waning of parasitaemia and is sometimes disproportionate to the degree of parasitaemia in animal models.[19]

Haemolysis of non-parasitized red cells by an immune or autoimmune mechanism has been suggested as a cause of severe anaemia in malaria. Although the direct antiglobulin test has been found to be positive in a substantial number of children with malaria in some populations, there is no evidence that this is a cause of haemolysis of non-parasitized cells in the majority of cases.[20,21]

Impairment of marrow function has also been proposed as a mechanism for the slow recovery from anaemia following malaria. This is thought to be due to either hypocellularity of the marrow and decreased iron incorporation[22-25] or dyserythropoiesis and ineffective erythropoiesis[26] (Fig. 58.3). The latter was observed in marrows of children in The Gambia where ineffective erythropoiesis was demonstrated by the lack of appropriate reticulocytosis despite the presence of gross erythroid hyperplasia.

deficiency or that it is an immune drug-induced haemolysis due to quinine, as it has not been described during the period when quinine ceased to be the major antimalarial in use; both these causes have been excluded in some patients in recent studies in Thailand. Recent evidence suggests that blackwater fever is being seen more frequently.

Whatever the cause of anaemia in malaria it responds to the successful treatment of malaria and any interference with marrow function seems easily reversible as brisk reticulocytosis

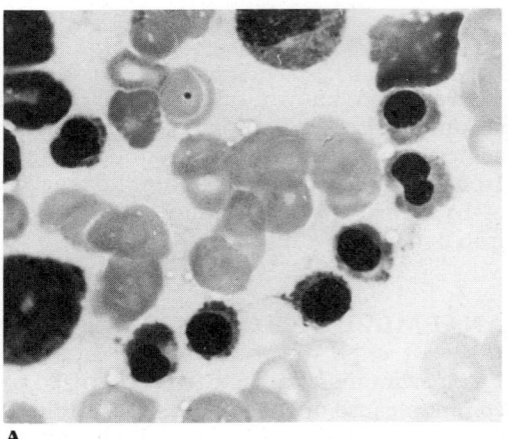
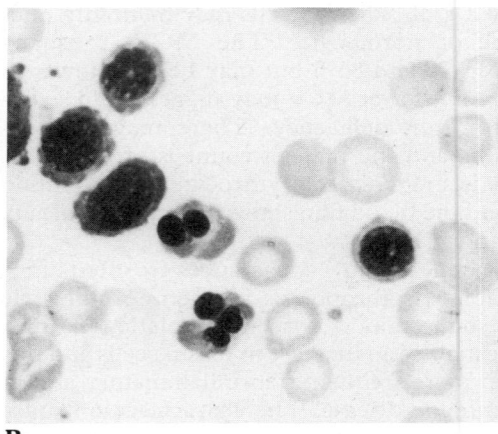

A   B

Fig. 58.3 A and B, Dyserythropoiesis: a term used to describe specific morphological changes in bone marrow which usually denotes ineffective erythropoiesis. These changes include cytoplasmic vacuolation, basophilic stippling, intracytoplasmic bridges, nuclear fragmentation (karyorrhexis), incomplete and unequal nuclear division and multinuclearity. Dyserythropoiesis occurs to a variable degree in many anaemias.

In non-immune adults anaemia is sometimes severe and may accompany other complications such as renal failure where other mechanisms contribute to anaemia.[27]

Severe anaemia following malaria is most commonly seen in endemic areas in young children below the age of five years and in pregnant women. It is also seen in non-immune adults who visit a malarious area and also in populations where there is unstable malaria.

Blackwater fever is a condition characterized by severe haemolysis during an attack of malaria with massive intravascular haemolysis and haemoglobinaemia and haemoglobinuria. It has been suggested that blackwater fever may be due to malaria-associated haemolysis in patients with glucose-6-phosphate dehydrogenase (G-6-PD)

follows with a consequent rise in haemoglobin. Although treatment with folic acid has been advocated[28] because of the increased red cell production there is no evidence that folate deficiency plays a major role in anaemia in malaria[29]. It has also been suggested that administration of iron to iron-deficient subjects may lead to recrudescence of severe malaria in these subjects[16] (see also section on disseminated intravascular coagulation (DIC), p. 983).

HAEMATOLOGICAL FEATURES OF KALA-AZAR (VISCERAL LEISHMANIASIS) (Chapter 4)

Pancytopenia is a common feature of visceral

leishmaniasis. The anaemia is usually normocytic, normochromic and moderate. In young children it may be very severe with a picture suggestive of acute haemolysis. Because splenomegaly is a major feature of kala-azar, anaemia is thought to be due to hypersplenism (p. 972). The severity of the pancytopenia is related to the size of the spleen, which in turn is directly related to the duration of the disease.[30] A recent study in Kenya has shown that dyserythropoitic changes are commonly found in bone marrows of patients with kala-azar and that ineffective erythropoiesis may therefore play a part in the pathogenesis of anaemia in this condition.[30a]

Further evidence for the role of the spleen in pancytopenia in kala-azar was demonstrated by Bada et al[31] who described a patient with kala-azar who had been previously splenectomized and who did not become anaemic.

There is a shortening of the mean red cell life-span with increased sequestration of red cells in the spleen.[32,33] and an increase in plasma volume.

There have been several reports of the presence of complement components[32,34] and of IgG and complement components[35] on erythrocytes of patients with kala-azar. However, there is no direct evidence that autoimmune haemolysis contributes to the severity of the anaemia in kala-azar.

Neutropenia can sometimes become very severe[36] predisposing to severe bacterial infection, but neutrophil function is normal.

Thrombocytopenia may occasionally be severe enough to cause mucous membrane bleeding but purpura is said to be rare.

The bone marrow is usually grossly hypercellular with hyperplasia of all marrow cells. Macrophage hyperplasia may be prominent and many of these cells may contain *Leishmania donovani* parasites bodies. Ferrokinetic studies have shown an increased plasma clearance of ^{59}Fe but with reduced iron incorporation into circulating red cells.[37] Further studies suggest that this may be due to removal of reticulocytes by the spleen rather than ineffective erythropoiesis.[33]

The pancytopenia of kala-azar responds to specific antiparasitic therapy. If anaemia is severe then transfusion may be needed. Thrombocytopenia is rarely severe enough to require platelet transfusions. Antibiotic therapy may be needed to treat infections which may occur due to severe neutropenia.

TRYPANOSOMIASIS (Chapter 2)

Moderate or occasionally severe anaemia has been described in African trypanosomiasis. The most important mechanism appears to be haemolysis of red cells. There is a reduction in the mean red cell life-span,[38] as measured by the ^{51}Cr method. Several mechanisms have been proposed for the haemolysis including a lysin produced by trypanosomes,[39,40] coating of red cells with complement possibly as a result of the presence of circulating immune complexes[38] and hypersplenism.[41,42] Other haematological changes include leukocytosis but usually with relative neutropenia, and thrombocytopenia. The thrombocytopenia is usually moderate to severe.[43] It is thought to be due to platelet pooling in the enlarged spleen. A factor which produces platelet damage and aggregation has been described in experimental trypanosomiasis.[44] Some cases of overt DIC have been described in infections with *Trypanosoma rhodesiense* and this is thought to be triggered by endothelial damage and haemolysis.[43,45,46]

The haematological changes usually revert to normal when the disease is treated.

TUBERCULOSIS (Chapter 59)

A variety of haematological problems are associated with tuberculosis and its treatment. Anaemia in patients with tuberculosis is common and has a multiplicity of causes. The anaemia of chronic disorders, with a block in iron-incorporation into erythroblasts, is seen frequently (p. 953). However, several workers have shown that true iron deficiency is common in patients with tuberculosis at presentation[47] and also during treatment.[48] Although several studies have shown significantly lower levels of serum folate in patients with active tuberculosis when compared with controls[49] the incidence of significant megaloblastic anaemia is low.[50] It has been postulated that the deficiencies may be due to poor nutrition, to anorexia and debility, to over-utilization especially of folate and to malabsorption in intestinal tuberculosis.

A variety of other haematological abnormalities have been described in association with tuberculosis. These include leukaemoid reactions, pancytopenia, myelofibrosis, leukaemias and lymphomas (reviewed by Cameron[51]). These dyscrasias have often been described in cases with florid areactive tuberculosis. It appears, however, that in many of these cases the haematological abnormality is the primary lesion and that disseminated tuberculosis occurs as an opportunistic infection in the presence of reduced cell-mediated immunity.[52]

Drug therapy for tuberculosis is also associated with numerous haematological side-effects. Isoniazid, cycloserine and pyrazinamide are pyridoxine antagonists. A high rate of acquired sideroblastic anaemia is seen in patients treated with these drugs.[53] The anaemia is reversible if the drugs are stopped and pyridoxine is administered.

Other side-effects of antituberculous drugs are haemolytic anaemia and autoimmune thrombocytopenia (para-aminosalicylic acid (PAS) and rifampicin) and aplastic anaemia and agranulocytosis (PAS, streptomycin, thiacetazone). It was also suggested that PAS therapy may lead to B_{12} malabsorption[54] but this has not been confirmed by other observers.[55]

SCHISTOSOMIASIS (Chapter 22)

The cause of anaemia in schistosomiasis depends on the species of worm. Several mechanisms are involved. In *Schistosoma mansoni* and *S. japonicum* infestation the ova in the intestinal wall lead to the formation of ulcers, polyps and fibrosis. These result in blood loss from the colon which has been estimated to be 2.3–25.9 ml per day (equivalent to 0.6–7.7 mg of iron per day).[56,57] This leads to iron deficiency when chronic. The severity of the anaemia depends on the age of the patients and the intensity of infestation.

In more advanced cases liver fibrosis occurs and this leads to portal hypertension and consequently oesophageal varices and splenomegaly. Bleeding from varices increases the loss of iron and if severe may lead to an acute anaemia due to blood loss. Splenomegaly may also lead to hypersplenism with varying degrees of pancytopenia.[58] Red cell life-span is shortened and there is compensatory marrow hyperplasia.[41] Liver failure may also lead to defects in the hae-

mostatic mechanism with a prolongation of the prothrombin time[59] (p. 979).

Infestations with *S. haematobium* affects the urinary tract. Urinary blood loss has been estimated at 2.6–12.6 ml per day (0.6–37.3 mg iron).[56] Hepatic fibrosis is rare. Ureteric fibrosis may lead to attacks of pyelonephritis with the picture of anaemia of chronic disorder developing. Renal failure complicates late cases and further increases the anaemia.

HOOKWORM (Chapter 21)

Hookworms attach themselves to the intestinal mucosa of the host and feed on these cells. This leads to blood loss which has been estimated as 0.03–0.05 ml per day per worm for *Necator americanus* and 0.16–0.34 ml per day in *Ancylostoma duodenale*.[60] As a rough guide it is estimated that for both species the average daily loss is 1 mg of iron per 1000 ova per gram of faeces.[61]

The type and onset of anaemia is related to the worm load and the state of iron repletion of the infected individual and the availability of iron in the diet. Thus a very large worm load in an iron replete individual may cause a normocytic, normochromic anaemia due to haemorrhage[62] whilst a lesser worm load in an individual with an inadequate supply of iron may lead to an iron deficiency anaemia. In addition to iron depletion hookworm infestation leads to the loss of a great amount of protein from the intestines.[63] In addition it has been suggested that following the treatment of severe iron deficiency anaemia, the resulting marrow hyperplasia may lead to folate deficiency and the use of folic acid has been advocated in the treatment of these patients.[64]

Hookworm infestation is a rural disease and in any one community, the prevalence of the infection in the different sexes and age groups depends on local farming practice (reviewed by Fleming[61]). Treatment with iron supplementation may diminish the incidence of anaemia in highly endemic areas where the feasibility of treatment of infestation is low in view of the high rate of reinfection.

Haemolytic Anaemias

This is a group of anaemias in which there is an increase of red cell turnover due to a shortening of the red cell life-span from the normal range of

100–120 days. The clinical and laboratory features of haemolytic anaemias are due to the increased breakdown of haemoglobin and of compensatory mechanisms of increased red cell production (Table 58.4).

Table 58.4 Features of haemolytic anaemias.

Features of increased haemolysis:
  Jaundice
  Hyperbilirubinaemia (unconjugated)
  Increased urobilinogen and stercobilinogen excretion
  Reduced haptoglobin
  Reduced RBC life-span
  Increased serum lactate dehydrogenase (LDH)

Features of increased RBC production:
  Reticulocytosis
  Bone marrow hyperplasia
  Erythroid hyperplasia

Patients with chronic haemolytic anaemia of any cause may present with aplastic crises. There is a shutdown in erythropoiesis with reticulocytopenia and a drastic drop in haemoglobin. Recent work has implicated parvoviruses as the cause of these crises. This is usually transient but transfusion may be life-saving.

Another important complication in patients with chronic haemolysis is folate deficiency which may lead to worsening of the anaemia. Folate supplements should be given to all patients with chronic haemolytic anaemias.

Table 58.5 Causes of haemolytic anaemias.

Intracorpuscular defects
Haemoglobinopathies and thalassaemias

Metabolic disorders:	G-6-PD deficiency (common) (Fig. 58.4B)
	Pyruvate kinase deficiency (rare)
	Other enzyme deficiencies (extremely rare)
Membrane disorders:	Spherocytosis (Fig. 58.4C)
	Elliptocytosis (Fig. 58.1A)
	Ovalocytosis

Extracorpuscular defects

Immune mechanisms:	Haemolytic disease of the newborn
	Immune drug-induced haemolytic anaemia
	Autoimmune haemolytic anaemia
Drug induced:	Immune
	G-6-PD deficiency
	Oxidative drugs: i.e. dapsone
Other causes	Malaria
	Bartonellosis
	Fragmentation haemolytic anaemia (heart valves)
	Severe burns
	Hypersplenism
	Disseminated intravascular coagulation

The main causes of haemolytic anaemia in the tropics are G-6-PD deficiency and the haemoglobinopathies and thalassaemias. The reader is referred to standard haematological textbooks for a detailed description of other causes of haemolysis (see also Table 58.5).

GLUCOSE–6–PHOSPHATE DEHYDROGENASE (G–6–PD) DEFICIENCY

This is by far the most common cause of nonspherocytic haemolytic anaemia in tropical and subtropical countries, excluding the haemoglobinopathies. The condition was first described by Carson et al in 1956.[65]

G-6-PD function and variants

Erythrocytes obtain energy from the breakdown of glucose, 95% of which is metabolized by anaerobic glycolysis to lactate and in the process adenosine triphosphate (ATP) is produced. Five per cent of the glucose is broken down via the pentose phosphate shunt to produce reduced NADP the function of which is to protect the red cell from oxidative stress. G-6-PD is the first and rate-limiting enzyme in this pathway.

There are over 200 variants of G-6-PD described and many of the variants reach polymorphic frequencies in different populations. Variants are determined by their activity using a spectrophotometric assay of enzyme activity or by their electrophoretic mobility and by a study of enzyme kinetics (Michaelis–Menton constant, pH optimum, substrate specificity and thermostability). Many of the variants described are of normal or marginally reduced activity and are of no clinical significance.

In African and American blacks the commonest G-6-PD variant is designated type A$^+$. This isoenzyme has a faster electrophoretic mobility than the commonest type found in Caucasian populations which is designated type B. The second most common variant in blacks is the A$^-$ type which varies in frequency between 10% and 20% (reviewed by Bienzle[66]).

In Asia other variants are present; the most important from a clinical point of view are called Mahidol, Canton and Union. The Mediterranean type of G-6-PD is the commonest abnormal type in the Middle East but occurs sporadically elsewhere.

The G-6-PD gene is located on the X chromosome. In variants with low levels of activity haemolysis occurs following the appropriate challenge, most commonly in hemizygous males and homozygous females and rarely in heterozygous females.

Clinical picture

The major feature of G-6-PD deficiency is haemolysis. The severity of the haemolysis varies according to the type of enzyme. The following in order of importance are the clinical syndromes.

1 *Drug induced haemolysis.* A variety of oxidant drugs may precipitate haemolysis even in relatively mild G-6-PD deficiency such as the Negro type A⁻. A list of the most important drugs that have been implicated in causing haemolysis is given in Table 58.6. (See also below.)

2 *Haemolysis associated with infection.* The vast majority of patients with G-6-PD variants with a mild or moderate deficiency will haemolyse only in the presence of a severe infectious illness. The commonest infections implicated are typhoid fever, other bacterial infections,[68,69] viral hepatitis[70] and malaria. It has been suggested that blackwater fever may be produced by a severe attack of malaria in patients with G-6-PD deficiency[71] although recent studies in Thailand do not confirm this. Some of the drugs used in treatment of infection may also precipitate haemolysis.

3 *Neonatal jaundice.* This is common in South-East Asia and the Mediterranean type of G-6-PD deficiencies. Although it is less frequent in the black A⁻ types of G-6-PD variant it is said to be the single most important cause of severe neonatal jaundice in a survey in Nigerians.[72]

4 *Favism* (Chapter 49). This is characterized by severe haemolysis of acute onset following the ingestion of broad beans or inhalation of pollen from the plants. This syndrome is seen most commonly in the Mediterranean type of G-6-PD deficiency found in the Middle East and amongst Parsees in India.

5 *Chronic non-spherocytic congenital haemolytic anaemia.* This is a rare condition. Numerous variants have been described usually in non-

Table 58.6 Drugs and other agents commonly associated with oxidative damage to red cells.

Drugs and chemicals which cause oxidative damage to red cells in normal subjects and more severe haemolysis in G-6-PD deficient subjects:
  Phenylhydrazine
  Dapsone and other sulphones
  Naphthalene (moth balls)
  Phenacetin and acetanilide (in large doses only)
  Sulphasalazine (Salazopyrin)

Drugs and chemicals which are shown to cause haemolysis in G-6-PD deficient subjects:
  Acetanilide and phenacetin (therapeutic doses)
  Methylene blue
  Nalidixic acid
  Niridazole (Ambilhar)
  Nitrofurantoins
  Orange RN (red Suya food colouring)[a]
  Pamaquin
  Primaquine
  Pentaquine
  Sulphonamides: sulphacetamide
                 sulphamethoxazole
                 sulphanilamide
                 sulphapyridine
  Thiazosulphone
  Toluidine blue
  Trinitrotoluene (TNT)

Drugs and chemicals that may cause haemolysis in some types of G-6-PD deficient subjects but not shown to be haemolytic in A⁻ type in Negroes[b]:
  Aspirin (in large doses)
  Chloroquine
  Quinine
  Quinidine
  Vitamin K analogues
  Chloramphenicol
  Dimercaprol (BAL)
  Vicia faba (broad beans)

[a] Akinyanju and Odusote.[67]
[b] This list is not comprehensive. In addition there are many isolated unconfirmed reports of other drugs causing haemolysis in G-6-PD deficiency.

blacks. Clinically the condition may vary in severity from severe intermittent haemolysis precipitated by infections to a transfusion dependent anaemia (examples of variants: G-6-PD Bangkok).

DIAGNOSIS

The diagnosis of G-6-PD deficiency can be suspected in populations where it is known to be common when there is severe anaemia accompanied by jaundice especially in the presence of a precipitating factor such as infection or use of drugs and food additives. Confirmation can be obtained by the demonstration of haemolysis (reticulocytosis, raised bilirubin and lactate dehydrogenase in serum) and specifically by the assay of enzyme activity. The red cells usually show typical morphological changes of oxidative damage during a haemolytic episode (Fig. 58.4B). A simple screening test is available using the decolorization of brilliant cresyl blue in the presence of G-6-PD activity.[73] Diagnosis may be difficult to confirm in females as the level of activity may vary from very low to low normal levels in heterozygous females. Also diagnosis is difficult to establish in the less severe forms such as the A⁻ type during a haemolytic episode as young cells (reticulocytes) produced in response to haemolysis have a raised level of enzyme. An enzyme assay using a spectrophotometric method to measure the reduction of NADP to NADPH can be used for confirmation but it may be best to await the return to a steady state before performing this test.

Management

The most important aspect of management is immediate discontinuation of a drug or agent implicated in precipitating haemolysis. Infections must be treated vigorously with the appropriate antibiotics or antimalarials if malaria is suspected (see below). The patient must be discouraged from self-medication in future and all drugs that may cause haemolysis should be avoided (Table 58.6). Once haemolysis has

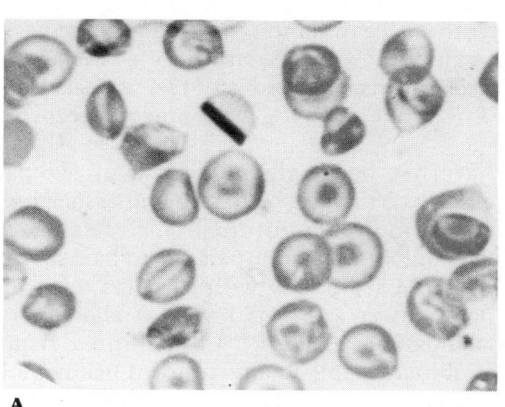

A

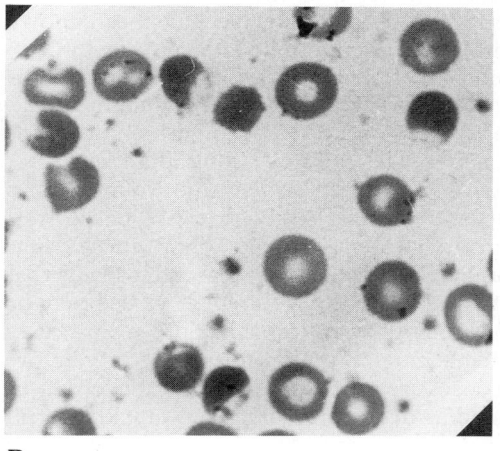

B

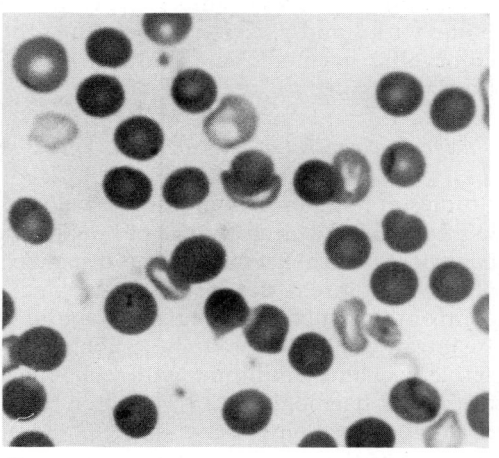

C

Fig. 58.4 A, Haemoglobin C disease: there are numerous target cells and one red cell shows intracellular crystal formation. B, G-6-PD deficiency: red cells showing oxidative damage. The haemoglobin seems to be separated from the membrane of the cells in certain areas and the rest of the cell looks dense. These changes occur only during a haemolytic episode. C, Spherocytosis: many red cells are round and very dark-staining with loss of central area of pallor. Most of the cells showing central pallor in this film were polychromatic red cells. Spherocytosis occurs in hereditary spherocytosis, autoimmune haemolytic anaemia and isoimmune haemolysis.

occurred in G-6-PD deficiency there is no means of stopping it. In very severe cases death may ensue from anaemia or renal failure. Fortunately in most cases of mild or moderately severe deficiency, haemolysis is self-limiting. This is because the older cells with less enzyme activity are preferentially haemolysed and the new cells produced are rich in enzymes and are more resistant to oxidative stress.

In severe cases transfusion may be needed if the haemoglobin falls to dangerously low levels.

G-6-PD deficiency and treatment of malaria

Apart from the posssible selective pressure of malaria on the presence of numerous G-6-PD variants (the malaria hypothesis) (Chapter 1) another important interaction between the two conditions causes a clinical dilemma. Many of the drugs used to treat malaria have been known to cause a certain amount of haemolysis in G-6-PD deficient subjects. This is usually of no clinical importance in the African A$^-$ type, but fatalities have been described even with chloroquine given prophylactically in Cambodian soldiers[74] and with quinine. Primaquine, which is a stronger oxidant, is likely to cause haemolysis even in the milder A$^-$ type. Where these drugs have to be given for clinical reasons it seems that there is no real choice. A small test dose may be given at the outset in less clinically severe cases and the haemoglobin monitored carefully before larger doses are given. The choice in severe cases is limited as drugs must be given quickly in full doses.

In the case of primaquine the problem usually arises in subjects who have frequent troublesome relapses of non-falciparum malaria after leaving a malarious area. In such cases the benefits of a radical cure must be weighed carefully against the possibility of a catastrophic haemolysis. Such therapy must be conducted under close supervision of a clinician with frequent monitoring of haematological parameters. Continuous prophylaxis with a non-provocative drug is an alternative.

HAEMOGLOBINOPATHIES

The inherited disorders of haemoglobin synthesis, the haemoglobinopathies, are by far the largest group of genetic anaemias. Although these conditions are found most frequently in the Mediterranean region, Africa and parts of Asia, they have been encountered in every racial group.

The clinical classification and our present understanding of the pathophysiology of these conditions is based on knowledge of the structure and genetic control of normal haemoglobin.

Normal human haemoglobin

Structure

In adult life human haemoglobin is a mixture of proteins, consisting of a major component, haemoglobin A, and a minor fraction which makes up about 2.5% of the total, haemoglobin A$_2$. In intrauterine life fetal haemoglobin is the main respiratory pigment while in the embryo, up to about eight weeks, several embryonic haemoglobins make up a variable proportion of the total haemoglobin. At birth fetal haemoglobin synthesis ceases and by the age of one year haemoglobins A and A$_2$ are fully established. The mechanisms which control this remarkable series of adaptive changes have not yet been worked out.

Normal haemoglobin consists of two pairs of peptide chains, each chain being associated with a haem molecule. All the human fetal and adult haemoglobins have a pair of α chains. In adult life these are paired with β chains to form haemoglobin A ($\alpha_2\beta_2$) and with δ chains to form haemoglobin A$_2$ ($\alpha_2\delta_2$). In fetal life α chains are combined with γ chains to form haemoglobin F ($\alpha_2\gamma_2$) and with ε chains to form embryonic (or Gower 2) haemoglobin ($\alpha_2\varepsilon_2$). There is also an embryonic α chain called a ζ chain which combined with ε and γ chains to form the other two embryonic haemoglobins, Gower 1 ($\zeta_2\varepsilon_2$) and Portland ($\zeta_2\gamma_2$).

The genetic control of haemoglobin synthesis

Studies of families with abnormal haemoglobins have provided a clear picture of how the genetic control of normal haemoglobin is organized (Fig. 58.5). Separate pairs of allelomorphic genes control the structure of the α, β, γ and δ chains. In intrauterine life the α and γ chain genes are active, α chains combining with γ chain genes to form fetal haemoglobin ($\alpha_2\gamma_2$). After birth the γ chain genes are repressed and the β and δ chain genes activated; α chains now combine with β

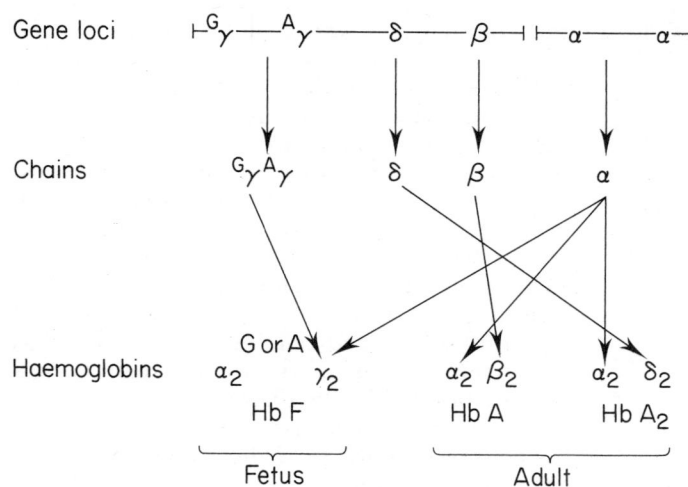

Gene loci

Chains

Haemoglobins

Fig. 58.5 Genetic control of normal haemoglobin. For the sake of simplicity the embryonic haemoglobins are not included.

chains and δ chains to form haemoglobins A ($\alpha_2\beta_2$) and A$_2$ ($\alpha_2\delta_2$) respectively. This explains why inherited disorders of the α chains affect both fetal and adult haemoglobin whilst abnormal β chain production only affects adult haemoglobin.

There are three groups of inherited disorders of haemoglobin synthesis (Table 58.7). First there are those which result from a genetically determined alteration in the *structure* of haemoglobin which may modify its stability or function. A second and larger group is comprised of disorders which result from an inherited defect in the *rate* of synthesis of one of the globin chains, the structure of which may or may not be normal. These are known collectively as the thalassaemia syndromes. Finally there are heterogeneous groups of conditions characterized by the persistence of fetal haemoglobin synthesis into adult life, hereditary persistence of fetal haemoglobin. The latter group is of no clinical importance.

Table 58.7 Classification of the haemoglobinopathies.

Structural haemoglobin variants:
   α chain
   β chain
   γ chain
   δ chain

Defects in the rate of globin production:
   α thalassaemia
   β thalassaemia
   δ-β thalassaemia
   δ thalassaemia
   γ-δ-β thalassaemia

Developmental changes in haemoglobin production:
   hereditary persistence of fetal haemoglobin, chromosomal abnormalities

STRUCTURAL HAEMOGLOBINOPATHIES

Most of the structural haemoglobin variants differ from haemoglobin A by the substitution of a single amino acid in one of the globin chains. A few variants have one or more amino acids missing or deleted. All these disorders are inherited in a Mendelian codominant fashion.

The majority of haemoglobin variants have been discovered by electrophoresis, the amino acid substitution altering the charge of the molecule so that it moves differently from haemoglobin A in an electric field. Originally letters of the alphabet were used to designate a new haemoglobin variant, but since these have long been used up, the place of origin of the affected individuals is now used. The heterozygous carrier state for a haemoglobin variant is called the 'trait', e.g. haemoglobin S trait, while the homozygous condition is designated 'disease', e.g. haemoglobin S disease.

Many of the haemoglobin variants have no clinical significance and have been found during population surveys. However, some amino acid substitutions, because they occur at critical sites in the molecule, result in deformation of the red cells, lack of molecular stability or abnormal oxygen transport, and hence disease. The clinical disorders which result from structural haemoglobinopathies are summarized in Table 58.8. The sickling disorders and haemoglobin C disease are very common in parts of Africa, while haemoglobin E disease occurs frequently in South-East Asia. The other structural haemoglobin variants are rare, are not restricted to

Table 58.8 Disorders resulting from structural haemoglobin variants.

Haemolytic anaemia:
 Haemoglobin S disorders
 Haemoglobin C disease
 Haemoglobin D disease
 Haemoglobin E disease
 The unstable haemoglobin disorders
Congenital methaemoglobinaemia:
 Haemoglobin M disorders
Congenital polycythaemia:
 Haemoglobins with increased oxygen affinity
Congenital hypochromic anaemia (thalassaemia-like disorder):
 Haemoglobin Lepore syndromes
 Haemoglobin Constant Spring

any particular racial group, and are associated with conditions such as familial polycythaemia, congenital methaemoglobinaemia and congenital non-spherocytic haemolytic anaemia.

Sickling disorders

The sickling disorders result from the inheritance of haemoglobin S, either alone or in combination with other abnormal haemoglobins (Table 58.9).[75,76] They consist of homozygous sickle cell anaemia and the compound heterozygous states for haemoglobin S and other structural haemoglobin variants or thalassaemia. Sickle cell anaemia is most frequently encountered in Africa where it occurs in a broad belt across the middle third of the continent. The carrier rate in this area is 10–30% of the population and the disease accounts for approximately 80 000 infant deaths per year. It also occurs with a much lower incidence in parts of Italy, Greece, the Middle East and India. The high frequency of this gene in Africa has arisen because heterozygous carriers are more resistant than normal to *Plasmodium falciparum* malaria during early childhood.

Haemoglobin S differs from haemoglobin A by the substitution of valine for glutamic acid in the sixth position along the β-chain. This causes fundamental differences in the physical properties of sickle haemoglobin as compared with haemoglobin A. In conditions of reduced oxygen tension haemoglobin S is relatively insoluble, the haemoglobin molecules forming linear stacks or tactoids. These produce the typical sickled deformity of the red cell (Fig. 58.6) which has two main consequences. First, small vessels become blocked by aggregations of sickled erythrocytes resulting in tissue infarction. Second, the deformity of the sickled cells results in their shortened survival and hence in a severe haemolytic anaemia.

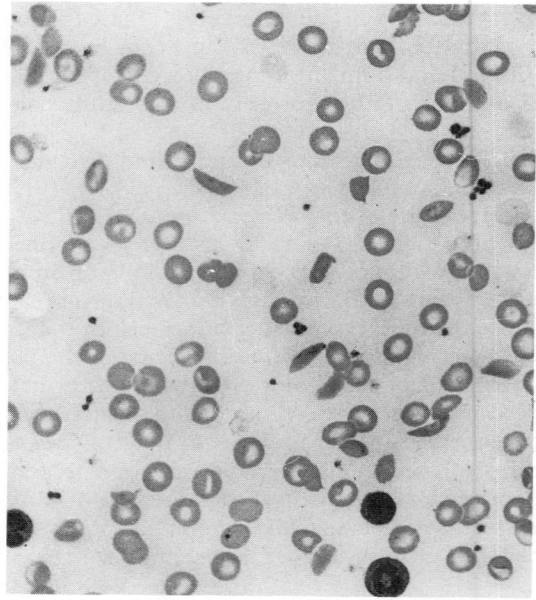

Fig. 58.6 Peripheral blood film in sickle cell anaemia.

Table 58.9 The common[a] sickling disorders.

Disorder	Genotype	Clinical findings
Sickle cell disease	$\alpha\alpha\,\beta^S\beta^S$	Severe haemolytic anaemia[b]
S–C disease	$\alpha\alpha\,\beta^S\beta^C$	Moderate haemolytic anaemia
S–D (Punjab) disease	$\alpha\alpha\,\beta^S\beta^D$	Moderate haemolytic anaemia
S-hereditary persistence of HbF heterozygosity	$\alpha\alpha\,\beta^S\beta^-$	No clinical abnormality
S–O disease	$\alpha\alpha\,\beta^S\beta^O$	Moderate haemolytic anaemia
Sickle cell β thalassaemia	$\alpha\alpha\,\beta^S\beta^{thal}$	Variable—depending on type of associated thalassaemia gene (see text)

[a] The sickle gene has been found in association with many other rare structural variants (see Huehns[79]).
[b] Mild cases may be encountered. In racial groups like the Shiite Arabs the condition is uniformly mild.

The clinical manifestations of the sickling disorders depend on the number of cells capable of sickling, the level of haemoglobin S in each red cell, the amount of interaction between haemoglobin S and other haemoglobin variants which may be present and the packed cell volume. Thus in sickle cell trait where there is only 30–40% haemoglobin S, symptoms are rare. Haemoglobin S interacts with haemoglobin C and D to produce a severe clinical disorder, whereas large amounts of haemoglobin F appear to protect against sickling. Owing to the sickling phenomena, the blood viscosity in sickle cell anaemia increases as deoxygenation occurs. This effect is much more marked when the packed cell volume rises above 30%.

Sickle cell anaemia: homozygous haemoglobin S disease

Clinical picture

The disease usually presents after the third month of life. The earliest symptom is often symmetrical painful swelling of the hands and feet, the 'hand and foot' syndrome. Alternatively the affected infant may present with failure to thrive or with a severe infection. At this stage of development the infant is noticed to be pale and slightly icteric. Other symptoms during early childhood include those of chronic anaemia made worse by infection. This chronic ill-health is interspersed with acute episodes or crises which are described in detail below.

On clinical examination affected children are pale and mildly jaundiced. Recurrent leg ulcers may leave characteristic scars over the antero-medial tibial regions. Splenomegaly is commonly observed during early childhood but, due to repeated episodes of infarction, it rapidly regresses and it is quite exceptional to find a palpable spleen at puberty. The liver is sometimes enlarged. The heart is also commonly enlarged and a variety of murmurs may be heard. In some cases bone marrow expansion results in deformity of the skull very similar to that observed in thalassaemia (Fig. 58.8, p. 968).

The blood picture in sickle cell anaemia is very characteristic. There is nearly always a marked degree of anaemia with a packed cell volume in the 20–25% range. The peripheral blood film is characterized by marked variation in size, shape and colour of the red cells and usually sickled forms are present (Fig. 58.6). In older patients

Howell–Jolly bodies due to hyposplenism are frequently seen. The reticulocyte count is elevated in the 15–20% range. The serum bilirubin level is raised and haptoglobins are absent. The white cell count is normal except in crises when it may be markedly elevated. There is often a moderate elevation in the platelet count. Sickling can be demonstrated by incubating the cells in 2% sodium metabisulphite under a coverslip sealed by petroleum jelly or by one of the tests which relies on the reduced solubility of haemoglobin S. Several commercial 'kits' make use of the latter approach. The diagnosis is confirmed by haemoglobin electrophoresis which shows only haemoglobin S with an elevation of fetal haemoglobin, usually in the 5–10% range, and by finding the sickle cell trait, i.e. haemoglobins A and S, in both parents (Fig. 58.7).

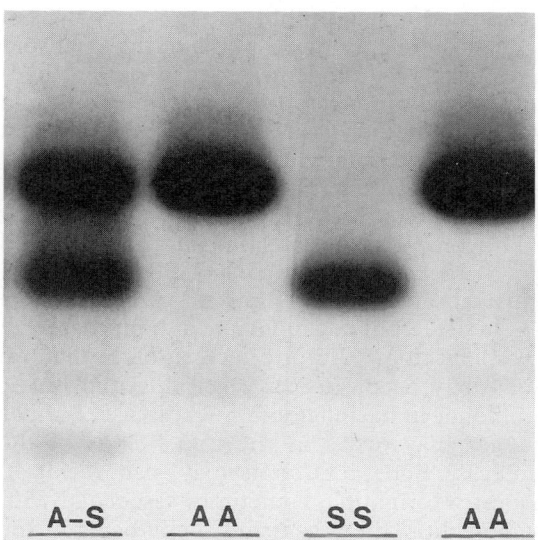

A–S   A A   S S   A A

Fig. 58.7 Haemoglobin electrophoresis, showing the sickle cell trait and sickle cell disease.

Complications

Patients with sickle cell anaemia are very susceptible to all types of *infection*. They are particularly prone to pneumococcal infections including meningitis and to *Salmonella* infections of bone. *P. falciparum* malaria infection is probably an important cause of mortality in Africa. Infection is an important precipitating factor in the production of crises.

Several types of *crises* occur in the sickling disorders. The so-called painful crisis is characterized by severe pain in the back, limbs and abdomen associated with a high fever and prostration. Any organ may be infarcted but pulmonary vascular occlusion (lung syndrome) and involvement of the cerebral vessels leading to convulsions with or without focal neurological signs are particularly serious. In young children massive sequestration of sickled erythrocytes in the liver and spleen may result in rapid enlargement of these organs associated with a dramatic fall in the packed cell volume, the sequestration crisis. In some crises there may be a marked increase in the rate of haemolysis resulting in a rapid fall in the haemoglobin level. Another mechanism for sudden worsening of the anaemia is erythroid hypoplasia. Such 'aplastic' crises commonly occur in more than one family member at the same time, have a distinct seasonal and geographical incidence and hence are thought to follow infections, probably viral. Recent studies have implicated the parvovirus in many of these episodes. Aplasia of the erythroid series may occur together with increased haemolysis and produce a life-threatening anaemia over a few hours. Exacerbation of the anaemia may also be brought about by folic acid deficiency resulting from a rapid turnover of erythroid precursors.

The complications which result from repeated *infarctions* may involve practically any organ. Thus repeated splenic infarcts result in severe pain in the left hypochondrium and ultimately in autosplenectomy. Aseptic necrosis of the femoral heads may occur in sickle cell anaemia but is commoner in haemoglobin S–C disease. Similar changes may occur in the upper ends of the humerus. Bone infarction may also result in sequestra formation, sometimes associated with osteomyelitis, the organism usually being of the *Salmonella* group. Chronic leg ulceration is common. The gradual cardiac enlargement which occurs in sickle cell anaemia probably results from a combination of factors including multiple small infarcts, chronic anaemia, siderosis of the myocardium and pulmonary hypertension secondary to multiple small pulmonary thrombotic episodes. Focal neurological signs, recurrent attacks of haematuria and priapism also result from small vessel blockage. Chronic liver damage and liver failure may occur. Many children with the disorder have diminished ability to produce a concentrated urine which is corrected by transfusion of normal blood. This abnormality cannot be corrected in adult sicklers. A true nephrotic picture and/or chronic renal

failure may develop. Renal failure is an important cause of death in adults with this condition in Jamaica.

Ocular manifestations occasionally occur in sickle cell anaemia and take the form of a remarkable tortuosity of the retinal vessels. These changes are more marked in haemoglobin S–C disease where there is often a gross proliferation of the retinal vessels with a tendency to intraocular haemorrhage, retinal detachment and permanent visual disturbance.

Pregnancy in sickle cell anaemia is associated with a high incidence of folic acid deficiency and also, in some cases, an increased frequency of crises. There is an increased incidence of fetal mortality and morbidity.

Treatment

The treatment of sickle cell anaemia presents two distinct problems: the management in between crises, including their prevention, and the management of the established crisis.

In between crises patients should be maintained on folic acid supplements and iron should be avoided. They usually manage quite well with a packed cell volume in the region of 20–25% and on no account should they receive blood transfusions to try and raise the haemoglobin to a higher level. Transfusions that raise the packed cell volume into the 30% range bring the blood viscosity up to a dangerous level without reducing the number of sickle cells and tend to precipitate crises. Malarial prophylactics should be taken regularly in tropical areas and there is some evidence that the taking of prophylactic antibiotics in the winter months may be helpful for those who live in Europe or North America. Certainly many crises are precipitated by mild upper respiratory tract infections and the patient should be warned of this danger. The use of pneumococcal vaccines is under investigation; their value is not yet established.

Crises should be managed by adequate analgesia, rehydration, warmth, oxygen and antibiotics with frequent estimations of the packed cell volume and reticulocyte count. It should be remembered that these patients can become profoundly anaemic over the period of a few hours. Transfusion should be withheld unless the packed cell volume falls to a dangerously low level but sometimes the use of a plasma volume expander may be helpful. In some patients with sickling crises there may be a high titre of cold agglutinins and thus blood for cross matching should be taken into a container at 37°C. Regimens using alkalis, magnesium, low molecular weight dextrans, phenothiazines, hyperbaric oxygen, urea and many other forms of therapy have been advocated for the treatment or prevention of crises. Because of the natural tendency for crises to settle, it has been extremely hard to assess the value of such agents and where they have been exposed to adequate trial none has been shown to be of any benefit.

Another approach to the management of sickle cell anaemia has followed the observation that carbamylation of haemoglobin S by cyanate increases its oxygen affinity. Blood treated in this way in vitro has a longer red cell survival and the administration of cyanate to patients with sickle cell anaemia also prolongs their red cell life-span. However, neurotoxicity has been observed with this therapy and it is not safe to use this agent over a long period.

If there are repeated crises over a short period of time or if major surgery is contemplated for such complications as chronic leg ulceration or osteomyelitis, exchange transfusion or hypertransfusion if the initial haemoglobin is between 5 and 6 g/dl are the most reliable methods of management. The aim should be to lower the number of sickle cells to less than 50% of the total cell mass. Once this is achieved it is possible to maintain the patient in this state by frequent small transfusions which depress the patient's own red cell production. It is possible to prevent crises for many months using this technique.

Anaesthesia is hazardous in patients with sickling disorders unless a high oxygen concentration is maintained. Nitrous oxide anaesthesia for minor operations is particularly dangerous. All Negro patients or those from other at-risk populations should have a sickle cell preparation performed before being anaesthetized.

Pregnancy in sickle cell anaemia is associated with increased risk to both mother and fetus. Although the sickling disorders are not an indication for termination, affected mothers require careful antenatal care. Folic acid supplements are vital and, if frequent crises occur, exchange transfusion is indicated.[77]

Sickle cell anaemia can now be diagnosed in utero by either fetal blood sampling or analysis of the DNA of amniotic fluid fibroblasts or after chorion villus sampling.[78] Thus it is possible to offer therapeutic abortion to mothers carrying homozygous fetuses.

Prognosis

The prognosis in sickle cell anaemia depends on the socioeconomic background of the patient. In Africa it has been unusual for patients with this disorder to survive early childhood. With earlier treatment of infection and anaemia and improved facilities for diagnosis, this picture is changing and there are increasing numbers of adult patients with sickle cell anaemia in Africa. In the USA it is quite common for patients to reach adolescence and adult life, although few of them survive over the age of 50. The commonest cause of death at all ages is infection. In some populations, such as the Shiite Saudi Arabians, the disease is unusually mild, probably because of the large amounts of fetal haemoglobin which are produced by affected individuals.

Other sickling disorders

The sickle cell trait does not usually cause any symptoms. There is an increased incidence of haematuria and serious organ infarction, e.g. spleen, may follow exposure to very low oxygen tensions such as occur in unpressurized aircraft.

The other sickling disorders result from a double heterozygosity for the sickle cell gene and for another haemoglobin variant (Table 58.9). The clinical picture depends on the degree of interaction of the particular variant with haemoglobin S. Thus haemoglobins C or D interact with haemoglobin S to produce a variable haemolytic anaemia with sickling crises, while haemoglobin J shows no such interaction; haemoglobin S–J disease is a very mild disorder. The reason for these different interactions is unknown but they probably depend on the physical properties of the particular haemoglobin variants and their ability to potentiate or reduce the rate of tactoid formation.

Haemoglobin S–C disease results from the inheritance of both haemoglobins S and C. It is characterized by a mild haemolytic anaemia associated with splenomegaly and a variable number of sickling crises. The blood film shows numerous target cells, sickled erythrocytes and intracellular crystals. This condition is important because it may present for the first time in adult life with serious thromboembolic episodes particularly during pregnancy. Massive pulmonary infarction occurring late in pregnancy is a particular hazard. If symptoms suggestive of a sickling crisis occur in a pregnant woman with this disorder exchange transfusion is indicated. Patients with haemoglobin S–C disease are also prone to aseptic necrosis of the femoral heads, haematuria and progressive deterioration of vision due to retinal vascular disease.

Haemoglobin S–D disease is usually associated with a clinical picture indistinguishable from that of sickle cell anaemia. Sickle cell thalassaemia is of variable severity depending on the type of thalassaemia gene. In the most severe cases the clinical picture is very similar to homozygous sickle cell anaemia.

All these variants of sickle cell anaemia can be diagnosed by haemoglobin electrophoresis combined with a family study. The treatment, where required, is similar to that of sickle cell anaemia.

Other haemoglobinopathies associated with haemolytic anaemia

The other common haemolytic haemoglobin disorders are haemoglobin C, D and E diseases.

Haemoglobin C disease occurs commonly in West Africa, the carrier rate being highest in north Ghana with an incidence of 16–28%. The homozygous disorder is characterized by a mild haemolytic anaemia and splenomegaly. It can be recognized by examination of a blood film which shows up to 100% target cell formation with intracellular crystals (Fig. 58.4A). Mild microcytosis is a common but not universal feature of haemoglobin C trait and disease. The diagnosis can be confirmed by haemoglobin electrophoresis.

Haemoglobin D disease has been found in several racial groups. The clinical picture is that of a moderately severe haemolytic anaemia with splenomegaly. The blood film usually shows moderate numbers of target cells. There are several different types of haemoglobin D, all of which have the same rate of electrophoretic migration as haemoglobin S but do not result in sickling. Haemoglobin D (Punjab) is the one which is associated with the most marked clinical symptoms.

Haemoglobin E disease is extremely common in South-East Asia and also occurs in India, Burma and Pakistan. It is characterized by a very mild haemolytic anaemia with hypochromic red cells and is occasionally associated with splenomegaly. Haemoglobin E is easily recognized on haemoglobin electrophoresis, migrating in the same position as haemoglobin A_2.

Other disorders due to structural haemoglobin variants

The other clinical disorders due to structural haemoglobin variants are rare. They include congenital cyanosis due to methaemoglobinaemia, congenital non-spherocytic haemolytic anaemia and congenital polycythaemia. They are reviewed in detail by Huehns.[79]

THALASSAEMIA SYNDROMES

The thalassaemias are inherited abnormalities of the rate of synthesis of the globin chains of haemoglobin.

Thalassaemia was first described by Thomas Cooley of Detroit in 1925. He described a series of children with severe anaemia and splenomegaly who usually died within the first years of life. The term 'thalassaemia' (from Greek $\theta\alpha\lambda\alpha\sigma\sigma\alpha$ = the sea) was invented when it was noted that these early American patients all came from the Mediterranean region. Some years later it was realized that thalassaemia is inherited and that Cooley's anaemia is the homozygous state for a partially dominant mendelian gene. This became known as 'thalassaemia major' and the heterozygous carrier state as 'thalassaemia minor'. It is now known that the clinical picture of thalassaemia can result from many different inherited abnormalities of haemoglobin synthesis which are now grouped together as the thalassaemia syndromes (Table 58.10).[80] Furthermore, thalassaemia is not localized to the Mediterranean. It also occurs with a high frequency, i.e. a carrier rate of 2–10%, in the Far East, parts of India, Burma and Pakistan, and in the Middle East and West Africa. Sporadic cases have been described in practically every racial group. It has been estimated that there are more than 100 000 children with homozygous thalassaemia in the world population.

Thalassaemia can result from an inherited defect of either α or β chain production and therefore is classified into two main types; the α thalassaemias and the β thalassaemias (Table 58.10).

Each form of thalassaemia is characterized by unbalanced globin chain synthesis. In the case of β thalassaemia this results in an excess of α chains which are unstable and precipitate in the red cell precursors to produce large inclusion bodies. It is the latter which cause intramedullary death of

Table 58.10 The common thalassaemias.[a]

Type	Homozygous state	Heterozygous state
β thalassaemia (with haemoglobin A production) β^+ thalassaemia	Classical Cooley's anaemia. High level of haemoglobin F	Increased level of haemoglobin A_2
β thalassaemia (with no haemoglobin A production) β^0 thalassaemia	Similar clinical picture to above. Haemoglobin consists of F and A_2 only	As above
δ-β thalassaemia	Moderate anaemia. Haemoglobin consists of F only	Normal level of haemoglobin A_2. Haemoglobin F in 5–20% range
Haemoglobin Lepore thalassaemia	Classical Cooley's anaemia. Haemoglobin consists of Lepore and F only	Low level of haemoglobin A_2. Haemoglobins F and Lepore present
α^0 thalassaemia	Haemoglobin Bart's hydrops syndrome	Mild thalassaemic changes in blood. Normal levels of haemoglobin F and A_2; 5% haemoglobin Bart's in infancy
α^+ thalassaemia	Same as heterozygous α^+ thalassaemia	No haematological abnormality. Normal haemoglobin pattern. 1–2% haemoglobin Bart's in infancy
Haemoglobin Constant Spring	Mild thalassaemia disorder with about 5% haemoglobin Constant Spring	Normal. Above 0.5–1% haemoglobin Constant Spring

[a] Other forms of α thalassaemia are probably common in Africa and Asia but the genetic transmission is not yet determined. The heterozygous states for α thalassaemia 1 and 2, or α thalassaemia 1 and haemoglobin Constant Spring produce haemoglobin H disease (see text).

red cell precursors and the ineffective erythropoiesis characteristic of this disorder. Those cells which do reach the peripheral blood are damaged, also because of the inclusion bodies, and this results in a haemolytic process. The ineffective erythropoiesis and haemolysis combine to produce a profound degree of anaemia which stimulates erythropoietin production and further expansion of the ineffective erythroid mass. This in turn produces the bony deformities and hypermetabolic state characteristic of the thalassaemia disorders. In the case of α thalassaemia, the excess β chains which are produced are able to produce a haemoglobin molecule, β_4 or haemoglobin H, albeit unstable, and thus the degree of ineffective erythropoiesis is less in α thalassaemia than in β thalassaemia.

The molecular basis for the defective production of α and β chains has been worked out in the last few years.[80,81] At least some of the α thalassaemias result from deletions (i.e. loss) of the α chain genes. Normal individuals inherit two such genes from each parent, four in all. Some forms of α thalassaemia (α^0 thalassaemia) result from the loss of both genes on one chromosome, others (α^+ thalassaemia) from one of them. In some forms of α^+ thalassaemia the α genes are intact but there is a base change which inactivates them or reduces their output. An example which is particularly common in South-East Asia is haemoglobin Constant Spring which results from a single base change in the α globin

gene termination codon. There are at least 40 different molecular defects which can produce the clinical phenotype of β thalassaemia. There is only one deletion form which is found in a localized region of northern India. Many cases result from so-called nonsense or frameshift mutations which are due to single base changes which produce premature stop codons or scramble the reading frame of the genetic code. In the last few years it has been found that the globin genes, like other mammalian genes, are interrupted by regions called intervening sequences or introns. When the genes are transcribed both the coding regions, or exons, and the introns appear in the initial messenger RNA transcript, while in the nucleus the introns have to be excised and the exons spliced together. It turns out that many forms of β thalassaemia are due to defects in the splicing mechanism so that no normal messenger RNA is produced. Finally, some forms of β thalassaemia result from single base changes in the regulatory sequences for the β globin genes. In most cases these cause a slightly reduced level of transcription of the affected gene and hence a mild form of β^+ thalassaemia, i.e. a form of β thalassaemia in which some globin chain is produced, as compared with β^0 thalassaemia where there is a complete absence of gene product.

There are many different forms of both α and β thalassaemia but only the main clinical disorders produced by these genetic defects are described here. For more extensive coverage the reader is referred to recent reviews.[80,81]

β Thalassaemia

Clinical and haematological features

The homozygous state for β thalassaemia results in the clinical picture first described by Thomas Cooley. Affected children are well at birth but become anaemic from about the third month of life. There is increasing hepatosplenomegaly and retardation of growth. Characteristic bone changes develop which include 'bossing' of the skull, overgrowth of the maxillary regions and a tendency for spontaneous fracture. The skull changes cause the typical 'mongoloid' facies which characterize this entire group of anaemias. Radiographs of the skull show a typical 'hair on end' appearance (Fig. 58.8). If inadequately

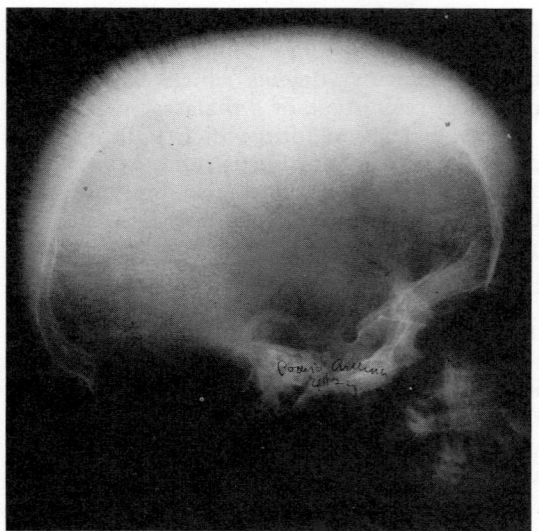

Fig. 58.8　Skull radiograph in β thalassaemia, showing the hair-on-end appearance.

treated these children become wasted, pot-bellied and hypermetabolic. They suffer from spontaneous fractures, bleeding and hyper-splenism, i.e. discomfort from a large spleen and worsening of their anaemia. Most of these children require regular blood transfusion if they are to survive. They are particularly prone to infection, folic acid deficiency and transfusional iron overload and, if they survive early childhood, usually die during the second decade of cardiac failure following iron deposition in the myocardium. If transfused they grow and develop normally but develop signs of iron overload in their late teens with liver, endocrine and cardiac failure.

The blood picture is characterized by anaemia, gross hypochromia and variation in size and shape of the red cells with variable numbers of target cells and nucleated red cells (Fig. 58.9). The reticulocyte count is only moderately elevated but the bone marrow shows striking erythroid hyperplasia. Erythropoiesis is 'ineffective' with a large amount of haemoglobin, i.e. excess α chain, destroyed in the bone marrow.

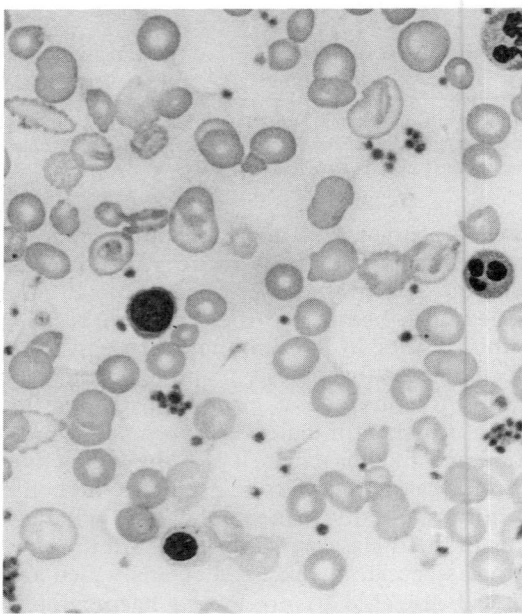

Fig. 58.9　Peripheral blood film in β thalassaemia, showing gross hypochromia, numerous target cells and nucleated red cells.

After the red cells have been stained with methyl violet many irregular inclusion bodies can be demonstrated, particularly after splenectomy. The haemoglobin pattern is characterized by a variable increase of fetal haemoglobin ranging from 20% to over 90% of the total. The diagnosis is confirmed by finding heterozygous β thalassaemia in both parents.

β Thalassaemia minor or heterozygous β thalassaemia is associated with mild anaemia and morphological changes of the red cells. The anaemia of thalassaemia minor is made worse by infection or stresses such as pregnancy. The haematological changes are characterized by variation in size and shape of the red cells with variable hypochromia. The red cell indices are always abnormal with characteristically low MCH and MCV values. Haemoglobin electrophoresis shows an increase in the level of the minor haemoglobin component, haemoglobin A_2, from the normal range (1.5–3.3%) to a level of about 5%. Fetal haemoglobin is slightly elevated (2.5%) in about half the cases.

There are certain well-defined variants of β thalassaemia. In some cases there may be a deficiency of both β and δ chain production and the haemoglobin pattern of heterozygotes is characterized by high levels of haemoglobin F without any increase in the amount of haemoglobin A_2. The clinical findings are the same as in true β thalassaemia. An example of this type of disorder is haemoglobin Lepore thalassaemia (Table 58.10) (see also Weatherall and Clegg[80]).

β Thalassaemia may occur in association with structural haemoglobin variants, i.e. thalassaemia is inherited from one parent and the variant from the other. The commonest of these combinations are sickle cell thalassaemia, haemoglobin C/thalassaemia and haemoglobin E/thalassaemia. The clinical findings in sickle cell thalassaemia vary, in some cases being as mild as those in thalassaemia minor, in others resembling sickle cell anaemia. This variability depends on the severity of the associated thalassaemia gene. Haemoglobin E/thalassaemia is extremely common in South-East Asia and the clinical picture is very similar to homozygous β thalassaemia. The condition can be distinguished from the latter by the finding of one parent with thalassaemia minor and the other with haemoglobin E.

Course, complications and prognosis

The course of the illness in β thalassaemia major depends on whether adequate transfusions facilities are available. If so, many survive well into the second decade. At this time death due to cardiac failure following siderosis of the myocardium is common. At puberty there is usually retardation of growth and secondary sexual development, with multiple endocrine deficiencies. Pancreatic insufficiency with diabetes is particularly common.

During the course of the illness the spleen may become grossly enlarged leading to worsening of the anaemia and a haemorrhagic tendency. Due to expansion of the bone marrow cavity pathological fracture is not uncommon and massive extramedullary erythropoiesis may result in tumour-like masses in the chest or skull. Some patients with β thalassaemia have an illness intermediate between that of β thalassaemia major and minor. Such cases of 'intermediate β thalassaemia' may result from a variety of genetic variants of thalassaemia. There are several specific forms of β thalassaemia which are particularly mild, and the simultaneous inheritance of an α thalassaemia may ameliorate β thalassaemia.

Treatment

Patients with severe β thalassaemia require constant hospital supervision in a centre with a special experience of this disease. The parents must be interviewed as soon as the diagnosis is properly established and the problem fully explained to them.

The children's haemoglobin should be maintained at a level of about 10–12 g/dl by repeated blood transfusions. The intervals between transfusions vary greatly but are usually about six to eight weeks. Where available washed or frozen red cells should be used; there is no place for whole blood. Despite careful crossmatching, transfusion reactions may occur; these include transient pyrexias, urticarial rashes and the development of antibodies against minor blood groups. All donors should be screened for hepatitis antigens. Regular folic acid supplements should be given, but other haematinics, particularly iron, should be avoided. If hypersplenism develops, splenectomy is indicated but not until after the age of five years because of the risk of infection. Persistent leukopenia, thrombocytopenia or increasing transfusion requirements are useful guides to whether splenectomy should be considered.

If available, chelating agents should be used to try to prevent iron overloading. A regimen using desferrioxamine by 12-hour overnight subcutaneous infusion will remove as much iron as is administered with an average transfusion regimen. The parents can be taught to give desferrioxamine infusions in this way. It is important to study iron excretion patterns from time to time to see how well the chelating regimen is working. It is still too early to be sure whether regular chelation from early in life will prevent the deaths of thalassaemic patients due to the cardiac effects of iron loading. However, it is already clear that if the regimen is adhered to rigidly children may enter a normal puberty and it is quite possible that they will have a much longer survival than was hitherto possible. Recent evidence suggests that even if they are already iron loaded they may be 'rescued' to some degree by intensive chelation therapy. There has been a recent interest in the application of bone marrow transplantation to treatment of β thalassaemia. While early results are promising the problem of graft-versus-host disease has not yet been overcome and hence this approach cannot be widely recommended as yet.

In the last few years there have been major advances in the prenatal diagnosis of β thalassaemia.[78] Originally, this required fetal blood sampling and measurement of globin chain synthesis but more recently direct analysis of fetal DNA, obtained either by amniocentesis or chorion villus sampling, has been applied to the early intrauterine diagnosis of this condition. These advances have been used widely in Europe and the USA and already have markedly reduced the incidence of new cases. Whether they can be applied widely in the developing countries remains to be determined.

α Thalassaemia

Alpha chains are shared by both fetal and adult haemoglobin. For this reason inherited abnormalities of α chain synthesis result in defective haemoglobin production both in fetal and adult life and a severe defect in α chain synthesis is incompatible with fetal survival.

If there is a deficiency of α chains an excess of γ chains and β chains are produced in infancy and adult life respectively. In infancy the excess of γ chains form molecules with the formula γ_4 called haemoglobin Bart's. Similarly, excess β chains form molecules with the formula β_4, called haemoglobin H. Thus the α thalassaemias are disorders which are characterized by a thalassaemia-like blood picture associated with the presence of haemoglobins Bart's and/or H.

The clinical disorders associated with α thalassaemia result from the interaction of three distinct types of α thalassaemia determinants. These are called α^0 thalassaemia, α^+ thalassaemia, and haemoglobin Constant Spring. α^0 Thalassaemia results from the loss of both α chain genes from one chromosome, α^+ thalassaemia from the loss of one of a pair of α chain genes and haemoglobin Constant Spring is a curious haemoglobin variant which has an elongated α chain. The latter

has arisen by an abnormality of termination of globin chain production. Haemoglobin Constant Spring is produced at a reduced rate and produces the clinical picture of α^+ thalassaemia.

The homozygous state for α^0 thalassaemia produces the haemoglobin Bart's hydrops syndrome. The heterozygous state for α^0 thalassaemia and either α^+ thalassaemia or haemoglobin Constant Spring produces haemoglobin H disease.

Haemoglobin Bart's hydrops syndrome

This condition results from the homozygous state for α^0 thalassaemia. It is characterized by intrauterine death usually at about the thirty-fourth week, although affected infants may survive until term and live for a few hours. The condition is common in South-East Asia and has been observed in Greece and Cyprus.

The clinical picture is of severe hydrops fetalis with massive oedema and enlargement of the liver and spleen. The blood picture is characterized by severe anaemia with gross abnormalities in size and shape of the red cells and numerous nucleated red cells in the peripheral blood. The haemoglobin pattern consists almost entirely of haemoglobin Bart's with no haemoglobins F, A or A_2. There is no treatment for the infants who do survive until term. Mothers who carry these hydropic infants have a high incidence of toxaemia and postpartum haemorrhage.

The parents usually show moderate abnormalities in size and shape of the red cells with no changes on haemoglobin electrophoresis, i.e. the carrier state for α^0 thalassaemia.

Haemoglobin H disease

Haemoglobin H disease is a milder form of α thalassaemia which is compatible with survival into adult life. The clinical severity is very variable ranging from an incapacitating anaemia like that of homozygous β thalassaemia to a very mild disorder associated with low grade haemolytic anaemia. The clinical findings are anaemia and splenomegaly. The haematological changes are similar to those of a β thalassaemia of intermediate severity. Incubation of the red cells with brilliant cresyl blue results in ragged inclusion bodies which consist of precipitated haemoglobin H. The diagnosis can be confirmed by haemoglobin electrophoresis which shows the presence of a rapidly migrating haemoglobin component. In those cases where haemoglobin H disease has resulted from the heterozygous state for α^0 and haemoglobin Constant Spring, traces of the latter may be observed migrating more slowly than haemoglobin A_2.

Usually one parent shows α^0 and the other α^+ or traces of haemoglobin Constant Spring.

Haemoglobin H disease requires no treatment unless the spleen is enlarged enough to cause hypersplenism when it should be removed. Oxidant drugs should be avoided since their administration results in the precipitation of haemoglobin H.

Heterozygous states for α thalassaemia

The α^0 thalassaemia trait is recognized by mild thalassaemic blood changes with normal levels of haemoglobins A_2 and F. In the neonatal period such carriers have about 5% haemoglobin Bart's. The α^+ thalassaemia trait is completely silent in adult life as is the haemoglobin Constant Spring carrier state although in the latter, trace amounts of abnormal variant can be observed in haemoglobin electrophoresis. The heterozygous state for both α^0 thalassaemia and haemoglobin Constant Spring is associated with the production of 1–2% haemoglobin Bart's at birth.

There are forms of α thalassaemia in the Middle East and Africa which do not conform with the patterns outlined above. The genetic transmittance of these disorders is not yet worked out.

DEVELOPMENTAL ABNORMALITIES OF HAEMOGLOBIN PRODUCTION

There are several well-defined developmental abnormalities of haemoglobin production. These are not of great clinical importance and, in fact, are probably very mild forms of thalassaemia. They are all associated with elevated levels of fetal haemoglobin after the neonatal period.

Hereditary persistence of fetal haemoglobin

This disorder is characterized by a genetic persistence of fetal haemoglobin synthesis beyond the neonatal period. For this reason it is usually called 'hereditary persistence of fetal haemoglobin'. It is inherited in a simple mendelian dominant fashion. The haematological picture varies considerably from race to race and has been best defined in the Negro and Greek populations.

Heterozygous carriers in the Negro population carry about 25% fetal haemoglobin in adult life while homozygous individuals have 100% fetal haemoglobin and no haemoglobins A or A_2. These individuals have no clinical abnormality except that the homozygotes have slight morphological abnormalities of the red cells and a tendency to a high packed cell volume.

In the Greek population the findings are similar to those in the African Negro except that the levels of the fetal haemoglobin in the heterozygotes are lower. There is another form of hereditary persistence of fetal haemoglobin, described first in Switzerland, in which affected persons have an inherited elevation of fetal haemoglobin in the 1–2% range. This is of no clinical importance except that again it may be mistaken for a thalassaemia carrier state. It occurs in about 2% of northern Europeans.

Several other forms of the condition have been reported and it is reviewed in detail by Weatherall and Clegg.[80]

DIAGNOSIS OF THE HAEMOGLOBINOPATHIES

These conditions must be suspected from the clinical history, racial background of the patient and physical examination with particular reference to such features as anaemia, icterus, cyanosis, polycythaemia, splenomegaly, abnormal body habitus, bone and joint deformities and the presence of scars from leg ulcers. The skull and facial deformities of thalassaemia are easily overlooked, particularly in the Oriental races.

Examination of a stained blood film is the single most useful laboratory investigation. Morphological appearances of a blood film can be diagnostic in thalassaemia and the various sickling and haemoglobin C disorders. The standard investigations for haemolysis and red cell osmotic fragility should be carried out. Structural haemoglobin variants are recognized by their electrophoretic behaviour on either filter paper, cellulose acetate or starch gel.

The diagnosis of thalassaemia can be confirmed by measuring the levels of haemoglobins F and A_2. If α thalassaemia is suspected the red cells should be incubated in brilliant cresyl blue and haemoglobin electrophoresis performed at an acid pH, both procedures being designated to demonstrate haemoglobin H. In difficult cases it is best to refer the patient to centres able to measure the in vitro rate of globin chain synthesis.[80]

If a haemoglobin variant is found it can be partially identified by its rate of migration as compared with known standards. However, this is insufficient to fully characterize a new haemoglobin and it should then be referred to a special centre for chemical studies designed to identify the altered amino acid residue.

Hypersplenism

This is a term used to describe a syndrome consisting of splenomegaly from any cause and varying degrees of pancytopenia. The degree of cytopenia is usually related to the size of the spleen. The anaemia is due to (a) shortened RBC life-span with evidence of increased destruction of red cells by the spleen, (b) increased red cell pooling in the spleen, and (c) haemodilution due to an increase in plasma volume. The mechanisms of leukopenia and thrombocytopenia are similar to that of anaemia.

The anaemia is usually normocytic and normochromic. The bone marrow shows hyperplasia and there is reticulocytosis.

Splenomegaly and hypersplenism is a frequent accompaniment of several chronic tropical diseases such as kala-azar (Chapter 4), chronic endemic malaria (Chapter 1), trypanosomiasis (Chapter 2) and schistosomiasis (Chapter 22). A specific type of chronic splenomegaly termed Tropical Splenomegaly Syndrome (TSS) has been described in tropical areas (Chapters 1 and 60).

TROPICAL SPLENOMEGALY SYNDROME (Chapters 1 and 60)

Splenomegaly is common in the tropics and may be due to malaria, visceral leishmaniasis, schistosomiasis or other conditions. The term tropical splenomegaly syndrome (TSS) is, however, now used to describe a distinct entity. The major feature of TSS is gross splenomegaly occurring mainly in young adults in certain parts of the tropics where there is a high malaria transmission rate. There is a high titre of antimalaria antibodies in the serum but malaria parasites and pigment are often difficult to find in the peripheral blood. The other major features of TSS are the high value for serum IgM (more than 1000 international units (IU)/ml) and a response to prolonged antimalarial therapy with

a reduction in splenomegaly and serum IgM. The IgM is polyclonal and there is no increase in IgG.

The other features of TSS apart from a massive spleen are as follows.

1 Characteristic liver biopsy changes consisting of sinusoidal dilatation with infiltration by lymphocytes and Kupffer cell hyperplasia with phagocytosis of cellular debris and erythrocytes. There is also patchy lymphocytic infiltration of the portal tracts and minimal hepatocellular changes. Malaria pigment is often absent (Fig. 60.4b, p. 1008).[82]

2 Other serological phenomena include cryoglobulinaemia and reduced serum level of C3,[83] the presence of rheumatoid factor but without the presence of joint involvement, and the presence of a low molecular weight IgM monomers and free light chains in the serum.[84]

3 The spleen is usually massive with greatly dilated sinusoids lined with reticulum cells showing marked erythrophagocytosis and sometimes prominent lymphocytic infiltration in the pulp (Fig. 60.4a, p. 1008). Various degrees of hypersplenism occur.

4 Blood changes: varying degrees of pancytopenia occur in TSS. The anaemia is normocytic, normochromic and does not respond to therapy with haematinics or deworming. Radiochromium erythrocyte survival studies show shortening of the life-span of the red cells due to sequestration of red cells in the spleen. The spleen red cell pool is greatly increased from the normal 20–30 ml to a massive 3–38% of the total red cell mass. There is usually a raised reticulocyte count. The anaemia is rendered more severe by haemodilution due to an increase in plasma volume.[85] Leukopenia is usually due to sequestration of granulocytes in the spleen as there is active granulopoiesis seen in bone marrow biopsy. In some cases in Nigeria marked infiltration of the bone marrow with lymphocytes together with peripheral blood lymphocytosis

may lead to a picture very similar to chronic lymphocytic leukaemia.[82] Thrombocytopenia is also due to increased trapping of platelets in the spleen but these are not damaged and recirculate.

Epidemiological studies implicate chronic malaria in the aetiology of TSS which occurs only in malarious areas and patients have high levels of antimalaria antibodies. Added proof is the response to prolonged antimalarial therapy. This is the case in the absence of demonstrable clinical malaria or parasitaemia. Relapse, however, often occurs after discontinuation of therapy.

TSS is thought to be an abnormal immunological response with malaria as the initial stimulus. Immune complexes are formed and these then lead to stimulation of macrophage proliferation and also suppressor T cell inhibition.[86] The reaction is maintained with only small amounts of antigen reinoculation.

The treatment of TSS is either splenectomy followed by antimalarial prophylaxis or antimalarial therapy alone. Splenectomy leads to alleviation of symptoms and reversal of haemodilution but has to be followed by antimalarial therapy. Antimalarial therapy alone is slower acting and may take up to a year to produce a response and has to be continued for life. There is evidence that genetic factors[87] play a part in TSS. The syndrome is most commonly seen in Papua New Guinea and East and West Africa.

Anaemia in children

Numerous studies have revealed that children are the largest group in the population who suffer from the effects of anaemia. The following is a brief outline of the common causes of anaemia according to age in tropical countries.

The first three months of life

Glucose-6-phosphate dehydrogenase deficiency is a very common, and often unrecognized, cause of neonatal jaundice and anaemia in the tropics.[72] Bacterial infections are an important cause of anaemia in normal children and lead to increased haemolysis in subjects with G-6-PD deficiency.

Other causes include blood loss from the umbilical cord stump during or soon after birth and circumcision where that is widely practised. Prematurity is another important cause of severe neonatal anaemia and is often due to inadequate iron stores.

Three months to two years

In areas of high falciparum malaria endemicity, malaria is a major cause of anaemia in this age group. Bacterial infections are also an important cause of anaemia.

In black Africans one of the other major causes of anaemia is sickle cell disease where the incidence of heterozygous carriers may be higher than 20%. Thalassaemias and other haemoglobinopathies such as haemoglobin E disease are important causes of anaemia in the Mediterranean and Far East, respectively.

Nutritional anaemia is next as a cause of anaemia. This is less likely to occur in countries where breastfeeding is continued until the second year of life.

Two to five years

This is the age group where malnutrition is an increasing cause of anaemia. PEM is an important cause, iron deficiency is common and folate deficiency less common. Infections are also important causes but as the child grows, malaria becomes less of an important cause of anaemia.

Five to 15 years

As children leave home and walk in the fields, they are more likely to become infested with hookworm. In addition, with the added demands of growth during adolescence and of menstruation in females there is a very high incidence of iron deficiency anaemia, which becomes the most important cause of anaemia.

Anaemia in pregnancy

In pregnancy there is an increase of plasma volume which leads to a fall in haemoglobin concentration. This is termed the 'physiological anaemia' of pregnancy. The haemoglobin reaches a nadir at about 32–36 weeks of pregnancy. The haemoglobin rarely falls below the level of 10–11 g/dl, however, unless there are other factors.

In pregnancy there is an increased demand for haematinics. The amount of iron consumed may be 500 mg or more and women in the child-bearing age are often in a precarious state of iron balance even in Western industrialized nations. In the tropics factors that increase the severity of iron deficiency are hookworm infestation, schistosomiasis and generally poor nutrition.

Folate deficiency is also fairly common in pregnancy but the rate is very variable in different populations. There is an increased demand for folate which is most marked during the third trimester.

Most obstetricians now advocate iron and folate supplementation therapy during pregnancy and this should be standard practice where antenatal follow-up of patients is available.

Malaria is an important cause of anaemia during pregnancy.[88] There is an increase in incidence and severity of malaria and this is thought to be due to diminution in immunity.[89]

There is an increase in the severity of anaemia in pregnant patients with sickle cell disease. This is due to an even higher demand on folate and an increased incidence of sequestration crises. In tropical Africa an added factor is malaria. It is advocated that patients with sickle cell anaemia should have regular malaria chemoprophylaxis during pregnancy in addition to haematinic supplements.[90] In cases where severe anaemia occurs transfusion may be considered. The topic of the value of regular prophylactic transfusion in patients with sickle cell disease is reviewed by Fleming[90] (see also p. 964).

The role of transfusion in the treatment of severe anaemia

Blood transfusion is a temporary but highly effective therapy for anaemia. Because of risks of adverse reactions and of transmission of infections such as viral hepatitis, syphilis, AIDS (acquired immunodeficiency syndrome) and malaria, blood transfusion must only be used when there are specific indications. However, in areas where there is a high carrier rate for malaria and hepatitis there may be no choice but to transfuse blood from affected donors. In some areas antimalarials may have to be administered prophylactically to all recipients of blood transfusion.

Blood transfusion is required following acute haemorrhage. The body can generally tolerate the loss of about 15% of the blood volume without undue cardiovascular embarrassment (equivalent to 750 ml of blood in an adult). Losses above this level may lead to postural hypotension and other related phenomena. Losses in excess of 30–40% of the total blood volume may lead to hypotension, collapse, shock and death. Loss of blood is less tolerated if initial anaemia is present.

Severe anaemia from any cause may require blood transfusion such as following acute hae-molysis, as occurs in G-6-PD deficiency or due to other causes. In sickle cell diseases transfusion may be needed in the following situations: (1) acute sequestration crises, (2) aplastic crises, (3) in late pregnancy where anaemia may be severe.[77]

In children with severe anaemia from any cause, such as malaria, blood transfusion may be life-saving. This is particularly the case when the haemoglobin is below 4–5 g/dl and there are signs of heart failure. In this case transfusion must be carried out very slowly and diuretics must be given.

Exchange transfusion is a technique whereby approximately an equal amount of blood is removed as is transfused.[91] It is the recommended method for treating severe anaemia during late pregnancy where delivery is imminent, in treatment of patients with sickle cell anaemia with repeated painful crises or cerebral symptoms and has also been advocated in cerebral malaria where there is a high parasitaemia.

Blood should not be transfused when anaemia is mild or moderate and where other simple measures such as administration of haematinics can be used.

OTHER HAEMATOLOGICAL PROBLEMS
Haematological malignancies

LYMPHOMAS

The distribution of different types of lymphomas follows a variable pattern in different parts of the world.[92] Thus Burkitt's lymphoma is the predominant tumour in black Africans and in Papua New Guinea, whereas Hodgkin's disease affects children and young adults more frequently in Egypt, Israel, Singapore and Brazil (Chapter 67).

In all the lymphoreticular tumours there may be involvement of the bone marrow, the manifestations of which are: (1) anaemia which may be that of chronic disease (p. 953), (2) anaemia due to poor nutrition and debility, (3) anaemia due to marrow infiltration, and (4) hypersplenism. Epidemic Burkitt's lymphoma rarely presents with a leukaemic picture (reviewed by Olweny[93]). Thrombocytopenia and leukopenia may also occur as a result of bone marrow infiltration or hypersplenism.

LEUKAEMIAS

The leukaemias are neoplastic processes of leukocytes characterized by purposeless proliferation of cells which may be at various stages of maturation. As a general rule the less differentiated the cell type, the faster the rate of proliferation and the more acute the disease. This, however, does not correspond to prognosis. Some acute leukaemias are sensitive to chemotherapy (e.g. acute lymphoblastic leukaemia) and longer survival can now be achieved in patients with this condition than with chronic granulocytic leukaemia.

The incidence of leukaemia is lower in blacks than in whites in the USA.[94] In Africa the true incidence has not been determined because of the lack of trained haematologists but where surveys have been carried out has been found to be low.[93] The pattern of leukaemias is also different and there is a higher prevalence of acute myeloid leukaemia and of chronic granulocytic leukaemia in children.[95]

In tropical America the incidence of reported leukaemia also appears to be lower in blacks than in whites, and this may be related to incomplete records, but the true incidence cannot be ascertained.[96] The commonest type is acute lymphoblastic leukaemia which constitutes 80% of cases whilst chronic myeloid leukaemia is very uncommon.

Types

The most common leukaemias are acute lymphoblastic, acute myeloblastic, chronic lymphocytic and chronic granulocytic leukaemias and their variants.

Acute leukaemias

Clinical features

The common presentation of acute leukaemia is related to the failure of production of one or more of the normal types of blood cells, because of crowding of the bone marrow by leukaemic cells. Anaemia is frequently present and leads to progressive weakness, listlessness, breathlessness and pallor. Haemorrhagic manifestations occur when the platelets fall to levels below 30×10^9/litre and may contribute to the anaemia. Bleeding from the skin and mucous membranes is the commonest presentation of thrombocytopenia. Infections occur commonly in acute leukaemias when there is neutropenia. Other clinical features of acute leukaemias are due to infiltration of specific organs. Bone infiltration may lead to bone pain and tenderness. Moderate hepatosplenomegaly may occur in both lymphoblastic and myeloblastic leukaemias. Lymph node enlargement is, however, commoner with lymphoblastic leukaemia. Massive mediastinal infiltration is commoner in T lymphoblastic leukaemia which usually presents with a higher peripheral blood blast count.

Haematological features

In most cases of leukaemia the white cell count is raised and there are many 'blast' cells in the blood. These may be distinguishable to an experienced haematologist on morphological features as 'lymphoblasts' or 'myeloblasts' or as other cell types. Quite often, however, further cytochemical stains or immunological membrane markers are needed to confirm the diagnosis.

In some cases of leukaemia there is no elevation

of white cell count and the number of circulating blasts may be low. In this case a bone marrow is essential to confirm the diagnosis. In all cases of leukaemia at presentation a bone marrow should be performed, even if the diagnosis is obvious from peripheral blood examination, in order to assess the remaining bone marrow reserve for comparison after treatment.

Treatment

Suggested drugs include 6-mercaptopurine, methotrexate, prednisolone, vincristine (Table 58.11). The effective treatment of acute myeloblastic leukaemia (AML) is myelotoxic. It is therefore difficult to treat without backup supportive blood component and intravenous antibiotic therapy and should only be attempted in a centre where these facilities are available.

Table 58.11 Outline of treatment of childhood ALL.

Remission induction
  Vincristine (1.5 mg/m² max. 2 mg) IV weekly for 4 weeks
  Prednisolone (40 mg/m²) daily for 4 weeks tailing off
  Bone marrow to confirm remission

Consolidation	
L-Asparaginase	These agents are usually
Cyclophosphamide	given in various
Cytosine arabamoside	combinations after
Anthracyclines	remission is achieved

CNS prophylaxis
  Cranial irradiation
  Intrathecal methotrexate

Maintenance chemotherapy	
Methotrexate	
6-mercaptopurine	In various
Vincristine	combinations
Prednisolone	

Problems in the treatment and management of acute leukaemias

Infections. In the presence of neutropenia severe infection can develop in a very short period of time. There may be poor localization of infective organisms and lack of clinical signs. Sustained fever of 38°C or more is therefore usually treated as presumptive evidence of an infection and intravenous antibiotic therapy consisting of an aminoglycoside and one of the wide-spectrum penicillins is instituted without delay. Buffy coat preparations when available may be given if the fever persists despite antibiotic therapy.

Haemorrhage. Platelet transfusions, where available, can be used to treat haemorrhage in a thrombocytopenic patient. Platelet transfusions may also be used prophylactically to prevent haemorrhage in certain situations (p. 978).

Metabolic complications

Hyperuricaemia. This may result from the destruction of a large number of leukaemic cells at remission induction, and may lead to acute renal failure. This can be avoided by the administration of allopurinol during induction therapy.

Electrolyte disturbances. Hypokalaemia and hyponatraemia may occur and are more commonly associated with some types of AML where there is monocytic differentiation. Destruction of blast cells during induction may lead to hyperkalaemia.

Liver abnormalities. A cholestatic or a hepatitic picture may be seen due to liver infiltration due to chemotherapy or due to infections such as cytomegalovirus and viral hepatitis associated with transfusion.

Other complications of chemotherapy. Apart from severe marrow suppression certain chemotherapeutic agents are associated with other side-effects. Vincristine may produce a peripheral neuropathy which may be severe. Anthracycline antibiotics have a severe vesicant effect and should be given in a fast running drip. Dose-related myocardial damage and subsequent heart failure may occur. Steroids in high doses may cause gastrointestinal ulceration and haemorrhage in susceptible individuals. In addition most of the chemotherapeutic agents cause alopecia and some may also cause mucositis (methotrexate) and haemorrhagic cystitis (high-dose cyclophosphamide).

Prognosis

Acute lymphoblastic leukaemia (ALL) in childhood carries a generally good prognosis if treated adequately. 'Common' ALL, which constitutes the majority of cases in Western countries, has a better prognosis than 'T' ALL. Bad prognostic features at presentation are a high blast count of more than 20×10^9/litre, age of more than 13 years and less than one year and the presence of T cell markers. These poor prognostic features are commoner in blacks. The prognosis is also worse in boys, who have a high rate of testicular relapse.

In AML the prognosis is generally poor. In large centres where intensive chemotherapy is given the remission rate is about 60%. The median survival after remission is usually 18 months to two years.

Chronic leukaemias

Chronic granulocytic leukaemia (CGL)

The major findings in CGL are a high leukocyte count with the presence of all stages of cells of the neutrophil series from blasts to neutrophils but with a preponderance of more mature forms. Splenomegaly is usually present. The majority of cases have a chromosomal abnormality of cells in their bone marrow which consists of translocation of the long arm of chromosome 22 to chromosome 9—the Philadelphia or Ph[1] chromosome. Some cases lack the Ph[1] chromosome and usually have other atypical features.

CLINICAL FEATURES
In the early phases the disease may not cause any symptoms. In more advanced cases splenomegaly is marked and there may be symptoms related to the enlarged spleen and hypermetabolic state. Anaemia and thrombocytopenia are only late complications of CGL in the chronic phase and usually portend progression of the disease to an accelerated phase.

NATURAL HISTORY
CGL may be looked upon as a preleukaemic condition. In many cases there is progression after a variable period of two to three years or more to either an accelerated phase or to acute leukaemia. This acute transformation may be to a common ALL phenotype which is then relatively sensitive to treatment for ALL but may be to the more resistant AML. The prognosis of acute leukaemia following CGL is generally poor.

TREATMENT
The indications for treatment of CGL are anaemia or the presence of symptoms related to splenomegaly or a hypermetabolic state. Treatment improves the quality of life but does not increase its duration or improve the final prognosis. Busulphan is the drug most commonly used, in doses of 0.065 mg/kg body weight orally daily until the white blood-cell count (WBC) falls to about 20×10^9/litre. The WBC may continue to fall for a few weeks after cessation of busulphan. Hydroxyurea is an alternative drug to use. It is less myelotoxic. Usual doses are 1–2.5 g daily orally.

Chronic lymphocytic leukaemia (CLL)

CLL is a lymphoproliferative disorder of B cells in the majority of cases. The cells are morphologically generally indistinguishable from mature small lymphocytes with scanty cytoplasm. Another feature is the presence of a large number of smear cells. Other lymphoproliferative disorders which may present with lymphocytosis include prolymphocytic leukaemia and Waldenström's macroglobulinaemia, but the morphology of the lymphocytes is distinctive.

DIAGNOSTIC FEATURES
A diagnosis of CLL is based on the presence of persistent lymphocytosis in the peripheral blood in the absence of any obvious cause and of bone marrow infiltration with lymphocytes. In many cases of CLL at presentation lymphadenopathy and splenomegaly may be minimal. Either or both of these features may, however, occur at any stage of the disease.

Immunoparesis is another feature of CLL and patients often suffer from repeated infections. The differential diagnosis is that of lymphocytosis with or without lymphadenopathy or hepatosplenomegaly, such as lymphocytic lymphoma, prolymphocytic leukaemia, hairy cell leukaemia and Waldenström's macroglobulinaemia. Some cases of tropical splenomegaly syndrome with persistent and marked lymphocytosis, indistinguishable from CLL have been described. To distinguish between the two it is essential to test whether the cells rosette with mouse red cells, which is characteristic of CLL, and whether they are mainly B cells with weak staining monoclonal surface immunoglobulin.

TREATMENT
The indication for treatment of CLL is usually bone marrow failure. Severe anaemia or thrombocytopenia are the usual effects of bone marrow infiltration by lymphocytes. Treatment usually improves bone marrow function but may increase the severity of immunosuppression.

Other beneficial effects of therapy are the reduction in size of lymph nodes and of the spleen if they are enlarged.

Autoimmune haemolytic anaemia may also occur in CLL without bone marrow failure. Similarly autoimmune thrombocytopenia may occur. Treatment with prednisolone alone may suffice in these cases.

The most widely used drugs for the treatment for CLL are chlorambucil or cyclophosphamide. These may be used alone or in conjunction with prednisolone. Prednisolone is often used initially when there is severe marrow failure as it is lympholytic without being myelotoxic. Response, however, may be limited and one of the other agents is then needed. Prednisolone may be used in doses of 40 mg daily. If chlorambucil is used, 10 mg is given daily, initially until the WBC starts to fall, when this may be reduced to 5 mg daily and discontinued when the WBC falls to about $10–15 \times 10^9$/litre. An alternative is to use high dose intermittent chlorambucil. The dose is 0.5 mg/kg daily for 4 successive days. This is then repeated every four weeks until an optimum response is achieved.

The aim of therapy in CLL is to improve bone marrow function and not to produce a cure. Therefore chemotherapy is usually continued until maximum benefit is obtained. Treatment should also be discontinued if no improvement is observed after four to six months of therapy.

PROGNOSIS

As CLL is a disease of elderly patients and is usually chronic, many patients may die of unrelated causes. The main causes of death are severe infections and uncontrolled disease with bone marrow failure. The majority of patients may live for many years without even the need for treatment.

Haemorrhagic disorders

The haemostatic mechanism has four major components: vascular, platelets, coagulation and fibrinolysis. Disturbance of function of any of these may result in either excessive haemorrhage or in generalized thrombosis. This section deals only with the haemorrhagic disorders. The most important aspect of investigation of a haemorrhagic disorder is careful history taking (Table 58.12). It is often easy to conclude from the history whether a disorder is most likely to be congenital or acquired and whether it is due to a platelet or a coagulation disorder. The following is a summary of the commonest causes of generalized haemorrhagic disease.

THROMBOCYTOPENIA

Thrombocytopenia is the most common cause of abnormal bleeding. It may be due to decreased platelet production or an increase in platelet destruction or splenic pooling. The normal range for the platelet count is $150–400 \times 10^9$/litre. The mean platelet counts may be lower in populations where splenomegaly associated with malaria is common. The major causes of thrombocytopenia are listed in Table 58.14.

Although severity of haemorrhage due to thrombocytopenia is not strictly related to the platelet count certain generalizations can be made. Spontaneous haemorrhage or bleeding after minor trauma is rare if the platelet count is in excess of 60×10^9/litre, but excessive bleeding may occur at this level with major trauma or surgery. When the platelet count is between $30–60 \times 10^9$/litre major life-threatening haemorrhage is unusual though minor degrees of haemorrhage may occur. Severe spontaneous haemorrhage is common when the platelet count falls below 20×10^9/litre.

Idiopathic thrombocytopenic purpura (ITP)

This is a disorder characterized by increased platelet sequestration due to immunological destruction of platelets. The clinical features differ with age. ITP in childhood is usually of sudden onset and associated with very low platelet counts. It often occurs about two to three weeks after an acute viral infection and there is a high rate of spontaneous remission. In adults ITP is usually of more gradual onset and is not associated with a preceding viral infection. Although usually less severe there is a lower rate of spontaneous remission.

The diagnosis is based on the finding of isolated thrombocytopenia in a previously healthy individual. The rest of the blood count is normal unless there has been severe haemorrhage when

Table 58.12   Investigation of haemorrhagic disorders.

I History	
Type of bleeding:	Petechiae: common in platelet and vascular disorders
	Haematomas and haemarthroses: common in coagulation disorders
Duration of bleeding and presence of rebleeding or of spontaneous bleeding:	Rebleeding is common in the coagulation disorders whilst prolonged initial bleeding is commoner in thrombocytopenia
Age at onset:	Early age suggests a congenital disorder, later onset suggests an acquired disorder
Drug history:	Drugs which may cause marrow damage (e.g. gold etc.)
	Drugs associated with immune thrombocytopenia (e.g. penicillin, quinine)
	Drugs which cause a platelet defect: e.g. aspirin and other non-steroidal anti-inflammatory drugs. Effect may last for about 1 week after a single dose
	Anticoagulants
Previous history:	Bleeding after surgery
	Epistaxis
	Minor wound bleeding
	Tooth extraction
	Tonsillectomy
	Circumcision
Coexistence of other conditions:	Liver disease
	Scurvy
	Pregnancy
	Severe illness
	haemorrhagic fevers
	carcinomas
	septicaemia and other conditions that may be associated with DIC
Examination:	Document extent and site and nature of bleeding, look for stigmata of liver disease, presence of bleeding from venepuncture site
II Laboratory tests	
Platelets	
Platelet count:	Thrombocytopenia
	Thrombocythaemia (may also be associated with abnormal bleeding)
Platelet morphology:	Abnormal morphology in certain inherited platelet disorders
Hb, FBC etc.:	Prolonged chronic bleeding may lead to an iron deficiency anaemia
Bleeding time:	Prolonged in vascular disorders, thrombocytopenia and von Willebrand's disease
Clotting time:	This is a simple bedside test which detects any major clotting derangement
Clot retraction:	This is a simple test for platelet function
Coagulation tests:	Prothrombin time
	Kaolin cephalin clotting time
	Thrombin time (see Table 58.14)

Table 58.13   Coagulation tests.

Prolongation of:	
Prothrombin time (PT) only	Factor VII deficiency (rare)
Kaolin cephalin clotting time (KCCT) only	Deficiency of factor VIII or IX (commonest causes) or II or XII (rare)
	Von Willebrand's disease (prolonged bleeding time as well)
	Factor VIII inhibitors (lupus etc.)
Both KCCT and PT prolonged	DIC
	Liver disease
	Vitamin K deficiency or antagonists
	Heparin therapy
	Dysfibrinogenaemia
	Hereditary deficiencies of factorsV, X or fibrinogen (rare)
Confirmatory tests	Individual clotting factor assays as indicated:
	Commonest are factor VIII and IX deficiencies

anaemia may also occur. The bone marrow is normal apart from an increase in megakaryocytes many of which may lack nuclear division and cytoplasmic granulation.

ITP is thought to be an autoimmune disorder. Confirmation of the diagnosis depends on the demonstration of an increase in platelet associated IgG. Platelet isoantibodies may also cause thrombocytopenia. This is of major importance in the neonatal period where children of mothers with ITP may have severe thrombocytopenia even if the mother is in remission. Maternal isoantibodies to infants' platelets may also cause thrombocytopenia in a mechanism similar to haemolytic disease of the newborn. In young adults, especially females, it is important to exclude the diagnosis of systemic lupus erythematosus when the diagnosis of ITP is made.

Treatment of ITP

In adults with a platelet count of more than 50×10^9/litre and in children who do not have severe haemorrhage, an expectant policy should be adopted. Steroids should be used in adult ITP when the platelet count is $<50 \times 10^9$/litre at a dose of 50–80 mg of prednisolone daily as spontaneous remission is not common. Steroids should be tailed off gradually when a response occurs or after five to six weeks if there is no response. They should not be used for a prolonged period. Some patients who respond to steroids may relapse after therapy is stopped. In children with more severe haemorrhage 0.5 mg/kg of prednisolone should be given daily and there is usually a high response rate. Relapse after tailing off of therapy is uncommon.

Intravenous immunoglobulin therapy can lead to a fairly rapid but usually transient rise in platelet counts in ITP. It is expensive and of limited value in long-term management. It is useful, however, to reduce bleeding in an episode of acute life-threatening haemorrhage or prior to planned surgery, such as splenectomy. Fresh frozen plasma has also been tried with some success. One unit given daily for 3 days may produce a modest rise in platelet counts. In view of its easier availability and lower cost it may be a useful form of treatment to attempt in the tropics.

Splenectomy is indicated in ITP in patients who do not respond to prednisolone therapy or who relapse after discontinuation of prednisolone and who continue to have severe haemorrhages. Splenectomy should be avoided in children especially under the age of five years. Splenectomy increases the susceptibility to pneumococcal septicaemia and malaria. Splenectomized patients should therefore be given prophylactic oral penicillin and antimalarials on a long-term basis. Platelet transfusions in ITP are only attempted when all other methods have failed in the presence of life-threatening haemorrhage.

Thrombocytopenia due to infection

Thrombocytopenia is very common in infections. The mechanisms which cause thrombocytopenia in infections include the following.

Splenomegaly. Varying degrees of splenomegaly occur in kala-azar, trypanosomiasis, schistosomiasis, tropical splenomegaly and malaria. Thrombocytopenia results from increased splenic platelet pooling but its severity depends on the degree of splenomegaly and the presence of other mechanisms leading to thrombocytopenia. In many of these conditions thrombocytopenia is usually moderate or mild and is not of any clinical consequence.

Immune mechanism. Immune thrombocytopenia is common in patients suffering from chickenpox, rubella, measles and other viral infections. ITP in children may also be classified under this category and may be due to the association of platelets with immune complexes formed by viral antigen–antibody reaction. Recent work suggests that this may also be a mechanism that contributes to thrombocytopenia in malaria.[97]

Bone marrow aplasia. This mechanism is most often implicated in aplastic anaemia following infectious hepatitis.

Disseminated intravascular coagulation (p. 983). This is the mechanism that may lead to thrombocytopenia in many conditions such as septicaemias, viral haemorrhagic fevers and in some cases of cerebral malaria.

Treatment of thrombocytopenia

In considering treatment, the clinical condition of the patient is of greater importance than the platelet count. In most of the above mentioned conditions thrombocytopenia is often not severe enough to cause haemorrhage. When haemorrhage occurs or in the presence of severe thrombocytopenia due to any cause other than ITP, platelet concentrates should be transfused. The use of fresh blood is usually not sufficient as platelet concentrates from 6–8 units of fresh blood are usually needed to arrest haemorrhage. This is needed daily whilst thrombocytopenia persists. In thrombocytopenia secondary to infection, platelet count often rises rapidly when the infective cause is treated. The treatment of DIC is discussed below.

DISORDERS OF BLOOD COAGULATION

These are not common disorders with an incidence of about $1 : 10^4$ subjects in Caucasians. The three commonest inherited disorders of coagulation are haemophilia (also known as haemophilia A; factor VIII deficiency), Christmas disease (also known as haemophilia B; factor IX deficiency) and von Willebrand's disease. Although the frequency of these disorders has not been fully worked out in the tropics, they do occur with sufficient frequency to warrant attention.

Haemophilia A

This is an inherited disorder of coagulation which is transmitted in a recessive sex-linked manner. This means that heterozygote females are carriers for the disorder which they pass on to half their male offspring who suffer from the disease. Female carriers have on average half the factor VIII level of normal individuals but do not suffer from a haemorrhagic disorder. Homozygous females are as severely affected as hemizygous males but are far less common. Although a history of a haemorrhagic tendency in the family can usually be elicited, previous family history may be lacking in some cases.

Clinical picture

(Normal factor VIII = 50–200 IU/dl, may be higher in Africans.[98])

Mild haemophilia with factor VIII level of 5%. These individuals suffer from severe haemorrhage only after major trauma, surgery or tooth extraction. They often present at an older age than more severe cases.

Moderate haemophilia with factor levels of 2–5%. These patients usually suffer from deep tissue haematomas or haemarthroses associated with trauma. Episodes of bleeding are therefore less frequent than in severe haemophilia.

Severe haemophilia. These present at an early age, even in infancy. There are repeated haemarthroses and deep muscle haematomas. These result in fibrosis and joint deformities if untreated at an early stage.

Diagnosis

The history is of prime importance (Table 58.12). Investigations reveal a prolonged kaolin cephalin clotting time (KCCT) and a normal prothrombin time. Factor VIII assay will yield the definitive diagnosis as well as define the level of deficiency. Factor VIII related antigen and ristocetin cofactor are normal (see von Willebrand's disease below) (Table 58.14).

Table 58.14 Major causes of thrombocytopenia.

I Due to increased platelet destruction	
Idiopathic thrombocytopenic purpura and immune thrombocytopenia	
Splenomegaly	
DIC:	viral haemorrhagic fevers etc. (Chapter 5)
II Due to decreased platelet production	
Bone marrow infiltration	
leukaemias	
lymphomas	
carcinomas	
Aplastic anaemia or	Drug damage
selective megakaryocytic aplasia:	Viral: infectious hepatitis
Defective platelet production:	Severe megaloblastic anaemia
	Acute alcoholic intoxication
III Due to several mechanisms (see text)	
Infections (with or without DIC):	Septicaemias
	Malaria
	Kala-azar
	Trypanosomiasis

Treatment

With the advent of blood component therapy concentrated factor VIII preparations are now widely available commercially. Alternatively cryoprecipitate may be used if concentrated factor VIII preparations are not available. The volume needed for treatment is higher than that required for factor VIII. Plasma, whether fresh or fresh-frozen, is of no value in treatment of haemorrhage in haemophilia as large amounts are needed. In cases of mild haemophilia or as an adjuvant to therapy with factor VIII concentrates tranexamic acid, an inhibitor of fibrinolysis, has been found to be useful. This is particularly so following dental extraction but is contraindicated if haematuria occurs as it may lead to obstruction of the urinary tract by clots. The dose is 1–1.5 g orally every 8 hours (25 mg/kg). The initial dose may be given by slow intravenous injection.

Major surgery and trauma. The aim is to increase factor VIII levels to 80–100% units/ml in the patient's plasma. (Amounts required are about 40–50 IU/kg.) The amount needed to maintain adequate levels should be assessed by monitoring the factor VIII levels produced or by performing a KCCT. Initially factor VIII may need to be given every 12 hours but after the first 3 days or so may be reduced to once daily until wound healing is complete.

Severe haemarthroses or minor surgery. A level of 20–40 IU in the patient's plasma is needed (10–20 IU/kg) and may need to be repeated for a few days.

Minor haemorrhage or haemarthroses. A single dose of 8–10 IU/kg body weight is usually sufficient to stop haemorrhage.

Haemophilia B (Christmas disease)

This disorder is similar in inheritance and in clinical manifestation to haemophilia A. The general guidelines to management also apply but factor IX preparations are needed instead of factor VIII. As factor IX is not precipitated in the cold, cryoprecipitate is very poor in factor IX and should not be used to treat Christmas disease.

The diagnosis is established by the demonstration of normal levels of factor VIII and low levels of factor IX.

Von Willebrand's disease (VWD)

It has been shown that the factor VIII functional coagulation complex is made of several components: factor VIII procoagulant activity and factor VIII related antigen.

Factor VIII procoagulant activity (VIIIc). This is measured by a clotting procedure and is the product of an X-linked gene. Deficiency leads to haemophilia A.

Factor VIII related antigen (VIIIRAg). This is a high molecular weight protein which is present in plasma from haemophiliacs but is low in plasma from patients with von Willebrand's disease. The level of this protein can be measured by the Laurel rocket technique using a rabbit antibody to the human antigen. Other methods of measuring the activity of this protein are by measurement of shortening of bleeding time after an infusion of normal plasma into patients with von Willebrand's disease or by measurement of aggregation of platelets by ristocetin (von Willebrand factor and ristocetin cofactor, respectively). These three activities are probably identical. Von Willebrand factor is a product of an autosomal gene. VWD is genetically heterogeneous and there are several modes of inheritance and a wide spectrum of severity.

Clinically von Willebrand's disease may present in a similar way to haemophilia. Unlike haemophilia, VWD occurs in females as well as in males. Mucous membrane bleeding, prolongation of bleeding from superficial skin lacerations and of the bleeding time are important clinical features that distinguish VWD from haemophilia.

Diagnosis

The diagnosis of von Willebrand's disease is based on the demonstration of a low factor VIII level, low VIII related antigen, a prolonged bleeding time and a low ristocetin cofactor.

Treatment

In mild cases it has been shown that treatment with 1-deamino-8-D-arginine-vasopressin (DDAVP) will reduce the incidence of haemorrhage following surgery or minor trauma. Tranexamic acid should also be used as DDAVP also stimulates the release of plasminogen activators.

In more severe cases an infusion of cryoprecipitate or even factor VIII concentrates may be needed. It must be remembered that factor VIII concentrates may not improve the bleeding time in von Willebrand's disease and that cryoprecipitate is usually preferable in the treatment of this disease.

ACQUIRED BLEEDING DISORDERS

The main causes of acquired disorders of haemostasis are vitamin K deficiency, liver disease and disseminated intravascular coagulation.

Vitamin K deficiency

The main causes are obstructive jaundice, severe malabsorption states and prematurity in infants. Vitamin K is a cofactor in the carboxylation of inactive forms of factors II, VII, IX and X into active clotting factors. Oral anticoagulants act by blocking this action. The prothrombin time is the most useful index of the severity of the deficiency. Spontaneous haemorrhage in vitamin K deficiency is unusual unless this is severe. Treatment is by administration of vitamin K 10 mg intramuscularly if the defect is not severe or intravenously if the defect is severe. The drug must be administered slowly as there is a risk of anaphylaxis.

Liver disease

In advanced hepatocellular disease there are several haemostatic defects as the liver is the main site of production of several of the clotting factors: the vitamin K dependent factors II, VII, IX, X and also of fibrinogen, factors V and XIII and of antithrombin III. In addition disseminated intravascular coagulation is common in hepatocellular disease due to impaired clearance of activated coagulation factors and reticuloendothelial block. The haemostatic defect in liver disease is therefore multifactorial. In mild deficiencies treatment with vitamin K may be sufficient but in more severe cases and where haemorrhage occurs infusions of fresh frozen plasma may be needed (see also DIC below).

In liver disease the prothrombin time, KCCT and thrombin time are all prolonged. The most sensitive index is the prothrombin time, which is used to monitor progress and response to therapy as it is sensitive to factor VII deficiency, which is the factor with the shortest half-life.

DISSEMINATED INTRAVASCULAR COAGULATION (DIC)

This is a disorder in haemostasis which occurs as a response to severe injury of any form. It is characterized by the widespread deposition of fibrin in tissues throughout the body. There is secondary activation of fibrinolysis and the production of a severe coagulation defect and thrombocytopenia.

DIC is an exaggeration of the normal haemostatic mechanisms. It occurs (a) when there is a sudden large production of thrombin due to release of substances which lead to thrombin formation (i.e. endotoxin, septicaemia, snake venom, amniotic fluid, embolism, crush injury, acute intravascular haemolysis etc.), (b) vascular injury (i.e. vasculitis), (c) inability to handle an excess of activated clotting factors (as in reticuloendothelial blockade, overwhelming infections and hepatocellular disease), (d) release of plasminogen or plasminogen activators (some carcinomas or sarcomas—rare).

Whatever the cause of DIC the picture is similar. The initial lesion is usually either vascular endothelial damage or direct activation of the clotting cascade. Platelet aggregation or coagulation factors activation may occur either directly or as a result of vascular endothelial damage by any injurious factor. There is a sudden generation of thromboplastin followed by tissue deposition of fibrin. This deposition may then lead to damage of various organs but quite often fibrin deposits may be cleared rapidly. Fibrin deposition in small vessels leads to fragmentation of red cells (microangiopathic haemolytic anaemia) and renal damage. The other major effect of DIC is depletion of coagulation factors and thrombocytopenia and secondary activation of fibrinolysis all of which may lead to haemorrhage.

Diagnosis of DIC

It is important to make a diagnosis as early as possible. DIC must be suspected in any severely ill patient. The important tests are: platelet count, thrombin time, prothrombin time and KCCT and measurement of fibrinogen degradation products (FDPs). These tests usually show prolongation of all three clotting tests, a low platelet count and a raised level of FDPs. Assay of fibrinogen in plasma may also show low fibrinogen levels. A very quick method for diagnosis which can be carried out by the bedside is to incubate some blood in a small glass tube at 37°C in a water bath. If the blood fails to clot or forms only small wisps of clot then the diagnosis can be made (Fig. 58.10).

Clinical features

DIC is a dynamic process and mild cases may progress to severe cases in a short period of time. The clinical picture may vary from that of mild derangement in clotting tests to severe coagu-

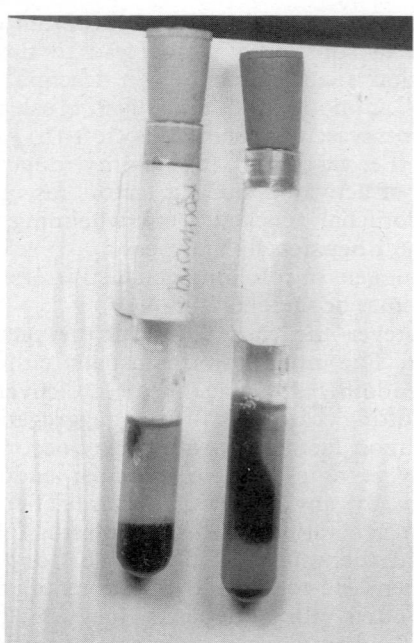

Fig. 58.10 A bedside test for DIC: the tube on the right contains blood from a normal person and shows a normal clot with clot retraction and a few red cells sedimented at the bottom. The tube on the left contains blood from a patient with DIC. There is a very small wispy clot and most of the red cells have sedimented to the bottom of the tube.

lation defects and haemorrhage. The most common clinical presentation is haemorrhage which may occur from mucous membranes or skin. A common feature is oozing from a venepuncture site. Clinical evidence of thrombosis is not common with DIC although neurological symptoms may occur (as in thrombotic thrombocytopenic purpura) or renal failure. Peripheral gangrene is another rare feature of thrombosis in DIC.

Common causes of DIC

Infections
    Bacterial: septicaemias, especially meningococcal and gram-negative sepsis.
    Viral: viral haemorrhagic fevers (Lassa fever, green monkey disease, dengue haemorrhagic fever, yellow fever), acute fulminant hepatitis of any sort.
    Others: malaria (usually occurs in severe fulminant cases only and in cerebral malaria), trypanosomiasis etc.

Snake bites. See Chapter 48.

Obstetric causes. These include septic abortion, abruptio placentae, amniotic fluid embolism.

Other causes. These include vasculitis, disseminated carcinomas, shock, incompatible transfusions.

Treatment

The important principles of treatment of DIC are:
1 removal of the cause where possible: treatment of infection, delivery or evacuation of a fetus in obstetric cases and treatment of shock;
2 treatment of haemorrhage: where this is severe the administration of platelets, fresh frozen plasma fibrinogen or fresh whole blood according to the severity of the deficiency of each factor or availability of products;
3 heparin: the use of heparin in DIC is controversial in most cases. There are some cases where its use is indicated such as in chronic DIC with a retained dead fetus and in certain carcinomas prior to surgical manipulation and in acute promyelocytic leukaemia. If heparin therapy is used then a low dose regimen for a short period of time should be given with frequent monitoring of the laboratory parameters.

REFERENCES

1 WHO Technical Reports Series (1968) *Nutritional Anaemias*. Report of a WHO scientific group. No. 405.
2 Gilles, H. M. (1981) *Clin. Haemat.* **10,** 697–706.
3 Abdalla, S. H., Corrah, P. T. & Mabey, D. C. W. (1986) *Trans. R. Soc. trop. Med. Hyg.* **80,** 557–562.
4 Chanarin, I. (1979) *The Megaloblastic Anaemias*, 2nd edn. Oxford: Blackwell Scientific Publications.
5 Baker, S. J. (1981) *Clin. Haemat.* **10,** 841–872.
6 Wickramasinghe, S. N. (1981) *Clin. Lab. Haemat.* **3,** 1–18.
7 Walt, F., Holman, S. & Hendrickse, R. G. (1956) *Br. med. J.* **i,** 1199–1203.
8 Sandstead, H. H., Gabr, M. K., Azzam, S. et al (1965) *Am. J. clin. Nutr.* **17,** 27–35.
9 Fondu, P., Kabeya-Mudiay, S., De Maertelaere-Laurent, E. et al (1973) *Biomedicine* **18,** 51–58.
10 Spector, I. & Metz, J. (1966) *Br. J. Haemat.* **12,** 737–746.
11 Khalil, M., Tanios, A., Moghazy, M. et al (1973) *Arch Dis. Childh.* **48,** 366–369.
12 Omer, A., El Shazali, H., El Karim, O. A. et al (1973) *J. trop. Ped. envir. Chld Hlth*, **19,** 91–97.
13 Wickramasinghe, S. N., Akinyanju, O. O., Grange, A. et al (1983) *Br. J. Haemat.* **53,** 135–143.

14 Wickramasinghe, S. N., Litwinczuk, R. A. C., Akinyanju, O. O. et al (1983) *Br. J. Haemat.* 55, 385–387.

15 Wickramasinghe, S. N., Cotes, P. M., Gill, D. S. et al (1985) *Br. J. Haemat.* 60, 515–524.

16 Murray, M. J., Murray, A. B., Murray, N. J. et al (1978) *Br. med. J.* ii, 1113–1115.

17 Cartwright, G. E. & Lee, G. R. (1971) *Br. J. Haemat.* 21, 147–152.

18 Samson, D. (1983) *Postgrad. med. J.* 59, 543–558.

19 Zuckerman, A. (1966) *Milit. Med.* 131, 1201–1216.

20 Abdalla, S. & Weatherall, D. J. (1982) *Br. J. Haemat.* 52, 415–425.

21 Abdalla, S. H. (1986) *Br. J. Haemat.* 62, 13–17.

22 Kuvin, S. F., Baye, H. K., Stohlman, F., Jr et al (1962) *J. Am. med. Ass.* 184, 1018–1020.

23 Srichaikul, T., Panikbutr, N. & Jeumtrakul, P. (1967) *Ann. trop. Med. Parasit.* 61, 40–51.

24 Srichaikul, T., Wasanosomsithi, M., Poshyachinda, V. (1969) *Arch intern. Med.* 124, 623–628.

25 Srichaikul, T., Siriasawakul, T., Poshyachinda, M. et al (1973) *Am. J. clin. Path.* 60, 166–174.

26 Abdalla, S., Weatherall, D. J., Wickramasinghe, S. N. et al (1980) *Br. J. Haemat.* 46, 171–183.

27 Weatherall, D. J., Abdalla, S. H. & Pippard. (1983) The anaemia of *Plasmodium falciparum* malaria. In *Malaria and the Red Cell*. Ciba Symposium no. 94, pp. 74–88. London: Pitman.

28 Topley, E. (1975) *Trop. Doct.* 5, 18–22.

29 Abdalla, S., Wickramsinghe, S. N. & Weatherall, D. J. (1984) *Trans. R. Soc. Trop. Med. Hyg.* 78, 60–63.

30 Cartwright, G. E., Chung, H. L. & Chang, A. (1948) *Blood* 3, 249–275.

30a Wickramasinghe, S. N., Abdalla, S. N. & Kasili, E.E.G. (1987) *J. Clin. Pathol.* 40, 267–275.

31 Bada, J. L., Arderiu, A., Gimenez, J. et al (1979) *Trans. R. Soc. trop. Med. Hyg.* 73, 256–257.

32 Woodruff, A. W., Topley, E., Knight, R. et al (1972) *Br. J. Haemat.* 22, 319–329.

33 Musumeci, S., Romereo, M. & D'Agata, A. (1974) *J. trop. Med. Hyg.* 77, 106–110.

34 Aikat, B. K., Mohanty, D., Pathania, A. G. S. et al (1979) *Ind. J. med. Res.* 70, 571–582.

35 Abdalla, S. H., Kasili, E. & Weatherall, D. J. (1983) *Trans. R. Soc. trop. Med Hyg.* 77, 99–102.

36 Chatterjea, J. B. & Sengupta, P. C. (1970) *J. Ind. med. Ass.* 54, 541–552.

37 Knight, R., Woodruff, D. W. & Pettit, C. E. (1967) *Trans. R. Soc. trop. Med. Hyg.* 61, 701–705.

38 Woodruff, A. W., Ziegler, J. C., Hathaway, A. et al (1973) *Trans. R. Soc. trop. Med. Hyg.* 74, 436–457.

39 Huan, C. N., Webb, C., Lambert, P. H. et al (1975) *Schweiz. med. Wochensch.* 105, 1582–1583.

40 O'Daly, J. & Aso, P. M. (1979) *Exp. Parasit.* 47, 222–231.

41 Woodruff, A. W. (1973) *Trans. R. Soc. trop. Med. Hyg.* 67, 313.

42 Jenkins, G. C. (1980) *Trans. R. Soc. trop. Med. Hyg.* 74, 268–270.

43 Robins-Browne, R. M., Schneider, J. & Metz, J. (1975) *Am. J. trop. Med. Hyg.* 24, 226–231.

44 Davis, C. E., Robbin, R. S., Weller, R. D. et al (1974). *J. clin. Invest.* 53, 1359–1367.

45 Boreham, P. F. C. & Facer, C. A. (1973) *Trans. R. Soc. trop. Med. Hyg.* 67, 279.

46 Barrett-Connor, E., Ugoretz, R. J. & Braude, A. I. (1973) *Arch. intern. Med.* 131, 574–577.

47 Cameron, S. J. & Horne, N. W. (1971) *Tubercle*, 52, 37–48.

48 Oluboyede, O. A. & Onadeko, B. O. (1978) *J. R. Soc. trop. Med. Hyg.* 81, 91–95.

49 Roberts, P. D., Hoffbrand, A. V. & Mollin, D. L. (1966) *B. med. J.* ii, 198–202.

50 Markannen, T., Levante, A., Sallinen, V. et al (1967) *Scandinav. J. Haem.* 4, 283–297.

51 Cameron, S. J. (1974) *Tubercle* 55, 55–72.

52 Coburn, R. J., England, J. M., Samson, D. M. et al (1973) *Br. J. Haemat.* 25, 793–799.

53 Verwilghen, R., Reybrouch, G., Callens, L. et al (1965) *Br. J. Haemat.* 11, 92–98.

54 Heinivaara, O. & Palva, I. P. (1964) *Acta med. Scandinav.* 175, 469–471.

55 Paaby, P. & Norvin, E. (1966) *Acta Med. Scandinav.* 180, 561–564.

56 Farid, Z., Bassily, S., Schulbert, A. R. et al (1967) *Trans. R. Soc. trop. Med. Hyg.* 61, 621–625.

57 Farid, Z., Patwardan, V. N. & Darby, W. J. (1969) *Am. J. clin. Nutr.* 22, 498–500.

58 Uamra, M., Maspes, V. & Meira, D. A. (1964) *Rev. Inst. Med. trop. São Paulo* 6, 126–136.

59 El-Attar, O., Shakeen, H., El-Saadani, A. M. et al (1972) *J. Egypt. med. Ass.* 55, 512–519.

60 Edington, G. M. & Giles, H. M. (1976) *Pathology in the Tropics*, 2nd edn. London: Edward Arnold.

61 Fleming, A. F. (1981) *Clin. Haemat.* 10, 983–1012.

62 Miller, T. A. (1979) *Adv. Parasit.* 17, 315–384.

63 Gilles, H. M., Watson-Williams, E. J. & Edington, G. M. (1964) *Q. J. Med.* 33, 1–24.

64 Werblinska, B. & Fleming, A. F. (1979) *Ann. trop. Med. Parasit.* 73, 149–159.

65 Carson, P. E., Flanagan, C. L., Ickes, C. E. et al (1956) *Science* 124, 484–485.

66 Bienzle, U. (1981) *Clin. Haemat.* 10, 785–799.

67 Akinyanju, O. O. & Odusote, K. A. (1983) *Br. med. J.* ii, 1314.

68 Lampe, R. M., Kirdpon, S., Mansuwan, P. et al (1975) *J. Paediat.* 87, 576–578.

69 Clark, M. & Root, R. K. (1979) *Yale J. Biol. Med.* 52, 169–179.

70 Na-Nakorn, S. & Panich, V. (1971) *Siriraj Hosp. Gaz.* 23, 109–119.

71 Benjabhongs, U. (1966) *Med. J.* (supplement) 15, 128–152.

72 Effiong, C. E., Aimaku, V. E., Bienzle, U. et al (1975) *J. Nat. med. Ass. (USA)* 67, 208–213.

73 Motulsky, A. G., Kraut, J. M., Thieme, W. J. et al (1959) *Clin. Res.* 7, 89.

74 Sicard, D., Kaplan, J. C. & Cabie, D. (1978) *Lancet* ii, 571–572.

75 Milner, P. F. (1974) *Clin. Haemat.* 3, 289.

76 Serjeant, G. R. (1974) *The Clinical Features of Sickle Cell Disease*. Amsterdam: North Holland.

77 Charache, S. & Niebyl, J. R. (1985) *Clin. Haemat.* 14, 729.

78 Weatherall, D. J. (1985) *Clin. Haemat.* 14, 747.

79 Huehns, E. R. (1982) Haemoglobin and the haemoglobinopathies. In *Blood and its Disorders*, ed. R. M. Hardisty & D. J. Weatherall, 3rd edn. Oxford: Blackwell Scientific Publications.

80 Weatherall, D. J. & Clegg, J. B. (1981) *The Thalassaemia Syndromes*, 3rd edn. Oxford: Blackwell Scientific Publications.

81 Weatherall, D. J. & Wainscoat, J. S. (1985) *Rec. Adv. Haematol.* 4, 63–88.

82 Pitney, W. R. (1968) *Trans. R. Soc. trop. Med. Hyg.* **62**, 717–728.

83 Ziegler, J. L. (1973) *Clin. exp. Immunol.* **15**, 65–78.

84 Fakunle, Y. M. & Greenwood, B. M. (1977) *Clin. exp. Immunol.* **28**, 153–156.

85 Pryor, D. A. (1967) *Q. J. Med.* **36**, 321–336.

86 Fakunle, Y. M. & Greenwood, B. M. (1976) *Lancet* **ii**, 608–609.

87 Ziegler, J. L. & Stuiver, P. C. (1972) *Br. med. J.* **iii**, 79–82.

88 Gilles, H. M., Lawson, J. B. & Sibelas, M. (1969) *Trans. R. Soc. trop. Med. Hyg.* **63**, 245–263.

89 Bray, R. S. & Anderson, M. J. (1979) *Trans. R. Soc. trop. Med. Hyg.* **73**, 427–431.

90 Fleming, A. F. (ed.) (1982) *Sickle Cell Disease. A Hand-book for the General Clinician.* London: Churchill Livingstone.

91 Fullerton, W. T. & Turner, A. G. (1962) *Lancet* **i**, 75–78.

92 Correa, P. & O'Connor, G. T. (1973) *J. Nat. Canc. Inst.* **50**, 1609–1617.

93 Olweny, C. L. M. (1981) *Clin. Haemat.* **10**, 873–893.

94 Browning, D. & Gross, S. (1968) *Am. J. Dis. Chldh.* **116**, 576–585.

95 Kasili, E. G. (1978) Leukaemia in Kenya. M. D. Thesis, University of Kenya.

96 Jimenez, G. (1981) *Clin. Haemat.* **10**, 864–915.

97 Kelton, J. G., Keystone, J., Moore, E. J. et al (1983) *J. Clin. Invest.* **71**, 832–836.

98 Essein, E. M. & Ayenio (1978) *Br. J. Haemat.* **39**, 225–231.

Chapter 59
Tuberculosis

P. Chaulet and D. Mulder

Tuberculosis is still rampant in tropical countries and, although the disease has receded in the technically advanced countries of Europe and North America over the last thirty years, the absolute number of tuberculous patients throughout the world is *still* increasing, owing to population growth in the more underprivileged population groups.

Today in 1986 there are some 15 million tuberculosis cases worldwide, including seven million infectious cases, 95% of whom live in Asia, Africa or Latin America (based on Rouillon,[1] Styblo and Rouillon[2]). By the year 2000 the absolute number will probably be still as high, with incidence rates in poorer regions manyfold those in the technically advanced countries— partly on account of the difficulties encountered in these regions in the implementation of modern and effective tuberculosis control programmes.[3]

AETIOLOGY, TRANSMISSION AND CONTROL MEASURES

Tuberculosis is due to *Mycobacterium tuberculosis* of the human type. The bovine organism has only a limited responsibility in human infection even in countries where cattle are infected. The occurrence in certain tropical countries of varieties of the organisms which, as *Mycobacterium africanum*, exhibit a natural resistance to thiacetazone is nowadays less important because of the advance of chemotherapy. Atypical mycobacteria may cause clinical disease but this occurs rarely and has no impact on the persistence of the tuberculosis problem.

The source of tuberculous infection is the diseased man, in particular the patient with pulmonary disease. The infectiousness of a patient is determined by his bacillary status: patients in whom tubercle bacilli can be demonstrated in the sputum by direct smear examination are highly infectious; in contrast, patients in whom tubercle bacilli can be demonstrated in the sputum by culture only, or who are culture negative, are relatively non-infectious.

The bacilli are transmitted to contacts of the patient through infectious aerosol droplets discharged by the patient when coughing, sneezing or talking. Transmission is all the more intense among close relatives since they are in contact with the patient several hours per day: in practice, those who live under the same roof and sleep in the same room as the infectious patient are at highest risk.

Bacilli penetrate the bronchi and lung of a healthy subject when the latter inhales the droplets a few minutes after their discharge from a diseased individual: in a healthy and as yet noninfected individual the initial penetration of bacilli causes a *primary infection,* usually latent but sometimes accompanied by clinical signs (fever, skin or mucous reactions) and/or radiological signs (primary focus and hilar lymphadenopathy: primary complex). Within a few weeks of infection the skin response to tuberculin becomes positive. Primary infection may be followed by early post-primary disease (miliary tuberculosis, meningitis, pleurisy) or by late manifestations such as other extrapulmonary localizations (lymph nodes, bones and joints, abdomen). Endogenous reactivation of a postprimary pulmonary focus (following weakening of immune defences) or exogenous reinfection (new infection facilitated by repeated infections) causes a caseous focus to occur in the lung. Together with its liquefaction there will be microbial proliferation. Once this liquefied focus has drained via the bronchi there remains a *tuberculous pulmonary cavity,* converting the individual into a new source of infection.

Tuberculosis will maintain itself in a human community provided (a) that one tuberculous person infects approximately twenty others, (b) that among those so infected at least two break down with the disease, and (c) that of these two at least one becomes in turn a source of infection. This is, in general, what happens under natural conditions of transmission, because an untreated pulmonary tuberculous patient remains infectious for two years on average and infects about ten persons each year, the latter figure varying according to housing conditions.

With the technical means available today to fight tuberculosis the chain of transmission can be interrupted. Sources of infection can be identified by direct smear examination of sputum from tuberculosis suspects and in this way the detected patients can be given effective chemotherapy, which renders them non-infectious in less than two weeks and ensures firm cure within six or eight months. Identification of sources of infection and modern chemotherapy radically influence the transmission of tuberculosis in the human population when compared with transmission under natural conditions. BCG vaccination of young non-infected children is actually an artificial and innocuous primary infection: it helps to protect these children (if at risk) against more serious post-primary lesions (acute miliary tuberculosis, meningitis) and to prevent a certain number of pulmonary cases from developing in children and teenagers. Yet, since the number of cases with infectious pulmonary tuberculosis among children and young adults represents only a small percentage of the total number of sources of infection within the community, BCG vaccination has little impact on the transmission of the disease in the community. Thus, while BCG vaccination is an important measure for protection of individual children and young adults from developing tuberculous disease, case-finding and treatment of infectious cases are understandably the two fundamental measures of all modern anti-tuberculosis programmes, both to alleviate human suffering and to influence the chain of transmission.

EPIDEMIOLOGY

A stigma of poverty and social precariousness, tuberculosis is a major health problem in tropical countries. Whereas the annual incidence of tuberculosis (all forms) ranges from 15 to 50 cases per 100 000 inhabitants in Europe and North America, it reaches 100 to 500 cases per 100 000 inhabitants in most tropical countries. Of these cases, 50–60% are highly infectious cases (pul-

monary tuberculosis, smear positive); the remaining cases are smear-negative pulmonary tuberculosis cases (of whom some are culture positive) or extrapulmonary tuberculosis cases.

Within each 'tropical' country, even in those enjoying a comparatively high standard of living, there are certain population groups with a high tuberculosis prevalence: impoverished peasants possessing neither land nor cattle; migrants in search of work; populations of the shanty towns fringing modern cities; refugees trying to escape war, famine or drought.

The incidence of tuberculosis cases notified in health services' statistics rarely mirrors the actual situation, as the notified incidence depends on the quality of these services and their accessibility to the population. The assessment of the annual risk of tuberculous infection (by means of tuberculin surveys in representative samples of the young non-BCG-vaccinated population) yields a more accurate picture (and one which is not influenced by the intensity of the health services assessment activities) of the real magnitude of tuberculosis within the community. The annual risk of tuberculous infection represents the percentage of subjects who, over a one-year span, become infected for the first time (or are reinfected) by tubercle bacilli. The risk of infection is therefore directly proportional to the number of sources of infection in the community, regardless of whether these sources are identified and notified or not. It has been estimated that an annual risk of infection of 1% corresponds to an annual incidence of infectious pulmonary tuberculosis (smear positive) of 50–60 cases per 100 000 population. In most tropical countries, the annual risk of infection lies between 1.5% and 4%. As these rates can now be assessed with accuracy quantitative objectives may be set out for case-finding and treatment activities in any country.[4,5]

DIAGNOSIS

Tuberculosis occurs in particular in young adults and is accompanied by clinical signs often recognizable in members of the community. Lungs are always the most common site involved but extrapulmonary involvements may account for up to 30% of notified tuberculosis cases. Because of the age structure of the population and the prevailing living and housing conditions child tuberculosis is unfortunately not a rare occurrence, and gives rise to specific problems.

Pulmonary tuberculosis

Pulmonary tuberculosis can occur at all ages, usually more frequently in males than in females. In countries with a high prevalence young adults from 20 to 35 years of age are most commonly affected. Persistent cough, often associated with such symptoms as fever, asthenia, anorexia, loss of weight and haemoptysis, constitutes the classical picture. These symptoms usually alarm the patient and his relatives.

How rapidly the condition is diagnosed depends on the health services' accessibility to the population and on the diagnostic facilities available to health services.

In urban areas endowed with a hospital or clinic equipped with radiological facilities tuberculosis suspects (i.e. attenders with symptoms suggestive of tuberculosis or with lesions suspect of being tuberculous) should be easily identified among clinic attenders with recent respiratory symptoms (acute bronchitis, pneumonia, abcess) or with chronic respiratory conditions (asthma, chronic bronchitis, bronchiectasis).

In remote rural areas, where health services are not equipped with radiological means and where patients cannot afford to visit the nearest hospital, it is necessary to interview and examine all tuberculosis suspects at least twice (the second examination after an interval of a week or two, during which symptomatic treatment is given) to ascertain the chronic and persistent nature of symptoms, the presence of purulent sputa, and to rule out the possibility of asthma or non-tuberculous, acute bronchopulmonary infection.

In either case a positive tuberculin test is of little value for diagnostic purposes, especially in adolescents and adults, as it may indicate nothing more than BCG vaccination or a harmless non-progressive primary infection at some time in the past. A negative test, however, rules out a diagnosis of tuberculosis except in certain well-recognized circumstances (moribund/cachectic individual, patient harbouring virus such as measles/pertussis, woman in third trimester of pregnancy or patient on corticosteroids).

Although radiological examination is of great value for discriminating between X-ray appearances suspect of tuberculosis and other pathologies on the one hand and normal appearances on the other, the specificity is low and shadows are often difficult to interpret for the inexperienced reader. Even in the hands of experienced readers radiological examination alone results in considerable overdiagnosis. Suspicion, based on X-ray, should as a rule be confirmed by bacteriological examination.

So, in both urban and rural situations for any tuberculosis suspect it is imperative to collect, in clean sputum containers (they need not be sterile), two sputum samples of some 2 ml each, making sure that the samples contain purulent material and to send them to the nearest microscopy laboratory. In more than two-thirds of all cases, the diagnosis of tuberculosis can be made by microscopy examination of sputum smears: if the first sputum examinations are negative, microscopy of two sputum samples should be repeated fortnightly for the next month; this will ensure the detection of the great majority of infectious cases.

Culture of sputa is feasible only in some laboratories duly equipped with the proper facilities and staffed by skilled technicians. Culture is useful in the diagnosis of tuberculosis in cases with relevant pulmonary shadows and with (at least six) negative microscopy examinations. In most tropical countries, however, it contributes to the diagnostic confirmation of only a small proportion of the cases admitted to treatment.

The procedures for diagnosis of pulmonary tuberculosis outlined above should be carried out as a top priority among all clinic attenders over 15 years old presenting with lasting symptoms and among children and adults living in contact with an identified tuberculous patient. Where health services meet the needs of tuberculosis case-finding in both these population groups it is recommended that the case-finding procedures be extended to other population groups 'at risk' which are easily identified and mustered, such as diabetics or miners exposed to silica dust.

A major problem arises when a patient with suspect pulmonary X-ray appearances is negative on repeated microscopy examination of sputum and especially when in addition there is no culture laboratory. If the clinical signs (high fever, severe asthenia) and radiological signs are quite suggestive of acute miliary tuberculosis, or if the patient's life is endangered (for instance, extensive pulmonary lesions in diabetic patients), it is justifiable to make a diagnosis of tuberculosis and to treat the patient despite the lack of bacteriological confirmation. In all other cases it is better to wait and to repeat microscopy examination of sputa on two specimens collected at weekly or fortnightly intervals and chest X-ray examination after a month. Spontaneous regression of lesions, or their non-evolution, indicates that these are not active tuberculous lesions. In case of radiological deterioration or dubious evolution, the best course is to refer to a consultant rather than to initiate treatment in the absence of bacteriological evidence of the disease.

Extrapulmonary tuberculosis

The most common manifestations of extrapulmonary tuberculosis are readily suspected, but difficult to confirm. Lesions usually contain a small bacterial population and firm evidence of tuberculosis can be produced only by cultivating pathological material or by histopathological examination of biopsy material.

Tuberculosis of peripheral lymph nodes (most commonly cervical). This typically produces hypertrophy followed by softening of the nodes involved and fistula formation. Before the fistula appears diagnosis can be difficult. The white cell count and morphology can help identify infection or severe blood disease. The tuberculin test is always strongly positive. Culture of pus taken from the node or histopathological examination of a node can provide the basis for diagnosis when qualified laboratories are available. In most cases, however, physical examination, tuberculin testing and blood examination provide the only available basis for diagnosis.

Isolated pleural tuberculosis (not associated with pulmonary tuberculosis). This produces suggestive physical and radiological signs. The presence of pleural effusion with clear lymphocytic fluid, the effusion progressing for more than a week or two, the absence of other causes of pleural effusion combined with a positive tuberculin test all contribute to confirmation of the diagnosis. Pleural biopsy or identification of bacilli after culture of pleural fluid are more accurate, but rarely feasible, examinations.

Tuberculous meningitis. This is an early post-primary event which occurs occasionally in non-BCG-vaccinated children. It induces lymphocytic meningitis, associated with oculomotor paralyses, mood lability, and neurovegetative disturbances. If neglected, this condition may lead to coma due to meningitis which can be cured only with difficulty and often at the expense of severe neurological sequelae. Its diagnosis rests on typical chemical and cytological alterations in the cerebrospinal fluid—increased protein, diminished glucose and chloride content, cells mainly lymphocytic; bacilli may be found on smear examination of the clot which sometimes forms on cooling of the fluid.

Tuberculosis of the peritoneum. When accompanied with ascites, it can easily be diagnosed in an adolescent with positive tuberculin test results presenting with no liver or spleen disease nor with any sign of portal hypertension. But in its fibro-adhesive form it produces misleading, pseudo-obstructive manifestations calling for a digestive tract X-ray examination or for laparoscopy/laparotomy.

Bone and joint tuberculosis. It essentially involves the vertebrae (Pott's disease) and large joints (hip, knee, ankle joint, shoulder, elbow), and sometimes the longer bones (isolated osteitis). It leads to functional disability and sometimes to swelling of joints and abscesses. Radiological examination reveals reduction of joint space or of intervertebral disc space and more or less extensive bone damage. The clinical signs, the typical radiological lesions and the slow progress and positive tuberculin test results are the basis for diagnosis, which can be confirmed by culture of caseous pus from the abscess, taken by puncture, or from a biopsy of the bone lesions.

Other extrapulmonary sites of tuberculous involvement (pericardium, kidney, genitalia, liver, brain, skin). These forms seldom occur. Whilst, in renal tuberculosis, bacteriological examination of urine contributes to detection of tubercle bacilli (occasionally also on direct microscopy), specialized diagnostic facilities are required to establish the diagnosis in all other localizations: electrocardiogram and pericardial puncture, laparoscopy and liver biopsy, coelioscopy, biopsy of the endometrium, brain scan, skin biopsy. Such facilities are only available in urban hospitals.

Tuberculosis in children

This is relatively frequent in tropical countries, where it accounts for some 10% of the total number of tuberculosis cases. The diagnosis is attended by much difficulty because malnourished children and those suffering from rickets have frequent and repeated acute respiratory infections. Active diagnosis of these cases indispensably rests on examination of all children living in close contact with a tuberculous patient, on their tuberculin test and their chest or bone X-ray examination, the latter according to clinical symptoms observed.

In somewhat less than half of the children with tuberculous disease, an obvious primary infection can be observed, with fever, clinical manifestations (erythema nodosum, phlyctenular keratoconjunctivitis) and unilateral mediastinal lymphadenopathy with or without lung shadows on X-ray examination. Tuberculin test results are strongly positive. In a smaller proportion of the cases true pulmonary tuberculosis can be found, with nodular or even cavitary forms (specially in older children); if cavitation is present, bacilli can be detected at microscopic examination of the sputum smear, just as in adults. The remaining cases present with extrapulmonary tuberculosis involving the same diagnostic problems as in adults.

Overdiagnosis sometimes occurs in children on the basis of primary infection sequelae (pulmonary or mediastinal calcifications, lobar or segmental atelectasis) discovered on the occasion of a common acute respiratory infection. Diagnosis of recent primary infection is sometimes overlooked in *apparently healthy children* living in close contact with a tuberculous relative. In such cases, if the child is under five years of age and has not been BCG vaccinated, tuberculin test results should be taken into consideration. If the test is positive, the child should be considered to have had a recent infection and should be given chemoprophylaxis with daily isoniazid for six months. If the tuberculin test is negative, the child should be BCG-vaccinated. A BCG-vaccinated child, whether or not living in close contact with a tuberculous relative, usually shows a positive tuberculin test reaction; if the child is healthy (i.e. presenting no symptom of pulmonary or extrapulmonary involvement) he should not be given chemotherapy even if he is under five years old.

TREATMENT

Treatment of tuberculosis (any form) rests on chemotherapy. Antituberculous drugs must be administered in combination in order to avoid selection of resistant mutant organisms. A patient who has never taken antituberculous drugs generally carries bacilli sensitive to these drugs. If he is given an adequate combination of drugs, at the proper dosages and for a sufficient period of time, he will recover. But if he is given only one antituberculous drug, due to an error in prescription or due to wrong information given to the patient at the time he starts treatment, selection of bacilli resistant to this particular drug will occur, producing an *acquired bacterial resistance*. A patient who discharges resistant bacilli may infect a person never treated before who may then develop pulmonary tuberculosis with initially resistant bacilli. The prime objective of modern chemotherapy regimens is to provide all patients with equal chances of cure, whether they harbour sensitive bacilli or initially resistant bacilli.

Of the *six main antituberculous drugs*,[6] two are major antimicrobial agents which destroy all bacillary populations (inside and outside macrophages) harboured by the patient: these are *isoniazid* and *rifampicin*. Their synergic combination can cure nearly all patients when given for six months. Two other drugs, namely pyrazinamide and streptomycin are companion bactericidal drugs. *Pyrazinamide*, which is especially active in acid environment, acts on intracellular bacilli: its prime role is to reduce the risk of relapse. It has been demonstrated recently that it also helps to reduce failures due to primary isoniazid resistance provided it is prescribed for two months or more from start of treatment.[7-9] *Streptomycin*, which was the first antituberculous drug discovered, is an aminoglycoside active against extracellular and rapidly growing bacilli in the cavity walls, but it does not penetrate the macrophages. It rapidly reduces the number of bacilli in a cavitary lesion at the onset of treatment and, when combined with isoniazid and pyrazinamide, it induces bacteriological conversion in cases where rifampicin cannot be administered.

Lastly, two minor drugs show a complementary role when combined with one of the major bactericidal drugs (isoniazid or rifampicin): these are *thiacetazone* (always with isoniazid in combined tablets of fixed proportions) and *ethambutol*. As previously with para-aminosalicylic acid, their main effect is to prevent the emergence of bacilli resistant to the major bactericidal drug used, when the two major drugs cannot be given combined (either on economical grounds, or on account of proven bacterial resistance to one drug or the other).

With these six essential drugs, administered at proper dosages, it is possible to devise nearly 100% effective short-course chemotherapy regimens which are well tolerated and have low risks of toxicity. Precise dosages according to patient's body weight have been recommended for each drug by the International Union Against Tuberculosis (IUAT) (Table 59.1).[10]

ment. During the first two months (or the first eight weeks), these drugs are administered daily with a daily supplement of pyrazinamide and a fourth companion drug: ethambutol or streptomycin. During the next four months, isoniazid and rifampicin can be given daily or intermittently (twice or three times weekly) with equal efficacy.

Another six-month regimen combining streptomycin, isoniazid and pyrazinamide twice weekly during the last four months, following a two-month initial phase of four drugs (including

Table 59.1 Essential antituberculosis drugs; dosages (mg) recommended by the Committee on Treatment of the International Union Against Tuberculosis.[10]

Drug	Common abbreviation	Administration			
		Daily		Intermittent	
		mg/kg	maximum	mg/kg	maximum
Isoniazid	H	8[a]	300	15	750
Rifampicin	R	10	600	10	600
Pyrazinamide	Z	30	2000	50	3500
Streptomycin	S	15	1000[b]	15	1000[b]
Ethambutol	E	25[c]	1200	40	2000
Thiacètazone	T	2.5	150	—	—

[a] 10 mg/kg in children.
[b] In patients aged 45 and over the maximum dose is 750 mg (addition 1986 by one of the present authors).
[c] 15 mg/kg after two months.

All these modern regimens comprise two phases:
1 an initial intensive phase of eight weeks, combining three or four drugs, generally administered daily under direct supervision;
2 a maintenance phase lasting four to six months according to the regimen, during which drugs can be taken daily (self-administration) or under direct supervision, on an intermittent basis, twice weekly.

The modern regimens of six or eight months' chemotherapy replace the former regimens of 12 or 18 months which were based on daily administration of isoniazid and thiacetazone (or ethambutol) throughout the 12- or 18-month course, with a daily supplement of streptomycin for the first six to eight weeks. The efficacy of these modern short-course regimens has been amply demonstrated in many countries and after long periods of follow-up.[11–13] Their efficacy surpasses that of the former 12- or 18-month regimens, both in cases with initially sensitive bacilli and in those with initially resistant baccilli.

The principal six-month regimen combines isoniazid and rifampicin throughout the treat-

rifampicin) given daily, is as effective as the former regimen.

The six-month regimens are the most effective chemotherapy regimens known today: cumulative failure and relapse rates over the three years following treatment termination is below 2%.

The eight-month regimen is a short-course regimen within the reach of all tropical countries, since the most expensive drugs, rifampicin and pyrazinamide, are prescribed for the first two months only. In fact, during these first two months, four drugs are administered daily under direct supervision: isoniazid, rifampicin, streptomycin and pyrazinamide. Thereafter isoniazid alone or isoniazid and thiacetazone are administered daily for six months, usually without direct supervision, yielding an identical success rate to that of the six-month regimen in sensitive cases, but one slightly weaker in cases with initially resistant bacilli.

The cost of some of the drugs used in the short-course regimens has long been an obstacle to the adoption of short-course chemotherapy in tropical countries. Recent changes in drug prices should make it possible to provide short-course chemotherapy to all patients suffering from pulmonary tuberculosis: the cost of chemotherapy of one patient on such a regimen equals that of two or three chest X-rays and is cheaper than a 2-day hospital stay.

In addition to the high success rates of the new regimens their reduced treatment duration shortens the required duration of service delivery by health staff and considerably alleviates the constraints caused by the treatment for the patient and his family. These benefits gradually coax many countries to adopt these short-course regimens (Table 59.2). It cannot be over-emphasized that the important thing in therapy

health staff so that they can detect and correct side-effects of chemotherapy (minor gastrointestinal disturbances or joint pains; skin hypersensitivity; jaundice; neurosensory disturbances)[14] and so that they can assess treatment efficacy.

Systematic testing pre-treatment of drug sensitivity of *M. tuberculosis* strains in patients who have had no previous treatment and determination of isoniazid inactivation phenotype are unnecessary investigations (and moreover rarely feasible in tropical countries) if one uses standard chemotherapy regimens at IUAT-recommended doses. Similarly, routine pre-treatment liver or kidney function tests are to be avoided.

Table 59.2 Standardized chemotherapy regimens applied in national tuberculosis control programmes.

	Duration (months)	Regimens[a]	Failure–relapse (%)		1985 price[b] of drugs in US $
			Sensitive cases	Initially resistant cases	
Former	12–18	2 STH/TH	5	50	8
Modern	8	2 SRHZ/TH	2	6–30	24
		2 SRHZ/H	2	6–30	24
	6	2 SRHZ/RH or RH$_2$	0–2	0–10	51 or 35
		2 ERHZ/RH or RH$_2$	0–2	0–10	51 or 35
		2 SRHZ/SHZ$_2$	2	0–10	36

[a] For abbreviations see Table 59.1. The subscript 2 in RH$_2$ and SHZ$_2$ means that the drug combinations RH and SHZ, respectively, are to be taken twice weekly; where no subscript is indicated, drugs are to be taken daily.
[b] Price of drugs supplied by producers to WHO or UNICEF in 1985.

is to ensure that every tuberculous patient adheres to one or other of the regimens of proven efficacy regularly and for the required duration.

Antituberculosis drugs and sputum smear examinations necessary for monitoring treatment should be provided totally *free of charge* to all patients under the responsibility of the authorities vested with health matters in the community: this is the prime requisite for health care accessibility to patients, who must already more often than not pay for their transport to and from the health centre and must shoulder any loss of income due to their illness.

Direct supervision of the patient's drug intake by health staff during the first eight weeks of treatment is the first organizational step to take, whatever the place chosen to administer chemotherapy to the patient, i.e. whether in the general hospital, the closest health facility or the patient's home.

Clear technical guidelines must be given to

Changes during treatment of the erythrocyte sedimentation rate or of chest X-ray appearance are of no prognostic value, and these procedures, too, should be avoided. Chest X-ray examination can be made at the end of treatment to assess the extent of sequelae.

The only examinations indispensable for monitoring treatment efficacy are the bacteriological examinations conducted at *the end of treatment*. Some 90% of bacillary pulmonary tuberculosis patients treated with standard short-course regimens are sputum negative on both smear and culture by the end of the second month, this percentage steadily increasing during the following months. Close observation of large numbers of patients through prolonged periods of follow-up after completion of treatment has indicated that occasional, sporadic, sputum positivity (whether of smear or culture) is of no prognostic significance. For practical purposes, therefore, *cure, failure* and *relapse* can be defined as follows. A patient may be considered as *cured* when two smear examinations are negative at a month's interval at completion of treatment (one at one month before and one at the end of treatment). Treatment *failure* can be defined as the presence of bacilli in the sputum at two consecutive smear microscopy examinations conducted at an interval of one month or more, in a compliant patient under treatment for over five months. *Relapse* (in a patient previously declared cured) can be defined as the presence of bacilli in the sputum demonstrated by smear microscopy at two consecutive examinations at any time after the end of adequate chemotherapy.

No further special surveillance measure is necessary after completion of treatment if patients have regularly complied with the prescribed regimen for the adequate duration. Every patient on completion of treatment should be instructed to return immediately for further investigation in the unlikely event of recurrence of symptoms.

In the event of failure or relapse after short-course chemotherapy the great majority of patients harbour bacilli which are still sensitive to the antituberculosis drugs included in the initial regimes; the initial regimen should, therefore, be restarted, and continued under strict supervision. In case of failure or relapse after chemotherapy with a 12- or 18-month traditional thiacetazone/isoniazid regimen patients often harbour bacilli which are isoniazid resistant: if so, a 12-month re-treatment regimen, including rifampicin and ethambutol (daily, or daily during the first two months and twice weekly thereafter) will ensure recovery.

The definitions of *cure, failure* and *relapse* outlined above hold only for pulmonary tuberculosis cases, since failure or relapse in cases of extrapulmonary tuberculosis is exceptional and is usually not induced by bacterial resistance. Complete or partial subsidence of symptoms and extent of sequelae can be judged by clinical (and if necessary radiological) examination.

Finally some specific problems deserve consideration.

1 *Corticosteroids* at low doses may be prescribed for four weeks or so as a supplement to the antituberculosis chemotherapy in certain localized involvements where inflammatory reactions are serious (meningitis, serofibrinous pleuritis, ascites, pericarditis, pulmonary primary infection with segmental or lobal shadow).

2 *Chemoprophylaxis* with isoniazid alone at 5 mg/kg body weight for a period of six months may be prescribed in case of recent infection without clinical or radiological manifestations in non-BCG-vaccinated children under five years of age, living in close contact with a tuberculous patient and presenting with a strong positive reaction to tuberculin.

3 *A complementary orthopaedic or surgical treatment* may be necessary in certain extrapulmonary involvements: chronic pleuritis, chronic constrictive pericarditis, cerebral tuberculoma, spinal or bone and joint tuberculosis. Under these circumstances, surgical intervention should be preceded and followed by a sufficiently long course of chemotherapy.

BCG VACCINATION

When vaccination is made with a BCG vaccine assessed for quality and applied under proper technical conditions (freeze-dried vaccine inoculated immediately after its dilution as a strictly intradermal injection of 0.05 ml for children aged less than one year and of 0.1 ml for children aged one year and more, of the reconstituted vaccine with a graduated non-leaking syringe), it protects children to a considerable degree against severe forms of tuberculosis.

In high prevalence countries, therefore, children should be BCG-vaccinated as soon as possible after birth, so as to reduce the number of severe primary infections and of cases with miliary tuberculosis and meningitis. In most countries BCG vaccination is an integral part of the Expanded Programme of Immunization.

HEALTH SERVICES PLANNING FOR THE DELIVERY OF ANTITUBERCULOSIS MEASURES

On account of its prevalence in tropical countries tuberculosis is a particular problem for health services to deal with. This problem cannot be solved by heavy and expensive specialized structures located in urban areas, but rather through the implementation of a health action programme in all health facilities right down to the primary health care level in every region of the country.

1 The basic technical component of the programme is the establishment of a *microscopy lab-*

oratory network. Each peripheral laboratory must be equipped with a good microscope and staffed by two technicians trained in sputum smear collection, fixation, staining and reading. In view of the reagent, slide and sputum container supply situation and in view of the problems both of technical maintenance and of exacting quality control, the laboratories should not—lest their efficiency deteriorate—be located in basic health units but at the intermediate level, so as to meet the demands of a population of about 100 000, and to ensure about 1500 microscopy examinations per year per microscopy technician.[15,16] The microscopy laboratory would normally be a section of the local hospital laboratory.

These figures indicate an order of magnitude: the presence of microscopy laboratories for smaller population groups raises insuperable problems for the maintenance of equipment and quality control on a national scale. In densely populated areas, or in large cities, one microscopy laboratory can prove sufficient for a population of 300 000.

2 *Health staff employed in basic health units* at primary health care level should have, as far as tuberculosis is concerned, as their most important task the identification of tuberculosis suspects among clinic attenders and in the general population, on the basis of the clinical symptoms (and possibly also of radiological signs) observed. The main problem at this level is that of sputum sample collection. If a microscopy laboratory is nearby the easiest and most reliable procedure is to refer the suspect case to the laboratory where staff will collect directly from the patient, and under the proper conditions, the two sputum samples required for examination. But if the basic health facility and the microscopy laboratory lie too far apart it is necessary to plan the transport of sputum samples collected at the periphery: these samples must be collected from patients in non-leaking containers, kept at low temperature and away from light from the moment specimens are collected until they reach the laboratory. Transport should not exceed one week, lest bacilli present in the sputum be destroyed through remaining for too long a time under field conditions. Collection, storage and transport conditions should be kept under constant review so that sputum microscopy examination maintains its significance both for the patients and the health staff.

Procedures developed for the diagnosis of pulmonary tuberculosis in the various health facilities also apply to bacteriological examinations required at completion of chemotherapy.

To ensure optimal conditions for the identification of suspect cases, so that as many infectious patients as possible are diagnosed, it is essential that the population should have confidence in its health service, both at the level of *basic health units* (or first aid units) and at the level of *reference centres*. These services must deal with all demands for health care, including all forms of acute and chronic respiratory diseases which always occur more frequently than tuberculosis in any human population. An important element contributing to confidence in the health service is the proper and well-organized case-management of tuberculous patients under treatment.

3 *Organization of the treatment of tuberculous patients* is the key to the success of chemotherapy.

Nationwide *standardization* of chemotherapeutic regimens is a prerequisite to any action programme: the choice of the regimen (six, eight or 12 months) depends on resources available to health services for drug purchase. Regimens need to be standardized in order to facilitate planning of regular supply of drugs to health units in charge of treatment and to facilitate the free distribution of drugs to patients by health staff, at all levels, in the health units closest to the patients' homes. Precise technical guidelines should help health workers to prescribe the drugs required (specifying dosage according to patient's body weight) and to monitor he efficacy and possible toxicity of the treatment.

Drug taking should be supervised during the first two months of treatment; thereafter drug collections should be checked and the patient should be given sufficient explanation to ensure that he understands the importance of regular treatment and of regular collection of his drugs on prescheduled dates.

The *schedule* for technical follow-up visits (at which sputum specimens are due for collection: end of second month if possible, and end of treatment compulsorily) should be decided well in advance and brought to the patient's attention at the start of treatment.

Special measures should be taken to ensure provision of regular and efficient treatment in tuberculosis patients unable to come to the health centre (e.g. paraplegic or disabled patients, pregnant women, nomads) or suffering from certain other health problems (such as diabetes mellitus, chronic renal insufficiency, psychopathy).

Hospitalization may be necessary for patients who are seriously ill and it may also be of use during the initial phase of treatment of rural patients living unduly far away from a health facility. It has only secondary bearing on the success of the treatment of tuberculosis.

Specialists working in urban hospitals or in specialized tuberculosis clinics may act as consultants and help solve particular problems or complications occurring during treatment. But tasks involved with the treatment of tuberculous patients are performed, for the main part, by *multipurpose* health workers, whether medical or non-medical: the success of the treatment programme in the community depends on the quality of these health workers' work.

Decentralization of tuberculosis treatment in order to facilitate access by patients is the one organizational step which helps to prevent premature discontinuation of treatment. It also facilitates retrieval of patients who fail to attend one of the scheduled appointments. This retrieval will be impossible unless *all* the patient's addresses have been registered at the very start of the treatment in the patient's individual file, i.e. his personal address, his family's, his parents', as well as where he works or studies and the address of two of his friends or close relatives.

4 *Assessment of the tuberculosis control programme activities* is one of the fundamental elements of such programme. There are two principal tools for this assessment.

   (a) *A notification register* for tuberculosis cases put on treatment in a given area. In this register, the following information on cases admitted to treatment is recorded chronologically: particulars: age, sex, address; diagnosis and initial bacteriological status; date on which treatment was started; treatment regimen; follow-up schedule; results of bacteriological examinations during and at end of treatment; outcome of treatment.

   (b) *An individual patient file* should be kept at the unit where patients are treated and followed up.

By analysing data contained in a notification register which is kept up to date it is possible to assess *case-finding results* by calculating the numbers of notified tuberculosis cases by type of disease.

The *efficacy* of a *case-finding programme* can be assessed by comparing the number of smear-positive previously untreated cases identified through one year with the expected number of cases. For example, in a region where the annual risk of tuberculous infection is known to be 2%, some 100 smear-positive cases per 100 000 population can be expected to occur each year. When, in this situation, only 20 such cases (per 100 000 population) are diagnosed in any one year the case-finding programme is in obvious need of overhaul; if on the other hand, this figure reaches 70 the programme performance can be regarded as approaching a satisfactory standard. The proportion of pulmonary tuberculosis cases admitted to treatment without bacteriological evidence (e.g. acute miliary tuberculosis or nodular tuberculosis in children or adolescents) should not exceed 10% of the total cases of pulmonary tuberculosis; a higher rate would mean that some non-tuberculous patients are being treated or those who had tuberculosis previously but who are not in need of treatment anymore.

The analysis of a cohort of consecutive patients who were initially positive by direct smear is the basis for evaluating after six months or preferably one year after the start of treatment the true fate of cases enrolled, in terms of cured cases, failure cases, cases deceased and lost sight of and, thus, for *assessing the efficacy of the treatment programme*.

In general, early death (within two months of start of treatment) of a patient sputum positive on diagnosis indicates failure (delay) of case-finding rather than of treatment; later death from the disease is uncommon when treatment has been adhered to throughout the prescribed course. The low failure and relapse rates found among compliant patients together with the higher such rates among patients with irregular drug ingestion patterns do not under good field conditions exceed 5%. With an efficient health care network patients lost sight of before the end of treatment (and who must, therefore, be classified as failures) should not amount to more than 10%. Thus, with supervision of a well-planned programme the treatment success rate should be of the order of 85%. But when programme planning and programme implementation are inadequate even the most expensive chemotherapy will have a much lower, quite unacceptable, success rate.

Evaluation of the *BCG vaccination coverage* can be made by administrative processes if there are vaccination registers, or by investigating the percentage of children with vaccination scars in a selected target population. The coverage is considered satisfactory if at least 70% of the target population is reached. However, the best criterion on which to evaluate BCG vaccination is that of its practical efficacy: a reduced incidence of meningitis and acute miliary tuberculosis in children under five years of age. Such evaluation is only possible when facilities to diagnose these conditions exist.

CONCLUSION

Tuberculosis is an epidemiological and organizational challenge to the health services. A health index of poverty, it also epitomizes the health services' capacity to honour the right to health of the least privileged strata in every country, since a reliable and inexpensive technology to combat tuberculosis does exist.

REFERENCES

1 Rouillon, A. (1982) *Méd. Hyg.*, **40**, 1474–1482.

2 Styblo, K. & Rouillon, A. (1981) *Bull. int. Un. against Tuberc.* **56**, 118–126.

3 Chaulet, P., Aît Khaled, N. & Amrane, R. (1983) *Rev. fr. Mal. resp.* **11**, 79–110.

4 Bleiker, M. A. & Styblo, K. (1978) *Bull. int. Un. against Tuberc.* **53**, 295–298.

5 Styblo, K. (1984) Epidemiology of tuberculosis. In *Infektions Krankheiten und ihre Erreger*, Band 4/VII, pp. 77–161. Jena: Gustav Fischer Verlag.

6 World Health Organization (1983) *Wld Hlth Org. tech. Rep. Ser.*, no. 685.

7 Mazouni, L., Tazir, M., Boulahbal, F. et al (1985) *Rev. fr. Mal. resp.* **2**, 209–214.

8 Grosset, J., Truffot-Pernot, Ch., Poggi, S. et al (1985) *Rev. fr. Mal. resp.* **2**, 205–208.

9 Singapore Tuberculosis Service/BMRC (1985) *Am. Rev. resp. Dis.* **132**, 374–378.

10 Committee on Treatment of the International Union Against Tuberculosis (1983) *Bull. int. Un. against Tuberc.* **58**, 164–167.

11 Fox, W. (1981) *Br. J. Dis. Chest* **75**, 331–357.

12 Fox, W. (1984) *Lung India* **2**, 161–174.

13 Chaulet, P. (1983) *Bull. int. Un. against Tuberc.* **58**, 26–36.

14 Ross, J. D. & Horne, N. W. (1983) *Modern Drug Treatment in Tuberculosis*. 6th edn. London: Chest, Heart and Stroke Association, Tavistock Square.

15 Mitchison, D. A. (1974) *Trop. Doc.* **4**, 147–153.

16 Mitchison, D. A. (1982) *Bull. int. Un. against Tuberc.* **57**, 142–147.

Chapter 60
Gastroenterological Problems

G. C. Cook

INTRODUCTION

The portals of entry of organisms responsible for most infections which dominate medicine in the 'Third World', as elsewhere, are the skin, and respiratory and intestinal tracts. Consequently a very high proportion of the infections of warm climes originate from the ingestion of contaminated water and foodstuffs, and many of the resulting diseases fall into the subspecialty of gastroenterology.

MOUTH AND PHARYNX

The mouth and rectum are the most accessible parts of the gastrointestinal tract from a clinical viewpoint; therefore, where endoscopic procedures are not possible, and that applies to most tropical and subtropical countries, as much information as possible should be derived from careful examination of these organs.[1]

Viral, bacterial, mycotic and parasitic infections give rise to oropharyngeal pathology, and this is often most pronounced in the presence of associated malnutrition. Herpes simplex, Epstein–Barr (EB) virus and many enteroviruses can produce a stomatitis; oral ulceration is a common manifestation in Behçet's syndrome—common in the Middle East and Japan.[2] Lassa fever and diphtheria are often characterized by severe pharyngeal involvement and in rabies, dysphagia caused by spasm of the pharyngeal muscles is an important feature of the disease. As well as acute bacterial infections, tuberculosis, leprosy, syphilis and yaws all have oral manifestations. Candidiasis (common in the African acquired immunodeficiency syndrome (AIDS)), histoplasmosis, South American blastomycosis and coccidioidomycosis can also produce buccal lesions. The acute pharyngitis caused by infection with young adult *Fasciola hepatica* (ingested

in raw sheep or goat liver, reported from the Middle East and India, and known locally as 'halzoun'[3] (Chapter 22), is also caused by pentastomids (Chapter 24). Therapeutic agents such as sulphonamides (included in some antimalarial prophylactics) can give rise to the Stevens–Johnson syndrome in which oral ulceration is common. The manifestations of specific malnutrition states: vitamin B and C deficiencies and iron deficiency anaemia, are obvious, whereas in kwashiorkor these are often combined with infective complications. Cancrum oris, a gangrenous condition involving the gums and cheeks, and associated with *Borrelia vincenti* and *Fusiformis fusiformis* infection is particularly common in malnourished children—especially in West Africa (Chapter 45). Descriptions of the mouth, especially the tongue, in tropical sprue (Chapter 19) were dominant in clinical accounts of this disease in the nineteenth century (i.e. before the advent of laboratory investigations).[1]

Periodontal disease and dental caries are common in 'Third World' countries. Oral submucous fibrosis is a chronic disease of unknown aetiology which may affect any part of the oral cavity—most reports are from the Indian subcontinent and South-East Asia.[4] Fibroelastosis of the submucous tissues with epithelial atrophy are important features and these are probably premalignant changes.

Of the malignant diseases, buccal carcinoma is numerically pre-eminent (Chapter 67); Burkitt's lymphoma, ameloblastoma and nasopharyngeal carcinoma[5] are other malignancies which have important geographical distributions in tropical countries.

Hypertrophy of the salivary glands is especially common in malnourished children (Chapter 45) and is also associated with ascariasis and chronic calcific pancreatitis (see below). Tumours of the salivary glands are probably no more common than in temperate regions.

OESOPHAGUS

The most important disease to involve this organ is oesophageal carcinoma (Chapter 67). Mega-oesophagus, a feature of chronic *Trypanosoma cruzi* infection (Chagas' disease), is described in Chapter 3. Table 60.1 lists some causes of dysphagia in a tropical environment.

Table 60.1 Some causes of dysphagia.

Trauma	Gastritis
	Foreign bodies
	Corrosive agents
Infection	South American trypanosomiasis (Chagas' disease)
	Candidiasis
	Rhizopus, Absidia (mucormycosis)
Neoplasia	Oesophageal carcinoma
Oesophageal varices	Macronodular cirrhosis
	Schistosomiasis
	Portal vein thrombosis
	Tropical splenomegaly syndrome
Others	Achalasia
	Peptic oesophagitis
	Hiatus hernia
Extrinsic pressure	Endemic goitre

Oesophageal varices usually result from advanced macronodular cirrhosis (see below); hepatic schistosomiasis (*Schistosoma mansoni, S. japonicum, S. intercalatum* and *S. mekongi*) accounts for other cases (Chapter 22). Portal vein obstruction is also common in some parts of Africa and Asia, probably resulting from umbilical sepsis in the neonatal period in most, but it is occasionally associated with hepatocellular carcinoma. The very high splenic blood flow associated with the tropical splenomegaly syndrome can also give rise to oesophageal varices (see below). Where and when available sclerotherapy is of value in the treatment of oesophageal varices,[6, 7] but the ideal method of managing bleeding varices remains unresolved.[8]

Oesophageal trauma is a major problem in some African countries; foreign bodies (e.g. kola nuts and fish bones) and corrosive agents—which can give rise to strictures are also common.[9] Achalasia, peptic oesophagitis and hiatus hernia all occur but are not particularly common.

In the African AIDS syndrome (Chapter 68) oesophageal candidiasis is common (Chapter 35); other systemic mycoses can also produce an oesophagitis.

STOMACH AND DUODENUM

Peptic ulceration was at one time considered to be an unusual cause of abdominal pain in the tropics and was in fact thought to be a rare condition. It is now clear, however, that this is not the case and many of the difficulties facing the clinical epidemiologist in the Third World are highlighted by studies of the geographical distribution of this disease.[1] Because sophisticated methods of diagnosis—barium meal and upper gastrointestinal endoscopy[10, 11]—have not until very recently been widely used in developing Third World countries, diagnosis and attempts at establishing incidence rates have depended upon recording incidence rates of complications, especially pyloric stenosis (haemorrhage seems to be unusual and that is probably because such patients do not get as far as hospital before exsanguination occurs). Thus, it is very difficult to have any reliable idea of the true frequency, and to be able to comment accurately on regional and rural/urban patterns, and also upon variations with time, i.e. as 'westernization' takes place.

As recently as the 1950s, duodenal ulcer was considered to be a rare disease in Africa;[12] that is now known with certainty not to be the case because good radiological, and more recently endoscopic, facilities have given some idea of the true prevalence rate. Duodenal ulcer frequency has been assessed by Tovey in Africa from the available literature;[13] high incidence areas have been reported in parts of West Africa, Rwanda, Burundi, eastern Zaire, western Tanzania, south-western Uganda and the Ethiopian highlands. In south India[14] and Papua New Guinea the disease is also relatively common. The disease is often post-bulbar, and presentation with pyloric obstruction is relatively usual; the disease has a marked male predominance. Genetic factors might well be important; the role of dietary factors is difficult to assess. Whether the low rate of presentation with haemorrhage and perforation is a true reflection of events or is biased by inability to get sick patients to hospital is very difficult to evaluate. Evidence for an infective basis is growing.[15] *Campylobacter pylori* has been incriminated, but so far not all of Koch's postulates have been satisfied.[16]

Overall, gastric ulcer is not common in Third World countries. When it does occur it is most common in the fifth and sixth decades and has a male predominance. Pyloric obstruction is a common presentation, due frequently to the late stage of disease when first seen.

The management of bleeding peptic ulcers has been reviewed.[17] Gastritis, often caused by alcohol and spicy foods is a major cause of abdominal pain (Table 60.2). Infective causes of

Table 60.2 Some causes of chronic abdominal pain or discomfort.

Peptic ulcer disease
Gastric carcinoma
Gastritis
Small intestinal infections:
  Ascaris lumbricoides
  Hookworm
  Strongyloides stercoralis
  Giardia lamblia
Colorectal disease: amoebic and schistosomal colitis. Severe
  trichuriasis
Chronic calcific pancreatitis
Liver disease: many forms of hepatitis—viral, bacterial and
  parasitic; hepatoma
Biliary disease:
  Ascaris lumbricoides
  Clonorchiasis
  Opisthorchiasis
Familial Mediterranean fever

---

gastritis, including tuberculosis seem to be rare, although they are occasionally encountered; infections which involve predominantly the lower intestinal tract (e.g. typhoid and shigellosis) can occasionally produce gastric pathology. With regard to treatment, if H_2 receptor antagonists are used in developing Third World countries, the possibility exists that they will allow proliferation of intestinal infections, both bacterial and parasitic, for the gastric acid defence mechanism will be removed; more data are required on this point. There have been many studies of gastric acid production in different groups; overall mean acid production probably varies little in different ethnic groups. However, hypochlorhydria is probably relatively common in the tropics and whether it is the cause or consequence of intestinal infection (both bacterial—including typhoid fever—and parasitic) is still far from clear.[18, 19]

Gastric carcinoma is not unduly common in tropical countries (Chapter 67).

SMALL INTESTINE

Diarrhoea resulting from disease of the small intestine is of two main types: profuse watery

(e.g. cholera) and steatorrhoeic (as in tropical sprue)[1, 20] (Chapters 12, 19 and 57). Table 60.3 summarizes the most important causes; most of those responsible for the former type are infective and they exert their pathogenic effect by enterotoxin (heat-stable or heat-liable) production; invasive disease involving the enterocyte is of lesser overall importance. The role of intestinal hormones, especially vasoactive intestinal peptide (VIP) in the production of watery diarrhoea is now appreciated. The pathogenesis of diarrhoea in African AIDS is by no means clear; some but not all cases are associated with opportunistic infections, especially *Cryptosporidium* spp. Other opportunistic infections in this disease include cytomegalovirus (CMV), *Mycobacterium avium intracellulare*, salmonellae, *Isospora belli, Sarcocystis hominis, Microsporidium* spp. and *Strongyloides stercoralis*. In addition, Kaposi's sarcoma sometimes invades the small intestine (Chapter 67).

In all cases, the basis of management is oral

Table 60.3 Small-intestinal diarrhoea.

(a) *Watery diarrhoea* (characteristically large volume, fluid
    stools)
      Travellers' diarrhoea (turista)
      Vibrio cholerae (and other vibrios)
      Escherichia coli (enterotoxigenic)
      Salmonella spp.
      Campylobacter jejuni
      Rotavirus (and other enteric viruses)
      Cryptosporidium spp.
      (Food poisoning—*Staphylococcus, Clostridium*
        perfringens)
      Hypolactasia (a) *primary*—genetically determined
              (b) *secondary*—resulting from enterocyte
                 damage

(b) *Fatty diarrhoea (malabsorption)* (characteristically large
    pale, fatty, offensive stools; microscopy often shows fat
    globules in faecal smears)
    Gluten-induced enteropathy (coeliac disease) seems to be
    uncommon or even rare in most tropical populations.
    Occasionally it can be made clinically obvious in visitors
    from Western countries to the tropics
    Tropical sprue (postinfective tropical malabsorption)
    Intestinal parasites:
      Giardia lamblia
      Strongyloides stercoralis
      Capillaria philippinensis
      Coccidia: *Cryptosporidium* spp.
              Isospora belli
              Sarcocystis hominis
    Trauma—short bowel syndrome (e.g. recovered 'pigbel'
    disease)
    Lymphoma—Burkitt's, Mediterranean lymphoma
    Ileocaecal tuberculosis
    Chronic calcific pancreatitis
    Acute and chronic liver disease

---

rehydration (Chapter 12). Only in exceptional cases should antibiotics be prescribed either prophylactically or therapeutically; side-effects can be severe and the production of further antibiotic-resistant organisms (frequently by plasmid transfer) is a major problem; anti-peristaltic agents should also be used as rarely as possible for they prevent excretion of the responsible pathogen and prolong the carrier state.

Throughout tropical countries, minor degrees of small-intestinal damage are common, and this seems to be related to recurrent small-intestinal infections, of viral, bacterial and parasitic origin. Morphological changes are mild and the term *tropical enteropathy* is usually applied; malabsorption too is only marginal, and overt evidence of failure to absorb dietary constituents is absent (only minor abnormalities in the xylose test, for example, are present) (Chapter 19).

The vast majority of small-intestinal parasitic infections do not produce signs or symptoms unless present at a very high concentration.[21] In heavy infection, hookworm is responsible for hypochromic anaemia, and *Ascaris lumbricoides* can rarely produce obstruction in the small intestine, and biliary and pancreatic ducts (Chapter 21). The major sequel resulting from tapeworm infection is cysticercosis (*Taenia solium*) which is unrelated to the intestinal tract (Chapter 23).

Apart from infective causes, *primary* hypolactasia (lactase deficiency) (Chapter 19) is a further cause of watery small-intestinal diarrhoea in people indigenous to tropical countries. It is now clear that a low concentration of this enzyme in the brush border region of the enterocyte is the usual state for adult *Homo sapiens* as it is for other species of the mammalian kingdom.[22] This is under genetic control. Only in a minority of our species, i.e. northern Europeans, Africans with a Hamitic ancestry, certain Middle Eastern populations (e.g. Saudi Arabians), and those in northern parts of the Indian subcontinent is a high concentration preserved into adult life.[22] *Secondary* hypolactasia is caused by brush border damage (Chapter 19); all disaccharidases (and other digestive enzymes located there) are reduced in concentration and recover slowly after the initiating insult has disappeared. Thus, whenever enterocyte destruction occurs (tropical sprue included) a proportion of cases develop hypolactasia. Following ingestion of milk or some other milk product (in which lactose is not completely hydrolysed), an osmotic diarrhoea results, with abdominal colic, distension and flatulence. This results from intact lactose remaining within the lumen. Lactic acid production from hydrolysis of lactose by colonic bacteria produces an irritative diarrhoea which contributes to the symptoms. The precise role of the colon in adaptation is still unclear, but it is now known that a considerable quantity of carbohydrate in the form of free fatty acids (and also nitrogen and electrolytes) can be absorbed from this organ. Investigation of hypolactasia most often utilizes the breath hydrogen test, although lactose tolerance tests and assay of the enzyme in jejunal biopsy specimens are also used. In treatment, milk and all dairy products containing lactose should be eliminated from the diet; many people in tropical countries with *primary* hypolactasia regulate bowel function by varying lactose ingestion. Yoghurt is usually well tolerated because it contains adequate bacterial lactase to hydrolyse the lactose contained therein.

Table 60.3 also summarizes some causes of steatorrhoea (small-intestinal diarrhoea resulting from *malabsorption*). Most of these diseases are dealt with in Section II, and chronic calcific pancreatitis and liver disease, below. The role of parasitic infection has been highlighted by AIDS in which prolonged diarrhoea with malabsorption and weight loss can be a very troublesome clinical feature. In this context, *Cryptosporidium* spp. and *Isospora belli* have recently come to the fore and it is now also clear that these organisms can produce a self-limiting illness simulating travellers' diarrhoea (Chapter 14) in immunocompetent adults and children (Chapter 17). Whilst *Giardia lamblia* is undoubtedly the most common cause of parasitic malabsorption (Chapter 17), *Strongyloides stercoralis*, which is widespread in tropical countries and is still present in approximately 15–30% of former prisoners of war in South East Asia during the Second World War, is an underdiagnosed cause (Chapter 21).

Of all causes of malabsorption in relation to tropical exposure, *intestinal tuberculosis*, usually involving the ileocaecal region, is probably the one with the lowest 'index of suspicion' amongst medical personnel. Abdominal tuberculosis can take several clinical forms; apart from the hypertrophic ileocaecal type, glandular (involving the mesenteric glands), peritoneal (sometimes with ascites) and hepatic involvement (with granulomatous disease) are relatively common.[23] With the first type weight loss and diarrhoea are often accompanied by a low grade febrile illness; in severe cases the stools are large, pale and bulky. Examination sometimes reveals an ileocaecal mass and occasionally enlargement of one or more lymph glands; however, there is often no clinical abnormality. Late presentation can be as 'adult kwashiorkor'. Anaemia is common. Chest X-ray is usually normal. Tests of absorption are frequently abnormal; fat and B_{12} absorption are affected principally. There may also be a protein-losing enteropathy. Pathologically, the disease results either from miliary disease or follows ileal ulceration. The malabsorption is caused by a chronic loss of bile salts, normally reabsorbed in the terminal ileum; unabsorbed bile salts in turn interfere with colonic absorption. Barium meal and follow-through shows ileal strictures in a high percentage of cases, frequently multiple; the ascending colon may be shortened. The main differential diagnosis is Crohn's disease, which is much less common statistically in people indigenous to the tropics. *Yersinia* infection should also be considered (Chapter 14). The tuberculin test is usually positive. Needle liver biopsy sometimes shows hepatic granulomas with caseation. Diagnostic laparotomy is often necessary to obtain a tissue diagnosis. Treatment is with antituberculous regimens. Resection of strictures and even hemicolectomy are often necessary; chemotherapy should be started before surgical intervention.

A further cause of malabsorption in a tropical environment is the Mediterranean (α-chain) lymphoma which occurs sporadically in many parts of the tropics (Chapter 67).[24] If started early tetracycline can give good results.

LARGE INTESTINE

The vast majority of colorectal diseases in tropical countries have an infective basis (Table 60.4).[1] Most are therefore dealt with in Section II and they include the bacterial (shigellosis, *Campylobacter* spp. and invasive *Escherichia coli* infections) and protozoal (amoebiasis (Fig. 60.1) and balantidiasis) infections. In African AIDS (Chapter 68) cytomegalovirus (CMV) colitis is common; although *Cryptosporidium* is usually a small-intestinal parasite, colonic involvement can also occur. In addition, megacolon resulting from South American trypanosomiasis (Chagas' disease) (Chapter 3) also gives rise to colonic pathology. Of problems localized to the anal region, lymphogranuloma (Chapter 68) is

Table 60.4   Large-intestinal diarrhoea.[a]

Bacterial infection
  Shigellosis
  Campylobacter spp.
  Escherichia coli (enteroinvasive)

Protozoal infection
  Entamoeba histolytica
  Balantidium coli
Schistosomiasis

Unusual causes of colonic disease
  Non-specific ulcerative colitis } inflammatory bowel disease[b]

  Crohn's disease
  Appendicitis
  Diverticulitis
  Haemorrhoids
  Colonic carcinoma
  Irritable bowel syndrome

[a] Characteristically: numerous small stools containing mucus, pus and blood; microscopy shows pus cells and/or red blood cells in faecal smears.

[b] Although these diseases are uncommon, or even rare, in most tropical populations, they can be made clinically obvious for the first time in visitors from Western countries to the tropics.

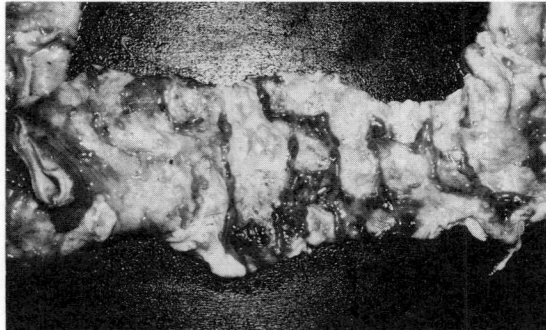

Fig. 60.1   Severe amoebic colitis; operative specimen from a patient misdiagnosed as having non-specific ulcerative colitis who deteriorated on corticosteroid management.

perhaps the most important, although other bacterial (including donovanosis, syphilis and gonorrhoea) and parasitic (including amoebiasis, schistosomiasis and enterobiasis) infections enter the list of differential diagnoses.[1]

The colorectal region is the part of the anatomy of *Homo sapiens* where there are *par excellence* major differences in disease incidence rates between Third World and westernized populations. The vast differences in incidence rates for colonic and rectal carcinoma for example, are covered in Chapter 67; overall these diseases are far less common in indigenous people in Third World developing countries compared with people in industrialized countries. Reasonable evidence now exists that their frequency is increasing with urbanization, in particular in Africa. Several theories have been put forward, including the greater consumption of dietary fibre in most tropical countries; however, these associations rarely have a proven cause–effect relationship.

Much has been written about bowel function in Third World countries; it seems probable that in Africa 24-hour stool weight and volume is higher, and that constipation is unusual. Overall, intestinal transit rate seems to be more rapid. There is some evidence that colorectal histology is mildly different in indigenous people in Third World countries, and is in some ways similar to tropical enteropathy.[25] Certainly in tropical sprue (see above) colonic functional abnormalities have been demonstrated in vivo in India.[26] Whether colonic pathology is important in a nutritional context is difficult to evaluate. There is now very good evidence that this organ is important in the absorption of nitrogen and free (volatile) fatty acids and it seems likely that colonic pathology must have some nutritional importance.[27, 28]

Inflammatory bowel disease (IBD) (non-specific ulcerative colitis (UC) (Fig. 60.2) and Crohn's disease (CD)) is far less common overall in indigenous people in the Third World than it is in the UK and other Western countries. There is only a small minority of reports of UC from African countries, with a few more from Asia; in people from the Caribbean and the Indian subcontinent in the UK the disease does exist, however. These differences apply to Crohn's disease probably to an even greater extent, although again the disease is also well recognized in Caribbean people in the UK. The aetiology of these diseases is completely unknown, although an infective basis has frequently been suggested; however sound evidence for a viral or bacterial (possibly mycobacterial) origin is at present lacking.[16] Although it behaves very much like tuberculosis of the intestinal tract in clinical practice, response to antituberculous therapy in Crohn's disease is extremely disappointing.[29] When IBD does occur it seems to behave in a similar way to that in the indigenous population of the UK. IBD is a common cause of bloody diarrhoea in travellers from temperate to tropical countries.[30] Similarly, appendicitis, diverticular disease and haemorrhoids are less common overall in developing country populations and again a higher 'fibre' intake has been implicated;

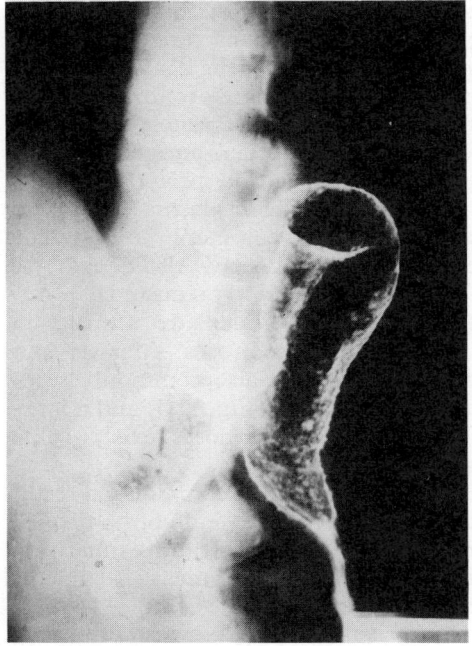

Fig. 60.2 Barium enema in a 35-year-old woman who experienced bloody diarrhoea during a visit to Africa; she had never previously had significant colonic problems. Non-specific ulcerative colitis was confirmed by tissue diagnosis at colonoscopy.

a causative association has not, however, been proved. Reasonable evidence exists that all of these diseases are increasing with urbanization in the Third World.

Although irritable bowel syndrome (IBS) (spastic colon) is a common problem in UK residents and others after an intestinal infection acquired in a tropical country it seems to be far less so in indigenous people in Africa and Asia. Whether that is a genuine difference is unclear because so many of the latter have more severe symptoms from different origins and these might mask symptoms of IBS. This syndrome is not a single entity and although some cases respond to mebeverine many do not.

Colonoscopy is a technique which is now available in some developing countries, albeit only at the teaching hospital and other centres of relative excellence.

LIVER AND BILIARY SYSTEM

The histology of the liver in indigenous people in tropical countries differs from that in an individual who has spent his/her life in a temperate part of the world.[1,31,32] First, it is subject to many systemic infections—viral, bacterial and parasitic—and secondly, it lies at the distal end of the portal circulation and is therefore 'bathed' with intestinal viruses, bacteria, parasites, ova, products of digestion and other antigens. Thus, Kupffer cell hyperplasia and periportal infiltration (with lymphocytes, plasma cells and eosinophils) are more common, and stellate fibrosis occurs more frequently. Also hepatocyte nuclear pleomorphism and sinusoidal lymphocytosis are features which are unusual in biopsies in temperate countries. Malaria and schistosomal pigment are also commonly seen. Granulomas are common (Fig. 60.3) and a large number of differential diagnoses exist; Table 60.5 lists some of them.[33,34]

Although jaundice is most commonly a result of viral hepatitis (types A, B, and non-A non-B) (Chapter 6), other important causes must also be considered. Table 60.6 summarizes some of them. An important cause is the jaundice of acute systemic bacterial infection,[35] most commonly caused by pneumococcal lobar pneumonia and pyomyositis. The mechanism of this type of jaundice is complex and consists of hepatocellular, cholestatic[36] and haemolytic elements, the importance of the latter depending to some

Table 60.5 Some of the more common causes of hepatic granulomas in tropical countries.

Infection:	
viral:	cytomegalovirus, EB virus
bacterial:	tuberculosis and atypical mycobacteria, leprosy, syphilis, Q fever, brucellosis
parasitic:	schistosomiasis, ascariasis, strongyloidiasis, toxocariasis, filariasis, enterobiasis, visceral leishmaniasis
fungi:	histoplasmosis, coccidioidomycosis, aspergillosis, actinomycosis, candidiasis
Neoplasms:	lymphomas, especially intra-abdominal Hodgkin's disease
Others:	(sarcoidosis) therapeutic agents: especially sulphonamides

Table 60.6 Some causes of jaundice in the tropics.

Jaundice of acute bacterial infection: pneumococcal lobar pneumonia, pyomyositis

Viruses:	hepatitis A, B and non-A, non-B yellow fever EB virus cytomegalovirus Marburg and Ebola diseases
Bacteria:	leptospirosis typhoid fever syphilis gonococcal disease bartonellosis
Parasites:	malaria (acute *Plasmodium falciparum* and *P. vivax*) schistosomiasis amoebiasis (rarely) toxoplasmosis trichinellosis fascioliasis ⎱ clonorchiasis ⎬ predominantly opisthorchiasis ⎰ large-duct ascariasis ⎰ obstructive jaundice hydatidosis (rarely)
Genetic:	sickle cell disease glucose-6-phosphate dehydrogenase deficiency Dubin–Johnson syndrome

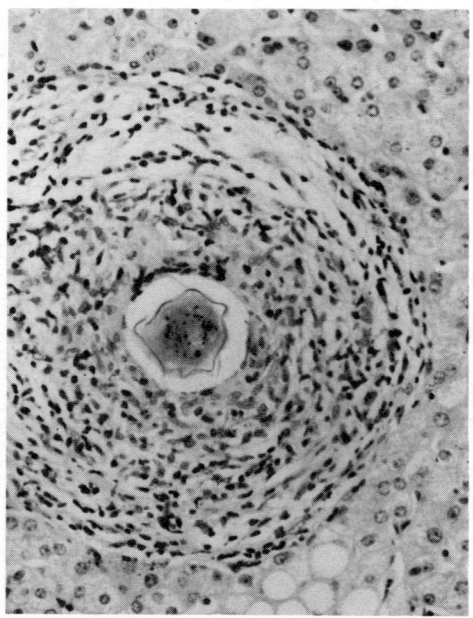

Fig. 60.3 Liver biopsy specimen from a 30-year-old Zambian woman showing a granuloma surrounding a degenerating egg of *Schistosoma mansoni*.

extent on the underlying incidence of glucose-6-phosphate dehydrogenase (G-6-PD) deficiency in the population under consideration (Chapter 58). It is important to differentiate this form of jaundice from viral hepatitis, otherwise the appropriate antibiotic will not be given for the underlying bacterial infection. Apart from the Marburg and Ebola viruses (Chapter 5), Lassa fever can produce a significant hepatitis; Dengue fever, Kyasanur Forest disease (Chapter 5), herpes simplex, EB and Coxsackie viruses are other causes.

In African AIDS (Chapter 68), the liver is affected by many opportunistic organisms including viruses; hepatitis B infections can be especially virulent. Liver biopsy may also yield evidence of CMV, *Mycobacterium tuberculosis*, *Mycobacterium avium intracellulare*, atypical mycobacteria, *Cryptosporidium* spp., *Pneumocystis carinii*, *Cryptococcus* and Kaposi's sarcoma. Cholestatic features are common.

Apart from septicaemia, several bacterial infections can produce jaundice; leptospirosis is usually accompanied by renal involvement (Chapter 32), whilst overt jaundice in typhoid fever is unusual. Melioidosis, plague, tularaemia (Chapter 27) and relapsing fever (Chapter 32) can also produce a hepatitis. Of parasitic causes, acute malaria is perhaps the most important. In acute (Katayama syndrome) and severe chronic schistosomiasis, and rarely (Chapter 22) in invasive amoebiasis, jaundice may be present. It is important, also to appreciate that most parasitic infections, including trypanosomiasis (Chapter 2) and visceral leishmaniasis (Chapter 4), can produce significant hepatitis and deranged hepatocellular function, often in the absence of clinical jaundice.

Several parasites (Table 60.6) can produce large duct biliary obstruction (see p. 1007); for practical reasons, ascariasis is probably the most important to recognize and treat (Chapter 21).

Of genetic causes, sickle cell disease and other haemoglobinopathies are important causes of haemolytic jaundice (Chapter 58). Jaundice in the presence of G-6-PD deficiency is frequently precipitated or worsened by therapeutic agents and toxins. In some parts of the tropics, especially Indonesia and Papua New Guinea, the Dubin–Johnson syndrome seems unusually common.[35]

Macronodular cirrhosis: there is now no doubt that most cases of this disease in tropical countries result from viral hepatitis—hepatitis B virus (HBV) most commonly, and to a lesser extent non-A non-B hepatitis. The sequence of events is: acute hepatitis→chronic active hepatitis→macronodular cirrhosis→hepatocellular carcinoma (hepatoma)[37] (acute viral hepatitis is dealt with in Chapter 6 and hepatoma in Chapter 67). Although HBV is undoubtedly the most important aetiological factor in hepatoma, the role of aflatoxin should not be completely disregarded.[38]

Most cases of chronic active hepatitis in tropical countries are therefore a result of HBV infection; in that form of the disease corticosteroids should not be administered for they exacerbate viral replication in the hepatocyte; interferon and adenine arabinoside have recently given encouraging results.[39] There is no good evidence that malnutrition (including kwashiorkor) or malaria are aetiologically important, although such beliefs still exist. Clinically, cutaneous stigmata of chronic hepatocellular disease are difficult to detect in brown or black skins. Similarly, other cutaneous stigmata of chronic liver disease may not be present. Diagnosis is by abnormal liver function tests, and a needle liver biopsy specimen is usually diagnostic. Peritoneoscopy is a technique which is relatively simple and underused in developing Third World countries; the more refined techniques are rarely available. When cirrhosis is established no treatment is of any avail. The major complications resulting from portal hypertension are: (i) haemorrhage from oesophageal varices, (ii) fluid retention and ascites, and (iii) hepatic encephalopathy. Pitressin (vasopressin) injection forms the basis of management of variceal haemorrhage; if and where available, upper gastrointestinal endoscopy with sclerotherapy is of value but this technique has usually to be repeated at intervals of six months or so. The Sengstaken tube, used for compressing varices, still has a place—especially in the Third World. Incidentally, haemorrhage is not a frequent presenting feature at most tropical hospitals, in many instances presumably because exsanguination occurs before the patient can reach hospital. Fluid retention is often a major problem, largely due to very low serum albumin concentrations. It is difficult to manage, partly because salt restriction is virtually impossible to impose; diuretics e.g. frusemide (Lasix) (40–120 mg daily) and spironolactone (Aldactone) (100 mg daily) usually achieve success. Paracentesis abdominis[40] should rarely be undertaken for as well as further depleting albumin stores, electrolyte balance can be seriously disturbed; 'tapping' ascitic fluid should be reserved for (i) diagnostic purposes—to determine whether tuberculous peritonitis or hepatocellular carcinoma has complicated an otherwise benign case of ascites; and (ii) management of tense ascites with respiratory embarrassment.[40] Hepatic encephalopathy[41] is managed by orthodox methods—oral neomycin (6 g daily) and/or lactulose (20–35 g three times a day); in the presence of hypolactasia lactose can be substituted for lactulose.

Other forms of cirrhosis include: alcoholic, veno-occlusive disease (Chapter 49) and Indian childhood cirrhosis. Wilson's disease (hepatolenticular degeneration) and other genetically determined forms of cirrhosis are of little or no importance numerically although they should enter the list of differential diagnoses.

Alcohol-related disease is common in both indigenous and expatriate populations in tropical countries. Genetic factors might be involved[42] and carriers of hepatitis B surface antigen (HBsAg) might also be especially vulnerable to disease. The actual quantity of alcohol ingestion per day required to produce this disease is still not known with accuracy and estimates vary widely; there is no doubt that a wide individual variation exists, and that women tolerate chronic alcohol ingestion less well than men. There are no major differences from the disease in temperate climates. Acute alcoholic hepatitis is underdiagnosed and has a high mortality rate; the role of corticosteroids in this condition is still disputed; if they are of any value at all it is marginal and they should probably be confined to severe, advanced cases. The liver in chronic alcoholic disease is classically micronodular but not always so; histology often shows characteristic Mallory's hyaline deposits and haemosiderin may be present in excess.

Indian childhood cirrhosis is largely confined to India, especially south India, Calcutta and the Punjab. Diagnosis is usually made between one and a half and three years of age and it is frequently familial; the upper strata of Hindu society are often affected. It can run fulminant, acute or subacute courses and carries a high mortality rate. Histologically there is progressive fibrosis with absence of regeneration; macro- and micronodular cirrhosis can result. Hepatocellular carcinoma is an uncommon complication. There now seems little doubt that the disease is associated with a high copper intake; epidemiological evidence suggests that early weaning and milk feeding from copper vessels gives rise to an excess copper intake.[43, 44] However, the possibility of an inherited defect resulting in excess copper absorption and/or metabolism has not been eliminated. The clinical course varies widely and is comparable to acute fulminant viral hepatitis at one extreme, and cir-

rhosis with one or all of its classical complications at the other extreme of the spectrum (see above). There is no adequate treatment but clearly milk for infant and childhood consumption should not be stored in copper-containing vessels.

Haemosiderosis (African siderosis) (see also Chapter 66) is confined to southern and to a lesser extent parts of East and West Africa. Whether it can proceed to a true cirrhosis is arguable; a heavy alcohol intake often takes place in areas where the disease is common and it is frequently impossible to exclude that as a factor in the aetiology of cirrhosis, as in haemochromatosis.[45] There is no doubt that iron-containing pots for cooking are commonly used in most areas where haemosiderosis is common, but other factors also seem to be involved. Also, chronic pancreatitis is often common in those areas, and there is good evidence that an excess of iron (and often fat also) in hepatocytes is common in that condition in several parts of Africa.

Portal hypertension can result from any form of chronic liver disease. Table 60.7 summarizes some of the causes of raised portal venous pressure in tropical countries. Coupled with cirrhosis is schistosomal liver disease ('pipe-stem' fibrosis) (Chapter 22); however, because hepatocellular function is preserved to a far greater extent and for longer than in cirrhosis, fluid retention and more importantly encephalopathy are not as common. A form of non-cirrhotic liver disease exists in India and that can be associated with portal hypertension; despite various suggestions

Table 60.7   Causes of portal hypertension in tropical countries.

Hepatic:	cirrhosis (macronodular, alcoholic, Indian childhood etc.) schistosomal ('pipe-stem') fibrosis veno-occlusive disease
Prehepatic:	tropical splenomegaly syndrome (TSS) portal vein occlusion splenic vein occlusion
Posthepatic:	cardiac failure (rheumatic cardiac disease) endomyocardial fibrosis (EMF) constrictive pericarditis

including arsenic poisoning, the aetiology is unknown. Veno-occlusive disease occurs in localized areas in the tropics (Chapter 49). Of prehepatic causes, the tropical splenomegaly syndrome (TSS) (p. 1008) is the most common; this gives rise to an increased splenic blood flow. Portal and splenic vein obstruction, probably resulting from umbilical sepsis in the neonatal period, are causes throughout tropical countries which are undoubtedly under-diagnosed; hepatocellular function is preserved. Other causes are: hepatocellular carcinoma, and various dehydrating diseases including dysentery and cholera. Posthepatic causes of portal hypertension include cardiac failure (usually resulting from chronic rheumatic cardiac disease), right-sided endomyocardial fibrosis, and constrictive pericarditis (Chapter 61) usually, but not always, resulting from tuberculosis. Clinically, splenomegaly is present in all forms of portal hypertension (that must be distinguished from other causes of splenomegaly in tropical countries). Barium swallow or upper gastrointestinal endoscopy usually demonstrates oesophageal varices. If available, ultrasonography is valuable especially in assessing patency of the portal vein.

The liver is also extensively involved in most chronic infective diseases but it is unusual for decompensation and liver failure to occur; tuberculosis, leprosy, syphilis, actinomycosis, visceral leishmaniasis and African histoplasmosis being examples. The major space-occupying lesions involving the liver are: amoebic 'abscess' (Chapter 17), pyogenic abscess, and hydatid disease[31,32] (Chapter 23); tuberculomas, cysticercosis and melioidosis (Chapter 27) can also give rise to such lesions. Of non-infective diseases, sickle cell disease, β-thalassaemia, haemoglobin H disease (Chapter 58), porphyria (Chapter 66) and α_1-antitrypsin deficiency can all produce hepatic pathology.

Biliary pathology in tropical countries is largely attributable to parasites—clonorchiasis, opisthorchiasis (Chapter 22) and ascariasis (Chapter 21)—although pigment stones (often intrahepatic) occasionally occur in sickle cell disease (Chapter 58). Overall, cholesterol stones and secondary infection associated with these are uncommon in Third World populations, especially in Africa. Typhoid involvement of the gallbladder can give rise to the typhoid carrier state, but most often the source of chronic infection is intrahepatic (Chapter 8). Carcinoma of the gallbladder is unusual. Ascariasis is an under-diagnosed cause of large-duct obstruction;[46] it must always be considered in this clinical situation in a tropical context, where it can be confused with pancreatic carcinoma. Endoscopy, if available, is of value; laparotomy may be necessary for diagnosis although medical treatment should always be tried first. Clonorchiasis and opisthorchiasis, acquired from eating raw freshwater fish can cause cholangiohepatitis and biliary obstruction; cholangiocarcinoma is a late complication of both of these infections (Chapters 22, 67). Fascioliasis can give rise to tender hepatomegaly and jaundice and occasionally produces a problem in diagnosis from viral hepatitis; an eosinophilia is, however, common with all biliary trematodes (Chapter 22).

PANCREAS

The two major diseases involving this organ in tropical countries and which differ from those in temperate ones are: (i) 'J-type' diabetes, which was first reported in Jamaica, and (ii) chronic calcific pancreatitis.

Diabetes which is not associated with pancreatic calcification in young people is seen throughout tropical countries; those affected are usually thin, and require high doses of insulin, but do not rapidly become ketotic when insulin is stopped. This entity was first described in Jamaica as 'J-type' diabetes[47] (Chapter 66) and might have a viral aetiology, possibly involving one of the Coxsackie group of viruses; an increased incidence of antibody to Coxsackie B_4 has been demonstrated in similarly affected patients in India. Suggestions have been made that these patients, especially in Africa, are less susceptible to diabetic complications than Europeans but this now seems unlikely.

A popular Indian and Chinese vegetable, karela (*Momordica charantia*), has hypoglycaemic properties; these are enhanced by chlorpropamide, a fact that must be taken into account in the management of diabetes in several Asian countries (Chapter 49).

A syndrome consisting of pancreatic calcification, associated with both exocrine and endocrine impairment is common in many tropical countries; most evidence comes from Africa (East and West), southern India and Indonesia. The aetiology of *chronic calcific pancreatitis* is still unknown. Pancreatic damage in kwashiorkor in childhood can be severe[1,48] and this could be relevant. Cassava has also been implicated.[49] It should not be forgotten, however, that permanent pancreatic damage can follow viral hepatitis.[50] A further suggestion is that the pancreatic ducts are blocked by secretions and inspissated mucus plugs which later calcify; this might be more common after starvation, gastroenteritis and dehydration.[51] Presentation is with weight-loss and malabsorption (in some parts of the tropics, especially Africa, this is the commonest cause of overt malabsorption); diabetes mellitus and pancreatic pain are also important features. Treatment consists of providing pancreatic supplements (e.g. pancreatin, BP, 6 g orally with meals) and control of the diabetes. The pain is often very difficult to manage and may be so severe that suicide is a sequel.

The pancreas can also be involved in infections caused by *Schistosoma mansoni*[52] and *S. japonicum*, trichinellosis, cysticercosis and hydatid disease.

Pancreatic duct obstruction with acute pancreatitis as a sequel is caused most commonly by *Ascaris lumbricoides*[53]; rarely tapeworms can also be implicated. Clonorchiasis and opisthorchiasis can similarly involve the pancreatic duct system.

SPLEEN

Table 60.8 summarizes some causes of splenomegaly in the tropics and Fig. 60.4 shows the clinical and histological appearances in the *tropical splenomegaly syndrome* (TSS). Most of the causes are covered in other chapters; portal hypertension has already been referred to (see above). The most extreme form of splenomegaly, TSS, is covered in Chapters 1 and 58, and the various viral, bacterial and parasitic causes under those respective headings.

The spleen is an extremely important defence organ against infections of many types, especially pneumococcal infection[54,55] and malaria. Thus splenectomized people in tropical countries should be given pneumococcal vaccine and carefully advised regarding malaria prophylaxis.

Splenic abscess is usually, but not always, a tropical disease. Most reports are from West

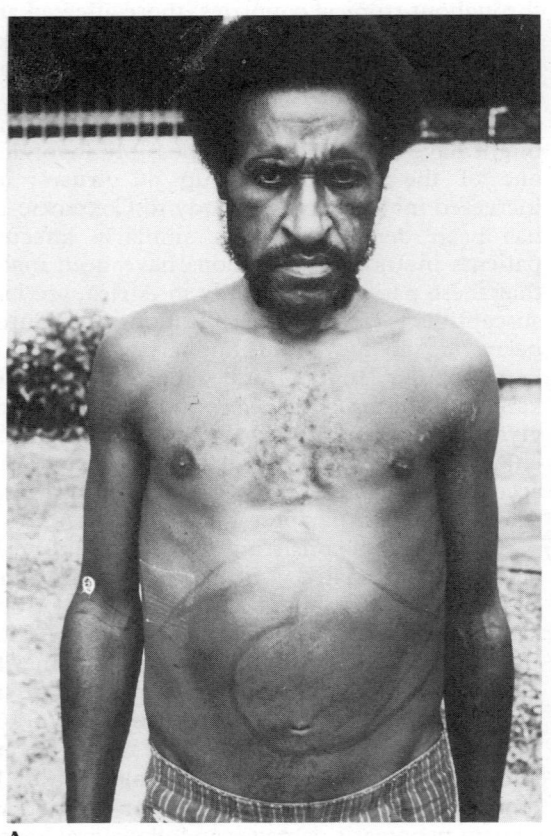
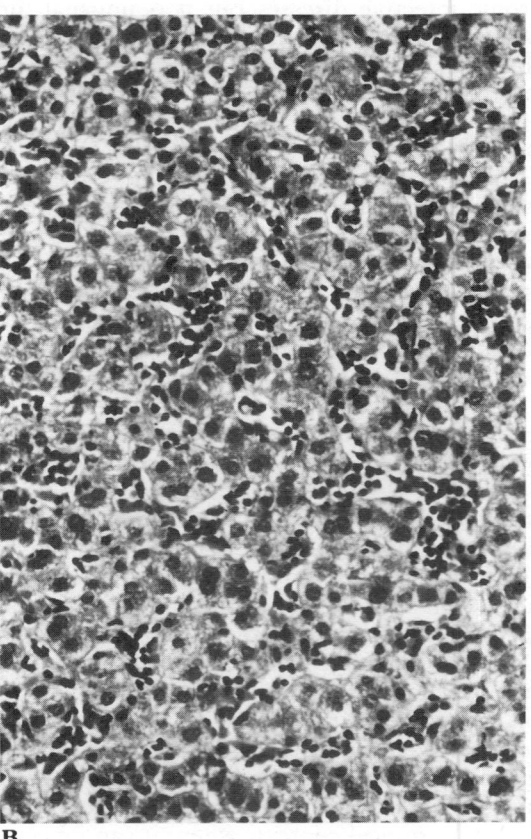

A **B**

Fig. 60.4 A, Papua New Guinean man with massive splenic enlargement. All of the features of the tropical splenomegaly syndrome (TSS) were present. B, Liver biopsy specimen from a patient with TSS showing marked hepatic sinusoidal infiltration with lymphocytes.

Table 60.8 Some causes of splenomegaly in the tropics.

Infections:	
Viral:	EB virus, cytomegalovirus, viral hepatitis and other virus diseases
Bacteria:	typhoid fever, brucellosis, tuberculosis
Parasites:	malaria (especially the tropical spleno-megaly syndrome), schistosomiasis, visceral leishmaniasis, trypanosomiasis

Portal hypertension

Haemopoietic diseases
   Sickle cell disease, thalassaemia

Reticuloendothelial diseases
   Burkitt's lymphoma, leukaemia, reticuloses

Cystic lesions
   Hydatid disease

Abscess
   Amoebic; unknown aetiology

Spontaneous haemorrhage and rupture

Metabolic
   Amyloidosis

Africa and Zimbabwe. In most, the cause is unknown but some are caused by *Salmonella typhi*.[56] The clinical history is usually one of two to three weeks' duration with pain and swelling in the left hypochondrium associated with pyrexia. The splenic swelling is tender, often exquisitely so, and fluctuant. Radiographs may show gas within the abscess. Untreated, these abscesses can rupture into the peritoneal cavity; splenectomy is therefore important in management. If the condition becomes chronic—an unusual sequel—splenectomy is also the correct management. The aetiology is unknown; viral and parasitic diseases have been suggested but not proved. A connection with carriers of the sickle cell gene has also been suggested but likewise not proved.

REFERENCES

1 Cook, G.C. (1980) *Tropical Gastroenterology*. Oxford: Oxford University Press.
2 Barnes, C.G. (1984) *Jl R. Soc. Med.* 77, 816.
3 Schacher, J.F., Saab, S., Germanos, R. et al (1969) *Trans. R. Soc. trop. Med. Hyg.* 63, 854.
4 Pindborg, J.J., Mehta, F.S., Gupta, P.C. et al (1968) *Br. J. Cancer* 22, 646.
5 Leading article (1984) *Lancet* ii, 20.
6 Westaby, D., Melia, W.M., MacDougall, B.R.D. et al (1984) *Gut* 25, 129.
7 Witzel, L., Wolbergs, E. & Merki, H. (1985) *Lancet* i, 773.
8 Leading article (1984) *Lancet* i, 139.
9 Martinson, F.D. (1978) *Trop. Doc.* 8, 123.
10 Cook, G.C. (1984) *Trop. Doc.* 14, 49.
11 Nicholls, J. (1984) *Br. med. J.* 289, 549.
12 *Br. med. J.* (1959) i, 1462.
13 Tovey, F.I. & Tunstall, M. (1975) *Gut* 16, 564.
14 Tovey, F.I. (1979) *Gut* 20, 329.
15 Pearson, A.D. (1986) *Advanced Medicine* 22, ed. D.R. Triger, pp. 167–186. London: Royal College of Physicians/Baillière Tindall.
16 Cook, G.C. (1986). *Curr. Opinion Gastroent.* 2, 81 & 83.
17 Leading article (1984) *Lancet* i, 715.
18 Bhalla, S., Vij, J.C., Anand, B.S. et al (1985) *Gut* 26, 491.
19 Cook, G.C. (1985) *Scand. J. Gastroent.* 20 (Supplement 111), 17.
20 Cook, G.C. (1984) *Lancet* i, 721.
21 Cook, G.C. (1986) *Trans. R. Soc. trop Med. Hyg.* 80, 675.
22 Cook, G.C. (1984) In *Critical Reviews in Tropical Medicine*, ed. R.K. Chandra, vol. 2, pp. 117–139. New York: Plenum Press.
23 Marks, I.N., Kottler, R.E. & Gilinsky, N.H. (1983) *Topics in Gastroenterology*, ed. D.P. Jewell & H.A. Shepherd, vol. 11, pp. 191–219. Oxford: Blackwell Scientific Publications.
24 Khojasteh, A., Haghshenass, M. & Haghighi, P. (1983) *New Engl. J. Med.* 308, 1401.
25 Mathan, M.M. & Mathan, V.I. (1985) *Gut* 26, 710.
26 Ramakrishna, B.S. & Mathan, V.I. (1982) *Gut* 23, 843.
27 Argenzio, R.A., Moon, H.W., Kemeny, L.J. et al (1984) *Gastroenterology* 86, 1501.
28 McNeil, N.I. (1984) *Am. J. clin. Nutr.* 39, 338.
29 Shaffer, J.L., Hughes, S., Linaker, B.D. et al (1984) *Gut* 25, 203.
30 Harries, A.D., Myers, B. & Cook, G.C. (1985) *Br. med. J.* 291, 1686.
31 Cook, G.C. (1983) In *Topics in Gastroenterology*, ed. D.P. Jewell & H.A. Shepherd, vol. 11, pp. 175–190. Oxford: Blackwell Scientific Publications.
32 Cook, G.C. (1986) In *Advanced Medicine* 22, ed. D.R. Triger, pp. 193–202. London: Royal College of Physicians/Baillière Tindall.
33 Ioachim, H.L. (1982) *Pathology of Granulomas*. New York: Raven Press.
34 Mills, P.R. & Russell, R.I. (1983) *J. R. Soc. Med.* 76, 393.
35 Cook, G.C. (1980) *Q. J. Med.* 49, 491.
36 Paton, A. (1984) *Br. med. J.* 289, 857.
37 Cook, G.C. (1985) *Q. J. Med.* 57, 705.
38 Enwonwu, C.O. (1984) *Lancet* ii, 956.
39 Weller, I.V.D., Lok, A.S.F., Mindel, A. et al (1985) *Gut* 26, 745.
40 Quintero, E., Ginés, P., Arroyo, V. et al (1985) *Lancet* i, 611.
41 Leading article (1984) *Lancet* i, 489.
42 Faizallah, R., Woodrow, J.C., Krasner, N.K. et al (1982) *Br. med. J.* 285, 533.
43 Tanner, M.S., Kantarjian, A.H., Bhave, S.A. et al (1983) *Lancet* ii, 992.
44 Lefkowitch, J.H., Honig, C.L., King, M.E. et al (1982) *New Engl. J. Med.* 307, 271.
45 LeSage, G.D., Baldus, W.P., Fairbanks, V.F. et al (1983) *Gastroenterology* 84, 1471.
46 Khuroo, M.S. & Zargar, S.A. (1985) *Gastroenterology* 88, 418.
47 Hugh-Jones, P. (1955) *Lancet* ii, 891.
48 Fedail, S.S., Karar, Z.A., Harvey, R.F. et al (1980) *Lancet* ii, 374.

49   Assan, R., Boukersi, H. & Clauser, E. (1984) *Lancet* **ii**, 1278.

50   Oli, J.M. & Nwokolo, C. (1979) *Br. med. J.* **i**, 926.

51   Nwokolo, C. & Oli, J. (1980) *Lancet* **i**, 456.

52   Fedail, S. S., Baher, Y. M. & Aboud, O. I. (1985) *Digestion* **32**, 132.

53   Choi, T. K., Wong, J. (1984) *J. trop. Med. Hyg.* **87**, 211.

54   Leading article (1985) *Lancet* **ii**, 928.

55   Padova, F.D., Dürig, M., Harder, F. et al (1984) *Br. med. J.* **290**, 14.

56   Kager, P.A. & Rietra, P.J.G.M. (1982) *Trop. geogr. Med.* **34**, 375.

Chapter 61
Cardiovascular Disease
Edmond Bertrand

INTRODUCTION

Cardiovascular disease is often regarded as an epidemiological problem which afflicts the wealthy countries of the temperate zone while sparing the developing countries in the tropics. Such a view is inaccurate; in fact, in many tropical regions cardiopathy is one of the major causes of adult illness and mortality. For example, in Mauritius, Sri Lanka, Singapore and Malaysia cardiovascular disease is the major cause of death. In the majority of other tropical regions cardiopathy ranks second or third among the causes of death; notably in Africa.

In the tropics cardiovascular pathology seems to reflect the stage of economic development. In underdeveloped areas endocardial and myocardial pathology is found as well as arterial hypertension. With economic development cardiovascular morbidity takes on a different shape as it becomes more prevalent and coronary artery disease becomes more prominent as endocardial and myocardial pathology decrease in frequency. Arterial hypertension, however, is still a major cause of morbidity.

The pattern of cardiovascular disease in the tropics deserves the attention of all doctors working there. This chapter therefore seeks: (a) to recall the cardiovascular features of the major endemic tropical diseases; (b) to describe briefly certain syndromes commonly encountered in the tropics but infrequently seen elsewhere, e.g. endomyocardial fibrosis and myocardial disease; and (c) to point out the manifestations of the more universal cardiovascular diseases as seen in the tropics. The chapter also includes a discussion of certain features of the normal electrocardiogram of the black African.

HEART DAMAGE IN THE MAJOR ENDEMIC PARASITIC DISEASES

The heart and trypanosomiasis

Cardiac involvement in American trypanosomiasis (Chagas' disease) is now fully recognized; that in African trypanosomiasis, however, has not been studied as fully.

American trypanosomiasis (Chapter 3)

Cardiopathic manifestations may be noted in the stage of invasive spread of the disease; for the most part, however, they are observed several years later in the chronic phase of the illness.

1 In the *acute invasive period* cardiac features are not always present; but in certain cases a severe acute myocarditis develops[1] with signs of heart failure including hepatic stasis, oedema of the lower limbs and breathlessness. At times the patient is in a state of collapse. Heart examination detects a tachycardia, dull heart sounds, gallop rhythm and at times a functional systolic murmur. The X-ray shows an enlarged heart. The ECG shows non-specific alterations of the ST segment and T wave. Disorders of rhythm and conduction may further complicate the picture and occasionally an acute pericarditis. About a tenth of the cases end fatally.

Diagnosis is established by detection of trypanosomes in the peripheral blood or pericardial fluid. Pathological changes include pseudocysts containing amastigotes in the heart muscle (Fig. 3.3), cytolysis of myocardial fibres and an interstitial inflammatory reaction.

2 After a latent phase lasting five, 10 or 20 years a *chronic cardiomyopathy* develops in some areas (Venezuela) in up to 50% of the cases. This

occurs most often among patients from the rural areas in their twenties and thirties. This stage is unlike the acute myocarditis seen in children. The signs are those of a failing heart with patients complaining of palpitations and precordial pain. The heart sounds are muffled; a gallop rhythm may be present or a functional atrioventricular insufficiency murmur can be heard. The X-ray shows an enlarged heart. Noteworthy is the marked frequency of arrhythmias and blocks which for the patient entail the risk of syncope or sudden death. Non-specific T wave irregularities may occur in the ECG which may also show signs of left ventricular hypertrophy. The histopathological picture includes interstitial fibrosis, cellular (lymphocytes, monocytes and plasmocytes) infiltrations and often the formation of a microaneurysm around the apex (Fig. 3.4, p. 78). At this stage no parasites can be demonstrated in the myocardium and the diagnosis is serological.

The disease is chronic. After the onset of heart failure the expectation of life is between seven months and two years. Treatment is symptomatic. Amiodarone may effectively control dysrhythmias.

African trypanosomiasis (Chapter 2)
Cardiac manifestations have been noted, particularly in the early blood stage, but occasionally also in the later cerebral stage of the malady. Diagnosis is based on finding the parasite in the blood, glands or cerebrospinal fluid. Serological findings may provide indirect evidence of the illness.

TRYPANOSOMIASIS DUE TO *T. BRUCEI*
RHODESIENSE (RHODESIAN SLEEPING SICKNESS)
Heart damage may cause death before the cerebral phase sets in. Myocardial damage is disclosed by pointers such as tachycardia, the muffling of the heart sounds, gallop rhythm and X-ray evidence of cardiac enlargement. At times an acute pericarditis occurs. The ECG is abnormal in half the cases[2, 3]—abnormal repolarization and AV block being particularly common. The development of heart failure has been reported[4] which can be cured by effective specific treatment of the trypanosomiasis.[5] Anatomical studies have found marked interstitial inflammatory infiltration of the myocardium and pericardium with disappearance of muscle fibres and fibrosis.

TRYPANOSOMIASIS DUE TO *T. BRUCEI GAMBIENSE*
(GAMBIAN SLEEPING SICKNESS)
The cardiological aspects of this disease were little known until recently.[6] They tend to be inconspicuous and are found in about 10–20% of the cases which present with palpitation, atypical precordial pain, muffling of the heart sounds and, at times, gallop rhythm or a systolic murmur. The pulse pressure is reduced especially on standing. A pericardial effusion may occur. X-rays may show a normal sized or enlarged heart. At times a reduction in the size of the heart is noted; angiocardiography then reveals a concentric muscular hypertrophy and a marked diminution of the size of the ventricular cavities. In about 35–40% of the cases the ECG shows ST and T abnormalities and, more rarely, signs of right or left ventricular hypertrophy. Rarer still are conduction changes (AV block 2.6%) which tend to respond to corticoid treatment.

Trypanocidal therapy with, if necessary, corticosteroids, may arrest the cardiopathy. On histological study of 11 cases (Fig. 61.1) histiocytic, lymphocytic and monocytic infiltration of myocardium, pericardium and even the pericardium

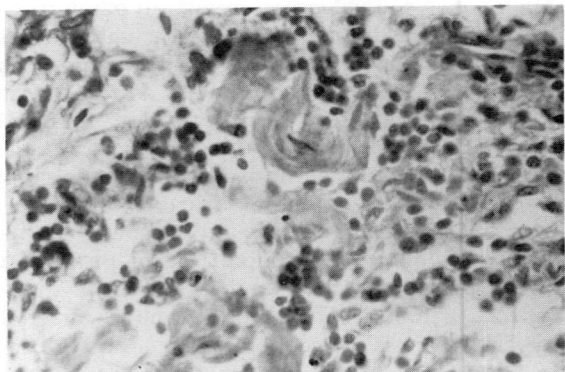

Fig. 61.1   African trypanosomiasis. Myocardial infiltration with lymphocytes and plasma cells.

were found. Patches of fibrosis may coexist and can compromise the conduction tissue.[7, 8]

The heart and schistosomiasis (Chapter 22)

In schistosomiasis cardiac manifestations may be the result of pulmonary arterial hypertension or they may have an indirect causation: iatrogenic, from anaemia or systemic hypertension. Schistosomal myocarditis is a less clearcut syndrome.

1   *Pulmonary arterial hypertension* is caused by the eggs of *Schistosoma haematobium*, *S. mansoni* or *S. japonicum* which migrate to the lungs and provoke an inflammatory or fibrous reaction in the pulmonary parenchyma and arterial walls

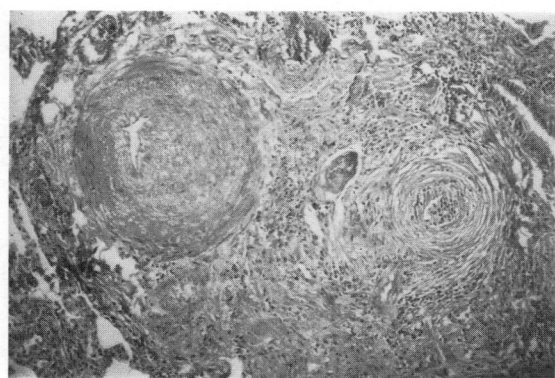

Fig. 61.2 Schistosomiasis haematobium. Pulmonary endarteritis obliterans. Schistosomal granulomas in lung.

(Fig. 61.2). The resulting hypertension is of the precapillary type. Sometimes shunts are formed which cause hypoxia. On routine examination of schistosomal patients 13%[9] and 21.6%[10] had pulmonary arterial hypertension. In other studies the same authors reported eliciting clinical signs in only 2.1% and 2.3% of the patients respectively. They believe that there can be a reversal of the inflammatory lesions in the course of the disease.

In symptomatic cases the X-ray shows a dilatation of the pulmonary artery and of its branches and sometimes a right-sided enlargement of the heart (cor pulmonale). The pulmonary parenchyma may be clear or present a micronodular or pseudomiliary appearance. On angiography the branches of the pulmonary artery resemble those of a dead tree. The ECG shows a right ventricle (RV) hypertrophy of the systolic type. In the presence of signs of heart damage it should be ensured that the drug treatment of bilharziasis will not affect the heart.

2 *Schistosomal myocarditis* in man is not well documented; in particular, direct myocardial damage by egg deposition is exceptional.[11] Experimental findings are controversial.[10] In general, myocardial lesions in schistosomiasis are poorly understood as to their existence, nature and mechanism. One may suspect a congestive myocarditis provoked by the parasite in young patients heavily infested by schistosomes. That suspicion gains ground when the ECG shows an abnormal T or ST or an AV block. Signs of stasis are exceptional. In the end diagnosis is a probability based on clinical grounds and ECG findings in the absence of pulmonary hypertension, and in the presence of active schistosomiasis and no sign of other causation. Certain antischistosomal drugs tend to exacerbate the cardiac damage such as niridazole and antimonials.

3 *Other cardiac features* are quite frequent in schistosomiasis. A cardiomyopathy of anaemic origin may follow haemorrhage from the urinary or the alimentary tracts or be caused by haemolytic or an iron deficiency anaemia. The frequency of hypertensive cardiomyopathy is not greater than that in the general population. A schistosomal acute cor pulmonale is a very rare complication.[12] An iatrogenic myocarditis occurred in 8% of patients on niridazole or dihydroemetine treatment. Newer drugs are not cardiotoxic. Lastly, in certain countries, e.g. Brazil and Ivory Coast, schistosomiasis is regarded as a possible cause of endomyocardial fibrosis (p. 1019).

The heart and malaria (Chapter 1)

Studies of the heart in malaria are rare.[13]
1 *Cardiac signs during the onset of malaria* include complaints of precordial pain or palpitations. Often one notices a pulse/temperature dissociation with a relative bradycardia. The T wave may be abnormal. Some cases of heart failure have been described.[14] It should not be confused with the pulmonary signs observed in 10% of the cases. In general, cardiac involvement does not influence the prognosis though Herrera[15] reported it as a cause of death in a child patient. The underlying pathology is vaguely described as 'myocardial lesions', microthromboses, altered capillary permeability and anaemia.
2 *The onset of malaria in a cardiac patient* is generally well-tolerated. A tachycardia faster than one warranted by the temperature and sometimes extrasystoles may be noted. These findings would seem to be produced by the haemodynamics of hyperthermia (analogous to an exercise test).
3 *The cardiac signs due to treatment with the aminoquinoline compounds* (e.g. quinine, chloroquine) should be pointed out. They exert a quinidine-like action. In the treatment of the onset of malaria normally one does not encounter iatrogenic cardiac signs beyond possibly a prolonged QT. Nevertheless, such treatment should be monitored especially in patients with nephropathy or hypokalaemia, or under treatment with analogous drugs for pre-existing cardiac illness. Numerous cases of self-poisoning with chloroquine bear witness to the drug's toxicity; such cases can die of heart block or from ventricular

fibrillation precipitated by secondary myocardial hyperexcitability.

4   *The antimalarial action of quinidine* has been the subject of recent studies.[16] The drug is very effective especially against chloroquine-resistant *Plasmodium falciparum*. It is well tolerated. A prolonged QT and a flattening of T have been noted but not dysrhythmia (p. 31).

The heart and amoebiasis (Chapter 19)

Heart involvement in amoebiasis[17] may occur as a result of an amoebic pericarditis; also as an iatrogenic complication; or as a repercussion in severe amoebic colitis.

1   *Amoebic pericarditis*[18] is a rare condition usually complicating amoebic liver abscess or pleuropulmonary pathology. The pericarditis may be a purulent one—amoebic pus being present in the pericardial sac. A tamponade syndrome may follow the sudden rupture of a hepatic or pulmonary abscess into the pericardium. This calls for surgical treatment in addition to specific antiamoebic therapy. A cure is achieved more often than was at one time believed possible. A reactionary pericarditis may occur with inflammation but without pus formation; the clinical signs are then less severe, often only an ECG/echocardiogram indicative of change. Specific antiamoebic therapy then suffices to secure a full recovery.

2   *Cardiac involvement in severe amoebic colitis* is for the most part disclosed by ST and T abnormalities, the reflection of metabolic changes or toxic shock.

3   *Iatrogenic cardiac complications* occur mostly in patients treated with emetine or dihydroemetine.[19] The toxicity is not dose dependent; sudden collapse or death may occur in severe cases. Most often cardiac involvement is deduced from a flattened T or altered ST level or a QT prolongation. Arrhythmias and blocks are seldom seen. Unless there has been a pre-existing cardiac condition these changes regress completely in a few days to a couple of weeks. The newer antiamoebic drugs, especially metronidazole and tinidazole are not cardiotoxic.

PRIMARY OR APPARENTLY PRIMARY MYOCARDIAL DISEASES

Idiopathic cardiomyopathy in the context of the total cardiovascular morbidity seems to occur more frequently in the tropics than in temperate regions. Lack of research facilities in many centres has precluded the ascertainment of its precise prevalence, statistically estimated at 5–20% of the total cardiovascular morbidity. In modern cardiological centres improvement in aetiological diagnosis has proportionately reduced the bulk of idiopathic cardiac pathology.

In our studies we have excluded cases of cardiomyopathy of known aetiology, such as arterial hypertension, valvular disease, congenital heart malformations or coronary artery heart disease. We have also omitted rare causes found in the tropics as elsewhere, such as haemochromatosis, amyloidosis and intoxication with tricyclic antidepressants. Endomyocardial fibrosis (p. 1019) has also been left out since it is an endocardial rather than a myocardial disease.

The apparently primary myocardial diseases considered below are outlined in a simple clinical order: first, the acute and subacute syndromes are studied, then the chronic ones. Finally, two more particularly tropical conditions are discussed: postpartum cardiomyopathy and the myocardial pathology of sickle cell disease.

Curable acute or subacute cardiopathies[20]

These are seen more often in the general medical wards than in the cardiological departments. They have to be remembered and looked for because they are either partially or completely curable.

1   *The metabolic cardiopathies* have four basic characteristics: (a) the lesions are congestive and consequently reversible; (b) they present a raised cardiac output before advanced failure sets in; (c) the aetiology is often identifiable; and (d) a cure can be achieved by treating the cause.

The *cardiopathy of anaemia* (Chapter 58) affects most often multipara inducing a moderate cardiomegaly but rarely signs of failure. The ST and T are abnormal but the QT interval is normal. With echocardiography and angiography one detects signs of a normotrophic, hyperkinetic cardiopathy. The heart muscle is deranged when the anaemia is chronic and the haemoglobin level falls below 7 g/litre. Correction of the anaemia reverses the cardiopathy (Fig. 61.3).

The *cardiopathy of beriberi* (Chapter 46) causes a global or left-sided heart failure. It occurs in patients whose diets are unbalanced consisting

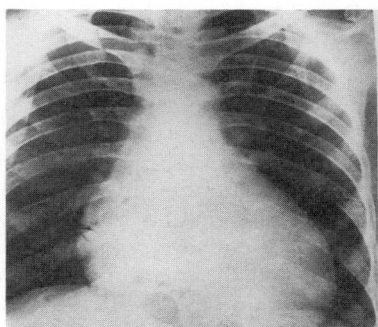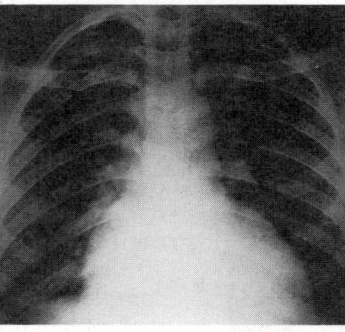

Fig. 61.3 Heart in anaemia. Decrease in heart size following treatment of the anaemia. Left: November 6. Right: November 28.

mainly of highly milled (polished) rice. They often present signs of polyneuritis, e.g. sluggish knee jerks. The diagnosis is based on finding a raised pyruvic acid level and a fall in that of thiamine in the blood. Also diagnostic is treatment with vitamin B₁ as it leads to a cure (Fig. 61.4). Subacute cases are given 250–500 mg thiamine intramuscularly every day followed by oral treatment. Acute cases require 500 mg thiamine in 500 ml glucosed serum intravenously over 12–24 hours. A thiamine shock syndrome is rare but should be borne in mind. Alcoholic

tious, parasitic or toxic context which may mask the cardiac features; (c) the possibility of detecting their cause; and (d) the feasibility of effecting a cure by treating the cause even if that cure is not invariably achieved. The clinical signs are not prominent; the heart is radiographically not much altered; the ECG is more helpful and may show low voltage, disorders of excitability, rhythm, conduction and even of repolarization.

Of the parasitic infestations we have already considered trypanosomiasis and schistosomiasis. It should be noted that kala-azar (Chapter 4),

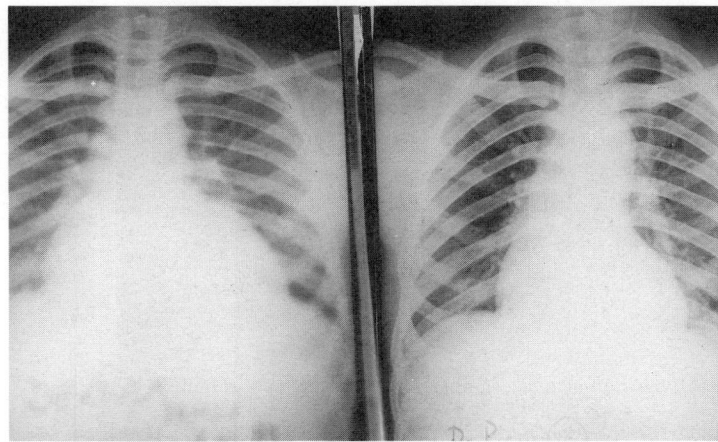

Fig. 61.4 Beriberi heart. Decrease in heart size 11 days after treatment with vitamin B¹. Left: before treatment. Right: after treatment.

beriberi necessitates abstinence in addition to vitamin therapy (see also Chapter 46).

Protein deficiency and hypokalaemia can both cause a myocarditis but in kwashiorkor myocarditis is a rarity.

2 *Infections, parasitic infestation and toxaemias* are causes of cardiopathy more frequently in the tropics than in temperate regions. These myocarditides are characterized by (a) interstitial inflammatory lesions and/or parenchymal involvement; (b) their occurrence in an infec-

toxoplasmosis (Chapter 9) and various infectious diseases, notably typhoid (Chapter 8) (frequently) and diphtheria (rarely) (Chapter 29) and the cocci can all have cardiac manifestations. Tuberculosis (Figs 61.5 and 61.6) affects the myocardium very frequently.[7] Certain viruses, e.g. measles, the arboviruses, poliovirus and the hepatitis viruses, have been incriminated as agents of myocardial damage. In rabies cardiopathy is terminal (see Chapter 42).[21] Other well-known cardiopathies are those due to group

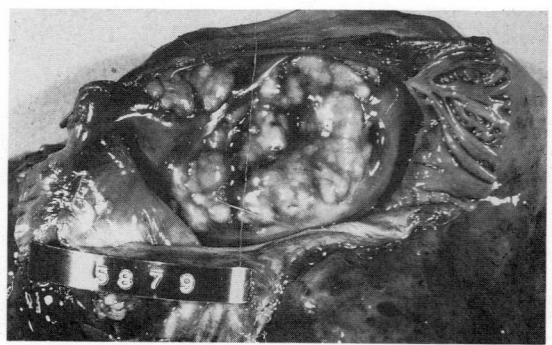

Fig. 61.5 Tuberculous carditis (to be distinguished from miliary tuberculosis). Pseudotumoral tuberculoma of myocardium.

Primary chronic cardiomyopathy

This section is brief since these conditions have similar features the world over.

1 *Chronic congestive cardiomyopathy* has been well studied.[22] In the tropics the importance of fibrotic lesions which cut up the myocardium in which evidence of inflammation is scarce is noticeable (Fig. 61.7). Patients are typically 30–50 years old, often in full heart failure. They complain of precordial pain which differs from that of angina in being less related to effort, duller, more prolonged and less radiating. The X-ray reveals a grossly hypokinetic heart difficult to differentiate from pericardial effusion. The

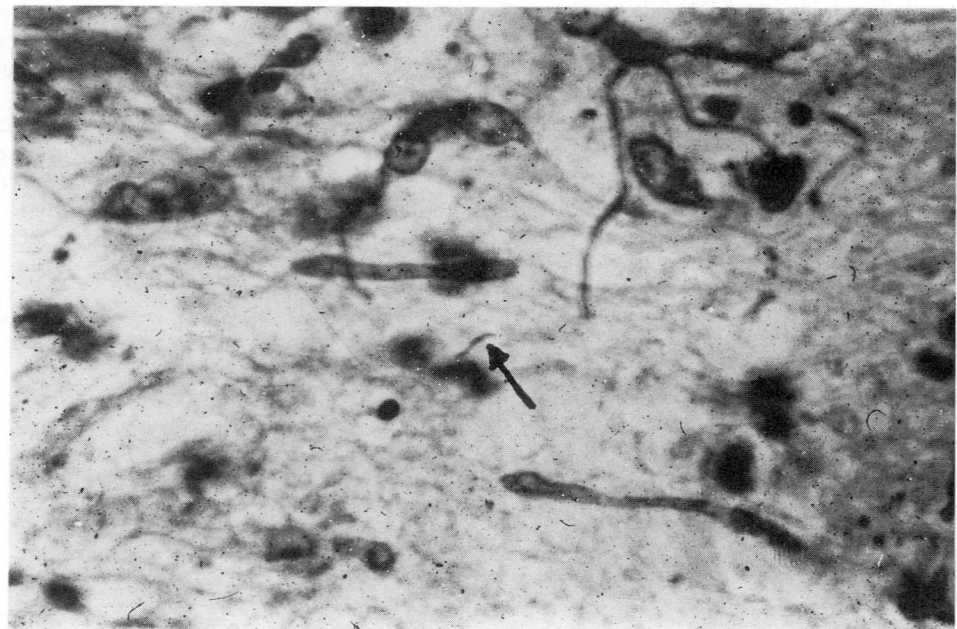

Fig. 61.6 Tuberculous carditis. *Mycobacterium tuberculosis* (arrowed) in the myocardium.

B Coxsackie viruses, to the *Rickettsia* (see Chapter 10) (often reversible) and to those provoked by a series of drugs—emetine and its derivatives, the antimony compounds, the phenothiazines, the tricyclic antidepressants and Antabuse.

3 *Allergic cardiopathies* can occur in the context of dermal or visceral allergies. They are frequently seen in the tropics as part of reactions to serum.

4 *Some cardiopathies of unknown aetiology* are still seen. A viral or an immunological aetiology is usually assumed.

ECG shows a QRS of reduced amplitude, numerous dysrhythmias, bundle branch block more often than AV block and a flat or negative T wave. Leads V1 to V3 in particular may show the Q or QS of 'fibrosis'. Echocardiography shows dilatation of the cavities, feeble contractility of the posterior and septal walls, a miniaturization of the mitral valve and a myocardium of normal size or hypotrophic. Angiography confirms the dilatation of the cavities with hypokinetic normal sized or hypotrophic walls. AV insufficiency is often detected.

Some cases are detected in the early phase by

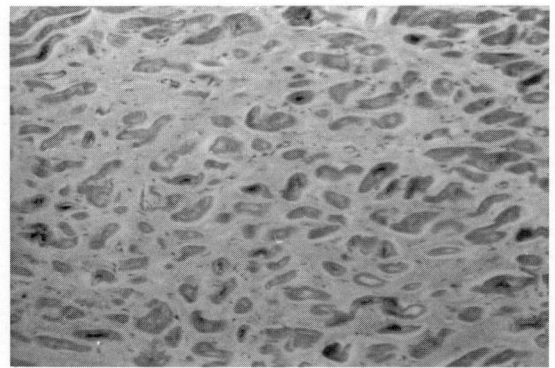

Fig. 61.7 Congestive primitive cardiomyopathy. Diffuse interstitial fibrosis of myocardium.

echocardiography undertaken for complaints of dyspnoea, palpitations, dysrhythmic ECG or radiographic cardiomegaly. The evolution is over several years of damage but it may be cut short by an embolus or dysrythmia. The treatment consists of administering digitalis combined with a diuretic. The addition of vasodilators taken regularly may be beneficial.

The cause remains elusive. There may be a multiple aetiology: genetic or an inadequately treated myocarditis, an immunological process; possibly a succession of myocardial insults cumulatively injure the muscle leading to its failure. A minority of the cases are alcoholics who present an analogous clinical picture in which, however, dysrhythmia is more frequent. Study of the duration of systole can disclose this damage early in the alcoholic patient.[23] Echocardiography shows up the initial parietal hypertrophy and in later stages the cavitary dilatation.[24] The regression which can follow abstention would confirm the alcoholic aetiology.

2 *Hypertrophic cardiomyopathy* used to be regarded as rare in Africa, probably for lack of investigative means such as echocardiography and angiography. Recently 31 cases have been observed at the Heart Institute of Abidjan.[25] In more than two-thirds of these patients an asymmetrical septal hypertrophy gave rise to the usual signs: syncope, chest pain, dysrhythmia, abnormal Q and T. In a fifth of the patients there was concentric myocardial hypertrophy and frequently heart failure. In one case, an elderly woman, there was an apical hypertrophy.

Postpartum cardiomyopathy (PPCM)

The *first description* of this condition was made by Ritchie in 1850 in Edinburgh. It was not until 1930 that it was again described; this time in American black women, notably in New Orleans. After 1960 several review studies were published.[26, 27] Recently studies were undertaken in Africa.[28–30] All these investigations lead to the conclusion that the black female is affected more often but the disease is also seen in other females in underprivileged environments.

These studies have included cases of heart failure of pregnancy and the peripartum as well as postpartum cases. To distinguish this group better it seems desirable to exclude all cases except postpartum ones; thus excluding all pregnancy-related cardiopathy. Also omitted are cases of hypertension, past or current.

An *epidemiological study* has revealed that 1 in 3000 after-delivery women in Africa are affected. The typical sufferer is about 25 years old, a multipara, occasionally has given birth to twins and comes from a low socioeconomic background. PPCM also occurs in primipara. The lesions are congestive and consequently potentially reversible (Fig. 61.8).

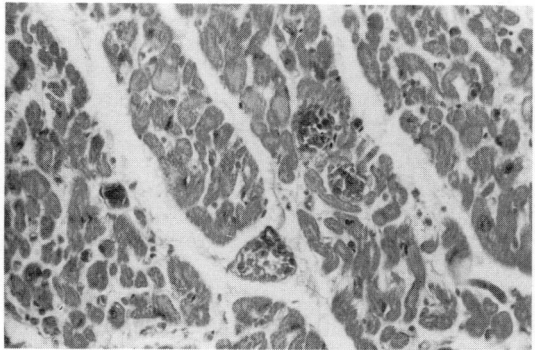

Fig. 61.8 Postpartum cardiomyopathy. Interstitial oedema of myocardium with arteriolar congestion.

The *onset* of PPMC is experienced in the second to the twentieth week after delivery. The symptomatology is that of heart failure with gross ventricular hypotrophy and hypotonicity detected by X-ray, echocardiography or angiography (Fig. 61.9). Pulmonary embolism is a frequent complication. A typical characteristic is the clinical evolution of the disease. Rest alone may lead to a complete recovery, or death may occur from embolism, or the disease may become chronic. A reserved prognosis should be maintained for about three months.

Treatment includes a prolonged rest—as much

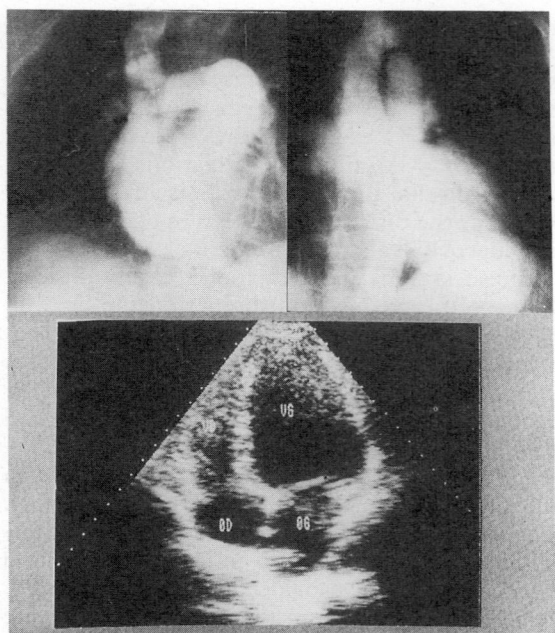

Fig. 61.9 Postpartum cardiomyopathy. Left ventricle dilated with a hypotrophic wall smaller than the right ventricle.

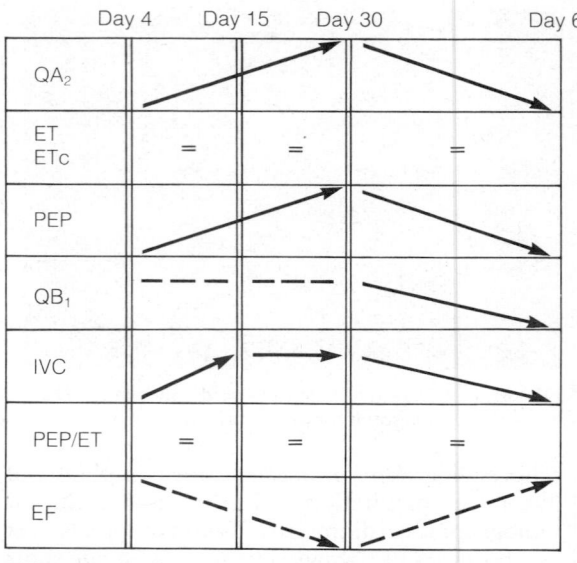

Fig. 61.10 Alterations of systolic time intervals during the puerperium on the fourth, fifteenth, thirtieth and sixtieth days postpartum. PEP, pre-ejection time; ET, ejection time; IVC, isovomumetric contraction; B₁, first heart sound; A₂, second aortic sound; EF, ejection fraction.

as feasible—for two to six months with sodium restriction; digitalis–diuretic administration may hasten recovery. Theoretically there is an indication for anticoagulant treatment. Prevention calls for systematic screening aimed at early diagnosis and early rest treatment.

How does one explain the occurrence of PPCM? Certain observations[31, 32] indicate that the normal postpartum is a period of reduced myocardial performance demonstrable by phonomecanography (Fig. 61.10). It is latent clinically and is the result of altered haemodynamics which obtain after delivery combined with a fall in the level of oestradiol (which has an inotropic action). This latent condition becomes manifest if certain risk factors prevail such as malnutrition, anaemia, excessive physical exertion, inordinate sodium intake (in Nigeria, see for example, Fillmore and Parry[29]); or extremes of environmental heat. The condition may or may not recur after subsequent pregnancy depending upon whether or not these risk factors persist. It should be noted that other explanations for the aetiology of PPCM have been put forward such as nutritional, immunologic and viral causes.[33]

Cardiomyopathy in sickle cell anaemia

Myocardial damage in the presence of sickle cell anaemia raises problems as yet unresolved. Ischaemia and even myocardial infarction have been described.[34] Histological proof, however, remains unconvincing. Chronic cor pulmonale and pulmonary infarction have been reported.[35] However, no difference in pulmonary pressures between anaemic patients with sickle cells or those without sickling was found in Abidjan. Cardiopathic manifestations attributed to the anaemia have been described in subjects with a haemoglobin level persistently below 7 g/litre.

The point at issue is whether or not a cardiomyopathy can exist in the sickle celled subject independently of the above cited pathogenesis and particularly of anaemia. Recently[36] evidence for an authentic cardiomyopathy in sickle cell subjects was forthcoming from studies of systolic intervals. In Abidjan[37] a catheterization and echographic study showed a reduced myocardial function in anaemic patients whether sickle celled or not. The only difference was a greater myocardial mass and RV volume in sickle cell patients, which presumably is attributable to their anaemia being of longer standing.

It has been demonstrated[38] that open heart

surgery under moderate hypothermia and haemodilution is well tolerated by individuals with sickling.

Subannular aneurysm of the left ventricle

This condition should be differentiated from postinfarction parietal aneurysm and that complicating infective endocarditis. Submitral, subaortic or subannular aneurysms are found more often in the tropics, especially in black Africa. They measure 1–8 cm and have fibrous or calcified walls (Fig. 61.11). They consist mainly of collagen fibres with some elements of inflammation and are found in about 3% of autopsies,[39] most often in men in their twenties. Black people, especially in the African forest, seem more prone but it is found in temperate southern Africa, in the USA, the Antilles and in France. Primary aneurysm is also found in Caucasians.

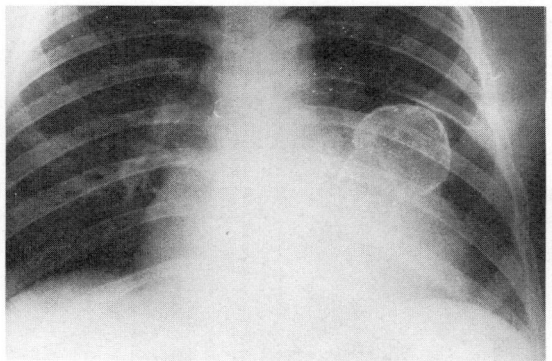

Fig. 61.11 Calcified submitral aneurysm of the left ventricle in a 29-year-old subject.

Clinically, the picture is varied and non-specific: left parasternal heaving, mediastinal compression, systemic emboli, dysrhythmias and complications from an extension of the aneurysm to the auricle or pericardium. ECG changes are those of ischaemia with elevated ST segment, frequently a prolonged QT, at times a Q of necrosis. The X-ray[40] may show the aneurysm's curved outline projecting from the left border of the heart, especially if calcified. An antero-posterior film may fail to reveal a posterior cardiac aneurysm which will show up on angiocardiography including at times an outline of its pockets.

The *aetiology* is not clear. A congenital defect is unlikely. Infection and rheumatism are sus-pected, particularly tuberculosis.[41] The aneurysm may be the sequel of myocarditis.

The only treatment possible is surgical.[38, 42] If tuberculosis coexists its specific treatment should precede and follow surgery.

CHRONIC PARIETAL ENDOCARDITIS (ENDOMYOCARDIAL FIBROSIS AND FIBROPLASTIC ENDOCARDITIS)

In 1936 Löffler described fibroplastic endo-carditis (FPE) in Switzerland. In 1948 Davies described endomyocardial fibrosis (EMF) in East Africa. In his first publication he had called it 'endocardial fibrosis'. It is thought that these two conditions represent two aspects of the same process: the first being an early inflammatory phase (FPE) and the second a late fibrous stage (EMF). The two may be combined under a single name of chronic parietal endocarditis (CPE).

CPE in the world

CPE has been described in Europe notably in Switzerland and in France where its possible filarial aetiology in patients from equatorial Africa had already been suggested. Indeed it is in black Africa that CPE has been most frequently observed and notably in Uganda[43, 44] and Nigeria.[39] Since 1969 at the Heart Institute in Abidjan, Ivory Coast, there have been 105 con-firmed cases of which over half were treated surg-ically. Other cases have been published in Africa: in Benin, in Central Africa, in Gabon and Zaire; that is in the forest region. Since 1950 and especially after 1960 the disease has been reported outside Africa and most often in the tropics in Colombia, Brazil, Venezuela, Mexico, in North America and in Asia, Sri Lanka, Indo-China and particularly in India. Recent advances have been made in the fields of echocar-diography, surgical treatment and in clarifying the causal role of eosinophils in the aetiology of the disease.

Pathology

The disease may be localized either in the left ventricle only (11–30%), the right ventricle only (10–38%) or affects both (50–60%). A serous or haemoserous pericarditis is common. The cor-onaries are normal. Peripheral arteries are often normal in the EMF form. They can be inflamed in the FPE form.

The left ventricle is moderately enlarged, the left atrium moderately dilated. The right ventricle is normal or reduced in size and notched at the apex when the fibrosis is of long standing. The right atrium shows marked dilatation which at times is aneurysmal. The tricuspid ring, too, is very dilated. The characteristic lesion is the endocardial parietal fibrosis; the heart lining shows mother-of-pearl plaques several millimetres thick which may be fibrotic or keloidal or calcified and occasionally ossified (Fig. 61.12). In the left ventricle this fibrosis may be limited to the base of one strand or to the apex but it can also affect the refilling chamber and even obliterate the ventricular cavity. In the right ventricle fibrosis is mainly in the apical and subtricuspid regions. The AV valves are damaged by fibrosis of the chordae or adherent to the fibrous wall.

Microscopically one can distinguish two endocardial layers: a superficial collagenous or hyaline stratum devoid of elastic fibres and poor in blood supply and cells, and a deeper juxtamyocardial layer, younger, rich in capillaries and fibroblasts and having few collagenous fibres and hardly any elastic fibres. There is no, or little, inflammatory reaction. Eosinophils are rare.

According to certain authors[45] the stage described above, generally observed in the tropics, is a terminal fibrotic one developing after an average period of $24\frac{1}{2}$ months. That stage would be the EMF one preceded by a necrotic phase with copious inflammatory cells and eosinophils giving way to a thrombotic phase. These two preceding phases would correspond to the FPE form.

Myocardial damage is more isolated and the muscle may be spared. It may develop sclerotic bands which from the endocardium interdigitate with subendocardial muscle fibres. Older cases develop deeper sclerotic lesions. In FPE the lesions are more inflammatory. The damage seems to start in the endocardium, as may be seen in the early cases. The forerunning and dominance of endocardial pathology justifies surgical treatment. This would be unsuccessful if the myocardial damage were substantial.

Physiopathology

Two processes are operative: parietal endocardial rigidity gives rise to constriction, while the

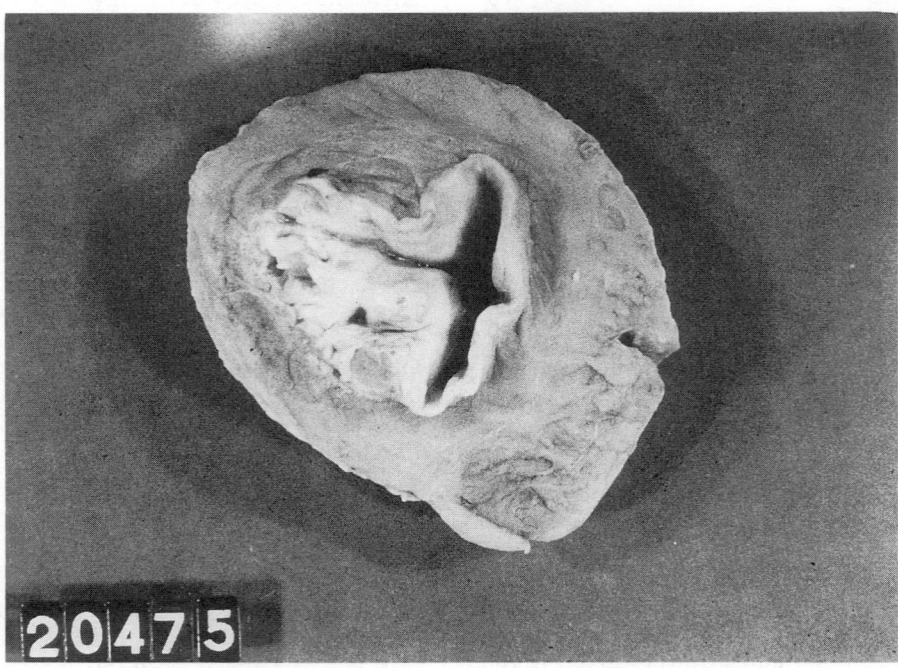

Fig. 61.12   Chronic parietal endocarditis. The endocardium forms a fibrous plaque 5 mm thick reducing the heart cavity. The myocardium is healthy beneath the subendocardial zone.

fibrosed valvular mechanism induces an AV insufficiency. In the left ventricle the valvular element predominates with early adverse effects of the pressure of the pulmonary circulation. In the right ventricle the dominating element is the constriction which engenders considerable stasis. Tricuspid insufficiency is more or less always present but hardly audible because of the slowing of blood flow and output.

Features common to all forms: right, left or bilateral

The disease occurs at any age. In the tropics the patient is often a child or adolescent about 15 years old on average. In such patients puberty can be retarded and weight and height below average. The temperature is normal or raised somewhat in febrile episodes, one of which may herald the onset of the disease (as reported from Nigeria). Effort breathlessness, palpitations and atypical pain are the usual symptoms.

Pathognomonic is a low frequency protodiastolic sound found in 80% which is called endocardial vibration. It may be followed by a short murmur. Dysrhythmias are common especially with right-sided lesions and include fibrillation, flutter and auricular tachycardias which vary spontaneously. AV and intraventricular blocks are common. In 8% of patients the X-ray shows a calcification of the left edge of the infundibulum in right-sided cases and around the apical region in left-sided ones. Echocardiography may reveal direct signs of intracavitary echoes or indirect signs from the septum which vary with lesion location.[12, 46]

The phonomecanogram[47, 48] registers the endocardial vibration; at times the characteristic features of the jugular venous pulse, and of the apex beat. Haemodynamic examination may reveal a 'square root sign' or less characteristic changes. Angiocardiography[49, 50] confirms the diagnosis, characteristically showing a shrunken deformed ventricular cavity especially at the apex, a dilatation of the rest of the ventricle and an irregular contour. Biopsy of the endocardium may aid the diagnosis if the number of specimens is adequate.

Features of the disease according to its location

1 *Right ventricular forms* give a picture of RV failure with marked stasis (enlarged liver, ascites, bloated facies) and tricuspid regurgitation. The ventricular beats are not palpable at the epigastric infrasternal hollow but an infundibular beat may be felt to the left of the sternal border. The lungs are clear. The ECG V1 leads show a Q or QS wave and an interesting right atrial hypertrophy without an RV hypertrophy. The haemodynamic 'square root sign' is usually evident and the JVP mecanographic signs are useful. Angiographic findings are described above. These forms may require a differential diagnosis from chronic constrictive pericarditis, Ebstein's disease and myocardial fibrosis or hypoplasia.

2 *Left ventricular forms* are more misleading. The clinical, X-ray and ECG findings are those of mitral disease or left ventricular failure. The left ventricle (LV) is at times relatively little dilated while the ECG shows no sign of ventricular hypertrophy. Echocardiography may elicit the direct intracavitary signs but often a rigid septal movement is detected with an M-like diastolic phase. On haemodynamic examination the typical plateau-dip is usually found but it may be absent or lack prominence. Angiocardiography reveals deformity of the heart (resembling a playing-card heart, a boxing glove or an apple's stalk distortion) and almost always a mitral insufficiency. The latter at times dominates the picture with few signs of constriction and little angiographic deformity making diagnostic differentiation from mitral disease very difficult. Sometimes even the diagnosis of a primary cardiomyopathy is questioned.

3 *Bilateral forms* are the most frequent. The commonest one is a combination of a right-sided marked stasis, moderate pulmonary hypertension and a mitral insufficiency. Specialized tests show that both ventricles are affected.

4 *Atypical forms* can be encountered such as dysrhythmic forms with alternating bradycardia and tachycardia which may be fatal or pseudo-cirrhotic forms with marked recurrent ascites and an enlarged fibrous liver. Forms with large pericardial effusion are difficult to diagnose. However, forms with a calcified endocardium are easier to diagnose. Nigerian authors have described a form with a febrile onset. Certain febrile forms are due to a supervening infectious endocarditis. There are also forms with a non-constrictive endocardial fibrosis.

Haematological findings

Eosinophilia is found more frequently in Europeans than in Africans. Parasites may be detected, e.g. filariae in Gabon and Nigeria, schistosomes in the Ivory Coast and Brazil and flukes in Europe. A high level of antistreptolysin noted in Uganda has not been reported from elsewhere. The erythrocyte sedimentation rate (ESR) is often raised and so are the beta and gamma globulins. Anti-heart antibodies have been found in central Africa.[51, 52] Coagulation data are lacking.

Evolution of the disease

On average death occurs within three to six years after the diagnosis with a survival of a few months to 10 years in range. The cause is a right-sided or bilateral failure or, at times, dysrhythmia or embolus and rarely pulmonary oedema. Exceptionally patients die from a supervening infection of the endocardium. However, in the adult the disease may be stabilized for years.

Treatment

The medical treatment is that of heart failure, i.e. sodium restriction, digitalis and diuretics. This is effective albeit for a limited period. Dysrhythmia requires constant attention. It has been observed that pacing stimulation by cardiac catheterization may fail if the contact is with a fibrosed endocardium. Anticoagulants are not used routinely.

The results of surgical treatment are interesting.[42, 53, 54] In a controlled study in Abidjan[55] an operated group fared better than a comparable non-operated one (Fig. 61.13). The indication

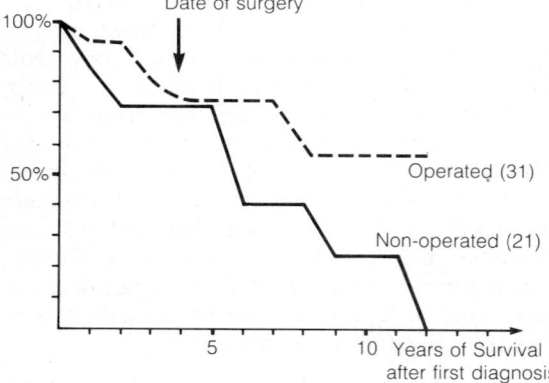

Fig. 61.13 Endomyocardial fibrosis. Actuarial survival curve showing the survival of 31 patients operated on compared with 21 patients who did not have an operation.

for surgery is a syndrome of severe cardiorestriction and/or a moderate to severe mitral regurgitation. Other cases, less frequent, can be monitored and treated medically. The only definite contraindication to surgery at present is the recurrence of ascites with hepatic fibrosis. The post-surgical fate of patients remains an open question. Meantime, no recurrence was noted in cases followed up for six years.

In the absence of a firm diagnosis treatment against the cause must necessarily be somewhat fortuitous. Existing parasitoses or infections require specific treatment. The therapeutic implications of a possible eosinophilic role in the aetiology are discussed in the following section.

Aetiology

Several hypotheses have been advanced to explain the aetiology. A hyperserotoninaemia due to the consumption of plantain bananas has been postulated. Streptococci have been held responsible for parietal as well as for valvular endocarditis. An immunological basis has been assumed in Kampala in patients with antibodies notably against malaria. Others have indicated certain parasites especially flukes, filariae and schistosomes. These speculations remain unconfirmed.

Current opinion favours the hypothesis that *eosinophils* cause the endocarditis. In some patients with a high eosinophilia these cells are alleged to become activated when immunoglobulins adhere to their surface. They then liberate proteolytic granules capable of lysing parasites but also at times of cytotoxicity against the body's epithelial, endothelial and nervous tissue in laboratory animals. It is supposed, but not yet confirmed, that this can happen in man in which case CPE would be the outcome of eosinophilic aggression in a continuum of eosinophilic syndromes: Löffler's syndrome, tropical eosinophilia (Chapter 20), leukaemia, FPE and EMF. This hypothesis could explain tropical EMF (in which eosinophilia is not invariably present) only if one accepts that it is a late diagnosis effected after high eosinophilic counts have disappeared.[56]

The eosinophilogenic hypothesis is particularly interesting in that a preventive approach then becomes possible. Screening of patients with high eosinophil counts or, better still, those with the proteolytic granules, would identify those at risk of developing CPE. Early discovery, possibly confirmed by biopsy, would then be followed by corticoid or hydroxyurea treatment capable of inducing the lesion to regress.[57]

Conclusion

EMF is now a disease of which the pathology, symptomatology, diagnosis and clinical evolution are well established. All points to a disease of the endocardium where the damage starts and predominates. The myocardium is affected in the subendocardial region only. It is this which justifies surgery for it would be useless, even dangerous, to operate if the myocardium was heavily implicated early on. The analogy with constrictive pericarditis is evident but the aetiology remains obscure, although the eosinophil hypothesis offers interesting preventive and therapeutic scope, if confirmed.

TROPICAL PROFILES OF THE UNIVERSAL MAJOR CARDIOVASCULAR DISEASES

Rheumatic valvulopathies

Whilst in developing countries rheumatic valvulopathy is becoming progressively rarer, it is still seen very frequently in the tropics.

The *epidemiology* of this condition in these regions still needs clarification,[58] particularly as the methodologies of the several surveys that have been carried out are hard to compare. A high level of antistreptolysin in the African population of school age surveyed was found in 19.5% in the Ivory Coast, 12–26% in Senegal and in 9.8–44.4% in Cameroon. In Egypt an estimated 30% of schoolchildren harbour group A *Streptococcus*. Analysis of the prevalence of this valvulopathy has brought out a distinct difference between the countries in black Africa with a rate of 1–3 per thousand and those in North Africa with a rate of 9.5–15 per thousand. Numerous studies of its hospital prevalence indicate that in the African forest and wet savannah regions it represents 10–20% of all cardiopathies whereas in regions to the north and to the south of this it is much greater: 26.7% in Senegal, 40.5% in Tunisia, 70% in Morocco, 36.6% in Madagascar and 20.8% in South Africa. A multicentre survey confirmed these data showing that rheumatic cardiopathy represents 43.8% of total cardiopathy in North Africa, 21.3% in the African savannah and 17.8% in the African forest

belt (Fig. 61.14). While socioeconomic factors may explain a prevalence difference between developed countries and underdeveloped ones, they do not account for differences within the underdeveloped zone or for those within the same country. Probably geoclimatic and genetic factors are involved epidemiologically.

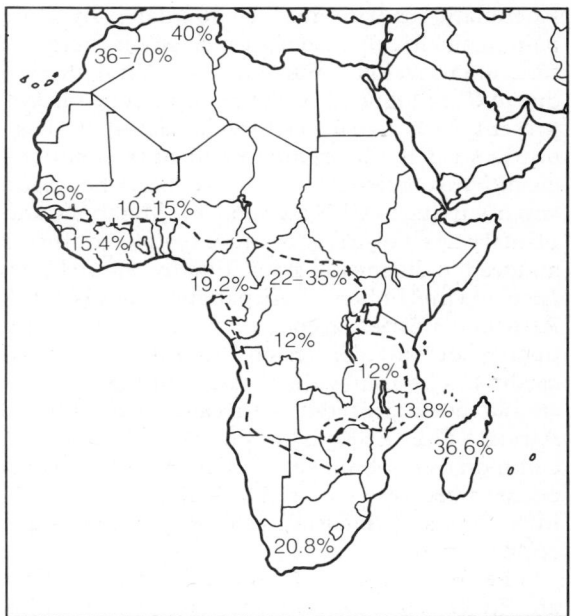

Fig. 61.14 Rheumatic valvular heart disease. Valvular disease as a percentage of all cardiovascular disease. Dotted line marks the border between forest and humid savannah.

Outside Africa[59] comparable valvulopathy studies of schoolchildren reported it at 1.8 per thousand in Brazil, 2–8 per thousand in Peru, 3–10 per thousand in India's different regions, 1–2 per thousand in the Philippines and also in Thailand, and 0.8 per thousand in Indonesia. In the Antilles the prevalence of rheumatic heart disease is very high.

Noteworthy is the youth of the average patient (average 23 years; one-third are less than 15 years old). The number and the promiscuity favouring spread in children are adduced to explain this streptococcal pathology prevalence but poor sanitary structures and weak health services in underprivileged areas are also operative. In terms of aetiology the rarity of articular rheumatism and chorea is worth noting.

Clinically, mitral stenosis is less frequent than insufficiency but statistics disagree on this point. Aortic regurgitation is less frequent than mitral lesions and aortic stenosis is even rarer. In about 25–65% of the cases seen for the first time heart failure is already present; such is the delay in medical intervention. The usual lack of prophylaxis leads to recurrences and thereby to a severe evolution of the illness. Embolism, however, is a rare complication.

Diagnostic problems may arise in the tropics. Rheumatic arthritis may be simulated by bone pain in sickle cell anaemia especially if there is a functional systolic murmur also. Viral disease due to Chikungunya and O'nyong-nyong viruses present with febrile arthralgia. Another diagnostic snag is the frequency of mitral and tricuspid insufficiency which are non-rheumatic and often due to CPE (see above). Metabolic and primary heart disease can cause systolic murmurs and lead to diagnostic error. Finally, at the Heart Institute in Abidjan where patients from 14 black African countries attend, we have noted the frequency of valvular lesions in infective endocarditis. The minor diagnostic criteria of Jones should be interpreted with caution in tropical Africa. The ESR is often high because of common dysglobulinaemia. Fever and arthralgia occur more often in sickle cell patients, viral infections and malarial onset. Cutaneous signs are hardly ever seen.

The inadequacies of regional health services are reflected in a lack of rigorous *treatment* which favours the development of valvular sequelae in patients. Meantime, surgical facilities are scarce; the Abidjan cardiology centre is the only one in black Africa where, in the last 10 years, cardiac surgery has been regularly available.

An effective *prophylaxis* of sore throats and rheumatic fever is needed. Admittedly, certain regions do not have adequate services to cover the whole population; in many countries, however, such a prophylaxis can be achieved at minimal costs by concentrating efforts on the school population.[60]

Infective endocarditis (IE)

In general IE is underestimated in tropical clinical statistics. According to pathological studies IE constitutes 20%[61] to 12%[39] of all cardiopathy. At the Heart Institute in Abidjan specialized investigation, notably echocardiography, detected IE in 1.5% of hospitalized patients. IE affects previously normal valves in 75% of cases; in the rest it complicated congenital cardiopathy or valvular prosthesis. Limited bacteriological

facilities in tropical areas impede the precise identification of causative organisms.

The incidence of complications is high. Over half the cases seen are in heart failure. Peripheral and cerebral emboli are common. Renal failure occurs very often. This high complication rate is due to the fact that by the time patients are first seen the disease in most is well advanced. In the rare studies published in Africa the prognosis has been very bad entailing a mortality ranging from 70%[62] to 92%.[63] Our series fared better, thanks to the availability of surgery. The overall mortality was 36% comprising 64% of non-operated and 14% of operated cases.

The frequency of IE is not surprising in regions where valvulopathy is common and infections numerous. Particular attention needs to be devoted to this illness.

Coronary disease

In the tropics coronary disease is still rare but, in the last 15–20 years, its establishment has become quite obvious. It is an important cause of death in Malaysia, Singapore, Sri Lanka and Mauritius.[64] In black Africa it figures in all epidemiological statistics. In the Ivory Coast it represented 2.2% of cardiovascular morbidity in the medical wards in 1965 and 5.3% in 1983. Two statistical pathological studies[65] in the same hospital showed that among South African blacks coronary disease occurred in 0.9% of autopsies made in 1959 but in 11.7% in those made in 1976. Among the indigenous population of the Ivory Coast acute myocardial infarction is reckoned to occur in 2.1 per 100 000.[66] Coronary pathology is more frequent in North Africa than in the African savannah or forest region[67] (Fig. 61.15).

The risk factors in the tropics are similar to everywhere else: male sex, sixth decade of life, smoking, hypertension, diabetes, overweight and lack of exercise. Most patients come from the middle class but a fifth have a poor background. Cholesterolaemia is higher than normal in patients—often more than 2.20 mg/litre. The reason for this is not clear since most follow a traditional diet poor in items such as butter and eggs. The reduction of endemic diseases is alleged to have caused a fall in globulins attended by a rise in cholesterol. Urban stress may be a factor; stress exists in rural areas, too, but is of a different nature. Acculturation—the interaction

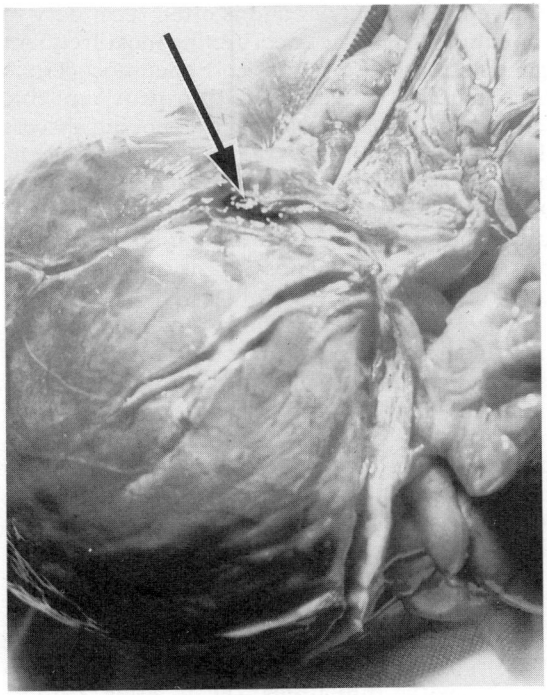

Fig. 61.15 Myocardial infarction in an African. Coronary artery atherosclerosis.

of distinctly different cultures, may be a possible factor in coronary disease.

One may ask *why coronary disease was and remains rare* in the tropics? Is it because of the low expectation of life (about 40 years)? Probably not; once the individual outlives the dangers of childhood his life expectation is equal to or greater than that which obtains in developed countries.[68] It is relevant to recall that by the year 2000 60% of those over 65 years old will be living in underdeveloped areas.[64] Is it then a matter of diet: long-chained glycosides rather than refined sugar, and alimentary fats mostly unsaturated? However, these food characteristics have never changed. Perhaps the reason lies in the rural way of life. This is possible even if not verifiable. It is also relevant to remember that by the year 2000 the population of the developing countries will be 41% urban.[64] Another explanation adduced is would-be peculiarity of the coronary network, but angiography has not confirmed this. We have noted that the pathology of thrombosis (arteritis, phlebitis, infarction and embolism) is rarer in developing countries. A recent study has shown that platelet aggregation is slower in the African than in the European, perhaps because of fish

consumption.[69] This important fact may have a bearing on the problem which, as yet, we cannot explain.

The *symptoms* are similar to those found elsewhere: angina pectoris and infarction have universal features. Angiography shows that the lesions tend to be more restricted involving preferentially the anterior interventricular branch.[70] The outcome of the infarct[71] is often fatal; in hospital 15% die. Death occurs in 20% by the second year and in 50% by the fifth. This fatality rate is attributable to inadequate health education of the public coupled with socioeconomic conditions which make long-term therapy exceedingly difficult. In any case, while the disease still remains relatively rare its evolution when it occurs is very serious indeed.

Treatment does not call for any particular comment were it not for the socioeconomic conditions and great distances that militate against it. Surgery is at present rarely practised because of the relative rarity of the disease. It seems certain that it will be increasingly developed in future in those centres adequately equipped for it.

Primary and secondary *prevention* are feasible in most countries. The rare occurrence of the disease in the tropics offers a good scope for primary prevention.[64] This entails national and international efforts to combat smoking, physical inactivity and hypertension. It would aim at maintaining the existing dietary habits which are healthy and should not be replaced by others less so. Urbanization should be planned to facilitate a healthier and happier way of life while health education of the young should aim at disease prevention. In fact, if preventive measures are not taken now, coronary disease will assume an increasing role in the morbidity of adults and will claim a progressively higher toll of their life.

Congenital cardiopathies

These present no special tropical characteristics. It should be pointed out, however, that the detection of cyanosis in black subjects is more difficult than in whites particularly when, as frequently happens, anaemia reduces the intensity of the discoloration. It is of particular importance then to examine the gums and nails carefully.

It is known that in Mexico and Peru the high altitude predisposes to a patent ductus and to pulmonary hypertension. Geoclimatic conditions in the tropics do not seem to have a role in the malformations of the heart, nor do the major endemic diseases or the haemo-globinopathies.

The frequency of the different congenital car-diopathies has been worked out in Central America, South-East Asia and in Africa. The commonest malformations are the same in trop-ical and in temperate regions: ventricular septal defect, atrial septal defect, Fallot's tetralogy, patent ductus arteriosus and pulmonary stenosis. Coarctation of the aorta and aortic stenosis were thought to be rarer in the tropics but catheter studies of 612 younger subjects have established only a narrower difference.[72] It is probable that congenital cardiopathies have the same dis-tribution throughout the world. Their treatment, too, is rarely undertaken in the tropics where they present no special features in either their presentation or outcome as observed in Abidjar.

Pericarditis

1 While *acute pericarditis* is common in the tropics it does not present any particular features clinically. In the absence of echocardiography or invasive exploratory means, diagnostic peri-cardial paracentesis is practised more often than in developed countries allowing the thick peri-cardium of tuberculous or purulent pericarditis, or the thin one of acute rheumatic or benign aetiology to be noted (Fig. 61.16).

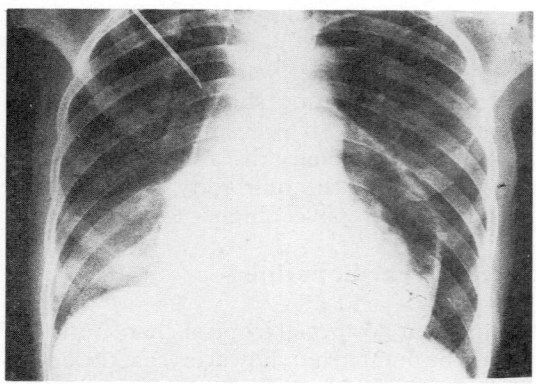

Fig. 61.16 Purulent pericarditis. Ragged pericardial shadow (after air injection).

What is particular about pericarditis in the tropics is the aetiology. In the causation of acute pericarditis, tuberculosis still ranks first and the benign varieties second. Third comes purulent pericarditis which is much more frequent than

in developed countries and is often secondary to a pneumopathy. The cocci are the most frequent agents (strepto-, staphylo- and pneumococci). A more tropical syndrome is purulent amoebic pericarditis, usually a sequel to amoebic abscess of the liver. Fourth in frequency are the rheu-matic lesions which can be quite misleading. Other causes include infarction, collagen disease, cancer and uraemia. As described above, Amer-ican and African trypanosomiasis can cause peri-cardial effusion.

2 *Chronic pericardial effusion* occurs more fre-quently in the tropics, not only that caused by cancer, amyloidosis, tuberculosis, collagen disease, X-rays or lymphatic block but also, and in particular, by endomyocardial fibrosis and primary chronic myocardiopathy. This means that effusion does not rule out these two diag-noses—this possibility of error is worth remem-bering.

3 *Chronic constrictive pericarditis* does not present unusual features. It is often the result of a long-standing tuberculous or purulent peri-carditis. The differential diagnosis from EMF is fraught with difficulties (even after cath-erization and echography) when the RV is crushed by the constriction. In general, however, it is these which clarify the diagnosis (see p. 1019).

Cardiac stimulation (pacemakers)

Cardiac stimulation is carried out in the tropics for the same reasons as in temperate regions but also for American trypanosomiasis (frequently) and in Africa for cardiomyopathies of diverse origin, mostly non-coronary. Patients in the tropics tend to be younger and generally to tol-erate the stimulation well both physiologically and psychologically. It should be noted that endocavitary stimulation may not be effective in patients with a fibrosed endocardium.

The cost of stimulators raises socioeconomic problems in addition to those of effecting adequate surveillance after implantation when patients live in remote areas. Therefore, at present the indications are restricted; mainly, pacemakers are used for AV block. For this reason in eight years only 120 have been implanted at the Heart Institute in Abidjan.

Arteritis

In the tropical zone arteritis is relatively rare. In Africa it makes up 0.55–4% of cardiovascular morbidity whereas in France, for example, it causes 6% of deaths.

The underlying pathology is usually atherosclerosis, while diabetes is an important factor in most studies and so is smoking. Males are more often affected but arteritis is also common in obese diabetic women. Other causes in the tropics may include collagen disease, Indian hemp toxicity (Morocco) and trauma. Typhoid and *Rickettsia* should be kept in mind as possible causes. Noteworthy is the frequent incidence of the Takayashu type of inflammatory arteritis. It affects the branches of the thoracic aorta and often the aorta itself inducing deformities of it which may be quite remarkable. The arteries of the lower limbs, too, may be affected.

The mainstays of treatment are the anticoagulants and the vasodilators. Surgery may be needed. The effect of anti-inflammatory drugs on inflammatory arteritis is not clear.

Phlebitis, pulmonary embolism

The rarity of phlebitis in the tropics is well documented in many countries. This is all the more surprising in that in some regions 15–25% of subjects have an abnormal haemoglobin. Surgical and gynaecological data show a prevalence of 0.04–0.7 per thousand of the patients seen. This in Europe is around 3–10 per thousand while pulmonary embolism complicates about 8% of surgical operations. The rarity of phlebitis and embolism in the tropics tends to induce physicians and surgeons to dispense with routine prophylaxis with anticoagulants, even in cases of expected high risk of thrombosis, e.g. bone or pelvic surgery or bedridden cardiac patients. It should be noted, however, that accidental pulmonary embolism (confirmed by angiopneumography) does occur[73] so that, even if the risks are smaller, it would be prudent to be cautious. Postpartum myocardiopathy and mitral stenosis with arterial fibrillation accentuate the risk.

Different causes can be noted, including cardiac, traumatic, gouty (Madagascar plateau, Polynesia) and haemopathic factors and anaemia (rare in spite of the frequency of anaemias). More likely causes are gynaecological, infections or sickle cell anaemia.

The clinical picture is that seen elsewhere and as elsewhere it can be quite misleading. Phlebography and ultrasonic examination of the blood flow (Doppler effect) as well as the distribution of injected ^{123}I-labelled fibrinogen may aid diagnosis appreciably. Treatment is based on anticoagulants with or without fibrinolytic therapy. Surgery may be indicated.

The rarity of thrombosis. Anticoagulant therapy

In various preceding sections it was stated that thrombotic lesions are rarer in the tropics.[74] It has been observed that the prevalence of myocardial infarction, arteritis, phlebitis and embolism is minimal. This leads to a certain laxity in anticoagulant therapy which is shortened, less strict and even omitted in cases in which elsewhere it would be rigorously prescribed. The cases of prophylaxis in surgery have already been cited. It is also known that certain North African authors[75] have noted few complications in patients with metallic valvular prostheses but without adequate anticoagulant therapy.

However, these findings would be more convincing if evidence were forthcoming of a reduced coagulability in the tropics, where its study showed it to be no different from that found in temperate zones. Nevertheless, there is growing evidence of an increased fibrinolytic activity and a reduced platelet activity in black Africans. In our laboratory[69] we have noted a distinct difference between Europeans and Africans, fibrinolysis in the latter being faster and more intense. Studies under way may bring to light fundamental biological data which would give the prevention and treatment of thrombosis in the tropics a more rational basis. One wonders whether these platelet modifications are genetic or acquired.[76] They may be correlated with high fish consumption.[69]

The 'tendency to coagulate less' should, one would have thought, entail an easier task for anticoagulant therapy and perhaps greater risks. Our experience, however, with heparin or antivitamin K treatment showed no difference in sensitivity or risk between whites and blacks as well as between subjects with sickling and those without it.

Arterial hypertension (AH)

Up to 1955–1960 arterial hypertension (AH) was considered a rarity in black Africa and in many underdeveloped tropical regions. Since then it has become common in numerous countries, its prevalence in blacks even exceeding that in whites according to some observers. Some now say that hypertension has become the commonest cardiovascular disease in black Africa and in many tropical countries.

Epidemiology

In tropical Africa AH affects about 10% of the population and up to 16–17% in certain countries. In a multicentre survey[77] AH was found to increase moving south from North Africa to the equator. Its occurrence is frequent in the elderly, less so in the young. About 4% of schoolchildren aged 10–16 years had blood pressures above the average by two standard deviations. Little information is available about the situation in tropical America. In tropical Asia the population prevalence is of a comparable order and higher in some areas.

Environmental factors play a role. In Africa and in the Pacific monitoring isolated populations has shown that their blood pressure (BP) rose but little with ageing. Once opened to exterior change these populations showed higher orders of blood pressure. The reasons for this development are not well understood. Altered salt consumption is a probable factor while others may be obesity, reduced activity, smoking, urinary infections and urban or rural stress.

In the Ivory Coast social class is seen to play a part: railway and bus workers have the highest BP figures, manual workers on agro-industrial plantations the second highest and peasants the lowest. Bilharziasis is not an important factor but acculturation stress in communities exposed to other cultures beside (and often in conflict with) their own is a likely operative factor.

Twin studies have revealed the importance of a genetic factor. A difference in sodium/potassium cellular transport and exchange is alleged to be a genetic factor predisposing the black more than the white to hypertension.

The BP is usually higher in men; for unknown reasons in women in the African savannah it is higher than in men. The fact that the women concerned regard stoutness and even obesity as aesthetically desirable may not be irrelevant.

General features and treatment

In tropical regions, notably in Africa, there are occasional excessively high BP figures—about 300 mmHg systolic and 150–200 mmHg diastolic. These extremes notwithstanding, the disease may be completely latent. Vertigo is the commonest complaint followed by headache or eye symptoms. Often the AH is disclosed by the onset of a complication. Cerebrovascular complications are more frequent perhaps than in temperate regions. Half the cases have signs of nephropathy. LV failure is very common but coronary complications are still rare. The varieties of AH seen are those one meets elsewhere and are attended by the same problems. The AH may be well tolerated, labile, malignant, paroxysmal or obstetrical. A syndrome to keep in mind is postpartum paroxysmal hypertension.

In *treatment* socioeconomic considerations dictate that costs be kept to a minimum. With this in mind an imposed sodium-free diet reduces by a third to a half the quantity of drugs required, even if it is not absolutely rigorous.[78] In the tropics many foods are poor in sodium, e.g. rice, banana, arrowroot and, notably, fruits. There are also 'sauces' poor in sodium and rich in potassium. Sodium restriction then is a feasible and essential element of treatment. Medical treatment may consist of diuretics but a certain resistance of blacks to beta-blockers has been described. In addition, diuretics are cheaper. If they fail, however, the other drugs may then have to be prescribed. Even where investigative means are modest an effort should be made to identify cases of secondary hypertension.

Hypertension as a public health problem[79]

In an African country like the Ivory Coast it has been calculated that surveillance and treatment of all hypertensives would consume one-fifth of the national budget or about half of the gross national product per inhabitant. This underlines the importance of the role of the physician in prescribing minimal cost treatment if he wants the patient to cooperate.

The disease imposes a heavy social burden. In the general medical wards AH accounts for 7% of the admissions, while AH-related conditions make up 9% of the deaths. The frequency and duration of absenteeism caused is difficult to estimate. It causes serious invalidity—over half the patients have heart and/or renal pathology whilst neurological complications are common.

Prevention is essential. Its target should be schoolchildren. It is necessary to seek 'borderline' cases (BP: average + 1 SD) and those at risk (BP: average + 2 SD) (Fig. 61.17). Surveillance of these children should be coupled

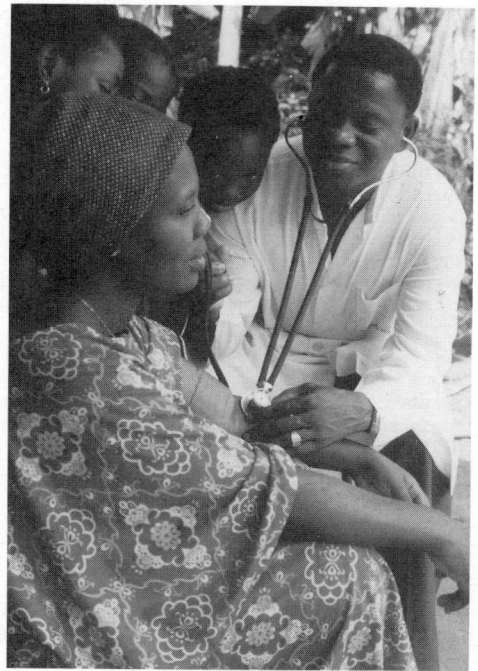

Fig. 61.17 Paramedical aide measuring arterial blood pressure during the course of a survey in a rural area.

with regimens of low salt, no smoking, weight control, sports activity and no oral contraceptives. This inexpensive strategy assumes that the adult follows the same BP corridor as the child. In any case it cannot be harmful but it is necessary to establish BP norms. In our experience weight-related norms are more satisfactory than those related to the height and age.[80]

THE ELECTROCARDIOGRAM OF BLACK AFRICANS

Since 1946 several surveys in the USA and in Africa have encouraged the notion that the ECG in the black differs from that of the white. Such a notion can have important diagnostic implications and needs careful analysis.

The departures from the norm which have been described are of three types:[81] (i) in right precordial leads a downshift of ST with a negative T; (ii) in the left precordial leads an elevation of ST with a broad T, and (iii) a rounded or flattened T in precordial leads. Other authors have noted an increased amplitude of R in V1 and of S in V6,[82] also a shortening of QRS.[83]

A characteristic of these 'normal' anomalies is

the enormous range of their occurrence according to different authors (0.7–60% of cases). They would seem to occur more often in lower social classes and in the young. No explanation has been put forward to account satisfactorily for these 'normal' deviations.

In a recent study we have compared matched, military, 20-year-old Africans and Europeans living in Abidjan.[84] Only two significant differences were found: Sokoloff's index was over 35 mm in 13.6% of Africans and in 7.1% of Europeans. In left precordial leads Africans had 'neurotonic' features (ST elevation; ample T) more often than Europeans. These differences do not seem to carry much weight. It is better to speak of 'anomalies of unexplained origin' rather than of 'normal ECG differences between black and white subjects'.

In practice the ECG of black Africans should be interpreted in the same way as one does that of the white, but perhaps in blacks more often one meets anomalies of undetermined origin which cannot be considered normal in either blacks or whites.

REFERENCES

1 Chapuis (1976) *Trop. Cardiol.* **2**, 179–183.
2 Jones I. C., Lowenthal, M.N. & Buyst, H. (1975) *Trans. Roy. Soc. Trop. Med. Hyg.* **69**, 388.
3 Schyns, C. & Janssen, P. (1965) *ISRAC (Kinsbasa)* **1**, 2–4.
4 De Raadt, P. & Koten, J.W. (1968) *East Afr. Med. J.* **45**, 128
5 Manson-Bahr, P.E.C. & Charters, A.D. (1963) *Trans. R. Soc. trop. Med. Hyg.* **69**, 388.
6 Bertrand, E., Serie, F., Rive, J. et al (1974) *Acta cardiol.* **29**, 363–381.
7 Bertrand, E., Loubiere, R., Barabe, P. et al (1969) *Presse Méd.* **77**, 1951–1952.
8 Poltera, A.A.H. (1976) *Br. Heart J.* **38**, 827–837.
9 Guimaraes, A.C. (1982) *Arq. Bras. Cardiol.* **38/4**, 301–309.
10 Bertrand, E., Dalger, J., Ramiara, J.P. et al (1978) *Arch. Mal. cœur* **71**, 216–221.
11 Gelfand, M. et al (1959) *Trans. R. Soc. trop. Med. Hyg.* **53**, 282–284.
12 Touze, J.E., Kacou, M., Bordahandy, R. et al (1984) *Bull. Soc. Path. éxot.* **77**, 666–672.
13 Charles, D. & Bertrand, E. (1982) *Méd. trop.* **42**, 405–409.
14 Sankale, M. (1969) *Vie Méd.* **50**, 2729–2734.
15 Herrera, J.M. (1960) *Arch. Inst. Cardiol. Mex.* **30**, 126.
16 Phillips, R.E., Warrell, D.A., White, N. J. et al (1985) *New Engl. J. Med.* **312**, 1273–1278.
17 Bertrand, E., Botreau Roussel, P. & Renambot, J. (1976) *Bull. Soc. Path. éxot.* **69**, 53–62.
18 Heller, R.F., Gorbach, S. L., Tatooless, C. J. et al (1972) *J. Am. med. Ass.* **220**, 988.

19 Ramachandraw, S. (1973) *Ceylon med. J.* 138–143.

20 Bertrand, E., Renambot, J., Chauvet, J. et al (1979) *Cœur* 3, 369–380.

21 Roux, F., Bourgeade, A., Salaun, J.J. et al (1976) *Cœur Méd. intern.* 15, 37–44.

22 Goodwin, S.F. (1982) *Br. Heart J.* 48, 1–18.

23 Askanas, A., Udoshi, M. & Sadjadi, S.A. (1980). *Am. Heart J.* 99, 9.

24 Matthews, E.C., Gardin, J.M., Henry, W.L. et al (1981) *Am. J. Cardiol.* 47, 570.

25 Touze, J.E., Ekro, A., Mardelle, T. et al (1986) *Cardiol. Trop.* 12, 17–24.

26 Meadows, W.R. (1960) *Am. J. Cardiol.* 6, 788–802.

27 Demakis, S.G., Shambudin, H., Rahim Toola, H. et al (1971) *Circulation* 44, 1053–1061.

28 Seftel, H. & Susser, M. (1961) *Br. Heart J.* 23, 43–52.

29 Fillmore, S.J. & Parry, E.H.D. (1977) *Circulation* 56, 1058–1061.

30 Bertrand, E., Langlois, J., Renambot, J. et al (1977) *Arch. Mal. cœur* 70, 169–178.

31 Burg, J.R., Dodek, A., Kloster, F.E. et al (1974) *Circulation* 49, 560.

32 Bertrand, E., Hanna, M., Levy, D. et al (1985) *Cardiol. trop.* 11, 57–69.

33 Melvin, K.R., Richardson, D.J., Olsen, E.G.J. et al (1982) *New Engl. J. Med.* 307, 731–734.

34 Botreau-Roussel, P., Drobinski, G., Levy, R. et al (1977) *Arch. Mal. cœur* 7, 141–148.

35 Moser, K.M. & Shea, J.G. (1957) *Am. J. Med.* 22, 561.

36 Balfour, I.C., Covitz, W., Davis, H. et al (1984) *Am. Heart J.* 108, 345–350.

37 Mardelle, T., Chauvet, J., Touze, J.E. et al (1986) *Cardiol. Trop.* 12, 31–40.

38 Metras, D., Coulibaly, A.P., Ouattara, K. et al (1982) *Thorax* 37, 486–491.

39 Brockington I.F. & Edington, G.M. (1972) *Am. Heart J.* 83, 27.

40 Cockshott, W.P., Antia, E.A., Ikeme, A.C. et al (1967) *Brit. J. Radiol.* 40, 424–435.

41 Lintermans, J.P. (1976) *Cardiol. trop.* 2, 13–27.

42 Metras, D., Ouattara, K., Coulibaly, A.O. et al (1982) *J. Thor. Cardio-vasc. Surg.* 83, 52–64.

43 Williams, A.O. (1974) In *Cardiovascular Disease in the Tropics*, ed. A.G. Shaper, M.S.R. Hutt & Z. Fejfar, pp. 314–323. London: British Medical Association.

44 D'Azbela, P.G., Patel, A.K., Grigg, L.G. et al (1974) In *Cardiovascular Disease in the Tropics*, ed. A.G. Shaper, M.S.R. Hutt & Z. Fejfar, pp. 58–69. London: British Medical Association.

45 Brockington I.F. & Olsen, E.G.J. (1973) *Am. Heart J.* 85, 308–322.

46 Dienot, B., Ekra, A. & Bertrand, E. (1981) *Cardiol. trop.* 9, 107–114.

47 Bertrand, E. & Renambot, J. (1975) *Acta cardiol.* 30, 405–418.

48 Carvalho, F.R., Matos, S., Victor, E.G. et al (1984) *Angiology* 35, 63–70.

49 Cockshott, W.P. (1965) *Br. J. Radiol.* 38, 192–200.

50 Bertrand, E., Cailleau, G., Ekra, A. et al (1980) *Cœur* 11, 15–25.

51 Van Der Geld, H., Petoom, F., Somers, K. et al (1966) *Lancet* ii, 1210–1214.

52 Shaper, A.G. (1967) *Scot. Med. J.* 12, 393–400.

53 Dubost, C.H. & Deloche, A. (1980) In *Actualités de chirurgie cardiovasculaire de l'Hôpital Broussais*, pp. 149–158. Paris: Masson.

54 Valiathan, M.S., Sankarkumar, R., Balakrishnan, K.G. et al (1983) *Thorax* 38, 421–427.

55 Bertrand, E., Chauvet, J., Odi Assamoi et al (1982) *Bull. Acad. Méd. Paris* 166, 1179–1186.

56 Olsen, E.G.J. & Spry, C.S.F. (1979) In *Progress in Cardiology*, ed. Yu & Goodwin, vol. 8, pp. 281–303. Philadelphia: Lea and Febiger.

57 Parrillo, J.E., Fauci, A.S. & Wolff, S.M. (1978) *Ann. intern. Med.* 89, 167–172.

58 Bertrand, E. & N'Dori, R. (1985) *Bordeaux Méd.* 87–110.

59 WHO meeting, New Delhi (1980) *Chronique OMS* 34, 357–367.

60 Strasser, R. & Rotta, J. (1973) *WHO Chron.* 27, 49.

61 Quenum, L. & Ndiaye, P.D. (1970) *Méd. Afr. Noire* 17, 877.

62 Falase, A.O., Jayesimi, F., Iyun, A.O. et al (1976) *Trop. geogr. Med.* 28, 9.

63 Koate, P., Wuenum, C. & Diouf, S. (1976) In *Cardiovascular Diseases in Africa*, ed. O.O. Akinkugbe, p. 259. Ibadan: Ciba-Geigy.

64 World Health Organization (1982) *WHO Tech. Rep.* No. 678.

65 Isaacson, C. (1977) *S. Afr. med. J.* 52, 793–798.

66 Bertrand, E., Kacou, G.M., Monkam Mbouende Y et al (1984) *Cardiol. Trop.* 10, 51–64.

67 Multaf-Cardio (1983) *Cardiol. trop.* 9, 105–112.

68 Walker, A.R.P. (1974) *Postgrad. med. J.* 50, 29–32.

69 Bertrand, E., Cloitre, B., Ticolat, R. et al (1986) *Cardiol. Trop.* 12, 95–96.

70 Touze, J.E., Ekra, A., Mardelle, T. et al (1986) *Cardiol. trop.* 12 (in press).

71 N'Dori, R., Kamara, M., Odi Assamoi, M. et al (1985) *Sem. Hôp. Paris* 61, 1057–1059.

72 Chauvet, J., Kacou, G.M. & Bertrand, E. (1987) *Cardiol. trop.* 11 (in press).

73 Touze, J.E., Moncany, G., Amonkou, A. et al (1985) *Med. trop.* 45, 43–46.

74 Bertrand, E. (1979) *Précis de pathologie cardio-vasculaire tropicale*. Sandoz: Rueil-Malmaison.

75 Ben Ismail, M., Abid,, F. & Mzah, N. (1983) *Ann. Cardiol. Angeiol.* 32, 165–169.

76 Buchanan, G.R., Holtkamp, C.A. & Levy, E.N. (1981) *Br. J. Haem.* 49, 455–464.

77 Multaf-Cardio (1983) *Cardiol. trop.* 9, 13–15.

78 Beard, R.C., Cooke, M.M. & Gray, W.R. (1982) *Lancet* 455–458.

79 Bertrand, E. (1983) *Bull. Soc. Path. éxot.* 76, 327–331.

80 Bertrand, E., Bertrand, C., Ravinet, L. et al (1982) *Cardiol. trop.* 8, 93–103.

81 Grusin, H. (1954) *Circulation* 9, 860.

82 Walker, A.R.P. & Walker, F. (1969) *Am. Heart J.* 77, 441.

83 Masica, D.N., Maron, B.J. & Krouetz, L.J. (1971) *Am. Heart J.* 84, 153.

84 Bertrand, E., Charles, D., Ravinet, L. et al (1982) *Cœur* 14, 325–331.

RECOMMENDED BOOKS

Akinkugbe, O.O. (1976) *Cardiovascular Diseases in Africa.* Ibadan: Ciba-Geigy.

Bertrand, E. (1979) *A Precis of Tropical Cardiovascular Pathology.* Rueil-Malmaison, France: Sandoz.

Shaper, A.G., Hutt, M.S.R. & Fejfar, Z. (1974) *Cardiovascular Diseases in the Tropics.* London: British Medical Association.

Chapter 62
Neurological and Psychiatric Problems
J. R. Billinghurst

NEUROLOGICAL PROBLEMS

INTRODUCTION

Doctors who write about tropical diseases tend to comment on the marked contrasts between the pattern of neurological disorders seen in developing countries and that found in the developed world. The more this is looked into the less true it seems to be. Nevertheless there are undoubted differences: in the tropics infections are more common, cerebral vascular disease less so, whilst tumours and degenerations are rare. The most plausible explanations for these contrasts are the differences in age distribution in the populations, the relative lack of wealth and maldistribution of what there is, the relative or absolute lack of highly specialized investigative procedures to assist in accurate diagnosis, and the way in which the natural history of some diseases is distorted by delayed diagnosis and delayed application of appropriate treatment.

Almost half of the patients in clinics and hospitals are children. Life expectancy is so much shorter that there are few elderly to manifest the diseases commonest at their advanced age, notably strokes, parkinsonism and senile

dementia. Poverty and ignorance increase the likelihood of nutritional neuropathies. The rich few, by contrast, show disease patterns more like those seen in temperate climes. Radioisotope and computerized X-ray scanning, neuroelectrical responses and specialized biochemical tests are beyond the means and expertise of most tropical centres. Many folk believe that local herbal remedies should be tried and local medicine men consulted in the first instance, falling back on 'Western medicine' only in the last resort and thus allowing some diseases to progress to an amazingly florid advanced stage.

For the epidemiologist prevalence rates are distorted by selection in that clinicians with expertise in neurology tend to work in referral centres with at least some specialized diagnostic equipment and treatment facilities.

In published series neurological diseases account for 5–10% of all medical admissions to hospital. Infections are common and include tetanus, meningitis, encephalitis, cerebral malaria, tuberculosis, leprosy and occasionally rabies, trypanosomiasis and worm infestations. One infection which has declined markedly over

Table 62.1 The changing pattern of neurosyphilis and neurovascular disorders at Mulago Hospital, Kampala (from Billinghurst, J.R. in Spillane: *Tropical Neurology*[1]).

	Adults and children			Adults only	
	1940–42 2 years	1947–52 6 years	1965–66 1 year	1957 1 year	1966–68 2 years
Total number included	165	681	594	256	648
Annual average	83	114	594	256	324
Annual rates for all vascular disorders except neurosyphilis	1 (1.2%)	11 (10%)	105 (18%)	30 (12%)	101 (31%)
Annual rates for neurosyphilis	33 (40%)	29 (26%)	9 (1.5%)	21 (8%)	13 (3.9%)

the years is neurosyphilis (Tables 62.1 and 62.2)[1] while the proportion of vascular disease has steadily risen.

Table 62.2 Manifestations of neurosyphilis in Uganda (from Billinghurst, J.R. in Spillane: *Tropical Neurology*[1]).

Manifestation	1937–41 5 years	1960–64 5 years	1966–68 2 years
Meningovascular (all)	69 (62%)	8 (42%)	12 (48%)
Dementia paralytica (general paralysis of the insane)	18 (16%)	4 (21%)	8 (32%)
Myelopathy	15 (14%)	5 (26%)	5 (20%)
Tabes dorsalis	—	1	—
All other cases	9 (8%)	1	—
Total	111	19	25
Total admissions	34 859	51 643	
Cases of neurosyphilis	0.3%	0.036%	

Epilepsy is widely feared and shunned and its prevalence is much underestimated in hospital statistics.

Myelopathies, nowhere common, constitute a most difficult diagnostic and therapeutic problem.

Amongst the nutritional neuropathies recent interest has particularly focused on the Nigerian tropical ataxic neuropathy, a chronic myelopathy somewhat resembling both subacute combined degeneration and tabes dorsalis, compounded by optic atrophy, sensorineural deafness and peripheral neuropathy, occurring in parts of southern Nigeria where cassava (manioc, manihot) is eaten as a staple, and probably due to chronic cyanide intoxication from the cassava inducing a conditioned vitamin B_{12} deficiency (Chapter 47).

In the course of time the discerning physician will recognize most of the rarer neurological diseases. He will diagnose multiple sclerosis in non-indigenous Europeans but virtually never in people who have been born and brought up in the tropics. This uniquely interesting phenomenon is reviewed in detail by Spillane,[2] whose book provides an invaluable conspectus of the patterns and peculiarities of neurology in the tropics.

SYMPTOMS AND SIGNS

Careful history taking is the foundation stone of clinical neurology. Duration, speed of onset and rate of progress, as well as the complaints themselves, are vital clues as to the likely pathological process. In some parts of tropical Africa the local medicine man, through his contacts with the spirit world, is expected to divine the nature of the disease so that any description of symptoms is unnecessary, even resisted. Even where such traditions do not exist, accuracy and completeness are seriously hampered by difficulties over language and comprehension, vagueness about disabilities of long duration, silence concerning feared conditions such as madness, epilepsy and leprosy, and falsification of other information brought about by a charming but mistaken intention to please. It is impossible to overestimate the value of statements made by relatives, friends, neighbours or onlookers where there is altered consciousness or behaviour.

Physical examination has three peculiarities worthy of mention: pupillary reactions, sensory testing and plantar responses. The reaction of the pupil to light is important, not for the detection of neurosyphilis, which is rare, but for the assessment of third cranial nerve function especially in suspected rapidly expanding intracranial lesions. Under those circumstances the reaction to accommodation is difficult or impossible to test. But as a true Argyll Robertson pupil is of the utmost rarity failure to test for accommodation does not matter anyway. The black pupil is not readily distinguished from a very dark brown iris and its reaction to light is more easily seen if observed through a simple hand lens.

In theory sensory testing can be of great diagnostic value; in practice it is liable to become time-consuming, exhausting and agonizingly inconclusive. The examiner must remain calm and gentle and rigorously resist the temptation to suspect the patient of being deliberately uncooperative.

The sensory modality least dependent on patient comprehension and cooperation is pain. Even in a drowsy or confused subject the response to the prick of a pin (preferable to a very sharp needle which too readily punctures the skin) is of lateralizing value in hemispheric (and lateral medullary) lesions and of great localizing value in assessing the level of a spinal cord lesion particularly when the transition from reduced or absent sensation to normal is marked by a band of hyperalgesia. The reaction at the level may be prompt and unmistakable. More cooperation is required when it comes to the 'glove and stocking' loss in suspected poly-neuropathy.

Appreciation of temperature is the first modality to be impaired in leprosy. A crude but simple method of testing is to exhale gently on to the area being examined (feeling of warmth) and then to blow out quickly between pursed lips (feeling of coolness induced by rapid evaporation of moisture on the skin). Needless to say, the latter is less cooling in a very humid atmosphere. Metal objects should feel cool unless already heated in the environment.

Vibrational sense is typically lost early in a polyneuropathy and should be a valuable diagnostic modality, but with an unsophisticated patient it is particularly important to ensure that it is the vibration and not the sensation of a hard metal object that is being enquired about. The tuning fork must vibrate at 128 Hz or thereabouts; conclusions based on using a fork at a higher frequency are likely to be invalid.

Loss of joint position sense, unless mild or dubious, should be associated with evidence of a sensory ataxia and a positive Romberg's sign.

To the clinician, intent on the earliest suspicious features of multiple sclerosis, the plantar response is of paramount importance. Not so in the tropics! Barefoot folk develop tough and unresponsive soles. As Spillane so aptly remarked, 'the great Babinski would never have discovered his famous sign if he had lived and practised neurology in Africa' (quoted by Osuntokun[3]). Perhaps he would have picked on neck stiffness instead.

MODES OF PRESENTATION

Matthews[4] did clinicians a great service in his book *Practical Neurology* by approaching the specialty along the lines of symptom presentation rather than the usual systematic analysis by anatomy or pathology. His approach is of enormous value to anyone having to cope with potential neurological problems in a busy outpatient clinic, casualty department or ward.

There are certain situations in the tropics sufficiently demanding and different from those in the developed world to merit special attention; they are considered below. The remainder are less dissimilar and need only be mentioned briefly.

Headache is a frequent complaint. Less serious causes include tension and anxiety (very common), migraine (rather uncommon), sinusitis, refractive errors and dental disease. Recent headache of increasing severity must arouse the suspicion of a low grade meningitis or meningoencephalitis; all forms of meningitis are much commoner in the tropics and most are potentially curable if treated and lethal if neglected. Raised intracranial pressure is a rare cause of headache; it is the accompanying apathy, drowsiness and vomiting which should alert the clinician, whether or not he can see papilloedema.

Giddiness is rarely due to neurological disease; anaemia is much more likely. The same applies to *weakness*. Unless physical examination supplies a vital clue an organic diagnosis remains elusive.

Paraesthesiae of the most bizarre description may be complained of; it is their distribution which can provide the important evidence of their significance. In endemic areas leprosy is greatly feared and the complaint of localized numbness may be an oblique call to prove or disprove that diagnosis.

Difficulty with walking, if due to a neurological cause, very probably indicates a myelopathy or peripheral neuropathy and is considered below.

Prolonged or permanent *physical handicap* because of neurological disease, of which leprosy and poliomyelitis are the commonest, throws a colossal burden on the family or local community when the government health services are inadequate. Voluntary agencies play an important part. Commendable improvements are occurring but they tend to be patchy.

Acute confusion and coma (toxic confusional states, acute brain syndrome)

Acute confusion and coma are two of the commonest presentations leading to hospital admission in the tropics. Since clouding of consciousness can progress rapidly to complete unconsciousness it is helpful to consider them under the single heading of acute brain syndrome. In this context 'acute' signifies a time interval between onset and presentation not exceeding 28 days; in most cases it is a matter of hours or days. Purely psychiatric disorders can present as apparent confusion, even coma. They are dealt with in Table 62.9.

In the initial and progressive assessment of patients the 'Glasgow coma scale' has proved to be of the greatest practical value.[5]

There are so many organic disorders to be

considered that they are divided into two tables. Table 62.3 lists likely systemic disorders which incidentally disturb brain function. Table 62.4 lists diseases having pathological processes primarily within the central nervous system.

A sustained body temperature of 40°C or more is likely to lead to disturbed brain function especially in children who are also more likely to have convulsions.

Hyperpyrexia, heat stroke and heat exhaustion are considered in Chapter 43. High fever occurs in tetanus, status epilepticus, drug reactions and mismatched blood transfusion. In the absence of such obvious causes a severe infection must be suspected, particularly malaria.

Mental function can also be deranged by dehydration induced by fluid deprivation, excessive sweating, vomiting or diarrhoea. Correction of fluid and electrolyte imbalance may lead to rapid improvement, even complete recovery.

Amongst the severe infections, in areas of endemicity for *Plasmodium falciparum*, malignant tertian malaria requires the most urgent consideration and treatment (see below and

Table 62.3 Acute brain syndrome (acute confusion, coma): likely causes in the tropics. Primarily extracerebral.

Hyperpyrexia, heat exhaustion, heat stroke
Dehydration; electrolyte imbalance
Infection especially: malaria
                 pneumonia
                 typhoid fever
                 typhus
                 urinary tract infection
Hypoglycaemia
Alcohol
Therapeutic drug
Drug of addiction
Poisoning
Heart failure, cardiac arrhythmia, hypotension, shock
Severe anaemia
Carbon monoxide poisoning
Liver failure, portal-systemic encephalopathy
Acute renal failure
Diabetic ketoacidosis
Hypothermia
Hypertensive encephalopathy

Table 62.4 Acute brain syndrome (acute confusion, coma): likely causes in the tropics. Intrinsically cerebral.

Head injury and post-traumatic states (including extradural haemorrhage, subdural haematoma)
Inflammatory disorders: Cerebral malaria
                      Meningitis
                      Encephalitis
                      Brain abscess
                      Tuberculoma
Vascular disorders: Haemorrhage: extradural
                              subarachnoid
                              intracerebral
                  Embolism
                  Non-embolic infarction (cerebral thrombosis)
                  Sickle cell crisis
                  Venous thrombosis
Epilepsy and post-epileptic states
Wernicke's encephalopathy
Intracranial space-occupying lesions: Tumour
                                     Abscess
                                       Tuberculoma
                                       Subdural haematoma
Raised intracranial pressure from whatever cause

Chapter 1). Pneumonia is common all over the world and remains one of the most frequent unsuspected causes of confusion and coma; typical signs may be missed and an X-ray may be unhelpful or unavailable. Typhoid fever is locally common (Chapter 8); apathetic clouding of consciousness in the second week is characteristic. Typhus is much more localized in its distribution (Chapter 10). Vomiting and abrupt onset of fever are typical of urinary tract infections which are quite common in young children.

The hazard of hypoglycaemia in diabetes is well known. Not so well recognized is the risk in alcoholics especially after a debauch. So frequently was this suspected in the casualty department at Mulago Hospital, the principal Government hospital in Uganda, that intravenous hypertonic glucose was routinely administered to confused and comatose patients, sometimes with dramatic results. Delay in the correction of hypoglycaemia can result in irreparable brain damage. A curious local cause in sparely nourished children in Jamaica is the fruit of the ackee tree[6] (Chapter 49).

Therapeutic drugs are well known as agents inducing disturbed consciousness. Haddock[7] mentions magnesium sulphate as a precipitant in small children in Ghana. Poisonous animals and plants are dealt with in Chapters 48 and 49. Atropine is a notable cause of acute confusion especially in small children; pupillary abnormalities are then of vital diagnostic value. Suicidal poisoning is most uncommon, homicidal poisoning can be a delusion of a paranoiac and accidental poisoning may be a 'diagnosis of exclusion' suspected by relatives or medical attendants when all other causes seem to be absent.

Carbon monoxide poisoning has been reported in settings where on cold nights people sleep in huts with a fire smouldering and ventilation blocked off.

In the usual case of liver failure several diagnostic clinical features are present. In some patients with portal hypertension and adequate liver cell function, however, portal-systemic bypass may result in confusion or coma (portal-systemic encephalopathy) together with marked rigidity and hyperreflexia of relatively sudden onset, but without jaundice, ascites, fetor, etc, thus confounding the unwary diagnostician.

A high blood urea is far more likely to be due to dehydration or shock than to intrinsic renal disease. Urethral stricture and vesical schistosomiasis are common causes of renal failure in relevant areas.

Head injuries are becoming commoner as the result of falls, brawls and road traffic accidents. A familiar scene in a casualty department is the arrival at night of a comatose patient, 'found unconscious on the road' and smelling of alcohol. The vital witnesses have a habit of vanishing into thin air, leaving a demanding diagnostic riddle to be solved. Falling from trees is a local hazard, notably in palm-wine tappers.

Cerebral malaria is commonest in small children but must be suspected at all ages especially in a person who has recently entered the endemic area from overseas *or even from a non-endemic area in the same country*. Failure to find malarial parasites in the blood does *not* exclude the diagnosis. Per contra, a positive blood film does not necessarily prove that a patient has cerebral malaria. This diagnostic dilemma is reflected in the widely varying incidences in published data. What is not open to doubt is the urgency of effective drug treatment in a suspected case. It is vital to act on reasonable suspicion, to act at once and to use a parenteral route if possible (Chapter 1, p. 32).

Meningitis, when acute, is characterized by neck stiffness, arguably the single most important sign in tropical neurology. Immediate lumbar puncture is mandatory since delay in diagnosis and in commencement of appropriate therapy is known to be a potently adverse factor in eventual outcome. Raised intracranial pressure is no contraindication, save possibly in the rare instance where meningitis is the result of the leakage or rupture of a cerebral abscess. In pyogenic meningitis the cerebrospinal fluid (CSF) is turbid or frankly purulent, the pleocytosis polymorphonuclear and the glucose reduced or absent. Gram stain may show an organism and culture should identify it. Frequently, however, such CSFs are sterile, usually because the patient has already received an inadequate amount of an antibiotic; the predominant cell may then be a lymphocyte. A sterile CSF may also be found in the occasional case when the primary infection is in the skull, paranasal sinuses or brain itself (cerebral abscess) and is causing secondary meningeal irritation. The pneumococcus is a common pathogen at all ages and in all places. The meningococcus is much more patchy in its distribution, being confined largely to dry savannah belts where it occurs in epidemics. *Haemophilus influenzae* is common only in small children and is hardly ever seen after the age of six years. Many other organisms are occasionally encountered.

Tuberculous meningitis varies unaccountably in incidence. Atypically the early pleocytosis may be polymorphonuclear before becoming lymphocytic. Meningitis is considered in detail in Chapter 30. The prognosis of pyogenic meningitis in the tropics is distressingly poor; adverse factors include delayed diagnosis, delayed appropriate drug treatment, early onset of coma, and the pneumococcus as causative agent.

Encephalitis is an ill-defined term and tends to be diagnosed when other causes of acute brain syndrome have been excluded. The matter is somewhat academic since no specific treatment is available. Virology studies may lead to the identification of a virus. The EEG sometimes shows distinctive abnormalities. Encephalitis occasionally complicates the recognized exanthemata and vaccination with a Semple-type rabies vaccine. Local outbreaks of other named virus infections have been reported. Herpes simplex encephalitis is of the utmost rarity.

Pyogenic brain abscess presents more like a fast-growing tumour than an infection. Tuberculoma is even more indolent. A few autopsy cases of amoebic abscess have been reported from South Africa. Theoretically the appropriate drugs should destroy the causative organism but in practice the lesion is so walled off that it is preferable to drain it (abscess) or shell it out (tuberculoma).

Vascular lesions, epilepsy and neoplasms are considered below and Wernicke's encephalopathy in Chapter 46.

Chronic brain syndrome (dementia) (Table 62.5)

Chronic brain syndrome, a useful term not widely used, is applied to states in which disturbances of consciousness, orientation, memory, intellect or behaviour have persisted for longer than a month. It is almost synonymous with dementia, but the latter term suggests an even longer duration and implies irreversibility. Most of the disorders mentioned in the tables of acute brain syndrome will have recovered or terminated the patient's life before a month is up; some leave enduring sequelae; others remain active, merging into a group of diseases with a more indolent natural history.

Chronic subdural haematoma is a recurring

Table 62.5 Chronic brain syndrome (dementia): likely causes in the tropics.

Prolongation of process mentioned in acute brain syndrome
Sequel of process mentioned in acute brain syndrome
Chronic alcoholism
Pellagra
Chronic renal failure
Chronic subdural haematoma
Low-grade meningitis, meningoencephalitis, encephalitis
Uncontrolled epilepsy
Intracranial space-occupying lesions
Occult hydrocephalus
Arteriosclerotic, multi-infarct dementia, Alzheimer's disease, other named dementias
Congenital, familial and degenerative disorders associated with dementia

therapeutic challenge where computerized scanning or angiography is unavailable. Focal signs are often subtle and may be falsely lateralizing because of the effect of tentorial herniation on the midbrain on the side opposite to the lesion. If burr holes on the suspected side result in a dry tap the most careful consideration should be given to doing burr holes on the opposite side. Sometimes haematoma is bilateral anyway. Relief of haematoma can be one of the most rewarding of neurosurgical procedures and does not require special expertise.

If low grade meningitis is not associated with characteristic signs of meningeal irritation its presence can easily be overlooked. Examination of the CSF should confirm or at least strongly suggest the presence of tuberculosis. *Cryptococcus neoformans* is a very uncommon yeast causing a somewhat similar low grade meningitis (Chapter 35). Malignant infiltration is unlikely except in Burkitt's tumour and where nasopharyngeal carcinoma is frequent (Chapter 67). Meningovascular syphilis and dementia paralytica once common, have shown a marked decline in frequency. Causes of low grade meningoencephalitis in relevant areas include African trypanosomiasis (Chapter 2), Chagas' disease (American trypanosomiasis) (Chapter 3), bartonellosis in Peru (Chapter 11), kuru in Papua New Guinea (Chapter 42) and cysticercosis (Chapter 23). Virus encephalitides are widespread (Chapter 5). An infantile tremor syndrome in India may possibly be a manifestation of such. Viral cerebellitis has been suspected in the tropics in some patients with cerebellar ataxia not otherwise explained. Kuru, a unique subacute progressive encephalitis, affects mainly the cerebellum and is confined to a Papua New

Guinea highland tribe which practises ritual cannibalism; it is due to a transmissible agent, a 'slow virus' (Chapter 42).

Of potentially sinister significance for East and central Africa, where clinical disease due to HIV (human immunodeficiency virus) is common, has been the recent accumulation of evidence, reviewed in the *New England Journal of Medicine*,[8] that the brain can be invaded by the organism, inducing a chronic meningitis, dementia or AIDS encephalopathy (Chapter 68).

Repeated attacks of temporal lobe epilepsy, especially in the absence of obvious grand mal seizures, must be considered amongst the possible causes of disturbed consciousness or behaviour often simulating an acute schizophreniform illness. Temporal lobe epilepsy is common in the tropics.

Spinal cord syndromes

For convenience acute and chronic myelopathies of peculiar tropical importance are considered separately (Tables 62.6 and 62.7). In an acute myelopathy the development of weakness is rapid, even sudden, and is typically flaccid and areflexic and associated with absent plantar responses. These are not the textbook features of an upper motor neurone lesion and may beguile the unwary into suspecting a different group of neurological diseases. Days or weeks may supervene before rigidity appears; in the most severe cases the limbs remain flaccid indefinitely. These devastating motor features are accompanied by marked or complete loss of sensation below a segmental (dermatomal) level (typically on the trunk) and by constipation and retention of urine with overflow incontinence. There is a risk of the early development of bedsores.

Most chronic myelopathies, by contrast, evince the expected upper motor neurone signs together with whatever other features are typical of the particular pathological process present. Few indeed are the spinal cord diseases which

Table 62.6 Acute myelopathy: tropical peculiarities.

Disorder	Clinical features	Locale	Cause
Burkitt's tumour (p. 1095)	Cord compression (tumour mass elsewhere)	Africa Papua New Guinea	Neoplasm
Lathyrism (p. 850)	Spastic myelopathy	Central India	Toxin in pea (*Lathyrus sativus*)
Gnathostomiasis (p. 558)	Myelopathy polyradiculopathy	South-East Asia	*Gnathostoma spinigerum*
Transverse myelitis (necrotic myelopathy)	Non-traumatic transection of cord	Widespread	Obscure

Table 62.7 Chronic myelopathy: tropical peculiarities.

Disorder	Clinical features	Locale	Cause
Pott's disease	Cord compression	Widespread	Tuberculosis
Adhesive arachnoiditis	Cord compression, spastic myelopathy or polyradiculopathy	Widespread	Tuberculosis in India, obscure elsewhere
Atlanto-axial dislocation	High cervical compression	India	Congenital
Fluorosis	Cord compression or polyradiculopathy	India	High fluoride content of drinking water
Schistosomiasis (pp. 472 and 488)	Low myelopathy or cauda equina syndrome	Africa South America	*Schistosoma mansoni* and *S. haematobium*
Cysticercosis (Chapter 23)	Myelopathy or cauda equina syndrome	Widespread	Cysticercus cellulosae, larval form of *Taenia solium*
Hydatidosis (Chapter 23)	Cord compression	Western South America	*Echinococcus granulosus*
Tropical spastic paraplegia	Myelopathy	Widespread	Obscure. HTLV-I virus?
Jamaican neuropathy (Strachan's syndrome) (p. 848)	Spastic or ataxic myelopathy, optic atrophy sensorineural deafness	Jamaica	Unknown nutritional factor
Tropical ataxic neuropathy (p. 849)	Ataxic myelopathy, optic atrophy, sensorineural deafness	South Nigeria, Mozambique	Cyanide in cassava (manioc)

do not touch the corticospinal (pyramidal) tracts.

Severe unremedied spinal cord damage is a major catastrophe leading to paraplegia (or tetraplegia), sensory loss, urinary and faecal incontinence, impotence in men and bedsores. Intractable bedsores and urinary infections are likely to bring a premature end to a wretched existence, for few homes or hospitals can cope with the great demands imposed by such disastrous disabilities. Moderate damage to the cord, on the other hand, can be compatible with some degree of independence; communities, especially in the rural setting, are usually very supportive of such cripples.

Spinal cord compression is the lesion most likely to be amenable to remedy. Cardinal features are the gradual onset and progress in one or both legs of weakness of upper motor neurone type (unless the lesion affects the lumbar enlargement), followed later by sensory impairment below a level on the trunk and still later by hesitancy of micturition. Depending on the nature of the lesion, root pains at its site may occur early in the process. Tuberculosis of the spine (Pott's disease) is common in much of the tropics and produces a gibbus deformity, cold abscess or other evidences of its presence. Plain X-ray of the spine provides useful information in tuberculosis and several other conditions characterized by spinal cord compression. It is important to remember that upper motor neurone lesions in the legs must be due to disease no lower than the thoracic region of the spine and that they can also be due to lesions in the neck (cervical myelopathy), preceding symptoms in the arms in the latter situation by weeks or months. In the absence of diagnostic disease seen in plain X-rays the next ideal procedure is myelography. If this is impracticable it is justifiable to carry out a lumbar puncture; the characteristic features of spinal block are xanthochromic CSF, low or unrecordable CSF pressure, no rise in CSF pressure on jugular vein compression, and high CSF protein content. If all or most of these features are present the patient must be referred to a centre where specialized investigation and surgery of the spinal cord can be carried out. Pott's disease has a good, even excellent prognosis. The outlook in many other diseases depends as much on the speed and expertise of action as on the nature of the lesion. Malignant infiltration (metastases uncommon in adults, Burkitt's tumour common in children) carries a grave prognosis.

Once it is established that cord compression is not present, a bewildering panorama of possibilities opens up. Most of the diseases occurring in developed countries have been reported at one time or another in the tropics. All are agreed about the extreme rarity of tabes dorsalis and subacute combined degeneration (combined system disease) and the unique rarity of multiple sclerosis. The writer believes that, despite some assertions to the contrary, typical motor neurone disease has an equal prevalence almost everywhere, suspects that markedly atypical manifestations indicate another diagnosis, and recognizes that there is a juvenile type seen in India with a distinctly better prognosis. The slow, almost imperceptible, progress of the purely atrophic form of motor neurone disease is already well attested anyway. Motor neurone disease is uniquely common among the Chamorros on the island of Guam in the Pacific (Chapter 47).

The reader is referred to specialized texts for details about the various tumours and other lesions causing spinal cord compression and the numerous non-compressive causes of myelopathy.

A most interesting recent discovery is the possible implication of the human T lymphotropic virus I (HTLV-I) in the type of tropical spastic paraplegia characterized by insidious onset and slow progress with or without systemic symptoms.[9] It appears that the spinal cord can also be involved in a subacute manner by the HIV virus in AIDS and the AIDS-related complex (Chapter 68).

Polyneuropathy

The causes, pathological processes and clinical features of (symmetrical, peripheral) polyneuropathy are so distinct from those of individual nerve lesions (p. 1041) that it is sensible to consider them completely separately. Whilst polyneuropathy has the same stigmata everywhere, there are some special problems in the tropics as regards both diagnosis and causation. A predominantly motor polyneuropathy can mimic an acute myelopathy. Motor polyneuropathy is more likely when paraesthesiae are present in all four limbs, reflexes are absent or markedly reduced in parts of limbs which are not weak, sensory impairment if present is of glove and stocking distribution rather than below a definite *segmental* (dermatomal) level, and sphincter involvement is mild, transient or absent. In both disorders CSF protein may be raised, even markedly so; in a polyneuropathy there are no features of spinal block, but such would not be present in a non-compressive myelopathy. In the Landry–Guillain–Barré syndrome, potentially the most dangerous motor polyneuropathy, weakness progresses or 'ascends' over several days whereas the full extent of loss in an acute myelopathy is often completed within hours or minutes.

A worker in the tropics has to consider the same formidable list of possible causative conditions as he would in temperate climes. Many are less common, notably diabetes mellitus. Others are more common, notably those caused by vitamin deficiencies and malnutrition (Chapter 46) and by isoniazid (INH). Isoniazid-induced polyneuropathy is more likely to occur in slow acetylators (about half the population in published series from Africa, India and the Far East) and in patients on high dosages for tuberculous meningitis. It can be prevented by pyridoxine 10 mg daily. Acute intermittent porphyria is curiously common in South Africa[10] (Chapter 66).

The commonest neuropathy in the world is that due to leprosy. In the strict sense of the term it is not a polyneuropathy. It is really a chronic 'mononeuritis multiplex'. The nerves implemented are always peripheral and near the surface. Tell-tale features include hypopigmented, hypalgesic and hypaesthetic skin patches; thickened superficial nerves; and motor, sensory and trophic changes resulting from damage to such nerves. The nerve trunks most commononly palpable are the great auricular in the neck, the ulnar just above the medial epicondyle, the median at the wrist, the lateral popliteal below the fibular head and the posterior tibial behind the medial malleolus. Trained paramedical staff become expert in detecting and confirming the presence of leprosy in suspects. The disease is considered in detail in Chapter 40. A very rare non-leprous hypertrophic polyneuritis (Déjérine and Sottas or primary amyloid) is a possible differential diagnosis. The author has seen a case of syringomyelia with its typical fleshy fingers referred from a leper colony because leprosy had been excluded on every other ground.

SPECIFIC DISORDERS

Many neurological diseases have already been referred to in this chapter or elsewhere. A few important groups remain, meriting more detailed attention.

Cerebral vascular disease

In most respects the pattern, natural history and possible causes of cerebral vascular disease are much the same everywhere. But there are some differences and peculiarities in the tropics, mostly relative rather than absolute. Vascular disorders, though often seen, are less common principally because of the paucity of elderly people. Atherosclerotic lesions, such as those responsible for transient ischaemic attacks, are less frequent, whereas uncontrolled hypertension assumes a greater importance. Observers are struck, nevertheless, by the numbers of comparatively young adults developing strokes for no apparent reason.

Tropical peculiarities include the haemoglobinopathies and non-syphilitic arteritis. In sickle cell disease (Chapter 58) and its variants the clumping of sickled cells in small vessels causes sluggish flow, stasis or actual occlusion. In the central nervous system this can lead to small but multiple areas of ischaemia, infarction, haemorrhage or even dural vein thrombosis, with a striking variety of focal neurological deficits. Confusion, fits and acute mental changes are, however, the features most commonly reported. The majority of patients are children.

An arteritis is occasionally encountered in young adults, not a sequel of tuberculous meningitis nor due to syphilis or giant-cell (temporal) arteritis. It involves the aortic arch and its large branches leading to occlusion of the latter and causing the pulse to become impalpable (pulseless disease, Takayasu's disease). Involvement of the nervous system can be mild to catastrophic. Reports emanate mainly from India, the Far East and Africa. The cause is unknown and the pathological process is not typically inflammatory. There may be several distinct disease entities waiting to be identified.

Epilepsy

Accurate information about the prevalence in the tropics of epilepsy and its variants is scanty but there are probably fewer global differences than had been thought in the past. Many workers, lacking any specialist investigative facilities, can only speculate on the likely underlying causes. Amongst tropical peculiarities is cysticercosis, the commonest cause of epilepsy of late onset in South-East Asia (Chapter 23). Precipitating factors include fever in children and alcohol-induced hypoglycaemia in adults; a south Indian peculiarity is 'hot water epilepsy', in which grand mal or temporal lobe fits occur when, as part of the traditional bathing practice, hot water is poured over the head. Nowadays photogenic epilepsy from flickering television sets is assuming a greater importance. Avoidance of the precipitating factor alone may be enough to stop the recurrence of fits.

The main challenges in epilepsy are its drug treatment and psychosocial aspects. A grand mal fit is the most dramatic and dreaded manifestation and treatment must be primarily directed towards preventing the recurrence of such attacks. The choice of drug is likely to be dictated by availability and cost. The aims are to achieve an effective blood level and to maintain it for years or indefinitely. The first aim may be frustrated by lack of facilities for measuring serum concentration and the second by failure of the patient or his relatives to acknowledge the necessity for long-term treatment. The most strenuous and persistent efforts must be made to convince the patient that fits can be prevented, often completely prevented, by the right dose of the right drug taken at the right time day after day and year after year. A special clinic is helpful. Drugs are prepared beforehand in suitable packages to last the patient till the next visit, indeed it is wise to be overgenerous so as to allow for delayed returns due to unexpected illness or transport problems.

Of all the available drugs phenobarbitone remains the cheapest and one of the most effective and its pharmacokinetics are such that it need be taken only once a day. Suicide is an extremely unlikely hazard and drowsiness is less of a disability in a rural setting than in a competitive urban or scholastic community. An adult starts with a nightly dose of 120 mg which is likely to be at least moderately effective and therefore to convince the patient that the tablets do work. In some the dose will have to be reduced, in others cautiously increased to a maximum of 300 mg nightly. Phenobarbitone may cause paradoxical restlessness and excitement in small children.

Phenytoin sodium is also very effective but not so cheap. It is less likely to cause drowsiness but more likely to cause ataxia, though this is actually very uncommon in practice. Protein binding in the serum explains the narrow dose range between effectiveness and toxicity. It is therefore helpful to have 25 mg as well as 100 mg preparations available especially if they are capsules. An adult starts with a daily dose of 200 mg and increases cautiously to a maximum of 600 mg. Twice daily dosing may be recommended if the timing of fits is unpredictable. A phenytoin sodium (100 mg) and phenobarbitone (50 mg) compound tablet is available, better for compliance but worse for flexible dosimetry of either drug.

Sodium valproate is considerably more costly and has to be taken in divided doses. It is effective in all forms of epilepsy and is usually free from side-effects apart from gastric irritation; rare hepatotoxicity is reported. Adult dose is 200 mg three times a day increasing by 200 mg/day at 3-day intervals to a maximum of 800 mg three times a day.

Carbamazepine is less costly than valproate and with fewer side-effects is particularly favoured in temporal lobe epilepsy. An adult starts with 200 mg once or twice daily and increases cautiously to a maximum daily dose of 1.6 g.

Children with petit mal but no grand mal seizures seldom find their way to a doctor. Ethosuximide is the drug of choice. To it must be added one of the above drugs if grand mal fits supervene as is likely when the petit mal is controlled or as the patient gets older.

The psychosocial disabilities suffered by epileptics in some tropical communities are truly appalling. They are graphically described in Nigeria by Osuntokun[11] and Dada,[12] in Uganda by Orley,[13] Billington[14] and Billinghurst,[15] in Ethiopia by Giel,[16] in Tanzania by Jilek[17] and in Senegal by Collomb.[18] Epileptics are likely to be excluded from communal feeding, school education, formal marriage, inheritance and employment. Such deprivations spring from the convictions that the disease is caused by evil spiritual forces, is not amenable to 'Western' medicine and tends to cause 'spoiling of the brain'. Hideous burns and scalds may occur when the onlookers flee from the unfortunate victim believing that body fluids are in some way contagious. Barbaric stimulants are sometimes used such as applying pepper to the eyes and dosing with cow's urine in Nigeria, the latter inducing hypoglycaemia which only compounds the tragic situation (Chapter 49). Gentle, intelligent and persistent effort is required to convince the sufferer, his family and his community that control is possible. It is here that effective drug therapy is so important.

Neoplasms

In contrast to the marked geographic differences in the incidence of cancer of the respiratory, gastrointestinal and genitourinary tracts, primary brain tumours are probably similar in incidence and type all over the world. In the tropics, however, there are more frequent intracranial space-occupying lesions of non-neoplastic pathology to consider: subdural haematoma (p. 1036), pyogenic abscess, tuberculoma, hydatid cysts and even the granulomas of *Schistosoma japonicum* in relevant endemic areas (p. 474). Whilst intracranial metastases are distinctly uncommon in the tropics, direct invasion of the skull contents is seen where Burkitt's tumour occurs and where carcinoma of the nasopharynx is common (Chapter 67, p. 1086).

The peculiar neoplasm of the tropics is Burkitt's tumour (Chapter 67, p. 1095). The nervous system is invaded in about one-third of cases, gravely worsening the prognosis. Involvement includes malignant CSF pleocytosis, multiple cranial neuropathies and acute myelitis. In parts of Africa it is the commonest cause of childhood paraplegia. Mental dullness, apathy, drowsiness, listlessness and irritability are among the most frequent of the symptoms, explicable by involvement of local meninges or actual microscopic invasion of the brain. Large intracranial masses are uncommon.

Individual nerve lesions

Table 62.8 outlines some known tropical peculiarities. Leprosy is individually considered in Chapter 40.

Optic neuritis, acute transverse myelitis, Devic's disease and the riddle of multiple sclerosis in the tropics

Acute optic neuritis, including the retrobulbar variety, is reported as being quite common in many tropical locations (Chapter 70). When recognizable causes have been excluded, methyl alcohol among them, there remains a group of obscure aetiology. The lesion is often bilateral. Prognosis for useful recovery is good though not invariably so. Recurrence is most unusual.

Acute transverse myelitis of obscure aetiology is also reported as being quite common. The features are those of a severe acute myelopathy and the prognosis for recovery is usually poor, but once the acute phase is over further progress or relapse does not occur and other system involvement is absent.

When the two conditions occur together, starting simultaneously or within an interval of not more than a few days, it is reasonable to talk of Devic's disease, which is less rare in the tropics than elsewhere. Since the cause of Devic's disease is not known, it cannot be proved or disproved that acute optic neuritis on the one hand and acute transverse myelitis on the other are each incomplete manifestations of the full picture as seen in Devic's disease itself. The pathological process in the spinal cord, where

Table 62.8 Individual nerve lesions: tropical peculiarities.

Nerve or nerves	Lesion	Locale	Cause
Cranial II	Acute papillitis (bilateral)	Widespread	Methyl alcohol
Cranial II	Acute neuritis (often bilateral)	Widespread	Devic's disease, obscure
Cranial III, IV and VI	Acute painful ophthalmoplegia, often recurrent, steroid responsive	South India, Africa	Obscure
Multiple cranials	Hydatid disease	Southern South America	*Echinococcus granulosus*
	Bartonellosis (Chapter 11)	Peru	
	Sickle cell disease	Africa	Homozygous Hb SS
	Sequel of meningitis, especially tuberculous	Widespread	
	Burkitt's tumour	Africa, Papua New Guinea	Malignant infiltration
	Nasopharyngeal carcinoma	South-East Asia	Malignant infiltration
Superficial nerve trunks	Tuberculoid leprosy	Widespread	*Mycobacterium leprae*

such scanty material is available, resembles that seen in the acute myelitis which follows rabies inoculation. So it is at least possible that an abnormal reaction to an as yet unidentified virus is the basis for the disorders mentioned above. What they do not in any way resemble is multiple sclerosis. They are severe acute events, once-only rather than remitting or relapsing, and the optic nerve involvement is often simultaneously bilateral.

Multiple sclerosis is so rare in the tropics that the diagnosis must remain suspect unless there is autopsy confirmation or, failing that, positive results from oligoclonal banding of the IgGs in the CSF and abnormal visual (and other) evoked responses. Accurate information about its world-wide distribution is of prime importance to the epidemiologist and is an essential item in the data required to explain the pathological process in this most baffling of neurological diseases.

PSYCHIATRIC PROBLEMS

INTRODUCTION

The general introductory remarks concerning neurology in the tropics apply also to psychiatry. The pattern of disorders is much more similar to that in the temperate zones than was once thought, but it is probably true to say that hysteria and mania are common and the compulsive-obsessive state rare at any rate in Africa. What are often starkly different are the various cultures with their beliefs, values and interpretations. Spiritual forces may be thought to exert an important, even a predominant role in the genesis of both bodily and mental disease. In a society which believes in witchcraft or the efficacy of other occult practices paranoid delusions in one sufferer and depression in another are seen potently to confirm and perpetuate such ideas. Understandably, help is first sought from local wise men, religious leaders or traditional healers rather than from a local hospital or medical clinic.

Not only does the doctor need to know something of the cultural background of each of his patients, he is also up against the ability of such patients to describe their problems in terms that are intelligible. Quite apart from difficulties with translation he has to cope with what to him appear to be purely psychiatric symptoms being described in graphic somatic terms as if the patient genuinely believed that it was his body which was at fault ('somatization of psychiatric symptoms'). Dizziness, palpitations, generalized or localized weakness, heat in the head or body, itching, pricking, numbness, bizarre exaggeration of pain, impotence, worms creeping from place to place, worms biting various parts in their stealthy progress: such are some of the common and curious complaints mentioned not only by rural people but also by the more sophisticated, especially students many of whom are under intolerable pressures to achieve more than they are academically capable of.

Nevertheless, every medical observer is struck by the frequency with which mental symptoms and disturbances do have an organic basis. In an acute psychiatric disorder it is particularly important to suspect the presence of physical disease. In a more chronic situation too, an organic cause must be carefully considered (see sections on modes of presentation, p. 1033, acute, confusion and coma, p. 1033, and chronic brain syndrome, p. 1036).

Technically speaking, an acute or chronic brain syndrome is an organic condition; but purely psychiatric disorders do have to be considered in the differential diagnosis.

For the main psychiatric diseases the reader is referred to a standard textbook. Special mention is made of three tropical peculiarities: mass hysteria, running amok and koro.

MODES OF PRESENTATION

Acute brain syndrome

Purely psychiatric disturbances (Table 62.9)

Emotional disturbances are very frequent as are undue exaggerations of bodily symptoms. The agitation and overactivity of both anxiety and hysteria can masquerade as acute confusion with or without hallucinations. The latter, together with delusions, are even more characteristic of acute schizophrenic and paranoid states and also of mania. Severe retarded depression, by contrast, may simulate stupor, as of course may hysteria. Hysterical trance is a well-recognized phenomenon. Aggressive outbursts, particularly in schizophrenia, are potentially dangerous.

Any of the above can present more than 28

Table 62.9 Acute brain syndrome: purely psychiatric disturbances.

Acute anxiety
Hysteria
Mania
Schizophrenic and paranoid states
Depression
Puerperal psychosis

days after onset and should therefore be considered again in the section on chronic brain syndrome (p. 1036). It is both important and difficult to distinguish between depression and dementia, especially in patients past the age of 50 years. Depression is quite common and often overlooked.

Even in what seems the most obvious psychiatric disorder the abuse of alcohol or drugs must always be borne in mind. Alcoholism can be both the cause and the result of mental disease and in parts of the tropics is a truly major psychosocial problem in all races. Restricted drugs are more readily available than in developed countries, notably amphetamine, the barbiturates and opium. Cannabis is easily obtained from local sources and is widely smoked. It is now well recognized as a precipitant of acute anxiety, confusion and manic and schizophreniform psychoses. Latent or overt schizophrenics can become dangerously violent and antisocial.

SPECIFIC DISORDERS

Mass hysteria

Hysteria is commonest in girls and young women. An amazing variety of local manifestations is recorded in the literature, both medical and 'secular'. Dramatic exhibitions include gross and bizarre involuntary movements, convulsive seizures simulating epilepsy, and apparent disturbances of consciousness ranging from overactivity to coma. In a relatively closed community, particularly a school or hostel, these manifestations, starting with one or two youngsters, quickly induce a high pitch of anxiety and are 'passed on' to many others, so as to mimic an epidemic. Typically the outbreak ceases as suddenly as it started. It is not difficult to detect or surmise what 'unconscious gain' the sufferers hoped to achieve.

Running amok

Technically this is a specific disorder of Malay men but its manifestations are so striking that it has found a permanent place in the English language. 'Amok in Malay means madness and the general idea conveyed by it is to die fighting.... The manic activity is short-lived and entirely murder-bent. A number of these patients have had to be shot during the furore.'[19] The murder weapon is typically a local knife.

Koro

Koro is a panic reaction in Chinese men induced by the belief that the penis is retracting into the abdominal cavity with potentially fatal results. The organ is gripped by hand or clamp.[19]

REFERENCES

1 Billinghurst, J. R. (1973) In *Tropical Neurology*, ed. J. D. Spillane, pp. 191–206. London: Oxford University Press.
2 Spillane, J. D. (1973) In *Tropical Neurology*, ed. J. D. Spillane, pp. 3–21. London: Oxford University Press.
3 Osuntokun, B. O. (1973) In *Tropical Neurology*, ed. J. D. Spillane, pp. 161–190. London: Oxford University Press.
4 Matthews, W. B. (1975) *Practical Neurology*, 4th edn. Oxford: Blackwell Scientific Publications.
5 Teasdale, G. & Jennett, B. (1974) *Lancet*, **ii**, 81.
6 Cruickshank, E. K. (1973) In *Tropical Neurology*, ed. J. D. Spillane, pp. 421–434. London: Oxford University Press.
7 Haddock, D. R. W. (1973) In *Tropical Neurology*, ed. J. D. Spillane, pp. 143–160. London: Oxford University Press.
8 Black, P. H. (1985) *New England Journal of Medicine* **313**, 1538–1540.
9 Gessain, A., Vernant, J. C., Maurs, L. et al (1985) *Lancet* **ii**, 407–410.
10 Dean, G. (1973) In *Tropical Neurology*, ed. J. D. Spillane, pp. 273–280. London: Oxford University Press.
11 Osuntokun, B. O. & Odeku, E. L. (1970) *Afr. J. med. Sci.* **1**, 185–200.
12 Dada, T. O. & Odeku, E. L. (1966) *W. Afr. med. J.* **15**, 153–163.
13 Orley, J. H. (1970) *Afr. J. med. Sci.* **1**, 155.
14 Billington, W. R. (1968) *E. Afr. med. J.* **45**, 563.
15 Billinghurst, J. R., German, G. A. & Orley, J. H. (1973) *Trop. Geog. Med.* **25**, 226–232.
16 Giel, R. (1968) *E. Afr. med. J.* **45**, 27–31.
17 Jilek, W. G. & Jilek-Aall, L. M. (1970) *Afr. J. med. Sci.* **1**, 305–307.
18 Collomb, H., Sankale, B., Courson, G. et al (1970) *Afr. J. med. Sci* **1**, 125.
19 Gwee, A. L. & Ransome, G. A. (1973) In *Tropical Neurology*, ed. J. D. Spillane, pp. 283–298. London: Oxford University Press.

Chapter 63
Renal and Urinary Tract Disease

In most tropical countries there is insufficient statistically valid information on disease prevalence to allow scientific comparisons to be made with disease patterns in developed countries, so reliance must be placed on clinical experience and impression. There appear to be five main areas where tropical urology differs from urology in the West.

1 A greater prevalence of glomerulonephritis.

2 A greater prevalence of immune complex-mediated renal disease.

3 A greater prevalence of obstructive uropathy affecting the upper urinary tract as a result of tuberculosis and schistosomiasis.

4 In some areas only, a vastly greater prevalence of bladder stone, reminiscent of the situation in Western Europe 100 years ago.

5 A predominance of postgonococcal urethral stricture over prostatism as a cause of lower renal tract obstruction.

CHRONIC RENAL DISEASE IN THE TROPICS

The general picture seems to be[1] that the major cause of chronic renal failure in the tropics is chronic glomerulonephritis, rather than chronic pyelonephritis, and that much of this chronic disease is related to malaria. It seems very likely that other causes of antigenaemia contribute to glomerular damage, and a report from Vellore, India[2] of 50 cases of membranoproliferative nephritis mentions eosinophilia as being present in more than one-third of patients with type 1 disease. Evidence of streptococcal infection was found in less than one-third of the patients, and other causes of antigenaemia included bancroftian filariasis, haemoglobin S antigenaemia, tropical pulmonary eosinophilia and lepromatous leprosy. The establishment of a direct causal relationship in these cases is, of course, extremely difficult.

In another report from India,[3] 74% of 576 renal biopsies were reported as showing features suggesting primary glomerulopathy.

Reports from different parts of the tropics vary, but the overall picture of a predominance of glomerular disease is virtually universal. One factor contributing to this is undoubtedly the extra exposure to streptococcal antigens from secondarily infected skin lesions, especially scabies.[4]

Other significant causes of chronic renal disease in the tropics include interstitial nephritis, hypertensive nephrosclerosis, diabetic glomerulosclerosis, renal amyloidosis and systemic lupus erythematosus.

Any physician taking up work in the tropics will soon be impressed by the importance of chronic renal failure, and often equally dismayed by his inability to cope with the situation with the resources available to him.

THE NEPHROTIC SYNDROME IN THE TROPICS

Particularly tropical causes of this are the nephrotic syndrome of children associated with chronic *Plasmodium malariae* infection and the nephrotic syndrome associated with schistosomiasis, most commonly *Schistosoma mansoni* (Chapters 1 and 22).

In both these conditions, deposits of specific immune complex can be demonstrated in the glomeruli on renal biopsy, and the main difference between them is in the prognosis: the *P. malariae* immune complexes are tightly bound to the basement membrane and remain attached even after antigenaemia has been terminated by specific chemotherapy. In contrast, the schistosomal immune complexes are relatively loosely bound, and sometimes complex disappears after antischistosomal chemotherapy, with remission of the renal disease especially in *S. haematobium* infection.

Amyloidosis can, of course, cause the nephrotic syndrome, and may complicate virtually any severe and prolonged infection. It is perhaps best known as a feature complicating a prolonged erythema nodosum leprosum (ENL) reaction in lepromatous leprosy,[5] but it can also complicate *S. mansoni* infection (Chapter 22) and kala azar (Chapter 4).

OBSTRUCTION OF THE URETERS

The two main causes are tuberculosis and urinary schistosomiasis due to *S. haematobium*.

It remains mysterious[6] why renal tuberculosis is relatively uncommon in those parts of the tropical world where pulmonary tuberculosis is highly prevalent, but it is so. But when renal tuberculosis does occur, ureteric involvement is common. Its main importance is that during antituberculous treatment, healing of the lesions is often accompanied by the rapid formation of a tight fibrous stricture which may seriously impair renal drainage and function. The progress of such cases whilst on treatment should, for this reason, be carefully monitored by repeated urography.

In contrast, the behaviour of schistosomal ureteric lesions is quite different,[7] and certainly in the earlier stages of the disease, treatment is often followed by resolution of the obstruction. An actual *increase* in obstruction, following treatment of schistosomiasis, is virtually unknown, and there is no need to repeat the urogram in such cases until three months after treatment is completed. If serious obstruction persists then, provided parasitological tests show that the infection has indeed been eradicated, it must be assumed that the residual obstruction is due to fibrous tissue, and appropriate surgical action must be taken.

BLADDER STONES IN THE TROPICS

Bladder stones in young boys were once common in Europe,[8] but largely disappeared from northern Europe in the late nineteenth century, and from southern Europe soon after the middle of this century. The outstanding change that accompanied the disappearance of the disease was an improvement in child nutrition, and it now seems certain that an infant diet which is low in protein but high in carbohydrate conduces to stone formation. In one of the areas of highest prevalence, north Thailand, mothers feed their babies with premasticated glutinous rice,[9] and in another high prevalence area in Indonesia, infants are fed with rice or wheat-flour pap from

an early age.[10] Similar patterns have been reported from Egypt and Turkey where bladder stone is common. The disease seems to disappear when animal protein consumption exceeds about 40 g/day. The stones are made of ammonium acid urate, mixed with calcium oxalate in Thailand. The basic cause is an acidogenic, low phosphate diet, excess production of ammonia by the kidney to buffer the acid, stasis accompanying a low fluid intake and, in the Thai cases, a high oxalate intake.[11] The reasons why stones affect mainly boys seem to be anatomical[12] rather than biochemical.

This disease should disappear from the present endemic areas, just as it has from Europe, with improvements in child feeding practices.

URETHRAL STRICTURES

Urethral stricture is a vastly more important cause of bladder outflow obstruction than prostatic disease in tropical countries. Although some strictures are post-traumatic, the vast majority follow gonorrhoea—untreated or inadequately treated. Stricture of the urethra may follow female circumcision in Africa, and inexpert male circumcision. These 'terminal' strictures are best treated with meatoplasty.[13]

Before strictures are treated by bougienage or plastic surgery it is essential to ensure that no residual gonococcal infection remains, as not only local reactivation of infection but also gonococcal septicaemia may follow failure to do so (see Chapter 68 for details of chemotherapy).

A full and detailed account of the up to date management of urethral strictures is available.[14]

REFERENCES

1 Kibukamusoke, J. W. (1984) In *Tropical Urology and Renal Disease*. Edinburgh: Churchill Livingstone.
2 Date, A. et al (1983) *Ann. Trop. Med. Parasitl.* 77(3), 279.
3 Mani, M. K. et al (1980) *Emirates med. J.* 1, 277.
4 Whittle, H. C. et al (1973) *Trans. R. Soc. trop. Med. Hyg.* 67, 349.
5 Shire, T. (1972) *Lepr. Rev.*, 42, 282.
6 Awunnor-Renner, C. & Smith, E. K. M. (1984) The kidney. In *Principles of Medicine in Africa*, ed. W. H. O. Parry. Oxford, Nairobi: Oxford University Press.
7 Oyediran, A. B. O. O. (1979) *Kidney Int.* 16, 15.
8 Ellis, H. (1969) *A History of Bladder Stone*. Oxford: Blackwell.
9 Halstead, S. B. et al (1967) *Am. J. clin. Nutr.* 20, 1352.

10 Kamardi, T. et al (1981) *Urinary Calculus*. Littleton, Mass: PSG.

11 Robertson, W. G. (1977) In *Idiopathic Urinary Bladder Stone Disease*, ed. R. Reen. US Department of Health Education and Welfare, Washington.

12 Halstead, S. B. (1977) In *Idiopathic Urinary Bladder Stone Disease*, ed. R. Reen, pp. 121–134. US Department of Health Education and Welfare, Washington.

13 Blandy, J. P. & Tresidder, G. C. (1967) *Br. J. Urol.* **39**, 261.

14 Manmeet Singh (1984) In *Tropical Urology and Renal Disease*, ed. I. Husain, pp. 325–342. Edinburgh: Churchill Livingstone.

I am indebted to Messrs Blackwell for permission to reproduce here some material that previously appeared in *Lecture Notes on Tropical Medicine*, 2nd edition (Blackwell, Oxford, 1985).

Chapter 64
Respiratory Problems

M. E. Molyneux

Most clinicians in the tropics have to deal with a large number of patients with chest complaints, and must do so without the armamentarium of diagnostic devices available to those working in richer nations. Fortunately a great deal can be achieved through careful history-taking and physical examination, judicious choice of which tests to do and (especially) which not to do, and a thorough knowledge of which diseases are important in the patient's environment.

In an average outpatient department 20–40% of patients have come with respiratory complaints, and 20–30% of hospital medical admissions are for disorders predominantly affecting the lungs. Many patients are suffering from conditions such as chronic obstructive airways disease that might occur anywhere in the world; others have diseases that are much commoner in, or peculiar to, tropical areas, e.g. pulmonary schistosomiasis: and within the tropics patterns differ greatly from one region to another.

Because tuberculosis is so common throughout the world, many people with other causes of chronic cough suffer unwarranted lengthy therapeutic trials of antituberculous drugs. The therapeutic trial for 'possible TB' is sometimes sensible, but must only be embarked upon when other diagnoses have been carefully sought. In 430 cases of 'unresponsive pulmonary tuberculosis' referred from district hospitals to a tuberculosis unit in South Africa, over half did not have tuberculosis at all.[1] The correct diagnoses in these were various, including nontuberculous bronchiectasis, lung abscess, foreign body, congenital cystic lung, hydatid disease, mitral stenosis, bronchial carcinoma, and sarcoidosis.

In a busy clinic a quick diagnosis may have to be made for patients with mild acute disease. But in any who are very sick or who have recurrent, chronic or unresponsive symptoms a full clinical assessment is essential.

The history may give useful clues. Ask about previous antituberculosis treatment and the adequacy thereof: this may not be mentioned by the patient and is easily neglected by the doctor. If there is a history of tuberculosis, it would help to know whether it was proven tuberculosis or merely suspected. Look for any history of an episode of unconsciousness preceding the symptoms, e.g. general anaesthesia, epilepsy, alcoholic coma, trauma; inhalation at such a time is a common cause of localized pulmonary infection or lung abscess. Enquire about place and conditions of work, with particular emphasis on dusts and the relation of symptoms to the time of work. Work in mines, even in the distant past, may have been responsible for fibrotic lung disease. A patient who works with animals or birds may be exposed to zoonotic diseases that sometimes have a pulmonary component—tularaemia, Q fever, leptospirosis or psittacosis. Smoking has increased in many countries (see section on smoking, below) and should be carefully asked about: it may be responsible for or exacerbate the patient's illness. Remember that bronchial asthma and left ventricular failure may each give rise to cough as the major symptom, or the only one the patient mentions: other clues if sought will usually point to the diagnosis. Mitral stenosis is much more common in developing than in industrial countries. In a patient with cough, associated symptoms may help with diagnosis or management: haemoptysis, breathlessness, night sweats, weight loss. In areas where gnathostomiasis occurs enquire about eating habits; where schistosomiasis is prevalent consider the lifestyle and likelihood of contact with schistosomal water.

The environmental or family context may suggest important possibilities: pneumonic plague is caught by inhalation from a close contact dying of septicaemic plague. Ask about contacts known to have tuberculosis; but also about any close contact known to have died recently of undiagnosed disease—tuberculosis is a strong possibility.

In the *physical examination* note the general condition and look carefully for evidence of cardiac or abdominal abnormalities. It is easy to miss pericardial constriction or effusion, which may mimic or complicate pulmonary disease. Right ventricular hypertrophy may develop in chronic pulmonary disease; it is sometimes a feature of pulmonary schistosomiasis. Palpable lymph nodes in the axillae or supraclavicular fossae may provide a source of diagnostic material, and should therefore be sought routinely and carefully. Because so many patients have advanced disease by the time they reach medical attention, a variety of physical signs are encountered that are seldom seen in industrial countries. Abnormalities of chest movement or shape, and mediastinal (tracheal) shift may indicate contraction from chronic fibrosis within the chest. A hydropneumothorax or pyopneumothorax can be identified clinically by the succussion splash and shifting dullness (percussion over the 5th intercostal space anteriorly is dull with the patient erect and hollow when he is supine). Amphoric breathing and post-tussive crackles may be heard over a large cavity. Amoebic liver abscess may present as cough and haemoptysis, which may be acute or chronic; this possibility should be deliberately looked for by palpating for intercostal tenderness over the right lower chest (the liver below the costal margin may be non-tender and is sometimes not palpable, especially when an abscess has discharged some of its contents upwards). A diagnosis of lung abscess can often be made from the characteristic pungent fetor that may fill a ward. Hepatosplenomegaly in a schistosomal area, or the presence of a caput medusae, increases the possibility of schistosomal lung disease and cor pulmonale. Chronic obstructive airways disease (COAD) is common everywhere; the characteristic physical signs should indicate the diagnosis, but remember that other pulmonary disease may be difficult to detect in the presence of COAD. In particular, any evidence of tuberculosis should be searched for carefully as the two conditions quite commonly coexist.

A number of *tests* can contribute to diagnosis and follow-up. A peak flowmeter provides an index of airways obstruction, both for diagnosis and for observing changes and response to treatment; a small portable version such as the Wright Peak Flow Mini-meter makes a useful addition to the doctor's bag, and there should be one on every ward. The mainstay of diagnosis in tuberculosis is microscopy of the stained sputum smear, but good sputum samples may yield a lot of other information. Note the quantity and appearance; microscopy may occasionally reveal larval helminths, *Paragonimus* ova, hydatid scolices or fungal hyphae (aspergilloma). Bacterial culture is of limited value because of the plentiful commensal flora in the pharynx. Culture for tubercle bacilli yields a delayed diagnosis in a small proportion of smear-negative subjects. The likelihood of getting useful information from the sputum is proportional to the quality of sputum sampling. Improved samples can be obtained by physiotherapy or by initiating a deep cough by spraying the vocal cords with a fine saline spray or by injecting 1 ml of sterile saline direct into the trachea through a fine needle inserted between the thyroid and cricoid cartilages.

Chest radiographs are important but expensive. (In a poor country one chest X-ray may cost as much as the entire health budget for a year for four people.) They should therefore be used with discretion, and with a clear idea of what they can and cannot do. Never use an X-ray as a short cut to the correct diagnosis, as it is highly susceptible to misinterpretation and is, anyway, often rendered unnecessary by proper clinical evaluation of the patient. Toman[2] has summarized several studies indicating how commonly one expert may differ from another, or from himself on different occasions, in the interpretation of chest films. There is no point in taking a chest X-ray to demonstrate what is clearly deducible from clinical features, as in lobar pneumonia, massive pleural effusion or sputum-positive tuberculosis, unless there is a definite indication that the picture may contribute to management. Follow-up pictures in a patient clinically improving on treatment for pneumonia or tuberculosis are rarely warranted. It is better to reserve X-rays for circumstances in which they can be most useful, as in the management of pneumothorax or the investigation of unresolving pneumonia.

If available, fibreoptic bronchoscopy may provide useful information towards diagnosis in a number of circumstances. The instrument is expensive, but each procedure then costs almost nothing. A physician, surgeon or radiologist may quite readily acquire the ability to use it after a period of instruction by an expert. The instrument is valuable for identifying causes of local bronchial obstruction (including small foreign bodies, tumours, etc.), for obtaining secretions from a local site by brushings or lavage (e.g. to look for acid-fast bacilli in the sputum-negative patient), and for obtaining transbronchial lung biopsies (highly effective in identifying *Pneumocystis carinii* pneumonia, but less effective for tumours distant from the hilum). The value of fibreoptic bronchoscopy is limited by the quality of laboratory facilities which can be applied to fluid or tissues obtained.

ACUTE LOBAR PNEUMONIA

Lobar pneumonia is common in all tropical countries and is a major cause of death, especially in children (see section on acute respiratory infection in children, below). Evidence suggests that bacterial pneumonias are often preceded by a viral infection that presumably alters the susceptibility of the host or damages local defence mechanisms. The circumstances of an individual's illness should be noted: 'primary' pneumonia occurs in the previously healthy, 'secondary' pneumonia as a complication of another disorder (e.g. structural defect) or circumstances (e.g. period of unconsciousness with aspiration or atelectasis). Note also the immune status of the host: the autosplenectomized sickler, the post-splenectomy patient, the pregnant woman, the alcoholic, the diabetic and the malnourished all have an increased susceptibility to bacterial infection.

The symptoms and signs of lobar pneumonia are well known but sometimes confusing. In early pneumonia, the diagnosis may have to be deduced from the symptoms and presence of fever, shallow tachypnoea and reduced chest movement, in the absence of any auscultatory signs. In one study in Africa it was shown that the site of consolidation could be more reliably predicted by the 'pointing sign' than by auscultation: the patient is asked to cough and point to the place where this causes pain. When pleurisy is diaphragmatic an abdominal cause may be suspected by patient or physician. In some populations a considerable proportion of patients with lobar pneumonia develop jaundice. This may be deep, but usually fades rapidly with treatment of the pneumonia (more rapidly than jaundice fades in acute viral hepatitis). This jaundice of pneumonia is hepatocellular in type and does not seem to be associated with pre-existing chronic liver disease or hepatitis B carrier status; in one study there was a significant association with glucose-6-phosphate dehydrogenase deficiency,[3] but others have not found this. Characteristic but minor changes of liver histology have been demonstrated.

Pneumococci and *Haemophilus influenzae* have been the commonest bacterial agents identified in most studies of lobar pneumonia. The organism may be identified by blood culture in about one-third of patients, or by detecting bacterial antigen in blood or urine. Direct needle aspiration from consolidated lung improves the yield but there is a considerable risk of pneumothorax.

Other bacterial causes of lobar consolidation may be difficult to distinguish, on the basis of the clinical features, from pneumococcal disease, but may be suspected in some circumstances. In legionella pneumonia there may be mental confusion, diarrhoea or hypotension; hyponatraemia and haematuria are common: these features, together with failure to respond to initial antibiotic treatment, should indicate the possibility of this diagnosis, for which erythromycin is the drug of choice. The incidence of legionella pneumonia in the tropics is not yet well known, but the propensity of the organism to multiply in water that is perpetually above a temperature of 25°C, and the fact that about a third of UK cases have acquired the infection after travel in southern Europe, suggests that *Legionella* may be responsible for more of the pneumonia occurring in the tropics than is generally recognized.

A proportion of pneumonias in any series prove to be due to *Mycoplasma pneumoniae*, although these organisms more commonly cause a mild upper respiratory tract infection. The illness cannot be distinguished from other pneumonias by clinical features, but may be suspected in the small percentage of patients who develop extrapulmonary complications, especially arthritis or haemolytic anaemia. Tetracycline is the drug of choice but erythromycin is effective.

A severely ill patient may have staphylococcal pneumonia, in which multiple lung cavities may develop. Many such patients are assumed to have sputum-negative tuberculosis and are given antituberculous drugs. The severity of illness and the presence of scattered, small, thin-walled cavities may alert the clinician to the correct diagnosis, when cloxacillin or a cephalosporin may be appropriate treatment. Chloramphenicol is usually as effective and a lot less expensive.

It is important in areas where tuberculosis is common, to remember that post-primary tuberculosis may present with a clinical syndrome indistinguishable from acute bacterial pneumonia. William Osler recognized this when working in Boston in 1900, where tuberculosis was as common as it is in many tropical areas today. He taught that every patient with lobar pneumonia should be considered to have tuberculosis until clinical progress proved otherwise. This advice is much more important today when specific therapy is available.

In some areas, particularly South-East Asia, melioidosis should be considered as a possible cause both of acute and of unresolving pneumonia, especially in the debilitated or immunocompromised. Appropriate media are needed to culture the organism and to indicate the correct therapy (Chapter 27).

Viral pneumonia cannot reliably be distinguished from bacterial: the latter may complicate upper respiratory tract viral infections; so that in both there may be preceding malaise, fever and upper respiratory symptoms. In children in particular so much pneumonia is viral that much of the antibiotic prescribed is needless. Careful studies in various localities are needed to provide guidelines for routine therapy.

A diagnosis that may have to be considered in patients with cough and dyspnoea, especially in the context of malnutrition or any of the conditions associated with impaired immunity, is *Pneumocystis carinii* pneumonia. Studies of the aetiology of pneumonia in patients with the acquired immune deficiency syndrome (AIDS) so far suggest that pneumocystis is less commonly responsible for this complication in Africa than it is in Europe and North America. Further observations are needed. Pneumocystis has also been recognized as the cause of a proportion of cases of acute pneumonia in otherwise healthy children and as a cause of epidemic interstitial pneumonitis. The clinical features are non-specific; dry cough, fever and dyspnoea are usual, and there are characteristically few signs on auscultation. X-rays usually show scattered reticulonodular shadows in both lungs, especially around the hila, progressing to larger areas of consolidation, but the picture is very variable. Diagnosis is most reliably made by transbronchial biopsy through a fibreoptic bronchoscope, but promising methods of detecting antigen in sputum may lead to readier diagnosis and a better appreciation of the role of this agent in pneumonia in tropical communities. Co-trimoxazole is the treatment of choice, as it is safer than pentamidine, which may be tried if co-trimoxazole fails.

There is no generally applicable standard treatment for pneumonia. Once the particular circumstances of an individual's illness have been carefully assessed, a policy derived from local studies of aetiological agents and drug sensitivity patterns should be applied. In some areas, particularly Papua New Guinea and South Africa, pneumococci resistant to penicillin have become common enough to alter the treatment policy. In a study in Papua New Guinea chloramphenicol was found to be effective as a routine treatment for childhood pneumonia and shown to be just as effective alone as when combined with penicillin.[4] Whatever drug treatment is given, the patient should be carefully observed for response to treatment and for the development of any complications: lung abscess, empyema, or metastatic (including cerebral) abscess.

PLEURAL EFFUSION

Patients may develop symptoms only when a pleural effusion has become massive, with no detectable resonance on the affected side, and shift of the trachea and mediastinum towards the opposite side. Such huge effusions are quite common, especially in young adults with post-primary tuberculosis. There may be a history of pleuritic pain on the affected side some days or weeks before, and breathlessness has usually ensued only recently. In addition to the classical stony dullness on percussion, bronchial breathing is usually heard over the affected hemithorax, but it is quiet and distant, heard only when the patient breathes deeply, unlike the bronchial breathing of consolidation which usually augments quiet breath sounds. A careful examination is required to look for evidence of other disease, and for abnormal lymph nodes. A sample of pleural fluid should be allowed to stand for half an hour on the bench: if a coagulum or 'web' appears the fluid is likely to be an exudate. The high protein content will be confirmed in the laboratory, but if this is not possible there is a simple bedside test that can indicate approximately the protein content of the fluid. This test depends on the fact that there is a fairly close correlation between the specific gravity and the protein content of effusion fluid (or serum). Having taken the fluid sample from the patient, expel one small drop of the fluid, from a height of about 1 cm, into a solution of copper sulphate.

If the drop sinks to the bottom, it has a higher specific gravity than the copper sulphate, if it floats, it is of lower specific gravity. The copper sulphate solution, which can be used several times, must be prepared in such a concentration (2.37 g of $CuSO_4 \cdot 5H_2O$ dried crystals dissolved in water to a volume of 100 ml) that its specific gravity is 1.016, because this is about the same as the specific gravity of an effusion containing 3.0–3.5 g/dl of protein. If the drop of fluid sinks in this, it is probably an exudate, if it floats it is probably a transudate. A test of this kind can only be a rough guide, but may help immediate decisions concerning further investigations or management.

When drawing fluid from an exudate it is wise to take a pleural biopsy at the same time, using an Abrams needle. If two or three specimens of pleura are taken in different directions at the same site there is a 70% chance of making a histological diagnosis, which in the young is usually tuberculosis, and in older patients may be tuberculous or malignant disease. Removing a litre of fluid will allow the lung to expand and may relieve discomfort; this can be repeated on later occasions but it is unnecessary to attempt to remove it all; a tuberculous effusion will resolve with drug treatment. Occasionally an effusion can become loculated in an unusual site, such as the anterior part of a pleural space, and may be associated with persisting fever or localized pain; the fluid must be identified by careful percussion and auscultation, with radiographic help if necessary, as removing the effusion may abolish the symptoms.

ASTHMA

This is common in the tropics and there are some differences in the pattern of disease from that seen in temperate countries. In a study in Nigeria[5] most adults with asthma had first developed symptoms in adult life; a minority of patients gave a history of rhinitis, and none had suffered from eczema; most patients suffered more at night than by day; about half could relate symptoms to exposure to house dust. In most studies nearly all patients have positive skin tests to one or more allergens, most commonly house dust mites[5,6] (such tests are also positive in a large proportion of the non-asthmatic population; control groups are essential in such studies). Where staffing allows, it can be useful to hold a regular asthma clinic[7] to which patients have ready access and at which good home therapy can be taught, problems discussed and drugs dependably supplied. Another value of such a clinic is that it can be the setting for good teaching on asthma for auxiliaries, students, nurses and doctors. Each patient should be assessed for possible precipitating factors or circumstances: season, time of day, exercise, dust, drugs (e.g. salicylates, present in innumerable mixtures and tablets available from grocery stores), animals, bedding. At a clinic all patients can be taught about the need for keeping home and bedding as clean as possible, about the dangers of smoking and the possible dangers of aspirin and other drugs, and the need for early treatment of attacks. Progress can be monitored by symptom indices and measurements of the peak flow rate.

Treatment should be appropriate to the frequency and severity of attacks, with beta$_2$-agonists (salbutamol or terbutaline) as the first line for mild attacks; cromoglycate may be assessed for prophylactic efficacy over a period of weeks for those suffering frequent attacks; severe episodes can be usefully treated with short courses or oral corticosteroids (e.g. prednisolone 60 mg daily for 3–5 days) with nebulized beta$_2$-agonists by inhalation initially. Long-term regular steroid treatment should be rarely necessary; if embarked upon the usual dangers must be considered; antimalarial and anti-tuberculous prophylaxis may be warranted. Although aerosol inhalers are of great value in asthma, many patients find them difficult or impossible to use; they are expensive, and should only be dispensed to those patients who demonstrate that they can inhale properly from them. This requires painstaking teaching by clinic staff.

In some areas patients with cough or wheeze may have tropical pulmonary eosinophilia—in which gross eosinophilia and lung shadows on X-ray are associated with a positive filarial complement fixation test; the condition improves rapidly with antifilarial treatment (Chapter 20). This possibility should be looked for in the asthma clinic especially in areas where *Wuchereria bancrofti* and *Brugia malayi* are common. The condition is uncommon in Africa, but a similar combination of cough, wheeze and eosinophilia may occur due to the migrating larval stages of ascaris, hookworm or strongyloides infection (Chapter 21).

SARCOIDOSIS

In many tropical countries sarcoidosis has never been identified. Studies in some areas suggest that the apparent dearth of cases may be due to the fact that most are misdiagnosed as sputum-negative tuberculosis or other chronic infections. In temperate countries Africans, West Indians and Asians have a much higher incidence of sarcoidosis than do Caucasians living in the same vicinity. In one UK study West Indians had an incidence of sarcoidosis that was over 14 times that in Caucasians living in the same part of London.[8] Caucasians are also found to have less severe disease, with less systemic manifestations, than the other racial groups. Nevertheless the condition remains uncommon in the tropics: a special unit in Delhi has detected increasing numbers of cases in recent years,[9] but the total number identified in the entire country in the years 1957 to 1982 was only 90. The possibility of sarcoidosis should be considered in patients with unresolving lung disease, especially if there are accompanying extrathoracic features such as iridocyclitis, lymphadenopathy, central nervous system complications or hypercalcaemia.

PULMONARY PROBLEMS IN COMMON PARASITIC DISEASES

Those working in a tropical area, or having to deal with travellers, must be aware of pulmonary aspects of most of the common parasitic diseases; lung involvement may complicate other more usual features of those infections, or may sometimes be the major mode of presentation. In some parasitic diseases, the lung is the predominant territory involved: paragonimiasis (Chapter 22) must be considered in patients with cough, haemoptysis and cavitating lung disease, often mistaken for tuberculosis; hydatid cysts (Chapter 23) may produce a variety of lung problems as a result of mechanical compression of intrathoracic structures. In a number of helminth infections (hookworm, *Ascaris, Strongyloides*) a larval stage of the parasite migrates through the lungs when it may cause cough, fever, dyspnoea and sometimes wheeze or haemoptysis (Chapter 21).

The severity of the illness probably depends on how many larvae are migrating at one time; the classical self-experiment of Koino[10] illustrated this. He swallowed two thousand viable ascaris eggs, and within a week suffered a severe illness with high fever, dyspnoea, cyanosis, severe cough and frothy, bloodstained sputum lasting for 7 days. There was eosinophilia, and many ascaris larvae were recovered from his sputum. It would be unusual for such a large number of eggs to be ingested simultaneously in natural circumstances. In schistosomiasis, especially where portal hypertension has led to venous shunts bypassing the liver, eggs may be deposited in pulmonary capillaries and arterioles, eliciting a granulomatous reaction resulting either in pulmonary hypertension or the accumulation of large masses of granulation tissue (Chapter 22).

Malaria may be complicated by pulmonary problems; cough is not uncommonly a symptom even in moderately severe malaria, and in severe falciparum malaria pulmonary problems have been reported in 5–15% of cases. Although pulmonary oedema due to therapeutic fluid overload, or bronchopneumonia complicating deep coma, may occur, a more specific malarial lesion has been recognized in which there is septal oedema, endothelial cell swelling and hyaline membrane formation within the alveoli (Chapter 1).

SMOKING IN THE TROPICS

Over 100 developing countries have a tobacco industry that contributes to revenue, employment and trade. The end product is, however, increasingly finding its way back to the countries of its origin, where the practice of smoking has increased steadily over the past decade. This increase has been estimated at 32% in Africa and 24% in South America between 1970 and 1980, but is much greater within certain sections of the population. In Nigeria 41% of adult men smoke. Particularly alarming are figures from secondary schools; 30–40% of pupils in some areas have been found to be regular smokers. Smoking-related diseases appear to have increased: the incidence of carcinoma of the bronchus in China increased sixfold between 1970 and 1980, and emphysema and lung cancer are becoming rapidly more common in Nigeria, India and Malaysia. Because of the delayed effects of smoking a great increase of these and other smoking-related diseases can be expected within the coming decade.

ACUTE RESPIRATORY INFECTION (ARI) IN CHILDREN

Respiratory diseases, particularly bacterial pneumonia, tuberculosis, measles and pertussis are major causes of death throughout the world. Children are at particular risk: at least two million and probably over five million die every year of respiratory infections. Only recently have these problems begun to receive the kind of attention that has been devoted to diarrhoeal disease and malnutrition, the other major killers in children.

The urban child whether in the tropics or non-tropics suffers an average of five to eight episodes of acute respiratory infection (ARI) per year. Of these, lower respiratory infections are the most lethal particularly in the tropics, where the risk of death from pneumonia in children aged one to four years has been recorded as 50 times as great as in comparable groups in USA and Canada.[11] Malnourished children are at special risk; in a study in Costa Rica the mortality of ARI was 12 times higher in malnourished infants than in those of normal weight.[12]

Upper respiratory infections are usually viral, but the causative agent is rarely identified. Upper respiratory viral infections may progress to viral pneumonia or may be complicated by bacterial pneumonia. Of the responsible viruses measles, respiratory syncytial virus (RSV) and the influenza and parainfluenza viruses are numerically most important. The commonest bacteria causing pneumonia are *Streptococcus pneumoniae* and *Haemophilus influenzae*, but staphylococci are important especially in infants and complicating measles or influenza. In about half of all cases of bacterial pneumonia there is clinical or serological evidence of a preceding virus infection.

Because of the enormous mortality from ARI, the World Health Organization has urged that each nation should embark on a national programme aimed at the study and control of ARI, particularly in children.[11] The programme should include a study of aetiological agents and their relation to clinical disease pattern and prognosis—important in deciding on vaccination policies. From studies of local disease patterns, clinicians should try to draw up standard treatment and referral flow charts for the use of primary health workers and rural hospital staff in an attempt to improve on the currently disastrous failure to save the lives of millions of children with treatable disease. Several simple measures in addition to clinical ones might have an important impact: the continued promotion of breastfeeding, which is known to halve the risk of RSV infection in infants;[13] timely vaccination in infancy against tuberculosis, measles, diphtheria, and pertussis; special vigilance for those children at greatest risk of death from respiratory infection: those with low birth weight, diarrhoeal disease, and malnutrition; and insistence on continued or increased hydration and feeding during respiratory illness. Each locality will have to decide at what level staff should be allowed to give antibiotic treatment and what that treatment should be in the light of bacterial agents and their drug sensitivities known to prevail locally.

Meanwhile there is urgent need for new and additional vaccines, particularly against RSV, pneumococci and *Haemophilus influenzae*. These too will need effective primary health and maternal–child health services if they are to be deployed effectively.

REFERENCES

1 Collins, T.F.B. Personal communication.
2 Toman, K. (1979) *Tuberculosis: Case Findings and Chemotherapy: Questions and Answers*. World Health Organization. Geneva.
3 Tugwell, P. (1973) *Lancet* 1, 968–970.
4 Shann, F., Barker, J. & Poore, P. (1985) *Lancet* 2, 684–688.
5 Warrell, D.A., Fawcett, I.W., Harrison, B.D.W. et al (1975) *Q.J.Med.* 174, 325–347.
6 Shao, J.F. & Shayo, A. (1985) *E. Afr. Med. J.* 62, 387–390.
7 Gill, G.V. (1979) *Trop. Doct.* 9, 155–157.
8 McNicol, M.W. & Luce, P.J. (1985) *J.R. Coll. Phys. Lond.* 19, 179–183.
9 Gupta, S.K., Mitra, K., Chatterjee, S. et al (1985) *Br. J. Dis. Chest* 79, 275–280.
10 Koino, R. (1922) *Japanese Medical World* 2, 317 (quoted in Woodruff, A.W. (ed.) (1974) *Medicine in The Tropics*, p. 159. Churchill Livingstone.
11 Memorandum (1984) *Bull WHO* 62, 47–58.
12 James, J.W. (1972) *Am. J. clin. Nutr.* 25, 690–694.
13 Pullan, C.R., Toms, G.L., Martin, A.J. et al (1980) *Br. med. J.* 281, 1034–1036.

Chapter 65
Dermatological Problems
J. H. S. Pettit

Most doctors working in tropical areas are unable to avoid patients who demand treatment for their skin ailments. The diseases for which these patients seek attention fall into three groups.

1 Common dermatoses of worldwide incidence whose presentation and treatment do not vary according to geography (e.g. warts, molluscum contagiosum, scleroderma, dermatitis herpetiformis, mycosis fungoides).

2 Diseases also of worldwide distribution which have different presentation or require a different approach to treatment (e.g. acne vulgaris, lupus vulgaris, psoriasis).

3 Dermatoses, the acquisition of which is dependent on residence, permanent or temporary, in tropical areas (e.g. Buruli ulcer, leishmaniasis, rhinoscleroma, Brazilian pemphigus).

No effort is made here to cover diseases falling in the first group; many suitable textbooks are available to advise on the diagnosis and treatment of such cases (see e.g. Pettit,[1] Pettit and Parish,[2] Hall-Smith and Cairns,[3] Rook et al[4]). Diseases discussed in this chapter will fall into one of the two other groups mentioned above.

REGIONAL VARIANTS OF WORLDWIDE DERMATOSES

ACNE VULGARIS

This common disease of adolescence usually presents as a combination of a greasy skin with comedones and pustules most frequently on the face but, in more severe cases, also affecting the chest and upper back. The condition may vary from a mild scattering of a few blackheads on the temples or forehead to a severe eruption in which the face is covered with pustulocystic lesions which leave deforming crateriform scars when finally the patient (with the doctor's assistance) manages to shake off the disease (Fig. 65.1). It is mainly because of these cosmetic deformities that it is worthwhile undertaking treatment to prevent patients being scarred for life.

Tropical variants of presentation

Greasiness is a necessary feature of acne and it necessarily follows that when patients move from a temperate to a tropical zone they will not only perspire more but will produce an increased greasiness of the skin. This means that those whose acne starts in a temperate climate may find on transfer to the tropics that they get worse—some authorities have used such phrases as 'tropical acne' or 'summer acne' for such a situation. It is also possible that young people who have been fortunate enough to avoid the development of acne when living in a cool climate will find that a holiday in a warmer country will precipitate the eruption of acne.

A high proportion of races living in the tropics (e.g. those of the Amazon valley and South-East Asia) are relatively less hirsute than their Caucasian brothers and consequently have less sebaceous glands and show a tendency for their acne to be less severe.

Treatment in the tropics

Routine therapy consists of degreasing the skin either with 1% cetrimide lotion or a suitably medicated soap and the application of a keratolytic—sulphur 6% in calamine lotion, 5% benzoyl peroxide lotion or 0.05% retinoic acid lotion—will usually be sufficient for the comedone type of acne. Patients with a predominance of pustules will need 500 mg of tetracycline once or twice daily for several months to suppress

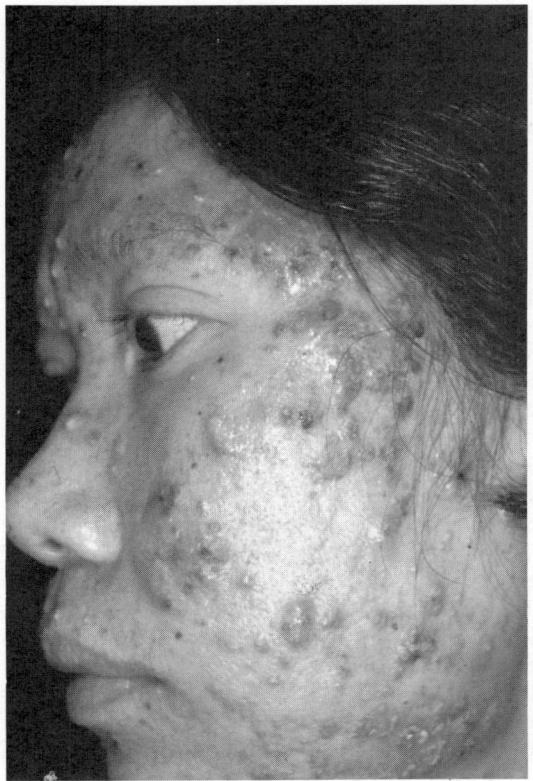

Fig. 65.1 Acne vulgaris. Severe nodulocystic pustular acne; in such cases the back is often affected.

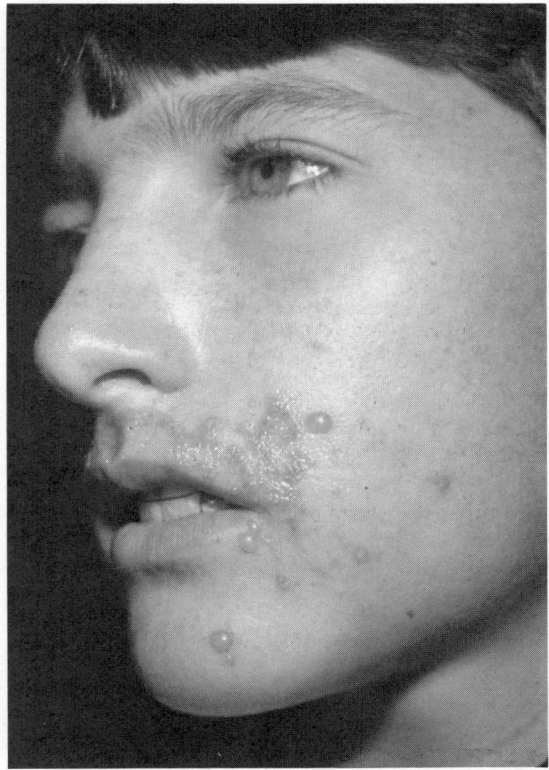

Fig. 65.2 Impetigo. Lesions usually start as bullae which break and cause crusts.

formation of pustules and so reduce the number of resultant scars.

13-*cis*-retinoic acid, recently popular for severe pustular acne, is only rarely needed for patients living in the tropics.

BACTERIAL DISEASES OF THE SKIN

Pyococcal infections

Impetigo contagiosa and ecthyma are the commonest forms of pyococcal infections of the skin. Impetigo is classically described as consisting of bullous or crusted lesions on exposed areas usually caused by staphylococci or streptococci (Fig. 65.2); studies from various parts of the world seem unable to agree as to which form of disease is caused by which organism.

Ecthyma is a rather deeper crusted infection often penetrating the basal layer and leaving a scar when it is healed, a finding which is not characteristic of impetigo.

Tropical variants of presentation

Barefoot or barelegged children in the fields or gardens of rural areas are exposed to all sorts of additional superficial lesions of the skin (boils, scratches, grazes, bites, etc.) which when secondarily infected by pyococcal organisms produce a spectrum of infection which is best called pyoderma. If left untreated these infections result in the development of hypopigmented scars which stay visible on the shins for many years.

Treatment in the tropics

Mild cases of pyoderma (Fig. 65.3) usually respond well to washing twice daily with warm water and soap followed by the local application of an antibiotic cream such as topical bacitracin, neosporin or sodium fusidate; but in areas where such sophisticated products are either too expensive or not available a satisfactory sub-

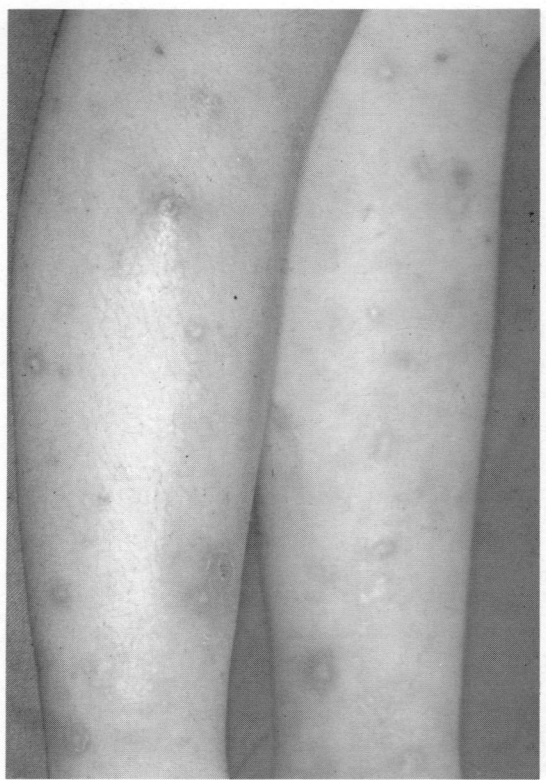

Fig. 65.3 Pyoderma. A mixture of infected scratches and impetiginized sores on a child's legs. (Courtesy Dr Radzi bin Jaafar.)

stitute may be made by mixing the contents of a 250 mg capsule of tetracycline with 25 g of a simple cream. Severe and extensive cases will respond more rapidly to systemic antibiotic therapy but it should be remembered that penicillin is often unsuccessful. In the tropics bacteriological studies are frequently not available and in such cases erythromycin or flucloxacillin are usually helpful.

Some authorities hold that all cases of pyoderma should be treated systemically because of the possibility that children may develop acute glomerulonephritis due to a nephritogenic *Streptococcus*. This problem has diminished in recent years[5] although by 1981 it had not entirely disappeared from Trinidad.[6] As systemic therapy has not been convincingly proved to prevent acute glomerulonephritis[7] it is suggested that such treatment need only be given for extensive cases of pyoderma and not used for milder infection.

Tuberculosis of the skin

Whether due to improved treatment or to the widespread use of BCG it is undoubtedly true that tuberculous infections are much less of a problem in temperate zones than they used to be. The varied clinical manifestations that used to be easily recognized are now less often seen in Europe or North America. These different presentations are usually caused by the patient's past experience of tuberculosis and the consequent underlying immunity. Those who have never previously been infected by *Mycobacterium tuberculosis* will produce a primary chancre if the organism is inoculated into the skin. A small, slowly growing nodule breaks down to form a painless ulcer not infrequently associated with a similarly painless regional lymphadenopathy. This often takes a long time to heal and if the patient cannot develop a high resistance one of the other forms of skin tuberculosis may appear at the site of initial infection.

All other forms of skin tuberculosis are associated with some deeper form of infection. Scrofuloderma overlies a colliquative necrosis of tuberculous glands (usually in the neck) and shows a combination of fluctuant nodules and discharging sinuses (Plate VII.4); tuberculous osteitis (knee, wrist, rib etc.) sometimes spreads to the overlying skin to cause a tuberculous ulcer in which the chronic granulation tissue on the floor of the ulcer is surrounded by a delicate bluish-white edge.

Lupus vulgaris occurs when an organism lodges in the skin of a patient who already has a positive Mantoux reaction. It causes a tuberculoid granuloma in the dermis which manifests itself initially as small brownish-red nodules which on vitropression are supposed to appear as translucent greenish-yellow 'apple-jelly' nodules (Plate VII.5). They extend centrifugally leaving in the centre an atrophic epidermis which may ulcerate or ultimately even become malignant. In the past lupus vulgaris was particularly common round the face and nose.

Tropical variants of presentation

In those parts of the world where individuals are exempted from the need to wear thick or any clothing superficial skin trauma is more easily experienced. In such areas pulmonary tuberculosis is by no means uncommon and it follows that previously uninfected children may develop a primary tuberculous chancre anywhere on the body where trauma has been associated with penetration by tubercle bacilli. A high index of suspicion must be maintained as otherwise these small painless ulcers may be treated lightly and the disease not diagnosed until one of the more extensive forms of tuberculosis has appeared.

Tuberculosis verrucosa cutis (Plate VII.6) is the most common form of tuberculosis in many parts of the Third World. It is somewhat similar to lupus vulgaris with a chronic tuberculoid granuloma appearing in the dermis after traumatic inoculation in a patient with high immunity but, in addition to the granuloma in the dermis, a reactive hyperplasia of the epidermis causes the lesions to be markedly warty. They will usually produce roughly concentric rings on the buttocks, elbows or ankles, and these sites are probably due to the fact that in some parts of the world people sitting on a wooden floor may be damaged by a splinter that has been contaminated by infected sputum from another member of the family.

Treatment in the tropics

In those parts of the world where there is a continuing high incidence of tuberculosis of the lung it is not surprising that skin tuberculosis is seen more often than in the more affluent regions. It has, however, been pointed out from Kenya that skin manifestations are less common than might have been expected. It must be remembered that before the discovery of specific antituberculous drugs in the late 1940s various forms of ultraviolet light and vitamin D (calciferol) were used for the treatment of skin tuberculosis and it is possible that numerous patients with a fairly high resistance do not develop an infection following inoculation, as they are exposed for hours a day to preventative doses of sunshine.

Such treatment cannot, however, be relied on and some form of antituberculous therapy must be used. Care should always be taken to investigate the probability of tuberculosis simultaneously infecting other sites and, even if such complications remain undiscovered, it is wise to treat the patient as if there is a hidden infection. The initial treatment should consist of isoniazid 200–300 mg daily and two other first-line drugs (rifampicin, streptomycin or ethambutol) in suitable doses followed by a period of six months to a year when the patient continues isoniazid with one of the other drugs (see Chapter 59).

In many parts of the tropics skin tuberculosis is often treated by isoniazid (INH) alone; this treatment is often dermatologically effective but should only be undertaken if it is certain there is no other active manifestation of tuberculosis in the body. INH resistance may develop.

ECZEMA–DERMATITIS

Throughout the world about half the people who seek treatment for a skin condition are suffering from various infections—bacterial, fungal, viral, parasitic, etc. The eczema–dermatitis complex makes up about 30% of all the other dermatoses put together. In the past the words 'eczema' and 'dermatitis' have been used interchangeably for a group of physical signs which start with a mildly pruritic erythema and soon develop a scattering of vesicles throughout the lesion associated with an increasing pruritus. Later the vesicles rupture, often as a result of scratching, and the consequent combination of oozing and scaliness produces a sticky crusted patch which can become secondarily infected. More recently it has become the custom in many centres to use the word 'eczema' to describe those cases that have an endogenous cause and the word 'dermatitis' to describe a similar clinical picture produced as a reaction to some extrinsic irritant or sensitizing application to the skin.

Endogenous eczema

Most often eczema presents in a discoid or nummular form mainly affecting young people in their late teens or early twenties. Scattered on the arms and legs are well-defined circular mixtures of erythema vesicles and crusts, usually less than 2 cm in diameter (Plate VIII.1) which are often mistaken for small patches of tinea corporis—potassium hydroxide preparations will show that no fungus is present. This is an exceedingly chronic condition and at any one time the patient has a combination of newly erupting and slowly healing circular patches which may continue for several years. No one has any idea as to the cause of this troublesome condition which may need small (5–15 mg) doses of prednisolone daily to keep the patient comfortable. This manifestation of eczema is found rather more frequently in the tropics than in temperate zones and as patients in warm countries do not take kindly to persistent use of creams and ointments the best treatment may be a combination of systemic corticosteroids and 1% hydrocortisone lotion. In Hawaii it has been found that a single deep intramuscular injection of 40 units of triamcinolone acetonide every four to six weeks is both effective and acceptable.

Pompholyx

When a potentially vesicular eruption affects the hands and the fingers the thickness of the keratin layer effectively modifies the clinical appearance and patients complain less of redness and crusting and more of itching and deeply sited vesicles. The condition often starts along the sides of the fingers and is particularly common in hot weather, so being usually limited to the summer months in temperate zones but occurring year round in the tropics.

Some patients develop this clinical picture as a sensitization phenomenon associated with a badly treated athlete's foot but in most cases the cause is unknown; the not infrequent association of pompholyx with discoid eczema leads some dermatologists to suspect that the same unknown aetiology may precipitate either clinical condition. Increased perspiration exacerbates pompholyx but is not the cause.

A proprietary preparation known as Bellergal (consisting of belladonna, ergotamine and phenobarbitone) is useful for these patients but not available in many countries and it is often necessary to treat them with small doses of oral prednisolone. Local applications of corticosteroids are not very helpful unless the affected part is occluded by a plastic glove or finger-stall; such dressings should be kept airtight and need be changed only once a day.

Contact dermatitis

Certain materials (soaps, strong acids or alkalies, etc.) will irritate any skin to produce reddening, vesiculation, exudation and scaliness (Plate VIII.2). Persistent use of such irritants will cause a condition often called 'housewife's dermatitis' or 'dish-pan hands'.

Other more unfortunate individuals develop a similar group of symptoms as an allergic reaction to a material to which they have become sensitized. The list of these sensitizers is pretty well unending: medicaments, preservatives, fragrances, metals, chemicals, may all cause sensitization.[8]

In the less developed parts of the world where industrialization has not yet attained unwelcome proportions contact dermatitis is inexorably spreading and industrial medical officers should learn not only to recognize the arrival of these allergic industrial dermatoses but also how to investigate them by the use of suitable patch-testing equipment.[9]

It must also be remembered that various foods, fruits and plants are potential sensitizers but in such cases the patient (frequently a housewife or shop assistant) will usually be aware of the cause and take necessary avoiding action.

A short course of oral prednisolone combined with local application of a corticosteroid will satisfactorily relieve the patients of their symptoms but it must be emphasized that *all* sources of the sensitizer should be eliminated from the patient's environment before a cure can be expected.

Atopic eczema

This unpleasant condition, frequently found in association with asthma and hay fever, is not a

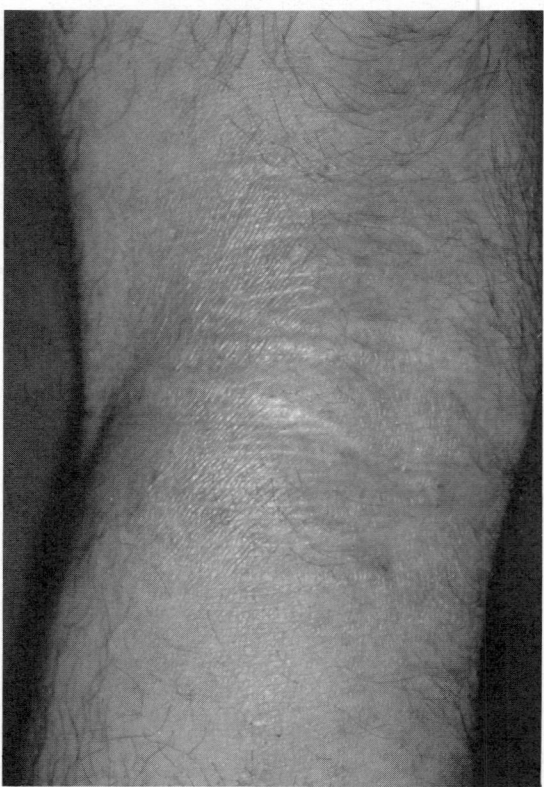

Fig. 65.4 Atopic eczema. Lichenification of popliteal space in an adult with atopic eczema since infancy.

true eczema and vesicles are rarely seen in any of the dermatological presentations: the skin is abnormally pruritic and reacts to scratching by the development of thick patches of the skin variously called lichenification or neurodermatitis (Fig. 65.4).

In the tropics patients or their parents often blame various forms of fish, crustacea, eggs or dairy products for the exacerbations of this condition and dermatologists seem to be slowly recognizing that atopic patients may indeed be sensitive to ingested allergens. Despite this relatively few children are cured by modifications of their diet. Stresses such as teething, illness, school, family or work problems often seem to play an important part in precipitating periods of exacerbation of the atopic diathesis.

Long-term use of weak steroid cream is necessary and this can sometimes be usefully combined with 2–3% liquor picis carbonis or 2–3% salicylic acid. Oral steroids should be avoided as much as possible as it is often difficult to stop such medication once it has begun.

FUNGUS DISEASES OF THE SKIN

Many fungi infect the skin usually having invaded it following superficial or deep trauma. These conditions are described in Chapter 33.

KAPOSI'S SARCOMA (Chapter 67)

First described by Kaposi in the 1890s under the name of 'idiopathic multiple pigment sarcoma' this condition was initially mainly found in central Europe and northern Italy. Reddish-brown or blue nodules varying in size from a pinhead to a pea or bean occurring mainly on the lower limbs gradually enlarged to form infiltrated plaques which, often extending along the veins, finally produced a marked board-like swelling of the extremity (Fig. 67.5). Purpuric lesions and thromboses also occurred. The lesions were often painful, lymph nodes became involved and although Kaposi originally said the disease was fatal in two to three years, it was often found to take a longer course.

It was not until the 1930s that the disease was recognized in central Africa at which time it was said to occur almost always in men.

Acquired immunodeficiency syndrome (AIDS) (Chapter 68)

The recent unhappy explosion of this frightening disease has drawn worldwide attention to Kaposi's sarcoma. Initially recognized in the homosexual communities in North America[10] it is now realized that AIDS is by no means uncommon in central and East Africa where it now affects men and women in about equal numbers. Kaposi's sarcoma affects about half the American cases of AIDS but it occurs less frequently (15–20%) in African cases.

Nowadays the presentation varies somewhat from the original description, the initial lesions, frequently symmetrical, being somewhat paler and more widely scattered and even appearing behind the ears and on the mucosae and gingivae, and later spreading to the internal organs (Chapter 67).

KELOIDS

Surgeons, physicians and even dermatologists seem to be easily confused by the strange spontaneously developing lesions which are seen far more commonly in central Africa than in other parts of the world. The not infrequent development of hypertrophic scars of the skin, usually following trauma, surgery or even inoculations (particularly BCG) are mistaken for keloids but, although keloids may be triggered off by trauma, the classical keloid lesion appears spontaneously often occurring on the chest wall over the sternomanubrial area, which is probably one of the least frequently damaged parts of the body (Fig. 65.5).

Starting as a small, hard nodule which extends peripherally to give a firm, very pruritic plaque it can be differentiated from an ordinary hypertrophic scar (which does not spread) by the characteristic pseudopodial extensions typical of a true keloid.

Differentiation is important as a hypertrophic scar in a non-keloidal patient can be excised with little danger of recurrence, while a true keloid whether starting spontaneously or following trauma reacts badly to surgical excision in the scar and a larger lesion will return.

Many patients with true keloids seek treatment, sometimes because of the intractable pruritus and sometimes for cosmetic reasons. The best form of treatment is to inject a corticosteroid

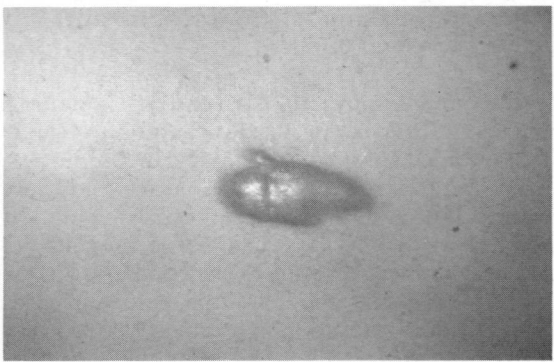

Fig. 65.5 Keloid. Hard, smooth, fibrotic lesion which had appeared spontaneously; no history of trauma or injection.

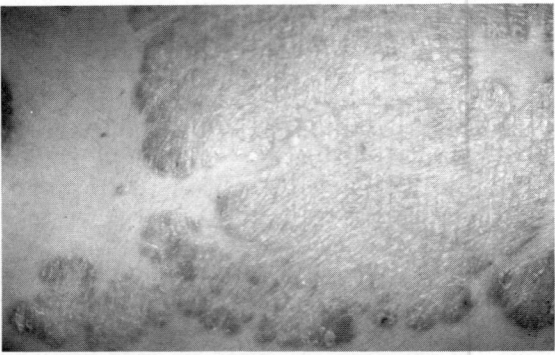

Fig. 65.6 Psoriasis. Well-demarcated erythematosquamous lesion on the back of a patient with seven-year history.

into the lesion but these injections are extremely painful and local anaesthetic must be injected under the keloid prior to actual treatment. It is best to use a corticosteroid which has been formulated for intra-articular use.

Although it is not easily available in the tropics, superficial X-irradiation is sometimes effective with or without simultaneous surgical excision; the dosage should be left in the hands of the radiotherapist.

PSORIASIS

There was a time when European dermatologists taught that psoriasis was less common in the warmer parts of the world; they were wrong. Reports from various parts of the tropics show that some 3–5% of all patients seen in skin clinics are suffering from psoriasis. It is, however, true that most patients (of whatever race) are less severely affected than those who live in cooler areas, probably because they have a much greater exposure to sunlight and are less affected because of this accidental therapeutic irradiation.

These well-demarcated erythematosquamous lesions can easily be recognized by an average medical student and are seen anywhere on the body (Fig. 65.6). They occur in small guttate lesions in children while in adults psoriasis occurs in larger plaques on the trunk, limbs and scalp. When it appears in the groins or other relatively moist flexures the appearance will be modified—well demarcated and erythematous but not scaly.

Treatment in the tropics

The wide range of medications and applications used throughout the world is regrettable evidence that a cure is not possible. Details of routine therapy can be obtained from a more specialized dermatological textbook but certain features should be mentioned here. Guttate psoriasis has been treated with success, particularly in South America and Malaysia by the use of dapsone 100 mg orally each day; smaller doses should be given to children. It is now recognized that haemolysis of red blood cells is dose related and this rarely occurs in adults taking less than 200 mg daily.

It is obvious that in the tropics those who have widespread psoriasis will be unwilling to cover large areas of their bodies with sticky or malodorous applications and, ideally, treatment should be administered systemically rather than locally, but the considerable value of dithranol ointment (anthralin in the USA) should not be overlooked.

A recent acceptable change in approach has led to the use of 0.5% dithranol in Lassar's paste being applied to the patches for no more than an hour each evening. This treatment does not stain the skin to anything like the extent caused by longer application and will often be accepted by patients who will otherwise reject dithranol.

In some of the more sophisticated parts of the world the use of oral psoralens associated with ultraviolet A light (PUVA therapy) has attained a high degree of popularity. This time-consuming and expensive therapy is rarely necessary in the tropics but patients who wish to spend the money may take two capsules of methoxsalen at 11 a.m. and spend their lunch-time from 1 to 2 p.m. sitting in the sun as completely unclothed as local tradition permits.

When patients are severely affected it may be necessary to resort to the oral administration of etretinate (1 mg/kg daily) for three to six months but this is not only expensive but has a number of side-effects which diminish the enthusiasm of many of its users.

The use of antimetabolites—methotrexate, hydroxyurea, etc.—should not be attempted by the non-specialist.

SCABIES (Chapter 53 and Appendix III, p. 1381)

This infestation by *Acarus scabiei* is found throughout the world, being readily spread from person to person and consequently more than one member of the family is usually affected at the same time. Pruritic papules first appear on the finger-webs and the fronts of the wrists and spread from there to the axillae, areola and around the umbilicus, later involving the genitalia, particularly the scrotum (Fig. 65.7). It is seen more frequently in children where the itching is often so badly scratched that patients become secondarily infected and complain of a pyoderma (Plate VIII.3).

In addition to having infected papules it is not unknown for patients to become sensitized to the presence of acari and consequently to develop a widespread papular urticaria looking somewhat like chickenpox. This may cause diagnostic confusion as the urticarial papules do not contain acari and scrapings will be negative. In any case, and contrary to the classical teaching, presence of the acarus is usually difficult to demonstrate in the tropics and diagnosis will often have to depend on the classical distribution of the lesions, combined with a history of nocturnal pruritus affecting several members of the family at the same time.

It is often not realized that patients who have been infected for the first time do not itch for the first three to four weeks and, because of this, some members of the patient's household may not know they have the disease: despite their protests *all* the members of the household should be treated at the same time (including the servants). According to availability, treatment can be benzyl benzoate emulsion 25%, malathion

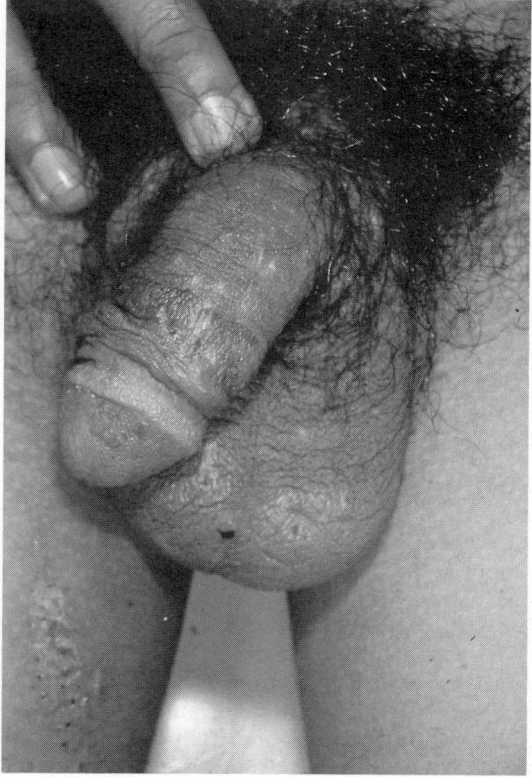

Fig. 65.7 Nodular scabies. Pruritic erythematous nodules on scrotum and penile shaft—acari present in skin scraping.

lotion 0.5% or monosulfiram 25% diluted with 2 or 3 parts of water. Any one of these lotions should be applied all over the body (omitting the head and neck which are rarely affected in adults), left on for 24 hours and then washed off. The treatment should be repeated on two or three consecutive nights. For children the same routine should be used although the lotion should be diluted to half-strength for those between eight and 12 years of age and a quarter-strength for those between four and eight years. Children under four should not be treated by these lotions; instead 6% sulphur ointment or 10% crotamiton can be used twice daily.

Crusted scabies

Although it was first recognized in Norway more than 100 years ago the condition now known as crusted scabies is still seen intermittently in the tropics, particularly being found in leprosaria or children's homes. It seems that patients with lepromatous leprosy or with Down's syndrome are particularly susceptible to invasion by the *Acarus scabiei* and do not react to such infections in the usual way. A massive proliferation of the acari stimulates an enormous non-pruritic scaliness of the skin which may be taken for an erythroderma. Not infrequently the presence of such cases in a ward is only recognized when an epidemic of scabies affects other patients, nurses, doctors, ward attendants and laundry assistants. All contacts must be treated with routine anti-scabies treatment but the index case often needs several weeks of daily treatment carefully applied.

SOLAR DERMATOSES AND EPIDERMAL MALIGNANCIES

Although Africans, Indians and other deeply pigmented races are usually careful to protect themselves from the sun's rays as much as possible, Caucasians often seem to imagine that despite their lack of protective pigmentation they can expose themselves to the dangers of solar irradiation with impunity. Because of this there is a high incidence of abnormalities of the skin caused by sunlight in Australia, the southern parts of the USA and other areas where a white population lives in an unsuitable geographical situation.

Photodermatitis

While it is obvious that excessive exposure to the sun may be expected to damage the cells of the epidermis to give various degrees of sunburn it is often forgotten that certain individuals, hypersensitive to the sun's rays, may develop skin lesions from no more than ordinary exposure. Such patients show a diffuse eczematous reaction limited to the exposed areas of the skin: forehead, nose, cheeks, V of the neck, forearms and hands (Fig. 65.8).

Drugs that produce this clinical picture include tetracyclines, phenothiazines, thiazides and the sulpha drugs, while among local applications that may sensitize the patient are buclosamide, topical antihistamines and the halogenated salicylanilides which have all been easily available to the public at various times and in various places.

Treatment is primarily directed at recognizing the cause of solar sensitivity but, unfortunately,

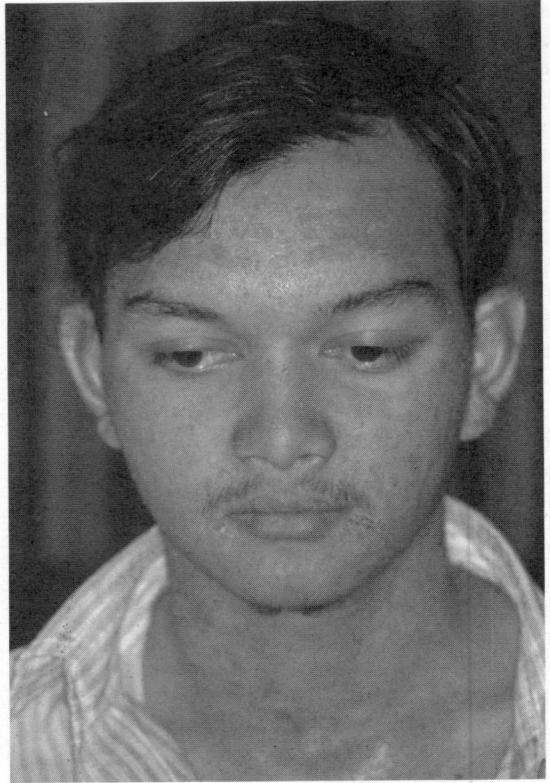

Fig. 65.8 Photodermatitis. Red pruritic skin of exposed areas in patient under treatment with chlorothiazide. (Courtesy Dr Radzi bin Jaafar.)

the elimination of the cause is not always followed by an amelioration of the dermatitis, in which case not only are systemic steroids necessary in small doses but a sun-barrier lotion or cream should be used on the exposed parts of the skin in the daylight hours. A large number of barriers are available, the simplest and cheapest being made with 10% para-aminobenzoic acid in 60% alcohol.

The porphyrias (Chapter 66)

Sometimes patients (either in childhood or adult life) develop a bullous sun sensitivity associated with scarring of the skin. If there is no evidence of the use of either local or systemic sun sensitizers it may be suspected that the patient has one of the forms of porphyria that affects the skin.[11] Expert biochemical assistance should be obtained.

Epidermal malignancies

Actinic keratoses

Long-term exposure to sunlight is now recognized as being the most frequent cause of epidermal cancer. Paler-skinned individuals are much more prone to these malignancies, which are therefore most common in Caucasians who spend long hours in the direct sunlight in oil fields, tin mines, rubber plantations, farms, golf courses etc. The first sign of trouble is an increased dryness and wrinkling of the skin associated with histological evidence of damage to the elastic tissue in the dermis (solar elastosis) and this is later followed by the appearance on the exposed areas of small scaly lesions with a bright erythematous base (Plate VIII.4) which show histologically that cells in the epidermis are undergoing malignant change. These actinic keratoses are potentially premalignant and, although patients report that some keratoses fall off, others ultimately change into one of the forms of cancer mentioned below. It is advisable to treat the keratoses before transformation occurs.

In places where liquid nitrogen or other forms of cryotherapy are available dermatologists often freeze individual lesions; other forms of direct destruction are not recommended. The best method of treatment is the use of 5-fluorouracil; a 5% cream is usually needed for keratoses on the dorsum of the hands, the arms and legs but this is often too strong for the face and a 1% lotion can be used which is made by adding the contents of a 5 ml ampoule of 5-fluorouracil (containing 250 mg) to 20 ml of propylene glycol. This lotion should be applied all over the face, the ears and the neck twice daily for three weeks, by which time there will be a strong reaction in all the visible lesions, perhaps even some erosions. The reaction will not only affect the previously visible keratoses but will also appear in unexpected sites where presumably sub-clinical lesions are in the early stages of development. Patients find this an uncomfortable treatment and may need to spend most of the daylight hours indoors during the last half of the three-week course but, after that, the use of 1% hydrocortisone lotion will clear the irritated skin and with any luck there will be no recurrences for at least four years.

Basal cell carcinoma (Chapter 67)

Most doctors can recognize these skin-coloured papules which slowly enlarge producing a pearly rolled edge (Plate VIII.5). Later the centre breaks down to form a typical rodent ulcer, a locally malignant tumour which extends remorselessly but almost never metastasizes. These lesions need to be taken seriously (especially if they are close to the eye) but there are various schools of thought concerning the best method of therapy. Many dermatologists curette the lesions extensively under local anaesthesia and cauterize the base; others use liquid nitrogen or radiotherapy. All treatments seem to be successful 80–90% of times but it is recommended here that treatment should consist of a thorough curettage under a local anaesthetic with the subsequent application of 5% 5-fluorouracil ointment to the residual ulceration; this will satisfactorily kill off any malignant cells which have escaped the curette. Such a therapy takes longer than the others but may be expected to produce a higher percentage of cures.

Squamous cell carcinoma

This condition also appears in light-exposed areas, the tumour being particularly common on the lip. Starting as a rapidly growing fleshy nodule it soon breaks down to give a mixture of crusting, ulceration and proliferation (Fig. 65.9). They are truly malignant and must always be treated seriously.

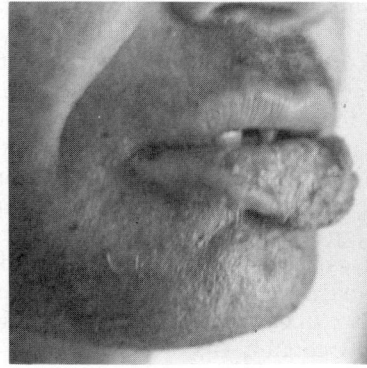

Fig. 65.9 Squamous cell carcinoma. Proliferating and ulcerating tumour on lower lip of an Iranian villager.

Similar malignancy may occur in any chronic ulcer of the skin seen in the tropics (tropical ulcer (Chapter 36), Buruli ulcer (Chapter 38), leprosy etc.); sometimes it is difficult to decide whether the proliferating tissue at the edge of an ulcer is truly malignant or whether the patient simply has a pseudoepitheliomatous hyperplasia.

All cases of squamous cell carcinoma should be treated by the combined attention of a surgeon and a radiotherapist.

Malignant melanoma (Chapter 67)

These highly invasive malignancies arise from melanocytes which normally live in the basal layer producing melanin and injecting it into nearby basal cells, thereby helping to protect the epidermal cells against solar damage. In Australia the incidence of melanoma rises in direct relationship to the nearness to the equator and the risk of melanoma has been shown to increase with accumulated sun exposure throughout life.[12]

Any new growth showing varied colours—black, brown, red or even blue—should be viewed with suspicion and, although melanomas do not always develop in a previously existing cellular naevus, patients with numerous moles should be warned to seek urgent medical attention if such lesions change their shape or their colour or if they start to bleed spontaneously (Fig. 67.4).

Malignancies in achromic skin lesions

Most skin malignancies occur in Caucasians, Japanese and the paler Chinese skins but Asians and Africans, whose normal skin colour provides a reasonably effective protection against the depredations of ultraviolet light, may have trouble if they suffer from any form of dermatosis which takes the form of a hypopigmented or achromic patch. Patients with long-standing vitiligo or albinism will find that after 10 or more years actinic keratoses and other forms of superficial skin malignancies may develop in the unprotected areas; consequently they should always use sun-barrier lotions during the daytime. When they occur the epidermal malignancies should be treated in the ordinary way.

URTICARIA

Every adult at one time or another experiences an attack of acute urticaria. This usually starts as a sudden eruption of raised white oedematous wheals on an erythematous base which are usually pruritic enough to prevent sleep (Fig. 65.10). Most cases of acute urticaria are manifestations of food sensitivity (shellfish, fish, dairy products etc.). In the tropics urticaria is seen in all countries but the causes may vary according to local habits of eating.

Fig. 65.10 Urticaria. Raised red wheals—pruritic following penicillin injections. Patient not previously known to be penicillin sensitive.

Chronic urticaria

This is usually defined as the persistence of urticarial attacks for more than two months. It is rarely due to food allergens for even the least observant individual will slowly recognize the association between an item of diet and a further attack and take suitable steps to avoid recurrence. Ingested drugs, particularly aspirin and other salicylates and benzoates and the yellow colouring known as tartrazine, are often unrecognized causes of chronic urticaria.[13]

In the tropics all the usual causes of chronic urticaria may be recognized but it must not be forgotten that many patients are reacting to parasitic infestations. All long-standing cases should have their stools examined for hookworm, tapeworms and roundworms and the patient should be carefully examined for evidence of trichiniasis (Chapter 21), onchocerciasis, dracunculosis and filariasis (Chapter 20) and strongyloidiasis (Chapter 21).

Treatment is aimed at removing any recognized cause but it should be remembered that a dermatosis as common as urticaria may exist coincidentally with some parasitosis without there necessarily being an aetiological connection.

A single daily tablet of astemizole (a non-sedating antihistamine) will usually be sufficient to suppress the symptoms.

DERMATOSES CHIEFLY LIMITED TO THE TROPICS

Residents of countries in or adjacent to the tropics not only develop the diseases that are found uniformly throughout the world but are also liable to acquire other conditions usually infective, the causative organisms of which can only exist in warmer or moister zones. Such diseases may be bacterial (e.g. anthrax, Buruli ulcer, leprosy and yaws), superficial and deep fungus infections (e.g. blastomycosis, paracoccidioidomycosis and rhinosporidiosis) or parasitic (e.g. amoebiasis, dracunculosis, filariasis, leishmaniasis, onchocerciasis, schistosomiasis). They are all discussed in their appropriate chapters.

There are, however, a number of other dermatoses, not of infective origin, whose incidence is much higher in the tropics; some of the more frequently occurring are discussed below.

ARSENISM

In the first half of the twentieth century the medical profession gradually and apparently somewhat reluctantly abandoned the habit of prescribing arsenic but there remain a number of other ways in which individuals may be poisoned by arsenic.

In some countries such as Argentina and the USA certain rivers are known to contain a higher than usual amount of arsenic and in several parts of the world communities living in the neighbourhood of tin mines have been poisoned by arsenic seeping into nearby wells to give a concentration of more than 0.1 mg/litre, the level which is usually considered dangerous. Another source, recognized in Iran, was the contamination of wells by a leaking drainpipe which led from the local public baths in which bathers had used an arsenical paste as a depilatory during bathing. In Thailand and Malaysia capsules containing up to 25% of arsenious trioxide have been sold in rural communities as an all-purpose tonic.

Dermatological manifestations due to arsenic are always slow to appear—acute arsenical poisoning does not have any time to produce skin lesions. After some years of persistent low grade ingestion changes appear starting with an abnormality of pigmentation particularly affecting the trunk; there is a diffuse hyperpigmentation of a rather slaty-grey colour scattered throughout

which are small areas of normal skin which have in the past been described as 'raindrop hypopigmentation' (Fig. 65.11). This is often the only manifestation of chronic arsenical poisoning but

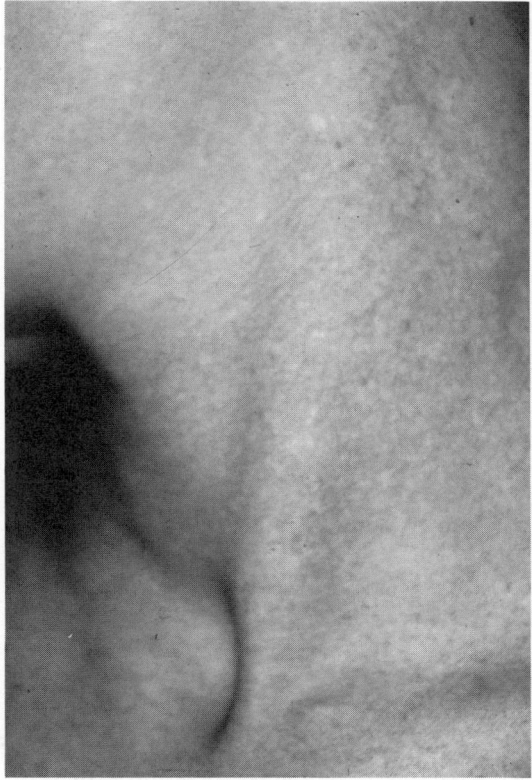

Fig. 65.11 Arsenism. Speckled reddish-brown macules on the neck of a Malay youth taking a folk remedy for leprosy which contained 23% arsenious trioxide.

sometimes, usually a few years later (small hard callus-like keratoses appear, particularly on the palms and soles (Fig. 65.12). These protrude from the surface and so do not particularly resemble plantar warts but may be mistaken for verruca vulgaris, although usually they are more numerous. Patients seek treatment if walking is painful but the recognized therapies for warts or actinic keratoses do not usually succeed and patients often resort to the use of pumice stone or a similar dermabrasive.

Despite a reputation to the contrary arsenical keratoses rarely, if ever, turn malignant but the concomitant development of skin malignancies

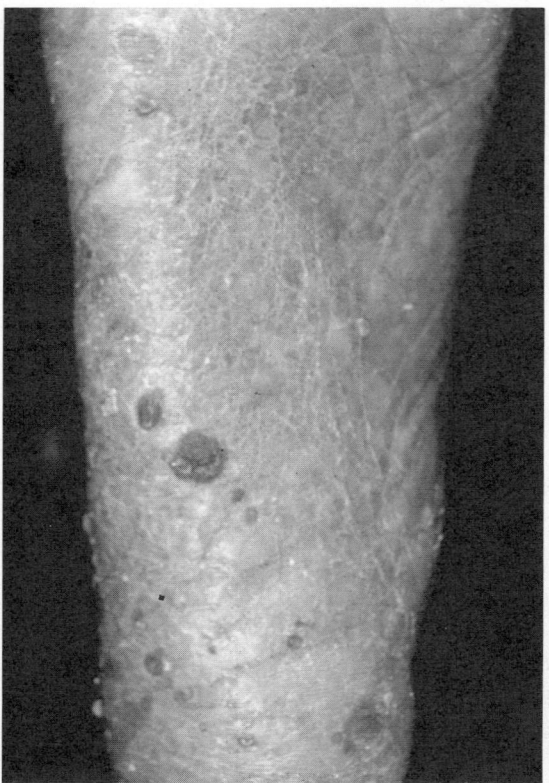

Fig. 65.12 Arsenism. Same patient as Fig. 65.11: multiple dark warty keratoses on soles, also present on the palms.

(especially Bowen's disease) is not uncommon.[14] Bowen's disease is a form of intraepidermal premalignancy looking somewhat like a patch of psoriasis; it often occurs in association with internal malignancies, particularly of the lungs and the stomach. As it is known that chronic arsenism is frequently associated with such neoplasms it is not clear whether the bowenoid lesions are a direct result of arsenical poisoning or a manifestation of an arsenically caused internal malignancy. All patients should be regularly examined for evidence of neoplasia and any recognized lesion must be treated in the normal way. At the same time tests should be made to ensure that the water supply is safe. It is wise to remind communities whose water is contaminated that boiling it does not make it safe.

BRAZILIAN PEMPHIGUS FOLIACEUS

The group of bullous eruptions which jointly share the name of pemphigus are autoimmune diseases characterized by histological presence of acantholysis in which disruption of intercellular bridges permits separation of epidermal cells. Consequent development of intraepidermal bullae develop, the type of pemphigus being determined by the site of the blister. If the intercellular split is low down in the epidermis or just above the basal layer the disease is called pemphigus vulgaris, while if it is higher (at or near the granular layer) the diagnosis of pemphigus erythematosus or pemphigus foliaceus is made. In these cases the blister roof will be more easily rubbed off and the patients will have less intact bullae and more erosions. These pemphigus diseases occur worldwide and, until recent improvements in therapy, were usually fatal. All these diseases occur in middle or later life and their aetiology is not known.

A strange variant of pemphigus is apparently limited to certain areas in Brazil (particularly the state of Goiás). This is in many ways indistinguishable from true pemphigus foliaceus but there are some features that are startlingly different. Almost half the cases start before the age of 21 and in many there is a family history. Clinically, however, the appearance is much the same, the eruption usually starting on the face and scalp and then spreading to the presternal regions as a scaly crusted redness in which only a few intact bullae are visible at any one time. The condition may persist for years but sometimes resolves spontaneously. In most cases the skin is increasingly involved by a scaly oozing erythema, the scalp hair becomes matted and this is followed by a widespread diffuse alopecia, while a combination of blistering and papillomatous lesions may affect the flexures.[15, 16]

It is not unusual for the bullae to be particularly sited around the edges of the erythematous patches. The disease is often complicated by bacterial superinfection and sometimes a viral contamination will cause a widespread varicelliform eruption of the type originally described by Kaposi (p. 1059).

Treatment

Whether the Brazilian disease is the same as ordinary pemphigus foliaceus remains uncertain but usually the same treatment is successful. Initial high doses of oral corticosteroids (up to 250 mg of prednisolone daily) rapidly suppress the appearance of new bullae and the dosage can quickly be reduced until further bullae erupt. The addition of small doses of methotrexate or azathioprine may permit the further reduction of steroids until only one or two 5 mg tablets are necessary each day. Quinacrine 0.3–0.6 g daily or dapsone 100 mg daily are also useful as supplementary medications.

As many cases of Brazilian pemphigus foliaceus suffer from pulmonary tuberculosis it may be necessary to avoid the use of steroids until the tuberculosis is under control; in this case quinacrine and dapsone may be particularly helpful.

LICHEN AMYLOIDOSUS

The systemic forms of amyloidosis whether primary or secondary occur rarely but widely throughout the world. Primary systemic amyloidosis usually shows cutaneous, subcutaneous and systemic masses of amyloid deposited widely to produce cutaneous plaques, alopecia, macroglossia, etc. Sometimes found in a family distribution, other cases are associated with plasma cell myeloma but in most patients there is no recognizable cause. Secondary systemic disease which rarely, if ever, involves the skin is usually the manifestation of some underlying chronic disease such as ulcerative colitis, tuberculosis or erythema nodosum leprosum (Chapter 40).

A third form of amyloidosis is localized to the skin and is called lichen amyloidosus. This has a worldwide distribution but is seen much more commonly in Asia, being particularly frequent in Indonesia, Malaysia and south India. It is not associated with the forms of systemic disease mentioned above. Starting as a pruritus of the shins it occurs less commonly on the arms and rarely on the trunk. The area slowing becomes hyperpigmented and rows of small maculopapules appear which gradually get darker, more raised and dome-shaped and finally appear somewhat like the ripples seen on a sandy shore at the sea's edge (Fig. 65.13). Histologically amyloid can be found deposited in the dermal papillae.

In severe cases the papular lichenoid eruption of the shins is associated with a macular hyperpigmentation on the back of the shoulders and between the scapulae but, although this discoloration is often quite extensive, it rarely changes into the dome-shaped papules that are

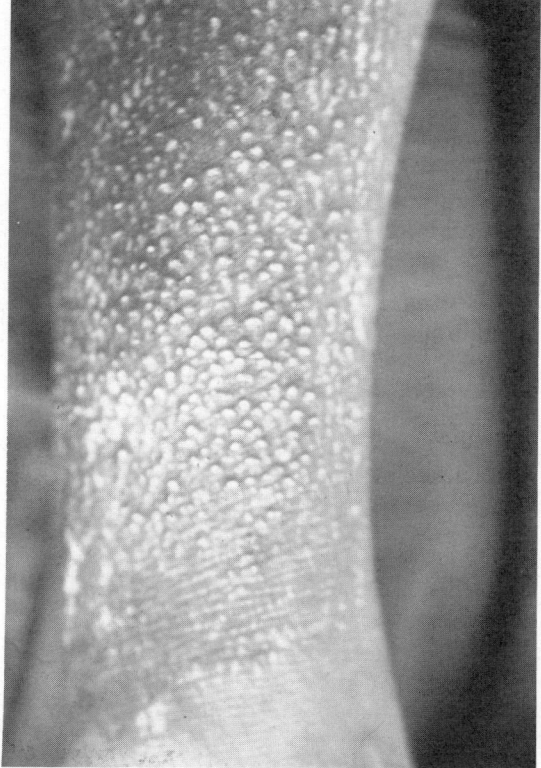

Fig. 65.13 Lichen amyloidosus. Extensive involvement of the shins by warty papules—very pruritic.

diagnostic on the shins. The macular amyloidosis is usually not pruritic.

Treatment

Patients are often more distressed by the itching than the appearance and local use of corticosteroid ointment (applied once a day and occluded by a plastic sheet) will often help the pruritus but prolonged use of this or of intralesional corticosteroid injections lead to atrophy of the skin and an increasingly unpleasant mottled appearance of the shins.

Triamcinolone A intramuscularly every six weeks often markedly diminishes the itching but produces relatively little change in appearance. Patients with only mild pruritus sometimes respond to one of the more sedative antihistamines: chlorpheniramine maleate in the daytime or promethazine hydrochloride at night.

Retinoic acid cream or lotion (0.05%) applied locally may soften the keratotic papules.

LICHEN PLANUS AND LICHENOID ERUPTIONS

Lichen planus is a relatively uncommon disease, the typical lesions being flat-topped, shiny, pruritic papules which often in Caucasians have a violaceous colouring. Although seen most frequently on the fronts of the wrists they can also be found scattered across the body, on the genitalia and even on the buccal mucosa where the condition takes the form of bluish-white streaks inside the cheeks or on the tongue or palate. Histology shows the epidermis to have a thickening of the granular and keratin layers as well as liquefaction degeneration of the basal layer, while a heavy infiltrate of T lymphocytes is present in the upper part of the dermis.

During the Second World War Caucasians fighting in the tropics not infrequently developed a papular pruritic eruption which was called 'tropical lichen planus'. As time went on it was realized that this was a drug eruption following the use of mepacrine (Atabrine) as an antimalarial. Routine treatment was changed to chloroquine; this drug did not produce a skin reaction and tropical lichen planus disappeared.

Hypertrophic lichen planus

Although lichen planus occasionally shows hypertrophic lesions, inhabitants of southern India and Sri Lanka often develop an eruption in which hypertrophic lesions are the only ones seen. Most common around the lower leg and the ankle, thick warty deeply pigmented and highly pruritic nodules may last for years (Fig. 65.14). Frequent intralesional injections of corticosteroids are liable to cause atrophy of the skin and it is better to give intramuscular injections of triamcinolone acetonide once every four to six weeks or ACTH 40 units weekly for six to eight weeks. Some workers have recently claimed that griseofulvin 500 mg twice daily for three months is effective but this should be tried only as a last resort.

Actinic lichen planus

This condition has sometimes, rather confusingly, been called 'lichen planus tropicus' but the name 'actinic lichen planus' is preferred for this peculiar lichenoid eruption[17] which occurs particularly on the face and forehead and is probably due to excess exposure to the sun. Itching, mildly

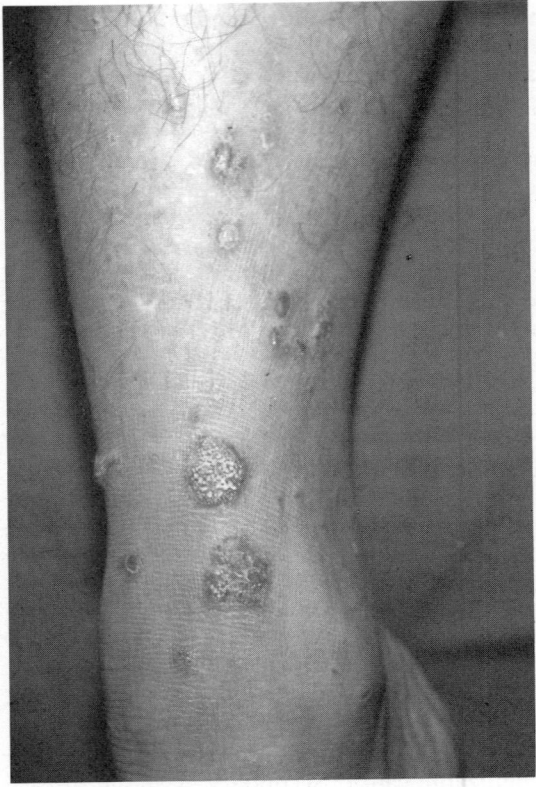

Fig. 65.14 Lichen planus (hypertrophic). Numerous dark warty patches on shins of a patient with ordinary lichen planus in the mouth.

hyperpigmented papules gradually extend and take on an annular appearance with a central depression; as they enlarge they may coalesce.

It seems to occur particularly along the north coast of Africa, in Egypt and the Near East. It is highly pruritic and takes two to three years to go away responding slowly, if at all, to the usual therapies given for lichen planus.

A slightly different condition described from Kenya as lichenoid melanodermatitis seems much the same as other forms of actinic lichen planus but it apparently runs a quicker and less pruritic course.[18]

PIGMENTARY PROBLEMS

Vitiligo

It is not known why so many people develop this cosmetically disquieting abnormality in which areas of skin in any part of the body suddenly lose all their colour and become not simply hypopigmented but totally achromic (Plate VIII.6); if it occurs on the scalp, hairs in the affected area usually lose their pigment. The darker skinned races are more particularly alarmed by this condition especially if it appears on the face or other uncovered areas of the body, and seem to seek attention more frequently than Caucasians. Whether this is because the disease is cosmetically less acceptable in pigmented peoples or whether such communities have a higher incidence of vitiligo is not certain. Patients, dreading the possibility of vitiligo, often consult their doctors urgently for hypopigmented lesions such as pityriasis alba, pityriasis versicolor or the early stages of leprosy.

Treatment

It is very difficult to know what advice to give to dark-skinned patients who have vitiligo. A few fortunates find the condition gets better, particularly if it has only been present for a few weeks, but the longer the condition lasts the less likelihood there will be of satisfactory treatment. Repigmentation appears initially around hair follicles and patients are frequently cheered by the appearance of these dark dots on the skin of the shins or trunk. Unfortunately, the repigmentation only rarely extends fully across the lesions and, after a year or so of expensive treatment, vitiligo often remains visible. It must be realized that pigmentation returning as it does from the depths of the hair follicles will not occur on the lips, areola, glans penis, palms or soles and patients must never be allowed to believe that colour will return to these sites.

It is necessary, therefore, to tell patients that treatment is successful in 25% of cases at most but many are so distressed by the condition that they press for treatment even if little success is anticipated. It is unfair to allow patients to pay large sums of money for medications whose success is not guaranteed and therapy should not be continued for more than three months, unless greater than usual success is being obtained.

Various psoralens are the most frequently prescribed medications sensitizing the skin to sunlight and, theoretically, encouraging the achromic areas to repigment. It is usually suggested that two 10 mg tablets of ammoidin or two 10 mg capsules of methoxsalen should be taken 2 hours before exposure to natural sunlight; the treatment known as PUVA is a combination of psoralens and carefully graded doses of UVA light. It should be remembered that vitiliginous patches which were previously heavily pigmented will be exceedingly susceptible to the side-effects of these treatments (elastosis, increased risk of 'non-fatal' cancer) and the long-term use of PUVA therapy is unwise unless it is producing dramatic results.

In some of the more sophisticated parts of the world it is possible to obtain various waterproof camouflaging preparations; Covermark, Dermocover and Keromask are proprietary products which all have various shades of masking and toning creams and finishing powders which can in experienced hands be very effective in covering areas of discoloration and so alleviating the patient's embarrassment. Where these preparations are not obtainable potassium permanganate 0.1% or even walnut juice may be used to mask the patches. In any case all patients should be advised to cover the achromic areas with a sun-barrier preparation as it is not unknown for actinic keratoses or lupus erythematosus to develop in these unprotected areas.

Melasma

The appearance of a brownish-black macular pigmentation over the cheek bones, the nose, the upper lip and the forehead has for many years been attributed to the combination of multiple pregnancies and exposure to the sun, the disease attaining its highest incidence in the Middle East, North Africa, India and Central America. In the past the condition was called 'chloasma uterinum' but, as it is now realized that it may also be due to a combination of sunlight and the prolonged use of oral contraceptive pills, it is better known as 'melasma'.

Mono-benzyl ether of hydroquinone is available in various strengths from 2 to 10% and when applied to the pigmented areas will slowly lighten the skin; a similarly effective application is of para-methyloxyphenol 10% in a water-soluble base. The best prophylaxis is for the patient or her partner to use a non-hormonal form of contraception.

PHRYNODERMA

In 1933 two papers were published associating the appearance of dome-shaped follicular hyperkeratotic papules with deficiency of vitamin A. At that time numerous associated symptoms were described including severe or fatal diarrhoea, peripheral neuritis and extensive oedema. It is now realized that these patients had multiple dietary deficiencies, the condition being most frequently found in severely malnourished prisoners or indentured labourers. This symptom complex is nowadays rarely seen except under famine conditions.

The skin lesions now known as phrynoderma (toad-skin) continue unabated in children and adolescents, being rare over the age of 18. Scattered raised papules with a hyperkeratotic punctum are grouped in areas 5–6 cm in diameter most often over the knees and elbows and often having a clearly visible hypopigmented background (Fig. 65.15).

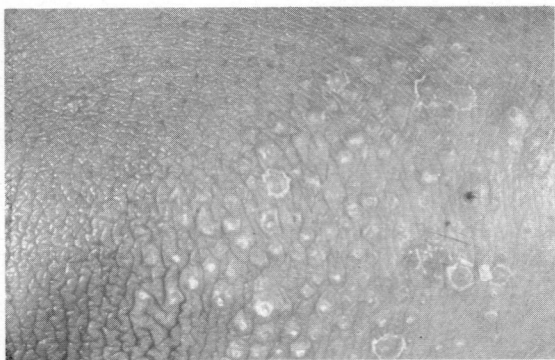

Fig. 65.15 Phrynoderma. Grouped dome-shaped papules with a central follicular hyperkeratosis.

Treatment

Despite occasional claims to the contrary vitamin supplements do not have much effect on this condition which responds best to emollient soap and various keratolytic creams. Retinoic acid 0.05% is often quite helpful, while if younger children (6–10 years old) find this to be too irritating, it may be advisable to mix the retinoic acid cream with an equal amount of hydrocortisone ointment.

The condition rarely, if ever, persists into adult life and should be thought of as a follicular disorder of keratin formation and not as a vitamin deficiency.[19]

REFERENCES

1   Pettit, J.H.S. (1983) *Manual of Practical Dermatology.* Edinburgh: Churchill Livingstone and E.L.B.S. edn, 1985.
2   Pettit, J.H.S. & Parish, L.C. (1984) *Manual of Tropical Dermatology.* New York: Springer Verlag.
3   Hall-Smith, P. & Cairns, R.J. (1981) *Dermatology.* London: Butterworth.
4   Rook, A., Wilkinson, D.S., Ebling, F.J.G. et al (1986) *Textbook of Dermatology*, 4th edn. Oxford: Blackwell Scientific Publications.
5   Dillon, H.C., Jr (1979) *Rev. infect. Dis.* **1**, 935.
6   Dillon, H.C., Jr (1981) *Int. J. Derm.* **20**, 396.
7   Dillon, H.C., Jr (1980) *Int. J. Derm.* **19**, 443.
8   Cronin, E. (1981) *Contact Dermatitis.* New York: Churchill Livingstone.
9   American Academy of Dermatology (1984) *Patch-testing in Allergic Contact Dermatitis*, 7th edn. AAD, Evanston, Ill.
10   Jaffe, H.W., Choi, K., Thomas, P.A. et al (1983) *Ann. intern. Med.* **99**, 145.
11   Bhutani, L.K. & Kumar, A.S. (1981) *Int. J. Derm.* **20**, 380.
12   Green, A. (1984) *Aust. J. Derm.* **25**, 99.
13   Warin, R.P. & Smith, R.J. (1975) *Br. J. Derm.* **93** (supplement II), 19.
14   Reymann, F., Moller, R. & Nielson, A. (1978) *Archs Derm.* **114**, 378.
15   Azulay, R.D. (1982) *Int. J. Derm.* **21**, 122.
16   Beutner, E.H., Prigenzi, L.S., Hale, E.W. et al (1968) *Proc. Soc. exp. Biol. Med.* **127**, 81.
17   Zanca, A. & Zanca, A. (1978) *Int. J. Derm.* **17**, 506.
18   Verhagen, A.R.H.B. & Koten, J.W. (1979) *Br. J. Derm.* **101**, 651.
19   Pettit, J.H.S. (1983) *Int. J. Derm.* **22**, 117.

Chapter 66
Metabolic Diseases

G. V. Gill

DIABETES MELLITUS

General considerations

Diabetes mellitus can be loosely defined as a state of chronic hyperglycaemia. It is important because:

1 it is common;
2 it is incurable;
3 treatment is difficult;
4 serious acute and chronic complications occur;
5 these complications reduce the quality and duration of life.

A modern classification of diabetes is shown in Table 66.1. 'Malnutrition-related' diabetes is naturally of great tropical interest and will be discussed later. All over the world, however, the commonest types of diabetes are simple insulin-dependent (IDDM, type 1) and non-insulin-dependent (NIDDM, type 2) disease. Type 2 diabetics outnumber their type 1 counterparts by 3 or 4 to 1.

Table 66.1 Classification of diabetes mellitus (World Health Organization Expert Committee[2]).

1 Insulin-dependent diabetes mellitus (IDDM, type 1)
2 Non-insulin-dependent diabetes mellitus (NIDDM, type 2)
  (a) obese
  (b) non-obese
3 Malnutrition-related diabetes mellitus (MRDM, type 3)
4 Secondary diabetes mellitus
  (a) pancreatic disease
  (b) endocrine disorders
  (c) receptor abnormalities
  (d) drug-induced
  (e) genetic syndromes
5 Gestational diabetes mellitus
6 Impaired glucose tolerance (IGT)

The aetiology of both types of diabetes remains largely obscure. Genetic susceptibility is important, and in type 1 diabetes a 'trigger-factor' such as autoimmunity or viral infection is thought to precipitate pancreatic beta cell loss.[1] The pathogenesis of type 2 diabetes is more difficult to understand. The deficiency of insulin is only relative (indeed, many obese patients are actually hyperinsulinaemic) and peripheral resistance to insulin action is important.

Diagnosis

Symptoms of diabetes are usually obvious, and the blood glucose (BG) level unequivocally raised. There will always be borderline cases, however, and Table 66.2 shows present diagnostic criteria. Note the difference between capillary and venous blood, particularly at higher BG levels. Laboratories should always report which specimen has been analysed, or important diagnostic mistakes will be made. The glucose tolerance test (GTT) should be rarely needed (see Table 66.2 for further details). If it is done, a normal response is for both fasting and 2-hour levels to be < 6.7 mmol/litre. Two-hour levels of 6.7–10.0 (capillary) or 6.7–11.1 (venous) mmol/litre are not diagnostic of diabetes, but they denote 'impaired glucose tolerance' (IGT). The

Table 66.2 Diagnostic criteria for diabetes (World Health Organization Expert Committee[2]).

	Capillary blood	Venous blood
Fasting blood glucose (mmol/litre)	> 6.7	> 6.7
Random blood glucose (mmol/litre)	> 10.0	> 11.1

1 Asymptomatic patients should have at least two abnormal values before final diagnosis.
2 The glucose tolerance test (GTT) is needed only for rare borderline cases, or to confirm renal glycosuria. A 75 g glucose load is used, and only 0- and 2-hour blood glucose levels are measured. The cut-off values are the same as for fasting and random levels respectively.
3 A 2-hour level on a GTT of 6.7–10.0 (capillary) or 6.7–11.1 (venous) mmol/litre denotes 'impaired glucose tolerance' (IGT).

significance of this state is that it carries a greatly increased risk for the development of diabetes later in life; and it is also an independent 'risk factor' for atherosclerosis.[2]

Prevalence

About 1.5% of Western populations have diabetes, but prevalence appears lower in tropical countries (Table 66.3).[3–8] This may be due to under-reporting or under-diagnosis. Certainly many quoted prevalence surveys are rather dated, and used crude diagnostic tests (e.g. urinary glucose). Even modern and well-constructed surveys are difficult to carry out in developing countries where populations are frequently mobile and always unnumbered. Nevertheless, reports from Africa continue to suggest a genuinely low overall prevalence, in the order of 0.1–0.2%.[9] There are also suggestions that diabetes is more common in urban compared with rural environments,[7,10] and that it is also very rare in the first decade of life.[9,11–13]

Table 66.3   Some studies of diabetes prevalence in Africa.

Location	Prevalence	Reference
Ghana	0.6%	Dodu[3]
Lesotho	0.2%	Politzer and Schneider[4]
Zimbabwe	0.1%	Carr and Gelfland[5]
Malawi	0.1%	Davidson[6]
Uganda	0.2%	Tulloch[7]
Nigeria	0.3%	Osuntokun et al[8]

The differences between urban and rural tropical areas; and between Western and developing countries, may reflect dietary patterns.[4] A further possibility is that it is due to the relative frequency of breastfeeding in these respective environments,[14] as there is evidence that the rate of breastfeeding is inversely related to diabetes prevalence.[15]

It must be recognized that there are considerable variations in diabetes prevalence throughout tropical countries. For example, diabetes is very frequently seen in the Asian subcontinent,[16] and it is exceedingly common amongst Asian immigrants, both in tropical[10] and non-tropical[17] countries, where rates of 5–10% or more are not uncommon.

Tropical diabetes

In 1955, a report from Jamaica suggested that some tropical diabetics could not be easily subdivided into the usual type 1 and type 2 categories.[18] These patients were young, lean, and insulin-resistant; but they were not ketosis-prone, and indeed could survive without insulin in many cases. 'J-type' diabetes, as it came to be known, was subsequently reported from wide areas of the tropical world (see Abu-Bakare et al[19] for an exhaustive review of this and other aspects of tropical diabetes). Some years later, the situation was complicated by a report from Zuidema in Indonesia[20] who described 'tropical pancreatic diabetes', or as it has widely become known—'Z-type' diabetes. As the name suggests, diabetes here is due to pancreatic fibrosis and/or calcification, and exocrine function of the gland is also disturbed. Although many cases of pancreatic diabetes in the developing world are alcoholic in origin, true Z-type diabetes is not. Like J-type diabetes it has also been widely reported from various tropical countries.[19]

The growth of interest in tropical diabetes has been reflected by a confusing growth in the terms used to describe it (Table 66.4)! Malnutrition in the past is widely felt to be important aetiologically, and the latest World Health Organization Expert Committee Report on Diabetes[2] has accepted this concept (Table 66.1). This may be a little premature, however, as the association is by no means proved. For the present, 'tropical diabetes' may be the best overall descriptive term.

Table 66.4   The confusing nomenclature of tropical diabetes.

J-type diabetes
Z-type diabetes
K-type diabetes
M-type diabetes
Type 3 diabetes
Malnutrition-related diabetes mellitus (MRDM)
Tropical pancreatic diabetes
Third syndrome
Phasic insulin-dependence (PID)
Protein-deficient pancreatic diabetes
Juvenile tropical pancreatitis
Fibrocalculous pancreatic diabetes
Pancreatic fibrosis and calcification (PFC) syndrome
Ketosis-resistant diabetes of the young

A further problem is that much of the literature on the subject is uncritical and anecdotal. Thus a later follow-up of the original cohort of patients with J-type diabetes,[18] revealed that many had become controllable on oral agents.[21]

At least some J-type diabetics may thus be young type 2 patients, and this may explain reports of 'phasic insulin-dependence'.[22]

Despite these considerations, the J and Z types of tropical diabetes have been widely recognized, and their similar and dissimilar features are outlined in Table 66.5. The important characteristic of Z-type diabetes is its association with areas where cassava is the staple food[23] (Fig. 66.1). Cassava contains small amounts of cyanide, and in the presence of malnutrition, this can accumulate and cause pancreatic damage.[24] The cassava hypothesis is an attractive answer to the puzzle of tropical diabetes, though a number of questions still remain and the subject will hopefully excite further vigorous research.

Table 66.5 The major syndromes of tropical diabetes.

	'J-type' diabetes	'Z-type' diabetes
Similarities		
Age at onset	young	young
Socioeconomic status	poor	poor
Sex	M > F	M > F
Weight	lean	lean
Malnutrition (past or present)	common	common
Ketosis	rare	rare
Insulin requirements	often high	often high
Endogenous insulin secretion	present	present
Differences		
Cassava consumption	rare	common
Abdominal pain	rare	common
Steatorrhoea	rare	common
Pancreatic calcification	rare	common

Management of diabetes

One of the aims of modern diabetic care is good blood glucose control. This is because it is now widely believed that glycaemic control is closely related to the risk of complications, particularly the microvascular problems of retinopathy and nephropathy. Both prospective,[25] retrospective[26] and interventional[27,28] studies support this hypothesis, though *absolute* proof is lacking.

In general terms, the treatment of type 1 diabetes can be considered to be primarily insulin, with diet of secondary importance. In type 2 diabetes, however, diet is of *prime* importance, with drugs taking a secondary role. Type 2 disease can be therapeutically divided into 'obese' and 'non-obese', and it can be seen from Table 66.6 that both the diets and drugs used are

Table 66.6 Simple management of type 2 diabetes.

	Obese type 2 diabetes	Non-obese type 2 diabetes
Primary treatment	Weight-reducing sugar-free diet	Sugar-free diet
Secondary treatment	Metformin	Sulphonylureas

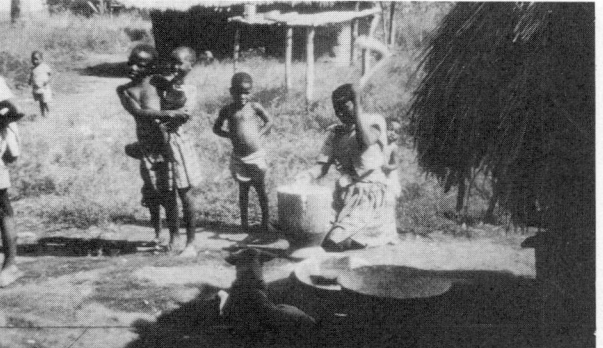
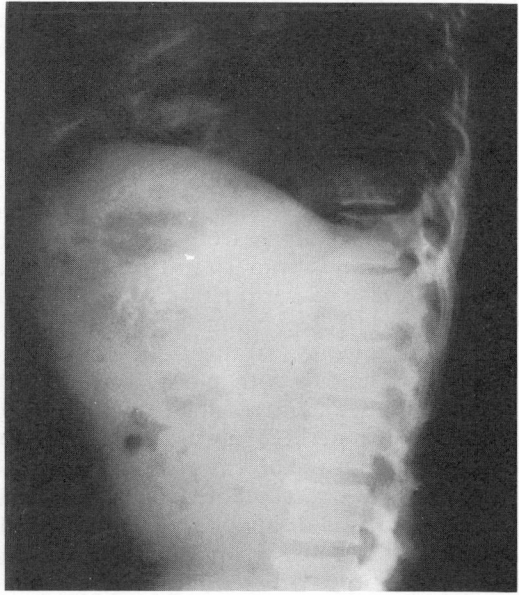

Fig. 66.1 The cassava hypothesis for the aetiology of tropical pancreatic ('Z-type') diabetes. On the left a rural Ugandan mother is beating dried cassava, which is their staple food. In malnourished people, long-term cassava ingestion can lead to cyanide accumulation which may cause pancreatic fibrosis and calcification (see lateral abdominal X-ray on right), with diabetes and steatorrhoea.

different. These will be discussed in more detail below.

Dietary treatment

A major problem in tropical countries is the lack of dieticians, and even of dietetic information (e.g. carbohydrate and calorie content) on local foodstuffs. However, for type 2 diabetics at least, simple diets can be prescribed by doctors, as suggested in Table 66.6. The non-obese patient should simply be advised to eat fairly regularly and to avoid all foods containing sugar. The obese patient should receive similar advice regarding sugar, but should also be told to reduce his usual helpings of staple carbohydrate food (e.g. rice, potato, tapioca, porridge, etc.) by a half, a quarter, etc., depending on the size of the patient and the urgency of the situation!

Dietary advice for the patient on insulin is harder, as ideally a gram-controlled carbohydrate diet with a system of exchanges is needed. As a compromise, patients can be instructed to *always* take regular meals and preferably snacks, to avoid sugar-containing foods, and to keep the amount of carbohydrate food at each meal and snack approximately equal.

Fortunately, the tropical diet is naturally high in fibre and low in fat, and this is now widely believed to be beneficial to diabetic control.[29]

Drug treatment

Oral hypoglycaemic agents (OHAs) are reserved for diet-failures. Obese type 2 diabetics who have failed to respond, or only partially responded to adequate dietary advice, may be given metformin (Glucophage). This is a biguanide drug whose main action is to suppress appetite and increase glucose uptake by peripheral tissues. The major side-effect is nausea, vomiting and/or diarrhoea; but the frequency of these problems can be reduced by starting with a low dose (e.g. 500 mg twice a day) before increasing to maximum doses of 850–1000 mg three times a day. The other biguanide drug phenformin should be avoided because of its unacceptable risk of lactic acidosis;[30] indeed it is disappointing to see this drug still available in many tropical countries. Lactic acidosis can occur with metformin, but it is much less common, and virtually always occurs only in the presence of hepatic or renal dysfunction. Metformin must therefore not be used in patients such as this.

Sulphonylureas are used for non-obese type 2 patients who are imperfectly controlled on diet alone. They work mainly by stimulating endogenous pancreatic insulin release. Many preparations exist, but the most popular are chlorpropamide (Diabinese), tolbutamide (Rastinon) and glibenclamide (Euglucon). Because of its low cost, widespread availability and once daily dosage, chlorpropamide is the most popular sulphonylurea in tropical countries. In Europe, however, it has fallen from favour because its very long duration of action can lead to severe hypoglycaemia. However, provided sensible precautions are taken (see Table 66.11) the drug can still be successfully used. The dose is 125–375 mg (if the 250 mg strength tablet is used), or 100–400 mg (for the 100 mg tablet)—both once daily. Glibenclamide is shorter-acting, but is quite potent and does have some hypoglycaemic risks, particularly in the elderly or those with renal impairment. Nevertheless, it is probably now the most popular sulphonylurea in the Western world, though its cost excludes wider tropical use. The dose of glibenclamide is 2.5–15 mg daily, with larger doses preferably given divided with meals. Tolbutamide is a generally underused drug, as it is cheap, safe and effective. Unfortunately the dose is a rather awkward 500–1000 mg two or three times a day.

Insulin treatment

Traditional beef insulins are now giving way to pork and human varieties which are purer and more easily manufactured. All insulins should very soon be standardized at U100 (100 units/ml). Purity, species of origin, method of production, and strength, are however relatively unimportant features compared with *duration of action* which is the vital property of any insulin to understand. All insulins can be divided into short-, intermediate- and long-acting (Table 66.7); and though there is considerable individual variation in response, this categorization allows sensible insulin regimens to be constructed. A variety of insulin 'mixtures' are also now available (Table 66.7); for example, Mixtard which is 30% short- and 70% intermediate-acting insulin. The present long and confusing list of available insulins is likely to become shorter and simpler in the not too distant future, when human insulins only will be available. There are no particular therapeutic advan-

Table 66.7 Insulins classified by duration of action (note the lists are not exhaustive).

Short-acting	Intermediate-acting	Long-acting	Mixtures
Soluble	Lente	PZI	Mixtard
Neusulin	Isophane	Ultralente	Initard
Actrapid	Monotard	Ultratard	Actraphane
Velosulin	Insulatard		
Humulin S	Humulin I		
	Neuphane		
	Protaphane		

tages with human insulin,[31] but its production by genetic engineering methods is becoming cheaper and easier than older extraction and semisynthetic methods.

The major insulin regimens in use at present are as follows.

1 *Twice daily short- and intermediate-acting insulin* remains the standard method, in which a mixed injection of e.g. Soluble and Isophane insulin, Actrapid and Monotard, etc. is given before breakfast and evening meal.

2 *Twice daily insulin mixtures*, of which Mixtard is the most popular. Although a little inflexible, this method removes the potential inaccuracies associated with mixed insulin injections, and studies suggest that the control achieved with twice daily Mixtard is just as good.[32]

3 *Once daily insulin* must be generally regarded as suboptimal. Some older-onset insulin-requiring patients can achieve reasonable control on such a regimen, but those who have no endogenous insulin never do so. When used, an insulin such as Lente or Monotard is to be given each morning, preferably with a small amount of Soluble insulin or Actrapid.

4 *'Intensified' insulin regimens* can be used when optimal blood glucose control is needed, and also particularly when overnight control is a problem. In its simplest form, the evening short/intermediate mixed injection is split so that the short-acting insulin is given with the evening meal, and the intermediate-acting at bedtime.[33] More elaborate methods involve short-acting insulins with each of the three meals, and intermediate- or long-acting insulins in the evening. Injection 'pens' have been devised to make such regimens easier,[34] and these seem likely to grow in popularity. They are certainly cheaper and easier to use than insulin infusion pumps, which after an initial surge of interest, are now declining in popularity.[35]

Application of the above principles in the tropics is frequently made difficult by precarious supplies of insulins—which are often of inappropriate and outdated types. Thus, Lester[36] reported that 40% of type 1 diabetics in Addis Ababa had major control problems due to erratic insulin supply. Even when supplies are good, diabetics in developing countries may be consigned to once daily regimens for 'social' or 'cultural' reasons. Thus, of 66 young type 1 patients in Soweto, South Africa, complications were found to be frequent (33%) and glycaemic control poor (mean glycosylated haemoglobin 10.5%), yet 44% were on non-ideal regimens of treatment.[37]. There is little excuse for not treating the majority of tropical type 1 diabetics with twice daily insulin. It is readily accepted, and gives improved control usually on lower total daily doses of insulin. There is also a smaller hypoglycaemic risk than with large single daily doses. Even if twice daily intermediate insulin only (e.g. Isophane, Monotard) can be regularly provided, the results will be good.

A final practical note concerns insulin bottles and syringes. Though insulin is ideally stored in a refrigerator, failure to do so in the tropics is not of great practical importance. Glass non-disposable syringes are clumsy, inaccurate, difficult to use and prone to breakage. Reused plastic disposable syringes are cheaper, easier and safer; and their use should be widely encouraged.[38]

Monitoring diabetic control

If blood glucose levels are to be as good as possible, reliable indicators of control are needed. Because BG levels fluctuate considerably, and clinic attendances are relatively infrequent; control parameters both *at home* and *at clinic* are used (Table 66.8).

Self monitoring is traditionally by urine testing, but though this is of use in non-insulin-treated patients, it is now widely accepted that home blood glucose monitoring is required for

Table 66.8 Assessing diabetic control.

At home	1	Urine glucose testing
	2	Blood glucose testing
At clinic	1	Blood glucose
	2	Glycosylated haemoglobin

diabetics on insulin. Though portable blood glucose meters are available, simple visually read strips such as BM-Test 1/44 (Boehringer) are sufficient. These can be introduced successfully to type 1 diabetics in developing countries,[39] and with care their cost may be comparable to urine testing (for example, by cutting the strips in half, by limiting their frequency of use, and by omitting urine testing).

In clinic, the random BG level may be of some use in type 2 patients, but it is of almost no value in assessing the control of type 1 diabetics. The glycosylated haemoglobin (HbA_1) has been a major recent advance in solving this problem, and it is now regarded as the 'gold standard' control parameter for all types of diabetics.[40] The HbA_1 reflects *mean* blood glucose over the preceding two to three months. Its usual normal range of 5.0–8.0% is particularly useful as it is almost identical to that of random BG levels. Thus, the HbA_1 tells the clinician approximately what the mean BG has recently been, by converting % of HbA_1 directly to mmol/litre of BG. Unfortunately, HbA_1 is not an easy biochemical assay, neither is it cheap. Nevertheless, its value is established and it will undoubtedly become more widely used worldwide in the future. In the absence of this test, the best policy for assessing control is:

1 use sensible and well-taught methods of home urine testing or (if possible) blood glucose monitoring;

2 check fasting (preferably) or random BG at clinic visits for type 2 diabetics;

3 bring type 1 diabetics to hospital as 'day cases' occasionally to measure BG levels three or four times throughout the day, on their usual insulin treatment.

Diabetes education

Of all the strategies of diabetes management, education is probably the most important. The philosophy of modern diabetes care is to train patients to look after themselves, and this requires a vigorous and structured programme of education. Some methods available are listed in Table 66.9, and these can be adapted to the

Table 66.9 Some methods of diabetes education.

1 'One-to-one' teaching
2 Poster displays
3 Handouts and leaflets
4 Group sessions
5 Tapes and slides
6 Videos

needs and facilities of different areas. They vary from the very expensive and sophisticated (e.g. video tapes) to the very simple and cheap (e.g. the doctor spending a few extra minutes talking to his patient). Fig. 66.2 shows a simple poster display for patients waiting in clinic—the writing is in the local language, but the nurses explain the posters to emphasize important points, and to allow participation by those who cannot read.

There is evidence that education programmes improve diabetic control, and are cost-effective to health services.[41] Because of this, Western countries have introduced the 'Diabetes Sister' as a vital part of diabetes care.[42]. Her specific job is to educate diabetic patients, essentially with a view to caring for themselves (e.g. injection and monitoring techniques, dealing with illness, exercise, etc.). Though such full time staff will be difficult to obtain in most tropical hospitals, it should be possible to allocate one or two nurses

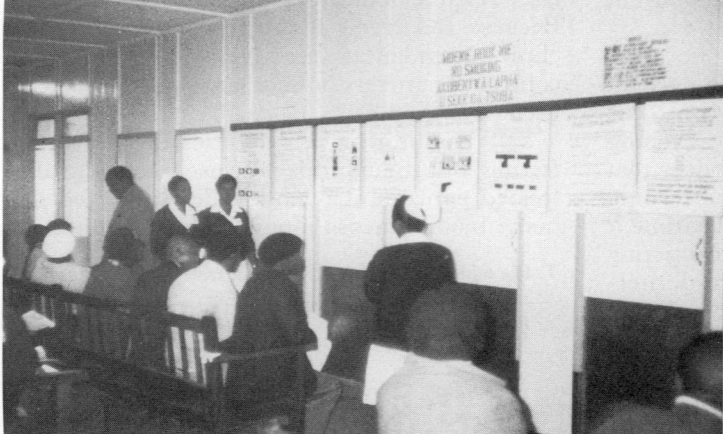

Fig. 66.2 Simple education in progress at the diabetic clinic at Baragwanath Hospital, Soweto, South Africa. While patients wait to see the doctors, the nursing staff explain the principles of diet, drugs, insulin and monitoring. They use illustrated posters in the Zulu language.

to be responsible for this work. These nurses can be taught the necessary skills, and can then attend outpatient clinics, and see diabetics who are admitted to the wards.

Hypoglycaemia

The acute complications of diabetes are essentially hypoglycaemia and diabetic ketoacidosis (DKA). Of the two, hypoglycaemia is by far the most common.[43] Most diabetic hypoglycaemia represents a failure of patient education (e.g. problems of diet, exercise etc.), or of inappropriate insulin regimens, (e.g. excessive doses, once-daily insulin, etc.). Guidelines for management are given in Table 66.10.

Table 66.10   Guidelines for treating hypoglycaemia.

1   If possible give sugary food or drink by mouth.
2   Otherwise give intravenous glucose (e.g. 50 ml of 50% dextrose), repeated if necessary.
3   Glucagon 1 mg intramuscularly may be useful for violent patients in whom intravenous injection is difficult.
4   After recovery give a carbohydrate-rich snack.
5   Hypoglycaemia due to sulphonylureas or alcohol may be severe and prolonged. Admit the patients and give an intravenous 5% or 10% glucose infusion for 24 hours.
6   Very severe hypoglycaemia may require hydrocortisone (100–200 mg) and/or glucagon (1–2 mg) intravenously, repeated 6-hourly if necessary.
7   After treating hypoglycaemia, review the patient's diabetic therapy to prevent recurrences.

A particular problem in the tropics is chlorpropamide-induced hypoglycaemia, as this drug is the most popular sulphonylurea in developing countries (p. 1074). The hypoglycaemia may be profound and prolonged, and deaths and brain damage can and do occur. Shorter-acting sulphonylureas are much less prone to hypoglycaemic problems, but if chlorpropamide is used properly it too is reasonably safe. Table 66.11 outlines simple strategies to prevent chlorpropamide hypoglycaemia. The main faults are

Table 66.11   Avoiding hypoglycaemia with chlorpropamide.

1   As with other sulphonylureas, use only in non-obese type 2 diabetics inadequately controlled on diet alone.
2   Observe maximum doses of 400 mg (for 100 mg tablets), or 375 mg (for 250 mg tablets).
3   Avoid in the elderly, alcoholics, and those with renal dysfunction.
4   Tell patients to maintain food intake at all times. If illness makes this difficult, they must seek medical advice.

the use of the drug in the elderly, prescription of excessive doses, and failure to warn patients never to stop eating regular meals.

Ketoacidosis

Ketoacidosis (DKA) is primarily a problem of type 1 diabetics, who have absolute insulin deficiency. It may be the presenting feature of diabetes, but more commonly it occurs in previously diagnosed patients who develop an intercurrent infection. Hyperosmolar non-ketotic coma (HONK) is less common, and occurs in older type 2 diabetics. Here, endogenous insulin prevents uncontrolled lipolysis and resultant ketogenesis, but is not sufficient to prevent severe hyperglycaemia and dehydration. These two types of acute hyperglycaemic emergencies may be difficult to distinguish clinically, but this can be done with the aid of simple 'bedside biochemistry' (Table 66.12). A visually read blood glucose strip (e.g. BM-Test strip, Boehringer) will rapidly confirm marked hyperglycaemia. Heparinized blood is then taken and tested with Ketostix strips or Ketotest tablets. This result will differentiate between DKA and HONK.

Table 66.12   Bedside diagnosis of diabetic comas.

	Ketoacidosis	Hyperosmolar non-ketotic coma
BM strip	High	High
Plasma Ketostix	Heavily positive	Negative or trace positive

Hyperglycaemic emergencies are common in the tropics, and mortality rates are high—often in the region of 20–30% or more.[44] The reasons for this include the tendency of tropical patients to present to hospital late, and the severity of underlying infections. A further cause, however, is delayed diagnosis and suboptimal treatment.[45] Modern methods of treating DKA and HONK are simpler than previous regimens, and can be easily and successfully adopted in the tropics.[46] Sophisticated laboratory support is also not essential; simple vigorous treatment may achieve mortality figures below 10% despite grossly inadequate biochemical back-up.[47]

Modern management of DKA is shown in Table 66.13. Infusion pumps for insulin delivery are rarely available in tropical countries, but the

Table 66.13 Modern treatment of ketoacidosis.

1 *Insulin* (soluble, Actrapid Velosulin, etc.)	*Either 'IV infusion'*	6 units/hour initially, adjusting as necessary. Use infusion pump, or simply put insulin into infusion bags or bottles.
	Or 'hourly IM'	20 units IM at once, then 10 units IM hourly. If glucose level does not fall in 2 hours, change to IV method.
2 *Fluids*		Normal (0.9%) saline 1 litre fast, then 1 litre hourly x 3–5 hours as necessary.
3 *Potassium*		Await initial plasma K level. As long as it is not high, start replacement at 10–30 mmol/h of KCl with saline infusion. Alter according to plasma K.
4 *Bicarbonate*		Only give if pH < 7.0. Then, give 50–100 mmol sodium bicarbonate, repeated as necessary till pH > 7.0.
5 *Monitoring*		Initial pH, BG and U & E. Repeat plasma K and BG 2-hourly. Later use BM strips.
6 *Later treatment*		When BG < 15 mmol/litre start glucose–potassium–insulin ('GKI') infusion; i.e. 500 ml 10% dextrose + 20 units soluble insulin and 20 mmol KCl 4–6-hourly. Adjust as necessary. When patient can eat revert to subcutaneous insulin.

'hourly intramuscular IM' system is simple and effective. An 'intravenous IV infusion' system can also be achieved by simply adding the insulin to the saline being infused. Saline should be 0.9% sodium chloride, and vigorous rehydration is needed—undertreatment with fluids is a common mistake. Bicarbonate is rarely required, but copious potassium chloride is always necessary (often 100 mmol or more). As BG levels fall below 15 mmol/litre, patients should be transferred to a 'GKI' regimen (glucose–potassium–insulin infusion, see Table 66.13). The constituents are altered as necessary according to BG and plasma potassium levels, and when the patient is able to eat, subcutaneous insulin can be restarted. The 'GKI' system is useful for type 1 diabetics undergoing surgery, or if food intake is difficult due to acute infections. Here the insulin used is generally a little lower (15 units per 500 ml 10% dextrose initially), as there will be less ketosis-induced insulin resistance. GKI with 5% dextrose can be used, with half the usual potassium and insulin.

As always in the field of tropical medicine, it is important to adapt therapy to situations of limited drugs or resources. Table 66.14 gives a schedule for DKA treatment which can be used when only bedside BG measurements are available (together with clinical judgement and meticulous care and observation). Other insulins and fluids can if necessary be used. Potassium phosphate will substitute for potassium chloride. If 0.9% saline is unavailable, 'half-normal' saline or even Darrow's or Hartmann's solutions may be used (Chapter 72). Even intermediate-acting insulins (in higher doses than usual) have been used when soluble insulin is 'out of stock'.

Table 66.14 'Blind' treatment of ketoacidosis.

1 *Insulin*	'Hourly IM' or 'IV infusion' as in Table 66.13; check response with BM strips.
2 *Fluids*	0.9% saline 1 litre fast, then 1 litre hourly for 3–5 hours.
3 *Potassium*	After first litre of saline, give 20 mmol KCl with each litre, up to 80 mmol total.
4 *Bicarbonate*	Give 50 mmol only if patient is *very* ill. Repeat once only if necessary.
5 *Later treatment*	When BM strip 15 mmol/litre or less, convert to GKI infusion as in Table 66.13. Revert to subcutaneous insulin when patient able to eat.

HONK is treated similarly to DKA with the following exceptions.
1 Dehydration is more severe, and rehydration will need to be more vigorous.
2 Bicarbonate is never needed.
3 Half-normal saline should be used if the patient is hypernatraemic.
4 Death due to stroke is very common, and low-dose heparin (5000 units subcutaneously, twice a day) may reduce the risk of such thrombotic complications.

Chronic complications

Specific diabetic complications. These include cataract, neuropathy, retinopathy and nephropathy. Cataract appears particularly common in African diabetics, and is treated by lens extraction (Chapter 70). Retinopathy is more of a problem in the tropics as laser therapy is very rarely available. Prevention by good glycaemic control is therefore the best policy. Nephropathy is fortunately a rarer complication and tends to occur late in the course of diabetes. Once established, improved glycaemic control does not delay the progression of renal dysfunction, but control of blood pressure and possibly protein restriction are valuable. When renal failure becomes severe, dialysis and/or transplantation are the only options. Neuropathy is very common, and is usually asymptomatic, but painful varieties affecting the legs can be very debilitating, as can autonomic neuropathy which may cause diarrhoea, postural hypotension and impotence. Most symptomatic neuropathies improve spontaneously with time, and this may be accelerated by improved diabetic control. Impotence is usually permanent, but 'diabetic diarrhoea' may be helped with tetracycline (it is presumably due to bacterial bowel overgrowth, caused by impaired gut motility). Painful neuropathic syndromes are usually helped by carbamazepine with or without imipramine.

A recently described and interesting complication is 'limited joint mobility' or 'cheiroarthropathy'[48] (Fig. 66.3). This affects some 30% of type 1 diabetics, both in tropical and non-tropical areas, and is associated with retinopathy. Limited joint mobility is a particularly interesting complication, as it is due to glycosylation of collagen overlying the joint. The earliest microscopic lesion in diabetic microangiopathy is basement membrane thickening, which appears to be due to protein glycosylation.[49] Interestingly, this basic process seems related to the degree of glycaemia, and can be retarded by improved control.[50]

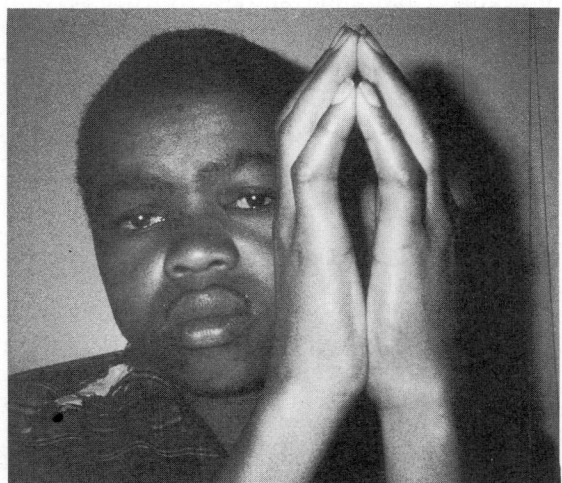

Fig. 66.3 Limited joint mobility in an African diabetic patient. This picture shows a positive 'prayer sign'.

Large vessel disease. This includes ischaemic heart disease, cerebrovascular disease and peripheral vascular disease. These conditions are of course not specific for diabetes, but they do occur more frequently, more severely, and earlier than in non-diabetics. In most areas of the tropics (especially Africa), however, such large vessel complications are generally uncommon (with the exception of stroke disease). This rarity is also seen in diabetic populations,[9,51] despite a very high prevalence of hypertension in African diabetics.[9,52] In Western countries, macroangiopathy is the main killer in type 2 diabetes, but the tropical diabetic is fortunately usually protected from this major scourge.

The diabetic foot. This well-known problem is due to varying degrees of neuropathy, ischaemia and infection. A typical example is shown in Fig. 66.4, here due mainly to neuropathy and infection (as in most tropical areas). Barefoot walking and poor hygiene greatly exacerbate the problem. Diabetic feet need vigorous treatment if amputation is to be avoided. Admission to hospital is needed for rest, dressings, antibiotics and optimization of diabetic control. Early limited surgery (e.g. toe, 'wedge' or 'ray' excisions) may prevent later more radical loss of limb. As with many diabetic problems, education in foot care is vital if problems are not to recur.

HYPOGLYCAEMIA

The treatment of diabetes (with insulin or sulphonylureas) is the most important cause of hypoglycaemia worldwide,[43,53] and this is discussed in detail in the previous section on Diabetes Mellitus. There are however, other non-diabetic causes which are of considerable tropical interest[54] (Table 66.15).

Hypoadrenalism in the tropics is usually due to tuberculosis involving the adrenal glands. Radiological calcification may be present. Symptoms are often vague; for example dizziness (due to hypotension) or hyperpigmentation. The latter feature is often dismissed as nonsensical in black patients, but it does occur. If proper biochemical evaluation with a short Synacthen test is not available, then a trial of hydrocortisone or cortisone treatment may be worthwhile.

Alcohol is an extremely important cause of tropical hypoglycaemia. Ethanol inhibits hepatic gluconeogenesis, and tends to cause hypo-

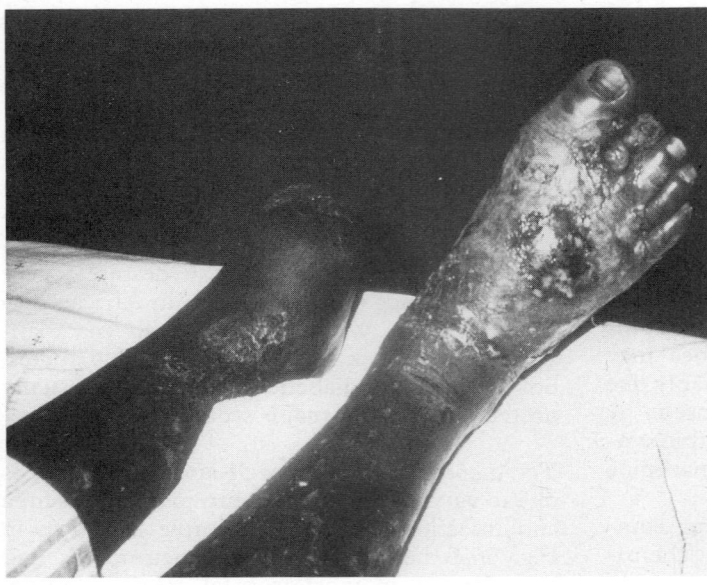

Fig. 66.4   A typical 'diabetic foot' showing gross sepsis, due to underlying neuropathy with unperceived trauma.

Table 66.15   Causes of hypoglycaemia.

Important tropical causes	Other causes
Diabetes treatment	Insulinoma
Liver failure	Other tumours
Alcohol	Dumping syndrome
Hypoadrenalism	Glycogen storage diseases
Malnutrition	Drugs and poisons
Cerebral malaria	'Essential' post-prandial
	hypoglycaemia

glycaemia particularly when food has not been taken for some time. In Africa, and other tropical areas, the scenario is usually that of a prolonged and vigorous beer party (often of the home-brewed type) in which food intake is forgotten! Such binges tend to occur when money is plentiful ('the end of the month' syndrome), and very profound hypoglycaemia may result, requiring admission to hospital and prolonged glucose infusion. The diagnosis may of course be masked by the features of drunkenness, and such patients always require a 'bedside blood glucose' estimation to exclude hypoglycaemia. Full details of the management of hypoglycaemia are given in Table 66.10.

HAEMOSIDEROSIS

'Bantu siderosis' was described many years ago, as a form of acquired iron overload due to the use of iron cooking vessels for making home-brewed beers.[55] The condition appeared to be almost entirely confined to Johannesburg blacks, of whom about a quarter had marked hepatic siderosis at autopsy. Acquired haemosiderosis in Africa is now known to be more complex than was previously thought. Thus, although the Transvaal area of South Africa is the main focus, the condition does occur elsewhere.[56,57] Factors influencing the absorption of iron are also now known to be important. For example, absorption is greatly enhanced by alcohol (which increases its degree of ionization) and also by fructose (with which it forms readily absorbable chelates). The epidemiology and pathophysiology of this interesting condition has been extensively studied by Bothwell et al[58] (Chapter 60, p. 1006).

From the clinical point of view, patients are usually male, and nearly all abuse alcohol. Indeed, it is often the features of alcoholism which bring these patients to medical attention. Alternatively, hepatomegaly or hepatosplenomegaly may be incidentally discovered, and subsequent liver biopsy may show the typical pattern of iron overload. Biochemically, serum iron and ferritin levels are considerably raised. A final possible presentation is with the features of osteoporosis—notably back pain and/or vertebral collapse. Haemosiderosis in Johannesburg is closely associated with vitamin C deficiency—a link which is believed to be causal.[59] This form of scurvy often leads to severe osteoporosis ('in the city of gold, the men of steel, have bones of clay').

Haemosiderosis in the tropics should be treated by venesection and vitamin C supplementation, together of course with advice to refrain from (or at least reduce) alcohol consumption. The prognosis is, however, rather poor. Fortunately the condition is now seen less frequently, presumably as patterns of beer drinking move from the iron pot to the glass bottle.

PORPHYRIA CUTANEA TARDA

This form of porphyria is peculiarly common in South Africa, particularly in the Transvaal area. Over 90% of patients abuse alcohol, and most have hepatomegaly and/or abnormal liver function tests. Porphyria cutanea tarda (PCT) can in fact to some extent be regarded as an acquired hepatic form of porphyria.[58] The underlying biochemical disorder is an underactivity of hepatic uroporphyrinogen decarboxylase. Although acquired liver disease appears necessary for the clinical expression of PCT, there does also seem to be some degree of genetic susceptibility.

Patients are usually male, generally drink alcohol excessively, and frequently have some degree of associated acquired haemosiderosis. Typical clinical features include blistering of light-exposed areas, hyperpigmentation, and hypertrichosis of the face. High levels of uroporphyrin are present in the urine, which may turn red on standing. Episodes of abdominal pain and vomiting may occur, but they are uncommon, and the general course of the disease is relatively benign.

Treatment of PCT is with venesection, as well as advice to avoid alcohol. Such treatment usually causes prompt remission of the bullous eruption.

South Africa is also well known for a further type of porphyria, 'variegate porphyria'.[60] This affects whites of Afrikaaner origin, and it is clinically a mixture of PCT and acute intermittent porphyria. It is inherited as a mendelian dominant, and the present South African pedigree can be traced back to Dutch settlers in the Cape in the late fifteenth century.

REFERENCES

1 Wilkin, T. & Armitage, M. (1986) *Br. Med. J.* **293**, 1323–1326.

2 World Health Organization Expert Committee (1985) *Wld Hlth Org. tech. Rep. Ser.*, 727.

3 Dodu, S. R. A. (1958) *W. Afr. med. J.* **7**, 129–134.

4 Politzer, W. M. & Schneider, T. (1960) *S. Afr. med. J.* **34**, 1037–1039.

5 Carr, W. R. & Gelfland, M. (1961) *Cent. Afr. med. J.* **7**, 332–335.

6 Davidson, J. C. (1963) *Cent. Afr. J. Med.* **9**, 92–94.

7 Tulloch, J. A. (1964) *E. Afr. med. J.* **41**, 572–580.

8 Osuntokun, B. O., Akinkugbe, F. M., Francis, T. I. et al (1971) *W. Afr. med. J.* **20**, 295–312.

9 Gill, G. V. & Huddle, K. R. (1984) *Cent. Afr. J. Med.* **30**, 189–195.

10 Campbell, G. D. (1963) *S. Afr. med. J.* **37**, 1195–1208.

11 Gelfland, M. & Forbes J. I. (1963) *S. Afr. med. J.* **37**, 1208–1213.

12 Seftel, H. C., Keeley, K. J. & Walker, A. R. P. (1963) *S. Afr. med. J.* **37**, 1213–1216.

13 Steel, J. M. & Mngola, E. N. (1974) *Trop. Doc.* **4**, 184–187.

14 Gill, G. V. (1984) *Lancet* **ii**, 1283.

15 Borch-Johnsen, K., Joner, G., Mandrup-Poulsen, T. et al (1984) *Lancet* **ii**, 1083–1086.

16 Verma, N. P. S., Mehta, S. P., Madhu, S. et al (1986) *Br. med. J.* **293**, 423–424.

17 Mather, H. M. & Keen, H. (1985) *Br. med. J.* **291**, 1081–1084.

18 Hugh-Jones, P. (1955) *Lancet* **ii**, 891–897.

19 Abu-Bakare, A., Taylor, R., Gill, G. V. et al (1986) *Lancet* **i**, 1135–1138.

20 Zuidema, P. J. (1959) *Trop. geogr. Med.* **11**, 70–74.

21 Tulloch, J. A. & McIntosh, D. (1961) *Lancet* **ii**, 119–121.

22 Ahren, B. & Corrigan, C. B. (1985) *Diab. Med.* **2**, 262–264.

23 McGlashan, N. D. (1967) *Trop. geogr. Med.* **19**, 333–343.

24 McMillen, D. E. & Geevarghese, P. H. (1979) *Diab. Care* **2**, 202–208.

25 Pirart, J. (1978) *Diab. Care* **1**, 168–188.

26 Dornan, T., Mann, J. I., & Turner, R. (1982) *Br. med. J.* **285**, 1073–1077.

27 Watkins, P. J. (1984) *Br. med. J.* **288**, 168–169.

28 Leading article (1985) *Lancet* **i**, 961–962.

29 Mann, J. I. (1984) *Diab. Med.* **1**, 191–198.

30 Gill, G. V. & Alberti, K. G. M. M. (1985) *Pract. Diab.* **2**(4), 15–19.

31 Home, P. D. & Alberti, K. G. M. M. (1982) *Clin. Endocrin. Metab.* **11**, 453–483.

32 Roland, J. M. (1984) *Diab. Med.* **1**, 51–53.

33 Francis, A. J., Home, P. D., Hanning, I. et al (1983) *Br. med. J.* **286**, 1173–1176.

34 Walters, D. P., Smith, P. A., Marteau, T. M. et al (1985) *Diab. Med.* **2**, 496–497.

35 Watkins, P. J. (1985) *Br. med. J.* **290**, 655–656.

36 Lester, F. T. (1985) *Diab. Med.* **2**, 405–407.

37 Gill, G. V., Huddle, K. R. & Krige, L. P. (1984) *S. Afr. med. J.* **65**, 815–816.

38 Bloom, A. (1985) *Br. med. J.* **290**, 727–728.

39 Gill, G. V., Huddle, K. R. & Krige, L. P. (1986) *Diab. Res.* **3**, 145–148.

40 Peacock, I. (1984) *J. clin. Path.* **37**, 841–851.

41 Connor, H. (1984) In *Diabetes Education*, ed. A. K. Baksi, D. W. Hide and G. Giles, pp. 3–10. Chichester: John Wiley.

42 Leading article (1982) *Lancet* **i**, 145–146.

43 Gill, G. V. & Alberti, K. G. M. M. (1985) *Prac. Diab.* **2**(5), 5–10.

44 Buch, E., Irwig, L. M., Huddle, K. R. L. et al (1983) *S. Afr. med. J.* **64,** 705–709.
45 Rwiza, H. T., Swai, A. B. M. & McLarty, D. G. (1986) *Diab. Med.* **3,** 181–183.
46 Pallangyo, K. J., Yusufali, A. M., Salim, S. S. et al (1984) *Trop. Doc.* **14,** 72–75.
47 Lester, F. T. (1980) *Diabetologia* **18,** 375–377.
48 Huddle, K. R., Gill, G. V. & Krige, L. P. (1983) *S. Afr. med. J.* **64,** 579–581.
49 Leading article (1984) *Lancet* **ii,** 19–20.
50 Siperstein, M. D. (1983) *New Engl. J. Med.* **309,** 1577–1579.
51 Seftel, H. C. & Walker, A. R. P. (1966) *Diabetologia* **2,** 286–290.
52 Oli, J. M. & Ikeh, V. O. (1986) *J. R. Coll. Physns* **20,** 32–35.

53 Potter, J., Clarke, P., Gale, E. A. M. et al (1982) *Br. med. J.* **285,** 1180–1182.
54 Baylis, P. H. (1985) *Pract. Diab.* **2**(6), 18–20.
55 Higginson, J., Gerritsen, T. & Walker, A. R. P. (1953) *Am. J. Path.* **29,** 779–815.
56 Speight, A. N. P. & Cliff, J. (1974) *E. Afr. med. J.* **51,** 695–702.
57 Gordeuk, V. R., Devee Boyd, R. & Brittenham, G. M. (1986) *Lancet* **i,** 1310–1313.
58 Bothwell, T. H., Charlton, R. W., Cook, J. D. et al (1979) *Iron Metabolism in Man.* Oxford: Blackwell Scientific Publications.
59 Seftel, H. C., Malkin, C., Schmaman, A. et al (1966) *Br. med. J.* **i,** 642–646.
60 Goldberg, A. & Moore, M. R. (eds.) (1980) *Clin. Haemat.* **9.**

Chapter 67
Cancer

M. S. R. Hutt and P. Clifford

INTRODUCTION

Any account of the problem of cancer in the tropics must take into consideration several accepted generalizations about tumours. The term cancer is used to describe a group of conditions which are characterized by an abnormal proliferation of particular cells. Each tumour is classified according to its cell of origin, anatomical site and biological behaviour, and each is due to a specific factor or constellation of factors, the majority of which are determined by geographical, social, economic or cultural influences, acting through physical, chemical or biological (viral) agents. Tumours due to direct genetic mechanisms are very rare, though genetic factors may render individuals or groups of people susceptible to particular environmental influences. The majority of malignant tumours show an age-related incidence which reflects length of exposure to carcinogenic factors in the environment.

As the age structure of most tropical populations is pyramidal with few old people, the numerical burden of cancer cases is lower than in developed countries, and the tumours that occur in early life are relatively more important. Cancer occurs in every ethnic group and in every part of the world but, as might be expected from our knowledge of the dominant role of environmental factors, the incidence of individual types of cancer varies greatly and some tumours show over 100-fold differences between different populations.[1] Comparisons of all-site age-adjusted incidence rates in many different countries reveals up to a fourfold difference between those with the highest and those with the lowest overall rates. These all-site rates hide important information. For example, India, which has one of the lowest overall rates (about 140 per 100 000 annually in men and 120 per 100 000 in women) has the highest rate for oropharyngeal cancer in the world.

Cancer incidence and cancer registration in the tropics

During the first half of this century little was known or published about cancer in tropical countries though individuals had recognized differences in the incidence and behaviour of certain tumours in different geographical regions. There was known to be a high incidence of nasopharyngeal cancer in the Far East; oropharyngeal cancer in the Indian subcontinent, squamous cell carcinoma of the bladder in Egypt and a peculiar tumour of the jaw in children living in sub-Saharan Africa.

In the post Second World War period cancer registries were established in many of the new medical schools and hospitals throughout the developing world and these were able to obtain for the first time age-specific cancer incidence rates in a few localized areas, usually around the teaching hospitals.[2,3] Proportional frequencies (frequency of individual tumours as a percentage of the whole) which are not dependent on a population census, showed that there were wide differences in the incidence of specific tumours within many developing countries as well as differences from the European and North American patterns.[4,5] Some of the most important aetiological discoveries in the cancer field have stemmed from epidemiological studies within tropical countries and between them and their immediate neighbours. The geographical mapping of each cancer type in the countries of the tropics and subtropics still contains many gaps though atlases of cancer incidence rates are now available from many regions such as China.[6]

Comparisons of individual cancer site-incidence rates have been made between the countries of the tropics (and subtropics) and those of Europe and North America.[7]

There are a group of cancers which are much more common in Western countries than in the general populations of any tropical region. These include carcinoma of the colon and rectum, the breast, the prostate, the endometrium and the lung. These tumours account for a high proportion of the incidence of all tumours in Western populations and also, with the exception of endometrium, for a high proportion of mortality rates. The incidence of these five tumours in the countries of the tropics appears to be directly related to the degree of westernization of each population and the lowest rates are found in the subsistence farmers and nomadic populations of the tropics. Although several aetiological factors are involved in the aetiology of large bowel, breast, prostatic and endometrial cancers, there is evidence that Western diets play an important role in their aetiology. Studies on immigrant groups in the USA who have adopted Western customs, and diets, show a rising incidence rate of all these tumours. The association of lung cancer with smoking is born out by the very low incidence of this tumour in most tropical countries where, as yet, smoking is mainly a habit of the affluent few. However, the rates are rising rapidly in countries such as Bangladesh and Zimbabwe where smoking cigarettes has become widespread in the population.

Although stomach cancer has a high incidence in Western populations and is relatively uncommon in most tropical and subtropical regions of Africa, India and the Far East, there are focal areas of high incidence in the tropics such as that found around Mount Kilimanjaro in Tanzania, the adjacent parts of Kenya, near Lake Kivu in Zaire and in the countries of Rwanda and Burundi. High rates are also found in the mountainous regions of Colombia, and in Chile. In the Far East stomach cancer is common in many areas of the Republic of China and Japan. Carcinoma of the pancreas appears to be increasing in frequency in Western populations but is as yet uncommon in tropical countries.

Malignant tumours in the tropics

Every clinicopathological form of cancer will be encountered in the tropics so it is proposed to concentrate on those which are particularly common in some tropical countries or are rare in

the Western world and those which have unusual clinical or aetiological features.

Although many countries of the tropics have centres of excellence with some of the recent methodology for diagnosis and management, it is recognized that in most countries these facilities are only available to a small proportion of the total population, mostly those who live in urban or peri-urban areas. For the predominant poorer section of the populations preventive measures, early diagnosis and modern therapeutic methods are rarely available.

A national or institutional plan for the treatment of cancer will depend on the human and economic resources available. Three avenues of treatment are available, used either singly or in combination.

1 Surgery

While for many tumours surgical excision is a first approach to treatment, survival rates are closely related to accurate staging. It must also be remembered that if excisive surgery removes a functioning part of the body, i.e. tongue or penis, interstitial or external irradiation in stage 1 or 2 tumours may be preferable.

2 Radiotherapy

Various forms of ionizing radiation are available in some regions of the tropics but their effective use depends on the presence of a team of highly trained personnel. Interstitial radiation using radium seeds or needles or iridium wire also requires skilled operators.

3 Chemotherapy

Of the large number of drugs used for cancer therapy less than 20 have been shown to be therapeutically effective. The newer drugs, such as cis-platinum compounds, are very expensive and often beyond the economic resources of the country.

In many tropical countries, where patients present with advanced disease there is a crying need for better palliative treatment. It is better to concentrate limited resources on improving early diagnosis when cancer can be controlled by early surgery, limiting the use of cytotoxins to those cancers where long-term survival has been convincingly shown and channelling other resources into relief of pain and other distressing symptoms.

ORAL AND OROPHARYNGEAL CARCINOMA

Squamous cell carcinoma of the mucosa of the oral cavity and the oropharynx is a tumour whose incidence is closely related to particular cultural habits. There is a high incidence in most of the population in the Indian subcontinent and in peoples of Indian extraction living in other countries of the Far East. Oral and oropharyngeal carcinoma accounts for nearly 50% of cancer patients registered at the Tata Memorial Hospital in Bombay and incidence rates of over 20 per 100 000 per year have been recorded in some districts of India.[8] In Malaysia these tumours account for 30% of all malignancies in the Indian population with low rates in the Chinese and an intermediate pattern in Malays.[9] A high incidence of palatal cancer is found in Andhra Pradesh, South-east India. This is due to the practice of smoking "Chutta" cheroots with the burning end in the mouth.

AETIOLOGY

The high incidence of oropharyngeal carcinoma in these populations is related to the cultural practice of chewing betel quid and/or the smoking of locally made cheroots called bidi. Betel quid consists of the young leaf of betel vine (*Piper betle*) mixed with slices of areca nut and varying quantities of slaked lime. Tobacco and spices may be added to the mixtures. The quid is held in the buccal sulcus for long periods of time and this leads to precancerous changes in the buccal epithelium which eventually progress to an infiltrating squamous cell carcinoma (Chapters 49, p. 903). A high alcohol intake, vitamin A deficiency, dental caries and sepsis may also be contributory factors in some patients.

CLINICAL FEATURES AND TREATMENT

Most surveys of high incidence populations show a male dominance which varies from 2 : 1 to over 10 : 1 according to the anatomical site of the lesion and the particular population. These differences probably reflect local preferences for the composition of the quid and the pattern of tobacco use. Cancer of the oropharynx initially presents as a red or white plaque. With time the plaque thickens and may bleed. At an early stage, it is not fixed to underlying structures and is curable by local excision. Later, the tumour will spread to involve adjacent structures and more extensive surgery may require transposition into the mouth of large full-thickness skin flaps which will restore function and improve the cosmetic result.[10] If there is clinical evidence of lymph node involvement, the Crile block dissection of regional nodes and adjacent structures should be performed. If surgery is undertaken following radiotherapy, a six-week period should be allowed for the early effects of irradiation to subside before operating. For inoperable cases symptomatic relief may follow the use of systemic or intra-arterial cytotoxic drugs such as vincristine, bleomycin and methotrexate.

PREVENTION

Oropharyngeal cancer, like lung cancer, is a largely preventable disease. Reduction in the use of betel quid and modification in its composition, particularly by the exclusion of tobacco, together with improved oral hygiene, should be a major part of health educational programmes among high incidence populations.

CARCINOMA OF THE OESOPHAGUS

GEOGRAPHICAL DISTRIBUTION

Squamous cell carcinoma of the middle or lower third of the oesophagus is a tumour which shows large variations in incidence throughout the world. In some regions the high incidence is quite localized with 20-fold differences in rates over distances of less than 100 miles. Within the tropics and subtropics there are high rates in many countries of sub-Saharan Africa, northern Iran adjacent to the Caspian Sea and northern China. The high incidence in the African continent was first recorded in the peoples of the Transkei in South Africa and later in other areas of the Republic. In recent years a high proportional frequency has been noted in Zimbabwe, Malawi, parts of Zambia, Tanzania and western Kenya. By contrast oesophageal carcinoma is uncommon in West Africa.[11] The evidence suggests that the present pattern is of recent development. Although the tumour is more common in men in all countries in Africa it is now becoming more frequent in women in the Republic of South Africa. In contrast to Africa and other parts of the world, the sex ratios are equal or women predominate in Iran.[12]

AETIOLOGY

The scattered regions of high oesophageal cancer incidence in different parts of the tropics show great variations in race and environment though most populations are rural and poor. Studies in endemic areas of Africa, Iran and China suggest that predisposition to oesophageal cancer may depend on the development of a susceptible epithelial lining combined with exposure to exogenous ingested agents. Dietary analyses have shown deficiencies in a variety of trace elements and vitamins, including molybdenum, zinc, manganese, riboflavine and nicotinic acid in some high incidence areas; such deficiencies may affect epithelial integrity. Alcohol per se does not appear to be a significant factor though in Africa contamination of home-brewed beers and the use of beers distilled from maize have been suggested as sources of carcinogens.[11] In China the people in high incidence areas consume large quantities of pickled vegetables which have been shown to be contaminated with the fungus *Geotrichum candidum* and also contain nitrosamines. Pyrolysed substances from opium smoking have also been suggested as carcinogenic factors in northern Iran.

CLINICAL FEATURES AND MANAGEMENT

In areas with a very high incidence it is not unusual to see cases presenting in the fourth or fifth decade though it is mostly a disease of elderly men (except in northern Iran where women predominate). The clinical features are similar to those seen anywhere with progressive dysphagia and wasting. In the vast majority of patients with carcinoma of the oesophagus seen in the tropics, resection of the tumour is impossible and attempts at heroic surgery will only add to the patient's discomfort. In those patients whose general condition permits, symptomatic relief may be obtained by the judicious use of radiotherapy, if it is available. Tumour reduction to improve obstruction may also be attempted by passing a 1 g radium tube down an oesophageal tube, provided its position can be frequently checked by radiography and the irradiation dose carefully assessed. For most patients, palliative measures, with the careful use of oesophageal tubes to bypass obstruction, are all that can be offered.

NASOPHARYNGEAL CARCINOMA (NPC)

GEOGRAPHICAL DISTRIBUTION

Carcinoma of the nasopharynx (NPC) is an uncommon tumour in the white populations of Europe and North America but has long been recognized as a major problem in parts of the Far East, particularly southern China.[13] In regions with a high incidence, such as China, NPCs are poorly differentiated or non-keratinizing squamous cell carcinomas, and often show a heavy stromal infiltration of lymphocytes, a feature which gave rise to the old term lymphoepithelioma. Such tumours appear to be aetiologically distinct from the well-differentiated squamous carcinomas that may occur anywhere in old people. The highest incidence rates are found in the southern provinces of China, particularly around Guangdong, and in Hong Kong and Singapore where rates of between 12 and 20 per 100 000 per year are recorded. There is also a high incidence in Malaysia, Thailand, Indonesia and Hawaii. NPC is twenty times more common in the Chinese population of Malaysia than in Indians and about six times as common as in Malays. The incidence of NPC in the different populations in South-East Asia is directly related to the degree of inbreeding with immigrants from Southern China.[14]

Regions of intermediate incidence (from 1.5 to 9 per 100 000 per year) are found in Africa. These include the highland areas of Kenya, the Sudan, Tunisia, Morocco and Algeria. In these areas the age distribution shows two peaks with the first occurring between 10 and 20 years. This contrasts with other high incidence regions which show a steady increase in incidence with age.

AETIOLOGY

The high incidence in peoples of southern Chinese (Cantonese) descent who live in very different environments, often contrasting with a low incidence in neighbouring ethnic groups, suggests a genetic susceptibility. HLA typing has shown that Cantonese Chinese with A2BW46 and AW19BW17 haplotypes have an increased risk of developing NPC.[15]

The association of NPC with Epstein–Barr virus (EBV) infection has now been confirmed in different ethnic groups throughout the world and appears to hold true for high, intermediate and low incidence areas,[16] an exception being some of the high keratinizing tumours of the elderly. The association was first noted by the finding of high mean IgA antibody titre to EB viral capsid antigen (EBVCA) and to early antigen antibody diffuse component (EA-D) in patients with NPC.[17] High IgA-VCA antibodies have also been detected before clinical features of the disease are present and may be used as a screening technique for tumour development in high incidence populations. EBV-DNA sequences have been shown in NPC tumour cells and tumour cells express EBV-associated nuclear antigen.[18] Although these findings strongly support the role of EBV in the causation of NPC they do not explain the geographical and racial distribution. While the latter may, in part, be accounted for by genetic susceptibility, it is probable that other carcinogenic factors are involved. The high intake of salted marine fish and pork, using sodium nitrate as a preservative and colour enhancing agent by the Chinese, has long been suspected as an aetiological factor in NPC. These foods have been found to contain appreciable amounts of dimethylnitrosamine. Case-control studies in Chinese Malays have also suggested that inhaled and ingested carcinogens may be cofactors.[19] Present evidence suggests that EBV and ingested or inhaled carcinogens in genetically susceptible populations may explain the curious geographical distribution of this tumour.

CLINICAL FEATURES

Nasopharyngeal carcinoma has a great variety of clinical manifestations; 95% of patients present with enlarged, often massive, cervical lymph nodes, which may be mistaken for tuberculosis or malignant lymphoma (Fig. 67.1). In 45% this

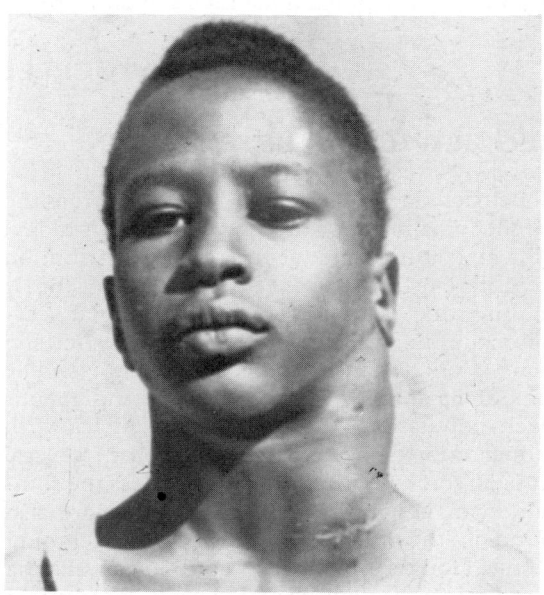

Fig. 67.1 Nasopharyngeal carcinoma with massive cervical lymphadenopathy. (Courtesy Professor M.A.O. Malik.)

is associated with some cranial nerve involvement with paresis or pain due to extension of the tumour throughout the base of the skull; in 5% the only symptom is cranial nerve paralysis.[20] Other symptoms, related to the anatomical situation of the tumour, are epistaxis, uni- or bilateral nasal obstruction, deafness due to eustachian tube obstruction, otalgia, proptosis and broadening of the root of the nose. A firm diagnosis is made by histological examination of tissue taken from the nose and/or from a cervical node metastases. The extent of bone erosion of the midcranial fossa can be estimated by radiological examination of the skull base; such examination should also include the cervical vertebrae and pulmonary fields.

TREATMENT

If the facilities are available, high dose megavoltage external irradiation is the treatment of choice. The fields should include regional lymph nodes as well as the primary site. The results of treatment are influenced by the clinical state when the disease is diagnosed. Lederman[21] noted that 90% of patients presenting with cranial nerve lesions died with uncontrolled disease and that the prognosis was not altered by the presence or absence of regional node metastases. In those patients whose disease is confined to the nasopharynx a 54% survival is reported, 40% in those with cervical node involvement and only 16% in those with neurological involvement. Chemotherapy, using the alkylating agent nitrogen mustard, with aortic abdominal occlusion, has been shown to be useful in palliating painful disease.[22]

HEPATOCELLULAR CARCINOMA

GEOGRAPHICAL DISTRIBUTION

Hepatocellular carcinoma (HCC) arises from the parenchymal cells of the liver and its aetiology, clinical features and geographical distribution are different from intrahepatic cholangiocellular or bile duct carcinoma. Hepatocellular carcinoma is one of the commonest malignancies in many countries and regions of the tropics. The tumour has a high incidence in the indigenous black populations of sub-Saharan Africa with annual rates of over 50 per 100 000 in several areas; in some African countries HCC is the commonest malignancy in men. High rates are also found in the Far East and Oceania including China, Hong Kong, Malaysia, Taiwan, Papua New Guinea, Indonesia and Hawaii. By contrast HCC is uncommon in northern India (1.4 per 100 000 annually in Bombay), though proportional frequencies are higher in south India and in Sri Lanka. Rates intermediate between those of the tropics and those of Europe and North America are recorded in countries of the Middle East, the Caribbean and South America.

AETIOLOGY (Fig. 67.2)

The great majority of hepatocellular carcinomas arise in patients with cirrhosis of the liver.[23] This is usually macronodular in type and the risk of developing a tumour is much greater in patients with this morphological type than in micronodular cirrhosis, which is usually associated with an alcoholic aetiology. In high incidence areas of HCC there is a high prevalence of hepatitis B surface antigenaemia in the general population (5–20%) and 50–70% of patients with cirrhosis and HCC are hepatitis B surface antigen (HBsAg) positive;[24] nearly all the negative cases have antibodies to hepatitis B indicating previous infection with the virus. Antigenaemia is

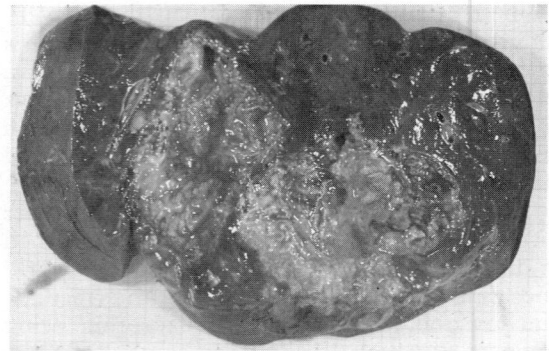

Fig. 67.2 Hepatocellular carcinoma. Mass in liver.

common in the mothers and siblings of patients[25] and follow-up studies on individuals with antigenaemia indicate an attributable risk of over 50%. Further support for implicating hepatitis B infection in the genesis of the tumour comes from the demonstration of the integrated DNA sequence of hepatitis B in cell lines of the tumour.[26] The virus also has many common characteristics with a virus that causes hepatomas in woodchucks and ground squirrels.[27] (See Chapter 6, p. 173.)

Various mycotoxins, which are capable of causing liver necrosis and hepatoma in a variety of animals including primates, are known to be present in the environment of countries with a high incidence of HCC. Aflatoxin, a product of the fungus *Aspergillus flavus*, which contaminates foodstuffs such as peanuts, has been shown to be present in high quantities in several countries with a high incidence of HCC and there appears to be some relationship between the degree of food contamination and the incidence of the tumour.[28] The role of aflatoxin in the genesis of HCC remains uncertain.[29] It may act as a cofactor with hepatitis B or have an effect through its immunosuppressive properties (Chapter 49, p. 907).

CLINICAL FEATURES AND MANAGEMENT

In Europe and North America HCC usually develops as a complication in an elderly man who has been known to have cirrhosis for several years. In high incidence areas the symptoms of the tumour often antedate those of the cirrhosis and patients are more often seen in the third or fourth decade, or even younger. The tumour is commoner in men than in women as in other parts of the world. In the rural tropics patients often present late in the disease complaining of wasting, abdominal distension, which may be due to the enlarged tumorous liver and/or to ascites, and persistent right hypochondriac pain; jaundice is uncommon.[30] A palpable liver mass is usually felt and the diagnosis confirmed by direct needle biopsy. If no mass is present a standard liver biopsy may reveal tumour deep in the liver. If a liver biopsy cannot be performed the presence of the bloodstained ascites is very suggestive. In high incidence areas the serum alphafetoprotein is positive in about 60–90% of cases. The prognosis in patients with HCC is very poor. Most patients have advanced tumour when first seen (Fig. 67.2) and the underlying cirrhosis precludes the possibility of restoration to a normal liver, even if an effective chemotherapeutic agent was available. Nevertheless, an attempt to control tumour growth, with symptomatic relief, may be valuable in appropriate circumstances, and Olweny et al[31] using intra-arterial Adriamycin have obtained subjective remission in 44% and a complete response in 10% of selected cases of HCC in Uganda. Survival rates with all forms of treatment remain very poor and a palliative approach is appropriate for most cases.

PREVENTION

It is to be hoped that prophylactic inoculation with hepatitis B vaccines will eventually reduce the incidence of this common malignant tumour (Chapter 6, p. 177).

BILE DUCT CARCINOMA (CHOLANGIOCARCINOMA)

Adenocarcinoma may arise from the intra- or extrahepatic bile ducts. The former location is often classified as a primary liver tumour though these tumours differ in geographical distribution, aetiology and clinical features from hepatocellular carcinomas. Bile duct carcinomas are rare tumours but have a relatively high incidence in parts of the Far East, such as Hong Kong and Thailand, where clonorchiasis and opisthorchiasis are prevalent. These oriental forms of distomiasis are associated with hyperplasia and metaplasia of the lining epithelial cells of the ducts and, after many years, this may give rise to malignant transformation of the epithelium (Chapter 22, p. 496). Most patients present over 50 years of age and are often jaundiced in contradistinction from patients with hepatocellular carcinoma.

CARCINOMA OF THE BLADDER

GEOGRAPHICAL DISTRIBUTION

Throughout most of the world the common histological type of bladder cancer is transitional cell carcinoma; this accounts for about 98% of all epithelial malignancies. These tumours have a higher incidence rate in the countries of North America and Europe than in most developing countries in the tropics. Well-differentiated transitional carcinomas are very uncommon in the rural populations of sub-Saharan Africa.

By contrast there are several countries in North, East, central and southern Africa, and in the Middle East, where the predominant epithelial malignancy is squamous cell carcinoma. In some of these countries, particularly Egypt, the Sudan, Malawi, Iraq, Zimbabwe, Saudi Arabia and parts of Nigeria, Guinea, and Ghana, Tanzania, Zambia and the Republic of South Africa, the proportional frequency of these tumours is high.[32] At the Cairo Cancer Institute bladder cancer contributes to 38.5% of all cancers in men and 11.3% in women.[33]

AETIOLOGY

The low incidence of well-differentiated transitional cell carcinomas in many tropical countries and the high incidence of the squamous type suggests that the latter are aetiologically distinct. The association with *Schistosoma haematobium* in Egypt has been recognized since the early part of this century[34] and the relation of this infection to the development of squamous cell carcinoma is borne out by a comparison of the geographical distribution of the parasitic disease and the proportional frequency of bladder cancer. This association is particularly marked if cancer frequency is related to intensity of infection and egg load in the population (Chapter 22).

Many theories have been advanced to explain the relationship between bladder schistosomiasis and cancer. Epithelial hyperplasia is a constant histological feature of the schistosomal bladder and such epithelium is particularly susceptible to carcinogenic stimuli. It is unlikely that there is a direct effect of the schistosome ova in the neoplastic process. A constant feature of a heavy parasitic infection is impairment of bladder function with imperfect emptying and resultant repeated bacterial infections, often mixed in type. Such infections may result in the conversion of ingested nitrates to carcinogenic nitrosamines within the bladder.[35,36] This hypothesis is also consistent with the observation that squamous cell carcinoma of the bladder is also seen in some non-schistosomal tropical regions associated with urethral stricture, a lesion that produces similar dysfunction of the bladder and recurrent infections. It has also been suggested that abnormal tryptophan metabolites, which have been conjugated in the liver as glucuronides, may be released into the bladder as a result of the high quantity of beta-glucuronidase in the bladder urine derived from schistosome eggs and inflammatory cells.[37] (See also Chapter 22, p. 461.)

CLINICAL FEATURES AND MANAGEMENT

Unfortunately the cardinal early sign of a bladder tumour in the developed world—painless haematuria—is often ignored in an area of endemic schistosomiasis, for most of the population have had haematuria from childhood. The great majority of bladder cancers seen in the rural tropics present late,[38] often with severe urinary obstruction and it is not uncommon to find a bladder almost full of a highly keratinizing tumour. The extensive damage to the non-tumorous mucosa of the bladder, which may show precancerous changes, also limits any chance of a radical cure in schistosomal bladder cancer. An account of the surgical aspects of this tumour can be found in *Tropical Urology and Renal Disease*.[39]

CARCINOMA OF THE CERVIX

GEOGRAPHICAL DISTRIBUTION

In most populations living in the tropics and subtropics carcinoma of the cervix is not only the commonest malignant tumour in women but it also exeeds any other form of malignancy as a cause of mortality. High incidence rates (20–60 per 100 000 annually) are found in the Indian subcontinent, Africa, the Far East, the Caribbean and in many countries of South America.[1,40] In some of these countries cervical carcinoma accounts for 35–50% of all malignant tumours in women. There is a considerable variation in the frequency of the tumour within population groups living in the same region, though it is always more common in women from lower socioeconomic groups.

AETIOLOGY

Epidemiological evidence suggests that cervical carcinoma is the result of a sexually transmitted infection and that the risk is highest in those populations where sexual intercourse occurs regularly at, or near, the time of puberty, particularly if this is with multiple sexual partners.[41] It follows that very high rates are found in young prostitutes in several tropical countries. The role of specific, venereally transmitted, infections in the aetiology of cervical carcinoma is still not clear. There is an association with herpes simplex virus (HSV) (type 2)[42] and also with human papillomaviruses (HPV) both in invasive cancer and in individuals with premalignant cervical dysplasia.[43,44] Current evidence suggests that the development of the tumour is multiphasic over a long period of time and that several exogenous factors, including specific viruses such as HSV and HPV, are responsible for inducing the initial and subsequent changes in the epithelial lining.[45]

CLINICAL FEATURES AND MANAGEMENT

The clinical and histopathological features of cervical carcinoma are similar throughout the world. However, in the tropics where there is a very high incidence, patients often present at an earlier age (second or third decades), and at a later stage than in Europe. In Africa over 50% of cases are in stage 3 or 4 when first seen. Clinical management of cervical carcinoma should be no different in the tropical environment, but fre-

quently facilities for radium treatment and other modern radiotherapeutic techniques are not available. In such circumstances radical or palliative surgery is the only treatment available.

Exfoliative cytology

Widespread screening of young women using cervical cytology would seem to be indicated as a priority preventive measure for this commonest form of cancer in the tropics, but the logistics and financing of screening on a large scale preclude its use in many countries. Selected screening of high risk groups, particularly young women attending clinics of genitourinary medicine, gynaecological outpatients, family planning and obstetric clinics, should be available when the medical services can provide such facilities without depleting other resources.

CARCINOMA OF THE PENIS

GEOGRAPHICAL DISTRIBUTION

Squamous cell carcinoma of the penis is a tumour whose incidence is closely related to poverty and poor social conditions. For this reason the tumour is seen more commonly in the populations of the tropics than in those of Europe or North America. High rates (over 4 per 100 000 annually) have been described in the countries of the Caribbean, South America and many countries of sub-Saharan Africa. The tumour is more common in the Hindu population of the Indian subcontinent than in Muslims. Considerable variations in frequency are recorded in different tribal groups and geographical areas from within these continents and regions. In East Africa the proportional frequency of carcinoma of the penis is lower in Kenya than in Uganda. Within Uganda there are large differences in proportional frequency, often over quite short distances; in some districts carcinoma of the penis is the commonest malignancy in men while in others it is not common.[46]

AETIOLOGY

All the epidemiological evidence suggests that carcinoma of the penis is related to sexual activity and to personal hygiene. Under similar socio-

economic conditions the tumour is less frequent in populations who circumcise. This is most apparent in those who practise infantile circumcision, such as the Jews, but is also found in groups who circumcise as a pubertal rite. This explains the lower incidence in Kenya than in Uganda and in the Muslim population of India than in Hindus. Within uncircumcised groups there are, however, large differences in frequency. This may be explained by differences in hygiene and sexual mores. There is increasing evidence that the tumour is due to a sexually transmitted viral infection.[47] Viral DNA from human papilloma virus (HPV type 2) has been reported in patients with verrucous carcinoma[48] and it has been suggested that condyloma acuminatum may be a precancerous lesion.[49,50]

CLINICAL FEATURES AND MANAGEMENT

Unfortunately in many areas of the tropics where carcinoma of the penis is common patients present late in the state of their disease, often with large fungating tumours and extensive necrosis of much of the organ. However, most tumours are very slow growing and metastasize late to the inguinal and later the internal iliac glands. Bloodstream spread with distant metastases is rarely seen even in patients with extensive and destructive disease.

TREATMENT

If the lesion is localized to the prepuce, local excision may be adequate. For extensive lesions, penile excision, at least 2 cm proximal to the proximal area of induration is essential. For those with metastases to the inguinal lymph nodes, bilateral inguinal node resection is necessary. Radiotherapy has been used successfully in treating small early lesions but may be followed by urethral stricture. Chemotherapy, using methotrexate, cis-platinum or bleomycin have

been used in combination, with or without radiotherapy, in attempts to avoid mutilating surgery.

PREVENTION

The decline in frequency of carcinoma of the penis in the Western world and in higher socioeconomic groups in the tropics suggests that improved social conditions and better personal hygiene will result in a decrease in the importance of this tumour. Improved education should also result in cases being seen earlier at a time when surgery can offer a high cure rate.

MALIGNANT TUMOURS OF THE SKIN (see also Chapter 65, p. 1063)

SQUAMOUS AND BASAL CELL CARCINOMA

The high incidence of squamous and basal cell carcinomas in Europe, North America and Australia is due to the prolonged effects of solar ultraviolet light on lightly pigmented skin. By contrast individuals with deeply pigmented skins, as are found in the 'black' populations of the world, are resistant to this effect and solar cancers are very rare except in albinos who all die as a result of multiple squamous carcinomas of the skin. People of Indian extraction with 'light brown' skins are also relatively resistant to solar damage. In many tropical regions, however, squamous cell carcinomas of the skin are quite common.[51] These arise in an area of damaged skin, most frequently in long-standing tropical ulcers (Fig. 67.3), the scars of old burns or

epithelialized skin sinuses. Some, like the Kangri cancer of India, are related to skin damage connected with specific cultural habits.

Tropical ulcers are considered in Chapter 36. They occur in the poorer members of rural communities who are often on the verge of malnutrition. Early treatment by simple techniques has been shown to reduce the later development of malignant change in the ulcers.

MALIGNANT MELANOMA

Malignant melanoma of the skin is less common in coloured and black populations and when it occurs the lesions are nearly always on the non-pigmented sole of the foot (Fig. 67.4) or on the palmar side of the fingers or hand. There is evi-

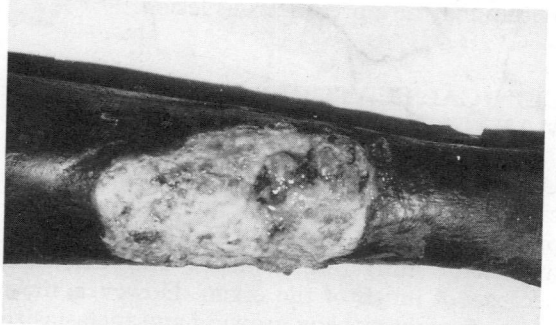

Fig. 67.3 Squamous cell carcinoma in long-standing tropical ulcer. (Courtesy Dr E.H. Williams.)

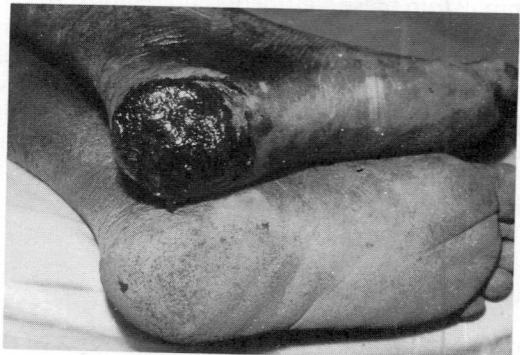

Fig. 67.4 Malignant melanoma on sole of foot. (Courtesy Dr E.H. Williams.)

dence that such tumours are more common in those who go barefoot and that they arise in junctional naevi which are activated by trauma.[52]

The principles for treatment are similar to those seen in temperate climates and are governed by the site of origin.

MALIGNANT TUMOURS OF CONNECTIVE TISSUES

The high proportional frequency of sarcomas of the connective tissues in some parts of the tropics, particularly sub-Saharan Africa,[53] is largely due to the high incidence of Kaposi's sarcoma in this region, but also reflects the tendency for these tumours to occur in younger age groups which form the majority of the population in these countries.

KAPOSI'S SARCOMA (see also Chapter 65, p. 1059)

GEOGRAPHICAL DISTRIBUTION

Kaposi's sarcoma is a malignant tumour of undifferentiated angioformative cells, usually starting in the skin, but occasionally involving many other organs of the body.

It occurs in three epidemiological forms.[54] Sporadic Kaposi's sarcoma, first described in Austria by Moricz Kaposi in 1872, is a rare tumour occurring in many different parts of the world but slightly more common in people of Jewish extraction and in southern Europeans. The occurrence of an endemic region of Kaposi's sarcoma in sub-Saharan Africa was first noted by Smith and Elmes in Nigeria in 1935.[55] They drew attention to 10 cases in a series of 500 malignancies in the indigenous population of Nigeria. Since that time Kaposi's sarcoma has been recognized as endemic in sub-Saharan Africa with an epicentre of high frequency in eastern Zaire and western Uganda[56,57] where proportional frequencies of over 15% are recorded. Kaposi's sarcoma has reached epidemic proportions in parts of North America and Europe with the outbreak of the acquired immunodeficiency syndrome (AIDS) first described in 1981.[58] Over 50% of patients dying of AIDS have Kaposi's sarcoma. The tumour may be the only manifestation of AIDS or may occur with a variety of opportunistic infections. AIDS is now known to be due to the human T cell lymphotropic virus type III (HTLV-III) also designated as lymphadenopathy associated virus (LAV) (Chapter 68).[59,60]

AETIOLOGY

The geographical and other epidemiological features of the various forms of Kaposi's sarcoma suggest that both genetic and environmental factors are involved in the aetiology. The major histocompatibility antigen HLA-DR5 occurs with a significantly higher frequency in patients with epidemic (AIDS) and sporadic forms of the tumour. HLA-DR5 has a higher frequency in blacks, Jews and Italians than in whites who live in New York.[61] The association of Kaposi's sarcoma with AIDS which is characterized by immunosuppression due to a deficiency in T lymphocyte helper cells, and the relatively high frequency in patients on long-term immunosuppressive therapy, such as renal transplant cases, suggests that a depressed immune system is important in the aetiology. Although HTLV-III is known to be the causative agent of AIDS, there is no evidence that it is directly implicated in the development of Kaposi's sarcoma. All patients with T lymphocyte deficiency, particularly those with AIDS, are susceptible to other virus infections and cytomegalic virus (CMV) has been regarded as a possible carcinogenic agent in Kaposi's sarcoma. CMV-related antigens have been demonstrated in tumour biopsies and CMV-DNA and CMV-RNA sequences have also been described in the tumour.[63] The relationship of AIDS to endemic Kaposi's sarcoma remains uncertain. AIDS has been reported both in expatriates and in the indigenous populations of central Africa, particularly in eastern Zaire, Rwanda, Burundi and Zambia, and HTLV-III antibodies are prevalent in these populations.[64] There is also evidence that the clinical features of Kaposi's sarcoma (see below) have changed in recent years in some parts of Africa and that the tumour is more aggressive like the epidemic, AIDS-related form of the disease.[65] The widespread immunosuppression in African populations due to the heavy infectious load, virus and parasitic, from an early age, may also be a significant factor in the aetiology of the endemic tumour. However, it is still difficult to explain the curious geographical distribution in Africa on these factors, nor do they explain the marked male dominance of the tumour.

CLINICAL FEATURES[66]

Sporadic (classical) Kaposi's sarcoma usually presents with multiple small nodules on the extremities of the limb in elderly males. It runs a benign course but occasionally the viscera are affected.

Endemic Kaposi's sarcoma of Africa

The majority of patients are men who present with tumour nodules on the extremities, particularly the lower legs and feet. This may be associated with, or preceded by oedema of one or both limbs (Figs. 67.5 and 67.6). The tumour also occurs on the skin in a plaque form. Such cases run an indolent course and many are alive 10 to 20 years later. Spontaneous regression of nodules can occur. A more florid form of the disease may develop in some of these patients who develop large ulcerating tumours and extensive local invasion which may involve bone. A few present with these aggressive skin lesions. These patients run a progressive course and often develop systemic lesions that may involve many different internal organs; local lymph node metastases also occur. At autopsy such patients often have extensive mucosal tumours throughout the length of their gastrointestinal tract as well as secondaries in many internal organs. Kaposi's sarcoma may also affect the mucous membranes of the eye, mouth, penis and vulva. Such patients are usually in younger age groups and run a more aggressive course. In young children, usually under eight years of age, Kaposi's sarcoma presents with widespread lymphadenopathy without skin lesions. Unlike the adult form of the disease this lymphadenopathic variety does not show a male predominance.[53, 56, 57] The condition is rapidly progressive and tumour spreads to the viscera. Such cases rarely survive more than six months. Recently, aggressive and atypical types of Kaposi's sarcoma have been reported

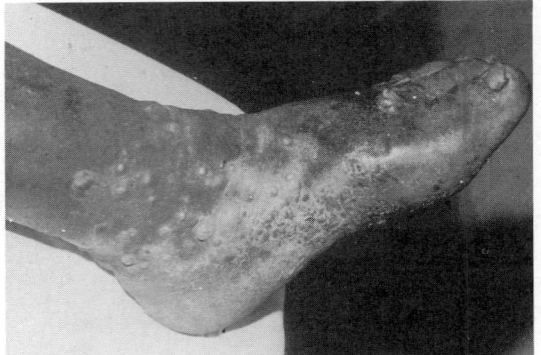

Fig. 67.5 Endemic Kaposi's sarcoma. Tumour nodule on foot with oedema. (Courtesy Dr E.H. Williams.)

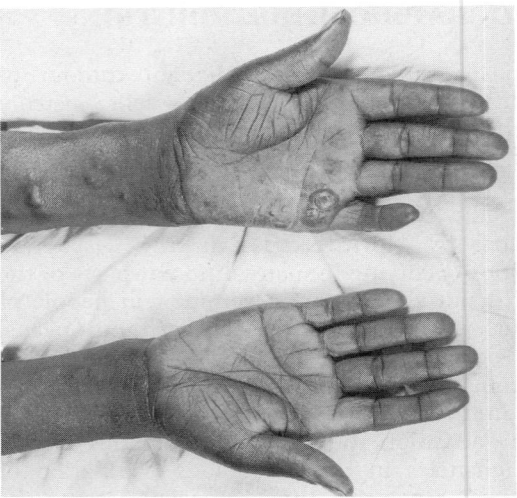

Fig. 67.6 Endemic Kaposi's sarcoma of the hands showing tumour nodules. (Courtesy Dr E.H. Williams.)

as occurring with greater frequency in adults in Zambia.[65, 67] Some of these patients have had unusual features such as lymphadenopathy, lung involvement and diffuse invasion of soft tissues. These cases are associated with HTLV-III (AIDS) infection, whereas the endemic form is not usually HTLV-III seropositive,[67, 68] nor is it associated with immunodeficiency.[69]

TREATMENT OF ENDEMIC (AFRICAN) KAPOSI'S SARCOMA

As Kaposi's sarcoma is a multifocal tumour which often presents with several, serparate lesions chemotherapy is the treatment of choice. There are two situations when surgery may be appropriate. The first is partial or complete amputation of a limb because of a gross, disabling deformity, and the second is tumour-bulk reduction as an adjuvant to other forms of treatment.[70, 71] If radiotherapy is available it can be used prior to surgical removement of large tumours, or as an alternative to surgical excision, but is not a curative procedure.

Chemotherapy is the treatment of choice and Kaposi's sarcoma has been shown to be responsive to several different agents given singly or in combination.[72] Using a three-drug combination[73] of actinomycin D, vincristine and imidazole carboxamide, 30 out of 32 (94%) patients had complete tumour regression, one had partial and one had no response. Other regimens, using BCNU (Carmustine) and bleomycin, have also given a high regression rate.[72, 73]

MALIGNANT LYMPHOMAS AND LEUKAEMIAS

Three forms of non-Hodgkin's lymphoma—Burkitt's lymphoma, Mediterranean lymphoma and histiocytic medullary reticulosis—have an unusual frequency in different regions of the tropical world and are described in detail.

Large cell, aggressive non-Hodgkin's lymphoma, formerly called reticulum cell sarcoma or histiocytic lymphoma, is proportionately more common in the countries of the Middle East, Africa, Central and South America, than the well-differentiated follicular lymphomas. Some of these cases are associated with human T cell leukaemia/lymphoma virus (HTLV-I) which has a high incidence in the Caribbean as well as Japan[74,75] and also occurs in Africa.

Hodgkin's disease in the tropics tends to occur in much younger age groups than in Europe or North America; nearly 50% under the age of 20 years and a few even before five years.[76,77] Also the proportion of histological subtypes that carry a poor prognosis are more common.

Acute lymphoid leukaemia of early childhood is much less common in the tropics than in Europe, though acute myeloid leukaemia in older children and adults is not rare.[78,79] Chronic myeloid and lymphatic leukaemia show similar features to those seen elsewhere.

Burkitt's lymphoma (BL)

In 1958 Denis Burkitt described a tumour syndrome in African children characterized by the presence of tumours of the jaw, abdomen and other extralymphopoietic sites.[80] The tumour was shown to be a non-Hodgkin's lymphoma and has been identified as originating from B lymphocytes.

GEOGRAPHICAL DISTRIBUTION

Burkitt's lymphoma is endemic throughout a large belt across sub-Saharan Africa. This belt lies approximately between 10° north and 10° south of the equator with a tail running down the east coast as far as southern Mozambique. In the Sudan the tumour is confined to the southern part of the country, and east and west of the Sudan to the regions below the deserts. Within the belt there are areas where the tumour is less common or rare. These include the highlands of Rwanda, Burundi and parts of eastern Zaire, south-western Uganda and the Kenya highlands. The apparent altitude barrier to the tumour falls progressively with distance from the equator and appears to be temperature related as most cases of the tumour are seen in river valleys, near lake shores and on coastal plains. In West Africa the tumour is rare where rainfall is less than 20 inches.

BL accounts for over 50% of all malignant tumours of childhood in tropical Africa.[81] In Ibadan in Nigeria, the tumour accounts for 70% of all neoplasms of childhood. In that country the incidence has been estimated as 15 cases per 100 000 children between the ages of five and nine years.[82]

BL is also endemic in the lowland regions of Papua New Guinea where similar climatic and geographical conditions prevail.[83]

The tumour is very rare in the populations of Europe and North America and the clinical features are also different. Although the tumour is not endemic in the Far East, the Middle East or South America, proportional frequencies of childhood tumours from several countries such as Malaysia, Iraq, Iran and Brazil indicate that BL is more common in these regions than in temperate climates.

AETIOLOGY

The geographical distribution of endemic BL in sub-Saharan Africa and Papua New Guinea corresponds closely to that of holoendemic malaria[84,85] and an association with malaria would explain the low incidence of the tumour in high altitude areas and also its rarity in the islands of Zanzibar and Pemba where there is effective malarial control. There are several possible ways in which recurrent malaria might play a role in tumour development in young children. *Plasmodium falciparum* is known to be mitogenic for B lymphocytes[86] and stimulates their proliferation, and recurrent malaria leads to immunodepression and an altered cellular response to other infective agents.[87,88]

In 1964 Epstein and his co-workers isolated a new virus, the Epstein–Barr virus (EBV) from a tissue culture of BL cells.[89] All African children with BL have been shown to have antibodies to the virus. In 1970 Zur Hausen et al[90] showed that BL biopsies from endemic areas contained EBV genome by nucleic acid hybridization. Later studies demonstrated that 96% of BL biopsies from endemic areas contained an average of 30 EBV equivalents per tumour cell.[91,92] In a prospective study of 42 000 children from the West Nile region of Uganda it was found that 16 developed BL within seven months to six years after an initial blood sample had been taken. These 16 children who developed the tumour all exhibited higher EBVCA titres than age/sex/locally-matched controls. Twelve of 13 cases had higher VCA titres than any of the controls and EB-NA and EBV-DNA sequences were established in nine of 10 cases during this study.[93] It is postulated that in endemic populations EBV infection occurs soon after birth and that in some individuals it is an initiating event in a multistep carcinogenic process.[92] This process is enhanced by the effect of recurrent malaria on the immature lymphoreticular system which also occurs in the first year of life.

CLINICAL FEATURES[94]

In endemic regions the highest incidence of the tumour is in children between four and seven years. Between eight and 16 years the incidence declines sharply. No cases have been reported under two years of age. Rare cases have been recorded over the age of 20; the majority of these have been in pregnant women who have presented with breast tumours. The male to female ratio is approximately 2 : 1 irrespective of the site of the tumour. Jaw tumours, which may affect one or more quadrants of the mandible or maxilla, occur more frequently in males. Jaw localization is found in nearly 100% of children who present at three years of age and is progressively less common over five years (Fig. 67.7). Other common presenting sites are the abdominal retroperitoneal lymph nodes and, in young girls, bilateral ovarian tumours. However, the incidence of abdominal tumours (including ovarian) is equal between males and females. Abdominal lymph node involvement is sometimes associated with paraplegia, which is initially flaccid, and in endemic areas of BL this is the commonest cause of paraplegia. Other tumour sites include the thyroid, testis, bones and soft tissues. The mediastinal and peripheral nodes are rarely affected.

Before the days of chemotherapy most patients

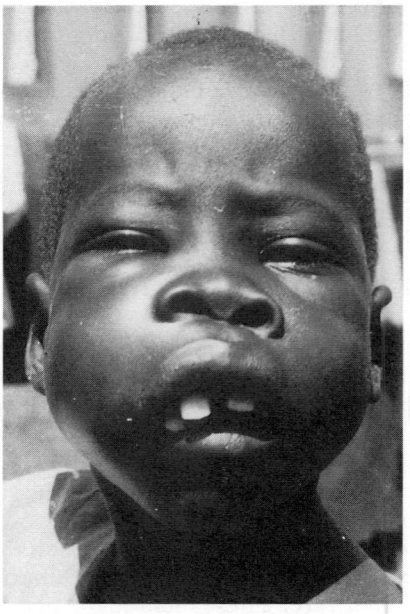

Fig. 67.7   Burkitt's lymphoma. Jaw tumour.

with BL died within a few months of initial diagnosis. At post-mortem they showed widespread metastases in the liver, kidneys and retroperitoneal lymph nodes as well as at the presenting sites.[95] With the advent of effective chemotherapy recurrence of the tumour, particularly in those children with jaw tumours, is often due to invasion of the brain and meninges which results in a variety of central nervous system (CNS) symptoms and signs.

The diagnosis of Burkitt's lymphoma is often evident from the peculiar distribution of lesions in a child from an endemic area. However, histological confirmation should always be sought as other tumours, such an embryonal rhabdomyosarcoma or neuroblastoma may mimic the picture. Histologically, the classical starry sky picture (Fig. 67.8) is highly suggestive of BL and is due to the presence of large numbers of phagocytic macrophages among the tumour cells.[96] The latter have a characteristic appearance in good sections with two or three indistinct nucleoli and basophilic cytoplasm. Where facilities for histological diagnosis are not available

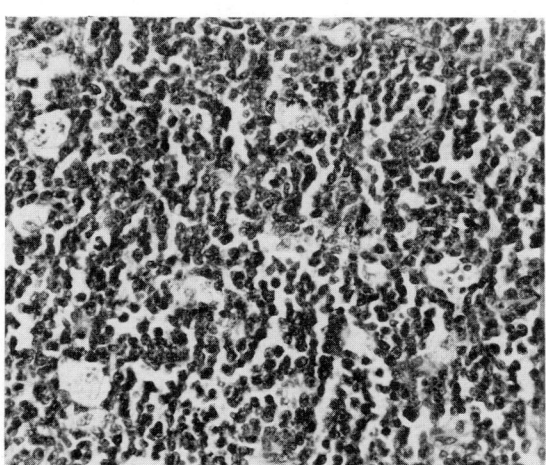

Fig. 67.8 Burkitt's lymphoma. 'Starry sky' picture.

imprint cytology is valuable and with some practice can be carried out and interpreted in small peripheral hospitals.

TREATMENT

Burkitt's lymphoma is extremely sensitive to chemotherapy and the initial results with cyclophosphamide were a turning point in the use of these agents for solid tumours. As a single drug cyclophosphamide should be given intravenously at a dose of 40 mg/kg and repeated after two weeks, this dose continued at two-weekly intervals for six weeks.[97] Very rapid remission of tumours follows this treatment and it may be followed by high uric acid levels in the blood and renal complications. For this reason it is necessary to give plenty of fluids and keep the urine alkaline with sodium bicarbonate. Combination therapy is now advised for patients with BL if the drugs are available. Ziegler et al[98] using a combination of vincristine 1.4 mg/m^2 intravenously on day 1; methotrexate 15 mg/m^2 days 1–4 followed after two weeks by cytosine arabinoside 250 mg/m^2 by continuous intravenous infusion for 3 days led to 90% remissions in patients who had failed to respond to cyclophosphamide treatment. Randomized trials of single-agent versus combination therapies are described by Olweny et al.[99] Chemotherapy in stage A (solitary extra-abdominal tumour) gives a survival rate of 87% at 10 years; for B and C (multiple extra-abdominal sites and intra-abdominal tumour with or without facial tumours) the 10-year survival falls to 50% and for stage D (intra-abdominal tumour with sites other than facial) it is only 25%.[100] Relapse is often associated with CNS development. Attempts to prevent CNS involvement by prophylactic irradiation have proved unsuccessful and trials by prophylactic intrathecal methotrexate are being assessed.[100]

Primary upper small intestinal lymphoma (PUSIL) (Mediterranean lymphoma)

These tumours of the upper part of the small intestinal mucosa occur endemically in some subtropical regions of the world and should be distinguished from the rare primary intestinal lymphomas seen in temperate climates or from involvement of bowel in the late stages of systemic lymphoma. Malignant change in the

lymphoid cells is often preceded by proliferation of plasma cells and lymphocytes associated with mucosal atrophy (immunoproliferative small intestinal disease) (IPSID). This may be associated with the production of alpha heavy chains which can be detected in the serum, and have given rise to the term alpha heavy chain disease.

GEOGRAPHICAL DISTRIBUTION

The term Mediterranean lymphoma was coined because of its frequency in Israel, Lebanon, Iran, Iraq, Syria, Algeria and Tunisia.[101,102] However, the first cases were described in Peru[103] and the condition has also been reported in other South American countries and in the coloured population of South Africa.

AETIOLOGY

The majority of patients with PUSIL come from a very poor socioeconomic background and give a history of repeated attacks of diarrhoea and accompanying malnutrition in the first year of life. In such children small-intestinal mucosal atrophy is common as is lymphoplasmacytic proliferation in the lamina propria (IPSID). These intestinal features are associated with thymic atrophy and persistent cell-mediated immune deficiency. It is postulated that the prolonged B cell and plasmacytic hyperplasia associated with depression of cellular immunity may lead to mutation of lymphocytes and the development of malignant lymphoma in adult life.[104]

CLINICAL FEATURES

Most cases begin insidiously with abdominal discomfort, diarrhoea and weight loss. Clubbing of the fingers and hypoproteinaemic oedema are also quite common. Diagnosis of tumour depends on obtaining an adequate small intestinal biopsy but it may be difficult to distinguish between the pretumorous proliferation of lymphocytes and plasma cells and the definite development of malignant lymphoma. The presence of alpha chains, which has given rise to the term alpha heavy chain disease, in the blood assists in the diagnosis but does not distinguish between non-neoplastic and neoplastic proliferation. The prognosis in patients with established tumour is poor and there is no specific therapy.

Histiocytic Medullary Reticulosis (HMR)

HMR is a very rare form of lymphoma in Europe and North America but occurs with an unusual frequency in some countries of sub-Saharan Africa; these include Uganda, Kenya, Zambia and Malawi.[100,105] Clinically patients with HMR, usually present with anorexia, fever, weakness and abdominal swelling. They are anaemic, with moderate generalized lymphadenopathy and hepatosplenomegaly. The anaemia is haemolytic in nature and is accompanied by neutropenia and thrombocytopenia. Most patients are labelled as PUO (pyrexia of unknown origin) but all laboratory tests are negative for infectious agents and the patients deteriorate rapidly. Diagnosis is rarely made in life and depends on the finding of the atypical malignant cells in the sinusoids of a liver specimen obtained by needle biopsy. There is no satisfactory treatment for this tumour though temporary responses have been obtained with steroids.

REFERENCES

1 Waterhouse, J.A.H., Muir, C.S., Correa, P. et al (eds) (1976) *Cancer Incidence in Five Continents,* vol. III, IARC Scientific Publication No. 15, Lyon.

2 Higginson, J. & Oettlé, A.G. (1960) *J. natn. Cancer Inst.* **24**, 589–671.

3 Davies, J.N.P., Knoweldon, J. & Wilson, B.A. (1965) *J. natn. Cancer Inst.* **35**, 789–821.

4 Hutt, M.S.R. & Burkitt, D.P. (1965)*Br. med. J.* **ii**, 719–722.

5 Templeton, A.C. & Hutt, M.S.R. (1973) Introduction. Distribution of tumours in Uganda. In *Tumours in a Tropical Country,* ed. A.C. Templeton, pp. 1–22. Berlin: Springer-Verlag.

6 Kaplan, H.S. & Tsuchitani, P.S. (1978) *Cancer in China.* New York: Alan R. Liss.

7 Doll, R., Muir, C.S. & Waterhouse, J.A.H. (eds) (1970) *Cancer Incidence in Five Continents,* vol. II, UICC. Berlin: Springer-Verlag.

8 Jussawala, D.J. (1976) The problem of cancer in India: An epidemiological assessment. In *Cancer in Asia,* ed. T. Hirayama, pp. 265–274. Baltimore: University Park Press.

9 Ramanathan, K. & Lakshimi, S. (1976) Oral carcinoma in Peninsular Malaysia: Racial variations in the Indians, Malays, Chinese and Caucasians. In *Cancer in Asia,* Ed. T. Hirayama, pp. 27–36. Baltimore: University Park Press.

10 Cook, R.R. (1976) Cancer of the lower alveolus. In *Cancer in Asia,* ed. T. Hirayama, pp. 37–48. Baltimore: University Park Press.

11 Cook, P. (1971) *Br. J. Cancer* **25**, 853–880.

12 Kmet, J. & Mahboubi, E. (1972) *Science* **175**, 846–853.

13 Clifford, P. (1970) *Int. J. Cancer* **5**, 287–309.

14 Ho, H.C. (1976) Epidemiology of NPC. In *Cancer in*

Asia, ed. T. Hirayama, pp. 49–61. Baltimore: University Park Press.

15 Simons, M.J., Chan, S.H., Wee, K. et al (1978) Nasopharyngeal carcinoma and histocompatability antigens. In *Nasopharyngeal Carcinoma: Etiology and Control*, ed. G. de Thé & Y. Ito, p. 271. IARC Scientific Publications No. 20, Lyon.

16 de Thé, G. & Geser, A. (1974) *Cancer Res.* **34**, 1196–1206.

17 Henle, G. & Henle, W. (1976) *Int. J. Cancer* **17**, 1–7.

18 Desgranges, C., Bornkamm, G.W., Zeng, Y. et al (1982) *Int. J. Cancer* **29**, 187–191.

19 Armstrong, R.W. & Armstrong, M.J. (1983) *Ecol. Dis.* **2**, 185–198.

20 Clifford, P. (1979) Tumours of the nasopharynx. In *Clinical Otorhinolaryngology*, ed. A.G.D. Maran & P.M. Stell, pp. 315–327 Oxford: Blackwell Scientific Publications.

21 Lederman, M. (1961) *Cancer of the Nasopharynx*. Springfield, Illinois: Charles C. Thomas.

22 Clifford, P., Bhardwaj, B.V. & Whittaker, L.R. (1965) *Br. J. Cancer* **9**, 51.

23 Anthony, P.P. (1979) Hepatic neoplasms. In *Pathology of the Liver*, ed. R.N.M. MacSween, P.P. Anthony & P.J. Scheuer, pp. 387–413. Edinburgh: Churchill Livingstone.

24 Tabor, E., Gerety, R.J., Vogel, C.L. et al (1977) *J. Nat. Cancer Inst.* **58**, 1197–1200.

25 Stevens, C.E., Beasley, R.P., Tsui, J. et al (1975) *New Engl. J. Med.* **292**, 771–774.

26 Shafritz, D.A. & Kew, M.C. (1981) *Hepatology* **1**, 1–8.

27 Summers, J., Smolec, J.M. & Snyder, R. (1978) *Proc. Natn. Acad. Sci., USA* **75**, 4533–4537.

28 Peers, A.G. & Linsell, C.A. (1973) *Br. J. Cancer* **27**, 473–484.

29 McGlashan, N.D. (1982). *Ecol. Dis.* **1**, 37–41.

30 Alpert, M.E., Hutt, M.S.R. & Davidson, C.S. (1968) *Am. J. Med.* **46**, 794–802.

31 Olweny, C.L.M., Katongole-Mbidde, E., Bahendeka, S. et al (1980) *J. Cancer* **46**, 2717.

32 El-Bolkainy, M.N. (1982) Bladder cancer and Bilharziasis in Egypt. In *Geographical Pathology in Cancer Epidemiology*, ed. E. Grundmann, J. Clemmesen & C.S. Muir, pp. 41–56. Stuttgart: Gustav Fischer Verlag.

33 El-Sebai, I., El-Bolkainy, M.N. & Hussein, M.H. (1973) *Med. J. Cairo Univ.* **41**, 175–181.

34 Fergusson, A.R. (1911) *J. Path. Bact.* **16**, 76–94.

35 El-Merzabani, M., El-Aaser, A.A. & Zakhary, N.I. (1979) *Eur. J. Cancer* **15**, 287–291.

36 Hicks, R.M., Walters, C.L., El-Sebai, I. et al (1977) *Proc. R. Soc. Med.* **70**, 413–417.

37 El-Aaser, A.A., El-Merzabani, M.M., Higgy, N.A. et al (1979) *Eur. J. Cancer* **15**, 573–583.

38 Ghoneim M.A., Mansour, M.A. & El-Bolkainy, M.N. (1974) *Urology* **3**, 40–42.

39 Husain, I. (ed.) (1984) *Tropical Urology and Renal Disease*. London: Churchill Livingstone.

40 Persaud, V. (1977) *Trop. geogr. Med.* **29**, 335–345.

41 Rotkin, I.D. (1973) *Cancer Res.* **33**, 1353–1361.

42 Mendis, L.N., Best, J.M., Senarath, L. et al (1981) *Int. J. Cancer* **28**, 535–542.

43 Durst, M., Gissman, L., Ikenberg, H. et al (1983) *Proc. Natn. Acad. Sci. USA* **80**, 3812–3815.

44 McCance, D.J., Walker, P.G., Dyson, J.L. et al (1983) *Br. med. J.* **287**, 784–788.

45 Zur Hausen, H. (1982) *Lancet* **iv**, 1370–1372.

46 Dodge, O.G. & Linsell, M.D. (1963) *Cancer* **16**, 1255–1263.

47 Zur Hausen, H. (1977) *Current Topics in Microbiology and Immunology* **78**, 1.

48 Ubben, K., Kryzek, R., Ostrow, R., et al (1979) *J. invest. Derm.* **72**, 15.

49 Schmauz, R. & Owor, R. (1980) *J. clin. Path.* **33**, 1039–1046.

50 Schmauz, R. & Schahter, A. (1982) Geographical clues from Israel for a relationship between *Condyloma acuminatia* and cancer. *In Geographical Pathology in Cancer Epidemiology*, ed. E. Grundmann, J. Clemmesen & C.S. Muir. Struttgart, New York: Gustav Fischer.

51 Iversen, V. & Iversen, O.H. (1973) Tumours of the skin. In *Tumours in a Tropical Country*, ed. A.C. Templeton, pp. 180–199. Berlin: Springer-Verlag.

52 Lewis, M.G. (1973) Melanoma. In *Tumours in a Tropical Country*, ed. A.C. Templeton, pp. 171–180. Berlin: Springer-Verlag.

53 Templeton, A.C. (1973) Soft tissue tumours. In *Tumours in a Tropical Country*, ed. A.C. Templeton, pp. 234–269. Berlin: Springer-Verlag.

54 Hutt, M.S.R. (1984) *Br. med. Bull.* **40**, 355–358.

55 Smith, E.C. & Elmes,. B.G.T. (1934) *Ann. trop. med. Parasit.* **28**, 461–512.

56 Ackerman, L.V. & Murray, J.F. (ed.) (1962) *Symposium on Kaposi's sarcoma*. Unio Internationalis Contra Cancrum. Basel: Karger.

57 Olweny, C.L.M., Hutt, M.S.R. & Owor, R. (eds) (1981) *Kaposi's Sarcoma: 2nd Kaposi's Sarcoma Symposium. Antibiotics and Chemotherapy*, Vol. 29. Basel: Karger.

58 Göttlieb, G.J., Ragaz, A., Vogel, J.V. et al (1981) *Am. J. Dermatopath.* **3**, 111–114.

59 Gallo, R.C., Salahuddin, S.Z., Popovic, M. et al (1984) *Science* **234**, 500–503.

60 Brun-Vezinet, F., Rouziu, C., Barré-Sinoussi, F. et al (1984) *Lancet* **i**, 1253–1256.

61 Friedman-Kien, A.E., Laubenstein, L.J., Rubenstein, P. et al (1984) *Ann. Intern. Med.* **96**, 777–779.

62 Giraldo, G., Beth, E. & Huang, E.S. (1980) *Int. J. Cancer* **26**, 23–29.

63 Boldogh, J., Beth, E., Huang, E.S. et al (1981) *Int. J. Cancer* **28**, 469–474.

64 Colebunders, R., Taelman, H. & Piot, P. (1985) *Trop. Doctor* **15**, 9–12.

65 Bayley, A.C. (1984) *Lancet* **i**, 1318–1320.

66 Taylor, J.F. & Kyalwazi, S.K. (1972) Kaposi's sarcoma. In *Medicine in a Tropical Environment*, ed. A.G. Shaper, J.W. Kibukamusoke & M.S.R. Hutt, pp. 213–226. London: BMA.

67 Bayley, A.C., Cheingsong-Popov, R., Dalgleish, A.G. et al (1985) *Lancet* **i**, 359–361.

68 Biggar, R.J., Melbye, M., Kestens, L. et al (1984) *New Engl. J. Med.* **311**, 1051–1052.

69 Kesten, L., Melbye, M., Biggar, R.J. et al (1985) *Int. J. Cancer* **36**, 49–54.

70 Hiza, P.R. (1981) Surgical treatment of Kaposi's sarcoma. In *Kaposi's Sarcoma*, ed. C.L.M. Olweny, M.S.R. Hutt & R. Owor, pp. 70–72. Antibiotics and Chemotherapy 29. Basel: Karger.

71 Bayley, A.C. (1981) Role of surgery in the management of Kaposi's sarcoma in Lusaka, Zambia. In *Kaposi's Sarcoma*, ed. C.L.M. Olweny, M.S.R. Hutt & R.

Owor. pp. 73–81. Antibiotics and Chemotherapy 29, Basel: Karger.

72 Vogel, C.L. (1981) Management of Kaposi's sarcoma. In *Kaposi's Sarcoma*, ed. C.L.M. Olweny, M.S.R. Hutt & R. Owor pp. 82–87. Antibiotics and Chemotherapy 29. Basel: Karger.

73 Olweny, C.L.M. (1981) Management of Kaposi's sarcoma. In *Kaposi's Sarcoma* ed. C.L.M. Olweny, M.S.R. Hutt & R. Owor. pp. 88–95. Antibiotics and Chemotherapy 29. Basel: Karger.

74 Blattner, W.A., Saxinger, C., Clark, J. et al (1982) *Lancet* **iii**, 61–64.

75 Blattner, W.A., Blayney, D.W., Robert-Guroff, M. et al (1983) *J. inf. Dis.* **147**, 406–416.

76 O'Conor, G.T. (1982) Environmental influences on lymphoma incidence. In *Geographical Pathology in Cancer Epidemiology*, ed. E. Grundmann, J. Clemmesen & C.S. Muir, pp. 183–189. Stuttgart: Gustav Fischer Verlag.

77 Ziegler, J.L., Morrow, R.H., Fass, L. et al (1970) *E. Afr. med. J.* **47**, 191–192.

78 Kasili, E.G. (1981) *Postgrad. Doc.* **3**, 126–129.

79 Williams, C.K.O., Folami, A.O., Laditan, A.A.O. et al (1982). *Br. J. Cancer* **46**, 89–94.

80 Burkitt, D.P. (1958) *Br. J. Surg.* **46**, 218–223.

81 Burkitt, D.P. (1970) Geographical distribution. In *Burkitt's Lymphoma*, ed. D.P. Burkitt & D.H. Wright, pp. 186–197. Edinburgh: Livingstone.

82 Edington, G.M. & MacLean, C.M.V. (1964) *Br. med. J.* **i**, 264–266.

83 Booth, K., Burkitt, D.P., Bassett, D.J. et al (1967) *Br. J. Cancer*, **31**, 657.

84 Dalldorf, G., Linsell, C.A., Barnhart, F.E. et al (1964) *Perspectives in med. Biol.* **7**, 435–449.

85 Burkitt, D.P. (1969) *J. natn. Cancer Inst.* **42**, 19–28.

86 Greenwood, B.M., Oduloju, A.J. & Platts-Mill, T.A.E. (1979) *Trans. R. Soc. trop. Med. Hyg.* **73**, 178–182.

87 Wedderburn, N. (1970) *Lancet* **ii**, 1114–1116.

88 Whittle, H.C., Brown, J., Marsh, K. et al (1984) *Nature* **312**, 449–450.

89 Epstein, M.A., Achong, B.G. & Barr, Y.M. (1964) *Lancet* **i**, 702–703.

90 Zur Hausen, H., Schulte-Holthausen, H., Klein, G. et al (1970) *Nature* **228**, 1056–1058.

91 Nonoyama, M., Huang, D.P., Pagano, J.S. et al. (1973) *Proc. Natn. Acad. Sci. USA* **70**, 3265–3268.

92 de Thé, G. (1982) Epidemiology of Epstein-Barr virus and associated diseases in man. In *The Herpes Viruses*, ed. B. Roizman, vol. 1, New York: Plenum Publishing.

93 Geser, A., de-Thé, G., Lenoir, G. et al (1982) *Int. J. Cancer* **29**, 397–400.

94 Burkitt, D.P. (1970) General features and facial tumours. In *Burkitt's Lymphoma*, ed. D.P. Burkitt & D.H. Wright, pp. 6–15. Edinburgh: Livingstone.

95 Wright, D.H. (1970) Gross distribution and haematology. In *Burkitt's Lymphoma*, ed. D.P. Burkitt & D.H. Wright, pp. 64–81. Edinburgh: Livingstone.

96 Wright, D.H. (1970) Microscopic features, histochemistry, histogenesis and diagnosis. In *Burkitt's Lymphoma*, ed. D.P. Burkitt & D.H. Wright, pp. 82–102. Edinburgh: Livingstone.

97 Nkrumah, F.K. & Perkins, I.V. (1973) *Int. J. Cancer* **11**, 19.

98 Ziegler, J.L., Blumming, A.Z., Fass, L. et al (1972) *Cancer Res.* **321**, 267.

99 Olweny, C.L.M. et al (1976) *Int. J. Chemother.* **17**, 436–440.

100 Olweny, C.L.M. (1984) Cancer. In *Principles of Medicine in Africa*, ed. E.H.O., pp. 985. Parry. Oxford, Nairobi: Oxford University Press.

101 Ramot, B., Shahin, N. & Bubig, J.J. (1965) *Israel J. med. Sci.* **1**, 221–226.

102 Al-Saleem, T. & Zardawi, I.M. (1979) *Histopathology* **3**, 89–106.

103 Barna, R.L. & Quintanillo, E.R. (1964) *Gastroenterology* **46**, 521–522.

104 Borochovitz, D., Dutz, W., Kohout, E. et al (1979) *Israel J. med. Sci.* **15**, 397–404.

105 Serck-Hanssen, A. & Purohit, G.P. (1968) *Br. J. Cancer* **22**, 506–516.

Chapter 68
Sexually Transmitted Diseases

O. P. Arya

INTRODUCTION

The sexually transmitted diseases (STDs) are a group of contagious conditions in which the principal mode of transmission is by heterosexual or homosexual activity. This can involve a number of sites of contact including penis, vagina, cervix, lips, oropharynx, anus and rectum together with adjacent skin areas. The organisms involved can also be transmitted in ways other than sexual contact as for example: ophthalmia neonatorum where the gonococci or chlamydiae are inoculated into the conjunctivae by direct contact with infected secretions in the birth canal during delivery, congenital syphilis (transplacental), prepubertal vulvovaginitis (via fomites such as shared damp towels), transfusion

syphilis (via fresh blood), acquired immunodeficiency syndrome—AIDS (via fresh blood, blood products or contaminated needles), inclusion conjunctivitis (by contaminated fingers), and pubic lice (shared clothes, overcrowding and proximity, and possibly, toilet seats).

There are no reliable data on the national incidence of these diseases in the tropical countries. Nevertheless, studies among selected populations have shown alarmingly high rates of the classical venereal diseases, namely, gonorrhoea, syphilis and chancroid. Antimicrobial resistance of STD agents (e.g. penicillinase-producing *Neisseria gonorrhoeae*—PPNG) has become a major problem in some areas. Complicated forms such as urethral stricture, epididymitis, pelvic

Table 68.1 Aetiological classification of sexually transmitted diseases.

Group	Agent	Disease
Viruses	Herpes simplex virus	Genital herpes
	Papillomavirus	Genital warts
	Poxvirus	Molluscum contagiosum
	Hepatitis virus	Hepatitis A, B, D, possibly non-A, non-B
	Cytomegalovirus[a]	Congenital infection: birth defects; varied manifestations in immunosuppressed host
	Human immunodeficiency virus (HIV)	Acquired immunodeficiency syndrome (AIDS)
Bacteria	*Neisseria gonorrhoeae*	Gonococcal infections
	Chlamydia trachomatis	Non-gonococcal, 'non-specific' urogenital infections
		Lymphogranuloma venereum
	Ureaplasma urealyticum	Non-gonococcal urogenital infections
	Mycoplasma hominis[a]	
	Haemophilus ducreyi	Chancroid
	Treponema pallidum	Syphilis
	Various vaginal anaerobes[a]	'Non-specific' vaginitis, anaerobic vaginosis, bacterial vaginosis
	Calymmatobacterium granulomatis	Granuloma inguinale
	Shigella species	Shigellosis
	Group B *Streptococcus*[a]	Neonatal sepsis
Fungi	*Candida albicans*	Genital candidiasis
Protozoa	*Trichomonas vaginalis*	Trichomoniasis
	Entamoeba histolytica	Amoebiasis
	Giardia lamblia	Giardiasis
Helminths	*Enterobius vermicularis*	Enterobiasis
Arthropods	*Phthirus pubis*	Pediculosis
	Sarcoptes scabiei	Scabies

[a] Epidemiological importance in this context not yet established.

infection and ectopic pregnancy are common. High rates of infertility (up to 30%) in some parts of Africa are considered mainly to be the consequence of STD. Ophthalmia neonatorum (gonococcal and/or chlamydial) is frequently encountered. The two other classical venereal diseases, namely, granuloma inguinale (donovanosis) and lymphogranuloma venereum have a rather patchy distribution. More recently, AIDS in central Africa is thought to have reached epidemic proportions.

Sexually transmissible pathogens now comprise a wide spectrum of medical microbiology (Table 68.1). It follows that the diagnosis of most of these conditions, besides requiring a high index of suspicion and careful examination by appropriately trained personnel, can be confirmed only by laboratory methods necessitating proper collection of specimens, technical expertise and equipment. In the tropics the majority of the STD patients are dealt with (a) by medical or paramedical staff with inadequate or no training in the management of STDs, and, (b) at medical centres with shortage of drugs and nonexistent or less than minimum laboratory facilities. (Minimum laboratory facilities include a microscope, staining materials and possibly a screening test—such as rapid plasma reagin (RPR) or Venereal Disease Research Laboratory (VDRL) for syphilis.)

Except in those patients with anogenital warts, molluscum contagiosum, pediculosis and scabies, the use of clinical acumen alone will miss the correct diagnosis in a considerable proportion of cases (see later). Asymptomatic carriage of sexually transmissible pathogens is also common. These patients, as well as being potentially at risk of developing complications themselves, constitute an important reservoir of infection. In addition, a patient may have more than one STD at the same time.

This chapter provides guidelines to realistic and proper approaches in the management of some of the sexually transmitted diseases in terms of the common presenting syndromes including urethral discharge and epididymitis in males, vaginal discharge and pelvic infection in females, ophthalmia neonatorum, and genital ulcers in both sexes. For more detailed information on these and other conditions not dealt with in this chapter, the readers may consult literature recommended at the end of the chapter.

URETHRAL DISCHARGE IN MALES

Urethral discharge is the most common presenting symptom in STD clinics. In a young adult male it generally denotes sexually acquired urethritis.

Aetiology. Urethritis may be gonococcal due to *N. gonorrhoeae* or non-gonococcal. The aetiology in almost half of the cases of non-gonococcal urethritis (NGU) is *Chlamydia trachomatis*; about 5–10% of the cases are due to *Trichomonas vaginalis*; 10% due to *Ureaplasma urealyticum*, other bacteria, herpes simplex virus and *Candida albicans*. The cause in the remainder (30%) remains unknown.

Some patients acquire both the gonococcal and non-gonococcal (such as chlamydial) infection at the same time. The initial symptoms of these patients are usually those of gonorrhoea. If the patient is not treated or treated inadequately, he may develop complications such as epididymitis (see section on acute epididymitis, below), infertility, urethral stricture, prostatitis and conjunctivitis—the last by accidental contamination,

and more rarely, especially in the case of gonorrhoea, tysonitis, cowperitis, periurethral abscess and disseminated infection.

MANAGEMENT OF URETHRAL DISCHARGE IN MALES

1　If microscopy is available

In the absence of spontaneous discharge, the urethra should be massaged from below the root of the penis to the meatus. A urethral sample is obtained by a sterile disposable plastic loop or by cooled flamed platinum loop or cotton wool or calcium alginate swab passed 1–2 cm into the urethra and gently rotated. (A loop is especially useful for making smears when the discharge is minimal.) The loop or swab is then smeared on to the glass slide. The smear is dried, fixed by gentle heating, stained with Gram stain (which is preferred to methylene blue—see p. 1109) and examined under the microscope using the oil immersion lens.

If the urethral smear shows typical gram-negative bean-shaped intracellular diplococci, a presumptive diagnosis of gonorrhoea is made and the patient treated for gonorrhoea (p. 1104). (There is an agreement between the results of urethral smear and culture in over 95% of the males with urethral discharge.)

If gram-negative diplococci are not seen and the smear shows more than five polymorphonuclear leukocytes (PMN) in a high power field (HPF), then a diagnosis of NGU is made and the patient treated for NGU (p. 1104).

Follow-up. All patients should be followed up, one and two weeks after the completion of treatment and tests repeated. Patients who fail to respond, and after reinfection has been excluded, should be treated with an appropriate alternative regimen.

Most or all of the patients with combined infection (gonococcal and non-gonococcal/chlamydial) treated with penicillin or another therapeutic agent which has no effect on the causative organism of NGU, will develop post-gonococcal urethritis (PGU). However, once the gonococcal infection is eliminated, these patients may remain asymptomatic or have minimal symptoms which may be ignored by the patient. A careful examination, after the patient has held urine for about 4 hours, may reveal minimal greyish or clear discharge on massaging the urethra and urine will be turbid. If a gram-stained urethral smear shows more than 5 PMN/HPF, PGU should be diagnosed and the patient treated as for NGU.

Contacts. Sexual partners of all patients should be examined and if possible investigated. In the absence of facilities, however, they should be treated on an epidemiological basis with the treatment regimens similar to the ones administered to the index patient.

2 If microscopy is not available

The diagnosis will have to be made on a clinical basis. The patient with balanoposthitis should be examined carefully to ensure that the discharge is urethral and not subpreputial. Table 68.2 shows the distinguishing features between gonococcal and non-gonococcal urethritis. There is, however, an overlap, e.g. a proportion (20%) of the NGU cases may show a mucopurulent urethral discharge. Likewise, the discharge in up to 15% of gonorrhoea cases may be scanty or mucoid. Moreover, the quality and the quantity of discharge, and the appearance of urine may be affected by the interval since the patient last voided urine. In these circumstances, or, if the majority of the cases with urethral discharge in the area are due to gonorrhoea, it may be desirable to treat all such patients initially for gonorrhoea, followed by a course of treatment for NGU.

Sexual partners should be treated with similar treatment regimens.

All patients should be followed up, one and two weeks after completion of treatment. Those not responding to the treatment regimens suggested below should be referred to a specialist.

In the absence of facilities for microscopy, a significant proportion of the NGU cases who have minimal or no symptoms and minimal or no demonstrable discharge will be missed if not examined carefully and on a full bladder, i.e. if the patient has not held urine for 4 hours. *C.*

Table 68.2 Comparison of urethral discharge in males.

Clinical features	Gonococcal urethritis	Non-gonococcal urethritis
1 No symptoms In the majority of *symptomatic patients*:	≤5%	≥25%
2 Incubation period	2–5 days	5–20 days
3 Urinary symptoms (burning during micturition, discomfort in penis)	Moderate to severe	Mild to moderate
4 Urethral discharge quality	Thick, mucopurulent to purulent (Fig. 68.1)	Thin, mucoid to mucopurulent
quantity	Profuse	Scanty (often demonstrable only on massaging urethra)
5 Urine in first glass	Hazy	Hazy, or, clear with shreds
6 Course	See text	See text

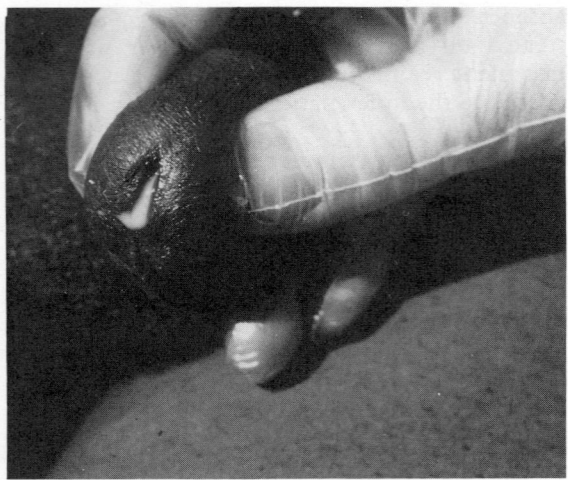

Fig. 68.1 Gonorrhoea: purulent urethral discharge in the male. (From Arya et al,[1] courtesy Churchill Livingstone.)

trachomatis has been isolated from urethral swabs of asymptomatic patients without overt discharge.

Treatment of uncomplicated gonococcal infections

Ideally, the treatment should be standardized. The choice of the standard regimen should be made with the full knowledge of the antimicrobial resistance patterns of the circulating strains. The situation should be monitored periodically by the specialists concerned.

1 If chromosomal gonococcal sensitivity is favourable,
AND prevalence of PPNG is less than 5%
AND the patient can be rechecked after 3–7 days, any of the following regimens may be used:

aqueous procaine penicillin G, 4.8 g (4.8 million units) intramuscularly plus 1 g probenecid by mouth,
OR amoxycillin, 3 g plus 1 g probenecid by mouth,*
OR ampicillin, 3.5 g plus 1 g probenecid by mouth,*
OR tetracycline hydrochloride, 500 mg by mouth, on an empty stomach half to one hour before food, four times daily for 7 days (this regimen will also prevent, in most cases, the development of PGU and cure concomitantly acquired chlamydial infection).

2 If chromosomal gonococcal resistance is high,
OR prevalence of PPNG more than 5%,
OR patient infected in an area of high resistance,
OR gonococcal resistance pattern unknown,
OR follow-up not ensured,
then the recommended choice is as follows:

spectinomycin, 2 g intramuscularly,*
OR cefotaxime 1 g intramuscularly plus 1 g probenecid by mouth,
OR cefoxitin, 2 g intramuscularly plus 1 g probenecid by mouth,
OR ceftizoxime, 1 g intramuscularly,
OR ceftriaxone, 250 mg intramuscularly,
OR kanamycin, 2 g intramuscularly,*
OR thiamphenicol, 2.5 g by mouth,*
OR trimethoprim (80 mg)/sulphamethoxazole (400 mg) four tablets twice daily for 2 days.

There is geographical variation in the efficacy of kanamycin, thiamphenicol and trimethoprim/sulphamethoxazole, and they are not recommended in pregnancy.

Ciprofloxacin (a new 4–quinolone derivative), in a single dose of 250 mg by mouth, has been found to be highly effective. However, this drug has not yet been extensively evaluated in the tropics: it is not recommended for children and is contraindicated in pregnancy and lactation.

Treatment of uncomplicated nongonococcal urethritis and chlamydial infection

Tetracycline hydrochloride, 250 mg by mouth, on empty stomach half to one hour before food, four times daily for 7–14 days (tetracycline is contraindicated in pregnancy),
OR erythromycin, 250 mg by mouth four times daily for 7–14 days.

For recurrent urethritis in males

Doxycycline, 100 mg by mouth twice daily for 10 days,
PLUS metronidazole, 400 mg twice daily for 5 days.

---

*These and possibly other single dose regimens may be ineffective against pharyngeal gonorrhoea.

ACUTE EPIDIDYMITIS

CLINICAL FEATURES

The patient generally presents with a painful scrotal swelling which is usually unilateral. The scrotal skin is hot and reddened. The epididymis is enlarged and intensely tender. The inflammation which is initially localized to one part of the epididymis may later become more generalized and involve the testicle as well. There may also be an associated hydrocele. Some patients may be febrile.

In most sexually active men the epididymitis will have been preceded by urethral discharge and/or dysuria. With the development of epididymitis the urethral discharge often becomes scanty. Nevertheless, careful examination will reveal evidence of urethritis.

AETIOLOGY

The causative organism is often *N. gonorrhoeae* or *C. trachomatis* in sexually active young men, and coliform or *Pseudomonas* infections in men over the age of 35 years. Other rare causes include *Brucella* spp. and *Streptococcus pneumoniae*. No pathogen may be isolated from some patients.

DIFFERENTIAL DIAGNOSIS

The important conditions to be differentiated include torsion of the testicle, strangulated hernia, filariasis, mumps, haematocele, tumour and tuberculous epididymitis which is usually subacute or chronic.

LABORATORY DIAGNOSIS

The urethral smear should be gram-stained and examined. Culture of the material obtained from urethra or of urine is usually adequate to detect the causative organism.

TREATMENT OF SEXUALLY ACQUIRED EPIDIDYMITIS

1 General measures: rest in bed, scrotal elevation, analgesics.
2 Single dose therapy for uncomplicated gonorrhoea (see above) if gonococcal infection cannot be excluded.
3 Tetracycline hydrochloride, 500 mg by mouth four times daily for at least 10 days, *OR* erythromycin, 500 mg by mouth four times daily for at least 10 days, *OR* doxycycline, 100 mg by mouth twice daily for at least 10 days.

The patient should be re-examined after 3 days to assess response to treatment, and then once weekly. If the swelling persists for longer than one month, possibilities of tuberculosis or a tumour should be considered and the patient referred or investigated appropriately.

VAGINAL DISCHARGE IN PREMENOPAUSAL ADULTS

Whereas urethral discharge in almost all young sexually active males denotes sexually acquired urethritis, vaginal discharge in many females may be unrelated to STD.

Excessive vaginal discharge may be due to physiological, non-physiological (non-infectious) and biological (infectious) causes.

1 Physiological causes

These include *puberty* (discharge due to hormonal changes), *premenstrual congestion*, *sexual activity* (pelvic congestion), and *pregnancy* (increased vascularity). These discharges are not usually associated with vulval soreness or irritation. The patient should be reassured after other causes have been excluded.

2 Non-physiological (non-infectious) causes

These include *foreign body:* symptoms resolve after the removal of offending object; *chemical vaginitis* as a result of use of disinfectants, antiseptics, deodorants; a careful history will identify the cause; *gynaecological causes* such as a large cervical erosion, polyp, neoplasm etc. which will need referral to a gynaecologist.

3 Biological (infectious) causes

The discharge may originate in the vagina, cervix, or higher up in the genital tract.

(a) *Vaginal causes* include vaginitis due to *Candida albicans* and other yeasts, *Trichomonas vaginalis*, *Gardnerella vaginalis* and other anaerobic bacteria. There may be an associated ectocervicitis.

(b) *Cervical causes* include cervicitis due to *N. gonorrhoeae*, *C. trachomatis* and herpes simplex virus.

Vaginal infections

Table 68.3 summarizes the cardinal symptoms, signs, diagnosis and treatment of vaginal infections due to yeasts, *T. vaginalis* and bacterial vaginosis. Although in many patients, these infections may manifest easily recognizable characteristic features (e.g. Fig. 68.2), proper assessment of the genital signs in females often requires considerable skill, experience and facili-

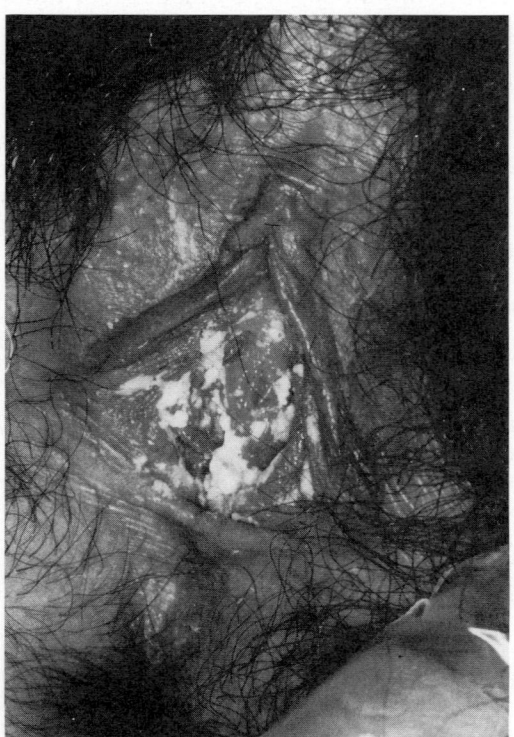

Fig. 68.2 Candida vulvovaginitis: curd-like exudate.

ties including an examination couch, light source, vaginal speculum and gloves. Moreover, any of the above organisms, singly or in combination, may be isolated from asymptomatic clinically normal women. They may also be associated with *N. gonorrhoeae* and/or *C. trachomatis* infection. Diagnosis based on clinical presentation, therefore, is often inaccurate. Consequently any treatment based on such diagnosis may be inappropriate.

Cervical infections

Cervicitis due to *N. gonorrhoeae* or *C. trachomatis* is potentially more serious (p. 1108) than the other causes of vaginal discharge and should first be excluded. Herpes simplex virus infection should be suspected in the presence of multiple painful vulval and/or cervical ulcers (p. 1108). Gonococcal or chlamydial infection may involve multiple sites including cervix, urethra, Bartholin's glands and ducts, oropharynx (as a result of oral sex) and rectum (as a result of secondary spread from the cervix or rectal intercourse).

STD screening

A full routine for STD screening of a female patient should comprise: (a) an adequate history including symptoms and their duration, whether on any medication or any treatment recently received, contraception, last menstrual period, sexual history, information on recent symptoms related to STD in the male partner, allergy to drugs and the relevant past history; (b) a full clinical examination and that of genitalia including vulva, urethra and urethral orifice, Bartholin's glands and duct orifices, speculum examination of the vagina and cervix followed by pelvic examination; (c) collection of specimens with cotton-wool-tipped swabs from the posterior fornix and vaginal walls for yeasts, *T. vaginalis* and other organisms, and material from the endocervix and possibly from urethra, rectum and if necessary also from the oropharynx for *N. gonorrhoeae*, and from the endocervix for *C. trachomatis*; and finally, blood sample for tests for syphilis.

Diagnosis of gonococcal and chlamydial infection in females

It is impossible to exclude or diagnose gonococcal or chlamydial infection simply on a clini-

Table 68.3 Comparison of vaginal infections.

	Yeast vaginitis	Trichomonal vaginitis	Bacterial vaginosis
Aetiology	*Candida albicans* and other yeasts	*Trichomonas vaginalis*	*Gardnerella vaginalis* and mixed anaerobes
Predisposing factors	Recent antibiotics, diabetes mellitus, pregnancy, oral contraceptives, general debility, steroids, immunosuppression, obesity, nylon underwear, tight jeans, deodorants	Recent partner change; often associated with gonococcal infection	Use of an intrauterine contraceptive device
Symptoms: (vulvar irritation, soreness, discharge, odour)	Vulvar irritation (prominent), vulvar soreness with or without increased discharge, external dysuria, dyspareunia	Vulvar irritation, vulvar soreness, foul smelling excessive discharge, dysuria, frequency of micturition	Vulvar irritation absent or not prominent, slightly increased discharge which is malodorous—likened to that of rotten fish
Signs: (inflammation of vulva or vaginal wall)	Vulvar congestion may extend to surrounding area, vaginal epithelium reddened	Vaginal walls red and inflamed, occasionally strawberry cervix	No erythema or minimal erythema of vulva or vagina
Amount of discharge	May or may not be increased	Profuse	Slightly increased
Colour of discharge	Watery white or creamy	Lime green	Greyish white
Consistency of discharge	Thin, watery or curdy or cheesy plaques which may be adherent to the inflamed vaginal wall and vulva (Fig. 68.2)	Watery, frothy	Homogeneous, often adherent to the vaginal wall rather than pooling in the posterior fornix, occasionally thin, frothy
pH of vaginal fluid	≤4.5	≥5.0	≥5.0
Amine test[a]	Negative	Often positive	Always positive
Lab. diagnosis: Smear	Gram-positive yeast spores and pseudomycelia in the gram-stained vaginal smear of up to 80% of patients with positive culture	Motile trichomonads can be recognized by their jerky movements, abundant polymorphonuclear leukocytes (smear alone may miss 20% of cases)	Wet mount may show curved rods (*Mobiluncus* sp.); gram-stained vaginal smear shows mixed gram-variable bacterial flora and clue cells (vaginal epithelial cells covered by coccobacilli), pus cells are scanty and lactobacilli absent or scanty
Culture		Vaginal swab should be sent to the laboratory in a suitable transport medium	
Treatment	*Clotrimazole*, 100 mg intravaginally for 6 days OR 200 mg intravaginally for 3 days OR 500 mg intravaginally once; OR *nystatin* (100 000 units) 2 pessaries intravaginally for 14 days; OR 1% gentian violet, one good application to vaginal walls. For vulvitis—clotrimazole or nystatin cream twice daily for 7–14 days	Metronidazole, 400 mg orally twice daily for 7 days, OR 2.0 g in a single oral dose (avoid alcohol during treatment); lactating women to interrupt breastfeeding for 24 hours after single dose therapy	Same as for trichomonal vaginitis
		If pregnant: avoid metronidazole; treat with clotrimazole, 100 mg intravaginally for 7 days (symptomatic improvement but failure rate high)	*If pregnant*: Ampicillin, 500 mg by mouth four times daily for 7 days (cure rate lower than with metronidazole)
Treatment of male partner	Clotrimazole or nystatin cream if female is experiencing recurrent candidiasis or if male has candidal balanitis	Examine for other STD and treat with metronidazole	Examine for other STD; no treatment if no other STD detected.

[a] Mix with a wooden stick 1–2 drops of vaginal discharge with 1–2 drops of 10% potassium hydroxide on a glass slide; transient release of ammoniacal odour denotes positive amine test.

cal basis. The majority of these patients have no symptoms. Only 30% or so may show macroscopic cervicitis, i.e. mucopurulent discharge exuding from the congested endocervix (Fig. 68.3). However, if mucopurulent discharge in the endocervix is present, then *N. gonorrhoeae* and/or *C. trachomatis* may be isolated from over

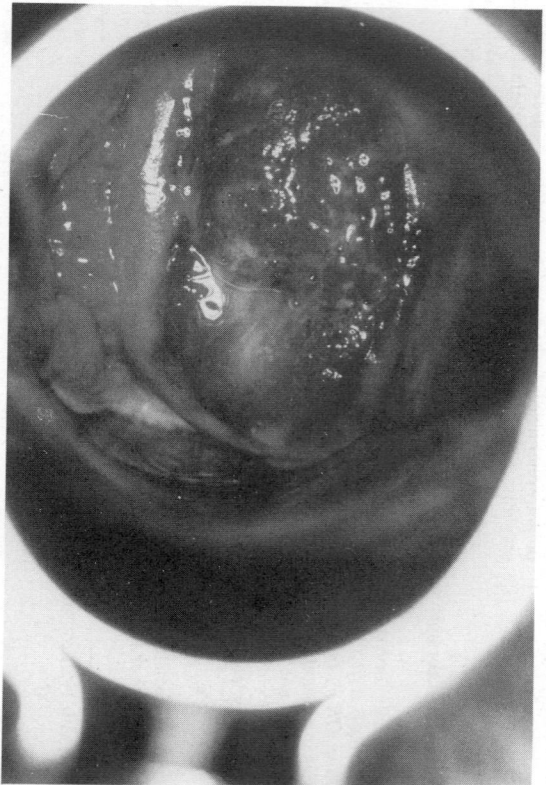

Fig. 68.3 Cervicitis showing endocervical mucopus and cervical oedematous ectopy.

70% of such women. Almost half of those infected with *N. gonorrhoeae* may also be infected with *C. trachomatis*. *If laboratory facilities are not available*, then these infections, singly or in combination, should be suspected if the patient has lower abdominal pain (p. 1110) or mucopurulent cervicitis or if the partner has recently experienced urethral discharge and/or dysuria.

Laboratory diagnosis

Gonococcal or chlamydial infection may involve multiple sites (mentioned above) but if only one site is to be sampled, then the cervix is the preferred site. However, unlike the very high cor-

relation between the urethral smear and culture in the diagnosis of gonococcal urethritis in the males, a gram-stained cervical smear alone will be positive in not more than 55% of cases (see below). The yield on smear alone could be increased by about 5% if urethral smears were also made and another 2% if rectal smears were taken from the consorts of men with gonorrhoea. Lack of a culture facility will therefore result in almost half of the cases being missed. In this situation it is mandatory to treat the female consorts of men with gonorrhoea on a presumptive basis.

Chlamydial infection cannot be confirmed or excluded without culture or fluorescent monoclonal antibody staining (pp. 1109, 1110).

The comprehensive routine for STD screening (described above) can be carried out fully in only a few large centres in the tropics. In most other areas/situations, depending upon the facilities available, compromises have to be made. Thus, in the absence of even microscopy, patients will have to be diagnosed on clinical and epidemiological information. Moreover, if high frequencies of certain conditions associated with vaginal discharge can be demonstrated, such as over 10–20% of women with vaginal discharge found to be harbouring *N. gonorrhoeae*, and/or *T. vaginalis* in some tropical areas, then simple treatment protocols could be formulated by the experts for use at local level. An example of a protocol for the situation just mentioned would include gonorrhoea treatment of all women with vaginal discharge (without abdominal pain) as the first management step. These protocols can be made even more 'scientific' by incorporating (a) clinical signs if examination of the patient by an appropriately trained person is possible, and (b) whatever laboratory tests are possible. The effectiveness of these protocols should be periodically monitored. Changes in STD pattern and in antimicrobial susceptibility may render them obsolete. It must be emphasized that the protocols not backed by appropriate clinical and laboratory findings should be considered as stopgaps while efforts to achieve improved standards are continuing.

LABORATORY METHODS FOR THE DIAGNOSIS OF GONOCOCCAL AND CHLAMYDIAL INFECTIONS

Gonococcal infections

Gram-stained urethral smears detect the characteristic intracellular diplococci accurately in over

95% of males with gonococcal urethral discharge. However, the sensitivity of the gram-staining method for material from other sites such as the cervix and rectum even in experienced hands is reduced to less than 65%. Cultures are, therefore, essential to confirm or exclude gonococcal infection in females and passive homosexuals. Culture and further identification are also essential to diagnose gonococcal infection of the pharynx which may harbour other commensal *Neisseria* species.

Smear

GRAM-STAINING METHOD

Stain the fixed smear with 1% crystal violet for 20 seconds; rinse with tap water; pour on Gram's iodine and leave for 20 seconds; rinse with tap water; decolorize with acetone or alcohol for a few seconds until the fluid flowing out is colourless; wash with tap water; counterstain with safranine or carbol fuchsin for 10 seconds or with neutral red for 60 seconds; blot dry and examine under a microscope using the oil immersion lens. Gonococci appear as gram-negative bean-shaped intracellular diplococci. The smear should be reported as inconclusive if only extracellular diplococci are found.

METHYLENE BLUE STAINING METHOD

The air-dried and fixed smear is covered with the methylene blue stain for one minute; the slide is then washed with water, allowed to dry and examined under the microscope using the oil immersion lens. This method is quicker than gram-staining but the disadvantages are that (a) the methylene blue solution has to be kept in darkness at 4°C until use, and (b) it does not allow the determination of gram-staining characteristic of gonococci.

Culture

The material for *N. gonorrhoeae* is obtained with an appropriate loop or swab inserted into the required site(s) and the swab rotated several times.

Modified Thayer–Martin medium is the one most commonly used. The immediate direct inoculation of a specimen on to the culture plates is the most satisfactory procedure. The plate is then incubated at 35–37°C for 24–48 hours in an atmosphere of 3–10% carbon dioxide—the former level can be achieved by using a candle jar. A moistened pad kept in the jar will ensure the maintenance of moisture, an essential requirement.

When direct inoculation is not possible or the laboratory is some distance from the health centre, the material for culture should be obtained on a charcoal impregnated swab which should be sent to the laboratory in Stuart's transport medium. The bottles or the tubes containing the swab in the transport medium should preferably be stored at 4°C until despatched to the laboratory, so as to allow the isolation of gonococci from over 90% of the cases provided the delay of cultivation is not longer than 24 hours.

Colonies are positively identified by colonial morphology, the oxidase test and fermentation reactions.

Slide agglutination methods using antigonococcal antibodies are replacing the tedious fermentation reactions in some laboratories.

Penicillinase (or β-lactamase) production can be tested by using the starch paper method or by the chromogenic cephalosporin test.

Chlamydial infections

Culture

Isolation of *C. trachomatis* is the best method for the diagnosis of chlamydial infections. The procedure is possible only where the facilities for tissue culture are available. The samples are obtained by rotating a swab against the infected mucous membrane such as the endocervix, urethra, rectum, lower tarsal conjunctivae and nasopharynx. In the case of suspected lymphogranuloma venereum, the material is obtained from a genital ulcer and/or bubo aspirate. Culture swabs in the transport medium are stored at −70°C until inoculated into cycloheximide treated McCoy cell monolayers on coverslips in universal containers. (If swabs are refrigerated at 4°C they should be cultured within 24 hours.) After centrifugation and appropriate incubation the infected coverslips are stained with Giemsa reagent and examined for inclusions.

Smear

Direct staining is only useful (with claims of success in 60–95% of cases) in diagnosing acute ophthalmia neonatorum. The scrapings are obtained from the conjunctival epithelium, stained with Giemsa's stain and examined with a microscope for dark purple chlamydial inclusions.

Serology

The microimmunofluorescence test (MIF) is much more sensitive than the complement fixation test (CFT). These tests are often helpful in the diagnosis of lymphogranuloma venereum (p. 1114) and they are useful in epidemiological studies. However, because of the high back-ground prevalence rate of antibody in sexually active populations, they are of little use as a routine diagnostic tool.

Newer non-culture tests, using monoclonal antibody, for *C. trachomatis* and *N. gonorrhoeae* are being evaluated for wider application.

(The direct immunofluorescent tests using monoclonal antibody for the rapid detection of *C. trachomatis* takes only up to 30 minutes, but the cost may be high. Other problems include those of interpreting fluorescence, and mental fatigue if a large number of slides have to be examined.)

PELVIC INFECTION

Pelvic infection is a microbial inflammatory process involving the uterine endometrium, fallopian tubes, ovaries, parametria and pelvic peritoneum. The other names for this condition include pelvic inflammatory disease (PID), salpingitis, salpingo-oophoritis, adnexitis, and pelvic sepsis.

Pelvic infection is a major cause of ectopic pregnancy, infertility and chronic pelvic pain. A high proportion of gynaecological admissions to hospitals in tropical countries are caused by pelvic infection.

PATHOGENESIS AND AETIOLOGY OF SEXUALLY TRANSMITTED PELVIC INFECTION

The infection originates in the cervix and ascends along the surface of the endometrium into the fallopian tubes resulting in endosalpingitis. In some cases the damaged tissue may subsequently be invaded by the endogenous cervicovaginal bacteria. Thus the aetiology is often poly-microbial and the organisms include:

1 *Sexually transmitted agents: N. gonorrhoeae, C. trachomatis,* and *Mycoplasma hominis.*
2 *Endogenous bacteria* (usually implicated in the more severe cases of pelvic infection): *Bacteroides, Peptococcus,* anaerobic streptococcus, *Escherichia coli.*

Predisposing factors include a past history of pelvic infection, young age, multiple sex partners, intrauterine contraceptive device (IUCD), dilatation and curettage, hysterosalpingography and primitive midwifery.

(Postpartum and postabortion ascending infections are usually related to lack of hygiene and poor obstetrical care, and cause exosalpingitis.)

CLINICAL FEATURES

The presenting symptoms include lower abdominal pain, menstrual disturbances, dyspareunia, fever, vaginal discharge, and backache. An occasional patient may complain of pain in the right hypochondrium associated with perihepatitis as a result of retrocolic or transperitoneal spread of infection from the fallopian tubes.

Clinical examination should include general physical, genital and pelvic examination.

DIAGNOSIS

The classic clinical criteria for diagnosis of pelvic infection include lower abdominal pain, fever, mucopurulent endocervical discharge, cervical motion tenderness, adnexal tenderness and leukocytosis. In the absence of confirmation by laparoscopy, possible in only a few large centres, overdiagnosis and underdiagnosis will occur. Insistence on rigid clinical diagnostic criteria will miss some of the subacute cases.

The main conditions to be considered in the differential diagnosis are: ectopic pregnancy, cystitis, appendicitis, torsion or rupture of an ovarian cyst, peptic ulcer, ovarian tumour, endometriosis and diverticulitis as well as filariasis, schistosomiasis, typhoid and dysentery. Peri-hepatitis will have to be differentiated from cholecystitis, subphrenic abscess, pleurisy, pneumonia, acute pyelonephritis, pancreatitis and perforated peptic ulcer. In a patient with perihepatitis, laparoscopy will show violin-string adhesions between the anterior surface of the liver and the anterior abdominal wall.

Laboratory tests

Depending upon the facilities available, the material is collected from the endocervix, urethra, and rectum with cotton-wool-tipped swabs, and if at all possible from the fimbrial end of the fallopian tubes. Some workers also perform culdocentesis. Gram-stained smears are examined for gram-negative intracellular diplo-cocci and cultures are made for *N. gonorrhoeae*, *C. trachomatis* and other organisms.

The blood count may show poly-morphonuclear leukocytosis and the erythrocyte sedimentation rate is raised.

TREATMENT

The patient should be admitted if: severely ill; oral therapy is not possible; pelvic abscess is suspected; diagnosis is in doubt; response to out-patient therapy is not satisfactory.

Treatment should be started immediately without waiting for the results of laboratory tests, and modified, if necessary, after the laboratory results are available. The aetiology being poly-microbial in many cases, a combination of anti-biotics is used.

Mild cases (patients not requiring hospitalization)

Treat as for gonococcal infection with a single dose (p. 1104), followed by:
doxycycline, 100 mg by mouth twice daily, for 10–14 days;
OR tetracycline hydrochloride, 500 mg by mouth four times daily, for 10–14 days.

Moderately severe cases (patient febrile and/or with palpable adnexal swelling)

Treat as above,
PLUS metronidazole, 400 mg by mouth three times daily for 10 days.

Severely ill patients (patient appears toxic, has peritonitis, oral therapy not possible)

(General measures include rest, analgesics, maintenance of fluid and electrolyte balance.)

Doxycycline, 100 mg intravenously twice daily,
PLUS cefoxitin, 2 g intravenously four times daily,* for 3–4 days;
OR metronidazole, 1 g intravenously twice daily, for 3–4 days;
followed by: doxycycline 100 mg orally twice daily for 10 days, and metronidazole, 400 mg orally thrice daily for 7 days.

Many physicians advocate removal of any IUCD 24–48 hours after the antimicrobial therapy is commenced. Others recommend its removal only if response to treatment is unsat-isfactory. The removal of the IUCD will necessi-tate contraceptive counselling.

Severely ill patients should be observed care-fully to assess response to treatment, and to detect complications, such as pelvic abscess, requiring surgery. Those found initially to be harbouring gonococci should be re-examined 3 days, 7 days, and 14 days after the start of therapy and swabs repeated to ensure eradication of gonococci.

Patients should be advised to abstain from sexual intercourse for three weeks. Male partners who may often be asymptomatic should be exam-ined and appropriately treated for gonococcal and/or non-gonococcal (such as chlamydial) infection.

---

* Cefoxitin (which is also active against *Bacteroides fragilis*) or an alternative cephalosporin is to be preferred if the incidence of penicillinase-producing *N. gonorrhoeae* in the area is high.

OPHTHALMIA NEONATORUM (see also Chapter 70, p. 1146)

Ophthalmia neonatorum (or conjunctivitis in the newborn) is defined as any conjunctivitis with discharge from the eyes during the first 28 days of life.

AETIOLOGY AND INCIDENCE

N. gonorrhoeae is the most serious cause of con-junctivitis in the newborn, and is considered to be more common than the other sexually transmitted agent, *C. trachomatis*, in the tropics. The two infections may coexist. The true incidence of gonococcal or chlamydial conjunctivitis is unknown, but has been estimated to be 5–50 per 1000 live births in some African countries. The infection with either of these agents occurs by direct contact with infected cervical secretions during delivery.

Other bacterial causes, often acquired in the hospital or from the infant's skin or bowel, include *Staphylococcus aureus*, *Streptococcus pneumoniae*, *Escherichia coli*, *Haemophilus*, *Klebsiella*, *Proteus* and *Pseudomonas* spp.

CLINICAL FEATURES

Gonococcal ophthalmia

The incubation period is usually less than 7 days. The condition is often bilateral, starting with watery or slightly bloodstained discharge which rapidly becomes mucopurulent or frankly purulent. There is severe inflammation and swelling of the eyelids (Fig. 68.4). The pus which is under tension behind the oedematous eyelids may spurt out when the lids are separated. Hence the medical attendants should protect their own eyes when opening these infants' lids for examination.

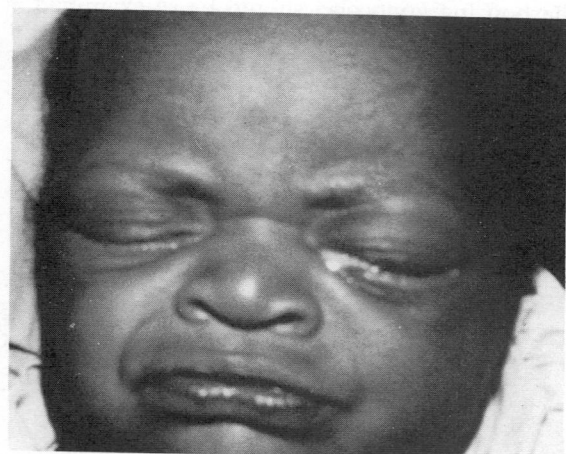

Fig. 68.4   Gonococcal ophthalmia neonatorum.

The severity varies considerably. If untreated, the condition may progress to corneal ulceration, perforation and eventually blindness. Gonococcal septicaemia is a rare complication.

Chlamydial ophthalmia

The incubation period is 5–14 days. The condition is unilateral in almost half of the cases, and usually less severe than gonococcal opthalmia. The infant develops sticky eyes followed by oedema of the lids and conjunctival inflammation (Fig. 68.5). The discharge is thin, watery or mucoid, sometimes mucopurulent which may become purulent especially in the presence of secondary infection. In some cases the condition may resolve spontaneously after several weeks while others may eventually develop trachoma-like changes. Infection may also spread to other tissues and result in neonatal pneumonia.

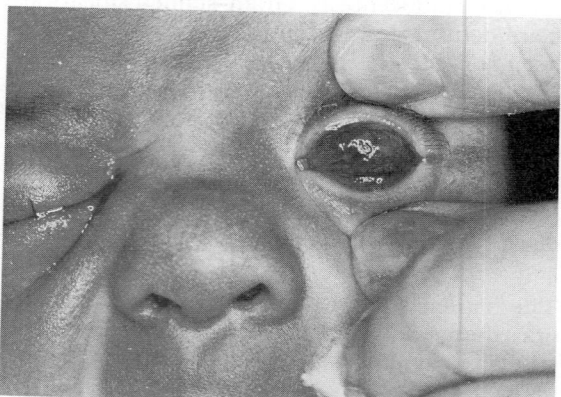

Fig. 68.5   Chlamydial ophthalmia. (Courtesy Dr Elisabeth Rees.)

MANAGEMENT

The background information necessary to plan appropriate management policy includes the prevalence of gonococcal and chlamydial infections in pregnant women and sensitivity of local strains to antimicrobials.

Diagnosis (with laboratory facilities)

A gram-stained smear of conjunctival exudate will show numerous polymorphonuclear leukocytes and will help to differentiate gonococcal from non-gonococcal aetiology depending upon the presence or absence of gram-negative intracellular diplococci. Some use methylene blue stain (p. 1109).

A diagnosis of chlamydial infection may be made by the demonstration of intracytoplasmic inclusions in a smear of conjunctival scrapings (from the lower tarsal conjunctiva) stained with Giemsa. Adequate sample of epithelial cells is essential (see also p. 1108).

Swabs for culturing *N. gonorrhoeae*, *C. trachomatis* (p. 1109) and other organisms should also be obtained. For the isolation of *N. gonorrhoeae* from cases of ophthalmia neonatorum, selective media are not necessary; a non-selective medium such as an enriched chocolate agar is satisfactory.

Treatment of gonococcal ophthalmia (or presumed gonococcal ophthalmia)

1 Hospitalize and isolate for 24 hours.

2a If prevalence of PPNG is less than 1%:
aqueous crystalline penicillin G (30 mg/kg), intramuscularly divided into two doses daily for 3 days,
OR aqueous procaine penicillin G (50 mg/kg), intramuscularly once daily for 3 days.
PLUS after swabbing away pus:
flood conjunctivae with crystalline penicillin eye drops, 1 mega unit/ml, repeat after 15 minutes and then after each feed for 3 days;[2]
OR apply tetracycline 1% eye ointment to both eyes (placed on the exposed conjunctiva of the lower lid) every hour for 24 hours, every 3 hours during the second day and then four times daily for 8 days.[3]

2b If prevalence of PPNG is more than 1% or gonococcal resistance pattern is unknown:
cefotaxime, 100 mg/kg intramuscularly (single dose),
OR kanamycin 25 mg/kg intramuscularly (single dose).
PLUS tetracycline 1% eye ointment four times daily for 7 days.

2c The following regimen has been found to be effective against ocular as well as extraocular gonococcal infection concurrent in some cases:
ceftriaxone, 125 mg intramuscularly (single dose) plus ocular washes with cooled, boiled water four times daily until the eyes are free of discharge.[4]

Treatment of chlamydial ophthalmia (or presumed chlamydial ophthalmia)

Erythromycin syrup, 50 mg/kg in two to four divided doses daily for 14 days,
PLUS tetracycline 1% eye ointment into both eyes, four times daily for 14 days.

Diagnosis and treatment without laboratory facilities

In the absence of laboratory facilities, the diagnosis will have to be made on clinical and epidemiological evidence. However, such diagnosis may not be accurate. Mixed infections may also occur. Hence in these circumstances, treatment should first be directed to the potentially more serious aetiological agent, i.e. *N. gonorrhoeae* (see above).

Treatment of parents

Both parents should be examined, investigated and treated. If left untreated, the mother may develop puerperal complications such as pelvic infection. The father, who may also be asymptomatic, may still have demonstrable urethral discharge and thus provide circumstantial evidence of the sexually acquired infection.

Follow-up tests should be performed between 3 and 7 days after completion of treatment.

PREVENTION OF OPHTHALMIA NEONATORUM

1 Routine screening for gonococcal and chlamydial infection in the antenatal clinics (of all or selected women) may not be possible if culture facilities are not available.

2 Disinfection of the infant's conjunctivae at birth:

(a) *Credé's method.* After the head is born, the eyes are cleaned before they are opened; one to two drops of 1% aqueous silver nitrate solution are then instilled into each conjunctival sac. Its limitations are: it is not effective against *C. trachomatis*; the protection against gonococcal infection is not 100% but probably better than erythromycin or tetracycline for the penicillinase-producing *N. gonorrhoeae*; it may cause chemical conjunctivitis.

(b) *Benzylpenicillin solution* may sensitize, may promote penicillin resistance, and is ineffective against penicillin-resistant strains as well as *C. trachomatis*.

(c) *Tetracycline (1%) eye ointment.*

(d) *Erythromycin (0.5%) eye ointment.*

Although highly effective in the prevention of chlamydial ophthalmia, (c) and (d) may not prevent nasopharyngeal colonization of *C. trachomatis*; some gonococcal strains may be resistant.

GENITAL ULCER DISEASE

AETIOLOGY AND DISTRIBUTION

Genital ulcer(s) is a presenting symptom in 20–70% of patients seen in clinics for STDs in some tropical countries. The aetiology, which may be infectious or non-infectious (e.g. various traumatic and septic lesions and fixed drug eruption), varies with geographic areas. The main sexually transmitted agents which cause genital ulcers are: *Haemophilus ducreyi*, *Treponema pallidum*, herpes simplex virus, *Chlamydia trachomatis* (L1, L2, L3 strains) and *Calymmatobacterium granulomatis*. A variety of aerobic and anaerobic bacteria may also be isolated from the genital ulcers but their significance is unknown. However, erosive balanitis, usually seen in uncircumcised men, presenting with oedematous phimotic prepuce and foul smelling purulent subpreputial discharge, is often associated with *Bacteroides* spp, fusobacteria and non-syphilitic spirochaetes. The condition will respond to metronidazole or co-trimoxazole tablets together with clo-trimazole cream or subpreputial irrigation with saline. Spirochaetal balanoposthitis may be treated with benzathine penicillin using the same dose as that for primary syphilis (p. 1120).

In almost 25% of the patients with genital ulcers no specific cause may be found.

Chancroid is the most common cause of genital ulcers in South-East Asia and Africa. Syphilis, herpes and lymphogranuloma venereum (LGV) are encountered in all tropical areas but generally less frequently than chancroid. Granuloma inguinale (donovanosis) is more commonly seen in Papua New Guinea and India than in Africa and the Caribbean.

Most genital ulcer cases presenting to the clinic are heterosexual males, perhaps because the lesions (which may be painless) in many of the homosexuals who practise anal intercourse and in females are out of sight.

usually disappeared by the time the patient attends the clinic. The lesion may occur anywhere in the genital and anorectal area. In men the most common site of occurrence is the coronal sulcus. If in the meatus or urethra, the lesion may be asymptomatic or the patient may notice scanty urethral discharge. In women, the sites commonly affected include the fourchette, the posterior vaginal wall and the posterior lip of the cervix. Some patients, particularly women, may present with lower abdominal pain because of the involvement of pelvic and lumbar lymph glands. Rectal infection may cause anal pruritus and rectal discharge.

The most frequent manifestation, and more common in males than in females (because of the site involved and lymphatic drainage), is inguinal lymphadenopathy. It begins as a firm mass involving several groups of lymph nodes, soon becoming attached to the skin and subcutaneous tissue. The swelling then becomes fluctuant and painful. This stage may be associated with systemic spread of the lymphogranuloma venereum organisms.

The involvement of the lymph glands above and below the inguinal ligament may produce a characteristic groove sign.

Untreated, the condition may continue to progress in some cases and involve deeper tissues. The external genitalia may become swollen due to an active chronic inflammatory process as well as lymphatic stasis. The sequelae include elephantiasis of the external genitalia, ulceration, sinuses and fistula formation, chronic proctitis and rectal stricture.

The differential diagnosis, in addition to the conditions in Table 68.4, will include consideration of inguinal hernia, tuberculosis, filariasis, actinomycosis, amoebiasis, schistosomiasis, Crohn's disease, ulcerative colitis, malignancy, Hodgkin's disease and other lymphomas.

CLINICAL ASPECTS OF LYMPHOGRANULOMA VENEREUM
(Figs. 68.11 and 68.12)

The incubation period in most cases is 7 to 28 days. The primary lesion, which is a vesicle or a papule, later becoming a shallow ulcer, has

CLINICAL ASPECTS OF DONOVANOSIS (Figs. 68.13 and 68.14)

After an incubation period ranging from a few days to several weeks, the primary lesion starts as an indurated painless papule which progresses to form a beefy granulomatous ulcer with hyper-

Table 68.4 Comparison of infectious genital ulcer disease.

	Syphilis	Chancroid	Herpes	Lymphogranuloma venereum	Granuloma inguinale (donovanosis)
1 Causative agent	*Treponema pallidum*	*Haemophilus ducreyi*	Herpes simplex virus	*Chlamydia trachomatis* (L1, L2, L3 strains)	*Calymmatobacterium granulomatis*
2 Incubation period	9–90 days	1–15 days	2–7 days	7–28 days	7–90 days
3 Description of lesion:					
(a) Initial appearance	Papule	Papule/pustule	Grouped vesicles	Papule/vesicle	Papule
(b) Developed appearance of ulcer(s) (number, consistency, shape and edges) (Retract prepuce to detect concealed ulcers)	Usually single, firm, circular or oval, well defined (Fig. 68.6)	Usually multiple soft, circular or oval, edges undermined and ragged (Fig. 68.7)	Usually multiple, non-indurated, coalesce to form large lesions with polycyclic borders (Figs 68.8, 9, 10)	Usually single, non-indurated, herpetiform	Single or multiple, firm, beefy, granulomatous, well-defined and raised above surrounding skin surface (Fig. 68.13)
Pain	Painless, not tender (unless secondary infection)	Usually very painful[a] and tender	Pain and tenderness[a] more often experienced in initial attack than in recurrences	Usually painless	Usually painless (unless secondary infection)
Tenderness					
Secretion	Clear serum	Haemorrhagic, purulent, sticky	Clear serum	Rare	Rare, may be haemorrhagic
4 Inguinal lymphadenopathy ('bubo') unilateral or bilateral	Painless, non-tender, discrete, firm (unless secondary infection)	Painful, tender, matted, overlying skin red, may progress to suppuration, sinus formation and spreading ulcer	Slightly painful and tender in about 50% of cases of initial infection	Initially firm, discrete, tender and later matted; may resolve or progress to softening and suppuration; 'sign of the groove' (adenopathy above and below the ligament) seen in some (Fig. 68.11)	Lymph glands not involved; inguinal swelling is subcutaneous granulomatous process (pseudo bubo)
5 Course	Spontaneous healing with or without scarring followed by latency, secondary syphilis, and further manifestations in some cases in later years	Slow healing, relapse common, lesions may progress to phagedenic ulceration in some cases; and ulcerated bubo as mentioned above	Spontaneous healing usually within 1–3 wks; recurrences common	Primary lesion transient and often escapes notice; the disease may progress to sinus and fistula formation, lymphatic obstruction and systemic changes in some cases	Lesions enlarge by local extension followed by fibrosis, tissue destruction, lymphatic obstruction, neoplastic change and metastatic spread reported
6 Diagnosis	See text (p. 1118)	See text (p. 1118)	See text (p. 1119)	See text (p. 1119)	See text (p. 1119)
7 Treatment	See text (p. 1120)	See text (p. 1120)	See text (p. 1120)	See text (p. 1120)	See text (p. 1121)

[a]Females with ulcers on the vulva may complain of burning sensation on urination.

trophic velvety granulation tissue and characteristic rolled edges. The lesion, which is well defined and elevated, often looks more like a growth than an ulcer, and bleeds easily with trauma. Occasionally, a female patient may present with vaginal bleeding because of intravaginal lesions.

The commonly affected sites include the anogenital area, the thighs and perineum. Extragenital involvement is rare and metastatic spread to bones, thorax, liver and spleen has been reported.

The inguinal lymph glands are not involved unless there is secondary infection. However, a subcutaneous granuloma in the inguinal region may be mistaken for inguinal adenopathy (pseudobubo); this may proceed to an abscess which may later rupture resulting in open ulcers.

Untreated, the lesions spread slowly. The secondary infection may contribute to large, painful, foul smelling, destructive lesions. Healing takes place by intense fibrosis and there may be elephantoid enlargement of the external genitalia

CLINICAL COMPARISON OF GENITAL ULCER DISEASE

Typical clinical and distinguishing features of the different genital ulcer diseases are shown in

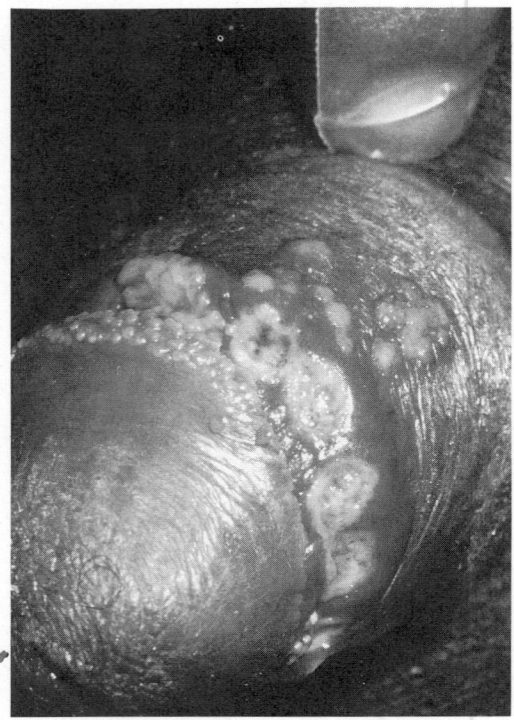

Fig. 68.7 Chancroid (mixed with herpes): multiple chancroidal ulcers and herpetic lesions on coronal sulcus and prepuce.

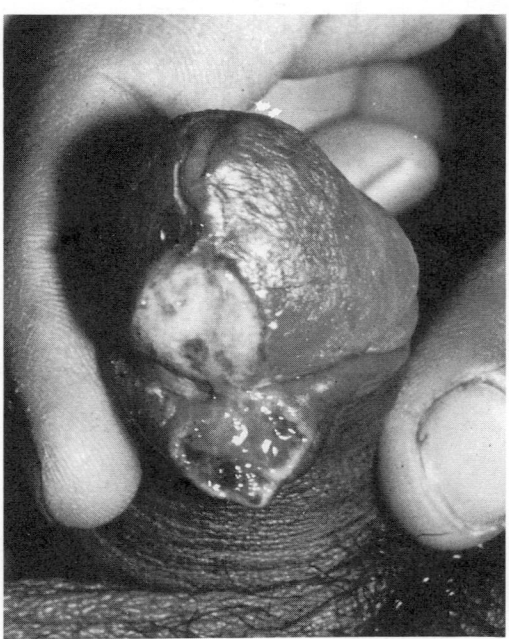

Fig. 68.6 Primary syphilis: chancre on the penis.

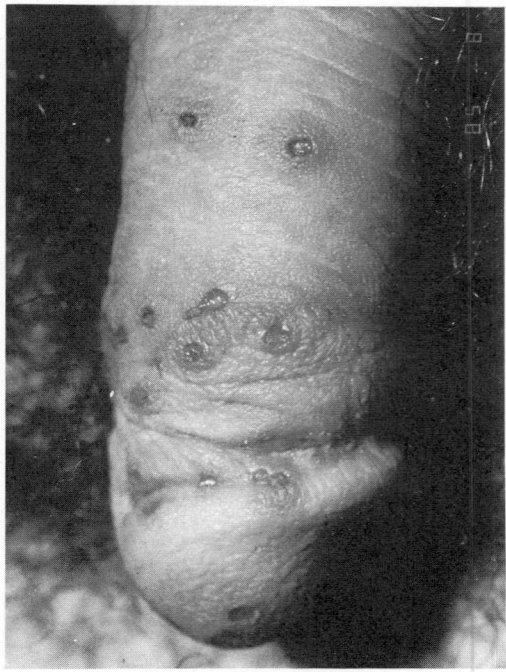

Fig. 68.8 Genital herpes: multiple lesions on the penile shaft and glans.

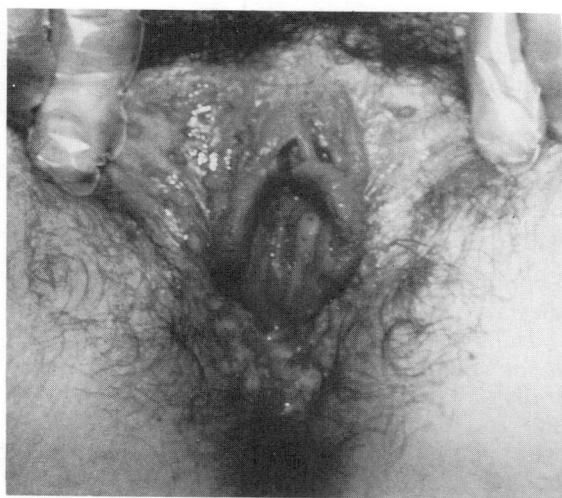

Fig. 68.9 Genital herpes: multiple lesions on the vulva. (From Arya et al,[1] courtesy Churchill Livingstone.)

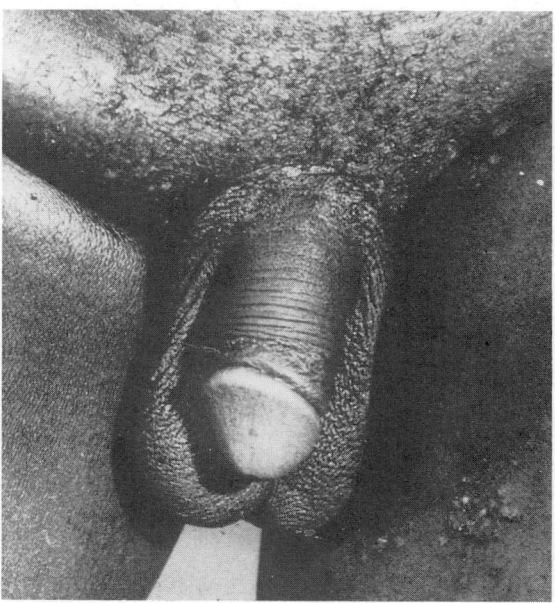

Fig. 68.11 Lymphogranuloma venereum: showing 'sign of the groove'. (From Arya et al,[1] courtesy Churchill Livingstone.)

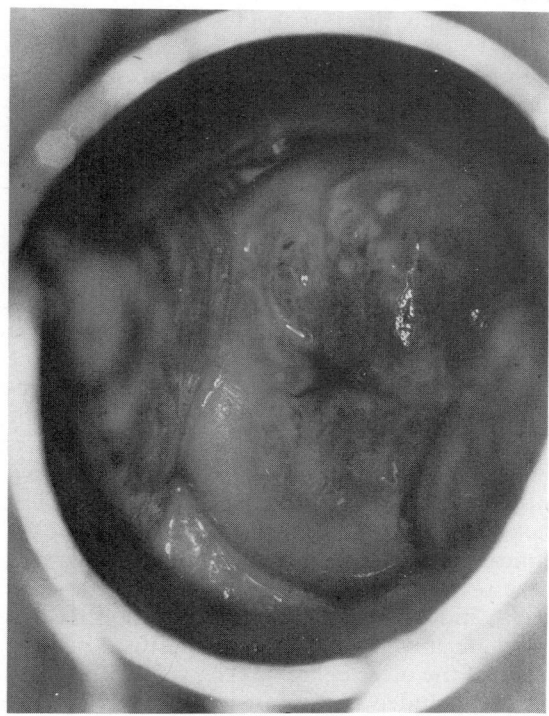

Fig. 68.10 Genital herpes: multiple lesions on the ectocervix.

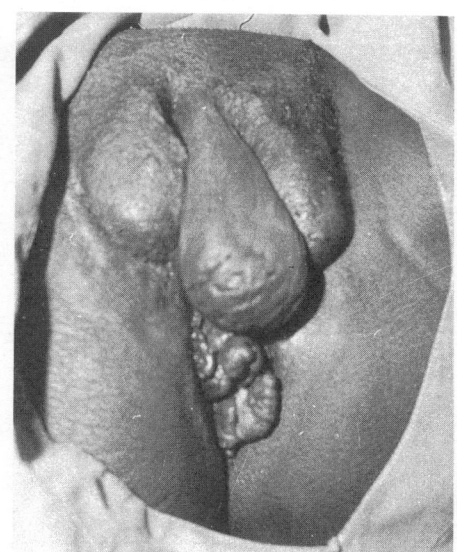

Fig. 68.12 Lymphogranuloma venereum: elephantiasis of labia majora and clitoris, and hypertrophic perineal skin tags. (From Arya et al,[1] courtesy Churchill Livingstone.)

Figs. 68.6–14 and a summary is given in Table 68.4. However, the appearance of the lesion may be affected by any treatment received, presence of secondary infection and variability in response to infection. In clinical practice atypical lesions are commonly seen. In the case of syphilis multiple lesions may occur, lesions may become painful as a result of secondary infection, and induration is not a constant feature. Syphilitic infections mixed with herpes and/or chancroid

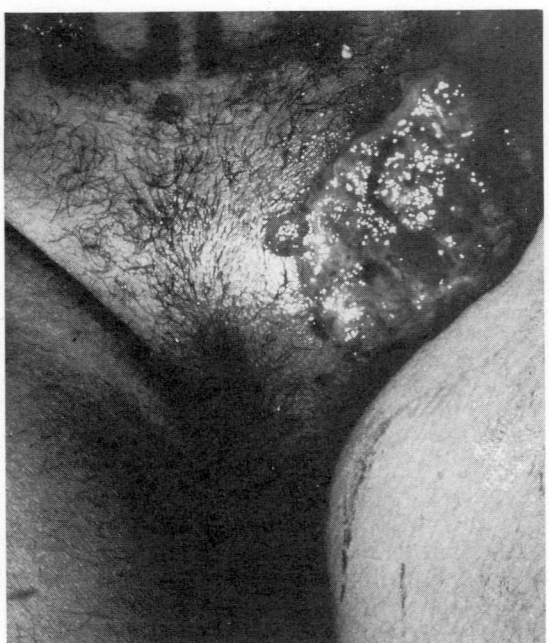

Fig. 68.13 Donovanosis: typical beefy granuloma. (Courtesy Dr I. Maddocks.)

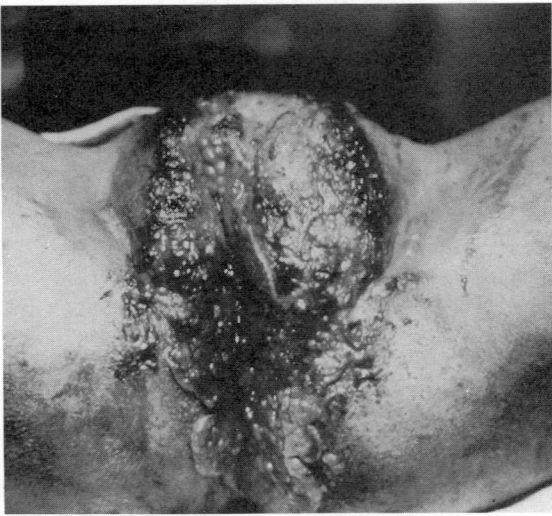

Fig. 68.14 Donovanosis: vulval lesions in the female. (Courtesy Dr J. Richens.)

are common. Primary lesions and regional adenitis may then assume different characteristics. Moreover, clinical differentiation of herpes from chancroid is often impossible. It must, therefore, be emphasized that the appearance of the lesion can only give rise to the suspicion of the aeti-

ological agent. Final diagnosis rests on the demonstration/isolation of the pathogen concerned.

LABORATORY DIAGNOSIS OF GENITAL ULCER DISEASE

Syphilis

Syphilis must be considered in all cases of genital ulcers.

Dark-field examination to demonstrate *T. pallidum* should be carried out repeatedly in clinically suspicious cases. This procedure requires skill and experience. The ulcer is gently cleansed with gauze soaked in water or saline before obtaining the serum. Rubber gloves should be worn when squeezing the lesion with the thumb and index finger. The clear serum is touched with a coverslip which is then placed on a microscope slide. *T. pallidum* will have to be differentiated from saprophytic spirochaetes which are recognized by their shape and movements. When attempts are being made to demonstrate *T. pallidum*, no topical medication other than normal saline should be applied. The only permissible systemic treatment is a sulphonamide which is non-treponemicidal, will clear many non-syphilitic lesions and facilitate dark-field examination.

Gland puncture to demonstrate *T. pallidum* should be considered if on presentation the ulcer has healed or has been treated with an antiseptic.

Serological tests for syphilis become positive at different times after the development of the initial lesion. The FTA-ABS (fluorescent treponemal antibody-absorption) test, likely to be available in only a few large teaching hospitals, is usually the first to become positive. A cardiolipin antigen test such as the RPR or VDRL test should be performed at the first attendance. If clinical or epidemiological suspicion is strong, these tests, should be repeated weekly for four weeks and then monthly for two months. An initial negative test becoming positive is diagnostic of the ulcer being due to syphilis. Syphilis can be excluded if the tests are negative at the end of three months.

Chancroid

Direct smear. The ulcer is carefully cleansed with saline-soaked gauze and the material is obtained from beneath the undermined edge and/or pus is aspirated from the bubo. The smear is then stained with Gram stain and examined under a microscope. *H. ducreyi* is a gram-negative fine short rod with rounded ends. In stained smears the organisms are often seen in a typical 'shoal of fish' or a 'rail-road track' formation. The demonstration of the causative agent by this method is not always easy because of contamination due to secondary organisms.

Culture. A definitive diagnosis can only be made by isolating *H. ducreyi* from the lesion. A useful medium is Mueller–Hinton agar base with chocolate horse blood 5%, fetal calf serum 5%, isovitalex 2%, and vancomycin 3 mg/litre. Other requirements are: high humidity, 5–10% carbon dioxide, and incubation at 33–35°C. The yellow–grey smooth dome-shaped colonies appearing 2–7 days after incubation can be pushed intact across the plate. The organisms are then easily recognized in gram-stained smears, and their identity confirmed by their positive tests for alkaline phosphatase and nitrate reduction, and negative test for porphyrin. In parts of Africa and the Far East many of the strains of *H. ducreyi* produce a plasmid mediated β-lactamase.

Herpes

Smear. The slides prepared from the scrapings of the lesions are examined for herpes simplex virus particles by an electron microscope and by fluorescent or peroxidase antibody staining.

Culture. The swab is sent to the laboratory in a viral transport medium for viral isolation in tissue culture.

Serology. Demonstration of seroconversion or fourfold rise in the serum antibody titre of the convalescent sample taken two to three weeks after the acute sample will support the diagnosis of a primary infection.

Lymphogranuloma venereum

The diagnosis is confirmed either: (a) by the isolation of lymphogranuloma venereum strains of *C. trachomatis* from the bubo aspirate or from the genital lesion (for culture method see p. 1109), or (b) by the demonstration of fourfold or greater increase in MIF or complement-fixing antibody titres. In chronic cases in whom rising titres are seldom demonstrated, the diagnosis

may be supported by high levels of MIF ($\geqslant 512$) or complement-fixing antibodies ($\geqslant 1 : 64$).

Granuloma inguinale (donovanosis)

Smear. The definitive diagnosis depends on the demonstration of the large mononuclear cells filled with intracytoplasmic gram-negative rods which have a closed safety-pin appearance (Donovan bodies) due to the characteristic bipolar staining (Fig. 68.15). A piece of granulation tissue from the edge of the lesion is crushed between two slides. The smear is air-dried and stained with Giemsa, Wright, Leishman or Gram stain, to detect Donovan bodies.

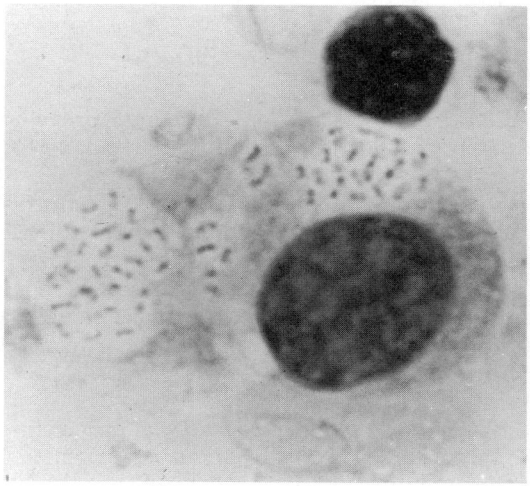

Fig. 68.15 Donovanosis: a stained biopsy specimen showing intracytoplasmic Donovan bodies. (Courtesy Dr A. Wisdom.)

MANAGEMENT OF GENITAL ULCER DISEASE IN THE ABSENCE OF LABORATORY FACILITIES

If laboratory facilities are not available, the diagnosis will have to be made on a clinical basis. Accordingly, management protocols in the form of flow charts have been proposed using typical clinical features (summarized in Table 68.4) to serve as guides in the process of differential diagnosis, leading on to the final diagnosis and thence the treatment. In this situation the margin of error, even in the hands of experienced physicians, may be considerable. Thus the accuracy of clinical diagnosis has varied from approximately

40% to 80% for syphilis, 45% to 65% for herpes and 35% to 75% for chancroid. To improve the diagnostic accuracy, and to make the management more realistic, it is advisable to validate the protocols locally, correlating epidemiological, clinical and microbiological findings. For example, if the validating study in an area showed that *H. ducreyi* was isolated from 40% of the patients with painful genital ulcers, but that over 10% of these patients also had syphilis, then it may be logical to treat all cases of genital ulcers in that area initially for both chancroid and syphilis. Clearly, the situation needs to be monitored periodically.

TREATMENT OF GENITAL ULCER DISEASE (and follow-up and treatment of contacts)

Syphilis (primary)

Treatment with penicillin. Aqueous procaine penicillin G (600 mg), intramuscularly daily for 10 days,
OR benzathine penicillin G (1.8 g), intramuscularly (900 mg into each buttock) at a single session. If the patient is thought to have a mixed infection, i.e. syphilis and chancroid, then chancroid should be treated first, otherwise penicillin administered for syphilis may be destroyed by the β-lactamase produced by *H. ducreyi*.

If the patient is allergic to penicillin. Tetracycline hydrochloride,★ 500 mg by mouth four times a day, on an empty stomach, for 15 days,
OR erythromycin,† 500 mg by mouth, four times a day for 15 days.

Follow-up. Sexual intercourse should be forbidden until treatment has been completed. If possible, the patient should be followed up and VDRL or RPR carried out at the end of three months, six months and 12 months. In a successfully treated case, the titres fall by the end of three months and the tests become negative within six months in most cases of seropositive primary syphilis.

Contacts. All contacts within the past three months should be sought out and examined.

★ Tetracycline is contraindicated in pregnancy.
† Transplacental penetration of erythromycin may be inadequate.

Those found infected should be treated. If surveillance of the others is not possible for up to three months following exposure then they should also be offered treatment (with the regimen similar to that administered to the index patient) after appropriate explanation.

Chancroid

1 Locally, use only saline until dark-field examinations for *T. pallidum* have been carried out.
2 Trimethoprim (80 mg)/sulphamethoxazole (400 mg), two tablets twice daily for 7 days. Treatment failures have been observed with this regimen in some areas.
OR erythromycin, 500 mg by mouth four times daily for 7 days,
OR trimethoprim/sulfametrole, 8 tablets (640/3200 mg) at a single session,
OR thiamphenicol, 2.5 g by mouth daily for 2 days,
OR ceftriaxone, 250 mg by intramuscular injection.
(There are limited data on the efficacy of trimethoprim/sulfametrole, thiamphenicol and ceftriaxone.)
3 Aspiration of fluctuant bubo through healthy skin using a wide-bore needle.
4 Examine and treat sexual partners.

Herpes

Symptomatic treatment. Application of salt solution, analgesics, treat concomitant candidiasis which aggravates symptoms in females, suprapubic catheterization if patient develops retention of urine (more common in females).

Antiviral treatment (consider only for patients with severe initial episode). *Acyclovir*: topical cream five times a day for 5–10 days,
OR oral—one tablet (200 mg), five times a day for 5 days (preferred treatment for most patients),
OR parenteral—5 mg/kg 8-hourly for 5 days (by slow intravenous infusion).

Lymphogranuloma venereum

1 Tetracycline hydrochloride, 500 mg by mouth on empty stomach, four times daily for 14 days,
OR erythromycin, 500 mg by mouth, four times daily for 14 days,

OR doxycycline, 100 mg by mouth, twice daily for 14 days.
2 Aspirate fluctuant lymph nodes through healthy adjacent skin.
3 Examine and treat sexual partners.

Granuloma inguinale (donovanosis)

Trimethoprim (80 mg)/sulphamethoxazole (400 mg), two tablets by mouth twice daily for 14 days,

OR tetracycline hydrochloride, 500 mg by mouth on an empty stomach four times daily for 14 days,
OR chloramphenicol, 500 mg by mouth four times daily for 21 days,
OR gentamicin, 1 mg/kg intramuscularly three times daily for 21 days.
(A combination of lincomycin, 500 mg by mouth four times daily, and erythromycin, 500 mg by mouth four times daily for 14 days, has been found to be satisfactory for pregnant patients.)

SEXUALLY TRANSMITTED DISEASES IN HOMOSEXUALS

In most large cities male homosexuals and bisexuals are of epidemiological importance in the spread of STDs, because: (a) often a variety of sexual practices and a large number of sexual partners are involved, and (b) some of the sites of infection may produce few or no symptoms. Anorectal and pharyngeal chancres, and gonococcal and non-gonococcal infection of the pharynx and rectum may be asymptomatic. On the other hand, in some patients gonococcal pharyngitis may cause sore throat, rectal infection may be associated with tenesmus, mucopus and blood, and anorectal herpes may cause severe discomfort. Homosexuals are susceptible to all STDs and particularly at risk of hepatitis, intestinal infections (*Entamoeba histolytica*, *Giardia lamblia*, *Enterobius vermicularis*, *Salmonella typhi*

and *Shigella sonnei*) and AIDS. Anal warts in them are more common than penile warts.

Quite clearly, it is important to obtain an accurate history as regards sexual orientation and sexual practices. This is followed by careful examination, obtaining swabs from all of the appropriate anatomical sites and other samples including blood for serological tests.

ACKNOWLEDGEMENTS

I am indebted to Churchill Livingstone for permission to reproduce Figs. 68.1, 9, 11 and 12 and to draw material from *Tropical Venereology* (Arya, Osoba and Bennett, 1st edn, 1980; 2nd edn in press). I am grateful to Dr Elisabeth Rees for Fig. 68.5, Dr I. Maddocks for Fig. 68.13, Dr J. Richens for Fig. 68.14 and Dr A. Wisdom for Fig. 68.15.

INFECTION WITH HUMAN IMMUNODEFICIENCY VIRUS (HIV) AND ACQUIRED IMMUNODEFICIENCY SYNDROME (AIDS) IN THE TROPICS

Peter Piot

INTRODUCTION

The acquired immunodeficiency syndrome (AIDS) was first described in the USA in 1981.[5] By the end of 1986, over 30 000 cases have been reported from all continents. These figures grossly underestimate the extent of the problem, particularly in some parts of Africa, where several thousands of cases are not being recognized or reported. AIDS has now become an international health concern involving the industrialized and the developing countries.

AIDS is an infectious disease caused by human immunodeficiency virus (HIV). For surveillance purposes AIDS is defined as an illness characterized by the presence of a reliably diagnosed disease at least moderately predictive of cellular immunodeficiency, and by the absence of an underlying cause for immunodeficiency or any defined cause for reduced resistance to the disease.[6] Diseases at least moderately predictive of cellular immunodeficiency are listed in Table 68.5. In addition to AIDS, HIV causes a broad spectrum of clinical diseases as described below.

Table 68.5 Opportunistic infections at least moderately predictive of cellular immunodeficiency.[6]

1 *Protozoal and helminthic infections*
  Intestinal cryptosporidiosis (for over 1 month)
  Pneumocystis carinii pneumonia
  Strongyloidosis: pneumonia, central nervous system infection or disseminated infection
  Toxoplasmosis: infection in internal organs other than liver, spleen, or lymph nodes
2 *Fungal infections*
  Candidiasis: oesophagitis
  Cryptococcosis: central nervous system or disseminated infection
3 *Viral infections*
  Cytomegalovirus causing infection in internal organs other than liver, spleen, or lymph nodes
  Herpes simplex virus causing chronic mucocutaneous infection with ulcers (for over 1 month), or pulmonary, gastrointestinal or disseminated infection
4 Progressive multifocal leukoencephalopathy
5 *Cancer*
  Kaposi's sarcoma
  Lymphoma limited to the brain
6 *Other opportunistic infections with positive tests for HIV*
  In the absence of the above opportunistic diseases, any of the following is indicative of AIDS if the patient has a positive test for HIV:
    disseminated histoplasmosis
    bronchial or pulmonary candidiasis
    isosporiasis (for over 1 month)
7 *Chronic lymphoid interstitial pneumonia* (in children <13 years)

GEOGRAPHICAL DISTRIBUTION

Infection with HIV is occurring in all continents, but the major foci are in North America, the Caribbean, Europe and Africa.

The intensity of AIDS and HIV infection in the Caribbean and Africa is difficult to assess, because surveillance for the syndrome is poorly developed and because diagnostic capabilities for AIDS and associated opportunistic diseases are often limited.

Among Haitian immigrants entering the USA after 1977, the cumulative incidence rate of AIDS was 101 per 100 000 population in 1984.[7] The major cities of central Africa and to a lesser degree of adjacent East Africa, are most severely affected, but the disease is said to be also common in rural Uganda and north-west Tanzania.[8, 9] AIDS has now become a public health problem in these countries. Thus, the estimated annual AIDS incidence rates in Kinshasa, Zaire (1983, 1984), and Kigali, Rwanda (1983) were 170 to 500 per million, and 800 per million population,

respectively.[10–12] In Kinshasa in 1984–1985, peak incidence rates were 786/million and 601/million for 30–39-year-old men and women (Table 68.6).[11] In Haiti and Africa the male-to-female ratios are 1.8 : 1 and approximately 1 : 1, respectively. Women with AIDS are generally younger than men.[11, 13, 14]

Table 68.6 Annual incidence rates of AIDS among adult Kinshasa residents (1984–1985) (From Mann et al).[11]

Age group	Cases/million adults	
	Men	Women
20–29	155	417
30–39	786	601
40–49	748	180
50–59	337	83
>60	168	0
Total	365	394

(Reproduced with permission from the author from *J. Am. med. Assoc.* (1986) **255**, 3255–3259.)

Seroprevalence rates among the general population in Africa range from 0.5% to 18% among blood donors, and are as high as 27% to 88% in high risk groups such as prostitutes.[15–17] Among the healthy population of Kinshasa the age specific seroprevalence rates exhibit a bimodal curve with a peak prevalence under one year and between 16 and 29 years of age—a pattern suggestive of a sexually transmitted infection and of passive antibody transfer and transmission of virus from mother to child. The seroprevalence rate in the age group 16 to 29 years was significantly higher in women than in men.[17]

The seroprevalence rates among the general population in Nairobi and Kinshasa increased slowly, but steadily over time, with an annual incidence rate of HIV antibody of 0.75% in Kinshasa.[17, 18] However, the fulminant rise in HIV seropositivity among prostitutes in Nairobi from 4% to 59% between 1981 and 1985 demonstrates the rapid dissemination in a high risk population of heterosexuals, similar to that observed among homosexual men in the USA.[16]

It is difficult, if not impossible, to define when HIV appeared in Africa or Haiti. Whereas isolated case reports and the results of some retrospective serum surveys suggest that HIV may have existed earlier in Africa,[17, 19] it is clear from the study of hospital records in Africa and Europe, and of some sentinel markers of AIDS such as cryptococcosis and generalized Kaposi's sarcoma, that the current epidemic of AIDS in central Africa started also during the late 1970s and early 1980s.[17, 20] There is evidence for recent geographic spread of HIV infection from the central African focus to other parts of Africa.[17]

HUMAN IMMUNODEFICIENCY VIRUS

The cause of AIDS, HIV (previously designated as lymphadenopathy associated virus (LAV) or human T lymphotropic virus type III (HTLV-III)), is a retrovirus which belongs to the Lentiviridae as based on morphology, reverse transcriptase production and nucleic acid composition.[21] Important biological properties of HIV include the presence of a reverse transcriptase, an enzyme enabling this RNA virus to make a DNA copy of its genome, the integration of viral DNA into the genome of the host cell, and the preferential infection of T lymphocytes with the helper phenotype (OKT4/Leu 3a$^+$).[21, 22] HIV infection of helper T lymphocytes may result in cell destruction, but the virus may also remain in a state of latency in the lymphocytes or replicate without causing any obvious cell damage or clinical disease. It is thought that infected individuals carry the virus for life.

HIV has been isolated from lymphocytes, cell-free blood, semen, cervicovaginal secretions, brain tissue, cerebrospinal fluid, saliva, tears, breast milk, urine and bone marrow, and can probably be isolated from other tissues, body fluids, secretions and excretions.

Typical HIV strains have been isolated from African patients with AIDS or AIDS-related complex (ARC).[23] However, when compared with isolates from Europe and North America, African isolates as a group were more heterogeneous by restriction map analysis.[24, 25] African strains had more unique genomic restriction sites and 40% less conserved sites, with most of the genomic variability occurring in the *env* region encoding for the envelope glycoproteins.

Retroviruses related to, but clearly distinct from HIV by protein analysis, were isolated from West Africans. Viral isolates designated as HTLV-IV were recovered from healthy Senegalese prostitutes, and cross reacted serologically with HIV, but more strongly with STLV-III$_{AGM}$, a retrovirus found in *Cercopithecus* sp. (green monkey).[26] Another retrovirus referred to as LAV2 was isolated from AIDS patients from Cape Verde and Guinea-Bissau, whose sera cross reacted more strongly with STLV-III$_{MAC}$, a retrovirus isolated from macaques with immunodeficiency, than with HIV.[27] Preliminary results from protein analysis suggest further divergence among HIV, LAV-2 and HTLV-IV within the envelope gene.

TRANSMISSION

HIV is transmitted by sexual contact (heterosexual or homosexual), administration of infected blood or blood products, contaminated injections, and from infected mothers to their infants.[7] In contrast to North America and Europe where the overwhelming majority of AIDS cases acquired the disease by homosexual contact or were intravenous drug addicts, bidirectional heterosexual transmission is the major mode of infection in Africa.[9, 10, 12, 19] In Haiti, a shift in risk factors has been observed between 1983 and 1986, with significantly less cases being homosexual, bisexual or intravenous drug abusers in 1983, and proportionally more being women in 1986.[14]

In case control studies, AIDS cases had a higher number of heterosexual partners than controls and had sex more often with female prostitutes. The risk of seropositivity increased with the number of different sex partners and with a history of sexually transmitted diseases.[17, 28] Prostitutes probably play an important role in the spread of the infection.[15, 29] Specific sexual practices such as anal intercourse were not associated with HIV infection. However, disruption of genital epithelial integrity (such as by genital infections or trauma) was a risk factor for HIV infection.[29, 30]

Other risk factors for HIV infection in the developing world include blood transfusions, injections with contaminated needles and syringes, scarifications, and perinatal mother-to-infant transmission. Male homosexuality and intravenous drug abuse seem to be much less important routes of HIV transmission. As a result of HIV infection in women, perinatal transmission is increasingly occurring in Africa. In one study among hospitalized children between two and 14 years of age, 11% were seropositive.[11] The efficiency of perinatal transmission is estimated at 25–50%. The infection may be acquired in utero, or during or shortly after birth. The natural history of perinatal infection is not known.

The potential risk to transfusion recipients in

central Africa is high compared with Europe, as estimated from HIV seropositivity rates among blood donors. Between 9% and 31% of adult and paediatric AIDS patients had a history of blood transfusion.[11,17] Because they need frequent transfusions, patients with sickle cell anaemia may be at high risk for AIDS.[31] Injections with contaminated needles and syringes, and scarifications may play a significant role in the transmission of HIV in Africa, since they were consistently a risk factor in seroprevalence studies both among adults and children in Kinshasa.[11,13,17,32]

As in Europe and the US, there is no evidence for HIV transmission in the tropics by casual contact, by arthropods or within household and occupational settings such as the hospital.[13,33]

IMMUNITY

The basic clinical features of AIDS and ARC originate from the critical injury of the immune system, due to the selective infection of helper T lymphocytes. As a result of this, the host becomes susceptible to life-threatening opportunistic infections and malignancies. Functional defects can be identified in almost every part of the immune system, including cellular and humoral immunity. Thus, the main immunological disorders include lymphopenia, a decrease in helper T lymphocytes, T cell dysfunction, defective monocyte cytotoxic function, polyclonal B cell activation, non-specific antilymphocyte antibodies, increased levels of beta-2-microglobulin and defective delayed hypersensitivity (cutaneous anergy).[34]

Whereas immunological abnormalities were very similar among AIDS cases of different geographic origin, healthy African controls also exhibited an increased circulation of activated lymphocytes and increased levels of immune complexes, suggesting that the immune systems of African heterosexuals are in a chronically activated state secondary to chronic antigenic exposure.[35]

It is not known whether HIV infection has any effect on other endemic diseases in which T cell-mediated immunity plays an important role, such as malaria, tuberculosis and leishmaniasis, but it seems likely.

Serum antibodies against HIV (IgG and IgM) can be demonstrated by several serological assays (see section on diagnosis, below).

CLINICAL FEATURES

The clinical expression of HIV infection is very diverse, varying from a healthy carrier state to potentially fatal opportunistic diseases. The clinical manifestations associated with HIV infection vary also in different populations, possibly due to the relative frequency of endemic infections. This brief review will focus on the particular aspects of the disease as occurring in Africa and Haiti where gastrointestinal and dermatological manifestations seem to be more common than in Europeans and Americans with AIDS.

AIDS-related complex (ARC)

Patients with ARC present with similar signs and symptoms, and immunological defects as AIDS cases, but the clinical manifestations are generally less severe. In contrast with AIDS patients there are no opportunistic infections or malignancies.

Clinical manifestations of ARC in adults include profound weight loss, malaise and lethargy, anorexia, abdominal discomfort, diarrhoea, fever, night sweating, headache, itching, amenorrhoea, lymphadenopathy and splenomegaly. These signs and symptoms are often intermittent and can disappear spontaneously during variable periods.

Lymphadenopathy involving two or more extra-inguinal sites is found in the majority of ARC patients. Lymphadenopathy occurs most frequently in the cervical and axillary regions. Lymph nodes are firm, mobile, non-tender and generally do not exceed 6 cm in diameter. Lymph nodes larger than 6 cm in diameter in HIV-infected patients are often of tuberculous origin in Africans. They can regress during progression of the disease.

Mucocutaneous manifestations are common in patients with ARC or AIDS. A characteristic generalized papular pruritic eruption is found in approximately 20–60% of African and Haitian patients with HIV infection.[36,37] It is often seen in the early stages of illness but is generally found intermittently throughout the course of the disease. Its aetiology is unknown. The initial lesion is a small firm and very pruritic papule, which releases a small drop of fluid when scratched. The papules become hyperpigmented macules. They are symmetrically distributed over the body, but are most frequently found on the extremities. Histological features are non-specific and include perivascular infiltration of the skin and subcutaneous tissue with mononuclear cells with a variable number of eosinophils.

Recurrent mucocutaneous herpes simplex infections are found in 5–10% of African patients with HIV infection. Ten per cent of patients with HIV infection experience a varicella zoster infection which is recurrent in one-quarter of the cases.[36] The initial episode of varicella zoster infection is often the first manifestation of HIV associated illness.

Oral candidiasis in the absence of antimicrobial immunosuppressive therapy or an immunosuppressive illness, is highly associated with HIV infection. Its occurrence in an ARC patient is often a bad prognostic sign and an indication of progression towards 'full blown' AIDS.

AIDS

Approximately 20% of patients with ARC progress to 'full blown' AIDS.

The same manifestations as described for ARC occur in cases with AIDS, but they become more pronounced. In addition, symptoms and signs caused by the associated opportunistic illnesses are present. The clinical course is characterized by recurrent opportunistic infections. The case fatality rate of AIDS is high, with an average time of survival of three to six months from the date of diagnosis among Haitian patients and a mortality rate of *42%* at three months after diagnosis in Kinshasa.[10, 38]

Table 68.7 summarizes the clinical characteristics of AIDS among African and Haitian patients. Profound weight loss, progressive fatigue, chronic and intermittent diarrhoea, anorexia, and low grade fever were the most common manifestations in both patient populations.

The predominant clinical presentation of AIDS in adults in the tropics is a diarrhoea–wasting syndrome.[36, 37, 39] Patients may lose several litres of liquid stool a day sometimes leading to severe dehydration. The cause of this secretory diarrhoea is not known, and established intestinal pathogens can be detected in only a minority of patients. Thus, *Cryptosporidium* and *Isospora belli* are found in 22–51% and 1–15%, respectively, of African and Haitian patients with AIDS.[40, 41] Treatment of AIDS-associated diar-

Table 68.7 Clinical manifestations in patients with AIDS in Kinshasa, Zaire, and Haiti. (From Colebunders et al,[36] Pape et al,[37] Malebranche et al.[39])

Signs or symptoms	% of patients with manifestations		
	Zaire	Haiti	
		Pape et al	Malebranche et al
	$N = 196$	$N = 61$	$N = 27$
Weight loss (>10% of body weight)	99	100	93
Asthenia	91	NA	93
Anorexia	NA	NA	100
Fever (>1 month)	54	89	97
Diarrhoea (>1 month)	41	91	93
Cough	37	NA	55
Dyspnoea	23	NA	NA
Headache (>1 month)	33	NA	NA
Pruritus	30	NA	NA
Amenorrhoea (women only)	42	NA	NA
Dysphagia	35	72	NA
Oral thrush	47	NA	93
Pruriginous papular eruption	20	61	59
Generalized lymphadenopathy	11	9	31
Lesions of shingles	9	NA	NA
Convulsions or neurological abnormalities	6	NA	NA

NA = information not available.

rhoea is particularly difficult, though trimethoprim–sulphamethoxazole is effective to control episodes of isosporiasis.[40]

Neurological syndromes such as chronic and acute meningitis, myelopathy, encephalopathy with dementia and peripheral neuropathy complicate the clinical course of a majority of AIDS cases. The most common neurological disorder is a progressive change in behaviour associated with dementia, which usually progresses towards severe dementia.

Cough in AIDS patients with *Pneumocystis carinii* pneumonia or with lymphoid interstitial pneumonitis is usually non-productive and frequently associated with dyspnoea. Haemoptysis and pleural effusion are mainly caused by tuberculosis or Kaposi's sarcoma.

Most *infants* with AIDS present within the first six months of life. Clinical disorders include failure to thrive, persistent oral candidiasis, persistent pulmonary infiltrates, hepatosplenomegaly, and recurrent diarrhoea.[38] Among children between one and 14 years of age in Kinshasa, HIV serum antibody was significantly associated with a diagnosis of malnutrition, pneumonia and anaemia. The in-hospital mortality rate of seropositive children was over three times higher than for seronegative children.[33]

The most commonly identified opportunistic diseases in African and Haitian patients with AIDS are listed in Table 68.8.

headache, confusion, focal neurological signs, fever and grand mal seizures. Serum antibody titres against *Toxoplasma gondii* are of little use for diagnosis and difficult to interpret.

Tuberculosis is frequently found in African and Haitian patients with HIV infection. Thus in Florida, 60% of Haitians with AIDS had tuberculosis as compared with only 3% of non-

Table 68.8　Opportunistic diseases in African, Haitian and American patients with AIDS (from Colebunders et al,[36] Pape et al,[37] Fischl and Scott,[38] Sonnet and Taelman,[42] Peterman et al[43]).

	% of patients with opportunistic disease				
	Africans Country of diagnosis		Haitians Country of diagnosis		Americans
	Zaire	Belgium	Haiti	USA	USA
Number of patients studied	196	42	61	65	NA
Candidal oesophagitis	27	21	67	51	10
Pneumocystis carinii pneumonia[a]	17	24	20	42	61
Diarrhoea for over 1 month					
with *Cryptosporidium*	6	7	5	3	3
with *Isospora belli*	1	5	NA	10	NA
Cryptococcosis	5	29	3	10	6
Herpetic ulceration (>1 month)	3	33	8	17	4
Toxoplasma encephalitis	NA	17	3	27	3
Atypical mycobacterial infection	NA	10	NA	4	4
Generalized cytomegalovirus infection	NA	20	10	13	5
Progressive multifocal					
leukoencephalitis	NA	2	NA	1	0.6
Tuberculosis	13	12	24	52	NA
Salmonella bacteraemia	NA	NA	NA	4	NA
Kaposi's sarcoma	4	26	26	12	26
Cerebral lymphoma	NA	0	0	NA	0.5

[a] In Zaire: bilateral pneumonia of unknown aetiology.
NA = information not available.

Patients with cryptococcal meningitis often present with mild headache, low grade fever and weight loss. In Kinshasa a generally mild neck stiffness occurred in only 60% of cases during the course of the disease. Therefore, a lumbar puncture is always indicated whenever an HIV-infected patient develops headache.

P. carinii pneumonia was less frequent among Africans with AIDS seen in Europe than among Europeans. Studies are presently underway to define the aetiology of pneumonia in African AIDS patients.

Toxoplasma encephalitis was diagnosed by biopsy or at autopsy in 27% of Haitian patients in Miami and 17% of African patients in Europe, indicating that this is a significantly more common opportunistic infection than among American AIDS cases.[36, 38] It is characterized by

Haitian patients with the syndrome.[44] In 78% of AIDS cases with tuberculosis the disease was disseminated, including both miliary and generalized lymphatic tuberculosis.[38] Extrapulmonary tuberculosis was significantly associated with AIDS in this population. Tuberculous lymph nodes in AIDS patients frequently show no granulomas, due to an inadequate cellular response. In Zaire, 33% of hospitalized tuberculosis patients were HIV seropositive, including 67% of patients with extrapulmonary tuberculosis. Seropositivity was significantly associated with anergy to tuberculin and receiving a blood transfusion during the previous five years, but not with the extent of radiographic lesions, duration of disease, or initial response to treatment.[32] HIV infection may complicate the management of individual patients, as well as tuberculosis

control programmes in HIV endemic areas. In contrast to tuberculosis, generalized infection with atypical mycobacteria such as *Mycobacterium avium* and *M. intracellulare* is as frequent among African and Haitian patients with AIDS, as among Europeans.

Kaposi's sarcoma, an angioproliferative disorder of endothelial origin, is found in 4–15% of African patients with AIDS, as compared with nearly half of American and European homosexual men with AIDS. In contrast to the 'classic' endemic form of Kaposi's sarcoma in central Africa (Chapters 65, 67), which is not associated with HIV infection or immunosuppression,[20,45,46] it presents as a generalized aggressive disease, with involvement of the skin, lymph nodes and various organs, particularly the pulmonary and gastrointestinal systems. In general, lesions appear as hyperpigmented black plaques on the black skin, and as purple plaques on the white skin. Some lesions may be infiltrative or present as nodules or tumours (ulcerated or not). Lesions may be surrounded by oedema as in the classic type of Kaposi's sarcoma. They appear on all parts of the body. In the mouth, lesions are mainly found on the hard palate.

DIAGNOSIS

The diagnosis of AIDS is a clinical one, and is based on the identification of an opportunistic infection or a malignancy listed in Table 68.5. Whenever possible, the presence of serum antibody to HIV should be demonstrated by a well-evaluated serological test. However, in many developing countries, diagnostic and laboratory facilities may be insufficient to reliably diagnose most opportunistic diseases associated with AIDS. Therefore a provisional clinical case definition of AIDS was developed by the World Health Organization (Table 68.9). The specificity of this definition for the diagnosis of HIV infection in one hospital in Kinshasa was 94%, the sensitivity 62% and the positive predictive value 84%.[36] Tuberculosis represents one of the major problems in the differential diagnosis. Cutaneous anergy to tuberculin, even in the presence of tuberculosis was significantly associated with AIDS in Kinshasa.[32] Clinical definitions which optimize sensitivity and specificity for AIDS should be developed for epidemiological and diagnostic purposes.

Table 68.9 Provisional WHO clinical case definition for AIDS where diagnostic resources are limited. (Definition developed at WHO Workshop on AIDS in Bangui, Central African Republic.)

Adults

AIDS in an adult is defined by the existence of at least 2 of the major signs associated with at least 1 minor sign, in the absence of known causes of immunosuppression such as cancer or severe malnutrition or other recognized aetiologies.

1 Major signs
  (a) weight loss >10% of body weight;
  (b) chronic diarrhoea >1 month;
  (c) prolonged fever >1 month (intermittent or constant).
2 Minor signs
  (a) persistent cough for >1 month;
  (b) generalized pruritic dermatitis;
  (c) recurrent varicella zoster;
  (d) oropharyngeal candidiasis;
  (e) chronic progressive and disseminated herpes simplex infection;
  (f) generalized lymphadenopathy.

The presence of generalized Kaposi's sarcoma or cryptococcal meningitis are sufficient by themselves for the diagnosis of AIDS.

Children

Paediatric AIDS is suspected in an infant or child presenting with at least 2 major signs associated with at least 2 minor signs in the absence of known causes of immunosuppression.

1 Major signs
  (a) weight loss or abnormally slow growth;
  (b) chronic diarrhoea >1 month;
  (c) prolonged fever >1 month.
2 Minor signs
  (a) generalized lymphadenopathy;
  (b) oropharyngeal candidiasis;
  (c) repeated common infections (otitis, pharyngitis, etc.);
  (d) persistent cough;
  (e) generalized dermatitis;
  (f) confirmed maternal HIV infection.

An enzyme immunoassay (EIA) is usually used as a first line test for the demonstration of HIV antibody. Its sensitivity and specificity are approximately 95–99%. Other serological tests include an indirect immunofluorescence test, radio immunoprecipitation and immunoblotting ('Western' blot). All positive test results in the HIV EIA should be confirmed first by repeating the enzyme-linked immunosorbent assay (ELISA), and if positive again, by a well-evaluated serological assay, such as the Western Blot, since the predictive value of a positive EIA result is insufficient in low prevalence populations (even with a seroprevalence of 5–10%).

Since HIV can be isolated from up to 80% serum antibody positive individuals, persons carrying such antibody should also be considered as potentially infectious.[47]

TREATMENT, MANAGEMENT AND PREVENTION

Effective specific treatment for HIV infection is not available as yet (early 1987). The opportunistic diseases should be treated using recommended therapeutic schedules. The management of patients with AIDS requires no special facilities or quarantine. However, contact with mucosal surfaces, blood and other secretions and excretions of such patients should be avoided by wearing gloves when drawing blood, or examining mucous membranes. In general, gloves should always be used when assisting in delivery or performing invasive procedures since in some populations a considerable proportion of women are infected with HIV. Finally, taking care of AIDS patients may be a heavy psychological burden for health workers, as well as for their families. Hospital personnel should be thoroughly informed on HIV infection and on patient management.

AIDS has become a serious health problem in major parts of the Caribbean and Africa, where the number of infectious individuals is estimated to be several millions. Because of the rapid and continuous spread of HIV infection by sexual contact, perinatal transmission and exposure to blood, control of HIV infection should be considered a public health priority.

Since no effective therapy or vaccine is available, control of AIDS is of necessity based on prevention. The latter is complicated by social, economic and political constraints in many developing countries. The prevention of sexual transmission of HIV infection requires a reduction in the number of sex partners and the use of condoms. It is not clear what type of educational approaches will be successful to meet these goals in the developing world.

Transmission through blood transfusions can be drastically reduced by screening blood donors for HIV antibody and probably by using disposable or properly sterilized needles and syringes (or at least a reduction in the number of injections given). Interruption of perinatal transmission may be achieved by screening women of childbearing age and counselling on contraception for HIV seropositive women. All these measures would require a substantial financial and organizational effort which may be difficult to implement.

AIDS and HIV-infection now clearly represent one of the most dramatic challenges to the public health system in many developing countries. Unless control programmes are successful, HIV infection will have a growing negative impact on health and health care services in Africa and other areas of the developing world.

REFERENCES

1 Arya, O.P., Osoba, A.O. & Bennett, F.J. (1980) *Tropical Venereology*. Edinburgh: Churchill Livingstone. (2nd edn, 1987, in press).
2 Dunlop, E.M.C. (1977) *Clin. Obst. Gyn.* **4**, 451–477.
3 World Health Organization (1986) *Conjunctivitis of the newborn: prevention and treatment at the primary health care level*. WHO, Geneva.
4 Laga, M., Naamara, W., Brunham, R.C. et al (1986) *New Engl. J. Med.* **315**, 1382–1385.
5 Gottlieb, M.S., Schroff, R., Schanker, H.M. et al (1981) *New Engl. J. Med.* **305**, 1425.
6 World Health Organization (1986) *Weekly Epidemiological Record* **61**, 69.
7 Curran, J.W., Morgan, W.M., Hardy, A.M. et al (1985) *Science* **229**, 1352.
8 Forthal, D.N., Mhalu, F.S., Dahoma, A. et al (1986) *AIDS in Tanzania*. Abstract of the International Conference on AIDS, Paris, 1986.
9 Serwadda, D., Mugerwa, R.D., Sewankambo, N.K. et al (1985) *Lancet* **ii**, 849.
10 Piot, P., Quinn, T.C., Taelman, H. et al (1984) *Lancet* **ii**, 65.
11 Mann, J.M., Francis, H., Quinn, T. et al (1986) *J. Am. med. Ass.* **255**, 3255.
12 Van de Perre, P., Rouvroy, D., Lepage, P. et al (1984) *Lancet* **ii**, 62.
13 Mann, J.M., Kapita, B., Colebunders, R.L. et al (1986) *Lancet* **ii**, 707.
14 Johnson, W.D., Liautaud, B., Thomas, F. et al (1986) *Abstract of the 2nd World Congress on STD*, Paris, 1986.
15 Van de Perre, P., Clumeck, N., Carael, M. et al (1985) *Lancet* **ii**, 524.
16 Piot, P., Plummer, F.A., Rey, M.A. et al (1987) *J. Infect. Dis.* **155** (in press).
17 Quinn, T.C., Mann, J.M., Curran, J.W., et al (1986) *Science* **234**, 955.
18 Brun-Vézinet, F., Rouzioux, C., Montagnier, L. et al (1985) *Science* **226**, 453.
19 Biggar, R.J. (1986) *Lancet* **i**, 79.
20 Bayley, A.C. (1984) *Lancet* **i**, 1318.
21 Weiss, R.A. (1984) In *Molecular Biology of the Tumor Viruses: RNA Tumor Viruses*, ed. R. Weiss, N. Teich, H. Varmus et al, vol. II, supplement. New York: Cold Spring Harbor Laboratory.
22 Barré-Sinoussi, F., Chermann, J.C., Rey, F. et al (1983) *Science* **220**, 868.
23 McCormick, J.B., Krebs, J.W., Mitchell, S.W. et al (1986) *Am. J. trop. Med. Hyg.* (in press).
24 Benn, S., Rutledge, R., Folks, T. et al (1985) *Science* **230**, 949.
25 Alizon, M., Wain-Hobson, S., Montagnier, L. et al (1986) *Cell* **46**, 63.

26 Kanki, P.J., Barin, F., M'Boup, S. et al (1986) *Science* **232**, 238.

27 Clavel, F., Brun-Vézinet, F., Guétard, D. et al (1986) *Comp. Rend. Acad. Sci. Paris*, **302**, Série III, 485.

28 Clumeck, N., Van de Perre, P., Carael, M. et al (1985) *New Engl. J. Med.* **313**, 182 (letter).

29 Kreiss, J.K., Koech, D., Plummer, F.A. et al (1986) *New Engl. J. Med.* **314**, 414.

30 Mann, J.M., Quinn, T., Francis, H. et al (1986) Abstract of the International Conference on AIDS, Paris, 1986.

31 Izzia, K.W., Lepira, B., Kayembe, K. et al (1984) *Ann. Soc. belge Méd. trop.* **64**, 391.

32 Mann, J.M., Snider, D.E., Francis, H. et al (1986) *J. Am. med. Ass.* **256**, 346 (letter).

33 Mann, J.M., Francis, H., Davachi, F. et al (1986) *Lancet* **ii**, 654.

34 Lane, H.C. & Fauci, A.S. (1985) In *Advances in Host Defence Mechanisms*, ed. J.I. Gallin & A.S. Fauci, vol. 5, p. 131. New York: Raven Press.

35 Quinn, T.C., Piot, P., McCormick, J.B. et al (1987) *J. Am. med. Assoc.* **257** (in press).

36 Colebunders, R., Mann, J., Francis, H. et al (1986) *Méd. Mal. infect.* **15**, 350.

37 Pape, J., Liautaud, B., Thomas, F. et al (1983) *New Engl. J. Med.* **309**, 945.

38 Fischl, M.A., & Scott, G.B. (1985) In *Advances in Host Defense Mechanisms*, ed. J.I. Gallin & A.S. Franci, p. 109. New York: Raven Press.

39 Malebranche, R., Arnoux, E., Guérin, J.M. et al (1983) *Lancet* **ii**, 873.

40 De Hovitz, J.A., Pape, J.W., Boncy, M. et al (1986) *N. Engl. J. Med.* **315**, 87.

41 Coleblunders, R.C., Francis, H., Mann, J.M. et al unpublished.

42 Sonnet, J. & Taelman, H. (1986) In *Clinical Aspects of AIDS and AIDS-related Complex*, ed. M. Staquet, R. Hemmer, A. Baert, p. 78. Oxford: Oxford University Press.

43 Peterman, T.A., Drotman, D.P., Cussan, J.W. (1985) *Epidemiol. Rev.* **7**, 1.

44 Pitchenik, A., Cole, C., Russel, B.W. et al (1984) *Ann. intern. Med.* **101**, 641.

45 Biggar, R.J., Melbeye, M., Kestens, L. et al (1984) *New Engl. J. Med.* **311**, 1051.

46 Kestens, L., Melbye, M., Biggar, R.J. et al (1985) *Int. J. Cancer* **36**, 49.

47 Gallo, R.C. & Broder, S. (1984) *New Engl. J. Med.* **311**, 1292.

48 World Health Organization (1985) Workshop on AIDS in Central Africa. WHO/CDS/AIDS/85.1.

FURTHER READING

Holmes, K.K., Mardh, P.A., Sparling, P.F. et al (eds) (1984) *Sexually Transmitted Diseases*. New York: McGraw-Hill.

World Health Organization (1975) *The epidemiology of Infertility*. Report of a WHO Scientific Group, Technical Report Series, 582, WHO, Geneva.

World Health Organization (1978) *Neisseria gonorrhoeae and gonococcal infections*. Report of a WHO Scientific Group, Technical Report Series, 616, WHO, Geneva.

World Health Organization (1981) *Nongonococcal urethritis and other selected sexually transmitted diseases of public health importance*. Report of a WHO Scientific Group, Technical Report Series, 660, WHO, Geneva.

World Health Organization (1982) *Treponemal infections*. Report of a WHO Scientific Group, Technical Report Series, 674, WHO, Geneva.

World Health Organization (1985) *Control of Sexually Transmitted Diseases*. Report of a WHO Scientific Group. WHO, Geneva.

World Health Organization (1986) WHO Expert Committee on Venereal Diseases and Treponematoses, Sixth Report, Technical Report Series, 736, WHO, Geneva.

World Health Organization. *Simplified approaches for sexually transmitted disease (STD) control at the primary health care (PHC) level*. Report of a WHO Working Group (24–28 Sept 1984). Unpublished WHO document WHO/VDT/85.437.

Chapter 69
Musculoskeletal Disease

All the diseases of temperate climates occur in the tropics, although there are some differences in frequency, some of them difficult to explain. For example, rheumatoid arthritis is relatively uncommon in many tropical countries, but as we are still ignorant of its aetiology, speculation on the cause of the difference is largely idle. On the other hand, the doctor working in rural Africa will be scarcely surprised at the relative rarity of advanced osteoarthritis of the hip, when he remembers the small number of very old people he sees in his clinic. Neither will the doctor be surprised at the relatively high frequency of pyogenic arthritis when he is daily presented with enormous amounts of untreated sepsis. And the same goes for joint damage from guinea-worms, and the appalling deformities of childhood poliomyelitis, and local oddities may vary the clinical scene, such as the gross stiffness of the spine where calcification of the ligaments is produced by fluorosis.

But some strange absences of disease do really challenge the imagination. Why is it that, even in areas of tropics where people habitually carry huge loads on their heads, degenerative disease of the cervical spine is so rare?

There seems to be only one clearly defined musculoskeletal disease that is almost *peculiar* to the tropics, and that is pyomyositis.

PYOMYOSITIS

Pyomyositis is an acute inflammation of skeletal muscle, mainly confined to the tropics and subtropics. Muscular pain is usually the first symptom, followed within the next week by fever, localized induration and oedema. Any muscle group may be affected, but the most commonly involved are the gluteal and quadriceps muscles. There is often a minor degree of polymorphonuclear leukocytosis and a moderate eosinophilia of about 10% is common.

If untreated the condition will progress over the next four weeks until there is extensive muscle destruction. The appearance of the muscle in the late stage is 'a bag of pus'. From the induration that precedes this stage, pus can often be aspirated from 10 days onwards, and from this pus, *Staphylococcus aureus* can almost always be isolated. Diagnosis before the stage of pus formation is from the clinical features supported by the white cell changes described. Management in the early stages is by the administration of large doses of a β-lactamase resistant penicillin, and later, by the addition of adequate surgical incision. Despite the destruction of a large amount of muscle, functional and cosmetic recovery is usually remarkably good.

The aetiology is usually obscure. A small number of abscesses develop as part of a wider staphylococcal septicaemia, but this is unusual. Trauma, viral infection, various parasitic infections and malnutrition have all been postulated at various times, but none has been adequately substantiated. The odd clues—a marked male preponderance and the accompanying eosinophilia—have not yet led to the solution of the mystery.

For a review of pyomyositis with useful references see Chiedozi.[1]

AINHUM

This is a condition in which a stricture slowly develops between the fifth toe and the foot, leading to spontaneous amputation.

Geographical distribution

Ainhum has its highest incidence in Africa, especially the Transkei in South Africa[2] but it also occurs in people of Negro descent in the New World,[3] and has been described in whites,[4] Polynesians,[5] Indians[6] and Saudis.

Aetiology

The aetiology is obscure and leprosy, tuberculosis, syphilis and yaws are no longer considered causative. There are three currently suggested causes.

Abnormal fibrogenesis

Over-production of fibrous tissue in response to injury and infection such as an absence of shoes combined with rotational strain on the toe in persons with a tendency to keloid formation has been suggested as a factor.[7]

Angiodysplasia

Obstruction of the posterior tibial artery with the absence of the plantar arch and its branches, with a diminution in blood supply to the little toe has been demonstrated in cases of Ainhum[8] probably of genetic origin.

Toxic

In the Transkei, phocomelia is also frequent and a common toxic cause for both ainhum and phocomelia, possibly of plant origin, has been suggested.[2]

Pathology

No changes other than non-specific inflammation and fibrosis have been reported, and histology has thrown no light on the cause.

Clinical features

The patient notices the slow development of a constriction encircling the little toe at the level of the metatarsophalangeal joint (Figs. 69.1 and 69.2). Pain may occur, and the distal portion of the toe may swell. After some years the toe may remain attached to the foot by a fragile cutaneous pedicle only, and at this stage spontaneous or deliberate amputation usually occurs. If a long stump remains, this in turn may be affected by the same process later.

Diagnosis

This is clinical only.

Treatment

It has been suggested that division of the constricting band might delay evolution of the disease, but this has not been confirmed. When troublesome, the affected toe should be amputated.

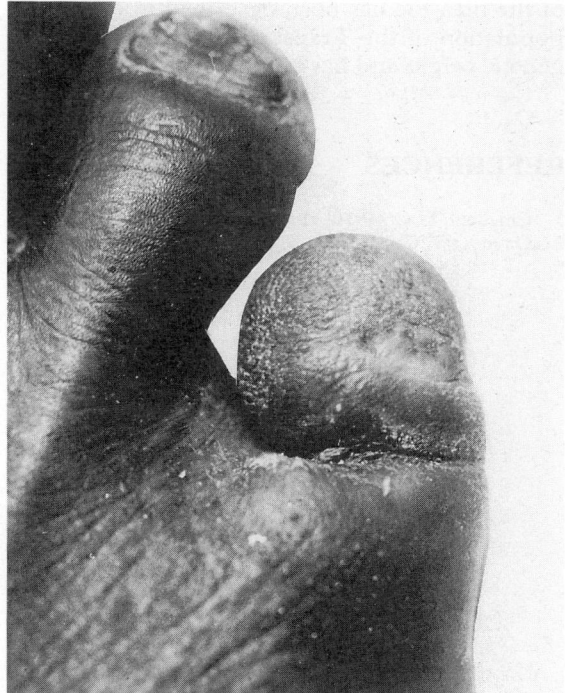

Fig. 69.1 Ainhum at its height. (Courtesy Dr W. M. Meyers.)

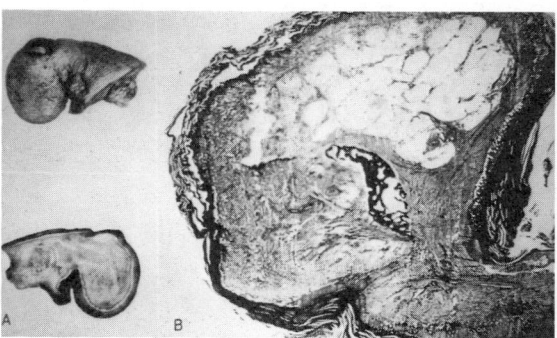

Fig. 69.2 An amputated toe from a patient suffering from ainhum, showing constriction at the base. (Courtesy Professor B. H. Kean.)

Epidemiology

In the Transkei where ainhum is common, it occurs six times more frequently in females than males,[2] and it is more common in people who habitually walk barefoot.

TRANSKEI FOOT

A disorder consisting of marked lateral deviation

of the fifth toe has been described in the Xhosa population of the Transkei which is possibly of genetic origin and has been called transkei foot.[9]

REFERENCES

1   Chiedozi, L. C. (1979) *Am. J. Surg.* **137,** 255.
2   Daynes, W. G. S. (1973) *S. Afr. med. J.* **47,** 320.
3   Kean, B. M., Tucker, H. A. & Miller, W. C. (1946) *Trans. R. Soc. trop. Med. Hyg.* **39,** 331.
4   Shaffer, L. J. O. (1947) *Archs Path.* **43,** 170.
5   Browne, S. G. (1961) *Ann. trop. Med. Parasit.* **55,** 314.
6   Aggarwal, N. D. & Singh, H. (1963) *J. Bone Jt Surg.* **45b,** 376.
7   Browne, S. G. (1965) *J. Bone Jt Surg.* **47,** 52.
8   Dent, D. M., Fataar, S. & Rose, A. G. (1981) *Lancet* **iii,** 396–397.
9   Schwartz, P. A., Shlugman, D., Daynes, G. et al (1974). *S. Afr. med. J.* **48,** 961–962.

Chapter 70
Eye Diseases
F. C. Rodger

GENERAL CONSIDERATIONS

The high incidence of eye disease in the tropics with its accompanying physical suffering, blindness and economic loss, both to the individual and the community, cannot be overstressed. (One is apt to forget that most eye diseases are painful.) Those who have no experience of tropical ophthalmology at first hand may be forgiven for thinking that ocular infections, infestations and aberrations follow the same clinical and pathological course in all parts of the world. This is not necessarily so for in the Third World lack of medical care and resources, a void in diagnostic procedures outside the large towns and the conditions of life generally, modify these processes. On top of this one is faced by diseases found exclusively in the tropics. In many respects, therefore, ophthalmology in the tropics is a more demanding discipline than in the Western world and one of the major problems facing a doctor in these parts.

SOCIOECONOMIC FACTORS

Poverty and malnutrition, particularly vitamin A and protein deficiency, housing and sanitary conditions, ignorance and lack of education, indifferent personal hygiene often associated with a poor water supply, the havoc wrought by unqualified and unskilled practitioners using unscientific methods of treatment, such as couching for cataract with an acacia thorn, all play their part. A peculiar and interesting factor is that which occurs in primitive and isolated communities by inbreeding. Examples of this are the high incidence of retinitis pigmentosa in Tristan da Cunha and albinism among the Cuna Indians of Panama. In the Pingelap Atoll in the eastern Caroline Islands 4–10% of the 900 inhabitants are blind from birth, manifesting nystagmus, night blindness, colour blindness and eventually cataract. The cause is attributed to a typhoon about 1780 which reduced the male population of this lonely island to nine!

PSYCHOLOGICAL FACTORS

Apathy and fatalism, superstitious beliefs, fear and suspicion of gratuitous outside help, or plain stupidity are frequently found among deprived people although they may to a lesser degree be found anywhere in the world. In such people there is a great dependence on traditional methods of treatment, some of which may do little harm but many of which are pernicious.

CLIMATIC FACTORS

Glare, heat, humidity, wind and dust are other adverse factors as are bacteria, fungi, parasites and insects, all abundant in the tropics and productive of eye trouble as well as systemic and cutaneous disease.

Pterygium

A good example of the effect of exposure and climatic irritants on the eye is the condition known as *pterygium*; here the basement membrane of the cornea is separated from Bowman's membrane by a large wedge of fibroblasts, the advancing head being narrower than the base. It occurs in the exposed areas on the nasal or temporal sides in the horizontal plane, one or both, and can grow across the cornea impairing sight. It should be sliced off the cornea with a knife and a V-shaped portion of its conjunctival base excised and cauterized, leaving the sclera bare to prevent regrowth.

Solar keratopathy

While it is possible that the rays of the sun play a part in the development of pterygium there is another condition where the evidence is very strong that it is the short ultraviolet waves alone which damage the cornea.

Nature has made adequate provision for protecting the cornea and inner eye from light; the brows, most pronounced in aborigines, screen the eye from above and the lids narrow to reduce the pencil of rays to a minimum. The pupil also cuts down the incident light and the uveoretinal pigment prevents the scatter of light within the eye itself. Eskimos make use of slotted strips of leather, bone or wood to cut out snow-reflected light. This in fact is the most potent factor, reflectance from a good reflecting surface. Within the range of 290–310 nm, short ultraviolet rays (SUVR), depending on the reflecting surface, the clarity of the atmosphere and the altitude, can burn the surface of the eye. In the tropics salt-spattered white coral sand gives the greatest reflectance after snow and ice at high altitudes and salt-pans. In people working in the open under such conditions the SUVR burn the lids, which swell, as well as burning the strip of cornea exposed through lids narrowed against the glare. This gives rise to what is called a band-shaped, climatic or solar keratopathy (Fig. 70.1). Strictly speaking, this is not a band-shaped lesion except in its early appearance for as the eyelids retract to allow better vision around the central opacity so the damaged (white) area gradually adopts an elliptical shape. The term 'band-shaped' is perhaps better restricted to that lesion where a primary or secondary calcinosis of the cornea occurs, a somewhat rare but long-established clinical entity (Fig. 70.2).

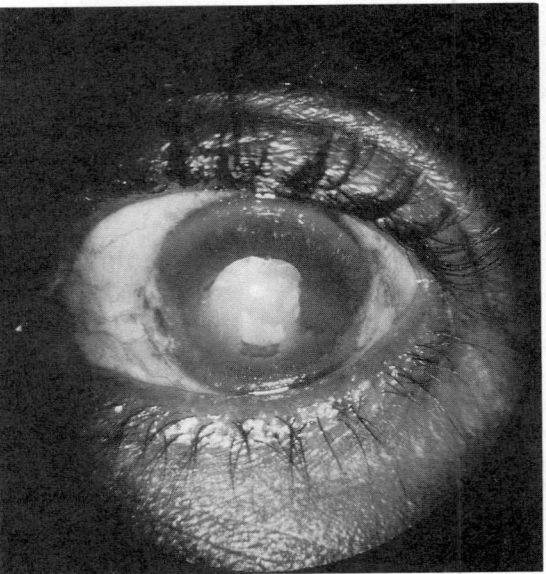

Fig. 70.2 Onchocercal sclerosing keratitis, early 'tongues', complicated cataract due to anterior uveitis and a partially transparent band-shaped opacity of cornea. (Courtesy Mr F. C. Rodger.)

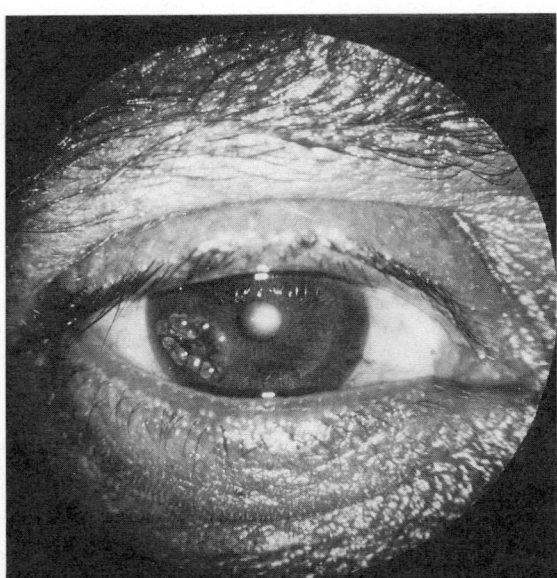

Fig. 70.1 Climatic keratopathy, cystic stage. (Courtesy Mr F. C. Rodger and *British Journal of Ophthalmology*.)

Solar keratophy consists of an alteration of the superficial corneal collagen *without calcinosis*. At the start the alteration is barely discernible; in time it is seen to be grey and ultimately white. The overlying epithelium becomes cystic quite early on (if you can say that of a condition which takes many years to develop). Some of the cysts have within them a core of brown debris, well described as looking like 'oil drops'. The writer[1] photographed this condition in all its many stages in the Red Sea islands. The 'oil drops' consist of aggregates of elastotic degeneration.[2] In further studies it has been demonstrated[3] that the droplets also contained a protein (diffusing plasma proteins, they believe) which does not have all the properties of elastic tissue. This spheroidal type of degeneration of the cornea also occurs as a secondary phenomenon in eyes where scarred corneas are uncovered by the lids; the eyes of the blind are often raised seeking the light, the SUVR having constant direct access; nevertheless, considering the vast number of scarred corneas in the tropics, it is not common (Plate IV.1). When spheroidal degeneration does occur as a secondary phenomenon, because the lesion takes so long to develop, it is invariably found in someone who has been blind for many years; 10 to 20 years may have to pass, the effect being cumulative. Where it is a primary condition it is invariably in a subject who works in areas of high reflectance, such as white coral sand, or salt-splattered beaches, day in and day out.

In high altitudes where the air is always purer and clearer—hence the marvellous vista photographs from the top of the Himalayan peaks—and in the presence of high reflectance from the snow and ice above the tropical valleys of Asia, SUVR quickly burn the corneal surface giving rise to classic snow blindness. In this condition the corneal changes are not permanent; the surface epithelium is eroded exposing and damaging the free pain endings which lie between the cells. There is intense photophobia, reflex lacrimation and pain, just as in 'welder's flash'. An acute keratopathy of this nature has been reported by the author from an area of high reflectance on a salt-coated sand spit used for observing fish traps in the Red Sea.

Solar retinopathy (*maculopathy*)

Although the eye usually reflexly evades the direct rays of the sun, in certain circumstances the gaze may linger too long. Watching an eclipse with the naked eye or through glasses that give inadequate protection is one example of this. Scanning the sky for aircraft during attack is another where so often aeroplanes attack out of the sun. Many mentally disturbed patients are known to have suffered retinal damage by obsessive sun-gazing.

Visible light consists of electromagnetic vibrations of wavelengths between 400 and 760 nm. Below 400 nm short ultraviolet radiations (SUVR) exist and those between 290 and 310 are the most harmful to the eye. The intense glare of the sun at the end of an eclipse can burn a hole in the macula which then has all the appearance of a ruptured cyst being accompanied by minute haemorrhages, radiating folds in the retina and a clear outline to the hole. If less severe, macular oedema and a localized detachment with temporary visual disturbance can result. It is possible that some eyes which appear to have had ruptured macular cysts in the past (it can be uniocular) are really examples of solar maculopathy.

Protection against solar damage

The wearing of correct sunglasses can protect against solar keratopathy. A large proportion of untinted spectacle lenses absorb UV radiation up to (at the least) 310 nm. The level of absorption is determined by the dioptric power on which the thickness of the lens depends; at least 2 mm of thickness is needed.

Up to 100% UV absorption below 400 nm is achieved by most manufacturers using simple filter or tinted lenses. To watch an eclipse in safety *indirect* observation projected on to a screen is the only truly safe method. Socrates knew this and advised watching the reflection of an eclipse in still water.

GENERAL HEALTH IN PEASANT FARMING COMMUNITIES

Finally, one must take into account the general health of the community in which one is working in the tropics. It varies a lot in different bioclimatic zones. These differences should be learned as soon as possible. What are the dominant diseases? Is traditional medicine practised? What is the state of nutrition? The possibility always exists that the subject with eye disease is also suffering from malnutrition although this may not be immediately obvious. The high incidence in the tropical world of such diseases as malaria, schistosomiasis, filariasis, sexually transmitted diseases, the dysenteries, and so on, further reduces the resistance of the patients one is trying to help. It is a poor ophthalmologist who concentrates only on the eyes.

THE RED EYE

Before discussing the various diseases which cause blindness in the tropics and the methods of treating them it would be as well to describe what one should be looking for when faced with a 'red eye'. The latter is more common than an eye with a scar or a healthy-looking but obviously blind eye—two other common clinical appearances. It is, moreover, the red eye which is most likely to be helped by treatment.

CONJUNCTIVITIS

Conjunctivitis, in one form or another, is one of the commonest conditions which occurs in the practice of ophthalmology in any country. The forms it assumes range from a simple catarrhal conjunctivitis to acute trachoma.

Signs and symptoms

Conjunctivitis in the absence of complications is not painful. Discomfort and a feeling of dryness or grittiness are common complaints and watering or running of the eye is often experienced. The sticking together of the eyelids on waking is a complaint frequently made. Photophobia is rarely present unless the cornea or iris is involved. In simple conjunctivitis there is no interference with vision though flecks of mucous secretion may cause transient blurring.

In the normal eye the transparent bulbar conjunctiva reveals the underlying white episclera on which branching blood vessels rest. The palpebral conjunctiva which lines the eyelids is a smooth, regularly pink-coloured, glistening, mucous membrane. Departure from these criteria is shown by increased vascularity or by irregularities of the smooth surface or both.

Increased vascularity may be generalized (the bloodshot eye) or localized when the eyeball is red in a particular sector, as in phlyctenular or angular conjunctivitis, or when there is a deeper red patch due to a subconjunctival haemorrhage or (epi-) scleritis.

Irregularities of the lid conjunctiva are seen in conditions such as vernal catarrh, folliculosis and trachoma, soon to be described.

Scrapings of the conjunctival epithelium stained with Giemsa can help identify the TRIC (trachoma inclusion conjunctivitis) virus, and is a useful technique.

Aetiology

The causes may be divided into four groups.
1 Infections with microorganisms through contact with fingers, towels, dust, dirt, house flies, birth canal.
2 Allergies.
3 Febrile diseases: influenza, measles, chickenpox, typhus, and so on. The first stage of Weil's disease exhibits intense congestion of the eyeball.
4 Trauma, adherent foreign bodies, irritant or corrosive fluids (from larvicides, adulticides, herbicides and defoliants), SUVR, snake venom and various insects (p. 1179).

In the first three groups the conjunctivitis is usually, but not always, bilateral. When only one eye is affected trauma, a foreign body in the cornea or in the fornix, or something other than conjunctivitis should be looked for—for example, a corneal ulcer.

Staining with 1% fluorescein is important to help identify a corneal lesion at this point. Less likely causes should be sought if a blank is drawn, such as the recent use of native medicine.

The more common forms of conjunctivitis are now given in some detail.

Angular conjunctivitis

This disease is probably becoming less common. The conjunctival infection is localized near the canthi, especially the inner, and a silvery secretion lodges there. The neighbouring skin is red, excoriated or eczematous. Polyavitaminosis may also play a part. It is generally found among the older and more feeble members of the community. The specific organism involved is a saprophyte, the diplobacillus of Morax–Axenfeld. It responds quite well to treatment with a zinc drop. *Staphylococcus aureus* is sometimes the cause.

Acute bacterial conjunctivitis

This, the commonest cause of a red eye, may be sporadic or epidemic; it may be moderate or severe. If possible the bacteria involved should be identified and, if not, a broad-spectrum antibiotic used freely. Any bacteria can cause conjunctivitis but in the tropics the commonest, often found associated with groups of infected children or in a family group, are *Diplococcus pneumoniae*, the Koch–Weeks bacillus (*Haemophilus aegyptius*), *Staphylococcus aureus*, *Streptococcus viridans*, the various *Neisseria*, and more rarely the influenza and diphtheria bacteria.

The acute catarrhal conjunctivitis typifying this disease usually does not become chronic. The eye is bright red and there is a profuse discharge which may be mucopurulent or purulent. The cornea can exhibit punctate opacities (as in staphylococcus); there may be subconjunctival haemorrhages (as in pneumococcus); it may be hyperacute leading to corneal ulceration in most of these infections (especially with gonococcus, meningococcus and the Koch–Weeks bacillus). The acute condition may be associated with membranes or pseudomembranes covering the bulbar conjunctiva (as in *Corynebacterium diphtheriae* and streptococcus). In the debilitated child in particular, corneal ulceration with loss of the eye is common. Other rarer causes of conjunctivitis are discussed towards the end of this chapter commencing on p. 1159.

In endemic trachoma areas an epidemic of bacterial conjunctivitis activates the TRIC infection with disastrous long-term results and so it is very important to treat the acute conjunctivitis not only as a therapeutic measure but as a prophylactic. Oral chemotherapy or antibiotics, even without topical treatment, can swiftly quash bacterial conjunctivitis provided the causative agent is known and treated correctly. In the case of bacteria this should always be possible. If one is completely isolated and does not have this knowledge the best approach is to treat as for acute trachoma (p. 1144).

Phlyctenular conjunctivitis

This condition occurs predominantly in undernourished children and is often associated with tonsil and adenoidal infection, otorrhoea and both cervical and hilar adenitis. Although the tubercle bacillus cannot be isolated from the conjunctiva the disease is caused by an endogenous protein allergen, which is frequently tuberculoprotein. The phlycten appears as a small (3 mm) yellow swelling in the conjunctiva close to the limbus surrounded by a localized spread of blood vessels. It may also be found on the palpebral conjunctiva. The phlycten can extend to the cornea where it breaks down to form an ulcer. When the latter heals an irregular semiopaque scar remains. If central, of course, vision is reduced. The greater the vascular invasion of the cornea in the wake of the phlycten, the harder the condition is to cure.

Topical steroid drops—used with care if the cornea is involved—a bactericidal drop and a supplementary diet with vitamins are indicated. The child should be examined for signs of pulmonary tuberculosis.

Vernal or spring catarrh

This is also an allergic reaction but to exogenous allergens. Here the eye is photophobic and painful. There are two clinical appearances: in one the undersurface of the upper lids is covered with large pale pink cobblestone follicles; in the other the limbus is swollen in its entirety (in pigmented races it is dark in colour). The use of topical steroids has revolutionized the treatment of vernal catarrh. In recalcitrant cases oral steroids in small doses usually dispel this highly uncomfortable or painful condition.

Follicular conjunctivitis

There is a condition called *folliculosis* which may confuse the diagnosis. In it there are rows of follicles of seed-pearl size, particularly in the lower fornix and palpebral conjunctivas, the surfaces of which are packed with them. There is a remarkable absence of symptoms and the eye is not red, which distinguishes it from a florid trachoma. The condition, a simple adenitis, is found in children and recovery (helped by steroid drops) follows improvement in general health. When follicles are present one has to be careful an underlying viral (kerato-) conjunctivitis is not the real cause. If it is, steroid drops will worsen rather than help and should be stopped.

Enteroviral haemorrhagic conjunctivitis (EV70 disease)

This acute conjunctivitis has been identified only in the last decade. Its global incidence by last year was assessed at between 70 and 80 million.[4] The causative agent is an enterovirus, EV70.[5] It is now known that it may be associated, although not necessarily, with a polio-like paralysis of the limbs or cranial nerves or both, with severe root pains at the onset. Vertigo and pyramidal signs may result from adjacent oedema. The combination of a haemorrhagic conjunctivitis, especially if in epidemic proportions, and an acute paralysis simulating classical poliomyelitis is caused by EV70 alone.

Within a few days of the onset of the ocular appearances, EV70 can be isolated from the conjunctival secretion. The ocular diagnosis is important as it may permit one to limit the spread of what could turn out to be an epidemic or worse; the 1981 pandemic in India was on a vast scale affecting perhaps 40 million people. Adult males predominantly contract the disease. The eye changes after a brief prodromal irritation consist of pain, marked swelling of the lids, lacrimation and a serous or mucopurulent discharge. It is highly contagious. Follicles on the lower palpebral conjunctiva occur in about half of those affected. There is no corneal involvement. The pre-auricular glands are enlarged and sore throat with a fever generally accompany the central nervous system (CNS) lesions. The distinctive clinical feature, however, is the rapid appearance of subconjunctival haemorrhages. Early on there is hyperaemia of the *upper* bulbar conjunctiva and fornix, the lower fornix seldom being involved. Haemorrhages which range from a few minute petechiae to gross extravasations occur in the upper part of the eyeball. They increase during the first 48 hours, fade from the fifth day onwards and in most cases are totally absorbed by the tenth day.

Facial nerve palsy is the most common cranial nerve complication. The upper lid descends somewhat owing to reciprocal inhibition of the levator but the lower lid sags and tears spill over the margin. The sixth nerve may also be affected with divergence weakness or, more probably, a convergent squint arises with diplopia. The vagus nerve is sometimes involved as well. Recovery from cranial nerve paralysis is more complete than spinal as a rule. Further precise knowledge about this disease is required. The enterovirus seems to grow in the first instance in the epithelial cells of the conjunctiva, infection of the CNS following. Occasionally the neurological disorders have appeared before the ocular, sometimes apparently without the ocular, and there have been several epidemics in which no CNS changes occurred whatsoever. In the first report of acute haemorrhagic conjunctivitis[6] 13 664 patients were seen in Ghana in 1969, none of whom suffered from cranial nerve or spinal cord involvement. There is no treatment for this disease.

Adenoviral (AV) punctate keratoconjunctivitis

This condition, generally seen in epidemic form, offers a wide variety of clinical features ranging from the very mild to the severe. That is why it is difficult to diagnose without identification of the viral agent, especially when seen as a sporadic case and not in an epidemic. The punctate opacities can be epithelial or subepithelial, depending on the severity of the infecting agent and the stage at which the condition is examined. It is a non-TRIC viral infection (it can somewhat resemble the TRIC); for practical purposes it is always adenoviral (although Coxsackie A24 has been shown to produce a very similar picture). The severity depends on which of several adenoviruses is causing the lesions. Since AV8 was first identified (1957 was a good year for adenoviral literature) the causative viral agents have been shown to include four subtypes of AV8 as well as AV1 to 11, AV13 to 15, AV19 and AV29. Those which produce the most severe clinical symptoms are AV5, 8 and 19. AV3, 4 and 7 are somewhat less severe and the remainder are generally mild in their effect.

The origin of the adenoviruses in the upper respiratory passages of man, not surprisingly, can cause some degree of rhinopharyngitis with pre-auricular lymphadenopathy. Malaise and a low fever generally are associated and in severe cases nausea and diarrhoea. From the reservoir in man's nose and throat infection reaches the external ocular membranes and from there can pass from eye to eye. At its mildest, epidemic punctate keratoconjunctivitis lasts three weeks and at its most severe perhaps three years. It can produce a very red eye.

As always when the cornea is involved the first indication is photophobia and lacrimation. The eye becomes increasingly hyperaemic and is associated with a watery or mucopurulent discharge. In severe cases (AV8 and 19 in particular) there may be a pseudomembrane seen lying in the lower part of a fiery, red eye, not closely adherent—as is the case in diphtheritic conjunctivitis where the membrane has to be torn off—but able to be lifted off (Plate IV.2). Papillae are profuse especially under the upper lid. Follicles can be moderately large and are seen in the fornices and may extend downwards on to the upper bulbar conjunctiva. One or two punctate or small haemorrhages have been noted in the *lower* half of the eye in severe cases. It is known that concurrent infection with EV70, the agent of haemorrhagic conjunctivitis, can occur in epidemic adenoviral conjunctivitis making it a difficult clinical diagnosis.[7] Most of the small haemorrhages in the adenoviral disease may be incidental or due to rubbing and are always in the lower eyeball.

There is nothing very specific about the types of corneal change found. As said at the start, the punctate opacities are superficial and subepithelial. There may be very few in mild cases and they will clear rapidly; in moderate cases they will disappear in about three months. In severe cases where conjunctival scarring may result by the time the acute phase starts to fade a chronic stage, during which the corneal opacities persist in diminishing numbers, lingers on. Even in the very late stages some opacities, more usually the subepithelial, can be seen generally in the centre of the cornea accompanied by prolonged mild watering of the eyes and slight photophobia. Antibiotics and steroids are ineffective but the former prevent secondary infection by bacteria or the TRIC virus.

Conjunctivitis is the commonest cause of red eye but corneal and uveal involvement, as we have seen, may be part and parcel of the same disease. Nevertheless, keratitis and uveitis can occur as separate entities, each giving rise to a painful red eye.

KERATITIS

The commonest explanation of a single sore red eye is a corneal foreign body or an ulcer, especially a herpes simplex (dendritic) ulcer. More than one may be present. Fluorescein staining will reveal the characteristic, tiny-branched shape, the *dendritic* ulcer (Fig. 70.3). If untreated or wrongly treated (steroids must be shunned) the herpetic ulcer can advance to chronic painful ulceration with secondary stromal changes which combined leave scarring. Simple débridement with a cotton-wool bud is an effective first treatment, with or without soaking the area with tincture of iodine (using a topical anaesthetic drop), care being taken to carry out the procedure gently. Débridement may be repeated, an eye drop or ointment being

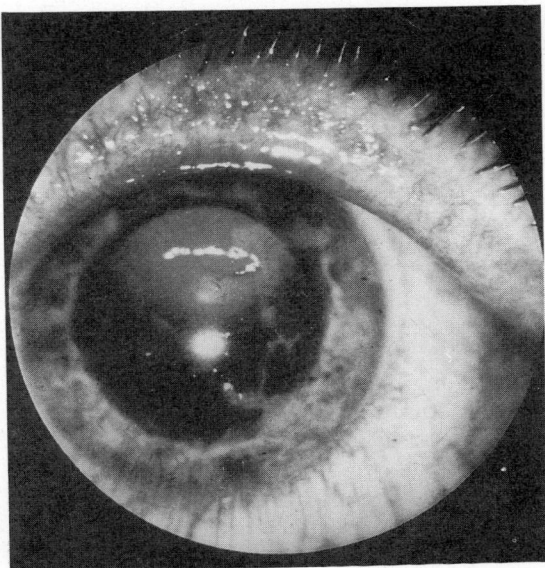

Fig. 70.3 Herpetic (dendritic) ulceration: a metaherpetic reaction below a new ulcer with scarring above. (Courtesy Mr F. C. Rodger.)

applied to avoid infection, and a mydriatic to inactivate the pull of the iris. Herpes simplex virus infections, types I and II, can be treated with idoxuridine 0.1%, the drops being instilled every hour during the day and every 2 hours at night. Alternatively, the 0.5% ointment requires to be inserted every 4 hours, day and night. This is not often going to be practical in the tropics. Vidarabine 3% eye ointment five times daily and acyclovir 3% four or five times daily, are alternatives, but the cost of one tube of these ointments is about the same as three months' income to a peasant farmer.

Corneal ulcers following herpes simplex infection, injury, malnutrition or bacterial infections may increase in size and become impossible to cure by reason of secondary fungal infection (p. 1161). A large amoeboid ulcer is suggestive of this and it is worth treating it as such (Chapter 24).

Mooren's (rodent) ulcer is seen in much younger age groups (20–40) in the tropics than in the West. It generally commences as a large arcuate ulcer advancing from the limbus and penetrating the stroma so that it has an advancing, overhanging edge. The whole cornea may be undermined in this process. The spread is slow but sure. The uninvolved cornea remains transparent. Hypopyon and perforation sometimes occur. Topical treatment will not cure Mooren's ulcer. General treatment of associated debility or diseases such as hookworm may help. Conjunctival excision with thermocautery at the site of the ulcer at the periphery may give some relief. Ulcers in general are difficult to cure. Mydriatics, a scraping for microscopic examination and building up the patient's general health, along with any specific therapy is the correct approach.

In its various forms of surface ulceration or deep infiltration, keratitis is accompanied by some degree of ciliary injection. Conjunctival vessels dilate; some pass over the surface of the cornea to ramify over and around the ulcer, as in phlyctenular disease; new vessels invade the stroma along with the infiltrating inflammatory cells, sometimes in characteristic 'brushes' as in luetic interstitial (stromal) keratitis, at others without a pattern, simply reaching out to vascularize inflammatory regions as in onchocerciasis where the stromal reaction arises around the place of death of the microfilariae. While surface keratitis should not be treated with topical steroids, deep keratitis often responds well.

Other forms of keratitis (fungal, gonococcal, luetic, TRIC, xerophthalmic are discussed under specific headings.

EPISCLERITIS AND SCLERITIS

Inflammatory lesions of the outer (white) coat of the eyeball may be superficial (episcleritis) or deep (scleritis). They are usually localized, sectorial, slightly elevated, nodular, generally but not always adjacent to the limbus. In the episcleral lesion when the conjunctiva is gently moved over the affected area, the vessels move with the membrane; in the deeper scleral lesion they do not move. The sclera proper is almost avascular but some vessels penetrate it to reach the uvea below. The mass of vessels is small and lies in the loose episcleral tissue. Inflammation in these structures may be bacterial, rarely fungal, and especially in Caucasians is most probably metabolic or due to a collagenous disorder. Usually episcleritis clears quickly with corticosteroids or other anti-inflammatory topical therapy. Scleritis takes longer and it is as well to make every effort to understand its pathogenesis. A biopsy should be considered if despite treatment it proves recalcitrant. Patches of inflammation can spread into the adjacent cornea to produce a sclerosing keratitis. This is the classic lesion of onchocerciasis, for micro-

filariae tend to die in numbers at the limbus whence further passage is not easy, the juncture of the conjunctiva and cornea impeding their movements. A sclerosing keratitis is also seen in leprosy.

IRIDOCYCLITIS (ANTERIOR UVEITIS)

When there is an iritis the ciliary body is usually also involved, hence iridocyclitis; these structures happen to form the anterior part of the uvea.

An acute bacterial conjunctivitis is the probable cause of a really red eye. An acute congestive glaucoma makes for a heavily congested blue-red eye with a dilated fixed pupil. An acute anterior uveitis associated with an acute secondary congestive glaucoma, as one would expect, is worst of all. However, an anterior uveitis by itself with a small or distorted pupil makes for a red eye; often the redness is confined to a circle of deep vessels around the limbus, the so-called *ciliary injection* or *rose blush* when only moderately marked. The dilated vessels are branches of the anterior ciliary vessels which pierce the sclera about 4 mm from the limbus to reach the uvea below. In the Negro eye the inlet holes are outlined by black chromatophores. Other signs of anterior uveitis confirm the diagnosis: dilated vessels on the iris surface, a small maybe distorted pupil (contracted with pain), pus in the anterior chamber (Fig. 70.4), cells on the back

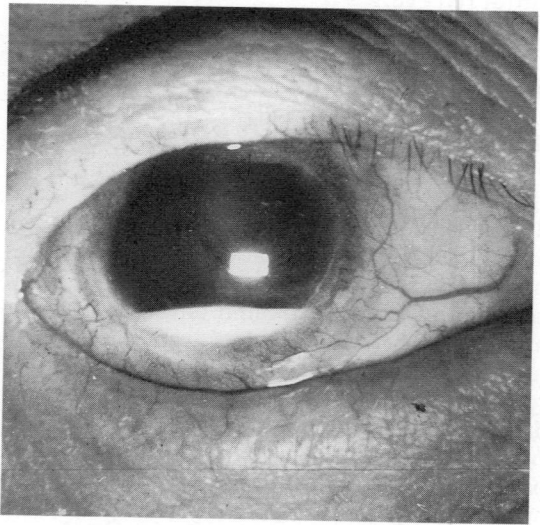

Fig. 70.4 A large hypopyon (pus in anterior chamber). (Courtesy Mr F.C. Rodger and Princess Margaret Hospital.)

of the cornea (keratitic precipitates—KP), small and pigmented maybe, or larger and fatty-looking, and adhesions binding some part or all of the pupillary margin to the underlying lens capsule (synechiae, seclusion) (Plate V. 5). A mydriatic and anti-inflammatory topical drop or ointment (such as hydrocortisone or 10% oxyphenbutazone) is the usual treatment. There is something to be said for leaving the steroid in reserve.

Iritis can be the complication of many systemic conditions; such a cause must be sought and if found specific treatment instituted. The uvea may be invaded by live pathogens, bacterial endotoxins, viral toxins or toxins from disintegrating elements, such as microfilaria (mf) volvulus. The cause of the uveitis may also be a rheumatoid factor or hypersensitivity to certain antigens. Under the conditions likely to be found in the tropics with an absence of laboratory backing, making a true diagnosis is very difficult. When the iris is grossly inflamed and exudation is liberal a secondary glaucoma may arise.

GLAUCOMA

The higher the ocular pressure the more congested become the vessels of the eyeball and the redder, then bluer, the colour. The cornea becomes less lustrous and oedematous. The pupil cannot contract because of the pressure on it and is forced to become ever wider. If the pressure is not released quickly it may remain permanently dilated. As raised pressure can result from blockage of the drainage angle or of part or all of the pupillary aperture (occlusion) by inflammatory debris derived from the anterior uvea (iris and ciliary body), the classic wide pupil of an acute narrow angle glaucoma described above may be concealed or absent. The raised pressure may then be missed. Such eyes are among the most congested one sees and the eyeball can be rock-hard. Surgery would prove disastrous. One is faced with the contradictory choice of using a meiotic for the raised pressure which would further close the pupil or a mydriatic for the anterior uveitis which, if it succeeds in opening the pupil, will further block the drainage angle. The correct approach is to use a systemic drug to reduce the intraocular pressure with topical anti-inflammatory drops or ointment, opening up the pupil as soon as seems safe. It may be necessary to inject Mydricaine under the bulbar conjunctiva to break down pupillary adhesions. A Diamox Sustet 6-hourly given with Slow-K and a subconjunctival injection of Depo-Medrone starts things off and then topical steroids and a mydriatic will be needed every half hour or so until some improvement shows. Nobody can do more than that. Only too often such terrible red eyes are seen too late for treatment to be of any good.

To return to the acute narrow or closed angle glaucoma *minus* the complication of an anterior uveitis the condition should respond quickly to 500 mg Diamox and Slow-K followed by 250 mg 6-hourly combined with regular applications (half-hourly at the least) of 1–2% pilocarpine nitrate. There may be cells in the anterior chamber expressed from the oedematous iris but this is no bar to surgery and the latter will be needed if the ocular pressure does not fall within 24 to 48 hours of diagnosis. Chronic open angle glaucoma does not cause a red eye unless the drainage angle in time is damaged by sporadic subacute attacks and becomes *ipso facto* closed. Chronic simple glaucoma requires the opinion of an eye surgeon. Pilocarpine 1% t.d.s. is standard.

Diagnosis of the cause of a red eye is not as forbidding as it may seem. A check list is helpful, especially in the absence of laboratory facilities.

By observing the type of *secretion*, if present, and by *staining* it with the simple Gram's technique (nearly all bacteria take up methyl violet, and most fungi), by judging the *eyeball pressure* with the finger tips or a small tonometer, by noting the size and shape and reaction to light of the *pupils*, by observing the distribution and degree of the *hyperaemia*, by searching carefully with a magnifying loupe for *cells* on the back of the cornea or in the anterior chamber, by paying attention to the *lustre* of the whole cornea and *staining* it with fluorescein, and by always looking for associated *physical symptoms*, most causes of a red eye will become clear.

MAJOR CAUSES OF BLINDNESS

The three major blinding diseases in the tropics are trachoma, malnutrition and onchocerciasis. So serious is the problem posed by the latter that if it were not restricted in its distribution because its preferred vectors are limited to a favoured ecology, blindness from this one disease would probably surpass the ravages of the other two together. There are other causes of blindness to be considered which are not quite as grave. These include vision impaired among others by leprosy, by cataract (which generally accounts for one-third of all blindness in any one place) and by diseases which lead to optic atrophy.

TRACHOMA

No disease of the eye causes more suffering and blindness—eight million at least—than trachoma. It is endemic, in some areas hyperendemic, in all developing countries except for one or two. The social and economic effects are considerable.

Aetiology

Although it is not confined to the tropics trachoma is found preferentially in such climates. In those parts of the world where protein is in short supply and malnutrition common, where habitations are squalid and overcrowded, where sanitary facilities are absent and where there is an inadequate supply of water, the disease is endemic. Dust, dirt and flies are ever present—pertinent factors all. Contagion and infection and reinfection by direct or indirect contact cannot be avoided under such circumstances. Epidemics of bacterial conjunctivitis (p. 1136) occur regularly; the latter, precipitated by repeated hatches of eye-seeking house flies, may activate a painful but bearable non-blinding trachoma into a hyperendemic blinding one (Plate IV.3). It is this combination of circumstances which has to be broken if control is to be achieved.

The species *Chlamydia trachomatis* includes the pathological agents of trachoma, inclusion conjunctivitis and keratoconjunctivitis and lymphogranuloma venereum (Chapter 68). TRIC virus spreads from eye to eye by transfer of ocular discharges produced almost invariably by the serotypes A, B and C of *C. trachomatis*. Inclusion conjunctivitis (the IC part of TRIC) is one of the few diseases grouped as paratrachomas which result from infection of the eye by sexually transmitted *C. trachomatis* (serotypes D to K); babies can be infected at birth. As a rule the paratrachomas produced by the TRIC virus do not progress to blindness but clinically they are sometimes indistinguishable from the milder inflammatory stage of endemic trachoma (Fig. 68.5, p. 1112).

Distribution

The World Health Organization (WHO) estimates that 500 million persons suffer from trachoma. In Europe the disease in the present century has been endemic in all the Balkan countries and even today there are areas in Bulgaria and Yugoslavia where it can be found. It is also found in small numbers in southern Spain. Trachoma is prevalent in the eastern Mediterranean particularly Lebanon and Jordan, as it is in North Africa in Morocco, Tunisia and Egypt, all heavily affected. There is a high endemic rate in Sudan[8] especially among preschool children. Throughout Africa there is scarcely a country in which it is not a problem. Interesting exceptions are Liberia and Zaire, countries surrounded by others in which the disease is heavy; a high proportion of the populations of Liberia and Zaire dwell in equatorial or rain forests with heavy falls of rain so that dust and sand are laid and do not pervade the air. Trachoma is also found to be endemic in Saudi Arabia, Iran and all other Arab countries. In India and in Pakistan it is a major public health problem. It is a well-known saying, although exaggerated, that 'every Punjabi suffers from trachoma'.

Statistics relating to eastern Russia and China are not available but in Singapore where socioeconomic conditions are good with abundant water and efficient medical services, of the relatively few persons suffering from the disease 77% had migrated from China. Trachoma is also prevalent in Indonesia, the Pacific archipelago and Japan. It has been recognized in Australia for over a century and was at one time the predominant form of eye disease.[9] A reservoir continues to exist among Aborigines but white Australians are now rarely affected. The disease started to decline before the inception of therapy, probably due to the higher living standards and good health education. It is still to be found among Aborigines who prefer to 'live rough'. With the influx of Asian and other migrants Western Europe has many such cases today entering their cities, although the improved conditions soon render the disease harmless.

Signs and symptoms

Stage I

In this early stage lacrimation and slight oedema of the eyelid may occur. The conjunctiva of the upper eyelid shows tufts of dilated capillaries, follicles and the formation of epithelial papillae. The follicles may be 2–3 mm in size and give the conjunctiva a granular appearance. With the slit lamp fine epithelial infiltrates may be seen at the margin of the cornea. The TRIC virus is found in epithelial scrapings. This stage may persist for many months. The upper lid is invariably the worst affected, the midtarsal area being significantly affected (Plate IV.4).

Stage II

Blood vessels, prolongations of the terminal vascular arcades, invade the cornea at its upper limbus, continuing as non-anastomosing brushes of fine vessels at whose tips there is a grey infiltrate between the epithelium and Bowman's membrane. The infiltrate later penetrates the

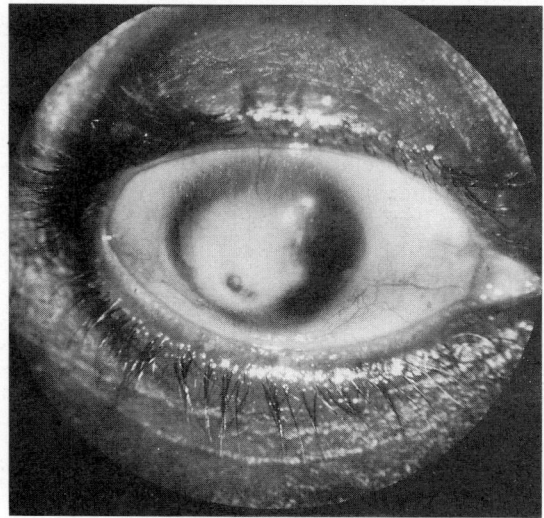

Fig. 70.5 Trachomatous pannus and leukoma adherens (scar from previous perforation).(Courtesy Mr F. C. Rodger and *American Journal of Ophthalmology.*)

substantia propria. This combination of new vessels and infiltrate, known as pannus, spreads from the periphery to involve the whole cornea. The subsequent loss of transparency can severely impair vision. Ulceration may occur especially if there is a secondary bacterial conjunctivitis. This may not end with corneal softening and rupture but, even if the cornea heals, loss of sight from the scar is great (Fig. 70.5). Stage II can last from six months to a year or more in untreated patients, during which the virus is recoverable from the tissues. Towards the end the telltale follicles become necrotic and less pronounced.

Stage III

In this stage, for trachoma is a self-limiting disease, linear cicatrization begins in the tarsal conjunctiva and in the subtarsal groove. Ruptured follicles are replaced by star-shaped white cicatrices forming a mosaic pattern. When active cicatrization has ceased the conjunctiva becomes smooth, white and avascular. The conjunctiva of the lower eyelid and the fornices may be covered with a bluish haze giving it a skimmed-milk appearance.

In the cornea also the follicles rupture or cicatrize. The craters of the ruptured follicles become lined with clear epithelium and produce at the limbus a series of lacunae called Herbert's pits.

In the cornea the invading vessels retrogress and infiltration is absorbed. Remnants of the vessels can always be seen with the loupe or slit lamp and a diffuse haze pervades the cornea. If a major disaster such as ectasia or rupture has not previously involved the cornea useful economic sight is often regained at this stage and persists.

Virus invasion is now less intense and is difficult to demonstrate.

The affected eye may remain in this state for many years.

Stage IV

At this stage the follicles have been replaced by scar tissue and active morbidity in the cornea has ceased. No virus is to be found. The active disease is now 'burnt out'. The leading role is assumed by an inexorable and progressive cicatrization of the scar tissue already present. The upper eyelid becomes grossly deformed due to scarring and buckling of the tarsal plate, and the margin of the eyelid is turned in towards the cornea, the condition of *entropion*. The lash-bearing area of the eyelid is distorted and irregular, secondary lines of eyelashes appear, thrusting out in all directions, the condition of *trichiasis*. Entropion-trichiasis (Fig. 70.6) is essentially an adult complication. The already damaged cornea is now excoriated by the continual impact of the inturned eyelashes and once more becomes vascularized and ulcerated. It loses its sensitivity and is laid open to further damage by particles of dust and sand.

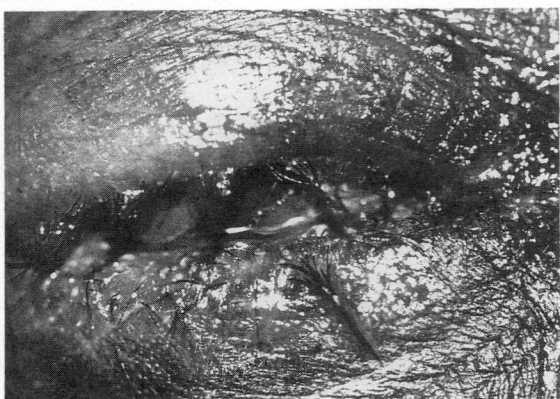

Fig. 70.6 Trichiasis–entropion in trachoma. (Courtesy Dr S. C. I. Sowa and *British Journal of Ophthalmology*.)

Cicatrization of the fornices leads to their obliteration and to the cutting off of lacrimal secretion. The condition of xerosis is established and cornea and conjunctiva are covered with a skin-like membrane. In long-standing cases, as the result of the blocking of lymphatics by scar tissue, the eyelid becomes swollen and heavy; this, combined with involvement of the levator muscle, causes trachoma ptosis.

The changes from stage to stage are a continuum and borderline cases present problems of clinical judgement. The World Health Organization has suggested that in order to attain reasonable uniformity in the results of field studies cases between stages I and II should be categorized as stage II; between II and III as stage III; and between III and IV as stage IV.

In the field where laboratory investigation is unavailable, *two* of the following signs must be present to establish a positive diagnosis:
1 follicles on the upper palpebral conjunctiva in the midtarsal area;
2 linear scarring of the tarsal conjunctiva of the upper lid, known as Arlt's line (Plate IV.5);

3 an active keratitis;
4 pannus in the upper third of the cornea.

In trachoma the maximum conjunctival involvement is in the upper lid, especially in the midtarsus, and the maximum pannus in the upper third of the cornea, whereas in inclusion conjunctivitis there is no pannus and the lower lid (like all the paratrachomas) is maximally involved and scarring absent.

Treatment

The association of trachoma with low socio-economic and sanitary levels and its tendency to disappear as a serious public health problem when living conditions improve are potent factors which must be taken into account at the same time as the individual treatment of the patient.

In the early stages local treatment with eye drops or ointments may be wholly effective but, if the conjunctiva is thickened with deep crypt formation, systemic therapy is indicated in addition to topical. This is also the approach if the response is poor. However, WHO stress 'Oral therapy . . . can be recommended only on a selective basis for severe and moderate intensity cases under medical supervision and only for children over 6–8 years of age and adult males.'

Topical treatment

Tetracycline (Achromycin) and oxytetracycline (Terramycin) are the antibiotics which have been most extensively used and give the best results; they are given by local application as solutions, suspensions or ointments at 1–3%, two to three times a day, over a period of six to eight weeks. Topical sulphacetamides given as a 30% drop or 6% ointment (Albucid) are also useful as an alternative and are cheaper. Whichever is used, treatment must be followed twice at monthly intervals by topical tetracyclines twice a day for 5 consecutive days or alternatively by using it once a day for 10 consecutive days every six months. This latter course is also recommended as prophylactic/preventive treatment for those living in an endemic area.

Oral treatment

When systemic chemicals or antibiotics are advised in severe or recalcitrant subjects in conjunction with topical treatment there may be limits placed on the prescriber by cost or availability, quite apart from the adverse effects. Tetracyclines and erythromycin are safer than sulphonamides which are now out of favour as they carry a substantial risk of hepatitis, crystalluria and blood dyscrasis, and put neonates, nursing and pregnant mothers at risk. Oral tetracyclines also harm little children, pregnant and nursing mothers and the elderly but not with such a long list of adverse effects as the sulphonamides. Erythromycin is much the safest. Apart from diarrhoea there are no serious side-effects although it is contraindicated in liver disease. Children require 125–250 mg every 6 hours and adults double that dose for 21 days. It is especially good in children and *Chlamydia trachomatis* has not developed a resistance against erythromycin. Rifampicin, which has a long list of adverse side-effects, is out of favour despite its efficacy.

Surgical treatment

Surgical treatment is indicated where there is deformity of the upper lid. When inturned (entropion) and when the lashes rub on the cornea (trichiasis) the end result is almost certainly going to be a severe reduction in acuity of vision. If the cornea is already scarred, to remedy entropion will eliminate pain. If caught early it could prevent blindness. One is dealing basically with thickening and deformity of the tarsal plate due to infection in the subconjunctival tissue overlying it. Several surgical procedures are possible and are described in textbooks of ophthalmic surgery, such as the very practical *Basic Eye Surgery* by J. E. K. Galbraith.[10]

The simplest operation is one described by Thommy:[11] the technique avoids vertical shortening of the upper lid with the risk of subsequent *ectropion*, the reverse of the condition being treated. It involves inserting a sheet of levator muscle from under the skin surface of the upper lid downwards under the lower part of the skin incision towards the eyelash margin where it is resutured. While no attempt to excise the lower part of the muscle sheet is made, some is lost in the procedure. This fact and the advancement of the levator largely correct the entropion.

PARATRACHOMAS

The link between blinding hyperendemic trachoma and the paratrachomas, as said earlier, is non-blinding meso- or hypoendemic trachoma. In the latter the factors which contribute to severe trachoma are either not all present or are much reduced.

Inclusion (kerato-) conjunctivitis

The responsible virus reaches the eye from the genital canal and then spreads from eye to eye. It does not lead to blindness. The eye becomes red and irritable and the discharge watery or mucopurulent. Large follicles can be seen especially in the lower fornix but also on the upper palpebral conjunctiva. However, the midtarsal area, so favoured by the trachoma agent (TR) is invariably clear with the inclusion conjunctival agent (IC). When the cornea is unaffected the disease causes moderate to severe discomfort for several months. The duration can be shortened if a course of topical tetracycline is given.

When the cornea is involved an added symptom is photophobia. Epithelial and subepithelial opacities can be revealed by staining but, once again, the midtarsal area of the upper lid is clear and there will be no pannus nor scarring. The condition takes a chronic course becoming gradually less acute. The corneal opacities and follicles have been seen after more than a year so vigorous tetracycline treatment is indicated. Nevertheless, untreated, this paratrachoma has been known to settle in the end without permanent scarring.

Blennorrhoea of the newborn (see also Chapter 68, p. 1111)

This condition occurs in the eyes of newborn babies, the infection coming from the birth canal or from dirty cloths used to wipe the infants' eyes. It starts as a gross swelling of the lids, the conjunctivae being infected by one of two organisms in particular. One is the TRIC virus (inclusion blennorrhoea); the other, the best known of the causative organisms, is the Gram-negative *Neisseria gonorrhoeae* (ophthalmia neonatorum). Pneumococci and streptococci may also be present. A WHO Working Group (1984) stated its concern over the worldwide increase in sexually transmitted diseases, blennorrhoeas being one group of them. Increased resistance of the gonococcus to penicillin and the abandonment of inserting silver nitrate eye drops or other medicaments into the eyes of the newborn as a routine were both blamed.

The TRIC virus takes longer to produce a reaction (21 days or thereabouts) than any of the bacteria; gonococcus takes the least (1–3 days). The lids in the TRIC infection may be slightly infected, the condition being catarrhal with a mucopurulent discharge. However, one is more liable to be faced in the tropics with gross swelling, the lids being under great pressure from the intense discharge within them. Inclusion blennorrhoea is soon controlled with sulphacetamide or tetracycline drops which require to be liberally inserted: one drop every minute for the first 30 minutes and then 10 times in the next hour and a half, then 2 hourly. Atropine 1% is instilled three times a day in case the cornea is damaged, for the greatest problem in treating severe blennorrhoeas is to force open the lids; retractors are needed and damage to the cornea is avoided with difficulty. Sometimes inclusion blennorrhoea is uniocular but cross infection can occur so, keeping in mind the long incubation period, treatment of the apparently unaffected eye should continue two or three times daily for three weeks. In those cases that have been neglected gross follicular formation on the palpebral conjunctiva will be seen and systemic antibiotic treatment with erythromycin should be given from the start.

It is convenient and appropriate to discuss *bacterial* infections of the eye in the newborn at this point. Here the blennorrhoea, especially with gonococcus infection, is excessively purulent and the cornea is at high risk (Fig. 68.4, p. 112). Only with secondary infection or following damage during treatment can the same be said in the case of TRIC infection. Corneal ulceration with rupture and loss of the eye can only be avoided if the infant eye is washed out thoroughly and repeatedly. It is essential to obtain access to do so and to insert antibiotic drops (such as gentamicin) and this may necessitate cutting open the outer canthus down to the bony margin with scissors. When the gonococcus is identified systemic ampicillin or paediatric suspension of Septrin (sulphamethoxazole with trimethoprim) is vital. If caught and treated early and thoroughly the speed and completeness of the cure in this dangerous condition is as dramatic as its onset (see also p. 1113).

MALNUTRITION AND THE EYE

Deficiency disease, apart from sheer starvation or deprivation of food of any kind, implies disease caused by ingestion of food below minimal requirements, defective utilization in the body of food substances or the absence in the food of protein, vitamins and amino acids and other essential chemicals, collectively or singly.

Nowhere in the body is the impact of deprivation more in evidence than in the eye and in the visual sense.

Distribution of malnutrition

At the present time the manifestations of deficiency disease are to be found mainly in underdeveloped countries. Protein deficiency arises where production of cattle is inadequate, for instance because of disease, such as trypanosome infection. In Africa between the southern limits of the Sahara down to latitude 20° south, 'nagana', the disease in animals caused by trypanosome infection, reduces the cattle-carrying capacity of the country by more than 50%. Wild animals and some breeds of cattle arrive at an understanding with the trypanosome risk to which they are exposed so as to be able to absorb it, not without being infected, but without clinical manifestations. If the mechanism were understood we would be in possession of a tool which could beyond any other available enlarge the production of available animal protein in the tropics.

Rinderpest and East Coast fever are other factors in this part of the world. In India religious restriction limits the amount of meat available as food, and in other parts of the world, Latin America and Asia, meat is simply too expensive.

Mankind through the ages has progressively acquired knowledge of improved methods of cultivation, animal breeding and animal health but, pari passu, adverse factors have arisen.

A good example of this is the clearance of bush in which tsetse flies breed thereby protecting the health of the animals which supply milk and beef and prolonging their lives. The unfortunate sequels are soil erosion following loss of the trees and subsequent overgrazing with failure of the crops. Soil erosion has been called a disease of civilization; it is preventable but continues unabated in those parts of the world where it should least happen. Clearance of trees to control insect vectors of disease or to supply fuel and building timber are the chief reasons for soil erosion. Other factors which increase the aridity of the land are the despoliation of anything green by wandering herds of goats and long-legged sheep, the use of animal manure as fuel instead of as fertilizer and the inadequacy of the water supply punctuated by periods of drought.

An uncontrollable birth rate adds to the competition for available protein and carbohydrate. Family customs and behaviour also play a part. The last born child in many parts of the world is suckled for a long time and then precipitously weaned, being placed on a wholly farinaceous diet without milk or protein or any vitamin A precursor. When meat or fowl is eaten the father has his fill, the mother next and the children in order of age. More usually the source of animal protein comes but rarely in the shape of a bird, frog, rat or snake in the family soup. It is a dismal picture. Despite these hardships in some places the harm is self-inflicted: in many countries potentially milk-yielding animals—cows, buffaloes, camels, sheep and goats—are kept as stock and are not milked. In disease-free areas, such as the highlands of Ethiopia—well above the tsetse belt and by no means all arid even in times of drought and, when rain falls, extremely fertile—indolence and lack of government concern prevent full use of the land for agriculture and the breeding of animals additional to those which satisfy immediate needs. As a result there is no reserve for times of famine in their own or other parts of their country. Vitamin rich fish livers are often regarded as poisonous and thrown to the pi-dogs. Stocks of green leaves rich in vitamins A, B and C, protein and minerals are ignored, even when the harvest store is used up and the people are hungry awaiting the rains.

The clinical syndromes of malnutrition are described in Chapter 45. They result from various combinations of dietary circumstance. Several vitamin deficiencies are involved, sometimes many at the same time (polyavitaminosis) (Chapter 46). The signs ascribable to deficiency of each are given at the end of this section but as a combined deficiency of vitamin A and protein is the greatest cause of malnutrition blindness, each will be described first.

Vitamin A

Derived from β-carotene this vitamin occurs in milk products, carrots, turnips, red palm nuts, leafy vegetables, egg yolks and liver from all sources. Vitamin A is mobilized by enzyme action to maintain a constant level in the plasma with a reserve in the liver which is only slowly depleted. It is found in rhodopsin, the visual purple of the rod receptors of the retina, essential to dark adaptation, and in iodopsin in the cones; it is vital in maintaining the health of the external ocular membranes. There is generally a plentiful supply of this vitamin except in sahel savannah and like places. The greener the leaf, the more red or yellow the fruit or vegetable or root, the more provitamin is present. The oil from the pulp of the red palm nut has a provitamin A value of 40 000–80 000 IU/100 g and forest dwellers in consequence where this tree grows benefit enormously.

Vitamin A deficiency is particularly devastating if it is combined with protein–energy malnutrition (PEM) especially when the latter is associated with a calorie *deficiency*. Kwashiorkor (Chapter 45) results from protein deficiency with calorie *sufficiency* (Plate IV.6). These are two opposite ends of a spectrum of disease confused by reason of intermediate appearances. In children with vitamin A, PEM and calorific deficiency, or some close variant of this, there arises *xerophthalmia*, a term which includes *xerosis* (dryness of the external eye) and *keratomalacia* (necrosis of the cornea). In such children the immunological defences are often reduced making the possibility of blindness even more assured by reason of secondary infection.

Ocular changes of xerophthalmia

Before the corneal changes reduce visual acuity night blindness can be demonstrated in those affected by measuring the threshold for light in the dark-adapted eye with one of several apparatuses available. The various transitory changes in the external eye vary from a small patch of wrinkled, dry bulbar conjunctiva lying between the limbus and the outer canthus usually (it may be nasal) to the horrific disaster of necrosis and rupture of the cornea. These changes do not necessarily occur progressively. They can be modified by the degree and persistence of the deficiencies. The speed of the damage thus varies. One eye may exhibit one feature, the other a different feature. Bearing this in mind, xerosis and keratomalacia will be described separately. As xerosis is a non-specific term, meaning dryness, it is more aptly called *nutritional* xerosis within the present context.

NUTRITIONAL XEROSIS
The initial change is in the conjunctiva,

especially the bulbar. If suspected, multiple conjunctival erosions can be revealed early on by vital staining with 1% rose bengal or 1% lissamine green. In time the cornea loses its lustre and transparency, thickens and wrinkles concentric to the limbus, loses its tone and becomes smokily pigmented.

Hyperkeratosis and desquamation of the epithelium with consequent destruction and loss of the mucus-secreting goblet cells is the underlying cause of these changes. The longer the patient remains untreated and the more severe the degree of malnutrition, the greater is the area affected. Sometimes the corneal epithelium is involved simultaneously; at others corneal changes follow the conjunctival. The lacrimal secretion is reduced and in the absence of mucus the tears are not retained on the corneal surface which accentuates the dryness of the external eye.

One of the most prominent features is the intense staining of the surface of the external eye with 1% rose bengal which demonstrates the punctate nature of the desquamation which occurs.

However, before leaving the conjunctival changes to describe the corneal there is one conjunctival xerotic change which for some reason remains restricted to a small region on the most protuberant part of the eyeball close to the limbus. This is called a *Bitot's spot* (Fig. 70.7) and may not be associated with a low serum vitamin A or carotenoid value, or indeed be related to any other sign of hypovitaminosis; further to confuse matters it does not always respond to vitamin A therapy. Nevertheless, Bitot's spots occur in situations where malnutrition exists or has existed in the recent past in the family circle, if not necessarily in the individual at the time of examination. The area may be coated with a pearly discharge (xerosis bacilli and gas bubbles) or with a mucoid material due to a (usually) mild infection. When the debris is wiped off a small xerotic patch is easily seen and any stain or material found in the fornices will adhere to the spot. That seems to be the end of the story.

To return to an established nutritional xerosis where the conjunctiva is densely involved and the cornea increasingly so, both structures will stain heavily with rose bengal. The corneal epithelium becomes ever more keratinized and flakes off in small, greasy patches. Infiltration of the stroma also occurs. It is at the apex usually that the degenerating epithelium first exhibits cracks or large erosions. As the affected area thins the adjacent cornea becomes opaque (blue-white) for the corneal metabolism is now disrupted. The tissue is wide open to bacterial infection so that ulcers with hypopyon can occur and may rupture. Alternatively, the eroded cornea may give way as the aqueous pressure pushes the iris outwards, often covered only by Descemet's endothelium (descemetocele). As in all perforations whether ulcerous or not once health is

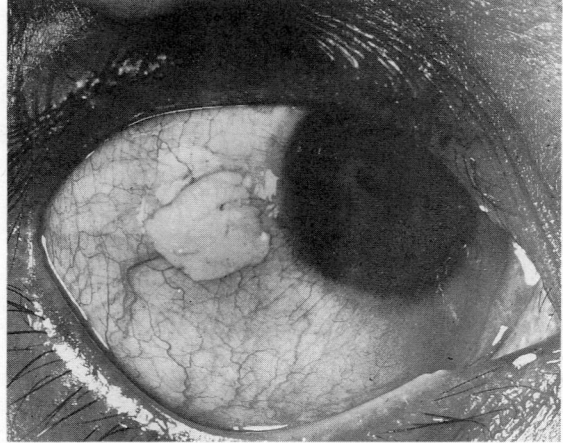

Fig. 70.7 Bitot's spot with mucopus caught on the xerotic area. (Courtesy Mr F. C. Rodger and *Journal of Nutrition*.)

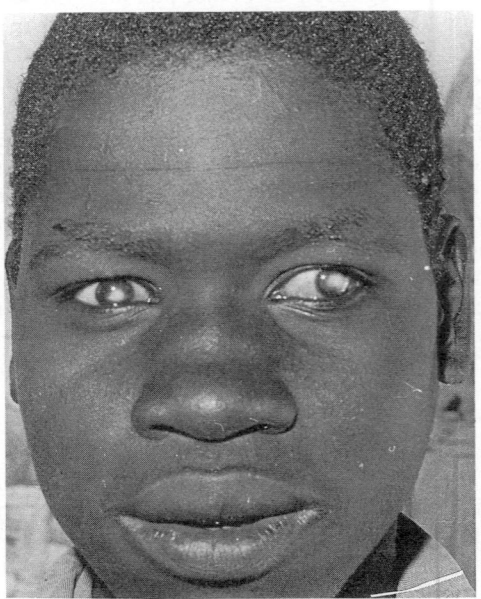

Fig. 70.8 Healed keratomalacia in Metabele boy. (Courtesy *Central African Medical Journal*.)

restored healing can occur leaving a scar known as a leukoma, which is also a finding in keratomalacia (Fig. 70.8). In the absence of treatment or an improvement in nutriture the eye ends as a disorganized phthisical mass, a non-specific picture.

KERATOMALACIA

Because the association between nutritional xerosis and keratomalacia is not always obvious it is as well to review the facts a bit more closely. Sauter[12] has written a masterly monograph in which he shows how xerophthalmia advances to rupture of the eyes in hospitalized children, severely ill with malnutrition, some with measles and some without. When examining less sick children in a village or outlying clinic, however, the relationship is not always so logical. Keratomalacia may be seen in one eye in the absence of any gross corneal change in the other and spontaneous dissolution of the cornea can occur in a clear cornea. This is one reason why keratomalacia is not yet fully understood. Recent work introduces other possibilities suggesting it has a pathogenesis differing from xerosis. Some have said it is tied in with a reduced concentration of the anticollagenase factor in the blood. It is not proven but it is difficult to disprove. The herpes simplex virus which constantly lurks in the tears and the virus of measles have both been put forward as aetiological factors in the causation of keratomalacia. The natural history of herpes simplex and the epidemiology of the disease as it affects the cornea would seem to exclude it as a factor.

As for measles, a much stronger case has been put forward by reason of the high incidence of keratomalacia when this disease is present in a tropical area. Sauter[12] in his 'in depth' study clarifies the relationship of measles to blindness. The invasion of the conjunctiva and cornea by the measles virus is so intense that the external eyes are photophobic, red, painful and with a mucopurulent discharge, whereas the most striking feature of xerophthalmia is the absence of such reactions: there is no congestion and no pain. Yet when malnutrition and secondary ocular infection were combined with measles, Sauter found the inflammatory response to the latter to be 'strikingly mild.'

In measles there is a subepithelial punctate keratitis and many surface erosions; the latter stain with rose bengal but the former do not, being best seen after soaking with a 1% fluorescein solution, subsequently washed off the surface. Thus the two most important differences between xerophthalmia and measles are the deep opacities in the latter, which do not stain with rose bengal, and the absence of pain in the former. It is not surprising that in measles where the eyes are so irritable and painful, secondary infection from rubbing occurs, which we know can advance to ulceration and rupture; the eye will then either heal, producing a leukoma, or become disorganized.

Sauter concludes that in the absence of malnutrition and/or secondary infection, measles does not lead to rupture of the eye; thus in the Third World measles has a non-specific contributory role. In addition, as with any fever, a dendritic ulcer can be a further complication, if somewhat rarely. Sauter's important conclusions substantiate a suggestion made 17 years earlier.[13]

In uncomplicated xerophthalmia, that is in the absence of measles or any other infectious disease, such as pneumonia, leading to extreme debilitation, it seems certain that signs of corneal change may be minor, or absent, prior to the development of keratomalacia. What are the clinical features of this lesion?

Although the cornea may be lustrous a localized depression or facet which does not stain, an indication of corneal thinning, may be the only sign. The bulbar conjunctiva may stain with rose bengal in the lower hemisphere and draw attention to the presence of a minor degree of nutritional xerosis; but staining is sometimes absent. The absence of corneal erosions that stain, of corneal infiltrates and dryness along with the localized crater is difficult to explain. A very small depression of this nature may perforate and a minute bleb of dark iris tissue protrude like the head of a fly (myocephalon), while the rest of the cornea remains quite transparent. A myocephalon is quite free from pain and there is no inflammatory reaction. This lesion may occur on a larger scale still without evidence of dryness and can advance to a descemetocele. In the end such a large area of keratomalacia consists of uvea behind Descemet's membrane, crossed by a few strands of collagen, the whole bound together by exudate, with the lens and vitreous pressing against this precarious barrier (Fig. 70.9). Such an eye, of course, is lost and is indistinguishable from the end picture of nutritional xerosis with corneal ulceration, rupture and dissolution described earlier.

It is these anomalies mentioned above which

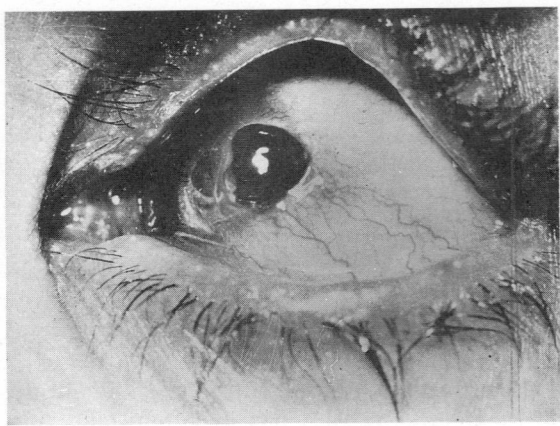

Fig. 70.9 Keratomalacia with part descemetocele. (Courtesy Mr F. C. Rodger and *Acta Ophthalmologica*.)

prompt the questions asked concerning the pathogenesis of keratomalacia. Nevertheless, the geographical distribution suggests all the variants described are due to vitamin A and/or protein lack, depending on whether it is acute or follows gradual deprivation of one or other or both.

Treatment

The following treatment is recommended for all cases of potential blinding malnutrition.[14]

VITAMIN A PREPARATIONS

On diagnosis, 200 000 IU by mouth (110 mg retinol palmitate) or, alternatively, 100 000 water-miscible IU by intramuscular injection (55 mg retinol palmitate). On the next day 200 000 IU (110 mg) should be given orally and the latter should be given again prior to discharge or if deterioration occurs (in a few days), or in the presence of kwashiorkor every two weeks because of the reduced absorption. Toxic effects of excess vitaminosis A (headache, pruritus and nausea) are unlikely with this dosage which can be tolerated for much longer. Thereafter a diet as rich in vitamin A as possible should be given and other hypovitaminoses treated as well.

It should be noted that spontaneous cures arise in both types of disorder, nutritional xerosis and keratomalacia, especially in a peasant farming community with pre-harvest starvation, where new supplies of essential foodstuffs may become available before xerophthalmia has advanced too far. Recovery often depends on whether the mother takes the trouble to feed and nurse her

child and she is much more likely to do so adequately if she herself is on a good diet. Evidence of healed xerophthalmia includes bulbar pigmentation, concentric scarring, leukomas (with iris inclusions in the white scars, leukoma adherens) or phthisis bulbi.

PROTEIN, CARBOHYDRATE AND MINERAL SUPPLEMENTS

In keratomalacia a high protein diet is required, milk being the basis. Glucose is added to the milk in the early stages of treatment as hypoglycaemia is invariably present. An intake of 1000 cal (4200 kJ)/kg should be the aim. At the start 2 g of potassium is needed daily. Although there is retention of sodium the level falls when treatment is under way and additional sodium chloride (1–2 g daily) is soon needed. In severe dehydrated cases a gastric or intravenous infusion may be necessary. Topical and/or systemic antibiotic therapy may be required for any coexisting infections of eye or body (such as the lungs or the bowels) and if possible should be given routinely. Intramuscular iron will cure anaemia and it is advisable also to treat routinely for malaria. It is the association of infections such as these which leads to the high mortality rate and the high incidence of blindness in such patients; hence the importance of using every possible aid.

In the event of prophylactic therapy being considered advisable oral retinol palmitate can be given at birth (50 000 IU), under a year (20 000 IU every four to six months), over a year (100 000 IU every four to six months). Further details in the management of those at risk in areas where malnutrition is known to exist or be a possible sequel to a bad harvest or drought are given in the WHO 1984 publication.[14]

Other vitamins

Vitamin B₁

The germ cells of cereals, milk, eggs, yeast, beef and leguminous vegetables are rich in vitamin B_1 (thiamine). Absence of vitamin B_1 is responsible for beriberi in which the ocular symptoms are a dry burning conjunctivitis, keratitis and ocular neuritis, progressing to optic atrophy. Wernicke's encephalopathy with its external rectus palsy together with cerebral symptoms is attributable to thiamine deficiency (Chapter 46).

Vitamin B₂

Vitamin B₂

Most of the foods with good B₂ (riboflavine) values are of animal origin (including fish) as well as pulses (dhals) and eggs. The evidence that the lack of B₂ produces peripheral corneal neovascularization, comparable to that found in experimental animals, is conflicting. Photophobia and keratitis have also been linked with riboflavine deficiency though somewhat indefinitely.

Vitamin PP (nicotinic acid)

The best sources are dried yeast, liver, wheat germ, lean meat and parboiled rice, in that order. The body can convert the amino acid tryptophan to nicotinic acid, so protein can be protective in those who are deficient in the vitamin. Deficiency classically causes pellagra, though B₁ and B₂ may also be involved, just as all three vitamins may play a combined role in the development of beri-beri and the orogenital syndrome.

Exposure to sunlight causes hyperpigmentation of the skin and this is manifested in the eyelids, the lid margins and the conjunctiva in pellagra. In the lens, powder-like opacities and peripheral tongue-shaped opacities are found. In the affected subject normal sunlight causes retinal hyperpigmentation and appearances at the macula similar to a burn, with hyperaemia and loss of the foveal reflex. The central changes result in a reduction of visual acuity.[15]

Vitamin B₁₂ (cyanocobalamin) and folic acid

The B₁₂ vitamin is the extrinsic factor of Castle. It contains a modified metalloporphyrin in the centre, linked to a nucleotide. Deficiency causes lesions in the spinal cord and optic nerve. Man gets most of his cyanocobalamin from animal sources, so the true vegetarian is at risk. Its absence leads to pernicious anaemia, tobacco amblyopia, Leber's optic atrophy and some toxic optic atrophies of doubtful nature. All these conditions respond to hydroxocobalamin, the form of choice of B₁₂ for treatment. Initially, it is given by intramuscular injection, 1 mg five times at intervals of 2–3 days; the maintenance dose is 1 mg every three months for adults and children.

Folic acid is present in abundance in dark green vegetables, liver and kidney and certain wheat preparations. Like vitamin B₁₂ it is involved in haematopoiesis and a deficiency produces macrocytic anaemia similar to that caused by B₁₂ deficiency but not the optic and peripheral neuritis and cord lesions. In developing countries folic acid deficiency, not B₁₂, is responsible for most macrocytic anaemias, particularly in the elderly, pernicious (addisonian) anaemia being rare.

It is not always possible to carry out sternal marrow punctures and so categorization of the anaemia as megaloblastic is impossible. Being so often accompanied by iron deficiency the blood picture is sometimes doubtful. Further doubts arise when the subject suffers from kwashiorkor, for the anaemia then discovered may result from a deficiency of folic acid, protein and iron (Chapter 58). In such a case it is better to treat with folic acid (5 mg daily) and ferrous salts (500 mg daily) until a response occurs when one then changes to small maintenance doses. Excess folic acid for a short spell is not harmful; it is cheap and a high dose may be effective by mouth even where there is malabsorption. With large and prolonged doses of folic acid, however, the blood B₁₂ will be lowered, and subacute combined degeneration of the cord precipitated with its concomitant optic neuropathy. If there is any suspicion of this, hydroxocobalamin must be given as well.

In addition to the simple optic atrophy one finds as a complication of vitamin B₁₂ deficiency, pernicious and other anaemias can lead to superficial flame-shaped haemorrhages in the retina. There may be only a few at the posterior pole but their possible significance should not be overlooked.

Vitamin C (ascorbic acid)

Vitamin C is found in many fruits, particularly citrus fruits, and leaves. The best sources are often the least palatable and vice versa. Meat and milk are poor sources. The classical lesion is scurvy. In this complaint which is distressing to the sufferer and beholder alike the patient often admits to an adherence to a starchy diet and an avoidance of fruit and green vegetables. Ocular lesions in scurvy are rare. Typical are haemorrhages in the eyelids, subconjunctiva and episcleral tissue and, rarely, in the iris and retina. Intracranial haemorrhages have been known to produce ptosis and external ophthalmoplegia. Repletion is important and should be quick. Vitamin C drops are said by many to promote healing of corneal ulceration.

Vitamin D (cholecalciferol)

Vitamin D is found in fish liver, milk, butter and eggs. Short waves in the sun activate the provitamin present in the skin to form vitamin D_3 so that as infants learn to walk in the sun any minor deficiency is soon corrected. The close link this vitamin has with calcium metabolism associates it with band-shaped keratopathy when in excess (a common condition in the tropics) and with infantile cataracts when deficient (tetany). The predominant systemic manifestation of deficiency is rickets.

Infantile cataract and rickets are rare in the tropics outside of the very largest cities.

ONCHOCERCIASIS

Onchocerciasis (river blindness) is found in Africa approximately from 15° north to 15° south as well as in Guatemala (where it was first described by Robles), Venezuela, Mexico and (lightly) in Colombia and Ecuador. There are in addition small foci in north Sudan and the Yemen. An account of this fascinating and terrible disease is given in Chapter 20. It is because the fly vector breeds in fast flowing rivers (riverine people are the first and worst affected) that the term 'river blindness' arose.

In the last few years it has emerged after intensive research organized by the WHO that the forms of *Onchocerca volvulus* in the West African rain forest and Sudan savannah are different, there being two physiologically distinct filariae. Moreover, transmission of each form, for so long believed to be by one species of *Simulium* fly in West Africa, another in East Africa and a third in Central America, is now known to be carried out by several flies, different cytospecies of the *Simulium damnosum* complex. Thus, it has slowly emerged that these different *Onchocerca/Simulium* complexes are associated with somewhat differing clinical patterns of eye disease. This is the explanation given for what has been known since 1956, namely that the microfilariae of Sudan savannah in West Africa cause far more blindness and, in particular, corneal blindness, than those in the forest. However, the tale is far from finished for this may not be the case elsewhere. In the equatorial forest of Zaire onchocerciasis is known to cause a great deal of blindness, somewhat more in fact than in the Zaire savannah. Although there are more cases of corneal blindness in Zaire savannah dwellers than in the forest (just as in West Africa) there is a great deal more blindness due to inner eye involvement (uvea and retina) in the forest and *from all causes* more blindness (19.0% in the equatorial forest and 14.3% in the savannah).[16] The problem is clearly huge and complex and requires to be worked out gradually in all the various onchocerciasis zones in Africa and the Americas.

Pathology

The microfilariae can and do reach the eye from under the skin over the lid margins, under the conjunctiva into the cornea and into the inner eye at the front via the loose adventitial sheaths of the perforating vessels.[17] Similarly, once in the orbit they can enter the eye from any quarter via the sheaths of perforating arteries as well as into the optic nerve. In this same paper[17] the first photomicrographs of mf volvulus in the sheath of a retinal vessel and within the retinal structure and the optic nerve are shown. The totality of the invasion of the eye is horrific.

Wherever microfilariae die the disintegrating bodies act as a toxin causing direct damage to adjacent tissues and vessels; closure of the latter giving rise to anoxia aggravates the pathological changes, as demonstrated in the skin. In the posterior segment of the eye the same processes probably account for all the retinal and choroidal changes depending on the number of microfilariae and foci involved, although the pathogenesis of the Hissette–Ridley fundus is not quite certain. The death in the retina—rather than in the choroid—of a few microfilariae, or even of small immature adult larvae in the absence of microfilariae has been suggested as the cause of the latter.

Ocular manifestations

Punctate keratitis and larvae in the anterior chamber

The most common early distribution is one of erratic dispersal of microfilariae within the entire cornea. When alive and moving, *O. volvulus* microfilariae are nearly impossible to see in the cornea unless close to the epithelium. The static appearance of linear and fluffy opacities up to 0.5 mm in length at all levels in the stroma results from the presence of dead larvae. If subepithelial these may be called a superficial punctate keratitis; an interstitial keratitis occurs when inflammatory cells surround dispersed groups of dead microfilariae in the stroma.

In a beam of light with a magnifying loupe the larvae in the anterior chamber are best seen in the line of the beam as minute, wriggling objects in the aqueous, their colour depending on the brightness of the incident light. Sometimes patients complain of entopic phenomena due to their lashing movements; usually around 50 microfilariae are present when such a complaint is received. *O. volvulus* microfilariae have been noted in the retrolental space of Berger and a few in the vitreous.

Nummular (larger coin-shaped) opacities are not uncommon in African eyes, two or three in a cornea, but also exist in areas where there is no onchocerciasis; they may be viral or due to trauma and need not be discussed further. They should not be considered as evidence of the presence of microfilariae.

Sclerosing keratitis

The classical corneal change in onchocerciasis is sclerosing keratitis (Fig. 70.2 and Plate V.1). The keratitis commences at three or nine o'clock from where 'tongues' of pannus onchocercosus invade the cornea; in the end they may meet at the centre. Another common appearance is as an 'apron' of pannus around the lower half of the cornea; this lesion also advances towards the pupillary area. Several tongues of pannus can appear at the same time in the lower half of the cornea, all becoming confluent in the end. When the condition is allowed to advance unchecked the end result is total involvement of the cornea.

The external appearance of the pannus onchocercosus is fairly characteristic: it lies at first between the epithelium and Bowman's membrane; subsequently, it may break through Bowman's membrane or appear well below it. It is often associated (when the cornea is invaded in force by microfilariae) with interstitial areas of fibrosis. The pannus consists of three zones: an advancing 'snowstorm' zone of separate grey dots; a middle, white zone, where the individual opacifications (infiltrates) are densely packed; and a basal pigmented zone. In the end the epithelial surface above the pannus may become entirely pigmented, although it can be seen under high magnification to fade off towards the upper pole of the cornea. Corneal neovascularization is

essentially restricted to the pannus, although in late cases new, large blood vessels may enter the stroma. In late stages of this condition one finds evidence of corneal degenerations, such as band-shaped and solar keratopathy. The keratitis is quite frequently associated with an anterior uveitis.

Anterior uveitis

About 60% of all defective sight resulting from onchocerciasis arises from anterior uveal inflammation and its complications. The condition is generally seen as an insidious, low grade, non-granulomatous infection, or, even when it has been severe, in a quiescent state; there seems little doubt that occasional short-lived bursts of acute or subacute uveal activity occur, as they have been witnessed in field surveys.

The iris changes are noticeable at the pupillary margin. There is loss of pigment from the frill, exudation in front of, across or behind the pupil, formation of posterior adhesions usually associated with entropion (inturning) of the pupil and keratic precipitates. The latter are pigmented and small, rarely lardaceous (mutton fat). A gelatinous exudate occasionally spills over into the anterior chamber at six o'clock, dragging the pupil margin down and outwards (hence the term ectropion of the pupillary margin); an oval or pear-shaped pupil may result. The exudate, when it has become organized becomes grey or white in colour. Not uncommonly circles or parts of circles, blue-white in colour, run round the pupillary margin or even cover the entire pupil. This appearance has been called 'flocculation' for convenience (Plate V.2). In an endemic area it is a specific sign. In severe anterior uveitis occlusion of the pupil or seclusion with secondary glaucoma is not uncommon; the iris crypts may be filled in giving a brown flat iris with the appearance of velvet. Complicated cataracts may be seen to have arisen and the choroid may also be affected.

Changes involving the posterior segment

The changes in the choroid are well established but frequently they are concealed by inflammatory membranes resulting from anterior uveitis, membranes covering either the front of the lens or, where the ciliary processes have been heavily involved, the back of the lens (cyclitic membrane). When a complicated cataract results without such membranes it has the same effect: the fundus is concealed and the choroidal changes go unrecorded unless the eye is examined under the microscope after excision. In such cases where *O. volvulus* microfilariae are found to be present throughout the entire uvea only a single *inflammatory* focus may be seen in the choroid but, generally, and probably ultimately, there are several scattered throughout the posterior segment. In all cases examined there has been the same underlying pathology: focal necrosis, oedema, cell infiltration (plasma, lymphocytes, eosinophils but no giant cells) associated with fragmented microfilariae, choroidoretinal scarring and fusion, and varying degrees of vascular closure of the adjacent choroidal vessels.

Optic atrophy is a common cause of blindness in onchocerciasis; how common it is not yet fully agreed. It is discussed elsewhere (p. 1158). It may be associated with disseminated posterior inflammatory foci (not necessarily parapapillary) but it can also occur as a primary lesion of the optic nerve, either resulting from closure of the nutrient vessels or from intoxication of the nerve fibres by the products of the disintegrating microfilarial bodies within or alongside the fasciculi of nerve fibres.

The classic posterior change in onchocerciasis, however, is the *Hissette–Ridley* (HR) fundus (Plate V.3); as the pupil is less commonly covered when this occurs, one sees with the ophthalmoscope far more examples of the HR fundus than of the disseminated lesion and so it is easy to get the wrong impression as to incidence. In order to understand why the pathogenesis of this lesion is so difficult, the histopathology of the disseminated choroidoretinitis described above has to be appreciated first, for neither the ophthalmoscopic nor the pathological pictures of the HR fundus are in accord with the former, unless one presupposes that it follows the repeated death in the choroid of only a few microfilariae at a time. The changes in the HR fundus, more comparable to a degeneration, are much less dramatic than in the disseminated variety but, despite the absence of severe or moderate inflammation, the lesion is as devastating. In this interesting condition the retinal pigment epithelium imperceptibly disappears here and there to expose the choroid. The choriocapillaris has gone, totally occluded at these points, the larger underlying vessels now being visible. In the latter some stage of developing sclerosis may

be evident in its varying coloration from healthy red to white (totally sclerosed). As has been said, at first these changes are patchy, the arteriosclerosed areas being separated from each other by healthy retina with sharp margins; in the end a proportion of the cases will become affected over the entire posterior pole. Clumping of pigment is invariably found somewhere in the affected zones. 'Comma-shaped' pigment figures are not infrequently found among the aggregates of pigment which, as has been suggested, may have engulfed dead larvae. By their size they cannot be microfilariae but they could be small immature adult larvae (growing worms). This suggestion raises the alternative that the HR fundus may depend on the death of a few such larvae or microfilariae or both in the retina as distinct from the choroid (uvea). In such an event they might well cause the degree of destruction found without producing much in the way of an inflammatory reaction in the choroid such as happens when multiple mf deaths occur in the latter.

Any one or all of the changes just described can be found at any one time. Not so frequent is the occurrence of bone corpusculation, resembling that seen in primary and secondary retinitis pigmentosa. It is far from being as common in the HR fundus as sometimes stated. The writer recently analysed 100 cases in his records and found that bone corpusculation existed in only seven. This clearly excludes retinitis pigmentosa from the diagnosis. It is harder to exclude familial choroidal sclerosis, but on statistical grounds it is highly unlikely.

Diagnostic criteria

In order for a diagnosis to be made with certainty residence in an endemic area and skin irritation with or without a rash are essential. In addition there should be at least *one* of the following: palpable nodules (a single nodule does not count), microfilariae in skin or conjunctival 'snips' and microfilariae in the cornea or an anterior chamber.

Treatment (see also Chapter 20, p. 382)

Over a period of time it is to be expected that in many of the nodules the adults will die and the nodule undergo fibrolipomatous degeneration. However, in a hyperendemic area new nodules are continuously coming into being, as is the presence of adult worms in deeper layers, unencapsulated, so that the supply of *O. volvulus* microfilariae is constantly being renewed and the overall total gradually increased. Theoretically, the best method of preventing the development of severe ocular lesions is by removing the microfilariae from the eye and skin by chemotherapy, for it will then take time for the mf population to build up to a dangerous level, that is to a level when there will be a spillover into the eye. This is true to a degree even where there are head nodules. Up to date diethylcarbamazine (DEC) has been administered to do just this. The usual treatment with DEC has been in the region of 3 g over 21 days, starting with a small dose for the first few days by reason of the severe reactions which immediately commence. There has always been some fear of the ocular complications of this effect, that is that it may tilt the balance and produce blindness in an eye with good vision. Corticosteroids and antihistamines have been used to prevent this but not with much effect. In the writer's experience, if the eye in a patient with a heavy skin infection, widely distributed over the body, has no evidence of a pathological change, it is not likely to react very much, if at all, to the effects of DEC therapy even when mf volvulus can be seen within the eye. On the other hand, where there already is an onchocercal eye lesion, even if quiescent, such an eye will react severely. (This is a personal observation of the author.)

DEC does not kill the adult worms and so, provided male and female adults are present—they are not always found together—the subject is certain to become reinfested and permanent damage to the eye merely postponed. (Nodulectomy reaches only a small proportion of the adult worms and achieves very little.) Moreover, during treatment with DEC, the severe systemic and ocular reactions are hard to bear.

In 1984 and 1985 work was carried out on a new microfilaricide, new in the field of human medicine. It has a broad spectrum of antiparasitic activity and has been used for some time in veterinary medicine. It is called *ivermectin* and is discussed fully in Chapter 20 and Chapter 72, p. 1213. It is not yet in general use. The great feature of ivermectin is its prolonged microfilaricidal activity and its surprisingly mild systemic reaction; there is minimal toxicity. Like DEC it does not affect the adult worms. From the promising results achieved with ivermectin it would seem that it is not just the heavy load of dead microfilariae which causes the violent reaction to DEC but that the latter must lead to other changes which produce the reaction.

Treatment of an eye with an active onchocercal lesion, whether selecting DEC or not, consists of using a mydriatic and topical steroid three or four times daily and keeping a watch on the intraocular pressure.

Antrypol (Suramin) is effective in killing microfilariae and adults but as the drug damages the kidney and there have been a few deaths it requires close supervision and is not a satisfactory treatment. No vaccine for diagnostic or therapeutic purposes has as yet been evolved, although it is under study.

As the output per day of one female *O. volvulus* has been found to average about 10 microfilariae in vitro (medium 199 and human sera), the chemotherapeutic battle, even if ivermectin proves to be as effective as is claimed, appears to be a losing one unless (until) the fly is eliminated. Prevention of onchocerciasis is not yet feasible; new drugs are awaited. Local fly control in areas where the prevalence of blindness is high is the best one can achieve at the moment.

LEPROSY

The clinical and pathological features are described in Chapter 40.

Ocular involvement

Great variations in the incidence of ocular lesions have been reported. Because people with leprosy tend to keep moving along (as in such vast countries as India) it is difficult to obtain statistical data. The prevalence rates of impaired vision are high. Some observers consider that ocular tissues are ultimately involved in all leprosy sufferers if untreated, or partially treated, which is commonplace. Other assessments range from 5% to 25%; we do not know precisely. This state of affairs is due not only to the migrant nature of those affected but also to difficulty in making a diagnosis unless one is an expert in tropical eye diseases; many people with leprosy in Africa have been blinded by onchocerciasis, for example, and not by leprosy.

Pathology

The clinical and pathological features are

described elsewhere in this volume, but as ocular involvement varies according to the type of this disease it may be recalled that in the tuberculoid type, epithelioid cells, lymphocytes and Langhans'-type giant cells are found in cutaneous nerve twigs. The relatively frequent invasion of the facial and trigeminal nerves results in ocular involvement. In the lepromatous type, *Mycobacterium leprae* are found in the cytoplasm of the Schwann cells which ensheath sensory nerves. The dermis is severely attacked and hair follicles and sweat and sebaceous glands are destroyed. The third method of attack is by participation of ocular tissues in the reactive phase which is a generalized allergic reaction.

Predominantly tuberculoid-type changes

In this instance the body reacts vigorously to the leprosy bacillus, the disease is essentially neural and on the whole is benign and stable. The nerve twigs are infiltrated leading to degeneration with widespread rashes and patches on the skin.

Lagophthalmos or imperfect closure of the eyelids due to paralysis of the seventh nerve, combined with swollen and stiff upper eyelids and over-action of the levator muscle, causes a wide-open eye and staring look which startles the observer. The paralysed lower eyelid falls away from the eye in what is called *paralytic ectropion* (Plate V.4). The punctum is everted and this leads to epiphora. The partially uncovered cornea becomes dry; keratitis and ulceration may occur and hypopyon, secondary glaucoma, endophthalmitis or even perforation may bring about the destruction of both eyes.

Predominantly lepromatous-type changes

These are characterized by the profuse development of granulation tissue containing the multinucleated giant cells called 'lepra' cells. These patients exhibit no defensive response. In the eye the commonest effects of this invasion by *M. leprae* are epibulbar nodules which may overgrow the cornea, keratitis, superficial punctate and deep (interstitial or stromal) and anterior uveitis (Plate V.5). Minute (miliary) lepromata are classically found among the iris leaves, being called 'leprous pearls', and are also found in the fundus. A peripheral choroiditis has also been (rarely) described. Associated with the superficial punctate keratitis is the ingrowth of new vessels which may be confused with the pannus

of trachoma. Typically, it is a sequel to limbal lepromata and therefore may arise anywhere on the corneal margin, unlike trachoma.

When the brows and lids are involved loss of the eyebrow (*madarosis*), especially the outer third, and of eyelashes arise; *tylosis* is the name given to the swollen, rolled appearance of the bare lid margins. Eye complications are much more common in tuberculoid leprosy.

Treatment

This is given, as it affects the general disease, in Chapter 40. There it will be learned that maximum doses must be given from the start and not changed if a lepra reaction occurs. It will also be seen that not one but three drugs must be administered for only in that way can drug resistance be prevented. This is most important if the eye complications are to be avoided. The treatment of the anterior uveitis is well worthwhile, being essentially the business of preventing adhesions between the pupil and the lens and thereby keeping exudate away from the optic axis. This is achieved by dilating the pupil widely either with atropine 1% or phenylephrine 10% or both. Synechiae can be broken down by subconjunctival injections of Mydricaine. Corticosteroids should also be given by this route, 0.15 ml of methyl prednisolone being injected under the conjunctiva in the lower fornix. This is as effective and is less painful than when given more deeply under Tenon's capsule. It takes three weeks to absorb, being active throughout this period. Steroid drops are more time-consuming and may even be less helpful if the patient resists.

In tuberculoid and lepromatous and all intermediate types of leprosy, acute general reaction to treatment may occur occasionally. These involve the skin (as erythema nodosum, painful) and the eye in an epibulbar and/or uveal inflammatory reaction, which may destroy it. Such reactions are not uncommon after dapsone therapy has commenced. The treatment is as for any primary inflammation as far as the eye is concerned.

Surgical treatment

In lagophthalmos, where the cornea is exposed and ulceration imminent, *lateral tarsorrhaphy* is indicated. Where the orbicularis is completely paralysed a nylon suture may be inserted along the margins of both lids in a purse-string fashion and drawn tight. The *temporalis sling operation* is more effective. Two strips of temporalis (or other) fascia are inserted into tunnels near the margins of the upper and lower eyelids and united at the medial tarsal ligament. Voluntary closure of the lids synchronizing with that of the other eye is brought about. The operation is described in detail by Somerset.[18]

The *Kuhnt operation* is also useful in tightening the flaccid lower eyelid but in the presence of active infection it is rather heroic. This is even more true for intraocular surgery and this should be delayed at least until treatment has reduced the virulence of infection.

When the pupil is occluded an *optical iridectomy* may be performed to make an artificial pupil. This operation is undertaken only in the later stages of disease when the iris is decongested, otherwise the new pupil immediately becomes blocked with haemorrhage.

When inflammation of the iris has been brought under control operations other than iridectomy can be tried. For example, cataract extraction and drainage for glaucoma can be successful. D.P. Choyce has demonstrated the effectiveness of the Choyce brown, haptic contact lens, Mark VIII, for the leprous iris tears easily and such a lens makes good the gaps in the iris.

CATARACT

Progressive lens opacities may advance in both eyes until the patient is blind. The writer has found in most of the villages he has visited in the tropics that about one-third of all blindness is due to this defect. The mature lens (rarely) may dislocate into the anterior or posterior chamber (Plate V.6). Where surgery is available sight can be restored but in developing countries many millions of people suffer blindness because of the lack of surgeons. The late Sir Henry Holland recognized this need and instituted the first Eye Camps in India; by a well-organized coordinated effort in the cool season on the part of the surgeons many hundreds of cataract operations are carried out weekly, the patients being nursed in tents by their relatives under supervision.

Couching a cataract is still practised in many countries, including the one in which it is believed to have originated—Egypt. Sometime later Egyptian migrations southwards of Hamitic people (mainly the Fulahs) brought couching as far as West Africa. Itinerant 'malams' still make quite a living out of it. The Indian method consists of puncturing the sclera behind the root of the iris and with a blunt spud pushing the lens downwards into the posterior chamber. In Africa a long acacia thorn is burned in fire until it is as hard as steel; the *malam* squats before his patient (also squatting, his head held) and places the thorn in the correct position; he then knocks the thorn sharply downwards and backwards, dislodging the cataract and clearing the pupil. Usually the capsule has only a single small hole and lens matter does not escape. The writer has several times seen cataractous lenses lying in the posterior chamber many years after couching in perfectly quiet eyes. If lens matter escapes, on the other hand, uveitis or endophthalmitis with destruction of the eye is the outcome.

As cataract is a surgical problem[10] it need not be discussed in detail here. In essence, the internal metabolism of the human lens has altered when opacities show. It is an ageing process, hence the term 'senile' cataract, an involutionary change which occurs to some degree in the majority of eyes. The metabolism of the lens is also affected when the surrounding structures are inflamed, in endocrinal disorders (secondary or complicated cataracts) or when the lens capsule is broken (traumatic cataract). Inflammatory exudate from the iris sometimes conceals a complicated cataract.

It is also found as a congenital change, the classical appearance being one of 'blue dots'. Several workers in the past have claimed that malnutrition and dehydration can lead to incipient cataract in young persons. However, neither cataract nor any other ocular abnormality was discovered in the thousands of prisoners-of-war in 1939–1946 apart from optic neuropathy. A search for early lens changes in the children of the African 'famine belt' of the eighties would be rewarding.

Opacities adopt different shapes. With a slit lamp, by frontal (direct) illumination and in optical section the position of the changes can be ascertained. Viewed through an ophthalmoscope (with a +10 lens in position) the opacities are seen as dark structures against a red background (the fundus). With the slit lamp, using direct focal illumination, the colour is white or yellow and often orange. The changes may be restricted to the nucleus (nuclear sclerosis) or to the cortex. Coloured crystals are sometimes seen in cataract, usually along the optic axis; they are largely made up of cholesterol. Water vacuoles in the cortex are very common. Cortical opacities may adopt the shape of the spokes of a wheel when viewed from the front but can adopt any formation. Usually nuclear sclerosis interferes with vision more severely and earlier than cortical changes, for acuity can be surprisingly good despite dense bars coming in from the periphery.

OPTIC ATROPHIES

In tropical countries optic atrophy is among the five most common findings among the blind. It poses many diagnostic problems.

In middle or old age arteritis is one of the commonest reasons in Europe for closure of the nutrient vessels of the optic nerves with the subsequent development of ischaemic optic atrophy, but its prevalence in the tropics is uncertain. Thrombosis of the central retinal veins is uncommon. Increased blood viscosity, as in sickle cell/haemoglobin C, and polycythaemia may also cause vascular occlusion of the nutrient vessels to the optic nerve but are also uncommon.

Increased resistance to aqueous outflow with pressure damage to the retina is the cause of chronic open-angle glaucoma. A reflex auto-regulatory mechanism opposes rises of intra-ocular pressure but has its limits and is less likely to be efficient the older the patient becomes, thus bringing in a second factor: ischaemia of the nerve head, which destroys the nerve fibres and aggravates the adverse pressurization of the retinal ganglion cells. In acute narrow-angle glaucoma optic atrophy is purely ischaemic following compression (by the high intraocular pressure) of the blood vessels nourishing the optic disc. However, primary narrow-angle glaucoma tends to be chronic in Negroes; that is to say high pressures are uncommon except as a secondary complication in acute (or repeated) attacks of iritis. Subclinical rises associated with narrow angles are believed to start early in life and continue till optic atrophy with deep cupping results. In South-East Asia primary narrow-angle glaucoma is more common than primary open-angle glaucoma. Optic atrophy following the glaucoma associated with epidemic dropsy is described in Chapter 49.

Mechanisms other than vascular ones also play a part in the production of optic atrophy, such as impairment of the cytoplasmic metabolism or of axon cylinders by poisons, malnutrition, metabolic disorders and infections. Apart from sanguinerine, the poison producing epidemic dropsy, chloroquine, lead, quinine, methanol and other alcohols (usually adulterated with methanol), tobacco, pentavalent organic arsenicals and certain poisonous glycosides all produce optic atrophy. Precipitating factors may coexist, such as malabsorption (common in strongyloidiasis), anaemias, protein–energy malnutrition (PEM) and a low intake of B complex vitamins, especially pyridoxine.

A toxic optic neuropathy occurs where there is a deficiency in certain sulphur amino acids associated with (or resulting in?) a defect of cyanide metabolism (Chapter 47). In these cases the cyanide detoxication mechanism breaks down. This does occur in people where malnutrition is known to exist. There is a link in this hypothesis with what is known to occur (for which there is some evidence) in the case of several plant foodstuffs containing cyanogenetic glycosides.

Linamarin is the glycoside of the dolichos and lima bean, sweet potato, gram and manioc (cassava), all staples. The enzyme which frees the prussic (hydrocyanic) acid contained in these foods is linase. The quantity released depends on the conditions under which the staple is harvested and prepared. Bruising or other injury brings about the enzyme action and hydrocyanic acid is set free from the glycoside. In most of these foodstuffs the glycosides are not likely to give rise to poisoning, either because they are present in too small amounts or in parts not eaten or because the risk is known and precautions taken in preparation. In Nigeria all six varieties of cassava grown there contain sufficient amounts of cyanogenetic glycoside to make them toxic and produce optic atrophy if care is not taken. Most of the poison lies in the outer coats of the manioc root and these parts may be easily peeled off. Bruising of the roots in preparation causes the hydrocyanic acid to spread through the substance. When the roots are boiled most of the toxin is dissolved and removed. The water is then thrown away. The value of cooking cassava in pots without lids lies in the fact that the volatile acid can escape with the steam. Inhalation of this steam, however, is as dangerous as consumption of the water. Repetitive small doses could be cumulative.

Nutritional amblyopia (retrobulbar neuritis) is not strictly speaking a *toxic* neuropathy. It is firmly established as a cause of optic atrophy resulting from a deficiency of one or more members of the B complex. Closely implicated are the three 'respiratory enzyme' vitamins, thiamine, riboflavine and nicotinic acid, administration of which can reverse the condition. There is a close link between beriberi and pellagra and nutritional optic atrophy (Chapters 46, 47).

The degree and duration of the deficiency of B complex and the age of the subject are important. Younger persons are more liable to develop an optic neuropathy. This was clearly demonstrated in Japanese prison camps. In West Africa school-children have been found with not inconsiderable defects of vision where the discs were red and swollen, recovering after taking the B complex. Similarly, students were reported with a degree of optic atrophy and ataxia whose symptoms disappeared after a course of B complex (Chapter 47).[19]

Optic atrophy from infections is more easily recognizable. It is seen at its most characteristic in cerebrospinal meningitis, trypanosomiasis and venereal syphilis. In onchocerciasis it can occur as a primary lesion but it is also commonly secondary to involvement of the retina and/or uvea.

OTHER EYE CONDITIONS

The most important diseases of the eye in tropical countries have been dealt with in the preceding pages, but there are others, in which the ocular condition is primary or secondary to general disease, that are not so prolific but must be understood. These are described in the remaining section of this chapter, which it is hoped will prove a useful reference compendium.

ACTINOMYCOSIS

The actinomycetes are discussed in Chapter 34 and are listed in Table 70.2. Although it grows in colonies like a fungus and forms hyphae, it tends to break up in the tissues and form free-living aerobic and anaerobic bacterial species, respectively of the genera *Nocardia* and *Streptomyces* (hence the term 'streptothricosis' which is now out of favour).

Involvement of the lids and orbit is invariably secondary to infection of the jaw and sinuses. Primary infection conveyed through an abrasion in the skin or by a thorn also occurs. The cutaneous lid lesions, at first nodular, soon discharge freely. The pus contains many soft, green or yellow clumps, which are colonies or 'grains' of the fungus, the latter term describing their size. The suppurating skin lesions multiply and interconnect and may burrow into the orbit; from here the infection may pass backwards into the posterior fossa and lead to a basal meningitis or forwards into the lacrimal sac or gland. Con-cretions are not infrequently found blocking the lacrimal canaliculus producing an intractable conjunctivitis and excessive lacrimation.

In mild ocular cases small scattered yellow nodules have been described on the palpebral conjunctiva, more usually on the bulbar conjunctiva near the limbus; both are associated with a watery, irritable eye. The conjunctival discharge is quite likely to become secondarily infected. The punctum is usually patulous and the lacrimal sac is very commonly involved (dacryocystitis) because the flow of tears takes the infection into it. These changes, if untreated, can become very troublesome. A superficial punctate keratitis with pannus formation, resembling trachoma, has been described by Jones.[20]

Primary corneal ulceration which can occur without lid involvement due to a *Nocardia* species is rare but has been recorded. Usually the infection does not penetrate far into the stroma and develops slowly. A corneal ulcer due to a *Streptomyces* species has been known not infrequently to follow injury. It advances steadily, has an associated hypopyon and may perforate the eye; an exogenous endophthalmitis follows with total loss of the eye.

ANCYLOSTOMIASIS

This disease and its treatment are given in Chapter 21 and Table 70.1. The two nematodes responsible, *Ancylostoma duodenale* and *Necator americanus*, produce the same symptoms in their

Table 70.1   Helminthic infections of the eye.

Helminths	Stage and size	Confirmed locations
NEMATODES		
Ancylostoma duodenale, Necator americanus and other hookworm spp. (Chapter 21)	3rd stage larva 700 μm at least	Vitreous, choroid, retina
Anisakis (herring worm) (Chapter 24)	3rd stage larva 1.5–2.6 cm	Choroid, retina
Ascaris lumbricoides and other ascaroids (Chapter 21)	3rd stage larva 1.3–2 mm	Subconjunctival, entire uvea, subretina
Angiostrongylus cantonensis (Chapter 24)	3rd stage larva 2 cm	Vitreous, subretina
Brugia malayi (Chapter 20)	Adult 2.5–5.5 cm and during growth	Subconjunctiva
Dirofilaria immitis, D. tenue and *D. repens* (Chapter 20)	Adult 8–15 cm and during growth	Lids, orbit
Dracunculus medinensis (Chapter 20)	Adult 60 cm (f) and 2 cm or less (m) and during growth	Upper lid into conjunctival sac and/or orbit
Gnathostoma spinigerum (Chapter 24)	3rd stage larva 5 mm	Penetrates anterior chamber and orbit
Loa loa (Chapter 20)	Adult 3–7 cm and during growth	Subconjunctiva, orbit
Onchocerca volvulus (Chapter 20)	Microfilaria 300 μm average. (Adult 2–4 cm and during growth, probable)	Lids, orbit, all ocular structures
Thelazia callipaeda (Appendix II, p. 1380)	Adult 4.5–17 mm and during growth	Subconjunctiva—damaging cornea, anterior chamber, uvea
Toxocara canis and *T. cati* (Chapter 21)	2nd stage larva 1–2 mm	Orbit, extraocular muscle, anterior chamber, subretina, choroid, optic nerve
Wuchereria bancrofti (Chapter 20)	Adult 4–6.5 cm and during growth	Orbit, subconjunctiva, anterior chamber, uvea, vitreous, subretina (rare)
CESTODES (Chapter 23)		
Diphyllobothrium spp. (sparganum)	Plerocercoid larva 3–12 mm	Lids, orbit, subconjunctiva, palpebral and bulbar conjunctiva
Echinococcus granulosus (hydatid). Maybe other spp.	Larval cyst with scolex, 1 mm to eyeball size	Orbit with oedema of conjunctiva, vitreous, subretina
Taenia brauni (coenurus cerebralis). *T. multiceps* (doubtful)	Larval cyst 2 mm to 2 cm	Subconjunctiva, anterior chamber, vitreous
Taenia solium (cysticercus cellulosae).	Larval cyst with scolex 5–20 mm	Orbit, extraocular muscle, subconjunctiva, anterior chamber, vitreous, subretina
PENTASTOMIDS (Chapter 24)		
Armillifer armillatus (*Porocephalus*)	Encysted nymphal stage 13–23 mm long	Subconjunctival space and posterior orbit
Linguatula serrata	Encysted nymphal stage 4–6 mm long	Anterior chamber of eye

respective geographical areas. When the hookworm is present in large numbers in the small intestine blood loss and chronic infections lead to anaemia. It is a most debilitating disease.

Perhaps as a result of the iron deficiency anaemia the parasites produce, *night blindness* is not infrequently associated with hookworm. Irritation due to endotoxins followed by hypersensitivity causes oedema of the lids which may be the first indication of infection. The eye has not been seen clinically invaded by larvae or adult worms but Wilder[21] found the larvae in the chorioretina of 24 out of 46 eyes enucleated from young children with a mistaken clinical diagnosis of retinoblastoma. Eosinophilic granulomas in the vitreous with central necrosis were found in some of the eyes which she examined to contain hookworm larvae, either entire or disintegrating; in others the larvae were those of *Toxocara canis*. Migration tracks in the choroid and retina have subsequently been demonstrated both histopathologically and by fluorescein angiography. The differential diagnosis of a local eosinophilic granuloma includes not only toxocara and retinoblastoma but cysticercosis, Coats' disease and bacterial endophthalmitis.

The clinical association between hookworm and an exudative haemorrhagic lesion of the retina had been noted for some time before the finding of Wilder but was considered to be due to an endotoxaemia, not the presence of hookworm larvae per se. Debilitation in children due to ancylostomiasis may trigger off xerophthalmia.

Strongyloides stercoralis (Chapter 21) is another extremely common nematode with a slightly different life history from the two described above. Mojon[22] by serodiagnosis using the indirect fluorescent antibody test (and excluding the lower dilutions where cross reactions may exist) found that just under 80% of her 281 patients revealed infection whereas in stool examinations of the same people the larvae were found in only 8%. Despite its frequency and wide distribution, especially where there is moisture in addition to heat, and despite the fact that the life history within man parallels *Ancylostoma* and *Necator* (none having any need of an intermediate host) and despite the fact that at all stages the larva is about the size of the common hookworm, it has never been seen to affect or invade the eye.

Table 70.2 Fungal infections of the eye.

Disease	Species	Confirmed ocular lesions	Topical treatment
Actinomycosis (Chapter 34)	*Nocardia* spp. and *Streptomyces* spp.	Purulent blepharitis. Orbital cellulitis. Dacryocystitis. Mucopurulent conjunctivitis. Nodules on palpebral and bulbar conjunctiva. Superficial punctate keratitis (SPK) with pannus (like trachoma). Corneal ulcers with or without hypopyon. Endophthalmitis (from small uveal abscesses).	Natamycin 5% drops or 1% oculentum. Penicillin drops, 5000 units in 5 ml. All 2-hourly.
Aspergillosis	*Aspergillus fumigatus, A. nigra* and *A. flavus*	Mucopurulent conjunctivitis. Dacryocystitis. Corneal ulcers. Orbital cellulitis. Endophthalmitis, preceded by 'white spots' on retina or vitreous (metastases).	Econazole 1–2% drops. Nystatin drops 10 000 units per ml in normal saline or oculentum. 100 000 units per g, both 3-hourly. Subconjunctival nystatin 5000 units in 0.5 ml normal saline, daily for 3 days.
Blastomycosis (Chapter 35)	*Blastomyces dermatitidis*	Lid ulceration. Blepharoconjunctivitis. Mucopurulent conjunctivitis. Dacryocystitis. Orbital cellulitis. Corneal ulcers. Nodules on iris with hypopyon. Blastomycetes in anterior chamber. Nodules on optic nerve with neuritis.	Nil effective. Systemic treatment only.
Candidiasis (Chapter 35)	*Candida albicans* and spp.	Mild conjunctivitis. Infection of lacrimal puncta. Dacryocystitis. Mucopurulent conjunctivitis maybe with pseudomembrane. Corneal ulcers. Extraocular myositis (post-surgical). Iridocyclitis. 'White spots' restricted to retina (metastases). Panophthalmitis.	Flucystosine 1.5% drops 3-hourly. Nystatin oculentum 100 000 units per g 3-hourly.
Cladosporiasis	*Cladosporium* and *Cladosporoides* spp.	Corneal ulcers	As above.

Table 70.2 —*cont.*

Disease	Species	Confirmed ocular lesions	Topical treatment
Cephalosporiasis (Chapter 34)	*Cephalosporium* spp.	Mild conjunctivitis and infection of puncta. Rarely corneal ulcers and iridocyclitis.	As above.
Coccidioidomycosis (Chapter 35)	*Coccidioides immitis*	Granulomas on lids, conjunctiva or in orbit. Rarely on optic nerve. Chorioretinitis and endophthalmitis.	Flucystosine 1.5% drops. Clotrimazole or miconazole 1–2% drops, all 2-hourly.
Cryptococcosis (Chapter 35)	*Cryptococcus neoformans*	Corneal ulcers with or without hypopyon. Rarely iridocyclitis. Chorioretinitis. Papilloedema and optic atrophy. 6th nerve palsy.	As above.
Fusariosis (Chapter 34)	*Fusarium oxysporum, F. solani* and *F. moniliforme*	Corneal ulcers with or without hypopyon, often with oedema of cornea as feature, and rarely panophthalmitis.	Econazole 1–2% drops 3-hourly. Natamycin 10% drops or 1% oculentum 2-hourly.
Histoplasmosis (Chapter 35)	*Histoplasma capsulatum*	Granulomatous disseminated choroidoretinitis, active or healed scars, sometimes involving macula. Focal reaction later at macula: oedema with haemorrhages. Panophthalmitis. Mild iridocyclitis and chorioretinitis suspected.	Nil effective. Systemic treatment only.
	Histoplasma duboisii	A few cases of orbital cyst (*H. duboisii* only).	
Mucormycosis (Chapter 34)	*Mucor corymbifer* and other Mucoraceae rarely, e.g. *M. mucedo*	Orbital cellulitis (via antrum). Blepharitis. Blepharoconjunctivitis. Keratitis. Dacryocystitis.	Nil effective. Systemic treatment only.
Paracoccidioidomycosis (Chapter 35)	*Paracoccidioides brasiliensis*	Lid ulceration. Orbital cellulitis. Blepharitis. Palpebral and bulbar conjunctivitis. Corneal ulcers. Dacryocystitis. Anterior and posterior uveitis.	Nil effective. Systemic treatment only.
Penicilliosis	*Penicillium citrinum* and spp.	Corneal ulcers with hypopyon. Iridocyclitis. Panophthalmitis.	Clotrimazole 1–2% cream.
Rhinosporidiosis (Chapter 34)	*Rhinosporidium seeberi*	Blepharitis. Palpebral and bulbar conjunctivitis. Episcleritis. Scleritis. Dacryocystitis.	By excision.
Sporotrichosis (Chapter 34)	*Sporothrix schenckii*	Blepharoconjunctivitis. Scleritis. Keratitis. One case of panophthalmitis.	Nil effective. Systemic treatment only.
Trichophytosis (Chapter 33)	*Trichophyton* spp.	Lid surfaces. Blepharoconjunctivitis.	Clotrimazole 1–2% cream.
Trichosporosis (piedra) (Chapter 33)	*Trichosporon* spp. *Piedraia hortai*	Panophthalmitis (rare).	Nil effective. Systemic treatment only.

BLASTOMYCOSES (INCLUDING PARACOCCIDIOIDOMYCOSIS)

The two varieties of *Blastomycosis* are described in Chapter 35 and shown in Table 70.2. Both are dimorphic fungi reproducing by budding. The North American infection (*Blastomyces dermatitidis*) differs from the South American (*Paracoccidioides brasiliensis*) as far as some immunological and clinical features are concerned. Diagnostic serological tests, for example, for the North variety are only half as reliable as for the South. However, the pathologies are not too dissimilar, nor are the eye lesions, and so the two fungal infections may be taken together within that context. The general common denominator is abscess formation with secondary chronic inflammatory and granulomatous changes in the infected ocular tissue.

In both, infectious primary lesions are common on the skin; in the South American variety invasion of the mouth is a feature. Ulcerative granulomas of skin, lids, nose and mouth thus occur, spreading to the conjunctiva lining both upper and lower lids (Fig. 70.10). From the fornices the infection spreads on to the bulbar conjunctiva as bands of granulomatous tissue resembling pemphigoid. The lacrimal passages may be blocked, or invaded more deeply. Marginal ulcers of the cornea may also be found. Invasion from the lacrimal passage leads to orbital cellulitis.

Small nodules have been found near the ciliary border of the iris. These have been seen to break down and discharge purulent material into the anterior chamber from which the fungus has been identified. An endogenous anterior uveitis is perhaps less common than a posterior, but both are found; both are rare. Small nodules have also been seen on the optic nerve. In all the confirmed cases of intraocular infection the eyes were destroyed.

No topical treatment helps. This disease, as far as the eye is concerned, has been more commonly seen in South America.

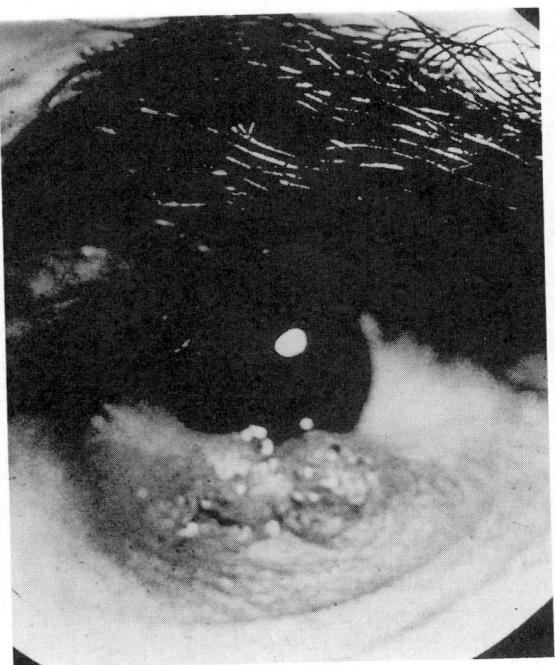

Fig. 70.10 Granuloma on lower lid spreading inwards due to *Paracoccidioides brasiliensis*. (Courtesy WTIM.)

BRUCELLOSIS

This disease and its treatment are described in Chapter 7. In the early stages pain on moving the eyes (due to a tenonitis, not an optic neuritis) is common. Invasion of the orbit leads to single oculomotor palsies. A basal meningoencephalitis is a less common complication. When it occurs bilateral sixth nerve paralysis can result. Pain on moving the eye will then be due to an optic neuritis with papilloedema and ultimately optic atrophy.

The *Brucella* organisms have never been conclusively demonstrated in the uvea. However, the serological, immunological and clinical evidence in those who have suffered from brucellosis associated with an anterior uveitis makes it highly probable. It is a recurrent granulomatous infection. Nodules are not seen on the iris surface but there is a strong suggestion they are present in the stroma. The lardaceous KP are small. Posterior uveitis with a similar coincidental history of brucellosis consists of several moderately sized areas of yellow exudate with little surrounding reaction, except perhaps a few minute superficial dot haemorrhages. The inflammation is self-limiting, leaving behind white glial scars. These inflammatory changes attributed to brucellosis rarely occur in the acute stages of the systemic infection, but months after they have subsided in the chronic stage. The uveal lesions are not infrequently recurrent—

sometimes, but not always, in association with recrudescences of the systemic disease.

Coin-shaped (nummular) subepithelial opacities in the cornea have been blamed on brucellosis but the evidence is thin.

CANDIDIASIS

This fungus infection is also known as 'moniliasis'. The infections caused by the genus *Candida* (*Monilia*) are characterized by their generally superficial nature and rather feeble invasive powers. This is not surprising as it is present in normal healthy eyes; in fact it is the second most common fungal flora, penicillium being the first. It is described with its treatment in Chapter 35 and is listed in Table 70.2.

Candida albicans can infect the eyelids, lacrimal canals, conjunctiva and cornea directly but it is invariably as a secondary infection following injury or surgery to the eyes that we see it. For example, an extraocular myositis with adhesions may follow squint surgery. A pseudomembrane has been described with a *Candida* conjunctivitis and increased ulceration not infrequently follows in the wake of a dendritic ulcer, forming a round circumscribed or amoeboid ulcer with a thin, dry membrane on the base. Endogenous invasion of the uvea and retina is not common but is known to occur: following candidaemia an anterior uveitis (iridocyclitis) can result with extension into the anterior chamber, a hypopyon and perhaps a further extension into the vitreous. A metastatic posterior uveitis (chorioretinitis) has also been described as have small metastases in the retina revealed as white spots.

CEREBROSPINAL MENINGITIS

Cerebrospinal meningitis and its treatment are described in Chapter 30. It is endemic throughout the world but is more frequently seen in the tropics because of epidemics. Thirty to forty years ago throughout West Africa whole villages were wiped out by epidemics of cerebrospinal meningitis, the few survivors leaving their deserted homes behind as they fled elsewhere. In Delhi in 1966 one-third of all infants below the age of one died in such an epidemic. Epidemics come in waves every so many years and thus it is important when first arriving in a new area to ascertain when the last one occurred.

Petechiae on the palpebral, rarely the bulbar, conjunctiva are common early on in the acute phase in about half the patients. An acute endogenous purulent conjunctivitis can be part of a *Neisseria meningitidis* septicaemia; episcleritis is a later manifestation (fifth to sixth day). Exogenous meningococcal conjunctivitis, which may be mild or mucopurulent, has been (rarely) reported in carriers in whom the organism has been isolated from the secretion of the eye as well as from the throat.

There are three serious ocular complications of cerebrospinal meningitis found in survivors. First, there may be an endogenous anterior uveitis, sometimes with hypopyon. Inflammatory exudate from the rim of the pupil may occlude it causing blindness. This membrane is particularly dense and more heavily pigmented after recovery than in any other uveitis, especially in the Negro eye. In some cases endophthalmitis follows uveitis leading to shrinkage of the eyeball. The inflammation of the iris and its complications may be treated by the insertion of a mydriatic and steroid ointment two or three times a day, as an adjuvant to systemic treatment.

The second serious complication leading to blindness in those who survive is a bilateral optic atrophy. This no doubt occurs because in the very young a basal meningitis is common; the simultaneous involvement of the brain stem explains the occurrence of various cranial nerve lesions: a sixth nerve palsy is the most common involvement. Nystagmus is hardly ever noted.

The third serious complication is a rarity: it occurs when the meninges in the occipital region are affected; complete blindness with normal fundi and pupillary reaction has been reported. Recovery is not likely but the return of central vision in one or two cases has been observed.

CHOLERA

This disease and its treatment are given in Chapter 13. An early ocular sign is a bluish discoloration of the skin of the eyelids. The general dehydration which characterizes the disease causes the lacrimal secretion to dry up and the eyeballs to sink into the orbits. The corneas become grey. There may be a catarrhal conjunctivitis with the risk of secondary infection although this rarely happens. When the patient is unconscious the eyelids are kept half open, the condition known as 'coma vigil'. The exposed dry cornea may then ulcerate; linear ulcers have been reported, leaving in those who recover a characteristic linear scar in the lower cornea. The retinal arteries in the severely ill are narrow and dark and the blood column in the veins broken. Cataract can develop rapidly in the stage of collapse. This is probably due to changes in the osmotic pressure or to loss of nutrients in the circumambient media of the lens. In lesser degrees of lens change transparency will be restored on recovery of the patient.

CYSTICERCOSIS

The pork tapeworm, *Taenia solium*, and its larva, cysticercus cellulosae, from which the name cysticercosis (larval taeniasis) is derived are described with the treatment required in Chapter 23 and in Table 70.1.

In 10% of cases with systemic cysticercosis the cysts are extraocular. They have been found in the upper lids and orbit; in the latter, attachment to the extraocular muscle cone leads to squint. Under the conjunctiva they appear as small, soft pea-shaped lumps. A great many of those with systemic infection may suffer from intraocular cysticercosis, usually in one eye; it is relatively frequent especially in Mexico and other Central and South American countries. A few cases have been found in the anterior chamber (Fig. 70.13) but in 90% of cases the cysticerci lie free in the vitreous-subretinal space and, more rarely, the subhyaloid space.

When present in the *vitreous* there may be a severe to mild anterior uveitis with pain and sudden or progressive visual loss. The cysticercus appears as a grey round vesicle up to 20 mm in diameter. A white spot on the surface is the site of the invaginated scolex. If more than one is present, one scolex at the least may be seen protruding outwards, swinging backwards and forwards while the vesicle undulates and contracts (Fig. 70.11). Crystals and yellow spots around the parasite probably represent its excretions (Liebreich's spots).

In *subretinal* and (rarer) *subhyaloid* lodgement of the cysticercus, there is less movement but a greater loss of sight which may be central or peripheral. The inflammatory effect on neighbouring tissues is more severe, moreover. Retinal detachment is quite a probability. Retinal haemorrhages are not a common finding nor is secondary glaucoma although both are seen. The

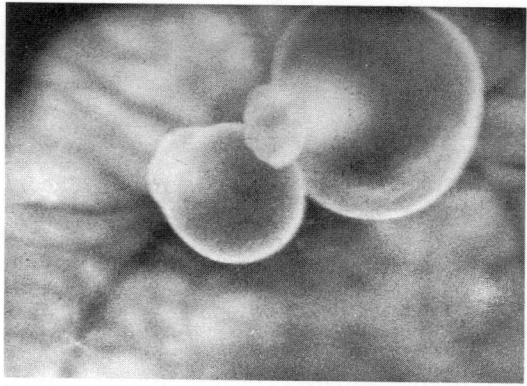

Fig. 70.11 Cysticerci cellulosae in the vitreous. Note protruding scolex in the nearer. (Courtesy Drs K. S. Zinn and Guillory, and *Acta Ophthalmologica, Chicago*.)

only treatment is to remove the parasites through a scleral incision and treat the reactions symptomatically.

THE DYSENTERIES

Amoebic dysentery and its treatment are described in Chapter 17. Anterior uveitis and chorioretinitis have been ascribed to this disease but some believe the association is fortuitous. It can be controlled by topical use of a mydriatic and steroid. Papilloedema may occur when an amoebic cerebral abscess develops, as in any space-occupying lesion. Retinal haemorrhages have been reported on several occasions.

Shigella dysentery and its treatment are described in Chapter 14. Conjunctival congestion occurs during the acute febrile stage. A true exogenous (shigellar) keratoconjunctivitis can occur after finger contamination of the external eye. An iridocyclitis associated with polyarthritis occurs within four weeks of the onset of the intestinal symptoms. Other causes such as Reiter's disease, Behçet's syndrome and lymphogranuloma venereum must be taken into account.

Treatment of the eye is symptomatic and in the iridocyclitis of *Yersinia* and *Salmonella* arthritis may have to be prolonged.

EPIDEMIC DROPSY

This condition, invariably observed in epidemic form, is described in Chapter 49 (p. 905).

The association of raised ocular pressure with epidemic dropsy was noted in 1877 but forgotten until Maynard's classic paper in 1909. The incidence of glaucoma has in fact never been recorded as great, ranging between 4% and 12%. It is only found in the most severely affected subjects. Ocular pain is unusual during the acute phase. It is the objective fundus findings which draw attention to the danger. The retinal veins are congested and there are retinal haemorrhages over and around the optic discs or alongside the veins, as in a toxic vasculitis (which it is). Nevertheless, although retinal venous changes are present in three-quarters of the subjects, only a small number exhibit raised pressures, generally high.[23] Unfortunately, there is no information concerning the appearance of the filtration angles.

In long-standing cases the fields of vision and acuity, as expected, are reduced and deep cupping by now may be present. Thirty years after an epidemic, survivors who may or may not have had glaucoma reveal evidence of chronic glaucoma, and in these blood histamines are raised. There seems little doubt that the toxic action of sanguinarine on blood vessels is the modus operandi of this particular glaucoma.

FILARIAL INFECTIONS OTHER THAN ONCHOCERCIASIS

Wuchereria bancrofti, Loa loa and *Brugia malayi* and their treatment are described in Chapter 20. Each can affect the eye as is shown in Table 70.1.

W. bancrofti adults have been found on a few occasions in the orbit causing proptosis (Fig. 20.11). They have also been seen pushing their way under the conjunctiva. Reports of their presence in the anterior chamber are increasing. Although the worm moves around like an eel, curiously little reaction occurs. Atropine causes its death; unfortunately, the dead worm excites a reaction leading to a keratitis and iridocyclitis and even a secondary glaucoma. It is better in consequence to remove the worm surgically while still alive. It has also been reported in the vitreous. Unlike *Onchocerca* the microfilariae of *W. bancrofti* do not affect the eye although they are blood-borne.

Loa loa adults are associated with allergic swellings under the skin presumably a reaction to their toxins (Calabar swellings). These have been noted on the eyelids and orbit (Fig. 70.12). The main invasion of the eye by the adult worm, however, is subconjunctivally. The worm passes at a fairly quick pace usually under the bulbar

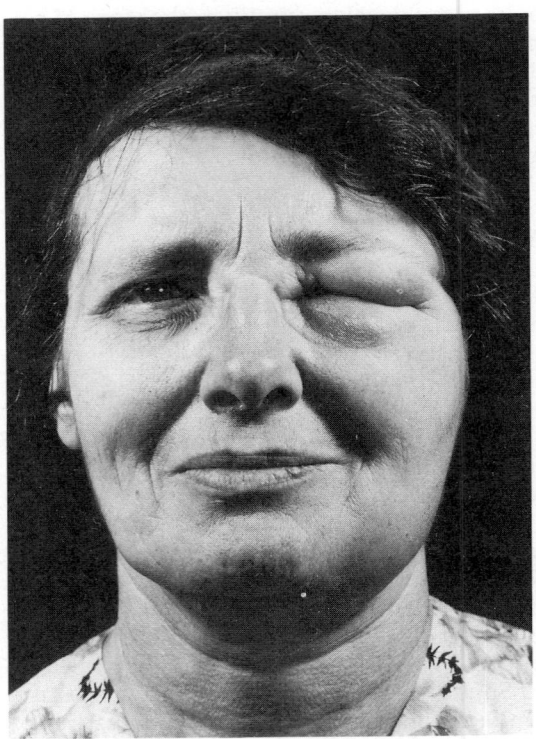

Fig. 70.12 Periorbital oedema and blepharospasm due to orbital loaiasis. (Courtesy Sir C. C. Chesterman.)

conjunctiva (Fig. 20.29 and Plate VI.3), but sometimes under the palpebral. It causes irritation and congestion and a sensation, which although not painful is frightening. If the facilities are immediately available its passage can be slowed up by instilling cocaine drops. The worm can then be held by a pair of forceps through the conjunctiva, an incision made in the thin membrane and, after releasing the first pair of forceps, the parasite can be easily withdrawn through the incision by a second pair. The mf *Loa loa* have not been associated with any ocular pathology. Simian *Loa loa* causes a subconjunctival granuloma known as the 'Owen–Hennesey granuloma' (Chapter 20) and is a cause of bung eye in Uganda (p. 389).

There have been several confirmed reports of the presence of *Brugia malayi* adults under the conjunctiva in Malaysia and, while on the subject

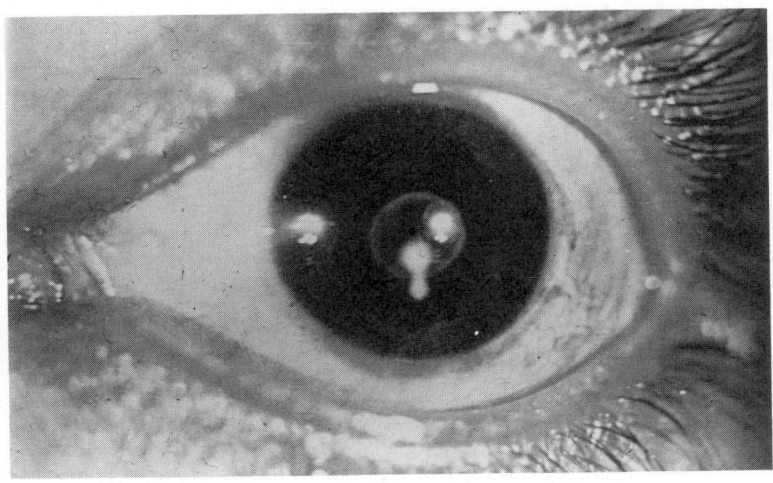

Fig. 70.13 Cysticercus in anterior chamber of eye. (Courtesy WTIM.)

of filarial worms, there have been a few accounts of *Dirofilaria repens* adult worms being recovered from eyelids in Thailand (Chapter 20).

HELMINTHIC INFECTIONS

Infections of the eye by nematode and cestode worms occur throughout the world with one species or another. Invasion may be by an adult, a larva at some stage in the life-cycle, or a microfilaria. The greatest destroyer of sight is the *Onchocerca* (p. 1152). Onchocerciasis is a highly complicated condition still under investigation, although we do know it is the dead larvae which cause the principal damage. Some of the other worm infections are also discussed separately, either because of their comparatively high prevalence or because of an interesting pathology. They include ancylostomiasis (Chapter 21), filariasis (Chapter 20) and toxocariasis (Chapter 21) among the nematodes and cysticercosis (Chapter 23) and sparganosis (Chapter 23) among the cestodes. The manner in which the pathological changes occur in these particular ocular conditions covers the entire spectrum of helminthic ocular pathology. Table 70.1 conveniently draws together all known infecting worms. It informs the reader of the stage in the life-cycle when each worm affects the eye, lists those parts of the eye likely to be invaded and (of some importance, this) the size of the invader.

In general, involvement of the lids and orbit produces localized inflammation which may involve the extraocular muscles or cause pressure symptoms. Protrusion from the orbit is a possibility and needs to be distinguished from a tumour. Microscopic microfilariae enter the inner eye through the loose sheaths of the penetrating vessels from the orbit or lid–conjunctiva route.

When the parasite dies under the conjunctiva, be it palpebral or bulbar, there is an itchy conjunctivitis with chemosis of the fornix. The thickened mucous membrane becomes raised in some instances into pea-shaped nodules. Pain and oedema of the lids is significant, producing ptosis (bung eye) (see also p. 389).

In those cases where the parasites reach the inner eye within the bloodstream they can escape from the choroidal capillaries into the choroidal stroma or enter the subretinal space; the smaller parasites can even bore into the retinal neural elements. Movements under the retina may be seen (larva migrans). The parasites can also pass from the anterior uveal capillaries into the iris or through the iris into the anterior chamber or vitreous. In the latter position the contracting, semitransparent vesicle of the cysticercus and hydatid is to be distinguished from a non-transparent, dense, grey retinal cyst, floating in a fluid vitreous. These parasites require to be removed surgically from the two humours.

If the offending parasite dies within the choroid or subretina when small it produces a granulomatous chorioretinitis with much scarring as it heals. On the other hand, if a small parasite is located more anteriorly it produces a second and less characteristic appearance with no sign of a parasite: a low grade iridocyclitis results or a chronic endophthalmitis, both with the usual complications of synechiae, cyclitic membranes and vitreoretinal adhesions which can cause detachment of the retina. Secondary glaucoma and cataract are two other probable complications. of inner eye disease caused by parasites.

When an adult worm or large larval stage occupies the anterior chamber or vitreous the sooner it is removed the better, for at a certain size the eye may be lost. It is undoubtedly lost when penetrated by a large worm such as *Dracunculus*. The worm has to be drawn out and the eye excised.

HISTOPLASMOSIS

This interesting disease is fully described along with its treatment in Chapter 35 and Table 70.2 (p. 1161).

Histoplasma capsulatum has now been twice isolated from the eye. This is not very strong evidence in itself but, before that, there was almost completely convincing clinical and circumstantial evidence indicating that this fungus was the most important of all the fungi in producing an endogenous uveitis.

The clinical evidence is very suggestive where small, discrete, multiple, peripheral areas of choroiditis, or the scars, exist with a clear vitreous and (later) a cystic macular lesion adjacent to which oedema and haemorrhages may be present. This picture has frequently been seen associated with the systemic disease and with the introduction of the histoplasmin test the link became even stronger. Woods[24] considered the central serous lesion with secondary haemorrhages around it a specific focal reaction in sensitized tissue. It is believed that this fungus may be sometimes of such low grade virulence that it produces no significant systemic symptoms apart from a chorioretinitis which adds to the difficulty in diagnosis.

A cystic swelling in the orbit due to *H. duboisii*, resembling a dermoid cyst, has been identified.

LEISHMANIASIS

This complex disease and its treatment are discussed in Chapters 4 and 37.

Cutaneous leishmaniasis is essentially a cutaneous but sometimes a mucosal infection and the lesion of the skin, known as *oriental sore* in Afro-Asia, and *espundia* in Central and South America, is a chronic infection. Sometimes it remains dry, as in oriental sore and, therefore, chronic; at other times it suppurates, as in espundia and in consequence becomes more extensive and destructive. In these conditions mutilations of the lids and face occur. The conjunctiva lining the lids is involved in many instances presenting as a granular, or papilliform, conjunctivitis.

Coin-shaped superficial and stromal opacities form in the cornea with new vessels growing in towards them. There is now pain, lacrimation and photophobia and a low grade iritis may accompany the keratitis.

In visceral leishmaniasis (kala-azar) despite the fact that the parasites have spread widely in the bloodstream into the viscera, there is some doubt as to their invasion of the inner eye. Retinal haemorrhages have, however, been frequently reported in kala-azar. As there is anaemia with leukopenia and fever they may be secondary. Retinal haemorrhages around areas of septic retinitis have also been recorded. Haemorrhages are the most common intraocular changes but thrombosis of the retinal vein has been seen and a disseminated choroiditis associated with post-kala-azar dermal leishmanoid, the latter disappearing after treatment for leishmaniasis.

MALARIA

This disease and its various treatments are fully described in Chapter 1.

The ocular affections which may be attributed to malaria are few. There are, nevertheless, certain important occurrences related to malaria and its treatment which must be known. The association of some of these changes may be fortuitous (blepharitis, pigmentation of the cornea, anterior and posterior uveitis and ocular palsies). Nevertheless, palsies involving the third, fourth and sixth cranial nerves, paralysis of accommodation and an Argyll Robertson pupil have been reported several times with cerebral malaria.

Following extensive haemolysis which results from severe repeated attacks of the fever, yellow pigmentation of the conjunctiva occurs. Post-malarial herpes simplex (febrilis) is more common than is usually recognized. The most important changes are retinal. Capillary obstruction brought about by leukocytic rouleaux or parasitic emboli can cause small peripheral, rarely larger, central haemorrhages which after absorption leave permanent pigmentary changes. In chronic, anaemic, cachectic patients, there may be widespread haemorrhages affecting the retina. These have been most frequently reported in association with falciparum infections and particularly with cerebral malaria, where they are of bad prognostic significance (p. 18). Round or flame-shaped (venous and arterial) haemorrhages, sometimes subhyaloid, occur. When round, exudates may also be present. It is likely that these patients had severe anaemia (e.g. from hookworm) before the attack of fever. Such haemorrhages are highly significant because if the patients are not yet comatose they are soon likely to be. Papilloedema may coexist. Papillitis has been seen in the absence of haemorrhages; in the hazy margin of an inflamed disc deposition of leukocytes causes a chestnut grey coloration. It is considered pathognomonic of malarial papillitis. Transient blindness (amaurosis fugax) may follow the comatose state after recovery. Sometimes it persists with signs of optic neuritis and eventually optic atrophy.

With the increasing importance of *quinine* in the treatment of severe malaria (due to the failure of other antimalarial drugs or their adverse effects), the complications of quinine, which are not common but can arrive like a bolt from the blue, have to be understood so that quick action can be taken to save sight.

Quinine amblyopia is due to a hypersensitivity to the drug and even small doses may bring on this condition in idiosyncratic people. The loss of vision may be absolute with no perception of light. The pupils are dilated and react sluggishly, if at all. The fundi show marked constriction of the retinal arteries; there is pallor of the disc and a cherry red spot at the macula, such as is seen in occlusion of the central artery. Vision may return in a few hours but may take days or weeks. When recovery occurs the fields of vision may be greatly contracted almost to tubular vision. If the case is seen at an early stage a retrobulbar injection of tolazoline hydrochloride may bring about vasodilatation.

An injection of 15 ml of 0.5% lignocaine with 1:300 000 adrenaline into the stellate ganglia can restore sight, even if incompletely. The author has experience of one such case where within a few days vision returned to 6/18. Other reports have been less promising.

Chloroquine (and hydroxychloroquine) are responsible in sensitive subjects for a variety of ocular side-effects.

Loss of sensitivity of the cornea is an early symptom associated with blurring of vision and the appearance of halos. Later, white granules appear in the epithelium which may become aggregated into bizarre curved lines below the centre of the cornea. Posterior subcapsular lens opacities can develop later.

As in the use of quinine the gravest changes occur in the inner eye. The patients often present themselves with depigmented patches on the face and lids. The macula exhibits a mottled appearance and pigment granules arise. An area of oedema envelops the macula (the 'doughnut' effect with a central dark ring). Narrowing of the vessels and peripheral pigmentation occur later. Toxic optic neuropathy is being increasingly reported.

The visual acuity should be noted at the start of treatment and at regular intervals throughout the course. Treatment must be discontinued if the acuity falls, even slightly, and particularly if any macular disorder is suspected. The retinal and optic nerve changes are irreversible.

MEASLES

Measles and its management are discussed in Chapter 6 and in this chapter on p. 1149 when malnutritional blindness is being described. Amplification of the eye changes are now necessary.

In the absence of a known deficiency of protein and vitamin A the eye changes commence in the incubation period with a characteristic catarrh (that is, redness and a mucopurulent secretion). The eyes in short reflect what is happening in the upper respiratory tract. When the skin eruptions occur minute superficial punctate erosions of the bulbar conjunctiva and cornea can be demonstrated with rose bengal; subepithelial opacities can be stained with fluorescein drops. The punctate keratoconjunctivitis of measles predisposes to secondary infections and ulceration of the cornea. The fever can lead to malnutrition with the added risk to sight which that means. There are no follicles or papillae on the palpebral conjunctiva and corneal vascularization, apart from limbal hyperaemia, is not seen. The eye is congested with dilated conjunctival vessels, some of which leak and give rise to the occasional small haemorrhage. Perforation of a secondary corneal ulcer as the child's condition deteriorates is common and the eye may be lost. If it heals, the iris is usually impacted in the white corneal scar (leukoma adherens). It is frequently bilateral. Such a scar is very suggestive of a past attack of measles when seen in a child, so much so that it is often called a 'measly' eye. Measles sufferers run the added risk of having herpes simplex (febrilis) follow or accompany the fever. Defective vision does not follow an uncomplicated attack of measles.

OCULOMYCOSES

Diseases caused by fungi are known as mycoses. Fungi belong to a group of plants (Thallophyta) which develop no roots, stems or leaves. The vegetative plant is the thallus or mycelium, the reproductive unit a spore. The terminology of the mycoses varies considerably with different authors but fairly well-recognized terms are the dermatophytoses or ringworm affections (the skin), otomycoses (the ear), onychomycoses (the fingernails), maduromycoses (usually the foot) and oculomycoses (the eye).

For further details and for systemic treatment the reader should refer to Table 70.2 which lists all proven fungal infections of the eye.

The mycoses flourish wherever the immunobiological functions of the invaded ocular tissues are depressed. This has been shown time and again since the introduction and use of steroids and other immunosuppressive substances. The cornea is particularly vulnerable in this respect. Excessive broad-spectrum antibiotic therapy has also been blamed for the increasing number of systemic and ocular fungal infections. Fortunately, steroid aids to infection are not common in the underdeveloped parts of the world where fungal infections flourish.

Fungi take every opportunity to invade abrasions or wounds, accidental or surgical and, being airborne, some of them are constantly present on the external ocular membranes. *Candida albicans, Aspergillus, Cladosporium* spp. and *Penicillium* are the most common fungal flora in normal healthy eyes which pose a threat when a wound or ulcer arises (Fig. 70.14). As with all fungi, however, these four also reach the eye from the air or soil or from contaminating trau-

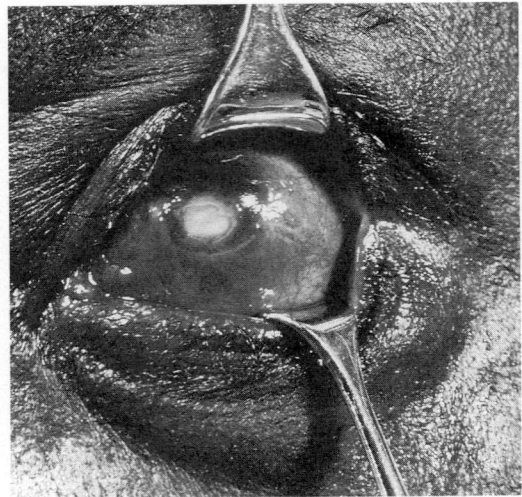

Fig. 70.14 Oculomycosis caused by *Cladosporium cladosporoides.* (Courtesy Dr H. C. Gugnani and *Mycopathologia.*)

matizing vegetation. Some will be inhaled into the sinuses and lungs whence they can enter the blood or lymph and so reach the inner eye, the orbit and lacrimal passages (retroversely). Some fungi prefer to remain on the surface of the eye or lids while others, passing by blood or lymph, have a preference for deeper structures. Despite the existence of hundreds of fungi only 15 to date have been identified in eye lesions. In the case of *Fusarium solani* a significant collagenase and other proteolytic enzyme activity has been shown which is probably the typical modus operandi.[25] Fusariosis (Fig. 70.15), first identified in the Americas, has been reported increasingly in Africa (*F. solani* and *F. moniliforme*). The various structures affected by the different fungi are shown in Table 70.2. Somewhat surprisingly the lesions produced by these different fungi in the

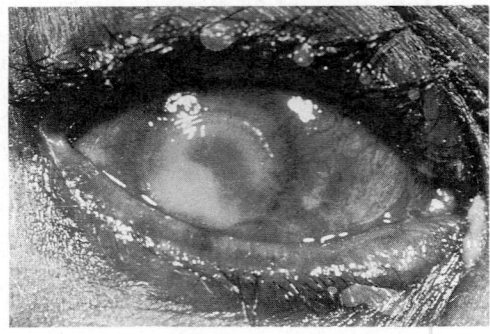

Fig. 70.15 Corneal ulcer due to *Fusarium moniliforme.* (Courtesy Dr H. C. Gugani and *Mycopathologia.*)

same tissue are not always identical. For example, *Actinomyces* produces multiple small abscesses in, or a generalized purulent infection of, the uvea whereas *Histoplasma capsulatum* leads to a mild granulomatous uveitis. This underlines the fact that some fungi are of lower virulence than others. Similarly, it is somewhat surprising to see that a uveitis (that is a chorioretinitis or iridocyclitis) has never apparently been caused by the Mucoraceaes whose activity is limited to the outer coats of the eye, although they are inhaled into the lungs, whereas *Histoplasma* also inhaled limits its activity entirely to the uvea. Why? *Aspergillus* and *Coccidioides*, on the other hand, can and do wantonly damage any part of the eye and its adnexa that they reach.

The four fungal infections most commonly linked with eye disease are actinomycosis, blastomycosis (with its South American counterpart, paracoccidioidomycosis), candidiasis and histoplasmosis; of the four, candidiasis is the only one that responds to treatment. In the others it is generally unsuccessful. Because of this and their frequency these diseases have been discussed at some length separately in this section.

The topical treatment of the eye, as distinct from the systemic, is hard—hard because antifungal drops are not readily available (although they may be obtained from some centres, such as Moorfield's in the UK) and hard because the drops or ointments used have to be inserted every 2 or 3 hours for several days. Yet this may be vital for often oral treatment has no effect on the ocular lesions. Full details of topical treatments are given in Table 70.2. It is advisable not to use steroid therapy at all.

OCULOMYIASIS

This is a term used to describe invasion of the human eye by maggots (larvae) which come from various flies in the order of Diptera. Known hosts include cattle, sheep, horses, deer and man himself, among others. They are as common in the West as they are in tropical countries. In addition to flies, vectors such as ticks and mosquitoes can convey the eggs of some of them to man. Man-to-man touch transmission is also important, especially in children.

The most common ocular lesions are associated with those flies which like the bots prefer to deposit their eggs on the moist lid margins whence they get into the conjunctival sac; they may even hatch between the eyelashes. Larval infestation of the external ocular membranes or the orbit is made easier where there are minor wounds. Some workers believe the parasites can be dropped on to the eye or the lids of a sleeper when the fly is in flight!

Apart from the usual signs of an irritable eye the maggots (which vary from 10 to 30 mm) can be found in the upper or lower fornices or the tear sac. They are quite difficult to remove for they usually are found to have burrowed beneath the conjunctiva forming small, undulating nodules; when dead they give rise to granulomas with an associated conjunctival hyperaemia. Pseudomembranes have been seen when the conjunctivitis is severe. They may also penetrate the sclera to enter the inner eye. The terms *external and internal oculomyiasis* are used to designate the location. Maggots are formidable invaders and have been seen in the anterior chamber giving rise to an anterior uveitis with the risk of an endophthalmitis. If they move round the uvea they can be seen through the retina. If subretinal, detachment is likely even if localized; when they die there they become encysted and reaction is less than one would expect but, if at the macula, sight will be lost. When free-floating in the vitreous there is little pain or distress despite their size. Table 70.3 lists the commoner maggots which invade the eye. The treatment is surgical.

Table 70.3   Maggot infections of the eye (oculomyiasis) (see also Chapter 51 and Appendix III, p. 1467).

1   Muscidae:
   (a) *Musca domestica* (the common house fly), worldwide
   (b) *Fannia canicularis* (the lesser house fly), worldwide
2   Cuterebridae:
   (a) *Dermatobia hominis* (tropical warble fly), found in tropical South and Central America (p. 1463, Figs. III.61 and III.62, p. 1465)
3   Calliphoridae:
   (a) *Cordylobia anthropophaga* (the tumbu fly), found in central Africa (p. 1462, Figs. III.59 and III.60B, p. 1463)
   (b) *Chrysomyia bezziana* (the screw-worm fly), found in Asia, Pacific, Africa and Australia (p. 1467)
   (c) *Wohlfahrtia magnifica* (the sheep maggot fly), found in western Asia and in Russia (p. 1465)
4   Gasterophilidae (horse bot or warble fly), various species, worldwide (p. 1467)
5   Oestridae
   (a) *Oestrus ovis* (sheep bot fly), found in Mediterranean littoral (including North Africa) and USSR (Fig. III.67, p. 1467)
   (b) *Hypoderma bovis* and *H. lineatum* (cattle bot, hornet or warble fly), found in western Asia and North Africa
   (c) *Rhinoestrus purpureus* (Russian gad fly) found in south and east Europe, western Asia and North Africa

PENTASTOMIASIS (Chapter 24, p. 562)

The pentastomids or 'tongue' worms are neither worms not typical arthropods although often considered to be the latter (Table 70.1). *Armillifer (Porocephalus) armillatus* is a member of the group and the encysted nymph, recognizable through its transparent capsule by the opaque annulated rings round the body, has been found in the subconjunctival space (Fig. 70.16) and posterior segment where it has been known to cause a retinal detachment.[26] The adult and encysted nymph are indistinguishable until recovered but only the nymph form is found in man.

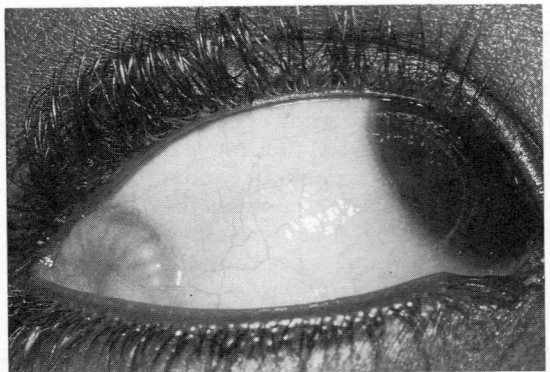

Fig. 70.16 Encysted nymph of *Armillifer (Porocephalus) armillatus* in the subconjunctival space. The annulations seen through the transparent capsule. (Courtesy Makerere College Medical Department.)

Another pentastomid, *Linguatula serrata*, has also been found in man's eye; the nymph form enclosed in its transparent capsule has been identified after removal from the anterior chamber.[27] It produces great pain if it enters the anterior chamber for an exudative iritis (anterior uveitis) occurs and a secondary glaucoma is an almost certain complication. It is fortunately rare to find a pentastomid in the eye. Treatment consists of surgical removal.

PROPTOSIS

Many benign primary or secondary malignant tumours, pseudotumours and developmental abnormalities may produce the clinical picture known as proptosis. Cancer is said to be twice as common in temperate zones than in the tropics. Orbital cancer is a cause of proptosis but it is one of the less likely (Fig. 70.17). In the event, although considering malignancy, it is as well to look for early signs of granulations or some parasitic infection, such as hydatid cyst. Congenital abnormalities are rare. Defects in the orbital walls giving rise to cephaloceles and meningocephaloceles are not, however, unknown. More cases have been reported from India and Pakistan than from elsewhere outside temperate zones. There can be no doubt that retinoblastoma is common in Africa although it is difficult to believe it is as common as the '8% of all blindness' reported by WHO in Malawi in 1979. The samples seem to have been too small but the figure should be noted. Retinoblastoma is an inherited, highly malignant congenital tumour of the posterior segment in which both eyes are involved in about 30% of cases (Plate VI.1). They are seen in small children as lemon-coloured masses behind the pupils. Up-country, without a doctor to turn to, these neoplasms push the eyeball outwards and ultimately destroy them. Malignant melanomas can do the same. Over many years the writer has only seen one proven case of malignant choroidal

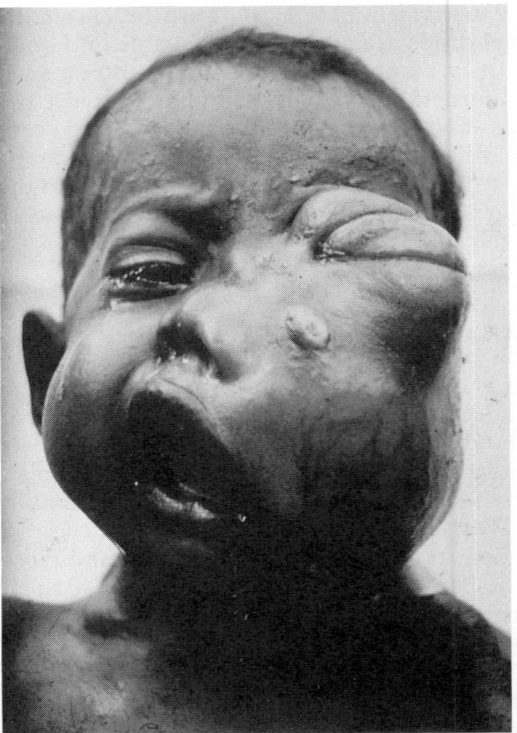

Fig. 70.17 Proptosis due to carcinoma of the maxilla. (Courtesy WTIM.)

melanoma so, although rare, they occur. After retinoblastomas, haemangiomas, chloromas and gliomas of the optic nerve are the most common tumours seen. Other (rare) causes include gumma and tuberculoma of the orbit, mucocele, sarcoma, endothelioma and possibly sarcoidosis —all associated with proptosis.

In the interior of Africa a highly malignant tumour syndrome affecting children up to about 14 years is the commonest cause of unilateral proptosis within certain defined areas. It is a lymphoma known as *Burkitt's tumour* (Fig. 70.18), first identified in Uganda. It is described along with the causative virus in Chapter 67. The peak age is said to be five. By far the commonest cause of proptosis, however, in the tropics resulting from an underlying orbital lesion is a pseudo-tumour due to healed endogenous inflammation of the soft tissue.

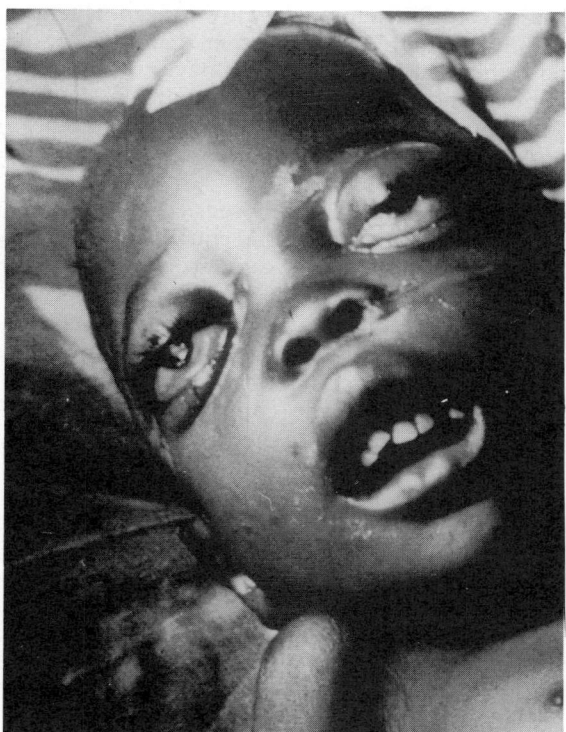

Fig. 70.18 Burkitt's lymphoma involving orbit. (Courtesy Mr D. P. Choyce and Churchill Livingstone.)

The orbit usually (in pseudotumours) has been infected secondarily, either from the paranasal sinuses (generally with *Staphylococcus aureus*) or by haematogenous transmission (usually by group A β-haemolytic streptococci). *Orbital cellulitis* is more common in children than in adults. The fretful patient is ill with a fever, sometimes slight, and a leukocytosis. The lids are swollen, red and oedematous. If an abscess is formed it can spread deeply and erode the bone. Thrombophlebitis of orbital veins advancing to *cavernous sinus thrombosis* is a serious complication. In the latter the fever becomes higher; there are rigors and oedema behind the ears over the mastoid processes. The patient now looks ill and is somnolent. Of course, cavernous sinus thrombosis can occur as a primary lesion following a blood-borne infection. When this occurs the lids are not fiery but otherwise the signs resemble an orbital cellulitis; the patient with orbital cellulitis is not so listless and somnolent as with thrombosis.

Pressure on the optic nerve arising from a gross untreated orbital cellulitis may destroy the nerve if it is not brought under quick control with an antibiotic. Orbital decompression surgery is not likely to be available everywhere. When the condition settles, becoming self-limiting, the proptosis is perpetuated by the subsequent organization and encapsulation of the inflamed tissues.

Erythromycin or the penicillins are the best antibiotics to try and should be given in large doses. If the patient is hypersensitive to the penicillins the cephalosporins should be tried. If the infection is known to be due to *Staphylococcus aureus* or some gram-negative bacteria erythromycin or the cephalosporins should cure the condition. A new cephalosporin, like cefuroxime, given by intramuscular or intravenous injection, 750 mg every 8 hours, or if severe, 1.5 g every 6–8 hours, is quite safe and most effective.

RUBELLA

German measles is a mild virus illness spread by droplet infection. No specific treatment is required. The distribution is worldwide but in the tropics so common is it in childhood that mothers are only rarely infected during pregnancy. The worst effect is on the defenceless fetus of a mother suffering from the disease. The virus strikes the fetus within the first three months of pregnancy. As it may persist for several months after infection a mother infected recently before pregnancy puts the fetus at risk although not as greatly as when actually suffering from rubella during the first three months of pregnancy. (For this reason the vaccine, being an attenuated living rubella, should not be given to pregnant women nor for three months *before* pregnancy if possible.)

It has been established that where the mother is infected during the first three months of pregnancy there is a 10–20% chance the child will be stillborn or born with a variety of teratogenic anomalies; the eye, ear, heart and brain are particularly affected. There is nothing that can be done if this situation presents itself before the child is born.

The ocular changes affecting one or both eyes include an embryopathic cataract (nuclear, atypical or total), frequently with a small pupil in a small eye (microphthalmos). Less commonly buphthalmos has also been reported, as has strabismus, iris deformities, corneal opacities and congenital glaucoma. It should be remembered that *high intraocular pressure is an epiphenomenon in the newborn for several weeks*. Another defect which can confuse where everything else seems in perfect order and where there is no positive history of rubella in the mother is a pigmentary degeneration of the retina which can simulate a luetic 'pepper and salt' fundus, a primary retinitis pigmentosa, secondary pigmentary degeneration after an arterial occlusion (usually sectorial), and any early central or paracentral macular change.

The classic finding in rubella is a centrally placed dispersal of fine pigment granules around the macular area with loss of central vision and nystagmus.

Surgery for cataract done within a year when the virus may still be present does badly; an anterior uveitis invariably complicates the operation. Treatment otherwise is symptomatic.

SCHISTOSOMIASIS AND THE KATAYAMA SYNDROME

Schistosomiasis (bilharziasis) and its treatment are described at length in Chapter 22.

The early phase of *S. japonicum* infection, known as the Katayama syndrome, is particularly associated with the ocular changes described below.

In the invasive stage urticaria and oedema of the face and eyelids may be observed. The conjunctiva is occasionally invaded and pinkish-yellow, soft, painless tumours may be seen in the palpebral conjunctiva of the upper eyelid and in the fornix.

Microscopic examination shows schistosome ova surrounded by endothelial cells, lymphocytes, plasma cells, eosinophils and giant cells. The adult fluke has been found in a dilated vein near the caruncle.

In the later stages intracranial involvement may occur with granulomatous swellings of the meninges and of the cerebral cortex. Ova have been demonstrated in these swellings. Visual disturbances up to total blindness may result from involvement of the optic tract and the visual cortex.

SICKLE CELL DISEASE

The sickling disorders are described with the treatment in Chapter 58. It is correct to say that the possession of the trait does not result in a lowered life expectancy and the incidence of ocular complications is very low indeed. Haemoglobin S is found in races other than the Negro; both the Middle and Far East have considerable populations affected. Approximately 25% of Africans reveal the presence of haemoglobin S; in America it is nearer 5% in the coloured population.

Classically small thromboses occur in the periphery of the retina at the equatorial-junction zone where the smallest capillaries exist. While these early changes, with or without associated haemorrhages, may regress in sickle cell anaemia leaving a scar with a pigmentary reaction, their presence in sickle cell haemoglobin C disease in which they are twice as common is much more likely to be persistent.

These changes stem from increased viscosity as sickling occurs in capillaries, arterioles and venules with increasingly low oxygen tensions. The circulation becomes slowed and small groups of sickle cells become impacted in various parts of the vessels which appear to collapse on either side. Small plugs of this nature can be seen in the conjunctival vessels as well as in the fundus. They have recently been noted on the optic nerve head, the appearance being one of small, dark red, round spots. There is no doubt that this is a helpful sign in an African (in whom diabetes is less likely). These red spots do not always remain but may clear; on the other hand, they can enlarge and lead to vascular blockages with haemorrhages around the optic nerve head (in about 5% of cases).

The most striking changes follow neovascularization; the anoxia of retinal vascular occlusion leads to the formation of an elaborate network of convoluted interanastomosing vessels with some arteriovenous fistulae. They occur within the retina in the first instance although they may eventually break out into the vitreous. The new vessels, attempting to compensate for the lack of oxygen, lie in a delicate matrix of mesenchymal cells, from which vascular endothelial elements and fibrous tissue arise. Such structures are called *sea fans*. When the sea fan grows into the vitreous it moves slowly with the movement of the vitreous, hence the use of that descriptive term. The vessels within the sea fan may leak into the matrix, ultimately to grow into the retina or through the retina into the vitreous, a condition known as *proliferating retinopathy* (Fig. 70.19). As a rule, however, the fibrous tissue element in the sea fan sooner or later becomes more dense and outweighs the vascular element so that the new vessels regress as a result of the increased fibrosis; the condition is then called *retinitis proliferans*.

The changes associated with the formation of a sea fan are more common in the peripheral retina and at the optic nerve head than in the central retina. They can appear in more than one site. Attachment of proliferating fibroblasts, whether in the vitreous or not, from one part of the retina to another may possibly lead to the development of holes or secondary detachments. However, healing and regression of a proliferating retinopathy, even when there is leakage into the vitreous, can occur without leaving anything other than a pigmented scar; this happens in about half of them. In sickle cell haemoglobin C disease about 5% exhibit in addition *angioid streaks*, although in no instance has the macula been reported damaged by the latter.

The complications of peripheral sickle cell retinopathy have been assessed as follows:

Vitreous haemorrhages	6–7%
Retinal traction bands (with or without detachment)	1–5%
Blindness in one eye	10–20%

As diabetic and hypertensive retinopathies are being increasingly reported from Africa and Asia the recognition of similarities between these diseases and sickle cell changes is important.

There is no ocular treatment outside a large hospital. Photocoagulation is used where available to burn up new tissue and seal leaking vessels but the results are disappointing.

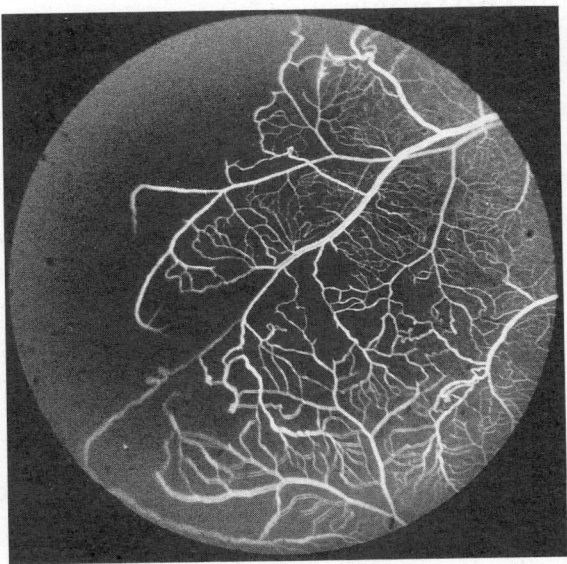

Fig. 70.19 Angiography of sickle cell proliferative retinopathy. Passage of dye is slow; none seen in choroid because of dense retinal pigment in negroid eye. (Courtesy Dr M. F. Goldberg and *Documenta Ophthalmologia*.)

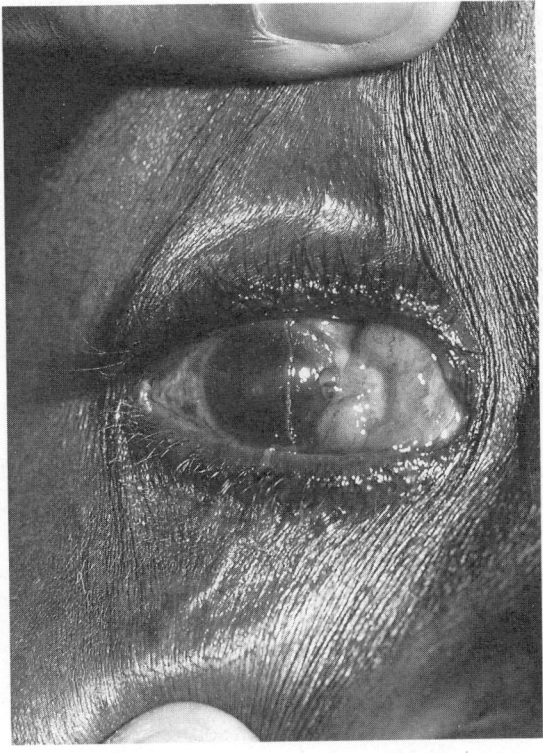

Fig. 70.20 Subconjunctival cyst containing sparganum. (Courtesy Dr D.W. Ellis-Jones and *British Journal of Ophthalmology*.)

SPARGANOSIS

This cestode larva infection is discussed in Chapter 23 (p. 554), and in listed Table 70.1.

The fully developed sparganum may enter the eye, as in other parts of the body, directly, or indirectly by emigrating from the alimentary tract. If it dies, or is held up by the tissue formation, it will produce a granulomatous nodule, which is red and painful. Such changes have been found and excised from the lid and the subconjunctiva (Fig. 70.20). From these locations they may be excised; it is harder to excise a sparganal nodule from the orbit. In the latter oedema of the lids occurs, and as the reaction increases as the parasites grow in situ, defective lid closure, proptosis and corneal ulceration can follow.

TOXOCARIASIS

This condition and its treatment are discussed in Chapter 21 and Table 70.1 (p. 1160). The second stage larva of this nematode is the one most commonly designated *larva migrans* although it is not the only migrating larva. Passing by the blood or lymph vessels the larvae can enter any tissue space around the eyeball, gaining access to the orbit and lids. They can also arrive within the uvea, rarely in the anterior segment as a rule. It is the dead larva (as it is the dead mf volvulus) which causes a severe reaction and in the eye this has been restricted to the posterior uvea giving rise to a severe chorioretinitis. This poses a clinical diagnostic problem as to the identity of the parasite. The early signs when the posterior segment of the eye is invaded by a living larva consist of linear reflexes which change position if viewed daily. After its death a raised pigmented lesion may be seen surrounded by oedema. Discrete deep retinal haemorrhages are sometimes associated. The elevated lesion in time settles and changes into a pale, circular, umbilicated mass into which a dilated vessel or vessels dip. The oedema settles after which pigment and gliotic scar tissue become increasingly obvious around the recent granulomatous lesion. The pigment later still becomes greatly heaped at the periphery of the affected part. Retinal detachment has been recorded in some of the cases when the final location was subretinal. While the macular area has been most frequently involved there have also been reports of larva migrans

dying further forwards in the uvea leading to a cyclitis.

Treatment of an active eye lesion (and this must be a rare finding) is a combination of a mydriatic and topical steroid with the systemic. Some people claim that some degree of vision can be saved by early treatment (Chapter 21, p. 417).

TOXOPLASMOSIS

For a description of this disease and its treatment the reader should refer to Chapter 9.

In the congenital form of the disease the organisms acquired by the fetus from maternal blood reach the choroid via the bloodstream. In most instances they enter the retina for which they have a liking and in that structure they are contained within a cyst. They produce a localized chorioretinitis which heals spontaneously but leaves a scar with destruction of the neuroretinal elements. Mothers are carriers without a symptomatology. Children having acquired the infection late in the mother's pregnancy seem to be those most affected. In some 80% of cases the focal chorioretinal scar is uniocular. It may be peripheral but, unfortunately, in many affects the macula. When a second lesion occurs at almost the same time it may overlap the first leaving a polyhedral scar (Plate VI.2). Such lesions should always be sought if an infant is seen to have a squint in a blind eye. Later damage due to the bursting of cysts with the spread of the infection and formation of secondary (daughter) lesions usually occurs, if at all, in the first and second decades. If they are seen in adults then the diagnosis is more questionable. *Late* secondary foci end up (close together but separate, unlike tubercular chorioretinitis) as rounded, well-circumscribed, pigmented scars of varying sizes, depths and degrees of pigmentation. Relapses cause acute oedematous reactions in the retina with vitreous haze (a choroiditis) which when they settle are seen to have adopted a characteristic almost round pigmented scar configuration.

In the acquired form in adults there may be a typhus-like fever suggestive of mononucleosis, mild but debilitating. There also may be signs of a mild meningoencephalitis. More usually there is simply a low grade fever with a lymphadenopathy, yet the uvea can be involved at this stage. The lesions attributed to acquired toxoplasmosis are a focal chorioretinitis (that is, a posterior uveitis) rather like the tuberculous lesion, a haemorrhagic perivasculitis of the retinal vessels, especially the veins, or an endophthalmitis. An anterior uveitis with large *fatty* KP and small nodules in the stroma has also been (rarely) described. Secondary (daughter) foci form around the posterior segmental lesion as in the congenital form.

Treatment is symptomatic in addition to the systemic treatment given in Chapter 9. Subconjunctival injections of steroid (Depo-Medrone) are more effective than drops.

THE TREPONEMATOSES

The various types of treponematoses and their treatment and management can be read about in Chapter 31. In this chapter yaws is discussed separately on p. 1181.

Involvement of the eye is found in both congenital and acquired syphilis. There is some doubt if it occurs in non-venereal endemic syphilis areas in the tropics—areas where yaws abounds; when seen it is almost certainly in those who have acquired syphilis elsewhere and settled later in bush villages. Although treponemes have been found in all parts of the eye, sometimes in great numbers in children, there is no reaction then; that comes later and so is considered to be the result of an antigen–antibody effect.

The classic ocular lesion of congenital syphilis occurring in about 10–15% of cases is *interstitial keratitis* (IK). It appears between the ages of two and 20 years; at first it may be unilateral but usually ends affecting both eyes with pain, lacrimation and photophobia. There is corneal haze as infiltrates and new vessels invade the stroma, especially in its posterior half. As with nearly all stromal inflammations there is an accompanying mild reactive iritis. At the outset the deep vessels entering the cornea invade most profusely in one sector giving rise to a characteristic dull, reddish-pink patch, known as a *salmon patch*. The condition is self-healing, becoming less and less troublesome; it is not destructive but, nevertheless, it leaves behind quite large, grey, polyhedral, deep scars with empty blood vessels (ghost vessels) adjacent to them. The interstitial keratitis of tuberculosis and trypanosomiasis somewhat resembles this.

The second ocular lesion in congenital syphilis which must be recognized is the *pepper and salt fundus*. Rarely isolated peripheral pigmented scars are found, probably never in the active stage; but this is rare. The usual form is a widely dispersed peripheral choroiditis consisting of a vast number of minute white and yellow exudates accompanied as they heal by fine pigment granules. It is always bilateral, heals of itself and does not recur. The name 'pepper and salt' describes the end result admirably.

Acquired syphilis is a comparatively rare cause of adult choroiditis. Early on in the disease in about 4% of cases the most common change is a severe *granulomatous anterior uveitis*. At first small capillary varicosities on the iris face arise (iritis roseata); later they become large enough to be defined as papules (iritis papulosa); later still they increase in size to become nodules (iritis nodosa). Aggregations of pigment in a densely pigmented eye may conceal these changes. The nodules usually disappear without trace but not before the iritis has produced adhesions between the pupil and back of the iris with the underlying lens and blocked the drainage angle with organized exudate, which leads to secondary glaucoma. However, with mydriasis and steroids and adequate specific systemic treatment these complications may be avoided.

The fourth important ocular manifestation of syphilis, also in the acquired condition, is a *diffuse chorioretinitis*. In about half the lesions are bilateral. It occurs any time after the primary stage—up to 10 years or longer. The early acute phase is non-specific with vitreous haze and choroidal exudates visible through the retina. They tend to occur around the disc and along arteries. Scattered superficial flame-shaped haemorrhages following the path of the vessels are a striking feature. Sometimes the exudate around the optic nerve head is so dense it conceals it. It resists treatment and runs a lengthy course. However, it is the final picture after healing which is most likely to present and this poses a problem in diagnosis for it can adopt a variety of appearances. Classically, there are many areas of pigment, partly concealing scars, some at least half the size of the optic disc. This pigment is retinal following involvement of the retina in the inflammatory process. These polymorphic pigment aggregations lie anywhere or everywhere over the fundi. When they coat blood vessels they look like retinitis pigmentosa at the first glance and then the pigment changes are seen to be too extensive. Sclerosis of the choroidal vessels may be seen through the retina when the pigment has migrated, and in an onchocercal area this can be mistaken for a Hissette–Ridley fundus until one weighs up the epidemiological data of both diseases.

TRYPANOSOMIASIS (INCLUDING CHAGAS' DISEASE)

African and South American trypanosomiasis and the systemic treatment are dealt with in Chapters 2 and 3 respectively.

In the African variety urticarial swellings of the eyelids occur soon after infection. Sometimes the lids are so swollen and oedematous they hang over the cheeks. The regional glands are enlarged.

Interstitial (stromal) keratitis with neo-vascularization of the affected areas of the cornea is due to invasion of the latter by trypanosomes. The parasites readily enter the anterior chamber in which small haemorrhages and exudates can be seen floating in the aqueous tide. The iris is involved as well, becoming oedematous and inflamed with small haemorrhages and exudates on the surface, the origin of those which fall into the aqueous. Similar localized areas of infiltration arise in the choroid affecting the retina on whose surface lie exudates in which trypanosomes have been identified.

Onchocerciasis, as already described in this chapter, exhibits a similar pathology and as the two diseases are found in the same bioclimatic zones a dual infection has to be considered. In the case of trypanosomiasis external ophthal-moplegias, ptosis, papilloedema and optic atrophy are later manifestations of involvement of the central nervous system. Apart from optic atrophy these are not accounted complications of onchocerciasis.

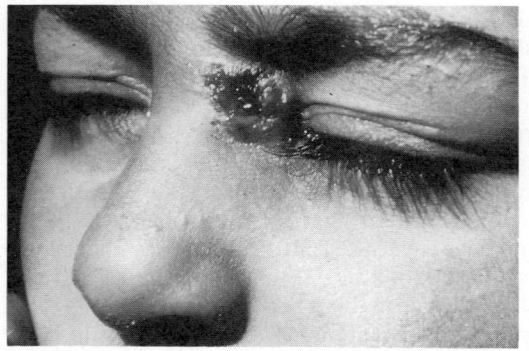

Fig. 70.21　Chagoma of inner canthus in Chagas' disease. (Courtesy Dr W. Crewe and Churchill Livingstone.)

In Chagas' disease (South American try-panosomiasis), after an incubation period of two weeks, a primary sore, the chagoma, develops in the skin and not infrequently on the eyelids (Fig. 70.21). In endemic areas oedema of the lids, known as Romaña's sign (Fig. 3.7, p. 80), as also seen in the African variety, is of diagnostic significance. The conjunctiva may be the initial port of entry. Dacryocystitis has been noted as a complication but intraocular manifestations have not been described.

TUBERCULOSIS

This historic disease and its treatment are described in Chapter 59.

In the tropics tuberculosis is far from being uncommon and the possibility of ocular disease being tuberculous is still as great as it used to be in Europe; it should be considered in every differential diagnosis. Phlyctenulosis (phlycten-ular keratoconjunctivitis) has been discussed on p. 1137. A granulomatous anterior uveitis is another manifestation with fatty KP, sometimes large. Rounded areas of chorioretinitis, usually contiguous, can arise which distinguish tuberculous from toxoplasmic chorioretinal 'daughter' lesions. Commencing, as acute chorioretinitis does, as a white oedematous patch of inflammatory exudate in the retina, treatment with steroids is essential. When the active stage settles and healing is completed the white, pigmented scars can be seen either as a solitary or disseminated phenomenon. In miliary tuberculosis the foci are small and widespread in the fundus. A solitary nodular tuberculoma is a rare finding. Nodular lesions are typical of tuberculosis of the eye. They can be found as solitary lesions on the palpebral conjunctiva as well as in the choroid and on the iris face.

Optic neuritis is a complication of a tuberculous basal meningitis, reflecting what happens in syphilis. Recurrent vitreous haemorrhages result from a tuberculous vasculitis and used to be common in Europe. It may be confused with sickle cell retinopathy and cerebral malaria.

TULARAEMIA

The disease is discussed with its treatment in Chapter 7.

In 1889 Parinaud described an infective conjunctivitis of animal origin, usually uniocular. Granules appear on the tarsal and bulbar conjunctiva and there is a mucofibrinous discharge. The ocular changes coincide with the acute systemic. The lids of the affected eye swell with oedema and the lymph glands on the same side are greatly enlarged and tender. Small lemon-drop ulcers may arise on the undersurfaces of both lids. Other smaller ulcers follow; as many as a dozen have been recorded. Eventually they are concealed by a necrotic membrane. Throughout, the discharge remains non-purulent. The eye changes can last over a month unless treated with the tetracyclines or chloramphenicol. The best regimen is to treat it like trachoma.

A somewhat similar lesion occurs in ocular *lymphogranuloma venereum* (p. 1112) but in the latter keratitis, uveitis and optic neuritis have been known to complicate the disease. The intradermal Frei test differentiates the two.

TYPHUS

Tropical (scrub) typhus and its treatment are described in Chapter 10.

The primary ulcer (eschar) has been seen many times on the lid. The ocular changes include a catarrhal conjunctivitis with photophobia in acute cases with slight corneal infiltration. In about 5% there may be subconjunctival haemorrhages which can be massive. A few cases of rather severe anterior (granulomatous) uveitis affecting both eyes have been reported.

By far the most frequent intraocular complications, however, are papilloedema, papillitis and optic neuritis. The retinal veins may become engorged with venous leaking. Invasion of the central nervous system in severe cases produces thrombotic lesions leading to oculomotor palsies in the febrile stage. These palsies often persist after recovery.

Topical treatment with mydriatics and tetracyclines and steroids are worth persevering with.

UNUSUAL OPHTHALMIAS

Various unusual ophthalmias continue to be reported although one might spend a lifetime in the tropics and not see any of them.

Blister beetles (cantharidiasis) (Chapter 55)

Several species of *Cantharida* are involved, some winged, some not. The wings, if they enter the eye, are well tolerated but if the toxic secretion of the blister beetle enters it produces a severe blepharoconjunctivitis, usually with subconjunctival haemorrhage (Nairobi eye) (Fig. 55.2). It takes some time to settle with symptomatic treatment. Unlike the haemorrhages in EV70 disease they are most commonly found in the lower part of the bulbar conjunctiva. The burning sensation produced is extremely painful.

Snake venom (Chapter 48)

In the African 'spitting' cobras the venom contains an active haemolytic and anticoagulant factor. The main effect on the eye is local necrosis. In Asia the cobras are generally only partly adapted for spitting. The *Naja* species and infamous South African *rinkals* are the danger. The venom can be ejected to hit an eye 10 feet away. Intense burning pain results. The lids should be forced open and the eye washed out as quickly as possible. This is not easy for oedema of the lids rapidly arises. The cornea becomes opaque and necrotic if untreated (Fig. 70.22). The sclera may be affected alone if the amount of venom which enters the eye is small or there may be only a small corneal ulcer, easy to heal but leaving a telltale white scar. This history is not uncommon when faced with such a scar in bush villagers.

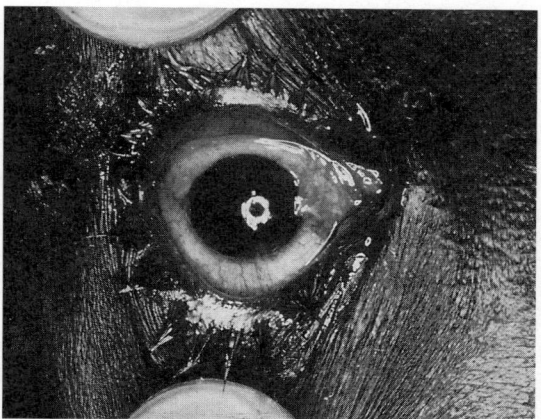

Fig. 70.22 Scleroconjunctivitis due to spitting cobra, *Naja nigricollis*. (Courtesy Dr D. A. Warrell and Churchill Livingstone.)

Wasp and bee stings (Chapter 55)

Wasps, being scavengers, may introduce bacteria or fungi into the eye. Bee stings have been reported mostly from India, wasp stings from South America, especially where the cornea has been penetrated. There is intense ocular pain, as one would expect, oedema and opacification of the cornea around the sting quickly following. An adjacent subconjunctival haemorrhage is a frequent finding. After 24 hours a large hypopyon may have developed. Raised pressure further complicates an already painful eye. If the sting has not penetrated the whole cornea, and not been left in situ, the eye will recover with symptomatic treatment. Where the sting has been left in the cornea or has driven through the cornea infection almost certainly will lead to an endophthalmitis and loss of the eye. When the lesion is on the lid or the bulbar conjunctiva the sting should always be sought and removed.

Caterpillar hairs (Chapter 55)

The caterpillars of certain *Lepidoptera* possess special hairs with poison gland cells located in the base. If these hairs become embedded in the eyelid an urticaria results. When they enter the eye accidentally they can penetrate the cornea; they have even been found in the anterior chamber. Usually they lodge in the bulbar conjunctiva where an intense conjunctivitis occurs. The reaction is focused on a small nodule as in a scleritis. Hairs should be removed and symptomatic eye treatment given.

Millipede and centipede toxins (Chapter 48)

This bizarre ophthalmia must be rare for millipedes (Diplopoda) are as a rule inoffensive. However, they do spray a caustic fluid from glands in the body which by contact may produce a violent urticaria of the lids. If this fluid is rubbed into the eye a keratoconjunctivitis can result. Centipedes (Chilopoda) are large in the tropics especially the poisonous *Scolopendra morsitans* which is 15 cm long. Bites are painful and a toxin is injected causing oedema of the eyelid, dizziness, headache and vomiting. If this poison reaches the external eye, a painful ophthalmia results.

Lice and mites

Certain ectoparasites of the lids (Chapter 54) cause a persistent itchy blepharoconjunctivitis. The itch mite of scabies, the mange mite and any of the lice causing pediculosis, even the pubic crab louse, can be found on the eyebrows or lashes feeding on the secretions of the lid margins.

General treatment for these ectoparasites should be given and if there is a blepharoconjunctivitis a cream consisting of triamcinolone acetonide 0.1% and chlortetracycline hydrochloride 3% may be rubbed along the lid margins. The results of local treatment with wood ash (Fig. 70.23) may suggest a faulty diagnosis of chronic trachoma, for the lids become swollen and the lashes fall out (tylosis).

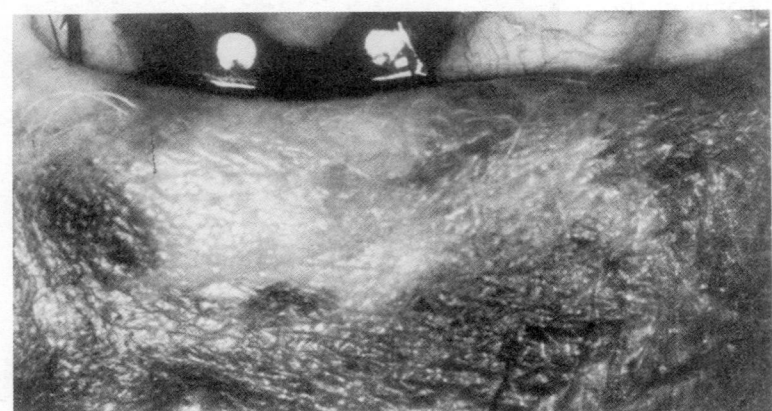

Fig. 70.23 Tylosis of lower lid after rubbing with wood ash to remove crab lice. (Courtesy Mr F. C. Rodger and Churchill Livingstone.)

VARIOLA RESIDUA

Smallpox has been eradicated but in the past the pustules spread over the lids to the external ocular membranes. Corneal ulceration, with or without secondary bacterial infection, was commonplace. If the patient survived, either the eye was lost or, if the perforation was small and blocked by iris tissue, the patient was blinded by the latter (leukoma adherens), or nearly so. There are many thousands of people walking about today with such eyes, the telltale pock marks on the face confirming the diagnosis. Such people are lucky to be alive. Corneal ulceration in smallpox was more frequently binocular than in measles. Accidental vaccination of the lids with *Poxvirus officinale* was not uncommon. It resulted in the development of one or more serpiginous ulcers, which could be as wide as a fingernail. These very often enlarged until they encroached on the lid margins and were confused with fungal infections but there were no serious systemic symptoms. The scars may still be seen in survivors.

WEIL'S DISEASE

Weil's disease is not synonymous with leptospirosis; although its ocular complications include, they go beyond, those of leptospirosis. Leptospirosis and its treatment are fully discussed and described in Chapter 32.

The causative organisms invade the eye during the febrile stage and may be found in the aqueous. Uveal inflammation usually occurs some weeks or months after the fever has gone, invariably involving both eyes. It is most commonly seen as an acute but fairly mild iridocyclitis but can appear as a more severe granulomatous uveitis. Clouding of the vitreous indicates involvement of the posterior uvea. The chorioretinal changes are as a result difficult to make out. Despite the disturbance of the vitreous (veils and membranes of fibrinous exudate have been described) the chorioretinitis runs a fairly mild course. Haemorrhages and exudates on the retinal surface have also been described. In Weil's disease at its most acute there is an intense congestion of the external eye with subconjunctival haemorrhage. Treatment of the eye is symptomatic.

YAWS

Yaws and its treatment are described in the section on treponematosis in Chapter 31.

Involvement of the eye has not been described in the early stage of yaws. In the widely distributed lesions of the later stage the eyebrows and eyelids are often affected and ulcerated granulomas or soft papillomas occur on the skin of the eyelids. Granulomas are not found on the conjunctiva but there may be an associated catarrhal conjunctivitis in the secretion of which *Treponema pertenue* may be found. Interstitial keratitis and iritis have been recorded, rarely.

Gangosa is regarded as a sequel of yaws. In this condition a destructive ulcerative rhinopharyngitis may spread through the nose to involve the eyelids and lead to cicatricial ectropion with exposure and consequent ulceration of the cornea (Fig. 31.20, p. 641).

Goundou (a form of yaws osteitis) is a symmetrical hyperostosis beginning in the nasal processes of the superior maxillae. The paranasal swellings increase to the size of an orange or larger, encroach upon the orbits, interfere with the fields of vision, displace the globes and may in extreme cases press upon and destroy the eyes (Fig. 31.12, p. 632).

REFERENCES

1 Rodger, F. C. (1973) *Brit. J. Ophthal.* **57,** 657.
2 Cursino, J. W. & Fine, B. S. (1976) *Am. J. Ophthal.* **82,** 395.
3 Johnson, G. J. & Overall, M. (1978) *Br. J. Ophthal.* **62,** 53.
4 Wadia, N. H., Wadia, P. N., Katrak, S. M. et al (1983) *J. Neurol. Neurosurg. Psychiat.* **46,** 599.
5 Kono, R., Sasagawa, A., Ishii, K. et al (1972) *Lancet* **i,** 1191.
6 Chatterjee, S., Quarcoopome, C. O. & Apenteng, A. (1970) *Br. J. Ophthal.* **54,** 628.
7 Lim, K. H. & Yin-Murphy, M. (1977) *Singapore med. J.* **18,** 41.
8 Majčuk, J. F. (1966) *Bull. Wld Hlth Org.* **35,** 262.
9 Hansman, D. (1969) *Med. J. Aust.* **1,** 151.
10 Galbraith, J. E. K. (1979) *Basic Eye Surgery.* Edinburgh: Churchill Livingstone.
11 Thommy, C. P. (1980) *Br. J. Ophthal.* **64,** 296.
12 Sauter, J. J. M. (1976) *Xerophthalmia and Measles in Kenya.* Groningen: van Denderen.
13 Rodger, F. C. (1959) *Blindness in West Africa*, p. 137. London: Lewis.
14 World Health Organization (1984) *Strategies for the Prevention of Blindness in National Programmes.* pp. 51 & 52. Publ. WHO.
15 Mathur, S. P. (1969) *Br. J. Ophthal.* **53,** 350.
16 Rodger, F. C. & Maertens, K. (1977) In *Onchocerciasis*

in Zaire, ed. F. C. Rodger, Chapt. 6. Oxford: Pergamon Press.

17 Rodger, F. C. (1959) *Trans. R. Soc. trop. Med. Hyg.* **53,** 138

18 Somerset, W. J. (1962) *Ophthalmology in the Tropics.* London: Baillière Tindall & Cassell.

19 Monekosso, G. L. & Ashby, P. H. (1963) *W. Afr. med. J.* **12,** 226

20 Jones, B. R. (1969) *Trans. Ophthal. Soc. UK* **89,** 819.

21 Wilder, H. C. (1951) *Trans. Acad. Ophthal. Otolaryng.* **55,** 99.

22 Mojon, M. (1977) In *Onchocerciasis in Zaire*, ed. F. C. Rodger, Chapt. 5, p. 85. Oxford: Pergamon Press.

23 Rathore, M. K. (1982) *Br. J. Ophthal.* **66,** 573.

24 Woods, A. C. (1961) *Endogenous Inflammations of the Uveal Tract.* Baltimore: Williams & Wilkins.

25 Gugnani, H. C., Gupta, S. & Talwar, R. S. (1978) *Mycopathologia* **65,** 155.

26 Reid, A. M. & Jones, D. E. W. (1963) *Br. J. Ophthal.* **47,** 169.

27 Rendtorff, R. C., Deweese, M. W. & Murrah, W. (1962) *Am. J. trop. Med. Hyg.* **7,** 62.

SECTION XVI
PROTECTING THE TRAVELLER

Chapter 71
Protecting the Traveller

This brief chapter aims to give guidance on protective inoculations for travellers to developing countries. Protecting the traveller is, of course, a much larger topic than inoculations alone, and travellers seeking more detailed advice than can be offered in the usual interview can be referred to the book *Travellers' Health* by Richard Dawood.[1] People going on expedition will find a rich source of information available from the Expeditionary Advisory Centre, 1 Kensington Grove, London SW7 2AR.

To immunize or not to immunize?

With immunization, as with chemoprophylaxis, the doctor has the problem of weighing risk and benefit, and usually neither is precisely quantifiable. I shall give my own views where appropriate, but freely admit that others just as well informed as I may have different opinions. But none of the vaccines I shall mention could reasonably be classed as dangerous, and it is discomfort rather than danger that weighs on the negative side in most cases.

Legal requirements

The physician dealing with immunization should have at his side the current World Health Organization (WHO) publication *Vaccination Certificate Requirements and Health Advice for International Travel*, WHO, Geneva, which is reissued annually in updated form. It gives the requirements for International Certificates and much other vital information, such as the malaria situation, country by country. There are only two types of International Certificate in current use, Yellow Fever and Cholera, now that smallpox has been officially eradicated from the world.

The main reasons for immunization

1 The traveller needs it for his own protection.
2 There is a legal requirement for an International Certificate.
3 The traveller needs an International Certificate to protect him from the depredations of corrupt immigration officials.

POLIOMYELITIS VACCINATION

This is recommended for all travellers. The disease occurs sporadically even in highly developed countries. Age alone does not protect against disease, despite the old name 'infantile paralysis'.

1 Poliomyelitis vaccine (oral), BP

This contains live attenuated poliomyelitis virus of strains 1, 2 and 3 and traces of antibiotics. It is given by mouth only.

2 Dose and administration

(a) To those previously immunized against polio: give a single dose (three drops) of oral vaccine (e.g. Pol/Vac(Oral)). This gives almost immediate protection by blocking virus receptor sites in the gut.
(b) To those not previously immunized against polio: give three doses, at intervals of at least four and preferably six weeks.

3 Risks

Vaccine-related paralysis: one in five million vaccinees; perhaps twice as high in contacts. Other risks are negligible.

4 Contraindications

(a) Pregnancy, unless there is a definite risk of polio. In the first trimester, give killed (Salk) vaccine instead, by injection.
(b) Diarrhoea and vomiting: wait until the condition has settled, or the vaccine might not 'take' in the gut.
(c) Extreme hypersensitivity to the antibiotics: polymyxin, neomycin, kanamycin, penicillin,

streptomycin. The amounts are so minute, they rarely cause trouble.

(d) Immunosuppression whether from disease or drugs. In such patients, used killed vaccine.

5 Precautions

Ensure vaccine is stored below 4°C, and so remains effective. Shake tube thoroughly before use. Hold vertically to deliver standard-sized drops. Vaccinate other unvaccinated members of the household simultaneously, to prevent transmission of virus of enhanced virulence to contacts.

6 Interaction with other vaccines

Oral poliomyelitis vaccine can be given at the same time as any other vaccine, living or dead.

7 Protection and duration of effect

Full vaccination gives a very high degree of protection against all strains of polio virus. Revaccination is not normally needed more often than every five years.

8 International Certificate

This is not applicable. No International Certificate exists, and no country requires one.

CHOLERA VACCINATION (Chapter 13, p. 271)

The currently available cholera vaccines are relatively ineffective, and their use is not justified in the usual holidaymaker. They are justified in those travelling extensively under arduous conditions in endemic areas, but the traveller must be told of the very incomplete protection given. A false sense of security may lead to a careless attitude to food and water, and an actual increase in the risk of infection from this.

The prospects for a much more effective *oral* vaccine seem good, but none is yet commercially available.

1 Cholera vaccine, BP

This contains heat-killed vibrios of the two pathogenic serotypes. Vaccination certificates are still required by some countries despite WHO recommendations to the contrary.

2 Dose and administration

A full primary course consists of two injections, the first of which must be subcutaneous, the second of which may be intradermal. Doses should preferably be more than four weeks apart, and not less than 7 days apart.

Subcutaneous dosage for cholera vaccine:

Age	First dose only
Children 1–5 years*	0.1 ml
Children 5–10 years	0.3 ml
Children over 10 years and adults	0.5 ml

Second and subsequent doses should be given *intradermally* which minimizes the local reaction without impairing the immune response.

Intradermal dosage for second and subsequent doses:

0.1 ml intradermally.

3 Risks

Local pain and tenderness are common but seldom serious. Severe reactions are more common in those vaccinated many times previously. Mild systemic effects sometimes occur. Reactions after intradermal boosters are usually slight.

4 Contraindications

None is absolute. It is best avoided in the presence of active infections.

5 Precautions

Store at 2–10°C, shake vial vigorously immediately before use.

6 Interaction with other vaccines

None is known.

7 Efficacy and duration of effect

It is not a potent vaccine: about 50% protection is conferred for up to six months. If cholera does develop despite vaccination, its severity is not reduced. There is no need to repeat the entire primary course, no matter how long since the last injection.

---

*The vaccination of infants aged less than one year is not recommended.

8 International Certificate

This can be issued after one injection only. It becomes valid 6 days after the first dose of vaccine, and immediately after a booster if given within six months.

TYPHOID VACCINATION

Typhoid is endemic in all developing countries and in much of southern Europe, but there is no general agreement on who should receive vaccination. British physicians tend to recommend typhoid vaccination for all travellers leaving Britain, but many Scandinavian physicians would advise it only for those at special risk such as those travelling overland in Asia. As with cholera vaccine, there are promising reports of oral vaccines with enhanced efficacy, but no such vaccine is yet commercially available in the U.K.

1 Typhoid vaccine, BP (monovalent)

This vaccine contains heat-killed *Salmonella typhi* preserved in phenol.

2 Dosage and administration

First dose:
   over the age of 10 years: 0.5 ml subcutaneously;
   age 1–10 years: 0.25 ml subcutaneously.
An initial dose of 0.2 ml intradermally for all ages is widely used.
Second and subsequent doses:
   0.1 ml intradermally for all age groups.
   Vaccination of children below the age of one year is not recommended.
   The full primary course consists of the initial subcutaneous dose, followed four to six weeks later by a booster dose given intradermally.

3 Risks

Local pain and tenderness occur, usually lasting a few days, and mild systemic reactions, in the form of fever and malaise. Reactions are minimized by intradermal administration. Rare neurological complications such as polyneuritis, myelitis and encephalitis have been reported.

4 Contraindications

Any concomitant infection is a contraindication.

5 Precautions

Store at 2–10°C. Shake vial vigorously immediately before use.

6 Interaction with other vaccines

None is known.

7 Efficacy and duration of effect

After the full primary course, there is 70–90% protection for three years. After a single injection, there is a similar degree of protection for up to six months. After a full primary course, boosters are needed every three years. It is never necessary to repeat a full primary course.

8 International Certificate

This is not applicable. No International Certificate exists and no country requires one, but it is a good idea for the patient to keep a record.

USE OF TYPHOID–PARATYPHOID A AND B VACCINE, BP (TAB)

This vaccine contains paratyphoid organisms in addition to those of typhoid, which increase the frequency and severity of reactions. The paratyphoid A component may provide some protection against this organism, found mainly in the Balkans and India. The paratyphoid B component has never been proved to be of any use.
   Dosage is exactly as for monovalent typhoid vaccine, which is normally preferred.

YELLOW FEVER VACCINATION
(Chapter 5, p. 142)

Yellow fever vaccine is required for their own protection by people going to places where yellow fever already exists, and for public health reasons, by people visiting areas which have mosquitoes capable of transmitting yellow fever, and who have come from areas where the disease is endemic. This is to prevent the establishment of yellow fever in areas where the infection did not occur before. Vaccination can only be carried out at designated vaccination centres.

1 Yellow fever vaccine

This is prepared from the living attenuated yellow fever virus, grown in chick embryos. Small amounts of neomycin and polymyxin are present.

2 Dosage and administration

Frozen lyophilized vaccine is freshly reconstituted and injected subcutaneously within half an hour. A French vaccine is inoculated by scarification.

3 Risks

Reactions to yellow fever vaccine are very uncommon. Rarely, encephalitis develops in children vaccinated under the age of nine months, so vaccination below this age is not normally recommended. The theoretical adverse effects of the vaccine in the fetus have never been demonstrated and in many cases vaccination in pregnancy is an obviously lesser risk than the danger of acquiring yellow fever.

4 Contraindications

Yellow fever vaccine is contraindicated in those who are immunosuppressed by disease or by drugs. In such a case the vaccine virus may multiply unrestrained by the host's immune response, and possibly produce an illness resembling yellow fever.

5 Precautions

The vaccine has special storage requirements and the reconstituted vaccine has a very short life; hence the restriction of vaccination to special centres.

6 Interaction with other vaccines

Yellow fever vaccination does not interfere with the effectiveness of oral polio vaccine, or with any killed vaccine.

7 Efficacy and duration of effect

Yellow fever is the most effective of all vaccines known. A single injection confers complete immunity for at least 10 years.

8 International Certificate

After the first vaccination, an International Certificate of yellow fever vaccination can be issued *at a designated yellow fever vaccination centre* only, and is valid for 10 years from the tenth day after vaccination. If revaccination takes place within 10 years, the Certificate is valid at once. It seems probable, although not as yet fully proved, that immunity may be lifelong.

MISCELLANEOUS VACCINATIONS

Smallpox vaccination

In 1980 the WHO officially declared that smallpox had been eradicated. The only *medical* reason for smallpox vaccination is to protect someone exposed to the virus in a laboratory.

Smallpox vaccine is now available in single dose vials, and is best given in vaccination centres. Those insisting on smallpox vaccination without medical reason should sign a disclaimer form before vaccination is carried out.

Death from vaccinia has occurred since smallpox was eradicated, due to unnecessary vaccination.

Measles vaccination

The same rule should be applied as to children living in Britain. Although measles is a more severe infection in children native to Africa, Asia and South America, this is because of lack of resistance to the infection. There is no evidence that measles acquired by *expatriate* children in tropical areas is more severe than measles acquired in Britain, so there is no need to modify the normal vaccination programme.

Triple vaccine for children proceeding abroad

Again, the normal British practice of vaccination should be observed, and no modifications are necessary for children who are proceeding abroad.

Tetanus

Although tetanus is more common in developing countries than in northern Europe, no special tetanus boosters are necessary for those proceeding on holiday to developing countries. The risk of developing tetanus is only increased in those with increased risk of exposure, such as those working in agriculture.

After a full primary course of three doses, a booster dose of tetanus (adsorbed tetanus vaccine, BP) is normally required once every 10 years. More frequent vaccination may result in a hyperimmune allergic reaction. The dose is 0.5 ml subcutaneously or intramuscularly, the subcutaneous route quite commonly causing a chronic tender induration.

Rabies vaccination

Effective pre-exposure vaccination to rabies can be achieved, safely, with three intradermal doses of human diploid cell vaccine. This is normally only recommended for those at special risk of exposure to infection, such as veterinary surgeons. It is expensive, but the cost can be greatly reduced by using the intradermal route Chapter 42), although people receiving chloroquine for malaria prophylaxis may have an impaired antibody response.

Gamma globulin for hepatitis A prevention

A single dose of 500 mg intramuscularly into the buttock or thigh will give passive immunity against hepatitis A for about four months. It does *not* protect against other types of hepatitis; 250 mg protects for about eight weeks, and 125 mg for four weeks.

It is usually given to those at high risk of exposure, such as overland travellers to Asia and Africa, but should ideally be given to all travellers to highly endemic areas. The use of the lower doses for shorter periods of protection (as above) helps to conserve material. Regular overseas travellers should have their hepatitis A IgG levels measured; if they have natural antibodies, lifelong immunity is assumed to exist.

BCG vaccine

This is advisable for Mantoux negative adults and children intending to *live* in areas highly endemic for tuberculosis.

Hepatitis B vaccine (Chapter 6, p. 177)

Vaccination is recommended for all medical workers in highly endemic areas including nurses, laboratory workers and doctors. A full course of three injections costs about £65.

European tick-borne encephalitis vaccine (Chapter 5, p. 163)

This vaccine is available on a named patient basis from Immuno Ltd., (tel: 0732 458101). Three spaced doses are needed for full protection, but 90% seroconversion occurs after the second dose. Cost about £8 per dose.

Meningitis vaccine (Chapter 30, p. 618)

Meningococcal vaccine types A and C are available on a named patient basis from Servier Laboratories (tel: 02816 2744) or SKF (tel: 0707 325111) from whom further details can be obtained. The vaccine is normally only given to those travelling in an area where an epidemic is in progress. A single dose gives two to three year's protection. Cost about £3.

Less common vaccines

These are mentioned in the text under the heading of the diseases to which they apply.

COMMON QUESTIONS ABOUT VACCINATION

Can I have four vaccinations all at the same time?

Yes.
It is common to give polio, yellow fever, typhoid and tetanus, for example, at the same session. But it would be sensible to give the tetanus and typhoid into one arm (the left arm for a right-handed person) and the yellow fever into the other. Polio and yellow fever vaccines do not interfere with each other if given *simultaneously* but they may interfere—because of interferon production—if given at different times close together. If one has been given already, the second vaccine should not be given until at least *three weeks* later.

Dead vaccines are not affected in this way.

When do I need to give a full primary course of immunization again?

Never.
For example: the patient had a course of three tetanus injections 30 years ago. Only one booster

dose is now needed to bring immunity up to date.

The same principle applies to polio and typhoid.

The patient is taking 10 mg prednisolone a day for ulcerative colitis. Can he go on holiday to Kenya?

Yes.

He can safely be given typhoid vaccine, a booster dose of killed (Salk) polio vaccine if he needs it and he does not need to have yellow fever vaccine. This is widely given to visitors to Kenya but is not required by Kenyan law, and despite the fact that Kenya is within the old 'yellow fever zone' in Africa, there has been no proven case there for over 40 years.

The patient is taking 10 mg prednisolone a day; can he go on holiday to The Gambia?

Not while he is taking the prednisolone, because of the danger of the live virus in an immu-nosuppressed subject. If medically feasible, the prednisolone should be gradually withdrawn and the yellow fever vaccine given at least two weeks after it has been stopped. If the patient cannot be weaned off prednisolone safely, he should choose somewhere else for his holiday.

Why is intradermal vaccine often more efficient than intramuscular or subcutaneous vaccine?

Because intradermal vaccine is absorbed via the lymphatics, and antigen is presented at high con-centration to immunoreactive cells in the regional lymph nodes. Repeat intradermal injec-tions should, for this reason, always be given into the same site. Also, specialized cells in the skin are very efficient at presenting antigen.

REFERENCE

Dawood, R. (1986) *Travellers' Health*. Oxford: Oxford University Press.

SECTION XVII
DRUGS

Chapter 72
Drugs

P. H. Rees

Dosages given are for the average 70 kg adult. Care should be taken to reduce the dose for children and small adults on a weight for weight basis. This is particularly so with the more toxic preparations, but is relatively unimportant with those drugs that are not absorbed (e.g. bephenium). It is rarely necessary and often unsafe (e.g.

niridazole) to increase the dose for heavier individuals.

Some drugs are included for their historic interest, and if they are but little used now, their dosages are not given. Dosages of newer drugs are also omitted where regimens are not yet established.

INDEX OF DRUGS AND PROCEDURES

HEAVY METALS

ANTIMONY

Organic compounds of trivalent antimony are more toxic to both host and parasite than pentavalent compounds. Trivalent compounds, already established as effective in trypanosomiasis and leishmaniasis, were introduced for the treatment of schistosomiasis immediately after the First World War and for the next 50 years they were by far the most important and most effective group of drugs for treating all three forms of human schistosomiasis. With the introduction of less toxic drugs with simpler administration schedules, it is now rarely, if ever, necessary to resort to the trivalent antimonials for treating schistosomiasis. Pentavalent compounds, however, remain most important in the treatment of leishmaniasis.

Trivalent antimony

Several compounds are available. In general, toxicity and efficacy are related to the total weight of antimony given. *Schistosoma haematobium* is the most susceptible to treatment and *S. mansoni* and *S. japonicum* progressively less so. Phosphofructokinase, an enzyme essential to schistosome glycolysis, is inhibited by antimony compounds. There is a hepatic shift of the adult worms and the production of eggs is disturbed.

Trivalent antimonials have also been used in trypanosomiasis, leishmaniasis, filariâsis, lymphogranuloma venereum, granuloma inguinale, mycosis fungoides and lepra reactions. Oral preparations have been used as emetics and as reflex expectorants.

Trivalent antimony is excreted slowly, mainly in the urine.

Toxicity

The important toxic effects are on the heart and liver. Sudden death may occur at any stage in treatment. Immediate symptoms of toxicity include cough, chest pain, pain in the arms, vomiting, abdominal colic, faintness and collapse which may be fatal but may be reversed by an injection of 1/1000 adrenaline. Those preparations that are given intravenously should be given slowly through a fine needle. Local leakage may cause great pain because of tissue damage. An anaphylactoid reaction may occur after the sixth or seventh intravenous injection with an urticarial rash, husky voice and collapse. Delayed reactions may occur during the course of treatment or later and include a multiplicity of symptoms, such as nausea, vomiting, anorexia, diarrhoea, pains in muscles and joints, arthritis, pneumonia, headache, fatigue, pruritus, back pain, excessive salivation, dizziness, a metallic taste in the mouth, skin rashes, constipation, fever, herpetic lesions and conjunctival injection. Electrocardiographic (ECG) changes with prolonged QT interval, and ST segment and T-wave changes are almost invariable, reverting to normal within about six weeks, but a fall in blood pressure or bradycardia necessitates discontinuation of treatment. Cardiovascular collapse or fatal arrhythmia may occur at any time. Haemolytic anaemia, sulphaemoglobinuria, retrobulbar neuritis and encephalopathy have been reported with some preparations. A rise in liver enzymes is common. Liver damage with hepatic failure and death is especially likely to occur in those with pre-existing liver disease.

Contraindications

Contraindications are liver, heart, renal and lung disease.

Route

Slow intravenous injection is required for most preparations but some (TWSb and stibophen) are given intramuscularly. Oral administration for schistosomiasis is not satisfactory because of the local emetic action and uncertain absorption.

Dose

The number of injections and the length of the course varies with preparations. In general a total dose of 0.5 g of trivalent antimony is given.

Preparations

Antimony lithium thiomalate (Anthiolimine, Anthiomaline). Available as a 6% solution for intramuscular injection, equivalent to 10 mg of antimony/ml, it is given over a period of 30 days on alternate days to a total of 40–60 ml.

Antimony potassium tartrate (tartar emetic, potassium antimonyl tartrate). The sodium salt of antimony tartrate is usually preferred, thus avoiding the intravenous administration of potassium ions.

Antimony sodium tartrate (sodium antimonyl tartrate). This contains 38% of trivalent antimony, and is given as a 2% solution by slow intravenous injection. An initial dose of 30 mg is increased on alternate days to a maximum dose of 150 mg and continued until a total of 2 g has been given.

```
        COO
         |
        CHO—Sb
         |   /
        CHO
         |
        COO Na
```

Sodium antimony tartrate

```
COONa                          COONa
 |                               |
CHS                             SCH
 |   \                       /   |
CHS —— Sb —— S         S —— Sb —— SCH
 |              \     /           |
COONa            CH—CH           COONa
                 |    |
              COONa  COONa
```

TWSb/6 (antimony sodium dimercaptosuccinate)

Antimony sodium thioglycollate.

Sodium antimonyl gluconate (Triostam). This contains approximately 36% of trivalent antimony; 190 mg are given intravenously daily for 6 days.

Stibocaptate (Astiban, antimony dimercaptosuccinate, Friedheim's TWSb). This is a combination form of trivalent antimony and a dimercaprol derivative analogous to melarsoprol (Mel B), it contains 25–26% of trivalent antimony. 500 mg are given on alternate days, twice weekly or weekly by intramuscular injection to a total of 2.5 g.

Stibophen (fouadin, fantorin, neoantimosan, reprodral). This contains approximately 16% of trivalent antimony. A 6.3% solution contains 8.5 mg of trivalent antimony/ml. Given intramuscularly, an initial dose of 2 ml is increased to a maximum of 5 ml and continued to a total course of 40–80 ml over a period of two to four weeks.

Pentavalent antimony

This remains the drug of choice in kala-azar. It is less useful in cutaneous and mucocutaneous leishmaniasis, and has also been used in schistosomiasis. It is possible that, as with pentavalent arsenic, it may be converted to the trivalent form in vivo.

Toxicity

It is less toxic than trivalent antimony. A single dose will be almost entirely excreted in the urine in 6 hours or less. There is no risk of cumulative toxicity, provided renal function is normal. If it is given intramuscularly there will be a dull pain at the injection site for several hours which may be aggravated by use of the muscle. In general, a course of treatment does not cause any side-effects though, rarely, unexplained reactions including fever, malaise, diarrhoea, nausea, generalized muscle and joint pains, and even sudden death, may occur. It is difficult to know whether to attribute such effects to the kala-azar itself, to the pentavalent antimony, or perhaps to a reaction precipitated by antimony damaged parasites. In such circumstances treatment should be interrupted until the cause of the symptoms is clear. Renal function should be checked. Even if it is probable that the antimony is responsible it is usually possible to restart treatment without any further toxic effects.

Contraindications

In kala-azar there are no absolute contraindications. In particular, pentavalent antimony should not be withheld because of pregnancy. In cutaneous and mucocutaneous leishmaniasis treatment is less urgent. Dosage should be adjusted in the presence of renal failure.

Route

The intramuscular or the intravenous route may be used with equal effect. The main objection to the intramuscular route is pain at the site of injection.

Dose

The dose of pentavalent antimony (Sb^V) used in treating kala-azar has varied from country to country and with different preparations. This has been partially due to apparent regional variation in the susceptibility of the parasites to pentavalent antimony and partially due to the recommendations of manufacturers. The regimen and dose used will often be dictated by local experience but 10 mg Sb^V/kg daily for 30 days is generally adequate, though children tolerate and require relatively more Sb^V and may be given 20 mg Sb^V/kg. As there is no cumulative toxicity there is no need for the rest periods previously employed, the duration of treatment being determined by parasitological and clinical response.

Preparations

Sodium stibogluconate (*sodium antimony gluconate, Pentostam*) contains 10% (100 mg/ml) Sb^V and may be given intramuscularly or by slow intravenous injection. At 10 mg Sb^V/kg, the daily dose of a 60 kg adult is 6 ml. At 20 mg Sb^V/kg, the daily dose for a 10 kg infant will be 2 ml.

Ethylstibamine (*Neostibosan, Neostam*) is given intravenously. It is no longer widely available.

Urea stibamine (*Stiburea*) is a compound of urea with stibamine but is no longer widely available.

Meglumine antimonate (*N-methylglucamine, Glucantime*) is supplied as a white powder containing 33–34% Sb^V. It is water soluble. Precise chemical structure is uncertain, but similar to Pentostam.

Sodium stibogluconate

ARSENIC

Trivalent arsenicals are more potent and more toxic than pentavalent arsenicals. Pentavalent arsenic owes its activity to its conversion to trivalent arsenic in vivo, and its relative non-toxicity to its ability to penetrate parasite cells more readily than host cells.

The main use of arsenicals is in the treatment of African trypanosomiasis. Sulphydryl enzyme systems of the trypanosomes are blocked. Arsenicals have also been used in spirochaetal infections (syphilis, yaws, relapsing fever, rat bite fever,

Vincent's angina), anthrax, protozoal diseases (malaria, amoebiasis, trichomoniasis) and in helminthic infections (pulmonary tropical eosinophilia, filariasis (effective against adult worms—macrofilaricidal), schistosomiasis and threadworm infection).

The pentavalent arsenical, diphetarsone, remains one of the most effective drugs against whipworm, *Trichuris trichiura*, and also against intestinal protozoa.

Toxicity

In general the more toxic preparations have been discarded and arsenicals themselves have been displaced as elective therapy in situations where less toxic drugs are available.

Immediate reactions include anaphylactoid arsenical shock, especially with tryparsamide. The face is flushed, with oedema of the tongue and eyelids, a burning taste in the mouth, nausea, vomiting, dyspnoea, cyanosis, precordial distress, sweating and coma. Herxheimer reactions may occur with fever and exacerbation of symptoms secondary to the effect on the trypanosomes.

Delayed toxicity includes rashes (particularly exfoliative dermatitis), nephritis, acute yellow atrophy of the liver, blood dyscrasias, peripheral neuritis, optic neuritis and encephalopathy. Arsenical encephalopathy which occurs in 10% of cases treated with melarsoprol is severe and often fatal. Melarsoprol should be used only when trypanosomes have invaded the central nervous system.

Sudden death may occur at any stage of treatment. The dose varies with the preparation but small initial dosages should be used, especially in debilitated patients. Arsenic is excreted slowly in the urine and faeces. It persists in certain tissues for long periods and may remain in a hair throughout its life.

Preparations of trivalent arsenic

Arsphenamine. Ehrlich's original 'therapia magna sterilisans' for relapsing fever. Replaced by less toxic neoarsphenamine.

Melarsen oxide. Replaced by less toxic melarsoprol.

Melarsonyl potassium (*Mel W*). Similar to melarsoprol, though water soluble and so can be given intramuscularly, but probably more toxic and less effective. It is a macrofilaricidal drug but is too toxic for general use in filariasis.

Melarsoprol (Mel B). A combination of melarsen oxide and dimercaprol (BAL), it is effective in Rhodesian and Gambian trypanosomiasis, on blood forms as well as those in the nervous system, and on trypanosomes resistant to other

Mel B (melarsoprol)

arsenicals. It is given by slow intravenous injection as a 3.6% solution in propylene glycol to a maximum daily dose of 5 ml (180 mg) and to a total dose of 30–40 ml over a period of three weeks.

Preparations of pentavalent arsenic

Carbarsone, introduced by Ehrlich, has an effect in non-invasive amoebiasis but is no longer used.

Diphetarsone (Bémarsal) is a very effective treatment of *T. trichiura* and intestinal protozoa, including *Entamoeba histolytica, E. coli, E. hart-manni, E. nana, Dientamoeba fragilis* and *Iodamoeba bütschlii.*[1] It appears to owe its useful luminal action to its poor absorption. Systemic toxicity is slight, but include transient changes in liver function tests and rashes. It is given by mouth in a dose of 30 mg/kg twice daily for 10 days.

Tryparsamide (Tryparsone, Novatoxyl) was used in African trypanosomiasis with central

Diphetarsone

nervous system involvement. It is no longer available, having been superseded by melarsoprol (see above).

HEAVY METAL ANTAGONISTS

Dimercaprol (BAL)

This is used in the treatment of poisoning with organic antimonials and arsenicals.

Dimercaprol (BAL)

Side-effects are common but the drug is not cumulative. A course of intramuscular injections is given at intervals of not less than 4 hours. The dose ranges from 1 to 3 mg/kg repeated every 6 hours for 3 days and thereafter twice daily until recovery.

Sodium calcium edetate

This is given intravenously in lead poisoning.

D-Penicillamine hydrochloride

This is administered orally in Wilson's disease, lead poisoning and haemosiderosis.

Desferrioxamine mesylate

This is given orally or by injection for acute or chronic iron intoxication.

PLANT DERIVATIVES AND RELATED DRUGS

EMETINE

This is an alkaloid present in the roots of the South American plant *Cephaelis ipecacuanha.* The crude preparation (ipecacuanha, Brasil root) was introduced into Europe in the seventeenth century for the treatment of dysentery, though the specific action of emetine against *Entamoeba*

histolytica was not appreciated until 1912. It has a direct amoebicidal action and parenteral emetine affords rapid symptomatic and clinical improvement in amoebic involvement of the liver, amoebic dysentery, amoeboma and other forms of invasive amoebiasis. When given by injection it does not affect *E. histolytica* in the intestinal lumen. However, the oral preparation, emetine

PLATE I

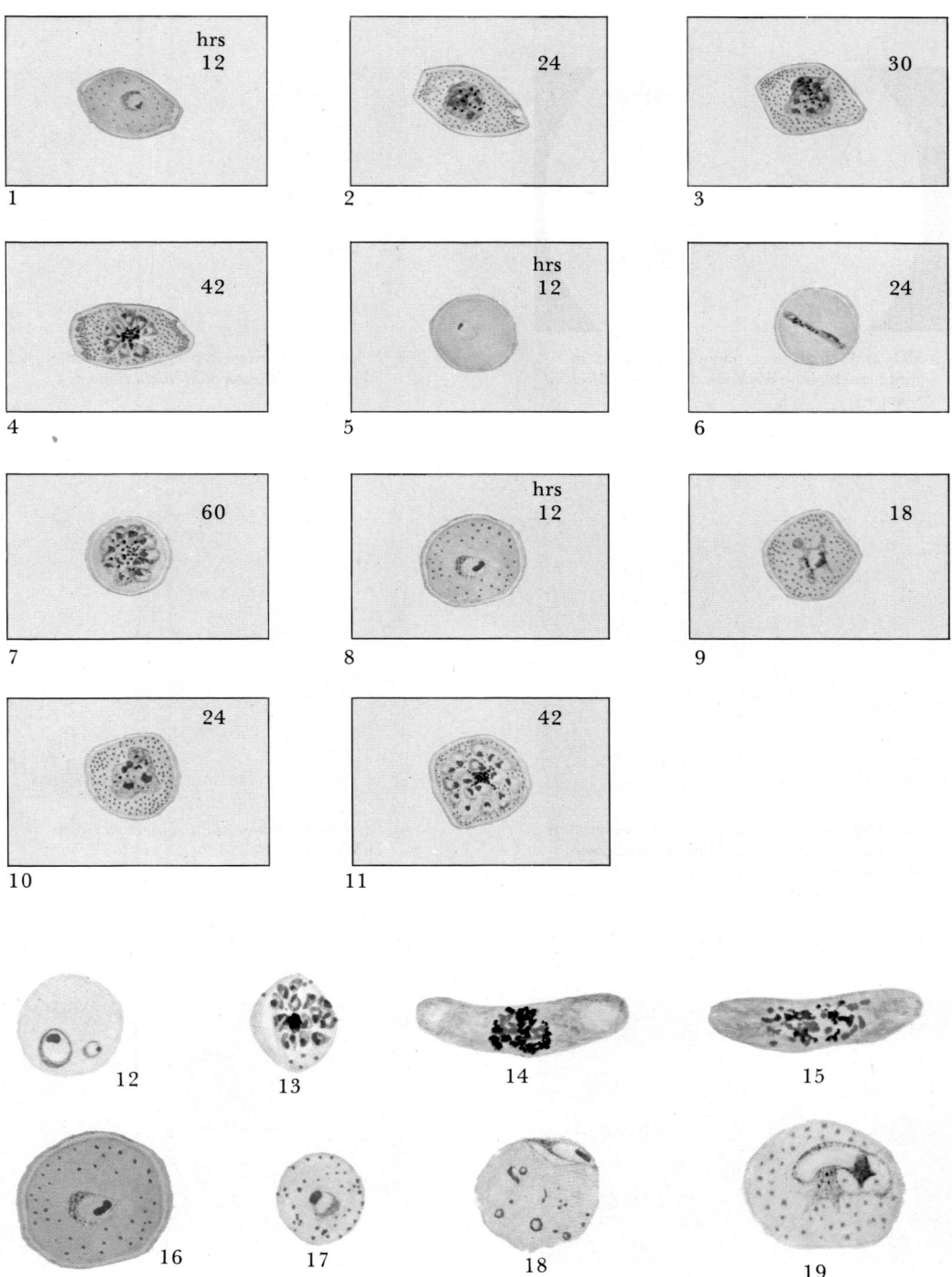

1. *P. ovale,* early trophozoite (12 hours), 2. *P. ovale,* half-grown trophozoite (24 hours), 3. *P. ovale,* schizont (30 hours), 4. *P. ovale,* mature schizont, eight merozoites (42 hours), 5. *P. malariae,* early trophozoite (12 hours), 6. *P. malariae,* band form (24 hours), 7. *P. malariae,* mature schizont (rosette) (60 hours), with eight merozoites, 8. *P. vivax,* early trophozoite (12 hours), 9. *P. vivax,* half-grown, trophozoite (18 hours), 10. *P. vivax,* late trophozoite (24 hours), 11. *P. vivax,* mature schizont (42 hours) with 16 merozoites, 12. *P. falciparum,* early trophozoite showing double infection, 13. *P. falciparum,* mature schizont, 14. *P. falciparum,* macrogametocyte, crescent, 15. *P. falciparum,* microgametocyte, crescent, 16. Host stippling in *P. vivax,* Schuffner's dots, 17. Host stippling in *P. malariae.* Ziemann's stippling, 18. Host stippling in *P. falciparum.* Maurer's spots, 19. Host stippling in *P. ovale.* James's stippling.

Painted by W. Cooper, Reproduced by courtesy of Professor P.C.C. Garnham and the Wellcome Museum of Medical Science

PLATE II

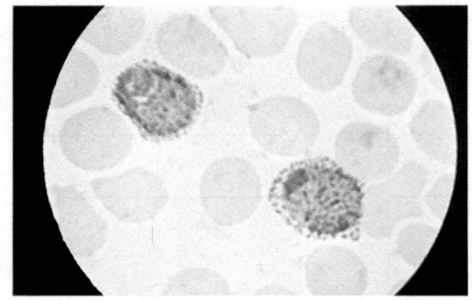

1. Male and female gametocytes of *P. vivax* in peripheral blood. (*Wellcome Museum of Medical Sciences*)

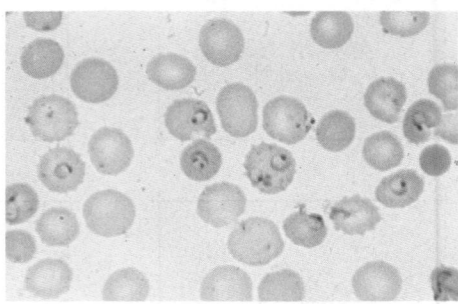

2. *P. falciparum* rings in peripheral blood. (*Wellcome Museum of Medical Science*)

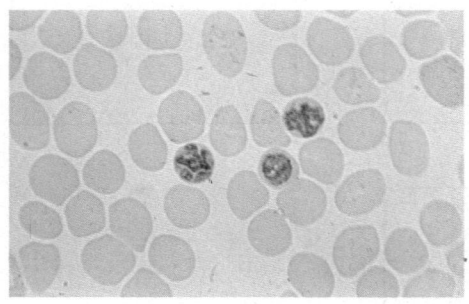

3. Late trophozoite and early and late schizont of *P. malariae* in peripheral blood. (*Wellcome Museum of Medical Science*)

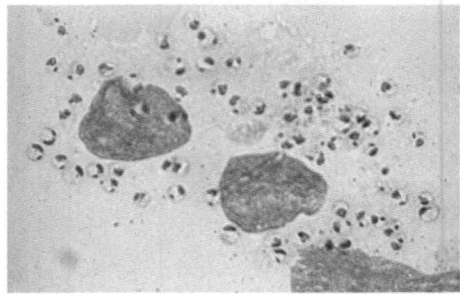

4. *Leishmania donovani* in a marrow smear, H & E x 1250

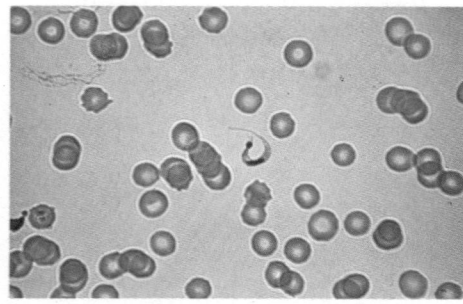

5. *Trypanosoma cruzi*, H & E x 1250

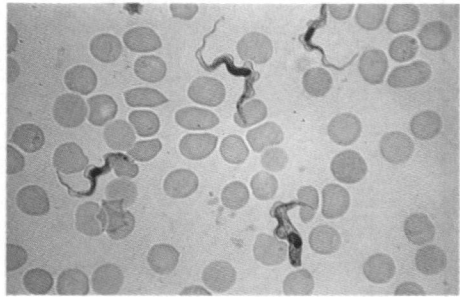

6. Long slender and short broad forms of *Trypanosoma rhodesiense*. H & E x 1250

PLATE III

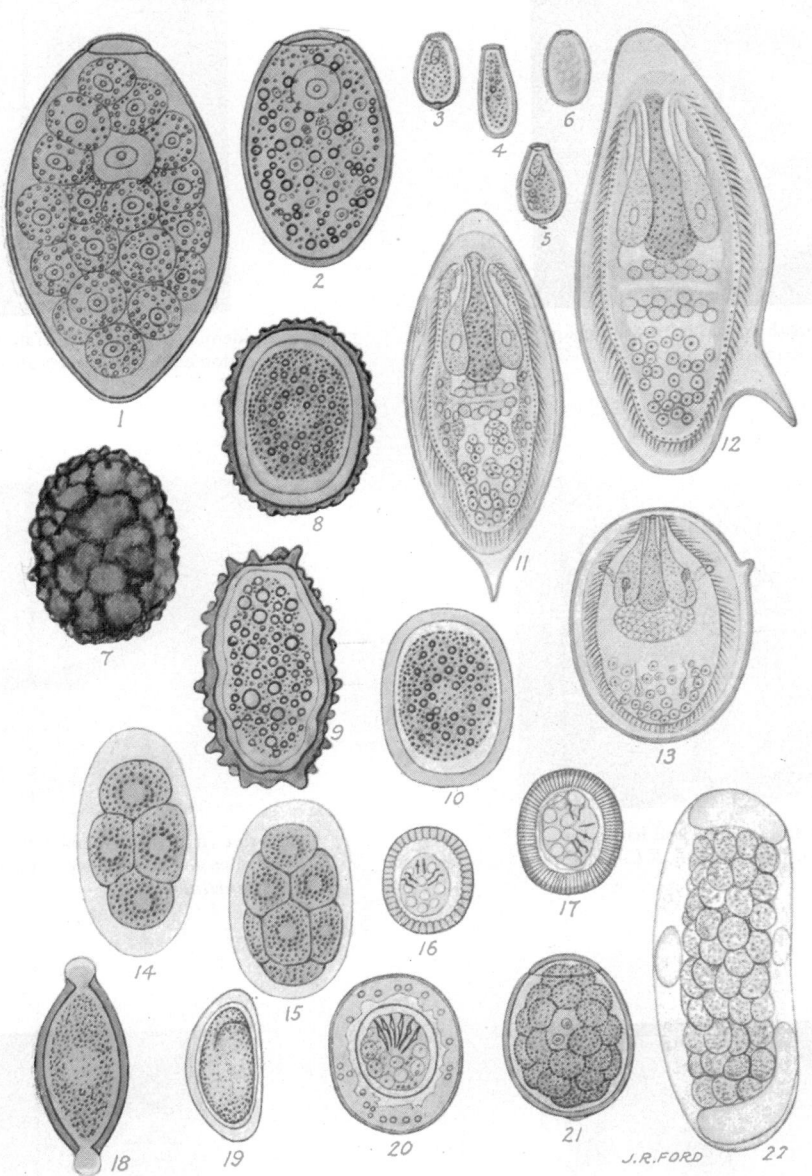

1. *Fasciolopsis buski.* 2, *Paragonimus westermani.* 3, *Heterophyes heterophyes.* 4, *Opisthorchis felineus.* 5, *Clonorchis sinensis.* 6, *Metagonimus yokogawai.* 7, 8, *Ascaris lumbricoides,* external aspect. 9, *Ascaris lumbricoides,* unfertilized egg. 10, *Ascaris lumbricoides,* decorticated egg. 11, *Schistosoma haematobium.* 12, *Schistosoma mansoni,* 13, *Schistosoma japonicum.* 14, *Ancylostoma duodenale.* 15, *Trichostrongylus colubriformis.* 16, *Taenia solium.* 17, *Taenia saginata.* 18, *Trichuris trichiura.* 19, *Enterobius vermicularis.* 20, *Hymenolepis nana.* 21, *Diphyllobothrium latum.* 22, *Heterodera radicicola,* non-parasitic, ingested with vegetables.

PLATE IV

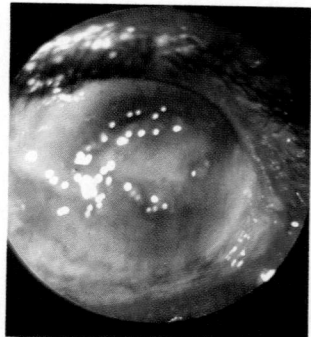

1. Solar keratopathy complicating an opaque cornea in onchocercal keratitis. (*Courtesy Mr F.C. Rodger*)

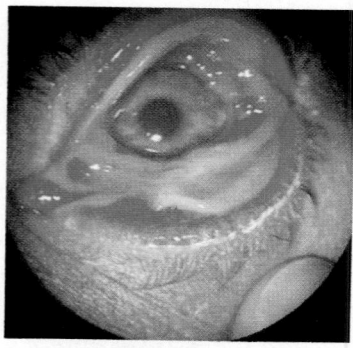

2. Epidemic (*adenoviral*) keratoconjunctivitis with pseudomembrane. (*Courtesy Mr. F.C. Rodger*)

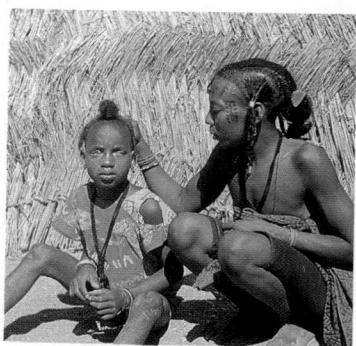

3. Fulani girl with trachoma and bacterial conjunctivitis. (*Courtesy Mr F.C. Rodger*)

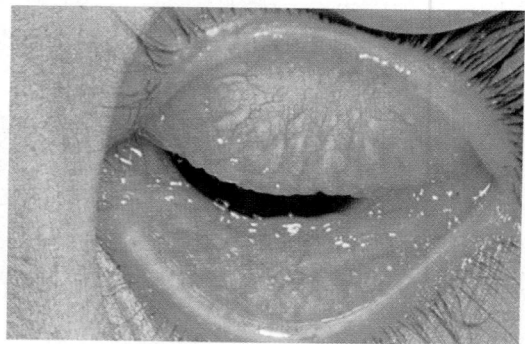

4. Active (florid) trachoma with multiple follicles and papillae and painful eyes. (*Courtesy World Health Organization*)

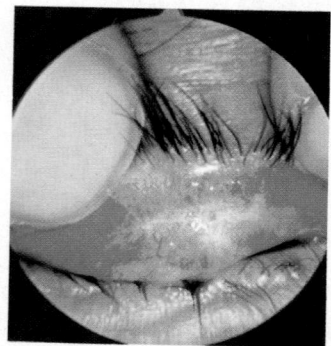

5. Trachomatous scarring of the upper lid conjunctiva (Arlt's line). (*Courtesy Mr D.P. Choyce*)

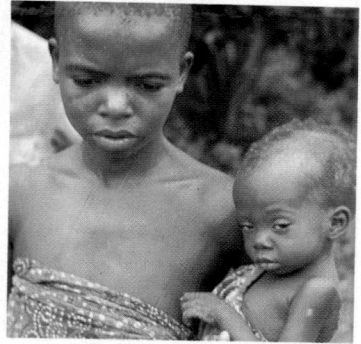

6. Zaireois child with kwashiorkor in area with some nutritional xerosis. The typical depigmentation of the hair is a warning. (*Courtesy Mr F.C. Rodger*)

PLATE V

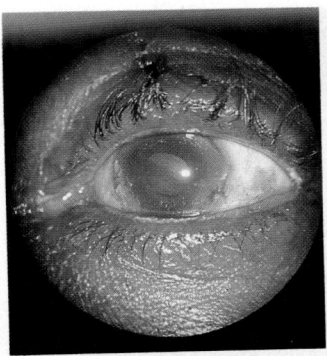

1. Onchocercal schlerosing keratitis. Note the three zones. Distortion of the pupil due to associated iritis. (*Courtesy Mr F.C. Rodger*)

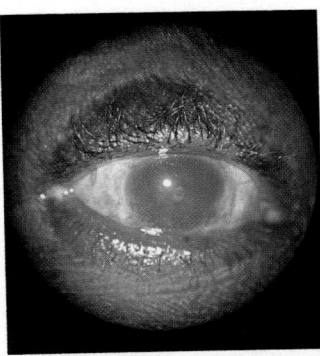

2. Small distorted pupil rimmed with flocculation indicating past onchocercal anterior uveitis. (*Courtesy Mr F.C. Rodger, and Pergamon Press*)

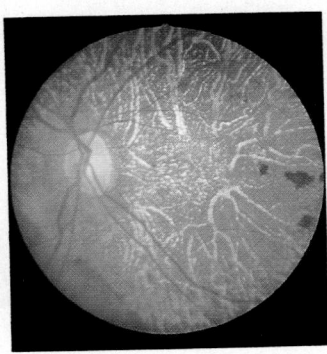

3. Hissette—Ridley fundus of onchocerciasis. (*Courtesy Mr F.C. Rodger*)

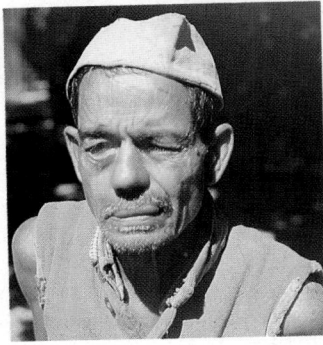

4. Ectropion in tuberculoid leprosy due to facial palsy. (*Courtesy Mr F.C. Rodger, and Churchill Livingstone*)

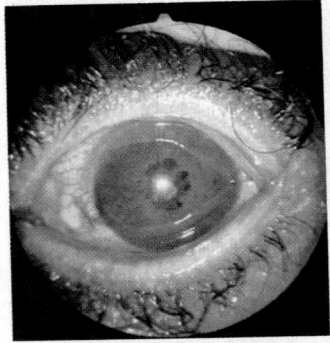

5. Lepromatous anterior uveitis with scalloped pupil margin due to adhesions at rim. (*Courtesy Mr D.P. Choyce*)

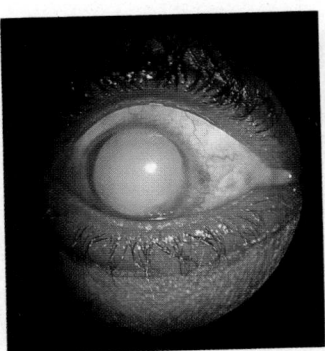

6. Hypermature cataract detached and dislocated into anterior chamber. (*Courtesy Mr F.C. Rodger, and Hutchinson*)

PLATE VI

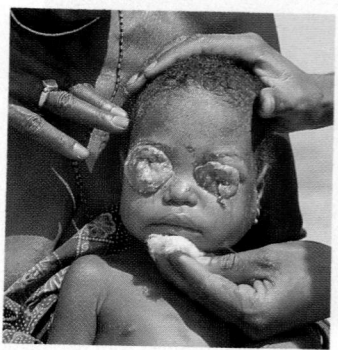

1. Bilateral retinoblastoma in Nigerian child. (*Courtesy Mr F.C. Rodger, and H.K. Lewis*)

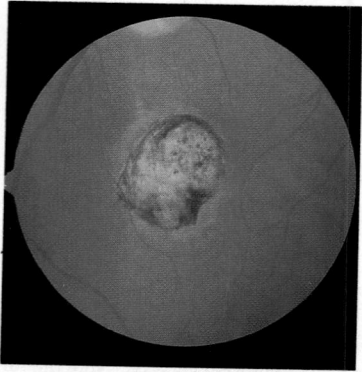

2. Acquired adult toxoplasmosis. The scars followed an acute focal choroiditis, confirmed serologically. (*Courtesy Mr F.C. Rodger, and Churchill Livingstone*)

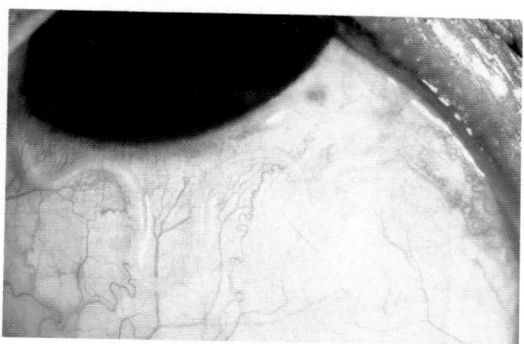

3. Adult *Loa Loa* beneath bulbar conjuctiva. (*Courtesy Dr J. Anderson*)

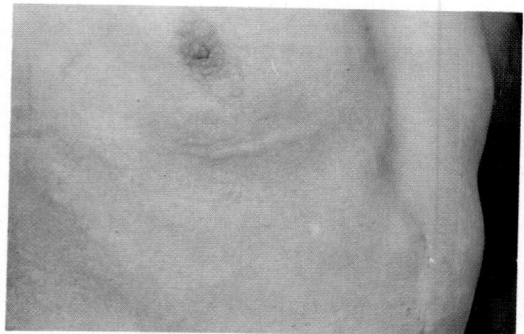

4. Skin rash (larva currens) of *Strongyloides*.

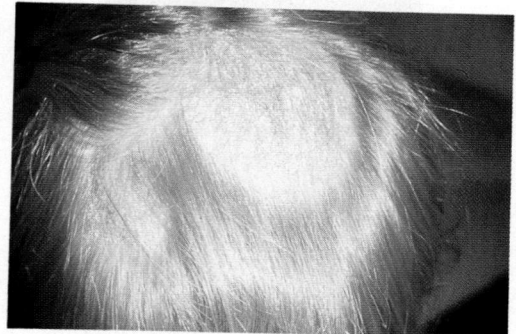

5. Tinea capitis. Circular patch of alopecia with distorted broken hairs and mildly inflamed scalp.

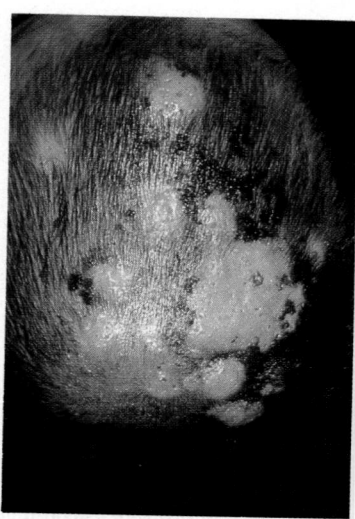

6. Kerion. Red, boggy inflammation affecting numerous areas of tinea capitis.

PLATE VII

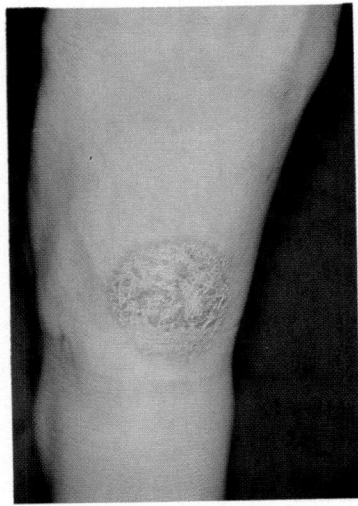

1. Tinea circinata. Round scaly patch with peripheral vesicles which may be seen on the trunk or limbs.

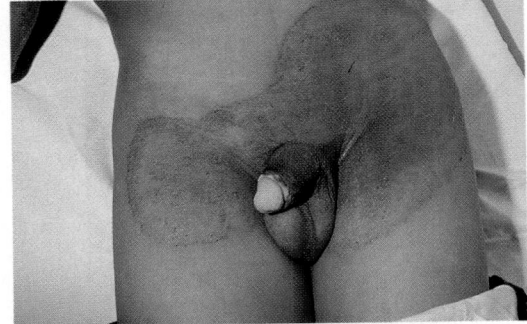

2. Tinea cruris. An extensive lesion with peripheral vesicles spreading from the groin on to the lower abdomen and upper thighs. (*Courtesy Dr Radzi bin Jaefar*)

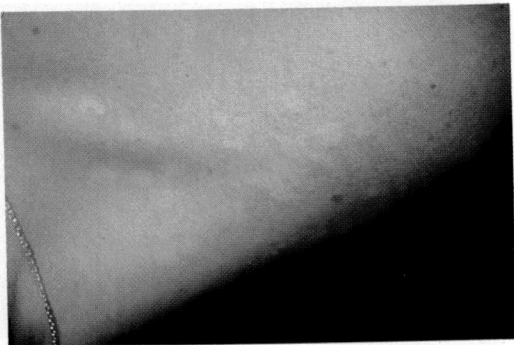

3. Pityriasis versicolor. (See Fig. 33.9   for Sellotape test.)

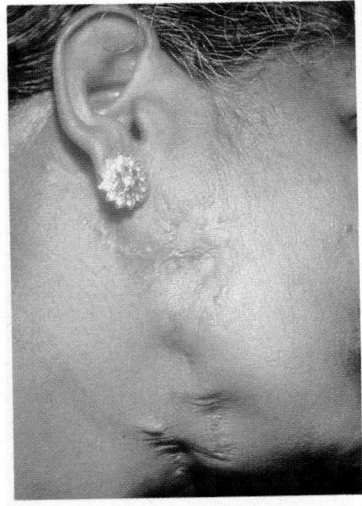

4. Scrophuloderma. Even when scrophuloderma has been treated there is usually marked deforming cicatrization.

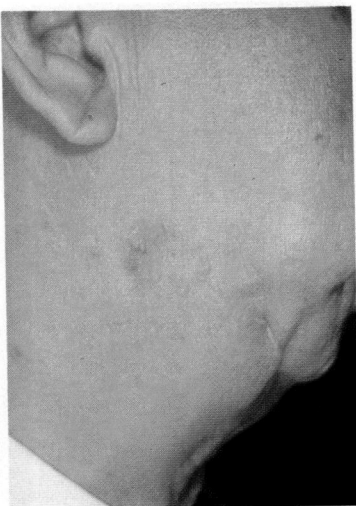

5. Lupus vulgaris. A reddish-brown granuloma with apple-jelly nodules clearing in the centre with residual scarring. The patient had tuberculosis of the mandible many years before.

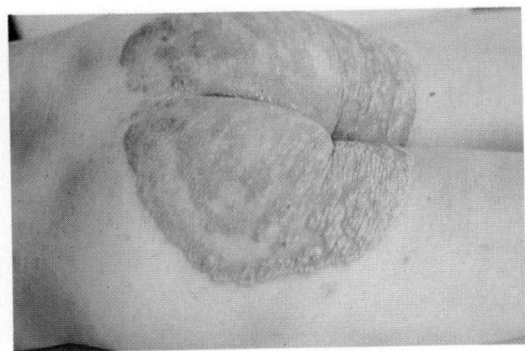

6. Tuberculosis verrucosa cutis. Waves of warty granulomas spreading centrifugally, responding rapidly to isonicotinic acid hydrazide.

PLATE VIII

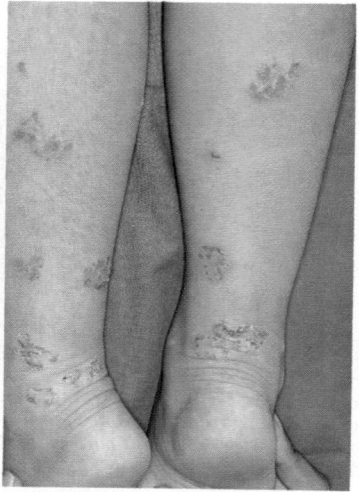

1. Discoid eczema. Several circular patches of acute eczematisation classically found predominantly on the lower limb. (*Courtesy Dr Radzi bin Jaefar*)

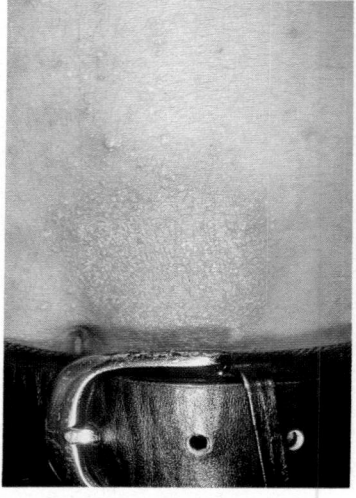

2. Contact dermatitis. Acute red vesicular lesion on abdomen due to sensitivity to nickel in a belt buckle.

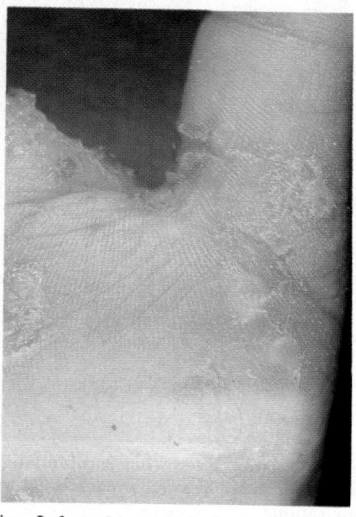

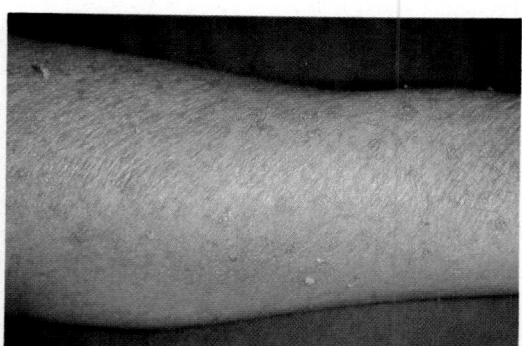

4. Actinic keratoses. Numerous small warty lesions on an erythematous base on a background of solar elastosis.

3. Scabies. Infected interdigital pustulopapules in a baby.

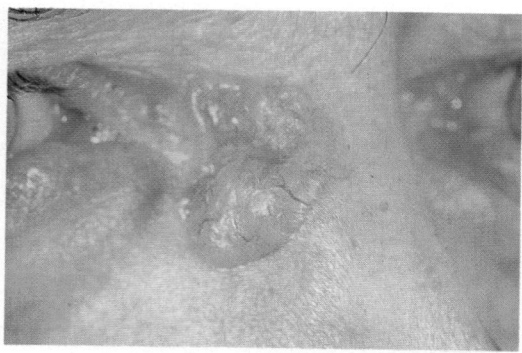

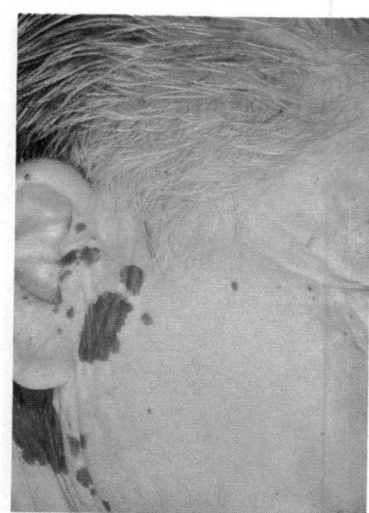

5. Basal cell carcinoma. Spreading pearly nodule with a rolled edge on the side of the nose.

6. Vitiligo. Most cases of vitiligo show patches of achromia. This patient, a Madrasi Indian, had only a few patches of normal skin; most of the body was depigmented.

Emetine

and bismuth iodide (EBI), is a most effective luminal amoebicide. Emetine injected locally relieves the pain of scorpion stings. It has been used for its emetic and expectorant properties and has an antibacterial action which has been utilized in the treatment of septic conditions.

Toxicity

Emetine is a protoplasmic poison. Damage to the heart is the most important side-effect. Full dosage of emetine almost inavariably produces changes in the electrocardiogram. Flattening or inversion of T waves and a prolonged QT interval are the main features. Reversion to normal may take several weeks. Tachycardia, which may be marked on the least exertion, hypotension, arrhythmias and precordial pain resembling a coronary thrombosis may occur. In deaths from emetine a degenerative myocarditis may be found. Weakness with muscle pain indicates myositis and both this and cardiac toxicity are aggravated by the hypokalaemia that may complicate invasive amoebiasis. Nerve involvement with motor and sensory loss is probably very rare. Pain due to local necrosis may occur at the site of injection. Other side-effects include nausea, vomiting, diarrhoea, depression, liver and renal damage and striation of the nails. Therefore emetine should only be given to patients on full bed-rest under constant supervision. Should signs of toxicity occur, especially in the cardiovascular system, treatment must be discontinued. The synthetic preparation dehydroemetine is weight for weight probably less toxic. The oral preparation EBI is less toxic but, as some of the emetine is absorbed, it is dangerous if given during or immediately after parenteral emetine. Emetine is slowly excreted, mainly by the kidneys, over a period of weeks, so that there is a risk of cumulative toxicity.

Contraindications

Heart, liver and renal disease and pregnancy are contraindications. Care should be taken to reduce the dose on a weight for weight basis in children and in adults who are debilitated and have lost weight.

Route

Emetine is given subcutaneously or intramuscularly but never intravenously.

Dosage

A maximum daily dose of 60 mg is given. In amoebic dysentery three daily injections may suffice but, in other forms of invasive amoebiasis, the injections should be continued for a maximum of 10 days. Relapses may occur after a 10-day course but, if the course is repeated three to four weeks later, the risk of relapse is virtually eliminated.

Preparations

Emetine hydrochloride injection. A sterile solution in water containing 60 mg/ml is the usual preparation but different concentrations are available.

Dehydroemetine hydrochloride. This is more rapidly excreted than emetine. Indications and cautions for use are similar to those of emetine. It has also been used in the treatment of schistosomiasis and cutaneous leishmaniasis.

Dehydroemetine

The injection is available in 2 ml ampoules (Mebadin) containing 30 mg/ml. There are tablets of dehydroemetine resinate containing 20 mg of the base, and of dehydroemetine and bismuth iodide.

Emetine and bismuth iodide tablets. Tablets of 60 mg. Emetine and bismuth iodide tablets are rarely used as a luminal amoebicide. The patient should be on bed-rest, since side-effects are almost invariable. A course consists of three 60 mg tablets daily for 10 days.

QINGHAOSU

Qinghaosu

The herb, qinghao (*Artemisia annua*), has been used as an antimalarial in China for over 1000 years. In 1972 the active principle, qinghaosu (artemisinine) was isolated. There is little experience of its use outside China, but it appears to be a rapidly acting schizonticide effective in chloroquine-resistant *Plasmodium falciparum* malaria, reducing parasitaemia faster than quinine, though it may be necessary to give prolonged courses or to use an additional drug to achieve total parasite clearance.

Toxicity

It is apparently less toxic than chloroquine; a potential problem is its embryo toxicity in rats.

Preparations and dosage (*qinghaosu, artemether methylether, artesunate hominsuccinate*)

Oral preparations are relatively ineffective and the best results have been achieved by the intramuscular injection of an oily solution of 900 mg quinghaosu over a 3-day period (600 mg artemether).

QUININE

An alkaloid prepared from the bark of various

Quinine

species of cinchona tree, quinine was introduced to Europe from South America in 1633. There are many other alkaloids in cinchona bark, one of which is quinidine, the D-isomer of quinine. The main use of quinine at present is in the treatment of *P. falciparum* infections resistant to 4-aminoquinolines. Quinine has been widely used as a prophylactic and for the treatment of acute attacks of all forms of malaria. It is a schizonticide, acting on early ring forms (trophozoites) with a rapid therapeutic response. The growth of the trophozoites is arrested, the cytoplasm may become clumped with loss of the vacuole and there may be disintegration of the nuclear chromatin. Such changes may be observed within hours of administering the drug. Damaged parasites may persist in the peripheral blood for 24–48 hours. Quinine is also gametocytocidal in the benign malarias. Its precise mode of action is uncertain but it may interfere with lysosome function or with nucleic acid synthesis.

Quinine is also used as a bitter. It is analgesic and an antipyretic and has a quinidine-like action on the heart. It increases the refractory period of skeletal muscle and depresses the excitability of the motor end-plate and thus is useful in the management of myotonia.

Quinidine is probably at least as effective and no more toxic than quinine. It may be used in the same way as quinine, both by mouth and by the intravenous route.[2]

Toxicity

This is related to dose, 8 g usually being fatal, but some individuals show intolerance, so that side-effects may occur at very low dosage. The combination of tinnitus, headache, nausea and visual disturbances is known as cinchonism and may also occur with salicylates and cinchophen. It is irritant, so that gastric discomfort may follow oral administration, sterile abscesses intramuscular injection and venous thrombosis intravenous injection. Peripheral vasodilatation occurs and may be useful in the treatment of night cramps. Unwanted cardiovascular effects include a fall in blood pressure and ventricular arrhythmias. It has an oxytocic action. However, the effect is not marked until late in pregnancy so that it is a poor abortifacient in early pregnancy. Toxic effects on the fetus include blindness (p. 1169) and deafness. In subjects with a glucose-6-phosphate dehydrogenase deficiency a haemolytic episode may be provoked. Hypersensitivity reactions may occur. Quinine bound to platelets may be antigenic and the subsequent production of platelet antibodies may lead to thrombocytopenia. Similarly, massive haemolysis may occur, especially in *P. falciparum* infections (blackwater fever) and in pregnancy. Agranulocytosis, anaphylactic shock, rashes and fever are further hypersensitivity reactions.

Administration

The oral route is satisfactory as it is rapidly absorbed. Excretion is rapid, mainly in the urine, so that frequent dosage is needed, 6- or 8-hourly. Parasite clearance is more rapid with intravenous quinine which should be used if the parasitaemia is heavy or if the patient is vomiting or comatose. Because of abscess formation the intramuscular route should be avoided if possible.

Dosage

Dosage is generally expressed in terms of the whole quinine salt; by mouth, 600 mg every 8 hours for 3–14 days depending on local experience and the immune status of the patient. If shorter courses are used tetracycline or another potentiating combination, such as Fansidar, should be used in addition to reduce the risk of short-term relapse (recrudescence). Intravenously the 600 mg may be given over a 6-hour period in a dextrose or dextrose saline infusion and continued 8-hourly until the clinical/parasitological response allows a switch to the oral route.

Preparations

Quinine bisulphate. Tablets of 300 mg containing 178 mg quinine base.

Quinine dihydrochloride. Tablets of 300 mg containing 246 mg quinine base. Ampoules for injection prepared at varying concentrations, typically 300 mg salt (246 mg quinine base)/ml.

Quinine hydrochloride. Tablets of 300 mg containing 246 mg quinine base.

Quinine sulphate. Tablets of 125 mg, 200 mg and 300 mg containing 103 mg, 165 mg and 248 mg quinine base respectively.

Quinidine sulphate. Tablets of 200 mg and 300 mg containing 165 mg and 248 mg quinidine base.

Quinidine bisulphate (Kinidin, Kiditard). Slow release tablets of 250 mg (165 mg quinidine base).

Quinidine hydrochloride or sulphate. Ampoules for injection. Available in USA. Various concentrations.

MEFLOQUINE

Mefloquine

Mefloquine is a new antimalarial developed by the Walter Reed Army Institute of Medical Research. It has the same basic quinoline methanol structure as quinine. It is rapidly absorbed but slowly excreted over a number of weeks. It is bound to plasma proteins and also to the cell membrane of red blood cells.

Toxicity

No major toxicity appears to have been described. Minor symptoms are similar to those of quinine and include nausea, vomiting, diarrhoea, dizziness, abdominal pain, sinus bradycardia, pruritus, rash and mental changes. Because of the long half-life, toxicity may become more of a problem when the drug becomes freely available with the consequent risk of overdose.

Dosage

In multidrug-resistant *P. falciparum* infections it may be best used in a single dose of 750 mg together with another drug such as Fansidar to reduce the risk of the parasite developing mefloquine resistance.

Preparations

Not yet generally released, but the indications are that it will be available as a compound tablet together with Fansidar.

DYES AND DYE DERIVATIVES

Some dye derivatives with particular actions, such as the sulphonamides (antifolate), will be described in other sections.

AMINOQUINOLINES

Chloroquine

A 4-aminoquinoline, chloroquine, has the quinoline nucleus in common with quinine and the side chain in common with mepacrine. Developed in the 1930s as a result of the intensive investigation into dyes and dye derivatives, it was not widely available until after the Second World War.

Quinoline

Choroquine

Its main use is in malaria. It is a schizonticide acting on the early ring forms. Growth is arrested, the cytoplasm becomes ragged and pigment granules are clumped. Damaged parasites may sometimes persist in the peripheral blood for 48 hours or more. It is effective against the gametocytes of *P. vivax, P. ovale* and *P. malariae*. Gametocytes of *P. falciparum* may be damaged but may remain viable. The precise action is unknown but it may be due to lysosome damage or to interference with nucleic acid synthesis. Chloroquine has no action on sporozoites or on the primary exo-erythrocytic (hepatic) stages, so is only suppressive in *P. vivax* and *P. ovale*. Its outstanding action against the ring forms of *P. falciparum* is increasingly diminished. Chloroquine-resistant strains are widely established in the Far East, South America and East Africa. Cross resistance occurs with mepa-

crine and amodiaquine. Chloroquine remains effective against the ring forms of *P. vivax, P. ovale* and *P. malariae*.

Chloroquine is also used in hepatic amoebiasis, in lung and liver fluke infections and in taeniasis and giardiasis. It has an anti-inflammatory action that has been used in lepra reactions, collagen diseases, sarcoidosis, urticaria and light-sensitive eruptions. It is a prostaglandin antagonist and this property may well be related to its anti-inflammatory action.

Toxicity

In malarial dosage side-effects are few, though deaths in children from cardiorespiratory collapse have been recorded after a few tablets (0.075–2 g) and from intravenous administration. Cardiac effects seen in acute toxicity include interference with cardiac muscle function, conduction and sinus node function. With prolonged administration cardiac effects are rarely reported but the possibility of myocardial damage, analogous to chloroquine myopathy, and conduction defects should be considered.

In adults, headache, visual disturbances, nausea, vomiting and pruritus may occur, especially if chloroquine is used for long-term prophylaxis. In the large dosages that are used for its anti-inflammatory effect, side-effects are more frequent. Difficulty in accommodation, diplopia, bleaching of the hair, changes in the electrocardiogram (T wave depression), skin rashes and weight loss occur.

Chloroquine is particularly deposited in melanin-containing tissues and persists for many months. A retinopathy (p. 1169) with a mottled appearance around the macula may be followed by pigmentary clumping with visual defects which may be permanent. Chloroquine is also deposited in the iris and in the cornea, in the latter causing opacities which usually resolve on cessation of treatment. The total cumulative dose needed to cause eye damage is probably greater than 100 g, but individuals, especially the elderly, may develop changes on less than this. At a normal prophylactic dose (300 mg/week, 15 g/year), it should thus be safe to take chloroquine for five years but, at the higher dose regimens used in some areas of the tropics, retinal damage might be anticipated in some individuals in two to three years. A myopathy may occur which is usually proximal. Psychotic behaviour, involuntary movements, agranulocytosis, thrombocytopenia and a blue–black pigmentation of the palatal mucosa and of the subungual tissues may occur. Marrow aplasia and leukaemia have been recorded following chloroquine therapy.[3]

Chloroquine is rapidly absorbed so that parenteral administration is unnecessary unless the patient is vomiting or comatose. Tissues, especially the liver, spleen, kidneys and eyes, are avid for the drug so that a loading dose is required. It is partially metabolized and excreted over a period of weeks or months in the urine.

Dosage

Various salts of chloroquine, the products of acids with the base chloroquine, are available so that the dosage is described in terms of the weight of chloroquine base rather than of the chloroquine salt.

MALARIA

For treatment of acute attack 600 mg of the base is given at once, followed by 300 mg 6 hours later and 300 mg daily for 2 days or more. Suppressive dose is 300 mg weekly.

CEREBRAL MALARIA

In areas of the world where chloroquine resistance is known or suspected, parenteral chloroquine should no longer be used for cerebral malaria. Treatment should be started with quinine. If the parasites are known to be fully sensitive to chloroquine, parenteral chloroquine, preferably intramuscular, may still be used.

Children. Intramuscular injection in a dose of 5 mg of the base/kg, repeated in 6 hours if necessary to a total of 25 mg/kg in four days. *For a warning on toxicity see p. 35.*

Adults. 200 mg of the base well diluted by very slow intravenous injection, or 200 mg intramuscularly, to a maximum of 900 mg in 24 hours.

Preparations

Chloroquine phosphate. Injection, usual strength 40 mg of chloroquine base/ml.

Chloroquine phosphate. Tablets (*Aralen, Avloclor, Resochin*) of 250 mg containing approximately 150 mg of chloroquine base.

Chloroquine sulphate. Injection, usual strength 40 mg of chloroquine base/ml.

Chloroquine sulphate. Tablets (*Nivaquine*) of 200 mg containing approximately 150 mg of chloroquine base.

Other 4-aminoquinolines

Although the uses and toxic effects are similar to those of chloroquine, in East Africa *P. falciparum* resistance to amodiaquine is less intense, so that amodiaquine may be used in preference to chloroquine in patients who are not critically ill, but it should not be used as a chemoprophylactic because of the risk of agranulocytosis.

Amodiaquine hydrochloride (Camoquin). Tablets of 200 mg.

Amopyroquine hydrochloride (Propoquin).

Hydroxychloroquine sulphate (Plaquenil).

Primaquine

The least toxic of many 8-aminoquinolines, primaquine is used for the radical cure of benign malarias (*P. vivax, P. ovale*) as it is effective against the liver forms (hypnozoites) of these parasites. It also has a weak schizonticidal action, a marked gametocytocidal action and some action against the pre-erythrocytic cycle of all species. It is rapidly absorbed.

Primaquine

Toxicity

In the recommended dosage side-effects are unusual but with higher dosage side-effects become increasingly severe. Abdominal pain, methaemoglobinaemia and haemolytic anaemia occur. In patients with a deficiency of the enzyme glucose-6-phosphate dehydrogenase, a haemolytic crisis may be precipitated.

Dosage

In the radical cure of benign malarias 7.5 mg of the base is given twice daily for 14 days. It is too weak a schizonticide for treating the acute attack, which should be controlled by the concurrent or previous administration of a powerful schizonticide such as a 4-aminoquinoline or quinine. A single dose of 45 mg primaquine base reduces the gametocyte count in *P. falciparum* considerably, and any surviving gametocytes will be incapable of development in mosquitoes.

Preparations

Primaquine phosphate. Tablets containing 7.5 mg of primaquine base. American tablets may contain 15 mg of primaquine base.

Other 8-aminoquinolines (pamaquin (plasmoquine), pentaquine, quinocide)

Various 8-aminoquinolines are being explored for the treatment of South American trypanosomiasis and for leishmaniasis.

Iodinated quinolines

These drugs are used in the treatment of amoebic cyst passers and to a less extent in amoebic dysentery. Toxic effects include diarrhoea, nausea, vomiting, pruritus, iodism, goitre and liver damage. In Japan one preparation, clioquinol, has been associated with two syndromes when clioquinol consumption exceeds the usual therapeutic dose: subacute myelo-optic atrophy in adults and optic atrophy with acrodermatitis enteropathica in children. A dose-related response has been established and all have recovered on stopping the drug. Clioquinol has now been banned and the practice of using iodinated quinolines for the prophylaxis of travellers' diarrhoea should now be stopped.

CLOFAZIMINE (B663)

This is an orange–red dye which has been used in the treatment of acid-fast infections. More useful in leprosy than in tuberculosis, it is one of the few drugs that appear to have some effect in Buruli ulcer (*Mycobacterium ulcerans*). It also has some anti-inflammatory action. A problem in light-skinned patients is the development of red and black pigmentation.

Dose

This is 100–400 mg daily (but see Chapter 40, p. 778).

Preparation

B663 (*Lamprene*). Capsules of 50 mg and 100 mg.

HYCANTHONE

A derivative of lucanthone, hycanthone is also a yellow dye. It is especially effective in *Schistosoma mansoni* infections, giving useful reductions in egg excretion and apparent cures at half (1.5 mg/kg) the dose at which it was initially

Hycanthone

introduced (3 mg/kg). However, it is not very effective against *S. haematobium* at the lower dose.

Toxicity

Side-effects are largely dose related. Nausea and vomiting, which can be very severe, are common at the 3 mg/kg dose, and the reports of liver failure and death have all been at this or a greater dosage. At 2 mg/kg or less nausea does not occur and side-effects are most unusual. Laboratory work has suggested that it may be mutagenic. It is contraindicated in pregnancy, active liver disease and in any severe coexisting illness. Other drugs, especially phenothiazines, should not be used concurrently.

Dose

This is 1.5 mg/kg by single intramuscular injection to a maximum of 100 mg. The higher dose of 3 mg/kg is not recommended.

PARAROSANILINE PAMOATE

This drug has been tried in the mass treatment of *Schistosoma japonicum* infestation.

MEPACRINE (ATEBRIN)

A yellow dye introduced for malaria therapy in the 1930s, and of great importance in the Second World War, it is now largely superseded. The side chain is identical with that of chloroquine. Its action in malaria is similar to that of chloroquine and quinine. It is also used in tapeworm infections and giardiasis and has anti-inflammatory properties similar to those of chloroquine.

Acridine

Mepacrine

Toxicity

The skin and urine are stained yellow. Dizziness, headache, nausea, vomiting and mental changes may occur. Skin rashes and corneal changes including oedema and vesiculation occur and deaths have been reported from exfoliative dermatitis and also from hepatitis. Toxicity is increased if an 8-aminoquinoline is administered concurrently.

Dosage

Malaria. Suppressive, 100 mg daily. Curative, 900 mg on the first day, 600 mg on the second day and 300 mg daily for 5 days, in divided doses.

Tapeworm. 1 g by duodenal tube.

Giardiasis. 100 mg thrice daily for one week.

Preparation

Mepacrine hydrochloride (Quinacrine). 100 mg tablets.

OXAMNIQUINE

A yellow dye, it has structural similarities both with quinine and hycanthone. It was first introduced for the treatment of a schistosomiasis as an intramuscular injection, but the injections caused so much pain that this route has been abandoned and it is now available only in tablet form. It is effective against *Schistosoma mansoni* at all stages of development, but it is not useful against *S. haematobium* or *S. japonicum*.

Oxamniquine

Toxicity

It seems to be singularly free from side-effects, though some drowsiness and other minor symptoms have been recorded. If given in the late evening no side-effects are noted. Parasite strains seem to vary in their sensitivity to the drug from one country to another. In East Africa and Brazil the parasites are sensitive but it is necessary to double the dose in Zimbabwe and Egypt. It has been used in severe infections with pulmonary and/or portal hypertension without ill effect.

Dose

This is 15–30 mg/kg at night for 2 days.

Preparation

Oxamniquine capsules (Vansil). Capsules containing 500 mg of oxamniquine.

OLTIPRAZ

This is an antischistosomal drug which is effective against all three species of schistosomes but has been withdrawn because of side effects.

PRAZIQUANTEL

Praziquantel is effective in a single oral dose against all three forms of schistosomiasis, *S. mansoni*, *S. haematobium* and *S. japonicum*, as well as *S. mekongi* and *S. intercalatum*. It is also effective against other trematodes, including lung and liver flukes and against intestinal cestodes, adult tapeworms, as well as some tissue stages of cestodes, such as cysticercosis (*Taenia solium*). As a veterinary taeniacide (Droncit), it is very effective in clearing adult *Taenia echinococcus* from dogs, but no effect on mature hydatid cysts in man has been shown.

Toxicity

Side-effects are few. Nausea, abdominal pain, headache, giddiness and drowsiness have been reported. In treating *S. japonicum* in China,

Praziquantel

occasional more severe effects, neuropsychiatric reactions, cardiovascular reactions, rashes, liver damage and asthenia, were noted.[4] In treating heavy *S. mansoni* infections in Zaire, bloody diarrhoea developed within an hour or so of taking the drug, but had ceased within 24 hours.[5]

Dose

A single dose of 40 mg/kg is given or 20–30 mg/kg on two occasions a few hours apart.

Preparation

Praziquantel (*Biltricide, Droncit Pyquiton (China)*). Tablets of 600 mg.

PYRVINIUM PAMOATE

This is a bright red dye used in the treatment of threadworm infections. The stools are stained bright red. Toxic effects include nausea, vomiting and diarrhoea, and it should be used with

caution in the presence of renal or hepatic disease.

Dose

A single dose of 5 mg of pyrvinium base/kg body weight is given.

Preparations

Pyrvinium pamoate. Tablets containing 50 mg of pyrvinium base.

Pyrvinium pamoate oral suspension (*viprynium mixture, Vanquin*). Contains 1% of pyrvinium base.

SURAMIN (BAYER 205, MORANYL)

A derivative of the trypan dyes, introduced in the 1920s for the treatment of African trypanosomiasis, it is also used in the treatment of onchocerciasis. Its mode of action in trypanosomiasis is unknown. It does not reach the cerebrospinal fluid so is of no value when the central nervous system is involved, though a single injection may usefully precede a course of Mel B in such cases. In onchocerciasis suramin's main action is on the adult worms (macrofilaricidal).

Toxicity

Immediate reactions include nausea and anaphylactic shock; 24 hours later photophobia and peripheral neuritis may occur. Albuminuria is a common late effect. Agranulocytosis and haemolytic anaemia are rare. The drug should be given under close medical supervision. If albuminuria is marked or casts appear, it should be stopped.

Route and dosage

It is given by slow intravenous injection. Only freshly prepared solutions should be used. The initial dose in trypanosomiasis, after a test dose of 0.1 g, is 0.5–1 g. Thereafter it is given weekly to a total dose of 7 g.

Preparation

Suramin injection (*Antrypol*). A sterile powder to be dissolved in water for injection immediately before use.

FOLATE INHIBITORS AND RELATED DRUGS

Differences in folate metabolism in man, protozoa and bacteria have led to the development of antiprotozoal and antibacterial antifolate drugs

PABA (para-aminobenzoic acid)

Folic acid

with limited human toxicity. The drugs act mainly by substrate inhibition, having structural similarities either to para-aminobenzoic acid (PABA) or to folic acid.

Block 1 is unimportant to human cells for they are permeable to preformed folic acid. Drugs acting at this point include sulphonamides, and probably also sulphones and para-aminosalicylic acid (p. 1208).

Block 2. Dihydrofolate reductases vary from order to order so that a drug may have a more marked effect in bacteria or protozoa than in man. Drugs acting at this point include pyrimethamine and proguanil (mainly protozoa especially plasmodium species), trimethoprim (bacteria and protozoa) and methotrexate (man).

SULPHONAMIDES

These drugs were developed from the azo dyes. Their mode of action is to block the synthesis of folic acid. They are bacteriostatic, but may be bactericidal when used in combination with dihydrofolate reductase inhibitors, and in such combinations have an antiprotozoal effect which has been used in malaria and toxoplasmosis. It has been suggested that high blood levels of sulphonamides may have a lethal effect on feeding mosquitoes.

Sulphonamides

Toxic effects

In general, the slowly excreted protein-bound sulphonamides are more likely to cause severe toxic effects. The poorly soluble sulphonamides have been largely superseded because of the risk of crystalluria and renal damage. General side-effects include nausea, vomiting, anorexia, fever, meth- and sulph-haemoglobinaemia, goitre, hypothyroidism, vertigo, tinnitus and ataxia. Skin rashes, of which the Stevens–Johnson syndrome, a severe form of erythema multiforme, is the most dangerous, acute haemolytic anaemia, agranulocytosis, thrombocytopenia and hepatitis may also occur.

Preparations

GROUP 1

These are well absorbed, relatively soluble, rapidly excreted—the drugs of choice for routine use.

Sulphadimidine. Tablets of 0.5 g; 0.5–1.5 g 6-hourly. Injection 1 g in 3 ml intramuscularly or intravenously.

Sulphadiazine. Tablets of 0.5 g; may be more effective than sulphadimidine in meningococcal meningitis.

Sulphasalazine (Salazopyrin). A compound of salicylic acid and sulphapyridine used in ulcerative colitis 0.5–1.5 g 6-hourly.

GROUP 2

These are poorly absorbed, previously used for bacillary dysentery, but now largely replaced by group 1 drugs: phthalylsulphathiazole, succinylsulphathiazole, sulphaguanidine.

GROUP 3

These are medium- to long-acting, bound to protein.

Sulphalene. Used in combination with trimethoprim.

Sulfadoxine (Fanasil). Tablets 500 mg. In combination with pyrimethamine (Fansidar, sulfadoxine 500 mg, and pyrimethamine 25 mg tablets), it may be used in malaria (see p. 1209). It is contraindicated in premature and newborn infants and during pregnancy, when possible risks should be balanced against the expected therapeutic effect. It should not be given during

Sulphalene

the week before the expected date of delivery. It is contraindicated in patients with known sulphonamide hypersensitivity or severe liver or kidney dysfunction. It is usually well tolerated. Side-effects in the form of skin rashes, gastrointestinal disturbance or allergotoxic skin reactions may occasionally occur as with other preparations containing sulphonamides or pyrimethamine. Blood dyscrasias may rarely occur over a long period and regular blood counts are recommended during long-term prophylaxis. Adverse reactions, however, are not normally more prolonged than those occurring after shorter-acting sulphonamides.

Sulphamethoxazole. Used in combination with trimethoprim (Septrin, Bactrim).

Sulphamethoxypyridazine (Lederkyn).

Sulphaphenazole (Orisulf, Orisul, Suta).

PARA-AMINOSALICYLIC ACID (PAS)

A weakly tuberculostatic drug, PAS is of little

value by itself, but useful in the prevention of the development of resistant organisms when combined with other antituberculous drugs. Structurally similar to *para*-aminobenzoic acid, its mode of action may be comparable to that of the sulphonamides. Side-effects resemble those of aspirin, and include anorexia, nausea, vomiting, diarrhoea, gastric haemorrhage and a possible association with peptic ulceration. Hypersensitivity may occur with fever, joint symptoms and skin rashes. Leukopenia, agranulocytosis, lymphocytosis, thrombocytopenia, liver damage, pancreatitis and nephritis may also occur. The prothrombin time is often prolonged and a number of patients develop a goitre and sometimes evidence of hypothyroidism.

PAS (Para-aminosalicylic acid)

The drug is well absorbed and is rapidly excreted by the kidneys. It should be used with caution in renal disease.

Dose

Six to 12 grams in single or divided doses is given daily, in conjunction with at least one other antituberculous drug.

Preparation

Sodium aminosalicylate. Cachets of 1.5 g. Many other preparations are available, particularly combined with isoniazid.

SULPHONES

Derivatives of diaminodiphenyl-sulphone (DDS, dapsone), their main use is in the treatment of leprosy, but they have also been used in combination with dihydrofolate reductase inhibitors in the treatment and prophylaxis of malaria. Many of the sulphones are metabolized to DDS in vivo. DDS is the most widely used preparation.

Sulphones

DDS (Dapsone)

Toxic effects

Reactional leprosy may be precipitated and this is the most important unwanted effect in the management of that disease. Other effects include fever, malaise, lymphadenopathy, skin rashes, anaemia, methaemoglobinaemia, depression, psychoses and hepatitis.

Dose

In leprosy 50–100 mg is given weekly in single or divided doses, but see p. 00.

Preparations

Diaminodiphenyl-sulphone (Dapsone, DDS). Tablets of 5 and 100 mg.

Diethyl dithiolisophthalate (Ditophal). A yellow viscous liquid with an odour of garlic. By inunction.

Sodium sulfoxone. No longer marketed.

Thiambutosine (Ciba 1906). Not a sulphone but a useful alternative in the management of leprosy. Tablets of 500 mg.

PYRIMETHAMINE

Pyrimethamine has structural similarities to folic acid, and acts by substrate inhibition, blocking the enzyme dihydrofolate reductase. The effect is most marked in malaria but is also useful in toxoplasmosis. In large doses an antifolate effect can be demonstrated in man with the production of a macrocytic anaemia. Pyrimethamine has been used in the treatment of polycythaemia vera. Its action in malaria is on the dividing schizonts and it has little action on the ring forms, so that its action is too slow for use in the acute attack.

Pyrimethamine

It has an action on the pre-erythrocytic stage of *P. falciparum* so that it is a causal prophylactic of *P. falciparum*. It is a suppressive prophylactic of the benign malarias. Some strains of *P. falciparum* are resistant to pyrimethamine, and in these there is a cross resistance to proguanil. However, combinations of pyrimethamine and sulphonamides exhibit synergism and have been used in the prophylaxis and treatment of chloroquine-resistant malaria. Pyrimethamine inactivates gametocytes so that they do not mature in the mosquito.

Toxic effects

These are rare in suppressive doses. The prolonged course used in treating toxoplasmosis may cause a macrocytic anaemia. Massive doses cause vomiting, collapse, convulsions and death.

Dose

Malaria prophylaxis. The dose is 25–50 mg weekly continued for two to four weeks after leaving the malarial zone.

Toxoplasmosis. The dose is 25–50 mg daily for three to six weeks, concurrently with sulphonamide.

Polycythaemia vera. The dose required to maintain a normal haemoglobin varies from patient to patient. Thrombocytopenia and leukopenia may occur.

Preparation

Pyrimethamine (Daraprim). Tablets of 25 mg. Also an elixir.

PYRIMETHAMINE/SULPHONAMIDE COMBINATIONS

Synergism against malaria parasites is exhibited by pyrimethamine and similar antifolates such as trimethoprim and proguanil when combined with sulphonamides. This appears to be so even if there already exists a degree of parasite resistance to pyrimethamine. Such combinations have been used both for prophylaxis and treatment, but because of increased reporting of serious side-effects, these combinations should probably now be reserved for treatment only.

Toxic effects

Unfortunately, there appears to be some synergism as regards the toxicity of these combinations. For example, the combination of proguanil and dapsone was associated with agranulocytosis in 1 in 10 000 persons per year. Reactions to Fansidar may occur after the third or fourth prophylactic dose and in general are similar to some of the severe reactions to sulphonamides. There have been several reports of a Stevens–Johnson syndrome and a number of fatalities have occurred. The incidence of serious side-effects has been roughly estimated at 1 per 20 000 persons at risk. Many reports have been of North American citizens where Fansidar is often advised for malaria prophylaxis in combination with chloroquine, whereas there have been few reports from Switzerland where Fansidar may be prescribed alone, so that a toxic synergism with chloroquine has been tentatively suggested.

Preparations

Fansidar. Tablets of pyrimethamine (25 mg) and sulfadoxine (500 mg). For prophylaxis, one tablet weekly continued for two to four weeks after leaving transmission zone; for treatment two to three tablets in a single dose.

Maloprim. Tablets of pyrimethamine (12.5 mg) and dapsone (100 mg). For prophylaxis, two tablets on first exposure, thereafter one tablet weekly, continued for two to four weeks after leaving transmission zone. Not normally used for treatment.

Metakelfin. Tablets of pyrimethamine (25 mg) and sulphalene (500 mg). Dosage as for Fansidar.

PROGUANIL

Developed from research into pyrimidine derivatives, it is much used for malarial prophylaxis. Probably with little antiplasmodial activity itself, it is metabolized in the body to cycloguanil, a triazine derivative. Cycloguanil has structural similarities with pyrimethamine and likewise is probably an inhibitor of dihydrofolate reductase in plasmodia. Like pyrimethamine its action is on the dividing schizonts, it is a causal prophylactic of *P. falciparum* malaria and a suppressive

Proguanil

Cycloguanil

prophylactic of the benign malarias and it inactivates gametocytes.

Cross resistance exists with pyrimethamine-resistant strains of *P. falciparum*. However, the metabolite, cycloguanil, is much more rapidly excreted than is pyrimethamine, so that daily administration is required. Proguanil is singularly free from toxic effects and appears to exert no antifolate activity in man. Loss of appetite, nausea, vomiting and diarrhoea may occur, perhaps owing to inhibition of gastric secretion. Large doses may cause haematuria.

Dose

For *malaria prophylaxis* 200 mg is given daily on arrival and continued for two to six weeks after leaving transmission zone. Formerly it had been used in a dose of 100 mg daily but this, for example in East Africa, is no longer effective.

Preparations

Proguanil hydrochloride (Paludrine). Tablets of 100 mg.

Chlorproguanil hydrochloride (Lapudrine). Slowly excreted. Tablets of 20 mg. Prophylactic dose 40 mg weekly or twice weekly.

Cycloguanil embonate (Camolar). The pamoate of the active metabolite of proguanil. Excreted very slowly so that a single intramuscular injection of 5–10 mg/kg may protect against malaria for three to six months. It has been used in the treatment of leishmaniasis.

TRIMETHOPRIM

Trimethoprim has a structural similarity to folates and thus acts as a spurious substrate for dihydrofolate reductase. The subsequent inhibition of tetrahydrofolic acid production is most marked in bacteria and plasmodia but is minimal in man in the therapeutic dose range. It exhibits synergism with sulphonamides so that whereas individually at a given concentration the drugs are feebly bacteriostatic, together they are bactericidal.

Combinations of trimethoprim and sulphonamides are used for their broad-spectrum bactericidal properties. It has also been shown that they are effective in malaria, and of possible use in chloroquine-resistant *P. falciparum* infections. Prolonged courses of several months are used in the treatment of mycetoma caused by higher bacteria (actinomycetoma), and in high dose 120 mg/kg daily for the treatment of *Pneumocystis carinii* infections.

Preparations

Co-trimoxazole. A mixture of trimethoprim 1 part, and sulphamethoxazole 5 parts. Tablets (Bactrim, Septrin) of 480 mg. Intramuscular injections of 320 mg/ml. Ampoules of 3 ml. Intravenous infusion of 96 mg/ml to be diluted. Ampoules of 5 ml.

Trimethoprim has been used with sulphalene in the treatment of malaria. A single administration of trimethoprim 10 mg/kg and sulphalene 20 mg/kg to a maximum of trimethoprim 0.5 g and sulphalene 1.0 g has been found effective.

Co-trimoxazole has been especially valuable in the treatment of typhoid. Its speed of action and effectiveness in typhoid are very similar to chloramphenicol.

Trimethoprim

DIAMIDINES

DIMINAZENE ACETURATE (BERENIL)

Widely used in veterinary medicine for the treatment of trypanosomiasis, babesiosis and bacterial infections, it has also been used for human trypanosomiasis due to *Trypanosoma gambiense* and *T. rhodesiense* in a dose of 2 mg/kg intramuscularly each day for 7 days. With difficulties in obtaining supplies of suramin, Berenil is likely to become increasingly important.

Diminazene (aceturate)

PENTAMIDINE ISETHIONATE, PENTAMIDINE METHANESULPHONATE (LOMIDINE)

A diamidine used as a second line drug in the treatment of African trypanosomiasis and visceral leishmaniasis, it is not effective in trypanosomiasis if the central nervous system is involved. It is excreted very slowly and single injections are used to give long-term prophylaxis in trypanosomiasis. The precise mode of action is unknown but it has been suggested that the glucose metabolism of the trypanosome may be disturbed. An alternative explanation is that the lysosomal enzymes may be affected. Rapid intravenous injection may cause hypotension. Other toxic effects include hypoglycaemia and pain at the site of intramuscular injection. The development of a temporary diabetic state after a course of pentamidine has also been noted. Its role in the treatment of *Pneumocystis carinii* has largely been replaced by co-trimoxazole.

Dose

For treatment of African trypanosomiasis 10 intramuscular injections of 4 mg/kg are given over a period of 10–20 days. For prophylaxis of

African trypanosomiasis, a single intramuscular injection of 4 mg/kg may protect for up to six months. Treatment of visceral leishmaniasis is similar to that used in African trypanosomiasis.

Preparations

Pentamidine injection (Lomidine). An ampoule, the contents of which should be dissolved in water for injection immediately before use.

HYDROXYSTILBAMIDINE ISETHIONATE

Hydroxystilbamidine isethionate is allied to pen-

tamidine and is used in the treatment of antimony-resistant kala-azar, and some deep mycoses. There is a fall in blood pressure after intravenous injection, and this must be counteracted by the simultaneous administration of an antihistaminic such as mepyramine maleate (Anthisan) 50–100 mg twice daily.

Dose

The dose is 250 mg daily by slow intravenous injection for 10 days, repeated after 7 days. The total number of courses for an adult in most forms of kala-azar is three, a total of 7.5 g of the drug.

MISCELLANEOUS

BITHIONOL

This drug has bactericidal properties but has also been shown to be useful in fluke infections including paragonimiasis and fascioliasis. Toxic effects include gastric irritation with nausea, vomiting and diarrhoea, urticarial skin rashes and transient albuminuria.

Dose

The dose is 30–50 mg/kg (orally) on alternate days for three or four weeks.

Preparation

Bithionol (2,2'-thiobis(4,6-dichlorophenol), Actamer, Bitin).

DILOXANIDE FUROATE

An effective luminal amoebicide, curing some 90% of *Entamoeba histolytica* cyst passers, it is used as a supplement to other drugs in invasive amoebiasis to ensure that the parasite is eradicated from the bowel lumen. It is free from serious side-effects but flatulence may occur.

Dose

The dose is 500 mg orally three times daily for 10 days.

Preparation

Diloxanide furoate (Furamide). Tablets of 500 mg.

DICHLOROPHEN

This drug is much used in veterinary medicine but it has also been used in the treatment of tapeworm infections in man. The worms are killed and part digested, so that it is impossible to identify the scolex and confirm the cure

Dichlorophen

immediately. It may be used in *Taenia saginata* infections but is contraindicated in *T. solium* because of the risk of autoinfection and subsequent cysticercosis. Toxic effects include nausea, vomiting, diarrhoea, urticaria, lassitude and jaundice. Rarely, fatalities have followed large doses.

Dose

The dose is 6 g (orally) daily for 2 days.

Preparation

Dichlorophen.   Tablets of 500 mg.

NICLOSAMIDE

This drug, widely employed as a molluscicide (Bayluscide), is effective in tapeworm infections, the worms being excreted in a partially digested or unrecognizable form. The drug is not absorbed and does not appear to irritate the gastrointestinal tract so that side-effects are minimal. There is no need for preliminary starvation or purgation.

Niclosamide

Dose

The dose is 1 g, chewed and washed down with water, followed one hour later by 1 g.

A 7-day course is sometimes used for *Hymenolepis nana* infection: 2 g are given on day one, and 1 g daily for the next 6 days.

Preparation

Niclosamide (*Yomesan*).   0.5 g tablets.

IVERMECTIN

Ivermectin is a new compound produced by the higher bacterium *Streptomyces avermitilis*. It has been extensively used in veterinary medicine and is specifically useful against nematodes, and also against some parasite arthropods. Its action is prolonged so that it may have a considerable value in controlling arthropod parasites in livestock, such as ticks and tsetse flies. Trials in man have been confined to *Onchocerca volvulus*. It appears to be superior to diethylcarbamazine in clearing microfilariae from the skin. Clearance is relatively slow but reactions are negligible. The action on adult worms is unclear. The dose used has been 0.1–0.2 mg/kg by mouth in a single dose.

NITROIMIDAZOLES AND RELATED DRUGS

There has been much recent development of a group of drugs based on the imidazole ring, largely following the discovery of 2-nitroimidazole in 1955 and the subsequent demonstration of its trichomonicidal properties.

Members of the imidazole group and related drugs are effective against helminths (e.g. thiabendazole, mebendazole), protozoa (e.g. metronidazole, benznidazole) fungi (e.g. miconazole), and bacteria (e.g. metronidazole).

A point of concern is the possession by many members of the group (cf. hycanthone, oxamniquine) of a nitro (NO_2) group which is theoretically carcinogenic. Although some members

2-Nitroimidazole

(e.g. niridazole, metronidazole) have been shown to be potentially carcinogenic in laboratory animals, there is as yet no evidence of carcinogenicity in man but they should be avoided in pregnancy. A point of interest, and perhaps of concern, is the realization that some members possess immunosuppressive and/or immunostimulant properties (e.g. niridazole, levamisole). Ketoconazole appears to be an antiandrogen.

ALBENDAZOLE

One of the most promising of the more recently introduced antiparasitic nitroimidazoles, it is effective against *Ascaris*, hookworm and threadworm in a single dose, but 3-day courses may be necessary in *Trichuris*, *Strongyloides*, *T. saginata* and *H. nana*. It is under trial in the treatment of hydatid cysts but high doses for prolonged periods will be needed. Albendazole is rapidly, but only partially, absorbed after oral administration and is metabolized in the liver so that only metabolites can be detected in the blood. Metabolites are largely excreted in 24 hours, mainly in the urine but also in faeces. Metabolites are concentrated in the liver and kidneys. Albendazole appears to block glucose uptake by worms and larvae.

Toxicity

Side-effects with a single dose seem to be very uncommon but there may rarely be some headache, nausea, diarrhoea and vomiting. Fever, transient elevation of liver enzymes and depression of neutrophils have been reported. In large doses in experimental animals embryotoxicity, teratogenicity and neutropenia have been described. Rats appear to be relatively susceptible but the absorption of albendazole may be much greater than in man. Sheep developed bone marrow depression with prolonged dosage at the relatively low dose of 10–20 mg/kg.

Dose

A single dose of 400 mg is given to adults and children over two years old.

Preparation

Albendazole (Zentel). Tablets of 200 mg. Suspension of 100 mg/5 ml.

Albendazole

BENZNIDAZOLE (Ro 7-1051, RADANIL)

This 2-nitroimidazole has shown considerable promise in the treatment of both acute and chronic Chagas' disease, being effective against intracellular as well as extracellular parasites. A dose of 5 mg/kg daily for 30 days has been shown to be effective. It may also have some value in cutaneous and mucocutaneous leishmaniasis. Toxic effects appear to be a problem if the dose of 5 mg/kg is exceeded and include skin rashes,

general malaise, nausea and a sensory neuropathy.

CLOTRIMAZOLE (CANESTEN) (1-(α-2-CHLOROTRITYL) IMIDAZOLE)

A topical fungicide similar to miconazole, it also has some action against *Trichomonas vaginalis.*

Preparations. Vaginal tablets, 100 mg; 1% cream.

ISONIAZID

This most effective and inexpensive tuberculostatic drug was developed as an intermediate product in the synthesis of the thiosemicarbazone of isonicotinaldehyde, which it was hoped would have useful antituberculous properties itself.

Toxic effects

These are not perhaps as frequent as with other antituberculous agents. Peripheral neuritis may occur but can be prevented by the concurrent administration of pyridoxine. Changes in mood may occur, and this observation led to the development of iproniazid and other monoamine oxidase inhibitors for the treatment of depression. Isoniazid is not a monoamine oxidase inhibitor itself.

Nausea, headache, anorexia, dry mouth, ataxia, drowsiness, tinnitus, fever, liver damage, skin rashes, pellagra, hesitancy and agranulocytosis may occur, but rarely unless high dosages are used. Some individuals have an inherited disposition governed by a recessive gene to inactivate isoniazid slowly.

Dose

The dose is 200–300 mg (by mouth) daily.

Preparations

Isoniazid. Tablets of 50 and 100 mg. A syrup and an injectable form are also available, as are many preparations combined with either para-aminosalicylic acid or thiacetazone.

KETOCONAZOLE

Ketoconazole is better absorbed than the other imidazoles introduced for the treatment of fungal infections. It is therefore theoretically useful in the systemic as well as the superficial mycoses. Experimentally it has been shown to have an action against a number of protozoa, including plasmodia, leishmania, trypanosomes and tissue stages of *E. histolytica*. It is an anti-androgen.

Toxicity

In short courses ketoconazole appears to be safe but it is hepatotoxic and this precludes its use systematically in other than life-threatening conditions.

Dose

The dose is 200 mg daily with food for at least one week after symptoms have cleared.

Preparations

Ketoconazole (*Nizoral*). Tablets of 200 mg. Cream 2%.

LEVAMISOLE

Levamisole is the laevo rotatory isomer of tetramisole, a drug introduced as a veterinary anthelmintic in 1966. The dextro isomer appears to be relatively ineffective both as an anthelmintic and as an immunostimulant. As an anthelmintic its main use is in the treatment of *Ascaris lumbricoides*. A single dose will give up to 100% cure rates. It has some action against *Necator americanus*. It has no useful action against *Trichuris trichiura*. It has been suggested that it may be effective against *Strongyloides stercoralis*. It acts by interfering with the carbohydrate metabolism of nematodes and inhibiting the production of succinate dehydrogenase; this produces muscular paralysis of the worms. Its action as an immunostimulant is on cellular immune responses and only if they are impaired. It has no action on humoral immunity. Its precise role

as an immunostimulant is not yet clear. It may be useful in aphthous stomatitis, herpes labialis, warts and other chronic infections with evidence of impaired cellular immunity, and also in Crohn's disease, collagen disorders and malignant disease. The value in these various conditions will be determined by controlled trials. It should be noted that under some circumstances it may be immunosuppressive, so that its use should be tempered with caution.

Side-effects with the single anthelmintic dose are unusual. With the more prolonged causes used in immunotherapy side-effects are more common though, particularly in collagen disease, it has been difficult to decide whether or not an effect is due to the drug or the disease. Nausea, vomiting, abdominal pain, dizziness, diarrhoea, skin rashes and a transient neutropenia have been described.

Dose

For ascariasis 2.5 mg/kg is given in a single dose.

Preparation

Levamisole (*Ketrax*). 40 mg tablets.

MEBENDAZOLE

Mebendazole has a wide range of anthelmintic activity against both cestodes and nematodes, and against tissue stages of the parasites as well as against worms in the lumen of the gut. A short course over 2–3 days is all that is required when used as a luminal anthelmintic but, as the drug is poorly absorbed, higher dosages and more prolonged courses are needed when it is used as a

Mebendazole

tissue anthelmintic. Side-effects are unusual with the lower shorter dosage regimens, but are much more common at higher dosages, and at very high dosages fatalities have occurred. Its full role is still being explored but it has a useful action against *Ascaris lumbricoides*, hookworm, *Enterobius vermicularis*, *Trichuris trichiura* and *Capil-*

laria. It is also likely to be useful against *Trichinella spiralis*, *Dracunculus medinensis* and *Strongyloides stercoralis*. It is effective against adult cestode worms such as *Taenia saginata* and *Taenia solium*. Although it is effective against hydatid cysts, large doses have to be given, and it may be necessary to continue the drug for years to prevent relapse.

Dose

Single dose of 100 mg is given for *Enterobius vermicularis*. Short course 100 mg daily or twice daily for 3 or 4 days. In these dose ranges the dose for children and adults is the same.

Preparation

Mebendazole (*Vermox*).   100 mg tablets.

METRONIDAZOLE

Introduced for the treatment of trichomoniasis, metronidazole has proved to be most effective in tissue amoebiasis and has largely replaced emetine as the first line of treatment. It is too well absorbed to be a good luminal amoebicide, though if the dose is high enough and the course is long enough, amoebae can usually be eliminated from the bowel. It is effective in giardiasis and dracontiasis. It has a valuable action against anaerobic bacteria and has been used in the treatment of Vincent's angina and also topically in

Metronidazole

chronic skin ulcers. There is some evidence that it may have an immunosuppressive action and this action has been explored in experimental transplant surgery. It has been used in alcoholism, the taste for alcohol being diminished, but if alcohol is taken concurrently a confusional state may occur. It is well absorbed after oral administration. An injectable form is now being made available.

Toxicity

Side-effects include nausea, vomiting, rashes and

mental changes. There may be some individual variability in absorption and/or metabolism. The urine becomes dark in some patients. A transient neutropenia may occur. Peripheral neuropathy has been reported occasionally.

Dose

The choice is between a single large dose (1.4 g) daily for 1–3 days or smaller doses (200–800 mg) three times daily for up to 10 days. There would seem to be advantages in the single large daily dose. A one-day course would be effective for trichomoniasis and a 3-day course, which can be repeated, is effective in tissue amoebiasis. Reports of metronidazole resistance of *E. histolytica* invariably concern the lower dose, three times daily in prolonged regimens.

Preparations

Metronidazole (*Flagyl*).   Tablets of 200 mg, 400 mg (UK) and 250 mg (USA). Intravenous infusion of 5 mg/ml. Ampoules/vials of 20–100 ml.

Entamizole tablets. A combination of metronidazole and diloxanide furoate (p. 1212).

METHISAZONE

A thiosemicarbazone used in the prophylaxis of smallpox, it is effective only if taken early in the incubation period. It has also been used in the treatment of eczema vaccinatum and vaccinia gangrenosum.

Toxic effects

These include nausea, vomiting, diarrhoea and fluid retention. These effects may be aggravated by alcohol.

Dose

This is 3 g (by mouth) twice daily.

Preparations

Methisazone (*Marboran*).   A chewable capsule of 1.5 g.

MICONAZOLE

Miconazole has a broad spectrum of activity against fungi. It has been used topically on the skin and vagina. It is not very well absorbed from the gut. Its value in systemic fungal infections has been disappointing.

Dosage

This is 15–20 mg/kg daily intravenously in divided dose, the maximum single dose not to exceed 600 mg. The miconazole is diluted with saline. Miconazole 60 ml with saline 40 ml will give a solution of 100 ml containing 600 mg

Miconazole

miconazole. This should be given by slow intravenous infusion over a period of 30 minutes, but experience suggests that it may be possible to reduce this period to 10–15 minutes. In cryptococcal meningitis 2 ml of undiluted miconazole may be given intrathecally daily. Treatment should continue until there is both clinical and mycological cure.

Preparations. Tablets of 250 mg. Oral gel, 25 mg/ml. Ampoules containing miconazole 1% solution for dilution before use.

NIFURTIMOX (LAMPIT, BAYER 2502)

Chemically related to nitrofurazone, this drug is effective in Chagas' disease. It is especially effective in acute infections. To obtain cures in chronic infections it may be necessary to give the drug for 120 days. Side-effects are common and often serious. Gastrointestinal symptoms and neurotoxicity are the major toxic effects. It is showing promise in the treatment of late stages of African trypanosomiasis refractory to trivalent arsenicals. Given by mouth, 500 mg 6-hourly for 14 days is usually successful.

Toxicity

Neurotoxicity and gastrointestinal symptoms are frequent.

Dose

In Chagas' disease the dose is 5 mg/kg rising to 15 mg/kg daily by week 10, the course continued for a further seven weeks.

Preparation

Nifurtimox (Lampit). Tablets of 100 mg.

Nifurtimox

NIRIDAZOLE

Useful in the treatment of schistosomiasis, it is also effective in amoebiasis and in guinea-worm infections. High cure rates are obtained in *S. haematobium* infections but in *S. mansoni* infections results are less good and side-effects are more frequent, particularly in the presence of portal hypertension. The drug has also been reported to be effective in *S. japonicum* infections. The mode of action in schistosomiasis is uncertain but may be related to an inhibitory action on the enzyme glucose-6-phosphate dehydrogenase of the adult worm. Niridazole is well absorbed and is metabolized rapidly by the liver so that it is necessary to give the drug twice daily. The metabolites are excreted in the urine, giving it the colour of Coca-Cola. The most important toxic effects are on the central nervous system and include changes in mood, confusional states and convulsions. Other side-effects include nausea, vomiting, anorexia, headache, drowsiness, urticarial rashes, a temporary haemolytic anaemia in subjects with glucose-6-phosphate dehydrogenase deficiency, tachycardia and ECG changes with flattening or inversion of T waves. In animals spermatogenesis may be inhibited but this has not been confirmed in man. It should not be used concurrently with isoniazid and with caution in those with liver, heart, renal or neurological diseases. It has been noted to have a suppressive effect on cellular immunity.

Dose

This is 25 mg/kg (by mouth) in divided doses

daily to a maximum of 1.5 g daily for 5–10 days. In *S. japonicum* infections 15 mg/kg is given daily for 24 days; or three 10-day courses with a month between each course have been used.

Preparation

Niridazole (*Ambilhar*).　500 and 100 mg tablets.

NITROFURAZONE

Related to the urinary antiseptic nitrofurantoin (Furadantin), this drug, besides similar antibacterial properties, has some value in the management of trypanosomiasis. It is not a first line drug but may be used in infections showing resistance to the usual trypanocidal drugs.

Toxic effects

Nausea, vomiting, headache, arthralgia, peripheral neuritis and haemolytic anaemia in subjects with a glucose-6-phosphate dehydrogenase deficiency have been reported.

Preparation

Nitrofurazone. Tablets containing 100 mg of nitrofurazone. (Furacin is a 0.2% ointment or solution.)

THIABENDAZOLE

A broad-spectrum anthelmintic which is particularly useful in the treatment of strongyloidiasis and creeping eruption, it also has some effect on hookworm, *Ascaris* and *Enterobius*. It is effective against *Capillaria* and the adult worms of *Trichinella spiralis*, but does not appear to be effective against the tissue parasite. It has no useful effect against *Trichuris trichiura*. Toxic effects include dizziness, anorexia, nausea and vomiting, pruritus, skin rashes, headache, drowsiness and a fall in blood pressure.

Dose

The dose is 25 mg/kg (by mouth) twice daily for 2 days.

Preparations

Thiabendazole (*Mintezol*).　500 mg tablets; also available as an emulsion.

THIACETAZONE

This drug is used in the treatment of tuberculosis, particularly in combination with isoniazid where economic considerations are paramount. It is also of some use in leprosy.

　　Toxic effects include nausea, vomiting, anorexia, headache, vertigo, blurred vision, urticaria and dermatitis, fever, anaemia, agranulocytosis, Stevens–Johnson syndrome and liver damage.

Preparations

Thiazina. Tablets containing thiacetazone and isoniazid. Varying combinations are available, including tablets of thiacetazone 150 mg and isoniazid 300 mg, and thiacetazone 75 mg and isoniazid 150 mg.

Thiacetazone (*TBI, Thioparamizone*). Tablets of 25 mg, 50 mg and 75 mg.

TINIDAZOLE

Tinidazole and several other compounds, such as nimorazole, are very similar to metronidazole and much of what has been said about metronidazole probably applies to tinidazole. It has been advanced as a single dose treatment of trichomoniasis and giardiasis and is also comparably as effective as metronidazole in large single daily dose therapy of tissue amoebiasis.

Dose

This is 2 g daily. A one-day course is adequate for *Trichomonas vaginalis*, but it should be continued for 3 days and repeated if necessary for tissue forms of amoebiasis, such as liver abscess or amoebic dysentery.

Preparation

Tinidazole (*Fasigyn*).　500 mg tablets.

CHLORINATED HYDROCARBONS

TETRACHLOROETHYLENE (TCE)

This is effective against hookworm, probably by causing a reversible paralysis. There is disagreement as to whether it is more effective in *Ancylostoma duodenale* or *Necator americanus* infections. In either case the worm load is likely to be reduced by half by a standard course of treatment.

Tetrachloroethylene

Toxic effects

It has a central action in some respects similar to that of chloroform ($CHCl_3$) but with proper administration little is absorbed or inhaled. However, headache, faintness, giddiness and loss of consciousness may occur. Local effects include nausea, vomiting and abdominal pain. The drug is hepatotoxic. It should not be administered to ill patients, particularly those with liver diseases. Its administration should be preceded by a low fat diet as its absorption is enhanced by fat. It may precipitate intestinal obstruction in patients with coexisting *Ascaris* infections.

Dosage

This is 2–3 ml of tetrachloroethylene. Side-effects are frequent with higher dosage.

Preparations

Tetrachloroethylene draught. 3 ml of tetrachloroethylene in 45 ml of flavoured water.

Tetrachloroethylene capsules. 1 ml.

NEUROMUSCULAR BLOCKING AGENTS

BEPHENIUM HYDROXYNAPHTHOATE

This drug was developed after investigation of the anthelmintic properties of quaternary ammonium compounds. It is used in the treatment of hookworm infections. It is thought to be more effective against *A. duodenale* than against *N. americanus*. It also has a useful action against roundworms and *Trichostrongylus*. Absorption is negligible, so that toxic effects are limited to the gastrointestinal tract and include nausea, vomiting and diarrhoea.

Bephenium

Dose

The dose is 5 g (2.5 g of base) daily for 3 days.

Preparation

Bephenium granules (Alcopar). Sachets containing 5 g of bephenium hydroxynaphthoate.

PYRANTEL PAMOATE

Pyrantel is effective against *Ascaris*, hookworm and *Enterobius vermicularis*. It is only slightly absorbed so that systemic side-effects are most unusual unless very large doses are given when neurotoxicity might be expected. The worms are paralysed by the depolarizing neuromuscular blocking action. Pyrantel also inhibits cholinesterases.

Pyrantel

Dose

For *Ascaris*, *Acylostoma* and *Enterobius* 10 mg/kg

in a single dose is given. For *Necator americanus* the drug should be given for 3 days.

Preparation

Pyrantel (*Combantrin*).   Tablets, 125 mg.

OXANTEL PAMOATE

Oxantel (1-methyl-1,4,5,6-tetrahydro-2-[2-(3-hydroxyphenyl(vinyl]pyrimidine), an *m*-oxyphenol analogue of pyrantel, is effective against *Trichuris trichiura*, but seems to have little if any action against other worms. The pamoate salt is but little absorbed, so that side-effects are rare. A dose of 10 mg/kg twice daily for 3 days is effective. The drug is available in a suspension combined with pyrantel.

PIPERAZINE

Piperazine was originally introduced for the treatment of gout as it is a good solvent of uric acid in vitro, but clinically it was found to be ineffective. It is now used for the treatment of roundworm and threadworm infections. Piperazine paralyses roundworms, probably by acetylcholine blockade. The worms, no longer able to maintain their position in the gut, are expelled by peristalsis.

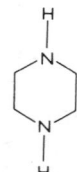

Piperazine

Toxicity

It is a safe drug, but excessive dosage in small children may cause vertigo, muscular incoordination and other neurological effects. Nausea, vomiting, diarrhoea and urticaria may occur. Rapidly absorbed, it is mainly excreted in the urine so that piperazine should not be given in renal disease.

Dosage

For *ascariasis* 3–6 g is given daily for 1–2 days.

For *enterobiasis*, 2 g is given daily for one week, or as for ascariasis.

Preparations

Piperazine adipate (*Entacyl*).   Tablets of 300 mg of piperazine adipate equivalent to 250 mg piperazine hydrate. Entacyl suspension contains 300 mg in 2 ml.

Piperazine citrate (*Antepar elixir*). The elixir containing equivalent of 750 mg of piperazine hydrate in 5 ml.

Piperazine hydrate.

Piperazine phosphate (*Antepar*). Tablets containing 520 mg of piperazine phosphate equivalent to 500 mg of piperazine hydrate.

Pripsen. A 10 g dose contains piperazine phosphate (4 g) and standard senna.

DIETHYLCARBAMAZINE

A derivative of piperazine, it is used in the treatment of filariasis and is more active against microfilariae (microfilaricidal) than against adult worms (macrofilaricidal). Its macrofilaricidal effect is most marked in *Loa loa* infections. It is usually effective in pulmonary tropical eosinophilia. Its action on microfilariae is probably to sensitize them, making them more susceptible to phagocytosis.

$CON(C_2H_5)_2$

CH_3

Diethylcarbamazine

Toxic effects

These are slight, but release of foreign protein following the death of microfilariae may lead to allergic reactions. This is especially so in onchocerciasis, and the subsequent skin reaction forms the basis of the Mazzotti test. Severe systemic reactions have been reported in heavy *Loa loa* infections. Reactions may be controlled by antihistamines or steroids.

Dosage

For *filariasis* the dose is initially 50 mg daily increased to a top dose of 150–450 mg in three divided doses daily for three weeks. For *pulmonary tropical eosinophilia*, the dose is 150 mg three-times daily for 5–10 days.

Preparation

Diethylcarbamazine (*Banocide, Hetrazan, Ethodryl*). 50 mg tablets of diethylcarbamazine citrate.

METRIPHONATE (DIPTEREX, BILARCIL)

An organophosphorus insecticide, it is especially valuable in the treatment of *Schistosoma haematobium*, though it has some action against intestinal nematodes. It acts by inhibiting cholinesterases and thus paralysing the worms.

$$
\begin{array}{c}
CCl_3 \\
| \\
CHOH \\
| \\
(CH_3O)_2 - P = O
\end{array}
$$

Metriphonate

Although it is effective against *S. mansoni* in vitro it has no useful action in vivo, except on *S. mansoni* worms in the bladder wall. It is not effective against rectal *S. haematobium*.

Toxic effects

Although the plasma cholinesterase falls and remains low for two weeks after treatment, side-effects are not severe. If the dose is increased above 10 mg/kg, abdominal pain, nausea and vomiting are frequent. There is a theoretical risk if muscle relaxants are used as part of general anaesthesia within two weeks of a course of metriphonate. If overdosage occurs, pralidoxime and atropine should be used as for other instances of organophosphorus poisoning. There is a drop in the sperm count and decreased viability after 24 hours.

Dose

The dose is 10 mg/kg to a maximum of 600 mg given on three occasions with a gap of three weeks between each dose. A single dose is reasonably effective and may be preferred in endemic areas. It has been used as a cream for creeping eruption.

Preparation

Metriphonate (*Bilarcil*). 100 mg tablets.

TOPICAL APPLICATIONS INCLUDING PARASITICIDES AND REPELLENTS

BENZYL BENZOATE

Effective in scabies as it is lethal to *Sarcoptes scabiei*, it is not so useful in pediculosis. It may cause skin eruptions, particularly in eczematous individuals.

Application

The patient is first scrubbed with soft soap. Immediately after drying benzyl benzoate is applied to the whole body below the neck. it is sometimes necessary to repeat the application.

Preparation

Benzyl benzoate application (*Ascabiol*). Benzyl benzoate 25% w/v with emulsifying wax and water.

CHLORBUTOL

This is antibacterial, antifungal and possibly antipruritic. It is used in many dusting powders and also as a preservative for injections and eye drops. It is related to chloral hydrate and has sedative and antiemetic actions.

DICOPHANE (DDT)

This is an insecticide which may be used to eradicate fleas and lice. Acute toxic signs include vomiting, diarrhoea, paraesthesiae, giddiness, tremors, anxiety and liver, bone marrow and renal damage.

DDT

Preparations

Dicophane. Available as an application and as a dusting powder.

DIBUTYL PHTHALATE

This is an insect repellent and mite repellent. Rubbed into clothes it may give protection for two weeks.

DIETHYL TOLUAMIDE

This is an insect repellent which may be applied direct to skin but the eyes and mouth must be avoided.

Preparation

Diethyl toluamide solution (Mylol). Available as 50% and 75% solutions in alcohol, and as a cream, a liquid and in pressurized containers.

DIMETHYL PHTHALATE

An insect, mite and tick repellent, it should be applied away from the eyes and mouth, and should not be allowed to come into contact with plastics and other synthetic materials.

Preparation

Dimethyl phthalate cream (Sketofax).

GAMMA BENZENE HEXACHLORIDE

This is used to eradicate lice and scabies. Toxic effects are similar to those of dicophane.

Preparations

Gamma benzene hexachloride (Lorexane). Avail-

able as a cream, dusting powder and application.

IDOXURIDINE (ACYCLOVIR)

This is an antimetabolite which disrupts DNA synthesis and thus prevents the replication of certain viruses. A 0.1% solution instilled into the conjunctival sac every one to two hours may control the keratitis of herpes simplex or vaccinia.

METHOXSALEN

This induces hypersensitivity to ultraviolet light. The subsequent stimulation of melanin pigments may be useful in idiopathic vitiligo, though not in secondary leukoderma. Side-effects including nausea and depression are common. It is toxic to the liver and may cause dermatitis.

Dose

This is 20 mg daily by mouth followed 2 hours later by exposure of vitiliginous area to ultraviolet light for 5 minutes increasing to 30 minutes. Alternatively a 1% lotion may be applied locally once a week and followed by a one-minute exposure to ultraviolet light. Treatment may need to be continued for months.

Preparations

Methoxsalen (Xanthotoxin, Meloxine, Meladinine, Methoxa-dome). 10 mg tablets.

Methoxsalen. 1% lotion.

ZINC UNDECENOATE

A topical fungicide, frequently combined with undecenoic acid, it is available as a dusting powder, spray or ointment (Mycota, Tineafax).

ELECTROLYTE AND FLUID REPLACEMENT AND REMOVAL (DIALYSIS)

Dehydration and the associated electrolyte loss must account for a great number of avoidable deaths in the tropics, and the unnecessary use of the intravenous route for the replacement of the deficit, for a large part of avoidable expenditure. Most dehydration, for example in cholera, can be corrected by the oral route.

ORAL REPLACEMENT

It is essential that glucose is included, for without glucose, absorption will be poor (cf. sea water). The simplest and most economical solution is:
    pinch of salt (thumb and 2 fingers) 1.5 g;
    scoop of sugar (3–4 finger scoop) 20–30 g;
    fruit (orange) juice—potassium;
    water—as clean as possible—1 pint/0.5 l.
Various preparations are available.

Sodium chloride and glucose oral powder. Na^+ 35 mmol, K^+ 20 mmol, Cl^- 37 mmol, HCO_3^- 18 mmol and glucose 200 mmol/litre when reconstituted. Available as 22 g packs to add to 0.5 litre.

Dextrolyte oral solution, Dioralyte oral powder, Electrosol tablets and Rehidrat oral powder are similarly constituted.

INTRAVENOUS REPLACEMENT FLUIDS

The following four solutions will cover most requirements. It may be useful in some circumstances to combine dextrose with either Hartmann's solution or half-strength Darrow's solution. This may be done by using a 'Y' junction and running both bottles simultaneously. Darrow's solution has a high potassium content and is specifically intended for the treatment of diarrhoea in infants. The precise electrolyte content of Hartmann's solution, and similar solutions, and half-strength Darrow's solution varies from manufacturer to manufacturer and from country to country. Contents should be checked locally.

Preparations

Glucose intravenous infusion 5%. 500 ml and 1000 ml packs. More concentrated solutions, 10%, 25%, 50% may be available for the provision of energy and for the treatment of hypoglycaemia. These hypertonic solutions may cause thrombophlebitis.

Sodium chloride intravenous infusion. 0.9% 500 ml and 1000 ml packs.

Sodium lactate intravenous infusion, compound.

(Ringer lactate, Hartmann's solution). Na^+ 131 mmol, K^+ 5 mmol, Ca^{2+} 2 mmol, lactate 29 mmol, Cl^- 111 mmol/litre.

Half-strength Darrow's solution. Na^+ 62 mmol, K^+ 17.5 mmol, Cl^- 52.6 mmol, lactate 27.5 mmol/litre.

FLUIDS FOR PERITONEAL DIALYSIS

Peritoneal dialysis may be used as an alternative to haemodialysis in acute renal failure and, in certain circumstances, in chronic renal failure. It may also be used in poisoning due to dialysable poisons, to remove fluid in resistant oedema, and in the management of pyogenic peritonitis.

A peritoneal catheter is inserted in the midline between the umbilicus and the symphysis pubis at the junction of the middle and lower thirds. The chosen peritoneal fluid is warmed to body temperature and 2 litres (1 litre for children) is run into the peritoneal cavity. After 20 minutes the fluid is siphoned out. The cycle may be repeated as necessary. In patients with normal or low levels of potassium it will be necessary to add 4 mmol K^+ to each litre of dialysis fluid.

There are two main fluids prepared by most companies, though the precise content varies from company to company. The first fluid is made slightly hypertonic by its glucose content ($\simeq 15$ g/litre) so that fluid is not absorbed from the peritoneal cavity, thus avoiding overhydration. It is useful for routine dialysis when there is no need to remove excessive fluid. The second fluid is much more hypertonic (40–60 g glucose/litre), enabling the rapid removal of large amounts of fluid from the body.

Preparations

Precise content of electrolyte varies with manufacturer.

	Routine solution		Hypertonic solution	
	mmol/litre	g/litre	mmol/litre	g/litre
Sodium	140		140	
Calcium	1.8		1.8	
Magnesium	0.75		0.75	
Chloride	100		100	
Lactate	45		45	
Dextrose	75	13.6	353	63.6

Other preparations may also be available, for example a low Na^+ solution for removal of excess Na^+ in chronic dialysis.

REFERENCES

1 Keystone, J.S. et al (1983) *Trans. R. Soc. trop. Med. Hyg.* 77, 84–86.

2 Phillips, R.E., Warrell, D.A., White, N.J. et al (1985) *New Engl. J. Med.* **312**, 1273–1278.

3 Nagaratnam, N., Chetiyawardana, A.D. & Rajujah, S. (1978) *Postgrad. Med. J.* **54**, 108.

4 Chen, M. et al (1983) *S.E. Asian J. trop. Med. Pub. Hlth* **14**, 495–500.

5 Polderman, A.M. et al (1984) *Trans. R. Soc. trop. Med. Hyg.* **78**, 752–754.

APPENDICES

Appendix I
Medical Protozoology

MALARIA PARASITES*
PHYLUM: PROTOZOA Goldfuss, 1818
SUBPHYLUM: APICOMPLEXA Levine, 1970
CLASS: SPOROZOA Leuckart, 1879
SUBCLASS: COCCIDIA Leuckart, 1879

ORDER: COCCIDIIDA Labbé, 1899
SUBORDER: HAEMOSPORINA Danilewsky, 1885
FAMILY: PLASMODIIDAE Mesnil, 1903

GENUS: *Plasmodium* Marchiafava & Celli, 1885
SUBGENERA: *Plasmodium, Laverania*

The genus *Plasmodium* includes the malaria parasites of man and animals (including birds). The species affecting man are:

Quartan group

P. (*Plasmodium*) *malariae* (Grassi & Feletti, 1892)
P. (*P.*) *brasilianum* (Gonder & von Berenberg-Gossler, 1908)

Benign tertian group

P. (*P.*) *vivax* (Grassi & Feletti, 1890)
P. (*P.*) *cynomolgi* Mayer, 1907
P. (*P.*) *cynomolgi bastianellii* Garnham, 1959

Malignant tertian group

P. (*Laverania*) *falciparum* (Welch, 1897)

Ovale group

P. (*P.*) *ovale* Stephens, 1922
P. (*P.*) *simium* Fonseca, 1951

Knowlesi group

P. (*P.*) *knowlesi* Sinton & Mulligan, 1932
Of these, *P. malariae, P. vivax, P. falciparum* and

* The information in the section on the malaria parasites has been revised, largely by reference to the authoritative descriptions contained in Professor Garnham's standard work.[1] This most comprehensive book contains references to the information collated from the work of vast numbers of scientists over the years, and of the distinguished author himself.

P. ovale are the most common and important. The others are primarily parasites of monkeys or apes, affecting man only incidentally and not seriously. *P. malariae* can exist in a man–mosquito–man cycle, but in parts of Africa there is evidence that a reservoir exists in chimpanzees, the parasite apparently passing backwards and forwards between these animals and man.

The life-cycles of these parasites have features in common. They are all carried from man to man or from animals to man by mosquitoes of the genus *Anopheles*, unlike the bird malaria parasites, which are carried by *Culex, Aedes* and other species. Rodent malaria parasites are also carried by *Anopheles* (e.g. *P. berghei* and *P. vinckei*).

LIFE-CYCLE OF THE MALARIA PARASITES OF MAN (Figs. I.1–I.6)[2]

The life-cycle, taking the sporozoite as the starting point, comprises several well-defined stages.

The *sporozoites* inoculated by the infected *Anopheles* enter the bloodstream, but cannot be found in it after about half an hour. Parasites reappear in the blood 5 to 15 days later, but in an altered form, having undergone profound developmental changes. Some sporozoites enter the parenchymal cells of the liver and there divide and multiply to form the *exo-erythrocytic (pre-erythrocytic) schizonts*, each developing within a liver cell and bounded by a limiting membrane. Multiplication takes place by division of the nucleus of the original sporozoite and continues until there are thousands of separate nucleated parasites in each schizont. These eventually burst the limiting membrane and are shed into the circulation as free individual *merozoites*, where they quickly invade erythrocytes.

As shown in Fig. I.2, some sporozoites (28) of *P. vivax* and *P. cynomolgi* penetrate parenchyma cells of the liver but remain *dormant* as *hypnozoites* (see below) for lengthy periods and then, as the result of an unknown trigger, become activated to resume growth (29–30). On maturity (31), merozoites are produced

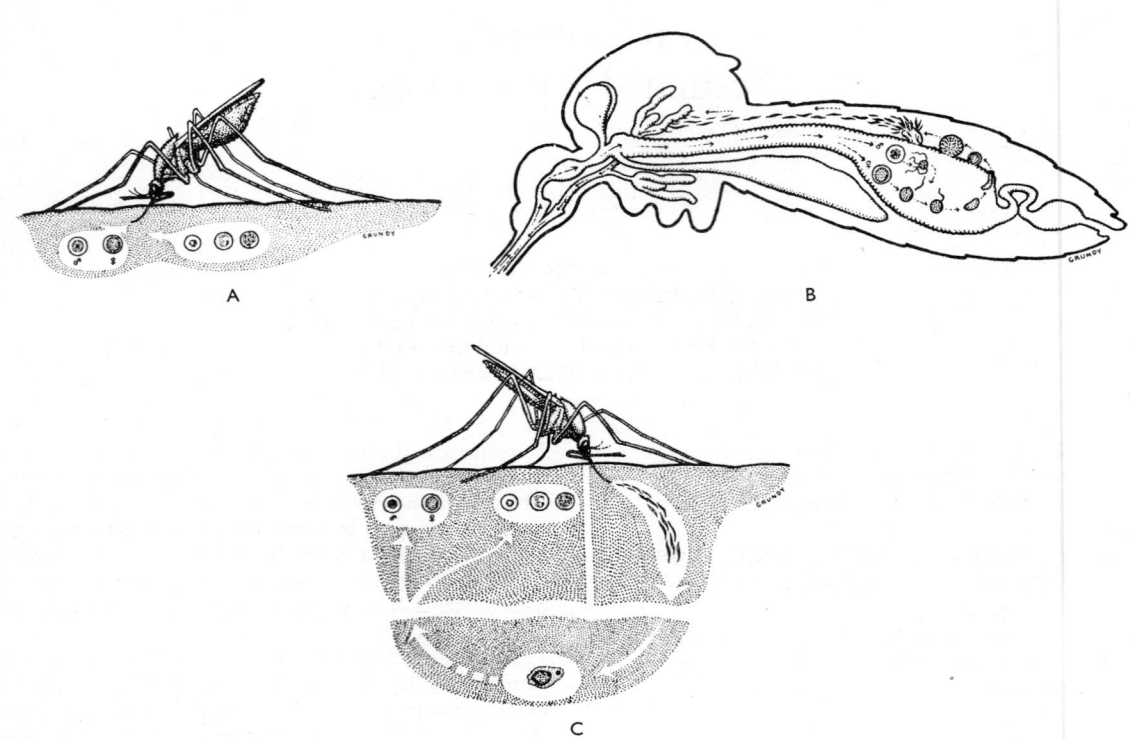

Fig. I.1 The malaria cycle. A, The female *Anopheles*, in feeding on a person with malaria, takes in blood containing the male and female gametocytes. B, The male gametocyte exflagellates to produce eight microgametes, one of which fuses with the freed macrogamete to give rise to the zygote. This develops on the stomach wall of the mosquito as an oöcyst, producing a large number of sporozoites, which make their way to the salivary glands. This cycle lasts 7 days or more. C, When, after the development of the sporozoites, the infected mosquito again feeds on man, she discharges sporozoites in the human tissues. These may be detected in the blood for not more than half an hour after the mosquito has bitten. Thereafter they develop in the cells of the liver, and the malaria parasites to which they give rise may be found in the blood 5–15 days after the bite of the infected mosquito. The clinical attack of malaria usually begins within a day or two of their appearance in the blood. Exceptionally, in *P. vivax* infections, this process of development may be delayed for several weeks or months. (The sizes of the mosquitoes and parasites are not in proportion.)

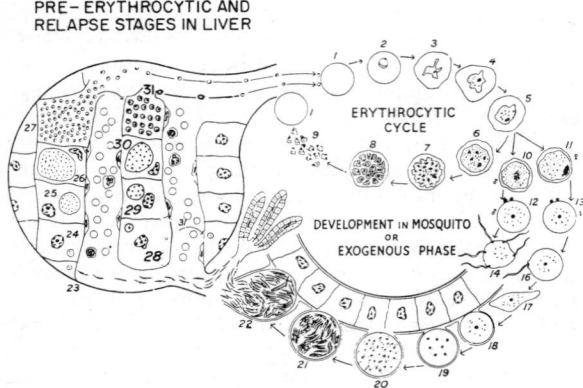

PRE- ERYTHROCYTIC AND
RELAPSE STAGES IN LIVER

ERYTHROCYTIC
CYCLE

DEVELOPMENT IN MOSQUITO
OR
EXOGENOUS PHASE

Fig. I.2 The complete life-cycle of the malaria parasite based on *P. vivax* and *P. malariae*. 1, Normal red cells. 2–5, Red cells containing young parasites (trophozoites). 6–8, Erythrocytic schizogony. 9, Liberation of erythrocytic merozoites into the blood. 10, 11, Development of male and female gametocytes in the circulating blood. 12, Mature male gametocyte. 13, Mature female gametocyte. 14, Exflagellation of male gametocyte producing male gametes (microgametes) in the stomach of the mosquito. 15, Female gamete, or macrogamete, being fertilized by the male to become a zygote. 16, Male gamete or microgamete. 17, Oökinete, or travelling vermicule, formed by elongation of zygote, about to penetrate the epithelial lining of the mosquito's stomach. 18–21, Oöcysts developing on the outer wall of the mosquito's stomach. 22, Mature oöcysts rupturing and liberating sporozoites, which enter the salivary glands. 23, Sporozoite from the salivary gland of the mosquito entering the liver cell of man. 24–26, Development of pre-erythrocytic schizont in liver cells. 27, Pre-erythrocytic schizont liberating pre-erythrocytic merozoites which enter red cells, to commence the erythrocytic cycle. 28–31, Relapse stages deriving from a special type of sporozoites. 28, Hypnozoite (remaining dormant for long periods in uninucleate condition). 29, 30, Resumed growth of exo-erythrocytic schizont (relapse bodies). 31, Mature relapse body, releasing merozoites into circulation to initiate relapse.

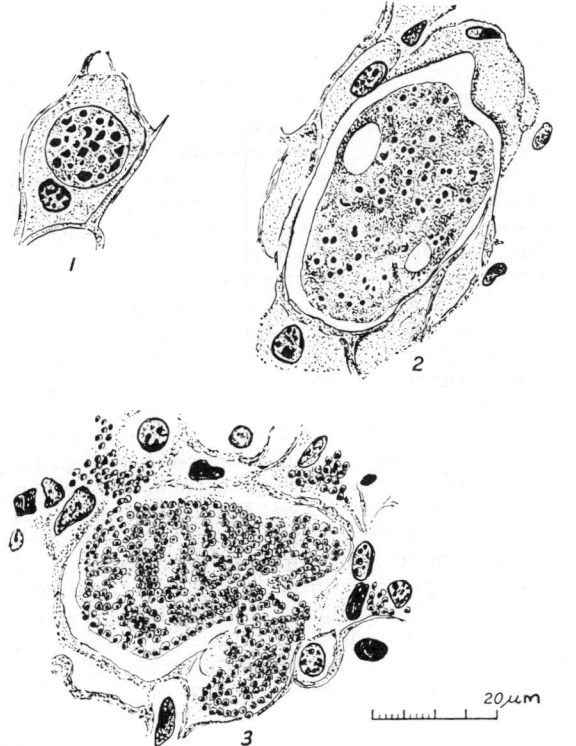

Fig. I.3 Pre-erythrocytic cycle of malaria parasites. 1, Pre-erythrocytic schizont of *P. cynomolgi* in a liver cell on the fifth day. 2, Pre-erythrocytic schizont of *P. vivax* in a liver cell on the seventh day, showing a form with two vacuoles. 3, A more advanced stage of (2) showing the formation and release of pre-erythrocytic merozoites.

20 μm

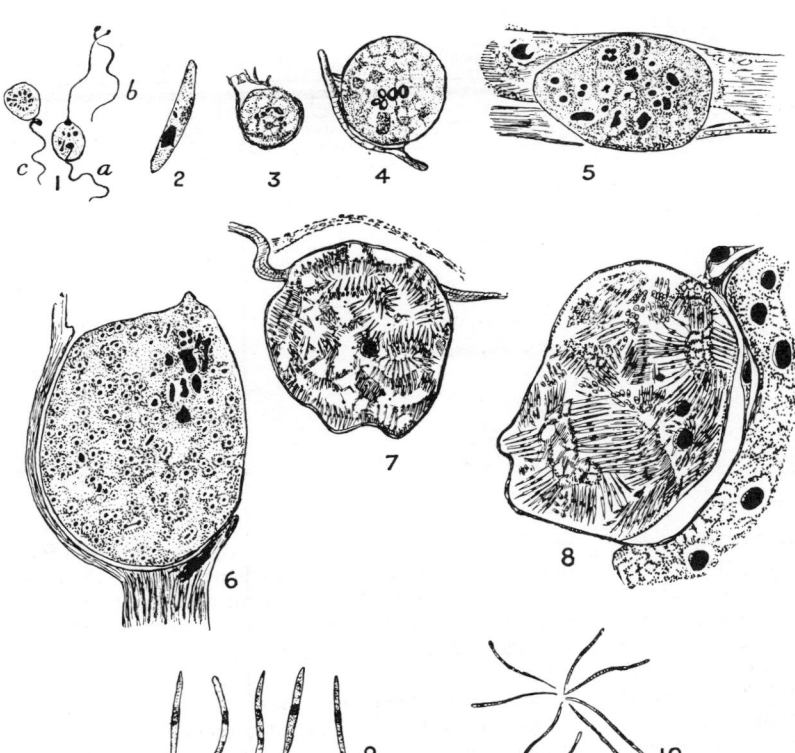

Fig. I.4 Stages in the development of *P. falciparum* in *Anopheles*. 1a, Exflagellation of male gametocyte of *P. vivax*. 1b, Free flagellum (male gamete). 1c, Fertilization of female gamete. 2, Oökinete. 3, Encysted zygote in the stomach wall. 4–6, Oöcysts showing reticulated cytoplasm. 7, Section of oöcyst showing sporozoite forming outgrowths from cytoplasmic reticulum. 8, Section of oöcyst into mature sporozoites. 9, Sporozoites from the salivary gland. 10, Sporozoites of *P. ovale*.

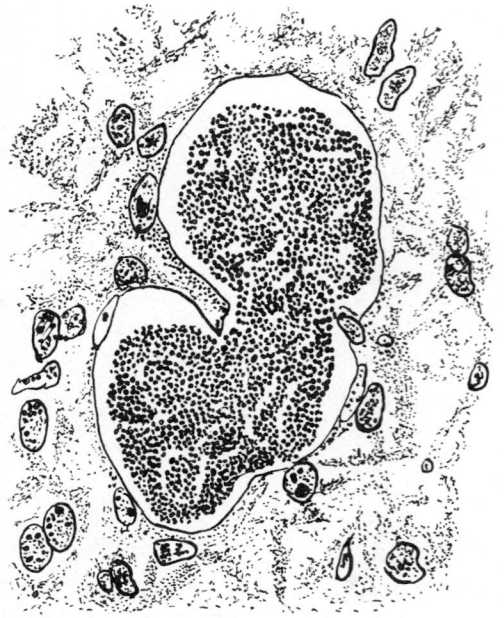

Fig. I.5 Pre-erythrocytic schizont of *P. falciparum* in human liver on the sixth day.

seen after inoculation of blood forms of the parasite. Moreover, latency is confined to *P. vivax*, *P. cynomolgi* and subspecies, *P. ovale* and *P. simium*. On the other hand, true relapses are absent in *P. falciparum*, *P. malariae* and *P. brasilianum* infections. There is evidence that the last two species (human and simian respectively) are identical. Thus, in the case of these three non-relapsing forms, exo-erythrocytic stages are solely of the pre-erythrocytic type and no hypnozoites are produced. The surprising longevity of *P. malariae* (and other quartan parasites) is due to the persistence of a small number of parasites in the bloodstream which occasionally increase in sufficient numbers to cause symptoms (recrudescences); in *P. malariae* they may occur for up to 50 years. In *P. falciparum*, the parasites persist in the blood for a much shorter period and recrudescences cause renewed bouts of fever for up to one or two years in persons in whom the infection is not completely eradicated. Thus, although *P. falciparum* is much more dangerous than *P. vivax* or *P. ovale*, it is more easily cured by the drugs we now possess, except where drug resistance has appeared. *P. malariae* exhibits a similar response to treatment.

Theories and studies on the cause of relapses in malaria have been advanced by the recent discovery

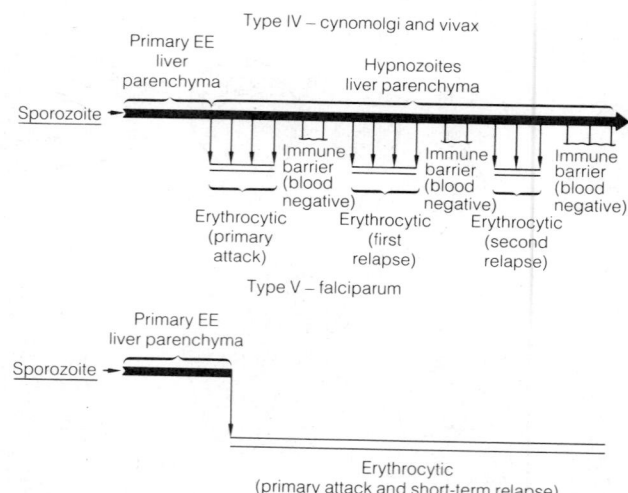

Fig. I.6 Types of erythrocytic schizogony. Above, *P. cynomolgi*. Below, *P. falciparum*. (After World Health Organization.[2])

which burst into the circulation, invade erythrocytes and give rise to a relapse. The latent period is of variable length; in *P. cynomolgi* infection it is about 100 days or less, while in *P. vivax* infection the length depends upon the strain of parasite. In some temperate strains the period is about 250 days. In other strains all the sporozoites become dormant and the prepatent or incubation period is delayed for 250 days or longer.

The relapse phenomenon, or delayed incubation, occurs only after infection by sporozoites; it is never

by Krotoski et al,[3] in a *P. cynomolgi bastianellii* infection in a monkey, of very small parasites within the parenchymal cells of the liver, in addition to normal schizonts. These parasites, in a biopsy specimen taken at 7 days, had a diameter ranging between 2.9 and 5.5 μm (average 4.5 μm), a single, reddish-purple nucleus surrounded by a clear or variegated bluish cytoplasm and a fine limiting membrane. Slightly larger forms were found in a later (day 50) biopsy specimen.

Relapses

It is now known that the forms 'hypnozoites'[4,5] are responsible for the relapses in relapsing malaria.

In relapsing vivax type parasites, the sporozoites invade the hepatocytes within 45 minutes of inoculation where they disappear until the earliest tissue schizonts can be found after 36 hours, when two different populations develop. One population develops, matures and discharges merozoites into the circulation causing an overt attack of malaria, the other remains dormant as a small single-cell structure (hypnozoite) for long periods of time until stimulated by some as yet unknown mechanism to mature and discharge merozoites into the circulation causing a relapse. Temperate and tropical strains of vivax differ in the proportion of these two forms. The temperate strains form few if any normal tissue schizonts but many hypnozoites, thus accounting for their tendency to relapse after long periods of time allowing them to survive by overwintering or resisting periods of drought. The tropical strains have no need for such forms and form mainly normal tissue schizonts.[6]

In *P. falciparum* infections the relapse phenomenon or delayed incubation does not occur and therefore recurrences of the type met with in the other species do not take place, though recrudescences due to persistence of the blood phase do occur and cause renewed bouts of fever for up to one to two years after first infection in persons in whom that infection is not completely eradicated. Thus, though *P. falciparum* is much more dangerous than the other three species, partly (probably) because it multiplies much more prolifically than them, it is more easily cured by the drugs we now possess—except where drug resistance has appeared. *P. falciparum* is not repeatedly locked away inside liver cells where 4-aminoquinolines do not reach it.

The merozoites are shed into the peripheral blood, in enormous numbers, from the bursting liver phases, and their function is to invade the red cells, particularly the young red cells, the reticulocytes. They enter these cells by a special mechanism. The merozoite organelles contact receptors on the red cell surface which consist of glycophorin A and B (sialoglycoproteins) the presence of which is necessary for entry (see section on natural immunity, Chapter 1, p. 12).[7] These organelles induce invagination of the red cell surface and the merozoite enters the red cell via the invagination maintaining contact between itself and the red cell membrane and two inner membranes, and slips into the cell. The merozoite has an envelope consisting of an outer plasma membrane and two inner membranes and acquires a surface coat in the plasma. On entering the red cell it loses the two inner membranes and sheds the surface coat.[8] Some *P. falciparum* parasites which seem to adhere to the outside of the red cells are known as *appliqué* forms. Once inside the red cell the parasites appear as *ring forms* each with a

nucleus and cytoplasm surrounding a vacuole. They then form *trophozoites* which feed on the haemoglobin of the red cell which is digested in food vacuoles with the production of typical yellow-brown to black pigment known as *haemazoin*. This dependence on the metabolism of haemoglobin is important in the action of chloroquine on the parasite and the development of chloroquine resistance (p. 36).

The malaria pigment appears as follows:

P. vivax	numerous fine, yellowish brown, golden dust-like particles;
P. ovale	numerous blackish-brown particles;
P. malariae	numerous coarse and dark brown particles;
P. falciparum	one, two or at most three solid blocks of black pigment (an important diagnostic feature);

When the red cell finally disrupts because the parasites burst out of it (see below) the pigment is shed into the blood and is taken up largely by cells of the reticuloendothelial system. It can be seen in those cells in the internal organs and is strong evidence of previous malarial infection, though similar pigment is seen in the liver in intestinal schistosomiasis.

It has repeatedly been noticed that infection by *P. falciparum* is less intense in children who carry sickle-cell haemoglobin (HbS) or other abnormal haemoglobins (e.g. HbC) than it is in carriers of normal adult Hb. The explanation may be that these abnormal haemoglobins do not effectively supply the nutrients needed by the parasites, but another explanation may be that the circulation, being slowed down in the capillaries, favours the sickling process of the red cells, which collapse and in which, therefore, the parasites die (p. 12).

The merozoites which invade the red cells grow in size for some hours and then begin to divide (*schizogony*), the nuclei splitting into daughter nuclei and forming the 'rosettes' characteristic of the *erythrocytic schizont* (or segmenter). Each daughter nucleus attracts its portion of the cytoplasm and eventually, in about 48 hours (*P. vivax* and *P. ovale*) or 72 hours (*P. malariae*), the daughter parasites (*merozoites*) burst out of the red cells, to invade other red cells and start this phase of the life-cycle all over again. In *P. falciparum* the periodicity is about 48 hours but is not so regular as in the other species. Moreover, although the dividing forms (*schizonts*, segmenters or rosettes) of *P. vivax*, *P. ovale* and *P. malariae* can be seen in the peripheral blood, in *P. falciparum* they are mostly present in the blood spaces of the internal organs; indeed, if they are found in the peripheral blood, this is a sign that the infection has become dangerous to life and is an indication for immediate and urgent treatment, especially in primary infections in non-immune persons.

The numbers of merozoites formed in red cells are:

P. vivax	8–24 (usually 12–18)
P. ovale	6–12 (usually 8)
P. malariae	6–12 (usually 8–10)
P. falciparum	8–32 (usually 8–18)

Although most merozoites invade red cells, to undergo the asexual cycle as described above, some develop quite differently, into male and female sexual forms (*gametocytes*). The mechanism which determines which merozoites become asexual trophozoites and which become sexual forms is not clear, but the sexual forms appear in the blood, each within a red cell, at a predetermined date.

The gametocytes, male (*microgametocytes*) and female (*macrogametocytes*), do not divide in the human or animal body. Their next stage of development takes place in the stomach of *Anopheles*.

Gametocytes of *P. vivax* (and probably of *P. ovale* and *P. malariae*) may originate from merozoites of exo-erythrocytic schizonts, but chiefly from merozoites of asexual erythrocytic schizonts, in successive waves. Gametocytes can appear 3 days after the beginning of parasitaemia following heavy sporozoite infection. It has usually been thought that gametocytes take twice as long as schizonts to reach maturity, becoming fully grown in 4 days and circulating in the blood for some time, reaching maximum numbers about 4–6 days after the peak density of asexual parasites.

Hawking et al,[9] however, have produced evidence which strongly suggests that gametocytes of *P. knowlesi*, *P. cynomolgi* (in monkeys) and *P. cathemerium* (in canaries) do not follow this pattern. They take a few hours longer than their asexual cycles to develop to the stage of infectivity for mosquitoes, remaining mature for only a few (5–12) hours and then quickly degenerate and disappear, to be followed by new gametocytes from each schizogony. This probably applies to all plasmodia which shows a synchronous asexual cycle, except perhaps to *P. falciparum*, in which gametocytes take 9–12 days to develop. This biological feature is assumed to be a mechanism which produces short-lived mature gametocytes in the blood to coincide with the biting habits of vector mosquitoes.

The gametocytes of *P. falciparum* when fully developed are crescentic bodies, longer than the diameter of the red cells in which they grow, with the result that the red cell membrane is stretched to accommodate this length. The name falciparum reflects this shape; it is derived from the Latin 'falx', a sickle or crescent, and 'parere', to bring forth.

In the other three species the gametocytes are round bodies which almost fill the red cells in which they grow; they differ from asexual forms in that the nucleus remains single. The pigment is scattered through the cytoplasm.

Gametocytes can persist in the blood after asexual forms have disappeared as a result of treatment (in *P.*

falciparum apparently as a result of a small but constant supply from internal organs). They are not affected by the antibodies which are active against the asexual forms.

When a thick drop of freshly drawn blood containing mature gametocytes is placed in a moist atmosphere, a remarkable change which takes place in the male gametocyte can be seen. The parasite sheds its erythrocyte envelope and throws out eight slender, active *flagella*, each containing nuclear material from the original nucleus. These flagella lash about vigorously, detaching themselves from the cell body, to swim free in the plasma. The process of *exflagellation* takes about 10–12 minutes. The function of these male elements is to fertilize female cells, after the fashion of spermatozoa in other forms of life.

Exflagellation can be achieved as follows.[10] A layer of filter paper is accurately cut to fit the bottom of a Petri dish and another to fit the lid. These papers are saturated with hot water, completely but without excess. A triangular piece of glass rod or tube is placed in the dish, which is immediately closed and kept for one hour. The operator then makes a thick film of blood on a slide, breathes on it and at once places it on the glass rod and replaces the lid. Exflagellation at a temperature of 25°C is complete in 15 minutes for *P. vivax* and *P. ovale* and in 15–30 minutes for *P. falciparum*.

The process of exflagellation and fertilization can take place in the stomach of any biting insect, but only in certain species of *Anopheles* can the parasites infecting man develop further. When a susceptible *Anopheles* takes in mature gametocytes at a blood meal, the male elements go through this process of exflagellation, the flagella moving vigorously in the fluid stomach contents. They are now known as *gametes*.

The female gametocyte has in the meantime freed itself from the erythrocyte membrane and is also known now as a *gamete*. If a flagellum (male gamete) now meets a female gamete, it enters it, thus fertilizing it, to form a *zygote*. This now elongates, becoming a *travelling vermicule* (*oökinete*) which is able to penetrate one of the epithelial cells lining the mosquito stomach. This done, the oökinete begins to develop, the fertilized nuclear material and the cytoplasm divide and subdivide continuously, forming a cyst (*oöcyst*) which grows and can be seen lying under the elastic membrane on the outer surface of the mosquito stomach if this is removed and examined. Mature oöcysts may number scores or hundreds in a single mosquito. Besides dividing forms, they contain pigment (Fig. I.7).

Division of the oöcyst contents continues until it is filled with masses of slender, pointed and nucleated individual forms known as *sporozoites*, about 9–14 μm in length. These finally burst out of the limiting membrane, flooding the body cavity and even the limbs of the mosquito. Masses of them find their way into the cells of the salivary glands of the mosquito and thence

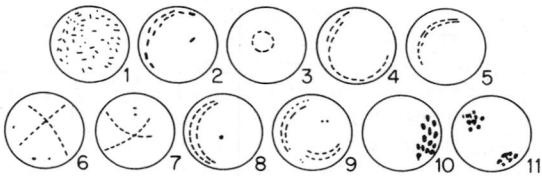

Fig. I.7 Typical arrangement of pigment granules in 3–4-day oöcysts. 1, *P. vivax* with golden-brown pigment. 2–5, *P. falciparum*, with black pigment. 6–9, *P. ovale* with dark brown pigment. 10, 11, *P. malariae*, with coarse black pigment.

into the saliva itself, which is injected into the next host on which the mosquito feeds.

Work on the electron microscopic examination of sporozoites at high magnifications has shown that their structure is complex. The outer coat is thick, giving a degree of rigidity. At the anterior end there is an organelle which probably produces a proteolytic enzyme to assist penetration of the tissues of the host. Fibrils probably have a supporting function and mitochondria provide a source of energy. There is a micropyle which is associated with the feeding mechanism.

Ross's 'black spores'

Sometimes the development of oöcysts is halted, with the formation of these 'black spores' (which are not true spores). They are banana-shaped bodies, dark brown or black, within the thickened oöcyst wall and occasionally in the thoracic muscles near the salivary glands; they are, presumably, chitinized sporozoites. The mechanism of their formation is obscure; it may be the result of unfavourable environmental or biological conditions and the deposition of dark material by some unknown biological action. Another view is that they are the result of the secretion of chitin around tracheoles or foreign bodies.

SUMMARY OF THE LIFE-CYCLE OF MALARIA PARASITES (Fig. I.2)

1 *Sporozoites* in the saliva of infected mosquitoes are injected into man and enter liver cells where they develop into *exo-erythrocytic schizonts*.
2 These produce *merozoites* which enter the circulation (*micromerozoites*).
3 In the circulation merozoites enter red cells to form: (*a*) asexual *trophozoites*, becoming *schizonts* which divide by *schizogony* to form new merozoites which again enter red cells and (*b*) sexual forms, male (*microgametocytes*) and female (*macrogametocytes*).
4 In the mosquito stomach male gametocytes become *gametes* and produce *flagella* which fertilize female *gametes*, forming *zygotes*, which become motile *oökinetes*.
5 The oökinetes traverse the mosquito stomach cells, producing *oöcyst* containing large numbers of *sporozoites* (*sporogony*).
6 Sporozoites enter the salivary glands, to be inoculated into man at subsequent mosquito feeds.

A *relapse* is a new manifestation of clinical symptoms or parasitaemia which is of two types: *short-term relapse* (the word recrudescence is now no longer used) due to an increase in the surviving population of erythrocytic forms which have persisted. This occurs in *P. falciparum* and *P. malariae* malaria. A *long-term relapse* is due to a multiplication of parasites in the blood from exo-erythrocytic forms in the liver, no erythrocytic schizogony occurring during the latent period (Fig. I.8). This is only possible in *P. vivax* and *P. ovale* malaria.

Malaria may be induced by means other than the bites of infected *Anopheles*.
1 Congenital malaria has been observed, but rarely, the parasites presumably having crossed the placenta.
2 By the inoculation of infected blood, as in transfusion of inadequately stored infected blood, in malaria therapy for syphilis, or accidentally in drug

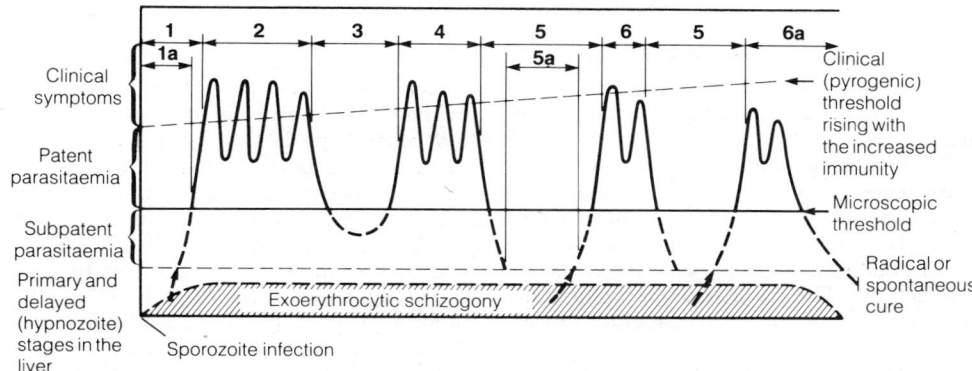

Fig. I.8 Phases of a malaria infection, showing relapses of the recurrent and recrudescent type. 1, Incubation period. 2, Primary attack composed of paroxysms. 3, Latent period (clinical latency). 4, Recrudescence (short-term relapse). 5, Latent period. 5a, Parasitic latency. 6, Clinical recurrence (long-term relapse) followed by parasitic relapse. 6a, Parasitic relapse.

addicts through the use of unsterilized syringes passed from one person to another. (Hepatitis and septicaemia are other common hazards of this practice.)

In such cases sporozoites are not involved and therefore the liver stages do not occur; true relapses are not possible, though short-term relapses from persisting parasites in the blood are possible. Malaria induced in these ways is easily curable by schizonticidal drugs.

FEATURES OF THE VARIOUS PARASITES OF MAN (Table I.1)

For a more detailed description of the morphology of all stages of malaria parasites both in man and the mosquito with electron microscope studies see Bannister and Sinden.[11]

The red cell is now enlarged to about $10 \mu m$ in diameter, is always heavily stippled and may be distorted; it ruptures to set free the merozoites and pigment. The pigment is taken up by phagocytes or by cells of the reticuloendothelial system. The merozoites measure about $1.5 \mu m$; they have no pigment.

Although the process of schizogony is never absolutely regular, maximum segmentation usually takes place in the afternoon.

In a mixed infection with *P. falciparum* the parasitaemia by *P. vivax* is likely to be inhibited because *P. falciparum* is dominant, overshadowing *P. vivax*, which may be missed. When the activity of *P. falciparum* subsides, *P. vivax* multiplies without hindrance and can be seen.

The asexual cycle in the blood is repeated until a peak occurs about two weeks after the first patency.

Table I.1 Tissue phase of human malaria.

Species	Duration of primary e-e schizogony (days)	Size of mature schizont (μm, approx.)	Number of merozoites	Size of merozoites (μm)	Special features	Delayed schizogony (hypnozoites)
P. vivax	8	45	over 10 000	1.2	Vacuoles	Present
P. ovale	9	70	15 000	1.8	Large nuclei	Present
P. malariae	15	56	15 000	2.0	Enlarged host cell nucleus	Nil
P. falciparum	$5\frac{1}{2}$	60	40 000	0.7	Small nuclei, cytomeres	Nil

Reproduced from WHO.[2]

Asexual forms

P. vivax (Plates I.8–I.11). The first stage is the ring stage, when a vacuole forms, surrounded by a loop of thin cytoplasm, and a small round nucleus, sometimes in the loop. The ring enlarges within a few hours and the cytoplasm becomes amoeboid, throwing out pseudopodia in rapid movements which justify the name vivax. Minute grains of light brown pigment appear in the cytoplasm.

The red cell enlarges and becomes pale, the whole cell developing the tiny spots known as Schüffner's dots, which stain red with Romanowsky stains at a suitably alkaline pH.

At about 24 hours the parasite occupies most of the red cell, the vacuole disappears and the cytoplasm becomes more dense. At about 36 hours a proportion of the parasitized red cells retreat into the blood spaces of the internal organs (though not so many as in *P. falciparum* infection). The nucleus divides and subdivides until, typically, there are 16 daughter nuclei (though the number varies), each attracting a portion of cytoplasm. This is the rosette stage. The pigment granules agglomerate and at maturity consist of a very few dark brown collections, though not so well coalesced or so big as in *P. falciparum*.

Parasites then become fewer until there is a short-term relapse in about a month. Short-term relapses are repeated a few times until a condition of latency occurs as immunity is established, when merozoites from the liver stages are taken up by phagocytes before they can do any harm. Immunity, which is stimulated by merozoites, then declines until, after a period, a relapse takes place.

P. ovale (Plates I.1–I.4). The development of this species in red cells resembles that of *P. vivax*; its periodicity is rather more than tertian, the merozoites taking 49–50 hours to grow to mature schizonts. The red cells show dots which stain more deeply than Schüffner's dots of *P. vivax* and have a violet tinge; they have been named James' dots. The cells become slightly enlarged, with weakening of the cell envelope, so that in thin films the cells (which are globular and stick to the side) are distorted by the process of spreading, and are seen as oval bodies with ragged or fimbriated edges. In humid conditions when films dry slowly this character may not be seen, but it is an important indication of a change in the physical state of the red cells.

A new form of *P. vivax* with a different pattern in the oöcysts has been described from China (*P. vivax multinucleatum*). It has a very long incubation period (312–322 days) and a time to primary relapse of 66–69 days.[12]

P. ovale often shows prolonged latency of months before the first attack and relapses tend to occur after intervals of about three months.

P. malariae (Plates I.5–I.7 and II.3). The asexual forms may be very scanty in the blood, even when the patient is experiencing definite attacks of fever every 72 hours. Trophozoites are seen in mature red cells, unlike the other species which favour reticulocytes, but cells harbouring very young rings have not been recorded. The trophozoites live longer in the red cells than the other species. They are less amoeboid than *P. vivax* and band forms are characteristic, reaching from side to side of the cells. This appearance may be an artefact, the parasite being distorted by the process of spreading thin films, as band forms do not occur in thick drops. The pigment is dark brown or black and tends to collect on one edge of the band; a linear nucleus is seen on the other edge.

The nucleus begins to divide after 48 hours and the rosette form is mature at 72 hours, usually giving eight merozoites, occasionally up to 12 but no more. The schizont usually ruptures in the morning or early afternoon.

P. malariae does not cause the red cell to enlarge, but after prolonged staining it produces characteristic (Ziemann) stippling with fine red-staining dots. This is difficult to demonstrate and is more important by its absence than by its presence, since in a well-stained film, parasites with undotted erythrocytes are almost certainly *P. malariae*.

P. falciparum (Plates I.12–I.15). This is vicious; it attacks both young and mature red cells, which then show a brassy coloration. The rings are small (1.2 μm) and hair-like, with thin cytoplasm, a prominent nucleus and a vacuole. The nucleus may be double. *Appliqué* forms are common, as is multiple infection of red cells. The trophozoites are very variable in shape and size. Except in pernicious attacks, however, only the ring forms and gametocytes are usually seen in routine examination in the peripheral blood, the developing stages and schizonts usually hiding in the blood spaces of internal organs—spleen, bone marrow, placenta, brain and others. This has long been recognized as a feature of this infection. Schizonts, however, can often be found very scantily in the peripheral blood after careful critical scrutiny—in 2% of light infections to 26–60% of heavy infections. They tend to be found in non-immune or susceptible persons in whom there has been fever for several days before administration of antimalarial drugs.

At 24 hours the parasite is a thick ring and the vacuole begins to disappear; at this time the retreat to the internal organs begins and consequently fewer may be seen in the peripheral blood.

The red cell begins to show six to 12 marks known as Maurer's clefts, which may be the result of loss of substance from the surface of the cell as a result of the attack by the parasite, and these show as red blotches if stained with a Romanowsky stain at pH 7.2–7.4, rather longer than usual. The red cell is now darker and purplish, with a red edging.

In the internal organs the nucleus of the schizont begins to divide and the pigment collects into a dark brown or black mass. The number of merozoites produced varies from eight to 32, but these extremes are rare. The periodicity is tertian, at about 48 hours.

Of peripheral red cells 25% or more may be infected and at this intensity a patient in his first attack, without acquired immunity (or passive from the mother in young infants), usually dies. Peak density is commonly reached in 10–14 days from the beginning of parasitaemia, after which the numbers quickly decline. In untreated cases short-term relapses can be expected once or twice a month for six to nine months, occasionally considerably longer.

Gametocytes (crescents) are never seen in the peripheral blood until about the tenth day of parasitaemia.

Gametocytes

P. vivax (Plate II.1). Mature gametocytes appear about the fifth day of a primary attack and immediately after a relapse. They are compact spherical bodies without vacuoles and with denser cytoplasm round a central nucleus. The red cells are enlarged and show Schüffner's dots. The fully grown gametocyte occupies most of the red cell, measuring 10–11 μm. The female stains bright blue with Romanowsky stains; the male is more grey. The male nucleus is larger than the female and stains more pink. In each the pigment is in the form of fine granules (coarser in the male) throughout the cytoplasm. The male gametocyte is smaller than the female.

The gametocytes take 4 days to mature, reaching their peak density 4–6 days after the peak of asexual forms. There are more females than males. Exceptionally, red cells may contain two gametocytes or a gametocyte and a schizont.

P. ovale. The gametocytes first appear, fully grown, on the fifth day of parasitaemia, becoming more numerous until in three weeks there are enough to infect mosquitoes effectively. They resemble solid asexual forms, but the scanty pigment is coarser and darker. They fill the red cells, measuring about 9 μm. Stained gametocytes have a lilac colour, less vivid in the males.

P. malariae. The gametocytes do not usually appear until late, about 5–23 days after the asexual forms. They are at peak density about 6 days after the peak of asexual forms and then they diminish. In endemic areas they are found only in young children.

The male has a large nucleus which stains pink, the cytoplasm being greenish-grey owing to fine black pigment granules. The parasite fills the red cell, which is not enlarged. The female is difficult to identify because it resembles the large uninucleate asexual form. It is spherical, about 7 μm, with a central nucleus and fine pigment granules. The cytoplasm stains deep blue.

P. falciparum (Plates I.14 and I.15). Elongated gametocytes are numerous in the peripheral blood of young children (maximum at nine months to two years of age) in endemic areas and after primary attacks, reaching 14.6×10^9/litre; they are rare in older children and adults. Young children are therefore the effective sources of mosquito infection.

The gametocytes appear in the peripheral blood in a wave, fully grown, 8–11 days after the asexual forms, rising to a peak and slowly falling until at about three weeks they have usually disappeared, though some may be found for several months. They are not numerous after the parasitaemia of short-term relapse, presumably because those of the first attack have provoked some immunity. If the first attack is aborted by quinine or Sulphamethazine, gametocytes appear 10–14 days later in enormous numbers.

The gametocytes are characteristically crescentic, but may be spindle-, diamond-, oat- or cigar-shaped, containing a few grains of pigment concentrated round the nucleus; the pigment does not clump as in the schizonts.

Occasionally certain inclusions known as Garnham bodies have been found in red cells harbouring developing gametocytes. These are thick filaments, loops or bars, staining deep red with Romanowsky stains. Their origin is uncertain.

Gametocytes of *P. falciparum* are not destroyed by the schizonticidal drugs, whereas gametocytes of *P. vivax* and probably also of *P. ovale* and *P. malariae* are destroyed by them.

INFECTION OF ANIMALS BY THE MALARIA PARASITES OF MAN

P. vivax. The chimpanzee is partially susceptible to sporozoites, which produce exo-erythrocytic schizonts pursuing a normal course, though blood infection is submicroscopic. If the spleen is removed the animal is much more vulnerable and parasitaemia is heavy, with the production of infective gametocytes and short-term relapses. *Aotus* monkeys are very susceptible, but rhesus monkeys are totally immune.

P. ovale. The chimpanzee has been infected with sporozoites, to the stage of exo-erythrocytic schizogony, but not further unless the spleen is removed, when the animal becomes completely susceptible, showing heavy parasitaemia, schizonts and gametocytes.

P. malariae. This is the only human parasite which occurs naturally in animals. In the chimpanzee it has repeatedly been found in nature in West Africa, though the incidence is low. It could conceivably be a natural source of infection for man. In the chimpanzee infection is light unless the spleen is removed, after which it flares up, with short-term relapses and the production of gametocytes.[13]

P. falciparum. Blood containing trophozoites has been shown to be infective to newborn mice and splenectomized gibbons and the gibbons have been infected by the bites of *Anopheles balabacensis*. *Aotus* monkeys are susceptible and young howler monkeys (*Alouatta palliata*) have also been infected by the injection of enormous numbers of blood forms. In the chimpanzee, sporozoites develop to exo-erythrocytic schizonts and merozoites invade red cells, but do not develop further unless the spleen is removed, when schizonts and gametocytes appear.

MALARIA PARASITES OF ANIMALS CAPABLE OF INFECTING MAN

Apart from *P. malariae* of chimpanzees, several other malaria parasites of primates can infect man.

Benign tertian type

P. cynomolgi is a tertian parasite of *Macaca irus*, *M. nemestrina*, *Presbytis* spp. and other monkeys of the Far East. It is capable of infecting a large variety of *Anopheles* and man is slightly susceptible to infection by sporozoites, though parasitaemia is light. Nevertheless, the clinical response may be quite severe and infections can last for some weeks.

P. cynomolgi bastianellii is a tertian parasite of *M. irus* in the Far East, transmitted by several species of *Anopheles*. Man has several times been infected accidentally in the laboratory when working with infected mosquitoes and, although parasitaemia is low, the clinical response with fever, enlargement of the spleen and liver and production of gametocytes is quite severe. In experimental work the red cells of Negroes are resistant whereas whites are susceptible; the red cells of New World monkeys are resistant, but liver stages have been found.

Ovale type

P. simium is a tertian parasite of ovale type, infecting *Alouatta fusca* in southern Brazil and, experimentally, *Saimiri sciureus* and *Callithrix jacchus*. Man has been infected in nature and can be infected by the bites of infected *Anopheles cruzi*.

Quartan type

P. brasilianum is a parasite of South American monkeys of the genera *Cacajao, Alouatta, Ateles, Cebus, Saimiri* and *Lagothrix*. It can be transmitted to man by the bite of infected *A. freeborni*, producing slight parasitaemia and quartan fever with splenomegaly. There is strong evidence that this species was derived from human infections of *P. malariae* in past centuries.

P. inui is normally a parasite of *Macaca irus* (formerly known as *M. inuus*, hence the name), *M. nemestrina, M. mulatta* and other monkeys. In the Far East it is transmitted by *A. stephensi* and can experimentally infect other *Anopheles*. Man can be infected experimentally by the blood forms, but parasitaemia and febrile reaction are slight.

P. shortti is a parasite of *M. radiata* and *M. sinica* of south India and Sri Lanka, probably transmitted by *A. stephensi*. Man has been infected experimentally with sporozoites, but the infection was mild.[14]

Knowlesi type

P. knowlesi is a quotidian (24-hour periodicity) parasite of *M. irus, M. nemestrina* and *Presbytis melalophos* in the Far East, in which it produces a low level of parasitaemia, though it is much more severe and fatal in *M. mulatta*. It is transmitted by *A. hackeri* and experimentally by several other species. Man is susceptible to inoculation of blood forms, which produce clinical effects varying from mild to severe; it has been used for malaria therapy of advanced syphilis. Chin et al[15] reported infection of man by mosquitoes in nature. *P. knowlesi* has been extensively used in studies on pathology and immunity in monkeys.

MALARIA PARASITES OF RODENTS AND BIRDS

The malaria parasites of rodents—*P. berghei, P. yoelii, P. vinckei* and *P. chabaudi*—have been much used in the study of parasites and their effects on vertebrate hosts. Man is not susceptible to them and they are therefore not described here. The same is true of the parasites of birds—*P. gallinaceum, P. relictum, P. cathemerium, P. circumflexum* and others.

Biologists who wish to study these parasites, or to use them for research are referred to the comprehensive book by Garnham.[1]

STAINING MALARIA PARASITES

The techniques briefly noted here are taken largely from a detailed paper by Shute;[15] readers are advised to consult the original.

Clean slides and neutral distilled water are essential for good results. Distilled water is usually too acid and if possible the pH should be tested. If this is not possible, a test can be made by adding a few drops of haematoxylin stain to 5 ml of water in a test-tube; if the solution remains reddish pink after shaking, the water is acid, and alkali (a few drops of saturated lithium carbonate or other alkali solution, after filtration) should be added—about five drops of alkali to 5 litres of distilled water is about right. Buffer salts are better:

potassium dihydrogen phosphate, KH_2PO_4	0.7 g
disodium hydrogen phosphate, Na_2HPO_4 (anhydrous)	1.0 g
distilled water	1000 ml

Alternatively buffer tablets may be used. The pH (normally 7.2) should be tested and necessary adjustments made. The solution keeps well for many months if well stoppered.

Thin films, Giemsa stain

Fix with 1–2 drops methanol; allow to evaporate. Make a 5% solution of the stain in the prepared distilled water, mix thoroughly and cover the film; leave for 20–30 minutes. Wash with distilled water from an aspirator.

Thin films, Leishman stain

With the slide on a level bench add 7–8 drops of stain. Leave for 20 seconds, *not more*, then add 12–15 drops of distilled water (pH 7.2). Mix thoroughly without spilling the stain; leave for 20 minutes and then wash off with distilled water from an aspirator.

Thick drops, Giemsa stain

The drops should be not too thick, about 10–15 leukocytes/field. They should be quite dry, having been protected against flies, which eat the blood. The slide should be placed in a plastic or glass staining jar, and the 5% stain (see above) should be gently poured on until the slide is submerged. Leave staining for 20 minutes and then gently run in distilled water at one end, from an aspirator, to wash off the stain. This stain diluted with distilled water stains the envelopes of erythrocytes; to overcome this, dilution with normal saline is advocated; it dissolves the envelopes and leaves a clear background. Good results are claimed if the thick drop is first lysed with 3 drops of 0.5 or 1% saponin solution for about 5 seconds (with gentle agitation); this is then drained off and the preparation is stained with Wright or Wright–Giemsa. The saponin does not appear to lyse the parasites and there is less background debris.[17]

To prepare Leishman stain

Into a clean, dry and securely stoppered polythene jar or hard glass flask, place about 50 large glass beads, 200 ml methanol (Analar) and 0.3 g of Leishman crystals. Stopper tightly and shake vigorously for a few minutes. Repeat the shaking at least six times at frequent intervals. The stain is ready in 24 hours.

Field's stain

Two solutions are used.

Solution A

Methylene blue (medicinal)	0.8 g
Azur 1	0.5 g
Disodium hydrogen phosphate (anhydrous)	5.0 g
Potassium dihydrogen phosphate	6.25 g
Distilled water	500 ml

Solution B

Eosin	1.0 g
Disodium hydrogen phosphate (anhydrous)	5.0 g
Potassium dihydrogen phosphate	6.25 g
Distilled water	500 ml

Dissolve the phosphate salts and then add the stain. Leave for 24 hours and then filter.

If the anhydrous salt is not available, sodium phosphate cryst. BP ($Na_2HPO_4.12H_2O$), 12.6 g, can be used.

In surveys of an infected population (preferably children) there may be heavy infections of 1000 parasites/mm^3 of blood. These can usually be found by examining a few fields of a thick film, but lighter infections of 100/mm^3 or less may be missed on such cursory examination.

The World Health organization[2] suggests that the standard time for examination of a thick blood film should be 5 minutes, during which the average microscopist can examine 100 fields, representing 0.1–0.2 mm^3 of blood. A thin film containing the same amount of blood will take 10–20 times as long to examine.

Disinfection of blood films where the possibility of arbovirus infection cannot be excluded

Thick and thin blood smears are made. Fix the thick smear on air dried slides directly in 10% buffered formalin for 15 minutes. Wash three times in buffered water at pH 7.0 and then stain with Giemsa. The thin smear should be fixed initially in methanol for 5 minutes before being fixed with formalin and treated as above for thick smears.

STAINING POST-MORTEM AND BIOPSY MATERIAL

Post-mortem material should be examined as soon as possible after death, because malaria parasites become unrecognizable within a few hours. Smears are better than sections because the parasites stain better, and smears can be made more quickly.[10]

Brain

A small portion no bigger than a pinhead is squashed between two dry slides, which are then dragged over each other, under pressure, to give two thin smears. When quite dry they are fixed for 5–10 minutes in methyl alcohol and stained with Giemsa (7 ml) in distilled water (100 ml) at pH 7–7.2 for 30 minutes, then flushed with distilled water and dried. They are soaked for 5 minutes in normal saline to remove most of the methylene blue from the tissue cells and washed with distilled water to remove all salt particles. In brain material the capillaries are well preserved. If a post-mortem cannot be conducted, material withdrawn in a large hollow needle inserted beneath the eyelid and through the orbital plate into the brain is satisfactory; suction is applied.

Spleen and other organs

A small piece of pulpy material from the spleen is broken down in a few drops of saline and thin films are prepared from this, fixed in methyl alcohol and stained with Giemsa. Material from the heart, liver, kidney and bone marrow can be treated in the same way.

CULTIVATION OF *P. FALCIPARUM* IN VITRO

About 10–20 ml of blood containing numerous rings of fairly large size (early rings do not grow well) are placed in a sterile test-tube and either defibrinated or prevented from clotting by the addition of heparin or sequestrene. The blood can be defibrinated with a thick wire passed through the cotton plug of the tube and with a loop at the lower end. The wire is rapidly rotated and then withdrawn with the clot, after which the tube is plugged. Then 0.2 ml of a 50% sterile solution of dextrose is added and mixed thoroughly. The tube is incubated upright at 37°C.

The erythrocytes quickly become sedimented below the buffy coat and the parasites grow in the erythrocytes immediately below the buffy coat. The tube must not be tilted when the upper erythrocytes are withdrawn by capillary pipette (with a little of the serum) for staining as thin films after incubation for various intervals up to 36–48 hours. Segmenting forms are usually most common after cultivation for 24–36 hours.

Trager has introduced a continuous culture method[18] which has been extremely valuable for the production of antigenic material from *P. falciparum*.

Growth medium RPMI 1640 supplemented with 25 mM Hepes buffer and 0.2% sodium carbonate, 10% AB human serum and a heparin solution (30 mg in 0.85% sodium chloride per 100 ml of blood) equivalent to 1/10 of the volume of red cells is allowed to flow from a reservoir over a thin layer of the stationary red cells into an overflow vessel at a rate of 50 ml per day in an atmosphere of 7% carbon dioxide or 5% oxygen and 95% nitrogen. Trophozoites are inoculated into the culture which is incubated at 38°C.

BABESIAE

FAMILY: BABESIIDAE (PIROPLASMS)

GENUS: *Babesia*

Members of this genus are parasites of cattle, dogs, rodents and other animals. Two species are known to infect man: *Babesia bovis* (*B. divergens*), a parasite of cattle found all over Europe and elsewhere, and *B. microti*, a parasite of rodents in North America and Europe. The parasites are intra-erythrocytic ring- and rod-shaped bodies which develop to become pear-shaped (piroplasms), resembling malaria parasites except that they contain no pigment and the cytoplasm remains pale (Fig. 1.19, Chapter 1). They multiply into two or into four bodies forming a tetrad, like a Maltese cross. Multiple invasion of the red cells is common. Garnham[19] finds that a useful distinction between *Babesia* and the malaria parasite is the presence, in *Babesia*, of 'what appears to be a white vacuole in some of the larger rings instead of the vacuole containing the pink stroma of the erythrocyte in the malaria ring'. A further means of distinguishing the

parasites is by culture, e.g. by Trager's method, when malaria pigment will appear in a malarial infection but not in one due to *Babesia*.

Transmission is transovarial, by ticks. *B. bovis* (*B. divergens*) is transmitted by *Boophilus* spp. and *B. microti* by a newly identified tick, *Ixodes dammini*, the reservoir hosts probably including deer mice and meadow voles. Diagnosis is made by the finding of the parasites in the peripheral blood or by the inoculation of blood into gerbils or hamsters for *B. microti* or into splenectomized calves for *B. bovis* (*B. divergens*). For the clinical features of infection (Chapter 1, p. 47).

The morphological features and classification of piroplasms and the taxonomy of the species infective to man have been reviewed by Hoare,[20] who holds that *B. divergens* should be regarded as a synonym of the older species, *B. bovis*. Others think that *B. divergens* is a valid species; Russian workers discard both in favour of *B. caucasica*, which, again, Hoare says is merely an intraspecific immunological strain (serodeme) and hence but another synonym of *B. bovis*.

COCCIDIA

ORDER: COCCIDIA

Coccidia are intracellular protozoa with a life-cycle consisting of an alternation of generations—an asexual cycle (*schizogony*) alternating with a sexual cycle (*sporogony*).

Life-cycle

The infective stage is the *oöcyst*, which contains two sporocysts each with four *sporozoites*, which is passed out in the stool to be ingested by a new host when the *sporozoites* are liberated to penetrate the epithelial cells of the bowel to develop into *schizonts*. The nucleus is divided by repeated fission until a number of daughter nuclei are produced and the schizont divides into as

many *merozoites*. When the cell bursts the merozoites are set free to enter other cells where they develop into schizonts. This is the asexual cycle or *schizogony*. In the sexual cycle (*sporogony*) the merozoites develop into male and female *gametocytes*. The male gametocyte divides further into small slender bodies (*microgametes*) which are liberated from the cell to enter the female cell (*macrogamete*) to form a fertilized cell (*zygote*). This secretes a tough membrane and becomes an *oöcyst*. Four coccidia are important in human disease: two, *Toxoplasma* and *Sarcocystis* have two hosts, one intermediate or prey (in which the asexual cycle is found) and the other definitive or predator in which the sexual cycle is found. The other two, *Isospora* and *Cryptosporidium*, have only one host, both cycles occurring in the one host.

GENUS: *Toxoplasma*

Life-cycle

Toxoplasma gondii has a sexual cycle (sporogony) of schizogony and gametogony in the intestinal epithelium of a definitive host (cat) and an asexual cycle of schizogony in the tissues of the intermediate or prey host—normally rodents, but also man.

Sexual cycle in the cat (enteric cycle)

Oöcysts ingested by the cat release *sporozoites* which enter the epithelial cells lining the intestine where they undergo *schizogony* to form *schizonts*. These in turn form *micro-* and *macrogametes* which fuse to form a *zygote* developing into an *oöcyst* which is passed out in the stool. The oöcyst contains two *sporocysts* each with four *sporozoites* ready to infect the new host.

Asexual cycle in man (toxoplasmic cycle)

Infection in man is from ingestion of oöcysts from infected cat faeces. The ingested sporozoites enter macrophages in the tissues in which they multiply as *endozoites* (Fig. I.9) forming a *pseudocyst*. The macro-

when they follow the enteric or toxoplasmic cycle as above, according to the type of host.

Morphology

In man only the asexual cycle has been observed, with endozoites and cystozoites.

Endozoites

Endozoites are typically curved or crescent-shaped organisms 4–6 μm in length and 2–3 μm in breadth with one end more rounded than the other. With Giemsa the cytoplasm stains blue and the nucleus is a red or purple mass. The ultrastructure as shown by electron microscopy reveals the organism to be a sporozoon. There is a distinct membrane surrounding a clump of densely staining material. A micropyle 100 nm thick is found in the centre of the organism inside of which are peripheral fibrils (toxonemes) terminating at the polar rim. The anterior tip is provided with a strong *conoid* or truncated cone in which are the anterior parts of the paired organelles which are the secreting *mitochondria*. A pseudocyst is small and contains up to 100 endozoites.

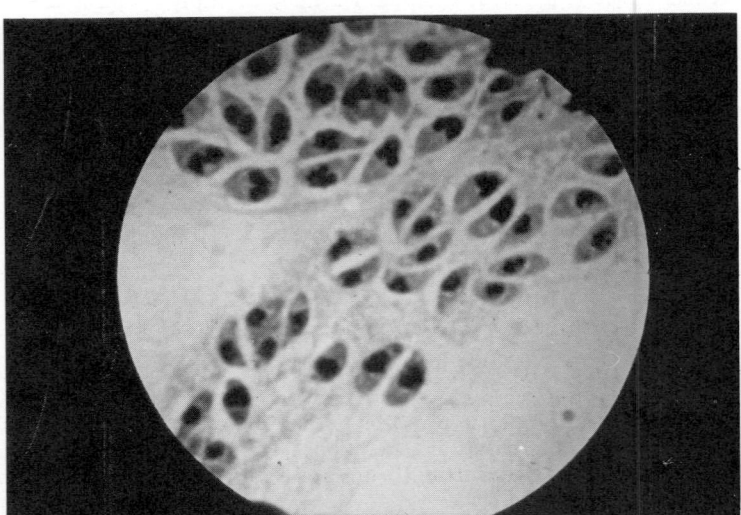

Fig. I.9 *Toxoplasma gondii* endozoites (trophozoites) in peritoneal exudate from a mouse. (Courtesy R. Lainson.)

phage walls rupture releasing the endozoites to infect fresh macrophages. As immunity develops true cysts, walled with parasite material, develop sealing off the contents from the immune defences of the host. These tissue cysts contain more numerous *cystozoites* which lie dormant, often for the whole of the host's life, until they are ingested by another intermediate or prey host

Cystozoites

Cystozoites are elongated sporozoite-like forms with a terminal nucleus each enclosed in a large red pellicle 6 μm in width. They are enclosed inside a tissue cyst which is larger—up to 100 μm in diameter—and contains thousands of cystozoites (Fig. I.10).

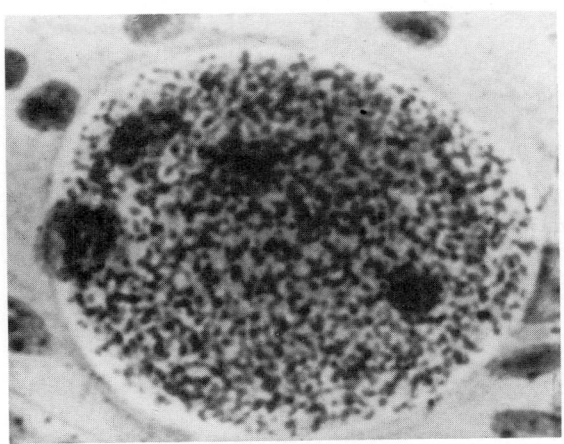

Fig. I.10 *Toxoplasma gondii* cystozoites in a cyst in mouse brain.

SUBORDER: SARCOSPORIDIA

GENUS: *Sarcocystis* (*Isospora*)
Isospora belli

Life-cycle

Isospora belli is a coccidian parasite with two cycles—asexual schizogony and sexual sporogony—in the epithelial mucosa of the human small intestine. Man is the only known host.

Asexual cycle (*schizogony*)

Mature oöcysts each containing two sporocysts each with four sporozoites excyst in the small intestine where the sporozoites invade the epithelial cells to form trophozoites. These mature into schizonts which then split up into merozoites to escape when the host cell ruptures and invade new cells.

Sexual cycle (*sporogony*)

Some merozoites develop into multicellular male gametocytes or unicellular female gametocytes. The male gametocyte ruptures liberating many microgametes which fertilize the macrogamete to form a zygote which is contained in an immature oöcyst to be passed out in the faeces where it sporulates to become infective after 48 hours.

Oöcyst

The immature oöcyst (Fig. I.11,1, and Fig. 17.23), which is seen in fresh faeces, is elongated with a tapering extremity ($12 \times 30 \mu$m in size) with a clear colourless wall containing an unsegmented zygote. After 48 hours further development takes place to form two ovoid sporoblasts each of which becomes enclosed to form two sporocysts (Fig. I.11,2) each containing four sporozoites. At this stage they are infective. For clinical features see Chapter 17.

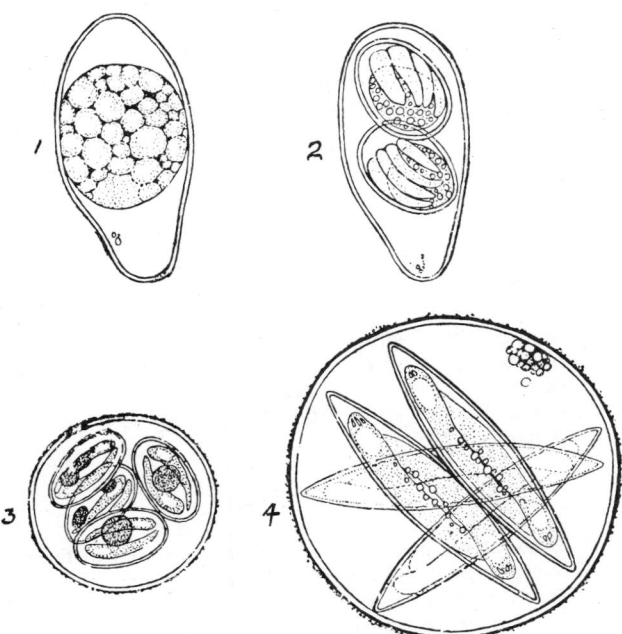

Fig. I.11 1, Immature oöcyst of *Isospora belli*. 2, Mature oöcyst of *Isospora belli* with sporocysts. 3, Fully developed oöcyst and spores of *Eimeria clupearum*. 4, Fully developed oöcyst and spores of *Eimeria sardinae*.

Sarcocystis bovihominis and S. suihominis

Sarcocystis is a coccidian parasite with two hosts, one intermediate or prey, the other definitive or predator. Man can be infected as a definitive host with two species; *S. bovihominis* and *S. suihominis* (*Isospora hominis*) and as an intermediate host by a number of as yet unidentified *Sarcocystis* species, probably of non-human primate origin.

Life-cycle in the definitive host man

Sarcocysts from beef or pork are eaten and burst in the small intestine to liberate numerous cystozoites which penetrate the epithelium of the intestinal mucosa to the subepithelial space where they undergo an asexual cycle (schizogony).

Asexual cycle (schizogony)

The cystozoites in the subepithelial tissues develop into further sarcocysts containing numerous merozoites which are released following rupture to form further sarcocysts.

Sexual cycle (sporogony)

After a period of time some merozoites enter the epithelial cells of the mucosa to form micro- and macrogametes. The microgametocytes break up into a number of microgametes which escape into the gut lumen where they fertilize the macrogametes to form oöcysts. The oöcyst develops two sporocysts each surrounded by a tough membrane and containing four sporozoites. At this time the sporocysts, which are passed out in the faeces, are infective.

Life-cycle in the intermediate host

(*S. suihominis* is specific for pigs and *S. bovihominis* for cattle.)

Infective sporocysts from the soil are eaten by pigs or cattle and sporozoites are released to enter vascular endothelium where they undergo schizogony forming numerous merozoites. After about a month the merozoites enter muscle cells (heart and oesophagus) where they secrete a cell wall inside which they multiply to form a sarcocyst containing numerous cystozoites (Fig. 17.24). The sarcocyst remains dormant in the tissues until eaten by the definitive host.

Sporocysts

Size: *S. bovihominis*: 13.1–17 μm × 7.7–10.8 μm. *S. suihominis*: 12.6 × 9.3 μm.

The sporocysts, which are usually shed singly, are fully sporulated containing sporozoites. In addition there is a *residual body* consisting of coarse loosely aggregated granules appearing polar in position and separate from the four sporozoites.

Sarcocyst

In muscle fibres the sarcocyst appears as an elongated cyst-like structure varying in size from a few micrometres to 325 μm in length. Within its covering membrane, which may be striated, the sarcocyst is divided by septa or trabeculae into numerous compartments containing many thousands of cystozoites.

Cystozoites

Cystozoites are uninuclear banana-shaped bodies with one rounded end and one pointed end measuring about 7 μm in length. Near the rounded end lies a vesicular nucleus (karyosome). The anterior third is occupied by a vacuole in which an apical complex structure can be recognized on electron microscopy.

GENUS: *Cryptosporidium*

Life-cycle

Cryptosporidium is a coccidian parasite with a life-cycle which takes place in the small intestine of man and other animals extracellularly in the mucoid material on the surface of the epithelial cells to which they attach themselves.

There is an asexual cycle (schizogony) and a sexual cycle (sporogony).

Asexual cycle

The *sporozoite*, which is liberated from the oöcyst, attaches itself to an epithelial cell and its nucleus divides to form a *schizont* 7 μm across containing eight nuclei. The schizont divides into eight *merozoites* each forming a new schizont (Fig. 17.25).

Sexual cycle

Merozoites form male and female gametocytes, the male fertilizing the female gamete to form an *oöcyst* containing four masses of cytoplasm each of which becomes a *sporozoite*. The oöcysts pass out in the faeces to be ingested by a new host in which they liberate sporozoites in the small intestine. Many oöcysts, however, liberate their sporozoites in the intestine while still in the host causing autoinfection (Chapter 17, Fig. 17.26).

GENUS: *Eimeria*

Cysts of the genus *Eimeria* have been seen in faeces but they are not really parasitic but are passed through the intestine after fish infected with *E. clupearum* or *E. sardinae* have been eaten (Fig. I.11,3 and 4).

AMOEBAE
Intestinal Amoebae
Class: Rhizopoda

Entamoeba histolytica Schaudinn, 1903

Entamoeba histolytica is a protozoon which normally lives and multiplies in the contents of the large intestine of man, but which can, in conditions which are not clear, invade the tissues, and in this pathogenic form can spread to the liver, brain, lungs, skin and other organs. The pathogenic forms can infect certain animals, especially kittens.

E. histolytica is closely related to *E. hartmanni*, which is considerably smaller and is never pathogenic.

There are several well-defined stages or forms: *trophozoites*, the vegetative, motile, dividing forms, which live either as commensals feeding on intestinal contents, or as pathogenic tissue-invading forms, ingesting erythrocytes, leukocytes and tissue debris, and producing necrosis in the bowel wall, liver, etc.

The commensal trophozoites are rather smaller than the pathogenic forms, and are therefore sometimes referred to as 'minuta' forms, but they are bigger than *E. hartmanni*. The dimensions are given in Table I.2.

The trophozoites (size 10–40 μm) have a characteristic nucleus (2.8–4.5 μm), a small central karyosome and peripheral chromatin in the form of fine granules (Figs. 17.8a and I.12,1). The cytoplasm has two zones—outer with clear ectoplasm, and inner with granular endoplasm, enclosing food vacuoles which, in pathogenic strains, usually contain ingested erythrocytes.

Trophozoites multiply by binary fission. In wet preparations they move sluggishly by suddenly thrusting out pseudopodia from the ectoplasm, into which the other contents of the cell flow. This has been described as like a slug moving at express speed.

Cysts

The trophozoites inhabit the crypts of the caecum and the first part of the colon, where they feed on mucus and its contents and probably live in symbiosis with intestinal bacteria. As they pass down the colon, and the faecal material becomes drier, the conditions are less favourable, and the trophozoites protect themselves by encysting, though what factors actually influence encystment are uncertain—one element seems to be the right bacterial flora. The cysts are quiescent and resist various environmental conditions which would be fatal to trophozoites. In this process the trophozoites discharge undigested food and condense into a spherical mass (the *precystic stage*) (Fig. 17.8g), with a tough wall and still a single nucleus. They may contain a mass of glycogen and chromatoid bodies which stain black with iron haematoxylin

The next stage is the development of the fully formed cyst. In the fresh state this has a greenish, refractile appearance. At 9.5–17.5 μm this is smaller than the trophozoite, and more compact. The nucleus divides by mitosis to produce two, then four nuclei, which have the same characteristics as the nucleus of the trophozoite, though they become smaller. Each nucleus has a central karyosome and peripheral chromatin granules, as in the trophozoite (Figs. I.12,2 and 3, and 17.18).

The cyst wall is relatively tough and within it there are one or more chromatoid bodies—oval bars staining black with iron haematoxylin—and in the early stages glycogen staining golden brown with iodine. The gly-

Table I.2 Differential characters of entamoebae of the *E. histolytica* complex.

	E. hartmanni	E. histolytica forms	
		Minuta	Large haematophagous
Trophozoite			
Body	3.0–10.5 μm	10.0–20.0 μm	20.0–40.0 μm
Nucleus	1.5– 3.2 μm	2.8–4.5 μm	
Cyst			
Body	3.8– 8.0 μm	9.5–17.5 μm	
Nuclei			
1	1.8– 3.0 μm	4.0– 5.5 μm	Absent (cysts produced only
2	1.3– 2.0 μm	2.0– 3.2 μm	by minuta forms)
4	0.7– 1.7 μm	1.4– 2.6 μm	
Glycogen	Small vacuoles	One large vacuole	

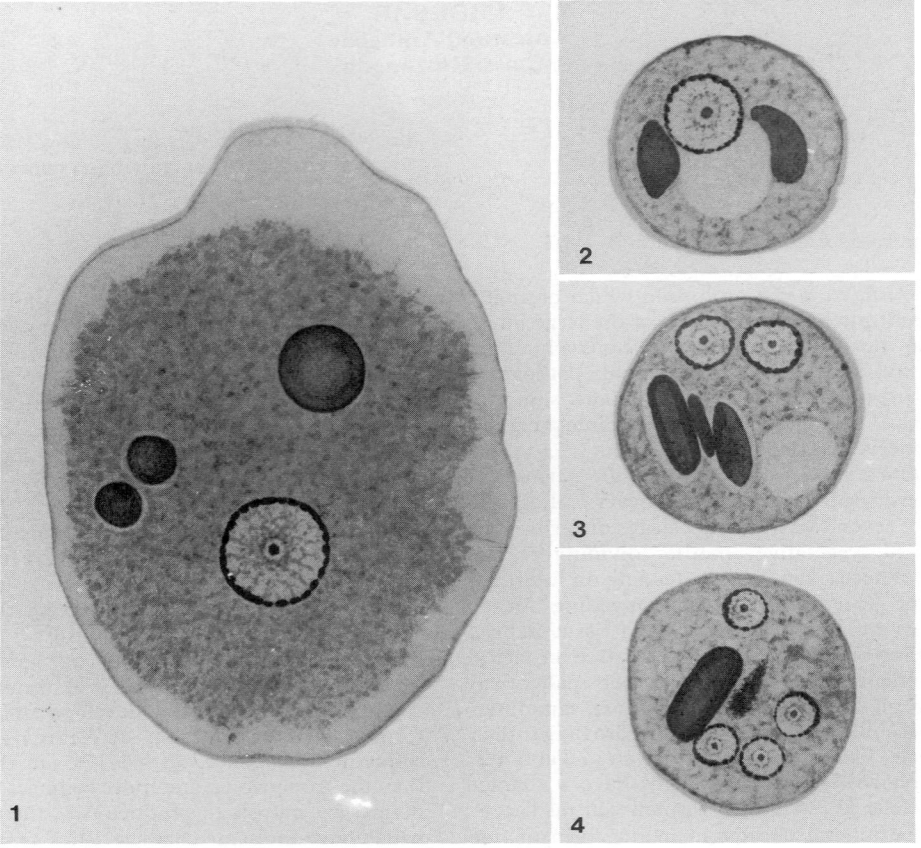

Fig. I.12 *Entamoeba histolytica.* 1, Active amoeboid form with ingested red blood cells. 2, Uninucleate cyst. 3, Binucleate cyst. 4, Quadrinucleate cyst.

cogen gradually disappears, presumably being metabolized, and the chromatoid bodies become less conspicuous.

Cysts are usually found without trophozoites in the faeces of infected persons not suffering from actual disease, but in such persons trophozoites can be demonstrated after a purgative has been given. Cysts are never found in liver abscesses or lesions of other organs; only the haematophagous trophozoites are found in such lesions.

Cysts are the only infective forms. They are passed in faeces and can resist external environmental conditions which are not too extreme—for instance they can remain viable in an ice box at 4–8°C for several days, in cool faeces for 12 days or more, in cool water for several weeks. They can withstand passage through the intestines of filth flies, and viable cysts and even trophozoites have been recovered from the vomit and faeces of flies. Cysts can pass through cockroaches and remain viable. They are sensitive, however, to desiccation and to temperatures above 50°C and below −5°C. They can resist 1 in 2500

mercury bichloride, 5% hydrochloric acid or 0.5% formalin for 30 minutes, and 1 in 500 potassium permanganate for 24–48 hours. They are killed by 1 in 20 cresol in 15 minutes, by 1% phenol in 30 minutes and by 5% acetic acid at 30°C in 15 minutes. They have considerable resistance to chlorine, but can be killed in drinking water by superchlorination and by iodine. Recorded experiments vary in the figures given for superchlorination. A *residual* of 2–3 ppm of chlorine kills over 99% of cysts in 20–30 minutes, but this is influenced by the organic content of the water. If the organic content is high, for instance through faecal contamination, the required concentration of chlorine is also high. Dechlorination is necessary in this process. Ozone at 0.5–1.0 ppm kills over 99% of cysts within 5 minutes, but ozone dissipates quickly and leaves no effective residual. Cysts pass through Mark O microstraining metal fabric (aperture 23 μm).[21] This is sometimes used as part of a treatment process for domestic water supplies. In relation to cysts coagulation and sand filtration are needed as well as chlorination.

When trophozoites are swallowed, they are destroyed in the acid contents of the stomach; cysts are not, and can therefore pass into the alkaline small intestine where excystation takes place, a mature cyst yielding eight small amoebae after metacystic development.[22,23] In this cycle there is normally no invasion of the intestinal wall, no ulceration and no spread beyond the intestinal lumen. The trophozoites and cysts in this cycle, though belonging to the large race (as distinct from *E. hartmanni*), may apparently be non-pathogenic (and worldwide) or pathogenic (mostly in hot countries). Yet the potentially pathogenic race can apparently live as non-pathogenic, commensal inhabitants of the intestinal lumen without invading the tissues, until some influence, at present obscure, causes the trophozoites to invade the intestinal mucosa and deeper tissues. These now pathogenic and invasive trophozoites destroy tissue, ingest red blood cells and tissue debris and, perhaps because of improved nutrition, become generally much larger than the commensal trophozoites. In faeces, active amoebae containing ingested red blood cells can confidently be diagnosed as *E. histolytica*.

The non-pathogenic entamoebae are sometimes called 'minuta' forms because, though belonging to the large race, they are smaller than the pathogenic invasive forms (Table I.3).[24] But they are not *E. hart-*

The virulent zymodemes are potentially pathogenic and in certain circumstances (as has been stated) can invade the tissues, causing disease. The mechanism by which pathogenic *E. histolytica* gains entry into the tissues is not clearly understood. It can hydrolyse casein, fibrin, haemoglobin and the epithelium of guinea-pig gut. It has tryptic and peptic activity and most pathogenic strains contain hyaluronidase and other enzymes. Trophozoites of various strains (pathogenic and non-pathogenic) are cytotoxic to leukocytes of some animals. Yet all these facts are not enough to explain invasiveness. These invasive entamoebae, causing disease, feed on erythrocytes both in the tissues and when they escape into the lumen of the bowel, and because they are in a better state of nutrition they increase in size to 20–40 μm. These large trophozoites (sometimes described as 'magna' forms) multiply and are passed out in the faeces, where they can be recognized by their morphology, movements and the presence of ingested erythrocytes.

Culture

E. histolytica may be cultured on special media to which *Trypanosoma cruzi* or *Escherichia coli* are added or axenically on diphasic medium.[26]

Table I.3 Aetiology of amoebiasis.

Hypotheses	Unicystic 1913	Dualistic 1925	Neodualistic 1957
Non-pathogenic amoebiasis	*E. histolytica* SMALL RACE LARGE RACE: Commensal phase ('minuta' form)	*E. hartmanni* *E. dispar*	*E. hartmanni* *E. histolytica* Avirulent large race ?
Pathogenic amoebiases			Virulent large race:
Subclinical		*E. dysenteriae*	Dormant in lumen of gut
Clinical	Virulent (tissue) phase ('magna' form)		Invading gut wall

After Hoare.[24]

manni, which is also non-pathogenic and even smaller, forming cysts with four nuclei, and which never invades the tissues (Fig. 17.2).

The aggressive pathogenic trophozoites which invade tissues do not give rise to cysts. They pass out in the faeces and, because they do not possess the defensive properties of cysts, they are a dead end in the chain of reproduction. Cysts are formed only by the commensal trophozoites.[25]

Criteria of pathogenicity

E. histolytica has been separated electrophoretically into a number of zymodemes which are populations of amoebae differing from each other in the electrophoretic mobility of their enzymes. Four enzymes are studied and to date 20 zymodemes have been described, distributed on a geographical basis of which only nine are pathogenic (invasive) (Figs. I.13 and

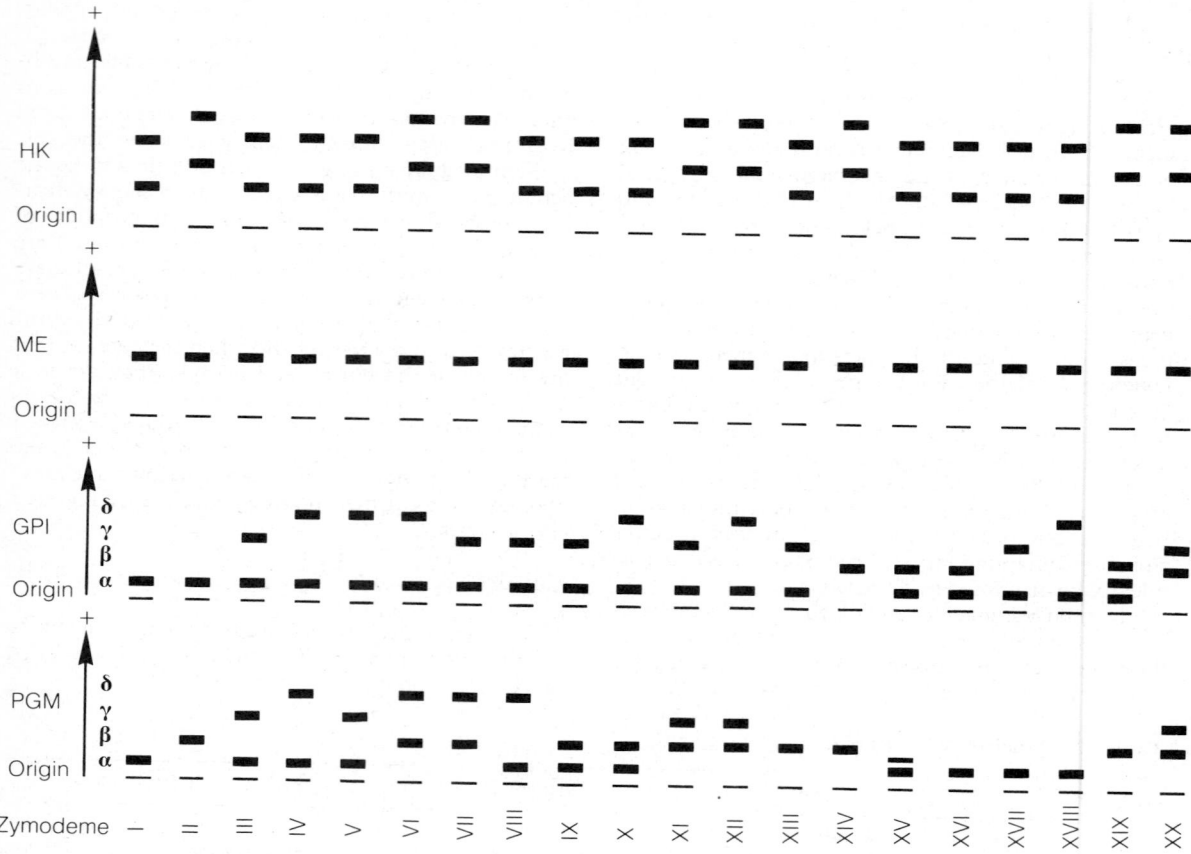

Fig. I.13 Zymodemes of *E. histolytica*[27] identified using EC 5.3.1.9 glucose phosphate isomerase (GPI); EC 1.1.1.40 L-malate : NADP + oxidoreductase (oxaloacetate decarboxylating) (ME); EC 2.7.5.1 phosphoglucomutase (PGM); and EC 2.7.1.1 hexokinase (HK). The markers for pathogenicity are the absence of the α band together with the presence of the β band in PGM. Advanced bands in HK confirm the PGM result. The only exception is zymodeme XIII which lacks advanced HK bands. There are six pathogenic (invasive) zymodemes distributed on a geographical basis: I, VI, VII, XII, XIII, XIV.

I.14).[27] Another criterion of pathogenicity is resistance to lysis by human serum, non-pathogenic strains being susceptible and pathogenic strains being resistant.[28]

Recognition and preservation of *E. histolytica*
(Chapter 17, Fig. 17.8 and Appendix IV, p. 1491)

Permanent preparations of *E. histolytica* in stools can be made using a fixative stain.

The Merthiolate–iodine–formaldehyde (MIF) fixative stain consists of 250 ml distilled water, 200 ml tincture of Merthiolate (1 in 1000), 25 ml formaldehyde and 5 ml glycerol, to which 10–15 parts of fresh Lugol's 5% iodine in 10% potassium iodide in distilled water are added. This may be used for direct smears or for preserving faeces. For preservation 0.15 ml of Lugol solution is placed in a tube, followed by 2.35 ml of the MIF solution, and 0.25 g of faeces is added and thoroughly mixed. The parasites are well preserved.

Trophozoites of *E. histolytica* can be detected in faecal specimens by the fluorescent antibody technique with the use of high titre antiamoebic sera.[29]

Entamoeba moshkovskii (Tshalaia, 1941)

This species resembles *E. histolytica* in both trophozoite and cystic stages and has been recovered from sewage in Moscow, USA, England and Brazil. Attempts to infect laboratory animals have been unsuccessful. *E. invadens*, a parasite of snakes, is also morphologically identical with *E. histolytica*.

Entamoeba coli (Grassi, 1879)

Unlike *E. histolytica*, this amoeba does not invade tissues; it is therefore a non-pathogenic species and a harmless commensal in the intestinal tract of man. A similar amoeba is found in monkeys and rats.

E. coli is a very common parasite in the tropics and

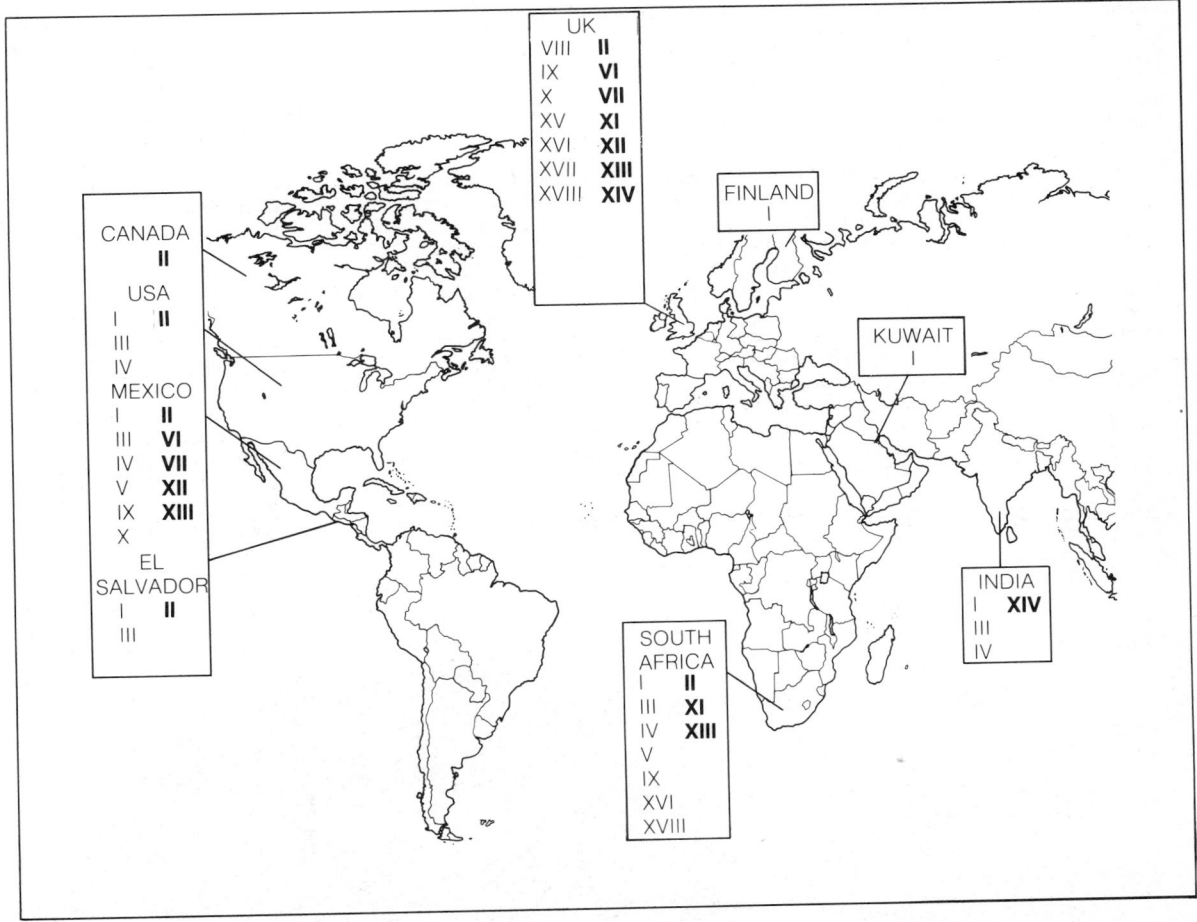

Fig. I.14 Geographical distribution of 18 *E. histolytica* zymodemes. Zymodeme number associated with clinical symptoms given a bold typeface, those not associated with clinical symptoms given in normal typeface. (From Sargeaunt et al.[27])

wherever sanitation is primitive it is probable that no individual escapes infection. On the average, *E. coli* is larger than *E. histolytica*, but varies greatly. The active vegetative stage measures from 10 to 40 μm, but is usually 20–30 μm in diameter. It normally lives in the large intestine, does not invade tissues, but develops in intestinal contents, where it ingests bacteria, yeasts and other material. *E. coli* can be differentiated from *E. histolytica* by means of the fluorescent antibody technique.

Generally speaking, movements are much more sluggish than those of *E. histolytica* and the individuals are less active (Table I.4 and Fig. 17.8b). The organism does not move across the slide, but remains stationary. The ectoplasm is not clearly defined but is represented by a superficial clearer area merging into the endoplasm. This is extensively vacuolated and food vacuoles contain bacteria, yeasts or even cysts of other protozoa, such as *E. histolytica*, *Giardia* and *Isospora*. Red blood corpuscles or tissue elements are not ingested. In general, *E. coli* is faintly grey, contrasting with the greenish tint and higher refractive index of *E. histolytica*. Sometimes individuals show various fissures or rectangular vacuoles representing degenerative changes.

The *nucleus*, compared with that of *E. histolytica*, is larger, coarser and more easily visible in the living organism (Fig. I.15). The chromatin granules on the nuclear membrane are relatively coarse, and there are others on the linin network. The karyosome, larger than that of *E. histolytica*, is usually eccentric in position, surrounded by a clear area intersected by linin network with chromatin granules. These nuclear characteristics are best seen in fresh specimens but are obscured in degenerate individuals. *E. coli* reproduces by binary fission.

Table I.4 Differential characters of the common intestinal amoebae.

Character	*Entamoeba coli*	*Entamoeba histolytica*	*Endolimax nana*
Size	10–40 μm	10–40 μm	6–12 μm
Morphology	No distinction between endo and ectoplasm	Granular endoplasm; clear ectoplasm	Granular and rather vacuolated cytoplasm
Ingests	Bacteria, other protozoa, etc.	Red cells, tissue cells, etc.	Bacteria and food granules
Nucleus	Distinct in fresh specimens. Coarse chromatin granules on nuclear membrane. Eccentric karyosome surrounded by coarse ring	Inconspicuous in fresh specimens. Fine chromatin granules on nuclear membrane. Central karyosome surrounded by delicate ring	Clear nuclear membrane and massive irregular karyosome
Movement	Sluggish movement with granular pseudopodia	Active movement with clear, blunt pseudopodia	Sluggish movement with clear pseudopodia
Multiplication	By binary fission in faeces. Encystment and formation of spherical cysts. 10–30 μm in diameter, with 1, 2, 4 or 8 nuclei	By binary fission. Encystment and formation of spherical cysts, 9.5–17.5 μm in diameter, with 1, 2 or 4 nuclei	By binary fission in faeces. Encystment and formation of nucleated oval cysts 8–10 μm in length by 4–5 μm in breadth, with 1, 2 or 4 nuclei
Chromatoid bodies	Typically not present in the mature cyst	Especially present in mature cyst	Not present in the cyst

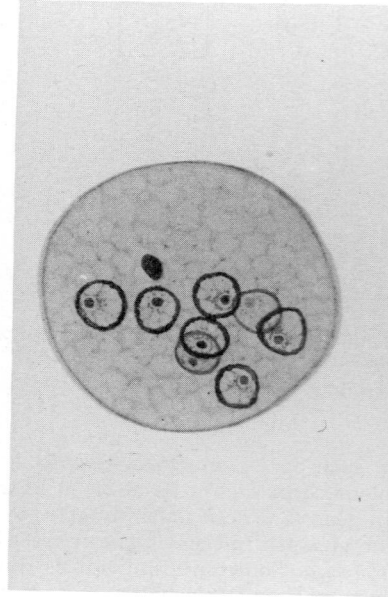 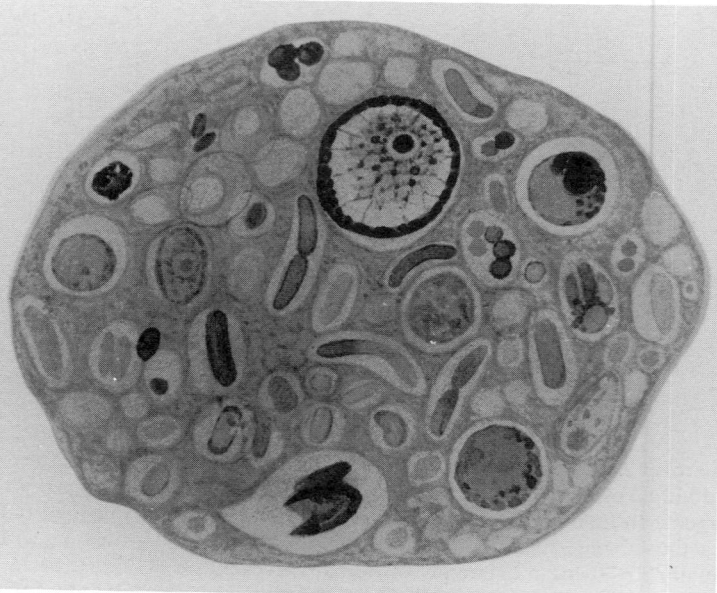

Fig. I.15 *Entamoeba coli. Left,* Cyst with eight nuclei. *Right,* Active amoeboid stage with ingested food material; note the characteristic nucleus with eccentric karyosome.

Precystic forms

Before encystment the amoebae undergo reduction in size, with the result that precystic forms are especially difficult to distinguish from those of *E. histolytica*, but are usually larger. Precystic forms are probably formed by division of larger individuals.

Cysts

The cyst wall is secreted round a spherical precystic amoeba. Individual cysts vary greatly in size, from 10 to 30 μm. Like *E. histolytica*, *E. coli* is a composite species consisting of a number of races distinguished by the dimensions of the cysts.

The cyst is at first uninucleate, the nucleus having the same characteristics as that of the active form. It divides repeatedly by mitosis, the nuclei progressively diminishing in size as their number increases. The quadrinucleate stage is passed through very rapidly and is therefore rarely seen. The mature cyst typically contains eight nuclei. Immature binucleate and quadrinucleate cysts are occasionally seen, even supernucleate cysts with 16 nuclei. The binucleate cyst frequently contains a large quantity of glycogen, which replaces almost the entire cytoplasm, but this usually disappears before the quadrinucleate stage is reached (Fig. 17.8d).

Chromatoid bodies are usually not present, but, when they are, they appear as small granular, spicular or rod-like bodies, more especially in the binucleate stage. In the mature octonucleate form they may occasionally be seen as pointed threads or splinters, thus differing from the stouter bodies with blunted ends common in *E. histolytica*. When hatching, an octonucleate amoeba escapes from the cyst and gives rise to eight uninucleate amoebulae.

The life-history of *E. coli* resembles that of *E. histolytica*, except that the vegetative forms inhabit only the faeces. This protozoan may be cultivated, but with difficulty, on the same media as are employed for *E. histolytica*. It is not affected by emetine. Cysts of *E. coli* can withstand drying while those of *E. histolytica* cannot. The cyst wall consists of two layers—a thick inner and a flexible outer wall measuring 1 μm in diameter.

Incidence

E. coli is common in man in temperate zones as well as in the tropics and found in about 15% of normal people. It is most readily seen in dysenteric cases with diarrhoea. Some monkeys harbour a parasite closely resembling it.

Entamoeba polecki

E. polecki is now known to be *E. histolytica*.

Entamoeba gingivalis (Gros, 1949)

This amoeba (Fig. I.16) is of interest, not only for its occurrence in the mouth, but also because it was the first to be discovered in man. The claim that it might prove to be the cause of pyorrhoea alveolaris has been disproved. This species has been found in pulmonary suppuration by bronchoscopy. The importance of this lies in its differentiation from *E. histolytica*. *E. gingivalis* may be found in the sputum where it can be mistaken for *E. histolytica* from a pulmonary abscess.

E. gingivalis is a small species with great variations in size, from 10 to 25 μm depending on its metabolic activity. As in *E. histolytica*, endoplasm and ectoplasm

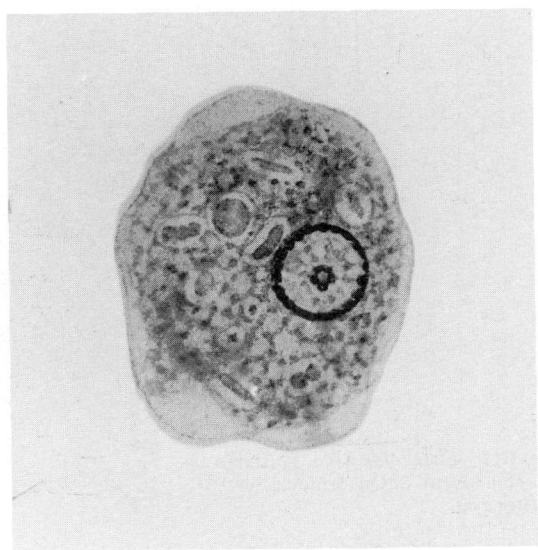

Fig. I.16 *Entamoeba gingivalis* in the active amoeboid form, with eccentric nucleus and ingested bodies.

are sharply differentiated. The cytoplasm is occupied by food vacuoles and peculiar inclusions of a greenish refractile appearance of undetermined nature, which may be the remains of salivary corpuscles or polymorphonuclear cells; there are also numbers of ingested bacteria.

The *nucleus* is similar to that of *E. coli*. It is 2.5–3 μm, spherical and vesicular but slightly smaller in proportion to the rest of the organism than in *E. histolytica* or *E. coli*. The nuclear membrane is a definite structure, and is lined with peripheral chromatic granules.

E. gingivalis probably reproduces by binary fission, although all intermediary stages have not been studied and it is probable also that it does not form cysts.

Endolimax nana (Wenyon & O'Connor, 1917)

This is a non-pathogenic species (Fig. I.17) commonly inhabiting the intestinal tract of man (mainly of the large and to a lesser extent of the small intestine), especially in the tropics, and it is of importance because the spherical quadrinucleate cysts resemble those of the small race of *E. histolytica*; moreover, it is found in 33% of dysenteric or diarrhoeic faeces, and is often very abundant indeed.

E. nana is a small species, 6–12 μm in diameter, it has a characteristic vesicular *nucleus* with a large irregularly shaped karyosome. It ingests food granules and bacteria, but not red blood corpuscles or cells. Its movements are sluggish, but it may become quite active on a warm stage.

The *cysts* (Figs. 17.8e and I.17) are of approximately the same size and appearance as the active form. When

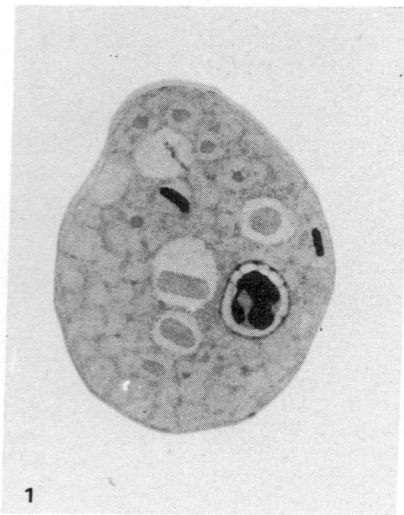 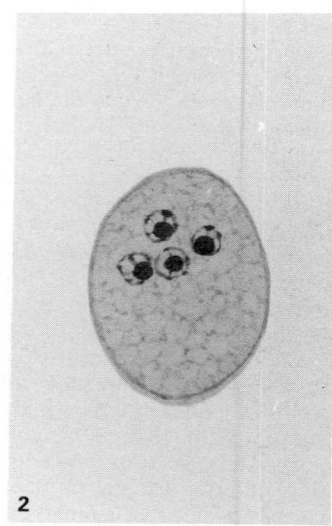

Fig. I.17 *Endolimax nana.* 1, Active amoeboid form. 2, Quadrinucleate mature cyst.

fully mature they have characteristic nuclei and contain a few refractile granules, but are devoid of vacuoles or chromatoid bodies. Sometimes they contain glycogen, especially the binucleate forms. In shape they vary from that of a typical oval to a sphere. Small individuals measure 6 μm in diameter. Occasionally, they contain small filamentous rods or granules.

E. nana is certainly non-pathogenic and is not amenable to emetine. This species has been successfully cultured on serum and egg media.

Iodamoeba bütschlii (Von Prowazek, 1912)
(Endolimax williamsi)

Cysts of this species have long been known in man as 'iodine', or 'I' cysts, and similar organisms are found in the faeces of monkeys and pigs.

I. bütschlii (Fig. I.18) is small, intermediate in size between *E. coli* and *E. nana*, measuring 9–20 μm in diameter, though smaller individuals, 5 μm in size, may occur. In form and habit it resembles small specimens of *E. coli*. The cytoplasm contains food vacuoles with bacteria and other food particles. There is no marked differentiation of ecto- and endoplasm. The movements are sluggish, like those of *E. coli*.

The *nucleus*, which is often indistinguishable in specimens containing many food granules, is large, being in diameter one-quarter to one-fifth of the whole organism. There is a large conspicuous karyosome which has a diameter of one-third to one-half of the nucleus.

The *cysts* are uninucleate, frequently irregular in outline, measuring 7–15 μm in diameter. There is a distinct cyst wall and inside the cyst is a rounded refractile body with a number of small *volutin* granules. There is usually a large and dense glycogen mass which shows up clearly in iodine solution and

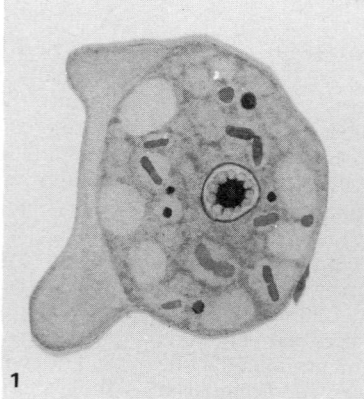 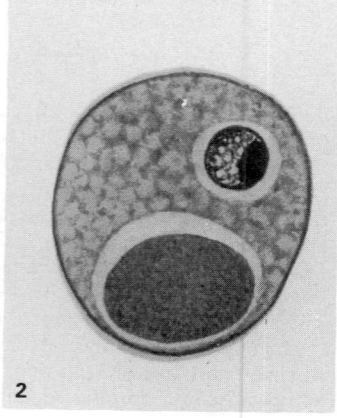

Fig. I.18 *Iodamoeba bütschlii.* 1, Active amoeboid form with ingested microorganisms. 2, Mature cyst (iodine cyst) containing a large iodine-staining glycogen mass.

sometimes even two or three separated masses may be observed within the same cyst (Fig. 17.8f).

The cyst nucleus, eccentrically placed, is comparatively large, 2–3 μm in diameter, while the karyosome, which is centrally placed in the nuclei of the precystic stage, gradually passes, during encystment, to the periphery, showing up as a large compact mass in close contact with the nuclear membrane.

It is remarkable that very large numbers of cysts may be present in the faeces without any evidence of free forms. The mature uninucleate cysts, save for the disappearance of the contained glycogen, do not undergo any further changes outside the human body.

It is estimated that *I. bütschlii* occurs in 5% of human faeces, most commonly in the tropics, and is found not infrequently in association with *E. histolytica*. Both the active forms as well as the cysts are amenable to emetine and emetine and bismuth iodide. This amoeba has been cultivated on egg medium and Locke's solution.

Dientamoeba fragilis (Jepps & Dobell, 1918)

This is a small species (Fig. I.19) which may measure 3.5 μm, but its usual size is 8–9 μm; it inhabits the large intestine of man and has also been found in monkeys (macaques in the Philippines). It is very actively motile, throwing out pseudopodia which are lobed and indented. Each amoeba is typically binucleate. The spherical *nucleus*, measuring 0.8–2.3 μm, contains six chromatin granules. The two nuclei are connected by a thread (*centrodesmose*). In fresh preparations the amoeba rapidly degenerates and vacuoles form. It lives exclusively on bacteria and small microorganisms, and is apparently amenable to emetine. No cystic stage is known.

There is evidence that this amoeba is closely related

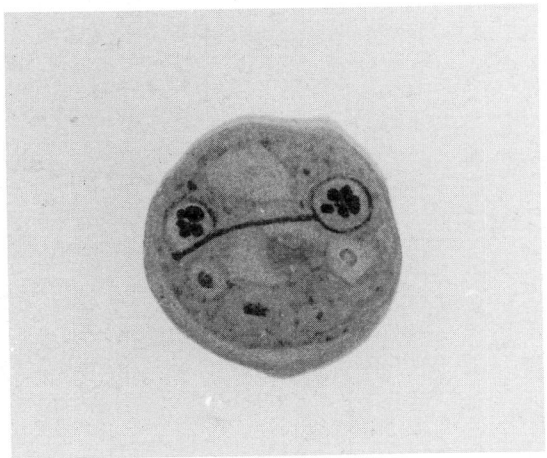

Fig. I.19 Binucleate forms of *Dientamoeba fragilis*.

to the flagellate *Histomonas meleagridis* (the parasite of 'blackhead of turkeys') which normally lives as a flagellate in the caecum, but can invade the liver, where it assumes the amoeboid form.

Burrows and Swerdlow[30] have recorded an abnormally high association between the incidence of *D. fragilis* and that of *Enterobius vermicularis*. Of 22 appendices harbouring *D. fragilis*, 12 were also infected with the pinworm. The association is supported to some extent by the supposed passage of *Histomonas meleagridis* of turkeys through the nematode, *Heterakis*.

Most human amoebae are liable to be parasitized by a fungus *Sphaerita*—consisting of a small spherical mass of coccus-like bodies, which are refractile and occur within vacuoles of the cytoplasm.

Free-living amoebae

GENUS: *Naegleria*

These free-living amoeba have been shown to cause primary amoebic meningoencephalitis (Chapter 24, p. 572). Their life-cycle is shown in Fig. I.20.

Morphology

Living amoebae in wet smears of cerebrospinal fluid.[31] The amoebae are slug-shaped, with one broad and one pointed extremity and are actively motile at 21°C. Movement is directional and quite brisk. Temporarily rounded forms, with diameters varying between 6 and 15 μm, may be found. A hyaline ectoplasmic layer is well differentiated from a finely granular endoplasm containing up to six small clear vacuoles. The nucleus

is distinctive, with a centrally located nucleolus. A few organisms undergo a transient flagellate transformation, which is a free-living form of the parasite.

Morphology in sections. When stained with haematoxylin and eosin the amoebae have a diameter between 6 and 9 μm, and may be as large as 12 μm. There is a very fine haematoxophilic cell membrane, usually giving rise to a circular occasionally oval, outline, which may be irregular. The cytoplasm has distinctive outer and inner zones, the outer packed with coarse magenta-stained granules and clear vacuoles, amorphous eosinophilic fragments and occasional red blood cells and granules of polymorphonuclear lymphocytes. The inner zone, up to half the diameter, consists of four to six vacuoles sur-

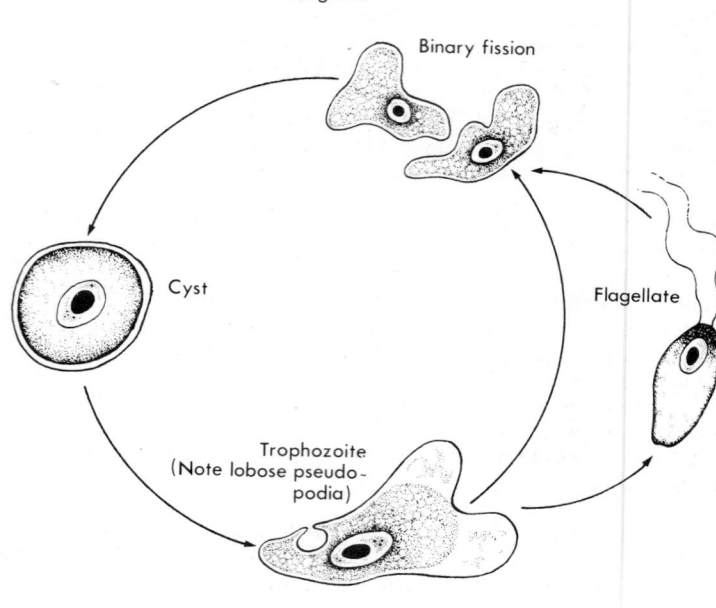

Naegleria

Binary fission

Cyst

Flagellate

Trophozoite
(Note lobose pseudo-podia)

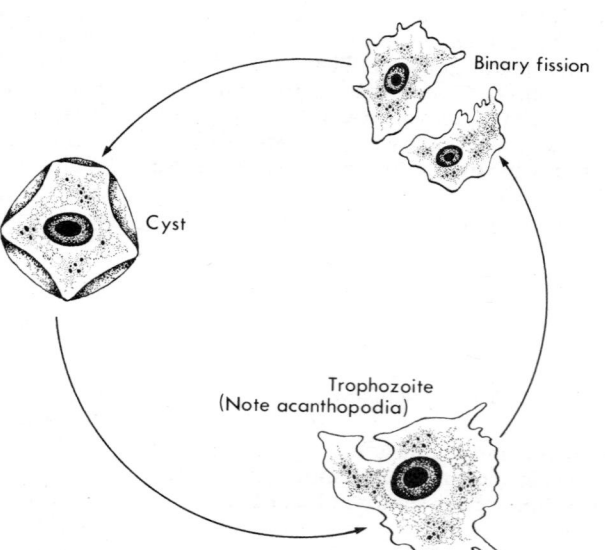

Acanthamoeba (Hartmannella)

Binary fission

Cyst

Trophozoite
(Note acanthopodia)

Fig. I.20   Life-cycles of *Naegleria* and *Acanthamoeba*. (Courtesy Dr D. C. Warhurst.)

rounding the nucleus, which is usually single, eccentrically situated and measures up to 2 μm in diameter. The nucleus contains a centrally located nucleolus 1 μm in diameter.

Culture

The amoebae may be cultured in a proteose–peptone–

glucose medium (PPG)[32] and the cultures, inoculated intranasally in to mice, cause fatal meningoencephalitis within 5 days.

The type species, *Naegleria gruberi*, is usually thought to be non-pathogenic to man, but that it is always so is not accepted by some authorities. Most human infections have been caused by *N. fowleri* which differs from *N. gruberi* in its fine structure, in the morphology and behaviour of its cysts (they do not resist freezing and desiccation as do those of *N. gruberi*) and in its greater cultural fastidiousness.[33]

GENUS: *Acanthamoeba* (*Hartmannella*)

The genera *Hartmannella* and *Acanthamoeba* are regarded as synonymous by some authorities, but others have found antigenic differences. Within *Acan-*

thamoeba (*Hartmannella*) there is much antigenic overlap between different species and strains. Morphologically they resemble *Naegleria* spp. but the trophozoites of *Acanthamoeba* move very slowly compared with those of *N. fowleri* and are furnished with thorn-like processes (acanthapodia). *Acanthamoeba* spp. have caused infections of the eye and also, rarely, primary amoebic meningoencephalitis.

INTESTINAL FLAGELLATES

ORDER: POLYMASTIGIDA
FAMILY: MONADIDAE

GENUS: *Enteromonas*

Enteromonas hominis (Da Fonseca, 1915)
Tricercomonas intestinalis (Wenyon & O'Connor, 1917)

This is a minute but very active pyriform flagellate, measuring $4–10 \times 3–6 \, \mu m$. The posterior end is attenuated to a fine point (Fig. I.21).

The *nucleus* is single and vesicular and three flagella of equal length arise from a blepharoplast. A fourth *flagellum* runs down the margin of the body to the posterior extremity and ends in a terminal lash. The combined movements of all these produce a sort of 'hovering effect' when in full action.

The *cysts* are small, oval, with a distinct cyst wall, resemble fungus spores, and contain iodophilic refractile bodies. This flagellate can be cultivated with comparative ease on Locke-egg medium. There is no evidence of pathogenicity.

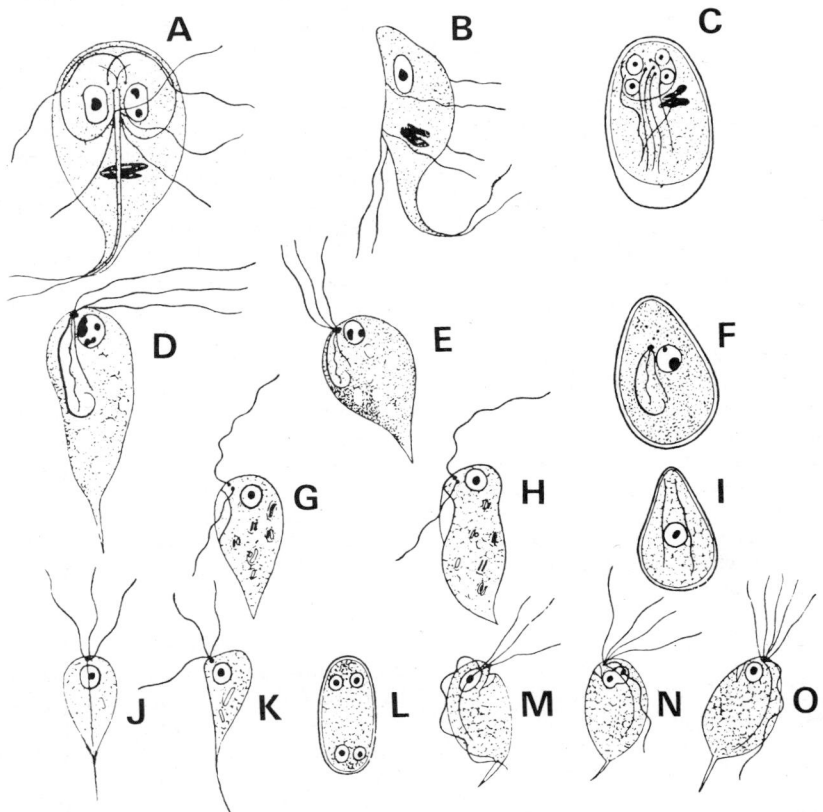

Fig. I.21 The flagellates of the human intestine, A–C, *Giardia intestinalis*, free and encysted forms. D–F, *Chilomastix mesnili*, free and encysted forms. G–I, *Embadomonas intestinalis*, free and encysted forms. J–L, *Tricercomonas intestinalis*, free and encysted forms. M–O, *Trichomonas hominis*, forms with three, four and five flagella.

FAMILY: EMBADOMONADIDAE

GENUS: *Embadomonas*

Embadomonas intestinalis (Wenyon & O'Connor, 1917)

A small but active flagellate, oval, 4–9 × 3–4 μm, which inhabits the intestinal tract (Fig. I.21G–I). There are two flagella: the anterior longer and thinner; the posterior projecting from a laterally situated mouth (cystostome), at the anterior extremity, supported by a ridge. The flagella act independently and thereby impart a peculiar jerky movement to the organism. The general shape is ovoid, with blunt anterior and pointed posterior extremities. The cytoplasm is vacuolated, containing ingested bacilli.

Cysts are pear-shaped, 4.5–6 μm in length, and appear structureless in the unstained state, but in iodine solution the *nucleus* can be discerned. This flagellate has been cultivated on egg medium. As in other members of this group, there is no evidence of pathogenicity.

FAMILY: CHILOMASTIGIDAE

GENUS: *Chilomastix*

Chilomastix mesnili (Wenyon, 1910) (*Tetramitus mesnili*)

This flagellate (Fig. I.21D–F) resembles *Trichomonas hominis* in general shape and size and occurs in the large intestine. There are three long flagella, but not undulating membrane or axostyle. There is a large mouth (cytostome), which occupies two-thirds of the body length, and contains a flagellum arising from a granule situated anteriorly to the spherical nucleus. The posterior extremity is attenuated. The cytoplasm contains numerous vacuoles and bacteria which form the main food supply. Division takes place by longitudinal fission. Individual organisms vary very much in length, but measure on an average 14 μm in length by 5–6 μm in breadth.

In freshly passed faeces, *Chilomastix* moves with active, jerky movements which distinguish it from the more deliberate rotatory action of *Trichomonas*.

Cysts

'Lemon-shaped' cysts appear in formed stools and are 7–10 μm in length; they contain a single nucleus and vestiges of a cytostome. In fresh preparations they have to be differentiated from yeasts.

Infections with this parasite are very persistent, but there is no evidence of pathogenicity.

C. mesnili has been cultured on artificial media.

FAMILY: TRICHOMONADIDAE

GENUS: *Trichomonas*

Trichomonas hominis (Davaine, 1860)

This is the most common intestinal flagellate of man, inhabiting the caecum and large intestine, often in enormous numbers (Fig. I.21M–O).

The body is pear-shaped, 10–15 μm in length by 7–10 μm in breadth. The spherical *nucleus* is at the anterior extremity and immediately in front of it are placed *blepharoplasts* from which three long flagella are directed forwards, while a fourth and stouter passes backwards to form the border of the undulating membrane, beyond which it is continued as a free flagellum. The cytostome is represented by a small aperture near the anterior end. A *stiffening rod*, arising from the blepharoplast, supports the undulating membrane. Running down the middle of the body is a second skeletal rod, or *axostyle*. The cytoplasm contains vacuoles with bacteria and food granules.

According to the number of flagella (three, four or five), three varieties are recognized, although the triflagellate is the most common. Dobell thought that these varieties were merely strains of the same species. This flagellate progresses by lashing movements from the three anterior flagella, and the undulating membrane causes it to revolve on a longitudinal axis. The parasite is also capable of amoeboid movement, especially evident in degenerate individuals. Reproduction is by longitudinal fission, by duplication of the various parts. No *cysts* are known.

The abundance of *T. hominis* in diarrhoeic stools in the tropics has induced some observers to consider it pathogenic and in one instance Wenyon found definite evidence of invasion of the intestinal mucosa by these organisms. Moreover, the closely allied *T. caviae* often causes ulceration of the large intestine in guinea-pigs.

On the whole, the pathogenicity of *T. hominis* in the intestinal tract of man is doubtful and its presence in diarrhoeic stools may be due to liquid faeces which constitute a congenial medium for this flagellate.

T. hominis can be artificially cultured on blood agar with Locke's fluid for many generations, but subinoculations are necessary every few days, but now bacteria-free cultures can be obtained with antibiotics on egg-slants overlaid with bouillon serum and yeast extract.

A somewhat similar species, *T. elongata*, is found in the mouth cavity, as well as on the tonsillar surface. A third form, *T. vaginalis*, is present in the vaginal cavity of 10% of women. *T. vaginalis* can be grown easily in bacteria-free culture and its requirements are less exacting than those of *T. hominis*.

Most gynaecologists now regard *T. vaginalis* as a definite clinical pathogen, responsible for vaginitis, and the human analogue of *T. foetus*, which causes inflammation of the genitalia of cattle. The two species are physiologically different. On serological grounds it has now been shown that *T. hominis* and *T. vaginalis* are distinct species. *T. vaginalis* is sometimes found in the male urethra and can invade the epithelium and prostate. The male is the most important transmitter of this infection. It flourishes mainly during the reproductive period, but not, as a rule, in young girls, or after the climacteric. It appears to multiply when the vaginal state is favourable, at pH 4, and a symbiotic association with a non-haemolytic streptococcus is suggested. The parasite disappears when the urine becomes alkaline. *T. vaginalis* is said to be considerably larger than *T. hominis*, reaching 27 × 18 μm. Four anterior flagella are of equal length, a fifth flagellum on the margin of the relatively short undulating membrane protruding a considerable distance beyond the posterior tip of the organism. *T. tenax* (*Tetratrichomonas buccalis*) Dobell, 1939, is probably a cosmopolitan parasite of man and has four anterior free flagella of equal length, a relatively short undulating membrane, a slender *axostyle* and a subspherical nucleus. On the average it is smaller than *T. hominis*. It inhabits the mouth, especially in diseased gums. It has been found in sputum from the lung and in pulmonary gangrene. It occurs in about 18% of individuals.

Trichomycin was obtained from a *Streptomyces* in soil in 1952. It is active against *Trichomonas* and is lethal in concentration of 2 μg/5 ml.

FAMILY: HEXAMITIDAE

GENUS: *Giardia*

Giardia intestinalis (Lambl, 1859) (*Giardia lamblia, Lamblia intestinalis*)

This remarkable parasite lives in the upper part of the small intestine, particularly the duodenum. In shape it resembles a half-pear, split longitudinally (Figs. 17.17 and I.21A–C). It measures 12–18 μm in length. The ventral surface is furnished with a concave sucking disc with a raised ridge at the anterior end, and the posterior extremity tapers into a fine tail and terminates in two flagella. There are altogether four pairs of flagella on the body, arising from as many blepharoplasts; the posterior three arise from the margins of the *axostyles*. There are two of these stiff supporting structures which pass down the centre of the body. The oval *nuclei* are situated within the sucking discs at the anterior end. The cytoplasm also contains a characteristically curved parabasal body in the lower half of the body. This flagellate swims rapidly, like a flat fish, swaying from side to side. *Giardia* reproduces itself by a complicated process of binary fission.

The *cysts*, which may occur in the faeces in enormous numbers, are characteristic structures. They are oval, measuring about 10.5 × 7.4 μm. The body of the flagellate becomes rounded, while the various inner structures (flagella, axostyle, etc.) become detached and cannot always be identified, except for the crescentic parabasal body. There are at first two nuclei, which divide, giving rise to four in the mature cyst. When examined in iodine solution, the cysts stain faint yellowish-brown and the cytoplasmic contents shrink back from the thick wall (Fig. 17.18).

The method of culture now used is Diamond's medium[26] modified by omitting the autoclaving step and sterilizing by membrane filtration. Subcultures are at weekly or biweekly intervals, by inoculation into 15 ml screw-capped test tubes and incubated at 37°C.

For pathology and treatment see Chapter 17.

Subphylum: Ciliophora
Class: Ciliata

GENUS: *Balantidium*

Balantidium coli (Malmsten, 1857)

This is a large protozoon belonging to the class Ciliata. Oval in shape and of variable size, it is 30–200 μm in length by 40–60 μm in breadth. The average is 50–70 μm. Various races are recognized by the size. The body is clothed with a thick covering of cilia arranged in longitudinal rows (Figs. 17.20 and I.22,1).

The *nucleus* is represented by a large kidney-shaped *macronucleus* with a small *micronucleus* closely approximated. The protoplasm contains two *contractile* and a number of *food vacuoles*. At the anterior end there is a *peristome*, leading into a mouth, or *cytostome*; posteriorly there is an anus or *cytopyge*. Nutrition is effected by ingestion of solid particles, leukocytes and red blood corpuscles.

B. coli reproduces asexually by transverse fission. Conjugation takes place by exchange of certain nuclear elements and, when once this has been effected, the conjugants once more separate.

The *cysts* (Figs. 17.21 and I.22,2) are ovoid, 45–60 μm in length, and are passed in the faeces. They contain the parasite which may be seen moving actively. The enclosed balantidium then loses its cilia, and sometimes two individuals are found in the same cyst. Transmission of infection takes place by means of cysts.

B. coli has been cultured in human serum diluted with saline. The presence of symbiotic bacteria is necessary, at 30–37°C, but frequent subinoculations have to be made.

For pathology and treatment see Chapter 17.

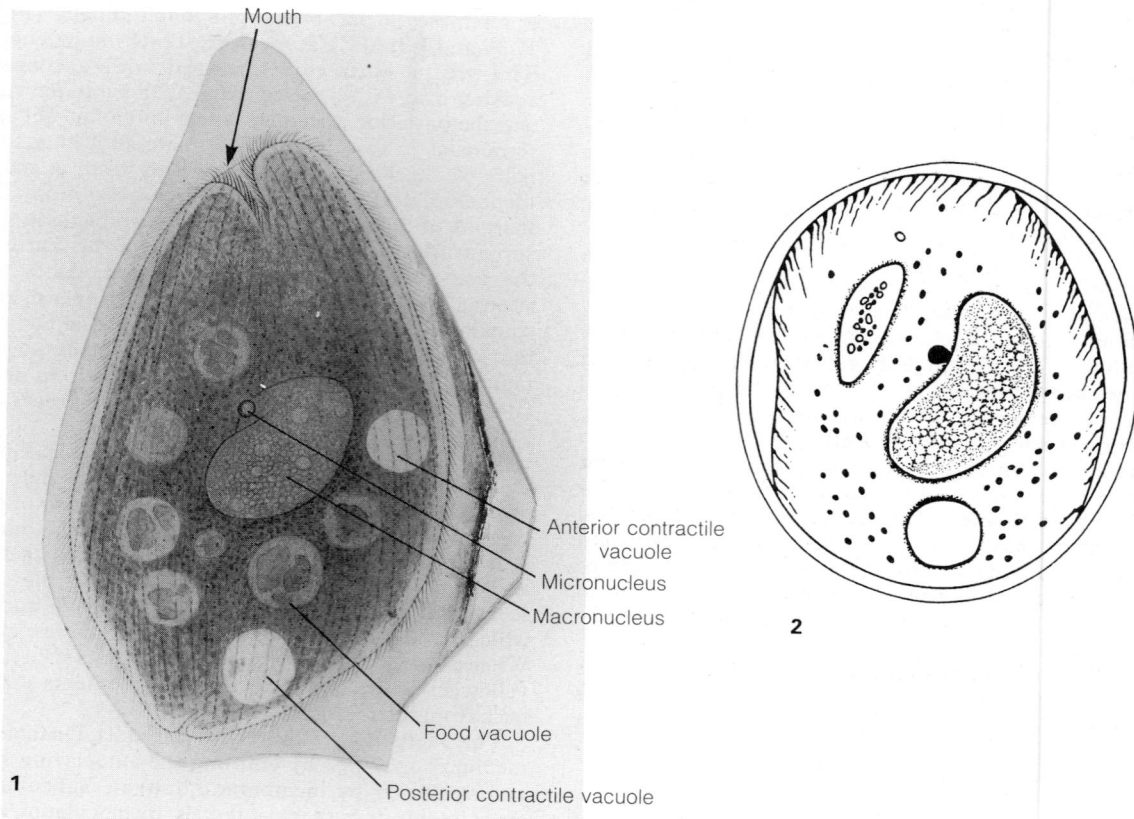

Fig. I.22 *Balantidium coli.* 1, trophoyoite. 2, Encysted form showing nuclei, posterior contractile vacuole and remains of cilia. × 1200.

THE TRYPANOSOMATID FLAGELLATES:
genera *Trypanosoma* and *Leishmania*

D. M. Minter

The order Kinetoplastida includes two sub-orders; the mainly free-living Bodonina and the entirely parasitic Trypanosomatina. The sub-order Trypanosomatina contains only one family, the Trypanosomatidae. This family includes the following nine genera: *Leptomonas, Herpetomonas, Blastocrithidia, Crithidia, Rhynchoidomonas, Phytomonas, Endotrypanum, Trypanosoma* and *Leishmania*. Only the genera *Trypanosoma* and *Leishmania* contain species which cause human disease.

Diagnosis of the order Kinetoplastida. Mainly parasitic flagellated protozoa, some species free-living, with one or two flagella; each flagellum composed of a paraxial rod (in the form of a filamentous lattice) alongside an axoneme (consisting of an outer ring of nine microtubule-doublets and an inner pair of unconnected microtubules). Flagella arise from an invaginated flagellar pocket or pit. A single mitochondrion typically extends the length of the cell, in the form of either a simple tube, a loop or a network of branched tubes, which contains the usually conspicuous kinetoplast (a DNA-containing organelle characteristic of the Kinetoplastida), close to the flagellar basal body; the latter (similar in structure to the centriole of other animal cells) is inserted on or near to the mitochondrial envelope. The cell body is supported mainly by pellicular microtubules, which envelop the cytopharynx found in many species (presumed to be lost secondarily in others, e.g. many *Trypanosoma* and all *Leishmania*).

No pseudopodia or plastids. Golgi apparatus typically near flagellar pocket, but not connected with basal bodies and flagella. Where present, the contractile vacuole discharges into the flagellar pocket.

Diagnosis of the family Trypanosomatidae. Kinetoplastida with a single locomotory flagellum, either free or attached to the pellicle as an undulating membrane. Second flagellum represented by a barren basal body. Kinetoplast relatively small and compact: DNA fibrils markedly anisotropic. All species parasitic, mainly in invertebrates or vertebrates, but plants in the case of *Phytomonas*.

Life-cycle stages in the family Trypanosomatidae

All trypanosomatids alternate between proliferative phases of binary fission (the establishment phase), which establish the parasites in a new environment, and non-proliferativeperiods (the transition phase), in which cell-division does not occur, associated with major environmental transitions (e.g. the alternation between vertebrate and invertebrate stages in the life-cycle).

Associated with these phase-changes, all trypanosomatids undergo morphological changes, mainly of shape, at different stages in the life-cycle of many species, particularly when members of the digenetic (heteroxenous) species change from one type of host to another, or during the course of their developmental cycle in a particular host.

Not every morphological form occurs in each of the nine genera. The nomenclature of the eight morphological variants generally recognized is based on the suffix '-mastigote', derived from the Greek word for whip, combined with various prefixes which refer to the origin, course and arrangement of the flagellum in relation to the position of the nucleus, and its point of emergence from the cell. The terms used are defined below and the characteristic morphology of each is shown in Fig. I.23.

1 *Amastigote* (all genera except *Herpetomonas*, *Rhynchoidomonas* and *Phytomonas*): an immobile and frequently intracellular stage, round or oval in shape, no flagellum visible by light microscopy, but stumpy interior flagellum seen by electron microscopy (EM); sometimes a short external prolongation is also visible by EM.

2 *Sphaeromastigote* (genus *Trypanosoma* only): motile rounded form with free flagellum, often a transitional stage from the amastigote.

3 *Promastigote* (all genera except *Crithidia* and *Rhynchoidomonas*): motile, elongated form with anteronuclear kinetoplast, near which the flagellum originates; free anterior flagellum. Promastigotes are usually long and slender, unattached and free-swimming: then known as nectomonads, to distinguish them from the attached and sessile forms (hap-

tomonads) also found, for example, in the genus *Leishmania* p. 1297).

4 *Paramastigote* (genera *Herpetomonas* and *Leishmania* only): motile non-dividing form with short free anterior flagellum, emerging from a long flagellar pocket which originates near the juxtanuclear kinetoplast. A transitional stage from the promastigote (to an opisthomastigote in *Herpetomonas*: to an infective promastigote in *Leishmania*).

5 *Opisthomastigote* (genus *Herpetomonas* only): elongated motile form with posteronuclear kinetoplast and emergent anterior free flagellum. Flagellum (and flagellar pocket) pass through the cell interior for most of the length of the body.

6 *Choanomastigote* (genus *Crithidia* only): pear-shaped ('barley-corn') motile stage with anteronuclear kinetoplast; free anterior flagellaum arises from a wide, conical flagellar pocket.

7 *Epimastigote* (genera *Blastocrithidia*, *Endotrypanum* and *Trypanosoma*): motile, elongated form with juxtanuclear kinetoplast; flagellum emerges laterally from body close to its origin and runs along the surface, sometimes in the form of an undulating membrane.

8 *Trypomastigote* (genera *Rhynchoidomonas*, *Endotrypanum* and *Trypanosoma*): elongated motile form with posteronuclear kinetoplast; emergent lateral flagellum runs along side of body as an undulating membrane; free anterior flagellum.

The Trypanosomatidae are parasitic flagellates which live in the tissues and/or body fluids of their hosts. The family is divided into nine genera, of which five are monogenetic parasites of invertebrates, particularly insects, and four genera are digenetic, alternating between an invertebrate intermediate host (often an arthropod) and a vertebrate animal (or plant; in *Phytomonas*). All members of the Trypanosomatidae have a single flagellum and kinetoplast.

Monogenetic (=monoxenous) genera. Parasites of arthropods, mainly of insects. Transmission contaminative, via amastigotes or trypomastigotes in faeces of the host.

1 *Leptomonas:* mainly parasites of insects, but also some other invertebrates; promastigote and amastigote (cystic) stages only. *Example: L. ctenocephali*, a parasite of the dog flea.

2 *Herpetomonas:* parasites of insects; promastigote, paramastigote and opisthomastigote stages. *Example: H. muscarum*, a parasite of the house fly, *Musca domestica*.

3 *Blastocrithidia:* parasites of insects and ticks; promastigote, epimastigote and amastigote (cystic) stages. *Example: B. triatomae* is a parasite of the medically important hemipteran insect *Triatoma infestans*, an important vector of *Trypanosoma cruzi*, the causative organism of American human trypanosomiasis. Both *B. triatomae* and *T. cruzi* occur in the hindgut and

Fig. I.23 Diagram of morphological forms in the Trypanosomatidae and their occurrence in monogenetic and digenetic genera.

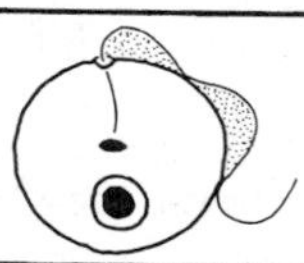

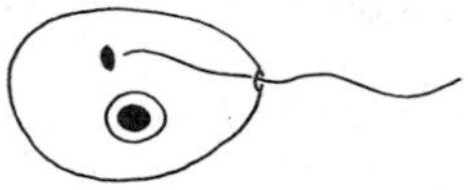

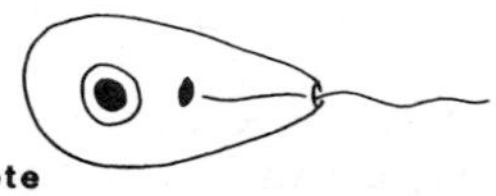

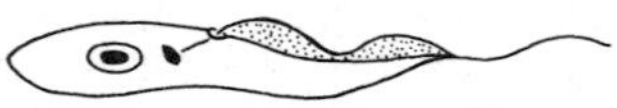

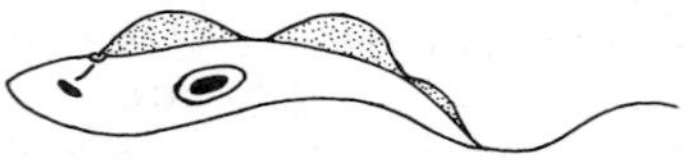

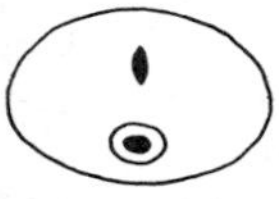

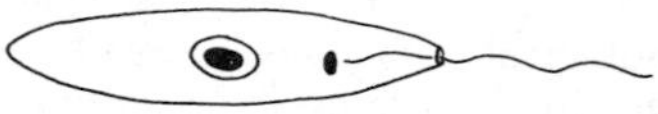

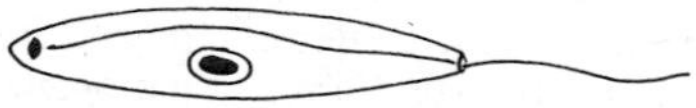

rectum of the triatomine, and this can lead to confusion when laboratory-reared bugs are used in xenodiagnosis of human infections with *T. cruzi* (Appendix III).

4 *Crithidia:* parasites of insects; amastigote and choanomastigote stages. *Example: C. fasciculata*, a cosmopolitan parasite of *Anopheles* and *Culex* mosquitoes.

5 *Rhynchoidomonas:* parasites of insects; trypomastigote stage only, which lack a free flagellum. Little is known of this genus; they are gut parasites of Diptera and frequently invade the malpighian tubules.

Digenetic (= *heteroxenous*) *genera.* Parasites of vertebrates or plants (*Phytomonas* only), with cyclical development in an invertebrate vector, commonly an insect; transmission to final host frequently inoculative, but sometimes contaminative (e.g. the medically important *Trypanosoma cruzi*, see below).

6 *Phytomonas:* parasites of plants; promastigote stage only, in both the final plant host and in the phytophagous bug vector (Hemiptera). *Example: Phytomonas* species are economically important parasites of coffee trees and coconut palms.

7 *Endotrypanum:* parasites of Neotropical sloths (Edentata); promastigote and amastigote stages in phlebotomine sandfly (*Lutzomyia*) vectors; intraerythrocytic epimastigotes (*E. schaudinni*) or bloodstream trypomastigote stages (*E. monterogeii*) in the mammalian host (sloths).

8 *Trypanosoma:* blood and/or tissue parasites of vertebrates (fish, amphibians, reptiles, birds and mammals); amastigote, promastigote, epimastigote, sphaeromastigote and trypomastigote stages. Bloodstream trypomastigotes or intracellular amastigote forms predominate in the vertebrate host (e.g. *T. cruzi*); epimastigotes are usually the predominant stage in the invertebrate, with amastigotes, trypomastigotes, promastigotes and sphaeromastigotes also found in the invertebrate hosts of some species. *Examples: T. brucei gambiense, T. brucei rhodesiense* and *T. cruzi* are respectively the causative organisms of African and American human trypanosomiasis. The Neotropical *T. rangeli* also infects man, but is not a human pathogen.

9 *Leishmania:* parasites of vertebrates, particularly mammals; promastigote and paramastigote stages in phlebotomine sandfly vectors (normally species of *Phlebotomus* or *Lutzomyia:* see also Appendix III, and p. 1294), in the vertebrate host intracellular amastigotes parasitize macrophages, rarely other celltypes. The status of *Leishmania* species described from reptiles (lizards), usually transmitted by phlebotomine vectors, often species of *Sergentomyia* in the Old World, is now in some doubt, since one species ascribed to *Leishmania* (*L. tarentolae*) recently was recognized to be a trypanosome, *Trypanosoma platydactyli. Trypanosoma* and *Leishmania* are the only trypanosomatid genera with species that cause disease in man.

Medically important trypanosomatid genera: systematic position (after Levine et al[34])

Kingdom:	Protista Haeckel, 1866
Subkingdom:	Protozoa Goldfuss, 1817
Phylum:	Sarcomastigophora Honigberg & Balamuth, 1963
Subphylum:	Mastigophora Deising, 1866
Class:	Zoomastigophora Calkins, 1909
Order:	Kinetoplastida Honigberg, 1963 *emend.* Vickerman, 1976
Suborder:	Trypanosomatina Kent, 1880
Family:	Trypanosomatidae Doflein, 1901 *emend.* Grobben, 1905
Genera:	*Trypanosoma* Gruby, 1843 *Leishmania* Ross, 1903

GENUS: *TRYPANOSOMA* GRUBY, 1843

Definition. Parasitic protozoa; life-cycle digenetic (heteroxenous); the requirement for cyclical development in an invertebrate has been lost secondarily in a few species (see below).

Vertebrate hosts in all major groups (fish, amphibia, reptiles, birds and mammals); in which *either* extracellular, leaf-like and motile trypomastigotes (with free flagellum) predominate, *or* immobile, intracellular, rounded amastigotes (without free flagellum).

Invertebrate hosts chiefly arthropods (insects or arachnids), but leeches (Hirudinea: Annelida) are vectors of many fish and amphibian trypanosomes. Epimastigote stages usually predominate in invertebrate hosts, but several other stages may also occur.

Medically important species of the subgenera *Trypanozoon* and *Schizotrypanum*, respectively, undergo cyclical development in tsetse flies (*Glossina* spp.) (Diptera: Glossinidae), or in several genera of triatomine bugs (Hemiptera, Heteroptera; family Reduviidae: subfamily Triatominae).

Multiplication in vertebrate and invertebrate hosts by binary fission: no known sexual cycle. Transmission to vertebrate host in most cases *either* by bite (species of the section Salivaria) *or* by faecal contamination of skin and mucosal surfaces (species of the section Stercoraria). (Distribution of the genus *Trypanosoma:* cosmopolitan.)

General features of trypanosomes

Some species of the Salivaria have secondarily lost the necessity for cyclical development in an invertebrate host. For example *T.* (*Trypanozoon*) *equiperdum*, the cause of dourine in equines, is transmitted by coitus; the related *T.* (*T.*) *evansi* (the cause of surra in camels, equines and bovines) is transmitted mechanically by biting flies, particularly Tabanidae and *Stomoxys*, and even (in the Neotropical region) by vampire bats, *Desmodus rotundus*.

Trypanosoma is the only genus of the Trypanosomatidae in which trypomastigotes are the predominant vertebrate life-cycle stage of most species; however, amastigote, promastigote, epimastigote and sphaeromastigote stages also occur in the invertebrate hosts of some species.

Except for the rounded, immobile and mainly intracellular amastigote stages which occur in the vertebrate host of relatively few species, the trypanosomes are typically motile, elongate, slender protozoa. Bloodstream trypomastigotes are extracellular, but some species also have trypomastigote or amastigote tissue stages.

Trypomastigotes are variable in size and morphology between species, but most species are monomorphic in the bloodstream of the vertebrate. A minority of species, however, exhibit some degree of polymorphism in the bloodstream trypomastigote stage, particularly species of the subgenus *Trypanozoon*. Bloodstream trypomastigotes are usually laterally flattened, with the body pointed anteriorly and the flagellum attached to the pellicle by an undulating membrane; the flagellum may be free anteriorly. Kinetoplast and basal body are posteronuclear, with the flagellum emergent laterally from an invaginated flagellar pocket. The detailed morphology of the bloodstream trypomastigotes is diagnostic for most species: intraspecific categories are often recognized on the basis of intrinsic biochemical characters, particularly by isoenzyme characterization (see also section on criteria for identification of *Trypanosoma* and *Leishmania*, below). Trypanosomes are common parasites of freshwater and marine fishes, amphibia, reptiles, birds and many groups of mammals. The account which follows, however, is restricted mainly to mammalian trypanosome parasites of economic and medical importance.

The mammalian trypanosomes are divided into two main groups; the section *Stercoraria*, in which development in the vector typically occurs in the posterior station (i.e. the posterior part of the alimentary canal) and transmission is by faecal contamination; and the section *Salivaria*, in which development in the vector is typically in the anterior station (i.e. the anterior part of the gut and the mouthparts, and/or salivary glands) and transmission is inoculative, by the bite of the vector.

Section Stercoraria

Trypanosomes with free flagellum; kinetoplast relatively large and not terminal. Posterior end of body pointed. Development of infective (metacyclic) nondividing trypomastigote stage in vector occurs in the posterior station (in *T. rangeli*, also in the anterior station, with possible inoculative transmission). Reproduction in the mammalian host is discontinuous, by binary fission, usually of amastigote or epimastigote stages. Typically not human pathogens (except *T. cruzi*). There are three subgenera, two of which contain species which infect man.

Megatrypanum. Type species is *T. (M.) theileri*, a generally harmless cosmopolitan parasite of cattle. No species of medical importance.

Herpetosoma. Type species is the flea-transmitted *T. (H.) lewisi* of rodents, particularly the genus *Rattus*, and lagomorphs. The subgenus includes the apathogenic, triatomine-transmitted *T. (H.) rangeli*, a common parasite of primates (including man), marsupials, rodents and other animals in Central America and northern parts of South America. *T. (H.) rangeli* has some characteristics of both Stercoraria and Salivaria.

Schizotrypanum. Type species is the triatomine-transmitted *T. (S.) cruzi*, the causative organism of American human trypanosomiasis (Chagas' disease) in the western hemisphere, where *T. (S.) cruzi* is a common and widespread parasite of wild mammals, particularly marsupials and rodents.

Section Salivaria

Trypanosomes with free flagellum or without; kinetoplast terminal or subterminal. Posterior end of body usually blunt. Development of infective (metacyclic) trypomastigote stages in the vector normally occurs in the anterior station (but mechanical transmission of bloodstream stages can occur in some species) and transmission is inoculative (except for coital transmission in *T. equiperdum*). Reproduction in the mammalian host is continuous, in the trypomastigote stage. There are four subgenera; three contain species of economic importance, but only *Trypanozoon* includes trypanosomes infective to man.

Duttonella. Type species is *T. (D.) vivax*, the economically important monomorphic parasite of livestock and wild animals in Africa, transmitted by tsetse flies (*Glossina*). Movement of infected cattle to Mauritius, the Caribbean and South America led to the introduction of the parasite to these areas, where the parasite is non-cyclically mechanically transmitted by other biting flies, particularly Tabanidae and *Stomoxys*. No species of medical importance.

Nannomonas. Type species is the pleomorphic *T. (N.) congolense*, also an economically important parasite of African livestock and transmitted cyclically by *Glossina*. *T. (N.) simiae*, also tsetse-transmitted, is of economic importance as a cause of serious outbreaks of trypanosomiasis in exotic breeds of pig in Africa. No species of medical importance.

Pycnomonas. Monotypic subgenus represented only by *T. (P.) suis,* a rare monomorphic and tsetse-transmitted parasite of pigs.

Trypanozoon. Type species is *T. (T.) brucei,* which is tsetse-transmitted, highly pleomorphic and usually considered to comprise three morphologically indistinguishable subspecies, of which two cause human disease. Other members of the subgenus are not tsetse-transmitted and do not infect man, although several species are of considerable veterinary importance, notably *T. (T.) evansi* (the cause of surra in equines and camels) and *T. (T.) equiperdum* (primarily a tissue parasite and the cause of dourine in equines). The name *T. (T.) brucei* is here used to refer to the species as a whole and to those stocks whose subspecific status has not been determined. The subspecies of *T. brucei* are:

1 *T. brucei brucei:* a parasite of mammals, defined as not infective to man. (Because this particular characteristic is very seldom known with certainty, the subspecific notation in *T. brucei* sensu lato is of doubtful taxonomic validity; it is therefore not universally accepted, and is used here largely for convenience rather than in any strictly taxonomic sense.)

2 *T. brucei gambiense:* causes, typically, chronic gambian sleeping sickness (SS) in man, mainly in western and central Africa. Isoenzyme characterization studies have revealed that evidently the same parasite is also sometimes found in dogs, pigs, sheep, hartebeest (*Alcelaphus* sp.) and kob (*Kobus* (*Adenota*) sp.).

3 *T. brucei rhodesiense* in man causes the typical acute, fulminating rhodesian sleeping sickness, but the parasite is also widespread in game animals in eastern areas of Africa. (*Note:* lower-case initial letters are used for the terms 'gambian' and 'rhodesian', to indicate that they have no geopolitical significance, but relate to the subspecific names of the causative organisms.)

Although the three subspecific names used above are widely used, many workers prefer to treat *T. brucei* as a single polytypic species, capable of causing a wide spectrum of human and animal diseases, ranging from a symptomless carrier state *via* chronic human disease (gambian SS) to a fulminating and fatal illness (rhodesian SS).

The economically important *Trypanozoon* species not transmitted cyclically by tsetse, *T. evansi* and *T. equiperdum,* are closely related to *T. brucei* sensu lato and many workers believe all three to be synonymous, on the evidence of isoenzyme and other intrinsic features. Mainly as a matter of practical convenience, however, it is useful to retain provisionally the specific and subspecific names used above.

Trypanosomes of mammals

These include many species pathogenic either to man or domestic livestock, as well as commonly non-pathogenic species which parasitize ruminants and many other mammalian groups. Only species which infect man and/or which cause economic loss among livestock are considered here: for a full treatment of mammalian trypanosomes the reader is referred to Hoare,[35] Kreier[36] and Lumsden and Evans.[37] Current literature on special topics can be traced very readily through the *Tropical Diseases Bulletin, Protozoological Abstracts* and the internationally sponsored *Tsetse and Trypanosomiasis Information Quarterly,* prepared by the Tropical Development and Research Institute (former Centre for Overseas Pest Research) in London.

CRITERIA FOR IDENTIFICATION OF *TRYPANOSOMA* AND *LEISHMANIA*

Morphological characteristics of vertebrate stages

These are the traditional means of diagnostic parasite identification, based upon size, shape and detailed morphology of parasites as seen in well-prepared thin films, carefully stained with Romanowsky stains, such as Giemsa. This requires little in the way of equipment or materials, and permits accurate determination to generic/subgeneric levels; often to species in the case of bloodstream stages of *Trypanosoma.* In combination with the site of parasite development in the insect vector, and the morphological stages of parasite involved, a similar level of certainty is possible also for the *Leishmania* subgenera.

1 Morphology of bloodstream stages of Trypanosoma species

Identification involves observation of size and proportions of the parasites, presence or not of a free flagellum and the position of nucleus, kinetoplast and flagellum in relation to the rest of the body. Observation of living parasites by phase-contrast and/or dark-ground microscopy is often a useful aid to identification, particularly of motile bloodstream forms whose movement may be characteristic: *Trypanosoma (Duttonella) vivax,* for example, is a large trypanosome which moves rapidly and in straight lines, with occasional short stops; *T. (Nannomonas) congolense* is comparatively sluggish in its movement in a wet blood film and frequently adheres to erythrocytes. *T. (Trypanozoon) brucei* subspecies are also of large size and very active, but their movement is generally not progressive or linear; rather, they tend to 'mark time' in rapid motion at one location.

Measurements of bloodstream stages, from drawings made with a camera lucida, are often used in descriptions and for identification of salivarian trypanosomes: the measurements and ratios used are as follows:

L = total length, inclusive of flagellum
F = length of free flagellum
PK = distance from kinetoplast to posterior end of parasite
PN = distance from nucleus to posterior end
KN = distance between nucleus and kinetoplast
NA = distance from nucleus to anterior end
NI = nuclear index: the ratio PN : NA
KI = kinetoplast index: the ratio PN divided by KN (if the kinetoplast is posterior the index is less than 2; if close to the nucleus the ratio is greater than 2; and when the kinetoplast is midway between nucleus and the posterior end, the ratio is 2).

2 *Morphology of Leishmania in the mammalian host*

Mammalian stages of *Leishmania* are intracellular, but in the preparation of tissue impression smears the macrophages, in which they are located, often burst open and parasites then appear to be extracellular. It is frequently stated that the amastigote stages of *Leishmania* in the vertebrate are morphologically indistinguishable. This is in fact erroneous, since often not only are there conspicuous differences in size and shape between amastigotes of various species, but there are also sometimes characteristic differences in morphology and/or ultrastructure. For example, *L. (L.) major* amastigotes are distinctly larger than those of *L. (L.) tropica*; *L. (L.) mexicana* complex amastigotes are always larger than those of the *L. (V.) braziliensis* complex. In the *L. (L.) hertigi* complex of Neotropical porcupines, amastigotes of *L. (L.) deanei* > *L. (L.) hertigi*; *L. (L.) deanei* also lacks the conspicuous cytoplasmic vacuoles characteristic of *L. (L.) hertigi*, and the morphology of the kinetoplast is different. The curious parasite of the guinea-pig, *L. (L.) enriettii*, has amastigotes of striking size, noticeably larger than those of any other member of the *L. (L.) mexicana* complex.

So-called 'refractile bodies' are noted consistently in the cytoplasm of amastigotes in some species of *Leishmania* (notably of *L. (V.) braziliensis* and *L. (L.) garnhami*; erroneously in *L. (L.) amazonensis*). These structures, of unknown nature and function, are visible in unfixed and unstained material, variable in colour (yellow, or amber, to black) and do not take up Romanowsky stains. In polarized light, refractile bodies resemble malaria pigment in appearance.

Nonetheless, it is true to say that *Leishmania* amastigotes have fewer useful morphological diagnostic characters than the bloodstream trypomastigotes of *Trypanosoma*, and they are more tedious to observe and measure, in view of their generally smaller size and overall structural similarity.

Site of parasite development in the invertebrate vector

The site of development in the vector, and the morphological forms encountered, are referred to elsewhere for both *Trypanosoma* and *Leishmania*; and are helpful diagnostic features, particularly at the subgeneric level.

Use of human volunteers

This is a matter mainly now of historical interest, since the use of volunteers is both unethical and is now also largely superseded by the introduction of new methods, mainly of a biochemical or biophysical nature. However, the use of human volunteers in the past, mainly for the identification of the *T. brucei* subspecies pathogenic for man (much less for the identification of man-infective *Leishmania*), has shown, for example, that *T. b. rhodesiense* maintained human infectivity during 20 years of cyclical transmission by *Glossina* to sheep and antelopes. The first demonstration that the bushbuck (*Tragelaphus scriptus*) is an epidemiologically important animal reservoir of *T. b. rhodesiense* was also made by the use of a human volunteer. Human volunteers were used in Zaire (then the Belgian Congo) to demonstrate that *T. b. gambiense* also retained its infectivity for man during more than 20 generations of cyclical transmission by *Glossina* to domestic livestock.

The blood incubation infectivity test (BIIT) for identification of potential man-infective *T. brucei* subspecies

This test, first developed in 1970, is based on the observation (made many years earlier) that normal human serum lyses *T. b. brucei* organisms, but not those of *T. b. rhodesiense* or *T. b. gambiense*. (The lytic factor in serum is due to a high-density lipoprotein fraction.) The lack of virulence of *T. b. gambiense* for normal laboratory rodents is a limitation of the BIIT for isolates from West and central Africa, but this has been to some extent overcome by the use of colonized multimammate rats (*Mastomys natalensis*), or of the American montane vole, *Microtus montanus*.

Unknown *T. brucei* subspecies isolates (= stocks) of bloodstream trypomastigotes are incubated at 37°C for 5 hours in human serum and then inoculated into mice or rats. Trypanosomes which survive the incubation in serum (i.e. are serum-insensitive) and infect the rodents are assumed to be potentially infective for man (= BIIT-positive result). Trypanosomes lysed by incubation in human serum (i.e. serum-sensitive), and which therefore fail to infect rodents in the bioassay, are regarded as not potentially infective to man (i.e. serum-sensitive: BIIT-negative result) and are assumed to be *T. b. brucei* by default. However, the test often fails to give a clearcut, unequivocal result;

probably as a result of variation in infectivity to man of the different antigenic types (VATs) which develop in succession during the course of infection in the mammalian host. There is also evidence that serum-sensitive stocks of *T. brucei brucei* can become serum-insensitive, and therefore potentially man-infective, if the stocks are passaged through *Glossina* fed on a mixture containing human serum; other tsetse fed on animal blood showed no such conversion of serum-sensitivity.

In spite of its limitations, the BIIT test is a useful one for practical purposes, since it can be carried out with minimal equipment and facilities. The BIIT is at present the only biological assay of potential man-infectivity available, in the absence (to date) of unequivocal biochemical or other indicators, apart from the use of human volunteers, no longer considered an acceptable practice. An in vitro version of the human serum resistance test has also been developed, in which laboratory rodents are replaced by a *Microtus* fibroblast cell-culture system, which permits the continuous growth of *T. b. rhodesiense* or *T. b. gambiense*, to which human serum is then added to carry out the test (see also p. 1319).

Immunological and serological methods of parasite identification (mainly for *Leishmania*)

1 *The Noguchi–Adler test.* This test has been in use for many years but is not widely used; it requires stringent sterility and great care and experience in the interpretation of the results. The test has been employed mainly to distinguish the Old World parasites *L. (L.) major*, *L. (L.) tropica*, *L. (L.) donovani* and *L. (L.) infantum*; also (less often) for the New World *L. (L.) mexicana* and *L. (Viannia) braziliensis*.

If *Leishmania* parasites are grown in a culture medium which includes a homologous antiserum, they aggregate to form immobile, living masses which resemble syncytia; EM micrographs show, however, that the cells remain intact but rounded-up and are separated by a precipitate (thought to be produced from the flagellar pocket). Endpoint dilution titres can be obtained with hyperimmune rabbit serum, at which no agglutination occurs, or at which free, mobile, promastigotes start to appear. If the endpoint dilution for two *Leishmania* stocks is identical when each is grown in the presence of antiserum to the other, the isolates can be considered antigenically identical; if the endpoints differ, the stocks are antigenically distinct. A complex system, developed in the USSR, can be employed to judge the degree of relatedness between stocks and isolates.

2 *Excreted factor ('EF') serotyping.* Culture promastigotes of *Leishmania* liberate metabolic products, functional exoantigens, into the surrounding medium; these are known as 'excreted factor' (EF) and accumulate in log-phase cultures. Their nature and composition is not fully known (see below), but they include antigenic determinants shared with the whole cultured promastigotes and react with antibody raised in rabbits against the homologous parasites. Promastigotes have a glycoconjugate-containing surface lipid (it functions primarily as a ligand for macrophage receptors). The glycoconjugate is released from the promastigote surface into culture media by the activity of an endogenous phospholipase; it is now known to be a major EF component.

Different *Leishmania* produce different EF serotypes; the EF antigens can be used in geldiffusion tests with homologous and heterologous hyperimmune rabbit antipromastigote sera, to serotype unknown isolates with reference to standard isolates of known provenance. Stocks of the same serotype cross react, those of a different serotype do not. Some *Leishmania* isolates produce EF which cross reacts with more than one type of serum and are known as 'mixed serotypes'. EF serotyping has largely been confined to Old World parasites, which comprise three major serotypes (A, B and mixed serotype AB). Based on incomplete or partial cross reactions of EFs with particular antisera, the types can be subdivided into various subserotypes (A^1, A^2, A^3, A^4, A^5, A^6; B^1, B^2B^3, A^1B^2, A^2B^2, A^3B^2 and A^4B^2). Although it is said the EF serotyping correlates well with other biological or biochemical characterization methods, some discrepancies (of unknown significance) have been noted, where EF serotypes differ among stocks not so far distinguished on the basis of isoenzyme profiles.

3 *Monoclonal antibodies (Mc Abs).* First used for identification of New World *Leishmania* isolates in the early 1980s, monoclonal antibodies were produced to promastigote membrane antigens, specific to *L. (L.) amazonensis* (with, however, some cross reactivity to the related non-human parasite *L. (L.) aristedesi*), *L. (V.) guyanensis*, *L. (V.) panamensis* and *L. (V.) braziliensis*. A variety of specific Mc Abs are now available for many of the New World parasites; these are in development for clinical use and for the identification of parasites in naturally infected sandflies. More recently, monoclonal antibodies have been produced which are specific for some *Leishmania* of the Old World. A solid-phase radioimmunoassay inhibition test has been developed utilizing a *L. (L.) major*-specific Mc Ab (WIC 79.3: Wellcome Research Laboratories); this will detect as few as six to 12 promastigotes of *L. (L.) major* in the gut of an infected sandfly; occasionally as few as three promastigotes are detectable with this system. With rapid developments taking place in this subject, it seems very likely that very sensitive and specific Mc Ab tests will soon be available for field typing of *Leishmania* in man, animals and infected sandflies.

A single Mc Ab (64B16: isotype IgG$_2$b), originally

raised against *L. (L) infantum*, recognizes an apparently common 70 kDa antigen of most (possibly all) *Leishmania*. The 64B16 Mc Ab inhibits growth and infectivity in mice (and in vitro amastigote multiplication), of *L. (L.) major*, *L. (L) mexicana*, *L. (L) amazonensis* and *L. (V) guyanensis*; the resultant antibody-mediated protection is possibly complement-dependent. The 64B16 Mc Ab may thus have important immunotherapeutic potential against systemic *Leishmania* infections. Such parasite-specific Mc Abs as 64B16 may eventually allow the identification of other *Leishmania* antigems responsible for protective immunity. This is in addition to their undoubtedly important future role in the rapid identification of parasites in patients, vectors and animal hosts at both clinical and field levels.

4 *Other serological methods.* Complement fixation tests (CFT) and the indirect immunofluorescence test (IFAT) have generally been of limited value to discriminate between the different *Leishmania* parasites. Passive haemagglutination tests use a soluble antigen adsorbed on to tanned mammalian erythrocytes; the method has been of limited use for Old World parasites, but does not seem suitable for those of the New World. Immunodiffusion methods, including immunoelectrophoresis (single- or two-dimensional), have also been used but depend on the quality of the necessary hyperimmune serum and the results are thus difficult to interpret and compare. It seems likely that serological approaches to *Leishmania* identification are likely to be superseded by either isoenzyme analysis or specific monoclonal antibodies; either alone or in combination.

5 *Methods based on cross immunity.* Little-used, because of the general lack of cross immunity between many of the parasites, although *L. (L.) major* immunizes against *L. (L.) tropica* (but not vice versa).

Biochemical methods

These have been developed and elaborated over the last two decades and the field is now in a phase of rapid expansion; it is probable that present methods will be both further refined and augmented by new and better ones.

The basis of the differences between one kind of organism and another is fundamentally a consequence of the information stored in the genome of each. If the DNA nucleotide sequence of an organism were known, its biochemical uniqueness would be explained. Trypanosomes and *Leishmania* are alike in the possession of a DNA-containing kinetoplast, in addition to nuclear DNA (nDNA); the maxicircles of kinetoplast DNA (kDNA) are equivalent to the mitochondrial DNA of other organisms, since the kinetoplast is merely a specialized region of the mitochondrion in Trypanosomatidae.

1 *DNA buoyant density*

DNA can be extracted from both the nucleus (nDNA) and the kinetoplast (kDNA) of either *Trypanosoma* or *Leishmania* organisms with comparative ease and in high purity, providing that the organisms can be grown and harvested in sufficient quantity.

The buoyant density of DNA (kDNA and nDNA), separately, can be measured in a caesium chloride (CsCl) density gradient. The buoyant density is a measure of the proportion of guanine–cytosine base pairs (and hence also that of the adenine–thymine base pairs), in any DNA sample measured.

At an early stage, it became apparent that kDNA and nDNA buoyant density measurements were mainly of value at the level of genera and subgenera, and were less sensitive to detect differences between species and subspecies.

2 *Isoenzyme electrophoresis*

At about the same time that the DNA buoyant density method was introduced, enzyme polymorphism was found to occur in trypanosomatids. Particular cellular enzymes occur in different molecular configurations, or isoenzymes (isozymes), which are characterized by differences in surface charge; these are reflected by different mobilities in an electric field. The occurrence of isoenzymes is determined by genetic factors, and thus different electrophoretic mobilities of isoenzymes reflect intrinsic genetic differences between populations of closely related organisms.

However, a few cautionary words are needed at this point, for the same or very similar mobilities of isoenzymes in an electrophoresis gel, do not *necessarily* mean a common molecular structure and, equally, molecular differences are not *necessarily* responsible for differences in surface electric charge; further, small charge differences may not always be resolved by gel electrophoresis.

Proteins on an electrophoresis plate through which an electric current is passed move towards either the anode or the cathode, at different rates dependent upon their surface charge. Following electrophoresis, bands of particular enzymes can be visualized on the plate by the use of staining techniques. Different isoenzyme mobilities imply genetic differences between parasite populations and, if sufficient enzymes are used (a dozen or more is common), then indistinguishable isoenzyme profiles from different isolates (stocks), imply a close relationship, or even identity, of the stocks. Starch-gel electrophoresis (SGE) and cellulose acetate electrophoresis (CAE) both permit the examination of large numbers of isoenzymes, and CAE can be adapted for use in a field laboratory. Isoelectric focusing is a further development; this allows the isoenzymes to be focused at their isoelectric points in a pH gradient, and can give greater discrimination of individual isoenzyme bands. Parasite populations that differ from others of the same species (or subspecies) in a number of specific isoenzyme mobilities are termed 'zymodemes'.

The application of isoenzyme analysis to both trypanosomes and *Leishmania* in recent years has been a powerful and valuable tool. For *Leishmania*, it has provided the most elegant and precise method of identification at the species and subspecific levels, at least until the more recent introduction of monoclonal antibody methods (see above). In the genus *Leishmania*, isoenzyme analysis has become an invaluable component among the various criteria available for parasite identification, and its use in studies of the epidemiology of leishmanial diseases of man and animals is equally important.

For African trypanosomiasis, however, the value of isoenzyme analysis for purposes of identification has been less, but it has facilitated the recognition of animal reservoirs of parasites which infect man, and has enabled the course of recent epidemics to be traced in detail and with precision. Together with the results of DNA analysis (see **3** below), it has nonetheless contributed to a greater understanding of speciation of trypanosomes (particularly, but not exclusively, those of the subgenus *Trypanozoon*, which cause African human trypanosomiasis, sleeping sickness). Unfortunately, no definite isoenzyme markers have been found which unequivocally indicate infectivity for man, although in the case of *T. b. gambiense*, a limited 'subset' of these parasites can now be recognized by isoenzyme characteristics, taken together with a low virulence for rodents and a particular variant surface glycoprotein (VSG) antigenic repertoire.

In the case of American trypanosomiasis, isoenzyme studies have disclosed the existence of three main, epidemiologically distinctive zymodemes of *T. (S.) cruzi*, each with some internal heterogeneity. All three zymodemes are man-infective, however, but they differ in geographical distribution (although with some overlap), and are associated variously with sylvatic or domiciliary transmission cycles. Isoenzyme patterns also suggest that *T. cruzi* is diploid, but no indication of genetic exchange, or of a sexual process, has yet come to light.

3 *Restriction-enzyme cleavage and DNA hybridization techniques*

A more recent DNA-based methodology is the comparison of restriction endonuclease 'finger prints', derived from the minicircle component of kDNA, of different populations of either trypanosomes or *Leishmania*. Particular fragments of kDNA can be separated and isolated, which are variously genus-, species-, subspecies- or strain-specific, and can be radioisotope or colorimetrically labelled for the production of probes used in the identification of quite small numbers of unknown organisms; by hybridization to

specific probes on nitrocellulose filters, or even on microscope slides. Paradoxically, one principal disadvantage of the method is its very sensitivity. The same principles can also be applied to nDNA, but less readily because of its greater complexity. Infraspecific groups of organisms based on kDNA diversity revealed by the above technique are termed 'schizodemes': for those *Trypanosoma* and *Leishmania* isolates so far examined, the number of different schizodemes identified among many local isolates has proved almost embarrassingly high, at least for the taxonomist to take into account. The epidemiological value of these very sensitive methods to detect small differences between populations of closely related organisms may well be much greater, but has yet to be fully evaluated. Similarly, the potential clinical value of methods based on specific hybridization of kDNA fragments (alone or cloned into plasmids, etc.), when fully developed and evaluated, is likely to be considerable, particularly for the unequivocal identification of *Leishmania* of both man and animals, as promastigotes in the gut of a sandfly and as amastigotes from cutaneous lesions or visceral infections. Undoubtedly, these methods will eventually prove to be of equal value also in African and American trypanosomiasis.

The recent combined application of restriction-enzyme cleavage, DNA hybridization (with three VSA-specific DNA probes and one probe of undefined genomic DNA) and gel electrophoresis methods, to 71 stocks of *Trypanozoon* (and one stock of *T. evansi*; isolated from a South American capybara, *Hydrochoerus hydrochaeris*) yielded interesting results.

All 34 stocks of *T. b. gambiense* were characterized by a conserved, specific DNA band pattern, regardless of the DNA probe used: this allowed the *T. b. gambiense* stocks to be unequivocally identified to subspecies (and also provided confirmation that pigs, dogs and sheep are potential reservoirs of *T. b. gambiense* in West Africa: see also p. 1278).

However, the 37 stocks ascribed variously to *T. b. brucei* and *T. b. rhodesiense* could not be distinguished by the same criteria; all 38 non-*gambiense* stocks (inclusive of the single stock of *T. evansi*) had highly variable DNA band patterns in regard to the number, size and labelling intensity of the genomic fragments. This indicates that VSA sequences in the non-*gambiense* stocks have diverged more rapidly than those of *T. b. gambiense*, but no specific pattern could be assigned either to the so-called *T. b. brucei* or *T. b. rhodesiense*, thus casting further doubt on their subspecific status, particularly that of *T. b. rhodesiense*. The similarity between stocks previously regarded as *T. b. brucei* and *T. b. rhodesiense* strongly implies that infectivity to man is not a character associated with a particular subspecies of *Trypanozoon*. Indeed, it remains to be seen if '*T. b. rhodesiense*' is really no more than one (or a few) human-serum resistant VSGs of *T. b. brucei*, as a variety of other studies also seem to suggest. The heterogenous non-*gambiense* stocks, on the basis of similarity indices, were grouped into five categories, some of which were correlated with the areas of origin. The single isolate of *T. evansi* was included within the fifth non-*gambiense* group. The same study showed also that *T. b. rhodesiense*-like trypansomes were found in man in West Africa (three stocks from the Ivory Coast) and confirmed earlier isoenzyme work with these stocks which, based on the BIIT (see above), previously also gave equivocal results for potential human infectivity.

The diversity thus demonstrated among the non-*gambiense* stocks lends further weight to the accumulated circumstantial evidence suggestive of genetic exchange (by a suggested, but so far unproved, process of sexual conjugation) between trypanosome stocks, with which the VSA-specific sequences seem to be particularly involved. The diversity between the non-*gambiense* stocks might then be explicable in terms of the presence of heterozygotes: genetic recombination would effectively contribute to the rapid evolution of antigen repertoires, which appears to have occurred in the non-*gambiense* group. However, there is no evidence to suggest that hybrid crosses between *T. b. gambiense* and non-*gambiense* actually occur: the generally invariable and specific DNA patterns of *T. b. gambiense* indeed suggests that hybrid forms are unlikely.

4 Radiorespirometry

Although specialized equipment and facilities are required, radiorespirometry is nonetheless a very sensitive and very rapid method to identify microorganisms. It was first used for identification of bacteria; later to screen for sensitivity to antibacterial drugs.

Known quantities of test organisms are incubated in the wells of microtitre plates (half an hour at 33°C), each well provided with a measured amount of a different radiolabelled source of metabolic carbon (commonly about a dozen sources are used, to provide a representative metabolic profile). The radiolabelled carbon dioxide evolved is allowed to react in a filter-paper disc moistened with a saturated solution of barium hydroxide, to result in a radiolabelled barium carbonate precipitate. The filter paper and precipitate are dried and the amount of radiocarbon determined in an argon : methane proportional spectrometer.

Radiorespirometry has been used mainly for *Leishmania*, but could also be used for trypanosomes. Each *Leishmania* stock studied has characteristic metabolic features which enable distinctions to be made at the species/subspecies level. The practical value of radiorespirometry remains to be seen, however; its very sensitivity may be a major limitation to interpretation. Parasites responsible for cutaneous lesions in man (*L. tropica, L. major, L. mexicana*) generally have high rates of metabolism for L-aspartic acid, L-asparagine, L-glutamic acid, L-glutamine and L-proline. Parasites which cause visceral infection in man (*L. donovani, L. infantum*) have high catabolic rates for L-aspartic acid and L-glutamic acid, but rather low rates for L-asparagine, L-glutamine and L-proline.

5 Protein and lipid composition

Lectins. Lectins are sugar-binding, cell-agglutinating proteins or glycoproteins (not of immune origin), found in the surface membranes of cells. Lectins are sugar-specific and can be used in agglutination tests to show the presence of membrane-bound carbohydrates. Lectins used to differentiate Old and New World *Leishmania* have given results that generally accord with those of other biochemical methods, although there are some unexplained discrepancies (such as a failure to distinguish *L. (L.) mexicana* from *L. (V.) braziliensis*). Lectins have also been used to discriminate between stocks or isolates of *T. cruzi*. Owing to the complicating factor of antigenic variation, however, lectins seem unlikely to be very useful for the medically-important salivarian trypanosomes.

Cyclopropane fatty acids (CFA). Some Trypanosomatidae contain high levels of a particular 19-carbon CFA, while others have little or none. Of *Leishmania* examined, the 19-carbon CFA was present in the *L. (L.) donovani* and *L. (L.) tropica* species-complexes, in *L. (V.) guyanensis* and *L. (V.) panamensis*, but totally absent from the *L. (L.) major* and *L. (L.) mexicana* species-complexes, from *L. (L.) aethiopica* and from the unnamed *L. (L.)* species of man, hyrax and sandflies in Namibia. Work so far suggests that the presence or absence of the 19-carbon CFA may be a useful trait to consider in addition to other biochemical criteria. Although not found in vertebrate or culture stages of different species of *Blastocrithidia* (1), *Endotrypanum* (2) or *Trypanosoma* (10), the same CFA was, however, found in '*Leishmania tarentolae*', now known to be *Trypanosoma platydactyli*.

ULTRASTRUCTURE OF THE TRYPANOSOMATIDAE

In spite of the morphological diversity of form in different species and stages of Trypanosomatidae, electron microscopy reveals an underlying similarity of cellular architecture, particularly among species of the genera *Trypanosoma* and *Leishmania*, since these have been the most extensively studied.

Morphology and ultrastructure of *Trypanosoma* species

In the vertebrate host (Fig. I.30a and c)

The surface membranes of *Trypanosoma* and *Leishmania* species, including that of the flagellum where present, are fundamentally similar and consist of a trilaminar pellicle or plasma membrane. The pellicle is a unit membrane 8–10 nm thick (it consists of two osmiophilic layers separated by an intervening clear layer). In metacyclic and bloodstream trypomastigotes of salivarian *Trypanosoma* only, this is often covered with an amorphous monomolecular coat of glycoprotein (12–15 nm thick) which is the source, at least in the subgenera *Trypanozoon* and *Nannomonas*, of antigenic variant surface glycoproteins (VSGs) by means of which the metacyclic and slender bloodstream trypomastigote stages (but not the non-dividing stumpy bloodstream forms) are able to evade the immune responses of the mammalian host (see also following section on antigenic variation). About 10 nm beneath the surface pellicle of all *Trypanosoma* and *Leishmania* species lies a network of longitudinal subpellicular microtubules, each about 20 nm in diameter and 10–25 nm apart, interconnected laterally at intervals; this network generally follows a spiral course in a single layer around the cell body. Among other functions, this elastic corselet of tubules maintains the shape of the cell. Where the flagellum is attached to the cell body there is a gap in the microtubule corselet and the flagellum is attached to the plasma membrane by desmosome-like attachment plaques, which act like rivets or spot-welds. The flagellar membrane covers the axoneme and joins the cell surface plasma membrane at the base of the flagellar pocket. The microtubules are present in the vicinity of the flagellar pocket or reservoir, but do not actually line it: only a special group of four tubules pass down to its inner end (see enlargement of flagellar basal complex in Fig. I.30). The plasma membrane in this area is modified for nutrient uptake by pinocytosis into membrane-bound vesicles which are pinched off, transported through the cytoplasm and later digested by lysosomal enzymes. Vesicles containing acid phosphatase similarly discharge waste metabolites by exocytosis to the exterior, through the flagellar pocket membrane.

All stages of *Trypanosoma* and *Leishmania* possess a flagellum, including the amastigotes, in which it is rudimentary and mainly internal. The flagellum arises from below the base of the flagellar pocket, a flask-like indentation of the plasma membrane. The flagellum originates internally from an organelle, the basal body (= kinetostome or blepharoplast) which lies near the base of the flagellar pocket. The basal body, in turn, is closely associated with the DNA-containing kinetoplast, characteristically present in all stages of the life-cycle of trypanosomatids, which is readily visible by light microscopy of stained specimens. After its emergence from the flagellar pocket the flagellum, covered also by the plasma membrane (and where present, the variant-specific glycoprotein coat), runs along the surface of the cell between two of the subpellicular microtubules, attached to the cell surface at regular intervals by a series of stud-like junctional complexes of the desmosome type. The flagellum often continues beyond the anterior end of the organism as a free flagellum and is itself capable of forming junctional complexes of the hemidesmosome/desmosome type with cells or other surfaces. The flagellum is supported throughout its length by the axoneme, a flexible rod-like structure composed of nine peripheral pairs of linked microtubules, together with a central unconnected pair, a structure common to the flagella and cilia of almost all animals and plants (Figs. I.25 and I.26). The axoneme originates in the basal body beneath the floor of the flagellar pocket; frequently a second basal body is located close to the first, and its presence is the first indication of impending binary fission.

The flagellum is further supported from the point at which it emerges from the flagellar pocket to near its anterior tip, by a paracrystalline rod with a lattice-like structure (Figs. I.24 and I.25). The flagellum is joined to the body surface of the trypomastigote by the characteristic undulating membrane which is clearly visible by light microscopy: this appears to be an elastic temporary distortion of the pellicle between two adjacent subpellicular microtubules and is therefore not a permanent structure.

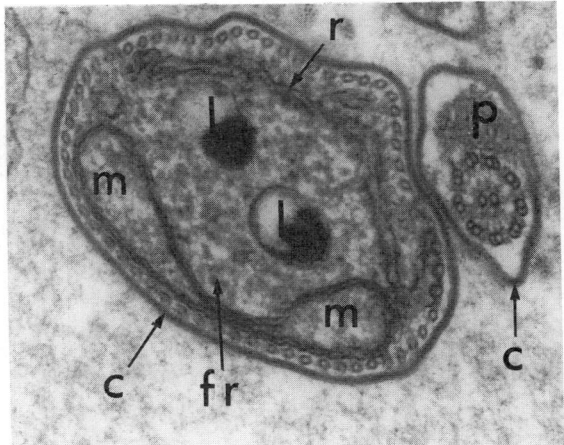

Fig. I.24   Cross-section of a trypanosome in a brain capillary. Note the secondary lysosomes (l) and the narrow mitochondrion (m) containing few or no cristae at this point in the life-cycle. The surface coat (c) around the pellicle and flagellum is arrowed. The subpellicular tubules (in cross-section) lie beneath the plasmalemma. Within the flagellar membrane are the axoneme and paraxial rod (p), the flagellar tubules of the former being arranged in the typical 9+2 pattern. fr = free ribosomes; r = rough endoplasmic reticulum. × 60 000. (Courtesy D. S. Ellis.)

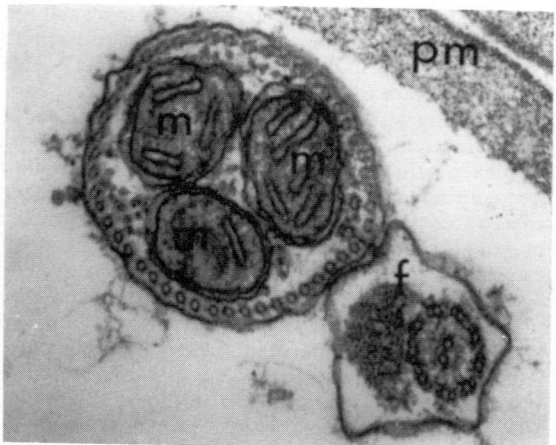

Fig. I.25 A trypanosome, cut at a similar point to that shown in Fig. I.24, lying within a tsetse fly midgut lumen, the peritrophic membrane (pm) upper right. Note the large mitochondria sections (m) containing many cristae, and the absence of any surface coat around the pellicle. The flagellum (f) contains paraxial rod and axoneme with the 9 + 2 tubule arrangement. × 60 000. (Courtesy D. S. Ellis.)

even the penetration of intact cells. Filamentous plasmanemes (or 'filopodium-like appendages') can be produced from the plasma membrane of bloodstream trypomastigotes of *Trypanozoon* species (mainly from long thin multiplicative forms) by various in vitro procedures, but it is doubtful if these long filaments occur in vivo. Shorter, thicker plasmanemes are found, not bounded by a cell membrane, particularly associated with short stumpy (non-dividing) forms in the blood and tissues of the mammalian host. They appear to be liberated from the flagellar pocket and are covered with the antigenic surface glycoprotein coat of the organism and are themselves highly immunogenic and contain also hydrolytic enzymes; their conjectural attachment to host cell surfaces provides a potentially rich source of antigen–antibody complexes, which may lead to vascular and other damage in the vertebrate host.

The ability, common among the salivarian metacyclic and bloodstream trypanosomes, to replace populations with one type of glycoprotein surface coat with a later wave of organisms with an antigenically different coat, reaches its peak in the *T. brucei* species (subgenus *Trypanozoon*) and gives rise to the well-known phenomenon of antigenic variation (see below). This process does not occur in the stercorarian trypanosomes (or in the genus *Leishmania*), in which the glycoprotein coat is less well developed.

Within the cell, the most prominent organelles are the nucleus and the kinetoplast, both visible by light microscopy of stained films (Fig. I.26). The ultrastructure of the nucleus reveals a central karyosome

Beating of the flagellum occurs by the passage of contractile waves between the flagellar tip and its base; this results in forward movement. Flagellar movement, together with the pellicular distortion evidenced by the undulating membrane, combine to give powerful swimming movements which also aid penetration between host cells and membrane surfaces;

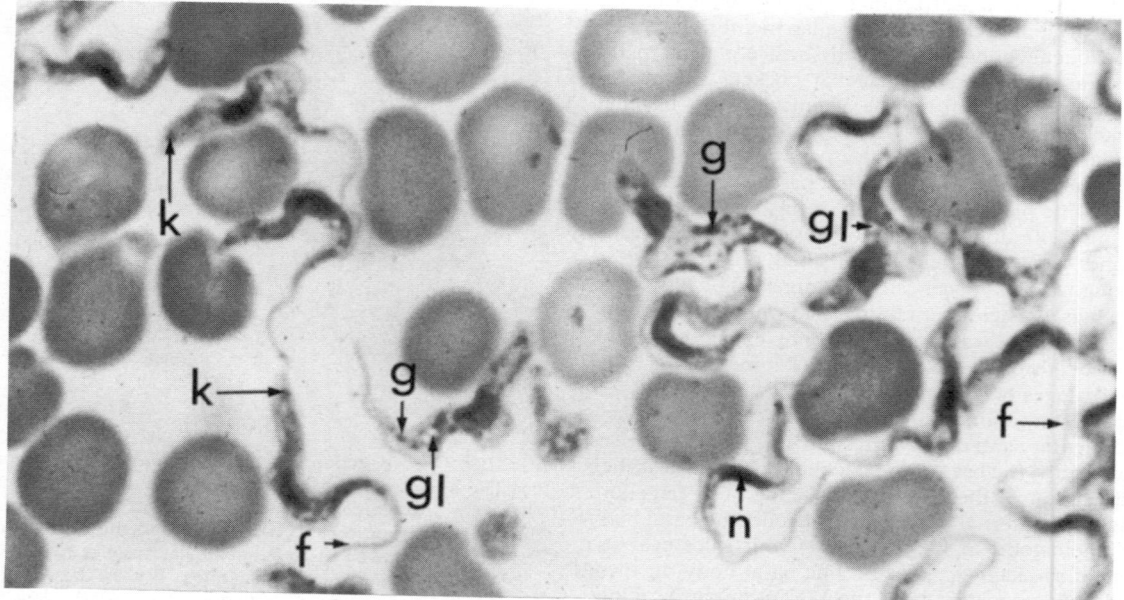

Fig. I.26 Long thin and stumpy forms of rhodesian sleeping sickness trypanosomes in a stained rat-brain blood film. The posterior kinetoplast (k), nucleus (n), dark staining granules (g), unstained lipid granules (gl) and flagellum (f) are arrowed. × 1400. (Courtesy W. E. Ormerod.)

or nucleolus and clumps of peripheral chromatin. The nucleus is bounded by a bilaminar envelope perforated by pores 80–100 nm across, which connect nucleoplasm and cytoplasm. The outer membrane of the nuclear envelope is continuous with a system of membranous cytoplasmic canals—the endoplasmic reticulum—which ramify through the ground cytoplasm (Figs. I.24 and I.27). Much of this endoplasmic reticulum (ER) is studded externally with ribosomes (contain ribonucleic acid: centres of protein synthesis) and is referred to as granular or rough ER (RER). Agranular or smooth ER (SER), is usually less extensive, has thicker membranes and lacks the attached ribosomes. In addition to their association with RER, ribosomes are frequently seen free in the ground cytoplasmic matrix (Figs. I.24, I.27). The ER is probably a functional mosaic with regions specialized for various biosynthetic and molecular transport purposes. Between the nucleus and the flagellar pocket region, a branch of RER is in close proximity to the Golgi apparatus (Figs. I.28 and I.29), a complex of laminar smooth-membraned (SER) sacs and cisternae, whose function is to enclose cellular secretions into membrane-bound vesicles, such as the lysosomes which contain the enzyme acid phosphatase. (The same enzyme is also found free in the flagellar pocket, whence it is discharged by the lysosomes, and probably is concerned with digestion of host materials in the flagellar pocket.) The flagellar pocket is also the site of protein endocytosis, in which clathrin-lined pinocytic vesicles are pinched off for transport through the cytoplasm.

Proteins, synthesized by the ribosomes and transported by the ER, undergo the addition of carbohydrate fractions in the Golgi apparatus before they are membrane-enclosed and discharged from the mature membrane face of the Golgi into the cytoplasm. The RER and the Golgi apparatus are also believed to be the source of the variant-specific glycoproteins discharged into the flagellar pocket, from whence they pass out over the plasma membrane to form the antigenic amorphous surface coat of the salivarian trypanosomes. The Salivaria have only a single Golgi apparatus; *T. (S.) cruzi*, however, sometimes has at least two.

A distinguishing feature of the kinetoplastid flagellates is the possession of a single mitochondrion provided with a concentration of mitochondrial DNA much greater than is found in other protozoa, and indeed all other cells. This mitochondrial DNA is found in the kinetoplast, a structure which itself is a capsular expansion of the mitochondrion: the DNA

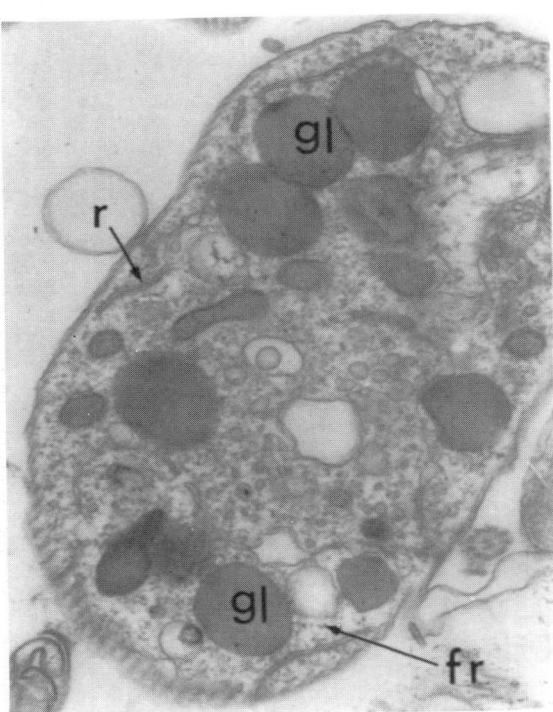

Fig. I.27 Cross-section of trypanosome (anterior to the nucleus) showing lipid granules (gl), sections of rough endoplasmic reticulum (r) and free ribosomes (fr). × 16 000. (Courtesy D. S. Ellis.)

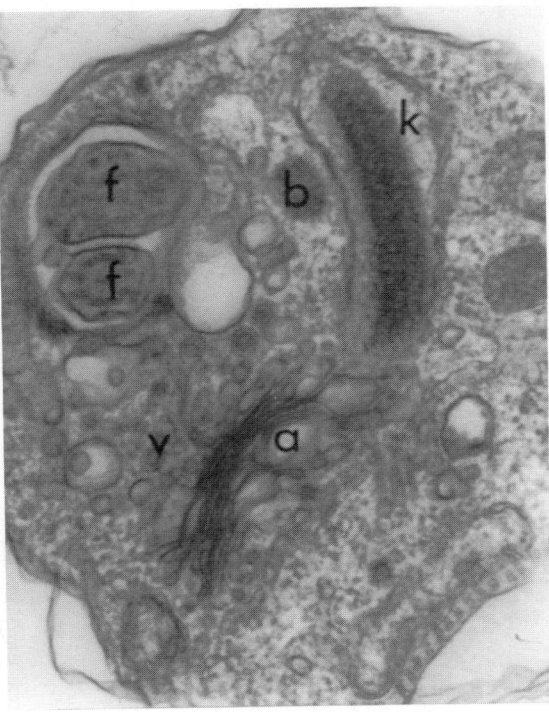

Fig. I.28 Cross-section of a dividing trypanosome (two flagella marked f lie within the flagellar pocket) showing the kinetoplast (k) containing the coiled DNA, next to a basal body (b). Beneath lies the Golgi apparatus (a) and associated vesicles (v). × 25 000. (Courtesy D. S. Ellis.)

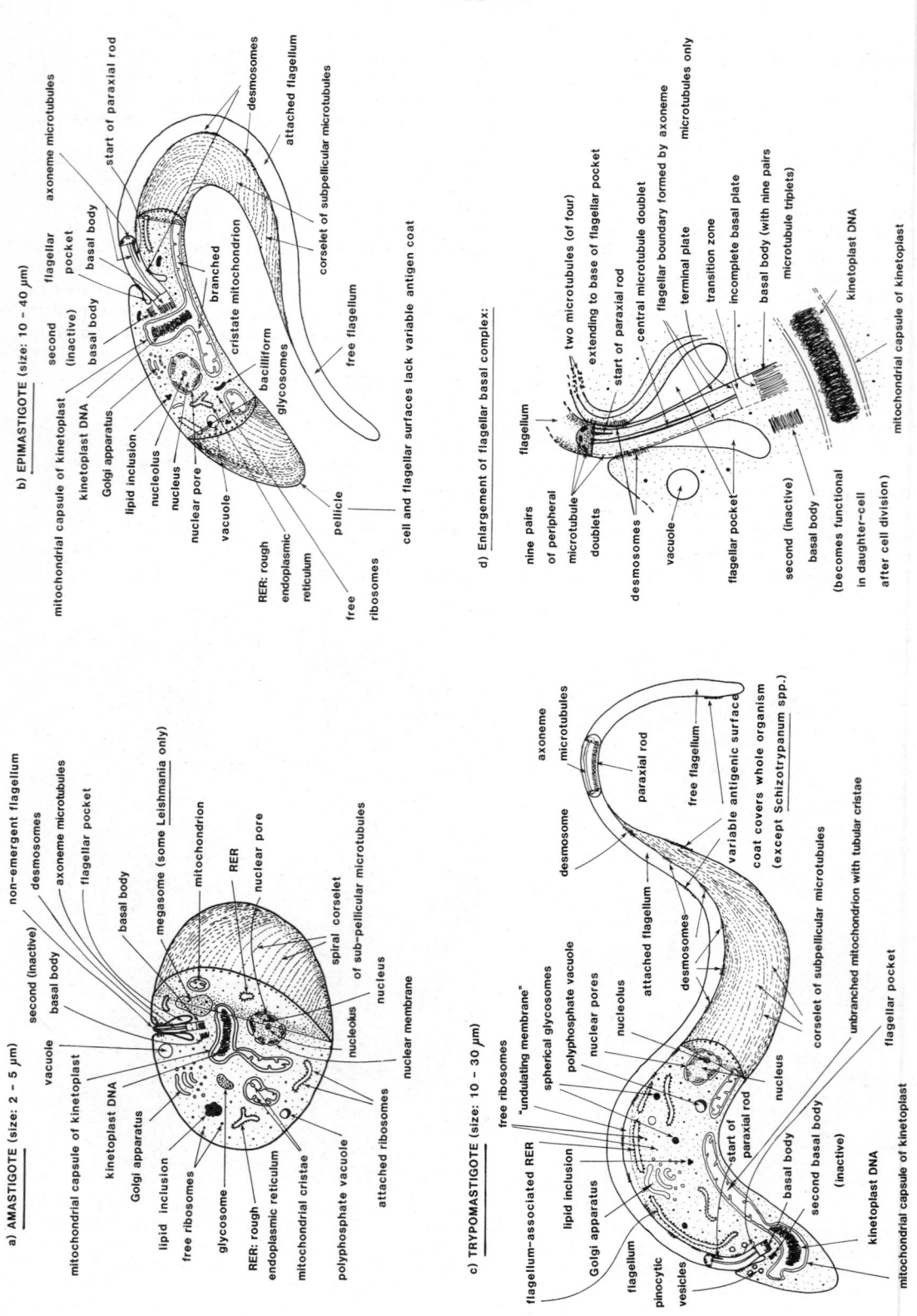

Fig. I.29 Internal ultrastructural architecture of trypanosomes and *Leishmania*: (a) amastigote; (b) epimastigote (the promastigote stage is similar, except for the anterior insertion of the flagellum); and (c) trypomastigote.

The "undulating membrane" of trypanosomatids is not a permanent anatomical structure, but a transient phenomenon produced by *temporary pellicular distortions* (between the intermittent desmosome-like junctional complexes which secure the flagellum to the cell-body), as contractile waves pass down the flagellum from its tip, to produce forward motion of the whole organism.

a) AMASTIGOTE (size: 2 – 5 μm)

- non-emergent flagellum
- desmosomes
- axoneme microtubules
- flagellar pocket
- basal body
- second (inactive) basal body
- vacuole
- mitochondrial capsule of kinetoplast
- kinetoplast DNA
- Golgi apparatus
- lipid inclusion
- free ribosomes
- glycosome
- RER: rough endoplasmic reticulum
- mitochondrial cristae
- polyphosphate vacuole
- attached ribosomes
- megasome (some *Leishmania* only)
- mitochondrion
- RER
- nuclear pore
- spiral corselet of sub-pellicular microtubules
- nucleus
- nucleolus
- nuclear membrane

b) EPIMASTIGOTE (size: 10 – 40 μm)

- axoneme microtubules
- start of paraxial rod
- desmosomes
- attached flagellum
- flagellar pocket
- basal body
- second (inactive) basal body
- corselet of subpellicular microtubules
- mitochondrial capsule of kinetoplast
- kinetoplast DNA
- Golgi apparatus
- lipid inclusion
- nucleolus
- nucleus
- nuclear pore
- vacuole
- branched cristate mitochondrion
- bacilliform glycosomes
- free flagellum
- pellicle
- RER: rough endoplasmic reticulum
- free ribosomes
- cell and flagellar surfaces lack variable antigen coat

c) TRYPOMASTIGOTE (size: 10 – 30 μm)

- free ribosomes
- "undulating membrane"
- spherical glycosomes
- polyphosphate vacuole
- nuclear pores
- nucleolus
- attached flagellum
- desmosomes
- corselet of subpellicular microtubules
- unbranched mitochondrion with tubular cristae
- flagellar pocket
- flagellum-associated RER
- lipid inclusion
- Golgi apparatus
- flagellum
- pinocytic vesicles
- start of paraxial rod
- second basal body (inactive)
- kinetoplast DNA
- mitochondrial capsule of kinetoplast
- nucleus
- basal body
- axoneme
- microtubules
- paraxial rod
- desmosome
- free flagellum
- variable antigenic surface coat covers whole organism (except *Schizotrypanum* spp.)

d) Enlargement of flagellar basal complex:

- nine pairs of peripheral microtubules
- flagellum
- two microtubules (of four)
- extending to base of flagellar pocket
- start of paraxial rod
- central microtubule doublet
- flagellar boundary formed by axoneme
- terminal plate
- transition zone
- incomplete basal plate
- basal body (with nine pairs microtubule triplets)
- microtubules only
- kinetoplast DNA
- mitochondrial capsule of kinetoplast
- doublets
- desmosomes
- vacuole
- flagellar pocket
- second (inactive) basal body (becomes functional in daughter-cell after cell division)

present consists of circular and linear molecules whose arrangement gives the kinetoplast its characteristic appearance by electron microscopy (Fig. I.28). Because of its staining characteristics, the kinetoplast DNA (kDNA; as distinct from nuclear DNA or nDNA) is also responsible for the appearance of the kinetoplast as a small round or oval body by light microscopy of Romanowsky-stained organisms (Fig. I.26), but the mitochondrion is visible only when cytochemical stains are used. Electron microscopy (EM) shows that the mitochondrion is a matrix-filled hollow structure bound by two membranes, which may occupy a large proportion of the cross-sectional area of the cell, particularly in some stages of the life-cycle of *Trypanozoon* (Fig. I.25). The inner mitochondrial membrane may be drawn out into disc-like, plate-like or tubular cristae, dependent upon mitochondrial activity at different stages of the life-cycle. During cell division the mitochondrion cleaves longitudinally, starting in the region of the nucleus, and the cleft then extends both forwards and backwards to divide the expanded kinetoplast capsule into two complete daughter-kinetoplasts. The form of the mitochondrion varies slightly from species to species, but commonly the most striking differences are observed from one stage of the life-cycle to another, within the same species.

The most dramatic, and most studied, mitochondrial changes are seen in the pleomorphic *Trypanozoon* species. In the multiplicative slender bloodstream trypomastigotes (in which endocytosis occurs via the flagellar pocket and the active glycosomes are spherical), the mitochondrion is in a repressed and inactive condition; by EM it is seen to be a narrow tube, with few or no cristae, which extends forward through the cell from the region of the kinetoplast (Fig. I.24), with a short posterior lobe. Slender bloodstream forms obtain energy from glycolysis of host glucose to pyruvate (the pyruvate is excreted, not oxidized in the mitochondrion), mainly in the glycosomes. (The trypanosomatids are unusual in that most of the glycolytic enzymes are localized in these organelles, found only in this group of the protozoa). Oxygen respiration is cyanide-insensitive, in the absence of a cytochrome-mediated electron transport chain at this stage of the life-cycle. As the slender trypomastigotes transform, first to the non-dividing intermediate form and then to the fly-infective short stumpy trypomastigote stage (Fig. I.26), the mitochondrion becomes activated and increases in girth, with the proliferation of further internal tubular cristae. In the stumpy trypomastigotes biochemical changes occur which herald a change to an amino acid based metabolism in the insect (*Glossina*) stages. Stumpy forms also show an increased pinocytic and lysosomal activity.

When ingested by a tsetse, the short stumpy trypomastigote begins to lose its glycoprotein coat and mitochondrial activation is enhanced during the transformation to the procyclic stage. This is accompanied by an increase in body length, extensive anterior and posterior ramification and branching of the mitochondrion, with the development of numerous discoid cristae (Fig. I.25); the relative mitochondrial volume is increased from about 5% to around 25%. These mitochondrial changes occur together with a cessation of endocytosis, a change in form of the glycosomes (to a bacilliform shape) and a change in the position of the kinetoplast (to a slightly more anterior location). These morphological and ultrastructural changes are associated with profound changes in cell respiration and metabolism, which occur in association with the change from the vertebrate to the invertebrate host (Figs. I.29, I.30, Table I.5).[38,39]

In the invertebrate (Glossina)

In the gut of *Glossina* glucose is no longer an available resource; most of the slender trypomastigotes die in the crop and midgut as the stumpy forms transform to the procyclic stage, in the endoperitrophic space of the posterior midgut (i.e., within the chitinous lining which separates the blood meal from the midgut epithelium).

Active division of the procyclics takes place during the first 3 days after ingestion of the stumpy bloodstream forms. In the absence of glucose, lost from the ingested blood meal within 15 minutes, proline is now utilized as the main energy source; it is the most abundant amino acid present in the tsetse midgut (proline is also the main source of energy for flight in *Glossina*). Mitochondrial activation, associated with the switch to proline metabolism, is also linked with a progressive change to cyanide-sensitive respiration, via a cytochrome chain. These respiratory changes may be related to the change in form (tubular to discoid) of the mitochondrial cristae.

From about day 4 after ingestion of the infected blood meal, procyclic trypomastigotes appear to penetrate the peritrophic membrane actively (rather than passing round its open posterior end) and enter the ectoperitrophic space as the more elongated, slenderer, 'established procyclic' stage, still in a state of active multiplication. Penetration of the peritrophic membrane sometimes occurs as far forward as the mycetome region of the tsetse midgut, but is more usually posterior to the mycetome. Moreover, penetration of adjacent midgut cells can subsequently occur; intracellular giant multinucleate forms are also observed. First seen by EM of experimental laboratory infections of tsetse, these observations were confirmed by more recent EM studies of natural *Trypanozoon* infections, in several tsetse species from West and central Africa. The importance of the multinucleate intracellular giant forms remains to be assessed, but active penetration of midgut cells by the established procyclic stage is further evidence for the occurrence of the postulated 'short-circuit' devel-

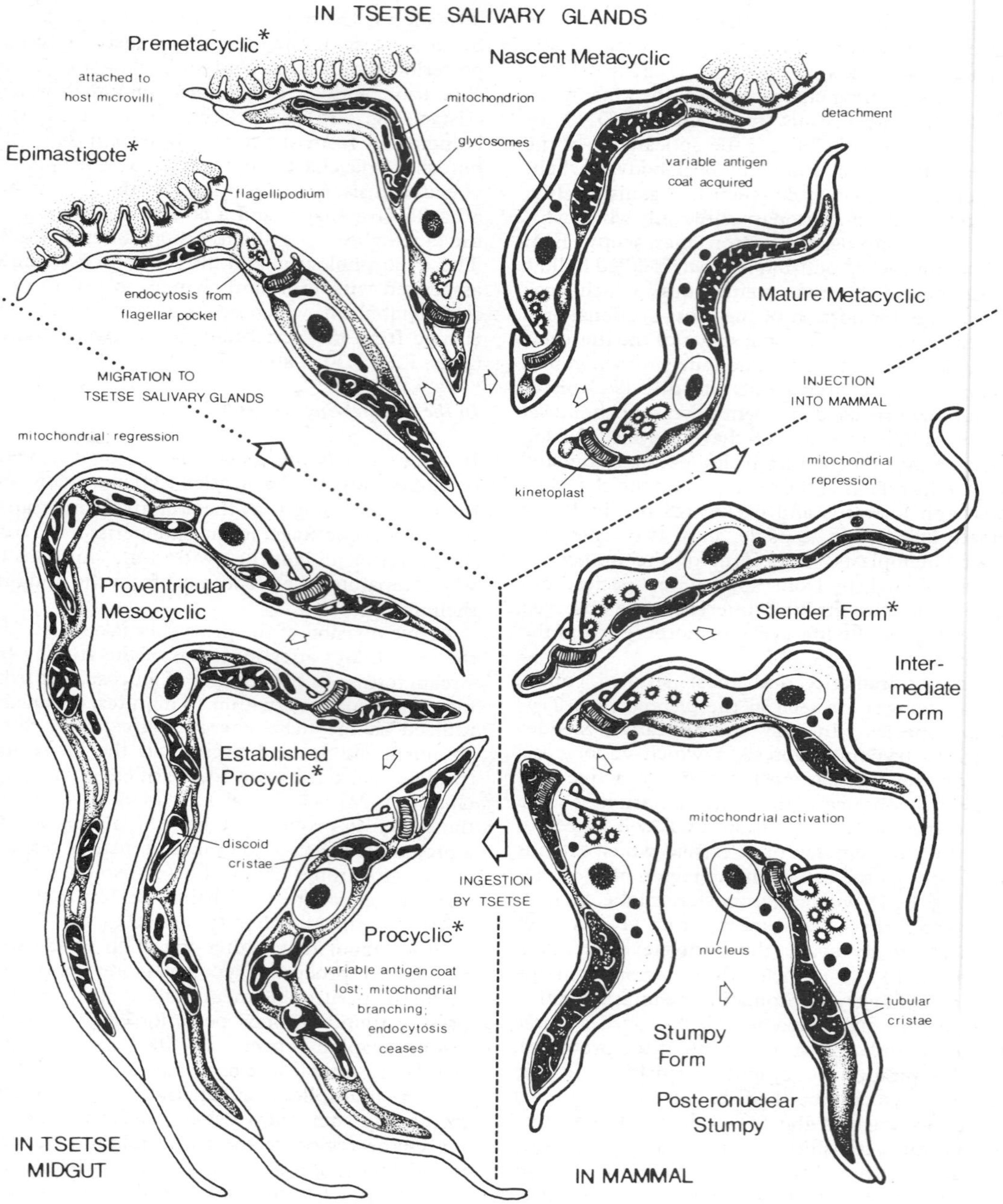

Fig. I.30 *Trypanosoma brucei*: developmental cycle in mammal and tsetse fly, showing changes in cell surface, mitochondrion, glycosomes and receptor-mediated endocytosis; also the relative size of different stages. Stages possessing the variable antigen coat lie to the right, uncoated stages to the left. The mitochondrion is depicted partly in section to show changes in the cristae. The posteronuclear stumpy form (bottom right) is included as an example of a form produced by some stocks, but which does not play an essential part in the cycle.

*Division occurs in these stages only.

(From Vickerman (1985);[38] with acknowledgements and thanks to the author, the British Council and the publishers of the *British Medical Bulletin*, Churchill Livingstone, London.)

Table I.5 The principal morphological changes which take place in the course of metacyclogenesis of *Trypanozoon* in the salivary glands of *Glossina*. (See Fig. I.30.)

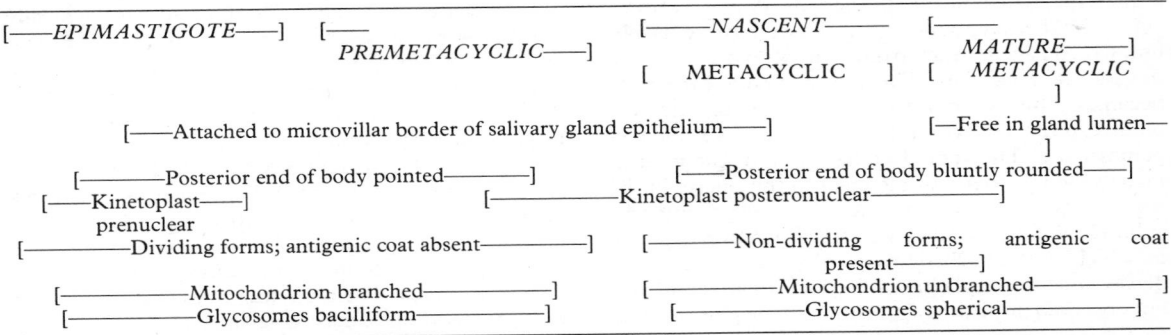

[——EPIMASTIGOTE——]	[—— PREMETACYCLIC——]	[——NASCENT——] [METACYCLIC]	[—— MATURE——] [METACYCLIC]
[——Attached to microvillar border of salivary gland epithelium——]			[—Free in gland lumen—]
[——Posterior end of body pointed——]		[——Posterior end of body bluntly rounded——]	
[——Kinetoplast——] prenuclear		[——Kinetoplast posteronuclear——]	
[——Dividing forms; antigenic coat absent——]		[——Non-dividing forms; antigenic coat present——]	
[——Mitochondrion branched——]		[——Mitochondrion unbranched——]	
[——Glycosomes bacilliform——]		[——Glycosomes spherical——]	

This table is based on part of a figure by Tetley and Vickerman (1985), with acknowledgements and thanks to the authors and publishers, the Company of Biologists Limited.[39]

opmental route for *Trypanozoon*, discussed in a later section and illustrated in Fig. I.32.

The ectoperitrophic established, procyclics migrate forward towards the region of the proventricular valve; they elongate even more (to about 60 μm) and cease division. A decrease in relative mitochondrial volume indicates the start of a phase of progressive mitochondrial repression, which continues for the remainder of the life-cycle, until reactivation again occurs in the stumpy bloodstream trypomastigote stage.

The elongated proventricular mesocyclics eventually migrate from the gut (whether by the 'classical' and/or 'short-circuit' routes is uncertain) and are next seen in the lumen of the salivary glands as shorter and stouter epimastigotes, now with an anteronuclear kinetoplast and again in a state of active division. The mitochondrion at this stage is divided into at least two branches, with many tubular cristae; the contents of the bacilliform glycosomes are homogeneous and dense. The epimastigotes are attached to the salivary gland epithelium by their flagella; dendritic outgrowths of the flagellum develop ('flagellipodia'), which interdigitate with the elongated (1–1.5 μm) microvilli of the salivary gland epithelial cells; multiple cup-shaped, hemidesmosome-like, attachment plaques are formed at points of contact between host and parasite (each about 100–130 nm in diameter) at regular intervals of 40–50 nm, but the electron-dense fibrillar material is formed only on the flagellar membrane side of the junctions (Fig. I.30). Between the junctional attachments there is a gap of about 20 nm between host and parasite membranes. The process of flagellar pocket endocytosis is resumed in the dividing attached epimastigotes, and continues during the subsequent period of metacyclogenesis in the salivary glands (summarized in Fig. I.30 and Table I.5).

Flagellar attachment to the salivary gland epithelium appears to be a necessary prerequisite for successful metacyclogenesis to take place in the subgenus *Trypanozoon*. However, in *T. (Duttonella) vivax* and *T. (Nannomonas) congolense*, epimastigotes undergo metacyclogenesis attached by their flagella to the chitinous internal surfaces of the proboscis of *Glossina*, by means of a continuous hemidesmosome-like junctional complex, but there is no distinctive flagellar expansion. *T. congolense* will form attachment plaques on inert (e.g. plastic) surfaces and undergo metacyclogenesis in vitro culture.

Among the attached epimastigotes of *Trypanozoon* in the salivary glands of *Glossina* are seen attached trypomastigotes, with posteronuclear kinetoplast and posterior flagellar emergence. These *premetacyclic stages* are still in active division and lack the external variant-specific glycoprotein coat. Attachment of the flagella to the microvillous epithelial surface by flagellar outgrowths and attachment plaques is continued, but the outgrowths are reduced in size compared with those of epimastigotes and the attachment zone is less extensive.

Other attached trypomastigotes are encountered, which now possess the external glycoprotein coat and whose flagella still retain attachment plaques, but which lack the flagellar outgrowths characteristic of the preceding epimastigote and premetacyclic stages. These are referred to as *nascent metacyclics*: they appear to be a non-dividing stage and the mitochondrion is now unbranched, with a reduced number of ampulliform cristae. The glycosomes have resumed a spherical form and their contents are less electron-dense; the process of flagellar pocket endocytosis is still evident. The reduction in mitochondrial size and complexity, and the return of the glycosomes to a spherical shape (both of which changes are synchronized with the reacquisition of the antigenic glycoprotein coat), appear to be preadaptive changes that prepare the organisms for the future metabolic and respiratory 'switch' which will accompany the change from an invertebrate to a vertebrate host. Other than by their continued attachment to the epithelial microvilli, the nascent metacyclics differ from the *mature metacyclics*, which lie free in the salivary gland lumen, chiefly by the retention of a short anterior free flagellum, which is very much truncated (or lost entirely) in the mature metacyclic. The posterior end of the body becomes bluntly rounded, as compared with the pointed posterior extremity of the premetacyclic trypomastigote. The short free flagellum of the nascent metacyclic is either still attached to the microvilli by focal plaques, or may be actually inserted into the submicrovillous apical cytoplasm of an epithelial cell, to which it is attached by evenly spaced, electron-dense, attachment plaques. This form of attachment is not observed until after acquisition of the glycoprotein coat.

The junctional attachment complexes of the flagellar region persist during acquisition of the glycoprotein surface coat by the nascent metacyclic trypomastigotes: either the development of the coat to maximum thickness finally breaks down the insect–parasite attachment, or it is disrupted by secretory products which result from the internal metabolic changes at this stage.

The mature metacyclic trypomastigotes liberated into the lumen of the salivary glands also appear to be incapable of division; they now entirely lack any indication of the junctional complexes by which they were previously attached to the gland epithelium. Their internal organization is unchanged from that of the preceding nascent metacyclic stage. Once injected with the saliva into a susceptible vertebrate, the metacyclic trypomastigotes undergo the final minor changes necessary for the transformation to the reproductive slender bloodstream trypomastigote stage; in which, however, there is some further repression of the mitochondrion, associated with the resumption of the glycolysis of glucose to pyruvate in the vertebrate.

Other cytoplasmic organelles of Trypanosomatidae

There is a large and confusing older literature concerned with 'cytoplasmic organelles' and the like in the Trypanosomatidae; the functional significance of many such cytoplasmic inclusions remains to be definitely established, together with their homology with comparable organelles of other eukaryotic cells.

In *Leishmania* and *Trypanosoma*, the membrane-bound lysosomes are products of the Golgi apparatus: the primary lysosomes formed by the Golgi cisternae contain acid hydrolases, particularly acid phosphatase, whose function is variously to digest ingested material (heterophagy), both unwanted products of the cell itself, which are first walled off by membranes (autophagy), or cell secretions (crinophagy). Primary lysosomes fuse with the vacuoles which contain material to be digested and the resultant vacuole is termed a secondary lysosome. These are discharged to the

exterior in the flagellar pocket region; it is thought that, in salivarian trypanosomes, this is the means by which the molecules of each of the antigenically distinctive variable glycoprotein 'coats' (the VSGs) are exposed on the surface of the trypomastigotes, after synthesis by the Golgi apparatus—RER system. The flagellar pocket region of some life-cycle stages in particular Stercoraria (but not Salivaria or *Leishmania*) may be structurally modified into a microtubule-lined cytostome and cytopharynx, in which materials ingested are initially digested and into which metabolic waste products can be discharged, but such a structure is not found in the salivarian bloodstream trypomastigotes. This structure does occur, however, in the intracellular amastigote stage of *T. (S.) cruzi* in the vertebrate host, and also in the epimastigote and sphaeromastigote stages in the gut of the triatomine vector. The flagellar pocket region, whether modified into a cytopharynx or not, is thus important in both the entry and exit of macromolecular materials. Residual bodies, the undigested remnants of secondary lysosomes, are cast out into the flagellar pocket together with the lysosomal enzymes. The residual bodies exocytosed by *T. brucei* are frequently large ($> 1\,\mu m$) and often have the structure of a liposome, with several concentric membrane layers, and may be covered with the surface coat glycoprotein. The residual bodies of Salivaria may be a source of the non-variable common antigens of bloodstream trypomastigotes; their discharge to the exterior as thick streamers from the flagellar pocket canal may be the source of the thick plasmanemes (see also p. 1268) and they, together with the lysosomal enzymes that accompany them, may play a role in the pathogenesis of African trypanosomiasis. Host serum proteins are endocytosed in the flagellar pocket region by the process of pinocytosis, in which spiny vesicles are formed and are pinched off internally from the pocket lining to enclose the host material. The spiny vesicles are budded off and transported to a specialized storage region of SER cisternae, with which they fuse. Primary lysosomes from the Golgi complex also fuse with this storage network, where heterophagic digestion is probably completed.

Glycosomes (formerly called microbodies or peroxisome-like organelles) contain oxidative metabolic enzymes which, in bloodstream salivarian trypomastigotes, break down host-derived glucose into pyruvate which is excreted into the bloodstream of the host, where its presence may cause pathogenic effects. Trypanosomes are unusual in that they lack carbohydrate reserves; since the salivarian bloodstream trypomastigotes metabolize glucose extensively, this is obtained in large amounts from the host. The invertebrate stages of Salivaria, where glucose is not available, switch their metabolic pathway to utilize amino acids, particularly proline, as respiratory substrates. This change is associated with a massive increase in the mitochondrial network and with changes of its internal structure, as described earlier. These mitochondrial changes occur to a lesser extent in Stercoraria (e.g. *T. (S.) cruzi*), in which (as also in *Leishmania*) the mitochondrial cristae are always plate-like; this probably correlates with the absence of any profound metabolic changes at any stage of the life-cycle, at least in *T. cruzi*.

Polyphosphate vacuoles occur in the Salivaria (very probably also in the Stercoraria and *Leishmania*) and are membrane-bound; their function may be to store energy-rich phosphate bonds or simply to serve as phosphate reserves. The polyphosphate vacuoles are one of a group of cytoplasmic inclusions collectively often referred to as 'volutin granules', particularly in earlier literature, because of their staining reaction with thiazine dyes.

The minute granular ribosomes are numerous, whether bound to the RER or free in the cytoplasm. They contain RNA and are active in protein synthesis throughout the cell.

Lipid inclusions are common in trypanosomes and *Leishmania*, either as membrane-bound liposomes or as free lipid droplets, whose function in cell metabolism is not always clear.

When the plasma membrane of salivarian and stercorarian trypanosomes, *Leishmania*, or other trypanosomatids, is ruptured by application of the freeze-fracture replica technique, the split often occurs along the middle of the lipid bilayer, passing over and under minute intramembranous particles (IMPs). The IMPs consist of proteins or lipoprotein complexes and, particularly in trypanosomes, they often are associated in linear clusters with the desmosome-like junctions between flagellum and cell surfaces. The number, density, location and arrangement of IMPs varies between the salivarian, stercorarian and *Leishmania* species; they probably represent functionally specialized regions of enzymes on the surface membrane. As in all cells, IMPs occur also in the plasma membranes of *Leishmania*, and all other kinetoplastids. Table I.6[40,41] gives details of IMP density and distribution (on the protoplasmic (PF) and exoplasmic faces (EF) of the freeze-fracture cleavage plane) for the stercorarian and salivarian trypanosome species, *Leishmania* spp. and other trypanosomatids so far investigated.

Mitochondrial changes in other trypanosomes (and in *Leishmania*)

The marked mitochondrial changes seen in the life-cycle of the salivarian subgenus *Trypanozoon* are much less pronounced in *T. (Duttonella) vivax* or the pleomorphic *T. (Nannomonas) congolense*; in both species there is little indication of mitochondrial repression; the bloodstream forms always have some tubular cristae and all vector stages have extensive cristae.

In the stercorarian *T. (Schizotrypanum) cruzi*, the plate-like cristae are found in all life-cycle stages,

although cyclical changes seem to occur also in the size of the mitochondrial network, minimal in the intracellular amastigote, larger in the bloodstream trypomastigote and maximal in the epimastigote stage in the triatomine vector. The most pronounced mitochondrial changes in *T. cruzi*, however, occur with the amplification of the kinetoplast capsule in the metacyclic and bloodstream trypomastigotes, where changes occur in the arrangement of the DNA molecules: in the trypomastigote there are several rows (three or four; sometimes six to eight) of looped fibrils arranged in tiers in the basket-shaped capsule, while in other stages there is only a double-layered array of fibrils in the discoid kinetoplast capsule, connected to the inner mitochondrial membrane by a loose felt of fine filaments.

Mitochondrial changes in *Leishmania* have been less well studied. However, there is an increase in the mitochondrial volume associated with the amastigote–promastigote transformation; but the total size of the parasite as a whole is also increased. Mitochondrial volume is greatest, in in vitro cultures, about 5 hours after transformation to the promastigote stage has started. (In the sandfly gut, amastigotes have been observed to divide at least once before transformation to the promastigote stage begins.) Throughout the life-cycle of *Leishmania*, the mitochondrial cristae are always plate-like and the mitochondrion is always cyanide-sensitive.

Dyskinetoplasty

A condition in which the kinetoplast DNA (kDNA) is irreversibly lost is known as dyskinetoplasty: the kinetoplast capsule is, however, retained and the term akinetoplasty is therefore not appropriate. Dyskinetoplasty may arise, apparently spontaneously, among a few trypanosomes in a population, or from the action of drugs with specific toxicity for the kinetoplast (e.g. acridines, phenanthridines or diamidines), which may produce totally dyskinetoplastic populations that breed true in the mammalian host. The dyskinetoplastic condition, however, precludes a digenetic life-cycle, since the presence of an intact kinetoplast (complete with kDNA) is essential for survival and reproduction in the insect vector. The mitochondrial kDNA is thus most likely to be absent in trypanosomes, such as *T. evansi*, which are not normally tsetse-transmitted.

Drug-induced dyskinetoplastic lines of *T. brucei* can live indefinitely in the mammal, probably because of mitochondrial repression at that stage of the life-cycle; with the continued production of stumpy trypomastigotes, although these are unable to survive if ingested by *Glossina*.

Unlike *T. brucei*, however, *T. (S.) cruzi* has no obvious phase of mitochondrial repression, and drug-induced dyskinetoplastic epimastigotes can continue to differentiate into metacyclic trypomastigotes; these are capable of invading mammalian cells and of further reproduction as intracellular amastigotes.

MITOSIS IN THE TRYPANOSOMATIDAE

Nuclear division in protozoan cells differs from that in the eukaryotes in several ways; the process (intranuclear mitosis) has been studied at the EM level mainly in the flagellate stages of some species of *Leishmania*, *Trypanosoma* and other trypanosomatids, in all of which the process is fundamentally similar. In none of the Protozoa are there centrioles and nuclear division occurs without disruption of the nuclear membrane.

However, it is noted elsewhere (see section on 'invertebrate life-cycles of *Leishmania*' below) that in the genus *Leishmania* the normal process of cell division is, at least sometimes, uncharacteristic of the remainder of the Kinetoplastida (in which division of the kinetoplast always occurs before division of the nucleus), since (in the invertebrate cycle of *L. (L.) infantum*), nuclear division can normally precede that of the kinetoplast. (In *L. infantum* the first indication of cell division among large nectomonad promastigotes in the abdominal midgut of the sandfly is actually the production of a second, and smaller flagellum: this is followed by nuclear division and then division of the kinetoplast.) But in spite of this anomaly in at any rate some species of *Leishmania*, or perhaps all, the process of nuclear division per se appears to be uniform throughout the Kinetoplastida.

Interphase. Nuclei are rounded in shape, with moderately dense chromatin associated with the nuclear membrane. The central nucleolus is spherical and composed of electron-dense granules. The remainder of the nucleus is homogeneous in texture.

Mitosis: preliminary phase. The first sign of incipient division is a decrease in size and electron density of the heterochromatin mass, together with a reduction in the density of the nucleolus. Microtubules develop in the still-spherical nucleus, to form the mitotic spindle.

Equatorial phase. As regions of heterochromatin begin to decondense they become less dense and homogeneous in appearance. The nucleolus is retained during the mitotic process, but at this stage it elongates to an oval shape. Electron-dense plaques appear in the equatorial region of the nucleus, attached to the 40–60 spindle microtubules, which originate near the nuclear membrane at both poles. The equatorial dense plaques appear to be the functional equivalent of the centromeres of higher organisms; their number is constant for each genus so far examined. There are six plaques in *Leishmania (L.) donovani*, *L. (L.) mexicana* and *L. (V.) braziliensis* (the number was not determined in *L. (L.) tropica* or *L. (L.) hertigi*, although the dense plaques were also seen). *Trypanosoma cruzi* has 10 plaques; *Crithidia (C. fasciculata)* and *Blastocrithidia (B. triatomae)* each have three plaques. As division proceeds, the dense plaques divide to form pairs of hemiplaques (karyomeres), at which some microtubules terminate (others run tangentially to the plane of the plaques).

Elongation phase. The nuclear outline changes from oval to dumbbell shaped as the equatorial hemiplaques, or karyomeres, begin to separate in a polar direction, along the spindle microtubules (with which they remain in contact). The nucleolus elongates and divides into two. A narrow connection between the dividing nuclei is occupied by the spindle microtubules; the nuclear membrane is still intact at this stage (see Fig. I.38).

Reorganization phase. The nuclear membrane heterochromatin pattern reappears, as the spindle microtubules and the dense hemiplaques disappear, and division into two rounded daughter cells (each with a spherical, dense nucleolus) is completed. There are indications of quantitative differences in the heterochromatin volume in some species: *L. (L.) donovani* promastigotes, for example, appear to contain more chromatin than those of *L. (L.) mexicana* and *L. (V.) braziliensis*.

LIFE-CYCLE AND TRANSMISSION OF TRYPANOSOMES

SALIVARIA

Except for *T. equiperdum*, directly transmitted between horses during coitus, the salivarian trypanosomes are transmitted by invertebrate vectors in which cyclical development normally occurs. Development is anterior and transmission is inoculative. The salivarian trypanosomes of economic and medical importance are transmitted either cyclically by species of tsetse flies, or mechanically by biting flies (e.g. *T.*

evansi, transmitted mainly by Tabanidae), where no cyclical development occurs in the vector.

SUBGENUS: *Duttonella*

T. vivax in Africa is transmitted by tsetse flies, but transmission can also occur mechanically; this is the normal method in many areas of Latin America and in Mauritius, where the parasite was introduced in imported livestock and *Glossina* spp. are absent. In the tsetse belts of Africa, however, *T. vivax* is cyclically transmitted by *Glossina*, principally by members of the *morsitans* group, and development and multiplication are confined to the biting mouthparts. Multiplication of epimastigotes occurs in the proboscis and gives rise to dense clusters of flagellates attached to the walls of the labrum and labium; these eventually detach and invade the hypopharynx, where they transform into trypomastigotes; eventually these mature into infective metatrypomastigotes which resemble the bloodstream trypanosomes, with rounded posterior end and a prominent subterminal kinetoplast (mean length $> 20 \mu m$). The cycle in the fly usually takes from 5 to 13 days, partly depending on temperature.

The bloodstream trypanosomes occur in wild ungulates and domestic livestock; extravascular trypanosomes are often numerous in the lymph glands. *T. vivax* is uninfective for man but is an important cause of economic losses in livestock; the effects of the parasite vary from chronic to acute, depending on the virulence of the trypanosome strain and the resistance of the host. *T. uniforme* is closely allied to *T. vivax* but is smaller and of lesser economic importance (mean length $< 18 \mu m$).

SUBGENUS: Nannomonas

T. congolense is more widespread and common than *T. simiae*, the other species of this subgenus. Neither species is infective to man but both are of great economic importance as pathogenic parasites of domestic livestock. Wild ruminants are generally symptom-free when infected with *T. congolense*, of which they are the natural hosts.

T. congolense is an economically important parasite of cattle, goats, sheep, camels, pigs, dogs and cats. Disease manifestations vary from chronic to acute, depending on the strain of parasite and other factors, but severe anaemia always occurs.

The related *T. simiae* has a life-cycle similar to *T. congolense* and is an important cause of economic loss in exotic domestic pigs, among which epidemics of a fulminating and fatal infection occur.

Bloodstream trypomastigotes of *T. congolense* are variable in size but are generally small ($8-24 \mu m$) and typically monomorphic, with an inconspicuous undulating membrane and usually no free flagellum. Extravascular stages have been demonstrated in rabbits but it is not clear whether these are a normal part of the vertebrate cycle.

In the tsetse, *T. congolense* undergoes cyclical development which takes 19–53 days to complete to the infective stage, depending on temperature and other factors. Trypanosomes pass with the blood meal into the gut and multiply as elongated trypomastigotes. These later enter the ectoperitrophic space and migrate forward through the oesophagus to the proboscis, where they transform into epimastigotes. Finally they enter the hypopharynx with the formation of infective metatrypomastigotes. *T. congolense* must complete its full developmental cycle in the tsetse before the trypanosomes are infective to mammals, but mechanical transmission of bloodstream trypanosomes can also occur.

SUBGENUS: Pycnomonas

T. suis is the only species and, because it causes acute disease in pigs, has often been confused with the unrelated *T. simiae*. The parasite is found in Tanzania and Burundi and is transmitted by *G. brevipalpis* and *G. vanhoofi*; its normal hosts are probably wild pigs. *T. suis* is a broad, short, monomorphic species in the bloodstream stage, with a small posterior kinetoplast. Development in *Glossina* resembles that of *Trypanozoon* spp. and takes about 28 days: slender trypomastigotes from the cardia region of the gut invade the salivary glands, where they transform into epimastigotes; these then pass through the salivary ducts into the hypopharynx, where infective (metacyclic) trypomastigotes finally develop.

The metacyclic trypomastigotes of *T. (P.) suis* in the fly can be distinguished, by the presence of a free flagellum, from metacyclics of all other species of *Trypanozoon*.

SUBGENUS: Trypanozoon

The best-known members of this subgenus are the tsetse-transmitted sleeping sickness trypanosomes of Africa, the cause of gambian and rhodesian disease in man, but the subgenus also includes *T. equiperdum*, a sexually transmitted parasite of horses (the cause of dourine), and *T. evansi* (the cause of surra), which is mechanically transmitted between camels, equines and other animals in North Africa, Asia and South America.

The subgenus *Trypanozoon* is the most homogeneous group of the salivarian trypanosomes, represented by species and/or subspecies that are morphologically indistinguishable but which differ in biological, nosological and biochemical characteristics and are also markedly pleomorphic in the vertebrate host.

The three subspecies of *T. brucei*—*T. b. brucei*, *T. b. gambiense* and *T. b. rhodesiense*—are confined to tropical Africa and are transmitted cyclically by *Glossina* spp. They are pathogenic for various vertebrates. *T. b. brucei* is by definition not pathogenic to man but is the cause of nagana in livestock, whilst *T. b. gambiense* and *T. b. rhodesiense* cause human sleeping sickness. Parasites causing rhodesian sleeping sickness in human volunteers have been isolated from bushbuck (*Tragelaphus scriptus*) and from domestic cattle in East Africa, as well as from ungulates and carnivores. Recent evidence also implicates pigs as peridomestic hosts of putative *T. b. rhodesiense* in Uganda (strains serum-resistant in the BIIT).

As indicated elsewhere (see p. 1265), *T. b. gambiense* in some areas of West Africa has been shown convincingly (by isoenzyme studies, in the main) to occur in domestic dogs, pigs and sheep, and in some wild ungulates also. At least the dogs and pigs, and perhaps the sheep, seem to constitute a peridomestic reservoir of parasites capable of causing human disease. The long-held 'classical' view that *T. b. gambiense* had no animal reservoir is clearly no longer tenable. However, it remains to be seen if domestic animals, or indeed, wild antelope are of general (rather than occasional) importance in the epidemiology of gambian sleeping sickness.

T. b. brucei is an important parasite of livestock and domestic pets; its normal hosts are mainly wild ungulates and, occasionally, carnivores. Infections with *T. b. brucei* are most serious in equines, camels, goats, sheep, dogs and cats; cattle and pigs are less susceptible. Economic loss due to *T. b. brucei* is most serious among horses, donkeys and mules and least in cattle. Bloodstream stages of all members of *Trypanozoon* are pleomorphic but are otherwise morphologically identical. The tsetse-transmitted metatrypanosomes are short and slender and these first transform in the subcutaneous tissues into long

slender forms (20–40 μm) and enter the blood; stumpy forms (15–25 μm) are also found in the blood and tissue fluids. Some of the stumpy forms have the nucleus near the posterior end and are often referred to as posteronuclear forms. Slender trypomastigotes have a long flagellum and a subterminal kinetoplast; stumpy forms have either no free flagellum or a very short one and the kinetoplast is posterior. Forms intermediate between slender and stumpy ones are also found. The long slender trypomastigotes are considered to be essentially multiplicative and the short stumpy ones to be the stage principally infective to *Glossina*, but the role of the different stages is still controversial (see below).

The considerable morphological variability of the bloodstream forms of *Trypanozoon* is termed variously 'polymorphism' or 'pleomorphism'; the latter term is preferable, since 'polymorphism' has the additional connotation of genetic variability, which is inappropriate in *Trypanozoon*; pleomorphism still occurs when infection is initiated with a single organism. The causes of the morphological diversity of the bloodstream (and tissue) phases of *Trypanozoon* have been a source of much interest and controversy for very many years and are still far from fully understood. Ormerod[42] discussed very fully the development of *T. brucei* organisms in the vertebrate host and advanced

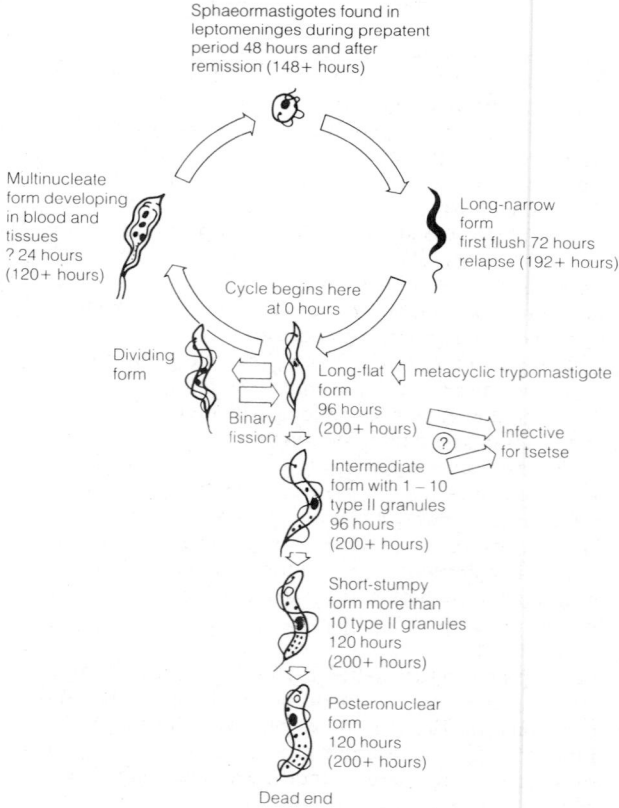

Fig. I.31 Life-cycle of *T. brucei* according to the 'multinucleate hypothesis'. The hourly figures in parentheses are for the second time around the cycle. (After Ormerod.[42])

some interesting new hypotheses on the significance of pleomorphism, the significance of 'aberrant' forms in the blood and tissues and the possible significance of tissue forms of the parasite in the mammalian stages of the life-cycle. Many of Ormerod's views are summarized in his postulated life-cycle diagram (Fig. I.31).

Ormerod and co-workers have recently (several papers published in 1986) indirectly demonstrated, by electron microscopy and selective drug treatment regimens, what they believe to be true intracellular vertebrate stages of *Trypanozoon* which occur, at least in mice, in ependymal cells of the choroid plexus and those which line the brain ventricles. They consider these stages truly intracellular, very probably anaerobic (in contrast to the aerobic bloodstream and tissue forms found elsewhere, e.g. in plasma cells) and that they possibly undergo multiple fission. The ependymal cells parasitized in the choroid plexus are destroyed, but appear to be rapidly replaced, and the choroid plexus maintains its integrity by regeneration of an outer layer of new ependymal cells. Replacement of ependymal cells in the ventricular linings, however, is very slow (if it occurs at all), which suggests this may be a factor in pathogenesis. Suramin failed to clear the intracellular forms from the ependymal cells, although this drug eliminated parasites from the cerebral cortex, which suggests that the intracellular

forms are functionally protected from the activity of at least some drugs in common therapeutic use. A suramin/metronidazole mixture, however, was effective in clearing the parasites from ependymal sites, although metronidazole alone was ineffective: this is the main evidence which suggests that intracellular stages may be anaerobic.

The life-cycle of *T. brucei* subspecies in *Glossina* was studied in detail by Robertson in 1913 and the 'classical' view which she proposed was essentially as follows (Fig. I.32,1–8). Once in the midgut of the tsetse the bloodstream trypomastigotes were imprisoned within the peritrophic membrane (the endoperitrophic space) until they reached its posterior extremity, where they could then escape into the ectoperitrophic space. In the ectoperitrophic space the trypomastigotes migrated forward until 10 or 20 days after infection, when they reached the region of the proventricular valve and developed into the more slender and elongated 'proventricular' forms, which then actively penetrated the newly-secreted and still fluid peritrophic membrane and escaped through the proventricular valve, first into the oesophagus and thence to the tip of the labrum. At the tip of the labrum the trypanosomes then entered the open end of the hypopharynx and from there passed into the salivary glands. Once in the salivary glands the proventricular forms change into epimastigotes; these first multiply

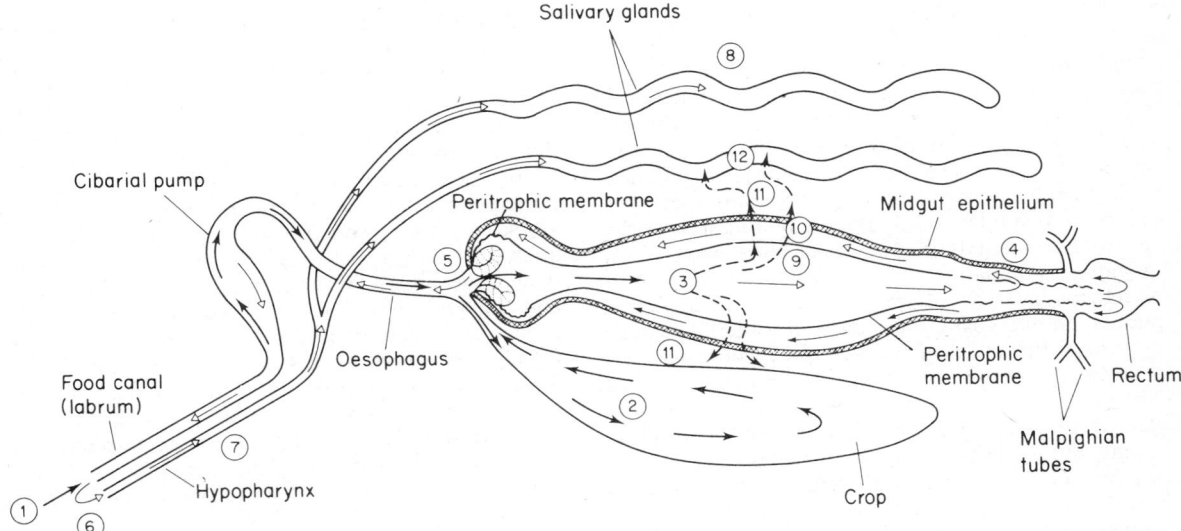

Fig. I.32 The alternative or concomitant developmental pathways of *Trypanosoma brucei* subspecies in *Glossina*: the 'classical' and 'short-circuit' routes. Solid arrows with black points ($\rightarrow$) show the passage of trypanosomes in the blood meal from the food canal (1), via the crop (2), to the midgut (3). From the midgut the 'classical' route is indicated by solid arrows with white points ($\longrightarrow$); trypanosomes escape from the peritrophic membrane only at its posterior extremity (4), move forward in the ectoperitrophic space to the proventricular valve (5), where they penetrate the still-fluid part of the peritrophic membrane to enter the oesophagus and thence pass forward to the tip of the labrum; here they turn round (6) and enter the hypopharynx (7), en route to the salivary glands (8). Dashed arrows with black points ($-\rightarrow$) show the direct 'short-circuit' route, by which trypanosomes actively penetrate the intact peritrophic membrane (9), enter midgut epithelial cells (10), in which they divide before passing into the haemocoel (11), then (probably) directly penetrate through the cellular walls of the salivary glands (12) to complete development to the metacyclic stage.

and finally give rise to the infective metatrypanosomes. The cycle in *Glossina* occupies a period of about one month, but can be variable.

Robertson's interpretation of her observations, however, has recently been opened to some doubt (Fig. I.32,9–12). First, trypanosomes were observed in the haemocoel of a proportion of naturally infected wild *Glossina* and this observation was confirmed with experimental flies. More recently, in flies infected experimentally 9 to 12 days earlier, electron microscopic studies have shown the presence of free ecto-peritrophic midgut trypomastigotes with extended mitochondria; these were found to penetrate and divide in midgut cells. Dividing forms from the midgut cells were sometimes accompanied by enigmatic multinucleate 'giant forms' whose significance is unresolved. Ribbon-like trypomastigotes and epimastigotes were then seen in the haemocoel (possibly after escape from the midgut cells) and these are now believed to be able to penetrate the salivary glands directly, although final proof of this is lacking. Fig. I.32 summarizes both the 'classical' pathway and the 'heretical' or 'short-circuit' pathway that now seems to occur, either as well as, or possibly instead of, the classical route.

Biochemical characterization of salivarian trypanosomes

Since the demonstration of isoenzyme polymorphism among populations of morphologically indistinguishable salivarian trypanosomes in the 1970s, much subsequent use was made of isoenzyme electrophoresis (on thin-layer starch gels or cellulose acetate), as a means to distinguish and delimit 'zymodemes' in trypanosomes. A zymodeme is a population of organisms (in this context, of trypanosomes) that differs from similar closely related populations in the electrophoretic mobilities of one or more isoenzymes; in short, a population with a specific combination of isoenzyme patterns. (A stock, on the other hand, is a population of trypanosomes derived by serial passage in vitro and/or in vivo from a primary isolate without characterization or any implication of homogeneity.) The newer and more discriminatory technique of iso-electric focusing in agarose gels is used to a lesser extent, and is useful mainly for enzymes which do not resolve well on starch gels. Enzyme electrophoresis is valuable also in the study of other morphologically similar groups of pathogenic organisms, among them *Entamoeba* and *Leishmania*. The principles and methodology of enzyme electrophoresis are now well known and the method is briefly considered in another section (see section on criteria for identification of *Trypanosoma* and *Leishmania*, above).

About 1000 stocks of *Trypanozoon* have been studied, variously ascribed on other criteria to *T. b. brucei*, *T. b. gambiense*, *T. b. rhodesiense* and *T. evansi*, together with many of *T. vivax* and *T. congolense*.

From 12 to 20 enzymes are commonly used, selected for their clear and consistent banding.

Well over 70 *Trypanozoon* zymodemes are now known: early hopes that enzyme electrophoresis would serve unequivocally to separate *T. b. brucei*, *T. b. gambiense* and *T. b. rhodesiense* were unfortunately not borne out. In particular, no isoenzyme marker was found which is associated with infectivity for man, and no unequivocal means has yet been discovered to distinguish stocks with certainty as *T. b. brucei*, *T. b. gambiense* or *T. b. rhodesiense*; whether based on zymodemes alone or in association with other methods of intrinsic characterization, such as kDNA analysis or the use of monoclonal antibodies.

Trypanozoon stocks separate into two broad geographical zymodeme groups; one principally West African, the other from eastern Africa, on the basis of distinctive patterns for phosphoglucomutase (PGM) and isocitrate dehydrogenase (ICD). This division suggests that *T. b. brucei* sensu stricto stocks from West and eastern Africa may be at least as distinct as those of *T. b. gambiense* and *T. b. rhodesiense*.

The East African stocks are further geographically divided on a north–south basis; stocks from Botswana, Zambia, Tanzania and Mozambique (which constitute a closely related group of zymodemes), have single-banded patterns for PGM and ICD, whilst those from the Lake Victoria area of Uganda and Kenya (a considerably more diverse zymodeme cluster) have multi-banded PGM and ICD patterns. This north–south division may possibly be a reflection of the differing patterns of epidemicity in the two regions: a more stable endemic situation in the south contrasts with a tendency for intense epidemics, and a greater intrinsic diversity among *Trypanozoon* organisms, in the Lake Victoria basin further north. Cluster analysis of East African stocks revealed a further zymodeme subgroup, kiboko, whose zymodemes are characterized by variation in the normally stable patterns of threonine dehydrogenase (TDH), nucleoside hydrolase (NH), and malate dehydrogenase (MDH). The kiboko group, also characterized by a distinctive kDNA, is largely restricted to tsetse–wild animal cycles in Kenya, Tanzania and Zambia, but three human infections with kiboko zymodemes are nonetheless reported from Zambia. The possession of a distinctive kDNA, and of enzyme markers, may indicate an isolation of the kiboko zymodemes from the main eastern African stocks of *Trypanozoon*.

A special subgroup of *Trypanozoon* zymodemes cause human sleeping sickness in parts of West Africa; this set of zymodemes combine a distinctive isoenzyme profile with a low virulence to rodents, a characteristic VAT repertoire and a specific coding sequence for a particular VSG gene, whether this is expressed or silent; they also lack one other VSG gene commonly possessed by the *T. brucei* subspecies. This group of stocks also apparently has fewer mini-chromosomes (see below) than other zymodeme groups in *Try-*

panozoon, and appears generally to correspond with the classical concept of *T. b. gambiense*. Other stocks from West Africa, which also cause chronic human (i.e. gambian) sleeping sickness, do not share these genetic characters, whose specificity to *T. b. gambiense* has yet to be tested with *T. b. brucei* from the same region.

Although chromosomes cannot be visualized directly in the Kinetoplastida (and cytogenetic analysis is therefore not possible), pulsed field gradient gel (PFG) electrophoresis can separate chromosome-sized fragments of DNA ('molecular karotypes'), in the size range 50–2000 kilobase pairs (kb). *T. congolense* and *T. b. brucei* have up to five large chromosomes (in the size range 1–2 megabase pairs, Mb), several of intermediate size (200–700 kb) and many mini-chromosomes (50–150 kb). *T. vivax*, however, differs from the former two species in its lack of mini-chromosomes. (Other Kinetoplastida are different yet again: *T. (S.) cruzi* and *Leishmania* each have 10–20 chromosomes, all in the intermediate size range, 700–2000 kb.)

Molecular karyotyping and kDNA analysis (particularly of the maxicircles, the equivalent of mitochondrial DNA in other organisms) may contribute in future to a solution of the taxonomic and other enigmas which still remain in the subgenus *Trypanozoon*, but it is presently uncertain whether or not kDNA is inherited independently of nuclear genotype. (If kDNA is indeed inherited independently, features of kDNA would not be suitable as markers for characterization.)

Despite their considerable value in epidemiological studies, isoenzymes and other methods of intrinsic characterization may yet prove fruitless for the practical purposes of the physician with patients, who needs to know if he is dealing with 'gambiense' or 'rhodesiense' parasites. The recent demonstration that hybrid enzyme variants arise, by some form of genetic interchange (possibly of a sexual nature), during cyclical transmission in *Glossina*, is not only further evidence for diploidy and of possible sexual processes in trypanosomes, but is also a further indication that the *T. brucei* 'subspecies' are indeed a human artefact, and *T. brucei* sensu lato probably a continuous and interbreeding population. The factors in *Trypanozoon* which confer human serum resistance, and hence infectivity and virulence for man, may in the end be found elsewhere. Some recent evidence suggests the key to this particular mystery may lie in a selection for serum-resistant (or serum-sensitive) individual *T. brucei* trypanosomes, in the course of their exposure to blood meals of differing origins in the alimentary canal of individual *Glossina*.

Antigenic variation in mammalian trypanosomes

Infections with the salivarian trypanosomes are char-acterized by periodic fluctuations in the peripheral parasitaemia, which rises and falls each few days during the course of infection, a feature not seen in infections with the Stercoraria or *Leishmania*, in which the vertebrate stages of the parasites are either principally (*T. cruzi*) or entirely (*Leishmania*) intra-cellular amastigotes. The appearance of each successive parasitaemic wave of the salivarian trypanosomes is related to changes in the antigenic composition of the trypanosome population following each peak of parasitaemia. This is a result of changes in the variant-specific glycoprotein (VSG) surface antigens, expressed on the surface coat of the bloodstream trypomastigotes; each trypanosome thus expresses a particular surface variant antigen type (VAT) at any one time. Host antibodies produced in response to one VSG (= VAT) are ineffective against the antigenically different VSGs (expressed as bloodstream VATs, or B-VATs) which appear in subsequent parasitaemic waves. Hence, each successive and antigenically distinctive trypanosome population which arises can evade the immune responses (i.e. VAT-specific antibodies) of the host to earlier VSGs.

This phenomenon is known as antigenic variation; each different VSG expressed on the trypomastigote surface coat causes successive variant antigenic types (VATs). Antigenic variation occurs in all the subgenera of the Salivaria (but is unknown, or at least very rare, in Stercoraria and *Leishmania*), but the process has been mainly studied in the tsetse-transmitted members of *Trypanozoon*. Antigenic variation in *Trypanozoon* is associated particularly with the dividing slender bloodstream trypomastigotes, rather than with the later mature, and non-dividing, stumpy stages.

On ingestion by the tsetse fly the surface coat, and thus the last VSG, is rapidly lost. Later in the developmental cycle in the fly (in the nascent metacyclic trypomastigote stage, still attached to the salivary gland epithelium (Fig. I.26)), the antigenic surface coat is reacquired and a new VSG is expressed on its surface, as a metacyclic VAT or M-VAT. Following cyclical transmission through *Glossina*, there is a tendency for subsequent reversion to one or a few common VATs, but this anamnestic response is not invariable and it was shown conclusively that metacyclics of individual flies are generally heterogeneous with regard to the VSG (and hence the M-VAT) expressed. The number of VSGs/VATs which can be expressed by a cloned trypanosome population is known as the VAT repertoire. The relatively limited M-VAT series seems to be a limited subset within the overall VAT repertoire; monoclonal antibody studies showed 12 M-VATs in a *T. congolense* stock, but 16 main M-VATs and numerous minor M-VATs (expressed sporadically and at a low level) in one of *T. b. rhodesiense*. Of the 1000 or more VSG genes of the *Trypanozoon* trypanosomes, only 1–2% produce the major M-VATS. Also a feature of M-VATs is their relative predictability (in comparison to the general unpredictability of the later and more numerous B-VATs). The M-VAT composition of the population does not include, and is not influenced by, the larger series of B-VATs (including the ingested VAT—the I-VAT—which initiated infection of the fly). Unfortunately for earlier hopes of effective vaccines based on M-VATs, major M-VATs are occasionally lost in sequential fly transmission of cloned stocks (and probably replaced by others) and the situation is further complicated by the unpredictable occurrence of numerous, sporadic, minor M-VATs.

When metacyclics enter the bloodstream of the mammal, they transform into bloodstream trypomastigotes, but continue to express M-VATs until these are eliminated by the antibody responses of the host. At this early stage, once the M-VATs have ceased, among the first of the B-VATs to appear is the I-VAT, which originated infection of the fly from a previous host. Throughout the cycle in the fly (i.e. in the uncoated stages), a high potential for reactivation of the I-VAT (the infecting B-VAT) is thus retained—a 'memory' of the last VSG expressed. Each bloodstream trypomastigote has a coat of about 10^7 VSG molecules on its surface: these account for about 10% of total cell proteins. Multiple expression of two VSGs at the same time is possible in vitro by bloodstream forms in culture; each VSG behaves as a separate entity on the cell surface, not as a hybrid protein. In the mammal host, however, any trypanosomes which may transiently express more than one VSG would rapidly be eliminated, by antibodies directed against the first VSG expressed. Available evidence strongly suggests that production of M-VATs and B-VATs is controlled by separate mechanisms. M-VSG genes, however, appear to be located only on the larger chromosomes. Most other VSG genes occur in tandem arrays within chromosomes, but a distinct subset (including those for B-VATs with the highest expression potential), occur at telomeres (chromosome ends); the numerous 'minichromosomes' of the trypanosome genome seem to function solely as a source of telomeres, as a repository for this set of VSG genes.

Antigenic variation is known to be antibody-independent, non-random and under genetic control; the number of possible VSGs (and hence first M-VATs, then B-VATs) is large, but not infinite. The role of each successive VAT-specific antibody produced by the host is selective rather than inductive; at any one time during infection a small number of new (heterotype) VATs are expressed by some few individual trypanosomes among the predominant homotype population. The production of host antibodies in response to the numerous, successive, homotypes results in their destruction, but allows the few new heterotypes to survive and proliferate in their place, thus producing a new parasitaemic wave. The greater the heterogeneity of VATs (i.e. VSGs), sequentially

expressed, the more likely is infection to persist; the response of individual trypanosomes to changing host conditions (antibodies) is far less important, if at all, than the cumulative response of the heterotype/homotype population as a whole.

Because of the implications of antigenic variation in regard to possible immunization against trypanosomal diseases, the subject has attracted much attention and, thanks to recent technological advances, the fundamental genetic mechanisms which control the process (and the biochemistry of its expression) are now understood relatively well, with rapid accumulation of new detailed information. (For a comprehensive recent review of the molecular biology of African trypanosomes with particular reference to antigenic variation, the interested reader is referred to Barry.[43])

Antigenic variation evidently is not the result of random, spontaneous mutation (since particular VATs tend to appear early in infection and others late). Cloned DNA sequence probes for VSG genes and their corresponding messenger RNA (mRNA), have indeed shown that most, if not all, VSG genes exist in the genome prior to antigenic variation. Further, only one VSG gene is normally expressed as mRNA at any one time. The VSGs are encoded by a multigene family and antigenic variation occurs when expression of one VSG gene is switched to that of another. At any time, only one VSG gene is active: expression of VSG genes occurs only at telomeres (chromosome ends). Each VSG gene exists in the genome as a non-transcribed *basic copy* (BC) gene; two main, and independent, processes of VSG BC gene activation occur. In the first of these (the duplicative transposition process; also known as a gene conversion), the BC is duplicated to produce an *expression-linked copy* (ELC), which is then transposed to a chromosome end (telomere) and there transcriptionally activated (the non-transcribed BC is retained during this process of gene conversion). In the second (non-duplicative) process, the BC is already located at a telomere, where it is activated without duplication, and apparently without transposition. (For telomeric VSG BC genes, located at chromosome ends, there are at least three different mechanisms by which gene activation can occur: telomeric conversion, reciprocal translocation and in situ activation.) Transcription of the VSG genes in trypanosomes is discontinuous, a distinctive and even unique feature, apparently confined to the Trypanosomatidae.

BC genes may be telomeric or lie within the length of the chromosome; both types can be activated by the duplicative transposition process, but only telomeric BC genes can be activated by the non-duplicative process. Hence, active transcribed VSG genes are always sited at telomeric locations, but this location per se is not sufficient for transcription to take place. Antigenic variation can occur by the duplicative process, in which one ELC is replaced by another, or it can occur when a telomeric BC is activated (and the previous telomeric VSG gene simultaneously inactivated). The anamnestic 'memory effect' of *Trypanozoon* trypanosomes referred to above, in which the I-VAT (the B-VAT which initiated infection of the fly) is re-expressed early in the B-VAT series, is due to the retention of the inactivated ex-ELC (or 'lingering ELC') of the last B-VAT through the uncoated stages of the insect cycle, and its subsequent reactivation in the next host. The balance of evidence suggests that VSG genes, of which only one is active at any one time, are activated and inactivated independently of each other; cells which do not express a VSG (or express multiple VSGs) fail to survive in the mammalian host and therefore are not detected.

As indicated in the section on ultrastructure of the Trypanosomatidae, above, four different morphological stages of *Trypanozoon* are found in the lumen of the tsetse salivary glands (epimastigotes; premetacyclic, nascent metacyclic and mature metacyclic trypomastigotes). Only epimastigotes and premetacyclic stages undergo binary fission in the gland; multiplication is mainly in the epimastigote stage, which generally outnumber the premetacyclics by about 10 to one. Premetacyclics become nascent metacyclics when they cease division and undergo the preparatory ultrastructural and physiological changes necessary for the alternation to a vertebrate environment (this includes reacquisition of the VSG surface coat), whilst still attached to the internal surface of the salivary gland wall. Although bloodstream trypanosomes in the mammal have a VSG (and hence B-VAT) repertoire of the order of 10^2–10^3, metacyclics exhibit one or another of a restricted series, probably in the range 10–20, of strain-specific metacyclic VATs (M-VATs). These originate from the activity of a correspondingly few M-genes functional at this stage, but the gland metacyclic population is nonetheless antigenically heterogeneous from the start (rather than of a single 'basic' antigenic type, as once thought). The genetic commitment to a particular M-VAT is probably decided at the premetacyclic stage, or perhaps even earlier. The number of M-VATs per serodeme is rather few (six for *T. vivax*, about 12 in *T. congolense* and apparently in the range 10–20 major M-VATs for *Trypanozoon*, although in the latter instance numerous minor M-VATs occur sporadically). This has again raised hopes for a possible 'cocktail' vaccine, composed of M-VAT antigens against local serodeme M-VAT repertoires, at least in the case of the economically important *T. vivax* and *T. congolense*, if not for the *Trypanozoon* subspecies which cause human disease.

It is still uncertain if the programmed genetic changes which result in both the expression of VSGs and in morphological type at different stages in the life-cycle, are unidirectional and immutable or otherwise. Some changes appear to be expressed as a result of environmental changes, such as the switching off of the currently expressed VSG/I-VAT gene, when the bloodstream trypanosomes transform in the fly midgut to the very different and uncoated procyclic stage. Such is clearly not the case, quite obviously, in the salivary glands of the fly, since several M-VAT heterotype metacyclics develop simultaneously, often in very close proximity.

Two aspects of differentiation in *Trypanozoon* as yet remain a particular mystery; the slender–stumpy bloodstream transformation, and the generally predictable sequence (for particular serodemes) of homotype B-VATs in the early infection of the mammal. In the latter instance, the regular succession of homotypes is apparently not merely the result of an orderly expression of different genes. The genotype-specific M-VATs predominate in the early parasitaemia, yet are followed by the anamnestic I-VAT (the 'memory', carried by the dormant ELC, of the particular B-VAT earlier ingested by the individual fly); the unknown factors that determine which of the concurrent heterotype B-VATs becomes the next homotype of the population also still await an explanation. Inter-VAT competition, of a nature still unknown, seems to play a decisive role at this point, or so it presently appears.

Among the other interesting and unusual features of trypanosomes, the mRNAs that code for the VSGs (and for some structural proteins, tubulins and calmodulin, and also a further set of proteins) in *Trypanozoon* species and subspecies, are characterized by a common 35-nucleotide leader sequence (or 'miniexon') at their 5′ ends. The mini-exon sequence is encoded in a repeated DNA sequence in the genome; in *T. brucei* subspecies the spliced leader (mini-exon) is transcribed from a 1.35 kilobase (kb) sequence, present as about 200 copies within tandem arrays. The initial transcript from these repeats is a 140–nucleotide RNA that contains the mini-exon, with a cap structure at the 5′ end. The same mini-exon sequence also occurs in some cDNAs of *T. cruzi* and in other trypanosomatids; it is thus not a feature only of trypanosomes which undergo antigenic variation. The mini-exon appears to have a fundamental role in the expression of most (perhaps all) structural genes of the Trypanosomatidae.

In no instance, however, is the real biological function of this characteristic mini-exon yet known with certainty. However, recent studies show that oligonucleotides complementary to the mini-exon can block translation of trypanosomal mRNAs in experimental systems. New advances in DNA synthesis suggest that it should be possible to test the potential therapeutic value of membrane-permeable complementary oligonucleotide analogues. These should be lethal to the trypanosomes, but would not affect protein synthesis by the host.

Little is known of the common surface antigens of *Trypanozoon*, exposed on the uncoated stages in the tsetse fly. These are conserved in different stocks of the same species, but differ between species. Some of the common antigens may be stage-specific: at least

25 surface proteins have been detected in procyclic stages. The common surface antigens of the fly stages offer potential for the development of a transmission-blocking vaccine, at least for animal trypanosomiasis (*T. vivax*, *T. congolense* and *T. b. brucei*) under ranch regimens, where flies have a very restricted range of potential hosts (mainly the cattle and a few game animals), and it may be feasible to inoculate the cattle with antibodies to the common fly-cycle exposed surface antigens, in order to inhibit later infections in tsetse which feed on the animals. However, since man is not a favoured host for tsetse, this approach is unlikely to be helpful in the case of human trypanosomiasis.

The complex processes of antigenic variation in salivarian trypanosomes are not without parallel, however. Antigenic variation occurs in other pathogenic organisms, such as *Neisseria gonorrhoeae*, species of *Plasmodium* and some viruses (influenza and some lentiviruses). The spirochaete genus *Borrelia*, in particular, has a mechanism of antigenic variation which resembles that of the Salivaria, in which the expression of variable major proteins (VMPs) on the cell surface is switched from one VMP to another, to avoid destruction of spirochaetes by the immune system of the host. Switching of VMPs in *Borrelia* involves transposition of a copy of a silent VMP gene from one plasmid to an expression site on another.

Inheritance of susceptibility to trypanosomes in *Glossina*

Despite their success as vectors of African trypanosomes to man and animals, natural infection rates in *Glossina* are generally remarkably low. In a series of field studies, about 9000 *G. morsitans* subspecies were dissected: overall infection rates were about 10%, with most infections of *T. (D.) vivax* (7%), fewer (2.6%) of *T. (N.) congolense* and only 0.3% of mature salivary gland infections with *T. (T.) brucei* subspecies. The infection rates with *T. vivax* in nature generally can be correlated with the proportion of feeds from Bovidae; there is no such apparent general correlation with host (blood meal) source in the case of *T. congolense* and *T. brucei* sensu lato, although the occurrence of mixed *T. congolense/T. brucei* infections was long ago noted to be more frequent than was explicable on the basis of chance alone. This observation was one of the first to indicate possible differences in the susceptibility of *Glossina* to trypanosome infection.

Experimental studies show that the proportion of tsetse which develop mature trypanosome infections, after feeding on an infected host, can be increased. The feeding of newly emerged flies in the first 24 hours of life was shown greatly to increase the number of *G. palpalis* which developed infections with *T. b. gambiense*. Environmental factors are also involved in susceptibility, as indicated by the higher rates of infection with *T. b. rhodesiense* obtained in flies whose puparia were previously incubated at an elevated temperature (30°C). The combination of raised puparial incubation temperature and subsequent feeding of *G. m. morsitans* within 4 hours of emergence produced even higher infection rates with some *T. brucei* stocks.

The development of in vitro systems, both for the maintenance of colonized *Glossina* and the culture of trypanosomes, enabled the conditions of infective feeds to be standardized for successive fly generations, each at an interval of about 60 days. Selection of two lines of *G. m. morsitans* was undertaken: a 'susceptible' line, from progeny of females which became infected with *T. congolense*; and a 'refractory' line, from progeny of those females which remained uninfected. A clearcut difference in susceptibility between the two lines was already seen in first-generation (F₁) family progeny. Backcrosses to males of the opposite phenotype, for over a dozen generations, excluded the possibility that non-inherited factors (e.g. maternal nutrition) were responsible for the observed differences in susceptibility; these backcrosses also showed that the susceptible/refractory traits were inherited entirely independently of male genotype. This unequivocally indicated the traits were inherited extrachromosomally, through the female parent. The susceptible and refractory traits were common to all *T. congolense* and *T. brucei* sensu lato stocks examined.

Rickettsia-like organisms (RLOs: of unknown nature and function) occur in many species of *Glossina* and are believed to be inherited maternally (since they occur in the ovaries as well as other tissues). Electron microscopy of the selected lines of *G. m. morsitans* showed that 'susceptible' females had ovaries full of RLOs, while ovaries of 'refractory' females had few or none at all. EM studies of wild-caught *G. pallidipes* and *G. m. morsitans* from Zimbabwe also showed the same close association between trypanosome infection and the occurrence of RLOs.

It remains uncertain how the presence of RLOs promotes the development of infection and their absence is inhibitory; but since the RLOs, when present, also occur in large numbers in the cells of the midgut, and especially in the mycetome region, this suggests that their effects may be mediated through digestion (since midgut cells secrete proteinases), and/or on bacterial symbionts in the mycetome (which produce vitamins), although digestion rates in susceptible and refractory *Glossina* lines do not noticeably differ.

Serum in the blood meal of *Glossina* is trypanocidal; reduction of blood meal serum levels enhances midgut infection with *T. b. rhodesiense*. This also indicates an involvement of midgut cell proteinases. The lipid elements of serum are particularly important to its trypanocidal effects; nearly all outbred susceptible flies develop midgut infections if fed a diet of blood from which the serum lipids only are removed, although these infections rarely mature beyond the midgut stage. This suggests, firstly, that serum lipid fractions may mediate disruption and lysis of trypanosomes in the midgut, and secondly that some factor in serum, probably lipid, is nonetheless necessary for infections to develop to maturity.

Just how the RLOs affect these different processes is not known; possibly by some indirect interaction with midgut cells and/or mycetome bacterial symbionts, perhaps involving lysozyme or lectin activities in the gut lumen. Trypanosome genotype, however, appears to be an overriding factor in maturation of infection in *Glossina*, since some stocks (particularly of *T. b. gambiense*) give high rates of midgut infection, but nonetheless fail to develop in the salivary glands.

The availability of susceptible and refractory lines of *Glossina* suggests the potential usefulness of the former in metacyclic production (for studies of antigenic variability in metacyclic stages, important in the development of any potential vaccine) and the value of the latter in sterile-male release control measures, which currently involve the release of potential vectors in large numbers.

The susceptibility status of regional and local *Glossina* populations is likely to be relevant in future assessments of risk ('trypanosome challenge') to animals or man, since this is based in part on natural *Glossina* infection rates observed in the field, and is therefore clearly influenced by any individual differences in susceptibility.

STERCORARIA

There are three subgenera of stercorarian trypanosomes: *Megatrypanum*, *Herpetosoma* and *Schizotrypanum*. The first two contain many species but *Schizotrypanum* has less than a dozen. *Megatrypanum* includes the cosmotropical triatomine-transmitted rat trypanosome *T. conorhini*, but has no species of medical importance and will not be considered further. Among *Herpetosoma*, *T. lewisi* is a well-known and cosmopolitan flea-transmitted parasite of *Rattus* spp.; rare reports of this trypanosome as a cause of human infection in South-East Asia are conjectural and almost certainly erroneous. (*T. lewisi* has a high degree of host specificity and cannot be transmitted even between rodents closely related to the genus *Rattus*. The reports of '*T. lewisi*' may not be unrelated to the widespread occurrence of several trypanosomes of uncertain provenance in Asian monkeys (*Macaca* spp.): whether the macaque and human infections are with some of the same trypanosomes is, however, unknown.)

The only *Herpetosoma* species regularly to infect man is *T. rangeli* (in the Neotropical region) and it is the only member of the subgenus to be considered further (see below).

Schizotrypanum contains the medically important *T. cruzi*, infective to both mammals and man. Other *Schizotrypanum* trypanosomes from mammals, including bats, generally resemble *T. cruzi* in morphology and it is possible some may be synonymous with *T. cruzi* or *T. cruzi* subspecies. Two *Schizotrypanum* species from bats, *T. vespertilionis* and *T. dionisii* (= *T. pipistrelli* of some authors) have a worldwide distribution; their vectors are unknown but are possibly arthropods, perhaps ectoparasites, since *T. vespertilionis* will infect *Cimex* spp. under experimental conditions.

All the Stercoraria develop in the posterior region of the alimentary canal of the invertebrate and transmission is characteristically by the faecal contaminative route, although in *T. rangeli* invasion of the salivary glands occurs and transmission is then inoculative.

T. (Schizotrypanum) cruzi

Unusually among the trypanosomes, this parasite was first found by Carlos Chagas in one of its invertebrate vectors, the blood-sucking *Panstrongylus megistus* of Brazil. Later, Chagas found the parasite in dogs and cats, then in a child with a febrile illness. In the decade following, Chagas also found the parasite in wild animals, studied the life-cycle and accurately defined the clinical manifestations of American trypanosomiasis; it is thus fitting that the disease is familiarly known as Chagas' disease.

Triatomine bugs are the invertebrate vectors of *T. cruzi* and become infected by ingesting bloodstream trypomastigotes from infected mammals (including man). Triatomines that are important vectors of the parasite to man are those which are able to colonize human habitations and which defecate before leaving the host. Among the domiciliary species, feeding of triatomines is nocturnal.

Trypomastigotes are taken with the blood meal into the expanded stomach of the triatomines and differentiate into forms amongst which epimastigotes and sphaeromastigotes usually predominate. Amastigotes also occur, sometimes singly or as small clusters, but syncytial agglomerates may occur. The significance of the latter is unknown, but they do not appear to give rise to further flagellated stages and may represent a dead end. Fusion, with possible exchange of cytoplasmic material, has been reported among amastigotes. Epimastigotes appear to differentiate both directly from the original bloodstream trypomastigotes and also from division of the sphaeromastigotes, which also occur as an intermediate stage in the differentiation of epimastigotes from trypomastigotes. Epimastigotes and sphaeromastigotes multiply in the stomach and then both forms are found in the long tubular intestine or posterior midgut. Intensive multiplication occurs anterior to the point at which the basal ampullae of the four malpighian tubules (the excretory organs of insects) arise and which marks the end of the endodermal midgut and the beginning of the ectodermal proctodeum. The proctodeum consists of an elastic rectal sac with an anterior glandular region close to the ampullae of the malpighian tubes. Numerous long epimastigotes, sphaeromastigotes and intermediate stages invade the rectal sac and further intensive epimastigote multiplication occurs. Attachment of epimastigotes to the rectal wall occurs, especially in the region of the rectal glands, with the formation of flagellar hemidesmosome-like junctional complexes. Further epimastigote divisions then give rise to slender infective metatrypanosomes, possibly chiefly by division of the attached epimastigotes. There is evidence to suggest that metacyclogenesis is influenced by the presence of uric acid or its salts, discharged periodically into the rectum from the malpighian tubules and also by lectins in the gut, but the mechanism by which this may occur requires clarification. When an infected triatomine defecates on a sleeping host trypanosomes (epimastigotes or trypomastigotes in variable proportions), are shed in large numbers in the liquid faecal material and the infective metatrypanosomes can enter the new host via abrasions of the skin or by direct penetration of the mucous membranes, such as the conjunctiva.

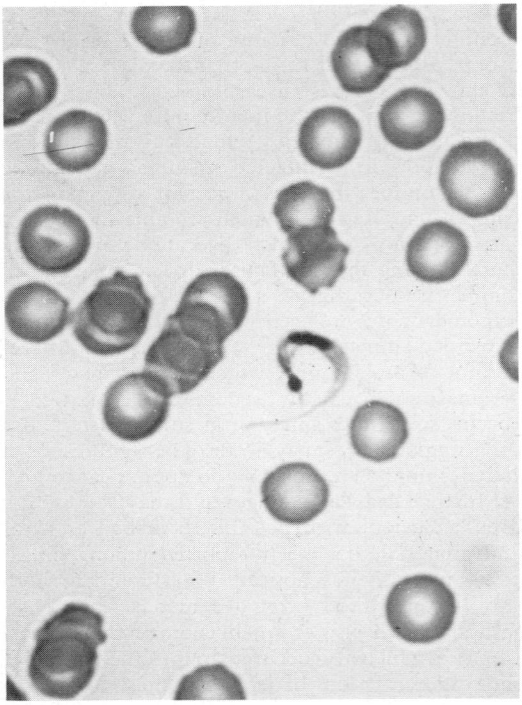

The triatomine starts to shed infective metacyclics in its faeces 6–15 days after an infecting feed; the period is shorter in the younger stages than in late-stage nymphs or adults. Once *T. cruzi* is established in the rectum of the triatomine the infection generally persists for the life of the insect.

There appears to be an interval of one or two weeks between the entry of the infective metatrypanosomes and the first appearance of circulatory bloodstream trypomastigotes; little is known of this early period of infection, but it is presumed that local multiplication occurs at the portal of entry of the parasite. In experimental animals, the trypanosomes found in the blood are pleomorphic, variously long and slender, broad or stout, in proportions which appear to be characteristic of different strains. The significance of this pleomorphism is not known, but slender forms seem generally to predominate in the early stages of infection and may be best adapted for cellular penetration. The bloodstream trypomastigotes have a typical appearance in stained smears, usually C- or S-shaped, with a long prominent posterior kinetoplast (Fig. I.33). The bloodstream trypanosomes do not multiply, but circulate until they ultimately penetrate a tissue cell and become intracellular. The body then shortens and the flagellum is retracted until the organism becomes a typical amastigote. Amastigotes are the multiplicative stages in the vertebrate host and a single intracellular amastigote rapidly gives rise to a dense mass of daughter-cells, usually termed a pseudocyst.

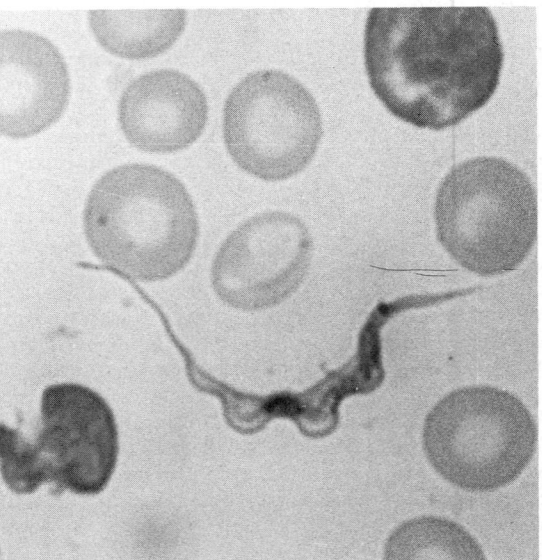

Fig. I.33 *Trypanosoma (Schizotrypanum) cruzi*, Giemsa-stained bloodstream trypomastigote. Note the typical 'C' shape, the large and prominent subterminal kinetoplast and the elongated central nucleus. The undulating membrane is characteristically not very obvious. (Courtesy of the Department of Medical Protozoology, London School of Hygiene and Tropical Medicine.)

Fig. I.34 *Trypanosoma (Herpetosoma) rangeli*, Giemsa-stained bloodstream trypomastigote. Note the prominent undulating membrane, the long pointed posterior end and the size and position of the kinetoplast, in comparison with that of *T. cruzi* (Fig. I.34). (Photograph by Dr Nestor Añez, Universidad de Los Andes, Mérida, Venezuela.)

As the host cell becomes full of parasites, first epimastigotes, then trypomastigotes, are produced. The
pseudocyst bursts and the trypomastigotes are liberated in the bloodstream, where the majority re-enter
the tissues and continue multiplication in the amastigote stage; the usually scanty circulatory trypomastigotes are available in the blood to infect
feeding triatomines. Only in the early stages of human
infection are trypanosomes sufficiently numerous in
the blood to be detectable in fresh or stained blood
films. The life-cycle of *T. cruzi* is summarized in Fig.
I.35. *T. cruzi* may parasitize any human or animal
cell type, but cellular parasitism is more frequent in
histiocytes, fibroblasts, central and peripheral neur-

oglia, smooth-muscle cells, cardiac muscle and skeletal
muscle. Different *T. cruzi* strains have different tissue
trophisms but the mechanisms by which this occurs
are unknown. Megaoesophagus and megacolon, for
example, are essentially confined to the southern areas
of Brazil and Argentina and are unknown in Venezuela
and Colombia (Chapter 3).

Intraspecific variation and characterization of *T. cruzi*

The technique of isoenzyme electrophoresis was
widely used in recent years for the characterization
of *T. cruzi* isolates from man, triatomines and wild

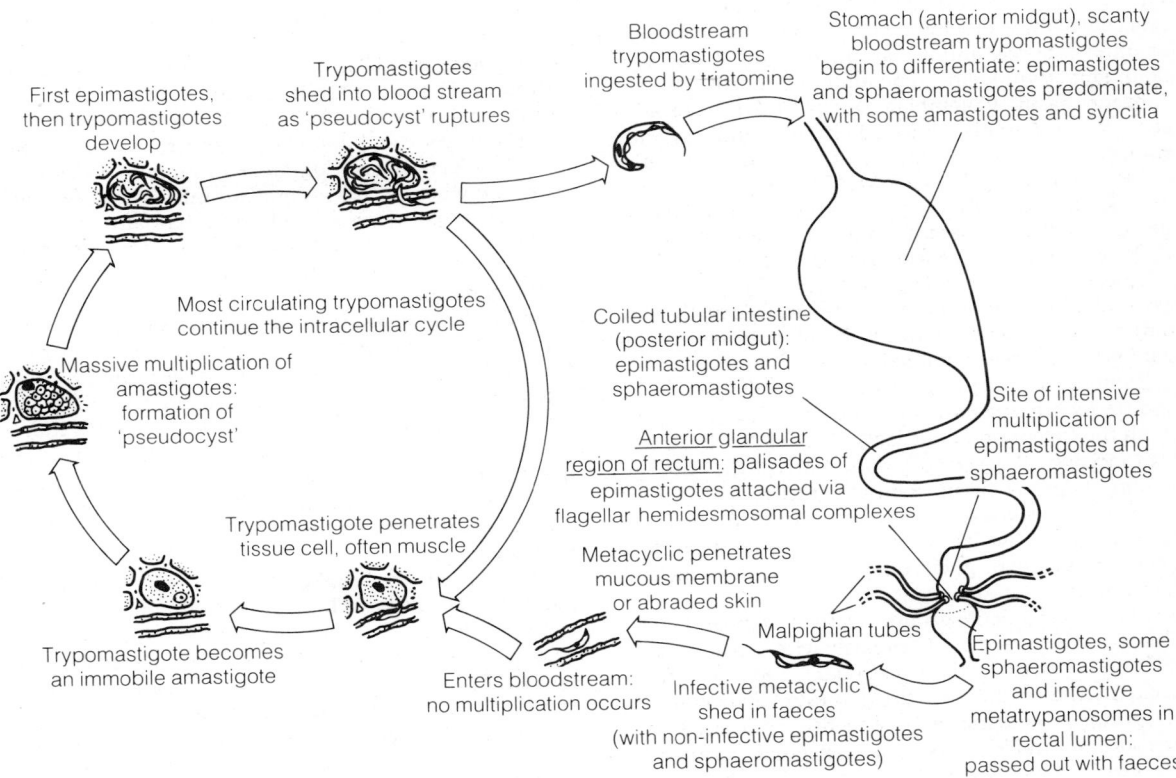

Fig. I.35 Developmental cycle of *T. cruzi* in arthropod and vertebrate hosts. *Insect cycle*: bloodstream trypomastigotes taken
in with the blood meal begin to differentiate in the anterior midgut ('stomach') of the triatomine into mainly epimastigotes and
sphaeromastigotes, with few amastigotes and occasional syncytial masses, but in both the stomach and the long tubular
intestine, parasites are not numerous. Intensive multiplication of epimastigotes and sphaeromastigotes occurs in the intestine
mainly at its posterior end, just before the point at which the malpighian tubes arise. Parasites pass into the rectum; in the
anterior glandular region dense masses of attached and dividing epimastigotes occur. Many epimastigotes and sphaeromastigotes
occur free in the rectal contents, together with a variable proportion of slender infective metacyclics. The latter are deposited
in the faeces of the bug. If deposited on abraded skin or on mucous membranes, contaminative transmission takes place.
Vertebrate cycle: after infection occurs there is probably local parasite multiplication before the non-multiplicative blood stream
trypomastigotes are liberated into the circulation. Most of these rapidly enter tissue or lymphoid-macrophage cells and
transform to intracellular amastigotes, which rapidly reproduce to form a *pseudocyst*. As the pseudocyst becomes filled with
parasites, epimastigotes and then trypomastigotes are produced; the latter are liberated into the blood when the pseudocyst
ruptures. Most trypomastigotes reinvade the tissues; those in the blood are available to infect further triatomines.

mammals, in many different areas of Central and South America. The source of characterized isolates ranges from the Yucatan peninsula of southern Mexico, El Salvador, Costa Rica and Panama, and from most of the South American countries.

Isolates from the various different biological and geographical sources all fall within three broad zymodeme groups, generally referred to as Z1, Z2, Z3; each with some internal variability. Variation among Z2-group stocks is particularly noticeable; multi-banded Z2 variants occur commonly in southern latitudes, generally in the context of domiciliary transmission (e.g. Chile, Bolivia, northern Argentina, Paraguay).

Zymodeme group Z1 occurs throughout the whole of Central and South America, associated with both sylvatic and domiciliary transmission cycles, especially where didelphine opossums (*Didelphis* spp.) or other arboreal animals are involved; it is the predominant zymodeme encountered north of the Amazon basin. Colombian stocks of Z1 were consistently separable into domestic and sylvatic subgroups, on the basis of variation in three enzymes (PEP: aminopeptidase; ALAT: alanine aminotransferase; G-6-PD: glucose-6-phosphate dehydrogenase). Similar variability in the enzymes ALAT and PEP was noted in Venezuelan isolates of Z1. Zymodeme group Z1 is primarily sylvatic; where found associated with household transmission (usually with outbreaks of recent origin), it is so far always accompanied by the major domiciliary zymodeme, Z2.

Zymodeme group Z2, found in all domiciliary cycles and frequently the only domestic zymodeme, is found (with the exception of one isolate from a North American raccoon, *Procyon* sp.), only south of the Amazon region. There is circumstantial evidence which indicates that Z2 sometimes may be derived from house-haunting bats, but it is far from clear if these animals are the main and original source of this zymodeme and its variants.

The Z3 zymodeme group, relatively rare and sporadic, is always associated primarily with sylvatic transmission cycles (with occasional, and essentially accidental, intrusion into the domestic environment). Z3-group zymodemes are frequently associated with armadillos (mainly the nine-banded armadillo, *Dasypus novemcinctus*, but also other burrowing animals), or with sylvatic triatomines particularly associated with armadillos and their burrows, such as the widespread *Panstrongylus geniculatus*.

The selection pressures which lead to the separation of *T. cruzi* into the three principal zymodeme groups are still far from clear. Adaptation to particular hosts and vectors, or repeated propagation within ecologically distinct transmission cycles, are two obvious but unproven mechanisms, which are not necessarily mutually exclusive.

Attempts have been made to correlate zymodemes with the clinical outcome of Chagas' disease in man, but the outcome of these studies is inconclusive. All three zymodemes can cause acute human disease, but infection with Z3 is rare. Z1 and Z2 cause acute human disease with identical symptomatology; there are indications that Z2 is more frequently associated with the mega syndromes, but the association remains a tenuous one. Most isolates from Brazilian patients with mega syndromes were identified as Z2, but the possibility of mixed original infections (in which Z2 outgrew any competitor in the course of parasite amplification in culture) cannot be excluded. Moreover, in Bolivia a survey indicated a link between mega syndromes and Z1-group zymodemes.

Much as in the salivarian subgenus *Trypanozoon*, the main contribution of isoenzyme studies of *T. cruzi* stocks has been to clarify the epidemiology of Chagas' disease and provide an insight into the distinctive ecological cycles of transmission, on a broadly regional basis. These are: (i) the discontinuous domiciliary and sylvatic cycles (as in Chile and much of Brazil south of the Amazon, often of Z2 and Z1, respectively); (ii) integral sylvatic and domiciliary transmission, mainly of Z1 (in Venezuela, Colombia and much of Central America; where *Rhodnius prolixus* infests both houses and nearby palm trees); and (iii) essentially enzootic cycles in which human infections are sporadic, accidental and generally rare (mainly Z3, e.g. in the Amazon basin).

Schizodeme analysis, based on the electrophoretic separation of kDNA fragments produced by restriction-endonucleases ('restriction fingerprints'), has also been used for *T. cruzi*. This has shown the existence of very many different schizodemes, which indicate an even deeper and more complex level of heterogeneity in this organism. The results of schizodeme analysis, and their epidemiological (or taxonomic) significance, have yet to be fully explained and evaluated.

Monoclonal antibodies (Mc ab) which identify parasite antigens have been produced which are species-specific for *T. cruzi*, and some evidently even zymodeme-specific; one of these may indeed have a potential practical application, as the basis for a Z2-specific enzyme-linked immunosorbent assay (ELISA) test. Mc abs specific to the immunodominant carbohydrate epitope of a *T. cruzi* surface glycoprotein (GP72: molecular weight 72 000), were used to compare the expression of this epitope among different zymodemes; it was particularly weak in Z1, as compared with Z2 and Z3. GP72 may be of particular importance in the differentiation of the insect stages of *T. cruzi* (from epimastigote to trypomastigote), since the epitope-specific Mc ab inhibits this transformation.

Isoenzymes of *T. rangeli* have been less intensively studied, but the profiles obtained clearly separate this species from *T. cruzi*; the two species are, however, also separated readily by their different morphology and life-cycle. However, isoenzyme profiles of trypanosome isolates from sylvatic triatomine species (e.g. *Rhodnius pictipes, R. robustus*) and the forest animals with which they are associated, have shown the distribution of *T. rangeli* in the Brazilian Amazon region to be far more extensive than was supposed. *R. pictipes*, particularly, is attracted from nearby palm trees into suburban houses by lights, and will occasionally transmit *T. rangeli* (or *T. cruzi*) to man under such circumstances.

As with other trypanosomatids, the question of ploidy and genetic exchange in *T. cruzi*, by sexual or other means, remains open and intriguing. The chromosomes of *T. cruzi*, as indicated by pulsed field gradient (PFG) electrophoresis, of which there are about 20 (of intermediate size, 200–700 kb; mini-chromosomes are apparently lacking), do not condense at mitosis and cytogenetic analysis is therefore not possible. However, indirect evidence again suggests (as with salivarian trypanosomes and *Leishmania*) that the organisms are probably diploid; but only rarely sexual, if indeed at all.

The answer to these questions, and probably others (e.g. whether *T. cruzi* is a single polytypic species or a species-complex) will probably emerge from future studies of the structure and function of its genome, by recombinant DNA techniques and molecular karyotyping by PFG electrophoresis.

Animal reservoirs of *T. cruzi*

T. cruzi naturally infects a very wide spectrum of wild animals and it seems probable that all mammals are susceptible to infection. Most widespread of the mammal hosts (from northern USA to southern Argentina), and very frequently infected, are the common opossums (*Didelphis* spp.). These cat-sized marsupials are nocturnal and omnivorous; they frequently visit human habitations in search of food. Much as the bushbuck of Africa, they are among the last of the wild fauna to be displaced by human activities and constitute an important and ever-present reservoir of *T. cruzi* in close proximity to man.

Hoare[35] gives a host–parasite checklist which includes most of the recorded natural hosts of *T. cruzi*, among which marsupials and rodents predominate.

Trypanosoma cruzi, other trypanosomes and Neotropical opossums (order Marsupialia: family Didelphidae)

An interesting recent discovery was made by workers in the south of Brazil, of an unusual dual developmental cycle of *T. cruzi*, in the anal scent glands of the didelphine common opossum, *Didelphis marsupialis*, already well known as an important natural host of the parasite and an animal which, by virtue of its synanthropic habits, is often a probable source of the introduction of *T. cruzi* into domiciliary cycles of transmission. All three species of the family Didel-

phidae in the Americas (*D. marsupialis, D. albiventris* and *D. virginiana*) are important and widespread hosts for *T. cruzi*.

The paired anal glands of opossums open into the rectum through a narrow duct: glands are present in both sexes and produce a sticky and wax-like substance with an offensive smell, ejected when the animals are attacked or suddenly disturbed.

The normal vertebrate *T. cruzi* life-cycle, with dividing intracellular tissue amastigotes and non-dividing bloodstream trypomastigotes, was shown to be accompanied by a concomitant cycle in the anal glands. Captive animals were infected with faeces of triatomines which had fed on other opossums, infected with *T. cruzi* derived from wild-caught animals of the same species. In the anal scent glands of the experimental animals large numbers of unattached *T. cruzi* epimastigote stages were found, together with metacyclic trypomastigotes (stages both typical of the invertebrate triatomine vector). These parasites were found to be of the same *T. cruzi* zymodeme and schizodeme as those isolated from the blood and normal tissues of the same animals: they thus apparently represent a subpopulation of the same organism as that found elsewhere in the body.

Organisms in the anal glands, moreover, were infective to experimental mice per os; this supports the probability that many unexplained localized outbreaks of Chagas' disease, in places where triatomines were apparently absent, may well have been due to the contamination of foodstuffs with the anal gland secretions of *Didelphis* species, rather than with their urine or faeces, as generally was suspected under such circumstances.

The body temperature of didelphine opossums is well below that of eutherian mammals (in the range 30–33°C) and this is thought to be the main reason for the presence of the invertebrate stages, rather than their protected intraluminal environment in the anal glands. *T. cruzi* grown in embryonated chicken eggs maintained at 32–34°C also has a similar double cycle; only intracellular amastigotes occur in eggs kept at 37.5–39°C. The bat trypanosome, *T. (S.) dionisii*, was cultivated in laboratory animals only in the testes of rabbits; also in the epimastigote stage characteristic of invertebrate cycles. This again probably was because the scrotal temperature is well below that of other regions of the body. (In the case of *T. dionisii*, the failure to obtain bloodstream stages in laboratory mammals was probably related, among other factors, also to body temperature; that of bats—except in periods of hibernation—is higher than that of many other mammals.)

More recently still, the same group of Brazilian parasitologists found a completely different trypanosome species in the anal glands of a wild-caught opossum (*D. marsupialis*) in the south of Brazil. This animal was not infected with *T. cruzi*, but with an entirely different trypanosome. No trypomastigotes were found (either in the anal glands or elsewhere in the animal), but extracellular dividing epimastigotes were numerous in the lumen of the anal glands. IFATs for *T. cruzi* were consistently negative; none of 91 laboratory-bred triatomines were infected after feeding on the opossum and the parasite was not infective for mice. Haemocultures from the animal were positive for trypanosomes on only three of five occasions; these cultures, however, yielded occasional metacyclic trypomastigote stages, but of very different morphology to those of *T. cruzi*. Both *T. cruzi* and *T. rangeli* were further excluded as candidate species, since the parasites failed to infect either triatomines or mice.

In the absence, to date, of the bloodstream trypomastigote stage of the organism concerned, its specific identity must remain open to doubt. But in regard to the lack of infectivity to mice or triatomines, it appears very probable that the parasite may be *T. (Megatrypanum) freitasi*, an apparently rare parasite of the opossum, which produces a scanty parasitaemia, grows poorly in usual culture media (NNN and LIT) and is also not infective to mice or triatomines.

Immunization prospects in Chagas' disease

These are not at present encouraging, despite the comforting absence of antigenic variation in *T. cruzi*. There are, however, presently no effective drugs for the treatment of Chagas' disease, once infection has passed from the initial acute stage. The prohibitive costs to poor countries, either to achieve effective vector control by insecticidal measures, or to reduce domiciliary triatomine populations by improvement of housing standards, on the necessarily massive scales required, leave the prospects of mass immunization as a tantalizing alternative. This attractive future prospect will no doubt continue to absorb the time and energy of many research workers for a considerable time to come.

Attempts so far to immunize animals with any of the available *T. cruzi* antigens have resulted in either only partial protection, or no protection at all on subsequent challenge. Antigens used include live attenuated or non-proliferating organisms, killed intact parasites, cell homogenates, subcellular fractions and purified surface glycoproteins. Further, there is no evidence that the severity of later cardiac or other lesions (which appear many years after infection) is in any way correlated with the severity, or other features, of the initial acute infection. Hence, only putative vaccines which afford total protection in animal models are likely to be further considered.

Two types of antibody are produced in Chagas' disease, with differing functional activities. One group are the protective (or lytic) antibodies, detected by complement-mediated lysis and immunofluorescence tests (based on live bloodstream or tissue culture trypomastigotes); these antibodies are associated with active resistance to infection. The second group of antibodies are those which form the basis of most serodiagnostic tests; these are not detected by complement-mediated lysis (CML) tests and are not associated with resistance to infection. Both types of antibody are produced by chronically infected patients or animals; but in immunized animals only the latter class are detectable.

From the above it is inferred that active infection induces protective (lytic) antibodies (PA), which recognize epitopes on living bloodstream (or tissue culture) trypomastigotes, and the non-protective antibodies (NPA) which recognize epitopes only of fixed, dead parasites. All immunization attempts to date have raised only the NPA. Since the NPA do not bind to living trypomastigotes, they are likely to be poor effectors of immune mechanisms which depend on the contact between antibodies and the target organism. Only sera of chronically infected animals or patients mediate parasite destruction by antibody-dependent cellular cytotoxicity (ADCC), while those of partially immunized animals (or the 'dissociated' sera of some treated acute patients), do not induce parasite lysis. Phagocytosis of bloodstream trypomastigotes by mouse peritoneal macrophages is enhanced significantly by sera of mice, rabbits or patients infected with *T. cruzi*, as compared with sera of immunized animals or the 'dissociated' sera of some treated acute patients (in which the NPA persist, but the PA are lost, possibly due to successful parasite destruction).

The reason that PA bind to viable trypomastigotes, but NPA do not, is unclear; it may be related to a different affinity for the target cells. The immune IgG fragments Fab and Fab' are as effective as intact IgG in the transformation of trypomastigotes into activators of the alternative complement pathway (ACP). This suggests that specific IgG binds to some trypomastigote surface component which normally inhibits complement activation, and induces parasite lysis by the ACP.

All experimental evidence to date suggests that surface antigens of trypomastigotes are responsible for host resistance to *T. cruzi*. This resistance may be strong enough to prevent a new outburst of parasitaemia on challenge, but it nonetheless allows a residual subpatent parasitaemia, a result of the superimposed infection, to persist.

Some recent studies have shown that sera from chronic patients, or mice, positive by CML in either case, are able to recognize (by immunoprecipitation) a 160 kDa surface polypeptide of *T. cruzi* trypomastigotes, while dissociated sera of treated patients, or of immunized mice (both without PA), do not. Isolation and identification of this important polypeptide might be crucial in future studies.

Immunization of mice with metacyclic trypomastigotes grown in an acellular medium, and killed by Merthiolate or heating to 50°C, promoted protection on challenge. Sera of the immunized mice were positive on CML and immunoprecipitation showed that they recognized surface proteins of 77, 82 and 88 kDa. This finding, if confirmed, might facilitate the production of protective antigens from cultured parasites, thought to have a less complex surface antigenic structure than the bloodstream trypomastigotes.

The use of isolated parasite antigens would enable tests to be made of the theory that only antigens which induce production of lytic PA are likely to achieve significant levels of protection. However, *T. cruzi* has evidently evolved several mechanisms to counter the immune responses of the mammalian host and there is therefore no certainty that PA would in any case accumulate to an effective level, or even that the PA detected by CML are not just indicators of further complex underlying events provoked by immunization with *T. cruzi* antigens.

If purified parasite antigens indeed were to produce a strong protection in an animal model, then the implications for human immunization are still far from resolved; since not only is it necessary to show a persistent and total protection against challenge, but the possibility of immune aggression must also be excluded.

Were a putative vaccine to reach the stage of a field trial, even in informed volunteers, many ethical and practical difficulties would have to be resolved; among these would be the morality of keeping 'vaccinated' individuals and unvaccinated controls exposed to the continued hazards of transmission.

T. (Herpetosoma) rangeli

T. rangeli is apathogenic to its vertebrate hosts, which include man, as well as a variety of wild and domestic animals, but it is unusual among trypanosomes in that it is markedly harmful to its invertebrate hosts, chiefly members of the genus *Rhodnius*, in Central and South America. Among the Stercoraria it is in many ways an aberrant species and to some extent appears to represent a link between the typical stercorarian species (such as *T. cruzi*) and the Salivaria, since in *T. rangeli* the haemolymph and the salivary glands are often invaded and inoculative transmission is the rule. Contaminative transmission by faecal forms is controversial and the majority of workers consider that it happens only rarely, if at all. Since double infection with *T. cruzi* and *T. rangeli* is common in man and animals in Central America, Colombia and Venezuela, the latter harmless species is nonetheless of practical importance since it must be distinguished from *T. cruzi* in the scanty bloodstream forms, in haemocultures and in the triatomines used in xenodiagnosis.

The bloodstream stages of *T. rangeli* resemble in size and form the bloodstream trypomastigotes of the congeneric rat parasite *T. lewisi*, but in *T. rangeli* the free flagellum is rather longer and the undulating membrane seen in fixed stained smears is more promi-

nent. Like *T. lewisi*, *T. rangeli* is slender with a long pointed posterior end, a central (or slightly anterior) nucleus and a kinetoplast which is some distance from the posterior end of the body.

Nothing is known of the site of reproduction of *T. rangeli* in the vertebrate host and it is probable that it does not reproduce at all, although some infections may persist for three years. However, this long duration is unusual; most experimental infections in laboratory animals seem to disappear in less than a year.

R. prolixus is geographically the main invertebrate host for *T. rangeli*; in Panama it is replaced by *R. pallescens* and in Peru by *R. ecuadorensis*. Panamanian and Peruvian *T. rangeli* strains do not infect *R. prolixus*. Other *Rhodnius* species reported as being naturally infected include *R. brethesi*, *R. robustus* (both in Colombia) and *R. domesticus*, *R. pictipes* and *R. robustus* in Brazil. *R. neglectus* is a good experimental vector, although not so far reported to be naturally infected. Among *Triatoma* spp., only *T. dimidiata* (in Colombia) has been found with a natural infection of the salivary glands; members of the genus *Triatoma* appear in general to be refractory hosts for *T. rangeli*.

Whilst the general course of development of *T. rangeli* in the invertebrate host is clear, there is some uncertainty in the interpretation of details of the cycle. It may be that there are some minor differences in the course of the cycle in different geographical parasite–vector combinations.

In the gut lumen epimastigotes and trypomastigotes predominate (the latter either long or short, with a posterior kinetoplast), but small round or oval forms, with or without flagella, also occur. Multiplication is mainly by division of epimastigotes; some of the long trypomastigotes also divide. It is uncertain if the short trypomastigotes found in the intestine and rectum are true metatrypanosomes; there are clear morphological differences between the rectal forms and the salivary gland metatrypanosomes. The intestinal flagellates are also found in the rectum and are expelled in the faeces, but do not form sessile colonies on the rectal walls (cf. *T. cruzi*).

Quite early in the gut infection, parasites actively penetrate the midgut epithelium and its muscular coat, mainly passing between the epithelial cells in light infections, but intracellular parasites, and obvious signs of damage to the muscular layers, have been seen in heavy experimental infections.

Parasites enter the haemolymph following penetration of the midgut wall; in very heavy experimental infections this occurs within less than a week and commonly in less than 50 days (range 15–183 days in *R. prolixus*). In the haemolymph epimastigotes and trypomastigotes again predominate, either free or engulfed by phagocytic haemocytes, in which they are probably ultimately destroyed. Other stages, such as sphaeromastigotes and metatrypanosomes, including dividing forms, have also been reported in the haemolymph. In late infections huge numbers of dividing epimastigotes may give a milky appearance to the haemolymph.

As early as 6 days after invasion of the haemocoel, trypanosomes actively penetrate the wall of the salivary glands and enter the lumen; prolific division of epimastigotes and long slender trypomastigotes then takes place, with the formation of short metatrypanosomes from around day 11 onwards. Before penetrating the salivary glands, the haemocoel trypanosomes align in dense parallel masses, flagellum foremost, against the outer wall of the gland, but there appears to be no formation of hemidesmosome-like junctional complexes. The trypanosomes penetrate the gland wall, flagellum foremost, and become enveloped in 'vacuoles' formed by invaginations in the gland cell plasmalemma, in which they cross the cytoplasm; near the internal brush border the vacuole is lost and the trypanosomes enter the lumen of the salivary gland. Among the outer layers of the limiting membranes of the salivary gland, but not within the gland proper, large multinucleate 'giant' or multiple division forms may be found in large numbers. The function of the giant forms (also observed on electron microscopy of *Glossina* infected with salivarian trypanosomes) is unclear, but is a possible opportunity for an exchange of genetic material. The process by which *T. rangeli* crosses the salivary gland cells, in a vacuole formed by invagination of the gland cell plasmalemma, is similar to the process by which *Trypanozoon* species cross the gut epithelial cells of *Glossina*: *T. rangeli* has one vacuole per parasite and loses the vacuole shortly before entering the gland lumen, whilst several *Trypanozoon* parasites crossing the tsetse gut epithelial cells may be found in one vacuole and the vacuole itself is generally discarded sooner, when the parasite is somewhere near the centre of the epithelial cell.

The salivary gland trypomastigotes of *T. rangeli* may be long, medium or short; long and medium trypomastigote forms have the kinetoplast far from the posterior end and are considered to be transitional stages to the short metatrypomastigote, with central nucleus and round subterminal kinetoplast and short flagellum.

Rates of infection of different sites (gut, haemolymph and salivary gland) of natural vectors are variable; in *R. prolixus* common rates are gut 2–47% and haemolymph and glands 1–15%. All stages and both sexes of the vector can be infected and the infection is not lost during moulting, generally persisting for life. Spontaneous loss of infection from either intestine and/or haemolymph and salivary glands can occur, either concomitantly or independently, in a variable proportion of infected insects. Mixed infections of *T. rangeli* and *T. cruzi* are common, in *Rhodnius*, animals and man.

Salivary gland infection with *T. rangeli* can be detected in bugs, much as in mature gland infections of *Glossina* by *Trypanozoon*, by persuading bugs to salivate on to a warmed slide. Gland infections of *T. rangeli* in *R. prolixus* may be sufficiently dense to give a white gross appearance to the normally pink salivary glands.

Transmission of *T. rangeli* to vertebrates is commonly and regularly achieved by the inoculative route, following development of the stout infective metatrypanosomes in the salivary glands, during either feeding or probing. Infection of experimental animals does not occur if bugs with metatrypomastigotes in the salivary glands are eaten, but does occur if glands containing infective forms are inoculated into the vertebrate host. Posterior station transmission, by the contaminative route, of infective stages in the faeces is, however, controversial and requires further study and clarification. The present balance of opinion is that if faecal contaminative transmission of *T. rangeli* does occur at all, it does so very uncommonly. This, and other aspects of the biology of *T. rangeli*, are considered by D'Alessandro.[44] The life-cycle of *T. rangeli* is summarized in Fig. I.36.

Animal hosts of *T. rangeli*

D'Alessandro[44] lists the known host range of biologically proven *T. rangeli*. This is much less extensive than the host range of *T. cruzi*, but again the common opossum (*Didelphis marsupialis*) is among the animals most frequently infected, together with the water opossum (*Philander opossum*), which is also frequently (often concomitantly) infected with *T. cruzi*. The recorded host range of '*T. rangeli*-like' parasites is more extensive, but marsupials and rodents are again prominent hosts. In addition to man, *T. rangeli* has been found naturally to infect six primate species (in the genera *Cebus*, *Saimiri* and *Leontocebus*). Other proven hosts are the raccoon (*Procyon lotor*), the guinea-pig (*Cavia porcellus*), the lesser ant-eater (*Tamandua tetradactyla*), the grey-headed tayra (*Eira barbara*) and the arboreal rice rat (*Oryzomys concolor*).

OTHER PROTOZOA NATURALLY INFECTING TRIATOMINES

Triatomines have been found infected with haemogregarines, usually of lizards, such as *Hepatozoon* spp. The stages found in the gut and haemolymph are gametes, sporoblasts, sporocysts and sporozoites. About 20% of *Triatoma arthurneavai* are found infected with *H. triatomae* (of trophidurid lizards) in parts of south Brazil and Uruguay. *Hepatozoon* spp. in bugs can be readily distinguished from *Trypanosoma* spp. in fixed stained films of gut contents and haemolymph.

Monoxenous insect trypanosomatids of the genera *Crithidia* and *Blastocrithidia* are uncommon in triatomines but natural infections with *Blastocrithidia*

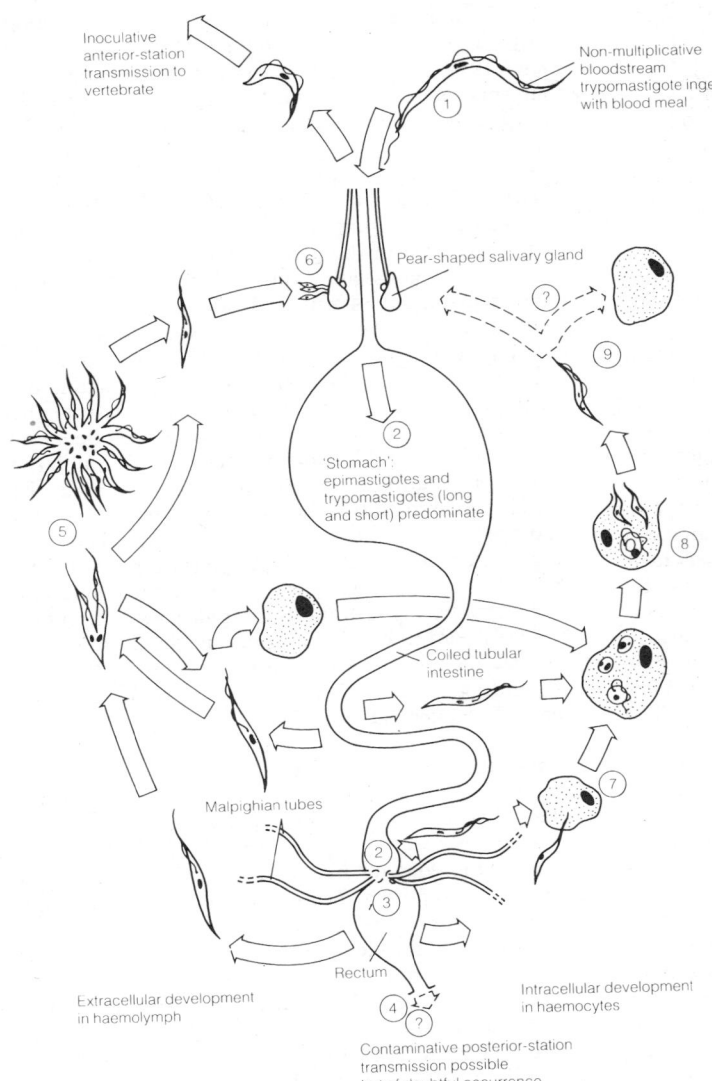

Inoculative anterior-station transmission to vertebrate

Non-multiplicative bloodstream trypomastigote ingested with blood meal

Pear-shaped salivary gland

'Stomach': epimastigotes and trypomastigotes (long and short) predominate

Coiled tubular intestine

Malpighian tubes

Rectum

Extracellular development in haemolymph

Intracellular development in haemocytes

Contaminative posterior-station transmission possible but of doubtful occurrence

Fig. I.36 Developmental pathways of *T. rangeli* in *Rhodnius* spp. The non-multiplicative bloodstream trypomastigotes (1) are drawn into the gut lumen (2) where multiplication occurs; epimastigotes and trypomastigotes (long and short) are the predominent morphological types. Similar forms occur in the rectum (3) and are discharged with the faeces, in which metatrypanosomes may also be found, leading to the possibility (4) of contaminative posterior-station transmission. No colonies of attached epimastigotes are found in the rectum. Parasites escape from the gut ((2) and (3)) into the haemolymph. Some parasites enter haemocytes and undergo intracellular development ((7) to (9)), in which dividing amastigotes and sphaeromastigotes are the predominant forms, but trypomastigotes arise from the unrolling of vacuolated sphaeromastigotes and are liberated when the haemocyte ruptures (8). The fate of the trypomastigotes is not known (9). Most parasites in the haemolymph are extracellular; epimastigotes and trypomastigotes again predominate. Binary division of epimastigotes may give way to multiple-division forms (5). Epimastigotes finally form a palisade along the outer membranes of the pyriform salivary glands, where giant multinucleate forms may also occur, before penetrating (6) the gland cells flagellum foremost to complete development to the infective metatrypanosomes, which are inoculated into a new vertebrate host in the saliva.

spp., although rare, are geographically widespread; they are reported from Venezuela, Brazil and Argentina and sometimes become established in laboratory colonies of triatomines kept for use in xenodiagnosis. Both genera lack trypomastigote flagellates and multiply as epimastigotes. Mixed infections of *Blastocrithidia* and *T. cruzi* occur and it is therefore important to bear in mind the possible presence of *Blastocrithidia* spp., both when wild triatomines are examined for trypanosome infection and when bugs used for xenodiagnosis are reared and used.

GENUS: *LEISHMANIA* ROSS, 1903

(The systematic position of the genus, after Levine et al,[34] is given on p. 1259.)

Definition (after Lainson and Shaw[45]). Parasitic protozoa of the order Kinetoplastida, family Trypanosomatidae; digenetic (heteroxenous), with promastigotes and paramastigotes (single free flagellum) in the alimentary tract of the insect host, and rounded amastigotes (no free flagellum) living and dividing in the macrophage cells of the vertebrate hosts; as far as is known, invertebrate hosts are limited to species of the blood-sucking phlebotomine sandflies (order Diptera: family Psychodidae: subfamily Phlebotominae) and the vertebrate hosts to a variety of mammals: there is no known sexual cycle, and multiplication in both the invertebrate and the vertebrate host is by binary fission: transmission among the mammalian reservoir hosts is predominantly by the bite of the infected insect.

Distribution. Throughout most of tropical and sub-tropical America, Africa, India and parts of eastern Asia (but unknown in Australasia); in central Asia; the Mediterranean basin, and some neighbouring European countries.

The intracellular amastigote stages of *Leishmania* parasitize the macrophages (histiocytes) of the vertebrate host, usually a mammal, where they are enclosed in the seemingly unfavourable environment of the phagolysosomes (formed from the original phagosome by fusion with secondary lysosomes), and bathed in lytic enzymes. Promastigotes, paramastigotes and occasional transitional amastigotes are found in the invertebrate vectors (various species of the phlebotomine subgenera *Phlebotomus* and *Lutzomyia*), and occupy a similarly hostile digestive environment in the alimentary tract of the insect host.

As noted previously, there is doubt about the status of the *Leishmania*-like organisms of reptiles; many workers now believe that these parasites form a sufficiently distinct group to include them provisionally in a separate genus, for which the name *Sauroleishmania* Ranque, 1973 was proposed. The genus *Sauroleishmania* differs from the genus *Leishmania* Ross, 1903 in the absence of a pronounced amastigote tissue phase in the vertebrate stage of the life-cycle, in the posterior-station development in the sandfly vector and the transmission of promastigotes from the sandfly vectors (members of the phlebotomine genus *Sergentomyia*) to reptiles *either* by bite *or* by ingestion of the whole infected insect. Parasites occur as amastigotes in the peripheral blood of the reptile host, with invasion of the thrombocytes in some species. There are ultrastructural differences in the spacing of subpellicular microtubules between *Sauroleishmania* and *Leishmania* (60–70 nm in the former and 30–40 nm in the latter). However, the fact that the proposed type species of *Sauroleishmania*, *Sauroleishmania tarentolae* (host: the gecko, *Tarentola mauritanica*), was shown to be a trypanosome (*Trypanosoma platydactyli*), casts serious doubt on the nature and status of all the other saurian parasites previously included in the genus *Leishmania*.

Some of the 'Sauroleishmania' ('*L. agamae*', '*L. gymnodactyli*' and '*L. ceramodactyli*') develop only in the hindgut of the vector (transmission by ingestion of infected insects by the reptile host) and were included in the section Hypopylaria ('under the gate') proposed for these species by Lainson and Shaw.[46] Other species ('*L. adleri*' and the former '*L. tarentolae*', now *Trypanosoma platydactyli*) retain hindgut development, but later migrate forward in the gut of the vector and are transmitted by bite. These species were included, with the New World mammalian parasites of the then '*L. braziliensis*' complex (= subgenus

Viannia of Lainson and Shaw, 1987) in the section Peripylaria ('on all sides of the gate') by Lainson and Shaw, 1979. All the other mammalian *Leishmania* (and four species of lizard parasites) were accommodated in the third section, the Suprapylaria ('above the gate').

The sections Hypopylaria, Peripylaria and Suprapylaria of Lainson and Shaw, 1979, are in many ways a convenient grouping but (like the sections Salivaria and Stercoraria in the genus *Trypanosoma*, to which they are analogous) at no time did these names have a defined taxonomic status and, for technical nomenclatural reasons (because no type species were designated), could not themselves be given taxonomic status, or be used as the basis of any formal taxonomic category (e.g. of genera or subgenera). Despite the elevation of the '*L. braziliensis* complex' to subgeneric rank (in *Viannia* Lainson & Shaw, 1987), and the doubts surrounding the nature and status of the saurian 'leishmanias', the sections Peripylaria and Suprapylaria still remain as a valid biological concept (the value of the section Hypopylaria for two of the 'Sauroleishmanias' is, however, more questionable). The terms Peripylaria and Suprapylaria will therefore probably continue to have a place in the literature on the classification of *Leishmania*, just as do the corresponding sections Salivaria and Stercoraria of the genus *Trypanosoma*.

Classification of the genus *Leishmania*

The classification of the genus *Leishmania* was reviewed recently by Lainson and Shaw,[45] who introduced some changes in status and nomenclature, as indicated above, which are expected to be generally adopted. Their 1987 classification is therefore used here (based on the elevation of the former '*Leishmania braziliensis*' complex of species as the new subgenus *Viannia* Lainson & Shaw, and the raising of former subspecies to specific rank); rather than their earlier but better-known (1979 up to 1986) nomenclature and grouping of species and subspecies referred to above (as three sections without taxonomic status: Hypopylaria, Peripylaria and Suprapylaria, within an undivided genus *Leishmania*). The new subgeneric classification of the genus *Leishmania* Ross, 1903 is given below, with parenthetic indication of subspecific names previously in use, where this may help to avoid confusion between the old and new terminologies.

1 *Subgenus Leishmania Saf'janova, 1982*

Definition (after Lainson and Shaw[45]). With the characters of the genus (as above): life-cycle in the insect host limited to the midgut and foregut of the alimentary tract: type-species *Leishmania* (*Leishmania*) *donovani* (Laveran & Mesnil, 1903) Ross, 1903. Old and New World.

   (a) The *Leishmania* (*L.*) *donovani* complex (= section Suprapylaria):

L. (L.) donovani (Laveran & Mesnil, 1903) Ross, 1903 (Old World)

(the former *L. d. donovani* of some authors).

L. (L.) infantum Nicolle, 1908 (Old World)

(the former *L. d. infantum* of some authors).

L. (L.) chagasi Cunha & Chagas, 1937 (New World)

(the former *L. d. chagasi* of some authors).

(b) Other possible (Old World) species of the *Leishmania (L.) donovani* complex (= section Suprapylaria). These comprise the following, at present undefined or of uncertain status:

L. (L.) archibaldi Castellani and Chalmers, 1919. Sudan: in rodents, the genet, the serval cat, and man.

Leishmania (L.) sp. Kenya: in man, and occasionally dogs.

Leishmania (L.) sp. Eastern Pyrenees: in man.

Leishmania (L.) sp. Italy: in foxes and dogs.

Leishmania (L.) sp. China (Gansu); Inner Mongolia: in man.

(c) Other Old World species, not of the *L. (L.) donovani* complex (= section Suprapylaria):

L. (L.) tropica (Wright, 1903) Luhe, 1906.

L. (L.) aethiopica Bray, Ashford & Bray, 1973.

L. (L.) gerbilli Wang, Qu & Guan, 1964.

L. (L.) major Yakimoff & Schokhor, 1914 *emend.* Bray, Ashford & Bray, 1973.

L. (L.) sp. Namibia: in man and the sandfly *Phlebotomus rossi*.

L. (L.) sp. Namibia: in the hyrax *Procavia capensis*.

L. (L.) sp. Ethiopia: in the rodent *Arvicanthis*.

(d) The *Leishmania (L.) mexicana* complex (New World) (= section Suprapylaria):

L. (L.) mexicana Biagi, 1953 *emend.* Garnham, 1962

(the former *L. m. mexicana*).

L. (L.) enriettii Muniz & Medina, 1948 (the former *L. enriettii*).

L. (L.) amazonensis Lainson & Shaw, 1979 (the former *L. m. amazonensis*).

L. (L.) aristedesi emend. Lainson & Shaw, 1979

(the former *L. m. aristedesi*).

L. (L.) venezuelensis Bonfante-Garrido, 1980 (the former *L. m. venezuelensis*).

Leishmania (L.) sp. Dominican Republic: man.

Leishmania (L.) sp. Belize, Central America: man.

(e) Possible additional members of the *L. (L.) mexicana* complex (section Suprapylaria):

L. (L.) pifanoi Medina & Romero, 1959 *emend.* Medina & Romero, 1962

(the former *L. m. pifanoi*).

L. (L.) garnhami Scorza et al, 1979

(the former *L. m. garnhami*).

Leishmania (L.) sp. Trinidad: in the sandfly *Lutzomyia flaviscutellata*, rodents and marsupials

(the former *L. mexicana* subspecies of Trinidad (Tikasingh, 1974)).

Leishmania (L.) sp. Vale do Ribeira, São Paulo state, Brazil: in man.

Leishmania (L.) sp. Caratinga, Minas Gerais state, Brazil: in the rodent *Proechimys dimidiatus*.

Leishmania (L.) sp. Caratinga, Minas Gerais state, Brazil: in man.

(f) The *Leishmania (L.) hertigi* complex (New World) (= section Suprapylaria):

L. (L.) hertigi Herrer, 1971 (the former *L. h. hertigi*).

L. (L.) deanei Lainson & Shaw, 1977 (the former *L. h. deanei*).

2 Subgenus Viannia Lainson & Shaw, 1987 (= section Peripylaria)

Definition (after Lainson and Shaw[45]). With the characters of the genus: life-cycle in the insect host includes a prolific and prolonged phase of development as rounded or stumpy paramastigotes and promastigotes, attached to the wall of the hindgut (pylorus and/or ileum) by flagellar hemidesmosomes, with later migration of flagellates to the midgut and foregut. Type-species: *Leishmania (Viannia) braziliensis* Vianna, 1911 *emend.* Matta, 1916. Distribution: the American tropics and subtropics.

(a) The *Leishmania (V.) braziliensis* complex (= section Peripylaria):

L. (V.) braziliensis Vianna, 1911 *emend.* Matta, 1916

(the former *L. braziliensis braziliensis*).

L. (V.) guyanensis Floch, 1954 (the former *L. b. guyanensis*).

L. (V.) panamensis Lainson & Shaw, 1972 (the former *L. b. panamensis*).

L. (V.) peruviana Velez, 1913 (the former *L. b. peruviana*).

(b) Unnamed species of the *L. (V.) braziliensis* complex (= section Peripylaria):

Leishmania (V.) sp. Belize, Central America: in man.

Leishmania (V.) sp. Pará state, Brazil (*south of the Amazon river*): in the sloth, *Choloepus didactylus*.

Leishmania (V.) sp. Itaituba, Pará state, Brazil: in the common opossum, *Didelphis marsupialis*.

(c) Other unnamed parasites of the subgenus *Viannia* (= section Peripylaria):

Leishmania (*V.*) sp. Pará state, Brazil: in the sandfly *Lutzomyia tuberculata*.

Leishmania (*V.*) sp. Pará state, Brazil: in an unidentified sandfly, *Lutzomyia* (*Psychodopygus*) sp.

Leishmania (*V.*) sp. Pará state, Brazil: in the sandfly *Lutzomyia ubiquitalis*.

Leishmania (*V.*) sp. Pará state, Brazil: in the nine-banded armadillo, *Dasypus novemcinctus*.

Leishmania (*V.*) sp. Pará state, Brazil: in man.

Leishmania (*V.*) sp. Pará state, Brazil: in man.

3 Doubtful leishmanial parasites

Leishmania herreri Zeledón, Ponce & Murillo, 1979. In the sandflies *Lutzomyia ylephiletor*, *Lutzomyia shannoni* and *Lutzomyia trapidoi*, and the sloths *Choloepus hoffmani* and *Bradypus griseus*. (There is no information on the development of this parasite in the sandfly, and it remains a dubious species.)

Leishmania sp. (Barbosa et al, 1976). From man, Mato Grosso state, Brazil.

Invertebrate life-cycles of *Leishmania*

The behaviour and life-cycles of different species of the genus *Leishmania* in their phlebotomine vectors are not uniform: the subgenera *Leishmania* (or section Suprapylaria) and *Viannia* (or section Peripylaria) differ notably in the initial site of parasite development in the vectors. The peripylarian subgenus *Viannia* alone has a hindgut developmental phase, which follows initial promastigote multiplication in the midgut; this precedes eventual forward migration, via

the oesophageal valve, into the head and mouthparts. The stage of posterior-station multiplication does not occur in the suprapylarian subgenus *Leishmania*.

For all *Leishmania*, the presence of other microorganisms in the gut of the sandfly is inimical to successful parasite multiplication and cyclical development. The effects of various blood sources on *Leishmania* development in sandflies require further study; the presence of turkey blood in the midgut of *P. papatasi* was shown to inhibit the development of *L.* (*L.*) *major*.

Plant-derived sugars, however, are an important factor in the promotion of infection in the sandfly gut, and are possibly essential for the eventual production of infective (metacyclic) promastigotes in the head and mouthparts.

Early development in the sandfly midgut (Fig. I.37)

There is reliable evidence that amastigotes, liberated from macrophages, and enclosed within the peritrophic membrane (secreted in the insect midgut, by the stomodaeal valve, soon after engorgement) normally undergo at least one cycle of multiplication before they transform to the promastigote stage. In *P. papatasi* infected with *L.* (*L.*) *major*, an intermediate stage has been observed (on or about the third day of infection); elongate (8–15 μm) amastigotes, with a conspicuous anterior flagellar reservoir but no emergent flagellum. Long slender nectomonad promastigotes were also present at the same time. Promastigotes eventually come to lie in the blood meal mass in tight clusters (often called 'nests' or 'nidi'), in the process of active division. As blood meal digestion proceeds further, the peritrophic membrane begins to disrupt and long, thin free-swimming (nectomonad)

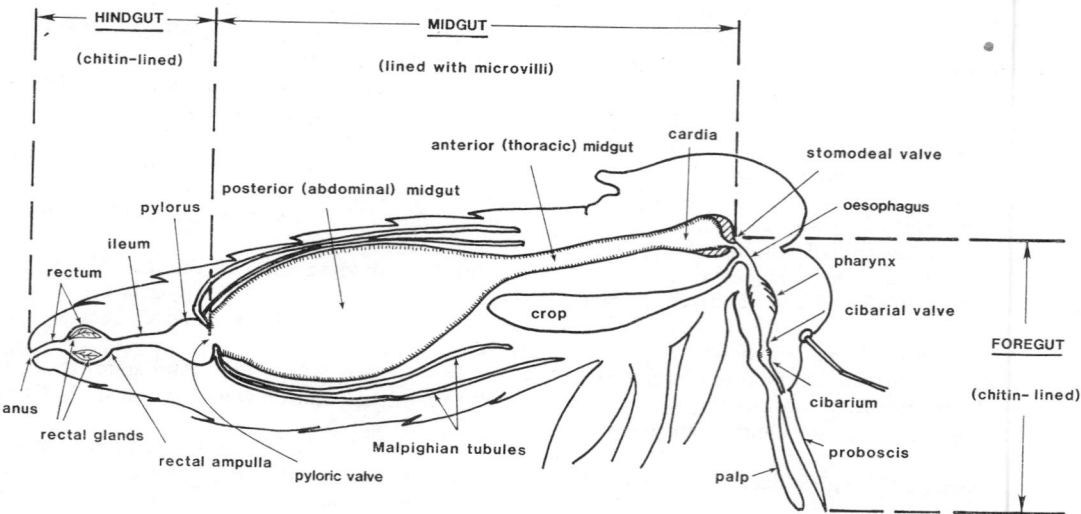

Fig. I.37 Diagrammatic sagittal section of a female phlebotomine sandfly to show the different regions of the alimentary canal.

promastigotes escape from it: either to colonize the anterior (thoracic) midgut (suprapylarian development: subgenus *Leishmania*), or to colonize, firstly, the pylorus and (later) the ileum (peripylarian development: subgenus *Viannia*). In *Viannia*, the early stages of midgut infection are not known sufficiently well, nor is the relation between parasites and peritrophic membrane (a factor in the development of *Leishmania* so far inadequately studied in any sandfly/*Leishmania* combination). Infections of *Viannia* are first recognized, about 4–5 days after the infecting blood meal, as small colonies of rounded paramastigotes (see below) in the pylorus and, subsequently, also the ileum.

The principal site of promastigote division in the sandfly midgut may vary from one *Leishmania* species to another. No evidence of division of stomodaeal (= oesophageal) valve haptomonads (see below) was seen in *L. (L.) amazonensis* developing in *Lutzomyia longipalpis*, but division continued in the case of haptomonads of *L. (L.) infantum*, after attachment to the valve of *P. ariasi*.

Almost all stages of *Leishmania* which occur in the sandfly alimentary tract are forms with a free flagellum, into which the amastigotes (ingested with the blood meal and enclosed within the chitinous peritrophic membrane) soon transform. Various forms of flagellate can be distinguished on the basis of their morphology and behaviour in the sandfly. Long, slender nectomonads usually predominate, either free-swimming or associated together as floating rosettes, attached together by their flagella. Short, stumpy haptomonads are a sessile promastigote stage, attached by flagellar hemidesmosomal plaques to the chitinous intima of the foregut (stomodaeal valve, oesophagus, pharynx) and/or the hindgut (pylorus, ileum). Paramastigotes are morphologically distinct from either type of promastigote, although probably derived from them. These different flagellate forms, encountered at different stages in the developmental cycles of *Leishmania* in sandflies, are considered in more detail below:

1 *Promastigotes.* The stage typical of the sandfly midgut, where two distinct forms usually occur (studied mainly in *L. (L.) amazonensis* and *L. (L.) major*); these are the nectomonad and haptomonad promastigotes referred to above.

Nectomonad: an elongated, spindle-like, form (12 μm × 2–3 μm: 15–20 μm × 1 μm in *L. major*), tapered to a point posteriorly, with central nucleus, anterior kinetoplast and emergent anterior flagellum (about as long as cell-body), free-swimming (sometimes in 'rosettes', with attached flagella: the result of rapid cell division), or attached to the midgut wall by unmodified flagella (10–20 μm in length), interdigitated between the midgut microvilli. Such nectomonad forms generally are predominant in the abdominal midgut region.

Haptomonad: short (5–10 μm) fat forms with an anterior kinetoplast; the free flagellum equals or slightly exceeds body length. Haptomonads are attached to the cuticular lining of the oesophageal (= stomodaeal) valve region of the abdominal midgut, secured by modified free, anterior flagella (up to 15 μm in length) with expanded ends, which develop attachments of the hemidesmosome type, formed within the flagellar sheath.

2 *Metacyclic promastigotes.* Very small, free-swimming promastigotes (of *L. (L.) major*) found in the sandfly thoracic midgut and proboscis (*Phlebotomus papatasi*) are believed to be the infective, metacyclic, stage of the parasite (although the mechanism of their transmission remains to be established). These small forms are highly motile and very narrow in comparison to the midgut promastigotes: they measure up to about 10 μm in length and 1–1.5 μm wide, with a pointed posterior end, nucleus slightly posterior of centre, anterior kinetoplast situated below the deep flagellar pocket; the free flagellum (ca 20 μm) is about twice as long as the cell body. The morphology of these stages has been studied so far mainly in experimental (and some natural) infections of *L. (L.) major*, in the sandfly *Phlebotomus (Phlebotomus) papatasi*, but they are clearly recognizable in illustrations (made in the 1940s) of the sandfly *Phlebotomus (Euphlebotomus) argentipes*, infected with the Indian *L. (L.) donovani*. In mature infections of *L. major* in *P. papatasi*, the oesophageal and stomodaeal valve flagellate population consists of attached haptomonads and promastigotes, together with unattached metacyclic forms. Although probably not transmitted, the attached stages are present in large numbers: in *L. major*, at least, they form a plug thought to impair the flow of ingested blood, and to favour the expulsion of the infective metacyclics into the bite-wound (see also p. 1317).

Similar infective stages have also been reported in *Leishmania* infections of Neotropical *Lutzomyia* species. Infective promastigotes are characterized also by the presence of a surface polypeptide of defined molecular weight (ca 116 000), absent from the non-infective promastigote stages. Studies with a Mc Ab which recognizes only the metacyclic promastigotes of *L. (L.) major*, indicate that carbohydrate determinants of a soluble acid phosphatase (with a transient membrane phase) are the key to recognition of the metacyclic stage by the monoclonal antibody.

3 *Paramastigote.* One flagellate form of *Leishmania* found in the sandfly anterior (= thoracic) midgut differs in its morphology (which is intermediate between promastigote and opisthomastigote), from the configuration of the promastigote (Fig. I.24); these are paramastigotes. Paramastigotes are round or oval in shape (5–10 μm × 4–6 μm or, in the case of *L. major*, only 2–3 μm in diameter when attached to the cuticle

of the oesophagus), found in the pylorus, ileum, oeso-phagus and pharynx of sandflies infected with species of the subgenus *Viannia*; but only in the stomodaeal valve region, oesophagus and pharynx of sandflies infected with members of the subgenus *Leishmania*. Paramastigotes have a juxtanuclear kinetoplast (just posterior or lateral of the nucleus) and a deep, pronounced flagellar pocket. The free flagella are variable in length (mostly 10–15 μm). Paramastigotes appear to be derived from promastigotes and are an essential developmental stage in the invertebrate cycle of many (perhaps all) *Leishmania* spp.; their presence in sand-flies infected with *L. (L.) donovani*, *L. (L.) infantum*, *L. (L.) major*, *L. (L.) amazonensis* and *L. (V.) braziliensis* at least, is incontrovertible. Paramastigotes in sandflies appear not to be a dividing stage (at least not those in the oesophagus and pharynx), in any species of *Leishmania* yet studied.

Cell division in Leishmania

Cell division in cultured promastigotes may begin with division of the kinetoplast and basal body (blepharoplast), prior to nuclear division. However, this appears to be uncharacteristic since, at least in the case of *L. (L.) infantum*, division of (large) promastigotes in the sandfly gut is initiated by the production of a second, smaller flagellum; this is followed by nuclear division and only then by division of the kinetoplast. (The process of division is finally completed by separation of the daughter cells, beginning from the anterior (flagellar) end.)

There is evidence that, in *Leishmania*, division of the nucleus prior to division of the kinetoplast is the norm in the invertebrate cycle, different as this is from other Kinetoplastida, where division of the kinetoplast always precedes that of the nucleus. By microscopy of Romanowsky-stained thin films, the kinetoplast, prior to its division, extends and appears diffuse, but without apparent structural change, and then it divides; details of the division of the basal body are not known, but one daughter-body is found at the base of the flagellum and another appears later, unassociated with the flagellum. One daughter-promastigote has a noticeably shorter flagellum than the other, at least in *L. (L.) infantum* in the midgut of one of its natural vectors, *P. (Larroussius) ariasi*. Nuclear division involves formation of a microtubule spindle, but the nuclear membrane structure remains unchanged during the process of division. (See also section on mitosis in the Trypanosomatidae, above.)

Ultrastructure of *Leishmania* (Figs. I.29a and I.38,1–3)

Promastigotes (nectomonad, haptomonad and metacyclic forms) and paramastigotes. These flagellate forms are all broadly similar in ultrastructure; but the mobile nectomonad promastigotes are more electron-dense than the relatively electron-lucid attached hapto-monads, due to their greater content of ribosomes. However, only haptomonads are able to develop junctional complexes within their expanded flagellar ends, for attachment to chitinous surfaces.

All insect stages (and amastigotes) are bounded by a smooth trilaminar unit plasma membrane, about 8–10 nm thick. Below the membrane, as in all trypanosomatids, is a structural corselet of longitudinal microtubules (external diameter 20–22 nm) made of tubulin, linked to the inner membrane by fibrils; the distance between microtubules is distinctive of some species, but not all. The microtubules lie in a cortical ribosome-free zone. As in the trypomastigotes of salivarian trypanosomes, a group of four additional microtubules (sometimes only three) occur in *Leishmania* promastigotes; parallel with the flagellar pocket, these have their own localized branch of RER, and are also associated with the desmosomal collar where the flagellum becomes free of the reservoir. This quartet (occasionally a triplet) of microtubules courses around in the cytoplasm surrounding the reservoir, as far as its base: the reservoir is not otherwise lined with microtubules. The uniformity of plasma membrane and subpellicular microtubules is interrupted in promastigotes, at the point where the flagellum exits from the flagellar reservoir; desmosomal attachment plaques form at points of apposition between the plasma membranes of flagellum and reservoir. These attachment-plaques are thought, together with the specialized quartet of circum-reservoir tubules, to be important in maintenance of the integrity of flagellum and cell body, in relation to the motility of the organism.

The flagellar pocket or reservoir is also, as in salivarian *Trypanosoma* species, the site of macromolecular ingestion by the process of pinocytosis, with the formation of internal spiny vesicles, but the processes involved have been less well studied in *Leishmania*. There is no cytostome demonstrable in the genus *Leishmania*. A contractile or pulsatile (membrane-bound) vacuole, contiguous to SER, is found close to the flagellar reservoir of promastigotes; although such contractile vacuoles are known in some other trypanosomatids, they are unusual and may have an osmoregulatory role.

The invertebrate stages of the genus *Leishmania* have flagella and basal bodies (or blepharoplasts), very similar in structure to those of *Trypanosoma*. (Amastigotes have the same structures, but the stumpy flagellum is usually wholly within the flagellar pocket.) There are nine peripheral axonemal doublets which enclose a separate (central) pair, distal to the basal body: the central doublet arises from the first basal plate. Proximal of the basal plate, the basal body consists of nine microtubule triplets, without the central pair; a structure analogous to that of the centriole of metazoan cells. Promastigotes with long flagella have a paraxial rod (of paracrystalline, lattice-like structure),

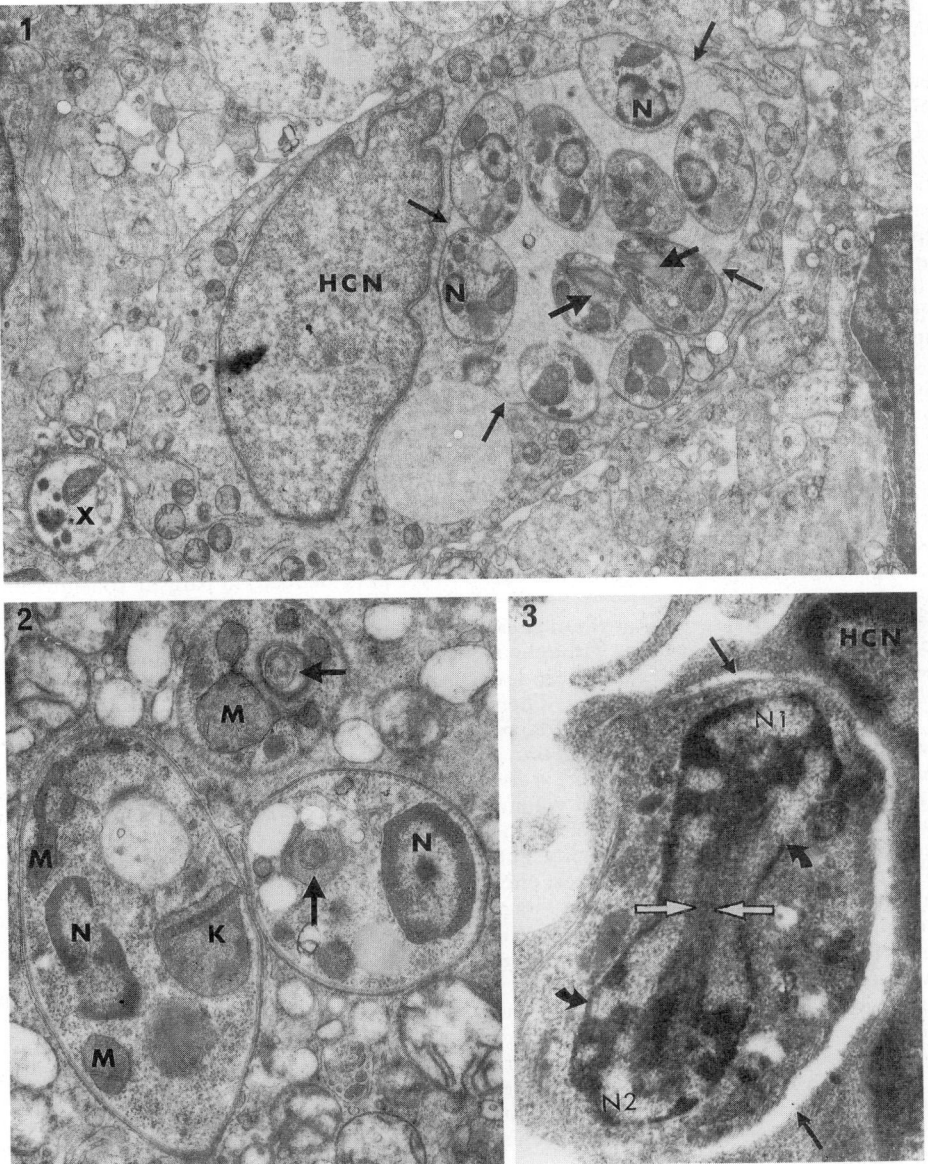

Fig. I.38 1, EM section of a human *Leishmania* (*L.*) *tropica* skin lesion. Ten intracellular amastigotes are seen in one macrophage. 'X' indicates a dying parasite, no longer within a host cell. Slender arrows indicate the membrane of the phagolysosome (parasitophorous vacuole). Broad arrows indicate the position of amastigote flagella (cut at different angles), within the flagellar pockets of two parasites. × 10 000. (Courtesy D. S. Ellis.) 2, Three amastigotes similar to those in 1, above, seen in greater detail at a higher magnification. Arrows indicate amastigote flagella in cross-section, each lying within the flagellar pocket. × 16 600. (Courtesy D. S. Ellis.) 3, A dividing *Leishmania* amastigote in a host macrophage. Protozoa lack centrioles, and division occurs within the intact nuclear membrane (*curved arrows*). Electron-dense hemi-plaques (karyomeres), attached to the spindle microtubules (*white arrows*), are seen in the process of separation to produce two daughter-amastigotes (N1 and N2). × 40 000. (Courtesy D. S. Ellis.)

Abbreviations: HCN: host cell nucleus; N: *Leishmania* parasite nucleus; K: kinetoplast; M: mitochondrion.

suspended by axonemal doublets 4 and 7; this lies in a plane which bisects the axoneme through the central pair of tubules. The structure of the paraxial rod closely parallels that of *Trypanosoma brucei*. The basal body (blepharoplast) of the flagellum in the invertebrate, and vertebrate, stages of *Leishmania* is also closely similar to that of *Trypanosoma* (and other trypanosomatids), with an inactive second basal body lateral and at right angles to the first, functional, body. As in trypanosomes, there is a constant spatial relationship between the kinetoplast and the basal body, but no obvious physical connection is detectable. The fibrous disc of kinetoplast DNA is enclosed within a capsular expansion of the mitochondrion, as in trypanosomes and other Kinetoplastida.

The endoplasmic reticulum (ER: SER and RER in *Trypanosoma*) is poorly developed in all stages of *Leishmania* by comparison with that of trypanosomes, but bears osmiophilic ribosome-like granules.

Cytoplasmic vacuoles occur, from 200 nm to 2 μm in diameter; there are also dense lipid inclusions of variable size. 'Volutin' granules (containing acid-insoluble polyphosphates and RNA) occur in old cultured promastigotes.

Large cristate mitochondrial sections are found near nucleus and kinetoplast; smaller sections throughout the cytoplasm. Mitochondrial changes have been less studied in *Leishmania* than in trypanosomes. There is, however, an increase in the mitochondrial volume associated with the amastigote–promastigote transformation, although the total size of the parasite is also increased. In in vitro cultures, mitochondrial volume is greatest about 5 hours after transformation to the promastigote stage has started. In the sandfly gut, amastigotes have been observed to divide at least once before transformation to the promastigote stage begins. Throughout the life-cycle of *Leishmania*, the mitochondrial cristae are always plate-like and the mitochondrion always cyanide-sensitive.

The Golgi apparatus is located between nucleus and kinetoplast and has a distinctive structure. Primary lysosomes (which contain acid phosphatase) are produced at the mouth of the densely packed Golgi cisternae. The nucleus is bounded by a double membrane with 60–80 nm pores; it contains the nucleolus, together with various granules and filaments.

The Feulgen-positive, DNA-containing, kinetoplast appears as a curved hollow bar, or is horseshoe-shaped, with longitudinal cristae attached to the posterior wall, and spirally coiled fibrils. Glycogen occurs in the kinetoplast. The basal body is anterior to the kinetoplast, isolated from it by a membrane. The part of the basal body remote from the flagellum has nine groups of three peripheral fibrils, lacking central fibrils; the latter appear only close to the flagellar base. The flagellum is bounded by a continuation of the cell membrane and contains nine pairs of peripheral fibrils and two central fibrils. The flagellar pocket is an invagination of the cell membrane at the point of attachment of the flagellum to the cell body and resembles a cytostome; it is the site of nutrient ingestion (probably by processes the same or similar to endocytosis in trypanosomes).

Amastigotes. Transformation of the infective promastigotes to amastigotes occurs within 12–24 hours of internalization by macrophage host cells, within the phagosome (parasitophorous vacuole), which after fusion with secondary lysosomes becomes the phagolysosome. The ultrastructure and morphology of the amastigote is similar to that of the promastigote, except for its overall shape and the absence of an emergent free flagellum. As indicated elsewhere, there are small but consistent differences of size and shape between the amastigotes of many *Leishmania* species.

There is no unequivocal evidence for a surface coat in *Leishmania*, of the kind found in the salivarian trypanosomes, although cytochemical and lectin-binding studies demonstrate the presence of surface polysaccharide components; these may play some role (yet to be defined) in parasite transmission.

The first computer-aided three-dimensional reconstructions from serial EM sections of two *L.* (*L.*) *mexicana* amastigotes (one nearly twice the size of the other; possibly each at a different physiological or developmental stage) clearly showed the internal architecture of the cells. The mitochondrion is large, basket-like and unitary, with plate-like cristae; its distribution is mainly peripheral, with broad and flat expanses linked by narrow strands and overall it occupies about 10% of the cell volume (about the same volume as the nucleus).

The most striking and abundant organelles (13–15% of cell volume) were lysosome-like 'megasomes' (18 and 34 in number in the two amastigotes). Megasomes, which have high levels of cysteine proteinase activity, have so far been reported only from amastigotes of *L.* (*L.*) *mexicana* and *L.* (*L.*) *amazonensis*; they are evidently absent or inconspicuous in amastigotes of most other *Leishmania* species (see below); they have not been observed in amastigotes of *Trypanosoma cruzi*, or other Stercoraria. (Megasomes are also not a noticeable feature of cultured promastigotes of *L.* (*L.*) *mexicana*, or other species.)

Megasomes of *L.* (*L.*) *mexicana* amastigotes are often larger than the nucleus and are so named for that reason. Megasomes appear to arise from the fusion of secondary lysosomes (these the product of coalescence of primary lysosomes and pinocytosis vesicles) with the phagosome (parasitophorous vacuole) of the host macrophage. In the two reconstructed *L. mexicana* amastigotes, the megasomes were variable in size (about 1 : 100, relatively), spherical, elongate or dumbbell shaped and bounded by a thick (10 nm) membrane. Megasomes contained electron-dense spherules, vesicles and occasional elongate crystalloid structures. The megasomes were packed together in the posterior parts of the cell, as far forward as the flagellar pocket.

The numerous (and voluminous) megasomes are similar to lysosomes in structure and enzyme contents, but their abundance suggests a special function in the amastigote; possibly they play some role in the survival of the amastigote in the macrophage host cell. Megasomes also occur in amastigotes of *L. (L.) amazonensis*, but are apparently lacking in amastigotes of *L. (L.) donovani* and *L. (L.) major*.

Thin-walled (6 nm) glycosomes were found (9–10 present) in the *L. (L.) mexicana* amastigotes, with no clear pattern to their distribution and no obvious association with each other or with any organelle. The inclusionless glycosomes, of irregular size and spherical to elongate in shape, occupied about 1% of the cell volume (about 10% of mitochondrial volume). There were a few (three and six; 1.6% and 2.7% of cell volume, respectively) rounded lipid storage globules, without bounding membranes, variable in size and noticeably anterior in position. Electron-dense vacuoles of variable size (11 or 12 in number; total volume about 0.5% of cell), with thick (10 nm) limiting membranes, had a random distribution and were identical in appearance to the polyphosphate vacuoles of trypanosomes.

The few glycosomes seen in *L. (L.) mexicana* amastigotes, and their variable size, contrasts with *T. brucei* bloodstream trypomastigotes, which contain 200–300 glycosomes, all of similar size. (*L. (L.) mexicana* promastigotes, however, have glycosomes of more variable size than *T. brucei*; while cultured promastigotes of *L. (L.) major* are said to contain as few as 50–100 glycosomes.) Since culture promastigotes are five to 10 times as large as amastigotes, glycosomes are of roughly similar abundance in the two stages. (The greater density of glycosomes in bloodstream *T. brucei*

trypomastigotes may partly reflect their greater reliance on glycolysis for energy production.)

The 'refractile bodies' in the cytoplasm of *L. (V.) braziliensis* and *L. (L.) garnhami* amastigotes (and erroneously reported for those of *L. (L.) amazonensis*) have not been studied at the EM level.

Intramembranous particles (IMPs), as revealed by the freeze-fracture replica method in trypanosomes, occur in both amastigote and promastigote stages of *Leishmania*, and are similarly believed to indicate specialized regions of integral proteins, and/or enzyme activity, in the plasma membrane. The IMPs are up to about 10 nm in diameter and occur on both the protoplasmic face (PF) and exoplasmic face (EF) of the plasma membrane freeze-fracture cleavage plane of all trypanosomatids. The number, density and distribution of IMPs are, however, not constant in the different stages or species of kinetoplastids examined (Table I.6).

In *Leishmania (L.) mexicana* and *L. (L.) amazonensis*, IMP density is greater in promastigotes (more abundant, but smaller, on PF than EF: density about 2000–3500, versus about 900/μm²) than it is in amastigotes of *L. (L.) mexicana*, where, in contrast to the promastigotes of both species, IMPs are more numerous on EF than PF (respective densities about 1400 and 750/μm²). The most common distribution of IMPs in trypanosomatids, and in eukaryote plasma membrane freeze-fracture surfaces generally, is that particle density is highest on the PF, as with the *L. (L.) mexicana* and *L. (L.) amazonensis* promastigotes. The reversed distribution in *L. (L.) mexicana* amastigotes may indicate a reduced plasma membrane enzyme content at this stage in the life-cycle. Amastigotes also have a greater concentration of plasma membrane surface sterols than is found in promastigotes; this is postulated to have some possible

Table I.6 IMPs in *Trypanosoma*, *Leishmania* and other Trypanosomatidae (based on Benchimol and de Souza,[40] and Tetley et al.[41]).

Trypanosomatid sp. (and -mastigote stage)	IMPs/μm²		Source
	P-face	E-face	
L. (L.) amazonensis (pro)	2040	890	Benchimol and de Souza, 1980
L. (L.) mexicana (pro)	3641	896	Tetley et al, 1986
(flagellar membrane)	650	543	
(amastigote)	761	1338	
T. brucei (trypo)	2500	1000	Smith et al, 1974
T. brucei (blood trypo)	2314	536	Vickerman and Tetley, 1977
T. brucei (48 h culture) (= ? procyclics)	3376	241	Vickerman and Tetley, 1977
T. cruzi (epi)	1830	1450	de Souza et al, 1978
T. cruzi (trypo)	122	126	de Souza et al, 1978
Herpetomonas samuelpessoai (pro)	1866	1875	de Souza et al, 1979
Leptomonas collosoma (pro)	1355	1476	Linder and Staehelm, 1977
Leptomonas samueli (pro)	1630	2350	Souto-Padron et al, 1980

Details of all sources can be found in Benchimol and de Souza[40] or Tetley et al.[41]

role in resistance to the parasiticidal activities of the host macrophage.

An incidental possibility is that the membrane surface may be a site of activity of *trypanothione*, the newly discovered kinetoplastid cofactor involved (in association with NADPH-dependent trypanothione reductase) in the maintenance of reduced glutathione levels, and hence of protection against hydrogen peroxide, by the vertebrate stages of *Leishmania*, *T. brucei* and *T. cruzi*; a biochemical mechanism quite different from that used by the cells of the vertebrate hosts. These trypanothione-dependent enzyme systems may protect the trypanosomatid parasites against the 'respiratory burst' of the host macrophage and the liberation of toxic oxygen radicals into the phagolysosome.

The promastigote flagellar membranes (of both *Leishmania* species) have few IMPs on PF and EF surfaces, but have an IMP 'collar' (clusters of particles, in both fracture surfaces) at the region of flagellar emergence. This collar may represent the junction of functionally distinct (though physically continuous) membrane domains, which cover respectively the cell body and flagellar surfaces, each with their separate physiological role in the life of the organism.

Factors in the infectivity of *Leishmania*

Infection of vertebrates with *Leishmania* metacyclic promastigotes is dependent on a process of recognition between host macrophages and parasites; this is necessary in order that first contact, then internalization and survival of the parasite (neutral in pH) can occur within the acidic environment of the phagolysosome. Surface molecules of both macrophage and promastigote are important in the recognition process, and probably their interaction triggers parasite ingestion and establishment.

In addition to a stage-specific polypeptide surface antigen (of molecular weight approximately 116 000), found only on the metacyclic forms, all *Leishmania* promastigotes have the same (or a very similar) mannose-containing surface glycoprotein (GP63), of molecular weight 63 kDa; this binds to complement factor C3 when the alternative complement pathway is activated.

GP63, involved in attachment to macrophages and their receptors, can also induce phagocytosis; it is fixed to the promastigote surface membrane by a phospholipid moiety, structurally akin to that which attaches the VSGs of *T. brucei*. GP63 is believed to interact with both the complement receptor type 3 and with mannose–fucose receptors on the surface of the macrophages. In addition to GP63, there is a surface glycolipid conjugate on promastigotes (of *L. (L.) major*), which acts as a ligand for macrophage receptors as yet not identified. The glycoconjugate is released from the promastigote surface by the activity of an endogenous phospholipase; when released into the culture medium in which promastigotes grow, the de-lipidized glycoconjugate is a major component of the specific 'excreted factor' (EF), the basis of EF serotyping of *Leishmania* (see also excreted factor serotyping, pp. 1263, 1303 and vaccination against leishmaniasis, below).

Macrophage receptors important in the binding and internalization of promastigotes have been studied mainly in murine models. Mannose–fucose receptors (MFR) and complement type 3 receptors (CR3) appear to be important; both are necessary for binding and ingestion to take place, in the case of mouse peritoneal macrophages. Only the MFR are of established importance in the case of human monocyte-derived macrophages. Infectivity may actually be enhanced after increased deposition of C3, by its facilitation of binding between parasite and macrophage receptors (CR3) (mediated by breakdown products of C3, rather than the activation of the lytic membrane attack complex, MAC). In the mouse model, at least, contact between promastigotes and mouse peritoneal macrophages can initiate the macrophage 'respiratory burst' (RB), which may seriously damage the parasites.

There are biochemical differences between amastigotes and promastigotes, which indicate corresponding differences in metabolic activity. Amastigotes contain more proteinases and hydrolases, catabolize fatty acids, peptides and some amino acids. They are able to synthesize pyrimidines and salvage purines (obtained from the host cell in the form of purine bases or nucleosides).

In amastigotes of *L. (L.) mexicana* and *L. (L.) amazonensis*, much of the proteinase activity is concentrated in the lysosome-like megasomes (so far known only in these two species), where large amounts of cysteine proteinase are found: it has been speculatively suggested that this enzyme may perhaps aid parasite survival in the phagolysosome, by in some way modulating this unfavourable environment. Metacyclic promastigotes are biochemically intermediate between the midgut promastigotes and amastigotes; this is suggestive of pre-adaptive metabolic changes, analogous to the more striking pre-adaptive metabolic switch of *T. brucei* metacyclic trypomastigotes, as discussed elsewhere.

Genetic factors in host resistance to infection with *Leishmania*

In the murine model, early host resistance (or susceptibility) to *L. (L.) donovani* is under the control of a single gene (*Lsh*) located on chromosome 1 and which appears identical to the genes *Bcg* and *Ity* that control infection with some mycobacteria and *Salmonella typhimurium*, respectively. It also has been demonstrated that polymorphism of other structural genes, encoding for class II molecules of the major histocompatibility complex (MHC), have a major effect on the later course of visceral *L.* (*L.*) *donovani* infection in the mouse. However, such polymorphism appears to have little effect on the evolution of skin lesions of *L.* (*L.*) *major*, or *L.* (*L.*) *mexicana*, but an H-11 linked genetic difference may override the MHC-controlled cure response to *L.* (*L.*) *donovani*, and it also has a dramatic effect on cutaneous infections of *L.* (*L.*) *major* (and on metastasis and visceralization of *L.* (*L.*) *mexicana*) in congeneric mice. The H-11 gene locus may therefore control a central mechanism of resistance to both visceral and cutaneous disease.

The extreme susceptibility of some strains of mice to *L.* (*L.*) *major* may depend on more than one gene; current evidence points to two loci, one possibly on chromosome 8, the other perhaps on chromosome 11. The importance of genetically controlled early events in *Leishmania* infection are illustrated by skin grafts from mice, infected with *L.* (*L.*) *major*, from susceptible or resistant mice to an uninfected F_1 hybrid intermediate: the disease phenotype in the recipients follows the pattern normal for the donor mouse strain.

Vaccination against leishmaniasis

A crucial factor for the possible development of a vaccine (or vaccines) against leishmaniasis is whether or not a protective immune response can be achieved in man. Infection with some *Leishmania* does induce a measure of cross protection. In the USSR, Iran and Israel 'leishmanization' with live, virulent cultures of *L.* (*L.*) *major* promastigotes protects against infection with *L.* (*L.*) *minor* (and gives some protection also against *L.* (*L.*) *infantum* and *L.* (*L.*) *mexicana*), but not vice versa; the same is true of some *L.* (*V.*) *braziliensis* sensu lato and *L.* (*L.*) *mexicana*. Amerindians have prolonged exposure to the Neotropical parasites, but rarely suffer patent disease. They show high levels of delayed-type hypersensitivity (DTH), but the nature and mechanism of this apparent acquired immunity is unknown. New methods are needed to evaluate the immune status of individuals in endemic areas, before vaccine development is able to proceed much beyond the theoretical stage. A simple and reliable field method to assess the immune state clearly would be invaluable also in the evaluation of any putative vaccination campaign.

Widespread leishmanization campaigns carried out in the past in the USSR and Israel have been discontinued, due to the large lesions which resulted, and because of secondary infections in some recipients. In Iran, however, a massive leishmanization campaign involves nearly a million people. Leishmanization is only successful when live, virulent *L.* (*L.*) *major* culture promastigotes are used; attenuated and avirulent promastigote strains always fail to give protection on natural challenge.

Killed vaccines, used occasionally in Latin America, have given results not always easy to evaluate, but some successes have been reported. High (nearly 90%)

rates of skin-test conversion are claimed, together with lower disease attack rates in the vaccinated groups, compared with unvaccinated controls (less than 2% among the vaccinated, versus *ca* 9% of control subjects).

Recent vaccine-directed studies have concentrated chiefly on the induction of protective immune mechanisms in murine models of leishmaniasis. High levels of long-lasting (> 150 days) immunity in mice are obtained by intravenous or intraperitoneal inoculation of heat-killed or irradiated (150 krad) *L.* (*L.*) *major* promastigotes. Subcutaneous inoculation, however, was counterprotective. Immunity was transferable via some T cell subsets (with either disease-inhibitory or disease-promotory effects), but not by B cells or antibody. Antibodies induced by vaccination, however, do not recognize on T cells the epitopes which transfer protection. BCG as an adjuvant to *L.* (*L.*) *major* vaccination in mice has given encouraging results.

Molecular characterization of parasite surface molecules is an area of study in rapid development generally: it is likely to contribute greatly to the identification of protective activity. A 46 kDa surface glycoprotein (recognized by a Mc Ab), a protease-resistant membrane protein with a single carbohydrate chain, is associated with protective antigenic activity, which is localized to a 22 kDa membrane-linked portion. The molecule appears to be specific to promastigotes. The *L.* (*L.*) *major* surface glycolipid which acts as a ligand for macrophage attachment (and which is a main component of EF when cleaved from the membrane surface by an endogenous phospholipase), also effectively immunizes mice against *L.* (*L.*) *major* (the first demonstration of a partially purified leishmanial antigen to stimulate a protective response), but it contains a carbohydrate fraction which, in isolation, exacerbates the cutaneous lesions. Protective molecules may therefore also contain components with counterproductive side-effects. It is postulated, in the mouse, that two different T cell subsets recognize different carbohydrate epitopes of the surface glycolipid, depending on the orientation of the molecule on the promastigote surface membrane. A disease-inhibitory ('suppressor') T cell group, it is suggested, can activate macrophages (possibly by production of gamma-interferon, leading to the macrophage respiratory burst and generation of parasiticidal oxygen intermediates) and recognize carbohydrate determinants of the glycolipid only when the lipid is bound to the macrophage membrane. The disease-promotory T cells are postulated to consume interleukin-2 and to recognize carbohydrate backbone determinants revealed only when the molecule is delipidated and oriented appropriately on the macrophage surface by receptors.

The immunoregulatory function of T and B cell subsets in the murine leishmaniasis models is an active area of research interest, and is likely to be of particular relevance to an understanding of protective immune mechanisms in the near future.

Molecular genetics of *Leishmania* are in a less advanced state of knowledge than is presently the case with trypanosomes, but the gaps are likely to be rapidly closed. The mini-exon of other kinetoplastids is a tandem repeat on chromosome 2 in the case of *L. (L.) major*, a simpler arrangement than in *T. brucei*; genes on other *L. major* chromosomes can also acquire a mini-exon sequence, suggestive that transcription of mature mRNA is discontinuous, at least in this species. Future studies in this field will certainly contribute to many areas of understanding in the biology, evolution and relationships of *Leishmania* species and may well have implications for the field of vaccine development, although perhaps the production of a cheap, stable and effective vaccine for field use is still at least a relatively distant prospect.

EPIDEMIOLOGY OF THE LEISHMANIASES

Parasites of the genus *Leishmania* are a biologically diverse (but morphologically similar) group of organisms, responsible for a wide spectrum of human disease. The genus contains more than 20 named forms, with many others still unnamed; about 15 named *Leishmania* parasites infect man in the warmer parts of the world. Most of the leishmanial diseases are zoonoses, with a wide variety of natural animal hosts (around 100 species); man is usually an accidental host, but in a few instances the human disease is secondarily anthroponotic. Natural wild hosts are normally little affected by the presence of the parasites and infections are often asymptomatic. The majority of the natural hosts are rodents or canids, but there are many exceptions.

The leishmanial parasites undergo cyclical development in tiny biting flies, the Phlebotomine sandflies, of which there are about 700 species, distributed throughout the tropics and warmer temperate areas of the world. Only female sandflies feed on blood: both sexes feed on sugary plant juices; these also appear to be essential for full parasite development in the female fly. Some 70 species of sandfly are implicated as vectors of leishmanial parasites; all belong to either the genus *Phlebotomus* (in the Old World) or to the genus *Lutzomyia* (New World only). Three other genera contain no vector species. There is normally a close specificity of vector and parasite species; but between parasite and vertebrate host the association is much less specific (governed largely by the behaviour and feeding preferences of the vector).

Sandflies are small cryptic insects with a crepuscular pattern of activity. With a few notable exceptions, they are seldom found in dwellings, but mainly rest and breed outdoors, in a variety of habitats (animal burrows, tree holes, etc.) which have in common the features of darkness and high humidity. Females feed on blood at 4–10 day intervals (depending on temperature, etc.) and mature batches of eggs after each full feed. Eggs, the four larval stages and the pupae are terrestrial but moisture-dependent; the larvae feed on organic detritus. The life-cycle from egg to adult usually takes 30–60 days; adult flies are short-lived by comparison and probably few survive for more than a few weeks. Some species survive unfavourable seasons (cold or drought) by diapause of egg or larval stages (usually the last larval instar).

When ingested by a susceptible female vector, the rounded and non-motile amastigote parasites contained in the blood meal transform into slender, motile promastigotes with an anterior flagellum. These undergo repeated division by binary fission in the sandfly midgut. After some further development, infective promastigote stages are found in the head and mouthparts; these are transmitted to a new host when the fly subsequently feeds.

In the vertebrate host, intracellular amastigotes parasitize macrophages and other phagocytic cells of the reticuloendothelial system. There is wide diversity in the clinical forms of human leishmaniasis and of the epidemiological situations in which they occur. There is no hard-and-fast distinction between visceral and cutaneous infection; often there is a spectrum which spans these extremes. Although for this reason imprecise, it is convenient to refer to cutaneous leishmaniasis (CL) or visceral leishmaniasis (VL) infections, parasites and vectors.

Further (geographical) subdivisions can be made, particularly in the case of CL, into 'Old World' (OW) and 'New World' (NW) forms. CL is further subdivided into simple CL (mainly self-limiting and cosmetic; often called oriental sores (OS) in the Old World), mucocutaneous—'mucosal' leishmaniasis is a more accurate term—(MCL: destructive and difficult to treat) and diffuse (anergic) cutaneous leishmaniasis (DCL: very disfiguring, difficult to treat). CL, MCL and DCL are caused by a variety of different parasites.

Old World CL (OS, or OWCL) includes the following main forms.

1 Anthroponotic CL (ACL: dry, urban; due to *L.(L.) tropica*, Middle East to the Indus basin). The same parasite causes the infrequent cases with tuberculoid, long-lasting, lesions of leishmaniasis recidivans (LR: very slow treatment response).

2 Zoonotic CL (ZCL: wet, rural; due to *L.(L.) major*, in lowland zones of Asia, the Middle East and Africa).

3 The unrelated *L. (L.) aethiopica* causes ZCL in highland areas of eastern Africa, particularly Ethiopia.

VISCERAL LEISHMANIASIS (Chapter 4)

VL parasites of the *L.* (*Leishmania*) *donovani* complex (OW and NW) cause a systemic infection and predominantly visceral lesions, with a grave prognosis and high mortality if untreated; cutaneous or mucosal manifestations nonetheless also can occur and subclinical VL infections appear to be frequent in some areas (e.g. Mediterranean basin; sub-saharan Africa).

Human VL in most foci is endemic or sporadic, but the occurrence of periodic epidemics is a feature of VL in several regions. The general features of VL outbreaks are as follows.

1 *Endemic VL*: age less than 10 years, incubation 10 days to one year, slow onset, males/females = 2 : 1. Most foci in the Mediterranean region, south-west Asia, India, China, South and Central America.

2 *Sporadic VL*: any age, affects mainly non-indigenous people. Abrupt onset. Mainly Asia, Middle East and Africa.

3 *Epidemic VL*: all ages, males : females = 4 : 3. Mainly Asia, especially the north-east of the Indian subcontinent.

4 *Post-kala-azar dermal leishmaniasis* (*PKADL*): a cutaneous post-treatment manifestation, usually more than one year after successful treatment. Mainly seen in India; uncommon in E. Africa and China, not reported elsewhere.

Old World VL foci (Fig. 4.3a)

1 Mediterranean basin to south-west Asia (L. (L.) infantum)

Reservoirs are:

Dogs; everywhere the common (secondary) synanthropic hosts;

Sylvatic (and probably primary) hosts are wild canids, as follows:

foxes, *Vulpes vulpes*; France, Italy, Spain, Iran; jackals, *Canis aureus*; Iran, USSR; wolves, *Cania lupus*; USSR.

Occasional reports of infection in species of the synanthropic genus *Rattus* (*R. rattus* and *R. norvegicus*) from Spain, Italy and Yugoslavia may represent accidental infections, or indicate the former existence of a primary rodent reservoir.

In this temperate to subtropical area, *Leishmania* (*L.*) *infantum* is the cause of infantile kala-azar; the many vectors are mainly species of the subgenus *Larroussius*. Domestic dogs and wild foxes are the most common animal hosts, but occasional infections of synanthropic *Rattus* spp. are also reported in Mediterranean VL areas (laboratory transmission of *L.* (*L.*) *infantum* to *R. rattus* by the bite of *P.* (*Larroussius*) *perniciosus* has been demonstrated).

North African vectors (west to east) are *P.* (*Larroussius*) *perniciosus* and *P.* (*Larroussius*) *longicuspis*, with *P.* (*Larroussius*) *langeroni* distributed from Morocco to Egypt, and suspected to be a VL vector near Alexandria. VL vectors in countries north of the Mediterranean (west to east) include *P.* (*Larroussius*) *perniciosus* in the Iberian peninsula, *P.* (*Larroussius*) *ariasi* (in southern France west of the Rhone valley), *P.* (*Larroussius*) *perniciosus* (east of the Rhone valley), *P.* (*Larroussius*) *perfiliewi* and *P.* (*Larroussius*) *major* subspp. Other *Larroussius* vectors, in the eastern Mediterranean area, are *P.* (*Larroussius*) *major* and *P.* (*Larroussius*) *tobbi*; *P.* (*Larroussius*) *smirnovi* is considered a VL vector near rivers in the south-eastern USSR (Kazakhstan) and the more endophilic *P.* (*Adlerius*) *longiductus* in towns and foothill zones of the same area. *P.* (*Adlerius*) *halepensis* and *P.* (*Paraphlebotomus*) *caucasicus* are implicated as main VL vectors in Transcaucasia, central Asia and Kazakhstan; *P.* (*Larroussius*) *kandelakii* is believed to be a vector in Georgia and Transcaucasia. *P.* (*Adlerius*) *brevis* is also a suspected VL vector in the USSR. Among 67 isolates characterized from most of the main Old World foci, 36 isolates from Portugal, Italy, Greece, Tunisia and Georgia (USSR) were indistinguishable by isoenzymes (= zymodeme LON-49), whether from man, domestic dogs, foxes (*V. vulpes*) or *R. rattus*, and conformed to a *L. infantum* WHO reference strain. A characterized strain from a dog in Kenya (LON-45) was similar to LON-49 in all but two of 13 enzyme patterns, but differed from Indian *L. donovani* sensu stricto (LON-41) in three (different) enzymes; most characterized human isolates from Kenya (with one from *P.* (*Synphlebotomus*) *martini*, a known vector), Sudan (with one from *Arvicanthis* sp.) and Ethiopia, fell into a group of six zymodemes (LON-44, LON-46, LON-48, LON-50, LON-51 and LON-56) which more closely resembled the Indian *L. donovani* sensu stricto, LON-41. Eight (mainly human) isolates from Iraq (one from a dog), Saudi Arabia and Ethiopia formed a separate (minor) subgroup of three zymodemes (LON-42, LON-43 and LON-52), which differed in five enzymes from *L. donovani* sensu stricto (LON-41) and from the *L. infantum* reference strain (LON-49) in six enzymes.

2 African sub-saharan VL foci

(Some probable *L.* (*L.*) *infantum*, characterized *L.* (*L.*) *donovani* (at least six zymodemes) and/or other uncharacterized members of the *L.* (*L.*) *donovani* complex.)

Reservoirs are:

Rodents and felines (Sudan, see below), unknown (e.g. Somalia, south Ethiopia, and Kenya Rift Valley) or none (anthroponotic foci: e.g. east Kenya);

Dogs; sometimes, as an accidental host (e.g. Kenya Rift Valley);

[Rodents, e.g. *Arvicanthis niloticus*, *Acomys albigena* and *R. rattus* were reported with VL parasites in Sudan (parasite identity requires confirmation); infected Sudan carnivores (genet cat, *Genetta genetta*; serval cat, *Felis serval*) which may have been accidentally infected by the oral route.]

The true reservoir remains unknown in most areas.

A diffuse area of low endemicity runs across Africa west of Lake Chad; human VL is rare (e.g. a few cases in Gambia; none in Senegal), canine VL may be common (as in Senegal: up to 50% of dogs in some areas) or not; parasites are generally thought to be *L. (L.) infantum*. Vectors and reservoirs are not known. Human CL (characterized *L. (L.) major*; rodent reservoir, vector *P. (Phlebotomus) duboscqi*) and canine VL coexist in Senegal, but canine VL and human CL infections are mutually exclusive.

East of Lake Chad, VL foci become more discrete and parasites are ascribed to *L. (L.) donovani*, or to closely related zymodemes, in most instances, with only one enzyme pattern in common with *L. (L.) tropica* and *L. (L.) aethiopica*; two patterns are common to *L. (L.) major*. Most characterized zymodemes (nine of 12 zymodemes, among 67 Old World stocks) are from Sudan, Kenya and Ethiopia; most differ only in one or a few enzymes from the Indian *L. (L.) donovani* sensu stricto reference strain (LON-41). A few are of zymodemes less closely related to LON-41.

Epidemic outbreaks occur (e.g. Sudan, Kenya), against a diffuse background of sporadic or low-level endemic VL in many lowland areas eastward to Djibouti and the Horn of Africa. Rare cases are reported as far south as Malawi, Zambia and Zaire; nothing is known of either the vector(s), the wild hosts or the parasite(s) responsible in these little-known southerly foci.

In eastern Africa, VL epidemics have occurred in Sudan and neighbouring lowland areas of western Ethiopia (between the Atbara (Takazze) river and the White Nile at Malakal), where another species of *Larroussius* (*P. orientalis*) is the established vector in wooded savannah areas (*Acacia–Balanites* woodland 'forests'). *L. (L.) donovani* parasites occur in several wild rodents and in serval and genet cats, but their role as reservoirs requires clarification. Human MCL occurs in some VL endemic areas of Sudan and Ethiopia, but has not been adequately studied; one human MCL isolate (from east Sudan) has, however, proved to be due to *L. major* on the basis of isoenzymes (and was very distinct from *L. donovani* by monoclonal antibodies).

Dogs are occasionally infected in the northern Kenya Rift Valley and in east Kenya, but so infrequently that they are probably accidental hosts and unlikely to be an effective reservoir: the real reservoir in these areas is unknown.

One species of the subgenus *Synphlebotomus*, *P. (Synphlebotomus) martini*, is the main vector in the sporadic/endemic area of northern Kenya, contiguous areas of Uganda and (probably) of Somalia and southerly areas of Ethiopia. All the East African members of the subgenus *Synphlebotomus* have as their principal resting site the ventilation shafts of the very conspicuous termitaria constructed by mound-building species of *Macrotermes*.

To the south of the Tana river in eastern Kenya, apparent anthroponotic VL has occurred in epidemic form since the Second World War: the disease seems to have been introduced by demobilized African troops, infected whilst serving elsewhere in eastern Africa, in the absence of a natural reservoir and where the settled human population is sufficiently numerous to maintain the infection. In this area *P. (Synphlebotomus) martini* is focally and seasonally present in small numbers (but only in discrete microfoci associated with 'dead', very much weather-eroded termite hills), together with two sibling species, *P. celiae* and *P. vansomerenae*. *P. (Synphlebotomus) martini* is thought to be the main vector, but one or both of its two sibling species may also act as vectors, both in eastern Kenya, part of southern Ethiopia (east of the Omo river) and in southern Somalia, where one or other sibling species (particularly *P. (Synphlebotomus) celiae*) also occur in termite hills, usually together with *P. martini*.

Human VL is reported occasionally from Upper Volta, Zaire, Chad and Zambia; but has not been adequately studied in any of these areas.

3 VL Foci in India and China (*L. (L.) donovani* and *L. (L.) infantum*)

Reservoirs are:

India; none (anthroponotic *L. (L.) donovani* only);

China, *L. (L.) infantum* areas; dogs and/or raccoon dogs (*Nyctereutes procyonoides*);

China, *L. (L.) donovani* foci; no extra-human reservoir known, disease anthroponotic.

Kala-azar in the Indian subcontinent is anthroponotic (*L. (L.) donovani* sensu stricto); where characterized stocks have been studied, no distinguishing isoenzyme pattern separates VL and PKADL strains, which thus appear to be identical.

VL is endemic on the eastern seaboard and in the west (Gujarat), and highly epidemic in the northeast states of the lower Ganges–Brahmaputra valleys, immediately to the south of the Himalayas and the Tibetan plateau; the parasite is *L. (L.) donovani* and the vector a peridomestic species of the subgenus *Euphlebotomus*, *P. argentipes*. (*P. argentipes* is the only species of *Euphlebotomus* implicated in leishmaniasis transmission and, in terms of the number of human infections, is the most important of all sandfly VL vectors.)

North and east of the mountain ranges of the Tibetan plateau, kala-azar occurs in extensive areas of east and central China, between the 30° and 43° north parallels.

L. (L.) infantum with a canine reservoir and anthroponotic *L. (L.) donovani* occur, respectively, in large adjoining northern and southern zones of east China. Smaller VL foci, scattered and sporadic, also occur north of the Tibetan plateau in north-west China (the Autonomous Region of Sinkiang Uighur (Xinjiang Uygur) and northern Kan-Su (Gansu)).

Until the extensive canine and human VL control campaigns of the 1950s (which almost achieved eradication), VL infections of man and dogs (probably *L. (L.) infantum*) were common along the lower reaches of the Yellow (Huanghe) river, south to the Yangtze (Changjiang) river; the proven vector was *P. (Adlerius) chinensis* sensu lato. There still remains an extensive area of sporadic human and canine VL in east and central China, largely confined to the Loess Plateau, over 500 m: the region affected includes the province of Liaoning, the north of Hopeh (Hebei) and Shansi (Shanxi), most of Shensi (Shaanxi), the south and west of Ningsia (Ningxia), southern Kan-Su (Gangsu) and part of north Szechwan (Sichuan).

Anthroponotic VL due to *L. (L.) donovani* (but with an isoenzyme profile somewhat different from the Indian parasite) now occurs sporadically, without a canine reservoir, in a huge adjoining area of east China, mainly in the lowlands of the North China Plain (below 200 m: provinces of Hopei (Hebei), Shansi (Shanxi), Shan-Tung (Shandong), Ho-Ware (Henan); northern parts of Kiangsu (Jiangsu) and Anhwei (Anhui). The vector in this region is also *P. chinensis* sensu lato.

L. (L.) infantum also occurs in several small foci of north-west central China (northern Kan-Su (Gansu)), where the natural host is the raccoon dog, *Nyctereutes procyonoides*; the vector is believed to be *P. (Larroussius) major wui*. Unsubstantiated suggestions that rodents, particularly the great gerbil, *Rhombomys opimus*, are important natural hosts in this area would be of considerable interest if demonstrated beyond doubt. (*R. opimus* in the USSR, also in west and north-west China, has a distinctive leishmanial parasite, *L. (L.) gerbilli*, which is non-infective for man; the vector is thought to be *P.(Paraphlebotomus) mongolensis*); in the USSR (Uzbekistan) the same host also has an additional *Leishmania* taxon, as yet unnamed, which is clearly different in its isoenzyme profile (LON-61) and DNA from *L. (L.) gerbilli*, *L. (L.) major*, *L. (L.) arabica*, *L. (L.) tropica*, *L. (L.) donovani* and *L. (L.) infantum*.)

Natural infection of *N. procyonoides* with *L. (L.) infantum*, together with human VL, is also reported near the Great Wall in the mountains north of Peking (Beijing) (and in the suburbs of Peking), but the vector in this area is probably *P. chinensis* sensu lato.

Human VL in north Kan-Su (Gansu) (and inner Mongolia) almost invariably is associated with non-tender lymphadenopathy (207 of 210 patients examined), particularly of inguinal and axillary nodes (a frequent cause of misdiagnosis). It is uncertain if the parasite which causes lymph gland leishmaniasis in this part of China is *L. (L.) infantum* or another parasite. Generalized lymphadenopathy, mainly non-tender, was (for the first time) reported to affect 80% of 75 parasitologically confirmed cases of Indian kala-azar (*L. (L.) donovani* sensu stricto) in a village epidemic 20 km north of Calcutta. Parasites were demonstrated more frequently in epitrochlear nodes (90%) than cervical (60%) or inguinal (50%) nodes (60%). Non-tender generalized or localized lymphadenopathy—usually of the oropharyngeal region—is also a frequent feature of some outbreaks of African VL, especially in Sudan, but not of others.

In the mountainous areas of south-west China (Szechwan (Sichuan) province), over 900 m, human VL is transmitted by *P. (Adlerius) sichuanensis*, a close relative of *P. chinensis* sensu lato, which replaces the latter species above 900 m and transmits VL at over 2000 m (*P. sichuanensis* occurs from 900 m to 2800 m). It is not clear whether the parasite is *L. (L.) infantum* (with a canine reservoir) or anthroponotic VL due to *L. (L.) donovani*; the available maps indicate that both are present in different parts of northern Szechwan (Sichuan).

Immediately to the north of the Tibetan plateau is the desert basin of north-west China, in the Autonomous Region of Sinkiang (Xinjiang). The 600 000 square km of the arid Tarim basin (once an Ice-Age inland sea the size of the Caspian), is interrupted by the highlands of the eastern Tien Shan running west to east across it; this range separates the Takla Makan desert to the south from the northern desert of Dzungaria (Junggar). Sporadic human VL, apparently anthroponotic *L. (L.) donovani*, occurs in several small and scattered foci along the foothills which form the western and north-western margins of the two deserts (near the borders with the USSR and Kashmir, respectively), and in the easterly foothills of the Tien Shan mountains in east Sinkiang (Xinjiang). In Turfan county, one of several foci in eastern Sinkiang (Xinjiang), the anthropophilic *P. (Paraphlebotomus) alexandri* was demonstrated convincingly to be a VL vector (here presumptively of anthroponotic *L. (L.) donovani*): this is the first proven implication of a species of the subgenus *Paraphlebotomus* in VL transmission.

Workers in Sinkiang (Xinjiang) consider that three different species are putative vectors of VL in differing ecological zones of this region. This is based on aspects of landscape epidemiology, experimental infections of the three species (*P. (Adlerius) longiductus*, *P. (Larroussius) major wui* and *P. (Paraphlebotomus) alexandri*), and the occurrence of natural infections in *P. (Paraphlebotomus) alexandri*.

In the mountain zone, with brown calcareous soil, and the old oasis area (whitish oasis soil), *P. longiductus* is the predominant species (> 90% of sandfly catches); in the stony mountain foothill zones (with brown desert soils), *P. alexandri* predominates (>90% of catches). In some lowland areas of dry desert, meadow soil with *Populus diversifolia* and *Tamalix* sp. occurs; here neither *P. longiductus* nor *P. alexandri* is found, but *P. major wui* comprises about 60% of all sandflies collected.

VL Foci: the New World (*L. (L.) chagasi; American VL: AVL*) (Fig. 4.3b)

Reservoirs are:

Dogs, the synanthropic hosts in all foci;

Foxes (*Cerdocyon thous* and *Lycalopex vetulus*), infected in Brazil;

Opossums, *Didelphis albiventris*, small synanthropic scavenging marsupials; infected in parts of Brazil (and perhaps *D. marsupialis* may be involved elsewhere).

AVL occurs in extensive areas of the Americas, from Mexico to northern Argentina, in sporadic and often widely separated foci. Surprisingly, throughout this vast range there is only one apparent vector, the often peridomestic *Lutzomyia (Lutzomyia) longipalpis* sensu lato, probably a complex of closely related species. Dogs are the normal synanthropic reservoir and foxes are also infected; natural infection of the peridomestic didelphine marsupial, *Didelphis albiventris* (the common opossum) has also been reported. The Neotropical VL parasite, *L. (L.) chagasi*, may include *L. (L.) infantum*, accidentally imported from Europe in the Hispanic colonial period. (Old and New World VL parasites often cannot be distinguished with certainty on modern biochemical criteria.)

CUTANEOUS LEISHMANIASIS

CL Foci: Old World

1 Anthroponotic CL (ACL): L. (L.) tropica (Fig. 37.1)

General features of L. (L.) tropica infections: incubation two to eight months; dry painless ulcers become scars in one to two years. (But in leishmaniasis recidivans (LR), slowly progressive lesions result in scars with prolonged peripheral activity and few parasites. Response to treatment is slow.)

There are no reservoirs other than man.

Anthroponotic CL (ACL) is caused by *L. (L.) tropica* (= *L. tropica minor*) and occurs north and south of the Mediterranean and eastwards to the southern USSR, Afghanistan and the Indo-Pakistan borders. ACL is found in well-established human settlements, often under urban conditions; there is no known sylvatic reservoir and transmission is peridomestic. (Occasional infections of dogs and rats (*R. rattus*) are probably accidental; there is no entirely convincing evidence of an extra-human reservoir of *L. (L.) tropica*.) Eighteen different zymodemes of *L. (L.) tropica* were differentiated by isoenzyme analysis of 27 stocks from different hosts (man, dog, *R. rattus*) and various geographical sources. *L. (L.) tropica* is thus a very heterogeneous organism, particularly as compared with the homogeneity of *L. (L.) major* (see below).

The most important and widespread vectors of *L. (L.) tropica* are the endophilic *P. (Paraphlebotomus) sergenti* and *P. (Phlebotomus) papatasi*. *P. (Larroussius) perfiliewi* is considered to be the vector of ACL in Italy and is probably important in neighbouring countries: the same species is also a VL vector in southern Italy, Malta and Sicily; possibly also in Yugoslavia (Serbia), Roumania and (as a vector secondary to *P. (Larroussius) perniciosus* in Tunisia. The finding of genetic differences in populations of *P. (Larroussius) perfiliewi* from east and west of the Apennine mountains in Italy suggests that *P. perfiliewi* sensu lato may also prove to be a species-complex.

Human cutaneous lesions of the west Mediterranean area (southern France, Spain, Italy, Morocco, Algeria and Israel), are now known to be often (always?) a dermal manifestation of infection with isoenzyme variants of *L. (L.) infantum*, rather than the result of *L. (L.) tropica* (as was formerly thought).

2 Zoonotic CL: L. (L.) major (= L. tropica major) (Fig. 37.2).

General features of L. (L.) major infections: incubation less than four months; moist painless ulcers become scars in two to eight months (but multiple lesions often become confluent and slow to heal).

Reservoirs are various cricetid, murid and sciurid rodents, particularly gerbils and jirds (occasionally ground squirrels), as follows (with main reservoirs of Asiatic foci in bold):

Rhombomys opimus (Cricetidae: great gerbil): most foci of south USSR; Iran; North Afghanistan; Mongolia.

Meriones spp. (Cricetidae: jirds): a few foci of south USSR and Iran (***M. libycus***, syn. *M. erythrourus*); north-west India (*M. hurrianae*); Israel and Saudi Arabia (*M. crassus*); Morocco (*M. shawi*); Tunisia (*M. shawi*).[*]

Psammomys obesus (Cricetidae: fat sand rat): Israel; Saudi Arabia; north-west Libya; Algeria. (Until 1986, no reservoir detected in Tunisia, but *M. shawi* now clearly implicated;* although *P. obesus* also numerous in the same area, none of 106 were infected.)

Mastomys (=*Praomys*) *erythroleucus* (Muridae: multimammate rat): West Africa (Senegal).

Mastomys (=*Praomys*) *natalensis* (Muridae: multimammate rat): East Africa (Kenya).

Tatera gambiana (Cricetidae: gerbil): West Africa (Senegal).

Tatera robusta (Cricetidae: gerbil): East Africa (Kenya).

Taterillus emini (Cricetidae: pygmy gerbil): East Africa (Kenya).

Arvicanthis niloticus (Muridae: Nile grass rat): West Africa (Senegal); East Africa (Ethiopia, Kenya and Sudan).

Aethomys kaiseri (Muridae: grass rat): East Africa (Kenya).

Nesokia indica (Muridae: short-tailed mole rat): Israel.

Xerus rutilus (Sciuridae: African ground squirrel): East Africa (Kenya).

The most important and widespread cause of ZCL in the Old World is *L.* (*L.*) *major* (formerly *L. tropica major*). ZCL due to *L.* (*L.*) *major* is characteristic of a rural environment in arid lowland steppe and semidesert zones, with a hot and prolonged dry season, and loess or alluvial soils conducive to the activities of burrowing animals. This parasite has an extensive distribution in the Palaeartic faunal region, from the USSR and Iran, through the Mediterranean region to Iraq, Saudi Arabia, Yemen, Afghanistan, north-west India (Rajastan) and Pakistan. Throughout most of this region, the vector of *L.* (*L.*) *major* to man is *P.* (*Phlebotomus*) *papatasi*. *R. opimus* and *M. libycus* are the major reservoirs of *L.* (*L.*) *major* in the foci of Asia. In the lowland steppe and semidesert areas of the distribution of *R. opimus* in Asia, *Meriones libycus* is the only other maintenance host of epidemiological significance (among 12 mammalian species regularly or occasionally infected with *L.* (*L.*) *major*), both as a maintenance host for the parasite and as a source of infection for man-biting sandflies.

R. opimus occurs east of the shores of the Caspian Sea to about 45° north, south into Iran (east of the Zagros mountains), with a northern lowland 'panhandle' running eastward into north-west China (Sinkiang: Xinjiang) and Mongolia. *M. libycus* has a similar distribution in Asia to *R. opimus* (although without the northerly eastern 'panhandle'), but its distribution extends much further to the west; across to the east Mediterranean littoral, the north-east of the Arabian peninsula, the western Red Sea littoral and thence across the northern Sahara to Morocco.

A geographically separate, but ecologically similar, sub-saharan belt of *L.* (*L.*) *major* is found in the Afrotropical faunal region further south, where the vector is the related *P.* (*Phlebotomus*) *duboscqi* and human infections are uncommon, from Senegal to the Nile valley and northern Kenya.

P. (*Phlebotomus*) *salehi* transmits *L. major* among colonies of *Meriones hurrianae* in Rajastan (north-west India) and may also be a vector of human infections in that area.

Despite its very large geographical range, *L.* (*L.*) *major* is remarkably uniform in biochemical characteristics: 100 of 135 stocks from the USSR, Iran, various areas of the Mediterranean, Kuwait, Saudi Arabia, Senegal, Kenya and Ethiopia belonged to a single zymodeme (LON-1). The remaining 35 stocks belonged to several different zymodemes:

LON-2 and LON-3, Israel;

LON-4, Kuwait and Saudi Arabia;

LON-62, Saudi Arabia (from feral dog, Hofuf);

LON-65, Saudi Arabia (human lesion);

LON-64,† Saudi Arabia (man, *P. obesus* and feral dog);

LON-5 and LON-6; north-west India (Rajastan).

In some of the geographical foci listed above, there is a degree of correlation between different zymodemes and particular rodent hosts. Further studies may well show that *L.* (*L.*) *major* sensu lato is indeed a complex of cryptic taxa, sometimes sympatric, in the process of speciation.

Although the main vector of *L.* (*L.*) *major* to man in the Palaeartic foci is the endophilic *P.* (*Phlebotomus*) *papatasi*, *P.* (*Paraphlebotomus*) *caucasicus* (and other members of the same subgenus, *P.* (*Paraphlebotomus*) *andrejevi* and *P.* (*Paraphlebotomus*) *mongolensis*), are important in the maintenance of infection among colonies of wild *Rhombomys* and *Meriones* spp. in the USSR, Iran and Afghanistan. However, *P.* (*Paraphlebotomus*) *caucasicus* may be also the vector of the Asiatic gerbil parasite, *L.* (*L.*) *gerbilli* (of which *P.* (*Paraphlebotomus*) *mongolensis* is thought to be the vector in China, east of the known range of *P.* (*Paraphlebotomus*) *caucasicus*). *L.* (*L.*) *gerbilli* is a specific parasite of *Rhombomys* and apparently incapable of causing infection in man (see also above, in section on VL Foci in India and China). *P.* (*Paraphlebotomus*)

---

* Recent work now implicates *Meriones shawi* as the reservoir of *L.* (*L.*) *major* in Tunisia. Up to 4% of 125 *M. shawi* in the Maghreb were infected with *L. major*; parasites of three *M. shawi* isolates identified by isoenzyme analysis (13 enzymes) all belonged to the same zymodeme (MON 25) as parasites isolated from man in Tunisia, Algeria, Morocco, Libya, Senegal, Mali and France. The zymodeme MON 25 is a minor variant (in the enzyme MDH) of the very widespread LON-1 referred to below. None of 105 *Psammomys obesus* examined in the same area of the Tunisian Maghreb were infected with *Leishmania*.

† LON-64 has since been given specific status as *L.* (*L.*) *arabica* Peters, Elbihari and Evans, 1986. Although morphologically indistinguishable from *L. major* sensu lato (and sympatric with LON-4 in the Eastern province of Saudi Arabia), the new parasite has distinctive kDNA and isoenzyme profile characteristics. The vector of *L.* (*L.*) *arabica* is not yet known.

chabaudi is suspected to be a vector of *L. (L.) major* in north-west Africa.

In addition to the rodents listed above, other members of the Sciuridae are naturally infected with *Leishmania* (probably *L. (L.) major*) in the USSR and Iran (e.g. the jird *Meriones meridianus* and *Spermophilopsis leptodactylus*, the long-clawed ground squirrel). In the USSR the house-mouse *Mus musculus* and the jerboa *Allactaga severtzovi* are occasionally infected. Small numbers of weasels, polecats, hedgehogs and other animals—even a coypu—have also been reported infected by this or a similar, but uncharacterized parasite in the USSR.

The cricetid rodent genera *Rhombomys*, *Meriones* and *Psammomys* have *L. (L.) major* parasites in the skin; the cricetid genus *Tatera*, and most infected murids and sciurids (e.g. *Arvicanthis*, *Praomys*) appear to have parasites only in the viscera (and, presumably, also in the blood).

In Senegal the main reservoirs are *Praomys* (= *Mastomys*) *erythroleucus* and *Tatera gambiana*: *A. niloticus* is involved (as a secondary reservoir) only when its populations are large. The relative importance of the different animals infected in East Africa has yet to be firmly established.

3 African highland ZCL: L. (L.) aethiopica
(Fig. 37.2)

General features of L. (L.) aethiopica infections: oriental sore (OS) common, DCL and MCL rare. Slow evolution of lesions, ulceration late or absent; healing normally in one to three years. Forested (and recently felled) highland areas, 1500–2700 m, of Ethiopia and Kenya (Mount Elgon, Aberdares), mainly within the 800 mm isohyet.

Reservoirs are mainly species of hyrax (known also as dassies or conies); sometimes a murid rodent, the African giant pouched rat (probably the latter an accidental host), as follows:

Procavia capensis (rock hyrax): Ethiopia and Kenya.
Heterohyrax brucei (rock hyrax): Ethiopia.
Dendrohyrax arboreus (tree hyrax): Kenya.
Cricetomys gambianus (African giant pouched rat): Kenya.
(*P. capensis* and *H. brucei* are the main reservoirs, in which infection is benign.)

In contrast to *L. (L.) major* (the ZCL parasite associated with lowland, semidesert and steppe regions), *L. (L.) aethiopica* is a ZCL parasite found only at high altitudes (*ca.* 2000 m), mainly on the Ethiopian highland plateau, but also in limited foci in highland areas of Kenya (in the Aberdare range and on the slopes of Mount Elgon). The normal hosts are various species of rock and tree hyrax: in Ethiopia the main vector is *P. (Larroussius) longipes*, but the closely related *P. (Larroussius) pedifer* becomes important in the southern part of the Ethiopian highlands and is the main vector in the Kenya foci. (Note that species of

the subgenus *Larroussius* are more usually associated with transmission of VL.)

In the highlands of Ethiopia *L. (L.) aethiopica* is a common cause of self-limiting oriental sore (OS) and only rarely the cause of DCL. In the Mount Elgon and Aberdare foci of Kenya, OS is uncommon but DCL appears to be relatively frequent. Isoenzyme patterns of characterized *L. (L.) aethiopica* have a low level of heterogeneity, although 13 zymodemes were found among 28 stocks: ten zymodemes formed a closely related group (LON-27, LON-28, LON-29, LON-30, LON-32, LON-34, LON-36, LON-37, LON-38 and LON-39) and three others (LON-31, LON-33 and LON-35) showed rather more variation. Stocks from OS and DCL patients were indistinguishable and only one enzyme pattern was common to *L. (L.) tropica* (LON-7), and none with *L. (L.) major* (LON-1), as reference strains.

4 Other ZCL foci

Occasional cases of DCL occur in Tanzania, south of Lake Victoria; lesions resemble those seen in the Kenya and Ethiopian highlands, but nothing is known of the aetiology of these infections, or of possible vectors and reservoir hosts.

Two undescribed *Leishmania* species occur in hot, dry, lowland areas of Namibia. The ecological situation superficially is reminiscent of *L. aethiopica* in the highlands of eastern Africa, since the natural hosts of at least one species are also rock hyrax (*Procavia capensis*); the second species is the cause of occasional human infections (often of DCL), but both organisms are biochemically distinct from *L. aethiopica* and from each other. The vector of both the unnamed Namibian parasites is thought to be *P. (Synphlebotomus) rossi*, since parasites from this species in a hyrax habitat were identical to parasites isolated from man, although they differed from *Leishmania* isolated from *Procavia capensis* in the same area.

Human CL of unknown aetiology is common in western areas of Sudan, and along parts of the Nile north of Khartoum, but neither the parasites, the unknown normal vertebrate hosts, nor the possible vectors have been studied.

CL, MCL and DCL: New World

It is extremely difficult to summarize current knowledge of the distribution of the numerous parasites which cause human CL in the Neotropical region, of different degrees of severity, with their many vectors and natural vertebrate hosts.

1 L. (L.) mexicana complex of species: (Fig. 37.11)

Members of the *L. (L.) mexicana* complex are readily distinguished from all other Neotropical *Leishmania* species by their larger size (as amastigotes and promastigotes), particularly from the much smaller parasites of the subgenus *Viannia*. L. (L.) *mexicana* group parasites are separated from other Neotropical members of the subgenus *Leishmania* (e.g. *L.·(L.) chagasi* and the exclusively porcupine parasites *L. (L.) hertigi* and *L. (L.) deanei*), and from all members of the sub-genus *Viannia*, on the basis of isoenzyme profiles, DNA buoyant density, monoclonal antibodies, culture characteristics, behaviour in experimental hamsters and by kDNA hybridization probes. The different species of the *L. (L.) mexicana* complex are separated from each other principally by isoenzyme profiles, monoclonal antibodies and kDNA sequence homologies. At least three species of the *L. (L.) mexicana* complex are the cause of occasional DCL in man; a condition not known to be produced by any other Neotropical members of the genus *Leishmania*.

Parasites of the *L. (L.) mexicana* complex are transmitted to man, where the vectors are known, by *Lutzomyia* species of the subgenus *Nyssomyia*, such as *Lutzomyia flaviscutellata* and *Lutzomyia olmeca*. The principal *mexicana* parasites of medical importance are *L. (L.) mexicana* (= *L. m. mexicana*), the agent of chiclero's ulcer or bay sore in Central America, and *L. (L.) amazonensis* (=*L. m. amazonensis*), the cause of swamp-forest leishmaniasis (enzootic rodent leishmaniasis) in the Amazon basin. Although *L. amazonensis* is relatively uncommon in man, DCL may result in 30–40% of those infected; this parasite is the major cause of DCL in the New World.

(*i*) *L. (L.) mexicana* (=*L. m. mexicana*). Chiclero's ulcer, bay sore. Forested areas of northern Central America: Yucatan peninsula, Belize and Guatemala. Painless, mainly single ulcers (60% on the ear), these mostly heal in a few months, but chronic destructive lesions may also affect cartilage of the ear pinna.

The primary vertebrate host is a forest cricetid rodent (*Ototylomys phyllotis*: big-eared climbing rat). Three other forest rodents are secondary hosts (*Heteromys desmarestianus*, spiny pocket mouse; *Nyctomys sumichrasti*, vesper rat; *Sigmodon hispidus*, cotton rat). The only vector incriminated is *Lutzomyia (Nyssomyia) olmeca olmeca*. Parasites from northern Mexico and southern Texas, tentatively ascribed to *L. (L.) mexicana*, are also responsible for occasional human DCL. (Putative vectors are *Lu. (Dampfomyia) anthophora* (among wild rodents) and the anthropophilic *Lu. diabolica* (*cruciata* group of species) to man.)

(*ii*) *L. (L.) amazonensis* (=*L. m. amazonensis*). Amazonian CL and DCL; enzootic rodent leishmaniasis. Forests (including timber plantations of non-indigenous tree species) of the Amazon region, and south at least to the Atlantic littoral forest remnants of Bahia state, Brazil. Single or multiple lesions, which seldom heal. Rare in man, but about 30% become DCL. Not

associated with classical human MCL, although the nasopharynx may be involved in advanced DCL.

The primary host of this parasite is the spiny rat, *Proechimys guyannensis* sensu lato (which may be a species-complex). *Proechimys · cuvieri* is naturally infected in French Guiana and may also be a primary host.

Numerous secondary vertebrate hosts include several genera and species among both rodents and marsupials. These are listed below:

Rodents:
  Oryzomys capito, *O. concolor*, *O. macconnelli*: rice rats;
  Neacomys spinosus: spiny rice rat;
  Nectomys squamipes: water rat;
  Dasyprocta prymnolopha: agouti.

Marsupials:
  Marmosa murina and *M. cinerea*: murine opossums;
  Metachirus nudicaudatus: brown 'four-eyed' opossum;
  Didelphis marsupialis: common opossum;
  Philander opossum: grey 'four-eyed' opossum.
(Occasional hosts of *L. (L.) amazonensis* include man and the savannah fox, *Cerdocyon thous*.)

The established vector of *L. (L.) amazonensis* is *Lutzomyia flaviscutellata* (but a recently described subspecies of *Lutzomyia olmeca*, *Lutzomyia o. nociva*, possibly also may be involved). Both *Lutzomyia flaviscutellata* and *Proechimys guyannensis* continue to survive in large numbers in commercial timber plantations of non-indigenous species, when the original forest cover is replaced.

2 Other *L. (L.) mexicana* group parasites

Human infections due to various, distinct but unnamed, parasites of the *L. (L.) mexicana* complex occur in Bolivia, Brazil (states of Mato Grosso, Bahia, Minas Gerais (Rio Doce: see also *L. (V.) braziliensis* below) and São Paulo (Ribeira valley: see below)) and possibly Colombia. Insufficient is known of these parasites, or their normal hosts or vectors, to comment further on them here. (In the case of the Rio Doce and Ribeira valley areas of Brazil noted above, the poorly known *mexicana* parasites are a more important cause of human CL than the *L. (V.) braziliensis* complex organisms also found in man in the same two areas: see below, section 3 (iii).

Three species of, or allied to, the *L. (L.) mexicana* complex are also not considered here, since they are not associated with human disease and seem very unlikely ever to cause human infections. These parasites are: *L. (L.) enriettii*, undoubtedly a *mexicana* complex parasite and exclusive to domestic guinea pigs (*Cavia porcellus*), whose sylvatic host is not known (but could well be the presumed wild ancestor of the guinea pig, the cavy (or preá), *Cavia aperea*, among which *Lu. monticola* would be a candidate vector) and the distinctive parasites *L. (L.) hertigi*

(Panama and Costa Rica) and *L. (L.) deanei* (Brazil), both exclusive to Neotropical porcupines of the genus *Coendu*. *L. (L.) hertigi* and *L. (L.) deanei* form a separate species-complex of doubtful affinities.

Included under the present heading, however, are three human parasites from Venezuela and a number of others from Central America, the Caribbean and Brazil. Not all have so far been a known cause of human infection.

(i) Venezuelan lowland CL: L. (L.) venezuelensis (= L. m. venezuelensis). This is so far known from one small forest focus in the Venezuelan state of Lara. The focus is confined to a small and isolated patch of riverine gallery forest, in an area otherwise generally arid. In man *L. (L.) venezuelensis* is the cause of single indolent nodular lesions; the parasite is apparently confined to a very limited area. The natural vertebrate host is unknown, but the vector is thought to be *Lutzomyia (Nyssomyia) olmeca bicolor*, although other sandflies are found in the same small, isolated, patch of forest (*Lutzomyia ovallesi, Lutzomyia evansi* (both *verrucarum*-group species), *Lutzomyia migonei* (*migonei*-group) and *Lutzomyia gomezi* (*cruciata* group).

(ii) Venezuelan Andean CL: L. (L.) garnhami (= L. m. garnhami). This is a parasite of man, dogs and donkeys in the Venezuelan Andes at altitudes of 800–1800 m; in man the parasite is the cause of single or multiple lesions, which heal in about six months. The normal wild hosts and affinities of *L. (L.) garnhami* are uncertain, but it appears by biochemical criteria to be close to *L. (L.) amazonensis*: the likely vector is believed to be *Lutzomyia youngi* Felicangeli & Murillo, 1987, previously mis-identified as the related *Lu. townsendi* (a member of the *verrucarum* group), but firm evidence of this is lacking.

(iii) Venezuelan DCL: L. (L.) pifanoi (= L. m. pifanoi). This parasite was isolated from patients with diffuse cutaneous leishmaniasis in several areas of Venezuela (in the states of Yaracuy, Lara and Miranda). It is tentatively considered to be a member of the *L. (L.) mexicana* complex, but stocks so far isolated and ascribed to *L. (L.) pifanoi* may include a number of different organisms (e.g. *L. (L.) mexicana*, *L. (L.) amazonensis* and one the '*L. mexicana* type III stocks' which closely resemble *L. (L.) major* in isoenzyme profile and are mentioned under (vii) below), and its status is therefore a matter of contention. A parasite assigned to *L. (L.) pifanoi* was isolated from *Lutzomyia (Nyssomyia) flaviscutellata*; this particular parasite may well prove to be *L. (L.) amazonensis*, of which *Lutzomyia flaviscutellata* is the established vector. No other likely vectors have been associated with *L. (L.) pifanoi*.

(iv) DCL in the Dominican Republic. An unnamed

mexicana group parasite, mainly associated with diffuse cutaneous leishmaniasis, occurs in upland (200–500 m) forest areas, interplanted with coffee and other crop trees, in the eastern Cordilleras of the Dominican Republic. The parasite appears, on the basis of isoenzyme profiles, to belong to the mexicana group. The natural vertebrate host is not known, but in view of the paucity of the present-day indigenous fauna, the ubiquitous introduced black rat (*Rattus rattus*) is a strong candidate. The rare capromyid rodent, *Plagiodonta aedium*, the Hispaniolan hutia, is the only surviving native mammal (three other genera of hutias on the island of Hispaniola were probably hunted to extinction for food, variously in prehistoric times or early in the period of European colonization). The introduced Indian mongoose, *Herpestes auropunctatus*, is one of the few other mammals now found on the island.

The vector of the unnamed Dominican parasite is thought to be *Lutzomyia (Coromyia) christophei*; although firm evidence of this is lacking, this sandfly is closely associated with *R. rattus* and is found in its nests. The only other known Dominican sandfly species is *Lutzomyia (Micropygomyia) cayennensis hispaniolae*; this has been discounted as a likely vector. Human infections have so far almost all been of DCL.

(v) Rodent leishmaniasis in Trinidad. An unnamed *mexicana* parasite in Trinidad, from the skin of rodents, is transmitted also by *Lutzomyia (Nyssomyia) flaviscutellata*, but is not as yet associated with human disease. The primary rodent host is the rice rat, *Oryzomys capito*: secondary hosts include the spiny rat *Proechimys guyannensis* sensu lato and *Heteromys anomalus*, the forest spiny pocket mouse. Other secondary hosts are marsupials: *Caluromys philander*, grey 'four-eyed' opossum; *Marmosa fuscata* and *M. mitis*, murine opossums.

(vi) Panamanian enzootic leishmaniasis: L. (L.) aristedesi (= L. m. aristedesi) in the Sasardi region of Panama is a parasite of rodents and marsupials, but so far is not associated with human disease. The primary host is the rice rat, *Oryzomys capito*; secondary hosts include the rodents *Proechimys semispinosus* (spiny rat), *Dasyprocta punctata* (agouti) and the marsupial *Marmosa robinsoni* (murine opossum). *Lutzomyia (Nyssomyia) olmeca bicolor* is a suspect vector of this parasite among its small mammalian hosts.

(vii) Others. Other foci of unnamed *mexicana* group parasites which cause human CL are known from east and central Brazil, but the normal hosts and vectors are either unknown or poorly known. Some biochemically characterized isolates, termed '*L. mexicana* type III stocks', constitute a phenotypically uniform and distinct isoenzyme (zymodeme) group which closely resembles *L. (L.) major*. It remains uncertain whether these isolates represent accidental importations of the

Old World species, the result of laboratory mislabelling, or the presence of indigenous *L. major*-like parasites in the New World.

3 *L. (Viannia) braziliensis complex of species* (Fig. 37.12)

The species of the subgenus *Viannia* are all of small size (amastigotes and promastigotes), as compared with all other Neotropical *Leishmania* species except *L. (L.) chagasi*. Behaviour in experimental animals is distinctive, with the production of lesions notably smaller than those of the *L. (L.) mexicana* complex. Members of the subgenus *Viannia* are separated readily from the subgenus *Leishmania* on biochemical criteria (low buoyant DNA density, kDNA hybridization probes, monoclonal antibody serology and isoenzyme profiles). There is a general lack of cross immunity between the parasites of the two subgenera and members of *Viannia* are not associated with DCL in man, although at least one species of *Viannia* (*L. (V.) braziliensis*) is associated with human MCL (espundia). Normal mammalian hosts of two species (*L. (V) guyanensis* and *L. (V.) panamensis*) are principally edentates, but the normal hosts of *L. (V.) braziliensis* are largely unknown.

Members of the subgenus *Nyssomyia* are among the many vectors (such as *Lutzomyia umbratilis* and *Lutzomyia trapidoi*) of the distinct *L. (Viannia) braziliensis* complex of parasites, which in general are a more common cause of human CL than are the *L. (L.) mexicana* group; especially of the more destructive MCL espundia lesions. (This is largely because vectors of the *braziliensis* parasites are often more anthropophilic than those of the *mexicana* complex). The vectors of the *L. (V.) braziliensis* complex of parasites are taxonomically diverse, but vectors in the subgenera *Nyssomyia* (see above) and *Psychodopygus* (such as *Lutzomyia (Psychodopygus) wellcomei*), are among the most important. *Lutzomyia cruciata* and *Lutzomyia gomezi* are vectors which belong to the *cruciata* group, not allocated to any subgenus. *Lutzomyia diabolica* also belongs to the *cruciata* group; the species occurs in Mexico and the southern USA and is suspected to be the vector of the few cases of human CL recorded from Texas (parasites all of *mexicana* type): although *Lu. (Dampfomyia) anthrophora* is a good experimental vector of *L. (L.) mexicana*. This species is not anthropophilic. It may, however, be an enzootic vector among rodents in northern Mexico and south-central Texas.

(i) *Pian-bois; bush yaws*: *L. (V.) guyanensis* (= *L. b. guyanensis*). This is the causative organism of 'pian bois' or 'bush yaws' in forested areas of the Guyanas and the north of Amazonian Brazil (*L. (V.) guyanensis* is not known to occur south of the river Amazon). The parasite in man causes painless, persistent single or multiple dry lesions. Metastatic lymphatic dis-

semination often occurs and infection may perhaps sometimes cause espundia.

Primary hosts are edentates, the two-toed sloth *Choloepus didactylus* and the lesser anteater *Tamandua tetradactyla* (sloths have parasites mainly in the viscera, with little dermal involvement). Secondary hosts are the marsupial *Didelphis marsupialis* (common opossum), the rodent *Proechimys guyannensis* (spiny rat) and man. *Lutzomyia (Nyssomyia) umbratilis* is the principal vector: *Lutzomyia (Nyssomyia) whitmani* and *Lutzomyia (Nyssomyia) anduzei* may be secondary vectors, principally among animal hosts, since these species seldom bite man in endemic areas of pian bois. In the case of *L. (V.) guyanensis* (and *L. (V.) panamensis*, below) there is an arboreal enzootic transmission cycle and a ground-level zoonotic cycle.

(ii) *Panamanian cutaneous leishmaniasis*: *L. (V.) panamensis* (= *L. (b.) panamensis*). In Nicaragua, Costa Rica, Panama and parts of Colombia, this parasite in man is the cause of single or few non-healing ulcers; lymphatic involvement is frequent and the parasite may also possibly cause espundia, although many experienced workers believe occasional cases of espundia in this region are caused by a different parasite.

The two-toed sloth *Choloepus hoffmani* is the primary vertebrate host; occasional secondary hosts include the three-toed sloths *Bradypus infuscatus* and *B. griseus*, the procyonid carnivores *Nasua nasua* (coati), *Potos flavus* (kinkajou) and *Bassaricyon gabbii* (olingo); the primates *Aotos trivirgatus* (night monkey) and *Saguinus geoffroyi* (Geoffroy's tamarin). The rodents *Proechimys semispinosus* (spiny rat), *Hoplomys gymnuras* (armoured rat) and *Heteromys desmarestianus* (spiny pocket mouse) are infected with the same, or a closely similar, parasite. Man and domestic dogs are accidental hosts.

Incriminated vectors are *Lutzomyia (Nyssomyia) trapidoi* and *Lutzomyia (Nyssomyia) ylephiletor* (both of which feed predominantly on sloths); probable secondary vectors include *Lutzomyia gomezi* (*cruciata* group) and *Lutzomyia (Psychodopygus) panamensis*. *Lutzomyia (Psychodopygus) carrerai thula* (= *Lutzomyia (Psychodopygus) pessoana*) is also a suspected vector. An anthropophilic possible vector in endemic areas of Costa Rica is *Lu. youngi*, a member of the *verrucarum* group of species.

(iii) *American CL and MCL; espundia*: *L. (V.) braziliensis* sensu lato (= *L. b. braziliensis* sensu lato). Forested, generally hilly regions (over 300 m) of Brazil, Colombia, Venezuela, Peru, Ecuador, Bolivia and Paraguay. In man the cause of primary single or multiple ulcers which seldom heal; early lymphatic involvement is common. About 80% of untreated primary lesions result in later MCL (espundia, 'tapir nose'), up to 30 years after initial infection. The distribution of *L. (V.) braziliensis* is ill defined, but extends from south-east Brazil via the cocoa-growing Atlantic littoral area of Bahia state, northward through the Amazon basin forests into Venezuela and Central America; a closely related (unnamed) parasite is the cause of occasional human infections in the forests of south and central Belize. (Lesions are single or few, often with lymphatic spread, but no known mucosal involvement).

The normal vertebrate hosts of L. (V.) braziliensis sensu lato are poorly known; uncharacterized isolates attributed to L. (V.) braziliensis come from the rice-rats Oryzomys concolor, O. capito and O. nigripes, the South American field-mouse (Akodon arviculoides), the climbing mouse (Rhipidomys leucodactylus) and the spiny rat (Proechimys guyannensis). Other un-characterized L. braziliensis stocks come from a marsupial and an edentate; the common opossum, Didelphis marsupialis and the two-toed sloth, Choloepus didactylus. Uncharacterized isolates, tentatively attributed to L. (V.) braziliensis sensu lato, in areas of Ecuador west of the Andes were isolated by liver culture from a kinkajou (Potos flavus), a three-toed sloth (Bradypus variegatus ephippiger) and a tree-squirrel (Sciurus granatensis), but not by culture of spleen or cardiac blood; skin was not cultured, but impression smears were negative from both skin and viscera. Dogs and donkeys are also infected by unch-aracterized L. (V.) braziliensis in western Venezuela, but these (like man) are probably abnormal hosts. Dogs are also infected with parasites fully char-acterized as L. (V.) braziliensis in the state of Bahia, Brazil, where this parasite is an important cause of human MCL (L. (L.) amazonensis also causes occasional human infections in the same area).

The vectors of L. (V.) braziliensis are also poorly known: in the Amazon basin Lutzomyia (Psychodopygus) wellcomei is an important vector of the parasite to man at over 300 m altitude in the Serra dos Carajas, of Pará state, Brazil. Lutzomyia (Psychodopygus) wellcomei is known from areas in Brazil as far south of the Amazon basin as the state of Ceará; this vector may prove to be common in its preferred ecotope in many upland forest areas of the Brazilian Shield, wherever climate and vegetation are suitable. Other members of the subgenus Psychodopygus (regarded as a genus by some workers) probably also are important vectors elsewhere; for example, Lutzomyia (Psychodopygus) panamensis in Venezuela. Lutzomyia (Nyssomyia) intermedia and Lutzomyia (Pintomyia) pessoai are infected with a parasite ascribed to L. (V.) braziliensis sensu lato in southern Brazil (São Paulo state).

Some of the parasites isolated from man in south-east Brazil (Rio Doce region of Minas Gerais state, Espirito Santo, the greater Rio do Janeiro area and the Ribeira valley of São Paulo state) are now sufficiently well characterized on modern criteria to be considered as L. (V.) braziliensis: infected dogs in these areas are, like man, probably an accidental host. (It should be noted that mexicana group parasites are in fact the commonest cause of human leishmanial infections in the Rio Doce (Minas Gerais) and Ribeira valley (São Paulo) regions.) Anthropophilic sandflies in all these areas of south-east Brazil are: Lutzomyia (Nyssomyia) intermedia (usually the dominant house-haunting species), Lutzomyia (Nyssomyia) whitmani, Lutzomyia migonei (migonei group) (also an endophilic sandfly) and Lutzomyia (Pintomyia) fischeri. However, none of these species has yet been incriminated as a vector, although Lutzomyia intermedia is considered the most likely candidate on circumstantial grounds.

MCL, due to a parasite not yet fully characterized but thought to be close to or identical with L. (V.) braziliensis (the vector not yet known), occurs in steep-sided valleys on the forested eastern slopes of the Bolivian Andes, from 400 to 2500 m, in areas where both subsistence slash-and-burn and plantation agric-ulture are practised and where, particularly between 1100 and 1600 m, MCL coexists with AVL (uncom-mon) and canine VL (widespread), both of the latter transmitted by Lutzomyia longipalpis.

(iv) Peruvian CL; uta: L. (V.) peruviana (= L. (b.) peruviana). This is the cause of 'uta' in man, in the arid western Andean regions of Peru (from latitude 5° to 13° south: altitude 900 m to 3000 m) and, probably, neighbouring areas of Bolivia and Argentina. The simple cutaneous lesions are single or few, mainly affect children and heal in about four months. Lesions and scars are found on exposed parts of the body, principally the face.

Uta occurs on the arid, generally treeless and barren western slopes of the Peruvian Andes, where the veg-etation is sparse and consists mainly of open low shrubs, at best. Infection is most common between 1800 and 2700 m, particularly among schoolchildren, of whom up to 94% may have active lesions or scars. Because of its clinical similarity, the lesions of uta were once thought to be oriental sore, due to imported 'L. tropica', but the parasite has been demonstrated unequivocally to be a distinct species of the L. (V.) braziliensis complex. Up to 10% of dogs are infected, with inconspicuous skin lesions; parasites sometimes occur in normal skin. No parasites have been found in other domestic animals, rodents or opossums (although 5.4% of 93 Rattus rattus from one uta focus were infected with an unidentified Leishmania). Dogs are certainly a secondary reservoir of the infection, but the primary host of the parasite is unknown. Rice rats (Oryzomys spp.), opossums (Didelphis spp.) and pericotes (leaf-eared mice), Phyllotis darwini and Phyllotis sp., are the common small mammals, but these animals have not been studied sufficiently to be either excluded or implicated as primary hosts. Rodents are thought to be the most likely of possible primary hosts, largely because 48% of sentinel ham-sters exposed, in the presence of 'wild' Lutzomyia (Helocyrtomyia) peruensis and Lutzomyia (H.)

noguchii, in a man-made roadside 'cavern', became naturally infected over a two-year period. (It was noted that the *Lutzomyia noguchii* were numerous only in the immediate vicinity of a cage which contained laboratory-reared individuals of *Phyllotis* sp., on which they were observed to feed.)

The sandfly *Lutzomyia (Helocyrtomyia) peruensis* has the same altitudinal and general distribution as uta, is anthropophilic and peridomestic, and parasites isolated from this species were infective to hamsters. *Lutzomyia verrucarum* (*verrucarum* group) is also a man-biting domestic sandfly (it is the incriminated vector of Carrión's disease (bartonellosis: *Bartonella bacilliformis*), which has a distribution in Peru very much the same as uta. *Lutzomyia verrucarum* may possibly also transmit uta, since it is an endophilic species (and is found also in pig-pens and dry-stone walls), but it appears to be a much less important vector; if, indeed, it is a vector at all. As noted above, *Lutzomyia (Helocyrtomyia) noguchii* is a species closely associated with *Phyllotis* spp. (it feeds mainly on the pericotes and is often found in their nests; among these animals *Lutzomyia (H.) noguchii* transmits a trypanosome: *Trypanosoma (Megatrypanum) phyllotis*). *Lutzomyia noguchii*, however, does not appear to be involved in the transmission of uta. Other sandflies found in the montane foci where uta occurs, include *Lutzomyia (Lutzomyia) battistini*, *Lutzomyia (Helocyrtomyia) pescei* and the inadequately described large sandfly *Lutzomyia (Lutzomyia) imperatrix*; none of these species are believed to be involved in the transmission of either uta or bartonellosis, however.

Prior to the widespread DDT house-spraying campaigns of the 1950s (an anti-bartonellosis measure, which also radically reduced the occurrence of uta), uta was seen in adults mainly among agricultural workers in settled areas and transmission was peridomestic; in the 1980s, following the resurgence of uta as a human infection, the disease is more closely associated with uncultivated (or recently settled) areas, especially those used for the grazing of livestock. There are now relatively fewer infections among children and more among adults; transmission currently may be more sylvatic than peridomestic, a feature which would be in full accord with the known habits of *Lutzomyia (H.) peruensis*.

(*v*) *Unnamed L. (V.) braziliensis complex parasites causing human disease.* Two different parasites of the *L. (V.) braziliensis* complex cause uncomplicated human CL in various parts of Pará state in Amazonian Brazil. Nothing is known of their normal hosts or vectors. Other distinct *L. (V.) braziliensis* complex parasites, not so far associated with human disease, have been isolated from animals or sandflies in the Amazon basin, but have not been further studied. (The hosts from which these parasites were isolated are as follows: the opossum *Didelphis marsupialis*, the two-toed sloth *Choloepus didactylus* and the nine-

banded armadillo *Dasypus novemcinctus*; the sandflies *Lutzomyia (Psychodopygus)* sp. nr. *Lutzomyia (Psychodopygus) davisi*, *Lutzomyia (Trichophoromyia) ubiquitalis* and *Lutzomyia (Viannomyia) tuberculata*.)

4 Neotropical Leishmania of uncertain status

The final three parasites to be mentioned are of no known medical importance and are of questionable taxonomic status.

(*i*) *L. herreri Zeledón, Ponce & Murillo, 1979.* This is a parasite of sloths in Costa Rica (*Choloepus hoffmani*, two-toed sloth; *Bradypus griseus*, three-toed sloth) and is apparently transmitted by the sandflies *Lutzomyia (Nyssomyia) trapidoi*, *Lutzomyia (Nyssomyia) ylephiletor* and *Lutzomyia shannoni* (*shanonni* group). The site of development in sandflies is not reported, although the size of amastigotes in tissue culture is within the range for members of the *L. (L.) mexicana* complex.

(*ii*) *Leishmania spp. of Panamanian rodents.* Two unnamed *Leishmania* parasites, of no known medical importance, have been isolated from Panamanian rodents. Their taxonomic status is questionable and nothing is known of the site of their development in sandflies. One parasite was isolated from the blood of a spiny rat (*Proechimys semispinosus*) and the other from the skin of an arboreal soft-furred spiny rat, *Diplomys labilis*.

VECTOR–PARASITE INTERACTIONS IN TRYPANOSOMATIDAE OF MEDICAL IMPORTANCE

Recent evidence suggests that, in many cases, infection of insect vectors of the family Trypanosomatidae with their particular parasites tends, in the case of those where transmission is by bite (*Glossina* with salivarian trypanosomes, phlebotomine sandflies with *Leishmania* and *Rhodnius prolixus* with *Trypanosoma rangeli*), to interact with the vectors in a manner which, by its effects on the probing and feeding behaviour of infected insects, tends to enhance parasite transmission, as compared with the normal feeding activities of uninfected vectors.

Much of the evidence is, however, based on observations under laboratory conditions, of experimentally infected vectors and uninfected controls; there is clearly a need to investigate how important such vector–parasite interactions may be under field conditions. Field observations in this connection are of obvious importance, both for practical reasons and in the development of quantitative epidemiological models of parasite transmission.

Until recently, it was generally assumed that vector insects probed and fed, survived and reproduced, in much the same manner whether infected or not. If parasite-induced changes in physiology and behaviour are widespread, then such assumptions will have to be changed accordingly. The present evidence suggestive of the probable importance of vector–pathogen interactions between the trypanosomatid parasites and their vectors is summarized briefly below.

Glossina and salivarian trypanosomes

Studies of the effects of *Leishmania* on the behaviour of infected phlebotomines about a decade ago (which suggested that *Leishmania* could interfere with cibarial chemoreceptors and/or mechanoreceptors on the labrum), prompted the first investigation of comparable phenomena in infected *Glossina*.

Tsetse flies have 50–60 mechanoreceptor (LC1) sensilla in the proximal third of the labrum, the region colonized by *T. (Duttonella) vivax* and the infective stages of *T. (Nannomonas) congolense*. Several workers used scanning electron microscopy (SEM) to demonstrate that the flagellates of both species were closely associated or intertwined with, and sometimes attached to, the LC1 labral receptors of *Glossina*. Rosettes of trypanosomes sometimes completely covered the receptors; transmission EM showed that *T. congolense* epimastigotes developed hemidesmosomal flagellar attachments to the chitinous LC1 receptors, in the manner in which other trypanosomatids attach to the chitinous intima of foregut and hindgut in their insect hosts. Similar EM studies showed frequent association with, and attachment to, LC1 sensilla by large numbers of *T. vivax*. *T. brucei* trypomastigotes in the mouthparts of *Glossina*, although present in smaller numbers, were shown also to entwine around the LC1 receptors. More recently, similar associations were shown between *T. vivax* and *T. congolense* with cibarial mechanoreceptor sensilla (LC2), which like the LC1 sensilla in the mouthparts, monitor the passage of blood through the alimentary canal in the head region.

The probable effect of the association between trypanosomes and the flow-regulating LC1 and LC2 sensilla was considered likely to affect adversely the normal ingestion of blood by infected insects; this was confirmed by observation of *G. morsitans* infected with *T. brucei*, compared with uninfected control insects. Infected flies probed more frequently before feeding than uninfected flies and fewer of them successfully fed to engorgement. Similar effects were observed with *G. morsitans* infected with *T. congolense*; increased probing and longer engorgement times were recorded for infected tsetse, compared with uninfected controls. *T. b. brucei* was transmitted to six mice by repeated probes of a single infected fly before it fed successfully. Some workers, however, were unable to detect significant differences in the probing and feeding behaviour of tsetse infected with *T. brucei*, *T. vivax* or *T. congolense*, as compared with uninfected controls. The observed discrepancies remain to be fully explained, but may be the result of different numbers, or distribution, of parasites in different experimental groups of flies.

Other differences between infected and uninfected tsetse also recorded include a different distribution of acetylcholinesterase activity, and different levels of sugars and amino acids, in the salivary glands of infected and uninfected *Glossina*. Pathological effects on the salivary glands of infected flies may also influence feeding behaviour as compared with that of uninfected flies. The presence of parasites may also have deleterious effects in energy metabolism: calculations show that infection may result in an energy loss equivalent to at least a 15% reduction in daily flight activity.

Field observations of infected *Glossina* indeed suggest that infection with trypanosomes may well affect feeding frequency, nutritional condition and overall longevity.

Triatomine bugs and stercorarian trypanosomes

Since *Trypanosoma (Schizotrypanum) cruzi* metacyclic trypomastigotes are transmitted by the posterior-station faecal contaminative route, there is no vector–parasite interaction in regard to the feeding activities of the vector as such, of the kind seen with salivarian trypanosomes or *Leishmania*. Recent work suggests nonetheless that morphogenesis of *T. cruzi* in the vector is influenced, and possibly controlled, by exposure to lectins in different parts of the triatomine gut. Moreover, the normal behaviour of triatomines to defaecate on the skin of the host whilst feeding (or shortly after) clearly favours successful contaminative transmission of the parasite: but there is no known difference in this respect between infected and uninfected bugs.

In the case of *Trypanosoma (Herpetosoma) rangeli*, however, transmitted from the salivary glands of *Rhodnius* spp. by bite, there are indications that infected insects experience difficulty in feeding to repletion. This is attributed to heavy infections of the salivary glands and/or to possible damage to the pharyngeal musculature by the trypanosomes. Recent work on probing behaviour of infected *R. prolixus* and *R. robustus* showed a significant difference between infected and uninfected insects. Eleven infected bugs probed an average of 13 times (range: 2–28) before engorgement; two failed to feed at all but probed 12 and 28 times on mice, which were infected from these probes. Uninfected bugs fed after an average of two probes only, and reached engorgement much more rapidly than infected insects.

Leishmania and Phlebotomine sandflies

Whilst the mechanism of *Leishmania* transmission by phlebotomine sandflies is still not fully understood, the question has received much attention in recent years and is the subject of continuing study. It was noticed, first in the 1940s and confirmed in laboratory transmission studies about 30 years later, that sandflies infected with *Leishmania* parasites took second and subsequent blood meals only with great difficulty, and as a result of frequently unproductive probes which, nonetheless, often led to successful parasite transmission.

Uninfected flies have a significantly better chance of successful engorgement than those which are infected; this first led to the suggestion that the presence of parasites in the head region in some way interferes with the normal sensory processes by which blood meals are obtained. Sandflies, like *Glossina*, have sensory sensilla in the cibarium and mouthparts; these are mechanoreceptors which appear to monitor blood flow into the alimentary canal.

The presence of large numbers of parasites in the oesophageal and pharyngeal regions (where they may form a plug which constricts the gut lumen), are thought to have a feedback effect on the cibarial and proboscis sensory receptors. Recent studies, particularly of sandflies (*P. papatasi* and *P. duboscqi*) infected with *L. (L.) major*, but also of New World *Leishmania* and Neotropical sandflies, have shown infected flies to produce either multiple lesions on a single host as a result of successive and unsuccessful attempts to feed or, conversely, to infect a series of different hosts in the same manner. This behaviour may explain not only simultaneous multiple lesions in patients with CL, but also the occurrence of multiple cases (of CL or VL) in individual families, or among troops and others. The location of parasites in the gut of individual flies plays an important role: sandflies with parasites in the midgut only, or which are uninfected, usually probe only once or twice and achieve full engorgement within 10 minutes. Sandflies with cibarial infections, however, commonly probe three or more times (26 successive probes, on a small area of skin, are recorded for one *P. papatasi*, with the subsequent production of 11 *L. (L.) major* lesions). Such flies either fail to feed at all, or take only a small blood meal in 15–20 minutes.

The concept that heavy parasite concentrations in the anterior regions of the alimentary canal, which may interfere with mechanoreceptors that monitor blood flow, and/or cause total or partial blockage of the stomodeal valve (and hence the regurgitation of infective midgut metacyclics: see below) is not intrinsically at variance with that of transmission effected by small, highly motile, metacyclic promastigotes present in the mouthparts. Indeed, the likelihood of transmission by proboscis metacyclics is enhanced by the inability of many infected flies to engorge normally; either because of a direct interference with cibarial receptor function, the perception of reduced flow (caused by oesophageal or pharyngeal parasite blockage), or a combination of both factors.

The role of sandfly nutrition in the development of *Leishmania* infections is also the subject of renewed interest. It has been known for many years that sugar-feeds after an infective laboratory blood meal enhance sandfly infections, but experimental transmission is nonetheless notoriously and unpredictably difficult to achieve.

Sandflies are observed to pierce plant stems and leaves, to obtain sugar-containing plant juices directly; the feeding mechanism is then similar to that in the 'blood-feeding' mode, and fluids pass directly to the midgut. Sandflies also feed on nectar and the 'honeydew' secreted by many plant-feeding homopteran bugs. In this case, where piercing of tissue is not involved, a 'sugar-feeding' mode is adopted: fluids are directed first into the crop, where they are mixed with its bacteriostatic contents, before the mixture ultimately passes to the midgut. Plant sap, nectar and honeydew all contain amino acids in addition to sugars; the amino acids may be important also for the successful development of *Leishmania* in sandflies.

In experimental studies with colony *P. papatasi* (in which they were force-fed a mixture of blood and *L. (L.) major* culture promastigotes in capillary tubes), it was shown that the addition of protein (as 2% albumin) to postinfection sugar feeds significantly enhanced the proportion of female *P. papatasi* which subsequently emitted *L. (L.) major* metacyclic promastigotes into capillaries of a saline/blood mixture, when force-fed a second time 10–12 days later. A 2% albumin/10% sucrose mixture was more successful in this respect than either 10% sucrose, 10% trehalose, or 10% albumin alone. Infected flies were nonetheless found in each of the experimental groups, which implied that there is no single nutritional factor essential for successful development of *Leishmania* parasites.

Emission of parasites into capillaries was also positively correlated with an inability of infected females to engorge successfully; some 70% of flies which emitted metacyclics failed to engorge, and only 20% completed engorgement normally. Many females emitting metacyclics failed to feed at all, in spite of normal action of the cibarial pump.

Infective stages emitted into capillaries were typical metacyclic promastigotes; these were also seen in large numbers in the oesophagus and anterior thoracic midgut regions of infected flies. (About 75% of infected flies emitted 10 or fewer promastigotes into the capillaries; some 20% from 100 to 1000 and about 5% emitted more than 1000.)

Almost all emitting flies had metacyclic forms in the anterior midgut and stomodaeal valve regions; about half also had unattached pharyngeal metacyclics (seen also in the pharyngeal region of non-emitting insects), but only rarely were metacyclics seen (in small numbers) in the cibarial region of transmitting flies. The presence of metacyclic forms alone thus does not necessarily indicate an ability to transmit parasites successfully.

Taken together with the presence of infective *L. (L.) major* metacyclic promastigotes in the midgut of *P. papatasi* from day 3 after an infective feed (with a peak of infectivity on day 5), this reopens the question of possible infection of a new host by regurgitation of midgut metacyclics, in the manner that proventricular blockage by plague bacteria in fleas causes infection by passive regurgitation.

Other studies of *P. papatasi* infected with *L. (L.) major* showed that parasites in the anterior (thoracic) midgut, stomodaeal valve and oesophagus consist of a dense mat of attached haptomonad promastigotes and paramastigotes, together with short, highly motile, metacyclic forms with long flagella; often intertwined with the sessile stages in the oesophagus. Although attached haptomonads and paramastigotes were not emitted into the capillaries, their presence in the region of the stomodaeal valve may constrict the valve lumen sufficiently to reduce, or prevent entirely, the entry of blood from the oesophagus into the midgut during feeding.

These observations provide further support for the 'blocked fly' concept of *Leishmania* transmission referred to above, and first proposed by workers in India nearly 60 years ago. Flies with a partial or complete stomodaeal valve blockage will draw blood into the oesophagus (by the normal action of the cibarial and pharyngeal pumps) at a rate faster than it can pass through the stomodaeal valve into the midgut. This increases the internal pressure on the oesophageal wall and causes dilation of the oesophagus (as seen in normal feeding), until its elastic pressure exceeds that of the pharyngeal pump, when a fluid backflow will occur and thus passively regurgitate free midgut metacyclics forward into the pharynx, cibarium and mouthparts; whence they can pass·(either actively or passively) into the skin of a new host.

Present indications are that a sugar/protein mixture is the most suitable to promote the heavy parasite infection necessary to cause stomodaeal valve blockage. Passive regurgitation of midgut metacyclics into the bite wound, together with their frequent absence from the cibarium and proboscis of infected flies, seems in accord with many recent observations. However, the 'blocked fly' regurgitation of midgut metacyclics does not necessarily preclude active inoculation of free-swimming proboscis metacyclics: possibly both mechanisms are involved in the transmission of the various *Leishmania* parasites by different sandflies.

There is as yet no direct evidence to demonstrate any effect of *Leishmania* infection on sandfly longevity per se, but it seems very probable that the evident difficulty of infected flies to feed normally, and the increased time they spend (at great risk) on the host as a result, is likely to reduce the life-span of infected flies.

ISOLATION, MAINTENANCE AND PRESERVATION OF TRYPANOSOMES AND *LEISHMANIA* OF MEDICAL IMPORTANCE

(This section is concerned only with viable living organisms and excludes methods used solely in parasitological diagnosis.)

Salivaria (*Trypanozoon*): isolation from the vertebrate host

Useful direct methods include differential centrifugation of blood, including the microhaematocrit method, extraction on DEAE cellulose columns (a miniature column, made from a plastic disposable syringe, is used for field work) and the use of density gradients. Indirect methods include animal inoculation and haemoculture. Trypomastigotes can also be cultured from the cerebrospinal fluid of patients.

Maintenance and culture. Members of the subgenus *Trypanozoon* can be cultured in vitro in a wide variety of media. For details of main culture methods, see Brun and Jenni,[47] Jenni and Brun[48] and Gray et al.[49] When incubated at 28°C, culture forms resemble the *Glossina* midgut procyclic stages and are not infective to mammals. Infective metacyclic stages are produced at 28°C in the presence of *Glossina* salivary gland explants, or of mammalian cell lines (see below). Bloodstream stages can be cultured continuously at 37°C in the presence of mammalian feeder-layer cells (even axenically in their absence, if provided at regular intervals with thiols, such as cysteine; although the population doubling time is then approximately doubled).

In the vertebrate, in addition to the blood-borne trypomastigote stages, there are also extravascular sites for trypanosomes (some tissues, including the ependymal cells of choroid plexus and ventricular linings, in which true intracellular stages may occur; and the lymphatic system). It is not clear which stages are produced in cultures of what are usually referred to as 'bloodstream stages' and this term may eventually prove to be a misnomer. The first continuous culture system for 'bloodstream stages', achieved in the mid-1970s, employed a tissue-culture medium supplemented with 20% heat-inactivated fetal bovine serum (FBS) and a feeder layer of bovine fibroblast cells.

The co-cultivation of trypanosomes and mammalian cell lines (of various kinds) continues to be a necessity in most continuous cultures, except in the thiol-supplemented axenic system referred to above. The 'bloodstream stages' produced in continuous cultures are infective to *Glossina* and vertebrates, and undergo antigenic variation in vitro. Their ultrastructure is quite normal and in every respect they are very close, if not identical to, the forms produced in vivo. The nature of the essential role played by the obligatory mammalian feeder cells is still quite unknown.

An entirely in vitro serum-resistance test is possible with the continuous culture system: two parallel cultures are set up, one with 20% heat-inactivated horse or rabbit serum as a control and the other with 20% human serum instead. This system is sensitive enough to distinguish single serum-resistant (i.e. presumptively man-infective) trypanosomes among large numbers of serum-sensitive individuals. However, the yield of continuous in vitro culture systems is relatively low, in the order of 10^6/ml (probably because of accumulation of pyruvate); this hampers the use of in vitro cultivation systems for the production of parasites in sufficient numbers for experimental work (e.g. drug-testing, antigen production for serodiagnostic purposes and studies of immunization).

In vivo maintenance of *Trypanozoon* in laboratory mice and rats is normally straightforward, although some refractory stocks of *T. b. gambiense* in West Africa (notably Ivory Coast and Liberia) are difficult, often impossible, to establish in normal laboratory rodents; giant pouched rats (*Cricetomys gambianus*), multimammate rats (*Mastomys natalensis*) or exotic voles (*Microtus montanus*, a North American species) are then useful as isolation hosts (although lengthy periods of adaptation are still often necessary). However, the refractory *T. b. gambiense* stocks are also readily cultivable in RPMI 1640 or MEM tissue culture medium with 20% inactivated serum (human, horse or goat) and a feeder layer of human embryonic fibroblast cells, or of *M. montanus* embryo fibroblast cells. These systems permit the direct cultivation of the 'refactory' *T. b. gambiense* stocks directly from the blood or cerebrospinal fluid of sleeping sickness patients and avoids any necessity for passage in rodents.

Where parasitaemia in laboratory hosts is low, recourse can be had to xenodiagnosis with laboratory-bred *Glossina*, from which cultures of midgut procyclic stages are then easily established. Although procyclic culture stages lack the surface coat of the bloodstream trypomastigotes, culture procyclics nonetheless can be used for isoenzyme characterization and for DNA analysis.

The epimastigote stages, which in the fly follow after the midgut procyclic stage, have not been successfully cultivated, however. This is unfortunate, in that the epimastigote stage is probably a necessary precursor for the cultivation of the salivary gland metacyclic stages. Culture of the non-dividing metacyclic stages per se has also not been achieved to date, although when non-infective trypomastigotes are cultivated in vitro at 28°C in the presence of many salivary gland explants of *Glossina m. morsitans*, a small proportion of infective metacyclic forms are produced; but this is normally less than 0.1%. Ultrastructural

and other studies demonstrate that these are real metacyclic forms; these are also produced in similarly small numbers in the presence in vitro of tsetse gut tissues, or abdominal body wall explants. Infected salivary glands, incubated at 25°C or 30°C, with macerated (uninfected) salivary gland tissues and a bovine embryonic spleen cell feeder layer, will also produce antigenically stable infective stages, presumptively metacyclics, in some cultures. The developmental potential of metacyclic stages is obviously strictly limited: they cannot be induced to transform back to the midgut procyclic stage, they are incapable of reproduction, and transform promptly to bloodstream stages under in vitro conditions. If the presumed 'inhibitory factor' present in the salivary glands (and which prevents the transformation of metacyclics to bloodstream forms in the glands) could be isolated and synthesized, then some of the major outstanding problems might be resolved.

Cultivation in vitro of the economically important livestock trypanosomes, *T. (D.) vivax* and *T. (N.) congolense*, has progressed in recent years, particularly in the case of the latter. *T. congolense* procyclic stages can be grown in semidefined media, either with or without *Glossina* cells; densities of about 4.5×10^7/ml are reached.

If probosces of *Glossina* infected with *T. congolense* are excised and cultured with bovine dermal explants, mouse-infective metacyclics are produced, along with procyclics and epimastigotes. Subpassages in media without the dermal explants will continue to produce infective metacyclics. A modified system used Vitrogen in place of bovine explants and produced moderate numbers of metacyclics. Up to 10^6 metacyclics are produced in these relatively simple systems, an output which compares favourably with the few hundred produced by individual infected *Glossina*, although metacyclic stages represent only a small proportion of the forms present in the cultures.

Some success with cultivation of bloodstream forms of *T. congolense* was achieved by placing infected skin into a continuous culture system of RPMI 1640 medium and a feeder layer of bovine endothelial cells, together with serum supplementation (16% heat-inactivated adult goat serum + 4% fetal goat serum). The culture stages produced appear identical to normal bloodstream forms, including the antigenic surface coat.

T. (D.) vivax continues to be the most recalcitrant of the African trypanosomes to cultivate in vitro. Procyclic and metacyclic stages were produced in vitro lately by introduction of mouse-adapted bloodstream stages into MEM medium and a feeder layer of bovine fibroblasts and beads of Matrix Green Gel A at 25°C. Although the yield of metacyclics is not high (less than 1%), it represents a considerable advance on infected *Glossina*, which frequently extrude metacyclics only one at a time. Some progress with cultivation of bloodstream stages of *T. vivax* stocks from West Africa was made, with a culture system of *Microtus* embryonic fibroblast cells in MEM medium and supplemented by 20% inactivated adult goat serum. The system, similar to that for *T. brucei* subspecies, has not yet proved amenable to East African *T. vivax* stocks.

Preservation. Bloodstream, culture and *Glossina* stages of *Trypanozoon* can be indefinitely cryopreserved, with dimethylsulphoxide (DMSO) or glycerol (respectively 10% and 8% final concentrations) as cryoprotectants, without significant loss of viability or infectivity. Frozen stabilates are stored in 'dry ice' (solid carbon dioxide) at $-79°C$, in liquid nitrogen at $-196°C$, or in the vapour phase above liquid nitrogen. Vector stages in intact tsetse flies can be cryopreserved in situ under field conditions, for subsequent study.

A controlled slow-cooling rate (about 2°C/minute) to below $-40°C$ is essential for successful cryopreservation of trypanosomes (see also section on preservation of *Leishmania*, below, for references to methods).

Stercoraria (*T. cruzi* and *T. rangeli*): isolation from the vertebrate host

Direct methods, such as differential centrifugation (including microhaematocrit centrifugation) and density gradients can be used where parasitaemia is sufficiently high, e.g. in acute human Chagas' disease. Extraction on anion-exchange columns is generally not useful for primary isolation, because of the negative surface charge of Stercoraria but, if buffered to pH 8, columns will yield trypomastigote-enriched fractions from epimastigote/sphaeromastigote/ trypomastigote mixtures of *T. cruzi* from cell-line cultures.

Indirect methods (xenodiagnosis, haemoculture and animal inoculation) are more suitable for primary isolations where peripheral parasitaemia is not microscopically detectable (e.g. from patients in the chronic stage of Chagas' disease).

Maintenance and culture. *T. cruzi* and *T. rangeli* grow readily in a variety of culture media (for details see Evans,[50] D'Alessandro[44] and Bruni and Jenni[47]), in which epimastigotes predominate at 26–28°C, but cultures are nonetheless infective to mammals. Defined culture media with serum supplements, and even chemically defined media without supplements, are now successfully used in a number of research establishments. Metacyclogenesis in vitro is relatively easy with *T. cruzi* and is favoured particularly in some media (LMC medium and Grace's insect tissue culture medium at pH 6.6, for example), and by the co-cultivation of insect tissues (such as triatomine cell lines), or the addition of insect extracts (e.g. of *Triatoma* gut cells).

Continuous-flow culture systems were developed for *T. cruzi* with little difficulty; in vitro cloning of *T.*

cruzi on plates of solid media is also relatively simple to carry out.

In the presence of human diploid cell lines, culture of *T. cruzi* at a higher temperature (30–33°C) yields about 95% trypomastigotes and 5% amastigotes. A high proportion of amastigote stages can be obtained with the use of other culture media, even cell-free semidefined media (the amastigotes produced are able to penetrate muscle cells and reproduce within), and in several systems which combine the co-cultivation of mammalian cells. Broad *T. cruzi* trypomastigotes infect triatomines but do not infect vertebrate cells; slender trypomastigotes are therefore necessary for cell penetration and the subsequent production of intracellular amastigotes, in the different cell lines which were variously used (chick embryo cells, bovine embryo muscle cells, HeLa or Vero cells, fibroblasts and myocardial cells). Transformation of intracellular amastigotes to trypomastigotes is induced by the substitution of horse serum for fetal bovine serum (FBS) in the medium.

Metrizamide or Ficoll gradient centrifugation is useful for separation of amastigotes from trypomastigotes, feeder cells and cell debris. The non-dividing bloodstream trypomastigotes cannot be cultivated in vitro, and are obtainable only by in vitro transformation from amastigotes, after intracellular multiplication of the amastigotes is completed. Host cells can also be disrupted, before trypomastigotes are liberated, and the amastigotes separated by metrizamide gradient centrifugation. Different feeder cell types release amastigotes and trypomastigotes in different proportions: macrophage-like cells liberate mainly amastigotes; fibroblast cells produce predominantly trypomastigote forms. Either stage can be purified by metrizamide or Ficoll gradients (DEAE cellulose columns are effective for the same purpose, but also reduce parasite infectivity).

T. cruzi is easily maintained in vivo in laboratory rodents; this is less practicable for *T. rangeli*, since infection of vertebrates is often short-lived. When parasitaemia of rodents is low, xenodiagnosis or haemoculture are useful methods for recovery of parasites of both species.

Preservation. All stages of *T. cruzi* and *T. rangeli* may be cryopreserved, with either DMSO (10%) or glycerol (8%) as cryoprotectants. A controlled slow-cooling rate (about 2°C/minute) to below $-40°C$ is essential for successful cryopreservation of both trypanosomes and *Leishmania*. For references to slow-cooling methods, see section on preservation of *Leishmania*, below.

Leishmania species: isolation from the vertebrate host

Amastigotes from spleen, liver or bone marrow biopsies can be isolated by culture in a variety of biphasic or monophasic media, or by intraperitoneal inoculation of golden hamsters (intracardiac or intrasplenic inoculation, although more difficult, yields a positive result within a matter of weeks, compared to several months after intraperitoneal inoculation). Media based on insect tissue culture formulae (such as Schneider's or Grace's medium) are often more efficient in parasite isolation from biopsy material in the case of kala-azar. Addition of 15% defibrinated rabbit blood to Grace's medium +20% inactivated FBS, markedly improved the number of successful isolations from bone marrow aspirates in Bihar, India (to 90%: this in comparison with 73% for modified NNN, 30% in Grace's medium +30% FBS and 13% in Grace's +20% FBS). Haemoculture is often successful in Indian kala-azar, generally less so in other kala-azar areas.

Skin biopsy material for detection of cutaneous parasites, obtained by scalpel, skin biopsy punch or a dental broach, from the *edges* of cutaneous lesions (or the apparently normal skin of known or suspected reservoir hosts), is usually more difficult to establish in primary cultures, particularly where species of the *L. (Viannia) braziliensis* complex are concerned. In the Neotropics, inoculation of material from the margins of dermal lesions (or dermal tissue homogenate samples from animal reservoir hosts, best refrigerated overnight in a saline/antibiotic mixture), into nose-skin and foot-pads of golden hamsters is a generally safer procedure for the isolation of cutaneous parasites; this is followed in due course by parasite culture from the dermal lesions produced in the hamster, often only after a lapse of several months. Sandfly midgut promastigote stages are usually easily cultivated, if aseptic procedures are followed.

Maintenance and culture. Most *Leishmania* spp. grow prolifically and with ease in most culture media: some are, however, more fastidious or die out on subpassage (mainly Neotropical cutaneous parasites) and require considerable expertise and/or particular culture media to become satisfactorily established. Evans[51] and Schnur and Jacobson[52] are good sources of information on isolation and culture methods for *Leishmania*, the latter also for other parasitological techniques with *Leishmania*. Insect tissue-culture media (chiefly Schneider's, but also Grace's) are sometimes very useful for *Leishmania* cultivation, with or without additional supplements (such as FBS). Growth in insect tissue culture media is often more rapid than in media which contain blood, and growth of amastigotes occurs if the incubation temperature is raised, from 26–28°C to 34°C.

Preservation. Cryopreservation, with DMSO (final concentration 10%) or glycerol (final concentration 8%) as cryoprotectant, is suitable for all *Leishmania*. Field cryopreservation of the insect stages of *Leishmania* spp., in intact, potentially infected, sandflies is also successful. A controlled slow-cooling rate (about 2°C/minute) to below −40°C is essential for successful cryopreservation of *Leishmania*. This can be achieved by several simple methods, applicable under field conditions.[53-55]

REFERENCES

1 Garnham, P. C. C. (1966) *Malaria Parasites and Other Haemosporidia.* Oxford: Blackwell Scientific Publications.
2 World Health Organization (1963) *Terminology of Malaria and of Malaria Eradication.* Geneva.
3 Krotoski, W. A., Krotoski, D. M., Garnham, P. C. C. et al (1980) *Br. med. J.* i, 153.
4 Markus, M. B. (1976) *Trans. R. Soc. trop. Med. Hyg.* 70, 535.
5 Markus, M. B. (1978) *S. Afr. J. Sci.* 74, 105.
6 Krotoski et al (1982).
7 Pasvol, G. & Wilson, R. J. M. (1982) *Br. med. Bull.* 38, 133–140.
8 Bray, R. S. & Garnham, P. C. C. (1982) *Br. med. Bull.* 38, 117–122.
9 Hawking, F., Worms, M. J. & Gammage, K. (1968) *Trans. R. Soc. trop. Med. Hyg.* 62, 731.
10 Shute, P. G. & Maryon, M. (1966) *Laboratory Technique for the Study of Malaria.* London: Churchill.
11 Bannister, L. H. & Sinden, R. E. (1982) *Br. med. Bull.* 38, 141–145.
12 Jiang, J. B., Huang, J. C., Wang, D. S. et al (1982) *Trans. R. Soc. trop. Med. Hyg.* 76, 845–847.
13 Bray, R. S. (1965) *Am. J. trop. Med. Hyg.* 14, 455.
14 Coatney, G. R., Chin, W., Contacos, P. G. et al (1966) *J. Parasit.* 52, 660.
15 Chin, W., Contacos, P. G., Coatney, G. R. et al (1965) *Science, N.Y.* 149, 865.
16 Shute, P. G. (1966) *Trans. R. Soc. trop. Med. Hyg.* 60, 412.
17 Umlas, J. & Fallon, J. N. (1971) *Am. J. trop. Med. Hyg.* 20, 527.
18 Trager, W. & Jensen, J. B. (1976) *Science, N.Y.* 193, 673.
19 Garnham, P. C. C. (1980) *Trans. R. Soc. trop. Med. Hyg.* 74, 153.
20 Hoare, C. A. (1980) *Trans. R. Soc. trop. Med. Hyg.* 74, 153.
21 Upton, A. J. (1969) *Trans. R. Soc. trop. Med. Hyg.* 63, 527.
22 Dobell, C. (1928) *Parasitology* 20, 357–412.
23 Cleveland & Sanders (1931) *Arch. Protisterk.* 70, 223–226.
24 Hoare, C. A. (1961) *Bull. Soc. Path. exot.* 54, 429.
25 Hoare, C. A. (1957) *Trans. R. Soc. trop. Med. Hyg.* 51, 304.
26 Diamond, L. S. (1968) *J. Parasit.* 54, 715.
27 Sargeaunt, P. G., Baueja, V. K., Nanda, R. et al (1984) *Trans. R. Soc. trop. Med. Hyg.* 78, 96–101.
28 Reed, S. L., Sargeaunt, P. G. & Braude, A. I. (1983) *Trans. R. Soc. trop. Med. Hyg.* 77, 248–253.
29 Parelkar, S. N. & Stamm, W. P. (1973) *Trans. R. Soc. trop. Med. Hyg.* 67, 659.
30 Burrows, R. B. & Swerdlow, M. A. (1956) *Am. J. trop. Med. Hyg.* 5, 258.
31 Carter, R. F. (1968) *J. Path. Bact.* 96, 1.

32 Band, R. N. (1959) *J. gen. Microbiol.* **21**, 80.
33 Carter, R. F. (1972) *Trans. R. Soc. trop. Med. Hyg.* **66**, 193.
34 Levine et al (1980) *J. Protozool.* **27**: 37–58.
35 Hoare, C. A. (1972) *The Trypanosomes of Mammals*, pp. 749. Oxford: Blackwell Scientific Publications.
36 Kreier, J. P. (1977) *Parasitic Protozoa*, vol. 1, pp. 441. New York: Academic Press.
37 Lumsden, W. H. R. & Evans, D. A. (eds.) (1976, 1979) *Biology of the Kinetoplastida*, vols 1 & 2. London: Academic Press.
38 Vickerman, K. (1985) *Br. med. Bull.* **41**, 105–114.
39 Tetley, L. & Vickerman, K. (1985) *J. Cell Sci.* **74**, 1–19.
40 Benchimol, M. & De Souza, W. (1980) *J. Parasit.* **66**, 941–947.
41 Tetley, L., Coombs, G. H. & Vickerman, K. (1980) *J. Parasit.* **72**, 281–292.
42 Ormerod, E. E. (1979) In *Biology of the Kinetoplastida*, vol. II, ed. W. H. R. Lumsden & D. A. Evans, pp. 339–394. London: Academic Press.
43 Barry, J. D. (1986) The molecular biology of African trypanosomes. *Trop. Dis. Bull.* **83**(4), R1–R25.
44 D'Alessandro, A. (1976) In *Biology of the Kinetoplastida*, vol. I, ed. W. H. R. Lumsden & D. A. Evans, pp. 327–403. London: Academic Press.
45 Lainson, R. & Shaw, J. J. (1987) In *The Leishmaniases in Biology and Medicine*, vol. 1, ed. W. Peters & R. Killick-Kendrick, pp. 1–120. London & New York: Academic Press.
46 Lainson, R. & Shaw, J. J. (1979) In *Biology of the Kinetoplastida*, vol. II, ed. W. H. R. Lumsden & D. A. Evans, pp. 1–116. London: Academic Press..
47 Brun, R. & Jenni, L. (1985) *Br. med. Bull.* **41**, 122–129.
48 Jenni, L. & Brun, R. (1987) In *In vitro Methods for Parasite Cultivation*, ed. A. E. R. Taylor & J. R. Baker. London, New York & San Francisco: Academic Press (in press).
49 Gray, M. A., Hirumi, H. & Gardiner, P. R. (1987) In *In vitro Methods for Parasite Cultivation*, ed. A. E. R. Taylor & J. R. Baker. London, New York & San Francisco: Academic Press (in press).
50 Evans, D. A. (1978) In *Methods of Cultivating Parasites in vitro*, ed. A. E. R. Taylor & J. R. Baker, pp. 55–88. London, New York & San Francisco: Academic Press.
51 Evans, D. A. (1987) In *In vitro Methods for Parasite Cultivation*, ed. A. E. R. Taylor & J. R. Baker. London, New York & San Francisco: Academic Press (in press).
52 Schnur, L. F. & Jacobson, R. L. (1987) In *The Leishmaniases in Biology and Medicine*, vol. 1, ed. W. Peters & R. Killick-Kendrick, pp. 499–541. London & New York: Academic Press.
53 Minter, D. M. & Goedbloed, E. (1971) *Trans. R. Soc. trop. Med. Hyg.* **65**, 175–181.
54 Dar, F. K., Goedbloed, E., Ligthart, G. S. et al (1973) *Ann. trop. Med. Parasit.* **67**, 21–29.
55 World Health Organization (1984) The Leishmaniases. *Wld Hlth Org. tech. Rep. Ser.*, 701, pp. 140.

SELECTED SOURCES FOR FURTHER READING

Ashford, R. W. & Bettini, S. (1987) In *The Leishmaniases in Biology and Medicine*, vol. 1, ed. W. Peters & R. Killick-Kendrick, pp. 365–424. London & New York: Academic Press.
De Souza, W. (1984) *Int. Rev. Cytol.* **86**, 197–283.
Gibson, W. C. & Miles, M. A. (1985) *Br. med. Bull.* **41**, 115–121.
Lainson, R. (1983) *Trans. R. Soc. trop. Med. Hyg.* **77**, 569–596.
Lewis, D. J. & Ward, R. D. (1987) In *The Leishmaniases in Biology and Medicine*, vol. 1, ed. W. Peters & R. Killick-Kendrick, pp. 235–262. London & New York: Academic Press.
Jordan, A. M. (1986) *Trypanosomiasis Control and African Rural Development*. Harlow (UK): Longman.
Molyneux, D. H. & Ashford, R. W. (1983) *The Biology of Trypanosoma and Leishmania, Parasites of Man and Domestic Animals*. London: Taylor and Francis.
Molyneux, D. H. & Killick-Kendrick, R. (1987) In *The Leishmaniases in Biology and Medicine*, vol. 1, ed. W. Peters & R. Killick-Kendrick, pp. 121–176. London & New York: Academic Press.
Opperdoes, F. R. (1985) *Br. med. Bull.* **41**, 130–136.
Peters, W. & Killick-Kendrick, R. (eds.) (1987) *The Leishmaniases in Biology and Medicine*, vols. 1 & 2. London & New York: Academic Press (in press).
Shaw, J. J. & Lainson, R. (1987) In *The Leishmaniases in Biology and Medicine*, vol. 1, ed. W. Peters & R. Killick-Kendrick, pp. 291–363. London & New York: Academic Press.
Snary, D. (1985) *Br. med. Bull.* **41**, 144–148.
Snary, D. (1985) *Trans. R. Soc. trop. Med. Hyg.* **79**, 587–590.
Steinert, M. & Pays, E. (1985) *Br. med. Bull.* **41**, 149–155.
Turner, M. J. (1985) *Br. med. Bull.* **41**, 137–143.
Van Meirvenne, N. & Le Ray, D. (1985) *Br. med. Bull.* **41**, 156–161.
World Health Organization (1979–1981) Studies on leishmaniasis vectors/reservoirs and their control in the Old World; Parts I to V. (Compiled by A. R. Zahar.) WHO, Geneva: unpublished documents:
Parts I & II (1979) General Review, Europe & N. Africa. WHO/VBC/79.749.
Part III (1980a) Middle East. WHO/VBC/80.776.
Part IV (1980b) Asia & Pacific. WHO/VBC/80.786.
Part V (1981) Tropical Africa. WHO/VBC/81.825.
World Health Organization (1986) Report of a training seminar on epidemiological methods for the leishmaniases. WHO, Geneva. Mimeographed document: TDR/LEISH-SEM/80.3.
World Health Organization (1986) Epidemiology and control of African trypanosomiasis. WHO, Geneva. *Wld Hlth Org. tech. Rep. Ser.*, 739, pp. 127.

Appendix II
Medical Helmintology

TREMATODES
Subclass DIGENEA (Carus, 1863) (Digenetic trematodes)

Fasciola hepatica

Fasciola hepatica (Linnaeus, 1758) is a parasite of sheep causing 'liver rot'. It is also found in jack and cottontail rabbits in the USA and rats in the Old World.

Distribution

Worldwide.

Characters (Fig. 22.25)

Pale grey with dark borders, it measures 2.3 cm × 8–13 mm; large specimens in cattle (7.5 cm) are known as *F. gigantica*. The anterior extremity is narrow, containing the oral sucker; the ventral sucker is larger than the anterior and situated 3 mm from the anterior extremity. Branched intestinal caeca with diverticula are present. The ovary is racemose, placed anterior to the testes in the posterior end of the body. The uterus is short and anterior to the ovary. An exsertile cirrus is present and the genital pore is median.

The *egg* (Fig. 22.26) is operculated. 130–140 × 63–90 μm, ovoid, brown and bile-stained and contains the ovum and yolk cells. A ciliated eye-spotted miracidium develops in about three weeks and enters freshwater amphibious lymnaeid snails of the species detailed below.

Life-cycle (Fig. 22.27)

Snail hosts of F. hepatica

Lymnaea truncatula (Europe, western Asia and highland southern Africa), *L. viator*, *L. diaphana* (South America), *L. bulimoides*, *L. humilis* (North America), *L. columella* (Africa, also occasionally North and South America, Australia), *L. cubensis* (Caribbean) and *L. tormentosa* (Australasia). *L. columella* is a proven host for both *F. hepatica* and *F. gigantica* and, in recent years, *L. columella* has become established in South Africa, Australia, New Zealand and Hawaii. In these it becomes a sporocyst, daughter sporocysts, rediae (named after the Italian zoologist Redi) and cercariae. Development takes two months. The cercaria is blunt-tailed and settles in grass or on bark

where it secretes mucus to form a cyst with two prominent suckers (metacercariae). Then it is eaten by the mammalian host. Metacercariae excyst in the duodenum and migrate through the intestinal wall into the body cavity, then to the biliary passages where they grow to maturity.

F. gigantica, a liver fluke, similar but larger, is now known to cause human infections in the USSR, Indo-China, West Africa and Hawaii. It develops in fully aquatic lymnaeid snails.

Fasciolopsis buski (Lankester, 1857) (Odhner, 1902)

Fasciolopsis buski (Fig. II.1) is a parasite of the pig which constitutes a reservoir for man.

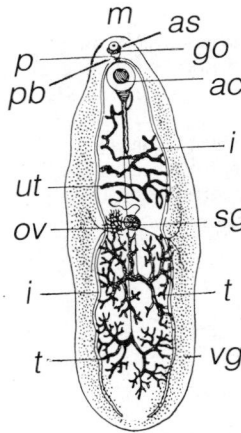

Fig. II.1 *Fasciolopsis buski.* The following key is used for the terminology of the anatomy of the trematodes in this and subsequent illustrations.

as	anterior sucker	va	vagina
m	mouth	oo	ootype
p	pharynx	ovd	oviduct
pb	pharyngeal bulb	vs	vesicula seminaris
ac	acetabulum or	oes	oesophagus
	ventral sucker	rs	receptaculum seminalis
go	genital opening	t	testis
ut	uterus	vd	vas deferens
vg	vitelline glands	i	intestine
ov	ovary	ic	branch intestine
sg	shell gland	lc	Laurer's canal
exp	excretory pore	gp	genital pore
nc	nerve cord		

Characters

F. buski inhabits the small intestine, rarely the stomach; only a small number of those infected show symptoms. This is the largest human trematode, measuring 3 cm × 12 mm and 2 mm thick. It is flesh-coloured, elongated and oval, with transverse rows of spines, especially numerous near the ventral sucker. The oral sucker is subterminal but ventral in position and is only quarter the size of the ventral which is placed close to the oral, and prolonged into the cavity dorsally and backwards, a feature peculiar to this species. (For details of the anatomy see Fig. 11.1.) The intestinal caeca are simple with two characteristic curves towards the midline. The genital pore is median, placed anterior to the ventral sucker. Branched testes are found in the posterior half of the body; there is a branched ovary and a fine, tortuous, Laurer's canal.

Development in the freshwater snail resembles that of *F. hepatica*.

The egg is operculated and yellow, measuring 130–140 × 80–85 μm (Plate III.1 and Fig. 22.36). Eggs are found in large numbers in the faeces, the egg capacity of each fluke being about 25 000/day.

Life-cycle (Fig. 22.37)

After three to seven weeks in water the eggs hatch a ciliated miracidium which develops in freshwater snails—*Segmentina hemisphaerula*, *Hippeutis umbilicalis* (Far East), *Hippeutis cantori* (Far East) and *Segmentina trochoidens* (India) (Fig. II.2). A sporocyst is formed in 3 days, followed by the rediae and daughter rediae, which eventually produce cercariae (the whole cycle takes two months).

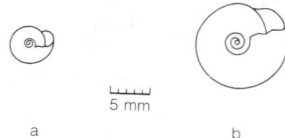

Fig. II.2 Molluscan hosts of *Fasciolopsis buski*. a, *Segmentina hemisphaerula*. b, *Hippeutis cantori*.

The cercariae, resembling those of *F. hepatica*, are oval, short-lived and lophocercous and measure 0.7 mm; they have a well-developed digestive tract with a muscular bladder and collecting tubules. They encyst, as *metacercariae*, on freshwater plants especially the outer cuticle of the water calthrop, *Trapa (Salvinia) natans* in China, *T. bicornis* in India, *T. bispinosa* in Taiwan. As many as 20 encysted metacercariae may be found on a single leaf. In south China the most important plant is the water chestnut, *Eliocharis tuberosa*, and water bamboo, *Zigania aqua-*

tica, in Chekiang and Canton, and the water hyacinth, *Eichornia crassipes*, in Taiwan. The outer layers of the plants are torn off by the teeth. All the plants are grown in ponds in China and fertilized by human faeces, thus affording an opportunity for infection; *F. buski* is therefore limited in distribution to that of these plants. The cysts when taken into the mouth pass through the stomach, excyst in the duodenum and become attached to the intestinal wall.

SUPERFAMILY: OPISTHORCHIOIDEA

GENUS: *Clonorchis*

Clonorchis sinensis (Figs. 22.28 and II.3) (also known as *Opisthorchis sinensis*)

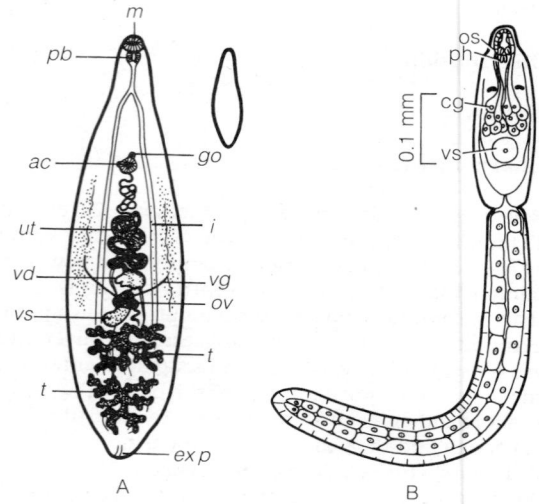

Fig. II.3 A, *Clonorchis sinensis*, magnified and natural size. B, Cercaria of *C. sinensis*.

os	oral sucker	cg	cephalic secretory gland
ph	pharynx	vs	ventral sucker

Distribution

Far East, especially China (Kwangtung province in south China, Indo-China and Okayama, Japan).

Characters

This is a common parasite of man and also of the biliary passages of the dog, cat, pig, rat, mouse, camel and badger, etc. It is found rarely in the gallbladder of man but often in the bile ducts, pancreas, pancreatic ducts and duodenum. It is spatulate, tapering anteriorly, reddish, semitransparent and measures 10–25 × 2–5 mm. The cuticle is smooth; the oral sucker is larger than the ventral; the intestinal caeca are simple.

The genital pore is median and placed anterior to the ventral sucker. The testes are branched and situated posteriorly one behind the other. The ovary is tri-lobate with coils anterior to the genital glands. Vitel-line glands are moderately developed in the mid-third of the body. Cross fertilization occurs; the sper-matozoa develop before the ova; the sperms enter the female genital pore, pass into the immature uterus and thence to the *spermatheca* (Fig. II.3) where they are stored; the ova are fertilized in the spermatheca and then pass on.

The egg measures 20–30 × 14–17 μm; it is opercu-lated, yellow-brown and one of the smallest trematode eggs found in man (Plate III.5 and Fig. 22.29). It is fully embryonated when discharged. It resembles an electric light bulb with the knob at the bottom. It withstands desiccation but not decomposition.

Life-cycle (Fig. 22.31)

The egg can remain viable in water for five weeks and is ingested by the snail before the escape of the miracidium which has a life-span of 20 minutes. Development continues in bythinid snails. The mira-cidium pierces the oesophagus of the mollusc, casts its cilia and soon becomes a sporocyst; later, the elongated rediae grow within the sporocysts and burst into the peri-oesophageal sinus and move tailwards into the liver, the whole process taking three to four weeks.

The cercariae (Fig. II.3B), 450–550 × 100–120 μm, escape from the rediae from the birthpore; they have two pigmented eyespots and a lophocercous blunt-ending tail, and burst through the space between the upper body surface and the shell, emerging into water. Within 24–48 hours they encys as metacercariae in the muscles and underscales of freshwater fish of families Cyprinidae and Anabantidae. Cercarial glands excrete a histolytic substance which dissolves the skin of the fish thus admitting percolating water. The meta-cercariae secrete a viscous fluid which forms an inner true cyst which in turn is encapsulated by a fibrous layer formed by the tissues of the fish. These are eaten half-raw, or pickled in soy sauce by the Chinese. The adolescercaria, the fully developed cyst, possesses a capsule protective against the gastric juice. In some species of fish—*Carassius auratus* (golden carp)—the parasite is found under the scales; in others it is in the flesh so that domestic animals which eat the offal may become heavily infected while man escapes. The cysts withstand a temperature of 50–70°C for 15 minutes. The cyst wall is digested by the succus entericus in the duodenum near the ampulla of Vater and the adolescercariae escape and attach themselves to the mucosa. The young distomes at first have spines but these are soon lost. They attain maturity in 26 days. Attracted by positive chemotaxis a small proportion of them reach the bile ducts but 95% are digested and destroyed. The size of the resulting fluke is determined by the calibre of the bile duct. Egg production is very large; in the cat 2400 eggs are produced daily but fewer in dogs. As many as 21 000 adults are found at autopsy.

Life-span is 12 years. Adult men are infected more than women.

The following is a list of the molluscs and fishes which may be intermediaries.

Hosts

First intermediate hosts (molluscs) (Fig. II.4)

The most important first intermediate (snail) hosts are *Bythinia (Parafossarulus) manchouricus* and *Bythinia fuchsiana*. Additional first intermediate hosts are *Bythinia longicornis*, *Assiminea lutea* and *Melanoides tuberculatus*.

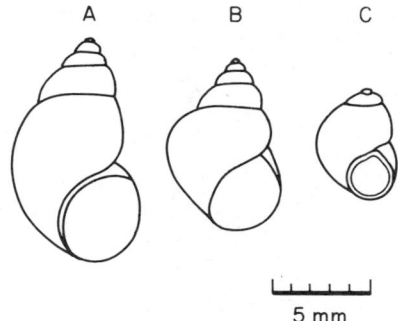

Fig. II.4 Molluscan hosts of *Clonorchis sinensis*. A, *Parafossarulus manchouricus*. B, *Bythinia fuschiana*. C, *Bythinia longicornis*.

Second intermediate hosts (fish)

More than 80 species of fish have been incriminated: 71 species of Cyprinidae, 2 species of Electridae. One species each of Bagridae, Cyprinodontidae, Clupeidae, Osmedipae, Cichlidae, Openocephalidae and Gobiidae. The most important cyprinoid fish are *Mylopharyngodon aethiops*, *Ctenopharyngodon idella* (Canton), *Cultur recurviceps* (Peking) and *Carassius auratus* (golden carp).

Major additional fish hosts are *Tribolodon hakonensis*, *Hemibarbus labes*, *Acanthorhodens asmussi*, *Pungtungia herzi*, *Pseudogobio esocinus*, *Gnathopogon atromaculatus*, *Cultriculus kneri*, *Macropodus chinensis*, *Opsariichthydis bidens*.

In addition in Fukien, China, freshwater shrimps (*Caridinia nilotica*, *Macrobrachium superboum*, *Palaeo-monetes sinensis*) are incriminated as sources of infec-tion in children.

Other fish hosts are *Hemicultur leucisculus*, *H. b. leekeri*, *Acanthorhodens chankaensis*, *A. gracilis*, *Abbotina rivularis*, *Pseudorasbora parva*, *Hyspeleotris swinhoensis*, *Philypus potamophilus*, *Rhodeus sinensis*, *Sarcocheilichthys nigripennis*, *S. sinensis*, *S. variegatus*, *Macropodus opercularis*, *Biwia zezera*, *Xenocypris davidi*, *Pseudiperilampus typus*, *Abbotina psegma*, *Paraleucogobio strigatus*, *Acheilognathus rhombea*, *A.*

lanceolata, A. limbata, A. cyanostigma, Labeo jordani, Hypophalmichthys nobilis.

GENUS: *Opisthorchis* (cat liver fluke)

There are two species of cat liver fluke: *Opisthorchis felineus* (Rivolta 1884), eastern Europe and USSR and *O. viverrini* (Poirier 1886) north-east Thailand, Laos.

Characters (*Opisthorchis felineus*)

It inhabits the liver, pancreas, bile ducts and lungs (in Russia). It is lanceolate and measures $8–11 \times 1.5–2$ mm. The cuticle is smooth, the suckers equal in size and separated by 2 mm (Fig. II.5). The egg measures $30 \times 12 \,\mu$m and is yellowish-brown with an operculum. At the posterior end there is a minute tubercular thickening (Plate III.4).

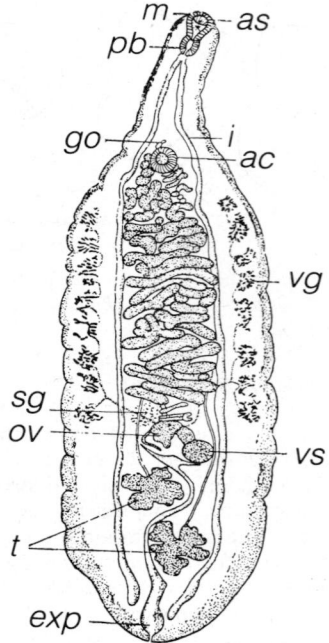

Fig. II.5 *Opisthorchis felineus*, $\times 9$.

Life-cycle (similar to *C. sinensis*, Fig. 22.31)

The definitive hosts are man and wild and domestic felines. The first intermediary host is a snail, usually

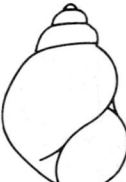

Fig. II.6 *Bythinia leachi*, the molluscan host of *Opisthorchis felineus*.

Bythinia leachi (Fig. II.6); an additional snail host is *Bythinia tentaculata*. The miracidium is fully formed in the egg and hatches in the snail forming a sporocyst in the intestine 1.2–1.85 mm. Rediae are formed in one month and then cercariae which mature in four months.

Cercariae, $430–670 \times 40–50 \,\mu$m, which leave the snail in daylight are phototactic and stimulated by agitation.

The second intermediary hosts are fish—the tench (*Tinca tinca*), the ide (*Leuciscus idus*), the barbel (*Barbus barbus*) and the roach (*Rutilus rutilus*). Additional second intermediary hosts are *Idus melanotus, Abramis brama, A. sapa, Cyprinus carpio, Blicca bjorkna, Alburnus lucidus, Aspilus aspilus, Scardinus erythrophthalmus*. The cercariae penetrate in 15 minutes and grow to three or four times their original size forming metacercariae $220 \times 160 \,\mu$m. When ingested by man they pass through the stomach, are freed by the succus entericus, attracted by the bile and travel up the bile duct in 5 hours. Infection is therefore contracted by eating raw fish. The entire life-cycle requires a minimum of four months. This fluke is not specially pathogenic, although 200 or more have been found in the body at autopsies.

Opisthorchis viverrini is the other species and is of importance in Thailand and India. It is morphologically similar.

Life-cycle of *O. viverrini* (similar to *C. sinensis*, Fig. 22.31)

The normal definitive hosts are the dog and civet cat. First intermediary hosts are snails, *Bythinia funiculata, B. siamensis, B. goniomphales* and *B. laevis*. Second intermediary hosts are fish, *Cyclocheilichthys siaja, Hampala dispar, Puntius orphoides, P. gonionotus, P. poctozyron, Labiobarbus lineatus* and *Osteochilus* sp.

GENUS: *Heterophyes*

Heterophyes heterophyes (Siebold, 1852)

Distribution

Egypt, China, Japan, Brazil, Korea, Spain and Greece.

Characters

Heterophyes heterophyes (Figs. II.7 and 22.39) inhabits the small intestine of man in large numbers and also that of the rat, fox, dog, wolf, jackal and cat; also in the black kite (*Milvus migrans aegyptius*) and a bat (*Rhinolophus divosus acrotis*) in the Yemen. It imparts a coffee grounds appearance to the intestinal wall. It is pyriform, grey and very small, measuring $1–1.7 \times 0.3–0.7$ mm. The uterus forms a brown patch in the centre. The oral sucker is subterminal and the

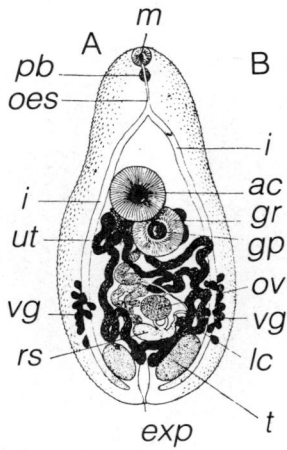

Fig. II.7 *Heterophyes heterophyes*, greatly magnified (A) and natural size (B).

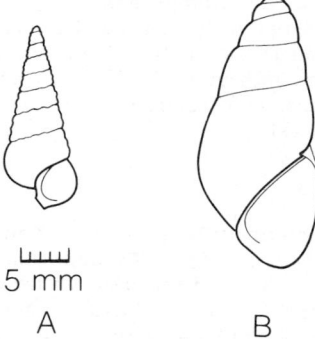

Fig. II.8 A, *Pirinella conica*, the molluscan host of *Heterophyes heterophyes*. B, *Semisulcospira libertina*, the molluscan host of *Metagonimus yokogawai*.

ventral sucker is three times the size of the oral sucker. The cuticle is thickly set with quadrate scales measuring $5 \times 4 \,\mu$m. There is a short prepharynx and long oesophagus. The intestinal caeca extend to the posterior extremity, converging close to the excretory vesicle. The vitelline glands are posterior, situated in two clumps; the genital pore is posterolateral in the vicinity of the ventral sucker and consists of a muscular ring armed with 70 chitinous cuticular teeth. The testes are oval and posterior, the ovary globular and median. There is a receptaculum seminis as large as the ovary; uterine coils are not numerous. Seminal vesicle and Laurer's canal are present.

The egg measures $20–30 \times 15–17 \,\mu$m, being the same size as that of *C. sinensis* (Plate III.3). Its greatest breadth is across the centre. There is no special ring to the operculum which is light-brown and contains a ciliated miracidium when deposited. It hatches after ingestion by the appropriate snail.

Life-cycle

H. heterophyes develops in brackish water snails. The proven hosts are *Pirinella conica* in the Middle East (Fig. II.8A), *Cerithidea cingulata* and *Tympanotomus micropterus* in the Far East. Additional recorded hosts include *Melanoides tuberculata* and *Cleopatra bulimoides*. The cercaria, which is eyed and has a membranous tail, enters the second intermediate host—a freshwater fish the mullet (*Mugil cephalus*) or in Japan a species of *Acanthogobius* in which metacercariae develop and encyst under the scales. Infection is acquired from eating raw fish.

In Africa two other species have been recognized—*H. brevicaeca* and *H. taihokui*. In Japan in the vicinity of Kobe a closely related species, *H. katsuradai*, is recognized which is stouter and has a relatively enor-

mous acetabulum. The eggs are smaller measuring $25–26 \times 14–15 \,\mu$m.

GENUS: *Metagonimus*
Metagonimus yokogawai (Katsurada, 1912)

Distribution

Korea, Taiwan, China, Japan, Philippines and Ukraine. Very common in the Far East.

Characters

Metagonimus yokogawai (Fig. II.9) is found in the small intestine of man, higher up than *H. heterophyes*, and also in the cat, dog, pig and fish-eating birds, such as the pelican. It is the smallest fluke parasitic in man with a mean size of 1.4×0.6 mm. The tegument is covered with small spines; the ventral sucker is deflected to the right with its long axis in the diagonal phase. There is a genital pore in front; the ovoid testes are posterior; the ovary and receptaculum seminis are situated medially in front of the testes. The yolk

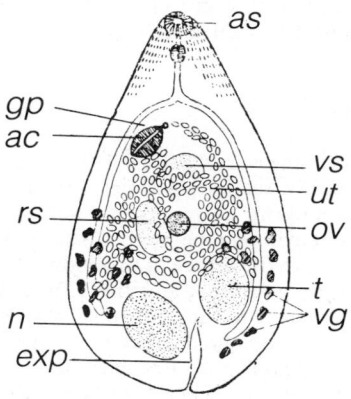

Fig. II.9 *Metagonimus yokogawai*, × 45.

glands are found in clumps in the posterior third. The uterus lies between the testes and the ventral sucker and the seminal vesicle in front of the ovary (Fig. II.9).

The egg measures 27–28 μm × 16–17 μm and resembles that of *C. sinensis* but is more regularly ovoid (Plate III.6).

Life-cycle

The first intermediate hosts are molluscs—*Semisulcospira libertina* (Fig. II.8B) and *Thiara granifera*. Sporocysts, rediae and cercariae are formed; the last has an anterior end provided with armament. The tail is long and membranous with lateral flutings and is discarded on entering the fish host. *Plecoglossus altivelis* is regarded as the most important source of infection of *M. yokogawai* in Japan. Other freshwater fish hosts recorded include *Carassius auratus*, *Cyprinus carpio*, *Zacco temminckii*, *Photimus steindachneri*, *Acheilognathus lanceolata* and *Pseudorasbora parva*. The metacercariae measure about 150 × 100 μm and encyst under the scales; infection results from eating raw fish.

SUPERFAMILY: PLAGIORCHIDEA

GENUS: *Paragonimus*

Many species of *Paragonimus* are found in nature and can be divided into four main groups by the nature of the cuticular spines and the ovary.
1 Westermani: *P. westermani*.
2 Compactus: *P. compactus*, *P. siamensis*.
3 Kellicotti-miyazaki: *P. kellicotti*, *P. miyazaki*, *P. heterotremus*, *P. caliensis*, *P. amazonicus*, *P. mexicanus* (*peruvianus*).
4 Ohirai-ilokstuensis: *P. ohirai*, *P. ilokstuenensis*.

Other species include *P. tuanshenensis*, *P. szechuanensis*, *P. hueitungensis* and the African species *P. africanus* and *P. uterobilateralis*.

Distribution

The Far East from Japan to India, Indonesia, Pacific Islands, West and central Africa and central South America.

Characters

P. westermani measures 8–20 × 5–9 mm and is oval (almost round in section), reddish-brown and translucent. The anterior extremity is rounded. The oral sucker is subterminal; the ventral sucker larger and placed anterior to the centre of the body. The pharynx and oesophagus are short and the bifurcation of the intestine is anterior to the ventral sucker (Figs. II.10 and 22.42). The intestinal caeca run a zigzag course; the common genital pore lies close to the posterior margin of the ventral sucker. The body is bisected by a large excretory vesicle. The testes are tubular and

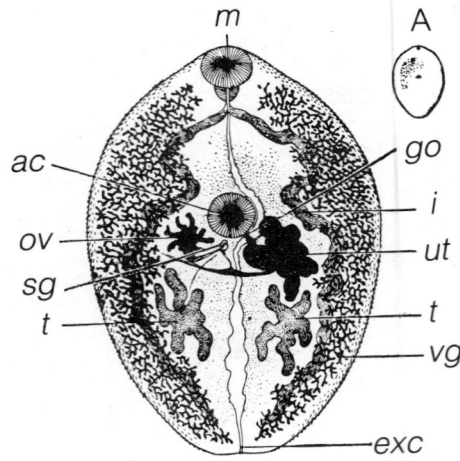

Fig. II.10 *Paragonimus westermani* (*ringeri*), natural size (A) and magnified.

racemose; the branched ovary may be to either the right or the left of the midline and posterior to the ventral sucker. The uterus is short, sac-like and lies opposite the ovary. The vitellaria are well developed extending through the whole body. Laurer's canal and shell-gland are present. The cuticle is studded with wedge-shaped spines which with the ovary are used to differentiate the four main types:
1 Westermani: cuticular spines singly spaced and ovary simple branched into four to six lobes.
2 Compactus: cuticular spines in groups and ovary simply branched into four to six lobes.
3 Kellicotti-miyazaki: cuticular spines singly spaced, ovary profusely branched.
4 Ohirai-iloktsuenensis: cuticular spines in groups, ovary profusely branched.

The egg is brown and operculated, measuring 90 × 55 μm. It shows a thickening at the pole opposite the operculum. The egg of *P. compactus* is smaller, 75 × 48 μm (Plate III.2 and Fig. 22.43).

Life-cycle (Figs. II.11 and 22.44)

The lung fluke can remain viable in the human body for 20 years. The eggs are first voided into cystic pockets in the lungs and then escape into water in the sputum and also in faeces from swallowed sputum. A ciliated miracidium hatches in 16 days to seven weeks and has distinctive characters. There is a ciliated covering in four rows at the anterior cone. The excretory pore forms a rosette. It enters the snail hosts (Table 22.2). It develops in about 60 days into sporocyst and rediae, each containing 20 cercariae; the latter, ellipsoid and microcercous, have a short knob-like tail and measure 200 × 70–80 μm with an anterior stylet and body covered with spines. The cercariae

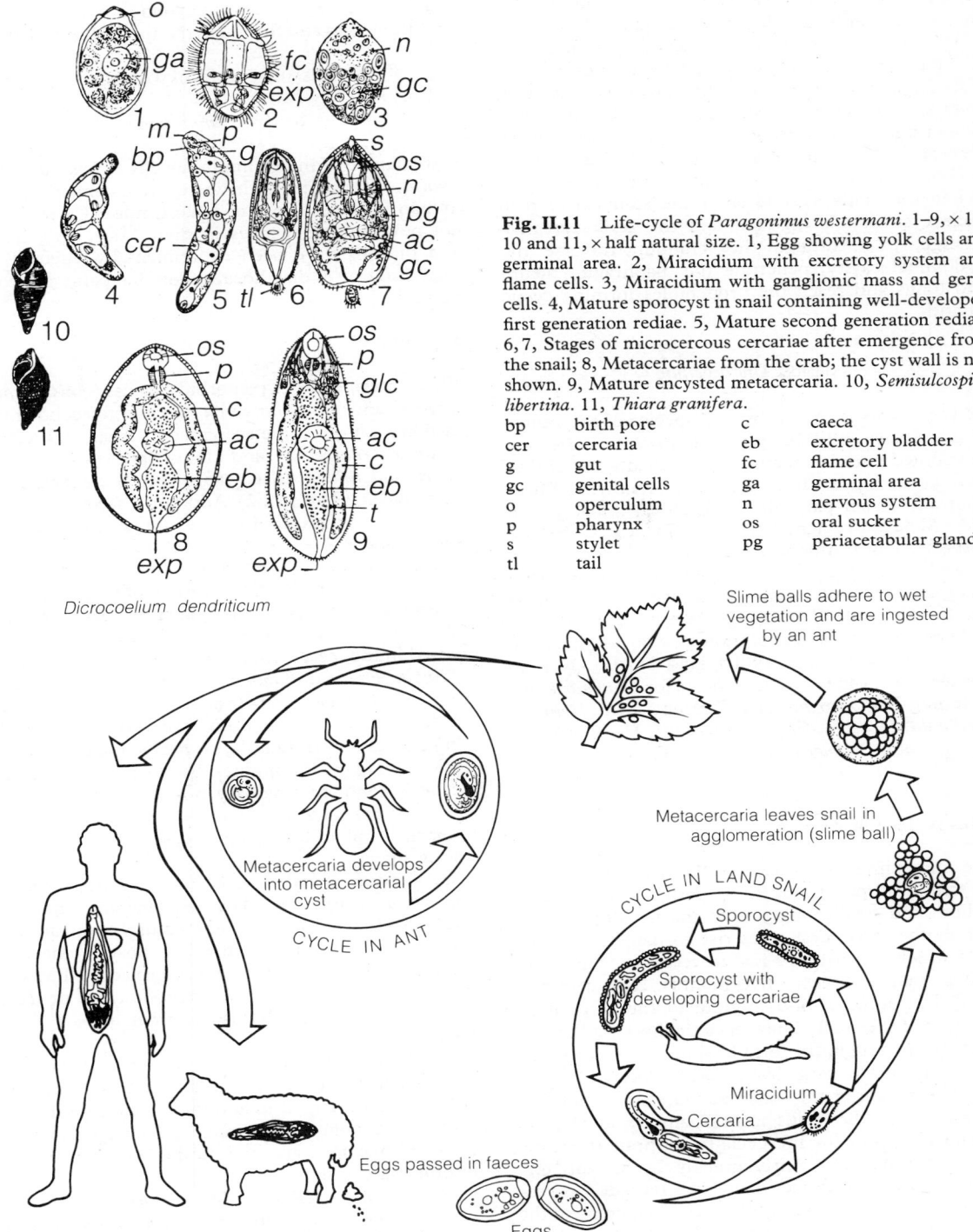

Fig. II.11 Life-cycle of *Paragonimus westermani*. 1–9, × 15; 10 and 11, × half natural size. 1, Egg showing yolk cells and germinal area. 2, Miracidium with excretory system and flame cells. 3, Miracidium with ganglionic mass and germ cells. 4, Mature sporocyst in snail containing well-developed first generation rediae. 5, Mature second generation rediae. 6, 7, Stages of microcercous cercariae after emergence from the snail; 8, Metacercariae from the crab; the cyst wall is not shown. 9, Mature encysted metacercaria. 10, *Semisulcospira libertina*. 11, *Thiara granifera*.

bp	birth pore	c	caeca
cer	cercaria	eb	excretory bladder
g	gut	fc	flame cell
gc	genital cells	ga	germinal area
o	operculum	n	nervous system
p	pharynx	os	oral sucker
s	stylet	pg	periacetabular glands
tl	tail		

Dicrocoelium dendriticum

Slime balls adhere to wet vegetation and are ingested by an ant

Metacercaria develops into metacercarial cyst

CYCLE IN ANT

Metacercaria leaves snail in agglomeration (slime ball)

CYCLE IN LAND SNAIL

Sporocyst

Sporocyst with developing cercariae

Miracidium

Cercaria

Eggs passed in faeces

Eggs

Man and reservoir host (sheep) infested by ingesting ant containing metacercariae. These migrate to the liver where the adult *Dicrocoelium dendriticum* develops

Fig. II.12 Life-cycle of *Dicrocoelium dendriticum*.

bore into freshwater crabs and become metacercariae in the crabs and crayfish shown in Table 22.2.

In the crustacean (the second intermediary) the metacercariae encyst in the liver, muscles and gills. In Japan crabs are eaten but in Korea and Taiwan they are not eaten; the supposition is that the crustacean phase is not always a biological necessity. In Venezuela the appropriate snails and crustacea are present and 30% of dogs are infected but man is not. When the metacercariae enter the stomach of man their cyst wall is digested and the adolescercariae emerge, pass through the jejunum, traverse the abdominal cavity, penetrate the diaphragm, pleura and lungs and reach the bronchioles forming cystic cavities.

GENUS: *Dicrocoelium*

Dicrocoeliosis is caused by two species of the genus: *D. dentriticum* and *D. hospes*. *D. dendriticum* is a widely distributed parasite, mainly of ruminants but also of man, occurring in all the European countries, European and Asian parts of the USSR, China, Japan, Indo-Malayan region, USA and Canada, Cuba and parts of South America, e.g. Brazil, Colombia. *D. hospes* has been recorded from many African countries, including Tanzania, Uganda, Sudan, Chad, Ghana and Sierra Leone. The eggs passed in faeces are fully embryonated, resist desiccation and do not hatch in water. They are ingested by land snails. Over 50 species have been recorded as hosts for *D. dendriticum* including *Theba carthusiana, Zebrina detrita, Helicella candidula, H. itala, Cepaea nemoralis, Helix vulgaris, Eulota lantzi, E. ruben,* and others (Table 22.2).

Life-cycle (Fig. II.12)

The miracidium is released in the digestive tract of the snail host, penetrates the glandular intestinal epithelium and finally migrates to the hepatopancreas. The mother sporocyst gives rise to daughter sporocysts which in turn give rise to cercariae, the whole process taking three to five months. The cercariae leave the sporocyst and migrate to the respiratory chamber of the snail. They leave the host via the respiratory opening in the form of slime balls, cemented by mucus originating from glands located in the posterior region of the cercariae. The slime balls are released from the snails individually or in clusters of four to 16; for the life-cycle to continue the slime balls must be eaten fairly quickly by an ant, e.g. *Formica fusca* (17 species have been recorded as secondary intermediate hosts, 14 species belonging to the genus *Formica*, plus *Proformica nasuta, Catagliphis bicolor* and *C. aenescens*). Penetration of the intestine occurs and metacercariae are formed in the abdominal cavity. If the infected ant is swallowed by man the

cyst wall is disrupted and the young flukes migrate to the bile system and the flukes mature in about 50 days.

SUPERFAMILY: ECHINOSTOMATOIDEA

GENUS: *Echinostoma*

A trematode of minor importance is *Echinostoma lindoensis*. Until recently it was quite commonly found in man in the environs of Lake Lindoe, Celebes, but not now due to changes in diet. Mice, rats, ducks and pigeons have been experimentally infected. *E. lindoensis* causes diarrhoea, abdominal pains and eosinophilia.

Life-cycle

First intermediary: planorbid snails (*Anisus sarasinorum* and *Gyraulus convexiusculus*); second intermediary hosts (metacercariae): snail (*Vivipara javanica rudipellis*) and four species of mussel (*Corbicula lindoensis, C. subplanta, C. celebensis* and *C. javanica*) (Table 22.2). Additional secondary intermediate hosts experimentally are snails and frogs and *E. lindoenssis* has been reported in *Biomphalaria glabrata* in Brazil. The cercariae have simple tails and a body resembling in miniature that of the adult worm. The eggs are straw-coloured, operculate and measure $92–124 \times 65–76 \, \mu m$ (Fig. 22.41). Immature when passed in the faeces, they mature in 6–15 days.

Euparyphium ilocanum is found in man in the Philippines, Celebes and Indonesia. The first intermediary hosts are *Gyraulus convexiusculus* in the Philippines and Indonesia, *G. prashadi* and *Hippeutis umbilicalis* in the Philippines. Fourteen species of snail act as second intermediary hosts, e.g. *G. prashadi, Vivipara burranghina, Planorbis umbilicatus* and *V. rudipellis* (Table 22.2). Human cases arise from people eating snails.

Echinostoma malayanum (syn. *Paraphostomum sufrartyfer*) is found in Malaysia, Thailand, India and the Sino-Tibetan border. The natural hosts are pigs and rats. The first intermediate host is the snail *Lymnaea leuteola*. The second intermediate hosts are snails (e.g. *L. leuteola, G. convexiusculus* or *Indoplanorbis exustus*) or the fish (*Barbus stigma*) (Table 22.2).

E. jassyense is found in Roumania and has been reported from the USA. The first intermediate host is *Stagnicola emargilatus* and the second intermediate host is a tadpole in Roumania and China. Normally the definitive hosts are mink, and trout are the second intermediate hosts.

E. recurvatum has been found once in a Japanese who had lived in Taiwan. The natural hosts are ducks etc.

E. revolutum is found in man in Thailand. The natural hosts are ducks and geese. At least 14 species of snail are known to act as first intermediate hosts

Table II.1 Differentiation of various species of *Schistosoma*.

Character	S. haematobium	S. mansoni	S. japonicum	S. intercalatum	S. mekongi
Habitat of adult	Vesical veins; occasionally veins of rectum and portal system	Inferior mesenteric and portal venous system	Superior and inferior mesenteric and portal venous system	Mesenteric and portal venous system	Superior mesenteric and portal veins
Adult male	10–15 × 0.75–1.0 mm	6–13 × 1.0 mm	12–20 × 0.5–0.55 mm	11–14 × 0.3–0.4 mm	6–15 mm
Cuticle	Fine tubercles	Conspicuous tubercle and microscopic tufts of hair	No tubercles; small acuminate spines	Tubercles and fine spines	No tubercles; spined from anterior level of gynaecophoric canal to posterior end of body
Oesophagus	Single bulb	Single bulb	Double bulb	Single bulb	Double bulb
Caeca	Unite in anterior half; posterior caecum short, one-third of body length	Unite in anterior half; posterior caecum long, two-thirds of body length	Unite in posterior half; posterior caecum medium, one-half of body length	Unite in posterior half; posterior caecum one-fifth to one-quarter of body length	Unite in posterior half; posterior caecum one-fifth to one-quarter of body length
Testes	4 or 5	2–14	6–8	4–6	6–7
Adult female	20–26 × 0.25 mm Darker than male, more blood pigment in gut	7–17 × 0.25 mm Darker than male, more blood pigment in gut	12–28 × 0.3 mm Darker than male, more blood pigment in gut	10–14 × 0.15–0.18 mm Darker than male, more blood pigment in gut	6–20 mm Darker than male, more blood pigment in gut
Cuticle	Transverse striations. Small tubercles at extremity	Transverse striations. Small tubercles at extremity	Transverse striations. Minute spines	Transverse striations, smooth	Transverse striations
Ovary	In posterior third	In anterior half	Central	In posterior half	In anterior 5/8 of body
Uterus	Anterior, long. Holds 10–100 eggs at one time. Produces 20–290 daily	Anterior, short. Holds 1–2 eggs only at one time. Produces 100–300 daily	Anterior, long. Holds 50 or more eggs at one time. Produces 1500–3500 daily	Anterior, long. Holds 5–50 eggs at one time	Anterior, long
Eggs	83–187 × 60 μm (Fig. II.16,3) Terminal spine	112–175 × 45–70 μm (Fig. II.16,1) Lateral spine	70–100 × 50–65 μm (Fig. II.16,2) Rudimentary lateral spine	140–240 × 50–85 μm (Fig. II.16,4) Long terminal spine	30–55 × 50–65 μm Small lateral knob
	Pass through bladder wall Discharged in urine	Pass through bowel wall Discharged in faeces	Pass through bowel wall Discharged in faeces	Pass through bowel wall Discharged in faeces	Pass through bowel wall Discharged in faeces
Shell	Non-acid-fast with Ziehl–Neelsen stain in tissues	Acid-fast with Ziehl–Neelsen stain in tissues	Acid-fast with Ziehl–Neelsen stain in tissues	Acid-fast with Ziehl–Neelsen stain in tissues	Acid-fast with Ziehl–Neelsen stain in tissues
Animal hosts	Occasionally baboons, monkeys, rats, pigs	(Occasional) baboons, rats	Rodents, dogs, cats, cattle, water buffalo, pigs, horses, sheep, goats	? Sheep, goats	Dogs

(e.g. *Indoplanorbis exustus, Lymnaea rubiginosa* and *L. stagnalis*). Numerous snails of the same species and others (including *Vivipara vivipara, Sphaerium corneum* and *Corbicula fluminea*), along with bivalves and tadpoles, are the second intermediate hosts. It is cosmopolitan in distribution in nature and is found in man in Taiwan and Indonesia where human infections result from eating salted or inadequately cooked clams.

Echinostoma hortense: the natural hosts are rats and mice in China, Korea and Japan. About 20 cases have been recorded in man in Japan and Manchuria. The first intermediate hosts are lymnaeid snails (*L. japonica, L. pervia* and *L. ollula*). Second intermediate hosts are tadpoles (frogs and newts) and fish (e.g. *Carassius* and *Cyprinus*).

Other human echinostomes are:

E. cinetorchis—in man in Japan (? syn. of *revolutum*)

E. macrorchis—in man in Japan (normally rats, *Caprella*)

Echinoparyphium paranlum—in man in USSR (? syn. of *revolutum*)

Echinocharmus perfoliatus—in man in Japan (normally cats, dogs)

E. japonicus—exp. in man, Japan (normally birds)

Himasthla muehlensis—a German who had lived six years in Columbia picked up this worm, but probably from raw clams (*Vems merceneria*) consumed in New York.

SUPERFAMILY: SCHISTOSOMATOIDEA (Stiles & Hassal, 1926)

FAMILY: SCHISTOSOMATIDAE (Looss, 1899)

GENUS: *Schistosoma* (Weinland, 1858)

The schistosomes commonly infecting man are:

Schistosoma haematobium (Bilharz, 1852) Weinland, 1858,

Schistosoma mansoni Sambon, 1907,

Schistosoma japonicum Katsurada, 1904,

Schistosoma intercalatum Fisher, 1934,

Schistosoma mekongi Voge, Bruckner & Bruse, 1978.

Differentiation of these five species is shown in Table II.1.

Infections of man have also been reported with:

Schistosoma mattheei Veglia & Le Roux, 1929,

Schistosoma bovis (Sonsino, 1876) Blanchard, 1895,

Schistosoma curassoni Brumpt, 1931.

Natural hybrids of *S. haematobium* and *S. intercalatum* and of *S. haematobium* and *S. mattheei* are known to occur in man in Cameroón and South Africa, respectively.[1,2] Although unequivocal evidence exists of *S. mattheei* in man[2] the evidence of *S. bovis* and *S. curassoni* occurring in man is less convincing.

The schistosomes are digenetic trematodes, their life histories consisting of alternating generations, each with its own range of hosts. The adult worms inhabit vertebrates; the larval stages inhabit snails which in the case of schistosomes pathogenic for man are freshwater snails.

The schistosomes are dioecious organisms, i.e. the sexes are separate. Adult schistosomes live in the veins of vertebrates; there is an oral cavity but no muscular pharynx; the eggs have no operculum; there is no encysted or metacercarial stage; the cercariae enter the definitive hosts through the skin.

Anatomy and physiology (Figs. II.13 and II.14)

Like other digenetic trematodes, the schistosomes are equipped with suckers. The *oral sucker* surrounds the mouth and is prehensile; the *ventral sucker* (*acetabulum*) is more posterior, on the ventral surface. With these suckers the worms can attach themselves to the walls of the vessels in which they live. The *mouth* itself is usually near the anterior extremity. The alimentary system consists of an *oral cavity* leading to the *oesophagus* and thence to the *gut* which soon divides into two *caeca* which reunite more posteriorly to form the *single posterior caecum* which ends blindly; there is no anus.

Food consists of the liquid material in which the worms live; unused material is rejected through the mouth. Schistosomes obtain oxygen from the blood in which they live.

The excretory system consists of two longitudinal canals opening posteriorly and fed by collecting tubules. There are flame cells whose function is to fan fluid wastes into the tubules by means of the vibratile cilia with which they are equipped.

There is a rudimentary *nervous system* with an oesophageal ganglion and commissure encircling the oesophagus and two longitudinal nerve cords running to the posterior end and intercommunicating by lateral branches.

The *male reproductive organs* consist of testes dorsal to and posterior to the ventral sucker. Each testis in which they live.

The excretory system consists of two longitudinal canals opening posteriorly and fed by collecting tubules. There are flame cells whose function is to fan fluid wastes into the tubules by means of the vibratile cilia with which they are equipped.

There is a rudimentary *nervous system* with an oesophageal ganglion and commissure encircling the oesophagus and two longitudinal nerve cords running to the posterior end and intercommunicating by lateral branches.

The *male reproductive organs* consist of testes dorsal to and posterior to the ventral sucker. Each testis discharges via a *vas efferens;* these unite to form the *vesicula seminalis* at the *genital pore* situated in the midline posterior to the ventral sucker.

The male worm is flat and leaf-like but is folded to form the *gynaecophoric canal,* enfolding the very

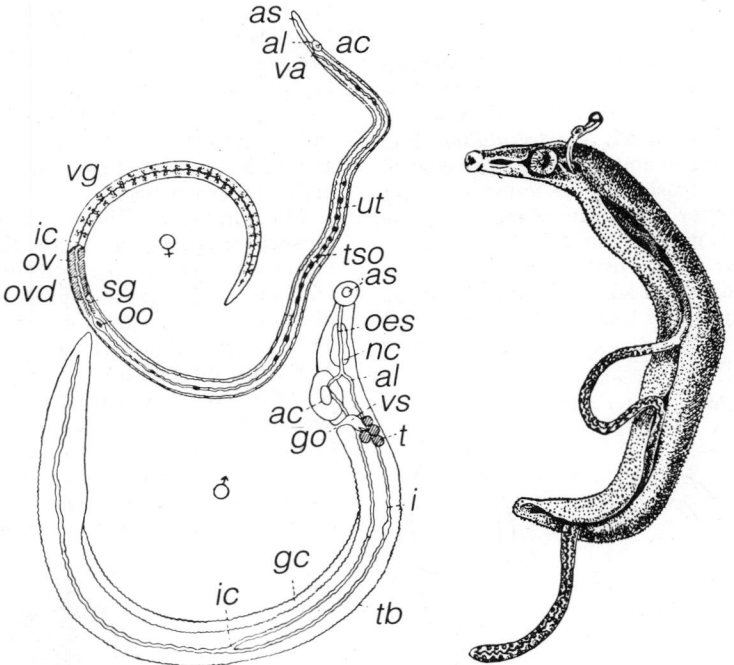

Fig. II.13   *Schistosoma haematobium,* × 10.

tso	terminal spined ovum	al	bifurcation of the alimentary canal	va	vagina
ic	union of intestinal caeca	gc	gynaecophoric canal	oo	oötype

     tb   tuberculations

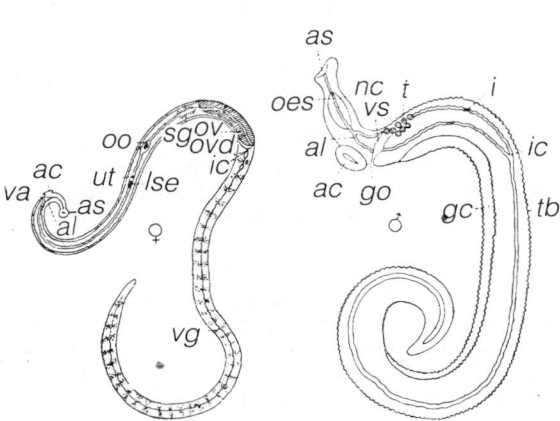

Fig. II.14   *Schistosoma mansoni* × 10. Key as Fig. II.13.
          lse   lateral spined egg

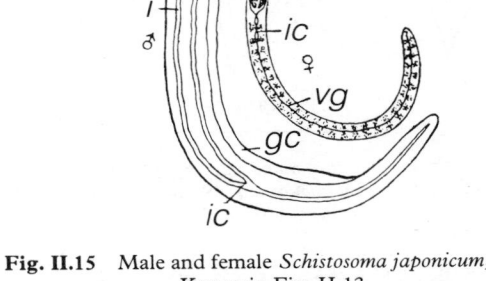

Fig. II.15   Male and female *Schistosoma japonicum,* × 10.
          Key as in Fig. II.13.

slender female for almost its entire length (Fig. II.15).

     The *female reproductive organs* consist of an elongated *ovary* in the posterior half, from which the *oviduct* passes forward, to be joined by the *vitelline duct* from the *vitellaria (yolk glands)*; the *shell gland* opens into the oviduct which passes forward to a straight *uterus*. This contains eggs and opens at the genital pore on the median surface posterior to the ventral sucker. The genital openings of both male and female face each other.

     S. mansoni has been cultivated in vitro.

Life-cycle (Fig. II.16)

The eggs of the schistosomes are passed by the definitive hosts (vertebrates) in urine (*S. haematobium*) (Fig. II.16,c) or faeces (*S. mansoni* (Fig. II.16,a), *S. japonicum* (Fig. II.16,b), *S. mekongi, S. intercalatum* (Fig. II.16,d)) but this is not an absolute rule since eggs of *S. haematobium* may occasionally be found in faeces and commonly in biopsy specimens of rectal mucosa and eggs of *S. mansoni* may be found in urine samples, especially in heavy infections. *S. mattheei* (Fig. II.16,e), a parasite of sheep and cattle which affects man in South Africa, is also found in both urine and faeces.

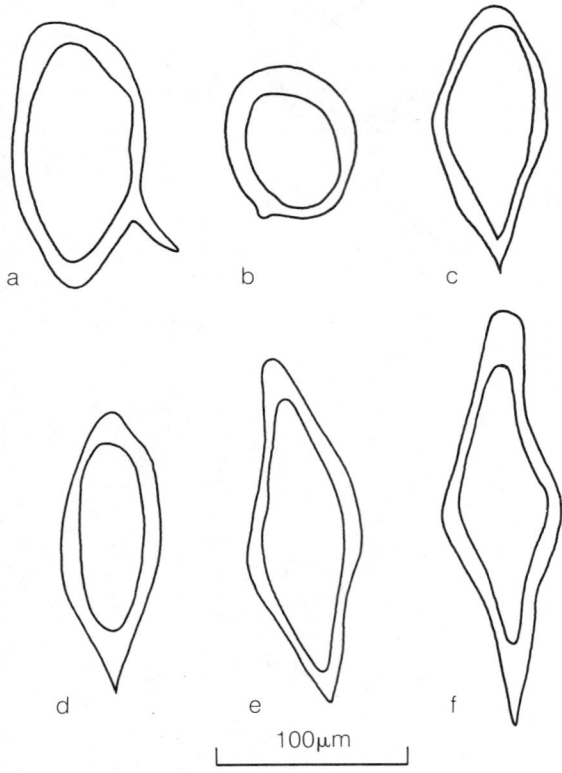

100μm

Fig. II.16 Eggs of *Schistosoma* spp. a, *S. mansoni*. b, *S. japonicum*. c, *S. haematobium*. d, *S. intercalatum*. e, *S. mattheei*. f, *S. bovis*.

Egg-shells of *S. mansoni, S. japonicum* and *S. intercalatum* (but not *S. haematobium* or *S. mattheei*) are acid-fast when stained by the Ziehl–Neelsen method.

When an egg reaches fresh water it contains a fully embryonated miracidium which hatches within a few minutes, partly as a result of osmosis, partly owing to its own movements. The miracidium swims actively by means of its ciliated epidermis for 6–8 hours searching for a snail host. Miracidia tend to move to the upper layers of water where many of their snail hosts live but in some circumstances they can infect snails inhabiting the bottoms of canals or lakes (e.g. Lake Victoria). These snails, however, frequently move up and down from the depths to the surface of such waters and miracidia have the opportunity of infecting them in the upper reaches.

The miracidium (Fig. II.17) has a complex array of sensory receptors which are considered to aid it in locating a snail host. Also the miracidium is endowed with a muscular apical papilla, apical gland and a pair of cephalic glands, all of which are considered to play a role in effecting penetration of the snail's epidermis. Miracidia do not appear to discriminate between species of snail and will sometimes enter the incorrect host thereby preventing further development. However, if a miracidium enters a compatible intermediate host, metamorphosis into the next stage—the mother sporocyst—takes place: the ciliated epidermis is cast off and is replaced by a syncytial tegument.

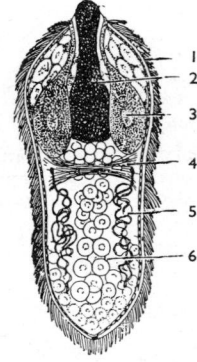

Fig. II.17 Miracidium of *Schistosoma haematobium*. 1, Cilia. 2, Papillary beak and primitive intestine. 3, Cephalic salivary gland. 4, Nerve centre. 5, Excretory tubules. 6, Primitive genital cells.

Within the elongated sac of the mother sporocyst germinal cells develop into daughter sporocysts. These leave the mother sporocyst after about 8 days and migrate to the digestive gland (liver) of the snail host, and within them further germinal cells develop into the next stage, the cercaria. Thousands of cercariae may result from one miracidium and all of these will be of the same sex. The cycle from penetration by the miracidium to the production of mature cercariae takes about three to four weeks for *S. intercalatum*, about four to five weeks for *S. mansoni*, five to six weeks for *S. haematobium* and *S. mekongi*, and seven weeks or more for *S. japonicum*.[3] The snails are damaged in the process and their life-span is shortened.

The mature cercaria (Fig. II.18) escapes from the daughter sporocyst, migrates through the tissues of

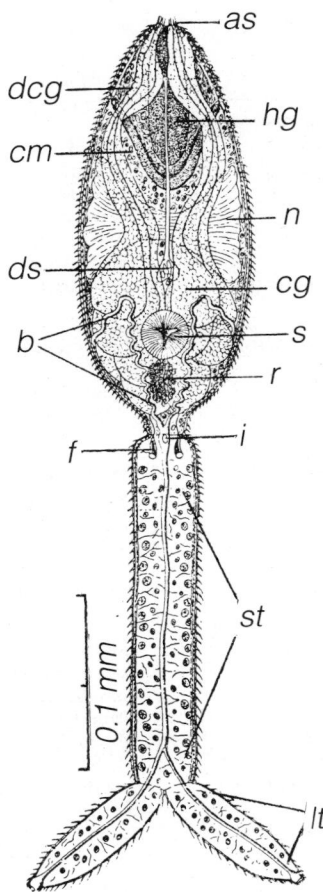

Fig. II.18 Cercaria of *Schistosoma japonicum*, ventral view.
× 240.

as	anterior spines	b	excretory bladder
cg	cephalic glands	cm	circular muscles
dcg	ducts of cephalic glands	ds	digestive system
exp	excretory pore	f	flame cell
hg	head gland	i	island in excretory bladder
lt	lobe of tail		
n	nervous system	m	mouth
r	rudimentary genital cells	st	stem of
		s	ventral sucker

secretion of the preacetabular glands helps to break down the skin barrier.

A snail may shed up to 3000 cercariae per day when in peak production; for example, *Biomphalaria glabrata* shedding *S. mansoni*. However, the number does vary day to day and some host parasite relationships are less productive; *Oncomelania hupensis* produces 15–160 cercariae per day of *S. japonicum*. Cercariae tend to swim up to the surface of water, sinking from time to time, and returning. They are influenced by the effect of light, gravity, agitation and touch. They are non-feeding and depend entirely upon their glycogen reserves when free swimming; consequently their life-span is short, up to 48 hours, but this depends upon external factors, such as turbulence and temperature. In many transmission areas the life-span will only be 8–12 hours.

A cercaria can penetrate the skin of a definitive host within a few minutes. In doing so it sheds its tail and in the tissues it becomes a *schistosomulum*. The trilaminate surface of the cercaria is replaced by a multilaminate surface of the schistosomulum and adult. The schistosomulum leaves the skin after about 2 days by the venous or lymphatic systems, to be transported to the lungs. In the lungs the schistosomulum becomes longer and thinner and then leaves the lungs via the pulmonary veins and passes through the heart to the systemic circulation. An individual schistosomulum may make several circuits of the pulmonary/systemic circulation before finding its way to the hepatic portal system. Growth takes place in the liver and paired worms may be found after about 26 days. Most worms leave the liver when they are sexually mature and have mated and migrate to the veins of the vesical plexus (*S. haematobium*) or the mesenteric veins (*S. mansoni*, *S. japonicum*, *S. mekongi* and *S. intercalatum*) where they begin to lay eggs. The period between penetration by the cercariae and egg-laying may be 30–50 days or more.

The mated worms move as far as possible towards the fine terminal vessels and the female then leaves the male progressing to the finest vessels where she deposits her eggs, retracting after having done so (Fig. II.19). The eggs escape from the venules into the tissues; those of *S. haematobium* largely into the wall of the bladder but occasionally into the wall of the lower bowel; those of *S. mansoni*, *S. japonicum*, *S.*

the snail and finally emerges to swim free in the water by means of its muscular, bifurcated tail, usually tail first. Its body length is less than 0.5 mm in length, with an oral organ and a smaller ventral sucker, a mouth, oesophagus and a pair of short caeca, and an excretory system of flame cells, tubules and excretory ducts leading into an excretory bladder at the posterior end of the body. It has ten glands, four preacetabular and six postacetabular glands. The secretion from the postacetabular glands is thought to help the cercaria attach itself to the skin of the vertebrate host, and the

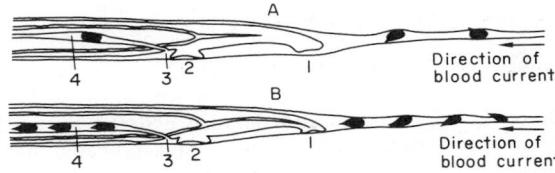

Fig. II.19 The deposition of eggs by *S. mansoni* (A) and *S. haematobium* (B) in the blood vessels and their passage to the exterior. 1, Anterior sucker. 2, Posterior sucker. 3, Vaginal orifice. 4, Uterus with contained eggs.

mekongi and *S. intercalatum* largely into the wall of the lower bowel. Many pass through the mucosa to be excreted in urine or faeces but some remain trapped in the tissues where they give rise to tissue reactions. Some eggs of all species are usually also found in the liver, genital tract, lungs, central nervous system and other organs. Eggs are responsible for most of the pathological effects of the infection.

Intermediate hosts (snails)

Strains of schistosomes which infect man vary in their ability to infect snail hosts. Usually this variation is associated with geographical area but the subject is complex. The following lists of proved and potential snail hosts have been constructed from Brown[4] and Jordan and Webbe.[3]

Snail hosts of S. haematobium *(Fig. II.20)*

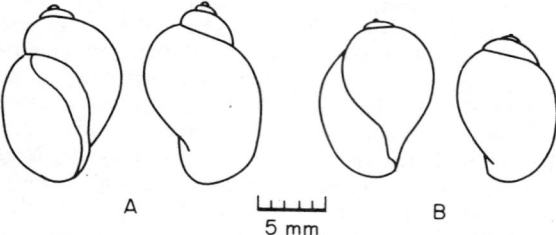

Fig. II.20 Molluscan hosts of *S. haematobium*. A, *Bulinus truncatus*. B, *B. africanus*.

S. haematobium is species complex and is transmitted throughout most of its range by species of the genus *Bulinus*. There is one possible exception: at Gimvi about 250 km south of Bombay, a schistosome considered to be *S. haematobium* is transmitted by *Ferrissia tenuis* but clearly further studies are required on this particular focus. A list of hosts and their distribution is given in Table II.2.

Snail hosts of S. intercalatum

These are shown in Table II.3.

Snail hosts of S. mansoni *(Fig. II.21)*

These are shown in Table II.4.

Snail hosts of S. japonicum *(Fig. II.22)*

Breeding experiments and detailed cytogenetic and biochemical studies in recent years have indicated that all of the proved hosts for *S. japonicum* should now be regarded as subspecies of a single widespread species, *Oncomelania hupensis*. A distinctive species in Japan, *O. minima*, appears to be resistant to infection. The hosts are listed in Table II.5.

Table II.2 Snail hosts of *S. haematobium*.

Snail species	Locality
Truncatus/tropicus complex	
Bulinus truncatus	Iran, Iraq, Near East, Yemen, North Africa (East Africa, potential), Egypt
B. rohlfsi	West Africa
B. guernei	West Africa
B. coulboisi (potential)	East Africa
Reticulatus group	
B. reticulatus (potential)	East, central and southern Africa
B. wrighti	Saudi Arabia, South Yemen
Forskalii group	
B. bavayi (potential)	Malagasy Republic
B. beccarii	North and South Yemen, Saudi Arabia
B. camerunensis	Cameroon
B. cernicus	Mauritius
B. senegalensis	Senegal, Gambia, Nigeria
Africanus group	
B. africanus	South and East Africa
B. globosus	Afrotropical region
B. nasutus	East Africa
B. abyssinicus	Ethiopia, Somalia
B. jousseaumei	West Africa
B. obtusispira	Malagasy Republic
B. hightoni (potential)	North-east Kenya
B. umbilicatus	Senegal
Ferrissia tenuis	India

Table II.3 Snail hosts of *S. intercalatum*.

Snail species	Locality
Bulinus globosus	Zaire
B. forskalii	Cameroon, Gabon

(Most species of the forskalii and reticulatus groups are capable of acting as hosts for the Cameroon strain of *S. intercalatum* but so far none has been implicated as a natural host.)

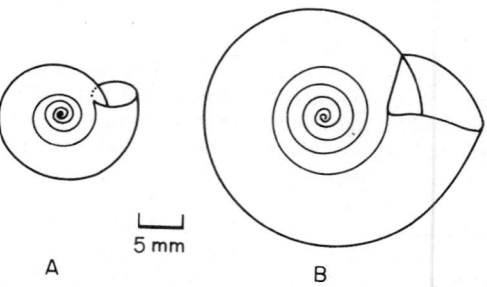

Fig. II.21 Molluscan hosts of *S. mansoni*. A, *Biomphalaria alexandrina*. B, *B. glabrata*.

Table II.4   Snail hosts of *S. mansoni*.

Snail (*Biomphalaria*) species	Locality
Biomphalaria pfeifferi	West, East and South Africa, Arabian Peninsula, Malagasy Republic
B. choanomphala *B. smithi* *B. stanleyi*	Great Lakes of East Africa
B. alexandrina	Egypt
B. angulosa	East and central Africa
B. sudanica	East and central Africa
B. camerunensis	West and central Africa
B. salinarum	South-western Africa
B. glabrata	West Indies, Venezuela, Surinam, French Guiana, Brazil
B. tenagophila	Brazil, Bolivia, Peru, Paraguay, Uruguay, Argentina
B. straminea (= *Tropicorbis centimetralis*)	Venezuela, Surinam, French Guiana, Brazil

The following neotropical species have been successfully infected with *S. mansoni* in the laboratory and must, therefore, be regarded as potential hosts.

B. chilensis	Chile
B. havanensis	Antilles, Mexico, Central America, northern South America
B. helphila	Puerto Rico, Cuba, Peru
B. peregrina	Ecuador, Bolivia, Chile, Paraguay, Argentina, Uruguay, Brazil
B. sericea	Ecuador

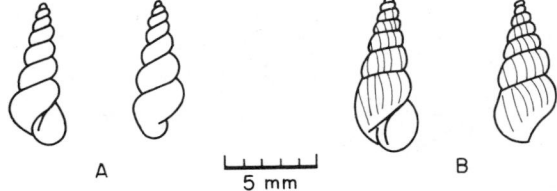

Fig. II.22   Molluscan hosts of *S. japonicum*. A, *Oncomelania hupensis nosophora*. B, *O. h. hupensis*.

Table II.5   Snail hosts of *S. japonicum*.

Snail species	Locality
Oncomelania hupensis hupensis	China
O. h. formosana	Taiwan*
O. h. chiui	Taiwan
O. h. nosophora	Japan
O. h. quadrasi	Philippines
O. h. lindoensis	Celebes

* The Taiwanese strain is not pathogenic to man.

Snail host of S. mekongi

The only recorded host is *Tricula aperta* which is endemic in the Mekong river, Laos and Cambodia. Three races of *T. aperta* are known: alpha, beta and gamma, and the last is considered to be the most important in transmission.

Interspecific antagonism between trematodes in snails

It has been reported[5] that if albino *Biomphalaria glabrata* is infected with *S. mansoni* and also with *Paryphostomum segregatum* (an echinostome from Brazil), the rediae of *P. segregatum* will attack and breach the thin wall of the early mother sporocyst of *S. mansoni* and ingest and destroy the daughter sporocysts within it. They fail, however, to destroy mature daughter sporocysts but they can cause degeneration of the schistosome sporocysts by other means. They can ingest whole cercariae. This biological antagonism between a dominant species and a subordinate species within a snail is also found with other trematodes and could conceivably be the basis of some form of biological control, but however that may be, it is an observation of great biological interest.

SUPERFAMILY: PARAMPHISTOMATOIDEA
(*amphistome trematodes*)

GENUS: *Gastrodiscoides*
Gastrodiscoides hominis (Lewis & MacConnell, 1876) Leiper, 1913

Distribution

Malaysia, Assam, India, Burma, South Vietnam, Guyana. In Kamrup district, Assam, 41% of the population are infected; in Burma 5%. The normal host is the pig or the mouse deer.

Characters

The fluke is reddish from haemoglobin pigment. When alive it is very expansile and can elongate to 1 cm. Preserved specimens measure $5-7 \times 3-4$ mm at the widest point. The anterior end is conical, the posterior discoidal, flattened ventrally to form a concave disc. Prominent genital papillae are seen and the common genital pore is 2.5 mm from the oral sucker. The ventral sucker (acetabulum) is ventrally situated in the caudal portion and measures 2 mm in diameter. The cuticle is smooth. The alimentary canal consists of a pharynx with two pear-shaped pharyngeal pouches. The oesophagus is 1 mm in length and ends in a muscular bulb where the bifurcation of the intestine takes place and caeca run back to the edge of the acetabulum. There are two lobulated testes placed diagonally between the intestinal caeca. A seminal vesicle is present but no cirrus. The ovary lies in the midline, posterior to the testes. An ovoid shell gland is placed near the ovary with a receptaculum seminis anterior to it. The uterus is short. Laurer's canal is present. The vitellaria lie in the mid-third. The ovoid egg measures $152 \times 60\,\mu$m and has an operculum.

Life-cycle (Fig. II.23)

The adult lives in the stomach of the definitive host (pig, deer, man). Eggs are passed in the stool which hatch into *Miracidia*. These enter a freshwater snail, *Helicorbis coenosus*, where they develop into sporocysts, and *rediae* forming *cercariae* which leave the snail host to encyst as metacercariae on vegetation which is then eaten by the definitive host.

GENUS: *Watsonius*

Watsonius watsoni has been found in large numbers in an African in South West Africa. Its normal hosts are monkeys of the genera *Cercopithecus* and *Papio* (baboon).

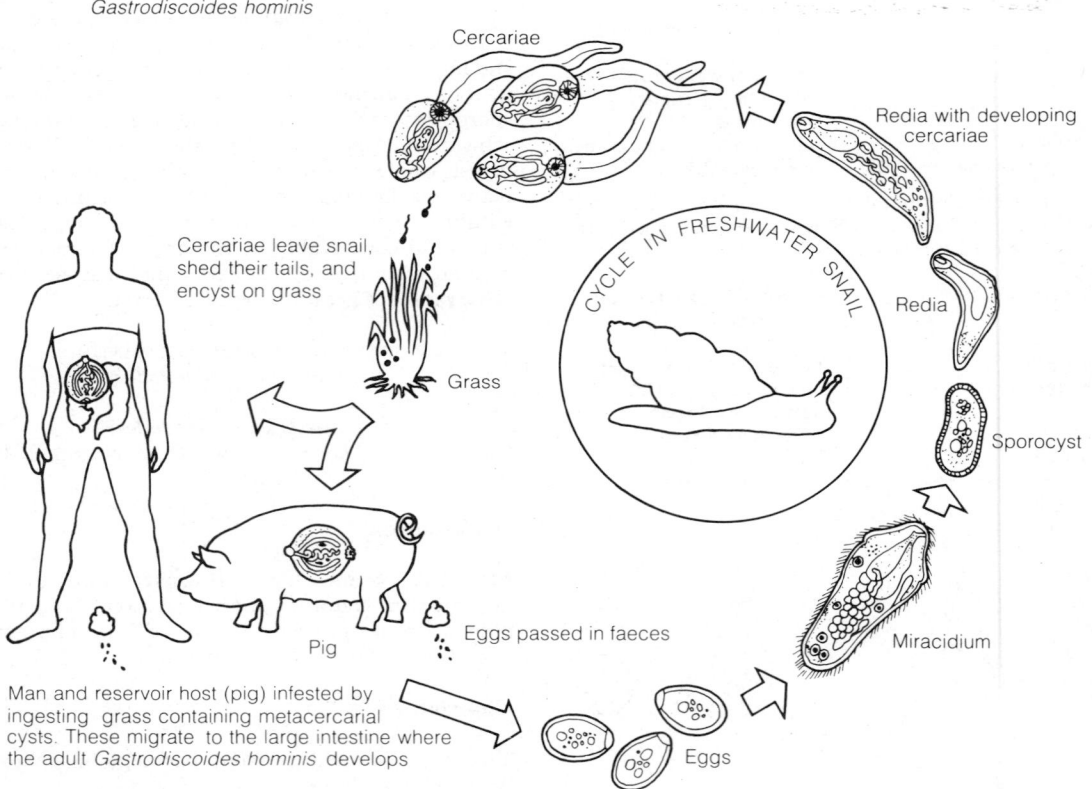

Gastrodiscoides hominis

Cercariae

Redia with developing cercariae

CYCLE IN FRESHWATER SNAIL

Redia

Cercariae leave snail, shed their tails, and encyst on grass

Grass

Sporocyst

Eggs passed in faeces

Miracidium

Pig

Man and reservoir host (pig) infested by ingesting grass containing metacercarial cysts. These migrate to the large intestine where the adult *Gastrodiscoides hominis* develops

Eggs

Fig. II.23 Life-cycle of *Gastrodiscoides hominis*.

CESTODES

Class: Cestoidea or tapeworms

The name cestode is derived from 'kestos' (Greek = a girdle). There is a head or *scolex* and the *strobila* or segments have their own musculature which relieves the strain on the head. The worms can live for several years and absorb nutriment through the tegument. They are hermaphroditic normally with male and female in each segment, the male fertilizing the adjacent female (with very few exceptions). Male organs often develop before the female. Human cestodes occur in two orders.

1 Pseudophyllidea with slit-like bothria, oval head (two long grooves with muscular walls), no hooks and the genital orifice on the flat surface.

2 Cyclophyllidea, cup-like or round suckers; genital orifice marginal.

ORDER: PSEUDOPHYLLIDEA

GENUS: *Diphyllobothrium*

Diphyllobothrium latum (Linnaeus, 1785)
(*Dibothriocephalus latus*, broad tapeworm)

Characters

It is greyish and more translucent and less fleshy than *Taenia* and may attain a length of 3–10 m, lying coiled up in the small intestine. Multiple infections are common. The scolex (3 mm) has no rostellum or hooklets but two slit-like suckers with longitudinal grooves (bothridia). The neck is thin; the proglottides number 3000–4000. The number of worms corresponds to the individual plerocercoids swallowed. Mature segments are broader than they are long. A single worm may discharge as many as from 36 000 to a million eggs each day. The worm may be discharged from the bowel naturally without treatment. (For details of anatomy of male and female elements, see Fig. II.24.)

The egg is operculated with a brown shell measuring $70 \times 45\,\mu$m (Plate III.21 and Fig. 23.19). No segments are passed in faeces (unlike *Taenia*).

Life-cycle (Figs. II.25 and 23.20)

If the egg is passed in water the operculum is lifted, the ciliated six-hooked coracidium emerges (Fig. II.25C); spherical (22.30 μm), it swims by means of its cilia but dies after 12 hours to 5 days depending on temperature. Normally it is swallowed by fresh water crusta-cea, the first intermediate host—*Cyclops strenuus, Diaptomus gracilis, D. graciloides* or *D. oregonensis, Cyclops brevisponosus,* and *C. prasenus* in the USA. The outer layer is then digested. The hooks tear a hole in the gut wall; the larva passes into the body cavity and may kill the cyclops. Lying outside the gut wall it becomes the *procercoid larva* (Fig. II.25D–G) which is ovoid, 50–60 μm long, with a terminal spherical appendix hearing six hooklets. At most two of these are found in one *Cyclops* which is then swallowed by freshwater fishes of many species—the second intermediate hosts—pike, perch, salmon, trout and grayling. In Africa, the barbel; in the USA the pike, wall-eye and burbot. Reaching the stomach of the fish the procercoid penetrates to the body cavity and after 3–4 days there encysts as a plerocercoid or *Spirometra* larva (6 mm) in the muscular and connective tissues (Fig. II.25H). Bothria, nervous and excretory systems are developed. It is then ingested by man with raw roe (caviar) or insufficiently cooked fish and the *plerocercoid* develops in five to six weeks into an adult *Diphyllobothrium*.

Freshwater fishes harbour other *Spirometra* larvae which are difficult to differentiate at this stage. The process of 'kippering' does not kill the plerocercoids and ordinary smoking is ineffectual but brine saturation is effective. The adult tapeworm can live as long as 29 years. *Diphyllobothrium dendriticum* (*minus*) is a small variety found in Lake Baikal and has a similar history. The second intermediate hosts are various species of salmon and grayling which are eaten frozen or salted by Mongolian peoples. *D. alascense* is a species found in Eskimos and can be differentiated by the form of the scolex. The plerocercoids occur in two species of fish—*Pungitus* and *Dallia*.

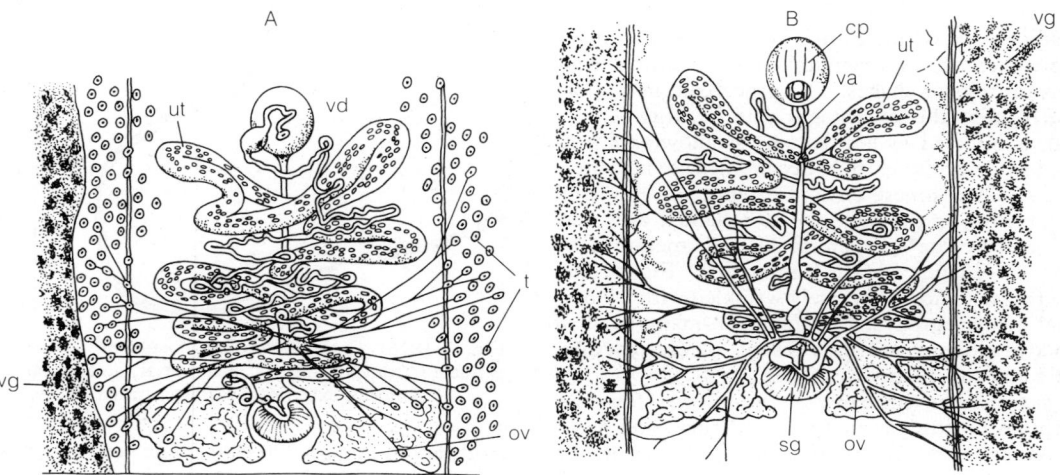

Fig. II.24 Mature segment of *Diphyllobothrium latum*. A, Dorsal or male aspect. B, Ventral or female aspect.

t	testes	vd	vas deferens	vg	vitelline glands	cp	cirrus pouch
ov	ovary	sg	shell gland	ut	uterus	va	vagina

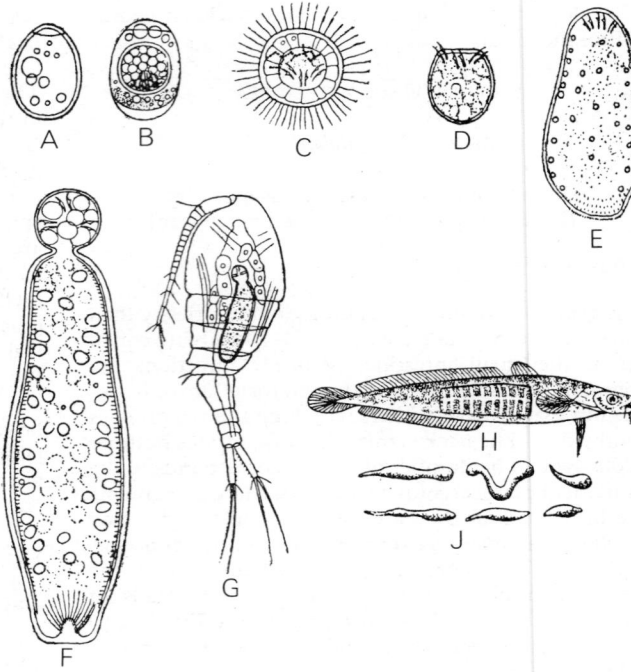

Fig. II.25 Life-cycle of
Diphyllobothrium latum (not to scale). A,
Egg of *D. latum*. B, Hexacanth embryo.
C, Ciliated oncosphere or coracidium.
D,E,F, Development of larvae or
procercoids in *Cyclops*.
G, Procercoid in the body cavity
of *Cyclops*. H, Development of
plerocercoids in fishes. J, Plerocercoids
of different shapes ingested by man, dog
or cat.

Spirometra mansoni (entracei) (Diphyllobothrium, Dibothriocephalus mansoni)

Characters

It resembles *D. latum*, is 6–10 m long and has a more
delicate structure with a narrower and more ellipsoid
egg than *D. latum*.

Life-cycle

The adult stage occurs in the dog and other animals,
the plerocercoid (sparganum) under natural conditions in frogs or snakes. The procercoid in *Cyclops
leuckarti* shows the same stages as in *D. latum*.

   Man is infected by accidentally swallowing a procercoid while drinking, thus becoming a second intermediary. The Chinese custom of applying raw split
frogs to sores on the hands or to inflamed eyes may
afford entry. The sparganum in man measures 8–
36 cm × 0.1–12 mm × 0.5–1.75 mm thick (Fig. II.26).
Its body is flat and transversely wrinkled with a longitudinal median groove. It is found in many parts of
the body: kidneys and iliac fossae, pleural cavities,
urethra and subcutaneous tissues.

   S. mansonoides (probably = *entracei*) was formerly
thought to be the parent form of *Sparganum proliferum*. It is found in the intestine of the cat in the
southern USA and is separable from *D. latum* and *D.
cordatum* by the scolex, uterine characteristics and
smaller size. Specimens vary from 20 to 60 cm in
length but may attain 1 mm × 8 mm. Immature pro-

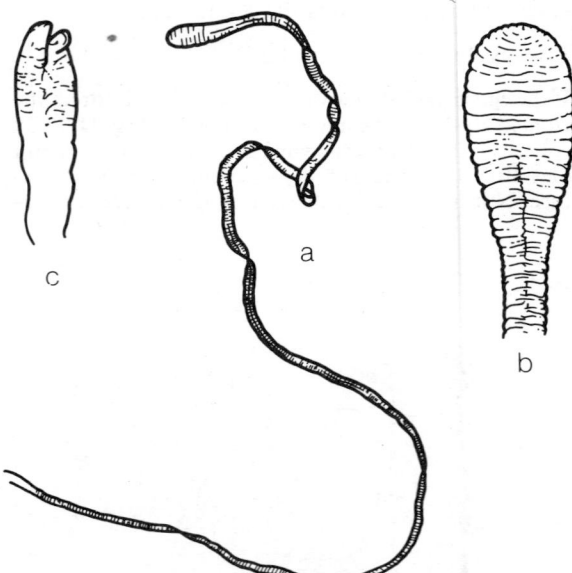

Fig.   II.26 *Diphyllobothrium   mansoni* plerocercoid,
extracted from an abscess in a Masai. a, Natural size. b,
Anterior extremity. c, Posterior extremity.

glottides number 200–300. The egg is pointed,
65 × 37 μm, with a conical operculum. The life-cycle
is as in *S. mansoni*.

   The   plerocercoids   (spargana)   measure   3–
12 × 2.5 mm (Figs. II.26 and II.27) and are contained

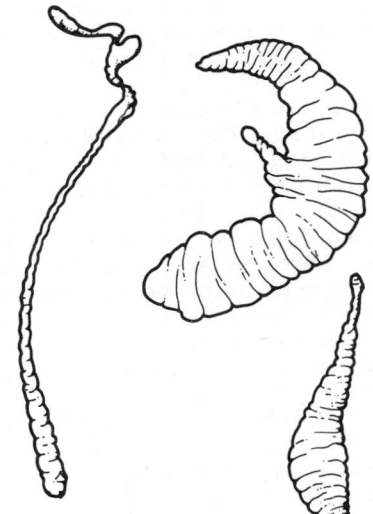

Fig. II.27 Different forms of sparganum proliferum.

in cysts which are found in man in Japan and Florida. The body contains calcareous corpuscles. The cysts may be disseminated throughout the body in the sub-cutaneous tissues, intra-muscular fasciae, walls of the alimentary canal, mesentery, kidney, lung, heart and brain. The prognosis in man is grave. Similar plerocercoids have been reproduced in macaque monkeys.

Sparganosis has been found in Korea and spargana, 23–50 cm in length, were removed from the muscles of the abdomen and chest. All patients had eaten raw snakes—*Dinodon rufozonatum*. It has also been found in abscess of the leg. The adult form is probably *Spirometra entracei*. Spargana are found near the central African lakes (generally in swellings in the chest) but also in Rwanda and Burundi. The adults are probably *S. theileri* or *S. pretoriensis*.

ORDER: CYCLOPHYLLIDEA

GENUS: *Taenia*

Taenia solium Linnaeus, 1758, pork tapeworm

Characters

T. solium (Figs. II.29 and 23.4) lives in the upper third of the small intestine. The name 'solium' is derived from the resemblance of the rostellum to the conventional figure of the sun. It attains a length of 2–3 m (exceptionally 8 m), having 800–1000 segments. The head is globular, quadrangular, 1 mm in diameter, and the rostellum short and pigmented, with a double row of 20–50 hooklets (Fig. II.28C). The four suckers project slightly and are circular, measuring 0.5 mm in diameter. The anterior proglottides are small, broader than they are long, the more mature ones measuring

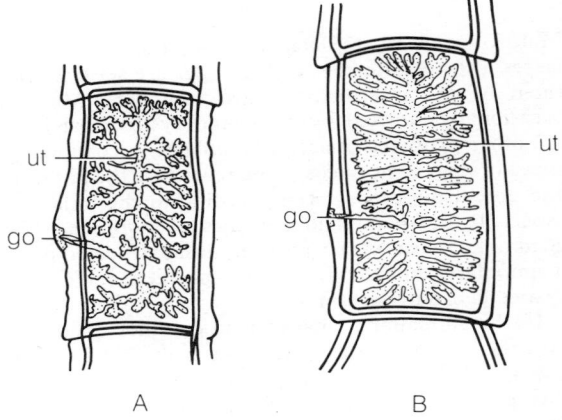

Fig. II.29 Segments of tapeworms, showing the characteristic branching of the uterus as seen in the mature segments. A, *Taenia solium*. B, *Taenia saginata*.

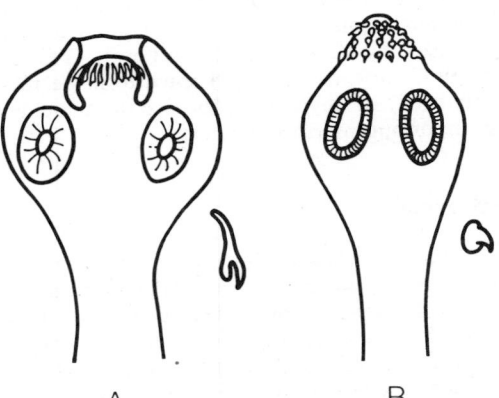

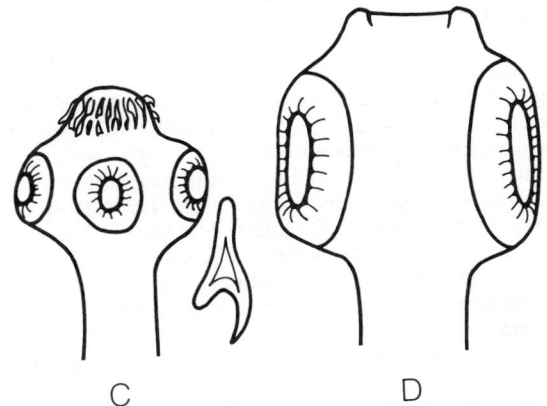

Fig. II.28 Heads of human cestodes, showing suckers and, when present, the arrangement of the hooklets. A, *Hymenolepis nana*. B, *Dipylidium caninum*. C, *Taenia solium*. D, *Taenia saginata*.

12 × 6 mm. Each proglottis has a marginal genital pore with thick lips; its situation alternates irregularly between the right and left margins. The uterus is median with seven to 13 stout diverticula (Fig. II.29A). The testes consist of 150–200 follicles, distributed throughout the dorsal plane. Proglottides number less than 1000. Terminal ripe segments pass out in the faeces and have an independent movement which enables them to migrate outside the anus. Each gravid segment contains 30 000–50 000 eggs.

The egg measures 31–56 μm in diameter and is round with no operculum (Plate III.16 and Fig. 23.6B). It has two radially striated shells, the inner formed by the embryo (thus differing from Pseudophyllidea), and a vitelline membrane when it is in the segment which is lost in the faeces. Small numbers of eggs are found in the faeces when the segments break. They contain the six-hooked oncosphere.

Life-cycle (Fig. 23.10)

Mature segments are detached and pass out with the faeces; they disintegrate and the eggs are set free and eaten by the intermediate host (the pig). Man is occasionally infected by cysticerci (cysticercosis); so are other primates (macaque monkeys), occasionally sheep or dogs. The oncosphere penetrates the gut wall and enters the bloodstream, settling in the muscles, especially the heart and becomes a *Cysticercus* (5–20 mm) known as cysticercus cellulosae. Infected pork is popularly known as 'measly pork'. At 0°C the cysticerci can persist for 70 days.

In the alimentary canal of man or other definitive host the bladder of the cysticercus is absorbed by the gastric juices; the scolex and head are evaginated and then pass to the small intestine, where the scolex fixes itself to the gut wall and forms proglottides.

Taenia saginata Goeze, 1782, beef tapeworm

Characters

T. saginata (Figs. II.28D, II.29B and 23.1) is whitish and semitransparent, measuring 4–10 m; when fully adult it may contain 20–2000 segments. The scolex is pear-shaped, cubical and 1–2 mm in diameter with four lateral suckers but no rostellum or hooks. The suckers and sucker-like organ (Fig. II.28D) at the apex are frequently pigmented. The neck is long and half the width of the scolex. The older proglottides are elongated; gravid individuals are three to four times longer than they are broad. The genital pore is single, marginally placed at the hinder end of the proglottis, alternating regularly between the right and left margins. There are 20–35 lateral branches on each side of the uterus which may ramify (Fig. II.29B). The genital organs in the mature proglottid differ from those of *T. solium* in having about twice the number

of testes (300–400) and in lacking the accessory ovarian lobe. Each gravid segment contains about 97 000 eggs. The total output per year is reckoned at 594 million.

T. saginata, like *Enterobius vermicularis*, oviposits on the perianal skin. The ova are expelled when the proglottid has detached itself from the strobila. The gravid uterus carries lateral branches terminating in blind club-shaped sacs. There they form a separate organ resembling a tassel (*thysanus*), which when it disintegrates leaves behind a mass of ova. The thysanus then becomes an aperture for oviposition (*protocostoma*). The stimulus is provided by thousands of eggs compressed within the uterus. The yolk mass which envelops the embryophores of the ova causes them to adhere to the perianal skin.

The egg is globular, 30–40 × 20–30 μm, with a double-shelled striated embryophore, which contains the oncosphere consists of an outer shell, chorionic membrane and two oncospheral membranes (Plate III.17 and Fig. 23.6A). *T. saginata* embryophores stain well with Ziehl–Neelsen stain whereas those of *T. solium* do not.[6]

Life-cycle

Gravid proglottides emerge in faeces or pass to the exterior independently; they then creep into grass or herbage, where they disintegrate. When the eggs are eaten by the ox, the oncospheres are set free and pass into the small intestine, where they bore through the wall and are carried to the muscles, especially the pterygoids and the fatty tissues round heart, diaphragm and tongue. Then cysticerci (cysticercus bovis) are formed, measuring 7.5–9 × 5.5 mm. They can be distinguished from other cysticerci by the absence of hooks on the scolices, other cysticerci having large hooks. They live for eight months in the ox and develop further in man, who constitutes the normal definitive host. The bladder is digested and the liberated scolex, passing to the small intestine, affixes itself by suckers to the gut wall. The cysts die at 48°C. Infected meat is known to inspectors as 'measly beef'. In Egypt and Morocco the camel is the most important intermediate host.

Cysticercus

The cysticercus has a small invaginated scolex (and a neck resembling an adult *Taenia*). The external tissue consists of hair-like processes, a peripheral collagenous fibrous layer, two muscle layers, peripheral cells, calcareous corpuscles, flame cells, a duct system embedded in a loose fibrous net and a central band of muscles. The different cestode larvae can be distinguished in human tissues by variations in these structures (Table II.6).[7]

Table II.6 Diagnostic characters of cestode larvae found in man.

	Cysticercus cellulosae	*Cysticercus bovis*	*Cysticercus cerebralis*	*Echinococcus granulosus*
Scolex	One	One	Several	Many
Hooks	Present	Absent	Present	Present
Bladder surface	Cuticle	Cuticle	Cuticle	Starified hyaloidine material
Superficial hair-like extensions	Hanging from 1 nm to 2.5 + μm	3–6 μm	1–2 μm	None
Subcuticular groups of muscles	Present	Absent	Absent	Absent
Make-up of wall	Wart-like processes	Rugae	Smooth and rugose	Smooth
Base of superficial protuberances	27–38 μm	50–70 μm	28–46 μm	None
Height of superficial protuberances	15–27 μm	23–27 μm	15–22 μm	None

After Slais.[7]

GENUS: *Echinococcus*

Echinococcus granulosus (Batsch, 1786)
E. multilocularis (Leuckart, 1863) Vogel, 1955
E. oligarthrus (Diesing, 1863)
E. vogeli (Rausch & Bernstein, 1972)
Synonym: *Taenia echinococcus* or hydatid

Characters

E. granulosus is very small, 3–8.5 mm long, with a pyriform scolex, 0.3 mm in diameter, provided at the apex with a projecting rostellum, four suckers and two circular rows of hooks, varying in size and number (Fig. II.30). The neck is short and thick; the pro-

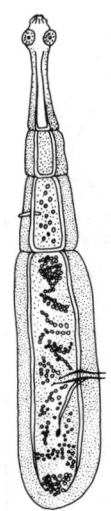

Fig. II.30 *Echinococcus granulosus.* × 15.

glottides usually four in number. The last one is the longest (2–3 mm); only one is sexually mature and this contains up to 5000 eggs. The genital apertures are marginal, one to each proglottis, in an alternating arrangement. The testes are spherical and numerous. The cirrus pouch is large and pear-shaped. The uterus is tubular and median with short unbranched lateral diverticula. The adult is difficult to remove from the small intestine of the dog without breaking its head. Eggs appear in the dog's faeces. Sometimes the fourth segment also comes away. Man is probably not a suitable intermediate host but is, of course, quite susceptible to hydatid infection.

The egg is spherical, 32–38 × 21–30 μm, and is double-shelled, the inner shell being thick. The egg is so similar to those of other tapeworms that it cannot be distinguished from them or from *Multiceps*. The oncosphere contains three pairs of embryonal hooklets.

Life-cycle (Fig. 23.7)

The egg is passed out in the dog's faeces until it is ingested by the intermediate host (sheep or man) either by eating contaminated grass or contaminated food. In the stomach the shell of the egg is digested and the oncosphere escapes. After 8 hours embryos can be found in the portal vein and liver whence they are filtered out. The next filter is the lung where a small number lodge. In three weeks the larval worm becomes vesicular and visible to the naked eye; in three months it attains a diameter of 5 cm and five weeks later has doubled that size. The hydatid cyst wall is composed of a fibrous laminated layer formed by the host, a thick median striated layer secreted by the cyst and an inner 'germinal' layer from which the brood capsules and daughter cysts arise. There are two types of proliferation: endogenous and exogenous. In the former, proliferation is inwards towards the cyst cavity; in the latter it is outwards. The varieties of hydatid are so striking that alveolar hydatid (*E. multilocularis*) has now been recognized as a distinct entity which has a limited geographical distribution.

The brood capsules are formed from small nuclear masses of the parenchymatous germinal layer; later, they become vacuolated to form vesicles. Larval scolices arise from a local thickening of the wall of the brood capsule; the wall evaginates to form a protective cup for the growing scolex. Near the head end the cuticle thickens and a circle of hooklets develops. The contractile part of the body of the scolex is capable of invaginating the head so that in the typical resting position the scolex has the hooklets inside. These hooklets may be strongly acid-fast, a characteristic which can be recognized in histological sections and reveal that the structure is a dead hydatid cyst. Free brood capsules and free scolices in the hydatid cyst cavity are known as 'hydatid sand'. In other cysts the brood capsules never produce scolices and are known as acephalocysts.

Daughter cysts may be produced by injury or by mechanical interference with the mother cyst, inside which they arise from the detached germinal layer and also from the brood-capsule cells; rarely by vesicular changes from the detached scolices. In the liver the daughter cysts are bile-stained. Intramuscular injection of scolices causes formation of new cysts and this accounts for the dissemination of hydatid cysts throughout the body which sometimes occurs after operation.

Exogenous daughter cysts in the omentum and bones are secondary caused by herniation or rupture of both germinal and laminated layers through weakened parts of the adventitia from intracystic pressure. By final exclusion of these herniations new cysts form.

Alveolar hydatid (*Echinococcus multilocularis*)

In the adult worm the differences are the position of the genital pore in front of the middle of the proglottis. The number of testes is 21–29 (as against 45–65). These lie behind the posterior end of the proglottis in the region of the cirrus sac. The uterus has no lateral branches. The length of the mature worm is 1.4–3.4 mm (as against 5–8 mm). The alveolar cyst grows by exógenous proliferation which invades the surrounding tissues and metastasizes. The cyst is solid with small irregular vesicles containing fluid and very rarely scolices.

Life-cycle

The definitive hosts of *E. multilocularis* are foxes and the intermediate hosts rodents.

E. oligarthrus and *E. vogeli* are about half the size of the other echinococci and the rostellar hooks are a means of identification of the protoscolices.

GENUS: *Multiceps*

Multiceps multiceps. The adult worm is 40–60 cm in length and has a pyriform scolex about 1 mm in diameter with four scolices and a rostellum armed with a double rank of 22–32 large and small hooks.

Multiceps brauni. The adult worm has a scolex armed with 30 rostellar hooklets. The coenurus differs from that of *M. multiceps* in its larger hooks with bilobed glands.

Life-cycle

The definitive hosts of *Multiceps* are canines and the intermediate hosts sheep and other herbivorous animals.

GENUS: *Hymenolepis*

Hymenolepis nana (Siebold, 1852)
(*Taenia nana, H. murina,* dwarf tapeworm)

Distribution

It is found in warm countries, Egypt, Sudan, Thailand, India, Japan, South America (Brazil, Argentine and especially Cuba), south Europe (Portugal, Spain and Sicily, where it affects 10% of the children). It lives in the small intestine (Fig. II.31).

Characters

H. nana is 25–45 mm long by 0.5–0.9 mm and has 100–200 proglottides. The scolex measures 139–480 μm, is subglobular with a well-developed rostellum, a single

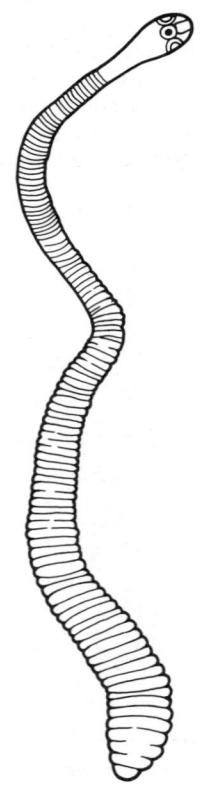

Fig. II.31 *Hymenolepis nana.* Magnified.

crown with 20–30 hooklets (14–18 μm) and four globular suckers (80–150 μm) (Fig. II.28A, Fig. II.31). The neck is long, the proglottides short anteriorly but the posterior ones increase in size and are broader than they are long. The genital pores are marginal and placed near the anterior border. There are three testes. The vas deferens widens into the seminal vesicle and the gravid uterus occupies the entire segment.

The egg is oval and there are 8–180 in each segment. It has two membranes—outer (vitelline), 40–60 μm and inner, 20–30 μm. There is a conspicuous mammillate projection at each pole, enclosing an oncosphere with three pairs of hooklets.

The segments when freed are partially digested and the eggs, set free in the faeces, are easily detected.

Life-cycle (Fig. II.32)

This worm forms an exception to other members of the group and does not necessarily have an intermediate host; the larva enters the villus of the intestine to become a cercocyst. In 40–70 hours after infestation the scolex appears; in 80–90 hours the rostellum has hooklets and then passes into the lumen of the intestine attached to the epithelium of the villus by a short neck. The rapidity of development varies greatly. Strobilization is rapid; the proglottides mature in 10–12 days and after 30 days eggs appear in the faeces to be ingested by another human host. *H. fraterna* of the rat is morphologically identical but its intermediate hosts are beetles and fleas (*Nosopsyllus fasciatus* and *Xenopsylla*).

Hymenolepis diminuta (Rudolphi, 1819)

This is a parasite of rats (*Rattus norvegicus* (*decumanus*), *R. alexandrinus*) and mice (*Mus musculus* and *M. sylvaticus*); it is found in man in Italy, South America, Zaire and the West Indies.

It measures 20–60 mm × 3.5 mm. The head is small and cuboidal. At the apex is a rudimentary rostellum with four small, unarmed suckers. The neck is shorter than the head. The proglottides increase in size as the tail is approached and are broader than they are long.

The egg is circular or ovoid, measuring 60–80 μm. Its outer shell is yellowish and thickened with indistinct radiations and contains a hexacanth oncosphere.

Life-cycle (Fig. II.33)

The cysticercus stages occur in the body cavity of insects and fleas during their larval stages: *Nosopsyllus* (*Ceratophyllus*) *fasciatus; Xenopsylla cheopis; Leptopsylla segnis* (mouse flea); *Pulex irritans;* in coleoptera and lepidoptera such as *Asopia farinalis, Anisolabis annulipes, Tinea pellionella, Akis spinosa* and *Scaurus striatus;* also in South America, in *Dermestes vulpinus, D. peruvianus, Ulosonia parvicornis* and *Embia argentina*.

The rat becomes parasitized by eating infected fleas or other insects. The cysticercoids, when ingested by the definitive host, become adult in 17 days.

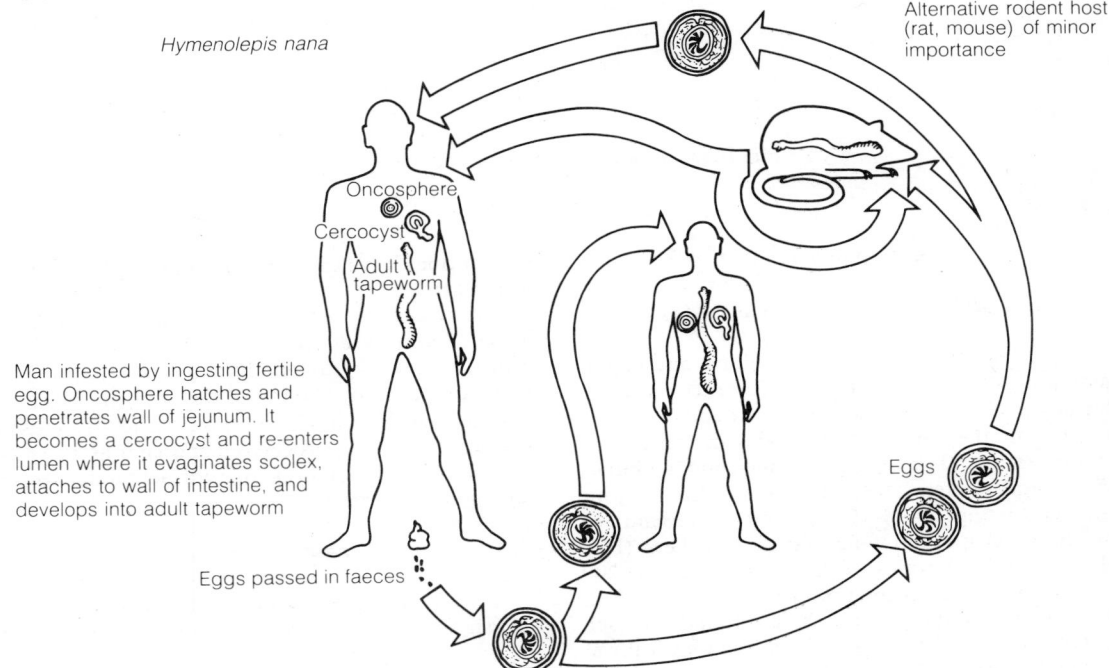

Hymenolepis nana

Oncosphere

Cercocyst

Adult tapeworm

Man infested by ingesting fertile egg. Oncosphere hatches and penetrates wall of jejunum. It becomes a cercocyst and re-enters lumen where it evaginates scolex, attaches to wall of intestine, and develops into adult tapeworm

Eggs passed in faeces

Alternative rodent host (rat, mouse) of minor importance

Eggs

Fig. II.32 Life-cycle of *Hymenolepis nana*.

Hymenolepis diminuta

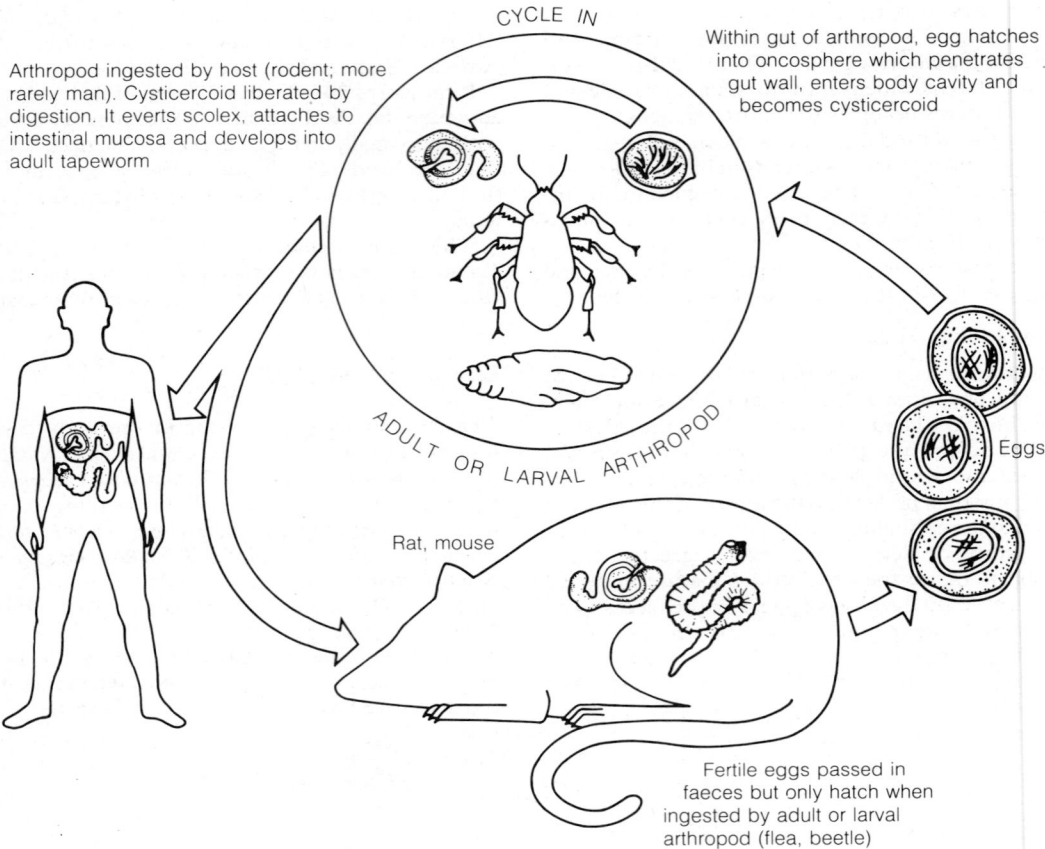

CYCLE *IN*

Arthropod ingested by host (rodent; more rarely man). Cysticercoid liberated by digestion. It everts scolex, attaches to intestinal mucosa and develops into adult tapeworm

Within gut of arthropod, egg hatches into oncosphere which penetrates gut wall, enters body cavity and becomes cysticercoid

ADULT OR LARVAL ARTHROPOD

Eggs

Rat, mouse

Fertile eggs passed in faeces but only hatch when ingested by adult or larval arthropod (flea, beetle)

Fig. II.33 Life-cycle of *Hymenolepis diminuta*.

GENUS: *Dipylidium*

Dipylidium caninum (Linnaeus, 1758)

This is a common parasite of the dog, cat and jackal. There are 200 records of its occurrence in man, especially in children in European countries.

It lives in the small intestine and measures 15–40 cm × 2–3 mm. The scolex is small and globular, 0.55 mm in diameter. The rostellum has three or four circles consisting of 28–30 hooklets (14–18 μm) of 'rose-thorn' shape and four elliptical suckers (Fig. II.28B). The proglottides are narrow and there are 200 or more of them. The segments measure 6–7 × 2.3 mm. Two sets of genital apparatus are found in each segment; the genital pores are placed symmetrically at the lateral margins. The uterine cavities contain egg-nests, each consisting of eight to fifteen eggs. Mature proglottides leave the intestine. The egg is round, 35–40 μm across.

The cysticercoid stage is passed through in the dog louse (*Trichodectes canis*), dog flea (*Ctenocephalides canis*), cat flea (*C. felis*) and human flea (*Pulex irritans*). Eggs are eaten by the larval flea and the hexacanth embryo develops in the adipose tissue and muscles, first appearing as a procercoid and later as a cysticercoid larva. Infection of man is accidental due to swallowing infected fleas.

GENUS: *Raillietina*

R. madagascariensis (formerly *Taenia madagascariensis*), *R. demerariensis*, *R. celebensis* etc.

These worms are found in Celebes, Thailand, Mauritius, Taiwan, Guyana and *R. demerariensis* has been reported in Ecuador and in Australia from *Rattus assimilis*, a race of *R. rattus*. Two cases were reported from Thailand as *R. siviragi*. They are characterized by numerous hooklets of 'coal-hammer' shape on the suckers and rostellum and by unilateral genital pores on the proglottides. Ripe segments contain egg capsules. The ovoid eggs possess conspicuously large hooklets. Usually they are parasites of birds, more rarely of rats. Their intermediary hosts are probably flies.

GENUS: *Bertiella*

Bertiella studeri has often been found in man and D'Alessandro et al[8] report a case of infection with *Bertiella mucronata*, a tapeworm of monkeys in a woman in Paraguay; three others have previously been reported.

GENUS: *Inermicapsifer*

This genus closely resembles the foregoing and cannot be distinguished from it by the ripe proglottides, but the head and the suckers are unarmed. *I. arvicanthidis*, a parasite normally of the field-rat, was found in a European child from Kenya; since then others have been reported in Ruanda-Urundi and in Arusha Tanzania. It is suggested that it is commoner than has been supposed. No fewer than 12 species of *Inermicapsifer* are parasites of hyraxes and rodents in Africa. *I. cubensis* appears to be common in Cuba where 76 cases in man have been described. It is identical with the foregoing; *I. madagascariensis* is also identical.

NEMATODES

Phylum: Nemathelminthes
Class: Nematoda or roundworms

The sexes of these worms are separate. They are cylindrical, non-segmented and taper at both ends. They are white or yellow, sometimes semitransparent and their eggs are characteristic.

SUPERFAMILY: ASCARIDOIDEA

GENUS: *Ascaris*

Ascaris lumbricoides Linnaeus, 1758 (roundworm)

Characters

Ascaris lumbricoides inhabits the intestine of man and allied species are found in the pig, cat, dog and horse.

The adult female worm measures 20–35 cm × 3–6 mm, the male 15–31 cm × 2–4 mm (Fig. 21.2). Both are pale yellow and brown with whitish longitudinal lines and round tapering ends. The mouth is at the anterior end and is guarded by thin lips with finely denticulated ridges (Fig. II.34). The anus is subterminal. In the female the vulva is anterior to the middle of the body. The vagina is directed backward and there are paired genital tubes each containing the uterus, receptaculum seminis, oviduct and ovary. The tubules and ducts attain a length of 12 cm and the capacity at any one time is 27 million eggs, the average daily output being 200 000. The male tail is conical without caudal alae and is curved in a semicircle with two rows of tactile papillae, mostly preanal but a few postanal. There are two chitinous spicules. The adults have a life-span of 10–12 months.

The egg measures 50–70 × 40–50 μm and is elliptical encased in a rough albuminous coat giving it a mam-

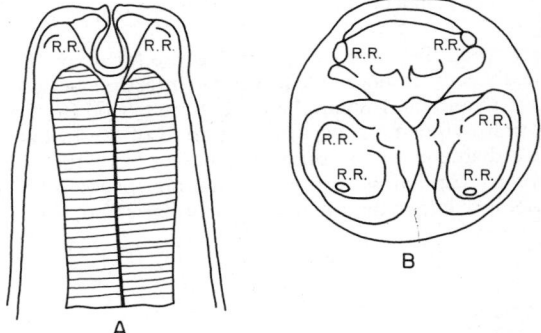

Fig. II.34 Head of *Ascaris lumbricoides*. A, Ventral view. B, Anterior view, showing the oral labia.

illated appearance. It is usually stained by faecal pigments (Plate III.9 and 10 and Fig. 21.3).

Life-cycle (Fig. 21.1)

When the eggs are passed in the faeces there is no segmentation or differentiated embryo. In water or in moist earth at 36–40°C within two to four months the embryo is seen coiled up and moving inside the egg-shell. The larva undergoes a moult before hatching and must be transformed into a second stage larva of the 'rhabditoid' type before it is infective. The embryo does not emerge from the egg until it is swallowed. The egg-shell is then softened by the gastric juice and hatches in the small intestine. The rhabditiform larva penetrates the mucous membrane, enters the blood via the heart and lungs and reaches the alveolar capillaries where it has a 'blood bath'. As the larvae cannot pass through they burrow through the wall of the alveolus and enter the respiratory tree, finally being carried up the trachea by ciliary action. Eventually, on reaching the vocal cords, the majority of the larvae are swallowed for the second time and reach the small intestine. The second invasion is often accompanied by severe allergic reactions, urticarial reactions and fall in blood pressure. The whole process occupies 10–14 days. During this time the larva moults twice (once after 5 or 6 days and the second time after the tenth day). The larvae measure 1.3–2 mm on the tenth day (Fig. II.35) and 1.75–2.37 mm on the fifteenth. Larvae

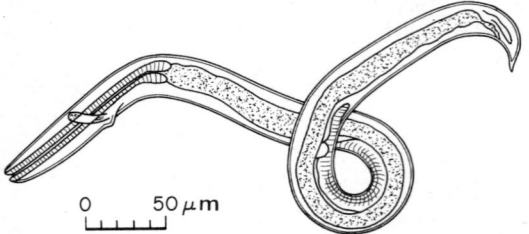

0   50 μm

Fig. II.35   Larva of *Ascaris lumbricoides* recovered from the trachea of a rat 8 days after ingestion of the eggs.

may reach the intestine as early as the fifth day. The fourth ecdysis takes place in the intestine between days 25 and 29. In man the incubation period (to time of first oviposition) occupies a period of 60–70 days. The diameter of the migrating larvae from the pulmonary capillaries to the terminal air spaces is considerably larger than that of the capillaries.

Ascaris suum

Ascaris suum of the pig is almost morphologically identical with *A. lumbricoides* except that the denticular ridges in the mouth are larger and have straight edges but these differences are not constant.

GENUS: *Toxocara*

Toxocara canis (Werner, 1782; Johnston, 1916)

Toxocara canis (the dog ascarid) is a cosmopolitan infection of dogs. The morphology is similar to that of *Ascaris*. The male worms are 4–6 cm long and the females 6.5–10 cm. In addition to the three characteristic lips of ascarids there are distinct cervical alae or wings which are much longer than they are broad and extend some distance from the anterior extremity along the lateral margins. The perianal papillae of the male worms are characteristic. The ova are pitted superficially and measure 85 × 75 μm. They are dark or greyish brown and unembryonated when passed.

The life-cycle is similar to that of *A. lumbricoides* with four larval stages. In pregnant bitches the pups

are infected transplacentally and are born infected with adult worms laying eggs. They may die within the first few weeks of life after which they acquire some immunity. Puppies are the main source of infection for children who develop toxocariasis.

Toxocara cati (Shrank, 1788; Brumpt, 1927)

This worm is the common ascarid of the domestic cat and some of its wild relatives. The male worms are 4–6 cm long and the females 4–12 cm. The anterior end has the characteristic ascarid lips and is provided with a pair of broad lateral cervical alae or wings which give a pyriform outline to the anterior end of the body. The eggs are similar to those of *T. canis*, as is the life-cycle.

GENUS: *Lagochilascaris*

Lagochilascaris minor (Leiper, 1909)

Lagochilascaris minor is a parasite of the opossum. Adult males measure 5–17 mm × 0.19–0.6 mm, females measure 20–60 mm × 0.2–0.81 mm. They are ascarid in morphology but the lips bear no denticles and they have a keel-like cuticular ledge along the entire extent of the lateral line. The eggs are spherical or slightly ovoid and measure 50 × 65 μm.

Life-cycle

Adult worms live in cavities in the submucosa of the small intestine of the opossum and eggs are passed out in the stool containing infective larvae which wait until they are ingested by mice and other small mammals when they hatch in the intestine and migrate to skeletal muscle to wait until the definitive host eats the prey.

SUPERFAMILY: SPIRUDOIDEA

GENUS: *Gnathostoma*

Gnathostoma spinigerum (Owen, 1838)

The adult worms are parasites of both wild and domestic felines and canines. Cats and dogs are important reservoirs.

Morphology

The adult worms in the feline host vary in length from 11 to 25 mm for males and 25 to 54 mm for females. They are stout, reddish-coloured, slightly transparent nematodes with a subglobose cephalic swelling separated from the remainder of the worm by a cervical constriction. One or more individuals are found in

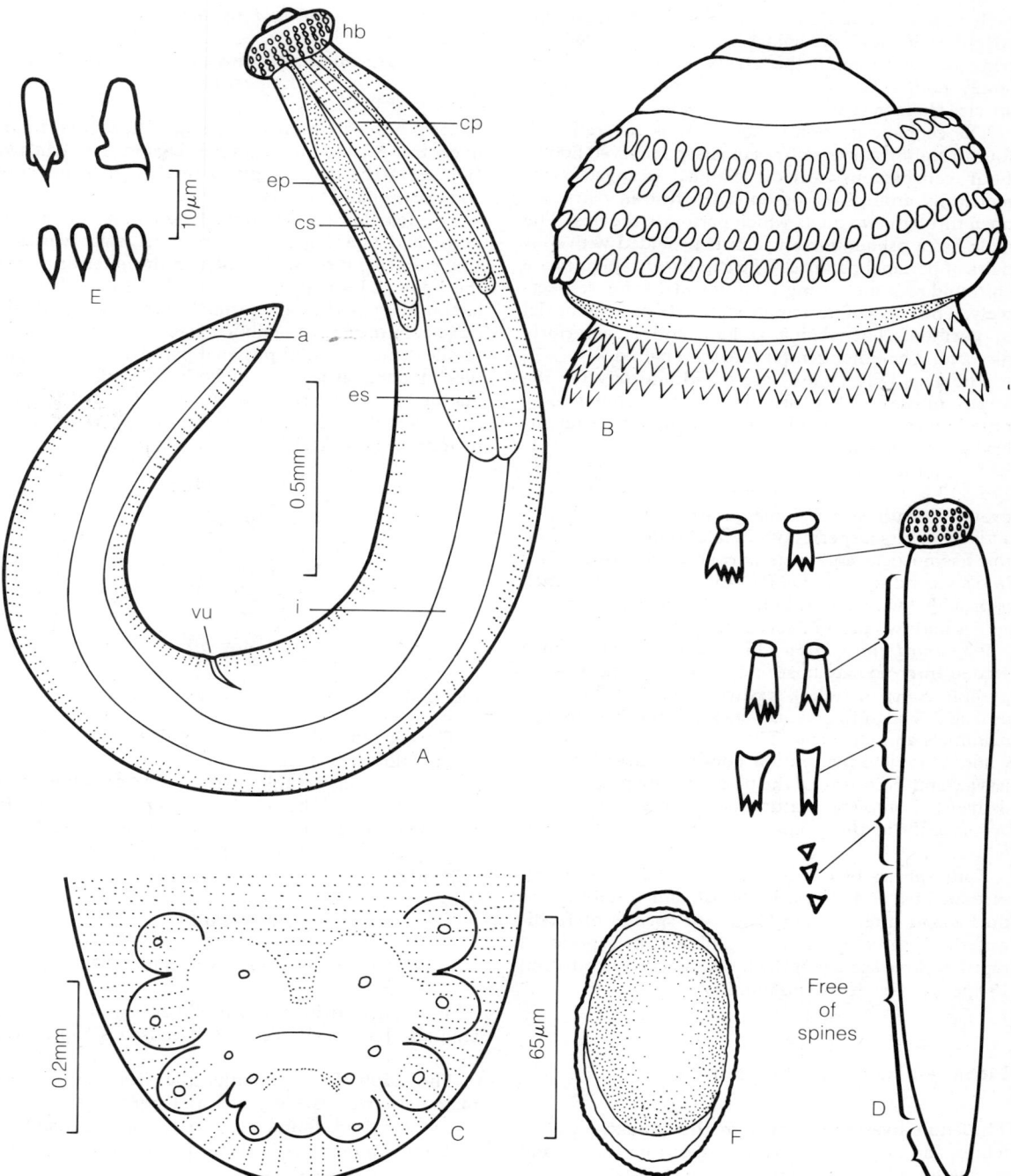

Fig II.36 *Gnathostoma spinigerum*. A, Lateral view of third stage larva. B, Head bulb of third stage larva with four rows of hooklets. C, Posterior end of male, ventral view, with minute cuticular spines omitted. D, Diagram of the types of spines at different levels of the body. E, Detail of the spines on the head bulb. F, Fertilized egg.

| a | anus | cp | cervical papilla | oes | oesophagus | hb | head bulb |
| cs | cervical sac (gland?) | ep | excretory pore | i | intestine | vu | vulva |

each tumour. The anterior half of the nematode is covered with leaf-like spines which are broader and tridented just behind the cervix and narrower and singly pointed more equatorially. These spines are species characteristic.

The cephalic portion of the body is covered with four to eight transverse rows of sharp recurved hooks. Four conspicuous cervical glands, arranged symmetrically around the oesophagus, fuse in pairs and open through two ducts which perforate the lips. The male has a pseudobursa which is provided with four pairs of perianal papillae. The copulatory spicules are chitinoid rods measuring 1.1 mm and 0.4 mm respectively. The vulva of the female is slightly postequatorial in position. The vagina is long and is anteriorly directed. The other genital tubes are paired.

The eggs (Fig. II.36F) are ovoid and $65-70 \times 38-40 \mu m$ in size. They are transparent, superficially pitted, have a mucoid plug at one end and are unembryonated when laid.

A motile first-stage larva, measuring $223-275 \times 13.4-17.4 \mu m$ and having a rounded anterior end provided with spines, emerges from the shell and actively enters a species of *Cyclops*, bores its way into the haemocoele and metamorphoses in 10–14 days into a second stage larva ($350-450 \times 60-65 \mu m$), which is provided with a head bulb armed with four rings of spines and two pairs of cervical glands.

The *third stage larva* (Fig. II.36) develops in a second intermediate host which can be a snake (rock python, cobra in India), freshwater fish (Philippines) or frog (Thailand), crayfish, crabs, amphibia, reptiles, mammals and chickens (Thailand) as well as man in whom complete maturation does not take place, the larva wandering around the body causing pathological damage. Complete maturation to the adult stage occurs only in the stomach of dogs, cats and other felines.

Four species of *Cyclops* can act as the first intermediate host and 28 species of fish and vertebrates as the second intermediate host: two species of freshwater fish, three species of amphibians, five species of reptiles, three species of fowl, two species of crabs and 13 species of rodents and monkeys.

Life-cycle in nature (Fig. 24.1)

The adult lives in tumours in the stomach wall of felines and dogs. Eggs are extruded from lesions and evacuated via the faeces into water where they embryonate and hatch. Larvae are ingested by *Cyclops*, which are then eaten by fish, frogs or snakes and the larvae develop into the third stage in the flesh of these animals. A dog or cat then eats the infected fish, frog or snake and the infection develops into maturity in the stomach wall in about six and a half months.

GENUS: *Physaloptera*

Physaloptera caucasica (Linstow, 1902) (*P. mordens*) (Leiper, 1907)

Normal hosts are monkeys. In man it has been found in central Africa, Mozambique, Uganda and Malawi. It lives in the oesophagus, stomach, small intestine and occasionally the liver.

The female ($2.4-10 \text{ cm} \times 1.14-2.8 \text{ mm}$) has a posterior end tapering to a sharp point, two ovaries, a single uterine tube, and a vulva in the anterior part of the body. The male ($1.4-5 \text{ cm} \times 0.7-1 \text{ mm}$) has two lateral alae on the tail, formed by expansion of the cuticle, four pairs of pedunculated papillae—six pairs sessile—one unpaired postanal papilla, and two spicules of unequal length. In both sexes the mouth is guarded by two large lips, armed with two papillae and rows of teeth, which serve to grip the mucous membrane (Fig. II.37).

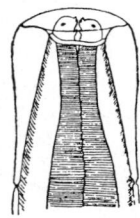

Fig. II.37 The head of *Physaloptera caucasica*.

The egg ($45 \times 35 \mu m$) has a double contour, smooth, thick, colourless shell.

The life-cycle is unknown; insects possibly act as intermediaries. The clinical symptoms are indeterminate. The worms live with heads embedded in the digestive tract from the oesophagus to the ileum (Chapter 24).

GENUS: *Anisakis*

Anisakis (*Eustoma*) (Van Thiel, 1962)

This is an ascarid parasite of herrings and marine animals. Its larval stages have caused symptoms in man.

The adult form inhabits the intestines of sea mammals (whales, dolphins and porpoises) and the larval stages are found in a variety of fish (haddock, mackerel, cod, pike, herring, bonita, squid, salmon and Alaskan pollack).

The infective larva, as seen in the infective stage, is slender and thread-like, measuring 1.5–2.6 cm long and 0.1 cm in diameter. Its outer surface is somewhat striated and there is a ventriculus between the oesophagus and the intestine, with the latter two structures meeting on an oblique plane. There is an excretion pore in the anterior part of the head, ventral to a small larval tooth, and there are three anal glands near the rectum. Transverse section shows the lateral cords arranged in a Y-shaped structure along the upper intestine or oesophagus or intestine. The cuticle consists of three layers and shows no alae.

GENUS: *Gonglyonema*

Gonglyonema pulchrum (Molin, 1857)

This is a spirurate nematode of a genus in which there are six species. It is a rare infection in man and pig but all ruminants are optimum hosts.

The worm lives most commonly in the upper portion of the digestive tract where it forms sinous galleries in the mucosa and submucosa of the oesophagus, buccal cavity and tongue.

The male is 62 × 0.15–0.3 mm and the female much larger, 145 × 0.2–0.5 mm. The anterior extremity is covered with a variable number of bosses or scutes arranged in eight longitudinal series.

The transparent thick-shelled oval eggs are embryonated when laid and are 50–70 μm in length by 25–37 μm. Development takes place in dung beetles of genera *Apodius* and *Onthophagus*, as well as in a small cockroach. (For infection in man see Chapter 24.)

SUPERFAMILY: STRONGYLOIDEA

GENUS: *Ancylostoma*

Ancylostoma duodenale Dubini, 1843
(Old World hookworm, miner's worm) (Fig. II.38)

Both sexes are cylindrical, white, grey or reddish-brown (from ingested blood). The female (1–1.3 cm × 0.6 mm), is cylindrical and slightly expanded posteriorly. The vagina is in the posterior third. The body cavity is occupied by the ovary and coiled uterine tubes packed with eggs. The maximum egg output occurs 15–18 months after infection. The male (0.8–1.1 cm × 0.4–0.5 mm) has a copulatory bursa consisting of an umbrella-like expansion of the cuticle; the dorsal ray is divided towards the distal end into smaller rays, which again divide into three unequal portions (Fig. II.39). There are two long delicate spicules. The genital papillae are tactile, finger-like projections near the anogenital opening. Owing to the situation of the genital openings in both sexes the worms in copulation assume a Y-shaped figure.

Two well-marked cephalic glands occupy the anterior third in both sexes and secrete an anti-coagulating ferment. The mouth end is bent dorsally. The excretory pore is ventral, placed at the level of the oesophagus. The buccal capsule is lined with chitin and contains two pairs of sharp teeth on its ventral aspect (Fig. II.40). The worm lives mostly in the jejunum and to a lesser extent in the duodenum but not in the ileum. The egg is ovoid (Figs. II.41, 22.12

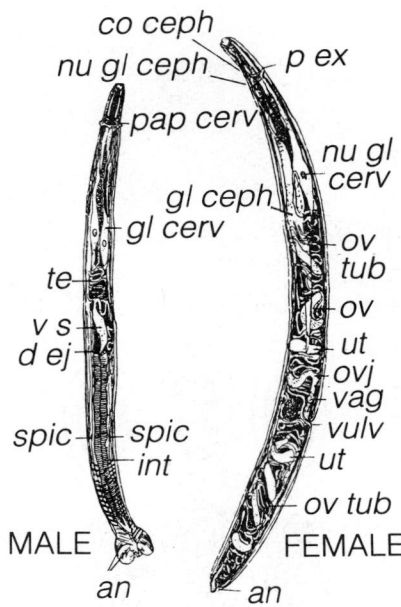

Fig. II.38 Male and female *Ancylostoma duodenale*. × 14.

an	anus	co ceph	cephalic nerve commissure
d ej	ejaculatory duct	gl cerv	cervical gland
int	intestine	nu gl cerv	nucleus of cervical gland
ov	ovary		
ovj	ovejector	ov tub	ovarian tubules
pap cerv	cervical papilla	p ex	excretory pore
te	testes	spic	spicules
vag	vagina	ut	uterus
vulv	vaginal opening	vs	vesicula seminalis

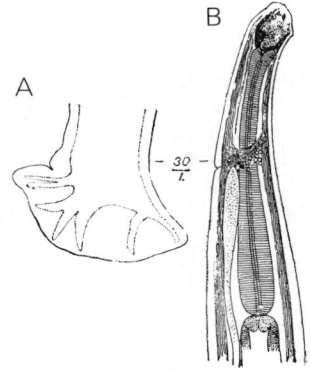

Fig. II.39 Bursa (A) and head (B) of male *Ancylostoma duodenale*.

and Plate III.14) measuring 60 × 40 μm, the shell is thin and hyaline and is passed in the early cleavage stage (Fig. II.41a–c). Outside the body it rapidly develops to the morula stage (Fig. II.41d) and hatches in 1–2 days.

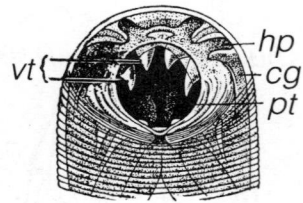

Fig. II.40 Head of *Ancylostoma duodenale*, showing the
hook-like teeth. × 50.

cg	cephalic gland	hp	head papillae
pt	pharyngeal teeth	vt	ventral teeth

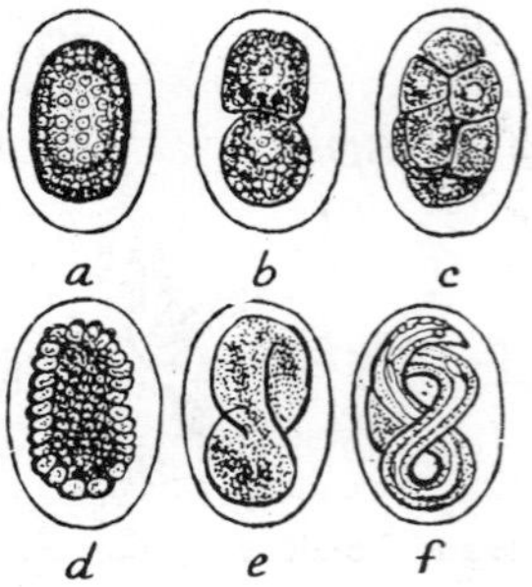

Fig. II.41 Development stages of *Ancylostoma duodenale* of
the larva in eggs; *a, b* and *c* are seen in fresh stools, and *d,
e* and *f* when the stools are stale. × 300.

At autopsy 500–1000 or more worms may be found.
They have a life-span of four to seven years. The
interval between active infection and the final disappearance of eggs from the faeces may be 76 months.
The female produces 25 000–35 000 eggs each day and
some 18–54 million eggs during its lifetime.

Ancylostoma braziliense De Faria, 1910

It is found in dogs and cats in Brazil. In Sri Lanka it
was described as *A. ceylanicum* from the civet cat.
  It is rarely found in the small intestine and then is
part of a mixed hookworm infection in man in India,
Malaysia and Thailand. It is smaller than *A. duodenale*
and the internal pair of ventral teeth are smaller than

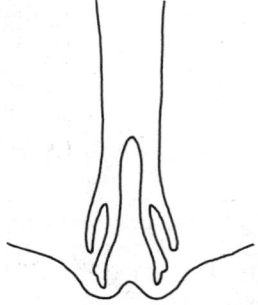

Fig. II.42 Dorsal ray of *Ancylostoma braziliense*.

the corresponding teeth of that species. The female
is 1 cm long and the male 8.5 mm. The rays in the
copulatory bursa differ (Fig. II.42) from those of *A.
duodenale* and are distinctive.
  The egg is indistinguishable from that of *A. duodenale*.
  The life-cycle is the same as *A. duodenale*. Man is
apparently an unsuitable host. The larva does not
penetrate into the bloodstream easily but wanders
under the skin causing irritation (larva migrans, see
p. 431).

GENUS: *Necator*

Necator americanus (Stiles, 1902), New World hookworm (Fig. II.43)

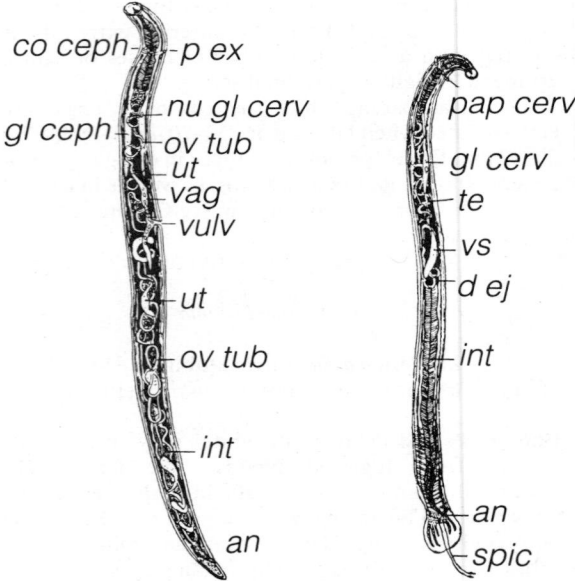

Fig. II.43 *Necator americanus.* × 12. Key as for Fig. II.36.

It is found in the small intestine of man and also of
the gorilla, patas monkey, rhinoceros, pangolin and a
rodent (*Caendu villosus*) and develops also in puppies.
On the whole, *N. americanus* is a shorter and more
slender worm than *A. duodenale*. The female (0.9–
1.1 cm × 0.4 mm) has the vulva placed slightly in front
of the middle of the body so that it copulates at a
Y-shaped angle, as in *A. duodenale*. The male (7–
9 × 0.3 mm) has the copulatory bursa closed and blunt
and a short dorsomedian lobe which appears as if
divided. The dorsal ray branches at the base into
divergent arms with bipartite tips (tridigitate in *A.
duodenale*). The base of the dorsal and dorsolateral
rays is short (Fig. II.44A). Two separate spicules unite
to form a single terminal 'fish-hook' barb. The living
worms are greyish-yellow, at times reddish.

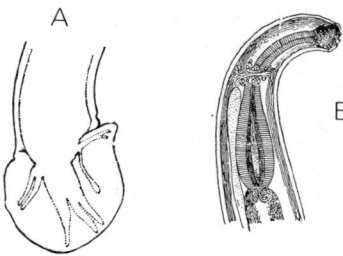

Fig. II.44 Bursa (A) and head (B) of *Necator americanus*.

The sudden dorsal bend of the head, especially in the female, is distinctive (Fig. II.44B). The buccal capsule is smaller than in *A. duodenale*, with an irregular border. In place of four hook-like teeth there is a ventral pair of cutting plates (Fig. II.45). The first pair of dorsal teeth are represented by chitinous plates. The outlet of the dorsal gland constitutes a 'dorsal rib' or tooth which projects into the oral cavity. Deeply placed in the capsule are one pair of dorsal and one pair of submedian lancets.

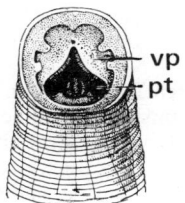

Fig. II.45 The head of *Necator americanus*, showing the pharyngeal teeth (pt) and the ventral plates (vp). × 50.

The egg is slightly larger than that of *A. duodenale* (64–75 × 36–40 μm) but otherwise similar. The infective (third stage) larva can be differentiated from that of *Strongyloides stercoralis* by the larger buccal vestibule and the intervening space between the oesophagus and midgut and from *A. duodenale* as shown in Table II.7. The presence of 44 eggs per gram of faeces is reckoned to represent one female worm. The

Table II.7 Differentiation of third stage larva of *Necator* and *Ancylostoma*.

	Necator	*Ancylostoma*
Oral capsule	Sharply defined; visible dorsally and ventrally	Hardly visible; more marked dorsally than ventrally
Tail	Rather blunt	Pointed
Zone of closing cells	Leaves only small space between oesophagus and intestine	Leaves considerable space

female lays from 6000–20 000 eggs/day. The estimated duration of life is about five years.

The life-cycle is identical with that of *A. duodenale* except that *Necator* infective larvae enter through the skin only whereas *Ancylostoma* can enter through the buccal mucous membrane as well and that the migrating larvae of *Necator* grow and develop in the lungs in contrast to those of *Ancylostoma*.

Life-cycle of hookworms (Fig. 21.13)

The eggs are deposited in the lumen of the intestine with two, four or eight blastomeres. They develop and hatch after expulsion in the faeces if they are deposited in damp, shaded soil.

1 The embryo moves about inside the shell and alters its shape, then escapes and gives rise to:

2 the rhabditiform larva which burrows into the faeces and feeds especially on bacteria. At first it has a double-bulbous oesophagus (Fig. II.46*b*). Feeding

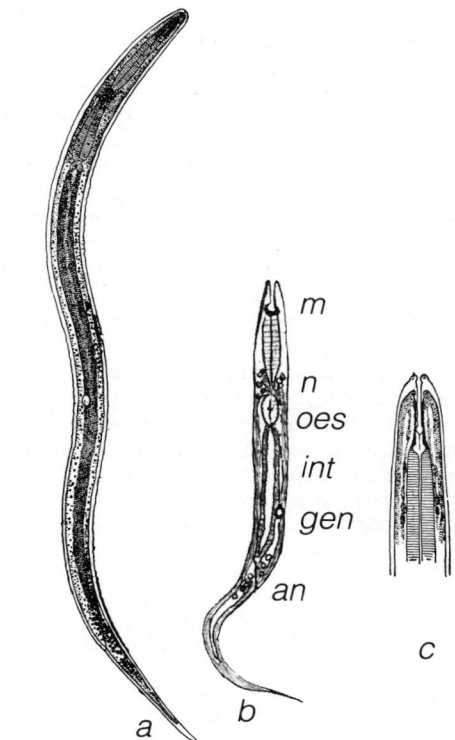

Fig. II.46 *Ancylostoma duodenale. a,* Mature infective larva. *b,* Rhabditiform larva. × 120. *c,* Head of larva.

voraciously, it stores oil globules in its intestinal wall. It moults on the third day; on the fifth the oesophageal bulb disappears and the larvae becomes elongated and fully developed at 20–30°C; the larva on the third day is 400 μm and on the fifth it is 500–700 μm long. It then moves away from the faeces into the earth, moults again and becomes:

3 the infective filariform, or third stage larva, with a well-developed mouth capsule, a simple muscular oesophagus and protective sheath, the walls of which are seen as two bright lines in the living specimen. It moves towards the oxygen supply but cannot swim in water. The larvae are most numerous in the upper 2.5 cm of the soil. They can ascend from deeper layers but lateral movements are limited. Attracted by warmth, it is quiescent in the cold; it moves along a thin film of water as well as in the earth. Enabled by the sheath to withstand a certain degree of desiccation, it can live in warm damp soil under optimum conditions for two years. This is the infective stage (Fig. II.46*a*). Direct sunlight, drying, flooding or salt water are fatal. On penetrating the skin of the host, the sheath is left behind and the larva then enters the lymphatics, gains the bloodstream and reaches the lungs on the third day. If pyogenic bacteria enter the skin with the larvae an open lesion may develop, producing 'ground itch'. *A. duodenale* can infect via the mucous membrane of the mouth, as well as the skin, whereas *N. americanus* infects via the skin. Breaking through the alveoli of the lungs, it enters the bronchioles and travels via trachea and oesophagus to the stomach. During this migration the third moult takes place and the buccal capsule is formed. Migrating larvae of *Necator* grow and develop in the lungs whereas those of *Ancylostoma* do not. On arrival in the intestine on the seventh day it undergoes its fourth moult; the terminal buccal capsule is changed into the 'provisional buccal capsule' with the mouth opening directed dorsally, as in the adult, but without teeth. On the fifteenth day the 'provisional buccal capsule' is cast off and it then assumes the adult form with adult buccal capsule and bursa in the male. In three to five weeks it becomes sexually mature, copulates and produces fertile eggs. Adult worms live from one to nine years and a female *Necator* lays 9000 eggs per day and *Ancylostoma* 30 000.

Hypobiosis

A phenomenon known as hypobiosis has been observed[10] in which there is arrested development of migrating *A. duodenale* larvae which migrate to the mammary gland, are secreted with the milk and infect the child. This is similar to that seen in *A. caninum* which infects puppies in the same way.

Cultivation of hookworm larvae

A small portion of faeces is rubbed over a petri dish with warm water, making a uniform layer like pea-soup. Inside the cover is placed a circle of wet blotting paper. This is kept moist and incubated at 23.9°C under a shade. If there is too much water the eggs will not develop. The larvae climb up the sides of the dish on to the blotting paper where they can be studied.

Differentiation of hookworms

The striation of the sheath is indistinct in *A. duodenale* but very distinct in *A. braziliense*. Rhabditiform ancylostome larvae are similar to those of *S. stercoralis* but are slightly more attenuated posteriorly and possess a much longer buccal vestibule. Infective (third stage) *A. duodenale* larvae are differentiated from *Necator* by the oesophageal shears which are unequal in thickness in *Ancylostoma* but equal in *Necator* and by the features shown in Table II.7.

GENUS: *Oesophagostomum*

Oesophagostomum apiostomum (Willach, 1891)
The female (1 cm × 0.325 mm) terminates posteriorly in a sharp point and has a vulva in its anterior half. The male (0.8–1 cm × 0.35 mm) has a copulatory bursa with a dorsal ray bifurcating into branches and forming a horseshoe-shaped structure, each limb giving off a short lateral horn near its base (Fig. II.47).

The egg (60 × 40 μm) closely resembles that of *Ancylostoma* but is passed in an advanced stage of development.

The larvae hatch from the eggs in the soil. When mature, they are unsheathed. The rhabditiform stage is swallowed and passes through the stomach and intestine. Then it invades the wall of the caecum where it forms nodules and, on occasions, it may penetrate the bowel and form intraperitoneal abscesses. The immature worms break out into the lumen, attach themselves to mucosa and become adult.

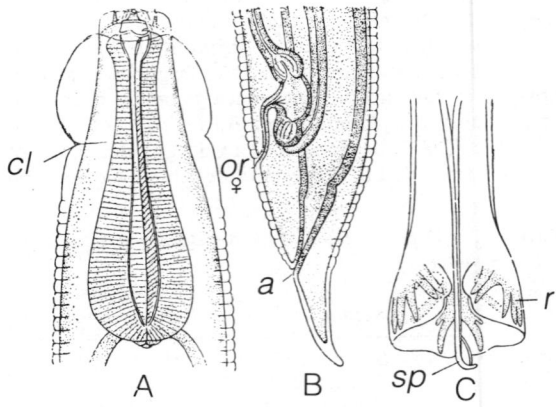

Fig. II.47 *Oesophagostomum apiostomum* (*brumpti*). A, Head, showing cuticular expansion and the oral vestibule. B, Tail of the female. C, Tail of the male, showing copulatory bursa.

a	anus	cl	ventral cleft
or	vaginal orifice	r	characteristic rays of bursa
sp	spicule		

Oesophagostomum stephanostomum var. *thomasi*
(Railliet & Henry, 1909)

This is a common parasite of monkeys (*Cercopithecus callitrichus*) and gorillas. The first case reported in man was in Brazil; the patient dies of dysenteric symptoms and peritonitis. It has also been reported in French Guiana and in northern Nigeria.

The morphology resembles that of *O. apiostomum* but both sexes are larger and it is distinguished by a corona radiata with 38 leaf-like spines.

The eggs in the faeces resemble those of *Ancylostoma*.

The life history is probably similar to that of *O. apiostomum*.

GENUS: *Ternidens*

Ternidens deminutus Railliet & Henry, 1905

The female (14–16 × 0.73 mm) has a genital orifice posterior and subterminal and a short vagina opening into two uterine tubes (Fig. II.48). The male (9.5 × 0.56 mm) has the dorsal ray of the copulatory bursa dividing into two distal extremities and each branch bifurcates again (Fig. II.49).

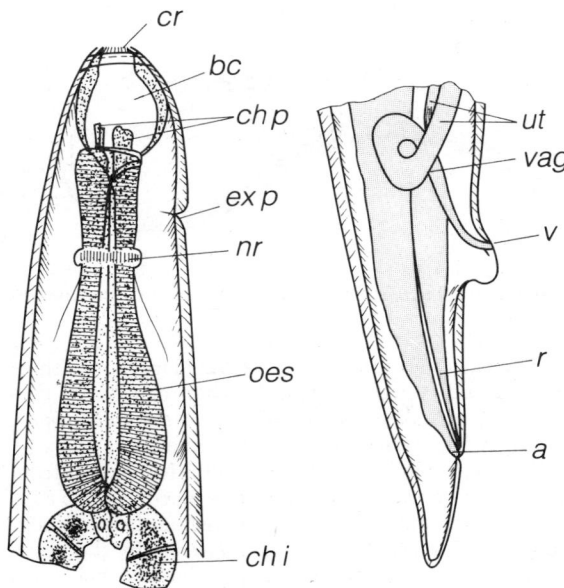

Fig. II.48 Female *Ternidens deminutus*. 1, Anterior extremity. 2, Posterior extremity.

a	anus	bc	buccal cavity
ch i	chyle intestine	cr	corona radiata
ch p	chitinous plates	nr	nerve ring
oes	oesophagus	r	rectum
ut	uterus	vag	vagina
v	vaginal opening		

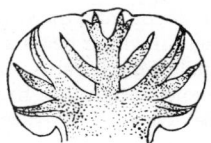

Fig. II.49 Bursa of male *Ternidens deminutus*.

The worm resembles a female ancylostome; its anterior extremity is not bent and the mouth capsule is terminal with a corona of setae. At the base of the cup-like buccal capsule three serrated teeth guard the entrance to the oesophagus; this is characteristic of the genus *Ternidens* (Fig. II.48).

The egg (84 × 40 µm) is delicate and transparent and in an advanced stage of segmentation resembles that of an ancylostome.

The rhabditiform larva (0.3 mm) with flagellar tail, hatches from the egg in soil, becomes sheathed and the infective filariform larva (0.6–0.7 mm) is formed. These can survive desiccation, reviving in water; thus they withstand drought.

The filariform infective larvae fail to penetrate human skin but gain entrance through the stomach and intestinal tract after the eggs are swallowed with soil-contaminated food or water.

SUPERFAMILY: METASTRONGYLIDAE

GENUS: *Angiostrongylus*

Angiostrongylus cantonensis (Chen, 1935)

The male is 15.5–22.0 mm in length by 0.25–0.35 mm in breadth. It is transparent and smooth with faint transverse striae. The head is smoothly rounded and the mouth is without lips. There are four pairs of minute, submedian papillae which are sometimes visible *en face* and two clearly defined minute triangular teeth present at the base of the oral cavity. There may possibly be a third which is difficult to define. The oesophagus is 0.29–0.33 mm long by 0.05 mm at maximum breadth at the posterior end. The intestine is a wide thin-walled tube. The excretory pore opens just posterior to the oesophageal–intestinal junction. The spicules are unequal, flexible and striated rods 1.2 mm in length. The bursa is well developed but the gubernaculum is absent and there is one pair of large adanal papillae.

The female is 18.5–33 mm long by 0.28–0.5 mm in maximum breadth. Cuticle, head, papillae, oesophagus and intestines are as in the male. In life, the spirally wound, milky white uterine tubules and the blood-filled intestine can be seen through the transparent cuticle and form a striking 'barber's pole' pattern. The uterine tubules unite about 2 mm from the posterior end to form the thin-walled vagina. The vulva is a transverse slit. The tail is obliquely truncated. The anus is 0.06 mm and the vulva 0.25–0.28 mm from the tip of the tail which bears a minute terminal projection. The male:female ratio is usually 2:3.

The eggs are ovoid with a thin hyaline shell measuring 46–48 × 68–74 μm. They are passed unembryonated.

The adult *A. cantonensis* lives in the pulmonary arteries of rats. Unsegmented ova are discharged into the bloodstream and lodge as emboli in the smaller vessels. The first stage larvae which hatch from these eggs break through the respiratory tract, migrate up the trachea and eventually pass out of the body in the faeces. In Hawaii the land snail *Achatina fulica*, the slug *Veronicella leydigi* and the land planarian *Geoplana septemlineata* have been found naturally infected.

Slugs (*Agriolimax laevis*) act as intermediary hosts. Two moults occur in the slug about the seventeenth day. The slugs are then eaten by rats (*R. rattus*) and the larvae remain in their cast skins until freed in the stomach of the rat by digestion. They then pass quickly along the gut as far as the ileum where they enter the bloodstream and congregate in the central nervous system some 17 hours after ingestion. The anterior part of the cerebrum is the favourite site and there the third moult takes place on the sixth or seventh days and the final one on the eleventh to thirteenth. Young adults emerge on the surface of the brain from the twelfth to fourteenth days and spread during the next two weeks on the arachnoid surface. From the twenty-eighth to thirty-first days they migrate to the lungs via the venous system, passing through the right side of the heart to their definitive site in the pulmonary arteries. The prepatent period in the rat usually lies between the forty-second and forty-fifth days.

Angiostrongylus costaricensis

Angiostrongylus costaricensis is larger than *A. cantonensis*. The male measures 22 mm × 140 μm and the female 42 mm × 350 μm and the morphology is similar. The eggs are ovoid and measure 90 μm with a thin hyaline shell and are passed unembryonated.

SUPERFAMILY: TRICHOSTRONGYLOIDEA

GENUS: *Trichostrongylus*

Trichostrongylus colubriformis (Giles, 1892) and allied species

Normally this is a parasite of the upper small intestine of the sheep and goat; it is not infrequently found in the duodenum and upper jejunum of man in agri-

cultural districts of India, central Africa, Egypt, Java, Australia, Japan, Korea and especially in Abadan (Iran) where 70% of inhabitants are infected. It has been found in Java in scrapings from the duodenum where the adults live with head embedded in the mucosa. By flotation technique the eggs of this species can be found in the faeces, together with ancylostomes, fairly frequently in India and Assam.

The females (4–6.5 mm) (Fig. II.50A) usually outnumber the males. They are very slender and pink with an attenuated anterior extremity and the vulva in the posterior quarter. The males (4–5 × 0.07 mm) have a bilobed copulatory bursa and two spicules (Fig. II.50B). These parasites are found a third to a half buried in mucus. When scraped on to a slide they appear as delicate red streaks. When the slide is shaken in saline in a petri dish they can be seen against a dark background. The adult worms are never found in faeces. The mouth is unarmed.

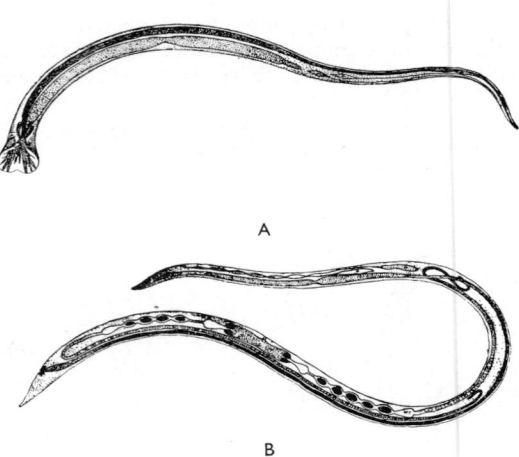

Fig. II.50 *Trichostrongylus colubriformis*. A, Female. B, Male. × 25.

The egg (85 × 115 μm) is relatively large, oval, thin-shelled and contains a morula when deposited. It is apt to be mistaken for that of *Ancylostoma duodenale*, is longer and narrower with more pointed ends.

The eggs hatch outside the body; the rhabditiform larvae metamorphose into infective filariform in 6 days at 22–25°C and can be distinguished from similar stages in *Strongyloides* and *Ancylostoma* by the bead-like swelling at the tip of the tail. The semifilariform third stage larvae are very resistant to desiccation. These enter the body via the skin or mouth, undergoing two ecdyses.

An eastern form has been separated in Japan (*T. orientalis*). *T. probolurus* (Railliet, 1896) is rarely seen in man; it is a natural infection of the gazelle and camel. *T. orientalis* is common in people who look after donkeys and goats.

SUPERFAMILY: RHABDITOIDEA

GENUS: *Strongyloides*

Strongyloides stercoralis (Bavay, 1876)

Characters

Formerly it was thought that embryos were produced by a parasitic, parthenogenetic female, in the absence of a male, but it is now known that a parasitic male exists, shorter and broader than the female. The oesophagus is characteristic, with a club-shaped anterior part and a post-central constriction and a posterior bulb (Fig. II.51). Later, two copulatory spicules and a gubernaculum are said to become apparent and, when developed, the adult male resembles the free-living form (Fig. II.52,3). Parasitic males are found in experimentally infected dogs but not in human infections owing to the fact that they do not invade the intestinal wall and so are eliminated from the bowel soon after the females begin to oviposit. Although adolescent parasitic females may be inseminated probably the majority are parthenogenetic. This is a process of *reversive metamorphosis*, in which it loses the ability of penetrating tissues and remains a lumen parasite.

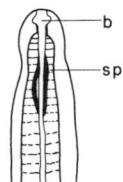

Fig. II.51 *Strongyloides stercoralis.* Anterior end of the parasitic male.

b   buccal chamber   sp   buccal spears

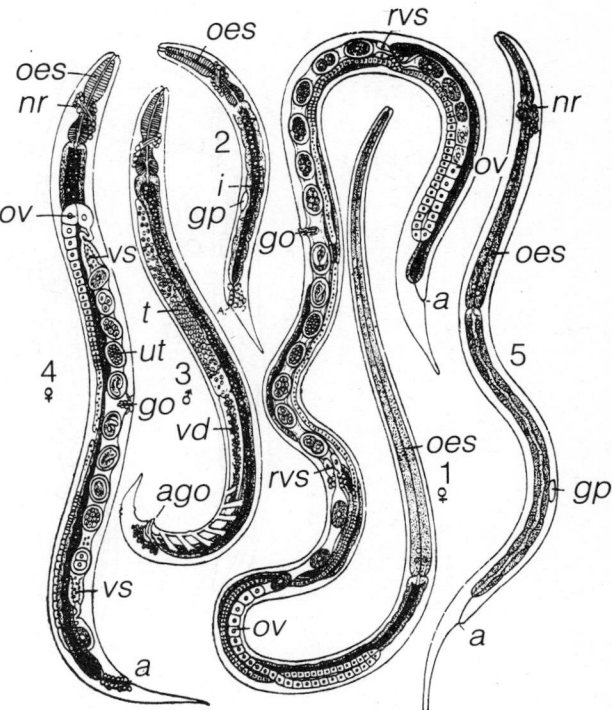

Fig. II.52 The life history of *Strongyloides stercoralis*. 1, Parasitic female. 2, Rhabditiform larva. 3, Fully grown male. 4, Fully grown female. 5, Fully developed filariform larva. × 30. (After Looss.)

a	anus	ago	combined anus and genital pore
go	genital opening		
i	Intestine	gp	primitive genital organs
oes	oesophagus		
rvs	rudimentary vesicula seminalis	nr	nerve ring
		ov	ovary
ut	uterus	t	testes
vs	vesicula seminalis	vd	vas deferens

The female (2.5 × 0.034 mm) (Fig. II.52,4) tapers anteriorly and ends in a conical tail. The mouth has three small lips and leads to an oesophagus occupying a quarter of the length of the body. The vulva lies in the posterior third. There is a prominent uterus containing 50 eggs (50–58 × 30–34 μm) which are laid in the lumen of the bowel in an advanced stage of development and may occasionally be found in the faeces. They hatch immediately to embryos (0.2–0.3 × 0.013 mm), which have a double-bulb oesophagus, apt to be confused with the rhabditiform stage of *Ancylostoma* and *Necator* (Fig. II.46b and c). They are passed active in faeces and in 3–5 days are converted into free-living male and female forms, both of which have a rhabditiform, double-bulb muscular oesophagus (Fig. II.52, 2). The male is a free-living form (0.7 × 0.035 mm) (Fig. II.53) with the tail curved ventrally, two spicules and an accessory piece. The free-living form of the female measures 1 × 0.05 mm. The vulva lies behind the middle of the body. The uterus contains thin-shelled eggs, measuring 70 × 40 μm (Fig. II.52,4).

Copulation between the sexes takes place in faeces. The rhabditoid larvae produced are indistinguishable from those derived from the parasitic female. After 3 or 4 days they develop into host-feeding, mature filariform larvae, which are the infective stage, and re-enter the definitive host via the skin or buccal mucosa, as in *Ancylostoma* or *Necator*, but remain alive in the soil for many weeks. The distinguishing feature is that the oesophagus in filariform larvae is half the length of the body (Fig. II.52,5); in *Ancylostoma* and *Necator* it occupies about a quarter. Filariform larvae find their way into the small intestine and develop into female parasitic forms. Under unsuitable climatic conditions the sexual phase in the faeces may be omitted and rhabditiform embryos produced by the parasitic

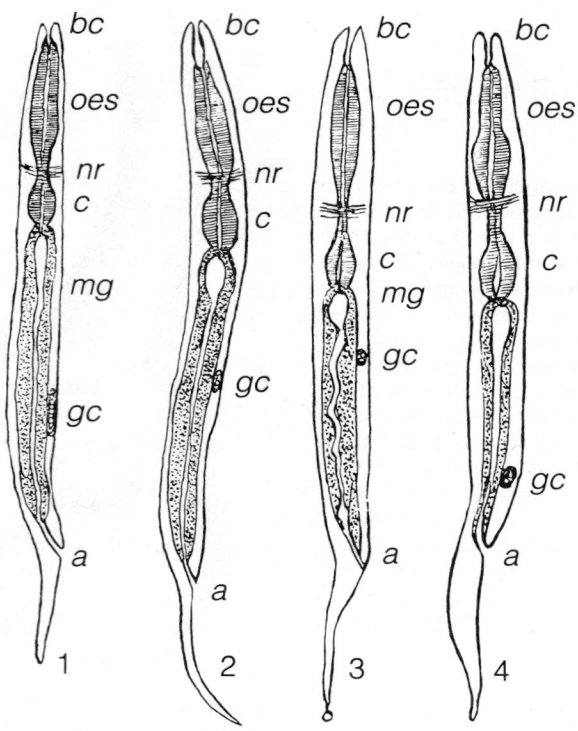

Fig. II.53 Distinguishing features of nematode larva in the faeces. 1, *Strongyloides stercoralis*. 2, *Ancylostoma duodenale*. 3, *Trichostrongylus colubriformis*. 4, *Rhabditis hominis*.

a	anus		bc	buccal cavity		oes	oesophagus		c	cardiac oesophageal bulb
mg	midgut		cg	genital cells		nr	nerve ring			

Characters	Strongyloides	Ancylostoma	Trichostrongylus	Rhabditis
Average size	$225 \times 16\,\mu$m	$275 \times 17\,\mu$m	$275 \times 15\,\mu$m	$240 \times 12\,\mu$m
Posterior tip	Blunt	Sharp	Sharp with bead-like swelling	Sharp
Buccal chamber	Shorter than width at tip of head	Longer than width at tip of head	Longer than width at tip of head	Longer than width at tip of head
Genital primordia	Fairly large	Small	Very small	Very small

female may develop directly into filariform larvae capable of infecting the definitive host (Fig. II.52,5). The larvae of *S. stercoralis* may be confused with those of *Rhabditis hominis*, a free-living worm which may gain entry by accident to the digestive tract of man. These larvae measure 240–360 μm in length by 12 μm in diameter and resemble the parent worm in shape and structure of the oesophagus and filariform larvae of *Ancylostoma duodenale*. The distinguishing features are given in Fig. II.53.

Life-cycle (Fig. 21.16)

There are two stages: parasitic and free-living in soil.

Parasitic stage

1 *Filariform* (infective) larvae from infective soil penetrate exposed skin or the mouth.
2 They may travel to the lungs via the intestine and copulate as male and female. Filariform larvae enter man by penetrating the skin or through the mouth, and migrate through the lungs to the oesophagus; on arrival in the pulmonary capillaries the larvae produce haemorrhages which form the avenue of escape into the alveoli; followed by cellular infiltration into the respiration passages with output of eosinophil cells. The changes result in *Strongyloides* pneumonitis. These develop in two weeks.

3 Females, with or without males, enter the mucosa (especially of the duodenum) and lay eggs.
4 Eggs hatch and larvae escape into the intestine. They may either (a) pass down and be evacuated or (b) become filariform larvae (infective) and re-enter the mucosa or perianal skin (autoinfection) and pass to the organs (e.g. lungs).

Free-living stage

Larvae from faeces in soil are either rhabditoid or filariform (infective). Rhabditoid larvae can either become filariform and invade exposed skin or become male and female and produce rhabditoid larvae which continue the cycle indefinitely.

Strongyloides fülleborni

S. fülleborni is a common parasite of monkeys and apes widely spread in human populations in tropical Africa, common in the rain forest and sporadic in the savannah, and is found in New Guinea. It may be identified by prominent vulvar lips and narrowing behind the vulva in the free-living females. The prominent oesophagus in the free-living stages is also characteristic. The eggs are passed in the stools in contrast to *S. stercoralis* and resemble hookworm ova for which they are commonly mistaken.

SUPERFAMILY: OXYUROIDEA

GENUS: *Enterobius*

Enterobius vermicularis (Linnaeus, 1758)
(threadworm or pinworm, *Oxyuris vermicularis*)

This is the only nematode of man with a double-bulb oesophagus in the adult. It is small and white, its mouth surrounded by a cuticular expansion, and its skin transversely striated. The male is seldom seen and does not migrate like the female. Much smaller than the female (2.5 mm), its posterior third is curved spirally and its caudal extremity blunt, with six sensory papillae and a single spicule, 70 μm (Fig. II.54B,C). The female (9–12 mm) has a long pointed tail, the anus 2 mm from the posterior extremity, and a transverse, slit-like vulva in the anterior fourth of the body (Fig. II.54A). The gravid female lays eggs in a stream of 10 000–15 000 in a few minutes and dies when egg-laying is completed.

The egg (50–54 × 20–27 μm) (Plate III.19 and Fig. 21.6) has a characteristic shape, flattened on one side, and is almost colourless, with a bean-shaped double-contour shell, which contains a more or less fully formed embryo.

Life-cycle (Fig. II.55)

There is no multiplication of worms inside the body.

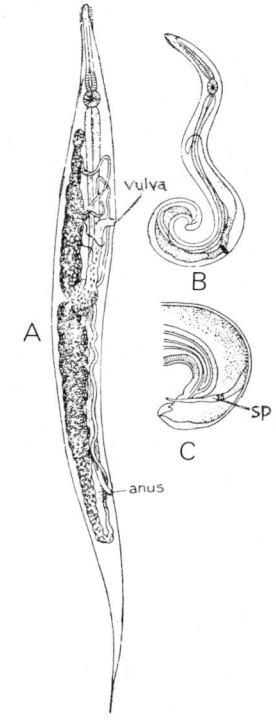

Fig. II.54 *Enterobius vermicularis.* A, Female. B, Male. C, Caudal extremity of male. × 12.

The egg-shell is weakened by the intestinal juices and the larva breaks out of the shell. Soon afterwards it invades the glandular crypts and penetrates into the glands and stroma, where it coils up, causing some liquefaction of the tissues, but no cellular reaction.

The life-span of *E. vermicularis* ranges from 37 to 93 days. As soon as the ovary becomes packed with eggs the female worm loosens her hold on the intestinal wall and lies passive in the faecal stream. The fertilized female migrates out of the anus to deposit her eggs in the perianal skin and perineum. The crawling of the gravid females produces intense pruritus. After a few hours the embryo develops rapidly and attains a length of 140–150 μm. The egg is ingested, generally as a result of deposits of faeces under the fingernails, conveyed to the mouth, and hatches in the digestive juices. Liberated larvae after two moults pass from the small into the large intestine, where they become mature. The whole cycle takes two to four weeks. Eggs can be inhaled through the nose from infected garments at some distance and embryonated eggs have been found in dust. Damp conditions with minimal ventilation are necessary for survival. The eggs require a 6-hour exposure to air before they can hatch.

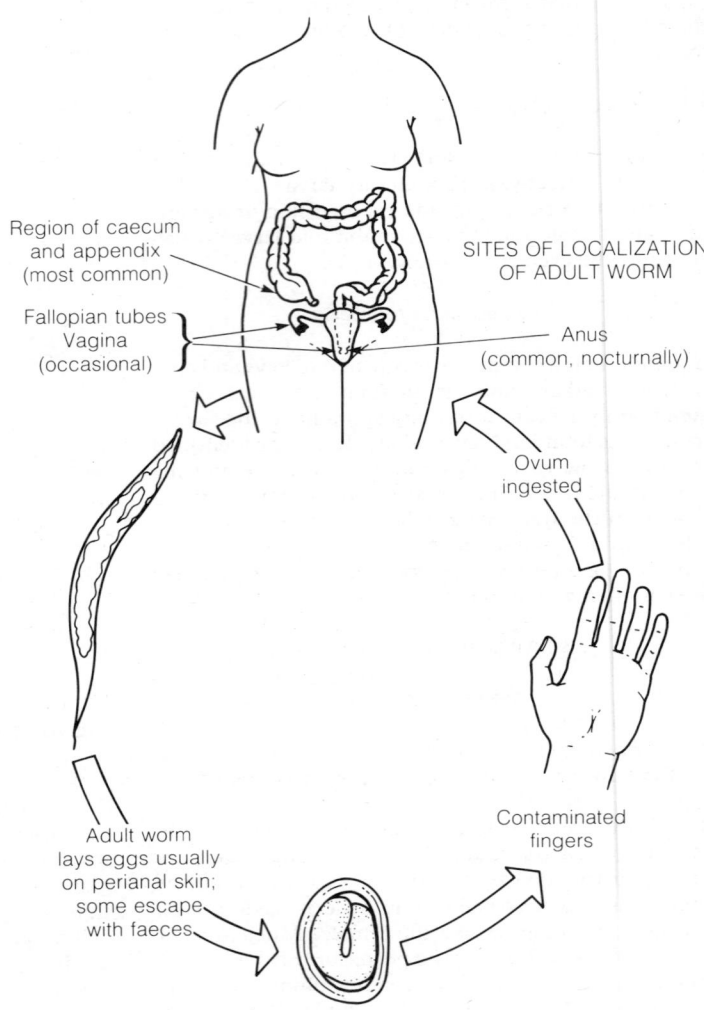

Enterobius (oxyuris) vermicularis
(Pinworm)

Region of caecum
and appendix
(most common)

SITES OF LOCALIZATION
OF ADULT WORM

Fallopian tubes
Vagina
(occasional)

Anus
(common, nocturnally)

Ovum
ingested

Contaminated
fingers

Adult worm
lays eggs usually
on perianal skin;
some escape
with faeces

Fig. II.55 Life-cycle of *Enterobius vermicularis*.

SUPERFAMILY: TRICHINELLOIDEA

GENUS: *Trichuris*

Trichuris trichiura (Linnaeus, 1771)
(*Trichocephalus dispar*, whipworm)

The male (30–45 mm) (Fig. II.56,1) has an anterior attenuated portion, containing the cellular oesophagus, which is half as long again as the thicker posterior portion. The caudal extremity is curved ventrally through 360° and there is a single spicule in the sheath, studded with spines (Fig. II.56,3).

The female (30–35 mm) (Fig. II.56,2) has an anterior attenuated portion, twice as long as the posterior half, which is occupied by a stout uterus, tightly packed with eggs. A sacculate tubular ovary runs forward from the posterior end for over half the thick part of the body. Females preponderate over males in a proportion of over 400 to 1.

The egg (50 × 22 μm) is brown and has a characteristic barrel shape and a single shell with a plug at each end. It contains an unsegmented embryo (Plate III.18 and Fig. 21.9).

The worm is greyish-white or slightly pink and lives in the caecum where it maintains its position by transfixing a superficial fold of mucous membrane

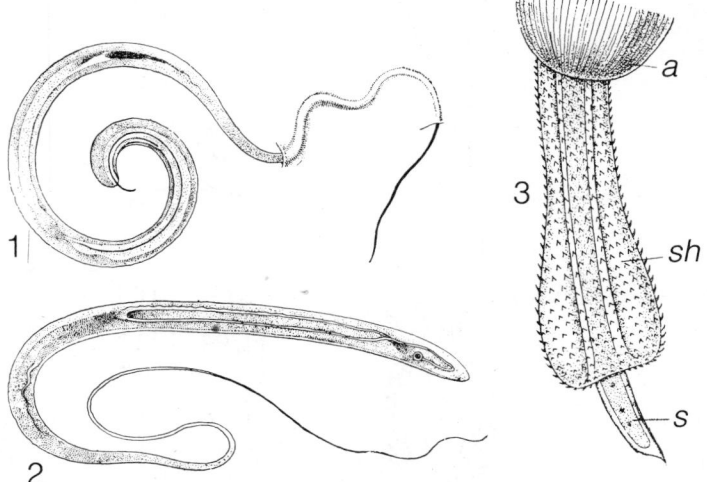

Fig. II.56 *Trichuris trichiura*. 1, Male partly embedded in the mucous membrane of the intestine. 2, Female. 3, Copulatory apparatus, greatly magnified. × 3.

a   posterior extremity of body   s   spicule   sh   sheath

with its slender neck, and lying embedded in mucus between the intestinal villi.

Life-cycle (Fig. II.57)

Infection is spread chiefly by stale faeces. The egg is unsegmented; embryonation takes at least 21 days. It can withstand a low temperature owing to its thick shell. Moisture is necessary and it cannot withstand desiccation. Development is direct. The embryo hatches only when the egg is swallowed: the egg-shell is digested by the intestinal juices, the larva emerges in the small intestine, penetrates the villi where it develops for a week and re-enters the lumen. It then passes to the caecum or large intestine, where it attaches itself to the mucosa and becomes adult.

 Trichuris suis of the pig, whose eggs are indistinguishable from those of *T. trichiura*, has been transmitted to man in an experiment in which 1000 infective eggs were swallowed. The volunteer had no symptoms but eggs appeared in the faeces in about 60 days and continued to be excreted for at least 10 weeks after maturation. *T. suis* may therefore be a cause of trichuriasis in man, especially if in contact with pigs.[11]

GENUS: Capillaria

Capillaria hepatica (Bancroft, 1893) (*Trichocephalus hepaticus, Hepaticola hepatica*)

Capillaria hepatica is a parasite of the liver of the rat. The adult worms are very similar to *Trichuris*; the female measures 2 mm × 10 mm, the male being half as long. The eggs resemble those of *T. trichiura* but

have an outer shell distinctly pitted and measuring 51–67.5 × 30–35 μm. It has a direct life-cycle like that of *Trichuris*.

Capillaria philippinensis

The adult worms resemble *C. hepatica*. The male worms measure 2.1–3.7 mm in length and the female worm 2.6–4.9 mm. The eggs measure 45 × 21 μm and are of two types: one typical bioperculate with a thick shell resembling a *Trichuris* ovum which is passed out in the stool unembryonated and the other atypical with a thin shell and embryonated resembling a *Strongyloides* ovum.

Life-cycle

The typical eggs pass out in the stool where they are taken up by an intermediate host (small fish) in which they hatch and locate in the mucosa of the small intestine. The atypical eggs hatch in the host's intestine and the larvae reinvade the bowel giving rise to intestinal autoinfection.

GENUS: Trichinella

Trichinella spiralis (Owen, 1835)

Trichinella spiralis (Fig. II.58) is a white worm just visible to the naked eye which inhabits the small intestine. The male (1.6 × 0.04 mm) has a cloaca situated posteriorly between two caudal appendages and two pairs of papillae. The female (3–4 × 0.06 mm) has a vulva in the anterior fifth, an ovary in the posterior

Fig. II.57 Life-cycle of *Trichuris trichiura*.

Trichuris trichiura (Whipworm)

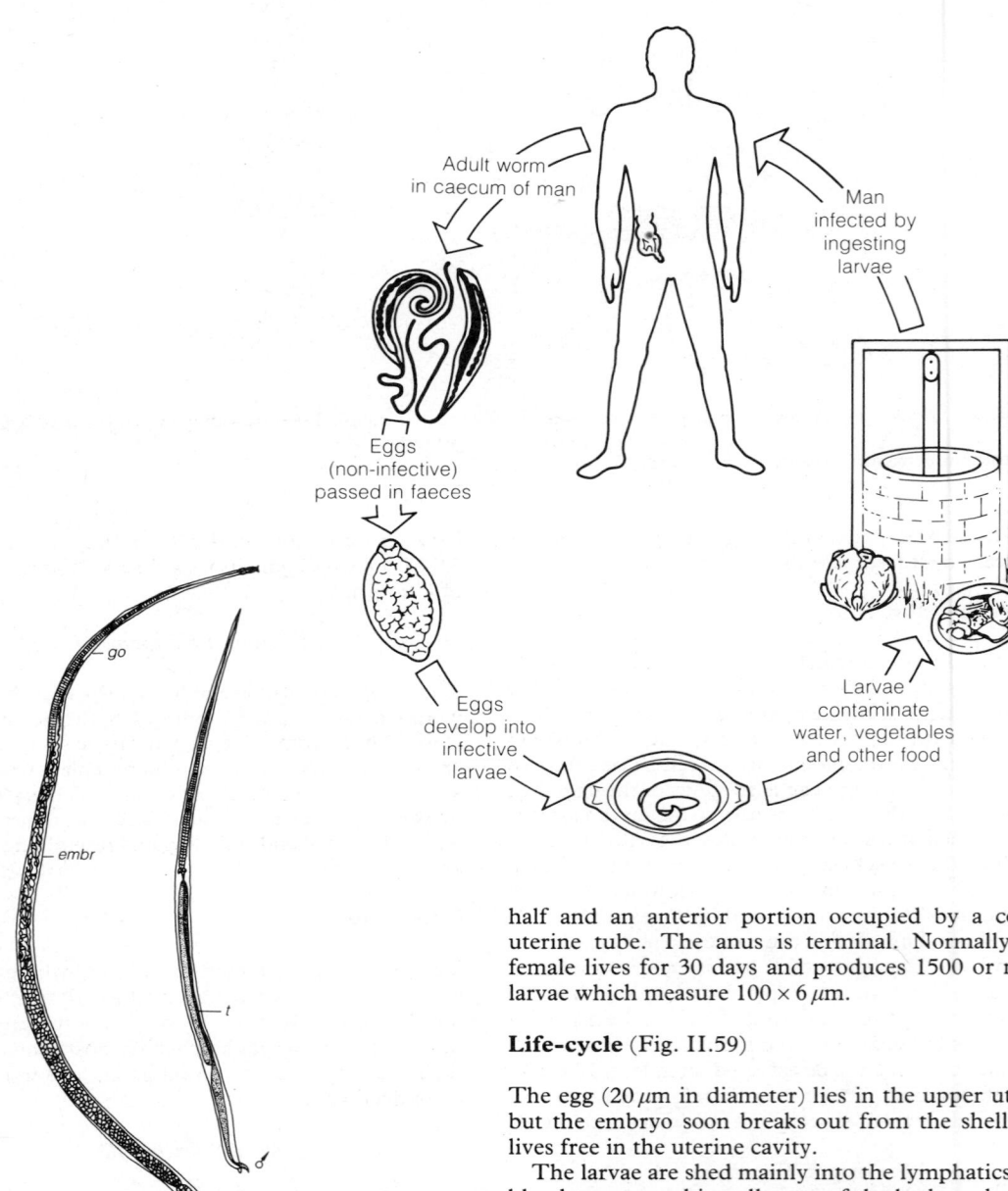

Adult worm in caecum of man

Man infected by ingesting larvae

Eggs (non-infective) passed in faeces

Eggs develop into infective larvae

Larvae contaminate water, vegetables and other food

Fig. II.58 Female and male *Trichinella spiralis*. × 45.

embr	embryos	go	genital opening
ov	ovary	t	testes

half and an anterior portion occupied by a coiled uterine tube. The anus is terminal. Normally the female lives for 30 days and produces 1500 or more larvae which measure $100 \times 6 \mu$m.

Life-cycle (Fig. II.59)

The egg (20μm in diameter) lies in the upper uterus but the embryo soon breaks out from the shell and lives free in the uterine cavity.

The larvae are shed mainly into the lymphatics and bloodstream reaching all parts of the body and encysting.

The cyst (Fig. II.60) is formed by a larva encapsulated by the host tissues. The capsule is an adventitious ellipsoidal sheath with blunt ends which results from round cell and eosinophilic infiltration round the tightly coiled larva. The long axis parallels that of the muscle fibres. Host amino acids can be transferred

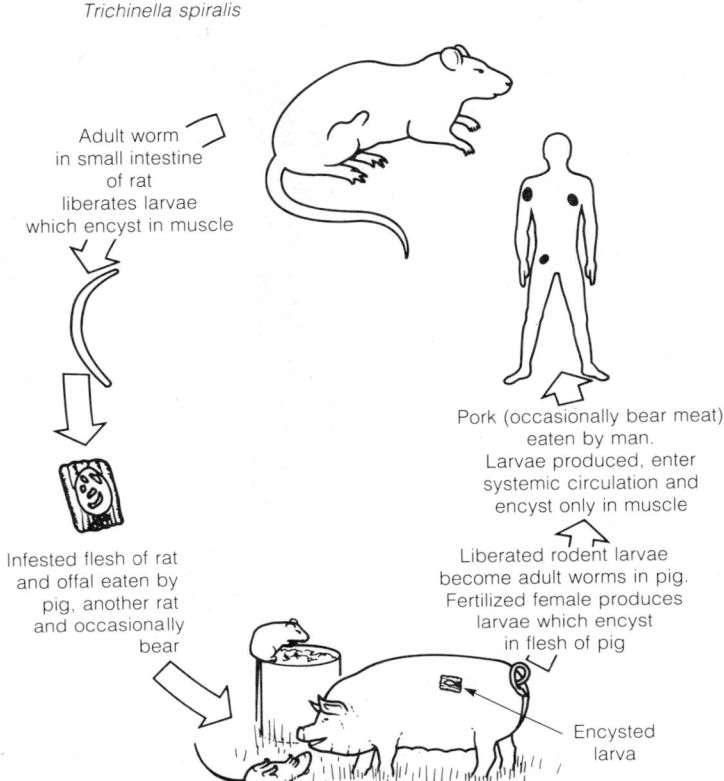

Trichinella spiralis

Adult worm
in small intestine
of rat
liberates larvae
which encyst in muscle

Infested flesh of rat
and offal eaten by
pig, another rat
and occasionally
bear

Encysted
larva

Liberated rodent larvae
become adult worms in pig.
Fertilized female produces
larvae which encyst
in flesh of pig

Pork (occasionally bear meat)
eaten by man.
Larvae produced, enter
systemic circulation and
encyst only in muscle

Fig. II.59   Life-cycle of *Trichinella spiralis*.

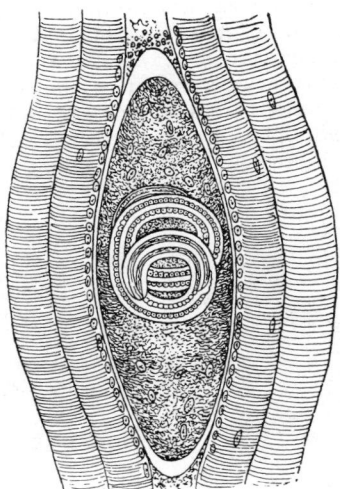

Fig. II.60   Encysted larva of *Trichinella spiralis* 15 days after entering muscle. × 300.

into the cyst and converted into larval protein so that an encysted larva remains viable for many years.

When consumed by a carnivorous host the cysts are digested in the stomach and, after excysting the larvae invade the duodenal and jejunal mucosa and develop through four ecdyses into adult males and females, which then enter the lumen of the bowel. Later they re-enter the mucosa and penetrate the villi, even reaching the mesenteric glands. Larviposition takes place over a period of from four to 16 weeks or more. The larvae are carried through the right heart and lungs to the arterial circulation which they reach between the ninth and thirteenth day finally reaching the striated muscles where they encyst.

There are three biological races of *Trichinella spiralis* distinguished by geography and ecology.

1 *T. s. spiralis* in the temperate zone involving wild and domestic pigs and temperate zone predators—rat, bear, fox, marten etc.

2 *T. s. nelsoni* in Africa involving bush-pig, wart-hog and African predators—hyena, leopard, lion, etc.

3 *T. s. nativa* in the Arctic involving walrus, seal and Arctic predators—polar bear, fox etc.

This group includes spirurate filiform nematodes adapted to inhabit the deeper tissues, such as the circulatory, lymphatic and connective tissue layers. Some insect intermediary is necessary to complete their development.

GENUS: *Wuchereria*

Wuchereria bancrofti (Cobbold, 1877) Seurat, 1921
(*Filaria bancrofti* (Cobbold, 1877))

Characters

Adult filaria

It is a thread-like white worm found in lymphatic vessels and glands. The sexes are coiled together and can be separated with difficulty. The cuticle is adorned with small cuticular bosses.

The male (4 cm × 0.1 mm) is coiled with a corkscrew-like tail and two spicules, the larger of which measures 500 μm. The smaller (300 μm) is grooved on its ventral aspect. There is a short, thick proximal and a whip-like distal portion, ending in a hook, and 15 pairs of minute sensory caudal papillae (Fig. II.61 *a,b*).

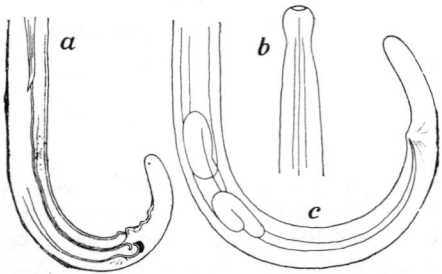

Fig. II.61   *Wuchereria bancrofti.* Magnified. *a,* Tail of male. *b,* Head and neck. *c,* Tail of female.

A saddle-shaped thickening of the cuticle on the posterior wall of the cloaca forms a shield, and there is an accessory piece peculiar to *W. bancrofti.* There are 12 pairs of circumanal papillae of which eight are preanal and four postanal in position. There are also two pairs of large sessile papillae and at the tail a solitary pair of minute size. The female (6.5 cm × 0.2–2.8 mm) has a tapering anterior end with a rounded swelling (Fig. II.62). There are sessile papillae on the head and an oral aperture leading to a cylindrical oesophagus. The mid-intestinal tube is one-third to one-fifth of the total diameter and opens into the rectum posteriorly. The caudal extremity is narrow and abruptly rounded (Fig. II.61*c*). The vulva is 0.8 mm behind the anterior extremity. A swollen vagina (0.25 mm in length) leads

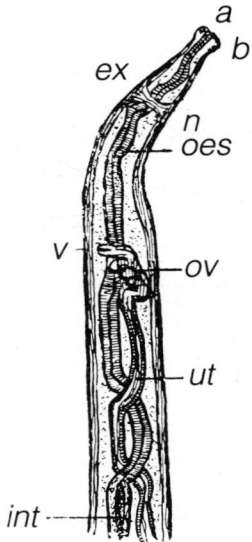

Fig. II.62   The head of *Wuchereria bancrofti,* female. × 50.

a	mouth	b	circumoral papillae
ex	excretory pore	int	intestine
n	nerve ring	oes	oesophagus
ov	oviduct	ut	uterus
v	vulva		

into the uterus which divides into two tubuli which are much coiled occupying the greater portion of the body with a diameter three times that of the midintestine (Fig. II.62). Two ovaries and ducts extend to within 1 mm of the tail.

The eggs lie in the upper uterus enclosed in a chorionic membrane which becomes a sheath to the living embryos (microfilariae) (Fig. II.63). They are emitted by the viviparous female and travel via the lymphatics into the bloodstream whence they are abstracted by various species of mosquito. Their size in the distal part of the uterus is 38 × 25 μm, but as they are pushed to the vagina they become more elongated. The microfilaria develops from an oval egg and measures at first 216 μm. The embryo often lies curled up in its shell which becomes lobed, resembling a Dutch twist or pretzel.

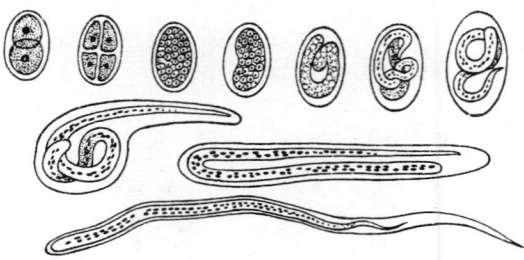

Fig. II.63   Evolution of sheathed microfilaria from the ovum in the uterus of the parent worm. The later stages may occasionally take place after emission from the vagina.

Microfilaria

The microfilaria ($280 \times 7\,\mu m$) (Figs. II.64, II.65 and II.73,2) in the living state appears structureless. With higher magnifications the entire microfilaria is seen to be enclosed in a sheath which is longer than the enclosed microfilaria and stains pale mauve with Giemsa, in contrast to microfilaria *Loa loa*, the sheath of which does not stain with Giemsa. In this sheath it can move backwards and forwards and the collapsed

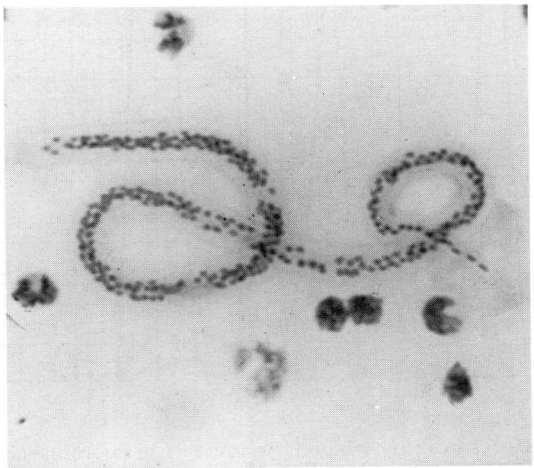

Fig. II.64 Sheathed microfilaria of *Wuchereria bancrofti* in a blood film. (Courtesy of Professor W. O'Connor.)

portion trails after the head or tail. The sheath has been the subject of controversy. It is generally held to be the outstretched vitelline membrane but in the microfilariae of *Litomosoides carinii* of the cotton rat it has been found that a true larval sheath is developed during its sojourn in the blood. In the middle third is some granular material or primitive gut (*Innenkörper*). There is transverse striation of the muscular layer throughout. At one-seventh of the length from the head there is a break which denotes the nerve ring (nr) and one-fifth of the length there is a triangular V-shaped patch, demonstrated by light staining with dilute haematoxylin, known as 'anterior V-spot', or the excretory pore and excretory cell (ep and ec). A short distance from the tail a second pore represents the anus, cloaca or terminal part of the primitive alimentary canal and is known as the 'posterior V-spot'. Deeply staining cells are known as genital cells (g¹–g⁴) (Fig. II.65). When stained, the body of the embryo is seen to be composed of closely packed cells and, by focusing when the movements of the living microfilaria have subsided, the head appears to be covered by a delicate prepuce. A short fang is from time to time shot out from the uncovered cephalic end and suddenly retracted.

Microfilariae pass with difficulty through the per-

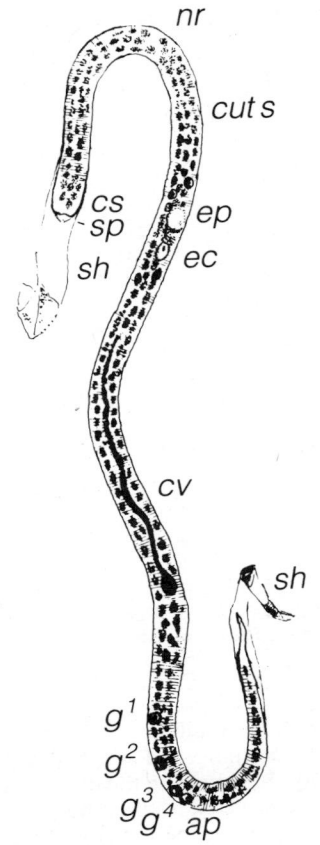

Fig. II.65 Morphology of microfilaria of *Wuchereria bancrofti*.

ap	anal pore	ep	excretory pore
cs	cephalic space	g¹–g⁴	'genital cells' of
cuts	cuticular striations		Rodenwaldt
cv	central viscus	nr	nerve ring
ec	excretory cell	sh	sheath
		sp	spicule and prepuce

ipheral capillaries and they are less active in day than in night blood. They are capable of movement and of transit from place to place.

Periodicity (Fig. II.66)

Microfilariae of *W. bancrofti* exhibit a nocturnal periodicity in certain parts of the world, in the West Indies, South America, North, West and East Africa, China, Indonesia, Papua New Guinea and Melanesia, i.e. they are present in peripheral blood in larger numbers during the night than during the day. The maximum concentration is from 22.00 to 02.00 hours. It appeared to Manson that this nocturnal periodicity was an adaptation to the habits of night-biting mosquitoes—*Culex quinquefasciatus, C. pipiens* and certain

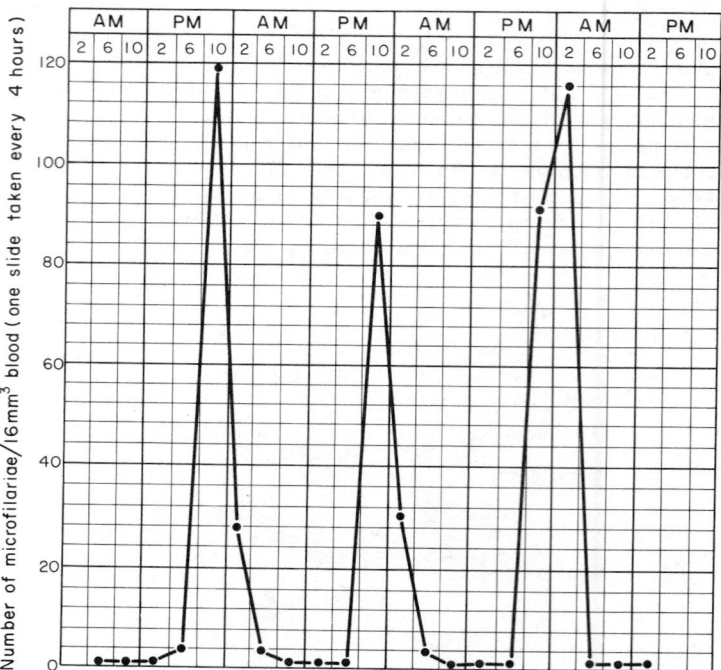

Fig. II.66 Filariasis due to *Wuchereria bancrofti*, showing the nocturnal periodicity.

Anophelines. The numbers of the microfilariae are influenced by sleeping and respond to waking and bodily activity. By reversing the hours of sleeping and waking the periodicity is disturbed for 3 days and then reversed to diurnal periodicity. Periodicity can be easily converted by a change in the rhythm of day and night and was found in emigrants from Okinawa (127° 40′ east, 28° 30′ north) to Bolivia (63° 30′ west, 17° 50′ south) to take 116 days.[12] Observations on microfilariae of animals (*Dirofilaria repens* of dog, filaria of American crow and that of Malayan monkey, *Macaca speciosa*) show that they also maintain nocturnal periodicity and reversal is easily established. Periodicity is probably a quality inherent in the microfilaria itself and persists unchanged in transfused blood. This was demonstrated in a patient injected with blood containing microfilariae and in whom a nocturnal periodicity was maintained for 14 days.

Many years ago Manson had an opportunity of ascertaining that during their diurnal absence from the peripheral circulation the microfilariae retire principally to the larger arteries and to the lungs where, during the daytime, they may be found in enormous numbers. Two mechanisms for periodicity have been suggested, alteration in oxygen tension of the blood and phototaxis on the part of the microfilariae.

Considerable light has been shed upon the mechanism of periodicity in general by the discovery of a non-sheathed microfilaria in a monkey (*Macaca speciosa*). In the animal, as in man, the curve of microfilarial density in the venous blood follows closely that of the capillary blood. An increase of microfilariae in the blood at night is due to the periodic liberation from accumulations in the small blood vessels of the lungs.

McFadzean and Hawking[13] proved that the microfilariae of *W. bancrofti* are affected by the oxygen concentration in inspired air and by muscular exercise. The periodicity of *W. bancrofti* and *B. malayi* may depend on changes in the difference of oxygen tension between venous and arterial blood by day and night. During the daytime the microfilariae accumulate in the lungs where the oxygen tension is high. They manage to hold themselves in the pulmonary capillaries by some force which is increased by the rise in the oxygen tension and decreased by its fall. This force seems to be switched on and off every 12 hours by some unknown mechanism inside the microfilariae.[14] A curious agglutinative phenomenon has been described on the injection of anticoagulant (heparin) to the drawn blood. Intravenous injection of this substance during daytime releases microfilariae of *W. bancrofti* into the peripheral blood for a short period. It is presumed that microfilariae gather together in the capillaries and other vessels of the lung during their absence from the peripheral blood by the power of agglutination and thigmotaxis. A different mechanism for periodicity has been suggested,[12] in which the microfilariae possess a photosensitive substance containing a vitamin-A-like carotenoid similar to visual pigments in fluorescent granules in the epidermis which causes them to leave the peripheral circulation in daylight and collect in the lungs. Periodic microfilariae possess numerous granules in contrast to subperiodic and aperiodic forms which have few or none.

A general anaesthetic does not affect the periodicity of *W. bancrofti* but markedly reduces the numbers of *L. loa* microfilariae in the peripheral blood.[14]

Formerly it was thought that nocturnal periodicity was uniformly observed by the microfilariae of *W. bancrofti* the world over but in 1896 it was remarked that in Tonga and Fiji the microfilariae were abundant in the blood both by day and by night; those in the western Pacific, the Solomon Islands, Papua New Guinea and Bismarck Archipelago are nocturnally periodic but in New Caledonia the microfilariae are non-periodic. The demarcating line between the two (Buxton's line) lies in longitude 170° east and this also coincides with the distribution of malaria. On the west of this line there are *Anopheles* and malaria, on the east there is neither. It was originally demonstrated that in Indian and Solomon Island immigrants in Fiji these microfilariae maintain their nocturnal periodicity amongst the non-periodic Fijians but, if they and the Europeans also contract the infection in Fiji, the microfilariae are non-periodic. An attempt was made to explain this anomaly by the day-biting habits of the mosquito intermediaries, *Aedes scutellans pseudo-scutellaris* and *Ae. s. polynesiensis* which have a regional distribution in the Pacific corresponding to that of the non-periodic filariae. As the microfilariae remain true to type after transfusion it was suggested that they are

the progeny of a parent distinct from *W. bancrofti*: this has been named *W. bancrofti* var. *pacifica*. The microfilariae of both varieties are morphologically indistinguishable. The non-periodic Pacific type in Fiji differs from that of periodic African *W. bancrofti* in that increased oxygen content of the blood brings about a *slight rise* of the microfilarial counts.

Periodicity is a biological rhythm inherent in the microfilariae but influenced by the rhythm of the host, which itself is influenced by the changes in body temperature which occur every 24 hours.

The two forms of *B. malayi* from Malaysia exhibit different periodicities which correspond with the biting habits of their chief vectors. Therefore attempts have been made to see whether it is possible to change periodicity by feeding mosquitoes by day on a nocturnal periodic infection and transmitting the few filarial larvae which develop in them to experimental animals. Thus when a human infection was transmitted to a cat it was found that the nocturnally periodic microfilariae became semiperiodic. By altering the feeding time and selective breeding of mosquitoes, successive transmission experiments have shown that it is possible to change the periodicity of the mosquito–filarial complex in a relatively small number of generations.

Life-cycle (Fig. II.67)

The life-cycle was first worked out by Manson in *Culex quinquefasciatus* in China in 1878. Within one

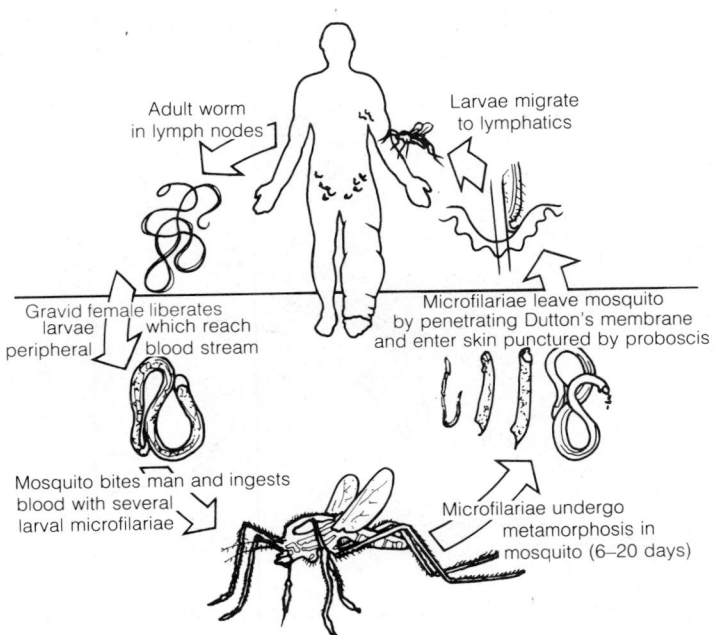

Filaria
Wuchereria bancrofti

Adult worm in lymph nodes

Larvae migrate to lymphatics

Gravid female liberates larvae which reach peripheral blood stream

Microfilariae leave mosquito by penetrating Dutton's membrane and enter skin punctured by proboscis

Mosquito bites man and ingests blood with several larval microfilariae

Microfilariae undergo metamorphosis in mosquito (6–20 days)

Fig. II.67 Life-cycle of lymphatic filaria (*Wuchereria bancrofti*).

hour of entering the mosquito's stomach the microfilariae cast the sheaths and bore through the stomach wall. At this stage the microfilariae may be damaged by the buccopharyngeal armature of the mosquito which may explain the differing infection rates of these vectors.[15] At the end of an infective feed the embryos collect at the anterior end of the stomach and then enter the anterior cylindrical portion of the midgut. Forward transportation is effected by reversed peristalsis until they are distributed over the whole of this cylinder. At the end of 16 hours they form a writhing mass behind the valve which prevents their progress into the foregut. The proboscis of the mosquito exerts positive chemotaxis upon microfilariae. Therefore vector female mosquitoes can abstract more embryos than would be present in a similar quantity of circulating blood. The mosquito abstracts 1 mm^3 of blood at each feed and, in so doing, concentrates the embryos tenfold. They next enter the thorax where they lie between the muscular fibres of the indirect or fibrillar flight muscle of the thorax and pharyngeal muscle of the head of the mosquito[16] (Fig. II.68). Within 2 days they increase in girth, the 'posterior V-spot' (or anal pore) enlarges and the excretory vesicle becomes more prominent. By rapid nuclear proliferation the larval filaria now assumes a squat 'sausage' form, the tail shrinks and is then absorbed (Fig. II.69). Mouth and oesophagus are apparent from the fifth day onwards. The g^2 and g^3 cells (Fig. II.65) divide several times and give rise to a column of cells which form the midintestine (large gut). The posterior intestine (rectum) is formed from four cells derived from the g^4 cell. The genital primordium is formed from the g^1 cell.

When the larva is 0.5 mm in length a bulbar oesophagus appears at the first and second fourths of the

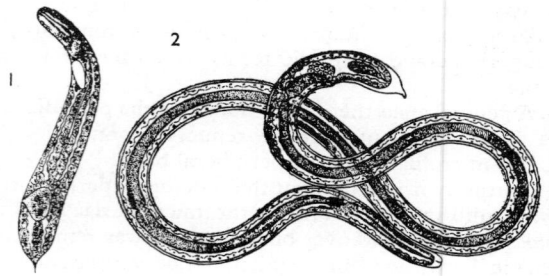

Fig. II.69 Stages of the larval forms of *Wuchereria bancrofti* from the thoracic muscles of *Culex quinquefasciatus*. × 150.

alimentary canal. Now elongated and worm-like the larva moves sluggishly about. Three caudal papillae develop which function in progression and facilitate penetration of human skin (Fig. II.70). About the tenth day (in favourable circumstances) the larval filaria, 1.4 mm long, travels forward into the head of

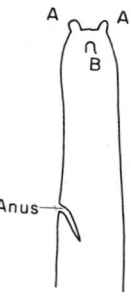

Fig. II.70 Larval filaria from the proboscis sheath of *Aedes pseudoscutellaris*. A, Terminal papilla. B, Postanal papilla.

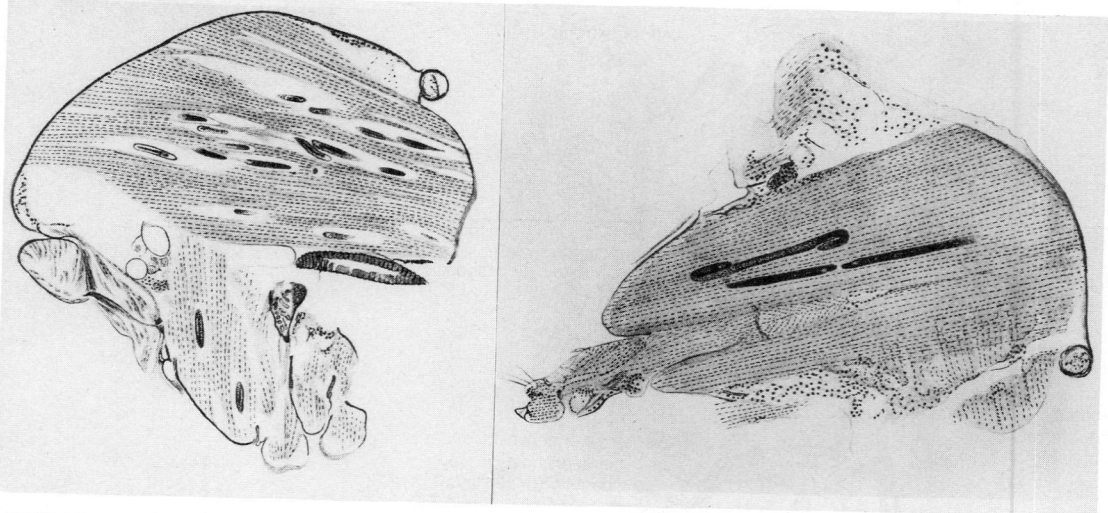

Fig. II.68 Section of the thoracic muscles of *Aedes pseudoscutellaris*. *Left,* The second day after feeding on a filaraemic patient. *Right,* The second week after feeding on a filaraemic patient.

the mosquito where it coils up and enters the proboscis sheath (Fig. II.71), but occasionally it may penetrate into the abdominal cavity and legs. Two or more ecdyses take place. At high temperatures and in moisture the complete cycle occupies 10–14 days but it is retarded to six weeks by cold. Sometimes the larvae die in the thoracic muscles and are enclosed in chitin producing a curious mummy-like structure. When an infected mosquito bites man, the larvae, attracted by warmth, break through the terminal portion of the proboscis sheath at the ligula at the central point of 'Dutton's membrane', wriggle out on to the skin, which they penetrate near the seat of the puncture caused by the stylets of the mosquito. A list of vectors is given in Table III.5, p. 1407.

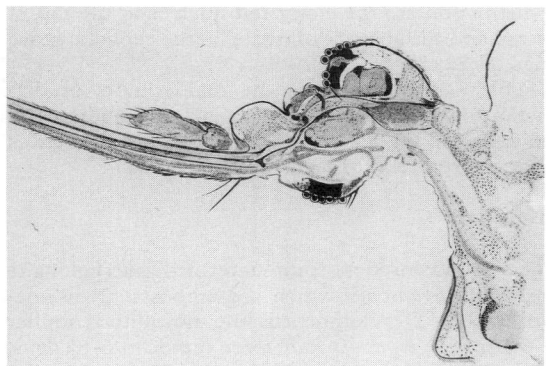

Fig. II.71 *Wuchereria bancrofti* in the head and proboscis of the mosquito.

In the human host the infective larvae pass through the peripheral blood vessels to the lymphatics where they become mature in an estimated period of three months to one year. Man is the only known definitive host.

In view of the fact that considerable confusion has been caused in recent years by the discovery of larval filariae in wild-caught mosquitoes, in the course of surveys upon the natural infection rate, it has become necessary to differentiate between the larval characters of human and allied species of animal origin. It has to be realized that the filariae of some animals, fruit bats and birds develop in those species of mosquitoes which normally transmit human filariasis.

The infective larva of *B. malayi* is 1–2 mm in length and has three poorly defined caudal papillae; that of *B. patei* is about the same length and has a marked dorsal protuberance resembling a dog's head, in lateral position. The larva of *Dirofilaria corynodes* of monkeys (*Cercopithecus* and *Colobus*) from *Aedes pembaensis* has the typical cigar-shaped tail but less pronounced narrowing between the anus and the extremity, with three small papillae. The larva of *D. repens* of the dog and cat resembles the foregoing but with only one terminal

papilla: it develops in *Aedes aegypti*, *Ae. pembaensis* and *Mansonia africanus;* that of *D. immitis* of the dog, from *Ae. aegypti* and *Culex quinquefasciatus*, cannot be distinguished from that of *D. repens*. The larva of *Setaria equina* of the horse, mule and donkey in *Ae. aegypti*, *Ae. pembaensis* and *Culex quinquefasciatus* is about the same length but can easily be distinguished by one large terminal papilla and two subterminal ones, looking like little ears. Distinguishing features are illustrated in a key by Nelson.[17]

Wuchereria bancrofti var. *pacifica*
(Manson-Bahr, 1941)

It has been suggested that the filaria found in the central and southern Pacific might be a separate species. As far as can be ascertained, embryos (microfilariae) are morphologically identical with those of *W. bancrofti*. Certain small differences have been noted in the adult morphology. The average length is smaller—females 58 mm, males 27 mm. The tail of the female lacks the bulbous swelling which characterizes those from Guyana. The anterior end of the Fijian specimens is oval in outline.

Microfilariae in Polynesians (Fiji, Samoa, Tonga, Cook Islands, New Caledonia) are non-periodic. In these islands as well as in Tokelau, Wallis, Ellice, Gilberts, Marquesas and those beyond 'Buxton's line' (longitude 170° east) they do not exhibit nocturnal periodicity but occur in equal numbers in the blood by day and night. Development of this filaria is confined to mosquitoes indigenous to the South Pacific islands of the *Aedes kochi*, *Ae. vigilax* and *Ae. scutellaris* groups which are adapted to coconut palms and bite by day (see Table III.3). The non-periodic microfilaria does not develop readily in *C. quinquefasciatus* which is the optimum host for the nocturnal periodic *W. bancrofti*.

GENUS: *Brugia* (Buckley, 1959)

The genus *Brugia* contains nine representatives: *B. malayi*, *B. pahangi*, *B. patei*, *B. beaveri*, *B. buckleyi*, *B. ceylonensis*, *B. guyanensis*, *B. tupiae* and *B. timori*.[18]

Brugia malayi (Brug, 1927;
Rao & Maplestone, 1940)

Distribution

This is the common form in Malaysia, Indonesia, Timor, central India, Sri Lanka, south China, Korea, Indo-China and Koshima Island (Japan). It has not been found in Africa, America, Australia or the Pacific Islands. *B. timori* is found in Timor and islands in south-east Indonesia (Sunda group).

Characters

The adults are practically identical with *W. bancrofti*

in nearly all characters; the females are indistinguishable. The female measures 55 mm in length by 160 μm. The vulva is situated 0.92 mm from the anterior extremity. The caudal end is bluntly rounded. The male is 22–23 mm in length by 88 μm in diameter. The posterior extremity has about three turns and the anus is 0.1–0.14 mm from the tip of the tail. One pair of large papillae are just in front of the cloaca and one behind. There are also two smaller pairs. There is a small naviculate gubernaculum and two spicules which are unlike in size and structure: the longer is 0.34–0.36 mm: the shorter 0.11–0.12 mm in length. There are morphological differences in the microfilariae and the mosquito intermediary is distinct—*Mansonia annulifera*. It is identical with the microfilaria of the 'kra' monkey (*Macaca irus*) which is transmitted by the same mosquitoes. It is common in domestic dogs and cats in Malaysia and has been found also in the slow loris (*Nycticebus coucang*), the banded leaf monkey (*Presbytis melalophos*) as well as in the pangolin (*Manis javanica*).

The microfilaria of *B. malayi* was first discovered by Lichtenstein in Celebes and was studied further by Brug in 1927. Brug and de Rook found natural infection in the mosquitoes, *Mansonia longipalpis* (also known as *dives*) and *M. annulata*.

Although the human form of *B. malayi* is common in dogs and cats in Malaysia and Indonesia, yet there is a species, *B. pahangi*, which is confined to these animals and which has distinctive morphological characters.

The human form of *B. malayi* can be transmitted to cats by the bite of *Mansonia longipalpis*. The period of full development of the adult filaria in this animal is about 65 days before microfilariae appear in the blood. The adult forms recovered from the cat correspond to the descriptions of *B. malayi* in man. *B. patei* microfilariae have been found in cats in Orissa, India, and in dogs and genet cats in Pate Island, Kenya. The nocturnal periodic form in Malaysia does not develop well in cats and is transmitted by species of *Anopheles* and *Mansonia*. A semiperiodic form occurs in man and commonly in cats, in freshwater swamps and forest. It is transmitted by *Mansonia annulata* and *M. uniformis*.

Microfilaria malayi has a nocturnal periodicity like that of *W. bancrofti* or may be semiperiodic. It is nocturnal on the west coast of the Malaysia peninsula but non-periodic in the Huantan district on the east coast. It measures 200–250 × 5–6 μm. Its chief points of distinction are the elongated nucleus at the top of the tail and the absence of nuclei in the cephalic space (Figs. II.72 and II.73,3).

Table II.8 summarizes the main points of distinction between microfilaria malayi and microfilaria bancrofti and Fig. II.73 with key shows the differences of the microfilariae of medical importance.

Life-cycle

The most favoured mosquito intermediaries belong to the genus *Mansonia* which are crepuscular or nocturnal feeds. Development in the mosquito is similar to that of *W. bancrofti* but more rapid, in 6–8½ days. Difficulties have been encountered in Malaysia in distinguishing larval forms of ornithofilariae of birds from those of human *B. malayi* in the routine dissection of mosquitoes.

The larval forms of *B. malayi* in *Mansonia* undergo two ecdyses. The buccal cavity is formed from the cephalic space; the oesophagus from the nuclei of the anterior part of the nuclear column; the rectum and anus from the four G cells of Rodenwaldt and the anal pore. The premature genital pore mass is derived from the nuclei of the *Innenkörper* and the muscles of the body wall from the 'subcuticular cells' of Rodenwaldt. The tail of the microfilaria, with its two nuclei (terminal nucleus in the tail—Fig. II.74), is shed with the first moult. As in the case of *W. bancrofti*, the larva, when in the thoracic muscles, feeds by absorbing food through the cuticle. It does not feed at the expense of these muscles as has been stated.

Brugia timori (David & Edeson, 1964)

The adult male *B. timori* differs from other *Brugia* spp. (except *B. malayi*) in having a spicular ratio of 3:1; it differs from *B. malayi* in having greater numbers of subventral adanal papillae (up to five on each side) that are loosely spaced and irregularly positioned about the cloaca, a greater diameter of the capitulum of the left spicule and greater length of the proximal section of the right spicule. The adult female

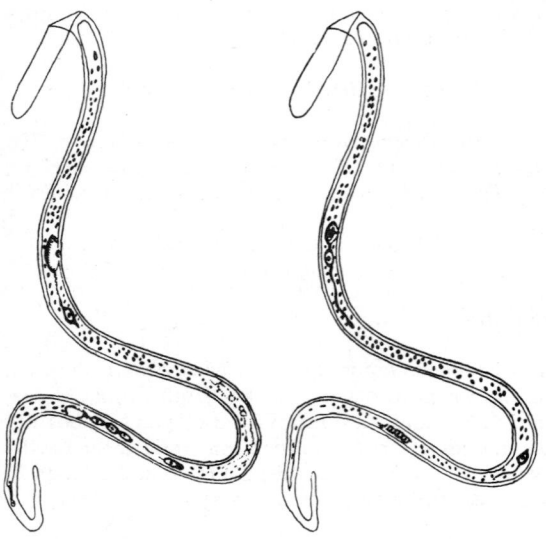

Fig. II.72 Comparative morphology of the microfilariae of *W. bancrofti* (left) and *B. malayi* (right).

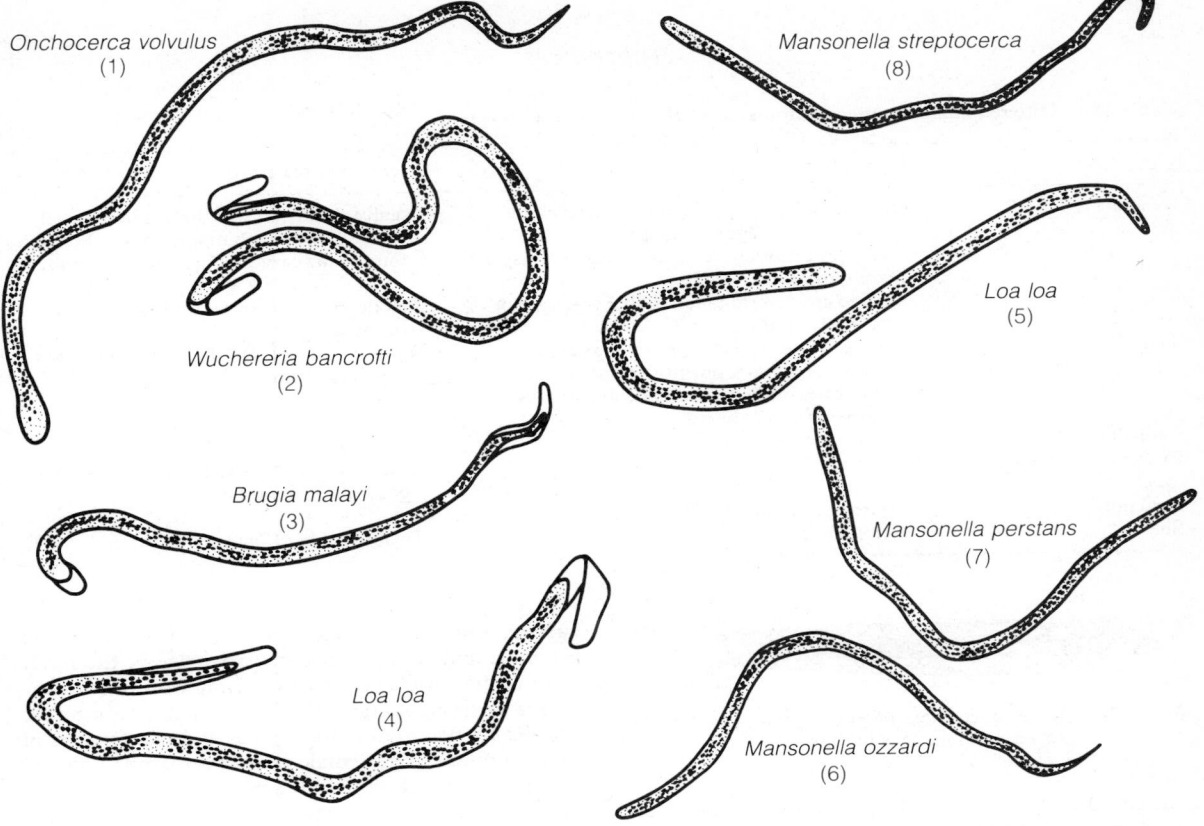

Onchocerca volvulus (1)

Mansonella streptocerca (8)

Wuchereria bancrofti (2)

Loa loa (5)

Brugia malayi (3)

Mansonella perstans (7)

Loa loa (4)

Mansonella ozzardi (6)

Fig. II.73 Microfilariae of medical importance. (Courtesy Professor D. A. Denham.)

Key to microfilariae found in human blood

Method 1. After staining with Mayer's haemalum

1(a)   Sheath present—*W. bancrofti*
  (b)   Sheath absent—*Loa loa* (5)
2(a)   Nuclei to tip of tail—*B. malayi*
  (b)   Nuclei not in tip of tail—*W. bancrofti*

3(a)   Two isolated nuclei in tail—*B. malayi*
  (b)   Solid column of nuclei in tail—*Loa loa* (4)
4(a)   Sheath loosely applied, worm over 250 μm long—*Loa loa* (4)
  (b)   Sheath very small, worm under 250 μm long—*Meningonema peruzzi*
5(a)   More than 275 μm in length—*M. ozzardi*

  (b)   Less than 250 μm in length—*M. perstans*

6(a)   Cephalic space longer than twice width of body—*O. volvulus*
  (b)   Cephalic space about width of body—*W. bancrofti* (with no sheath)
7(a)   Nuclei to tip of tail—*M. streptocerca*
  (b)   Nuclei not to tip of tail—*M. ozzardi*

8(a)   Tail straight with prominent terminal nucleus—*Dipetalonema perstans*
  (b)   Tail bent into crook shape—*Dipetalonema streptocerca*

Method 2. After staining with Giemsa

1(a)   Sheath present—*W. bancrofti*
  (b)   Sheath absent—*B. malayi*
2(a)   Sheath stained red, nuclei in tip of tail—*Brugia* spp.
  (b)   Sheath stained pale mauve, no nuclei in tip of tail—*W. bancrofti*

3(a)   Nuclei not extending to tip of tail—*Loa loa* (4)
  (b)   Nuclei to tip of tail—*M. ozzardi*
4(a)   Microfilariae about 300 μm long—*Loa loa* (5)

  (b)   Microfilariae 200–225 μm long—*M. ozzardi*

5(a)   Cephalic space more than 1½ times diameter of head—*O. volvulus*
  (b)   Cephalic space less than or equal to diameter of head—*W. bancrofti* (with no sheath)
6(a)   Microfilariae at least 260 μm long—*M. perstans*

  (b)   Microfilariae 200–225 μm long—*M. streptocerca*

7(a)   Tail with complete column of microfilariae—*Loa loa*
  (b)   Tail with two isolated nuclei—*Brugia* (with no sheath)
8(a)   Tail with prominent terminal nucleus—*Dipetalonema perstans*
  (b)   Tail with crook-shaped bend—*Dipetalonema streptocerca*

Notes 1 The sheath of *Loa loa* does not stain with Giemsa.
    2 While *O. volvulus* is normally in the skin appreciable numbers can be found in the blood.
    3 *B. malayi* periodic strain usually loses its sheath in blood smears.
    4 Any sheathed microfilaria may lose its sheath.
    5 The part of the tail of *M. ozzardi* which is free of nuclei is very fine and may not stain but there is no large terminal nucleus as in *D. perstans*.

Table II.8 Differentiation between microfilariae of *B. malayi* and *W. bancrofti*.

	Microfilaria malayi	Microfilaria bancrofti
General	Often found closely folded with head close to tail, and irregularly disposed for, besides major curves, minor angulations are typical	Usually seen lying with head and tail well separated, and commonly shows three or four major curves of graceful appearance
Nuclei	Blurred and intermingled so that they cannot be easily counted	Well defined and spaced and can easily be counted
Tail	Tapers to a fine point, continues as a fine thread. *Typically* one nucleus at the extremity of the tapered portion and two in the terminal thread	Tapers to a point and the terminal portion contains no nuclei
Cephalic space	Twice as long as broad	As long as broad
Excretory pore and cell	Separated	Close together. A thread of protoplasm runs posteriorly from the latter
Anal pore	Clear space about 40 μm from the tail end	
Sheath	Well stained	Hardly visible

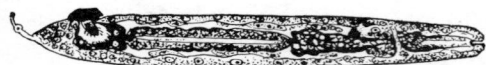

Fig. II.74 Development stage of *Brugia malayi* showing the terminal nucleus in the tail.

has an ovejector of greater length and width than that of *B. malayi*. Microfilariae typical of the Timor type have a greater length than other *Brugia* spp., length to width cephalic space ratio of 3 : 1 and a sheath which does not stain bright pink with Giemsa.[19] The vector is *Anopheles barbirostris*.

Fig. II.75 shows the differences between *Wuchereria* and *Brugia* forms of filaria.

GENUS: *Onchocerca*

Onchocerca volvulus (Leuckart, 1893) Railliet & Henry, 1910

Characters

The body is white and filiform, tapering at both ends. The head is rounded. The cuticle is marked by transverse ridges and raised with prominent angular and oblique thickenings, more distinct posteriorly. It is usually found in nodules but can reproduce outside them (Fig. 20.17). The male (2–4 cm × 0.2 mm) has a straight alimentary canal ending in a subterminal anus. The tail ends in a slight spiral and is bulbous at the tip. There are two pairs of preanal, two postanal, an intermediate large papilla, and two unequal spicules (82 μm, 77 μm) protruding from the cloaca (Fig. II.76); the former has a fluted end and the latter a narrow neck and knob. The female normally measures 60–70 cm × 0.4 mm but is often smaller, 35–40 cm. The head is round and truncated (0.04 mm), the vulva 0.85 mm from the anterior extremity and the tail

curved. Cuticular striations are not so marked as in the male and the presence of two striae in the inner layer of the cuticle is a distinguishing feature of onchocerca in tissue sections.[20] Usually males outnumber females by two to one (four males and two females in each tumour). The female is ovoviviparous and the egg has a striated shell with a pointed process at each pole (like an orange wrapped in tissue paper) measuring 30–50 μm in diameter. The microfilariae (300 × 8 μm) are sheathless and are found in the fluid of the nodule cavity and in the surrounding skin. The body tapers from the last fifth and ends in a sharply pointed, recurved tail (Fig. II.73,1). In the anterior fifth is a marked anterior V-spot. The cephalic cone is thickened at the commencement of the nuclear column. This microfilaria is non-periodic; it is found in skin in the femoral, inguinal and cervical lymph glands and in the expressed juice of tumours but sometimes in blood (2%) and also in urine. It is also present in the skin of widely separated portions of the body in apparently healthy people, without producing any nodules or tumours. Microfilariae are easily demonstrated in the skin by biopsy. They are often associated with eye symptoms in the absence of tumours and, by aid of the slit lamp, may be seen in the cornea.

Life-cycle

This was worked out in Sierra Leone. Development takes place in a 'black fly' or 'buffalo gnat' *Simulium damnosum* (*sensulatum*) in Africa and others in South and Central America (see Appendix III). The fly abstracts microfilariae from the deeper layers of the skin; they then enter the stomach, pierce its walls and pass to the thoracic muscles where they undergo further development. During growth two moults take place. At the seventh day the larva measures 0.65 mm. Development has been traced to the tenth day when the larva escapes from the proboscis; *Simulium* is a

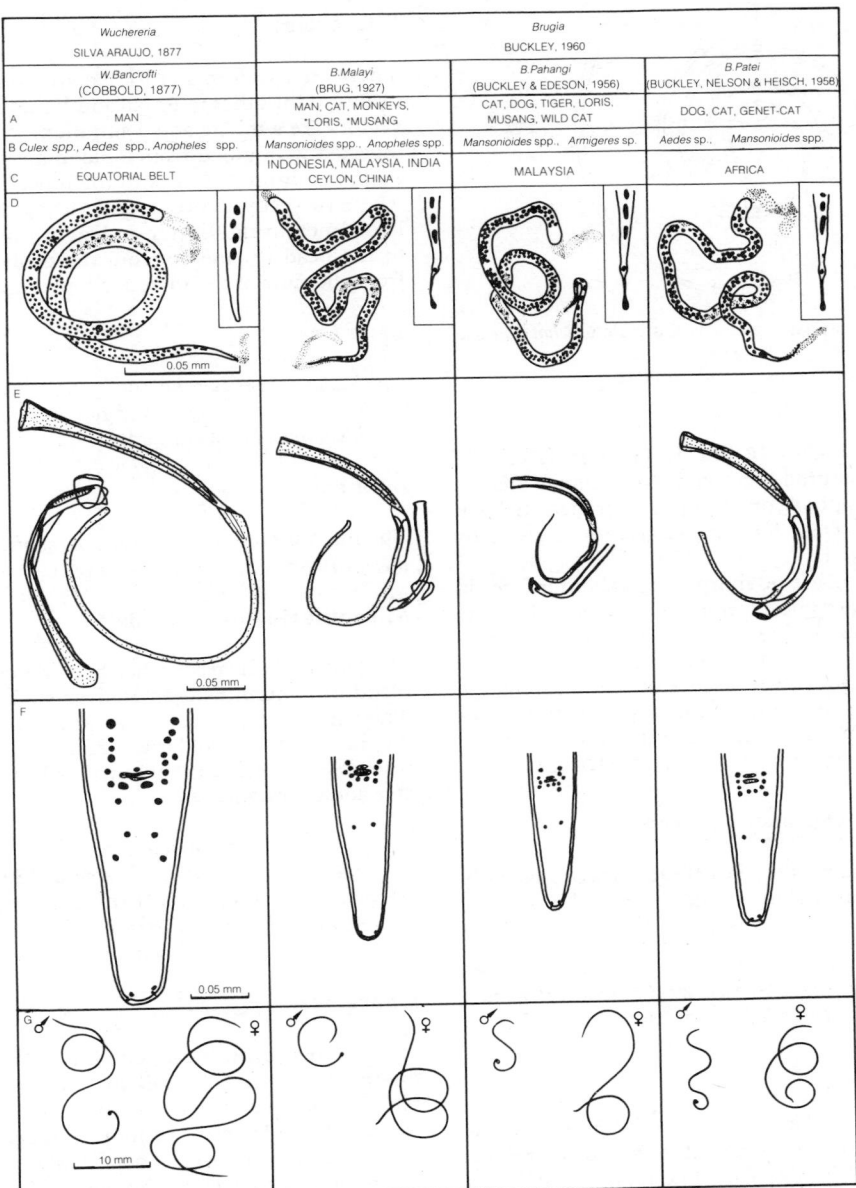

Wuchereria SILVA ARAUJO, 1877	*Brugia* BUCKLEY, 1960		
W.Bancrofti (COBBOLD, 1877)	*B.Malayi* (BRUG, 1927)	*B.Pahangi* (BUCKLEY & EDESON, 1956)	*B.Patei* (BUCKLEY, NELSON & HEISCH, 1958)
A MAN	MAN, CAT, MONKEYS, *LORIS, *MUSANG	CAT, DOG, TIGER, LORIS, MUSANG, WILD CAT	DOG, CAT, GENET-CAT
B *Culex* spp., *Aedes* spp., *Anopheles* spp.	*Mansonioides* spp., *Anopheles* spp.	*Mansonioides* spp., *Armigeres* sp.	*Aedes* sp., *Mansonioides* spp.
C EQUATORIAL BELT	INDONESIA, MALAYSIA, INDIA CEYLON, CHINA	MALAYSIA	AFRICA

Fig. II.75 The morphological distinctions between the genera *Wuchereria* and *Brugia*. A, Definitive hosts. B, Intermediate hosts. C, Geographical distribution. D, Microfilariae and (inset) tail nuclei of microfilariae. E, Spicules of male, lateral view. F, Tails of males, ventral view. G, Adult worms, actual size. * indicates experimental infection only. (After Bradley; by permission of *Annals of Tropical Medicine and Parasitology*.)

day-biting fly (06.00 to 18.00 hours) and 2.6% may be naturally infected. They probably attract and then abstract microfilariae by scraping the skin with their prestomal teeth.

In the South American form development is similar to that of the central African but occurs in *Simulium metallicum* (*avidum*), *S. ochraceum* and *S. callidum* (*mooseri*), which are common in endemic areas in Central America and other vectors in South American foci. Developing larvae are frequently found in the abdomen and malpighian tubules of these flies. Two caudal papillae are seen in fully developed larvae,

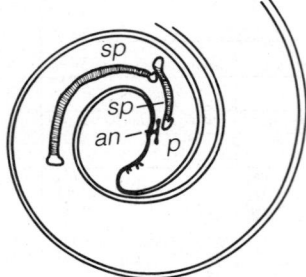

Fig. II.76   The caudal extremity of a male *Onchocerca vol-vulus*.
sp spicules   an anus   p papillae

which measure 0.45–1.14 mm. In Guatemala 11% of *Simulium* are naturally infected. Non-human filariae can occur in *Simulium*, and a key to their identification and distinction from human *Onchocerca* is given by Nelson and Pester.[21]

Although there are no morphological differences in the various geographical forms of *Onchocerca* there are at least six different *Onchocerca–Simulium* complexes which have their own clinical and biological attributes. Enzyme staining for the presence of acid phosphatase was found to show four distinct patterns in microfilariae from West Africa suggesting that a number of biological strains did exist in West Africa.[22]

Onchocerca gutturosa

O. gutturosa is a parasite of cattle and has occasionally been found to cause skin nodules in man.[23]

GENUS: *Mansonella*
Mansonella ozzardi (Faust, 1929) (*Tetrapetalonema* Faust, 1935 (*Filaria ozzardi* Manson, 1897)

Morphology[24]

The male is 24–28.4 mm long × 0.07–0.08 mm diameter. It is coiled in one and a half to two turns and has two spicules and caudal alae. The female is twice as long, 32.2–61.5 mm × 0.13–0.16 mm in diameter and has a vulva 0.76 mm from the caudal extremity. The vagina leads to paired uteri filling the body cavity with highly coiled ovaries in the posterior part of the body. The adult worms live in body cavities embedded in adipose tissues and in the mesentery. The microfilariae, which are unsheathed, are 207–232 μm long × 3–4 μm in diameter. The anterior end is round and they have an attenuated tail resembling *M. per-stans* but pointed and ending in a hook (Fig. II.73,6).

Transfusion experiments have shown that they can live in the blood of the recipient for more than two years.

Life-cycle

There are two forms of *M. ozzardi*, one in the Caribbean and the other in Brazil and Venezuela. The insect vectors are a midge and a simulium. Microfilariae are ingested with blood from a blood meal and the larvae migrate within 24 hours to the muscles of the thorax where two ecdyses occur, and the third stage infective larva, measuring 0.7 mm in length, migrates forward to the head to emerge from the proboscis in 8 days from the time of the infective blood meal.

In the Caribbean

Culicoides furens is a vector in St Vincent and Haiti, *C. paraensis* in Antigua and northern Argentina, and *C. phlebotomus* in Trinidad.

In Brazil

The main vector is *Simulium amazonicum* but *Culico-ides insinuatus* may also play a part.

Microfilaria bolivarensis[25]

Microfilaria bolivarensis has been described from the blood of Amerindians in Bolivar state in Venezuela. The microfilaria measures 256–300 × 7–8 μm and differs from microfilaria ozzardi. It superficially resembles microfilaria volvulus but has a greater diameter and a straighter tail.

Mansonella perstans
Dipetalonema perstans (Manson, 1891) Railliet,
Henry & Langeron, 1912 (*Filaria perstans,*
Acanthocheilonema perstans, Tetrapetalonema
perstans)

Characters

It has a long cylindrical, smooth body and a simple, unarmed mouth. The tail in both sexes is characteristic: incurvated, with a chitinous covering at the extreme tip split into two minute appendages, giving a mitred appearance. The female possesses four cuticular appendages at the posterior extremity, not two as hitherto believed. The male (4.5 cm × 0.06 mm) is smaller than the female. The head is 0.04 mm in diameter and the cloaca has four pairs of preanal and one pair of postanal papillae, and two unequal spicules (Fig. II.77). The female (7–8 cm × 0.12 mm) has a club-shaped head 0.07 mm in diameter, and a vulva situated 1.2 mm from the head. The anus opens at the apex of a papilla in the concavity of the curve formed by the tail; its diameter is 0.02 mm.

The microfilaria (200 × 4.5 μm) is unsheathed (Fig. II.73,7). It possesses in a remarkable degree the power of elongation and contraction. Therefore the measurements vary considerably. Long and short forms (90–

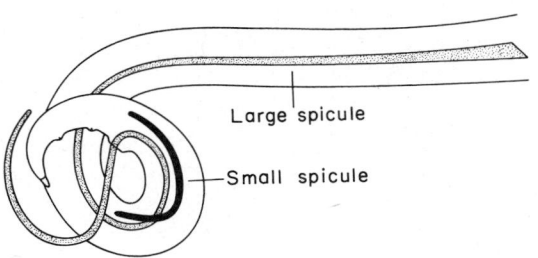

Fig. II.77 The tail of *Mansonella perstans,* showing two unequal spicules and papillae. (After Leiper.)

110 × 4 μm) have been described. It is smaller than microfilaria bancrofti or loa and its caudal end is truncated and abruptly rounded (Fig. II.78). The tapering tail extends two-thirds of the entire length. The anterior 'V-spot' is 30 μm from the anterior extremity. There is no marked tail spot, no central granular mass, and no cephalic prepuce. It moves freely in the blood.

The embryos occur in equal numbers both by day and night; according to the self-inflicted experiment of Gönnert this embryo can persist in the recipient three years after blood transfusion.

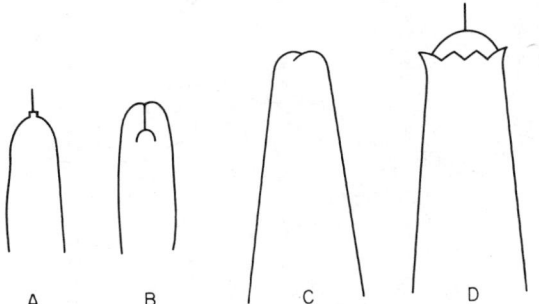

Fig. II.78 Structure of the head of microfilaria perstans (A, B) and microfilaria bancrofti (C, D).

Life-cycle

The insect vectors are species of *Culicoides.* Microfilariae are ingested and the larvae penetrate the stomach to develop in the thoracic muscles. Within 6–9 days third stage infective larvae 0.7 mm long emerge from the proboscis. Prior to emerging they cause a globular expansion of the labrum which then collapses, allowing the larvae to escape. There is confusion over the identity of the vector in Africa; originally it was described as *C. austeni* but it is more likely that *C. inornatipennis* and possibly *C. grahami* are the vectors. Transmission takes place at night.

Mansonella streptocerca
(Dipetalonema streptocerca) Macfie &
Corson, 1922)
Agamofilaria streptocerca (Macfie &
Corson, 1922)
(Acanthocheilonema streptocerca) (Stiles & Hassal,
1926)

This sheathless microfilaria is found commonly in the corium of the skin but not in the blood of people in Ghana (22 out of 50 in Accra). It has a wide distribution especially in Cameroon and other West African countries.

The microfilaria (Figs. II.79 and II.73,8) is 215 μm in length and is distinguished by the 'walking stick handle' of the tail extremity and an arrangement of nuclei in the head, and four prominent ones in the tail which has a bifid end[26] which distinguishes it from the microfilariae of *O. volvulus* and *M. perstans.*

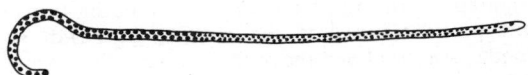

Fig. II.79 Microfilaria of *Mansonella streptocerca,* showing the characteristic curvature of the tail. × 200.

Life-cycle

The vector is *C. grahami* in which development takes place similar to that in *M. perstans.* Transmission takes place during the day.

Microfilariae were found in the skin of six of 11 chimpanzees (*Pan paniscus* and *P. satyrus*) in Zaire. Two adult female worms found in the connective tissue were closely similar to *M. perstans.* The microfilariae of this species, *D. vanhoofi,* closely resemble those of the latter. The incubation period of *D. streptocerca* is three to four months.

Mansonella berghei
(Tetrapetalonema berghei) (Chardome
& Peel, 1951)

This is found in Zaire together with *M. streptocerca.* It is a white nematode, 60.9 × 0.271 mm, with almost imperceptible striations. The head is hemispherical and a relatively large genital opening is situated anteriorly. The uterus divides into two branches. Microfilariae in all stages are visible in the uterus. There are several enlargements of the body at intervals. The caudal extremity narrows rapidly showing four excrescences. The tail is recurved. The microfilaria which is found in the skin resembles that of a small microfilaria perstans and measures 179 × 3.55 μm. The adult form may turn out to be similar to *M. perstans.*

Meningonema peruzzii (Orihel & Esslinger, 1972)

Adults are found in the subarachnoid space of *Cercopithecus* monkeys trapped in equatorial Guinea. The microfilariae resemble those of *M. perstans* but have an inconspicuous sheath. This worm is the same as that described by Peruzzi in 1928 in monkeys in Uganda and causes cerebral filariasis in Zimbabwe (Chapter 20).

GENUS: *Loa* (eye worm)
Loa loa (Guyot, 1778)

Adult *Loa loa* worms inhabit the subcutaneous connective tissues. Diurnal periodic sheathed microfilariae are shed into the peripheral blood.

Characters

The body is filiform, cylindrical, whitish and semi-transparent with numerous round, smooth, translucent protuberances of the cuticle, 12–16 μm in diameter, and 9–11 μm above the surface. These chitinous bosses are more numerous in females. Their distribution is irregular. In the male they are absent at the extremities; in the female they extend on the tail and also the cephalic end. The mouth is unarmed and destitute of papillae; there is no distinct neck but a shoulder 0.15 mm from the mouth where there are two papillae, one dorsal, the other ventral. The alimentary canal commences at a funnel-shaped mouth as a slender straight oesophagus, going on to an intestine 65 μm wide and a short attenuated rectum. The male (3–3.4 cm × 0.35–0.43 mm) (Fig. II.80) has its

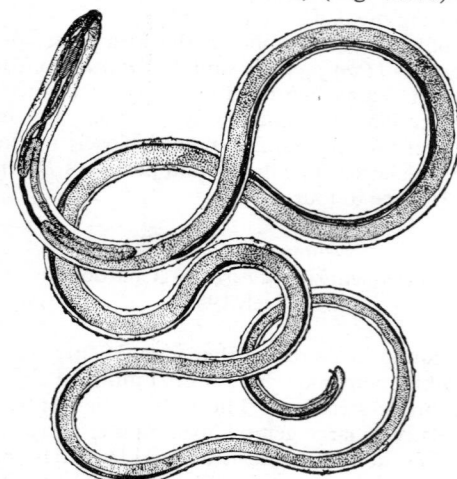

Fig. II.80 Male *Loa loa*. × 10.

maximum breadth anteriorly; posteriorly it tapers to a tail which is curved ventrally with two lateral expansions of the cuticle (0.7 × 0.029 mm) (Fig. II.81b). In the middle, 0.08 mm from the tail-tip is the opening

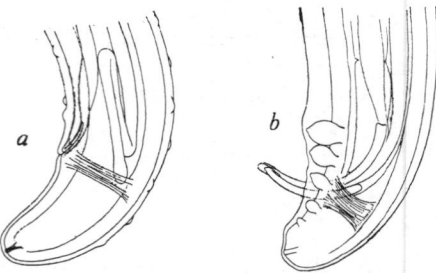

Fig. II.81 Posterior extremity of *Loa loa*. *a* Female. *b*, Male.

of the anogenital orifice with two unequal spicules (123–176 μm and 88–113 μm) surrounded by thick labia. There are four large globular, pedunculated papillae, decreasing in size anteroposteriorly, and a fifth pair of small postanal papillae. The female (5–7 cm × 0.5 mm) (Fig. II.82) has a straight, attenuated,

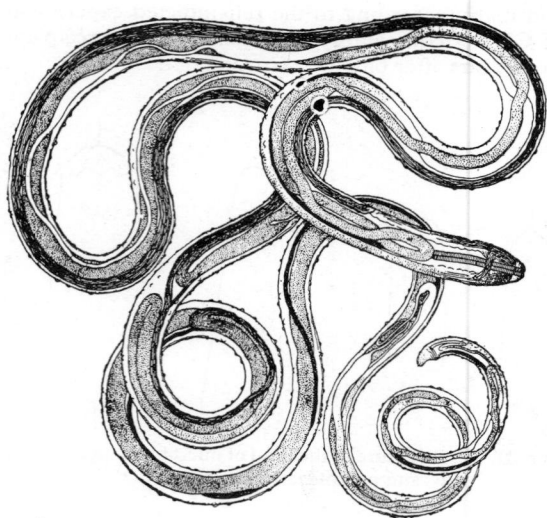

Fig. II.82 Female *Loa loa*. × 10.

broadly rounded posterior extremity and a vulva 2.5 mm from the anterior extremity placed on a small eminence (Fig. II.81a). The vagina, 9 mm long, branches off into long uterine tubes extending through the length of the body. At the narrow end are the ovaries with eggs in all stages. Reproduction is ovoviviparous; the embryos develop within the egg envelope and uncoil themselves on expulsion from the vagina. When dead the adult worm often becomes cretified.

The microfilaria (Fig. II.73,4 and 5) is similar in size (298 × 7.5 μm) and structure to microfilaria bancrofti but its sheath does not stain with Giemsa. In fresh blood it may be impossible to distinguish them.

In dried stained films it assumes a stiff angular attitude, the tail end is disposed in a series of sharp flexures, giving it a corkscrew appearance, with the extreme tip flexed, the nuclei of the central column of cells of microfilaria loa are larger and less deeply stained and the cephalic end of the column is more abruptly terminated (Fig. II.73,2 and 4). By special staining methods a large genital cell at the beginning of the posterior third constitutes a marked feature. Microfilaria loa takes up methylene blue (1 in 5000) in 10 minutes. In microfilaria bancrofti, absorption is much slower but it shows up the excretory pore. Microfilaria loa may not be found in the peripheral blood early after infection. It is strictly diurnal, from 08.00 to 20.00 hours—the reverse of microfilaria bancrofti. Inversion of periodicity takes place very gradually as, for instance, when daily observations are made on a voyage round the world. The periodicity of microfilaria loa is under circadian control by temperature and not by oxygen tension as in periodic *W. bancrofti*.

Life-cycle

There are two parallel and sympatric but ecologically separate cycles of *Loa loa* transmission in the West African rain forest. One cycle is that of the human *Loa loa* (*L. loa loa*) which is slightly smaller than the simian loa and has strictly diurnally periodic microfilariae with day-biting vectors (*Chrysops silacea* and *C. dimidiata*). The slightly larger simian parasite of drills *L. loa papionis* has nocturnally periodic microfilariae with tree-top *Chrysops* (*C. langi* and *C. centurionis*) vectors which feed early in the night.

Development in *Chrysops* (Fig. II.83)

Microfilariae are taken up with the blood meal and on entering the stomach the microfilaria casts its sheath in 3 hours and, piercing the stomach wall, enters the thoracic muscles and fat body of the thorax but principally that of the abdomen. Development is complete in 10 days. In 3 days it becomes broad and torpedo-shaped; on the fourth and fifth days the squat form lengthens to 0.8–1 mm; on the sixth day the corkscrew-like appearance is replaced by gentle curves. Then occurs the first ecdysis and the sharp tail is replaced by a rounded, trilobed extremity. By the tenth day it measures 2 × 0.025 mm and two moults have occurred, and infective third stage forms migrate forward into the head where they accumulate in large numbers, the majority at the root of the proboscis. At the next feed they break out of the labium and make their way on to the surface of the skin which they penetrate, and migrate along the interfascial planes.

Development of *L. loa* in *Chrysops* generally takes 10–12 days from the original infecting feed. *Chrysops* feeds to repletion once every 14 days and the gestation period is 12 days. It is a pool feeder, straining the

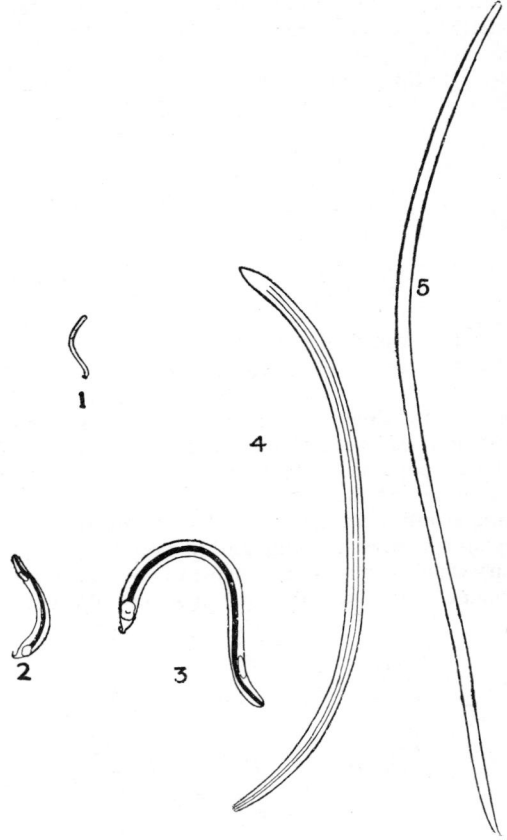

Fig. II.83 Development of *Loa loa* in *Chrysops*. × 30. 1, Larva, 24 hours old. 2, Fourth day, length 390 μm. 3, Fifth day. 4, Seventh day. 5, Tenth day, third stage infective larva. 2 × 0.025 mm.

blood from the subcutaneous haemorrhages caused by its bite.

SUPERFAMILY: DRACUNCULOIDEA

GENUS: *Dracunculus*

Dracunculus medinensis (Linnaeus 1758), guinea-worm

Characters

The female is the thickness of a knitting needle and usually 60 cm in length (60 cm × 1.5–1.7 mm; 90 cm is probably exceptional but 120 cm has been recorded). It lives in connective tissues and does not harm its host until about to produce its young when it exhibits 'geotropism', i.e. it is drawn towards earth, towards the limbs—to the fingers, if in the arms; to the scrotum or penis, if in the abdomen; to the breasts in the female, though 90% migrate to the legs and feet, especially behind the outer malleolus.

The body is cylindrical, white and smooth (Fig. II.84). The tip of the tail is pointed forming a blunt

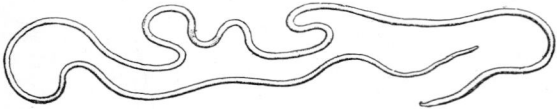

Fig. II.84 Female *Dracunculus medinensis*. One-third natural size.

hook which was formerly thought to be used for holding firm in tissues, but this is not correct. The head is rounded, terminating in a thickened cuticle cap or 'cephalic shield'. The mouth is triangular, small and surrounded by six papillae and an outer circle of four double papillae. A lateral pair of cervical papillae is situated behind the nerve ring (Fig. II.85A). There is a single-bulb oesophagus. The secretion from the head glands is very irritating and histiolytic. The alimentary canal is small and is thrust to one side by the branched uterus. There is no definite anus. The vulva

is difficult to see and has been only recently discovered as a very small tube in the centre of the worm. The whole worm is occupied by the double uterus packed with embryos (Fig. II.86). The coiled uteri, distended by three million larvae, fill the body. There is a double ovary and double oviducts at the posterior extremity (Fig. II.85B, C). When douched with water, waves of contraction force the uterine contents forward, the thickened cuticle gives way and the 'cap' is blown off. The uterus is extruded up to a length of 1.25 cm; this also bursts and the contained embryos are shed into the water. The worm dies when its nervous system is destroyed. The sinus containing the dead worm easily becomes septic, but it may coil itself round tendons and, if pulled upon, may break. It often becomes cretified and can then be demonstrated on radiography.

The male is known from a single specimen in man 40 mm in length but was discovered by Moorthy[27] in experimental dogs. It measures 1.2–2.9 cm × 0.4 mm, has subequal spicules (490–730 μm) and a gubernaculum (200 μm). The posterior end is coiled on itself one or more times. There are 10 pairs of caudal papillae, of which four are preanal and six postanal. The copulatory spicules are subequal, 490–730 μm in length. After copulation it dies and is absorbed. It lives in between the muscles of the groin. Copulation probably takes place in the deeper tissues.

The embryo (Fig. II.87) measures 500–750 × 17 μm and shows transverse striations of the cuticle. It is flattened, not cylindrical, with a long, slender tail and a rounded head. The alimentary canal has a rudimentary anus and a bulbous oesophagus. There are two glands at the root of the tail. In water the embryos cannot swim but sink and coil up and release again,

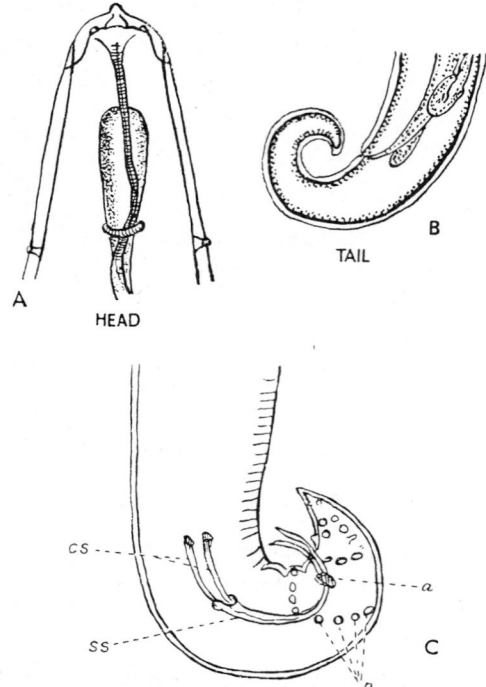

Fig. II.85 A, Anterior end of *Dracunculus medinensis*, female. B, Tail of *D. medinensis*, female. C, Posterior end of *D. medinensis*, male. Ventrolateral aspects. × 10.

a	anus	cs	copulatory spicules
p	preanal and postanal papillae	ss	spicular sheath

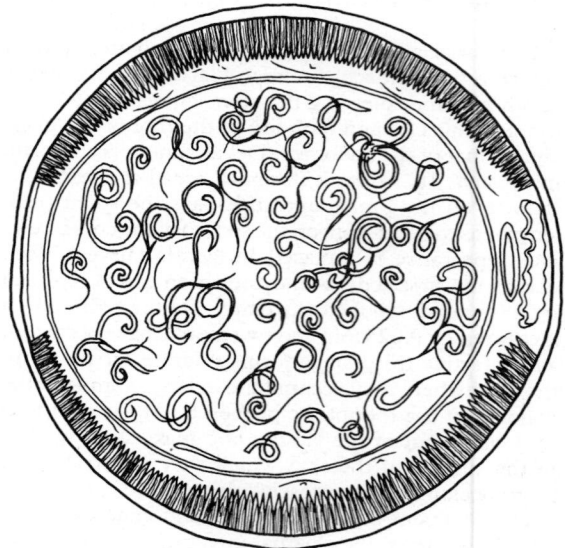

Fig. II.86 Transverse section of *Dracunculus medinensis*, showing the contained embryos.

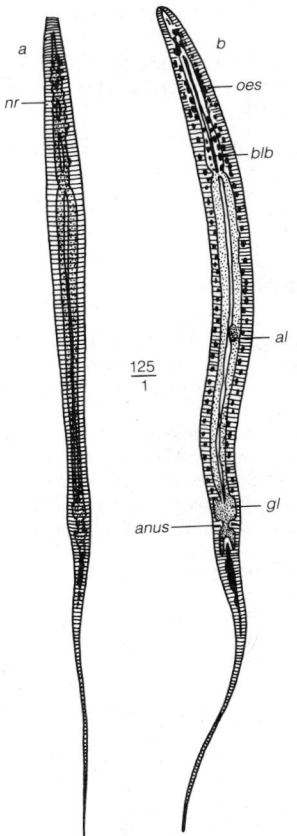

Fig. II.87 Embryo of *Dracunculus medinensis*. a, Side view.
b, Front view.

oes	oesophagus	blb	bulb
al	alimentary canal	gl	glands
nr	nerve ring		

moving by side-to-side lashing of the tail and tadpole-like movement of the body. Abnormal embryos, with prominences on the dorsal and ventral caudal surfaces, are not uncommon, but do not survive long.

Life-cycle (Fig. II.88)

In water they live for 6 days; in muddy water or moist earth for two or three weeks. If slowly desiccated they can be revived by water. They are swallowed by *Cyclops* (*Cyclops* has a very small mouth). The efficient intermediaries are *Cyclops quadricornis* or allied species (*C. strenuus, C. viridis, C. coronatus, C. bicuspidatus, Mesocyclops leuckarti* and *M. hyalinus*) but in the true tropics *Tropocyclops multicolor* and other species; in south Nigeria it is *Thermocyclops nigerianus*. Jerky movements of the embryo attract *Cyclops* as a trout is attracted by a fly. As many as 20 may be found in one crustacean but usually they die out when there are more than four (Fig. II.89). The pointed tail penetrates the gut wall; they then migrate into the body cavity and feed on the ovary or testes of the cyclops. There is no growth in size but two to three ecdyses take place. The tail is absorbed and they become cylindrical and the posterior extremity trilobed. Development takes four to six weeks but the

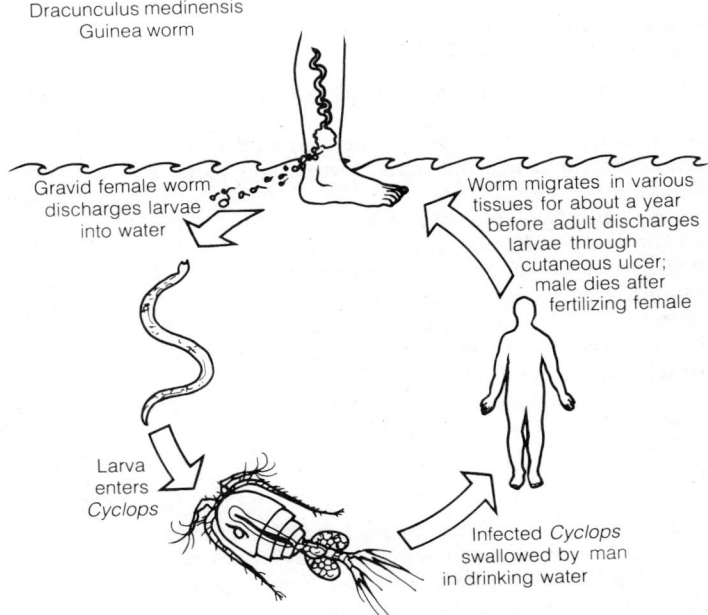

Dracunculus medinensis
Guinea worm

Gravid female worm discharges larvae into water

Worm migrates in various tissues for about a year before adult discharges larvae through cutaneous ulcer; male dies after fertilizing female

Larva enters *Cyclops*

Infected *Cyclops* swallowed by man in drinking water

Fig. II.88 Life-cycle of *Dracunculus medinensis*.

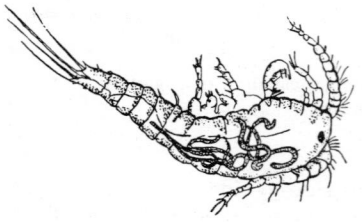

Fig. II.89 Larvae of *Dracunculus medinensis* in the body cavity of *Cyclops*.

larva may survive for four months. When 1 mm in length they acquire a simple muscular oesophagus (Fig. II.87) and the tail is truncated. This distinguishes the infective stage.

Cyclops is swallowed by man; in the gastric juice the body of the cyclops is dissolved and the larvae become active and burst out. The migration of the early stages in the mammalian host has been clarified.[28] It takes three to four months for the full development of both sexes. Immature stages were recovered 43–48 days while undergoing the fourth ecdysis. The route of the larvae from the alimentary canal to the subcutaneous tissues of the mammalian host takes place via the lymphatic system. The worms reach the subcutaneous tissues by the forty-third day. In this situation the sexes live in equal numbers and sexual differentiation is distinct, though the males have not developed spicules. The final ecdysis takes place in the subcutaneous tissues. The adult worm takes exactly one year to develop.

SUPERFAMILY: SPIRUROIDEA

GENUS: *Thelazia*

Thelazia callipaeda (oriental eye worm)

This nematode is a parasite of the conjunctiva of the dog, rabbit and man in India, Burma and parts of China.

The adult is a white thread-like worm (males 4.5–13 mm × 0.25–0.75 mm; females 6.2–17 mm × 0.3–0.85 mm) The oral end has a chitinized capsule with two circles of sessile papillae. The male has a recurved posterior end. The vulva of the female opens ventrally in the anterior half of the body. There is a single uterus which bifurcates into two ovaries.

The egg is ovoidal and measures 60 × 34–37 μm, is hyaline, thin-shelled and laid fully embryonated.

Life-cycle

Little is known of the life history but an insect intermediate host is probable since related species have *Musca* sp. as intermediate hosts and *Fannia* sp. have been shown to be susceptible larval hosts.[29]

Thelazia californiensis

T. californiensis has been found in man in California, the intermediate host of which is a species of Musca, *Fannia canicularis*.

REFERENCES

1 Southgate, V.R., Van Wijk, H.B. & Wright, C.A. (1976) *Feitschr. Parasit.* **49**, 145–159.
2 Wright, C.A. & Ross, G.C. (1980) *Trans. R. Soc. trop. Med. Hyg.* **74**, 326–332.
3 Jordan, P. & Webbe, G. (1982) *Human Schistosomiasis*, 2nd edn. London: Heinemann.
4 Brown, D.S. (1980) *Freshwater Snails of Africa and their Medical Importance*. London: Taylor & Francis.
5 Kian Joe Lie, Basch, P.W., Heynemann, D. et al (1968) *Trans. R. Soc. trop. Med. Hyg.* **62**, 299.
6 Brygoo, E.R. & Randrimalala, J.C. (1959) *Bull. Soc. Path. éxot.* **52**, 26.
7 Slais, J. (1970) cited in Dawes, B. (1972) *Advances in Parasitology*. London: Academic Press.
8 D'Alessandro, B.A., Beaver, P.C. & Pallares, R.M. (1963) *Am. J. trop. Med. Hyg.* **12**, 193.
9 Dismuke, J.C., Jun. & Routh, C.F. (1963) *Am. J. trop. Med. Hyg.* **12**, 73.
10 Schad, G.A. et al (1973) *Science* **180**, 502.
11 Beer, R.J.S. (1971) *Br. med. J.* **ii**, 44.
12 Masuya, T. (1976) *Jap. J. Parasit.* **25**, 283.
13 McFadzean, J.S. & Hawking, F. (1956) *Trans. R. Soc. trop. Med. Hyg.* **50**, 543.
14 Hawking, F. (1956) *Trans. R. Soc. trop. Med. Hyg.* **50**, 397.
15 Bryan, J.H., Oothman, P., Andrews, B.J. et al (1974) *Trans. R. Soc. trop. Med. Hyg.* **68**, 14.
16 Laurence, B.R. (1985) *Trans. R. Soc. trop. Med. Hyg.* **79**, 690–699.
17 Nelson, G.S. (1959) *J. Helminth.* **33**, 233.
18 David, L. & Edeson, J.F.B. (1964) *Ann. trop. Med. Parasit.* **59**, 103.
19 Partono, F., Purnomo, A.S. & Dennis, D.T. (1977) *J. Parasit.* **63**, 540.
20 Beaver, P.C., Horner, G.S. & Bilos, J.Z. (1974) *Am. J. trop. Med. Hyg.* **23**, 595.
21 Nelson, G.S. & Pester, F.N.R. (1962) *Bull. Wld Hlth Org.* **27**, 473.
22 Braun-Munziger, R.A. & Southgate, B.A. (1977) *Bull. Wld Hlth Org.* **55**, 569.
23 Collins, R.C. (1973) *J. Parasit.* **59**, 1016.
24 Orihel, T.C. & Eberhard, M.L. (1982) *Am. J. trop. Med. Hyg.* **31**, 1142–1147.
25 Godoy, G.A., Godoy, G., Oriheltic, C. & Volcan, G.S. (1980) *Am. J. trop. Med. Hyg.* **29**, 545–547.
26 Orihel, T.C. (1984) *Am. J. trop. Med. Hyg.* **33**, 1278.
27 Moorthy, U.N. (1937) *J. Parasit.* **23**, 220.
28 Onobamiro, S.D. (1956) *Ann. trop. Med. Parasit.* **50**, 157.
29 Burnett, H.S., Warren, E.P., Lee, R.D. (1957) *J. Parasit.* **43**, 433.

Appendix III
Medical Entomology

Edited by *D. M. Minter* and *G. B. White*

TICKS AND MITES
M.G.R. Varma

CLASS: ARACHNIDA

SUBCLASS: ACARI (TICKS AND MITES)

The arachnids include, besides ticks and mites, the scorpions and spiders. They differ from the true insects (Class Insecta) in possessing no wings or antennae and in having an unsegmented body. During the life-cycle they undergo incomplete metamorphosis; the eggs hatch into six-legged larvae which develop through the nymphal stage to the adults. The nymphs and adults have four pairs of legs. The acarine body is typically composed of an anterior gnathosoma or capitulum and a posterior idiosoma. The gnathosoma represents the head of a generalized arthropod and carries the paired palps, which are sensory in function, the paired chelicerae and the single ventrally situated hypostome, which together make up the cutting and blood-sucking apparatus. The idiosoma carries the paired legs.

There are about 30 000 species of acarines belonging to more than 2000 genera. The mites are usually much smaller than ticks. Of over 200 families of mites that have been described, only a few contain species that affect man.

FAMILY: SARCOPTIDAE

Sarcoptes scabiei (itch mite, scabies mite)

Sarcoptes scabiei causes scabies in man and mange in a variety of wild and domestic animals. Scabies mites of dogs and horses, which differ physiologically rather than morphologically from human scabies mites, can establish themselves briefly on humans and cause skin problems similar to scabies. Such infestations are usually mild and cure spontaneously. Increased incidence of human scabies tends to occur in 15–20 year cycles and the cycling is most probably due to changing levels of immunity in the human population.

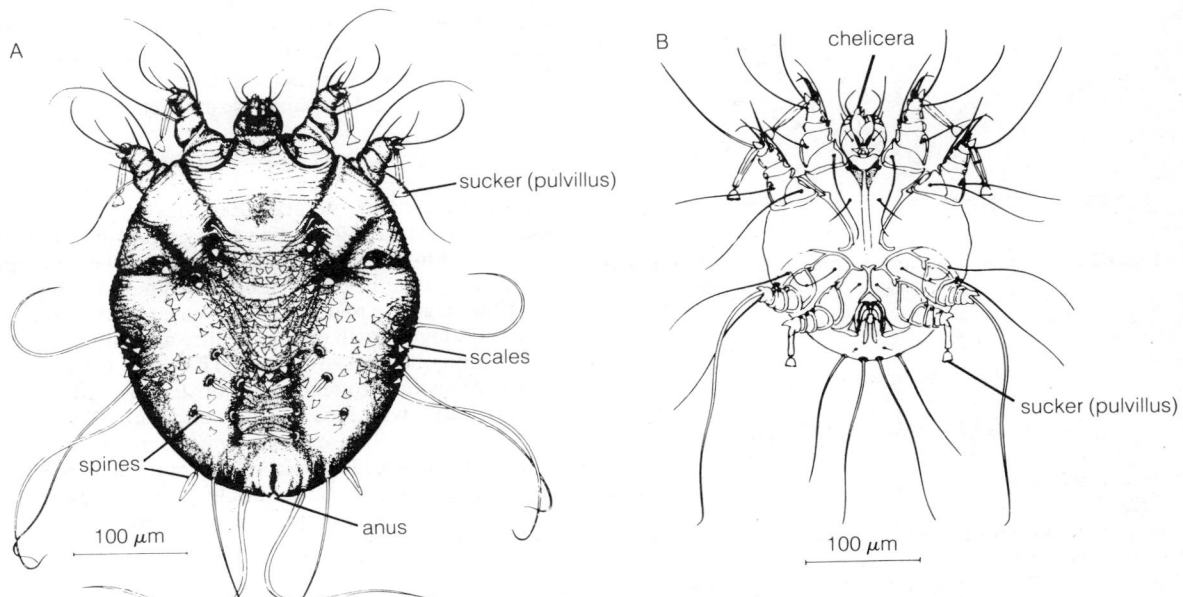

Fig. III.1   (A) Dorsal view of female *Sarcoptes scabiei* and (B) ventral view of male *Sarcoptes scabiei*. From Kettle.[1]

1381

Scabies is widespread in the tropics, although by no means confined to the tropics. It may disappear from one area for many years, only to reappear. It is thought that the recent resurgence in scabies is due to large population movements, insufficient or incorrect diagnosis by the medical profession and an altered lifestyle among younger persons in the developed Western countries, resulting in close personal contact. Infestation levels are highest in poorer communities and in children. Even in developed countries, infestation in schoolchildren can reach 5%.

The female of *S. scabiei* (0.3–0.4 mm) is bigger than the male (0.2 mm) (Fig. III.1).[1] The first and second pairs of legs of the female and the first, second and fourth pairs of legs of the male carry suckers. The surface of the female is covered with fine transverse striations and the dorsal surface bears a number of specialized spines and conical setae.

Both males and females make short burrows but it is only the fertilized females which make permanent winding burrows in the horny layers of the skin with the female at the end (Fig. III.2). The burrows contain faeces and the relatively large eggs. The majority of mite burrows are found in the interdigital skin, bends of the knees and elbows, the penis and breasts. The eggs hatch into larvae which find shelter and presumably food in the follicles. The larval stage is followed by two nymphal stages before the adult stage is reached. The whole life-cycle from egg to egg takes about 10–14 days during which there may be a mortality of about 90%. (For clinical features and treatment see Chapter 53.)

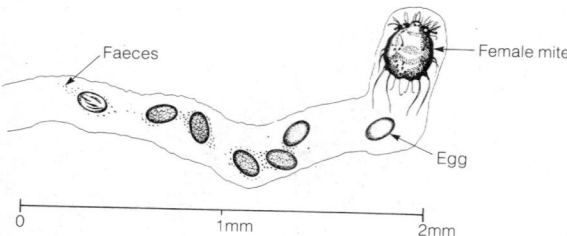

Fig. III.2   Burrow of *Sarcoptes scabiei* with female mite and eggs.

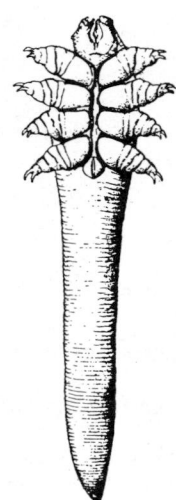

Fig. III.3   *Demodex folliculorum* the follicle mite. Ventral view. From Kettle.[2]

FAMILY: DEMODICIDAE

Demodex folliculorum (follicle mite

These mites are extremely small, 0.1–0.4 mm long (Fig. III.3). They have a worm-like transversely striated body with four pairs of stubby legs at the anterior part. They infest a wide variety of mammalian hosts but are highly host-specific. More than one species may occur on the same host but in different tissues. For example, *D. folliculorum* lives in the hair follicles of man and the stubby *D. brevis* is found in the sebaceous glands. The entire life-cycle is spent in the follicles. In man infestations occur mainly in the region of the eyelids, nose and facial area. Infestations are usually higher in aged persons in whom they may reach 100%. Diagnosis is by expressing sebum and examining it for mites. Since the mites are found on healthy and diseased hosts, it is difficult to assess their pathological significance. Infestations are usually benign, but dry erythema with follicular scaling, particularly in the region of the eyelids, may give rise to blepharitis. In the facial area there may be granulomatous acne. Gammexane (gamma benzene hexachloride) 0.5% in vanishing cream is effective.

FAMILY: TROMBICULIDAE

Of more than 1200 described species of trombiculid mites, only about 50 are known to attack humans or livestock. Only the larvae, popularly known as chiggers, are parasitic on vertebrates. They are widely distributed and in many countries cause a dermatitis in man, although not all chiggers cause an itchy reaction.

Trombiculid larvae (Figs. III.4 and III.5) normally parasitize rodents and birds but, given the opportunity, will feed readily on man. The nonparasitic female lays eggs in damp but well-drained soil. Typical breeding places are cultivated alluvial river banks in Japan, scrub jungle, grassy fields or untended gardens with a rank growth of grass and other vegetation.

Life-cycle (Fig. III.6)

On hatching, the six-legged larvae, which are creamy-

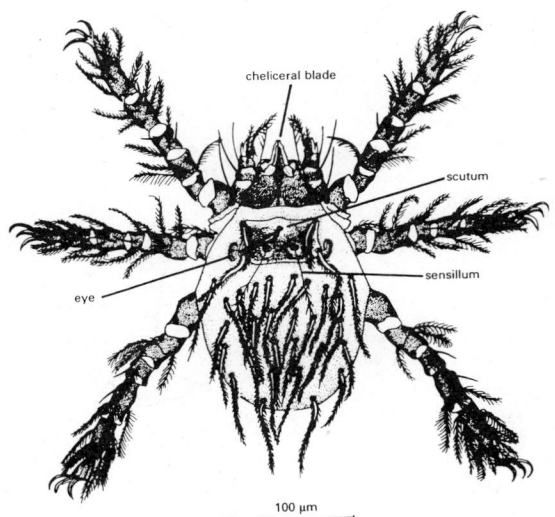

Fig. III.4 Dorsal view of *Leptotrombidium deliense*. From Kettle.[1]

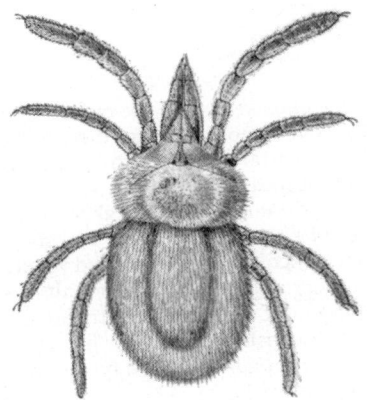

Fig. III.5 Fully grown imago of *Leptotrombidium akamushi*.

to the formation of a feeding tube or stylostome at the point of attachment. The commonest sites of attachment are inside the ears of rodents and around the eyes of birds. On man they tend to attach where clothing is tight, i.e. around the waist and on the scrotum. The larvae do not burrow into the skin nor do they feed on blood, although a few blood cells may be ingested. After feeding for several days (minimum 3 days), the larvae fall from the host and enter a quiescent stage before moulting into nymphs. The eight-legged nymphs have a figure-of-eight shape and a dense covering of red hairs which gives them a velvety appearance and the name 'velvet mites'. They are non-parasitic predators and feed on insect eggs or small inactive soil invertebrates. The nymph enters a further quiescent phase from which the adult moults. The adults are larger (about 1 mm long) than nymphs but resemble them in shape and habits. The males deposit stalked spermatophores containing sperms on the substrate and the females are inseminated by walking over them. In the warmer tropical regions the life-cycle may take about 40 days and breeding occurs continuously throughout the year. In the cooler temperate regions there is usually only one generation per year and the chiggers are seasonal, during summer and early autumn.

Chiggers and dermatitis

In parts of the world where the mites are present, persons who have been walking in vegetated areas may suffer from a severe itchy dermatitis consisting of pustules and wheals, 3–6 hours after exposure. The sudden appearance of these lesions should suggest attack by chiggers.

Neotrombicula autumnalis is the harvest mite, 'aoutat' or 'lepte autumnal' of Europe. The larvae normally parasitize voles, rabbits and hares as well as ground-frequenting birds and are active in summer and early autumn; hence the name 'harvest mite'.

Eutrombicula alfreddugesi, the common American chigger, feeds readily on man and is also known as 'thalzahuatl' and 'bicho colorado'. It extends from continental USA to South America and is most abundant in second growth, cut-over areas. Man is frequently attacked although the usual hosts are domestic and wild animals and birds.

Eutrombicula batatas ranges from the warmer southern states of the USA to Central and South America. It is not a serious pest of man in the USA but commonly attacks man in Panama and other tropical areas of its distribution.

Chiggers and scrub typhus

The vectors of scrub typhus (caused by *Rickettsia tsutsugamushi*) are trombiculid mites. The larvae usually infest rodents (*Rattus* spp.) and insectivores

white to bright red in colour and 0.25 mm long, ascend grass stems or the tips of fallen leaves and wait in clusters until carbon dioxide from a passing host activates them. The round or oval-shaped larvae have a prominent gnathosoma at the anterior end. The paired toothed chelicerae are flanked by stout palps. The penultimate segment of the palp has a claw which can be apposed to the last segment. Posterior to the gnathosoma on the dorsal side is a chitinized plate or scutum. The shape of the scutum and the shape and disposition of the setae (usually seven) on it are important characters in the generic and specific identification of the larvae.

The larvae attach in clusters and start feeding on the host's tissues by partially digesting them with saliva and sucking it up. The continual feeding leads

SUMMARIZED LIFECYCLE OF TROMBICULID MITES

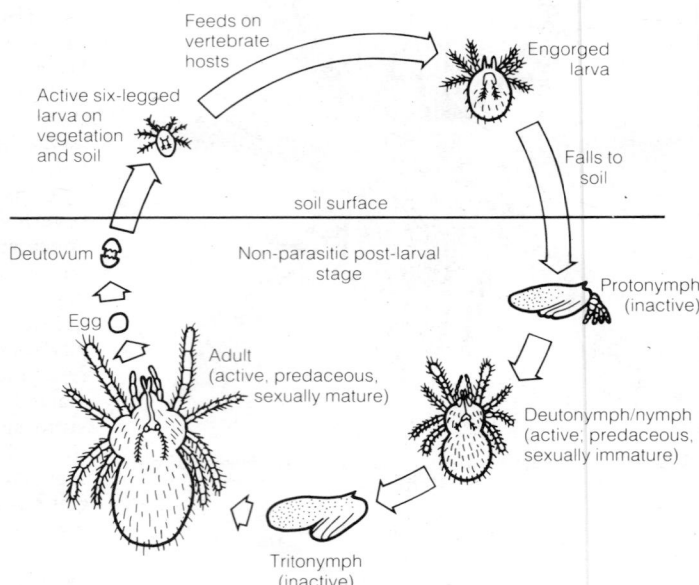

Fig. III.6 Summarized life-cycle of trombiculid mites.

which are the vertebrate reservoirs of the rickettsiae. The distribution of the mites on the ground is dependent on the home range of the hosts and, since the home ranges do not usually overlap, mite colonies have a restricted distribution and tend to be isolated from each other in the form of 'mite islands'. Man gets infected by intrusion into a rodent–mite cycle in infected 'mite islands'. Bird hosts of the larval mites can, however, disperse the mites into new areas where a fresh colony could be established.

The habits and life-cycle of scrub typhus vectors are similar to that of other trombiculid mites. The parasitic larvae attack man but seldom produce any noticeable itching or skin reaction; but the bite of an infected larva can produce a lesion—the eschar. Since only the larvae are parasitic and feed only once, only this stage can acquire and transmit the infection. This means that trans-stadial (stage to stage, i.e. from larva to nymph to adult) and transovarial (through eggs to next generation larvae) transmission are obligatory for maintenance of the infection in nature. Trombiculid mites therefore are the main reservoirs of scrub typhus rickettsiae. In the mites, the rickettsiae eventually localize in the larval salivary glands and transmission is by bite. All the important scrub typhus vectors belong to the genus *Leptotrombidium*, although the genus *Ascoschoengastia* may be involved in transmission among rodents.

Leptotrombidium akamushi is the vector in the classical areas of the disease (tsutsugamushi disease) in Japan. It is found in the cultivated flood plains of rivers.

Leptotrombidium deliense is the main—or an important—vector over most of the distribution of the disease, from coastal Queensland in the east through Papua New Guinea, Philippines, China, South-East Asia, Sri Lanka and India to Pakistan in the west. Over most of its range, *L. deliense* and the disease are associated with ecologically disturbed vegetation, such as secondary scrub and grass, the result of slash-and-burn cultivation of virgin forest. In South-East Asia and tropical Queensland the coarse fire-resistant kunai grass (*Imperata cylindrica*) is the typical habitat of the mite and its rodent hosts. The mites and the disease are also more likely to occur at the fringes of forests or scrub.

Leptotrombidium fletcheri is an important vector in Malaysia, Borneo, New Guinea and the Philippines.

Other important vectors are *L. arenicola* on sandy beaches in Malaysia, *L. pallidum* in limited areas of Japan, Korea and the Primorye region of Russia; *L. pavlovskyi* in Siberia and the Primorye region of Russia and *L. scutellare* in the Mount Fuji area of Japan (Fig. 10.12).

Protection against chigger mites

Personal protection is the best method of preventing attack by the mite larvae. If one has to go into mite-infested areas, impregnation of socks and trouser legs with a repellent, such as benzyl benzoate, dimethyl phthalate (DMP) or diethyltoluamide (DEET) will prevent mite attack. Dusting clothing with flowers of sulphur is not recommended.

Other mites of medical importance

Dermatophagoides pteronyssinus (house dust mite—(Family Pyroglyphidae) (Fig. III.7)

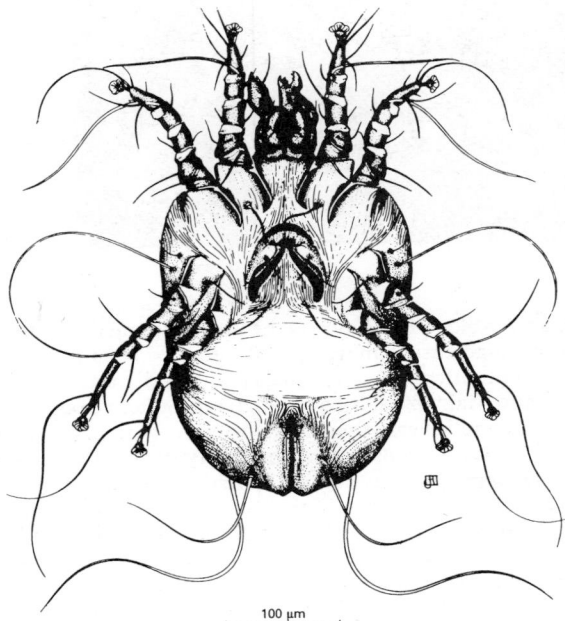

100 μm

Fig. III.7 *Dermatophagoides pteronyssinus* the house dust mite. Ventral view. From Kettle.[1]

This is a mite commonly found in house dust. It is widespread in the tropics and temperate regions. The mite can cause in sensitized individuals bronchial asthma, as well as extensive dermatitis. In house dust it feeds mainly on desquamated skin scales. The mites become airborne during bed-making and could then be inhaled; not only the living mites but also dead ones and mite faeces contain potent allergens. The best method of controlling the mites would appear to be treatment of beds and settees with insecticides followed by thorough vacuum cleaning to remove dead mites and faeces, as these could cause symptoms.

Dermanyssus gallinae (chicken mite—Family Dermanyssidae); *Ornithonyssus bacoti* (tropical rat mite), *O. sylviarum* (bird mite) and *O. bursa* (tropical poultry mite) (Family Macronyssidae)

These are blood-sucking mites and can cause dermatitis in man. In the absence of their natural hosts they will readily attack man. Rat mites are associated with groceries and warehouses. Bird mites are often found in the eaves of houses and in air-conditioning ducts and may be blown into houses when the air-conditioning is switched on.

Tyrophagus (forage mites—Family Acaridae)

These mites are pests of stored food products such as cheese, copra, vanilla pods, flour and macaroni. Persons handling such materials may be bitten or suffer from simple contact allergy, and various names, such as grocers' itch, copra itch and bakers' itch, indicate the occupational nature of these dermatoses. Some forage mites may be swallowed or inhaled and can cause gastric disturbances or respiratory symptoms. The mites do not breed in the body but may be recovered from faeces or sputum (see section on acarine dermatosis, Chapter 55).

SUBORDER: IXODIDA

SUPERFAMILY: IXODOIDEA (TICKS)

The ticks are bigger versions of the mites and lack the prominent hairs found on the mites. All species are obligate blood-sucking parasites of vertebrates. Originally parasites of reptiles, they adapted over the last 200 million years to the newly evolving warm-blooded birds and mammals; some ticks have retained a predilection for cold-blooded vertebrates. The gnathosoma or capitulum is well developed and the prominent ventrally situated median hypostome bears on its underside rows of backwardly directed teeth which help the tick in attaching firmly to the host and prevent it from being easily dislodged by the grooming activities of the host (Fig. III.8).

There are two basic types of ticks: the soft or argasid ticks (Family Argasidae) and the hard or ixodid ticks (Family Ixodidae). Most people are familiar with the slow-feeding ixodid ticks found on dogs, cattle and other domestic animals and which remain attached for several days. The argasids are rapid feeders and usually feed at night and are not familiar to many. Ticks are primarily parasites of wild animals; about 10% of the species feed on domestic animals but many will feed opportunistically on man, some of them more avidly than others. The soft tick *Ornithodoros moubata* of East, Central and South Africa is probably the only true man-biting tick; it is found in huts and feeds readily on man and chickens. Ticks parasitize a wide range of wild and domestic hosts and many appear to have a preferred host, although this apparent preference may be due to availability rather than choice. All ticks, particularly the slow-feeding ixodids, ingest considerable quantities of blood (a fully engorged female ixodid may reach a length of over 20 mm and weigh 2.0 g or more) and because of this are a threat to the health of domestic livestock with very heavy infestations. Apart from causing blood loss, ticks transmit a variety of pathogens among animals and are

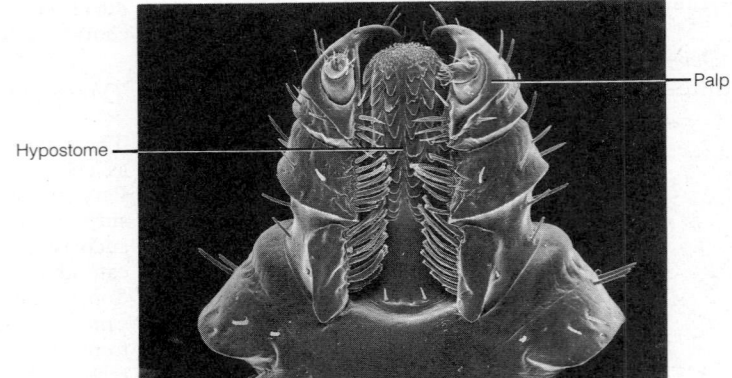

Fig. III.8 Electron micrograph view of ventral capitulum of ixodid tick. (Courtesy M. Nawar.)

therefore important in veterinary medicine. However, because of their indiscriminate feeding habits, many ticks can acquire an infection from animals and transmit it to man during the next blood feed.

Intercontinental and intracontinental movement of tick-infested animals, particularly of domestic livestock, has resulted in the introduction and establishment of exotic tick species in new areas. The cosmopolitan dog tick *Rhipicephalus sanguineus* is a carnivore parasite of Africa but is now a worldwide parasite found in kennels and households. Many tickborne diseases exist as silent foci and the pathogen, vertebrate host (usually a wild animal) and the tick have evolved to form a balanced relationship. The postwar years have produced a more affluent society with the time and money to undertake leisure activities, such as camping and walking in forests. Recreational parks with their rich fauna of wild animals and their tick parasites have become popular and there is an increasing demand for adventure holidays and safari tours in the tropical 'bush'. In developing countries, population increase and economic pressure have led to ecological changes brought about by clearance of forests for cultivation, or the growing of cash crops. The intrusion of man into such tick-infested areas and suburban encroachment into tick habitats with silent foci of infection have resulted in closer tick–man contact and an increase in the incidence of tick-transmitted diseases such as Rocky Mountain spotted fever in the eastern USA, tick-borne encephalitis in Europe, and the emergence of apparently 'new' diseases in man such as Kyasanur Forest disease in southern India and Lyme disease in the USA.

There are several factors which make ticks efficient vectors of pathogenic organisms. Firm attachment to the host prevents them from being easily dislodged. The slow feeding of ixodids not only gives them ample time to ingest large numbers of pathogens from an infected host and ample time to transmit them to a new host, but also allows dispersal of infected ticks into new areas while still attached to a host. The

multiple blood feeds during the life-cycle and the wide host range ensure more opportunities to acquire and transmit infections, and makes a blood meal more certain. Many ixodids have a high reproductive potential, laying several thousands of eggs, but this is to offset the very considerable mortality during the life-cycle. Some argasids can live for many years and starve for prolonged periods. This is of great survival value and gives them more opportunities to acquire and transmit pathogens during their long life. Transovarial transmission of many pathogens in ticks makes them true reservoirs of infection and some tick-borne infections can be maintained in nature in the absence of vertebrate hosts by transovarial passage through several generations of ticks.

Table III.1 Differences between argasid ticks and ixodid ticks.

	Argasidae	Ixodidae
Morphology		
Scutum	Absent	Present; anterior in larva, nymph and female, covering dorsal side in male
Capitulum	Ventral, not visible from above	Anterior, visible from above
Palps	Long, movable	Short, rigid
Life-cycle	Several nymphal stages	One nymphal stage
	Several batches of eggs, each batch (*ca* 200 eggs) after a blood meal	One batch of eggs (several 1000)
Habits	Rapid feeders, usually nocturnal; male and female feed repeatedly	Slow feeders, day and night, several days; only female feed once
	Restricted habitat, burrows or nests of hosts	Diffuse habitat, pasture, etc., where hosts forage

The Argasidae contain about 150 species in three genera of which *Argas* and *Ornithodoros*, which transmit tick-borne relapsing fever in man, are the most important. The Ixodidae have about 800 species in 13 genera. *Ixodes, Amblyomma, Hyalomma, Haemaphysalis, Dermacentor* and *Rhipicephalus* are the genera concerned in the transmission of diseases to man. *Boophilus* spp., the cattle ticks, are unimportant as parasites of man but are one of the most important tick parasites of domestic livestock. While there are similarities in the structure, habits and life-cycle of argasids and ixodids, there are important morphological and biological differences which distinguish the two families. These are summarized in Table III.1.

FAMILY: ARGASIDAE

Tough, leathery ticks, with the females ranging in size from small (4 mm) to large (15 mm); the males are smaller but otherwise very similar. In nymphs and adults the capitulum is ventral and not visible from above; in larvae, the capitulum projects anteriorly. The jointed palps are long and movable and in some species may be mistaken for an extra pair of legs. The surface of the integument is covered with mammillae or radially arranged depressions and discs, but the dorsal plate or scutum, characteristic of the Ixodidae is absent (Fig. III.9), hence the name 'soft ticks'. Eyes when present, are simple and situated laterally. Spiracles or breathing holes are present ventrally between the first segments (coxae) of the third and fourth pairs of legs. The genital opening is anterior and ventral, behind the capitulum, and the anal opening median and about a third of the distance from the posterior margin. There are two very small openings—the coxal openings—placed ventrally between the first and second pairs of legs. They are the external openings of the coxal glands which help to concentrate the blood meal by filtering off fluid from the blood and excreting it as two drops of coxal fluid. In many *Ornithodoros* vectors of relapsing fever and arboviruses the coxal glands are infected. Coxal fluid is excreted just before termination of a feed and pathogens in the fluid enter the bite wound. The glands therefore have an important role in disease transmission (Figs. III.10 and III.11).

The argasids are rapid feeders, the larvae of some species taking only 2–3 minutes to engorge; only the larvae of *Argas* remain attached to their hosts for several days. Soft ticks are usually nocturnal feeders and the house-haunting argasids (*O. moubata*) are not unlike bed bugs in their feeding and sheltering habits. They are ticks of restricted habitats and shelter in cracks and crevices in wood, stone or mud, in or near the surface of soil and in and around nesting or resting places of the host animals. Typical habitats are birds' nests in trees or on the ground, caves, burrows of wild animals, tree-shaded resting places of animals in semideserts, deer beds in forest, huts, log cabins, animal shelters such as chicken coops, pigeon lofts, goat sheds and pig sties. Access to a blood meal is therefore easy and the hazards in host finding considerably reduced. The six-legged larvae feed once; larvae of *Ornithodoros* do not feed but moult straight into nymphs. There are two to five or more nymphal stages; each stage feeds once and moults to the next stage. Adults mate off the host. Both males and females feed repeatedly, the females ovipositing after each blood meal, laying a batch of 100–150 eggs (Fig. III.12).

The two argasid genera *Argas* and *Ornithodoros* can be separated by the distinct flattened lateral margin of the body in *Argas* which is evident even when the tick is fully fed. *Argas* spp. feed on birds and bats, but some attack man and cause painful bites. *Ornithodoros* ticks have no distinct lateral margin. About seven species transmit relapsing fever to man (*Borrelia* spp.) (Table III.2). The tick vector, *Borrelia*, and distribution of tick borne relapsing fever are described in Chapter 32.

Foci of infection are usually restricted and include huts, caves, stables, pig pens, other animal shelters and resort cabins. There is a high rate of trans-stadial and transovarial transmission; this and the longevity and ability of the vector to starve for long periods lead to the perpetuation of natural foci in the absence of vertebrate hosts. The ticks therefore are the true reservoirs of infection and other animals, such as rodents, probably serve only as amplifiers of infection. Following an infecting feed, the ticks have a disseminated infection of practically all the internal organs. Transmission is usually through the salivary secretion containing the borrelias and/or through contamination of the bite wound through infective coxal fluid. Those species which do not excrete coxal fluid while still attached to the host transmit solely by bite.

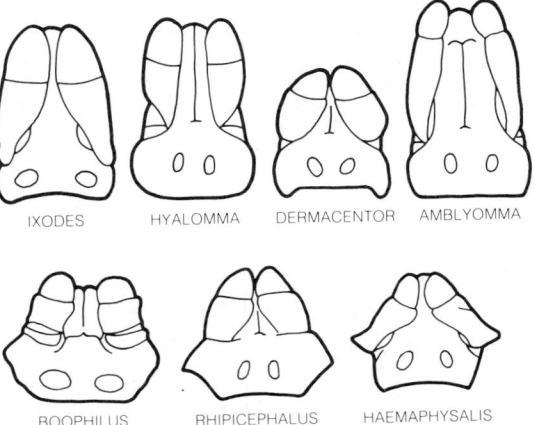

IXODES   HYALOMMA   DERMACENTOR   AMBLYOMMA

BOOPHILUS   RHIPICEPHALUS   HAEMAPHYSALIS

Fig. III.9 Dorsal view of capitulum of Ixodidae.

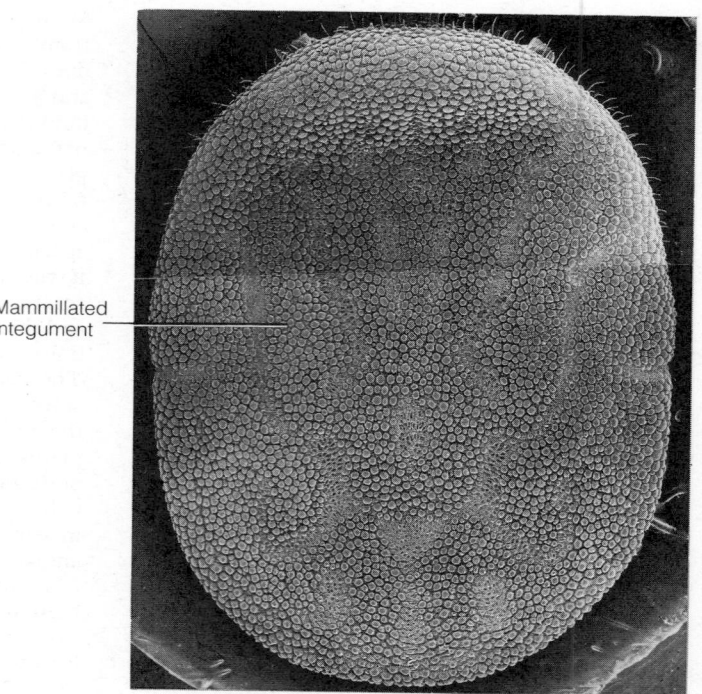

Mammillated
integument

Fig. III.10   Dorsal view of adult
female *Ornithodoros moubata*.
(Courtesy M. Nawar.)

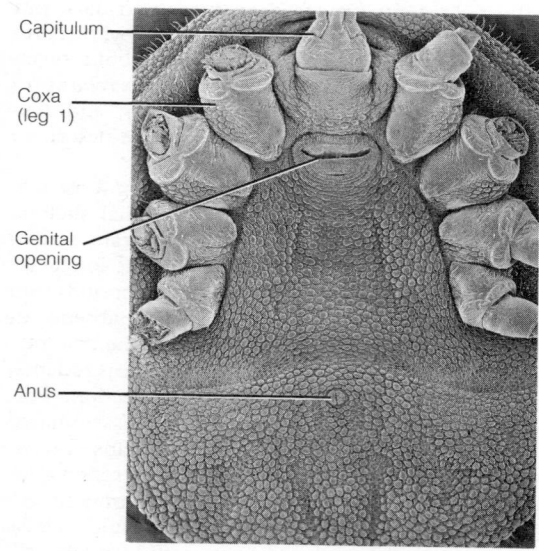

Capitulum

Coxa
(leg 1)

Genital
opening

Anus

Fig. III.11   Ventral view of adult female *O. moubata*.
(Courtesy M. Nawar.)

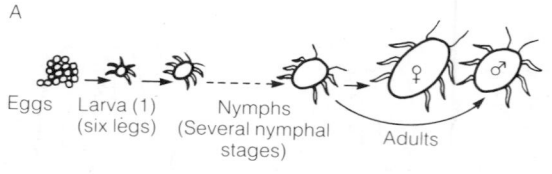

A

Eggs   Larva (1)
(six legs)

Nymphs
(Several nymphal
stages)

Adults

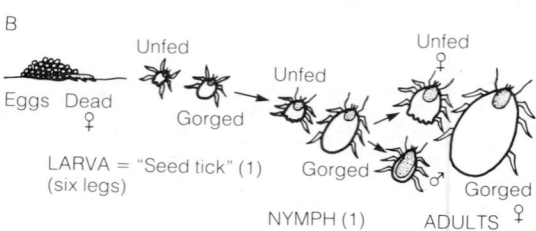

B

Unfed

Unfed

Unfed

Eggs   Dead
♀

Gorged

Unfed

Gorged

Gorged

LARVA = "Seed tick" (1)
(six legs)

NYMPH (1)   ADULTS ♀

Fig. III.12   Tick life-cycles: A, Argasidae; B, Ixodidae.

Table III. 2 Human tick-borne relapsing fever: the spirochaetes and the vectors (*Ornithodoros* spp.) which transmit them.

Tick vector	Spirochaete	Locality
O. moubata	*B. duttoni*	East, central and South Africa
O. erraticus	*B. hispanica*	Mediterranean region (part). Spain, North and north-west Africa
O. tholozani (=*papillipes*) including var. *crossi*	*B. persica*	Mediterranean region (part). Tobruk, Cyprus and Palestine, eastwards through Iran and central Asia to Kashmir and the Sinkiang (Xinjiang) province of western China
O. turicata	*B. turicatae*	Central and western USA, Mexico
O. parkeri	*B. parkeri*	
O. hermsi	*B hermsii*	
O. rudis (=*venezuelensis*)	*B. venezuelensis*	North, South and Central America; southwards to northern Argentina

Ornithodoros moubata

This is widely distributed in East, Central and South Africa, and is the vector of relapsing fever (*Borrelia duttoni*) in these areas. The integument is mamillated and is greenish-brown. The absence of eyes (hence the name 'eyeless tampan') helps to distinguish this species from the closely related and widely distributed sand tampan, *O. savignyi*, which has two pairs of eyes on the sides of the body. Both species are night feeders. *O. moubata* is found in huts including the occupants' possessions or in the burrows of wart-hogs. What was considered to be a single species is now believed to be more than one species, of which *O. moubata* sensu stricto with two subspecies is one. *O moubata moubata* feeds predominantly on man and chickens and *O. moubata porcinus* on wart-hogs, antbears and porcupines. In the cool wet habitats of the Kenya highlands and north-west Tanzania, 94% of *O. m. moubata* feed on man and 2% on chickens, but in hot moist habitats these percentages are reversed. Both subspecies have domestic and wild populations and it is the domestic populations which are important in disease transmission; no infected ticks have been found in wild populations. *O. moubata* is common on travel routes and may be carried long distances in mats and bed rolls. Rest houses are almost always infested. To prevent the risk of infection with relapsing fever old camping sites and mud houses should be avoided and it is advisable not to sleep on the floor. Since the ticks find shelter in cracks and crevices in mud walls and floors, better housing and the use of concrete and plaster in buildings will help to control the ticks. They can also be controlled by dusting the floors and walls of huts with gammexane powder.

Ornithodoros savignyi (eyed tampan or sand tampan)

This is widely distributed in arid and semi-arid areas from Sri Lanka westwards through India, Arabia, North, East and South Africa to Namibia. In certain parts of Africa the distributions of *O. savignyi* and *O. moubata* overlap. It is an outdoor tick found near the soil surface in the resting places of cattle, camels and other livestock in the shade of trees and stone fences. It will attack man given the opportunity and can transmit relapsing fever in the laboratory but is not involved in the transmission of the disease in nature.

Ornithodoros erraticus

This occurs in north-west Africa, Spain and Portugal. It usually lives in burrows feeding on rodents but considerable populations exist in pig sties where they feed on pigs. It is an important vector of relapsing fever in north-west Africa and Spain (*B. hispanica*).

Ornithodoros tholozani (= O. papillipes)

The area of distribution covers Libya, North-east Africa, the Mediterranean islands, northern Arabia, South-eastern Europe, southern USSR, northern India and western provinces of China. It is an important vector of relapsing fever (*B. persica*). Transmission is by bite. Typical habitats are caves and large burrows but the tick has successfully adapted to stables and rest houses. *O. tholozani* feeds on a variety of domestic livestock but also on birds and man.

Ornithodoros lahorensis

This occurs in Tibet, southern Soviet Republics, Pakistan, Turkey, Greece, Yugoslavia and Bulgaria. It is found in stables and human habitations and is suspected of transmitting relapsing fever.

Ornithodoros talaje

This is a South and Central American species extending northwards to the southern states of the USA. It feeds on wild rodents and domestic livestock as well as man and inflicts a very painful bite; relapsing fever vector in Guatemala, Panama and Colombia.

Ornithodoros rudis (= O. venezuelensis)

This is a Central and South American species and the most important vector (*B. venezuelensis*) in Panama, Colombia, Venezuela and Ecuador. It usually lives in the walls of huts and will feed avidly on man.

Ornithodoros hermsi

This is widespread in the Rocky Mountain and Pacific coast states of the USA. It is essentially a rodent parasite. It shelters in summer cabins at higher elevations and transmits relapsing fever (*B. hermsi*) to people occupying the cabins. Transmission is mainly by bite and injection of infected saliva.

Ornithodoros parkeri and Ornithodoros turicata

These have similar distribution occurring in the western USA but the range of *O. turicata* extends southwards into Mexico. They feed primarily on rodents and are vectors of relapsing fever (*B. parkeri* and *B. turicatae* respectively) to man. Transmission is solely by bite.

Ornithodoros coriaceus

This extends from California to Mexico. Known as the 'tlaaja' and the 'pajaroello', it is a large argasid and is notorious for attacking humans and cattle and deer in their bedding areas. The bites are reported to be painful. It is not a natural vector of relapsing fever.

Ornithodoros rostratus

Known also as the 'quanco' this occurs in southern

Brazil, Bolivia, Paraguay and north-eastern Argentina. It is an avid biter of man, domestic animals and wild animals, particularly peccaries. The bites are painful and pruritus and inflammation follow which may become secondarily infected. It is not a natural vector of relapsing fever.

Ornithodoros muesebecki

This is associated with marine birds on islands in the Arabian Gulf. The tick eagerly attacks humans and some dexterity is required to avoid being bitten. The bites may be numerous and irritant bullae develop at the bite sites with intense pruritus, headache and fever. A virus—Zirqa virus—(Bunyaviridae, Nairovirus) has been isolated from the tick and may be the cause of the illness associated with the bites.

FAMILY: IXODIDAE

The ixodids vary in size from small to large and the females are generally smaller than argasid females; but after a blood meal some ixodid females may exceed a length of 20 mm. The prominent capitulum projects anteriorly and is visible from above in all stages (Fig. III.13a). The mouthparts of some (*Ixodes* and *Amblyomma*) are long and can produce deep penetrating wounds in animals and man (Fig. III.13b). The shape of the basal plate of the capitulum is an important character in generic identification (Fig. III.9). The scutum is present in all stages, small and restricted to the anterior dorsum in larvae, nymphs and adults, but large and covering the entire dorsal surface in males; males and females can therefore be easily distinguished. Because of the large and hard scutum, male ixodids are unable to imbibe large quantities of

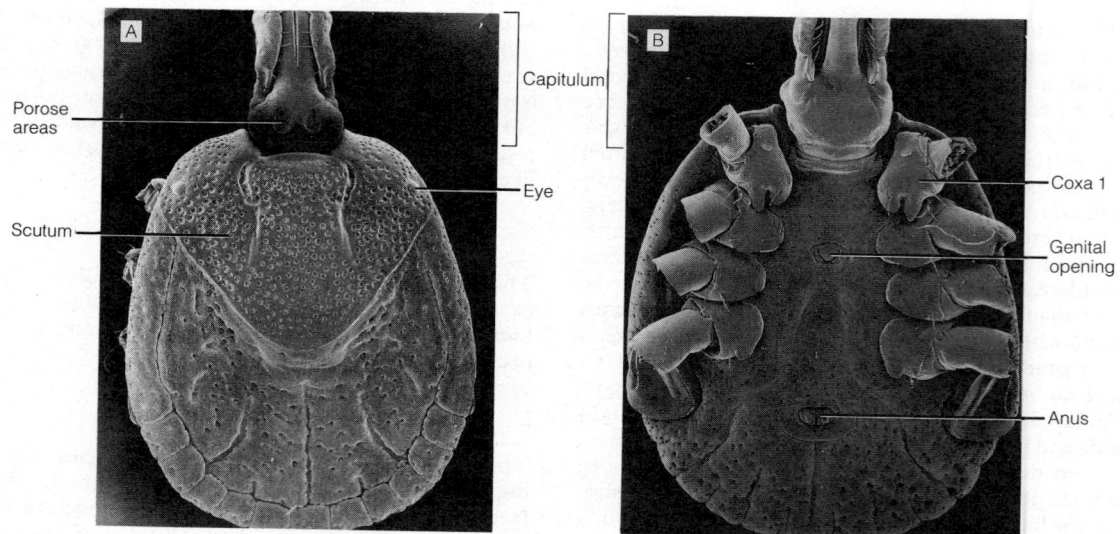

Fig. III.13 (A) Dorsal and (B) ventral view of *Amblyomma variegatum*. (Courtesy M. Nawar.)

blood. They do, however, ingest small amounts of blood. The scuta of some ixodids are ornamented with patterns of colours (*Amblyomma* spp.). Such ticks are called *ornate* ticks; those in which the scutum is not ornamented are called *inornate* ticks. Paired eyes when present are situated on either side of the scutum. The ventrally situated spiracles are behind the fourth pair of legs. Coxal glands are absent in ixodid ticks and the ingested blood is concentrated during the slow feeding by passage of fluid from the stomach into the body cavity from where it is processed through the salivary glands back into the host. During their slow feeding, ixodid ticks remain attached for several days, anchoring themselves firmly with the chelicerae and hypostome. They are helped in this by the secretion of a 'cement' by the salivary glands of most ixodids. Once attached great care should be taken in removing a tick because the mouthparts may be left behind in the host tissue and may become a source of irritation and secondary infection.

A few ticks, for example the cattle tick, are host-specific, but most utilize a wide range of hosts. Adult ixodids usually parasitize large mammals and the immatures, smaller mammals such as rodents and ground frequenting birds. Immatures of a few species of medical and veterinary importance have successfully adapted to feeding on small or large hosts. Man is only an occasional host for ixodids and it is usually the larvae and nymphs which attack man. Larvae or 'seed ticks' of some ixodids are avid feeders on man and are a bothersome nuisance in some outdoor areas in America and Africa. There are four stages in the life-cycle: the egg, and the three mobile stages, larva, nymph and adult. The fertilized and engorged female drops off the host on to the ground and lays a mass of several thousand eggs. The female dies after oviposition. The six-legged larvae after hatching climb to the tips of leaves, blades of grass or other vegetation to certain heights and gather in clusters questing for a host. They climb on to a passing host, feed for 4–6 days and drop to the ground and moult to the nymphal stage. Unlike the argasid ticks, ixodids have only one nymphal stage. The unfed nymphs quest for hosts like the larvae and after a blood meal (5–8 days) drop to the ground and moult into adults. Adults quest usually at a height greater than that of larvae and nymphs. Mating takes place on the host and the engorged female, after feeding for 6–12 days, drops off to lay a single batch of eggs.

The males may remain attached for many weeks or months, mating with several females. The whole life-cycle may take only two to four months in warm climates with continuous breeding throughout the year. In cold or temperate climates the life-cycle may take three to five years, the ticks being active or developing only in the warmer months. During the colder months and winter, one or more stages enter a diapause of several weeks or months. The parasitic feeding period of the different stages lasts from 4 to 12 days, which in the case of temperate climate ticks is a fraction of the time needed to complete the life-cycle (Fig. III.12). Most ixodid ticks have a three-host cycle in which each active stage (larva, nymph, adult) parasitizes a different animal of the same or different species. Hosts of immatures are smaller sized mammals or birds and of adults, large mammals. A few species of *Hyalomma* and *Rhipicephalus* have a two-host cycle. The fed larva moults on the host (not on the ground) into nymphs which drop to the ground and moult into adults. The adults seek a second host for a blood meal. *Boophilus* spp., the cattle ticks, have a one-host cycle. The larvae and nymphs feed and moult on the host. The stages found on the ground are unfed larvae and engorged females.

Ixodes dammini

The tick is widely distributed in the north-eastern USA and adjacent Canada and has also been recorded from Wisconsin; the range appears to be extending probably due to proliferation of deer, hosts of the adult ticks. Immature *I. dammini* parasitize rodents (particularly the white-footed mouse) as well as man, and adults appear to prefer feeding on the white-tailed deer; a few adults have been taken from man also. *I. dammini* is the vector of human babesiosis (*Babesia microti*) and of Lyme disease (a spirochaetal infection caused by *Borrelia burgdorferi*) in the eastern USA. Transmission of the babesia and the spirochaetes is by the bite of infected ticks.

Ixodes ricinus (European sheep tick or castor bean tick)

This tick is widely distributed in rough pasture and woodland in western Europe, extending from Ireland, Britain, southern Scandinavia to Spain, Portugal, Italy, Algeria, Morocco, central Europe and European USSR. Eastwards, the species extends to the Caspian Sea and northern Iran. *I. ricinus* is the vector of the flavivirus louping ill (primarily of sheep and cattle but affecting man also) in Great Britain and Ireland, and of tick-borne encephalitis (TBE) in Europe. Immature ticks are found on rodents and birds and adults attack sheep, cattle and also man. The life-cycle takes two to four years to complete. Transmission of infection is by bite. The tick also causes erythema chronicum migrans (ECM) and European Lyme disease similar to American Lyme disease.

Ixodes persulcatus (the taiga tick)

This tick is widespread in the USSR from the Baltic Sea to the Sea of Japan and also in Japan. It is more cold hardy than *I. ricinus*. The western distribution of the tick overlaps that of *I. ricinus*. In Russia, the tick is associated with the taiga forest. Feeding habits are similar to those of *I. ricinus*. The life-cycle extends over two to four years. It is the chief vector of Russian spring–summer encephalitis (flavivirus). Transovarial transmission occurs but the rate is variable.

Ixodes holocyclus

This occurs in the humid densely vegetated coastal areas of Queensland and New South Wales in Australia where it infests a variety of mammalian hosts. It causes tick paralysis in dogs and man. It is the vector of Queensland tick typhus (*Rickettsia australis*).

Haemaphysalis spinigera

This tick occurs in Sri Lanka and south India. It is abundant where cattle have been introduced into cleared forests. It is the chief vector of Kyasanur Forest disease in southern India (flavivirus). Immatures feed on small forest rodents, monkeys and man. Exposure of humans to the ticks and risk of infection are highest in the dry pre-monsoon period when villagers go into the forest to gather firewood. Transmission of infection to man is by bite of infected nymphs. There is no transovarial transmission in vector ticks.

Haemaphysalis leachi

This is a widely distributed carnivore tick. In South Africa urban cases of boutonneuse fever (*Rickettsia conori*) are associated with contamination of skin or of eyes from infected ticks crushed while de-ticking dogs.

Rhipicephalus appendiculatus

This is an African species found in wooded and shrubby grassland from southern Sudan to South Africa. It is absent in West Africa. In East Africa it is the vector of the protozoan disease East Coast fever in cattle. In the South African veld it is the chief vector of African tick typhus and an avid man biter.

Rhipicephalus sanguineus

This is a carnivore tick originating from Africa but now a cosmopolitan tick of dogs. In the Mediterranean basin it is the chief vector of boutonneuse fever to man.

Dermacentor andersoni (Rocky Mountain wood tick)

This is distributed from western Nebraska to the eastern slopes of the Cascades and from northern Arizona and New Mexico in the USA to British Columbia and Manitoba in Canada. It is the vector of Rocky Mountain spotted fever (*Rickettsia rickettsi*) in these areas. Larvae and nymphs feed on practically every rodent, adults parasitize wild and domestic herbivores and eagerly bite man. Transmission of the rickettsiae is by bite and trans-stadial and transovarial transmission occur. There may be an interval of some hours or a day before the attached tick can transmit the rickettsiae. If the tick is removed within a few hours the risk of infection is considerably reduced. This tick also transmits Colorado tick fever virus to man.

Dermacentor variabilis (American dog tick)

This tick occurs east of the Rocky Mountains and in California, Mexico and Canada. It is particularly abundant along the east coast of USA. Immatures feed on rodents, adults on wild and domestic carnivores, including dogs and also man. It is the vector of Rocky Mountain spotted fever in the eastern USA. Infestation of dogs with *D. variabilis* brings the disease close to homes and infections occur among women and children.

Dermacentor marginatus, D. silvarum and D. nuttalli

These are the chief vectors of Siberian tick typhus (*Rickettsia sibirica*). *D. marginatus* is found in shrubby areas and lowland forests from northern Kazakstan to central Europe. *D. silvarum* extends from the eastern limits of *D. marginatus* to western Siberia. *D. nuttalli* is widely distributed in central and eastern Siberia, Mongolia and China southwards to central Asia and Tibet. *R. sibirica* can survive for long periods in the ticks. Transmission is by bite and both trans-stadial and transovarial transmission have been demonstrated.

Dermacentor pictus

This tick has the same distribution as *D. marginatus* and occurs in mixed and deciduous forests. The arbovirus causing Omsk haemorrhagic fever infects this tick and has been isolated from it, but transmission to man is believed to be by contact with, or drinking water infected with, the urine and faeces of musk-rats.

Amblyomma hebraeum

Amblyomma ticks have long mouthparts. *A. hebraeum*, the South African bont tick, extends from South Africa into Zimbabwe and Mozambique. It is the vector of boutonneuse fever in the South African veld where immatures swarm and feed avidly on humans. Apart from man, immature stages feed on birds and small and large mammals while adults feed on large wild and domestic mammals. *Rickettsia conori* can be maintained for several generations in the tick by hereditary transmission.

Amblyomma americanum ('lone-star tick')

All stages attack man. It is widely distributed from South America into central and eastern USA. It is the vector of Rocky Mountain spotted fever in south-central and south-eastern USA. The attached feeding ticks are difficult to remove because of the long mouth-parts. But gentle traction, or previous application of 0.6% pyrethrin in methyl benzoate or of camphorated phenol to the skin makes detachment easier.

Amblyomma cajennense (Cayenne tick)

This tick extends from South America and the Carib-bean to southern Texas. Immatures attack man. It is the vector of Rocky Mountain spotted fever to man in Mexico, Panama, Colombia and Brazil.

Hyalomma marginatum marginatum

Hyalomma are hardy ticks adapted to living under arid or semi-arid conditions. They occur in the USSR and southern Europe. Birds are important hosts of the immature stages and the ticks have been carried to many parts of Europe and Africa by migrating birds. It is the vector of the tick-borne arbovirus causing Crimean-Congo haemorrhagic fever.

PENTASTOMIDS

J. Riley

Pentastomids, sometimes called linguatulids or 'tongue worms' are neither helminths nor typical arthropods. They possess a number of arthropod-like characters and there is evidence to suggest that they may be highly specialized endoparasitic crustaceans (see Riley,[2] for a review). However, most workers continue to treat pentastomids as a group of uncertain phylogenetic affinities. Four species, belonging to two genera, may affect man as dead-end infections: *Linguatula* which normally infects other mammals and *Armillifer* which infects snakes and mammals as intermediate hosts.

FAMILY: LINGUATULIDAE

GENUS: *Linguatula*

Linguatula serrata is found worldwide. The adults live in the nasal passages of dogs, foxes and wolves (family Canidae) which are the definitive hosts. Eggs are expelled by sneezing or in nasal discharges, or via the intestine where some premature hatching may occur. Eggs are infective to mammal intermediate hosts, including rodents and domestic animals such as sheep or goats. Primary larvae emerge, penetrate the gut wall and migrate to the viscera, particularly to the mesenteric lymph nodes, where they become encapsulated by host tissue. Within the cyst several moults eventually lead to the formation of an infective larva or nymph. Infection of the definitive host occurs when viscera containing the encysted infective stage is eaten. The epidemiology of *L. serrata* infections is complex, because both eggs and infective larvae can become established in man. When eggs are consumed, primary larvae encyst on the viscera producing visceral linguatulosis, whereas ingested infective larvae attempt to migrate to the nasal passages producing naso-pharyngeal linguatulosis or halzoun(Chapter 24).

Morphology

The body of adult *Linguatula* (Fig. III.14) is club-shaped, flattened ventrally, convex dorsally and transversely striated into about 90 superficial annulations. The cephalothorax bears the quadrangular mouth, which is flanked by two pairs of simple retractile hooks. Females are 80–130 mm in length, tapering from 8–10 mm anteriorly to 2 mm posteriorly. The uterine coils, full of reddish-brown eggs, occupy the median line of the body and the translucent flared lateral extensions of the anterior abdomen mould to the contours of the nasal sinuses. Living males are transparent in life but become white when fixed, measure 18–27 mm long and 3 mm broad anteriorly to 0.5 mm posteriorly. The oval eggs, measuring 70 by 100 μm are loosely enveloped by a thin hyaline outer capsule and contain mature primary larvae which have an anterior penetration stylet and four stumpy legs terminating in double claws. Infective nymphs (Fig. III.14) are worm-like, flattened and 4–6 mm in length;

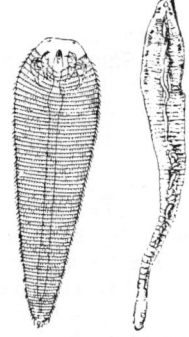

Fig. III.14 *Linguatula serrata.* Left, Nymph. ×6. Right, Adult. Natural size.

the posterior edge of each body annulus carries a row of prominent backward pointing spines which are sufficient to distinguish *Linguatula* spp. in any tissue section.

Infection in man

Cysts. Encysted infective nymphs are well tolerated and are frequently encountered in the mesenteric glands of domestic animals, as well as in rabbits and hares. Data on human infections arise only from incidental findings during autopsy and in the few instances where sample sizes were large nymphs were not uncommon.[3] Nymphs developing on visceral organs cause no symptoms but occasionally they penetrate the anterior chamber of the eye causing monocular uveitis. Following surgical removal of these parasites patients recover fully.

Clinical effects (halzoun; marrara syndrome).
See Chapter 24.

Diagnosis

In tissue sections, infective larvae of *Linguatula* are enclosed within a thin fibrotic capsule lined by the preceding cast nymphal cuticle. The spinous cuticle is distinctive and the spacious body cavity contains an obvious intestinal tract flanked by a pair of prominent glands composed of large individual gland cells. These characteristics will serve to distinguish them from sparganum (Fig. 23.40, p. 555).

FAMILY: ARMILLIFERIDAE

GENUS: *Armillifer*

Armillifer armillatus infects humans in tropical Africa. In Oriental regions *A. moniliformis* is the usual cause of human infections, which have been recorded from Malaysia, Java, Manila, Sumatra and China.

Morphology

Adult parasites inhabit the lungs of pythons, and in Africa large vipers; the larval forms encyst in the tissues of many mammal species, including monkeys and man. The parasite is cylindrical, vermiform, yellowish and translucent with conspicuous opaque annulated rings around the body, 1–2 mm apart (Fig. III.15). In females the uterine coils, filled with white

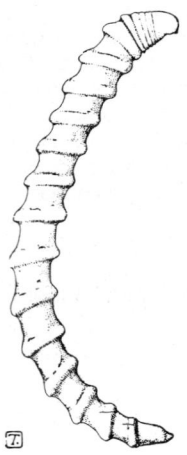

Fig. III.15 *Armillifer armillatus,* natural size.

or yellowish eggs, are easily visible through the cuticle. The female of *A. armillatus* is 70–140 mm long and 5–9 mm wide, the male 30–50 mm long and 3–4 mm wide: females possess up to 22 annuli and males up to 24. Both sexes of *A. moniliformis* are more slender and have more annuli (26 and above) than *A. armillatus*. The nymphs lie coiled within their cysts in a flat spiral, with the ventral surface corresponding to the convexity of the curve. In shape and structure they resemble the adult. A third species of *Armillifer* (*A. grandis*) has been reported from man in central Africa where nymphs are smaller (9–15 mm long) than those of *A. armillatus* (13–23 mm long): *A. moniliformis* nymphs are intermediate in size (12–20 mm).

Infection in man

The life-history of *Armillifer* is broadly similar to that of *Linguatula*, although man can act only as an intermediate host. Eggs remain viable on soil for at least three months and, when ingested, hatch in the intestine and the larvae immediately bore through the gut wall to lodge in any tissue. At least six moults occur over a period of six months to a year to form infective nymphs. Man acquires the infection by eating poorly cooked snake meat, or by drinking water contaminated by snake faeces. In man the infection comes to a dead end and the nymphs commonly encyst in or on the liver, intestinal tract and lungs.

For the clinical features of infection in man, see Chapter 24.

PHLEBOTOMINE SANDFLIES

R. P. Lane

FAMILY: PSYCHODIDAE

SUBFAMILY: PHLEBOTOMINAE

IMPORTANT GENERA:
Phlebotomus (Old World) and *Lutzomyia* (New World)

Phlebotomine sandflies are small, delicate, hairy flies (1.5–3.5 mm) with long, slender legs and filamentous antennae. Of the 700 species found throughout the tropics and subtropics, only a small proportion (*ca* 70 species) are thought to be involved in the transmission of disease to man. The flies are easily distinguished from other small Diptera when alive by the characteristic manner in which they hold their pointed wings above their body (like a vertical 'V'). In other blood-sucking Diptera the wings are held flat over the abdomen, either one on top of the other (Culicidae, Simuliidae, *Culicoides*) or slightly ajar (Tabanidae). It is important to differentiate phlebotomine sandflies from other small flies known colloquially as 'sandflies' in certain parts of the world, especially midges of the genus *Culicoides* (see p. 1435) which abound in coastal areas of the south-eastern USA, Central America and the Caribbean; and Simuliidae (see p. 1436) in Australasia.

Two genera contain anthropophagous species: *Phlebotomus* in the Old World and *Lutzomyia* in the New World. Rarely, some species of the genus *Sergentomyia*, which feed principally on reptiles, will bite man but there is no evidence to suggest they are capable of transmitting parasites on such occasions. There is relatively little external morphological difference between the females which suck blood and the males, which only feed on plant juices, other than the external genitalia.

Transmission of pathogens takes place during blood feeding. Phlebotomine sandflies are vectors of visceral leishmaniasis (VL: kala-azar; see Chapter 4), the various forms of cutaneous leishmaniasis (CL: oriental sore, espundia, etc.; see Chapter 37), bartonellosis (Oroya fever, Carrión's disease; Chapter 11) and sandfly fever (papataci or papatasi fever, three-day fever, etc.; see Chapter 5).

Sandflies are a difficult group to study in relation to disease, as the adults are small and can be hard to find; finding larvae is almost impossible. This has made the incrimination of vectors during epidemiological studies particularly difficult and, therefore, the vector status of many species remains uncertain.[4] (See also section on epidemiology of leishmaniasis p. 1304.) Compared with other vector groups (e.g. Culicidae and Simuliidae), the biology of sandflies is poorly known. However, a thorough understanding of the natural history of sandflies is essential, since the epidemiology of the diseases they transmit is largely determined by the ecology and behaviour of the vectors.

Distribution and ecology

Sandflies are found mainly in the tropics and subtropics, with a few species penetrating into temperate regions in both the northern (to 50° north) and southern hemispheres (to about 40° south). The distribution of leishmaniasis is not as extensive as that of sandflies, for reasons that are not entirely known: e.g. there is no human leishmaniasis recorded from South-East Asia and Australasia, although several potential vectors are present.

In the Old World, man-biting sandflies are confined to the subtropics, there being very few anthropophilic species in Africa south of the Sahara. Even in the visceral leishmaniasis areas of Kenya, man-biters are not conspicuous. In contrast, the transmission of leishmaniasis in the New World is principally in the tropics.

Sandflies occur in a very wide range of habitats, from sea level (a major focus of leishmaniasis around the Dead Sea is below sea level!) to altitudes of 2800 m or more in the Andes and Ethiopia, and from hot dry deserts, through savannahs and open woodland to dense tropical rain-forest. In general, each species has fairly specific ecological requirements and in a few cases these may encompass the conditions in and around the dwellings of man or his domestic animals and thus the species becomes peridomestic. The majority of peridomestic sandfly species are vectors of infections to man. The highly focal nature of many leishmaniases is undoubtedly a result of ecological constraints on the vectors and probably, to a lesser extent, on the mammalian reservoirs. In central Asia, sandflies are localized, restricted to the natural foci of gerbil colonies and by soil texture and moisture. Even in tropical rain-forests, sandflies are not uniformly distributed.

In the Old World most foci of leishmaniasis, particularly of cutaneous leishmaniasis, are in dry, semi-arid areas, in contrast to the New World where the disease is mainly transmitted in forests (although visceral leishmaniasis in South America is primarily in

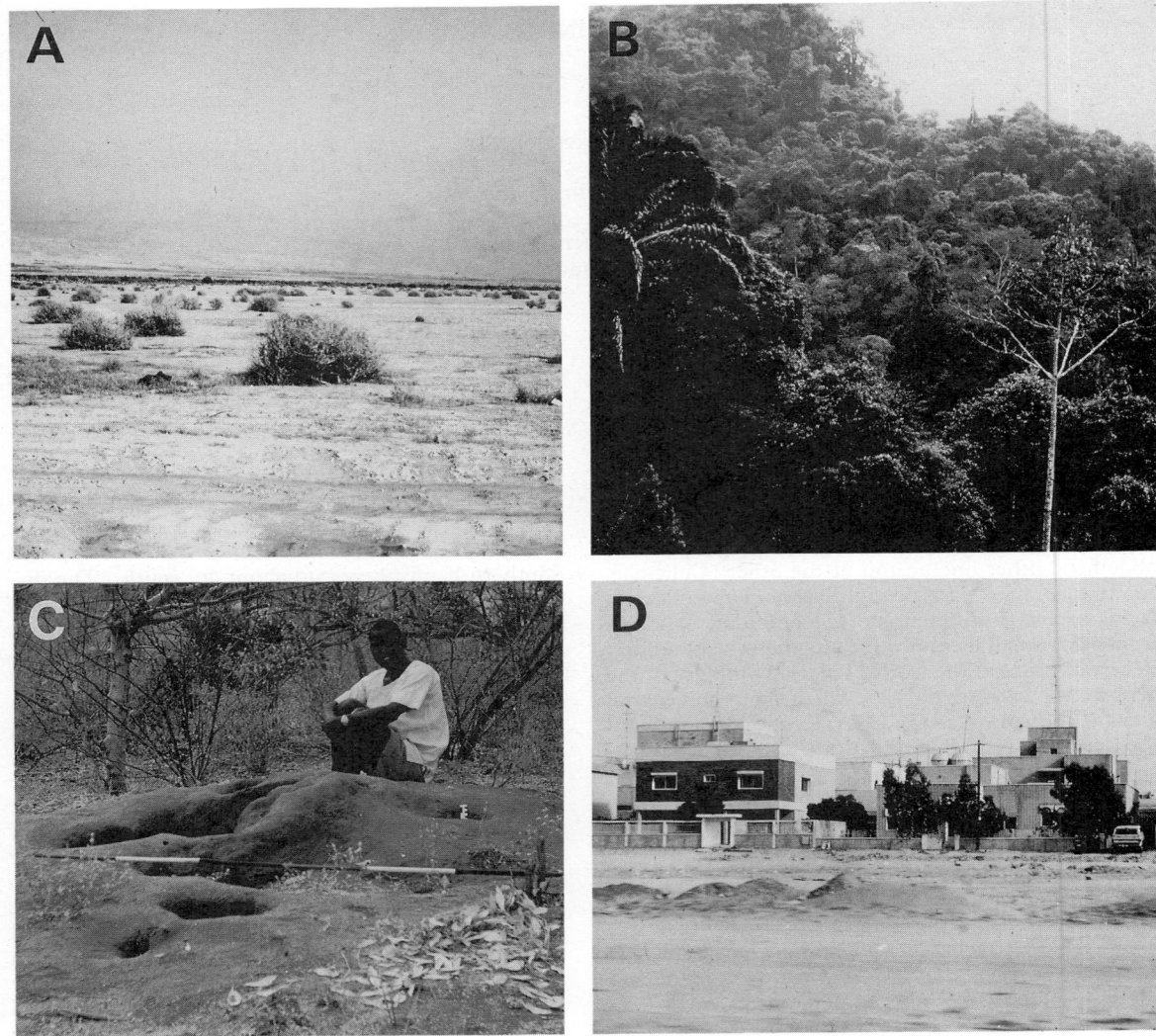

Fig. III.16 (A) A typical arid habitat of *Phlebotomus papatasi* (Jordan Valley), where this species transmits *L. (L.) major* from the fat sand-rat (*Psammomys obesus*) to man and causes cutaneous leishmaniasis. (B) Cutaneous leishmaniasis due to *L. (L.) mexicana* is transmitted from tree rats to man by *Lutzomyia olmeca olmeca* in wet forests of Central America (Belize). (C) Eroded termite hills are the preferred resting sites of the visceral leishmaniasis vector *Phlebotomus martini* in some areas of East Africa. (Courtesy D. M. Minter.) (D) Occupants of modern housing developments around expanding towns, particularly in the Middle East, may become infected by the bites of peridomestic sandflies.

savannah areas). Consequently, occupational differences exist between those acquiring infections; cutaneous disease in the Neotropics is primarily associated with working in or modifying the forest environment, whereas in the Old World the disease affects those in rural savannah and urban areas. The open nature of the savannah and steppe environments and the patchy distribution of suitable microclimates for sandflies, has prompted the application of landscape epidemiology in the investigation of many Old World foci of cutaneous leishmaniasis.

The distribution and abundance of sandflies can alter with changing land use. Deforestation in the New World has led to a marked reduction in cutaneous leishmaniasis (after the initial increase in disease during land clearance), but whether such areas will provide opportunities for the extension in the range of the VL vector *Lutzomyia longipalpis* and subsequent

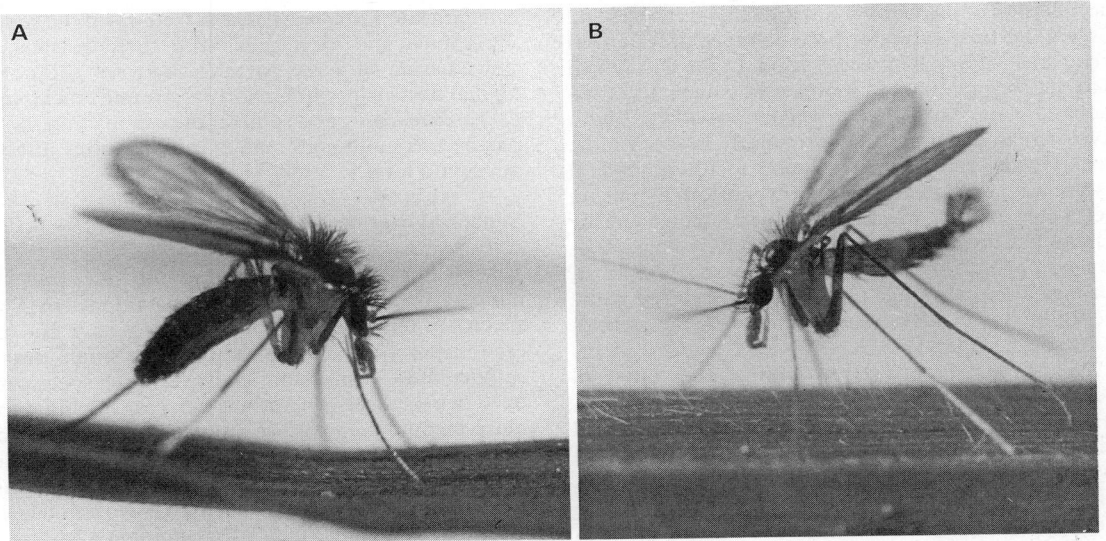

Fig. III.17 Living female (*left*) and male (*right*) phlebotomine sandflies (*Lutzomyia longipalpis*), showing the hairy body and wings, the generally mosquito-like stance and appearance except for the characteristic position of the wings, held in a V over the back. (Courtesy Mr C. J. Webb.)

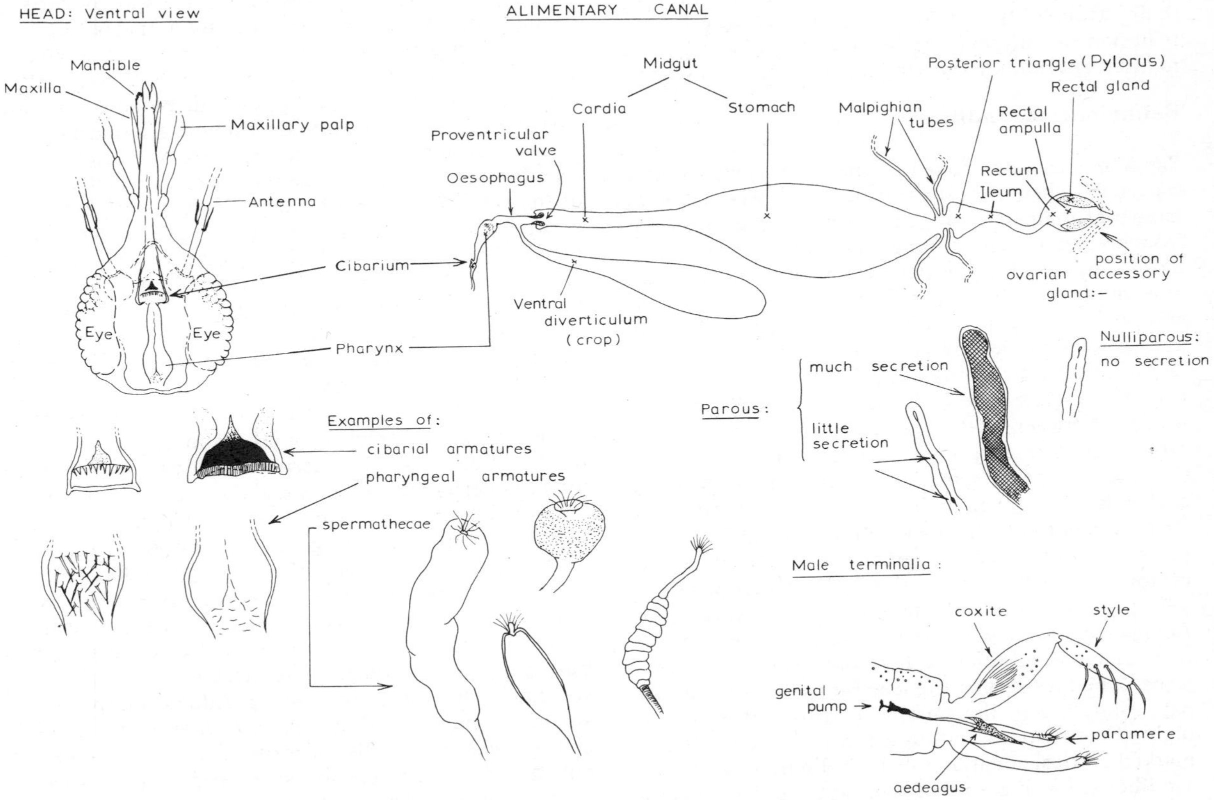

HEAD: Ventral view

ALIMENTARY CANAL

Maxilla
Mandible
Maxillary palp
Antenna
Cibarium
Eye
Eye
Pharynx

Midgut
Cardia
Stomach
Proventricular valve
Oesophagus
Ventral diverticulum (crop)

Posterior triangle (Pylorus)
Rectal gland
Malpighian tubes
Rectal ampulla
Rectum
Ileum
position of ovarian accessory gland:-

Parous:
much secretion
little secretion

Nulliparous:
no secretion

Examples of:
cibarial armatures
pharyngeal armatures
spermathecae

Male terminalia:
coxite
style
genital pump
aedeagus
paramere

Fig. III.18 The anatomy of the alimentary canal of sandflies, showing the ovarian glands and features of taxonomic importance.

transmission of the visceral disease remains to be seen. Visceral leishmaniasis has become more prevalent in urban areas of Brazil in recent years. In the Old World there has been a marked increase in cutaneous leishmaniasis (due to *L. (L.) major*) associated with development programmes, particularly in the Middle East. However, in Egypt a small focus of visceral disease was associated with town expansion. By raising the water table, irrigation projects considerably increase the breeding of some vector species, e.g. *Phlebotomus papatasi* but, in some circumstances at least, this may also discourage the rodent reservoir, e.g. the deeply burrowing *Rhombomys opimus* in the steppes of the southern USSR.

When they are not active, sandflies seek out cool and relatively humid (but not wet) dark niches. Resting sites such as caves, tree holes, tree trunks and the spaces between buttresses, cracks in rocks and cavities between boulders, fissures in the ground, buildings, termite hills and animal burrows are commonly used. By withdrawing to these daytime sites, sandflies are able to survive in very hot and dry climates, in conditions which would otherwise rapidly kill them, emerging at night when the ambient temperature drops and the humidity rises. Such resting sites are very important in the study of sandflies, as their availability determines the ecological distribution of different species: various traps are used to intercept sandflies moving to and from such places.

Behaviour of sandflies

Sandflies usually have a short hopping flight, especially when close to prospective hosts. Little is known of their long range movements (e.g. dispersal from breeding sites), although they can fly up to 2.2 km over a period of a few days in open habitats. They only fly at night and in a single night they may fly several hundred metres, in their search for a host and subsequent resting and breeding sites. Climatic factors affect activity markedly; biting does not usually take place below 20°C in tropical species; *P. papatasi* is active between 45–60% relative humidity, whereas other species require 75–85% relative humidity, and the flight range of some species (e.g. *P. sergenti*) is greater in humid than in dry climates. Although slight air movement aids the detection of hosts along odour plumes, wind speeds of greater than 1.5 m/second inhibit flight, which ceases altogether in light winds of 4–5 m/second. Forest sandflies, such as the Amazonian *Lutzomyia umbratilis*, often exhibit regular vertical movements in addition to horizontal movement patterns. The flies rest in the tree buttresses during the day, migrating to the canopy in search of a host at night. Furthermore, within a forest, there is often a marked vertical zonation in which different species of sandflies are active, so that some species remain close to the ground, feeding on ground-dwelling rodents (e.g. the South American vectors *Lutzomyia flavis-*

cutellata and *Lutzomyia olmeca* feeding on the rodents *Proechimys* and *Oryzomys*). For these reasons, the transmission of some parasites between the normal animal hosts is predominantly at ground level (e.g. *L. (L.) amazonensis*) and some in the canopy (e.g. *L. (V.) panamensis*), although man usually acquires infection at ground level.

Seasonal distribution

Several abiotic factors affect sandfly numbers, but temperature and rainfall are the most important. Some species in temperate regions may only have one generation per year, and consequently a single peak of activity and transmission. However, such species may have two or three generations per year in climatically more favourable areas. In tropical countries, species react more to rainfall cycles and may be more prevalent in either the wet or dry season. Several anthropophilic species may be present, each with its own annual cycle of activity and potential for transmission.

Blood feeding

Only females feed on blood, using the nutrients to develop eggs. feeding takes place on exposed parts of the body by thrusting the tiny mouthparts (0.15–0.57 mm) into the skin and, using minutely serated mandibles in a scissor-like manner, to create a small pool from which the blood is sucked. Blood taken in this manner is directed into the midgut. Liquids taken by other means (e.g. sugar feeding) are directed to the crop for sterilization and then to the midgut; infection of the sandfly gut with bacteria or yeasts appears to depress *Leishmania* development. Both males and females feed on sugars, which they obtain as honeydew or from plants, either passively (extrafloral nectaries, fallen fruits, etc.) or by actively piercing leaves or stems. The presence of sugars is essential for the full development of *Leishmania* (see section on invertebrate life-cycles of *Leishmania*, p. 1296).

The site of a bite determines the situation of pirmary lesions in cutaneous leishmaniasis, and may be influenced as much by the presence of clothes as by the intrinsic preferences of a vector. Consequently, sleeping outside in hot weather without bed-nets, or working in forests during the day without suitable clothing, increases the risk of acquiring an infection.

Sandflies are crepuscular; biting takes place at different times of the night according to the species. When disturbed, sandflies in dense forests, caves or buildings, may bite dutring the day. Only a few species are endophilic; these are mostly peridomestic species, such as *P. papatasi*, *P. chinensis*, *P. sergenti* and *Lutzomyia longipalpis*, the majority preferring to bite outside, often near their probable breeding and resting sites. It is a relatively small ecological step from rodent burrows and caves to human dwellings. The distinction between peridomestic and 'wild; species has little meaning in sparsely populated areas, where the buildings themselves are made of local materials, perhaps without solid walls. Equally, no species is entirely domestic.

The biting rates of sandflies vary greatly, up to a maximum of about 1000/h. Most species probably have a narrow range of preferred hosts. Species of *Sergentomyia* feed predominantly on reptiles, as do some species of *Lutzomyia* and *Phlebotomus*, but the latter genera feed mainly on homoiotherms, especially mammals. Several peridomestic, mammal-feeding sandflies (*P. papatasi*, *P. sergenti*, and *Lutzomyia longipalpis*), will readily feed on poultry, and chicken-coops may be a source of biting sandflies.

Most species are gonotrophically concordant, taking one blood meal for each batch of eggs matured. However, autogeny, the ability to lay eggs without a blood meal, is found in populations of some man-biting species. Some species will feed more than once per ovarian cycle, thus increasing man-fly contact. Oviposition usually takes place 5–10 days after a blood meal. The proportion of parous females within a population (i.e. those which have laid eggs and by inference have had a blood meal, with the concomitant risk of acquiring an infection) indicates the epidemiological potential of the population. The highest parous rates occur in populations towards the end of the 'sandfly season', when sandfly infection rates are maximal and subsequent transmission is most likely. Unfortunately, it is not easy to determine accurately the number of times a female sandfly has laid eggs, as in other vectors such as mosquitoes. The residual secretions in the accessory glands (at the base of the oviduct) have been used but are not always reliable. At present, the established method of searching for follicular relics in the ovarioles still needs to be developed, beyond simply distinguishing between parous and nulliparous sandflies.

Life-history

Relatively little is known about the immature stages of sandflies and their breeding sites, which are terrestrial, in striking contrast to other nematocerous flies such as Culicidae, Simuliidae, Ceratopogonidae, and Chironomidae. Breeding and resting often takes place in the same microhabitat; such as the soil accumulated in cracks in walls or among rocks, in animal burrows and shelters, caves, or in damp leaf litter in forests. The main requirements for breeding sites are moisture and the presence of organic detritus, etc. on which the larvae can feed.

The eggs are small, generally less than 0.7 mm, and elliptical with a fine chorionic pattern. Between 30 and 70 eggs are scattered about the potential breeding site by the ovipositing female. Hatching occurs one to two weeks later. The larvae are caterpillar-like and have a distinct dark head-capsule and the pale, cream-coloured body is sparsely covered with characteristic club-shaped hairs ('match-stick' hairs). There are four instars, the first with a single pair, and the remaining instars with two pairs, of long, highly characteristic, caudal bristles on the anal segment. The caudal bristles are almost as long as the body, Diapause occurs during the fourth instar of several species in areas where there are cool winters (e.g. Mediterranean basin). The pupa is inactive and usually hatches within 5–10 days. The duration of the larval instars varies greatly, both between and within species (in the laboratory at least), as it is regulated mainly by temperature. The period from oviposition to adult eclosion takes between 20 days and several months (in temperate or diapausing species and those living at high altitudes in the tropics, e.g. *P. longipes*).

Emergence takes place during the hours of darkness, often just before dawn. Males usually emerge first. Little is known of mating in sandflies. Although swarming does not generally take place, males may congregate on and around prospective hosts and mate with females there. Pheromones and auditory signals from wing beats are also probably involved. The life of adult flies is unlikely to exceed a few weeks in nature. Once the female becomes infected, perhaps at the first blood meal, parasites can be transmitted to new hosts at intervals throughout the rest of her life.

Transmission of disease organisms

Sandflies transmit viruses, bacteria and protozoa (*Leishmania*) to vertebrates, but not nematodes. It is tempting to suppose that their inability to transmit nematodes is the effect of the elaborate cibarial and pharyngeal armature, which many species possess, damaging the worms during ingestion. However, midges of the subgenus *Forcipomyia* (*Lasiohelea*) have similar structures, but effectively transmit species of cattle *Onchocerca*.

Leishmania

Phlebotomine sandflies are most widely known as vectors of several *Leishmania* species to man. There is a continual gradation between species which are common vectors of parasites (often peridomestic species), secondary vectors, and those which rarely come into contact with man at all. A species may transmit a particular parasite in one area, but not in another: no two areas or foci are the same. The degree of human involvement in leishmaniases is very variable; many are cycles of reservoir–fly–reservoir, with occasional, almost chance infections; others cause regular zoonotic infections and some anthroponotic cycles are thought to involve only flies and man. It is important to understand natural transmission cycles for two reasons. Enzootic cycles may pose an unknown threat in remote areas being developed (mining, agriculture, etc.) and secondly, transmission may be maintained by several species, only one of which transmits the infection to man, e.g. in the southern USSR, *L*(*L*.) *major* infections between rodents are maintained by *P. mongolensis*, *P. caucasicus* and *P. andrejevi*, but only *P. papatasi* transmits the parasite to man.

Incrimination of a sandfly species as a vector is difficult, as many criteria have to be satisfied before a species can be unambiguously incriminated. Remarkably few species fulfil all these criteria, which are based on the discovery of natural infections in wild-caught flies and experimental transmission studies, but also include evidence of contact between the sandfly and man, contact between the sandfly and the reservoir host (where known), and the life-cycle of the parasite in the fly. As there is often no sharp distinction between important and minor or occasional vectors, it is impossible to draw up a definitive list of vectors. Table III.3 gives a synopsis of the 'proven' vectors of *Leishmania*; further details of suspected vectors are given in the section on the epidemiology of leishmaniasis (see p. 1304).

Within the genus *Phlebotomus* the majority of subgenera contain vectors or suspected vectors. Species of *Phlebotomus* (*sensu stricto*) are associated with *L*. (*L*.) *major* transmission in arid environments of East Africa, the Middle East, and the USSR. The subgenus *Paraphlebotomus* contains many species living in rodent burrows in central Asia and transmitting *L*. (*L*.) *major* between rodents and occasionally to man. One species, the peridomestic *P. sergenti*, is a vector of *L*. (*L*.) *tropica* in western Asia and the Middle East. Vectors of visceral leishmaniasis in the Old World are distributed through several subgenera: *Larroussius* (Mediterranean basin and Sahel); *Synphlebotomus* (East Africa); *Euphlebotomus* (India); and

Table III.3 Synopsis of proven vectors of leishmaniasis.[a]

Parasite	Vector	Animal reservoir	Principal areas
L. (*Leishmania*) *donovani*	*P*. (*Euphlebotomus*) *argentipes*	? man	India
L. (*L*.) *infantum*	*P*. (*Larroussius*) *ariasi*	fox, dog	Southern France
	P. (*Larroussius*) *longicuspis*	dog	North Africa
	P. (*Larroussius*) *major syriacus*	dog	Eastern Mediterranean
	P. (*Larroussius*) *orientalis*	rodents and carnivores	Sudan
	P. (*Larroussius*) *perfiliewi*	fox; *Rattus*	Italy; Yugoslavia
	P. (*Larroussius*) *perniciosus*	dog	Western Mediterranean
	P. (*Larroussius*) *smirnovi*	wolves; jackals	USSR
	P. (*Larroussius*) *tobbi*	dog	Eastern Mediterranean
	P. (*Paraphlebotomus*) *alexandri*	? man	North-west China: Sinkiang (Xinjiang)
	P. (*Adlerius*) *sichuanensis*	?	South-west China: Szechwan (Sichuan)
	P. (*Adlerius*) *chinensis*	dog; raccoon dog	China
	P. (*Adlerius*) *longiductus*	dog; jackal	USSR
	P. (*Synphlebotomus*) *martini*	dog; man	East Africa
L. (*L*.) *chagasi*	*Lutzomyia* (*Lutzomyia*) *longipalpis*	dog; foxes (*Lycalopex*, *Cerdocyon*)	Brazil
L. (*L*.) *tropica*	*P*. (*Paraphlebotomus*) *sergenti*	? man	Middle East to Indus basin
L. (*L*.) *major*	*P*. (*Phlebotomus*) *papatasi*	burrowing rodents	North Africa, Middle East: USSR, North-west India
	P. (*Phlebotomus*) *duboscqi*	rodents	African Sahel (Senegal to East Africa)
	P. (*Phlebotomus*) *salehi*	rodents	North-west India
L. (*L*.) *aethiopica*	*P*. (*Larroussius*) *pedifer*	hyrax	Ethiopia, Kenya
L. (*L*.) *mexicana*	*Lutzomyia* (*Nyssomyia*) *olmeca olmeca*	forest rodents	Central America
L. (*L*.) *amazonensis*	*Lutzomyia* (*Nyssomyia*) *flaviscutellata*	forest rodents; agouti, opossum	Amazon basin (Brazil)
L. (*Viannia*) *brazilensis*	*Lutzomyia* (*Psychodopygus*) *wellcomei*	?	Brazil
L. (*V*.) *panamensis*	*Lutzomyia* (*Nyssomyia*) *trapidoi*	sloth (*Choloepus hoffmani*)	Panama
L. (*V*.) *guyanensis*	*Lutzomyia* (*Nyssomyia*) *umbratilis*	sloth (*Choloepus didactylus*)	Northern Brazil, Guyanas
L. (*V*.) *peruviana*	?	? (dog; as secondary host)	Western Andes (South America)

[a]Based on World Health Organization.[4] For further details, and for numerous species incriminated, but not conclusively proved as vectors, see also section on epidemiology of the leishmaniases, p. 735.

Adlerius (Near East, northern China). The genus *Lutzomyia* is much more diverse than its Old World counterpart; some subgenera contain several vector species (e.g. *Nyssomyia* and *Psychodopygus*), whereas many other subgenera and species-groups contain only one or two species which are involved in the transmission of *Leishmania*.

Leishmania in the sandfly. After ingestion, the parasites in an infected blood meal undergo metamorphosis to the promastigote form and multiply within the sandfly gut before they become infective. The site in which this development takes place varies between different groups of *Leishmania* and is related to the micromorphology and biochemistry of the sandfly gut. The attachment mechanisms of *Leishmania* are adapted to the surface structure (chitinous or membranous) of the section of the gut to which they adhere. Enzyme activity in the midgut, following blood meals from different hosts, will differentially affect the survival of *Leishmania*.

The location of the parasites in the gut during their development (relative to the pylorus; the sphincter between the mid- and hindgut), has been used in parasite classification (Fig. III.19).[5] This subject is discussed in detail in the section on the genus *Leishmania* (see p. 1294) and may be briefly summarized here as follows.

1 Peripylarian ('both sides of the gate') development takes place in the hindgut and then the parasites migrate forward before transmission by bite. Mainly parasites of New World mammals (members of the subgenus *L. (Viannia)*: *L. (V.) braziliensis, guyanensis, panamensis* and *peruviana*). Some parasites of Old World reptiles (e.g. the former *L. adleri*), whose taxonomic status (as '*Sauroleishmania*'; see p. 1294) is presently in doubt, also have a peripylarian form of development in sandflies.

2 Suprapylarian ('above the gate') development is entirely within the midgut prior to anterior migration and transmission by bite. Parasites of New and Old World mammals (members of the subgenus *Leishmania (sensu stricto)*: *L. (L.) donovani* group, *L. (L.) mexicana* group, *L. (L.) hertigi* group and *L. (L.) major* group).

The term hypopylarian ('under the gate') development was used for parasites of some Old World lizards formerly included in the genus *Leishmania*, but which are currently referred to as *Sauroleishmania* species (of uncertain status), e.g. the former *L. agamae* and *L. ceramodactyli*. Hypopylarian development is confined to the hindgut and transmission is by ingestion or crushing of the infected fly, when fed upon by lizards or other insectivorous vertebrates.

Although transmission occurs through the bite of a sandfly, the exact mechanism by which parasites are taken up or deposited in the skin of a new host is unclear (see the section on vector–parasite interactions, below). Infection with parasites changes the behaviour of a sandfly; a heavily infected fly probes much more frequently than an uninfected fly, in a manner analogous to a flea infected with *Yersinia*. *Leishmania* can be readily transmitted during each probe, which may only last a few seconds, and this is probably the origin of the multiple lesions seen in some patients (particularly those with *L. (L.) major* infections). Infection does not appreciably alter the dispersal of sandflies.

Vector–parasite specificity of sandflies and the *Leishmania* species they transmit is affected by several factors, including behaviour (e.g. propensity of a vector to bite a particular species of reservoir host), ecological factors and biochemical factors (e.g. enzyme activity) operating in the sandfly gut. Natural infection rates in wild flies are usually very low (below 1%), but exceptionally may be high in some foci (e.g. up to 20% in the Jordan Valley).

Viruses

Sandfly fever (papataci or papatasi fever, three-day fever) is caused by two distinct virus serotypes (Naples and Sicilian) and results in acute febrile illness in man, lasting 2 to 4 days although incapacitation may extend for much longer periods.[6] It is common during the summer months throughout the Mediterranean basin, the Middle East, Pakistan and parts of India and Central America. The disease is of considerable military importance because up to 75% of non-immune individuals arriving in an endemic area may be affected. In Mediterranean areas where the disease is endemic, most of the population is thought to be infected during childhood, possibly suffering only a mild illness (Chapter 5).

Phlebotomus papatasi was incriminated as the vector in Egypt and is generally thought to transmit sandfly fever throughout the Old World range of the disease (i.e. except Central America). Natural infection rates of sandflies are between 0.015 and 0.5%. No natural vertebrate reservoir is known, although infected humans can infect flies and thus have some amplifying effect during epidemics. It is most likely that the principal maintenance mechanism is by transovarial transmission along genetically susceptible lines of the vector.

Sandflies transmit several other phleboviruses; *Phlebotomus perniciosus* transmits Toscana virus in the northern Mediterranean and in the New World *Lutzomyia trapidoi* and *Lutzomyia ylephiletor* transmit Chagres and Punta Toro viruses. Viruses have been isolated from several other species.

Bacteria

Infections due to *Bartonella bacilliformis* (Oroya fever, verruga peruana) are found only in the central Andean Cordilleras of Peru, Colombia and Ecuador. The disease is endemic in valleys between 750 and 2700 m

Section of a Phlebotomine sandfly to show the different regions of the alimentary canal

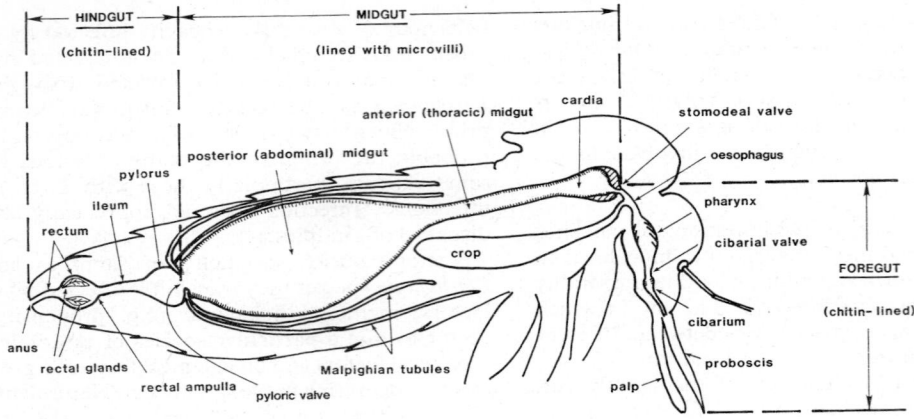

Section **SUPRAPYLARIA** ("above the gate")

Development in midgut only (no hindgut development). Transmission by bite

Parasites of Old and New World mammals: subgenus <u>Leishmania</u>:

1. Old & New World VL: <u>L. (L.) donovani</u> & <u>L. (L.) infantum</u> (OW)

<u>L. (L.) chagasi</u> (NW)

2. Old World CL: <u>L. (L.) tropica</u>, <u>L. (L.) major</u>, & <u>L. (L.) aethiopica</u>

3. New World CL (members of <u>L. (L.) mexicana</u> complex):

<u>L. (L.) mexicana</u>, <u>L. (L.) amazonensis</u>, <u>L. (L.) pifanoi</u>, <u>L.(L.) garnhami</u>,

<u>L. (L.) enriettii</u>, <u>L. (L.) aristedesi</u>, <u>L. (L.) hertigi</u>, <u>L. (L.) deanei</u>

Section **PERIPYLARIA** ("on all sides of the gate")

Initial phase of development in hindgut, with subsequent forward migration to

anterior station.   Transmission by bite.

Parasites of New World mammals: subgenus <u>Viannia</u>:

<u>L. (V.) braziliensis</u>, <u>L. (V.) guyanensis</u>, <u>L. (V.) panamensis</u>, <u>L. (V.) peruviana</u>

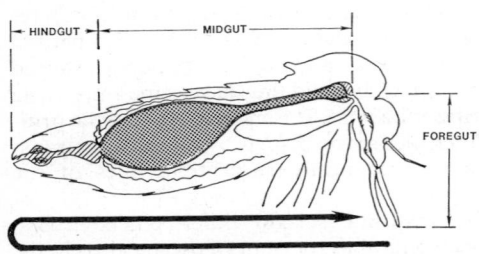

Note also the former Section <u>HYPOPYLARIA</u> ("under the gate"):

Development in hindgut only: no anterior migration. Transmission by ingestion

of infected insect. Parasites of Old World reptiles:

subgenus <u>Sauroleishmania</u>: (★) <u>L. (S.) agamae</u>, <u>L. (S.) ceramodactyli</u>

(★ organisms currently of uncertain status and affinity: some may be trypanosomes)

Fig. III.19 Classification of the *Leishmania* species based on their site of development in the phlebotomine host (after Lainson and Shaw[5]).

in altitude, apparently restricted by the ecological requirements of the vectors. Little detail is known of the transmission cycle; there are no known animal reservoirs, the sandfly vector acquires the pathogen from an infected human. The lack of a development cycle of *B. bacilliformis* in the vector (it occurs in the gut and on the mouthparts) suggests that transmission may be mechanical. In Peru, *Lutzomyia verrucarum* is considered the vector, although the disease exists in the absence of this species. The closely related *Lutzomyia colombiana* is thought to transmit the disease in Colombia (Chapter 11).

Reaction to sandfly bites: harara

Persons newly exposed to the bites of *P. papatasi* and other species in parts of the Middle East often experience a severe urticarial reaction to sandfly bites after a variable time. This period of sensitization may later be followed by desensitization. Such a reaction may also occur elsewhere in the world.

Control of sandflies

There is no general method of control for several reasons: the diversity of the habitats in which the diseases occur, behaviour of the vectors, and the public health importance of the disease they transmit. Several different strategies are used, principally aimed at reducing man–fly contact. Control of larvae is often impossible, as the breeding sites of many vectors are either unknown or inaccessible. However, in the USSR considerable success has been achieved by a combined method of pumping insecticides into rodent burrows (breeding and resting sites) and destruction of the rodent reservoirs (*Rhombomys opimus*).

Personal protection. Sandflies are able to penetrate the standard insect screens used in windows of houses and for normal bed-nets, and therefore fine sandfly bed-nets have to be used which are uncomfortable to sleep under in humid tropical climates. Chemical repellents (deet, DMP) applied to clothing and bed-nets are effective but when applied to the skin they are rapidly lost through perspiration. This is especially so when manual work is undertaken (agricultural labour, road building or military operations).

Insecticide control. Sandflies are susceptible to insecticides (only one instance of resistance to DDT has been reported) which are applied to resting and breeding sites, especially the interiors of buildings. Whilst there have been control programmes directed specifically at sandflies in several countries (Yugoslavia, Peru, USSR, China and, more recently, in Saudi Arabia and Egypt), effective control has occurred in some countries as a by-product of antimalarial spraying (e.g. India, Mediterranean). Leishmaniasis has increased with the cessation of such spraying.

Insecticide control of adults is only feasible where peridomestic transmission occurs in discrete and well-populated communities. Where sandflies are exophilic, or bite away from human habitations, insecticide control may not be effective: e.g. there has been little success with attempts to control forest sandflies in the Neotropics by barrier spraying.

Environmental. Changes have been effective in some areas (moving temporary buildings and camps away from microfoci, ploughing up breeding sites). Often, changing land use affects transmission in an unpredictable way. Sandflies in dense forest will rarely cross a clearing made around isolated houses or villages.

Collection of sandflies

The diverse biology of sandflies and their habitats means that special methods have to be used to catch them. Most methods rely on an understanding of sandfly behaviour, since they involve catching resting flies, attracting sandflies to a trap, or intercepting them during their nocturnal movements, and thus collecting efficiency will vary between methods and individuals.

The simplest method is to collect flies during the day from their resting sites, either catching them directly with an aspirator or with a fine-mesh net. This is useful for peridomestic flies and for forest flies resting on tree trunks and buttresses. Battery-operated aspirators avoid the risk of histoplasmosis (see Chapter 35, p. 699). A tent-like device (Damasceno trap) can be put over animal burrows or tree buttresses to catch resting sandflies. The most widely used method of collecting sandflies, at least in the Old World where sandflies live in relatively drier habitats, is setting sticky traps. These are sheets of paper (usually 10×17 cm) thinly coated in castor oil and fixed to sticks which are then placed near resting sites. Traps are set before sunset and collected the following morning. The adhering flies are removed with a needle, cleaned in dilute detergent and stored in 70% alcohol. Sticky traps are not usually effective in areas of high humidity. Several types of light traps can be used, although they are less effective in open habitats, such as deserts, than in woodland or forests. Similarly, a range of animal-baited traps have been devised for collecting sandflies. These traps are useful in areas where man-biting species are seldom caught by other means. Baiting such traps with a known reservoir host will help determine potential vector species. Light- and animal-bait methods are combined in the Shannon trap, a rectangular cloth trap with a central wall and an inverted box-like roof.

Man-biting catches provide an accurate method of finding which species are anthropophilic and assessing the extent of man–fly contact. Collecting larvae is enormously time-consuming and only rarely productive.

Preparation and preservation of specimens

Because many of the characters used to differentiate species are microscopic, correct preparation is of paramount importance. Flies can be cleaned in dilute detergent solutions to remove any adhering oil from sticky traps, rinsed in distilled water and mounted in Berlese medium. Other, more permanent, methods of clearing and mounting flies are also used. To display the diagnostic features most clearly, the head should be detached and mounted ventral side uppermost and the remainder of the body mounted laterally. Care must be taken in ringing such mounts to ensure they are permanent. Other mounting media based on Canada balsam are used, but do not show the spermathecae and antennal sensilla very clearly.

In the absence of proper equipment and facilities, sandflies can be preserved quite satisfactorily in a dry condition, in wisps of paper tissue (not cotton-wool), loosely packed in small tubes. Specimens stored dry are, naturally, rather brittle and easily damaged.

Classification and identification

There is no universal agreement on the ranking of taxa above the species level, although the proposals of Lewis *et al*[7] are generally accepted. Such differences in opinion can cause confusion, especially when they concern vector species; e.g. the South American *Psychodopygus* is treated as a genus by some, but as a subgenus of *Lutzomyia* by others. Of the five genera of Phlebotominae, only two contain vector species *Phlebotomus* (Old World) and *Lutzomyia* (New World). The remaining genera *Sergentomyia* (Old World), *Brumptomyia* and *Warileya* (both New World) rarely feed on man. There is a loose association between the subgenera of sandflies and the affinities of the parasites they transmit, and therefore deducing potential vectors from their taxonomic relationships with known vector species is important in the initial stages of an epidemiological study.

There is often considerable variation within species. This sometimes makes it difficult to determine the limits of particular taxa and indeed to distinguish some vector species. Recently, cryptic species and species complexes have been recognized.[8]

Identification of sandflies to species is difficult and requires specialist training. Species are differentiated by minute characters, many internal, such as details (teeth- or scale-like processes) of the cibarium and pharynx, and the structure of the spermatheca. External features of the male genitalia and the antennal sensilla are also used. Several new techniques (morphometrics, isoenzyme electrophoresis) are being used to differentiate some members of taxonomically intransigent species groups or complexes.

MOSQUITOES

G. B. White

FAMILY: CULICIDAE

Mosquitoes are not confined to tropical regions; the main genera *Anopheles*, *Aedes* and *Culex* are distributed worldwide, even above the Arctic Circle. Approximately 3200 species of Culicidae have been described, more being recognized each year. They are classified in three subfamilies and 35 genera, as follows:

Subfamily	Tribe	Principal genera
Anophelinae	—	*Anopheles*
Culicinae	Aedini	*Aedes*
		Armigeres
		Eretmapodites
		Haemagogus
	Culicini	*Culex*
	Culisetini	*Culiseta*
	Mansoniini	*Coquillettidia*
		Mansonia
	Sabethini	*Heizmannia*
		Limatus
		Sabethes
		Trichoprosopon
		Tripteroides
		Wyeomyia
Toxorhynchitinae	—	*Toxorhynchites*

Adult mosquitoes of both sexes feed on nectar and other fluids. Anopheline and culicine females also suck the blood of mammals, birds, frogs, etc., each species of mosquito tending to have particular host preferences. For blood-feeding, the proboscis stylets (Fig. III.20) are pushed into a blood capillary of the host skin. Localized sensitivity to saliva from the mosquito is what causes dermal reactions popularly known as 'mosquito bites'. Each blood meal generally provides enough nutrition for the female mosquito to produce a batch of eggs, 30–150 in number. Anophelines show the most regular cycles of blood-feeding and egg-laying. *Toxorhynchites* and some culicines produce eggs autogenously, i.e. without having fed on blood. Male and female mosquitoes may well live for several weeks, feeding repeatedly, under natural conditions. Through their regular attacks on man, female mosquitoes of certain species are important carriers of human diseases. All the vectors of human malaria belong to the genus *Anopheles* (Table III.4). The main morphological differences between anophelines and culicines are portrayed in Fig. III.21. Various anophelines and especially culicines transmit arboviruses and filariasis of man (Tables III.5, III.6). Mosquitoes also serve as the vectors of enzootic infections (i.e. restricted to animals or birds) and some

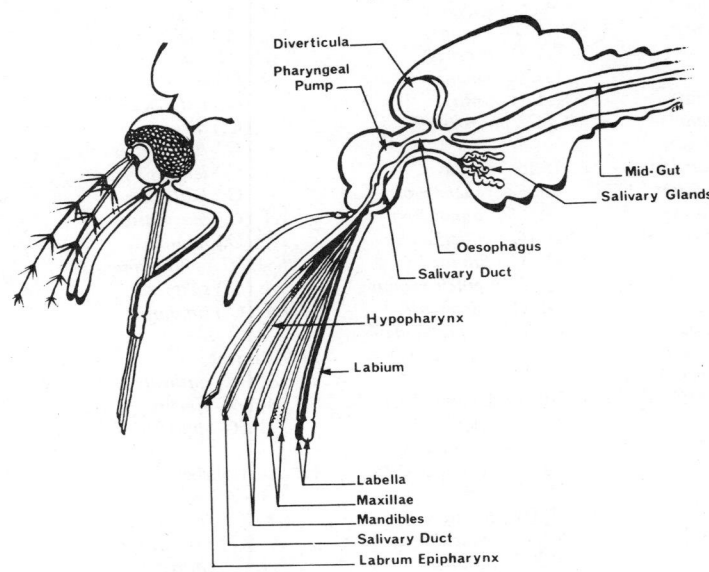

Fig. III.20 Anatomy of the proboscis of the female *Anopheles*.

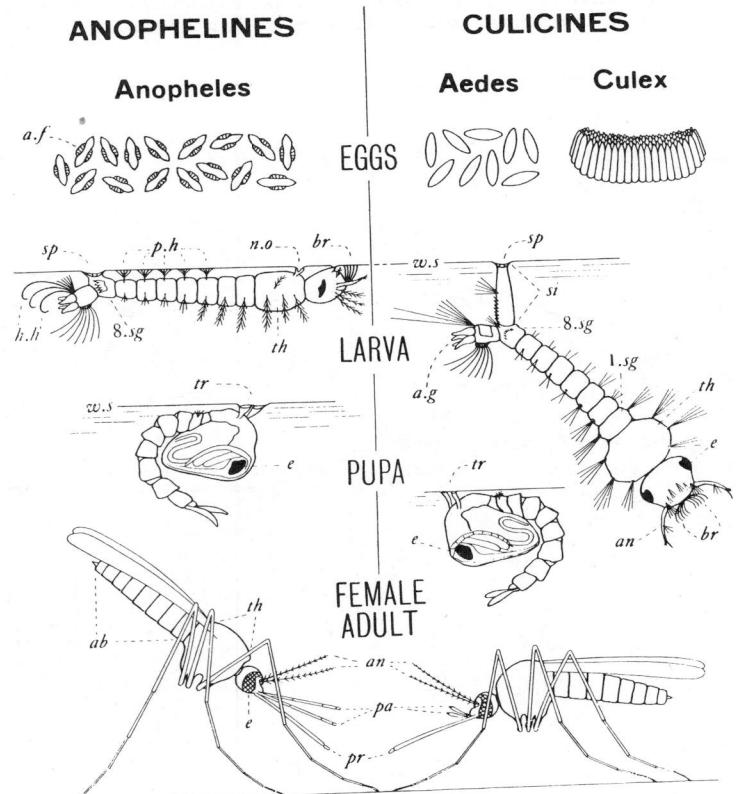

Fig. III.21 Chief distinguishing features of anophelines and culicines. *a.f.* air floats; *a.g.* anal gills; *ab* abdomen; *an* antenna; *br* mouth brushes; *e* eye; *h.h.* hooked hairs or caudal setae; *n.o.* notched organ; *pa* palps (maxillary palpi); *p.h* palmate hairs or float hairs; *pr* proboscis; 1.*sg* first abdominal segment; 8.*sg* eighth abdominal segment; *si* siphon; *sp* spiracles; *th* thorax; *tr* respiratory trumpets.

Table III.4 Epidemiological zones and vectors of human malaria.

1. North American
   A. (A.) freeborni
   A. (A.) quadrimaculatus
   (A.(N.) albimanus)

2. Central American
   (A. (A.) aztecus)
   (A.(A.) punctimacula)
   A. (N.) albimanus
   A. (N.) albitarsis)
   A. (N.) aquasalis
   A. (N.) argyritarsis
   A. (N.) darlingi

3. South American
   A. (A.) pseudopunctipennis
   A. (A.) punctimacula
   (A. (K.) bellator)
   (A. (K.) cruzii)
   A. (N.) albimanus
   A. (N.) albitarsis
   A. (N.) aquasalis
   A. (N.) argyritarsis
   A. (N.) darlingi
   (A. (N.) nuneztovari)
   (A. (N.) triannulatus)

4. North Eurasian
   A. (A.) atroparvus
   (A. (A.) messeae)
   (A. (A.) sacharovi)
   (A. (A.) sinensis)
   (A. (C.) pattoni)

5. Mediterranean
   A. (A.) atroparvus
   (A. (A.) claviger)
   A. (A.) labranchiae
   (A. (A.) messeae)
   A. (A.) sacharovi
   (A. (C.) hispaniola)
   (A. (C.) pattoni)

6. Afro-Arabian
   (A. (C.) hispaniola)
   (A. (C.) multicolor)
   A. (C.) pharoensis
   A. (C.) sergentii

7. Afrotropical
   A. (C.) arabiensis
   A. (C.) funestus
   A.(C.) gambiae
   (A. (C.) melas)
   (A. (C.) merus)
   (A. (C.) moucheti)
   (A. (C.) nili)
   (A. (C.) pharoensis)

8. Indo–Iranian
   (A. (A.) sacharovi)
   (A. (C.) annularis)
   A. (C.) culicifacies
   A. (C.) fluviatilis
   (A. (C.) pulcherrimus)
   A. (C.) stephensi
   (A. (C.) superpictus)
   (A. (C.) tessellatus)

9. Indo–Chinese Hills
   (A. (A.) nigerrimus)
   (A. (C.) annularis)
   (A. (C.) culicifacies)
   A. (C.) dirus
   A. (C.) fluviatilis
   (A. (C.) maculatus)
   A. (C.) minimus

10. Malaysian
    A. (A.) campestris
    A. (A.) donaldi
    A. (A.) letifer
    A. (A.) nigerrimus
    (A. (A.) whartoni)
    A. (C.) aconitus
    A. (C.) balabacensis
    A. (C.) dirus
    A. (C.) flavirostris
    A. (C.) leucosphyrus
    A. (C.) ludlowae
    A. (C.) maculatus
    A. (C.) minimus
    (A. (C.) philippinensis)
    A. (C.) subpictus
    A. (C.) sundaicus

11. Chinese
    A. (A.) anthropophagus
    A. (A.) sinensis
    (A. (C.) pattoni)

12. Australasian
    (A. (A.) bancroftii)
    A. (C.) farauti type 1
    A. (C.) farauti type 2
    (A. (C.) hilli)
    (A. (C.) karwari)
    A. (C.) koliensis
    A. (C.) punctulatus
    (A. (C.) subpictus)

Zonation according to the geographical distribution of the main vector species of *Anopheles*. In each zone (cf. map below) behaviour and ecology of *Anopheles* spp. governs transmission characteristics, e.g. indoor or outdoor transmission. Abbreviations: *A = Anopheles; C = Cellia; K = Kerteszia; N = Nyssorhynchus*. Bracketed names are those of local or secondary vectors.

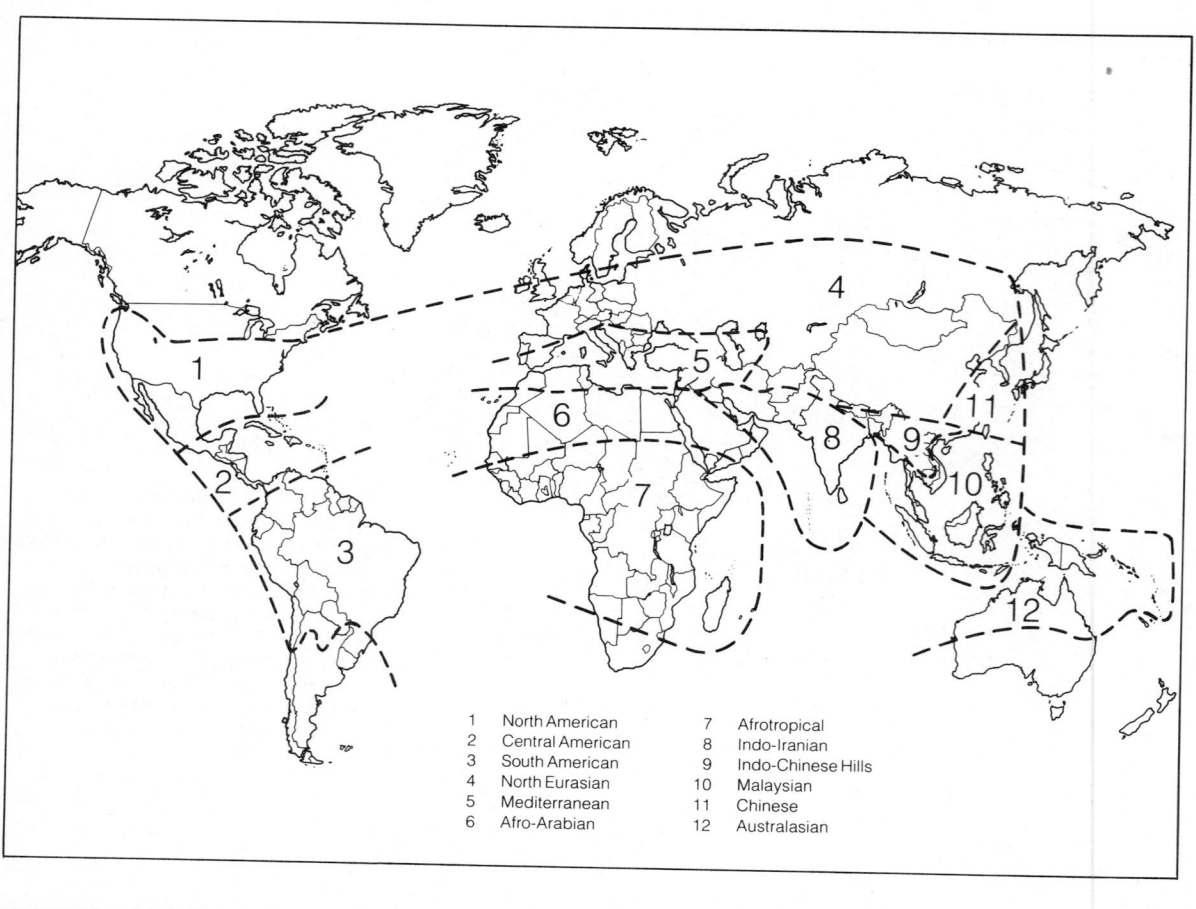

1	North American	7	Afrotropical
2	Central American	8	Indo-Iranian
3	South American	9	Indo-Chinese Hills
4	North Eurasian	10	Malaysian
5	Mediterranean	11	Chinese
6	Afro-Arabian	12	Australasian

Table III.5 The mosquito vectors of human filariasis

Mosquito groups and their general distribution	Vector species and places where incriminated	W. bancrofti np	W. bancrofti ns	W. bancrofti ds	B. malayi np	B. malayi ns	B. timori np
ANOPHELINAE							
Anopheles (Anopheles)							
bancroftii group: Australian and Papuan areas	*bancroftii* e.g. Papua New Guinea	+					
barbirostris group: Oriental region	*barbirostris*, e.g. Malaysia;	−			+	−	
	Sulawesi, Thailand; Flores				+		+
	campestris Malaysia	−			+	−	
	donaldi, e.g. Malaysia, Sarawak				+		
	anthropophagus, e.g. China	+			+		
	kewiyangensis, e.g. China				+		
hycanus group: Oriental and Palaearctic regions	*nigerrimus*, e.g. India, Sri Lanka, Thailand	+			+		
	sinensis complex, e.g. China, Korea,	+			+		
	Malaysia, Thailand				−	−	
umbrosus group: Indomalaysian area	*letifer*, e.g. Malaysia	+			−		
	whartoni, e.g. Malaysia	+			?		
Anopheles (Cellia)							
funestus-minimus group: Afrotropical and Oriental regions	*aconitus*, Flores	+					
	flavirostris, Philippines	+					
	funestus, e.g. Ghana, Kenya, Liberia, Malagasy, Nigeria, Senegal, Sierra Leone, Tanzania, Burkino Faso (Upper Volta), Zaire						
	minimus, Hong Kong	+					
gambiae complex: Afrotropical region	*arabiensis*, e.g. Burkino Faso (Upper Volta), Kenya, Malagasy, Nigeria, Tanzania	+					
	bwambae, Uganda	+					
	gambiae, e.g. Ivory Coast, Kenya, Malagasy, Nigeria, Tanzania, Zaire	+					
	melas, e.g. Gambia, Guinea, Ivory Coast, Liberia, Sierra Leone	+ +					
	merus, e.g. Tanzania						
jeyporiensis: Oriental region	*candidiensis*, e.g. China	+					
leucosphyrus group: Oriental region	*balabacensis*, e.g. Indonesia	+					
	leucosphyrus, e.g. Malaysia	+					
maculatus: Oriental region	*maculatus*, e.g. Malaysia	+					
nili: Afrotropical region	*nili*, e.g. Liberia	+					
pauliani: Madagascar	*pauliani*, Madagascar	+					
philippinensis: Oriental region	*philippinensis*, e.g. India	+					
punctulatus complex: Papuan area of Australia and western Pacific	*farauti*, e.g. Solomons Islands	+					
	koliensis, e.g. Papua New Guinea	+					
	punctulatus, e.g. Papua New Guinea	+					
subpictus group: Oriental region and Papuan area	*subpictus*, Flores	+					
tessellatus: Oriental region and Papuan area	*tessellatus*, e.g. Maldives	?					
vagus: Oriental region	*vagus*, e.g. Flores	+					
Anopheles (Kerteszia)							
bellator: South America	*bellator*, e.g. Brazil	+					

Table 111.5—*continued*

Mosquito groups and their general distribution	Vector species and places where incriminated	W. bancrofti np	ns	ds	B. malayi np	ns	B. timori np
Anopheles (Nyssorhynchus)							
albimanus group: South and Central America	*albimanus*, Caribbean	?					
	darlingi, e.g. Brazil, Guyana	+					
argyritarsis group: Neotropical region	*aquasalis*, e.g. Brazil, Guyana	+					
CULICINAE							
Aedes (Finlaya)							
kochi group: Indomalaysian, Papuan, North Australia and South Pacific	*fijiensis*, Fiji			+			
	oceanicus, e.g. Samoa, Tonga			+	+		+
	poicilius, Philippines	+					+
	samoanus, Samoa		+				?
	tutuilae, Samoa						
niveus group: Oriental region	*niveus*, e.g. Philippines	+					
	harinasutai, Thailand		+				
togoi: East and South-East Asia	*togoi*, e.g. China, Japan, Korea	+				+	
Aedes (Ochlerotatus)	*scapularis*, e.g. Brazil	+					
scapularis: Neotropical region							
taeniorhynchus group: USA and Neotropical region	*taeniorhynchus*, e.g. Virgin Islands	?					
vigilax group: East Africa, Australian, Indomalaysian, Papuan and South Pacific areas	*vigilax*, e.g. New Caledonia			+			
Aedes (Stegomyia)							
aegypti group: cosmotropical	*aegypti*, filaria susceptible genotypes occur at low frequency, especially in East Africa	−			−	−	
scutellaris group: North Australian, Indomalaysian Papuan and Pacific areas	*cooki*, Niue Islands		?				
	futunae, Horne Islands		+				
	kesseli, Tonga		?				
	polynesiensis, central and eastern Polynesia, e.g. Fiji, Samoa, Tahiti, Tuamotu		+				
	pseudoscutellaris, Fiji		+				
	rotumae, Rotuma Island		?				
	tabu, Haapai Tongatapu Island		+				
	tongae, Haapai Islands, Vavau Islands		+				
	upolensis, Samoa		+				
Culex (Culex)	*pipiens*, biotype *molestus*, e.g. Egypt, Turkey	+					
pipiens group: cosmopolitan	*pipiens*, form *pallens*, e.g. China, Japan	+					
	quinquefasciatus, tropical Africa, Asia, Caribbean and South America	+					
sitiens group: Afrotropical, Australian and Oriental regions	*annulirostris*, e.g. West Irian	+					
	bitaeniorhynchus, e.g. India, West Irian	+					
	gelidus, e.g. India	?					
	sitiens complex, e.g. India, Maldive Islands						
	tritaeniorhynchus, e.g. Bangladesh, India	?					
	vishnui complex, e.g. Bangladesh, India	?			?		
Mansonia (Mansonia)							
titillans: Neotropical region	*titillans*, e.g. Guyana	+					

Mansonia (Mansonioides)

dives group: Oriental region and Papua area	*bonneae*, e.g. Malaysia; Thailand	– +		+
		+		
	dives, e.g. Malaysia, Sumatra, Palawan	+		+
uniformis group: Afrotropical, Australian and Oriental regions	*annulata*, e.g. Kalimantan, Malaysia, Sri Lanka, Sumatra, Thailand	–	●+	
	annulifera, e.g. India, Kalimantan,[a] Sri Lanka, Thailand	+		
	indiana, e.g. India, Java, [a]Sri Lanka, Malaysia, Thailand	+		
	uniformis, e.g. Africa;	–		
	India, Kalimantan, Malaysia, [a]Sri Lanka;	–	+	+
	West Irian	+		

Abbreviations and symbols: np = nocturnally periodic; ns = nocturnally subperiodic or non-periodic; ds = diurnally subperiodic; + = proven vector; infective filarial larvae found repeatedly in wild mosquito female;— = non-vector: filarial larvae usually fail to develop; no entry = vector status undetermined or form of filariasis absent.

[a] *Brugia malayi* now virtually eradicated from Sri Lanka.

Zone 1: Neotropical
Anopheles albimanus, aquasalis, bellator, darlingi
Aedes scapularis, taeniorhynchus
Culex quinquefasciatus
Mansonia titellans
Zone 2: Afrotropical
Anopheles funestus, arabiensis, gambiae, melus, merus
Culex quinquefasciatus, sitiens
Zone 3: Middle Eastern
Culex pipiens, molestus
Zone 4: Oriental
Anopheles barbirostris, campestris, donaldi, nigerrimus, sinensis complex, *letifer, whartoni, aconitus, flavirostris, minimus, candidiensis, maculatus, philippinensis, subpictus, tesselatus*
Aedes niveus, harinasuti, togoi, poicilus
Culex bitaeniorhynchus, gelidus, sitiens complex, *tritaeniorhynchus, vishnui* complex
Mansonia uniformis, bonneae, annulata, annulifera, indiana
Zone 5: Western Pacific
Culex pipiens
Aedes togoi
Zone 6: Papuan
Anopheles bancrofti, punctulatus, farauti, koliensis, subpictus, tesselatus
Zone 7: South Pacific
Aedes (kochi group) *fijiensis, oceanicus, samoanus, tutuilae*
Vigilax (scutellaris group) *cooki, futanae, kesseli, polynesiensis, pseudoscutellaris, rotumae, tabu, tongae, upolensis*

zoonotic diseases due to pathogens transmitted from animals to man, e.g. yellow fever and subperiodic Brugian filariasis.

Breeding places of mosquitoes are always in water. Eggs may be deposited on damp soil or vegetation, in moist tree-holes or containers, and sometimes directly on to water. It is the choice of specific oviposition sites by female mosquitoes that determines the breeding places of each species. Eggs of the Aedini usually diapause, withstanding drought or winter, whereas other kinds of mosquito eggs hatch within a few days of being laid. Flooding and decreasing oxygen concentration trigger the hatching of eggs that have undergone diapause.

Larval development takes about a week for most tropical mosquitoes, but many temperate species overwinter as larvae. The fourth stage larva moults to the pupal stage, from which the adult mosquito emerges after a few days. Larvae breathe air via a pair of posterior dorsal spiracles mounted on a characteristic 'siphon' (Fig. III.21) which is not developed in anophelines. Pupae breathe via a pair of 'trumpets' on the thorax (Fig. III.22). Although some species have predacious larvae (e.g. *Toxorhynchites, Aedes* subgenus *Mucidus, Culex* subgenus *Lutzia*), the majority of mosquito larvae have mouthparts adapted for filter-feeding. Maxillary and palatal brushes sweep small food particles from the water, or from the substrate,

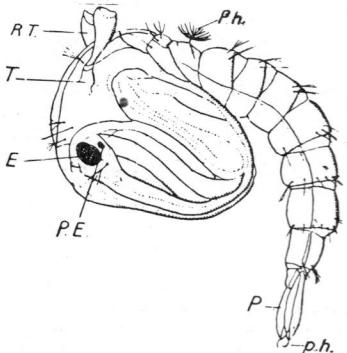

Fig. III.22   Pupa of *Anopheles maculipennis*.

E   eye of developing adult
P   paddle of pupa
PE   pupal eye
RT   respiratory trumpet
T   trachea leading to anterior thoracic spiracle

and pass them to mandibles flanking the larval mouth. The diet of most mosquito larvae comprises microorganisms and detritus. Rates of mosquito larval growth are influenced by such environmental factors as temperature, photoperiod, food supply and the degree of crowding. Aquatic predators, pathogenic fungi (e.g. *Coelomomyces, Lagenidium*) and protozoa (gregarines, microsporidians), viruses and bacteria, together with water effects such as flushing or drying out, combine to take a heavy toll of immature stages of mosquitoes. These natural agencies can be manipulated for mosquito control purposes.

Larvae and pupae of mosquitoes are sometimes called 'wrigglers' and 'tumblers' respectively, terms which express their vigorous movements in the water. When undisturbed, the pupa rests beneath the surface preparing for metamorphosis. Pupae do not feed. Eventually the pupal case splits along the back and the adult mosquito works its way out on to the water surface. Wings and legs become extended and the body cuticle begins to harden within half an hour of eclosion. The adult mosquito then flies to shelter and rests for several hours. Males are not able to copulate until their terminalia (external genitalia) have turned upside down, a process known as hypopygial circumversion, taking about one day for completion. Thereafter the males form swarms with specific characteristics at certain times daily. Female mosquitoes flying into or near a swarm are set upon by the males and copulation ensues. Once inseminated, a female mosquito carries in her spermathecae sufficient sperms for fertilization of all the eggs she may produce. Through the action of matrone, a hormone from male accessory glands, mated female mosquitoes normally become unwilling to accept sperms from additional males. Hibernation of mated females is a common way of overwintering among temperate species of mos-

quitoes, e.g. *Culex pipiens, Culiseta annulata, Anopheles maculipennis* complex. Seasonal changes in the duration of daylight govern the onset and finish of hibernation. Tropical mosquito adults are generally incapable of long-term quiescence.

When foraging, blood-thirsty female mosquitoes fly upwind searching for the scent trail of an attractive host. Sensilla on the palps and antennae serve to detect the host; eyes of the mosquito help to monitor ground speed, altitude, flight direction and details of host location. Intermittent downwind flights are also a feature of normal activity. The majority of mosquitoes hunt and feed at night, though many aedine mansoniine and sabethine species do so by day. Each species has a well-defined activity cycle: some attack at dusk, others around midnight or at other hours. Species showing strong attraction to man are said to be anthropophilic, or more strictly anthropophagic when man is bitten, as opposed to zoophilic or zoophagic species which attack other creatures. Endophilic mosquitoes are those which favour houses or animal sheds for resting indoors, whereas exophilic species prefer to remain outdoors. Outdoor biting behaviour is termed exophagy, as opposed to the endophagy of mosquitoes which enter dwellings to bite people or animals. It is important to realize that mosquitoes may rest outdoors after feeding indoors or vice versa. Male mosquitoes tend to be less endophilic than females of the same species, while many manbiting species seldom go indoors at all. Few species of mosquitoes have man as their principal host. In order to quantify amounts of man/mosquito contact for epidemiological purposes it is necessary to estimate (*a*) the number of bites per person per 24 hours, (*b*) the percentage of mosquito blood meals obtained from man, versus other animals and (*c*) the feeding interval, expressed as the mean number of days between times when successive blood meals are taken by a given species of mosquito. These data can be combined with the probability of mosquito daily survival, estimated from the proportion of parous females, in order to calculate an index of vectorial capacity.[9]

Male and female mosquitoes are good fliers and sometimes disperse over many kilometres. However, most kinds of mosquitoes remain in rather restricted habitats. Those breeding in saltmarshes include some notorious migrants, notably *Aedes taeniorhynchus* along the American east coast. It has been suggested that *Anopheles pharoensis* occasionally travels almost 300 km over desert in the Middle East. Adult mosquitoes can be accidentally transported alive overseas in ships and aeroplanes. For instance, at least six introduced species of mosquito have recently become established on the remote Pacific island of Guam. A survey of planes arriving at Nairobi during the mid 1960s revealed mosquitoes imported from several other countries, *Culex quinquefasciatus* being most frequently encountered, and one African *Anopheles* was found returning on a flight from India. It seems that

Aedes aegypti, Anopheles gambiae and possibly *C. quin-quefasciatus* have been inadvertently taken by man from the Old World to the New World, where these mosquitoes have caused inestimable troubles. *A. gambiae* was wiped out again in the 1930s before it had spread from the primary focus in Brazil, but introduced populations of *Aedes aegypti* and *C. quin-quefasciatus* are continually spreading throughout the tropics. Fortunately, not many species of mosquitoes readily become established in fresh situations.

Identification and taxonomy of mosquitoes are matters for specialists. The morphology of hairs, scales and other body structures must be studied in precise detail on adults of both sexes and on all the immature stages. This requires specimens in perfect condition as a basis for conventional identification. Where possible the larval and pupal skins should be preserved with the adult that emerges, so that the taxonomic characteristics of all life stages can be checked. Adult mosquito specimens should be kept on micro-pins, larvae and skins can be preserved in 60% alcohol or permanently mounted on a microscopic slide in chloral gum or Canada balsam for examination. Many species of mosquitoes show few points of distinction, although the characteristics of genera and subgenera can be recognized more easily. Most medically important species of mosquitoes have close similarities to other species which do not bite man. Specific identification may depend on minute features of the male, the larva or even the egg, often making it unreliable to identify individual female specimens. For some species of mosquitoes it may be necessary to look at their chromosomal characteristics, proteins or behaviour in order to distinguish between species which are morphologically identical, or nearly so. Groups of such closely related species are known as 'sibling species complexes'. Genetic evidence shows that these biologically distinct species do not normally interbreed in nature. The significance of species complexes is that some of the species are pests and vectors of disease while others are not.

Preliminary generic identification of mosquito specimens should be based on the information that follows.

Anatomy (Figs. III.20 and III.27)

The body of adult mosquitoes consists of three recognizable divisions: head, thorax and abdomen. The head is rounded and attached to the thorax by a slender neck. It is provided with large eyes, antennae and mouthparts. The antennae (Figs. III.25, 26) are composed of 15 segments. Each segment bears a whorl of hairs in the female, but in the male the hairs are profuse, giving a bristly or bottle-brush appearance. The mouthparts in the female consist of a proboscis fitted for piercing and sucking. The labium encloses the other mouthparts (Fig. III.20), except the maxillary palps, and ends distally in two pointed labella

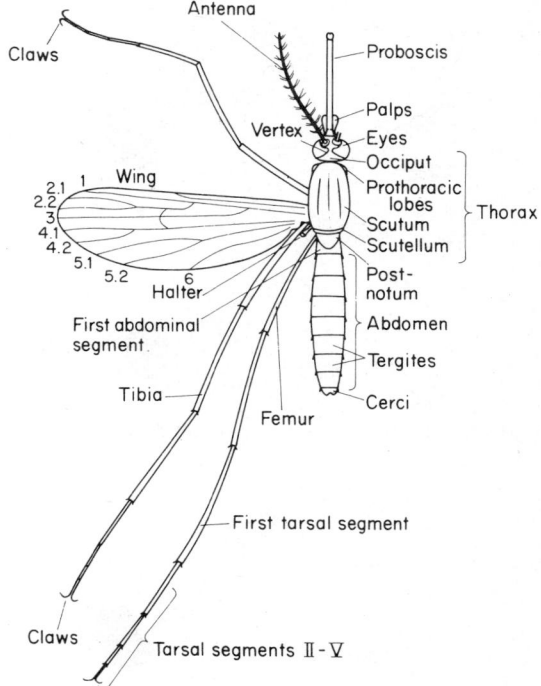

Fig. III.23 The anatomy of the female mosquito, showing wing veins 1 to 6.

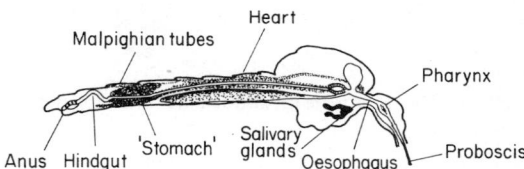

Fig. III.24 Longitudinal section of a female mosquito showing the anatomy.

lobes clothed with scales and hairs. In the act of biting, the labellae part and are applied to the surface of the skin, forming a sheath for the delicate piercing stylets, and do not enter the wound made for obtaining blood. Within is the labrum-epipharynx, forming a V-shaped channel open on the ventral surface. This extends along the whole length of the labium and ends in a sharp point. Lying directly beneath the labrum-epipharynx, closing the ventral slit, is the hypopharynx, consisting of a thin chitinous lamella, fitting closely to the ventral surface of the labrum-epipharynx, thus forming a tube through which the blood is sucked. In the longitudinal chitinous thickening runs a very fine channel extending from the base to the tip of the hypopharynx; through this the salivary secretion is poured into the wound (Fig. III.20). The mandibles form delicate chitinous stylets at the side

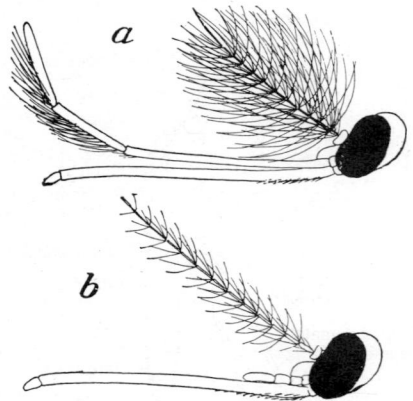

Fig. III.25 Heads of male (a) and female (b) culicine.

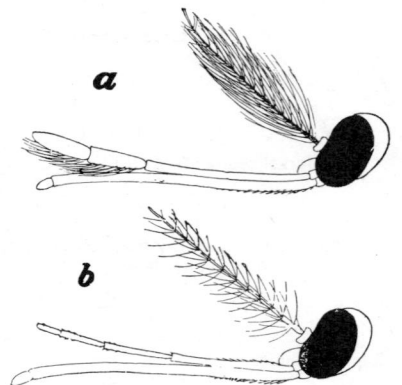

Fig. III.26 Heads of male (a) and female (b) anopheline.

of the hypopharynx. The labium buckles in the act of biting and the stylets emerge. Each of these tapers slightly, ending in a sharp point. The maxillary stylets are more robustly constructed, but have the same general form; the tip is generally supplied with a row of backwardly pointing teeth. The maxillary palps consist of five partially fused segments. In the male the mouthparts are not adapted for biting. The maxillary palps are elongated, extending above the proboscis, but the mandibles and maxillae are greatly reduced and may be lacking altogether.

In female anophelines the palps are as long as the proboscis and usually closely applied, but in female culicines the palps are short. In male mosquitoes, both culicine and anopheline, the palps are as long as the proboscis. The palps of the male culicines are bushy and the two terminal segments tend to turn upwards in *Culex*, downward in *Aedes*. Those of the male anophelines are rather club-shaped.

The thorax is wedge-shaped in side view; the sides form the pleura, with scale patches. The various sclerites composing the side of the thorax bear stiff setae or hairs, arranged in definite groups. The scutellum is separated by a transverse suture from the mesonotum. In all genera except *Anopheles*, it is trilobate and each lobe bears a group of stiff setae. In anophelines the scutellum is rounded and reduced. The region behind the scutellum is known as the postnotum and is generally nude. The wings are long and narrow, with venation; the scales are characteristic. Situated immediately posterior to the base of the wings is a pair of halteres or balancers, which have gyroscopic functions during flight.

The legs are long and slender, composed of coxa, trochanter, femur and tibia, as well as a tarsus of five long and slender tarsomeres. The last tarsomere bears

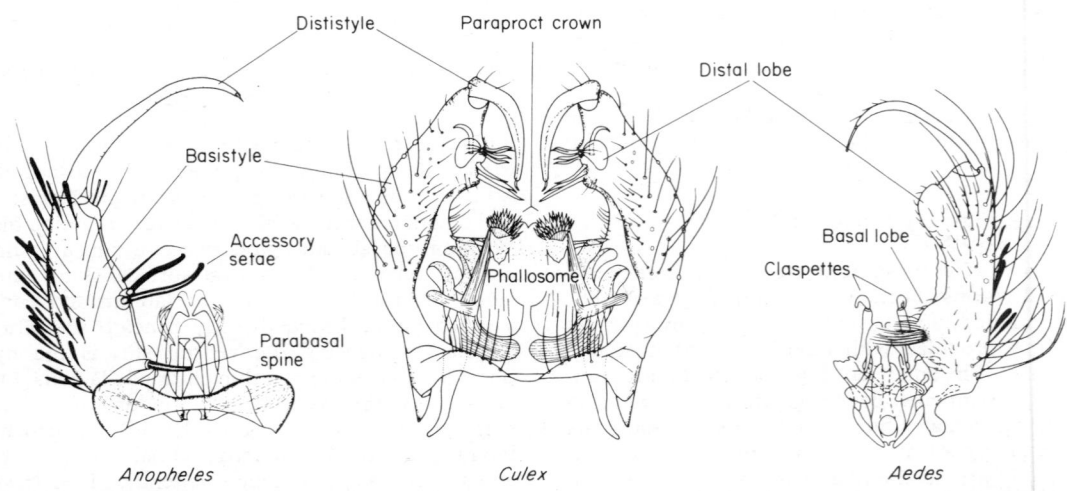

Fig. III.27 Male terminalia (external genitalia) of *Aedes*, *Anopheles* and *Culex* in ventral view, showing the main generic characteristics. These features show specific modifications that are useful for taxonomy and identification of species as well as genera.

a pair of claws (ungues), which vary greatly in size and shape; those of the hind legs are generally smaller than those of others. The abdomen is nearly cylindrical, narrow and elongated, consisting of 10 segments, the last two modified for sexual purposes. The terminal segment in the female is tapered. The ninth is reduced and in the intersegmental area between it and the eighth lies the opening of the reproductive organs. The tenth segment is greatly reduced and bears the anal opening and paired cerci. The abdomen of the male is slightly longer than that of the female. The terminal segments are greatly modified and bear paired claspers, between which lies the aedeagus, a complex organ for use in reproduction. Specific characteristics of these terminalia are the basis of much taxonomy (Fig. III.27).

SUBFAMILY: TOXORHYNCHITINAE

As they are larger than other mosquitoes, it is fortunate that *Toxorhynchites* cannot suck blood. The proboscis is strongly down-curved and suited only for imbibing nectar from plants or free fluids. About 60 species are known, all classified in a single genus. *Toxorhynchites* occur in all warmer regions of the world, between 35° north and 35° south approximately. Breeding places are flooded tree-holes, rock-holes and artificial containers such as buckets and discarded tyres. Female *Toxorhynchites* scatter their rounded buoyant eggs on to water while flying. Larvae soon hatch and become rapacious predators with mouth brushes composed of six to ten strong recurved teeth on each side for grasping prey. When the chance arises cannibalism occurs. A relatively short, dark, strongly chitinous respiratory siphon is present at the abdominal tip, as for larval Culicinae. Populations of some dangerous container-breeding Culicinae, notably *Aedes aegypti*, can be significantly reduced through larval predation by *Toxorhynchites*. This subfamily of mosquitoes should therefore be regarded as beneficial. Adult *Toxorhynchites* are colourful due to their iridescent and metallic scale patterns, with patches of purple, red, orange and green ornamentation on particular species. The lateral abdominal tail tufts and large size (up to 18 mm head to tail; wing span 12–24 mm) are distinctive. *Toxorhynchites* adults are diurnally active and sometimes venture into houses, where they may be found when trying to escape from windows.

SUBFAMILY: ANOPHELINAE

The palps in both sexes are as long, or nearly as long, as the proboscis. The scutellum is rounded. Wings of nearly all species have characteristic patterns of pale and dark spots of scales (Fig. III.28). The subfamily Anophelinae was divided by Edwards into three genera: *Chagasia* (scutellum slightly trilobed),

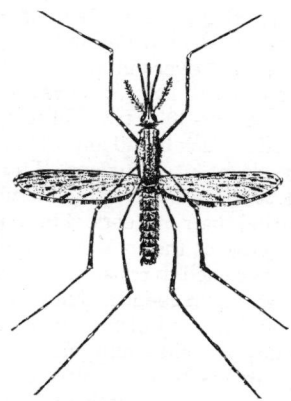

Fig. III.28 *Anopheles gambiae*. One of a series of drawings made by the late Sir Philip Manson-Bahr, showing the wing markings characteristic of *Anopheles*. × 6.

Bironella (scutellum evenly rounded, wing with stem of median fork wavy) and *Anopheles* (scutellum evenly rounded, wing with stem of median fork straight). The genus includes over 400 species. When settled, most *Anopheles* stand with the proboscis, head and abdomen in almost a straight line, usually resting on an upright surface at an angle of about 45°; exceptionally, as in *A. culicifacies*, the resting position adopted is more *Culex*-like (Fig. III.29). In flight the hum produced by *Anopheles* is low-pitched, almost inaudible unless close to the ear. Most species require large spaces for mating flights, rendering it difficult to

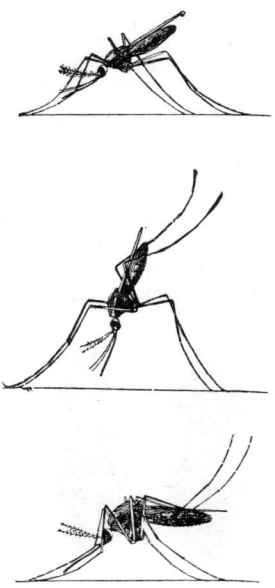

Fig. III.29 The resting positions of *Culex quinquefasciatus* (below), *Anopheles sinensis* (centre) and *Anopheles gambiae* (above).

propagate them in captivity. Overwintering females are fertilized before diapausing, but the males of temperate species cannot overwinter. For tropical species, both sexes are likely to live for several weeks, feeding intermittently. At 25–30°C tropical female *Anopheles* can be expected to suck blood and then lay eggs regularly at intervals of 2 or 3 days. The boat-shaped eggs (Fig. III.30) have an investing membrane inflated laterally to form a pair of floats. These represent air-filled spaces between the exochorion and the endochorion of the egg shell to resist submersion. Anopheline eggs are 1 mm in length. They are white when freshly laid, but tan to dull brown or black within a few hours. They are laid singly on the surface of the water, arrange themselves in a distinct pattern on the surface of the water, and hatch in 2 or 3 days. The larva feeds on small floating particles swept into its mouth by feeding brushes which can be folded under its head. When *Anopheles* larvae lie beneath the surface, the dorsal aspects of the thorax and abdomen face upward, but the head is rotated 180° so that its ventral surface lies upwards. Food consists of living organisms, bacteria and protozoa obtained beneath the surface, as well as particles of floating food such as dead insect fragments. The head of the larva is complex; the central portion is known as the clypeus, the anterior plaque as the preclypus. It has a pair of short antennae, eyes, a pair of feeding brushes and preclypeal and clypeal hairs. The respiratory opening is composed of two dorsally placed spiracles on the eighth abdominal segment. From the spiracles, the tracheae run the length of the body, conducting air to all regions for respiration.

The larva maintains itself under the surface film in a horizontal position by a row of dorsoabdominal plaques and a series of palmate hairs, known as float hairs. The terminal segment is provided with four anal papillae (gills), which have respiratory and excretory functions, but are mainly to absorb mineral salts. Above and below the anal gills are dorsal and ventral swimming-brushes (Fig. III.31). The eighth segment has a chitinous plate lying between the two openings of the spiracles; just below it there is a row of teeth arising from a chitinized base, known as the pecten.

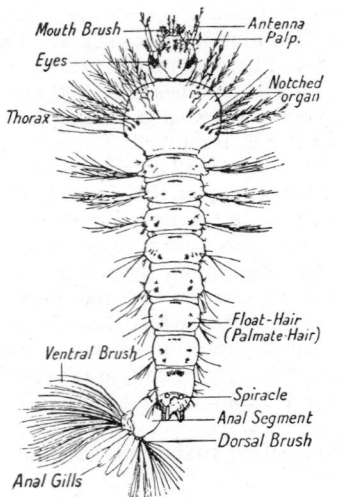

Fig. III.31 Larva of an anopheline (*A. maculipennis*) seen from above. The anal segment is twisted round to display the dorsal and ventral brushes.

Small glands secrete a waxy substance around the spiracles, which therefore cannot be wetted. (It is important to note this fact when oiling water to kill larvae.) Respiration also takes place through the cuticle but the oxygen intake from the water is not sufficient to maintain life, except when the temperature is low and metabolism is reduced.

The capabilities of any particular species of *Anopheles* to transmit malaria are regulated by a number of factors, such as the numbers present, the degree of anthropophily (human blood index), the probability of survival to a potentially infective age and whether the parasites of malaria can complete their development in the mosquito. A species proved to be a natural carrier in one situation does not necessarily play an important part somewhere else. There is a striking correlation between the incidence of malaria and of *Anopheles* as seen in the case of *A. punctulatus* complex, which occurs on some islands in the South

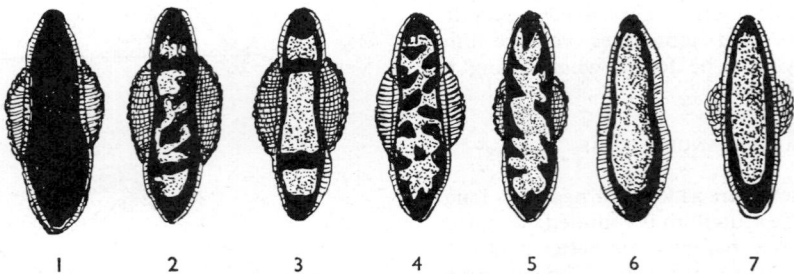

Fig. III.30 Eggs of the *Anopheles maculipennis* complex. 1, *melanoon*; 2, *messeae*; 3, *beklemishevi* or *maculipennis* sensu stricto; 4, *atroparvus*; 5, *labranchiae*; 6, *sacharovi* (summer); 7, *sacharovi* (winter). Species identification is based on the pattern on the deck (upper surface of egg) and the form of floats, i.e. size, number of ribs and striations.

Pacific, but not on others. Where these species occur there is malaria; where they do not, there is none. Malaria vector *Anopheles* spp. of the world are listed in Table III.4.

Nomenclature is a vexed question. A great many species have been renamed in recent years. In case of doubt recourse should be make to Knight and Stone.[10]

In making a malaria survey an attempt should be made to identify female anophelines; they should be collected and dissected to find out which species are infective. It is necessary to dissect at least several hundred insects and to examine the gut for oocysts and salivary glands for sporozoites. Immunological detection techniques (e.g. ELISA) are also now available for sporozoite detection. Infectivity rates are generally below 0.1%, though higher rates are often recorded, especially with *A. funestus* and the *A. gambiae* complex in Africa. Adults and larvae should be identified to determine whether known vector species are present. Any locality should be studied for at least a complete year. Seasonal transmission is important; one species may be responsible in spring and another during the autumn.

Identification of the many diverse species of *Anopheles* is specialized work. The following points are of specific importance: size, general coloration, colour of erect scales on the head, pattern of pale scales on the generally dark legs, wings and so on. The distal half of the proboscis may be pale, the palps may be smooth or shaggy, depending on the scales. The palps may be entirely dark or there may be pale bands. The general coloration of the thorax and scales on the mesonotum is helpful. These features are too intricate to be explained in detail here, and identification depends upon characters listed in the published keys (see p. 1432).

The distribution and importance of some species of *Anopheles* have been changed in recent years as a result of control or eradication programmes in which residual insecticides have been used. Formerly DDT was the insecticide of choice, being cheap and persistent, but to offset DDT-resistance some more costly organophosphate (e.g. malathion, fenitrothion, pirimiphos-methyl) and carbamate (e.g. bendiocarb, propoxur) insecticides are increasingly being utilized for house spraying.

Some species are less responsive than others to insecticides sprayed indoors because either they tend to leave buildings after feeding, without resting on treated walls, or they tend to bite and rest in the open and therefore do not come into contact with residual insecticides.

Much success has been achieved in eradication programmes in subtropical areas and in some parts of the tropics, but even where eradication has been almost complete, there have been renewed outbreaks of malaria, as in Sri Lanka, India and Guyana. Such outbreaks can occur if surveillance is insufficient, and mosquitoes are allowed to multiply enormously if conditions change so as to stimulate breeding.

In most parts of tropical Africa malaria transmission has hardly changed. Where intensive insecticide spraying has been carried out, *A. funestus* has been eliminated, though it could re-enter the area from the periphery when spraying is discontinued. The main vectors, members of the *A. gambiae* complex (*A. gambiae*, *A. arabiensis*, *A. melas*) breed so prolifically in so many collections of water, and bite man so voraciously indoors and in the open, that control by insecticides is extremely difficult.

In addition to malaria, *Anopheles* species transmit *Wuchereria bancrofti*, many of the malaria-carrying species being implicated (Table III.5). The newly recognized Timor filaria parasite of man, *Brugia timori*, has *A. barbirostris* as the only known vector, at least in the island of Flores.[11] *Anopheles* also transmit several arboviruses, for instance eastern equine encephalitis, western equine encephalitis, Venezuelan equine encephalitis, onyong-nyong, tataguine, and others listed in Table III.6.

Adult anopheline mosquitoes are active only at night when the females seek avidly to feed on the blood of vertebrates. Medically important anthropophilic species belong to the subgenera *Anopheles*, *Cellia*, *Kerteszia* and *Nyssorhynchus* of the genus *Anopheles*. Neither of the other two anopheline genera, *Bironella* and *Chagasia*, nor the *Anopheles* subgenera *Lophopodomyia* and *Stethomyia* are of any applied interest. Taxonomic separation of *Anopheles* subgenera is based upon the numbers and positions of certain spines on the male basistyle (see Fig. III.27), together with other features summarized well by Reid.[12]

Subgenus *Anopheles* predominates in the northern hemisphere, extending southwards with a few species found in Australia and through Africa. These mosquitoes are generally more robust and larger (wing span 8–12 mm) than those belonging to other anopheline subgenera. Taxonomists recognize six series of species within subgenus *Anopheles*. Vectors of human diseases belong to the *Myzorhynchus* series as well as series *Anopheles* sensu stricto.

Series *Myzorhynchus* occurs mainly in the Oriental region, the following species groups being involved in human disease transmission. *A. hyrcanus* group, mostly zoophilic species, but including *A. sinensis* the main vector of malaria in China, also implicated as a vector of rural filariasis (both *B. malayi* and *W. bancrofti*) in parts of South-East Asia; it thrives where paddy provides suitable breeding places. The closely related *A. nigerrimus*, which breeds in more permanent ponds, also contributes to malaria and filariasis transmission in South-East Asia (see Tables III.4 and III.5). *A. barbirostris* group of blackish species with shaggy palps includes two important Malaysian vectors of malaria: darker *A. campestris* associated with clay but not sandy soils, especially alluvial coastal areas, where the larvae occur in lightly shaded deep waters, and paler *A. donaldi* which breeds in swampy forests. These and other members of the *A. barbirostris*

Table III.6 Mosquitoes implicated as hosts involved in transmission of arboviruses affecting man.

Arbovirus and endemic area	Natural vector (*indicates principal species)	Arbovirus and endemic area	Natural vector (*indicates principal species)
Togaviridae		*Mucambo (MUC)*	
ALPHAVIRUS (= GROUP A)		South America	*Aedes* spp.
Chikungunya (CHIK)			*Aedes (Ochlerotatus) serratus*
Africa	*Aedes (Diceromyia) furcifer*		*Culex* spp.
	*Aedes (Stegomyia) aegypti		**Culex (Melanoconion) portesi*
	Aedes (Stegomyia) africanus		*Haemagogus* spp.
	Coquillettidia (Coquilletidia)		*Sabethis* spp.
	fuscopennata		*Wyeomyia* spp.
	Culex (Culex) quinquefasciatus	*O'nong-nyong (ONN)*	
		Africa	*Anopheles (Cellia) funestus*
	Mansonia (Mansonioides) africana		*Anopheles (Cellia) gambiae* sensu lato
	Mansonia (Mansonioides) uniformis	*Ross River (RR)*	
South-East Asia	**Aedes (Stegomyia) aegypti*	Australasia	*Aedes (Ochlerotatus) vigilax*
	Aedes (Stegomyia) albopictus?		*Culex (Culex) annulirostris*
	Culex (Culex) gelidus	*Semliki Forest (SF)*	
	Culex (Culex) quinquefasciatus	Africa	*Aedes (Aedimorphus) abnormalis* group
	Culex (Culex) tritaeniorhynchus		*Aedes (Aedimorphus)*
			argenteopunctatus
Eastern equine encephalitis (EEE)			*Aedes (Aedimorphus) dentatus*
North America	*Aedes (Aedimorphus) vexans*		*Aedes (Neomelaniconion) palpalis*
	Aedes (Ochlerotatus) atlanticus		*Anopheles (Cellia) funestus*
	Aedes (Ochlerotatus) fulvus		*Eretmapodites grahamii*
	Aedes (Ochlerotatus) mitchellae		
	*Aedes (Ochlerotatus) sollicitans	*Sindbis (SIN)*	
	Aedes (Ochlerotatus) sticticus	Africa	*Aedes (Aedimorphus) cumminsi*
	*Aedes (Ochlerotatus) taeniorhynchus		*Aedes (Neomelaniconion)*
	Anopheles (Anopheles) crucians		*circumluteolus*
	Coquillettidia (Coquillettidia)		*Anopheles (Cellia) pharoensis*
	perturbans		*Coquillettidia (Coquillettidia)*
	Culex (Culex) nigripalpus		*fuscopennata*
	Culex (Culex) quinquefasciatus		**Culex (Culex) antennatus*
	Culex (Culex) restuans		**Culex (Culex) perexiguus*
	Culex (Culex) salinarius		*Culex (Culex) pipiens* sensu lato
	*Culiseta (Climacura) melanura		**Culex (Culex) univittatus*
	*Culiseta (Culicella) morsitans		*Mansonia (Mansoniodes) africana*
South America	**Aedes (Ochlerotatus) taeniorhynchus*	Australasia	*Aedes (Ochlerotatus) normanensis*
	Culux (Culex) nigripalpus		*Aedes (Ochlerotatus) vigilax*
	Culex (Melanoconion) caudelli		**Culex (Culex) annulirostris*
	Culex (Melanoconion) spissipes		*Mansonia (Mansoniodes)*
	Culex (Melanoconion) taeniopus		*septempunctata*
Europe	*Culex (Culex) pipiens*	Orient	**Culex (Culex) bitaeniorhynchus*
			Culex (Culex) pseudovishnui
			*Culex (Culex) tritaeniorhynchus
Everglades (EVE)			
Florida	*Aedes (Ochlerotatus) atlanticus*	*Venezuelan equine encephalitis (VEE)*	
	Aedes (Ochlerotatus) taeniorhynchus	Tropical Americas	about 40 species implicated, including:
	Anopheles (Anopheles) crucians		*Aedes (Ochlerotatus) angustivittatus*
	Culex (Culex) nigripalpus		*Aedes (Ochlerotatus) scapularis*
	Culex (Melanoconion) spp.		**Aedes (Ochlerotatus) serratus*
			Aedes (Ochlerotatus) sollicitans
Mayaro (MAY)			**Aedes (Ochlerotatus) taeniorhynchus*
South and Central	*Culex* spp.		*Aedes (Ochlerotatus) thelcter*
America	**Haemagogus* spp.		*Aedes (Stegomyia) aegypti*
	Coquillettidia (Rhynchotaenia)		*Anopheles (Anopheles) aquasalis*
	venezuelensis		*Anopheles (Anopheles) crucians*
	Psorophora (Janthinosoma) ferox		*Anopheles (Anopheles) neomaculipalpus*
	Sabethini spp.		*Anopheles (Anopheles)*
			pseudopunctipennis

Arbovirus and endemic area	Natural vector (*indicates principal species)	Arbovirus and endemic area	Natural vector (*indicates principal species)
	Anopheles (Anopheles) punctimacula		*Aedes (Ochlerotatus) serratus*
	Culex (Culex) corniger		*Aedes (Stegomyia) aegypti*
	Culex (Culex) coronator		*Coquillettidia* sp.
	Culex (Culex) nigripalpus		*Culex (Culex) nigripalpus*
	Culex (Culex) tarsalis		*Culex (Culex) quinquefasciatus*
	*Culex (Melanoconion) spp.		*Culex (Melanoconion)* spp.
	Culex (Melanoconion) iolambdis		*Culex (Melanoconion) caudelli*
	Culex (Melanoconion) ocossa/panocossa		*Culex (Melanoconion) spissipes*
	Culex (Melanoconion) portesi		*Culex (Melanoconion) taeniopus*
	Culex (Melanoconion) taeniopus		*Haemagogus (Conopostegus)*
	Culex (Melanoconion) vomerifer		*leucocelaenus*
	Deinocerites pseudes		*Haemagogus (Haemagogus)*
	Haemagogus spp.		*janthinomys* (= *falco*)
	Limatus flavisetosus		*Psorophora (Janthinosoma) albipes*
	Mansonia (Mansonia) indubitans		**Psorophora (Janthinosoma) ferox*
	Mansonia (Mansonia) titillans		*Psorophora (Janthinosoma) lutzii*
	*Psorophora (Grabhamia) confinnis		*Sabethes (Sabethoides) chloropterus*
	Psorophora (Grabhamia) discolor		*Trichoprosopon* sp.
	Psorophora (Janthinosoma) albipes		*Wyeomyia* sp.
	Psorophora (Janthinosoma) cyanescens	*Japanese encephalitis (JE)*	
	*Psorophora (Janthinosoma) ferox	South-East Asia to	*Aedes (Aedimorphus) vexans*
	Psorophora (Psorophora) ciliata	India and Japan	*Aedes (Cancraedes) curtipes*
	Psorophora (Psorophora) cilipes	and USSR	*Aedes (Finlaya) koreicus*
	Sabethes spp.		*Aedes (Finlaya) togoi*
	Wyeomyia spp.		*Anopheles (Anopheles) barbirostris* group
Western equine encephalitis (WEE)			*Anopheles (Anopheles) hyrcanus* group
North and South America	mainly *Culex (Culex) tarsalis* in western USA *Culiseta (Climacura) melanura* in eastern USA occasionally *Aedes, Anopheles, Culex, Culiseta* and *Psorophora* spp.		*Culex (Culex) bitaeniorhynchus* group
			Culex (Culex) epidesmus
			Culex (Culex) gelidus
			Culex (Culex) pipiens group
			Culex (Culex) pseudovishnui
			*Culex (Culex) tritaeniorhynchus
FLAVIVIRUS (= GROUP B)			*Culex (Culex) vishnui* (= *annulus*)
Banzi (BAN)			*Culex (Culex) whitmorei*
Africa	*Culex (Culex) nakuruensis*	*Kunjin (KUN)*	
	*Culex (Eumelanomyia) rubinotus	Borneo, Australia	**Culex (Culex) annulirostris*
	Mansonia (Mansoniodes) africana		*Culex (Culex) pseudovishnui*
			Culex (Culex) squamosus
Bussuquara (BSQ)			
South and Central America	*Coquillettidia (Rhynchotaenia) venezuelensis*	*Murray Valley Encephalitis (MVE)*	
	*Culex (Melanoconion) spp.	Australasia	*Aedes (Ochlerotatus) normanensis*
	Culex (Melanoconion) epanatasis (= *crybda*)		**Culex (Culex) annulirostris*
			Culex (Culex) bitaeniorhynchus
	Culex (Melanoconion) taeniopus		
	Culex (Melanoconion) vomerifer	*Septik (SEP)*	
	Mansonia (Mansonia) titillans	Australasia	*Armigeres* sp.
	Trichoprosopon sp.		*Mansonia (Mansonioides) septempunctata*
			Mimomyia (Mimomyia) flavens
Dengue (DEN) types 1–4			
between 40° north and 40° south	*Aedes (Finlaya) niveus* group	*Spondweni (SPO)*	
	Aedes (Stegomyia) spp.	Africa	*Aedes (Aedimorphus) cumminsi*
	*Aedes (Stegomyia) aegypti		*Aedes (Aedimorphus) fowleri?*
	Aedes (Stegomyia) albopictus		**Aedes (Neomelaniconion) circumluteolus*
	Aedes (Stegomyia) polynesiensis		
	Aedes (Stegomyia) scutellaris		*Aedes (Ochlerotatus) fryeri?*
			Culex (Culex) univittatus
Ilheus (ILH)			*Eretmapodites* spp.
South and Central America	*Aedes (Ochlerotatus) angustivittatus*		*Eretmapodites silvestris*
	Aedes (Ochlerotatus) fulvus		*Mansonia (Mansonioides) africana*
	Aedes (Ochlerotatus) scapularis		*Mansonia (Mansonioides) uniformis*

Table III.6—*continued*

Arbovirus and endemic area	Natural vector (*indicates principal species)	Arbovirus and endemic area	Natural vector (*indicates principal species)
St Louis encephalitis (SLE) North America	*Aedes (Ochlerotatus) dorsalis/melanimon*	Asia	*Anopheles (Cellia) subpictus* *Culex (Culex) quinquefasciatus* *Culex (Culex) tritaeniorhynchus* *Culex (Culex) vishnui* group
Aedes (Ochlerotatus) scapularis		*Yellow fever (YF)* Africa	*Aedes (Aedimorphus) vittatus* *Aedes (Diceromyia) taylori*
	Aedes (Ochlerotatus) serratus *Anopheles (Anopheles) crucians* *Culex (Culex) nigripalpus* *Culex (Culex) peus* *Culex (Culex) pipiens* *Culex (Culex) quinquefasciatus* *Culex (Culex) restuans* *Culex (Culex) salinarius* *Culex (Culex) tarsalis*		★*Aedes (Stegomyia) aegypti* ★*Aedes (Stegomyia) africanus* *Aedes (Stegomyia) luteocephalus* *Aedes (Stegomyia) metallicus* ★*Aedes (Stegomyia) simpsoni*
South America	*Culex (Culex) coronator* *Culex (Culex) declarator* (as *virgultus*) *Culex (Culex) nigripalpus* *Culex (Melanoconion) caudelli* *Culex (Melanoconion) spissipes* *Culex (Melanoconion) taeniopus* *Psorophora (Janthinosoma) ferox* *Sabethes (Sabethes) belisarioi* *Sabethes (Sabethoides) chloropterus* *Trichoprosopon* sp. *Wyeomyia* sp.	South and Central America	★*Aedes (Stegomyia) aegypti* *Haemagogus (Conopostegus) leucocelaenus* *Haemagogus (Haemagogus) janthinomys* (= *falco*) ★*Haemagogus (Haemagogus) spegazzinii* *Sabethes (Sabethoides) chloropterus*
		Zika (ZIKA) Africa	★*Aedes (Stegomyia) africanus* *Aedes (Stegomyia) luteocephalus*
Wesselsbron (WSL) Africa	*Aedes (Aedimorphus) hisutus* *Aedes (Aedimorphus) minutus* *Aedes (Aedimorphus) tarsalis* group *Aedes (Neomelaniconion)* spp. *Aedes (Neomelaniconion) circumluteolus* *Aedes (Neomelaniconion) lineatopennis* *Aedes (Ochlerotatus) caballus* *Anopheles (Cellia) gambiae* sensu lato *Anopheles (Cellia) pharoensis* *Culex (Culex) telesilla* *Culex (Culex) univittatus* *Mansonia (Mansonioides) uniformis*	Malaysia	*Aedes (Stegomyia) aegypti*
		Bunyaviridae (Bunyavirus) BUNYAMWERA GROUP *Bunyamwera (BUN)* Africa	★*Aedes (Neomelaniconion) circumluteolus* *Aedes (Skusea) pembaensis* *Culex* sp. *Mansonia (Mansonioides) africana* *Mansonia (Mansonioides) uniformis*
Thailand	*Aedes (Aedimorphus) mediolineatus* *Aedes (Neomelaniconion) lineatopennis*	*Calovo (CVO)* Europe	*Anopheles (Anopheles) maculipennis* sensu lato *Coquillettidia (Coquillettidia) richiardii*
West Nile (WN) Africa	*Coquillettidia (Coquillettidia) metallica* *Culex (Culex) theileri* ★*Culex (Culex) univittatus* *Culex (Culex) weschei*	*Germiston (GER)* Africa	*Aedes (Neomelaniconion) circumluteolus* *Anopheles (Cellia) arabiensis* *Anopheles (Cellia) funestus* *Culex (Culex) theileri?* ★*Culex (Eumelanomyia) rubinotus*
Europe	*Culex (Barraudius) modestus*		
Middle East	*Anopheles (Anopheles) coustani* *Culex (Culex) antennatus* *Culex (Culex) perexiguus* (as *univittatus*) *Culex (Culex) pipiens* group	*Guaroa (GRO)* South America	*Anopheles (Kerteszia) neivai*
		Ilesha (ILE) Africa	*Anopheles (Cellia) gambiae* sensu lato *Mansonia (Mansonioides) uniformis*

Arbovirus and endemic area	Natural vector (*indicates principal species)	Arbovirus and endemic area	Natural vector (*indicates principal species)

Tensaw (*TEN*)
South-east USA
	Aedes (*Ochlerotatus*) *atlanticus*
	Aedes (*Ochlerotatus*) *infirmatus*
	Aedes (*Ochlerotatus*) *mitchellae*
	Anopheles (*Anopheles*) *crucians*
	Anopheles (*Anopheles*) *punctipennis*
	Anopheles (*Anopheles*) *quadrimaculatus*
	Coquillettidia (*Coquillettidia*)
	   perturbans
	Culex (*Culex*) *nigripalpus*
	Culex (*Culex*) *salinarius*
		Itaqui (*ITQ*)
		Brazil
		
		Madrid (*MAD*)
		Panama
		
		Marituba (*MTB*)
		Brazil
			Culex (*Melanoconion*) *spp.*
			Culex (*Melanoconion*) *portesi*
			Culex (*Melanoconion*) *vomerifer*
			
			Culex (*Melanoconion*) *vomerifer*
			
			Culex (*Melanoconion*) *ocossa*/*panocossa*
			   (= *aikenii*)
			Culex (*Melanoconion*) *portesi*

Wyeomyia (*WYO*)
South and
   Central America
	Aedes (*Howardina*) *septemstriatus*
	Aedes (*Howardina*) *sexlineatus*
	Aedes (*Ochlerotatus*) *fulvus*
	Aedes (*Ochlerotatus*) *scapularis*
	Aedes (*Ochlerotatus*) *serratus*
	Aedes (*Protomacleaya*) *argyrothorax*
	Anopheles spp.
	Anopheles (*Stethomyia*) *nimbus*
	Coquillettidia (*Rhynchotaenia*)
	   arribalzagae
	Culex (*Aedinus*) *amazonensis*
	Culex (*Culex*) *nigripalpus*
	Haemagogous (*Conopostegus*)
	   leucocelaenus
	Limatus durhamii
	Limatus flavisetosus
	Psorophora (*Grabhamia*) *cingulata*
	Psorophora (*Janthinosoma*) *albipes*
	Psorophora (*Janthinosoma*) *ferox*
	Trichoprosopon (*Runchomyia*) *leucopus*
	Trichoprosopon (*Runchomyia*) *longipes*
	Trichoprosopon (*Trichoprosopon*)
	   digitatum
	Wyeomyia (*Dendromyia*) *aporonoma*
	Wyeomyia (*Dendromyia*) *complosa*
	Wyeomyia (*Dendromyia*)
	   melanocephala
		Murutucu (*MUR*)
		South America
		
		Oriboca (*ORI*)
		South America
		
		Ossa (*OSSA*)
		Panama
		
		Restan (*RES*)
		South America
			Coquillettidia (*Rhychotaenia*)
			   venezuelensis
			Culex (*Melanoconion*) *ocossa*/*panocossa*
			   (= *aikenii*)
			Culex (*Melanoconion*) *portesi*
			other *Culex* spp. and *Sabethini*
			
			Aedes spp.
			Aedes (*Ochlerotatus*) *taeniorhynchus*
			Culex spp.
			Culex (*Melanoconion*) *portesi*
			Mansonia sp.
			Psorophora (*Janthinosoma*) *ferox*
			Sabethini
			
			Culex (*Melanoconion*) *taeniopus*
			Culex (*Melanoconion*) *vomerifer*
			
			Culex (*Melanoconion*) *portesi*

BWAMBA GROUP
Bwamba (*BWA*)
Africa
	Anopheles (*Cellia*) *funestus*
	Anopheles (*Cellia*) *gambiae* sensu lato
		CALIFORNIA GROUP
		California encephalitis (*CE*)
		South-western
		   USA
			
			Aedes (*Aedimorphus*) *vexans*
			Aedes (*Ochlerotatus*) *dorsalis*
			Aedes (*Ochlerotatus*) *melanimon*
			Aedes (*Ochlerotatus*) *nigromaculis*
			Anopheles (*Anopheles*)
			   pseudopunctipennis
			Culex (*Culex*) *tarsalis*
			Culiseta (*Culiseta*) *inornata*
			Psorophora (*Grabhamia*) *signipennis*

C GROUP *Apeu* (*APEU*) Brazil	*Aedes* (*Howardina*) *arborealis* *Aedes* (*Howardina*) *septemstriatus* *Aedes* (*Ochlerotatus*) *serratus* *Culex* (*Melanoconion*) *acossa*/*panocossa* (= *aikenii*)	*Inkoo* (*INK*) Finland	*Aedes* (*Ochlerotatus*) *communis*/*punctor*
		La Crosse (*LAC*) USA	*Aedes* (*Ochlerotatus*) *canadensis* *Aedes* (*Ochlerotatus*) *communis* *Aedes* (*Ochlerotatus*) *trivittatus* *Aedes* (*Protomacleaya*) *triseriatus* *Culex* (*Culex*) *pipiens*
Caraparu (*CAR*) South America	*Culex* (*Melanoconion*) *spp.* *Culex* (*Melanoconion*) *caudelli* *Culex* (*Melanoconion*) *portesi* *Culex* (*Melanoconion*) *spissipes* *Culex* (*Melanoconion*) *vomerifer* *Limatus durhamii* *Wyeomyia* sp.	*Melao* (*MEL*) South America	*Aedes* (*Ochlerotatus*) *scapularis* *Aedes* (*Ochlerotatus*) *serratus* *Psorophora* (*Janthinosoma*) *ferox*

Table III.6—*continued*

Arbovirus and endemic area	Natural vector (*indicates principal species)	Arbovirus and endemic area	Natural vector (*indicates principal species)
Tahyna (TAH)		*Rift Valley fever (RVF)*	
Africa	*Aedes (Skusea) pembaensis*	Africa	*Aedes (Aedimorphus) dentatus*
			Aedes (Aedimorphus) tarsalis
Europe	*Aedes (Aedimorphus) vexans*		*Aedes (Aedimorphus) triseriatus*
	Aedes (Ochlerotatus) cantans		*Aedes (Neomelaniconion) circumluteolus*
	Aedes (Ochlerotatus) caspius		*Aedes (Neomelaniconion) lineatopennis*
	Aedes (Ochlerotatus) cinereus		*Aedes (Ochlerotatus) caballus*
	Anopheles (Anopheles) hyrcanus sensu lato		*Aedes (Ochlerotatus) juppi*
	Anopheles (Anopheles) maculipennis sensu lato		*Aedes (Stegomyia) deboeri*
	Culex (Barraudius) modestus		*Aedes (Stegomyia) aegypti*
	Culex (Culex) pipiens sensu lato		*Aedes (Stegomyia) africanus*
	Caliseta (Culiseta) annulata		*Aedes (Stegomyia) dendrophilus*
			Anopheles (Anopheles) coustani
GUAMA GROUP			*Coquillettidia (Coquillettidia) fuscopennata*
Catu (CATU)			*Coquillettidia (Coquillettidia) microbannulata*
South America	*Anopheles (Stethomyia) nimbus*		*Coquillettidia (Coquillettidia) versicolor*
	Coquillettidia (Rhynchotaenia) venezuelensis		*Culex (Culex) neavei*
	Culex (Aedinus) mojuensis		*Culex (Culex) pipiens* sensu lato
	Culex (Culex) declarator (= virgultus)		*Culex (Culex) theileri*
	Culex (Melanoconion) portesi		*Culex (Culex) univittatus*
	Culex (Melanoconion) vomerifer		*Culex (Culex) zombaensis*
			Eretmapodites chrysogaster group
Guama (GMA)			*Mansonia (Mansonioides) africana*
South and	*Aedes (Howardina) sexlineatus*		*Mansonia (Mansonioides) uniformis?*
Central America	*Coquillettidia (Rhynchotaenia) venezuelensis*		
	Culex (Aedinus) mojuensis		
	Culex (Melanoconion) spp.		
	Culex (Melanoconion) epanatasis (= crybda)	**GANJAM GROUP**	
	Culex (Melanoconion) portesi	*Ganjam (GAN)*	
	Culex (Melanoconion) spissipes	India	*Culex (Culex) vishnui* group and ticks (Ixodidae)
	Culex (Melanoconion) taeniopus		
	Culex (Melanoconion) vomerifer		
	Culex (Tinolestes) sp.		
	Limatus durhamii	**ANOPHELES A GROUP**	
	Wyeomyia sp.	*Tataguine (TAT)*	
		Africa	*Anopheles (Cellia) funestus*
			Anopheles (Cellia) gambiae sensu lato
NYANDO GROUP			
Nyando (NDO)			
Africa	*Anopheles (Cellia) funestus*	**UNGROUPED**	
		Zinga (ZGA)	
SIMBU GROUP		Africa	*Aedes (Neomelaniconion) palpalis* group
Oropouche (ORO)			*Mansonia (Mansonioides) africana*
South America	*Aedes (Ochlerotatus) serratus*		
	Coquillettidia (Rhynchotaenia) venezuelensis		
	Culex (Culex) quinquefasciatus	***Poxviridae***	
Shuni (SHU)		*Cotia (COT)*	
South Africa	*Culex (Culex) theileri*	South America	*Aedes (Ochlerotatus) serratus*
			Coquillettidia (Rhynchotaenia) venezuelensis
PHLEBOTOMUS FEVER GROUP			*Culex (Melanoconion) portesi*
Chagres (CHG)			*Limatus pseudomethysticus*
Panama	*Sabethes (Sabethoides) chloropterus* and phlebotomine sandflies		*Psorophora (Janthinosoma) ferox*

group are important vectors of periodic *B. malayi*, but not of the subperiodic form or of *W. bancrofti* to which they are mostly refractory, although *A. donaldi* appears to transmit *W. bancrofti* in Borneo. The only known vector of Timor filariasis (*B. timori*) is said to be *A. barbirostris*,[11] but this mosquito might be the atypical form of *A. barbirostris* sensu lato regarded as a local vector of bancroftian filariasis in Sulawesi and perhaps other parts of Indonesia. In the closely related *A. bancroftii* group, the typical species transmits malaria and periodic bancroftian filariasis in New Guinea and Indonesia, formerly in Australia also. Finally in this series the *A. umbrosus* group, having larvae with reduced float hairs, includes two vectors of bancroftian filariasis and malaria in Malaysia: *A. letifer* and *A. whartoni*, both of which breed in partially shaded, acidic stagnant water. Much caution should be exercised in vector studies on mosquitoes belonging to the series *Myzorhynchus*, since they are frequently infected with zoonotic parasites (e.g. monkey malarias) and the taxonomic distinctions between many of the species require expert attention.

Series *Anopheles* includes the notorious *A. maculipennis* complex of a dozen species in the northern hemisphere.[13]) Specific patterns on the eggs (Fig. III.3) are the best means of distinguishing these sibling species (i.e. morphologically similar species) which have distinctive biological characteristics despite their anatomical similarities. Differences of the chromosomes and protein electromorphs are also useful for specific identification. Typical *A. maculipennis* sensu stricto seldom attacks man, so probably was never a malaria vector, although most malaria transmission in Europe was formerly due to *A. maculipennis* sensu lato, meaning all species combined in the complex. The most widespread member of the *A. maculipennis* complex is *A. messeae*, which is also mainly zoophilic. Arboviruses transmitted by the *A. maculipennis* complex (Table III.6) are usually associated with *A. messeae*. *A. labranchiae* and *A. sacharovi* around the Mediterranean and *A. atroparvus* in other parts of Europe were vectors of malaria, and still are in a few places. These three species tend to breed in brackish water, although they are not confined to coastal localities. Because *A. atroparvus* females spend the winter resting indoors, periodically biting people or livestock but not producing eggs until spring, they were responsible for the phenomenon of 'winter malaria' transmission in bygone days. The disappearance of malaria from Europe has been mainly due to the decline of these mosquitoes resulting from housing improvements, draining of marshes, breeding site pollution (soaps and detergents infiltrate the larval tracheae, causing them to drown) and through the application of chemical pesticides. Former malaria vectors in North America belonging to this group are the freshwater-breeding species *A. freeborni* and the more distinctive species *A. quadrimaculatus*.[14]One more medically important species belonging to this

series is *A. claviger* which overwinters as larvae and breeds in weedy ponds throughout Europe and the Middle East, where it still transmits a little malaria. *A. claviger* may also be involved with myxomatosis transmission among rabbits. Several arboviruses have been isolated from *Anopheles* spp. in Europe and North America (Table III.6) but it is doubtful if transmission depends upon these vectors in any case.

Subgenus *Cellia* has the majority of species in the genus *Anopheles*, with many complexes of sibling species including disease vectors that are extremely difficult to identify. The taxonomic literature is quite inadequate, except for the excellent monographs by Reid[12] covering Malaysian species and by Gillies and De Meillon[15] for African species. *Cellia* species are found almost exclusively in the Old World tropics, being classified into six series: *Cellia, Myzomyia, Neocellia, Neomyzomyia, Paramyzomyia* and *Pyretophorus*, according to the forms of pharyngeal teeth in females. Many *Cellia* spp. are attracted to man for blood meals and representatives of all six series have been implicated as vectors of human diseases.

Series *Cellia* is a group of about 10 distinctive savannah species in Africa and the Middle East. Adults differ from most other anophelines through having abdominal scales, those at the sides forming segmental tufts. The thorax and palps are unusually scaly also, the latter appearing shaggy. *A. pharoensis* is the dominant species, especially in Egypt where it is the main malaria vector. It also carries arbovirus and helminth infections to animals. The closely related *A. squamosus* is an incidental malaria vector in various parts of Africa.

Series *Myzomyia* includes the *A. funestus-minimus* complex, numbering about a score of small and delicate species with varied host preferences and breeding sites. Three of the most efficient malaria vectors in the world are *A. funestus*, which breeds in African swamps and mature paddy, *A. minimus* which breeds in streams of South-East Asia from the Himalayas to Hong Kong, with *A. flavirostris* doing likewise in the Philippines. These species are also important vectors of bancroftian filariasis. They are extremely endophilic in most areas, so usually respond well to control campaigns with residual insecticides sprayed inside houses. However, exophilic and insecticide-resistant populations of *A. minimus* are an intractable problem in Thailand. *A. fluviatilis* is another important exophilic member of this complex breeding in streams of southern Asia. *A. fluviatilis* maintains highly endemic malaria in localities where *A. minimus* has been eliminated. There is little evidence that these mosquitoes transmit arboviruses, although *A. funestus* has been involved with epidemic o'nyong-nyong fever in East Africa; *A. funestus* is also the type-host of Tanga virus. *A. aconitus* is closely related to the *A. funestus–minimus* complex, probably forming another complex of species in itself. It transmits malaria and possibly filariasis in Indonesia but not in Malaysia. Identification of all these species presents the utmost difficulty, but is vital if effort is not to be wasted in vain attempts to control the exophilic non-vector species in the complex.

A. culicifacies also belongs to series *Myzomyia*, being an opportunistic breeder in temporary pools, wells and other clean water sites from Arabia to China. It is not an efficient malaria vector, but is the only species implicated in Sri Lanka and clearly of importance in most parts of its range. Exophily makes control difficult and there is good evidence that several sibling species have been confused in what must therefore be regarded as the *A. culicifacies* complex. Similarly in the arid belt of North Africa and the Middle East, *A. sergentii* is an important but inefficient malaria vector, variations of which suggest that it comprises several taxonomic species.

Series *Neocellia* includes a number of Oriental malaria vectors, mostly having speckled legs and hind tarsi with white tips. *A. annularis* breeds abundantly in swamps of the kind covered with *Eichornia* weed (c.f. *Mansonia*) and in mature paddy, being a widespread and mainly zoophilic mosquito from India to the Philippines. In some situations *A. annularis* is a significant though inefficient malaria vector, often showing multiple resistance to insecticides. *A. karwari* is strongly zoophilic in South-East Asia, where it breeds in trickles of seepage water, but it has been reported to transmit human malaria in West Irian (Indonesian New Guinea) to where it was accidentally introduced. *A. maculatus* is an unusually variable species which also breeds commonly in seepages from Pakistan to Sri Lanka, China and the Philippines. Despite being mainly exophilic and zoophilic it serves as an important vector of malaria and contributes to *W. bancrofti* transmission in some places, especially where hilly countryside is being developed so that breeding sites for *A. maculatus* become plentiful. The African savannah species *A. rufipes,* also belongs to this series and was previously regarded as a secondary vector of malaria, because sporozoite infections are frequent, but it is now known that *A. rufipes* more often transmits antelope malaria.[16] Other local vectors of malaria to be mentioned here are *A. pattoni* in China, *A. pulcherrimus* in Afghanistan and *A. superpictus* in the eastern Mediterranean area (Table III.4). Finally in this series, *A. stephensi* is essentially a rural cattle-biting species in the Indian subcontinent. However, some populations have adapted to urban conditions in northern India and Pakistan, where they breed in wells and subsist largely on human blood, becoming important local vectors of urban malaria.[17]

Series *Neomyzomyia* has numerous species in Africa, Asia and Australasia, most of which are either dark and cave-dwelling or heavily spotted and forest-dwelling. *A. nili* breeds in African rivers and streams, being rather seasonal and locally important as an efficient vector of both malaria and bancroftian filariasis. *A. tessellatus* is widespread and usually zoophilic in South-East Asia, breeding in stagnant water.

It transmits malaria and filariasis in the Maldive Islands, where it is the only anopheline present. The *A. leucosphyrus* group extends from India to China and the Philippines, comprising at least 12 species several of which transmit monkey malarias (*P. cynomolgi, P. inui, P. knowlesi,* etc.) and sometimes infect man with these zoonotic parasites. *A. leucosphyrus* sensu stricto is also a regular vector of human malaria in Malaysia and Indonesia. The most important component of the *A. leucosphyrus* group is the *A. balabacensis* complex, which has not yet been analysed satisfactorily. The most widespread form in South-East Asia has been named *A. dirus,* but this seems to be four genetic species. In forests from Assam to Indonesia and China, '*A. dirus*' (formerly known as *A. balabacensis,* or simply as *A. leucosphyrus*) is an important vector of human malaria, including chloroquine-resistant *P. falciparum,* and of monkey malarias. True *A. balabacensis* is equally a vector where it occurs in Palawan and northern Borneo. Members of the *A. balabacensis* complex breed in fresh jungle pools; the adults are exophilic and elusive, but not difficult to control by home-spraying with insecticides or by means of forest clearance. Their possible involvement in transmission of arboviruses and filariae remains to be studied.

Also in series *Neomyzomyia,* the *A. punctulatus* complex comprises at least five sibling species which are vectors of malaria and nocturnally periodic bancroftian filariasis from the Moluccas, through New Guinea to the Solomon Islands and formerly in northern Australia. The true *A. punctulatus* is widespread, occurring together with *A. koliensis* and *A. farauti* in some islands. *A. farauti* itself comprises three or more genetic species in Australia and in Melanesia. Like the *A. balabacensis* complex, these vectors tend to rest among vegetation and to breed in small fresh pools, making it costly and difficult to attempt their control. However, house spraying with DDT has interrupted filariasis transmission in the Solomons, but malaria persists.[18]

Series *Paramyzomyia* has only four or five species, of which *A. hispaniola* and *A. multicolor* are regarded as malaria vectors in North Africa, although the evidence is equivocal. The latter species can tolerate strong salinity in the breeding places.

Series *Pyretophorus* also has several species adapted to brackish water breeding sites; the adults are characterized by banded tarsi and extensively pale wing markings. *A. sundaicus* is a mainly coastal and locally important vector of malaria in Indonesia, closely related to *A. litoralis* and *A. ludlowae* in the Philippines; the latter species extends to coastal Sulawesi where it joins in malaria transmission. *A. subpictus* ranges from the Middle East to New Guinea, tending to be more anthropophilic and associated with coastal salt-water habitats eastwards; it is a secondary vector of malaria and contributes to *W. bancrofti* transmission locally in Indonesia.

Of the greatest medical importance in Africa and southern Arabia is the *A. gambiae* complex, comprising two salt-water adapted species: *A. melas* in West Africa and *A. merus* in East Africa, *A. bwambae* restricted to mineral spring-water sites in the Rift Valley between Uganda and Zaire, and three widespread freshwater breeding species: *A. gambiae* sensu stricto (species A), *A. arabiensis* (species B) and *A. quadriannulatus* (species C). The last is essentially zoophilic, so not a vector, but the other five species transmit both malaria and bancroftian filariasis.[19] High rates of female mosquito longevity, coupled with marked preferences for human blood, give very high vectorial capacities to *A. arabiensis*, *A. gambiae* and to some extent *A. melas*. Wherever these species are found, malaria is highly endemic. House spraying with residual insecticides has not reduced malaria transmission to the expected degree, since members of the *A. gambiae* complex are capable of behavioural avoidance of the sprayed surfaces. Resistance to organochlorine and organophosphate insecticides is also spreading in populations of *A. arabiensis* and *A. gambiae*. Control of the salt-water species, *A. melas* and *A. Merus,* can be partially achieved by means of drainage and prevention of pool formation in coastal areas, through construction of dikes and bunds. Unfortunately, most breeding of *A. arabiensis* and *A. gambiae* occurs in temporary fresh rainwater pools, or irrigated furrows, which are impossible to prevent or treat adequately with larvicides. Separation of the six sibling species belonging to the *A. gambiae* complex depends upon the examination of chromosomal or protein characters. Adult females of *A. gambiae* sensu lato have the appearance shown in Fig. III.28, but could easily be confused with various other species in subgenus *Cellia*.

Subgenus *Kerteszia* is restricted to the American tropics, with about 10 species that breed exclusively in flooded axils of bromeliad plants or broken bamboos. Since they are found only in the forests of Central and South America, their medical importance is limited, although several species are sometimes abundant and strongly attracted to man. *A. cruzii* and *A. bellator* are significant vectors of malaria, and the latter sometimes contributes to filariasis transmission.[20]

Subgenus *Nyssorhynchus* forms the dominant anopheline fauna of the Neotropical region. Faran[21] has clarified the difficult taxonomy of the *A. albimanus* section, with species having small dark lateral scale tufts on each abdominal segment, including several vectors of diseases. *A. albimanus* itself is the main malaria vector in humid lowlands from southern USA to northern South America and in Caribbean islands. It breeds in stagnant water and the adults lack scale tufts on the first full abdominal segment. *A. albimanus* is insufficiently endophilic to be readily controlled by means of house spraying and has become widely resistant to all groups of insecticides. It may contribute to filariasis transmission and has been involved with epidemics of encephalitis and perhaps other arboviruses (Table III.6). Other malaria vectors closely related to *A. albimanus* are *A. aquasalis*, which also transmits Venezuelan equine encephalitis virus, and is mainly of importance in Trinidad, Tobago, The Guianas and coastal Brazil, usually breeding in brackish water; also *A. nuneztovari* is a primary malaria vector in parts of Colombia and Venezuela, probably comprising a complex of vector and nonvector species. Another section of subgenus *Nyssorhynchus* includes the malaria vectors *A. argyritarsis* and *A. darlingi*. The latter was eradicated from coastal Guyana, but remains of major importance in places from Brazil to Mexico. Infective larvae of *W. bancrofti* have occasionally been found in *A. darlingi* and *A. aquasalis*, suggesting that these species may contribute to periodic filariasis transmission.

SUBFAMILY: CULICINAE

This large and heterogeneous subfamily of mosquitoes contains over 2500 species and some 30 genera. The scutellum is trilobed, each lobe bearing bristles. The abdomen is blunt and completely clothed with broad flat scales. The eighth segment of the larva bears a patch of comb teeth on each side, used for cleaning the mouth brushes, and is drawn out into a respiratory siphon, with well-developed pecten teeth in a row on each side. There are no abdominal palmate hairs (cf. *Anopheles*). Below the siphon the anal segment of the larva bears a chitinous saddle, four gills, caudal setae and the ventral brush for swimming. Culicine pupae are similar to those of *Anopheles*, but the respiratory trumpets are not so flared distally.

The following are the main characteristics of culicines which distinguish them from anophelines (see Fig. III.21).

1 The eggs are not provided with air floats and are either laid separately (Aedini, Sabethini) or stacked in a floating raft (Culicini, Culisetini) or in a mass on floating vegetation (Mansoniini).

2 The larval spiracles are situated at the tip of a tail-like siphon, projecting dorsally from the eighth abdominal segment. Except for *Mansonia* and some other unimportant genera, which have larvae with the siphon modified for plugging into the air vessels of plant, the larvae hang head downwards from the water surface, supported by the capillary action of five hinged valves surrounding the tip of the siphon. They sweep suspended particles of food with mouth brushes below surface level (Fig. III.21) or else dive and scavenge at the bottom.

3 The adult has an abdomen densely covered with scales. The female has short and slender palps, from one-fifth to one-half as long as the proboscis. As a rule, the male has long hairy palps which have a plume-like appearance. These mosquitoes usually rest with proboscis and abdomen more or less parallel with the supporting surface (Fig. III.21).

TRIBE: AEDINI

GENUS: *Aedes*

Throughout the world, especially in temperate countries, a high proportion of mosquitoes belong to the genus *Aedes* in which there are more than 1000 species, classified as 40 subgenera. Many *Aedes* are vectors of arboviruses, including several of the most important mosquito-borne human diseases (see p. 1416, Table III.6). The genus is difficult to define precisely in morphological terms, although adults always possess bristles on the post-spiracular area (Fig. III.32) and the tip of the female abdomen is retractable. Separation from other genera in the tribe Aedini depends on characters given in Table II.7. *Aedes* larvae are characterized by having only a single pair of siphonal hairs, usually branched, in addition to pecten teeth. Many of the medically important *Aedes* species are active during daytime, although nocturnal activity is normal for most other species.

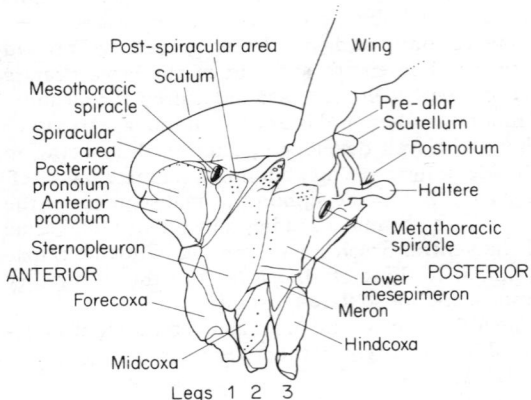

Fig. III.32 Mosquito thorax in side view, showing named components and sites of setae (bristles) referred to in the identification key (Table III.7).

Aedes eggs are especially capable of withstanding desiccation. They are laid on damp surfaces, such as soil or around the rim of water in a hole, in situations likely to be flooded causing the eggs to hatch after aequate rainfall. Most species of *Aedes* therefore breed seasonally in swamps and pools, with some significant groups adapted to smaller containers of water such as rock-holes, rot holes in trees, cut bamboo stumps, old snail shells, buckets and other artificial containers. Almost any kind of water can harbour some sorts of *Aedes*, from sea water to melted snow. It is to be expected that, after drought or winter, rainy seasons will cause the hatching of *Aedes* broods so that blood-thirsty females of these species become prevalent early in the season.

In an increasing number of cases, it has been demonstrated that arboviruses can be passed transovarially in *Aedes*, i.e. from mother to progeny via the egg. This is common with California group viruses[22] and has also been reported for yellow fever.[23] This phenomenon, a form of vertical transmission, is of great significance in epidemiology, as it can lead to long-term dormancy and reappearance of virus activity.

Representatives of three subgenera of *Aedes* are natural vectors of *Brugia malayi* and *Wuchereria bancrofti* causing human disease. Where transmission is due to nocturnally active *Aedes* and other mosquitoes, the microfilariae are normally nocturnally periodic in the human bloodstream. In Polynesia, Melanesia and a few areas in South-East Asia (parts of Thailand, Nicobar Islands) there are diurnally active *Aedes* which transmit strains of *W. bancrofti* that are subperiodic so that microfilariae circulate in the human bloodstream during the daytime, enabling their uptake by female mosquitoes which feed by day.

The majority of taxonomic subgenera of *Aedes* have few species and no medical or veterinary significance. Subgenera *Aedes* sensu stricto, *Aedimorphus*, *Mucidus*, *Neomelaniconion*, *Ochlerotatus* and *Verrallina* have numerous species which breed commonly in ground water, with many arbovirus vectors included (Table III.6). The habit of breeding in water-filled containers, holes and plant axils is a feature of the important subgenera *Diceromyia*, *Howardina*, *Protomacleaya*, *Finlaya* and *Stegomyia*; arboviruses are transmitted by all five of these subgenera and the last two include filariasis vectors (Table III.5).

Subgenus *Stegomyia* is probably of the greatest medical interest. More than 100 species have been described, all diurnally active and having beautiful specific patterns of black and white scales, especially noticeable on the scutum and banded tarsi. They are generally exophilic species which seldom shelter indoors. The *Ae. scutellaris* group numbers approximately 35 species in South-East Asia and the Pacific, including the main vectors of subperiodic *W. bancrofti* in Polynesia: *Ae. pseudoscutellaris* in Fiji, *Ae. cooki*, *Ae. kesseli* and *Ae. tongae* in Tonga, *Ae. upolensis* in Samoa and *Ae. polynesiensis* generally. Adults of the *Ae. scutellaris* group are characterized by having a single white line longitudinally on the middle of the scutum. They also transmit epidemic dengue viruses on many Pacific Islands and in parts of South-East Asia. However, the true *Ae. scutellaris* (sensu stricto) is confined to Seram and New Guinea, where it is zoophilic and not a vector. Breeding places of the *Ae. scutellaris* group are in coconut shells, crab holes, holes in trees and coral, axils of plants such as *Pandanus* and bananas, tyres, tins and other artificial containers. All species so far mentioned have complete stripes of broad scales along each side of the thorax, ending above the wing base. This distinguishes the *Ae. scutellaris* subgroup from the *Ae. albopictus* subgroup of species having an incomplete supra-alar stripe, with only narrow scales over the wing base. Species in the latter group are widespread vectors of dengue viruses,

Table III.7 Identification key to the genera of adult mosquitoes likely to be encountered indoors or attacking man.

1.	Large iridescent mosquitoes (wing span 12–24 mm); abdominal segments VI–VIII (but not I–V) with distinctive lateral tufts of scales; proboscis curved downwards approx. 90° in middle; feeders on nectar not blood; distribution 35° north to 35° south	*Toxorhynchites*
	Typical mosquitoes of various sizes (wing span 5–16 mm); abdomen usually without distinctive lateral scale-tufts; proboscis usually straight, or curved through no more than 40° downwards or upwards; females often suck blood	2
2.	Female palps as long as proboscis; male palps club-shaped (Fig. III.26); wing vein scales usually forming a conspicuous pattern of spots due to *either* clusters of scales at junctions of some veins *or* patches of pale scales and patches of dark scales alternating along some veins; scutellum evenly rounded posteriorly and lacking lateral lobes; abdomen usually not scale-covered, although some narrow scales may be mixed with the covering of fine hairs; worldwide distribution	*Anopheles*
	Female with short palps (Fig. III. 25b), usually one-third to one-fifth as long as proboscis; male palps not clubbed, although often apically thickened; wing vein scales usually not forming a distinct pattern of spots or pale and dark patches, although speckling may be due to mixtures of pale and dark scales on some veins; scutellum trilobed, i.e. with large mid-lobe and smaller lateral lobes; abdomen clothed with broad scales (powdery when rubbed) above and below (Culicinae)	3
3.	Female with tip of abdomen rounded, terminal segment non-retractable, cerci not conspicuous; postspiracular bristles absent (present in *Mansonia*, see no. 7)	4
	Female with tip of abdomen pointed, ending with a pair of prominent cerci, terminal abdominal segment retractable; postspiracular bristles present (Fig. III.32)	8
4.	Pre-alar bristles (Fig. III.32) usually numerous and at least one lower mesepimeral bristle present; postnotum normally without apical tuft; anterior pronotal lobes small; meron well developed, so that upper edge is dorsal to the base of hind coxa	5
	Pre-alar bristles usually absent, no more than four present; no lower mesepimeral bristles; postnotum with an apical tuft of small setae; anterior pronotal lobes large and conspicuously ornamented with scales; meron small, so that upper edge is in line with base of hind coxa or ventral to it; essentially sylvatic mosquitoes, i.e. found in jungle	12
5.	Tarsi with pulvilli (Fig. III.35) appearing as a pair of pale pads below the claws when examined at 50 × magnification or more; worldwide distribution	*Culex*
	Tarsi without pulvilli	6
6.	Bristles on spiracular area (Fig. III. 32) i.e. setae with roots in a vertical row just in front of the respiratory aperture on side of thorax (mesothoracic spiracle); worldwide distribution	*Culiseta*
	Spiracular bristles absent	7
7.	Bristles on spiracular area (Fig. III.32); wing vein scales very broad and forming a mottled pattern on all or most wing veins; ornamentation without any yellow scales; worldwide distribution	*Mansonia*
	Postspiracle bristles absent; wing vein scales narrow, not forming a mottled pattern on most veins; ornamentation mostly yellow, or with at least some bright yellow scales somewhere on body; worldwide distribution	*Coquillettidia*
8.	Scutum covered with broad, flat, metallic green scales; legs generally dark; anterior pronotal lobes very large, almost meeting anteriorly; small species (wing span 6–9 mm) active in daytime; Caribbean, South and Central America	*Haemagogus*
	Scutum not covered with shiny green scales; legs often with pale bands, especially on tarsi; anterior pronotal lobes not strongly developed; various sizes (wing span 6–16 mm), diurnal or nocturnal	9
9.	Broad silver scales on back of head, sides of thorax and hind corners of abdominal tergites; thoracic cuticle orange or reddish-brown; tropical Africa only	*Eretmapodites*
	Not with silvery scales in the places specified; although some of these areas bear white scales; thoracic cuticle pale or dark, but not orange or reddish; temperate or tropical regions worldwide	10
10.	Spiracular bristles present (Fig. III.32), i.e. setae with roots in a vertical row just in front of the respiratory aperture on side of thorax (mesothoracic spiracle); New World only	*Psorophora*
	Spiracular bristles absent	11

Table III.7—*continued*

11.	Abdomen more than 2 × length of thorax; normally one lower mesepimeral bristle present (Fig. III. 32); scales on top of head all broad, flat and decumbent; abdominal segment VIII partially retractile; distributed throughout southern Asia, from India to Japan, Philippines, Indonesia and Melanesia	*Armigeres*
	Abdomen not more than 2 × length of thorax; lower mesepimeral bristle usually absent; top of head with erect scales, seen best in side-view, forming a posterior tuft or more extensive 'crew cut' appearance (easily rubbed off), plus a layer of decumbent scales which are often curved and narrow along the midline but always broad and flat laterally; abdominal segment VIII almost completely retractile; worldwide distribution	*Aedes*
12.	Spiracular area bare, i.e. no scales or bristles on the small membranous area between the posterior pronotum and the main thoracic spiracle; South-East Asia only	*Heizmannia*
	Spiracular area with scales and/or at least one bristle	13
13.	Australasian or South-East Asian mosquitoes	*Tripteroides*
	New World mosquitoes	14
14.	Spiracular area with broad scales only, no bristles; proboscis shorter than fore-femur, thorax with some shiny golden scales; hind tarsi with single claw	*Limatus*
	Spiracular area with at least one spiracular bristle; thoracic scales various, none golden; proboscis longer than or equal to fore-femur; each hind tarsus with two claws	15
15	Scutum covered with broad, flat, shiny metallic scales; some tarsi with 'paddles' formed by inner and outer rows of long, mostly dark scales; Central and South America	*Sabethes*
	Scutal scales usually not shiny; tarsi without paddles	16
16.	Top of head often with erect scales; pronotal lobes widely separated anteriorly; membrane at wing base (squama) fringed with small setae; bristles on clypeus, i.e. bulbous area of the face between bases of antennae and palps; Central and South America	*Trichoprosopon*
	Top of head without erect scales; pronotal lobes very large and almost meeting anteriorly; membrane at wing base (squama) with no more than three small fringe setae; clypeal area of the face without bristles, although scales may be present; North and South America	*Wyeomyia*

notably dengue haemorrhagic fever in the Philippines and South-East Asian countries, but they are apparently refractory to filarial infection. These and other Pacific mosquitoes have been the subject of a monograph by Belkin[24] and a pictorial key provided by Huang.[25] A revision of Tongan species by Huang and Hitchcock[26] gives much recent information on bionomics and vector functions; vector genetics and speciation of *Ae. scutellaris* group were reviewed by Macdonald.[27]

Aedes (*Stegomyia*) *aegypti* is the most widespread and dangerous species in this subgenus.[28] In African forests, non-anthropophilic populations known as *Ae. aegypti formosus* are distinguished by their lack of pale scales on the abdominal tergites (i.e. the top of the abdomen is entirely dark). Presumably from this ancestral stock, man-biting populations have adapted to domestic breeding sites and become spread throughout the tropics within the 20°C isotherms, i.e. roughly between 35° north and 35° south. The general pattern on adult *Ae. aegypti* is depicted in Fig. III.33, showing the unique lyre-shaped pattern on the scutum, with narrow longitudinal lines flanked by curved silvery-white markings. *Ae. aegypti aegypti* has some white scales on all abdominal tergites, with *Ae.*

aegypti variety *queenslandensis* having the abdomen mainly pale-scaled dorsally.[29] Populations of *Ae. aegypti* breeding indoors in water pots, especially in eastern Africa, usually have the appearance of var. *queenslandensis*, whereas peridomestic populations are mainly of the type-form. Evolutionary relationships among various kinds of *Ae. aegypti* sensu lato are still the subject of much study and debate.[30] This is

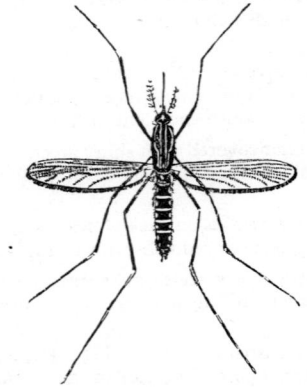

Fig. III.33   Female *Aedes aegypti*. × 4.

relevant to the fact that *A. aegypti* is the principal vector of chikungunya and dengue viruses in almost every outbreak. Urban yellow fever is also mainly transmitted by *Ae. aegypti* in Central and South America and in West Africa. *Ae. aegypti formosus* is probably involved in the sylvatic cycle of yellow fever in Africa. However, other *Stegomyia* species have more often been implicated as vectors of African enzootic yellow fever, especially *Ae. africanus* which also transmits Zika virus. In nature, these arboviruses affect monkeys in the jungle, being transmitted by mosquito species which seldom come into contact with man. At the forest edge, monkeys are likely to be bitten by *Aedes* (*Stegomyia*) *simpsoni* which breeds predominantly in water-filled axils of certain strains of banana plants, or rot holes in stems of paw-paw and candelabra *Euphorbia* (e.g. in Ethiopia). People working and living among such plantations in Africa are especially likely to become infected with yellow fever and other viruses transmitted from monkeys via *Ae. simpsoni*, some populations of which are strongly attracted to man. Man-to-man transmission may then be continued by *Ae. aegypti*. Thus the epidemiology of yellow fever in Africa conforms to the systems shown in Fig. III.34, depending on which species of *Stegomyia* and other mosquitoes are involved. Embryonated eggs of *Stegomyia* spp. can remain dormant for as long as a year and still hatch when flooded. The fact that *Ae. aegypti* eggs may be laid in portable containers allows this species to be inadvertently spread far and wide; continuously breeding populations often occur in water barrels on board ships and dhows.

Control of *Stegomyia* spp. presents great problems the world over, since breeding sites are small, scattered and usually inaccessible. In emergencies, as when an arbovirus epidemic is under way, periodic insecticidal fogging can be helpful in the vicinity of dwellings. Screening of houses and elimination of mosquito breeding places are desirable preventive measures.

Subgenus *Finlaya* has females with a conspicuous ventral scale tuft on the posterior abdomen; in both sexes the wings are usually spotted. The *Ae.*(*F.*) *kochi* group includes several local vectors of periodic *W. bancrofti*. *Ae. poicilius* is the most widespread, in Malaysia, Indonesia and the Philippines, breeding in axils of *Colocasia*, *Pandanus* and bananas (*Musa sapientum*). In parts of the Philippines, where *Musa textiles* (abaca or hemp) is intensively cultivated, *Ae. poicilius* is an important rural filariasis vector. Likewise in Fiji and Samoa, bancroftian filariasis is or was transmitted by several members of the *Ae. kochi* group (Table III.5) which breed in plant axils. Around the coasts of South-East Asia, the large, dark-winged species *Ae. (F.) togoi* often breeds in brackish water and contributes to transmission of periodic *B. malayi* and *W. bancrofti*. Finally in this subgenus, members of the *Ae. (F.) niveus* group transmit both periodic and subperiodic strains of *W. bancrofti* locally (Table III.5), but are probably of wider importance as vectors of jungle dengue and perhaps other arboviruses.

Subgenus *Diceromyia* of tree-hole breeding species resembling *Stegomyia* but having dark tarsi, includes the African *A. furcifer-taylori* group of species which have been occasionally implicated as vectors of yellow fever and chikungunya.[31]

Subgenus *Protomacleaya* has similarities in the New World, with *Ae. triseriatus* breeding in tree-holes of the eastern USA and being an important vector of California group encephalitides, with evidence of transovarial virus transmission. The closely related *Ae. hendersoni*, which may breed in the same tree-holes, is apparently incapable of virus transmission.

Subgenus *Neomelaniconion* is widespread in the Old World tropics and includes some commonly implicated vectors of arboviruses. These species are recognizable from yellowish stripes edging the scutum and some pale-scaled veins on the wings. They breed prolifically in temporary flood pans in savannahs and the adults shelter among grass. About 20 arboviruses have

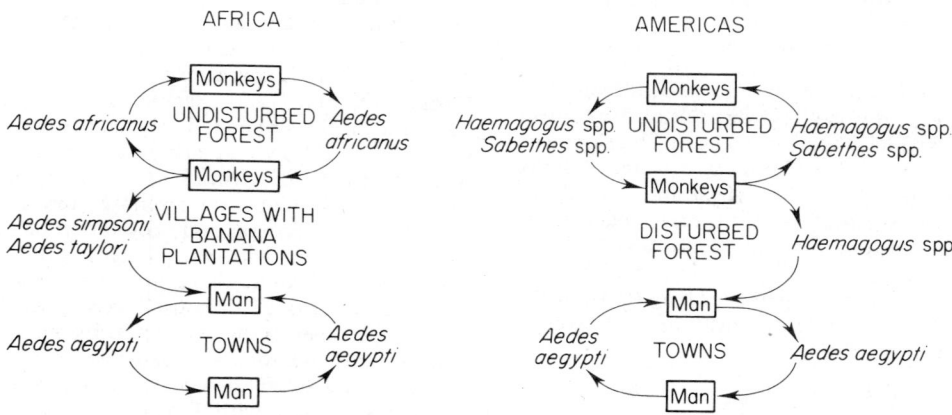

Fig. III.34 Yellow fever ecosystems in Africa and the Americas.

been isolated from *Neomelaniconion* spp., the most important to man being Rift Valley fever transmitted by *Ae. circumluteolus* and *Ae. lineatopennis* in southern Africa and probably elsewhere.

Subgenus *Ochlerotatus* is the dominant component of *Aedes* in terms of numbers of species and their distribution. They are ground pool breeders, mostly in temperate countries. Generally they bite mammals. In North America, *Ae. atlanticus* is an important vector of *D. immitis*, a filarial parasite affecting dogs and capable of causing dog heartworm disease in man. Rift Valley fever virus is commonly transmitted to livestock by *Ae. caballus* in southern Africa, although few *Ochlerotatus* spp. occur in Africa. *Ae. caspius* is widespread in Europe and North Africa, a fairly large speckled species that breeds commonly in brackish water, usually the vector of Inkoo virus in Scandinavia. Various North American *Ochlerotatus* spp. contribute sporadically to the transmission of encephalitides and are beyond the reach of economical control programmes. Species such as the salt-water-breeding *Ae. detritus* in Europe and *Ae. sollicitans* and *Ae. taeniorhynchus* in America are intolerable pests, and the latter has been implicated in *W. bancrofti* transmission. *Ae. (O.) vigilax* is another salt-water-breeding species locally responsible for periodic bancroftian filariasis transmission in New Caledonia (Table III.5) and for Ross River virus in Australia (Table III.6). This species and the closely related *Ae. fryeri* are so vicious and prolific as to make many islands uninhabitable in the Indian and Pacific Oceans.

Subgenus *Aedimorphus* and other subgenera of *Aedes* also include some species which are pests and vectors of arboviruses. In particular, *Ae. vexans* is probably the second or third most widespread mosquito in the world (after *C. pipiens* and perhaps *Ae. aegypti*). Seasonal breeding in grassland follows flooding and egg-hatching of broods which are immensely troublesome when the adult females attack; they bite during day and night, being especially numerous in late spring in northern latitudes.

GENUS: *Armigeres*

Widespread and common in the Australasian and Oriental regions, this genus is difficult to distinguish from *Aedes*, to which it is closely related. Development always occurs in small containers of water and the larvae grow very rapidly. *Armigeres subalbatus* (=*obturbans*) is a semidomestic species that breeds commonly in foul water, including latrines. This and several other species attack man during night and day. It has been suggested that they may transmit *W. bancrofti* and the encephalitis virus Sepik has been isolated from *Armigeres*.

GENUS: *Haemagogus*

This genus of forest mosquitoes is also closely related to *Aedes*. It occurs in Central and South America, breeding in flooded tree-holes. Adults are metallic blue and green due to their covering of scales on thorax and abdomen. Several species are vectors of sylvatic (jungle) yellow fever: *Haemagogus equinus*, *H. janthinomys*, *H. leucocelaenus*, *H. mesodentatus*, *H. spegazzinii* and *H. capricornii*. They are separable only on the characters of the male genitalia and not at all as larvae and pupae. The larvae of these vector species are 'hairy' and are thus distinguishable from some other species of *Haemogogus* which are not vectors. Adult females of *Haemagogus* seldom leave the forest and they attack man mainly during jungle clearance activities. Taxonomy of the genus has been revised by Arnell.[32]

GENUS: *Psorophora*

Three subgenera and almost 50 species are recognized, many of them vicious man-biters. Generic characters are the presence of spiracular *and* post-spiracular bristles, plus the retractable postabdomen as in other Aedini. Larvae of the typical subgenus are predacious. Eggs normally diapause before hatching and the breeding places are always in pools and marshes on the ground, not containers as used by some allied genera. Apart from their considerable significance as pests, *Psorophora* spp. are of widespread importance as vectors of arboviruses (Table III.6), especially Venezuelan equine encephalitis transmitted by *P. ferox* and *P. confinnis*, the latter being known as the dark rice-field mosquito. Taxonomy of this genus remains unsatisfactory, but Belkin et al[33] and Carpenter and LaCasse[14] give summaries.

TRIBE: CULICINI

GENUS: *Culex*

About 800 species of *Culex* are known, being classified in 21 subgenera, with many species acting as the vectors of enzootic arboviruses, protozoa and filariae. They bite at night and some species have much medical significance; many species can be pests when abundant. Generic characteristics are that eggs always form a raft (Fig. III.21), larvae have several pairs of hair tufts on the siphon, and the adults possess tarsal pulvilli (Fig. III.35) and lack post-spiracular bristles, with the tip of the female abdomen being bluntly rounded. Male palps are strongly curved upwards (Fig. III.25a). General body coloration of the adults is usually brown, with wings plain and vein scales dark. Unlike Aedini, the eggs cannot diapause, so *Culex* breeding is continuous, except when fertilized females hibernate as the overwintering mechanism for species found in temperate countries.

The typical subgenus *Culex* contains the majority of species, usually with a banded proboscis and/or basal pale bands on abdominal tergites. Japanese

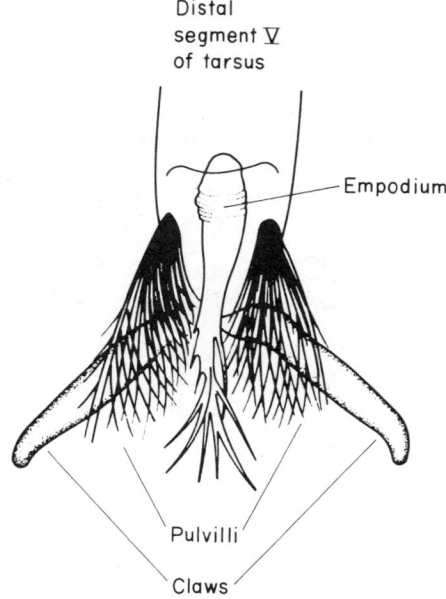

Distal
segment V
of tarsus

— Empodium

Pulvilli

Claws

Fig. III.35 Tip of tarsus of *Culex*, showing paired pulvilli below the claws. In life these pulvilli appear as pale pads, more conspicuous than the empodium which is present also in other mosquito genera.

encephalitis virus is mainly transmitted by *Culex* spp. in the Oriental region (for identification keys see Bram,[34] Sirivanakarn[35]), especially by the following species which breed prolifically in paddy and swamps: *C. tritaeniorhynchus*, *C. gelidus* and *C. vishnui*. Because they are abundant around villages wherever rice is grown in South-East Asia, and the adult females of these species attack various mammals by preference, they readily transfer Japanese encephalitis virus to man from pigs and other amplification hosts. *C. theileri* in southern Africa and members of the *C. pipiens* complex in Egypt are important vectors of Rift Valley fever virus from livestock to man. In Australia, *C. annulirostris* plays a similar role in the epidemiology of Murray Valley encephalitis, but the source of Murray Valley encephalitis virus remains a mystery. Like most other *Culex* spp., *C. annulirostris* feeds to some extent on birds and these may be responsible for virus dissemination. Eastern and Western Equine and St Louis encephalitis viruses in America are mainly found in birds (sparrows, pigeons), being transmitted by *C. nigripalpus*, *C. pipiens*, *C. restuans*, *C. salinarius*, *C. tarsalis* and other mosquitoes which occasionally pass infection to man and other mammals which serve as dead-end hosts. *C. pipiens* serves the same function for Eastern Equine encephalitis virus in Europe. West Nile virus has similar epidemiology in Africa, being transmitted from birds to man by members of the *C. univittatus* complex.

Culex-borne arboviruses can be carried through the

winter in hibernating female mosquitoes, although the ecological importance of this remains uncertain. The arrival of virus in migratory birds may set off seasonal transmission if it coincides with high densities of bird-biting mosquitoes. Investigations of arbovirus epidemiology are frequently hampered by difficulties of distinguishing and identifying the females of *Culex* spp., taxonomy of which is based on the morphology of male terminalia in many cases.

The *Culex pipiens* complex comprises several species, subspecies and forms, with representatives in all parts of the world. Typical *C. pipiens* occurs in temperate countries of the northern hemisphere, spreading through temperate highlands to southern Africa. Closely related species or subspecies are present in temperate parts of Australia and South America, but they seldom attack man in temperate countries. Whenever a man-biting infestation occurs to the north of the Mediterranean or equivalent latitude, it is likely to be a form usually known as *molestus* (*autogenicus*). This mosquito causes severe infestations due to prolific breeding indoors where circumstances are suitable. Although the females are autogenous (laying one egg batch without having fed on blood) they attack man viciously. Indoor infestations of *C. p. molestus*, or autogenous *C. pipiens*, occur as far north as Moscow. It seems that incapacity to hibernate is what keeps these mosquitoes indoors, breeding in flooded basements, cess pits, etc. Southwards, especially in North Africa, such populations are more often found breeding freely outdoors and it is unclear to what extent they may interbreed with anautogenous *C. pipiens*. In Egypt, the *C. pipiens* complex is responsible for bancroftian filariasis transmission[36] and has been implicated as the main vector in outbreaks of Rift Valley fever.

C. quinquefasciatus (=*C. p. fatigans*) is the main man-biting tropical member of the *C. pipiens* complex, distributed up to 38° north in USA, 30° north in Asia, but only 24° north in Africa. In the New World it interbreeds with *C. pipiens* sensu stricto, but they can generally be regarded as distinct species. Bancroftian filariasis is largely maintained in tropical villages and towns by *C. quinquefasciatus* alone, although West African strains of *W. bancrofti* do not develop in this species of mosquito. Elsewhere, *C. quinquefasciatus* is an efficient vector of *W. bancrofti* but refractory to *B. malayi*.

C. quinquefasciatus (Fig. III.36) is confined to domestic habitats, breeding abundantly in heavily polluted waters occurring in ditches, village ponds, soakage pits, cess pits and the like. Since these sites are inevitably associated with towns and urban development, *C. quinquefasciatus* thrives as a tropical pest in developing countries. Some breeding also occurs in rock holes, tree-holes and artificial containers such as tins, buckets and car tyres, where larvae of *Ae. aegypti* commonly mingle with those of *C. quinquefasciatus*. Control of both is best done by elimination of breeding

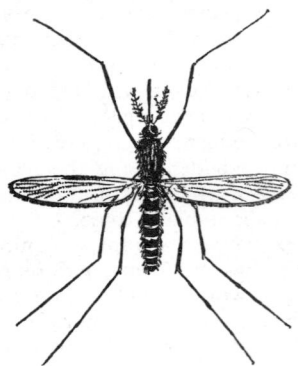

Fig. III.36 *Culex quinquefasciatus*. × 4. The name refers to the way that, when viewed from above with the naked eye, the abdomen seems to have five broad dark bands separated by pale bands (but so do many other species). The alternative name *Culex fatigans* (the mosquito that tends to make one fatigued) has been widely used, although *quinquefasciatus* has priority and is therefore correct.

Taxonomy of the *C. pipiens* complex is a matter of uncertainty and disagreement. Separation of species is traditionally based upon the morphology of male terminalia, as expressed by the ratio of distances between tips of the dorsal and ventral arms of the phallosome (D/V ratio) or the difference between these dimensions (D/DV ratio), as shown in Fig. III.37.

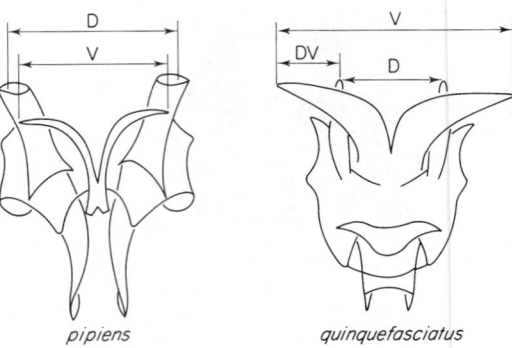

pipiens   *quinquefasciatus*

Fig. III.37 Male phallosomes of the *Culex pipiens* complex, ventral views. The shape and spread of the ventral arms is much wider in *C. quinquefasciatus* (= *C. p. fatigans*) than in typical *C. pipiens*. The ratio D/V can be used to express this contrast, sometimes given as DV/V. Members of the *C. pipiens* complex generally have the following values for D/V: *quinquefasciatus* 0.3, *pallens* 0.3–1.0, *pipiens* 0.8–1.0, *molestus* (= *autogenicus*) 0.8–1.2.

sites, putting covers on water pots, covering soakage pits and taking all possible precautions to prevent there being places where the female mosquitoes can lay their eggs on exposed water containing organic nutrients for the larvae. Larvicidal oils and insecticides have been widely employed, but they are increasingly uneconomical and in many countries *C. quinquefasciatus* has become resistant to both organochlorines and organophosphates. Nevertheless, it may be advisable to treat larger breeding places with emulsions of organophosphates or to employ costly carbamates, pyrethroids, biocides or mosquito growth inhibitors (e.g. diflubenzuron or methoprene) activity of which may be much reduced in polluted water. Minimal labour is needed if breeding sites are treated with briquettes or granular formulations, giving prolonged release of the chemical into solution.

As the bites of *C. quinquefasciatus* are painful, whether or not disease is likely to be transmitted, it is advisable to screen houses (plastic mesh, at least six strands per centimetre) and especially bedrooms, making them mosquito-proof. Cracks around ceilings and doors should be sealed. The use of bed-nets is highly desirable wherever *C. quinquefasciatus* occurs. Although several arboviruses have been reported from *C. quinquefasciatus*, it seems that this species is not usually an important vector of such infections. Adult males and females rest both indoors and outdoors during daytime; they are naturally quite tolerant of residual insecticides.

In the Far East, *C. pipiens pallens* seems to be biologically intermediate between *C. pipiens* and *C. quinquefasciatus*. It may be a distinct species or a hybrid. Formerly a filariasis vector in Japan[37] and still a pest there, the importance and distribution of *C. p. pallens* in South-East Asian countries is not well understood.

General recognition of the *C. pipiens* complex depends upon the following combination of characters: proboscis dark, not banded, paler below in middle; abdominal tergites with transverse pale bands basally and pale spots on hind corners; abdomen pale below, usually with median dark spots in a row; thorax reddish-brown dorsally, straw/pale brown coloured laterally without dark pleural markings, with dark bristles on scutum and whitish scales in patches on pleurae (sides) but without spiracular or post-spiracular scales; usually one lower mesepimeral bristle; wings with dark scales on all veins; tarsi entirely dark; mid femur dark anteriorly, without narrow longitudinal pale stripe as in some closely related species (which may also have spiracular or post-spiracular scale patches).

Apart from the species already mentioned, which all belong to subgenus *Culex*, some medically important species belong to subgenus *Melanoconion*. These small species are potent vectors of arboviruses in the American tropics (Table III.6). As distinct from subgenus *Culex* having narrow scales, species in subgenus *Melanconion* have a rim of broad scales above the eyes, and wing veins one and two with broader scales distally. It is difficult to identify females of *Melanoconion* specifically and breeding places are not easy to find. Usually the larvae occupy large, quiet, nonpolluted pools, often sheltering under vegetation.

Control is therefore impracticable without environmental damage. Adults of *Melanoconion* spp. shelter among vegetation and their attacks may be locally reduced by insecticidal fogging during the evening flight period. They prefer to feed upon a wide range of wild creatures, but man is often bitten. Taxonomic studies by Sirivanakarn[38] should pave the way to improved understanding of the vectorial significance of the various species.

GENUS: *Culiseta*

Distinctive features of this genus are the presence of spiracular bristles; the wing often has one or two dark spots in the middle (at base of vein three and sometimes vein two); the siphonal tuft is large, at the extreme base of the larval siphon; eggs are usually laid as a raft which is less well formed than in *Culex*. Approximately 35 species are classified in seven subgenera, some of which are given generic status by Maslov.[39] Most are harmless and found only in temperate countries. A few species are pests, notably *C. longiareolata* around the Mediterranean. This species inhabits arid terrain, breeding in wells and rock pools, whereas most other *Culiseta* spp. favour weedy ponds and marshes. In North America, both Eastern and Western Equine encephalitis circulate among birds through *C. inornata*, *C. melanura* and *C. morsitans*. The latter may also be involved as a vector in Old World situations. *Culiseta* spp. breed continuously throughout the year, females of some species (e.g. *C. annulata*) sheltering indoors feeding intermittently during winter in temperate countries.

TRIBE: MANSONIINI

GENUS: *Coquillettidia*

Most of these species are largely yellow, quite large and voracious biters, attacking by day and night. They lay egg masses on the surface of stagnant water or weedy ponds. Larvae and pupae have the respiratory siphon and trumpets pointed and strengthened for plugging into the air ducts of plant stems. The genus occurs in all continents; among 55 known species *C. perturbans* in North America and *C. venezuelensis* in South America are some of the most important pests, and the latter has been implicated as a vector of several arboviruses (Table III.6).

GENUS: *Mansonia*

This genus differs from the preceding one by characters given in the key (Table III.7) and because egg masses are deposited under floating leaves of certain aquatic plants. Like *Coquillettidia*, larvae and pupae of *Mansonia* breathe air from plant stems and have their respiratory appendages modified accordingly (Figs. III.38, III.39). Subgenus *Mansonia* has only a

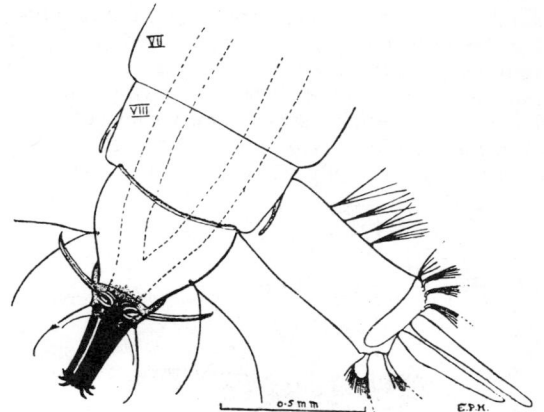

Fig. III.38 Respiratory siphon and terminal segment of the larva of *Mansonioides* (lateral view).

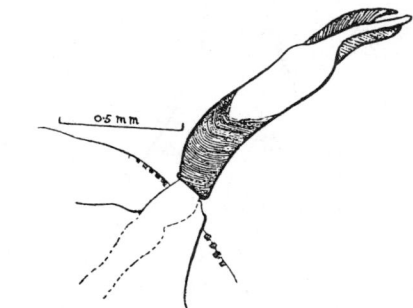

Fig. III.39 Respiratory horn of the pupa of *Mansonioides*.

dozen American species, notably the widespread pest *M. titillans* which breeds in swamps and marshes with floating water lettuce (*Pistia*) and water hyacinth (*Eichornia*) or rooted *Pontederia* and other plants favoured by the immature stages. *M. titillans* is an important vector of Venezuelan equine encephalitis and may contribute to transmission of *W. bancrofti*. As with other troublesome *Mansonia* and some *Coquillettidia*, *M. titillans* disperses far from the breeding sites in search of hosts to bite.

Subgenus *Mansonioides* also has a dozen species, endemic to the Old World tropics, being pests arising from breeding sites in water with plenty of *Eichornia*, *Pistia*, rooted *Isachne* (swamp grass), *Zuzania* and other suitable vegetation. When such well-aerated plants are removed, *Mansonioides* disappear. In parts of southern India (Kerala), Sri Lanka and elsewhere, *Mansonioides* populations thrive where flooded pits for soakage of coconut husks, from which rope is made, are allowed to provide breeding sites rich in organic food for the larvae. In some areas this problem has now been controlled by keeping the water free of floating plants.

Adult *Mansonioides* are strikingly marked (Fig. III.40), with banded legs and speckled wings having very broad scales on the veins. The tip of the female abdomen is curiously boat-shaped, to facilitate oviposition under floating leaves. Some arboviruses are transmitted by *Mansonioides* spp., but these species of mosquitoes are generally refractory to *W. bancrofti.*

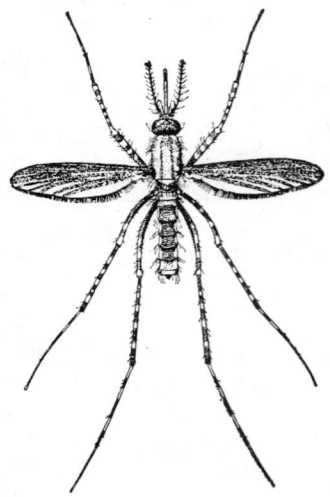

Fig. III.40　Female *Mansonia (Mansonioides) annulifera.* × 4.

In forested localities, or when weather is overcast, the females feed by day; they attack mainly at night outdoors, coming freely into houses, but not resting indoors during the daytime. The bites are more painful than for most other mosquitoes. *Mansonioides* spp. are of particular parasitological interest because, together with *Anopheles (Anopheles)* spp., they are the vectors of brugian filariasis (Table III.5). In South-East Asia, according to the work of Wharton[40] in Malaya, swamp-forest populations of *M. annulata, M. uniformis* and especially the sibling species *M. bonneae* and *M. dives* share the transmission of zoonotic subperiodic *B. malayi,* which they transmit to man from leaf monkeys and other wild animals. At the same time, *M. annulata, M. dives* and other *Mansonioides* spp. are vectors of *B. pahangi* from animal to animal, but rarely to man. Continuous biting activity, with peaks of attack at dusk and dawn, helps to make *Mansonioides* spp. in the forest suitable as vectors of these subperiodic parasites. In areas of paddy on the coastal plains, *M. uniformis* and *Anopheles* spp. (see p. 1409) are the principal vectors of periodic *B. malayi,* with some involvement of *M. annulata* and *M. dives.* However, *M. bonneae* is apparently refractory to the periodic strains of the parasite. In India and other parts of southern Asia, periodic *B. malayi* is or was generally transmitted by *M. annulata, M. annulifera, M. indiana* and *M. uniformis.* In eastern Africa, where

B. malayi is absent, *M. africana* and *M. uniformis* transmit *B. patei* among dogs and cats but rarely to people.

TRIBE: SABETHINI

GENUS: *Sabethes*

These are forest mosquitoes that transmit jungle yellow fever and other arboviruses (Table III.6) in South America. *S. chloropterus* is one of the most frequently involved vector species. About 30 species are known. This genus is very distinctive; its characters are given in Table III.7. The adults have a metallic lustre. The scales of all parts of the body are flat. There is a very large pair of procumbent bristles projecting from the crown of the head and a tuft of setae on the mesonotum. The antennae are similar in both sexes; the palps are short in the female and usually also in the male. The larvae are generally predaceous and live in the water which collects in the axils and bracts of leaves, in tree-holes, or which is secreted by pitchers or other modified parts of plants. They are usually rather hairy and have smooth or stumpy antennae. A siphon is present and a single row of scales on the side of the eighth abdominal segments. The pupae are characterized by the conspicuous fan of bristles at the posterolateral angles of the eighth and ninth abdominal segments and by the small tail-fins. *Sabethes* taxonomy is unsatisfactory and their control is impractical.

LITERATURE ON MOSQUITOES

Information on the many species of mosquitoes is voluminous, with about five or six publications on Culicidae appearing daily. Much of the literature on mosquito biology and identification is now obsolete, due to advances in knowledge. Some general references to be recommended are: Bates,[41] Gillett,[42] Harbach and Knight,[43] Harwood and James,[44] Horsfall,[45] Mattingly,[46] Service[47] and World Health Organization.[9]

For the identification of mosquito genera and species in each part of the world, the following publications contain the most up-to-date keys and/or other information on medically important species:

Africa: Anophelinae: Gillies and De Meillon.[15] Culicinae: Edwards;[48] Hopkins;[49] Mattingly;[50] Gerberg and Van Someren;[51] Cordellier et al.[52]

Americas: Lane;[53] Forratini;[54,55] Belkin et al;[33] Carpenter and LaCasse;[14] Wood et al;[56] Faran;[21] Darsie and Ward;[57] Sirivanakarn.[38]

Arabia: Mattingly and Knight.[58]

Australia: Lee;[59] Lee and Woodhill;[60] Dobrotworsky;[61] Marks.[62]

Cape Verde Islands: Ribeiro et al.[63]

Europe: Dahl and White.[64]

India: Anophelinae: Christophers;[65] Bhatia et al.[66] Culicinae: Barraud;[67] see also Oriental region.

Jamaica: Belkin et al.[33]

Japan: Tanaka et al.[68]

Madagascar: Grjebine;[69] Ravaonjanahary.[70]

Mediterranean: Rioux;[71] Senevet and Andarelli.[72]

New Guinea: Van den Assem and Bonne-Wepster.[73]

New Zealand: Belkin.[74]

Oriental: region: Anophelinae: Bonne-Wepster and Swellengrebel;[75] Reid;[12] Harrison and Scanlon;[76] Culicinae: Mattingly;[77] Bram;[34] Mattingly;[78] Reinert;[79] Sirivanakarn;[35] Huang.[80]

Pacific: Belkin;[24] Huang.[25]

Philippines: Delfinado;[81] Basio.[82]

Russia: Gutsevich et al.[82]

Seychelles: Mattingly and Brown.[84]

World: Foote and Cook[85] Mattingly;[86] Knight and Stone.[80]

Most recent advances in mosquito control are mentioned in the two volumes edited by Laird and Miles (1983, 1985).[87]

MOSQUITO PHYSIOLOGY

This subject is becoming more relevant to medical entomology. Some of the newer larvicides for mosquito control act as 'growth regulators'. One mode of action is to impair cuticle formation in the successive larval instars, the pupa and the adult through the application of chitin inhibitors (e.g. diflubenzuron). Another approach is to treat mosquito breeding places with compounds having activity like the juvenile hormones of insects; these 'juvenoids' (e.g. methoprene) prevent successful metamorphosis and maturation of the mosquito. So far there are no practical problems of resistance to these chemicals and there should be little cross resistance with conventional pesticides.

As for all other insects, the mosquito body is encased in an exoskeleton made of cuticle. Insecticides which act on the nervous system (i.e. organochlorines, organophosphates, carbamates, pyrethroids) must be readily absorbed through insect cuticle, but not through human skin. Cuticular hardness depends on the degree of chitinization. Mosquito larvae have a hard head capsule, siphon and many rigid bristles or setae and spines, but the thorax and abdomen are mostly covered by more flexible cuticle. Mosquito adults have strong and rigid cuticular plates forming

the head, thorax and abdomen, with flexible joints between them where necessary for articulation of limbs and segments. Respiratory spiracles on the larval siphon, pupal trumpets and on the adult sides (pairs on the mesothorax, metathorax and each abdominal segment) allow air to reach all internal organs via a network of tubes called tracheae. The use of larvicidal oils is intended to drown mosquito larvae by preventing them from reaching air when they try to open their spiracles at the water surface. However, Reiter,[88] working with monomolecular layers for anopheline control, has found that there may be sufficient dissolved oxygen for larval survival during much of the day and all of the night without access to free air. Oiling will therefore be most effective when an insecticide is included.

The body cavity or haemocoel of mosquitoes and other insects is filled with colourless haemolymph carrying haemocytes having some of the functions of blood corpuscles. There is an open circulatory system, with a dorsal aorta and heart in the abdomen. The mosquito brain is in the head, with neurosecretory ganglia and *corpus cardiacum* for hormone production. Other important sources of hormones controlling mosquito life processes are the ovaries and the thoracic *corpora allata*. A ventral nerve cord has segmental ganglia and paired lateral branches.

The mosquito gut (Fig. III.41) passes from the proboscis to the pharynx in the head, the oesophagus in the thorax, the midgut or stomach in the abdomen

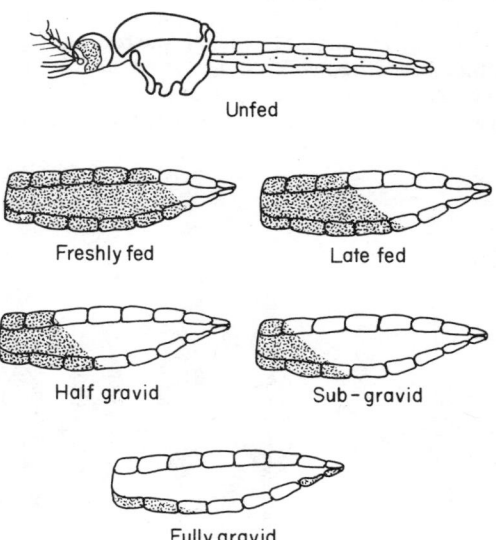

Unfed

Freshly fed

Late fed

Half gravid

Sub-gravid

Fully gravid

Fig. III.41 Classification of the abdominal conditions of female mosquitoes. The dark basal area of the abdomen contains the blood-meal in the stomach, decreasing as digestion proceeds. The pale posterior part of the abdomen contains the developing ovaries, increasing as the gonotrophic cycle proceeds. Unfed, fed and gravid female mosquitoes may be either nulliparous or parous.

and finally the rectum, where fluids are absorbed before defecation occurs through the anus below the tip of the abdomen. Within the foregut, especially of female anophelines, cuticular teeth protrude into the lumen of the gut; these are thought to have a primary function of rupturing blood corpuscles and they also inflict lethal damage on many ingested microfilariae. A large crop is formed by an oesophageal diverticulum; water and nectar are taken into the crop for digestion of sugars. Excretion is by means of a series of long white malpighian tubules in the abdomen, behind the stomach, with their ducts discharging into the midgut lumen.

When freshly engorged after biting, the abdomen of a female mosquito is swollen and reddened by the blood meal within the stomach. Paired ovaries, each with about 100 follicles for egg production, are situated posteriorly in the abdomen. In the terminal abdominal segment of females are spermathecae (three in culicines; one in anophelines) which receive and store sperms from males, so that mature oöcytes can be fertilized as eggs are laid.

As the blood meal becomes digested during the days after blood-feeding, the ovaries develop and fill the rear abdomen with whitish eggs. Fig. III.41 shows how the changes of abdominal condition can be classified as (*a*) unfed, (*b*) freshly fed, (*c*) one-third gravid or late stage fed, (*d*) half gravid, (*e*) two-thirds gravid or sub-gravid, (*f*) fully gravid. In parallel with these abdominal stages, it is customary to assess the progress of oögenesis by classifying the development of ovarian follicles. After emergence from the pupa, the follicles pass from stage I to stage II, which is the resting stage. After blood-feeding, yolk is deposited around the oöcyte nucleus, and stage III passes to stage IV when the clear nucleus is no longer visible when examined

in saline. Finally stage V represents formation of the full-sized egg, containing the unfertilized oöcyte. These categories of ovarian development in mosquitoes are generally known as 'Christophers' stages' (Fig. III.42).

At tropical temperatures, the eggs of mosquitoes become ready to lay (laying is termed oviposition) 2 or 3 days after ingestion of the blood meal. Blood-feeding and egg-laying are the first and last steps in what is called the gonotrophic cycle. Soon after having laid a batch of eggs, the female mosquito tries to feed again on blood. Thus there are regular and usually

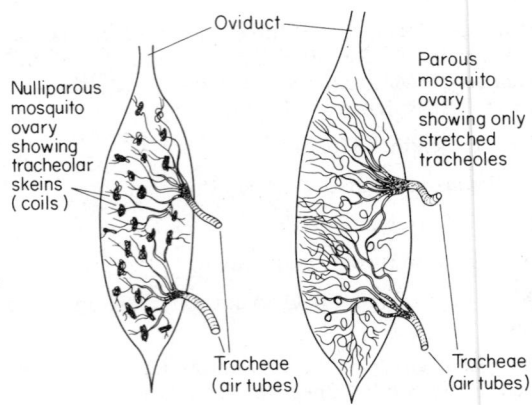

Fig. III.43 Mosquito ovaries, showing how the nulliparous female has coiled tracheolar 'skeins' in the ovary (left); tracheoles become permanently stretched in the parous ovary (right) due to previous growth of eggs. These features of the air tubes can only be seen in mosquito females with 'unfed' abdominal condition.

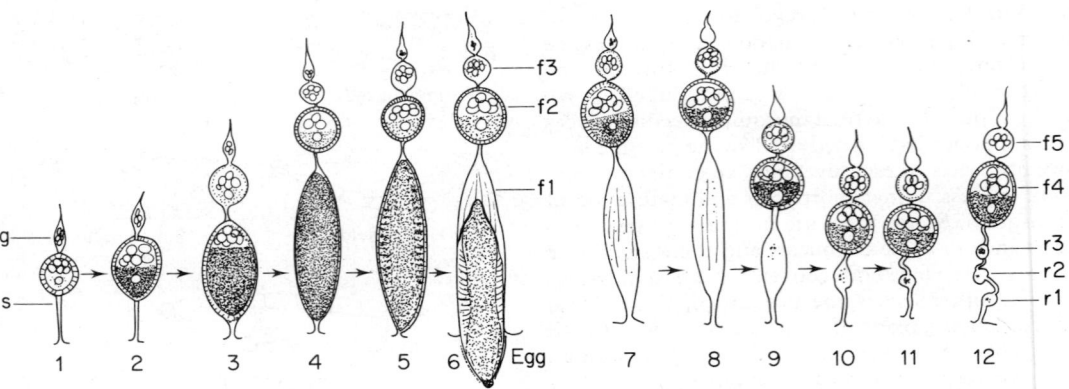

Fig. III.42 Christophers' stages of ovarian follicular development in mosquitoes. Each ovary contains approximately 100 ovarioles. Each ovariole consists of a hollow stalk (s), developing follicles (f1, f2, etc.) and a terminal germarium (g) from which successive follicles arise. Stages I to V of development of the first follicle are shown (1–5). The mature egg then passes from the stalk (6) to the common oviduct. A sac-like swelling of the ovariolar stalk contracts (7–10) to form a small persistent dilatation or follicular relic, which is slightly pigmented (11). Successive eggs formed in each ovariole leave a series of distinct relics (r1, r2 etc.) in the parous mosquito (12) from which the mosquito's age may be estimated in terms of the number of gonotrophic cycles.

continuous gonotrophic cycles. The feeding interval, or the duration of the gonotrophic cycle, measured in days, is an important factor affecting vectorial capacity. The more often a mosquito feeds on blood, the more likely it is to pick up infections and transmit them. Conversely, at cooler temperatures, the gonotrophic cycle takes longer, maybe 4 or 5 days, reducing the chances of transmission because (*a*) occasions when parasites can be acquired or transmitted are less frequent for each female mosquito, (*b*) the speed of development of parasites to the infective stage in the vectors is proportional to temperature and (*c*) mosquitoes are more likely to die before becoming infective. Clearly, if mosquito longevity is less than the time required for completion of parasite development, there is no likelihood of disease transmission. The aim

of spraying houses with residual insecticides is to kill the majority of adult female mosquitoes before they reach the age of infectivity, not to eliminate mosquitoes altogether.

One way to monitor the age composition and life expectancy of adult mosquito populations is to determine the proportion of females that are parous, i.e. have laid eggs at least once. This involves examination of the ovaries to see whether tracheal skeins are present implying nulliparity, or if follicular relics are present implying parity (Fig. III.43). It may be possible to count the number of relics on each follicular stalk in order to calculate the mosquito's age in terms of the number of gonotrophic cycles it has experienced.[9,89]

More general information on mosquito physiology has been reviewed by Clements.[90]

MIDGES

R. P. Lane

FAMILY: CERATOPOGONIDAE (BITING MIDGES)

GENERA: *Culicoides, Leptoconops* and *Forcipomyia* (subgenus *Lasiohelea*)

Biting midges are very small flies (1–4 mm long) called 'no-see-ums' in some parts of the world or, confusingly, sandflies in others such as the southern USA and Caribbean. They occur worldwide in habitats ranging from tropical forests and savannahs to agricultural districts, coastal and desert areas. The adults are compact, usually dark-brown or black flies, with the wings held flat over the back at rest. Only the females suck blood and often attack in huge numbers, their bites are painful and often elicit a prolonged reaction in sensitive individuals. The males, which can be distinguished by their plumose antennae, feed only on plant sugars. The larvae are small and wormlike, swimming in a sinusoidal manner through wet or moist habitats such as fresh or brackish water or mud, decomposing vegetation and wet bovine droppings.

The Ceratopogonidae (biting midges) are a large family of over 4000 species in 60 genera but only three contain species of medical significance: *Culicoides, Leptoconops* and *Forcipomyia* (subgenus *Lasiohelea*).[91] Their principal impact on man is as biting pests but species of *Culicoides* transmit filarial nematodes and are also of veterinary importance as virus and nematode vectors.

Leptoconops. Some species are serious pests, biting during the day. The flies are shiny black with milky white wings. Species of the subgenus *Styloconops* breed in sandy beaches surrounding the Indian Ocean (*L. spinosifrons; L. holoconops*), and are coastal pests in south-east USA, eastern Central America and the Caribbean (*L. becquaerti*); *Leptoconops* (*sensu stricto*)

breed in fine silt soils inland in south-east USA (*L. torrens*).

A few species of *Forcipomyia* subgenus *Lasiohelea* are serious pests: *F.* (*L*) *siberica* in the USSR, *F.* (*L.*) *taiwana* in Japan and China and *F.* (*L.*) *townsvillensis* in Australia.

Culicoides. These have a wing length of 2 mm; those of tropical species may be only 1 mm, and usually the wings are patterned (Fig. III.44). Of the 1000 species in this genus, many are biting pests in temperate and tropical countries and may have a significant effect on tourist based economies. Biting rates of 200–400 per hour are commonly recorded with a maximum of 3000 per hour on a single exposed limb! Attacks may cause severe discomfort, e.g. biting on the eyelids may induce sufficient swelling to prevent their opening for several days. New arrivals to tropical areas often suffer (or are worried) more than locals and subsequent scratching may produce deeply eroding secondary infections to the extent that skin grafting has been used. Dermatitis caused by *Culicoides* has been reported several times, e.g. *C. paraensis* in Bahia, Brazil.

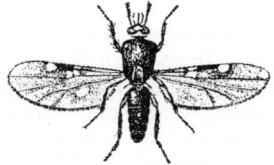

Fig. III.44 Female *Culicoides grahami*. × 50.

In the Caribbean and eastern Central America *Mansonella ozzardi* is transmitted by several species of *Culicoides*: *C. furens* in St Vincent, Haiti;[92] *C. phlebotomus* in Trinidad[93] and *C. paraensis* in Antigua and northern Argentina. Both *C. furens* and *C. phlebotomus* are coastal species the former breeding in mangrove swamps and the latter in streams crossing beaches. *C. paraensis* is a peridomestic species breeding in decaying fruits such as calabash or cacao pods. In the Brazilian and Colombian Amazon regions *M. ozzardi* is primarily transmitted by *Simulium*, but *C. insinuatus* may also play a role.

Culicoides are also vectors of *M. perstans* in Africa and believed to be the vector in the New World. There is considerable confusion over the identity of the species incriminated as the vector of *M. perstans* in West Africa. It was originally recorded as *C. austeni* (and later *C. milnei*), but it is more likely that *C. inornatipennis* (and possibly *C. grahami*) are responsible. The vectors breed in small pools of water in cut stems of bananas and plantains and therefore incidence of the disease is highest in and around plantations. Transmission takes place at night. In contrast, the transmission of *M. streptocerca* takes place during the day when the vector, *C. grahami*, bites man.

Culicoides paraensis, a domestic pest in many parts of Brazil, has been incriminated as the vector of Oropouche virus, which causes febrile illness in Amazonian Brazil. Several other viruses have been isolated from ceratopogonids: Japanese B encephalitis (*F.* (*L.*) *taiwana*); eastern equine encephalitis (pooled *Culicoides* in USA); Rift Valley fever (*Culicoides* in Kenya, Nigeria); Congo and Dugbe viruses (several pools of *Culicoides* in Nigeria). Although it is most unlikely that midges transmit these viruses, the question does remain open.

Control of ceratopogonids involves the use of insecticides, repellents and land management (draining and flooding).[94]

BLACK FLIES, BUFFALO GNATS, TURKEY GNATS

G. B. White

FAMILY: SIMULIIDAE

GENUS: *Simulium*

The Simuliidae are small, robust flies (1–5 mm long) (Fig. III.45); the females suck blood and have blade-like mouthparts; in the males these are more or less rudimentary. The flies have a characteristic humped thorax caused by the strong development of the scutum. The antennae are short and similar in both sexes.

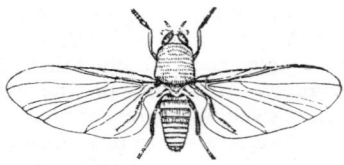

Fig. III.45 *Simulium damnosum.* × 10.

Black flies occur in enormous numbers in favourable localities during late spring and early summer in northern countries and are abundant in the north temperate and subarctic zones. They are also abundant in the tropics where man-biting species transmit *Onchocerca volvulus*. In addition to their role as transmitters of *Onchocerca*, they also act as intermediate hosts of other filariae and blood-borne protozoa of birds and mammals and are a severe biting nuisance when the flies are numerous. The females attack viciously in the open during the day but do not enter houses. Biting activity is known to be influenced by weather conditions and older (infected) flies may differ in their behaviour from newly emerged, unfed flies.

The females lay their triangular eggs in running (and therefore oxygenated) water, in masses of 300–500, which are attached to rocks, grass and other objects by a gelatinous fluid. The eggs hatch in one or two days and the emerging larvae attach themselves by the posterior end to a pad of silk spun from the salivary glands, on to submerged leaves and stones. The larvae and pupae of most species have specialized aquatic niches on stones, twigs or other substrates. Those of the *S. neavi* complex in tropical Africa always occur on freshwater arthropods, mainly crabs, prawns or mayfly nymphs. The larvae feed by straining fine particles from the water through fan-shaped mouth brushes. There are six to eight larval instars, ending in one to two weeks or more. Before pupation, the larva spins a tent-like, silken coccoon which protects the pupa inside it. The pupal period is 2 to 10 days and both larvae and pupae can be found in large numbers in the breeding places.

The following species are actual or potential vectors of *O. volvulus* in man:

Africa. The *Simulium damnosum* and *S. neavei* complexes are groups sibling species which have been separated into a number of different species by biological and chromosome studies. These species differ in their ecology and feeding preferences which affect their importance as vectors of human onchocerciasis. The *S. damnosum* complex (jinja fly) (see Table 20.3,

p. 385) contains at least 40 sibling species (identified chiefly by the pattern of chromosome banding), including forms that are found in the forest zone or in the savannah zone which are vectors only of the *O. volvulus* strain endemic to their own zones. Clinical manifestations of onchocerciasis in the savannah area are associated with lower biting densities and infection rates in the flies (annual transmission potential) compared to those found in the forest area. Different members of the complex breed in large or small rivers and in the outflow of dams, the larvae attaching to vegetation and stones in the river bed. Females are capable of long flights. In a control campaign using larvicides in West Africa, reinvasion of the controlled area was found over distances of 200–400 km.

The *S. neavei* complex is confined to small streams in hilly forest; its flight range is limited. The larvae and pupae are found attached to crabs of the genus *Potamonautes*. The chief vector species are *S. ethiopiense* in Ethiopia, *S. neavei* in Zaire and *S. woodi*; in Tanzania. Eradication of *S. neavei* and the interruption of transmission from man to man has been possible in highland foci in Kenya.

Central and South America. The *S. ochraceum* complex (orange/yellow species, unusual for a black fly) are the main vectors in Mexico and Guatemala. They breed in minute trickles of water, often under leaves, and in innumerable streams in rugged country with heavy vegetational cover; hence these species are difficult to control. They also breed close to villages in irrigated coffee plantations between 500 and 1200 m.

S. metallicum, S. callidum and *S. exiguum* are considered to be minor vectors in Central America but *S. exiguum* is the only anthropophilic species and therefore the principal vector in the endemic focus on the western slopes of the Andes in Colombia. *S. metallicum* is the main vector in Venezuela, breeding in small streams, and biting man avidly. In Mexico and Guatemala, however, this species does not feed on man so readily and is associated with larger streams.

In recently discovered foci of onchocerciasis in Amazonia (Brazil and Venezuela) the disease is transmitted by *S. limbatum* and *S. oyapockense* (formerly reported as *S. amazonicum*). The latter also transmits nonpathogenic *Mansonella ozzardi* in South America.

For control of Simuliidae see Chapter 20, p. 386.

TABANIDAE
Horse flies, Clegs, Deer flies

D. M. Minter

SUBORDER: BRACHYCERA
FAMILY: TABANIDAE
GENERA: *Tabanus, Haematopota* and *Chrysops*

The family Tabanidae belongs to the dipteran suborder Brachycera. The family (and to a large degree the suborder) is characterized in the adult stage most obviously by short, straight, forward-projecting, antennae that are shorter than the thorax. The three segments of the antennae (known also as the scape, pedicel and flagellum) differ in size and proportions in the three main genera, *Tabanus, Chrysops* and *Haematopota* (Fig. III.46b). The palps are short and consist of one or two segments only. The wing venation of tabanids is characteristic (Fig. III.46c), particularly the enclosed, nearly central, hexagonal discal cell and the open branch of the radial vein which encloses, in a submarginal cell, the wing tip of most species. There is also a second open submarginal cell anterior to the wing tip and five open posterior cells along the hind margin of the wing. The pattern of pigmentation of the wing, or its absence, is a useful feature for identification of the three genera of medical importance, in conjunction with the shape and proportion of the antennal segments (Fig. III.46b and c).

Other members of the suborder Brachycera are sometimes a severe biting nuisance, particularly in coastal and mountain regions of western North America. (They have a painful bite and are occasionally the cause of severe allergic manifestations.) These belong to the families Rhagionidae ('snipe-flies') and the closely related Athericidae. Although these two families have blood-sucking species, none have yet been associated with the transmission of pathogens. The rhagionid genus *Symphoromyia* is a vicious biter in the western USA; in Australia members of the genera *Spaniopsis* and *Austroleptis* are troublesome pests. Since they are of no known medical (or veterinary) importance, these two families are not considered further.

The family Tabanidae includes the largest blood-sucking flies known; some have a wing span of over 60 mm. Most species are stoutly built and robust insects, often brightly coloured in life, with large eyes and a body length from 5 to 25 mm. Viewed from above (Fig. III.46a), the eyes of females are widely separated (dichoptic), whilst the eyes of males are contiguous (holoptic). In life, the eyes of both sexes are often shot with species-specific iridescent bands, chevrons or spots of brilliant colours: these colours fade soon after death. Only females bite: because of their large size they take a large blood meal, from

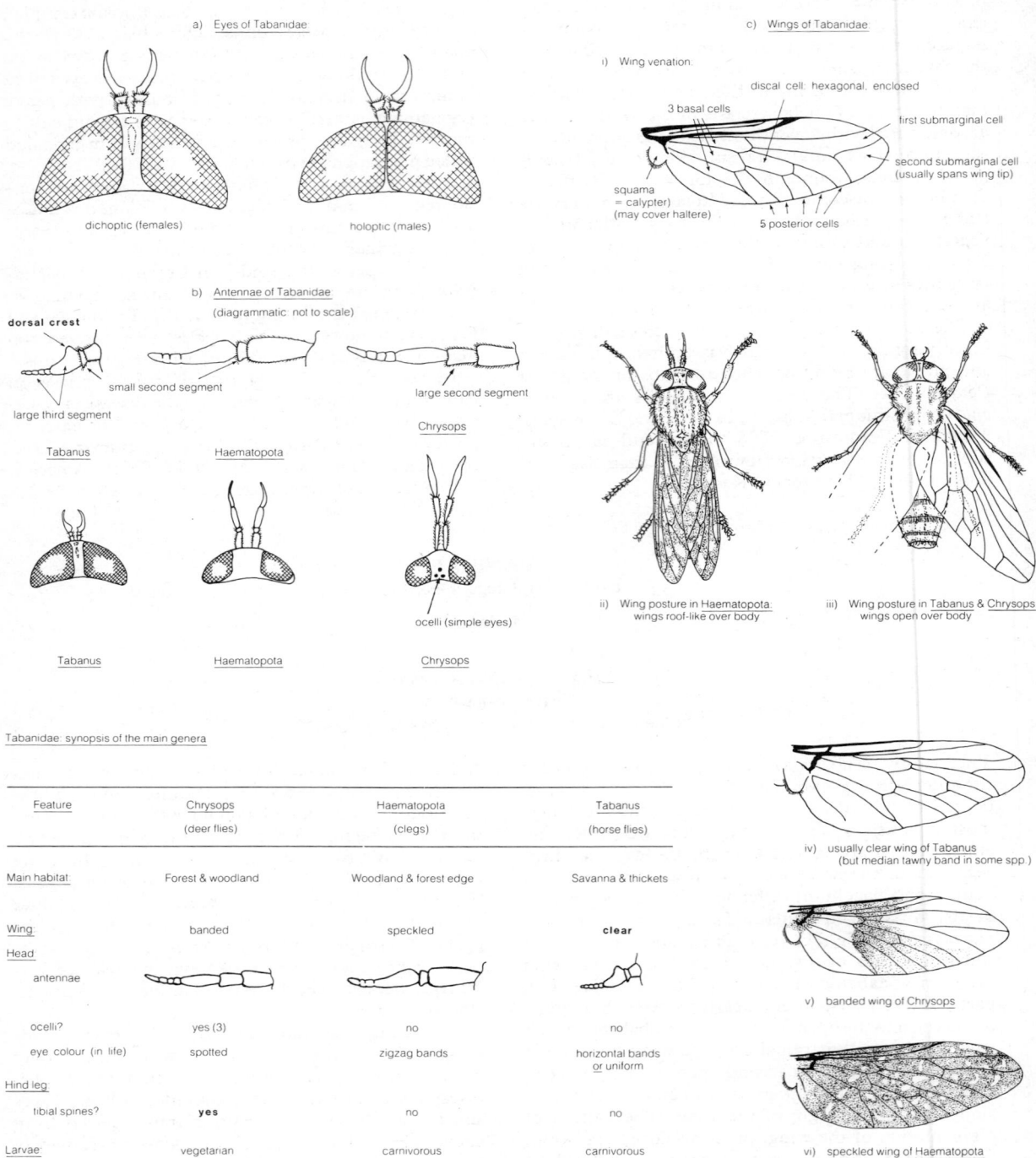

Fig. III.46 Characteristic features of the Tabanidae. (a) Holoptic and dichoptic condition of the head in male and female Tabanidae. (b) Antennae of adult Tabanidae: antennal features in the genera *Tabanus* (horse flies), *Chrysops* (deer flies) and *Haematopota* (clegs). (c) Wings of Tabanidae: (i) wing venation of Tabanidae; (ii) wing posture in *Haematopota* sp.; (iii) wing posture in *Tabanus* and *Chrysops* spp.; (iv) clear wing of *Tabanus* sp.; (v) banded wing of *Chrysops* sp.; (vi) speckled wing of *Haematopota* sp.

20 mg to 200 mg. The mouthparts are short and stout; they project downwards below the head and inflict a painful bite.

There are four subfamilies of Tabanidae (Scepsidinae, Pangoniinae, Chrysopsinae and Tabaninae). Medically important species are found only among the Chrysopsinae and Tabaninae. The Tabaninae is subdivided into three tribes (Haematopotini, Tabanini and Diachlorini), of which only the Haematopotini and Tabanini have species which normally bite man. There are about 3000 species of Tabanidae, in numerous genera, but medically important species occur only in the genera *Tabanus, Haematopota* (subfamily Tabaninae) and *Chrysops* (subfamily Chrysopsinae).

The Tabanidae are cosmopolitan; species of *Tabanus, Chrysops* and *Haematopota* occur in tropical, subtropical and temperate regions, but species of the genus *Haematopota*, although abundant in Africa, are absent from Australia and South America and are uncommon in North America.

The 'blue-tailed fly', celebrated in the well-known American ballad, is believed to be the widespread *Tabanus atratus* of eastern North America; the species is actually a uniform black colour, but there is a distinctly bluish tinge when the flies are covered with pollen or dust.

Recognition of the genera: *Chrysops, Tabanus* and *Haematopota*

The following notes, together with Fig. III.46, will facilitate recognition of the genera.

Chrysops (deer flies, greenheads, mango flies, mangrove flies). Fig. III.47. Medium size, 6–10 mm long. Wings held apart over the body, like a half-open pair of scissors. Wings usually with one or two brownish transverse bands. Antennae (Fig. III.46b) longer than those of *Tabanus* and *Haematopota*; the three segments are of similar length and project well in front of the head. Three spot-like, light-sensitive ocelli (simple eyes) present on the top of the head, behind the compound eyes. Tibia of hind legs spurred, with paired small distal spines, as well as the more prominent pair on the tibia of the middle legs (the latter found in all three genera). Eyes in life of iridescent colour, often of a golden hue. Mainly found in forest and woodlands, but often also common in marshy scrub and swampy woodlands.

Tabanus (horse flies, gad flies). Medium to large flies, 9–25 mm long, wings usually clear, held over back like a pair of half-open scissors (as in *Chrysops*). Antennae short (Fig. III.46b), first two segments small, the third segment long, with a pronounced dorsal 'hump' and an upturned tip. No ocelli. No spines on hind tibia. In life, eyes either of uniform colour or in a series of horizontal coloured bands. Mainly found in more open habitats, such as savannah and thicket vegetation.

Haematopota (clegs, stouts). Medium size, 6–10 mm long, wings folded over the back in a roof-like manner; in almost all species the wings have a complex mottled dark grey or brown pattern. Antennae (Fig. III.46b) with first and third segments markedly longer than the short second segment; third segment without dorsal 'hump' or upturned end. No ocelli. No spines on hind tibia. When alive, eyes have zigzag bands of iridescent colour. Mainly flies of woodlands and forest edges.

Biology and life-cycle

The family Tabanidae is believed to have evolved in close association with the ungulates, upon which they principally feed. Other mammals are also attacked, but seldom birds or reptiles. Most species are diurnal and hunt by sight; they are most active in bright sunlight; *Tabanus paradoxus* of central and southern Europe is unusual in that it is a nocturnal species.

Most tabanids inhabit woodland and forest; many

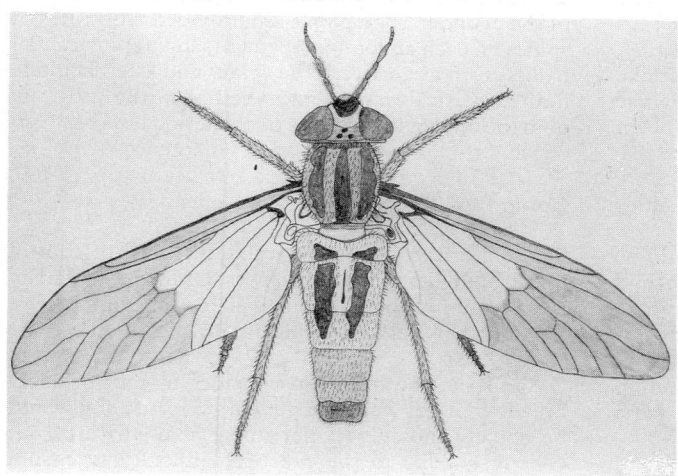

Fig. III.47 Female *Chrysops dimidiatus*. (Courtesy D. B. Thomas.)

species of *Chrysops* are found in waterlogged scrub and marshy woodlands: other species occupy more open areas of savannah woodland and grassland. Only females feed on blood; both sexes feed on sugary plant secretions. Because the female mouthparts are large and coarse, the bite is deep and painful; blood often continues to ooze from the wound for some time afterwards. Due to the painful bite, females are often forced, by defensive reactions of the human or animal host, to interrupt feeding and later resume on the same individual, or another, in order to feed to repletion. This behaviour considerably increases their efficiency as mechanical vectors of pathogens. Some individuals develop a severe allergic reaction to the large quantity of anticoagulant saliva pumped into the bite wound as the flies feed. With the exception of *Chrysops silaceus*, which will bite indoors, it is rare for tabanids to enter houses, although some species enter by accident and can be seen on windows, in an apparent attempt to escape.

The relatively short-lived adults are strictly seasonal in temperate climates, with biting confined to the warmest summer months. In tropical areas breeding is continuous, but biting activity of different species is very dependent on the rainy or dry season. The natural adult life-span of the important tropical species *Chrysops silaceus* is thought to be about three to four weeks.

In this respect rather like tsetse, tabanids are attracted to large, slow-moving dark objects (including vehicles: they may enter the windows to bite the occupants, or attack the warm tyres of stationary cars and trucks).

Gravid females are selective of particular plant species or other specific oviposition sites. Females lay lozenge-shaped egg masses, firmly cemented to the underside of grasses, other vegetation, rocks or stones, where these overhang suitable larval breeding places; either shallow water, mud or damp soil (even in tree-holes high above the ground). Egg batches consist of a few dozen, or more than a thousand slender, cigar-shaped eggs; each 1–2.5 mm long (Fig. III.48). The egg batches are coated with a waterproof layer; eggs are commonly off-white in colour, sometimes grey, brownish-black, or even orange. Eggs hatch after one to two weeks; the cream-coloured, grub-like larvae drop on to the water, mud or damp soil and soon begin to feed. Larvae of *Chrysops* feed on vegetable detritus, while those of most *Tabanus* and *Haematopota* are carnivorous; they feed on other invertebrates, including members of their own species.

Compared with the relatively short life of adults, the duration of larval life is long, for both tropical and temperate species. For most tropical species, four to five months is usual; one to two years is not uncommon, and some species in cooler climates may spend up to three years as larvae. When mature, after up to eight moults, larvae of different species measure from 10 to 60 mm in length.

Larval habitats differ between the genera and species, but are predominantly aquatic or semi-aquatic. *Chrysops* larvae generally live in the wettest places, such as the muddy margins of marshes (and salt-marshes), *Tabanus* spp. usually inhabit shallow seasonal pools, mud or wet soil near water, while *Haematopota* are most often found in drier habitats, such as damp soil.

Larvae are easy to recognize (Fig. III.48). They are cylindrical, with rather pointed extremities; at one end is the small head, which can be retracted into the thorax (the head has mouth-hooks like those of the Muscidae). At the other end of the body is the slightly upturned, conical, posterior respiratory siphon. There are tyre-like rings around the body, at the leading edge of each segment, most of which have a number of ventrolateral locomotory protuberances, known as 'pseudopods'.

Graber's organ is a structure unique to larval Tabanidae and of unknown function, possibly sensory or glandular. Visible in life through the integument on the dorsal side, near the base of the respiratory siphon, are a paired row of black, rounded structures (the number of which evidently is increased in older larvae). Together with an internal pyriform sac, which opens via a narrow tube to the exterior between the last two segments, these are the principal parts of Graber's organ that can be seen with a hand-lens or low-power microscope.

Population occurs in drier parts of the habitat: the brown-coloured pupae, 7–40 mm long (Fig. III.48), look rather similar to those of butterflies, but are partly buried, in an upright position, in soil or mud. Some *Tabanus* species whose larvae inhabit seasonal pools, protect the future pupa from exposure to predators or desiccation; the mature larva excavates a vertical spiral burrow to delimit a cylinder of mud, into the centre of which it then burrows before pupation takes place. When the mud of the pool finally dries out, the cylinder cracks free from the surrounding mud and the pupa is securely housed within. The adult eventually emerges, after the pupa has partly rasped away the top of the cylinder. The pupae are provided with rings of spines on each abdominal segment, and a spiny caudal pad (known as an aster); the spines and aster facilitate limited vertical movement, whether in the substrate or in the mud cylinder. The pupal period lasts between one and three weeks until adult emergence.

Control of Tabanidae

There are few or no practicable methods of control for tabanid flies in most instances. Drainage of marshy areas would probably limit available breeding places, although this seldom would be justifiable on a cost–benefit basis.

Similarly, the use of insecticides to control likely breeding places would be difficult to justify and would be equally difficult (if not impossible) to carry out effectively, due to the practical difficulty to ensure

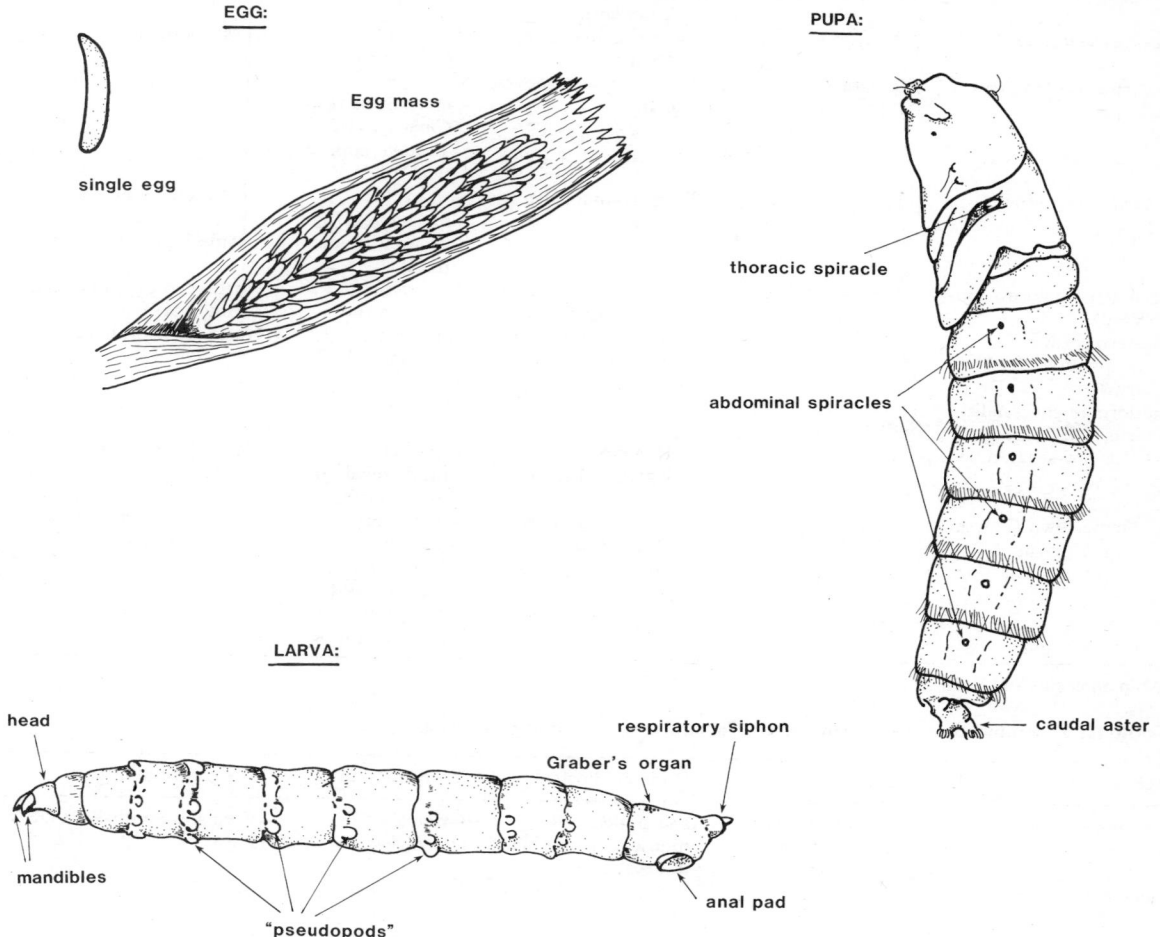

EGG:

single egg

Egg mass

PUPA:

thoracic spiracle

abdominal spiracles

caudal aster

LARVA:

head

mandibles

"pseudopods"

Graber's organ

respiratory siphon

anal pad

Fig. III.48   Egg, larva and pupa of Tabanidae.

adequate contact of insecticide with larval or pupal stages, often buried in wet soil or mud. Tabanid breeding places are in any event generally extensive and diffuse, difficult to delimit, and would be expensive to treat with insecticides. Insecticide-impregnated plastic collars and ear-tags have been developed to protect livestock from the attacks of ticks and various Diptera: they probably help also to reduce biting of tabanids.

Some success in reducing adult numbers of pest species of *Haematopota* has been achieved by the use of dark-coloured plates (about half a metre square) coated with a sticky adhesive, placed in open habitats where the flies are troublesome and the plates visible to the flies for some distance.

The wearing of open-mesh jackets impregnated with a synthetic pyrethroid insecticide (deltamethrin or permethrin), or a repellent such as deet (diethyl-

toluamide), would afford some personal protection from the attack of tabanids, in areas where they are sufficiently troublesome to warrant the inconvenience and expense of an additional garment.

Disease relationships of the Tabanidae (Tables III.8 and III.9)

Tabanidae can be a severe biting nuisance to people and livestock, to the extent that their attacks prevent all normal outdoor activities, affect the migration patterns of nomadic herdsmen and prevent the normal use of seasonal pastures by livestock (as in Sudan and parts of North America). In addition to the attacks of the adult flies, ricefield workers in Japan are sometimes attacked by the carnivorous aquatic larvae of *Tabanus* and *Chrysops*, which pierce feet or hands below the

Table III.8 Diseases transmitted to man by Tabanidae.

Agent	Disease	Principal hosts	Transmission	Distribution
Loa loa	Loiasis; Calabar swelling	Man, Drill (*Papio leucophaeus*)	Cyclical: *Chrysops* spp.	West and central Africa
Bacillus anthracis	Anthrax	Domestic livestock (man)[a]	Non-cyclic: mechanical	Cosmopolitan
Francisella tularensis	Tularaemia	Lagomorphs, rodents, man	Non-cyclic: mechanical (esp. *Chrysops* and *Tabanus* spp.: *also* ticks)	Cosmopolitan
Borrelia burgdorferi	Lyme disease	Deer, lagomorphs, (man)[a]	Non-cyclic: mechanical (main vectors: Ixodid ticks)	North temperate zone (Europe, North America) and Australia
Vesicular stomatitis virus (VSV)	Sore mouth (of cattle; horses)	Equines, bovines, pigs, (man)[a]	Non-cyclic: mechanical	North, central and South America
Western equine encephalitis (WEE) virus	—	Amphibia, reptiles, birds, (man)[a]	Non-cyclic: mechanical	North and South America
Californian encephalitis virus (CEV) group: La Crosse (LAC) virus	—	Rodents, lagomorphs, etc., (man)[a]	Non-cyclic: mechanical (*also* mosquitoes)	North America (USA)
Jamestown Canyon (JC) virus	—	White-tailed deer [*Odocoileus virginianus*], (man)[a]	Non-cyclic: mechanical (*Chrysops*, *Tabanus* and *Hybomitra* spp.; *also* mosquitoes)	North America (Alaska, Canada, USA)

[a] Man an accidental host.

Table III.9 Animal diseases transmitted by Tabanidae which rarely or never affect man.

Agent	Disease	Principal hosts	Transmission	Distribution
Elaeophora schneideri	Arterial worm disease (sheep)	sheep, deer, elk, moose (asymptomatic in deer)	Cyclical (*Tabanus* and *Hybomitra* spp.)	West and South-west USA; Italy
Dilofilaria roemeri	—	Wallaroo (*Macropus robustus*)	Cyclical (*Dasybasis hebes*)	Australia
Haemoproteus metchnikovi	—	Turtles	Cyclical (*Chrysops callidus*)	USA
Besnoitia besnoiti	Bovine besnoitiosis	Cattle (intermediate) Cat (definitive host)	Non-cyclic: mechanical (other mechanical vectors are *Glossina* and *Stomoxys*)	Africa, South America, Europe, USSR, Asia
Anaplasma marginale	Anaplasmosis	Bovines	Non-cyclic: mechanical (esp. *Tabanus* spp.)	Cosmopolitan
Trypanosoma (Trypanozoon) evansi	Surra (Old World) Derrengadera, Murina (New World)	Bovines, equines, camels, dogs	Non-cyclic: mechanical	Cosmopolitan; tropics and sub-tropics
Trypanosoma (Trypanozoon) equinum	Mal de Caderas	Equines, bovines	Non-cyclic: mechanical	South America
Trypanosoma (Duttonella) vivax	Souma	Bovines, sheep, goats, equines, dogs	Non-cyclic: mechanical	Mauritius, Antilles and South America
Trypanosoma (Megatrypanum) theileri	—	Bovines, antelopes	Cyclical (?)	Cosmopolitan
Equine infectious anaemia (EIA) virus	Swamp fever	Equines, pheasants	Non-cyclic: mechanical	Cosmopolitan
Hog cholera virus (HCV)	—	Pigs	Non-cyclic: mechanical	North America
Rinderpest virus	—	Ungulates	Non-cyclic (Tabanids are unproved, but potential mechanical vectors)	Cosmopolitan

water surface; a severe oedematous reaction may ensue from the painful bites of the larvae.

More exceptionally, there are instances where bites of tabanid flies have resulted in the mechanical transmission of anthrax bacilli (*Bacillus anthracis*) to man, but this evidently occurs only under very unusual circumstances, and must surely be a rare event. However, it is very probable that tabanids do play a significant role in the maintenance of anthrax epizootics.

Tularaemia. Of the two principal human diseases transmitted by tabanids, tularaemia is of lesser importance. Tularaemia is a zoonotic bacterial infection widespread in the northern hemisphere and caused by *Francisella tularensis*. In the Old World the disease occurs in most European countries, the USSR, Iran, Turkey, Tunisia, China and Japan. Ticks are thought to be the major vectors in most affected regions, but infection is contracted also in other ways; mechanically by the bite of various other arthropods, directly through the conjunctiva and via abrasions of the skin, and by the consumption of infected meat or contaminated water.

Tularaemia occurs also in Canada, the USA and Mexico, where it mainly is transmitted between rabbits, rodents, sheep, horses and man, by any of the routes above, including mechanical transmission by biting arthropods, notably ticks. However, in some areas, particularly the western USA, the disease occurs in summer outbreaks (with about 200 cases annually) in circumstances where rabbits are the most important reservoir of infection, and *Chrysops discalis* is certainly implicated as a mechanical vector of infection to man; the human disease is known locally as 'deer-fly fever'. *F. tularensis* bacteria have also been recovered from *C. fulvaster* and *C. aestuans*, but these species appear to play no part in the dissemination of tularaemia to man. (See also Chapter 7.)

Lyme disease and related disorders. For the role of Tabanidae as mechanical vectors of the spirochaete *Borrelia burgdorferi*, normally transmitted by hard ticks (mainly *Ixodes* spp.), see the section on Tabanidae as vectors of other pathogens, below.

Loiasis. The principal human disease transmitted by tabanids is loiasis, or Calabar swelling, caused by the filarial nematode *Loa loa*, and transmitted by species of *Chrysops,* notably by *C. silaceus* and *C. dimidiatus* (Bombe form), in which the worms undergo cyclical development. The disease is common and widespread in the rain-forest zones of West Africa, particularly Cameroon, and occurs sporadically across central Africa to the southern Sudan, Ethiopia and western Uganda. There are features of the epidemiology of loiasis which resemble the sylvatic cycles of yellow fever transmission.

Adult *Loa loa* worms inhabit subcutaneous con-

nective tissues; diurnal periodic sheathed microfilariae are shed into the peripheral blood, particularly during the morning hours, and are ingested by day-biting *Chrysops.* When infected people are bitten by *Chrysops,* particularly by *C. silaceus* and *C. dimidiatus* (which may enter houses to feed), a proportion of the exsheathed microfilariae survive digestion in the insect gut, penetrate into the haemocoel, invade the abdominal and thoracic fat-bodies, where they grow, moult twice and develop into infective third stage forms; these migrate forward into the head. Here the infective stages accumulate until the fly next feeds, when they break out of the labium into the mouthparts and infect a new host via the skin. Development of *L. loa* in *Chrysops* generally takes 10–12 days from the original infecting feed.

There are two parallel and sympatric, but ecologically separate, cycles of *Loa loa* transmission in the west African rain-forests (Fig. III.49). One cycle is that of the slightly smaller human parasite, often given subspecific status as *L. loa loa*. This has a strictly diurnal microfilarial periodicity and day-biting *Chrysops* vectors (*C. silaceus* and *C. dimidiatus*, Bombe form). The other cycle involves the slightly larger simian parasite, *L. loa papionis,* which infects only monkeys. *L. l. papionis* is a nocturnally periodic filarial parasite of drills (forest baboons), *Papio* (= *Mandrillus*) *leucophaeus* (infection rates of 96% and mean adult worm burdens of 17 are recorded in drills). *L. l. papionis* will also naturally infect at least two cercopithecine monkeys found in the same rain-forests, the putty-nosed guenon and the mona monkey, but the simian worm seems less well adapted to these two hosts. (Infection rates and mean adult worm burdens of 24%/6.3 and 12%/2.4, respectively.)

The vectors of the simian parasite (*L. l. papionis*) are two tree-top *Chrysops* species, both of which are active early in the night and feed on sleeping drills and other monkeys; these are *C. langi* and *C. centurionis.* The vectors of the human *Loa* (*C. silaceus* and *C. dimidiatus*) will bite both at canopy level and on the forest floor, but only in daylight hours, when they are seldom able to evade the vigorous response of the monkeys (Fig. III.49).

The obviously closely related parasites of man and monkeys are behaviourally and ecologically distinct; additionally, they are reproductively isolated, although experimental hybrids can be produced. There is evidence which indicates that the simian *Loa* is not transmissible to man, although drills are susceptible to experimental infection with the human *Loa,* and occasional natural infections of drills with the human *Loa* are known.

The day-biting vectors of the human *Loa* are active in the forest canopy, but especially they are attracted to descend to ground level both by some unknown component of wood-smoke (e.g. from cooking-fires) and by human movements. Thus human activities in general, and the scent of wood-fires in particular,

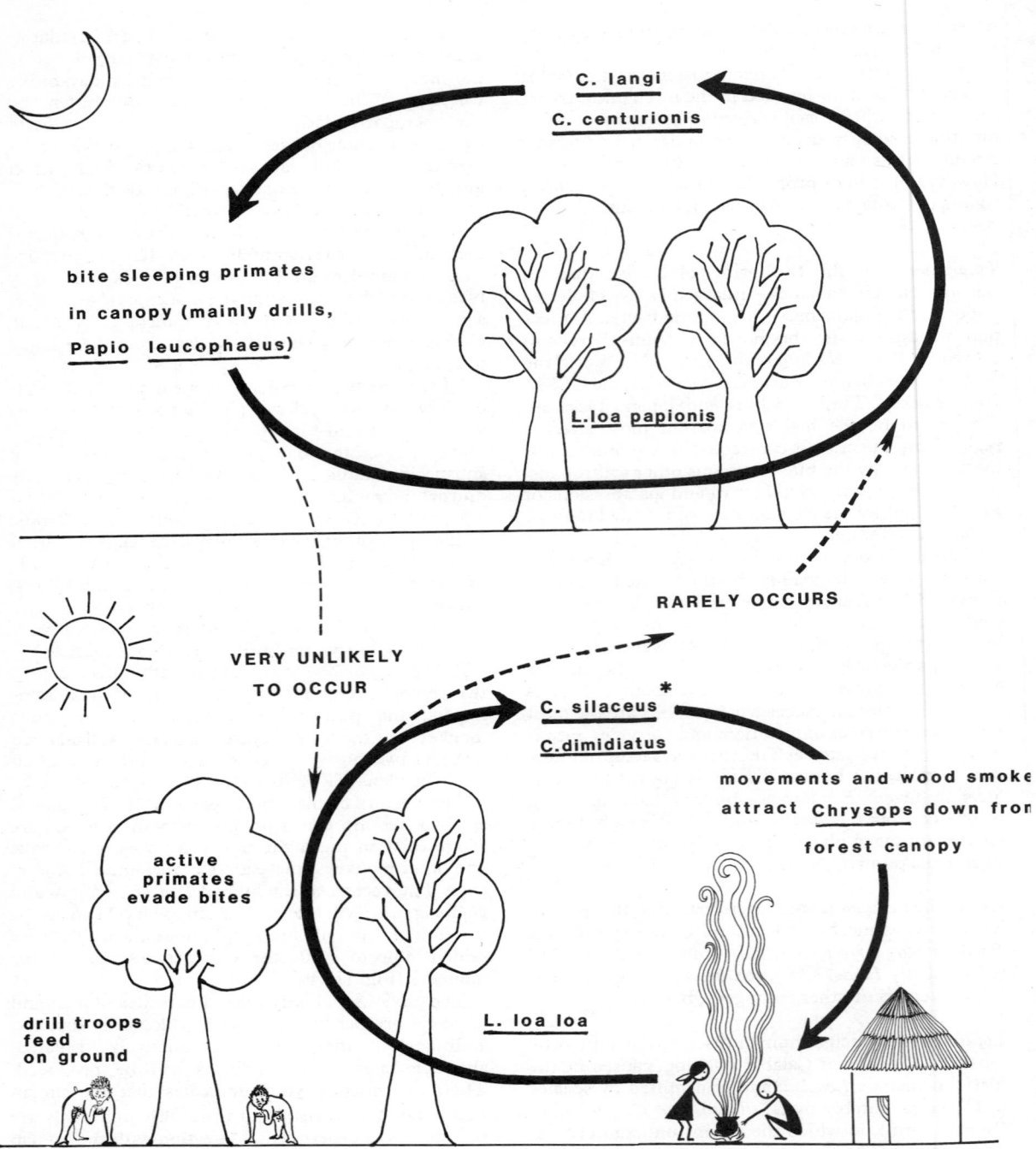

Fig. III.49   Diagram of transmission cycles of *Loa loa* to drills and to man in West African rain-forest.

combine to draw these canopy-dwellers to ground level and especially into houses in the forest, in order for the females to obtain a blood meal (Fig. III.49). These species will also emerge from the natural forest and enter teak or rubber plantations nearby, where these also have a high canopy.

There is at present no practicable method to reduce transmission of loiasis by means of vector control.

Other vectors of human loiasis

In the grassland and forest mosaic of the highland zone in the west of Cameroon, *C. zahrai* is implicated as a natural vector of local importance.

Chrysops distinctipennis and *C. longicornis* are believed to be vectors of human loiasis in southern Sudan, beyond the eastern limits of *C. silaceus* and C. *dimidiatus*. The widespread species *C. distinctipennis* may possibly be an occasional vector elsewhere in central Africa, since the range of all three main vectors shows considerable overlap. *C. streptobalius* is the probable vector of the few infections reported from Ethiopia. (See also Chapter 20).

Other filarial parasites transmitted by Tabanidae (Table III.8)

It is notable that human filarial parasites undergo early development in the fat-body of the abdomen and thorax of Tabanidae, and not in the musculature, as seen with human filarial nematodes whose vectors are Nematocera (whether these are mosquitoes, simuliids or biting midges). This pattern of larval development in the fat-body of the insect vector, with later forward migration of third stage larvae to the head, is seen also in two other tabanid-transmitted filarial nematodes, mentioned briefly below; neither are of medical or economic importance.

The first is *Dirofilaria roemeri* of Australian marsupials, particularly the wallaroo (*Macropus robustus*), the main vector of which is *Dasybasis hebes*, although other species of *Dasybasis* and of *Tabanus* assist in the maintenance of infection in nature. The remaining tabanid-transmitted filaria is the arterial worm, *Elaeophora schneideri*, whose normal definitive host is probably the mule deer, *Odocoileus hemionus*, of western North America. Other North American Cervidae, such as the moose (*Alces alces*), the black-tailed deer and the wapiti (*Cervus elephas*, syn. *C. canadensis*) are infected by this parasite; it is also the cause of a filarial dermatosis of sheep in the south-western USA. The vectors of *E. schneideri* are species of the tabanid genera *Hybomitra* and *Tabanus*.

Tabanidae as vectors of other pathogens (Tables III.8 and III.9)

Animal trypanosomiasis

1 Tabanidae have long been regarded as cyclic vectors of the cosmopolitan cattle trypanosome, *Trypanosoma (Megatrypanum) theileri*, although the evidence for this is largely circumstantial. *T. theileri* is a harmless parasite of cattle (and water buffalo), present in all continents except Antarctica, and the role of tabanids in natural transmission of the infection remains to be critically assessed. *Haematopota pluvialis* and *Tabanus glaucopis* are regarded as putative European vectors and *Tabanus striatus* as an important vector in Java.

2 *Trypanosoma (Trypanozoon) evansi* is closely related to the tsetse-transmitted *T. (T.) brucei*, from which it is indeed distinguished only by the fact that *T. evansi* is no longer transmitted cyclically by *Glossina*. *T. evansi* is the cause of surra, a frequently fatal disease of horses, camels and dogs. The parasite is normally not pathogenic to cattle and buffaloes, which serve as a reservoir of infection. Surra is widespread in Africa, mostly to the north of the tsetse belt, in much of southern Asia, including Indonesia and the Philippines, and both Central and South America. There is general agreement that there is no cyclical development of *T. evansi* in Tabanidae, but that this group of flies, particularly members of the genus *Tabanus*, are important mechanical vectors of the trypanosome. Site of feeding on, and disturbance of the host, may be important factors which influence the capacity of particular species to act as efficient mechanical vectors.

Almost all incriminated vectors are species of *Tabanus*; some species of *Chrysops* and *Haematopota* are also suspected, but members of these two genera appear to be rather poor mechanical vectors of *T. evansi*.

3 Tabanidae are important among the suspected mechanical vectors of the economically important animal trypanosome *T. (Duttonella) vivax* in tropical areas outside Africa, where this trypanosome has become established by human agency far beyond the tsetse belts (South America, the Antilles and Mauritius), as a parasite of cattle and water buffaloes. There is circumstantial evidence also that tabanids may play some minor, supplementary, role in the mechanical transmission of other, tsetse-transmitted, trypanosomiases in Africa, but specific incrimination is in all cases lacking.

Other pathogens

1 *Viruses.* Tabanids have been suspected, usually on tenuous and circumstantial evidence, as mechanical vectors of a variety of animal pathogens. These include in North America the viruses of equine infectious anaemia (EIA), vesicular stomatitis (VSV), hog cholera (HCV), equine encephalitis (EEV) and California encephalitis (CEV: Jamestown Canyon and La Crosse serotypes); rinderpest and tick-borne encephalitis (TBE) elsewhere. The role of tabanids in virus transmission remains uncertain in all cases, but these insects may amplify viral epizootics, in circumstances where infected and uninfected animals are in close proximity.

2   Bacteria. (Excepting spirochaetes; see following section **3.**) The implication of Tabanidae in the mechanical transmission of the tick-borne bacterial cattle pathogen, *Anaplasma marginale*, rests on rather more convincing evidence, particularly with regard to species of *Tabanus*, but the role of tabanids in the natural transmission of the parasite remains a matter of speculation. Other bacterial infections have been linked to tabanids as putative or possible vectors (in addition to *Anaplasma marginale*, *Bacillus anthracis* and *Francisella tularensis* referred to above); these are *Pasteurella multocida*, *Clostridium chauvoei*, *Brucella* species, *Listeria monocytogenes*, *Erysipelothrix rhusiopathiae* (the causative organism of swine erysipelas and human erysipeloid) and *Leptospira* species.

The relative importance of tabanids as vectors of these pathogens remains in most instances uncertain, although experimental transmission by tabanids has been demonstrated in the majority of cases.

3   Spirochaetes (*Borrelia burgdorferi*). Tabanid flies, members of the genera *Chrysops*, *Tabanus* and *Hybomitra*, were recently shown to be secondary (and probably purely mechanical) vectors of the newly recognized zoonotic spirochaetal pathogen of man and animals, described in 1984 as *Borrelia burgdorferi*, the causal organism of Lyme disease and related disorders in man.

Lyme disease is widely distributed in the USA, with closely related stocks of *B. burgdorferi* in Europe and parts of Australia. The disease was first recognized in the north-eastern USA in 1975, presenting as inflammatory arthritis (Lyme arthritis); Lyme disease was subsequently shown to be transmitted by hard ticks of the genera *Ixodes*, *Amblyomma* and *Dermacentor*. (*Ixodes dammini* and *I. pacificus* are particularly important in the USA: *I. ricinus* in Europe.) Lyme disease was later shown to be very similar, and of identical spirochaetal aetiology, to the dermatoses known previously in Europe as erythema chronica migrans (ECM: first described in 1910, the lesions then associated with the bites of ticks and insects) and erythema chronica atrophicans (ECA: also a tick- or insect-borne dermatosis). No aetiological agent has been found as yet for lymphadenosis cutis benigna (LCB), the third form of dermatosis associated with the bites of arthropods in Europe.

For recent brief reviews of clinical and other features of Lyme disease and related conditions, with their distribution and vectors, the reader is referred to Stanek,[95] Schmid,[96] and Magnarelli et al.[97]

In the period 1980–1986 there were more than 2700 cases of Lyme disease in the USA: some occurred outside the known areas of *I. dammini* and *I. pacificus*. In northern Europe, several cases are reported from southern England (the New Forest area and Suffolk); however, in Sweden 256 seropositive cases were recorded in 1985 alone, over half of which had neurological symptoms. Elsewhere in Europe the disease has been the subject of studies principally in Austria, Germany and Switzerland.

In the north-eastern USA, additional to ixodid ticks, known mechanical vectors of Lyme disease to man, domestic (horses, cattle) and wild animals currently include (as at the end of 1986: on the basis of dark-field microscopy of foregut tissues (oesophagus, pharynx, proventriculus and anterior parts of the salivary glands), direct immunofluorescence and indirect immunofluorescence tests with human serum or murine monoclonal antibody, H5322), the following species:

2 spp. of *Chrysops* (*C. callidus* and *C. vittatus*).
2 spp. of the genus *Tabanus* (*T. lineola* and *T. pumilis*).
4 spp. of the tabanid genus *Hybomitra* (These include *H. epistates*, *H. lasiopthalma* and *H. sodalis*).
3 spp. of *Aedes* mosquitoes (*Ae. canadensis*, *Ae. stimulans*, *Ae. vexans*).

(*C. callidus* and *H. lasiopthalma* are considered to be of particular importance as mechanical vectors in north-eastern USA.)

Wild hosts of *B. burgdorferi* in the USA are mainly woodland mammals and include the following:
white-tailed deer (*Odocoileus virginianus*)
white-footed mice (*Peromyscus leucopus*)
meadow voles (*Microtus pennsylvanicus*)
raccoons (*Procyon lotor*)
chipmunks (*Tamias striatus*)

Preliminary studies in Europe indicate that possibly mosquitoes and very probably the widespread tabanid *Chrysops caecutiens*, are mechanical vectors of *B. burgdorferi*. (*C. caecutiens* is recorded from all European countries, with the exception of Norway and Ireland.)

Mammals affected in Europe are little studied, but wild hares (20%: in Austria) have raised antibody titres. However, Austrian studies of tick-transmitted *B. burgdorferi* in laboratory rodents suggest that ixodid ticks themselves constitute the principal wild reservoir of infection, since patent parasitaemia in rodents does not persist for more than three weeks. Vertical transstadial transmission of the spirochaetes occurs in ticks; these can then be transmitted to man or animals at any stage in the tick life-cycle.

4   Protozoa. The role of Tabanidae in the mechanical

transmission of the protozoan *Besnoitia besnoiti*, the organism responsible for bovine besnoitiosis, is reasonably well established; but *Glossina* and *Stomoxys* also transmit the infection mechanically. A variety of different biting insects are likely to be involved as mechanical vectors, in the different geographical areas where bovine besnoitiosis occurs.

Without real evidence, tabanids have been speculatively postulated as ancillary vectors of the northern Eurasian reindeer piroplasm, *Theileria tarandi rangiferis*, although on circumstantial grounds ticks appear to be the most likely vectors.

Haemoproteus metchnikovi is a protozoan parasite of North American turtles (*Chrysemys picta*); this parasite is cyclically transmitted by *Chrysops callidus*, with the production of sporozoites in the salivary glands of the vector. The epizootiology and natural transmission of this unusual protozoan, however, remain to be elucidated.

TSETSE FLIES (*Glossina*)

D. M. Minter

FAMILY: GLOSSINIDAE

GENUS: *Glossina* Wiedemann 1830

The unique viviparous genus *Glossina* contains some 30 species and subspecies nowadays confined to tropical Africa between latitudes 15° north and 30° south. Until the early years of the twentieth century an isolated population (of *G. tachinoides*) still existed in the south-western part of the Arabian peninsula, but seems likely to have died out since then. Fossil tsetse flies occur in Oligocene deposits in North America (Colorado), suggesting that the distribution of the genus was once considerably wider.

Nonetheless, tsetse flies still occupy a very large area in Africa; about $10.4 \times 10^6 \, \text{km}^2$ are infested, roughly half of the surface of the continent.

The tsetse flies are large, brown to greyish, narrow-bodied flies, 6–15 mm long, with a stout proboscis projecting forward well in front of the head (Fig. III.50). The proboscis is adjoined laterally, except during the act of biting, by the paired labial palps. The mouthparts consist of a horny labrum, a slender hypopharynx (through which an anticoagulant saliva is injected into the bite wound) and a stout ventral labium (Fig. III.50). These three parts enclose a space, the food canal, through which blood is sucked by muscular action into the alimentary canal of the fly.

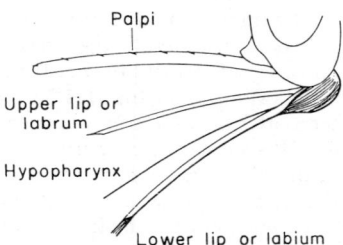

Fig. III.50 Mouthparts of *Glossina*.

During feeding the mouthparts, but not the palps, are lowered some 90° from the line of the body axis. Male and female tsetse feed exclusively on the blood of vertebrates.

Characteristic features which distinguish *Glossina* species (Fig. III.51) from other large biting flies, such as *Stomoxys*, *Haematobia*, *Lyperosia*, *Haematopota*, *Tabanus* and *Chrysops*, include the long straight proboscis with a basal bulb, the presence of branched hairs on the arista (Fig. III.52) (the prominent bristle on the largest, distal, segment of the antenna) and the length of the labial palps (as long as the proboscis in *Glossina*). The manner in which the wings are folded, scissors-like, over the back of the resting fly is also a very characteristic feature. The presence of the 'hatchet' or 'cleaver' cell, enclosed between the fourth and fifth longitudinal wing veins, is diagnostic of *Glossina* (Fig. III.53). This cell is clearly seen in the central area of the wings and contrasts with the triangular shape of the corresponding cell of related flies (e.g. *Stomoxys* (Fig. III.54)).

The genus *Glossina* is usually divided by modern taxonomists into three species–groups (Table III.10) (sometimes given subgeneric status) as follows:

1 The *fusca* group (subgenus *Austenina*).
2 The *palpalis* group (subgenus *Nemorhina*).
3 The *morsitans* group (subgenus *Glossina*).

This taxonomic separation is, in a general way, reflected in the ecological requirements and distribution of the species included in each group: characteristically, flies of the *fusca* group are associated with dense humid tropical forest or forest edges; members of the *palpalis* group are basically dependent on more or less dense riverine or lacustrine vegetation but their distribution extends into savannah zones well away from forested, or formerly forested, areas. Species of the *morsitans* group are the least hygrophilic and occupy vast areas of bushland and thicket vegetation often far from lakes and rivers. Strangely, however, one of the least hygrophilic species, occupying arid

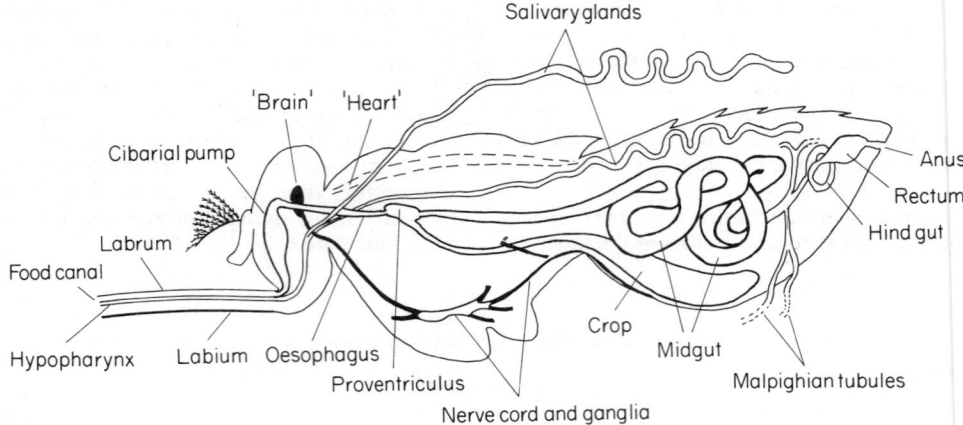

Fig. III.51   Schematic longitudinal section of *Glossina,* showing main features of the internal anatomy.

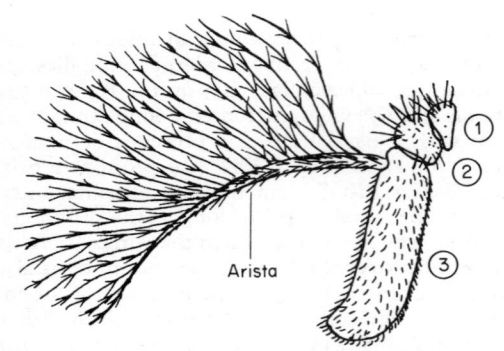

Fig. III.52   Antenna of Glossina showing the dorsal arista with branched hairs, which arises from the third antennal segment. In other flies the hairs of the arista are unbranched.

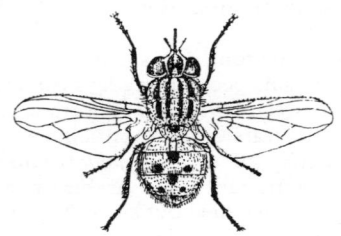

Fig. III.54   *Stomoxys calcitrans.* × 3.

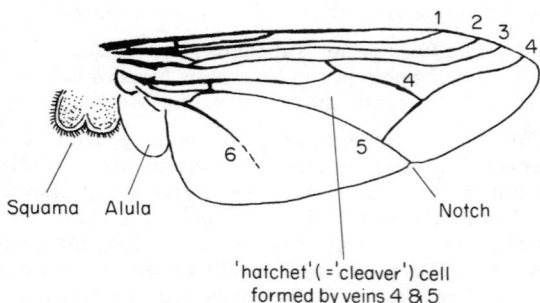

Fig. III.53   Wing of *Glossina* showing venation and the 'hatchet' (= 'cleaver') cell enclosed between veins 4 and 5. The shape of the 'hatchet' cell is unique to *Glossina*; in all other flies the corresponding cell is triangular. *Glossina* is also unusual among higher flies in that the wings are held scissor-like over the back at rest.

and semidesert areas, is *G. longipennis*, a member of the *fusca* group. *G. brevipalpis*, also a *fusca* group species, has a distribution which also extends into dry savannah zones. Though flies of the *fusca* group include important vectors of trypanosomes pathogenic to livestock, especially species of the *Trypanosoma vivax* group (subgenus *Duttonella*) and *T. congolense* group (subgenus *Nannomonas*), they have never been associated with the transmission of trypanosomiasis to man and will not be considered further in this section. Fig. III.55 indicates the distribution of the groups of main medical importance and Fig. III.56 shows the general characteristics of some *Glossina* species. Mulligan[98] and Ford[99] summarize modern views on the taxonomy and distribution of species and subspecies included in the *fusca, palpalis* and *morsitans* groups. Potts[100] gives a detailed key for the identification of all members of the genus and Pollock[101] gives simple regional keys.

Table III.10　Biotype, distribution and medical importance of *Glossina*.

Species group/subgenus	Habitat type	Distribution	Species of medical importance
fusca group (*Austenina*)	Mainly rain forest areas	Chiefly forest areas of West and central Africa, Relict species in dry areas ot East Africa	None. But several vectors of livestock trypanosomiasis
palpalis group (*Nemorhina*)	Mainly linear: shores of lakes and rivers in forested or formerly forested areas	15°N to 12°S, approx. 17°W to 15°E, approx.	*G. palpalis*, vector of *T. brucei gambiense* in West Africa
		10°N to 12°S, approx. 10°E to 40°E, approx.	*G. fuscipes* (and subspecies), vectors of *T. brucei gambiense* (West Africa, central Africa) and *T. brucei rhodesiense* (East Africa)
		12°N to 4°N, approx. 12°W to 40°E, approx.	*G. tachinoides*, vector of *T. b. gambiense* in West Africa and of *T. b. rhodesiense* in South-west Ethiopia
morsitans group (*Glossina*)	'Game' tsetse of the savannah zones; open woodland ('miombo'), bushland and thicket	15°N to 20°S, approx 17°W to 45°E, approx.	*G. morsitans* (and subspecies), vectors of *T. b. rhodesiense* in East and South-east Africa
		8°N to 20°S, approx. 25°E to 48°E approx.	*G. pallidipes*, vector of *T. b. rhodesiense* in East Africa
		Limited area south-east of Lake Victoria; mainly in Tanzania	*G. swynnertoni*, vector of *T. b. rhodesiense*

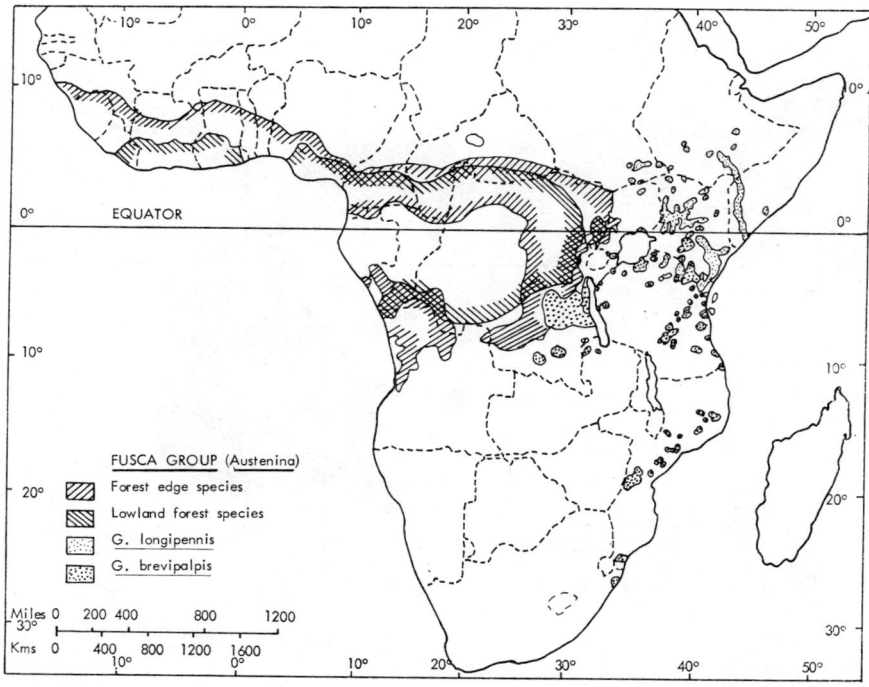

Fig. III.55A　Distribution of the important species of *Glossina*. A, *fusca* group; B, *palpalis* group (p. 1450); C, *morsitans* group (p. 1450).

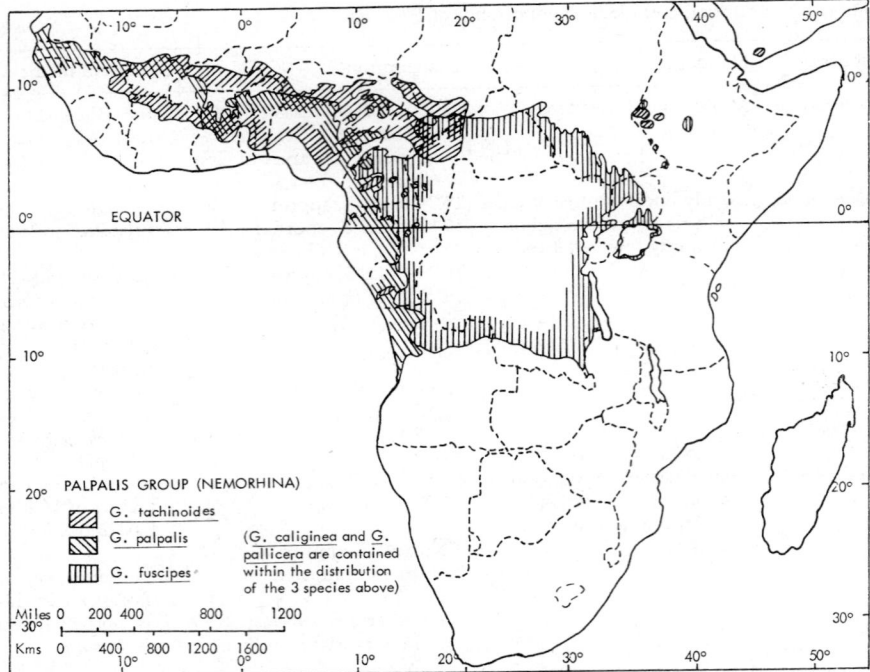

Fig. III.55B

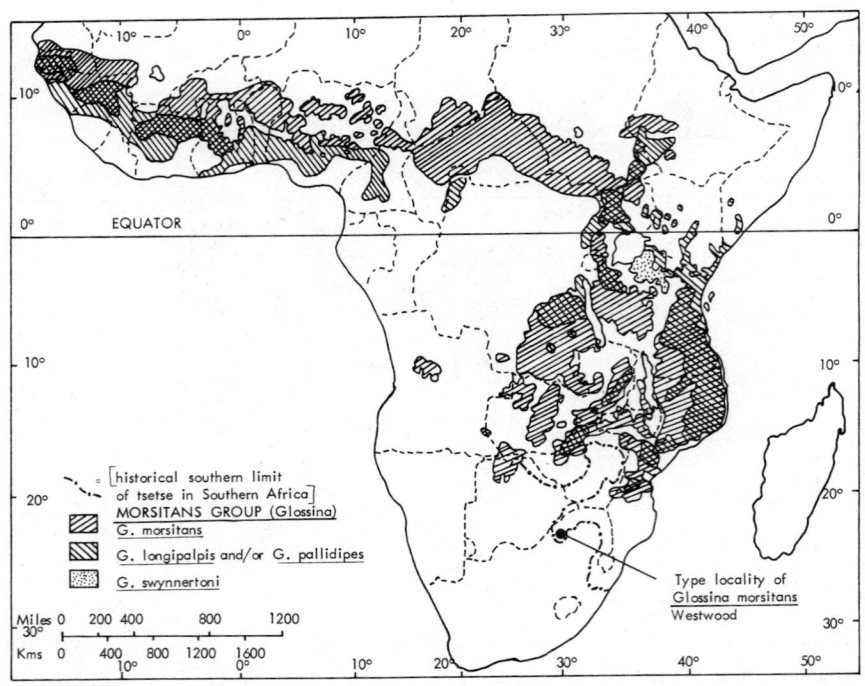

Fig. III.55C

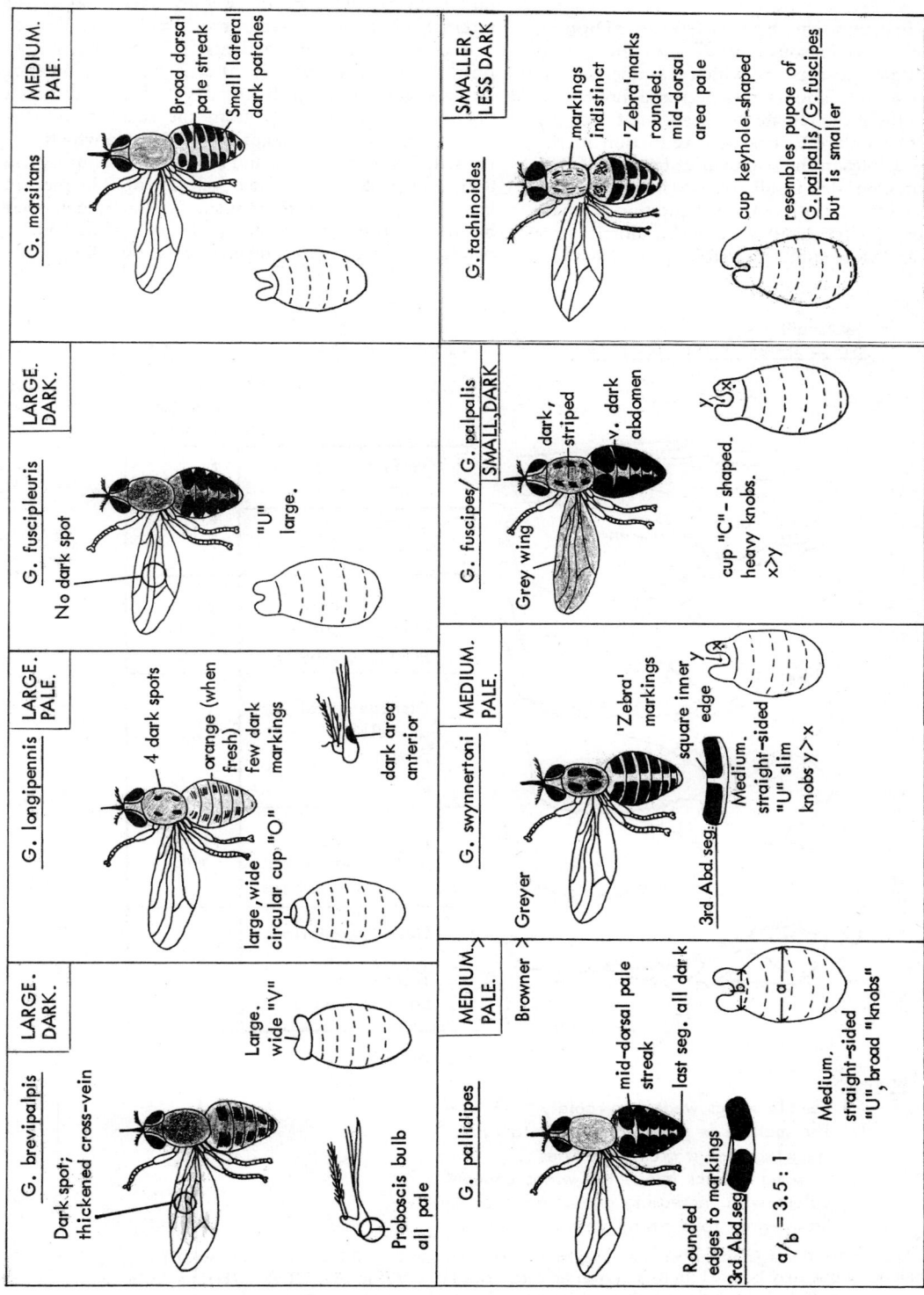

Fig. III.56 Outline guide to the identification of adults and pupae of some *Glossina* species, based on general characteristics visible to the naked eye or with the use of a simple hand-lens. The species illustrated are arranged in order of decreasing size, from top left to bottom right.

Life-history

Tsetse flies, in common with a very few other Diptera, have a method of viviparous reproduction uncommon among the higher insects, by which a single larva is produced at a time and is retained and nourished within the body of the female fly. Associated with the production of single offspring is a reduction in the number of ovarioles in the two ovaries to a single pair in each: four ovarioles in all, from which fertilized eggs pass into the uterus in a regular rotation. Female flies are normally fertilized only once, shortly after emergence, and store sufficient viable sperm from this single mating to last throughout life, during which, under favourable conditions, they may produce, at intervals of about 11 days, some 20 individual larvae.

Each successive fertilized egg (1.5 mm long) passes from the oviduct into the uterus where it hatches into a small, white, grub-like larva. The young larva obtains nutriment solely from the secretion of the uterine (or 'milk') glands of the mother, in which it is bathed. The larva grows, and twice moults, during the 8 to 12 days of intrauterine development. The mature larva, by now in the third instar, is finally extruded by the mother (by breech delivery) while she is perched on the ground, or on vegetation a few centi-

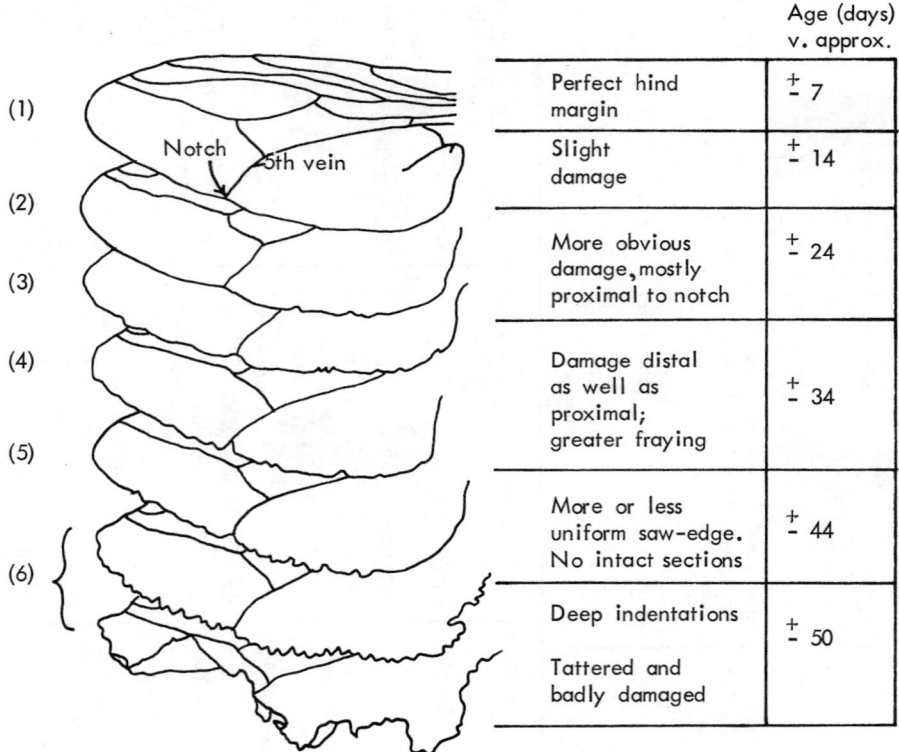

Glossina;
MALE WING FRAY DEGREES

		Age (days) v. approx.
(1)	Perfect hind margin	± 7
(2)	Slight damage	± 14
(3)	More obvious damage, mostly proximal to notch	± 24
(4)	Damage distal as well as proximal; greater fraying	± 34
(5)	More or less uniform saw-edge. No intact sections	± 44
(6)	Deep indentations Tattered and badly damaged	± 50

Notes:
(1) Female wings wear less rapidly
(2) The method is properly applied to find <u>mean</u> age for a <u>group</u> of males
(3) In some species (most) the wings change colour with increasing age, from a smoky brown-grey to a tawny yellow-brown.

Fig. III.57 Age estimation of *Glossina* using a wing fray chart for male flies. Wings of females wear less rapidly, but the degree of female wing fray may be used (in flies of ovarian categories IV to VII in Fig. III.58) to estimate whether flies are in an early or late stage. Based on Jackson[102] for *G. morsitans*.

metres above it, in a site selected for its shady situation and suitable soil texture. The newly deposited larva, creamy white in colour, with shiny black posterior polyneustic lobes through which it breathes, actively burrows below the surface soil to a depth of a few millimetres, using vigorous peristaltic movements. Having reached a point below the surface where conditions are suitable, it becomes immobile and begins to pupariate, still within the third larval skin, darkens and hardens. During emergence from the puparium, and in reaching the soil surface, the young fly is aided by an eversible bladder extruded from the front of the head and known as the *ptilinum*. During the first few days of life, this bladder can still be everted, while the body is still soft and 'soapy' in texture, if the young fly is carefully pressed between the fingers. Flies in this stage, so far unfed, are referred to as *teneral* flies: older flies as *non-teneral*, in which the head and body are hardened and horny and the ptilinum can no longer be everted. After the quiescent period, the young teneral flies seek their first blood meal. Flies of each sex normally feed at intervals of 3–4 days, sometimes less, and die of starvation if deprived of a blood meal for 10–12 days. The average life-span of female *Glossina* is two to three months: exceptionally, up to six or seven months. Male flies have a much shorter life-span.

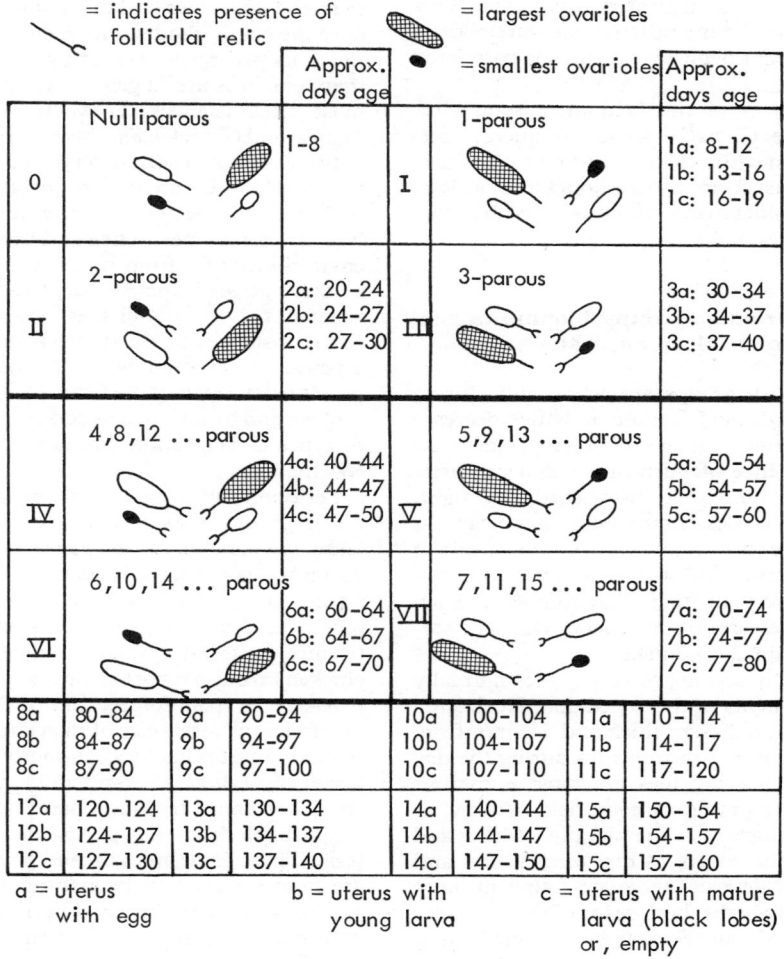

Glossina
OVARIAN AGE-GRADING

			a = uterus with egg		b = uterus with young larva		c = uterus with mature larva (black lobes) or, empty
8a	80-84	9a	90-94	10a	100-104	11a	110-114
8b	84-87	9b	94-97	10b	104-107	11b	114-117
8c	87-90	9c	97-100	10c	107-110	11c	117-120
12a	120-124	13a	130-134	14a	140-144	15a	150-154
12b	124-127	13b	134-137	14b	144-147	15b	154-157
12c	127-130	13c	137-140	14c	147-150	15c	157-160

Fig. III.58   Ovarian age grading chart for female *Glossina* as seen in dorsal view. From cycles 0 to III an accurate estimation is possible; from cycles IV to VII (between the heavy lines in the figures) the estimate is subject to error since the same configuration is found in flies of different ages (e.g. 4, 8, 12 parous; 5, 9, 13 parous). The degree of wing fray (see Fig. III.57) is often a useful guide as to which possible physiological age is the most probable. Modified from Saunders[103] and Challier.[104]

Male flies exhibit a progressive fraying of the trailing edge of the wings; this can be used to estimate the average age of *groups* of males from the same population. The wings of females also fray with age, usually less rapidly than those of males. With females, however, careful examination of the four ovarioles enables an estimation of the age of *individual* females to be made on a physiological basis. This method of 'ovarian ageing' is accurate to within a few days up to an age of about 40 days; with older flies there is a greater margin of possible error. For a fuller discussion of ageing methods, the reader is referred to Mulligan.[98] Fig. II.57 may be used to assess the degree of wing fray[102] and Fig. III.58 to estimate the age of individual females by examination of the ovarioles.[103,104] A new method to estimate age of *Glossina* (of both sexes) is suitable for laboratory automation, but requires sophisticated equipment. This method is based on the quantitative measurement of pteridine eye pigment deposition, which is correlated with age.

Female *G. fuscipes* in the field mate soon after emergence: female *G. pallidipes* are frequently fertilized near the host while seeking the first blood meal. Copulation may last from 2 to 24 hours and, at least in the laboratory, older males (about 14 days) are more potent than younger males.

Palpalis and *morsitans* groups: bionomics and ecology in relation to sleeping sickness

Species of these two groups are active only during daylight hours: flight and feeding activities decrease markedly even during dull and overcast weather; few species show evidence of purposive behaviour after dusk. Tsetse flies hunt their prey partly by sight, although scent becomes increasingly important at close range; the flies are often aware of movements at a considerable distance and will fly to investigate any large moving object in their environment. Such objects can include cars, trains, canoes and lake steamers as well as animals and man.

When not actively seeking food, the flies normally rest on woody elements of the vegetation. Horizontal or inclined branches, 2–5 cm thick and 1–3 mm from the ground, are favoured resting sites during the day for most species. Resting flies are most numerous where such perches provide a good field of view, as along the edge of thickets or the margins of lakes and streams. Flies in the course of digesting a meal and females seeking to deposit larvae are found in more sheltered places. By night, both sexes of those species so far investigated change from their daytime resting sites on the larger woody elements, to spend the hours of darkness on leaves and small twigs; the changeover takes place very rapidly, during the last few moments of twilight, and a reverse movement occurs at first light in the morning. The change of resting sites has,

perhaps, the function of protecting the flies from the activities of nocturnal predators. Challier[105] gives a valuable review of the ecology of tsetse; salient aspects are also dealt with by Molyneux and Ashford.[106]

Sleeping sickness vectors

G. palpalis, *G. fuscipes* and *G. tachinoides*. Until the closing years of the 1950s it was generally considered, firstly, that flies of the *palpalis* group were limited to, and dependent upon, the woody vegetation along streams and lake shores, and that the flies could not maintain themselves elsewhere except during limited sorties at favourable times of the year. Secondly, flies of the *palpalis* group were considered to be solely responsible for the transmission of gambian sleeping sickness; while flies of the *morsitans* group transmitted only the acute, rhodesian, type of disease. These distinctions are no longer completely tenable, though they remain as useful generalizations that apply under most circumstances. However, not only have *G. fuscipes* and *G. tachinoides* been implicated in epidemic outbreaks of the rhodesian type of disease (*G. fuscipes* in Kenya and Uganda; *G. tachinoides* in Ethiopia) but the same two species have been found (in Kenya and Nigeria) sometimes to live and breed in peridomestic environments far from water. It is now realized that neither species is quite so dependent upon particular vegetational associations as was formerly thought. Many instances of tsetse behaviour once labelled as atypical are now known to be quite commonplace: present-day views of the factors which influence tsetse ecology and behaviour, especially in relation to different types of vegetation, are now less rigid than once was the case.

Peridomestic pigs, sheep and dogs in West and central Africa harbour *T. brucei* trypanosomes apparently identical to *T. b. gambiense* (on biochemical grounds, particularly isoenzymes) and appear to be significant reservoirs of the disease. Domestic pigs, moreover, are attractive to tsetse and can act as maintenance hosts for *palpalis* group flies. West African chickens are also reported naturally infected with *Trypanozoon* trypanosomes, but their importance (or otherwise) as reservoirs of man-infective organisms is unclear. In Burkina Faso (formerly Upper Volta) both hartebeest (*Alcelaphus* sp.) and kob, *Kobus* (*Adenota*) sp., harbour trypanosomes which are indistinguishable from *T. b. gambiense* by biochemical criteria. These game animals, and possibly other species, are now believed to be natural reservoirs of *T. b. gambiense* in West Africa. These recent observations, with both domestic livestock and game animals, call for a reassessment of the long-held view that there are no animal reservoirs of gambian sleeping sickness; the evidence to the contrary is now incontrovertible and has obvious epidemiological implications.

In natural circumstances, where there is no close

contact with man and domestic animals, flies of the *palpalis* groups show a preference for feeding on large reptiles, such as monitor lizards and crocodiles. Reptiles form more than half of the feeds of wild flies in these conditions; bushbuck (*Tragelaphus scriptus*) account for about a quarter and other animals the remainder. Where man and domestic animals are available, they too are attacked readily by species of the *palpalis* group. In circumstances where man, domestic animals and flies of the *palpalis* group come into close proximity (such as at river-crossings, water-holes, etc.) people and their livestock become a major source of food for the flies, and sharp outbreaks of sleeping sickness are likely to occur, especially in the dry seasons when man, cattle and small populations of flies are likely to depend upon the same limited water sources.

G. morsitans, *G. pallidipes* and *G. swynnertoni*—the 'game' tsetse. Unlike flies of the *palpalis* group which commonly occupy waterside habitats of an essentially linear type, often intersected by patterns of human activity that may lead to close and personal contact, species of the *morsitans* group occupy vast areas of xerophytic woodland, dry bushland and thicket vegetation, particularly in the eastern parts of Africa. Under these conditions contact between man, his livestock and the wild fly populations is seldom close and intense. Species of the *morsitans* group obtain most of their blood meals from the wild game animals, especially Bovidae and Suidae, that roam the savannahs and 'miombo' woodlands, and amongst which trypanosomes of the *T. brucei* subgroup are circulated and maintained as a zoonosis. Some of the zoonotic strains are infective to man and give rise to symptoms, characteristically, of the acute, rhodesian type of disease. Human infections are, however, comparatively rare because of the infrequent and mainly accidental contact between the *morsitans* group and man. The number of cases of rhodesian sleeping sickness contracted in eastern Africa is very small in comparison with the number of mainly gambian cases in West Africa and the Congo basin, where man is a principal reservoir of infection, but almost certainly not the only one.

Exposure to *T. rhodesiense* strains is largely occupational: hunters, honey-gatherers, pole-cutters and charcoal burners are among groups likely to enter fly-infested bush. In recent years the rapid growth of the tourist 'package' industry in East Africa has put another large group of itinerants at risk: the tourists themselves. Although species of the *morsitans* group are relatively little interested in man as a source of food if game animals are locally abundant, they often attack in sufficient numbers to be a considerable nuisance. Flies of the *morsitans* group are likely to acquire strains pathogenic to man from prior feeds on bushbuck (the main proved reservoir) or other ungulates. In this latter category must be included domestic cattle; stocks of parasites which caused acute human disease in volunteers were first isolated during a localized outbreak in Kenya (Alego) some years ago. More recently, cattle isolates in Uganda (Busoga) were found to be indistinguishable from man-infective *T. b. rhodesiense* circulating in the human population during an epidemic outbreak, by isoenzymes and other intrinsic criteria. Cattle obviously act as temporary reservoirs, at any rate, under circumstances of human epidemic disease when challenge from animal trypanosomes is sufficiently low to permit survival of the animals. Movement of cattle under these circumstances might also result in the dissemination of man-infective trypanosomes to new foci. Cattle can seldom be kept long in the presence of heavy or moderate fly infestations, however, owing to the damaging incidence of infections with *T. vivax* and *T. congolense*.

Natural infection rates and methods of fly dissection

Infective metacyclic trypanosomes of the *T. brucei* subgroup (subgenus *Trypanozoon*) are found in the salivary glands of the tsetse fly. To reach their final station in the glands they undergo a complex migration in the fly that takes nearly three weeks to complete; hence it follows that only flies more than three weeks old can be infected with trypanosomes infective to man. Even among older flies, infection rates with the *T. brucei* subgroup are always low (commonly 0.1% or less: rarely more than 1%), especially when compared with infection rates with the *T. vivax* (= *Duttonella*) and *T. congolense* (= *Nannomonas*) groups in the same flies. The *T. vivax* group have a short and simple life cycle in the fly: infection rates may reach 75% or more. The *T. congolense* group have a longer and slightly more complex cycle in the fly: infection rates may reach 18–25%.

The full dissection of a tsetse involves the removal and microscopic examination of the elongate salivary glands, the midgut and the mouthparts. There are several possible methods of dissection, but given some practice there is probably little to choose between them. The method preferred by the writer is as follows.

1   The fly is killed (with ether, chloroform or by judicious finger pressure against the sides of the thorax), wings and legs may be removed at this stage, or left.

2   The fly is placed on a slide in a *small* amount of physiological saline (or 5% glucose solution).

3   The tough, membranous connection between head and thorax is 'frayed' carefully with the point of a needle to weaken it.

4   The proboscis is held (under a needle or with forceps) by the basal bulb and drawn slowly away from the head. With practice, the proboscis comes away from the head still attached to the salivary glands; continued slow, careful traction enables these to be

pulled gradually clear of the body. If the glands break at this stage they can be recovered later.

5 The labrum, hypopharynx and labium are preferably separated with needles and examined in saline under a coverslip. Or the intact semitransparent proboscis can be examined without separating the parts.

6 If removed with the mouthparts, the salivary glands are separated from the former and mounted in a small drop of saline under a coverslip.

7 If the salivary glands were broken during stage 4, the fly is now turned so that its abdomen lies flat on the slide, dorsal side uppermost. The thorax is pulled off and discarded and needles are inserted through the two anterolateral corners of the abdomen, at a point roughly halfway from the corners towards the long axis of the abdomen, with sufficient pressure to pierce well below the dorsal integument. Firm traction in the direction of the forward corners of the abdomen, to tear them open, will usually result in the recovery of the glands at this state: they may be recognized by their glass-like, refractile appearance. Continued

needle traction will normally pull the glands clear of the abdomen, for examination in a separate drop of fresh saline under a coverslip.

8 With a needle or scalpel the sides of the posterior tip of the abdomen are cut and the gut is extracted; the covering of fat-body is stripped off with a needle and the gut is placed in a drop of saline, teased open and examined under a coverslip for the presence of trypanosomes.

Trypanosome infections of tsetse are identified, in the organs dissected, by reference to their location and morphology. Infections of the mouthparts only are likely to be *T. vivax* group; infections in the mouthparts and gut only are likely to be *T. congolense* or a mixed infection of *T. vivax* and *T. congolense* groups. Infections involving the salivary glands, gut and mouthparts certainly include the *T. brucei* subgroup but may also be complicated by the presence of *T. vivax*, *T. congolese*, or both. Gut and mouthparts infections could also include immature infections with *T. brucei* subgroup (Table III.11).

Table III.11 Location of trypanosomes in tsetse flies.

Trypanosome species or group (subgenus)	Approx. time of development in *Glossina*	Usual range of infection rates in fly	Organs infected		
			Mouth parts	Salivary glands	Gut
T. vivax (*Duttonella*)	4–5 days	75–85%	+	−	−
T. congolense (*Nannomonas*)	8–10 days	18–25%	+	−	+
T. brucei subgroup[a] (*Trypanozoon*)	15–30 days	0.1–1.5%	+	+	+

[a] Includes the following parasites:
  T. brucei brucei—not infective to man.
  T. brucei gambiense—cause of gambian sleeping sickness in man (chronic).
  T. brucei rhodesiense—cause of rhodesian sleeping sickness in man (acute).

Control of tsetse flies

The subject of tsetse control is a large and complex one and any detailed treatment is beyond the scope of this section. The interested reader is referred to Molyneux[107] for a useful discussion of tsetse control in relation to prevention and control of sleeping sickness generally, to Allsopp[108] for an account of insecticidal control methods, to Jordan[109] for a review of non-insecticidal methods of tsetse control, and also to Jordan.[110]

In recent years there has been an increasing awareness that there is no single, ideal method of control for any arthropod pest or vector. For every vector-borne disease, an integrated strategy of vector and/or disease management is required, within the broader context of disease prevention and control; this must

take into account particular economic, biotic and other particular local circumstances. The strategy adopted may aim at vector eradication or, more usually, vector reduction, to the point at which disease transmission is interrupted, or at least reduced to a level at which it can be dealt with adequately within a prevailing system of health care.

Human trypanosomiasis in Africa is only rarely such a serious medical problem that large-scale vector control can be contemplated as an economically viable proposition, but the concurrent importance of animal trypanosomiasis nearly always alters the balance of the equation in favour of control or eradication of *Glossina*, on a topographically large scale, wherever technological and economic resources are sufficient to allow it. Large-scale tsetse control operations will probably continue to rely to an extent on the use of toxic chemicals, but these will increasingly be deployed in new ways and in amounts even less than is the current norm.

The recent development of simple, cheap and effective methods of tsetse population reduction, which can be operated and maintained by the local population on a self-help basis, for the first time now offers the prospect of effective local vector control (or even temporary eradication), to the point that human infection will virtually cease and at the same time trypanosomiasis in domestic livestock be greatly reduced, with a consequent economic benefit that itself provides an important motivation to keep the control measures in operation. Such simple and effective tsetse-control systems are already operational in some areas of West Africa, against vectors of the *palpalis* group with a linear habitat, and have proved very successful and cost-effective.

Research and development of similar simple methods for control of vectors of the *morsitans* group in East, West and central Africa, has now reached the stage of field trials. However, where very large areas are infested with tsetse of the *morsitans* group, and animal trypanosomiasis is a critical factor, it is probable that aerial application of non-residual insecticides at low doses will continue to be important for large-scale operations for some considerable time to come.

A 20-year project, supported by the European Economic Community, to eradicate animal trypanosomiasis (transmitted by species of the *morsitans* group) from Zimbabwe, Zambia, Mozambique and Malawi, is at the stage of advanced planning and large-scale field trials. It mainly will rely on a combination of non-residual insecticide application from fixed-wing aircraft, to provide an initial massive tsetse population reduction, and a simple 'traps and attractants' technology to maintain (and hopefully, further improve) fly control to the point at which eradication finally occurs.

A brief review follows of tsetse control methods in current use, or at a stage of development where they are likely to be applied widely in the field in the near or medium-term future.

Habitat alteration

All *Glossina* populations are highly dependent for their continued existence on microclimatic and other conditions provided by particular types of woodland vegetation or thicket, the precise nature of which varies from one species to another. The woody vegetation provides tsetse with shelter from climatic extremes, with appropriate breeding places and a source of the animal hosts from which they derive their sole nourishment.

It is possible to disturb the delicate balance between tsetse and their habitat in such a way that fly populations will decline or even disappear.

1 *Removal of woody vegetation.* This can be carried out by hand, as in the past or, increasingly nowadays, by mechanical means. Heavy tractors or bulldozers are used, often in pairs linked together by a heavy marine anchor chain; this smashes down a broad swathe of trees and bushes. Clearance of the tsetse habitat can be total (all woody vegetation removed) or partial (only selected elements removed, on which tsetse survival is known to depend). Formerly a very important indirect means of tsetse control, particularly for areas in which prompt settlement and agricultural development was intended after clearance, the method is now used less often (because of the escalating cost), and then mainly for the clearance of corridors or barrier zones, to protect villages, river-crossings, roads and cattle routes, or to isolate from reinvasion larger areas in which other forms of tsetse control are to be implemented. Vegetation is cut to below knee level, gathered into windrows and burned, after any more valuable or useful timber is removed. It is important that regeneration of woody vegetation is prevented by regular re-cutting as necessary, or by suitable land utilization. Pollock[101] describes the methodology of bush-clearance—and other forms of tsetse control—in a clear and practical way.

2 *Game exclusion and control.* This was formerly also an important form of indirect tsetse control, particularly in some countries of south-central Africa. The selective destruction of wild animals (usually by shooting, especially of wild Suidae, members of the pig family), which are important maintenance hosts for *Glossina* species of the *morsitans* group, resulted in a dramatic reduction of tsetse populations. The method has now been superseded for several reasons, among which are cost, conservation, the tourist industry and the development of better, more economical, alternative forms of control (particularly insecticides).

Game exclusion, by parallel game fences and stock fences about 5 km apart, is still used occasionally. This aims to reduce access of game animals to the intervening 5 km, from which livestock are also excluded. Vegetation clearance, selective shooting or insecticidal treatment of the barrier zone, can then be carried out in any required combination to maintain (on the far side of the stock fence), a cleared fly-free settlement area with livestock. Reinvasion along roads and tracks is reduced or prevented by the use of stationary pickets, who stop passing traffic to hand-catch tsetse from vehicles, cyclists and pedestrians. Vehicles can be sprayed with insecticides by the pickets, to kill any flies resting on inaccessible parts. Major traffic routes are further protected, where they cross the barrier zone, by clearance of woody vegetation for 1–2 km on either side of the road.

Insecticides

These are now the principal means of tsetse control

and eradication, particularly for the rapid clearance of large areas of woodland and thickets from infestation by tsetse of the *morsitans* group. It is now possible to eradicate tsetse from areas of more than 6000 square kilometres in a three-month operational campaign, by current methods which utilize several fixed-wing aircraft, flown in formation, and sophisticated navigational techniques. Very low doses of non-residual insecticide aerosols are applied in sequential cycles at fortnightly intervals. Doses as low as 6–20 g/ha/cycle of endosulfan (five to six applications needed), or even less of synthetic pyrethroids (e.g. deltamethrin at 12.5 g/ha), have been shown to give effective control (but, however, not complete eradication), with negligible or very minor undesirable environmental side-effects.

Originally DDT and BHC were the insecticides used for ground control operations, early in the post Second World War period; originally applied by hand-operated knapsack sprayers, nowadays often replaced by vehicle-mounted equipment for greater speed and mobility. Ground-level insecticide applications were the mainstay of tsetse control in most African countries for more than 30 years, and they still retain an important place. The East African *G. fuscipes fuscipes* was eradicated by this means from the Kenya shore, and offshore islands, of Lake Victoria. Impressively large areas of Nigeria were freed of tsetse in the same way, and there are many other examples of successful eradication and control in other countries.

DDT and BHC (as wettable powders) were followed later by the introduction of dieldrin (as a 2–3% emulsion concentrate). These, and other insecticides, were used initially to achieve persistent residual effects after a single application. The persistent insecticide formulations were, and still are, very effective when selectively applied only to known resting sites by hand-operated equipment. It is necessary to treat only about 10% of the total vegetation. Spraying is then normally both discriminative (only some specific elements of the woody vegetation are treated) and selective (only particular parts of the vegetation treated; such as the boles of trees and larger branches up to a specified height). For DDT, about 3–9 kg of active ingredient (a.i.) are used per hectare; with dieldrin, 2–6 kg a.i./ha is needed. Persistence of the residual deposit for a minimum of six to eight weeks is vital, since this is the maximum duration of puparial life of *Glossina* at the coolest time of year, and will therefore ensure death of any flies emerging from puparia in the soil.

For control of riverine species in fringing gallery forest, helicopter application (of once-only residual insecticide formulations, or sequential application of non-residual dosages) is possible in savannah zones, but extremely expensive. Advantages are the rapidity with which the operation is carried out, particularly in areas difficult to penetrate at ground level; disadvantages are the high operational cost and increased risk of river contamination. There are technical and operational reasons which largely preclude helicopter application in forest areas. Helicopters are best thought of as an expensive, but rapid, alternative to ground-based operations, and are normally used mainly for control of riverine tsetse species. Early helicopter operations used DDT, BHC or dieldrin, applied from boom-and-nozzle spraygear. Later operations utilized ultra-low-volume (ULV) formulations, dispersed by spinning-disc atomizers; endosulfan was the insecticide of choice in most cases, at rates of 800–1500 g/ha. In Ivory Coast, deltamethrin at 12 g/ha was combined with endosulfan at 267 g/ha; villages were treated with an aerosol of endosulfan at 10 g/ha. This combination, however, was not entirely successful. Two applications of deltamethrin at 0.2 g/ha, with a 14-day interval, gave a 95% reduction of *G. p. gambiensis* in 16 km of riverine vegetation in Burkina Faso prior to experimental release of sterile males (see following section). The impact of the spraying operation on the *G. tachinoides* population was rather less. However, deltamethrin alone at such a low dosage would be unlikely to give more than temporary control of *palpalis*-group flies.

Helicopter applications, although extremely costly, have generally not lived up to early expectation, and frequently have given rather disappointing results. Canopy penetration was often less effective than anticipated, although this was overcome to some extent (for narrow riverine vegetation) by the use of spraygear which emitted the spray obliquely, on one side of the helicopter only. This allowed insecticide application rates to be reduced (from 1000 g/ha to 200 g/ha for endosulfan: from 30 g/ha to 12.5 g/ha for deltamethrin). Helicopters and ULV techniques were used successfully in Nigeria to clear *G. palpalis* and *G. tachinoides* from riverine vegetation in an area of about 10 000 square kilometres. In the same country, helicopter treatment of savannah woodland infested by *G. morsitans*, with swathes flown on a grid pattern at 150–200 m intervals (insecticide applied only to 5–16% of the total area), was less successful. About a quarter of the area was recolonized by tsetse and required further treatment.

As yet, there are no reports of insecticide resistance in *Glossina*, but there are no reasons to suppose that this will not eventually occur.

Genetic control: release of sterile males

Tsetse have a low rate of reproduction and this is a feature of their biology which has aroused much interest in relation to control by the sterile insect release method (usually abbreviated as SIT: sterile insect technique). Reduction of the potential fecundity of *Glossina* populations by the release of sterile males is theoretically much more easily achieved than with the more typical oviparous insects, which produce offspring in large numbers. The SIT is strictly species-specific and relies on the periodic release of over-whelming numbers of colony-bred sterile males into the environment of the target population. Reared males are sterilized either by irradiation or by chemo-sterilants, usually the former. Sterile males necessarily must be fully competitive with wild males, in order to ensure that the maximum possible number of wild females are inseminated with sterile sperm and fail to reproduce. A succession of mass-releases is needed, in order that the fly population declines and finally is extinguished.

Effective methods were developed in European laboratories to colonize and mass-rear flies of most economically and medically important *Glossina* species, in numbers sufficient to ensure the production of sterile males en masse. An initial, small-scale field trial on an island in Lake Kariba (Zimbabwe), arti-ficially colonized with tsetse, yielded results from SIT sufficiently encouraging for two further field trials to be undertaken (in Burkina Faso—formerly Upper Volta—and in Tanzania).

The principal target species in Burkina Faso was *Glossina palpalis gambiensis*, with *G. tachinoides* in the same linear riverine habitat. The savannah woodland species *G. morsitans morsitans* was the target in Tan-zania, with *G. pallidipes* in the same area. In both trials, SIT releases were begun after aerial application of non-residual insecticides, to reduce initial wild fly populations as far as possible.

In Burkina Faso, about 650 000 sterile males were released in 32 km of riverine vegetation, in a total area of about 100 square kilometres; eradication of *G. p. gambiensis* was successfully achieved within two years. Populations of *G. tachinoides* were depressed by SIT, but recovered to their original level by the end of the trial.

The trial in Tanzania was rather less successful. This mainly was due to problems of reinvasion of tsetse from adjoining areas, beyond the 1 km totally cleared protective barrier zone around the exper-imental area. Some 350 000 sterile males were released in the 195 square kilometre trial area in Tanzania; *G. m. morsitans* populations were decreased in 15 months by about 80% of pretrial levels. *G. pallidipes* popu-lations initially fell, but later recovered.

The two trials demonstrated that SIT was effective after aerial insecticide treatment to achieve an initial population reduction, particularly in the linear riparian habitat of *palpalis*-group flies. The same com-bination of methods (insecticides, followed by SIT) is under trial in a 750 square kilometre area of Nigeria, for control of *G. p. palpalis* and *G. tachinoides*. *G. p. palpalis* was successfully eradicated from most of the area and attempts to eradicate *G. tachinoides* will follow.

In a more recent large-scale operation in Burkina Faso, in an area of approximately 3500 square kilo-metres, the insecticide/SIT combination was suc-cessfully modified, and made both more cost-effective and less damaging to the environment. For initial population reduction of *G. p. gambiensis* and *G. tach-inoides*, aerial application of insecticide was replaced by the use of static, insecticide-impregnated, coloured cloth screens, placed at intervals along the river banks. This was followed by release of sterile males. This combination of non-pollutant methods achieved eradication of both species from the entire area. The savannah species *G. m. submorsitans* also was suc-cessfully eradicated from that part of the same area where it occurred, by a combination of insecticidal screens and odour-baited traps (see below) for initial population reduction, followed by SIT. A cost–benefit comparison showed that integrated control with SIT as a final component is economically competitive with other methods of tsetse eradication.

The SIT is both most effective and least expensive when target populations are at minimal density and limited to circumscribed and well-defined habitats: the method seems most promising for *palpalis*-group flies in linear habitats, particularly for populations close to the climatic limits of their distribution. However, SIT has so far proved more difficult to operate with *morsitans*-group flies, dispersed over wide areas of woodland and thicket, where it is extremely difficult to prevent reinvasion from outside the treated area. SIT is nonetheless both a high-tech-nology and a high-cost method; it is likely to be most effective and least expensive to 'mop up' low-density populations which cannot be eradicated otherwise. It remains to be seen, however, whether or not the use of SIT on a large scale to achieve final eradication of tsetse will remain economically competitive in the longer term. Advances in the 'appropriate technology' field suggest that it may be superseded by develop-ment of other methods, equally effective but con-siderably cheaper, to bring about eradication of *Glossina* on a geographically wide scale within the foreseeable future. These methods are considered in the following section, set in an historical framework.

Traps, insecticidal screens, targets and odour attractants: application of 'appropriate technology' to tsetse control and eradication

Before the introduction of modern insecticides, much attention was devoted to passive systems to sample, or even control, tsetse populations. In the early years of the twentieth century *G. palpalis* was eradicated from the 125 square-kilometre island of Principe in the Gulf of Guinea, about 200 km offshore from Equatorial Guinea. Eradication was achieved, between 1906 and 1914, by an initial combination of vegetation clearance and destruction of maintenance hosts (these were chiefly domestic and feral pigs; thousands of stray dogs were also killed). There were no large wild mammals, crocodiles or large lizards on the island.

A decisive final contribution to the eradication pro-gramme was made by the use of men wearing a piece of black cloth on their backs, coated with sticky 'bird lime' to trap alighting flies. This technique was adopted after an astute plantation manager noticed that *G. palpalis* commonly landed on the backs of labourers as they stooped to cut crops. On the same plantation, some 130 000 flies were so trapped and destroyed in 18 months of 1906 and 1907. At the start of the later, island-wide, 'sticky-patch' campaign (in which 140 men were employed), it was not uncommon for one man to catch 500 flies a day. In January 1913, 21 000 flies were caught by 139 men, all dressed in white except for the sticky black patch on their backs. The last fly was trapped in April 1914; no flies at all were trapped in the following four months by 200 men with sticky black back-patches.

Principe remained tsetse-free until 1956, when a reinvasion of *G. palpalis* occurred (probably by the passive importation of mainland flies by trading vessels or fishing boats). The reinvasion of 1956 was successfully dealt with by the same 'sticky patch' method. It must be emphasized, however, that because of its isolation from the African mainland and its small size, the island of Principe constituted a special case: the same method would be unlikely to succeed anywhere on the African mainland. Indeed, a similar campaign by the then (1913) German colonial authorities, on a small island in Lake Victoria infested by *G. fuscipes*, was unsuccessful; this was probably because the island was not sufficiently isolated.

Several attempts to eradicate small mainland tsetse populations by means of hand-catching by parties of men with nets invariably met with failure; this was always due to reinvasion from surrounding areas, across cleared barrier zones. However, more than 30 000 tsetse were caught by villagers in Zaire when offered a 'per fly' payment, which showed that even this simple method is effective to some degree.

Traps for Glossina. The Harris trap, developed around 1930, was the first of a series of box-trap designs intended to simulate the outline of an animal. Flies are initially attracted to such traps by visual stimuli, and alight on the shaded underparts. They are then attracted, by the daylight above, to move up into a non-return cage at the top. Traps of this type were particularly successful to catch flies of the *morsitans* group, but were not effective for *palpalis*-group tsetse. This class of trap was intended primarily as a means to sample tsetse populations, rather than as a means of control. Although such traps will catch *morsitans*-group flies in large numbers, their use never resulted in the extinction of fly populations.

French workers in West Africa in the 1970s developed the now well-known biconical trap, widely used as a sampling system in many African countries. The vertical silhouette of the biconical trap, with a white upper cone and a blue one below (and an internal cruciform black cloth screen visible through vertical slits in the lower, blue cone) were shown by experiment to be the optimum combination of visual stimuli. The biconical trap was first developed to catch *palpalis*-group flies, but was found also to attract flies of the *morsitans* group.

Among the several advantages of the biconical trap are its portability, economy and ease of production. Later, simplified and cheaper versions on the same theme (based on a single inverted cone or pyramid), were shown to be equally effective for *palpalis*-group tsetse. Since more flies alight on such traps than actually enter them, impregnation of the fabric with small amounts of long-lasting persistent pyrethroid insecticides (e.g. deltamethrin) significantly enhances their effectiveness. Impregnated traps of this type are widely and successfully used for control of riverine tsetse (*G. palpalis* and *G. tachinoides*) in linear habitats of West and central Africa. Population reductions of the order of 95% or more are reported from several countries.

Screens and 'targets'. The success of the impregnated traps was followed, in West Africa, by the use of static rectangular blue fabric screens (about 120×90 cm), each impregnated with 100 mg of deltamethrin. These are cheaper than traps and, located along the margins of rivers and streams at intervals, were equally effective in dramatically reducing local populations of *palpalis*-group flies for several months without reimpregnation. Blue and black screens, with invisible (to tsetse) black netting at their lateral edges, are even more effective (about 2.5 times) than the plain blue screens. Biconical traps (together with simplified designs derived from them) and impregnated blue screens are both, generally, marginally more effective with *G. tachinoides* than with the *G. palpalis* subspecies. Unfortunately, however, neither biconical traps nor simple, static screens are very effective for flies of the *morsitans* group.

'Targets' were developed (in Zimbabwe; see below) for their attractiveness to flies of the *morsitans* group. They differ from screens in their greater complexity and the fact that their visual attractiveness is increased by an element of mobility; they are suspended about a rotating vertical axis and provided with a wind-vane which ensures a constant alignment in relation to local air movements. Flies are killed after contact with the insecticide-impregnated surfaces of the targets, not by entrapment. Targets are thus in many ways intermediate between simple, static screens and traps as such. The capacity to orient in line with wind direction makes them particularly suitable to combine with scent attractants.

Experimental studies in several parts of Africa have shown that both *palpalis*- and *morsitans*-group flies are attracted most strongly from a distance by blue surfaces (of a particular shade), but are stimulated more strongly to alight on a black surface than on a blue one. These characteristics of fly behaviour in relation to blue and black surfaces were incorporated in the design of a series of traps and insecticide-treated targets, developed in recent years by a small team in Zimbabwe, for the control of *morsitans*-group tsetse species (particularly of *G. morsitans* and *G. pallidipes*).

Odour attractants. It has been known for many years that components of host odour, particularly of pigs, have a powerful short-range attractant effect on tsetse. It has so far not been possible to isolate and synthesize a stable attractive compound from pigs. However, careful study of the components of cattle odour, also very attractive to *Glossina* species, showed that the exhaled breath of the animals provides the main olfactory stimulus; carbon dioxide and acetone are important attractants in breath odour, together with a further stable and powerful component. This is octenol (1-octen-3-ol), a relatively simple compound to synthesize.

The efficiency of the Zimbabwe trap and target designs was dramatically increased by the incorporation of some of these attractants; particularly acetone and synthetic octenol. The combination of odour attractants with an effective design of trap, treated screen or target will increase efficiency by 20–100 times. Carbon dioxide is inconvenient and expensive to use in the field, but acetone (100 mg/h) combined with octenol (0.5 mg/h) are convenient to use (dispensed at a controlled rate from bottles) and relatively inexpensive, and result in up to a tenfold increase in trap/target efficiency for *morsitans*-group flies (notably *G. m. submorsitans* in West Africa; *G. m. morsitans* and *G. m. pallidipes* in central Africa). Calculations show that use of impregnated targets, baited with acetone and octenol as odour attractants, deployed at the rate of 4–5 per square kilometre in an area of 1000 square kilometres, would probably eradicate *G. morsitans* and/or *G. pallidipes*.

Further developments in odour attractant technology may provide new, stable, cheap and even more potent attractants for the future. It still remains to be seen if the attractive components of pig odour, or of the urine of some wild animals (also known to be highly attractive to tsetse), can be used as the basis for practicable and more effective alternative scent attractants.

Important features of the improved and simplified odour-baited screens, targets and traps, are that they are simple and cheap to make, of materials available in most countries, require minimum maintenance over long periods and can be operated by unskilled local people. They do not require the application of toxic chemicals to the environment, or the corresponding expenditure of hard currency. They are, in a word, good examples of 'appropriate technology'.

Other control methods

One obvious way to prevent infection with African trypanosomes is to avoid the bites of tsetse. This is a neglected aspect of trypanosomiasis prevention, although it is known that the use of repellent-impregnated wide-mesh net jackets will reduce the number of bites received by 80–90%. Di-isopentyl malate was the most active repellent of several tested and was considerably more effective than deet (diethyltoluamide) in field tests.

Glossina have a number of known natural enemies, but no feasible system for their biological control has yet been devised.

Female tsetse have species-specific cuticular contact sex-recognition pheromones which stimulate copulatory behaviour in males of the same species; those of several species have been isolated and synthesized. It may prove possible to utilize these specific contact pheromones, in combination with chemosterilants, as a species-specific control method for field use, and field trials of this system are in progress.

Much research attention has been devoted to various compounds which regulate, or interfere with, the reproductive processes of *Glossina*. These include substances, such as phytosterols, sulphonamides, antibiotics and the trypanocidal drug isometamidium, which often exert their effects on reproduction by interference with the symbiotic bacterioids in the mycetome of the fly midgut. Flies fed on hosts injected with high doses of the anthelmintic drug Ivermectin® are killed, and injection of the drug into female flies markedly reduces their fecundity. The problem remains, however, of finding an appropriate delivery system, given the obligate blood-feeding habit of tsetse, to ensure ingestion by sufficient female flies to exert an effective control on the reproduction of populations. (Ivermectin® is one of the avermectins, a novel class of compounds obtained by fermentation of the soil organism *Streptomyces avermitilis*.)

Some compounds which interfere with reproduction can enter through the cuticle; these include juvenile hormone analogues, precocene and insect growth regulators (such as diflubenzuron analogues). The problems of topical administration of such compounds to tsetse in the field remain to be solved; moreover, on a cost-benefit basis it is unlikely that they would be competitive with established methods of insecticidal control, or with the community-based 'appropriate technology' methods described earlier.

FLIES CAUSING MYIASIS

R.P. Lane

Myiasis covers a variety of associations between dipterous larvae and mammals. The most comprehensive definition is 'the infestation of live human and vertebrate animals with dipterous larvae which, at least for a certain period, feed on the host's dead or living tissue, liquid body-substance, or ingested food'.[111] Such associations vary from complete endoparasitism, via casual or accidental myiasis, to the bizarre predation on human blood by free-living larvae. A wide range of families of flies are involved, but most are 'higher flies' (Cyclorrhapha) in which the larvae are either specialized endoparasites in other mammals or are scavengers and carrion feeders.

The numerous systems used to classify myiasis reflect the diversity of the subject and organisms involved. The two complementary classifications described here, clinical and parasitological, serve different objectives. From a medical standpoint the clinical classification is more important as it aids diagnosis and identification of the species responsible, but the second classification, based on the degree of the host–parasite relationship, assists in understanding the biological background and hence possible methods of prevention or control. Whilst a single incident can be remedied (e.g. by surgical removal) and the larva retrospectively identified, prevention of further attacks relies on a knowledge of the insects' biology.

Myiasis in man concerns a few common species (e.g. *Cordylobia*, *Dermatobia*, *Chrysomya*) and a large number of uncommon or rare examples. Numerous cases of myiasis have been published in which the identification of the larva responsible is doubtful.

Briefly, myiasis-producing larvae attack three main parts of the body.

1 Cutaneous tissue (which is subdivided into larvae producing furuncles, creeping myiasis and roving swellings, species invading sores and wounds). An additional category of 'sanguinivorous larvae' includes a single example in which the free-living larva feeds on blood.
2 Body cavities such as the nasopharynx, eyes and auditory canal.
3 Organs of the body; principally, the gut and urogenital system.

Parasitologically, myiasis producers can be divided into three categories.

1 Obligate parasites in which it is essential for the larvae to develop in living tissue; they are unable to develop elsewhere, unlike facultative parasites. Obligate parasites are highly specialized insects in which the larvae are endoparasitic and have developed sophisticated avoidance of the host's immune system. The adults do not normally feed.
2 Facultative myiasis producers, whose larvae usually develop on carrion but may invade wounds. This category can be further divided into primary flies which initiate myiasis (e.g. *Cochliomyia hominivorax*), secondary flies which enter the body only when an animal has become infested (e.g. *Cochliomyia macellaria*), and tertiary flies which become involved at a late stage, after decomposition is advanced (e.g. many carrion-breeding blow flies).[1]
3 Accidental myiasis producers whose eggs or larvae are accidentally ingested and are not killed in the intestine.

Larvae causing myiasis are similar in overall structure and are essentially hydrostatic bags against which the muscles work to produce movement. They do not have a recognizable head capsule (except *Psychoda*) but internally they have a small hard skeleton (cephalopharyngeal skeleton) composed of a pair of mouth-hooks to tear at the host's tissues, and a structure to anchor the muscles operating the mouth-hooks. The overall shape of the larvae varies from the wedge shape of blow flies (*Calliphora*, *Lucilia*, etc.), through the ovoid tumbu fly (*Cordylobia anthropophaga*) to the pyriform *Dermatobia hominis*. There is often a change of shape during larval development. Some species possess rows of hooks or spines to prevent their expulsion from the host. The distribution and shape of such spines, together with details of the spiracles and cephalopharyngeal skeleton, are used to identify the different species.

Myiasis of cutaneous tissue (Chapter 51)

This may be subdivided into four categories.

1 Larvae living in the skin and producing furuncles

These are usually specially adapted endoparasites and are the most commonly encountered by clinicians.

Cordylobia anthropophaga (Fig. III.59) (tumbu fly, mango fly or ver du cayor) is a large, robust, yellow-brown fly 7–12 mm long and resembling the adult of the Congo floor-maggot (*Auchmeromyia luteola*). It is fairly difficult to distinguish the adults of either from the numerous other species of the family Calliphoridae to which they belong. *C. anthropophaga* is an obligate parasite found throughout Africa south of the Sahara, although some areas are free from the fly. Recently it was recorded from a patient in southern Spain who had never visited Africa, thus indicating that it might

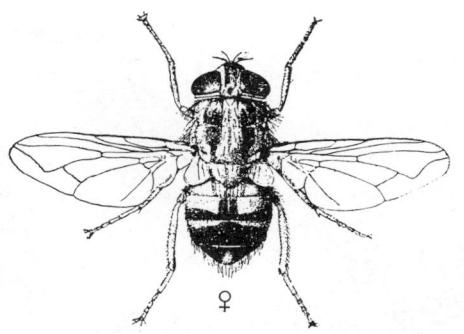

Fig. III.59 *Cordylobia anthropophaga*. Twice natural size.

be possible to establish foci outside endemic areas. Adults are active early morning and late afternoon and can be found resting in dark places in huts, etc. in the intervening periods.

The white, banana-shaped eggs are laid in two batches of 100–300 eggs. The female preferentially oviposits on sandy ground, particularly if contaminated with urine or faeces, but can also lay on clothing if similarly contaminated (although such clothing may appear clean to the human eye). Clothing laid on the ground to dry may also be affected, but not clothes hanging in bright sunlight since the eggs are only laid in shaded areas. The eggs are not laid directly on to skin, hairs or vegetation. On hatching the minute first instar larvae hold themselves erect, while waving the anterior part in search of a host and can remain alive without food for about 9 days. The larvae are sensitive to both heat and vibration and once they become attached to a host immediately begin to penetrate the unbroken skin, taking approximately one minute. Penetration is usually painless and may involve any part of the body, but most commonly on the back, neck and head in man. Larvae are acquired from lying on the ground or from clothing. They are commoner in children. *Cordylobia* breeds all the year

round but human cases are commoner in the wet season.

Initially, the small papule containing the larva may be itchy or pricking at intervals. As the papule increases in size the symptoms recur and may be painful enough to interfere with sleep. Serous fluid may be exuded and gland enlargement may occur, or even febrile reactions and malaise. The larvae are usually noticed when the third stage has been reached. During the time the larva is in the host (which lasts 8–12 days) the larva has its posterior segment, bearing the respiratory spiracles, protruding from the aperture which can be withdrawn when touched. The cavity containing the larva breaks down to form a swelling, resembling a boil, which bursts without much inflammation. The larvae emerge from the swellings, fall to the ground and pupate within 24 hours, and can be identified by its posterior spiracles (Fig. III.60B).[112] Pupal cases are commonly found in holes of black or brown rats, which, together with dogs, are the principal hosts other than man. The adult fly hatches out in 10–20 days according to temperature.

Larvae can be extracted by manipulation if mature or inducing the larvae to assist of their own accord by covering the aperture, through which they respire, with petroleum jelly. The larvae die when covered with adhesive dressing. All clothes in direct contact with the skin should be ironed on both sides. All drip dry clothes should be hung indoors with the windows closed, after checking for resting flies. Dogs act as an important reservoir. As a result of air travel, people infested with *C. anthropophaga* arrive in many parts of the world.

Dermatobia hominis (ver macaque, Berne, el tórsalo, beefworm, human bot fly) (Fig. III.61) is widely distributed throughout Central and South America, from Mexico to Argentina and Chile. It attacks a wide range of hosts and is a devastating pest of livestock in some areas. It even attacks fowls. The adult is a large bluish-grey fly, 1.5 cm long with a strong flight. *D. hominis* is primarily found on the edge of tropical forests,

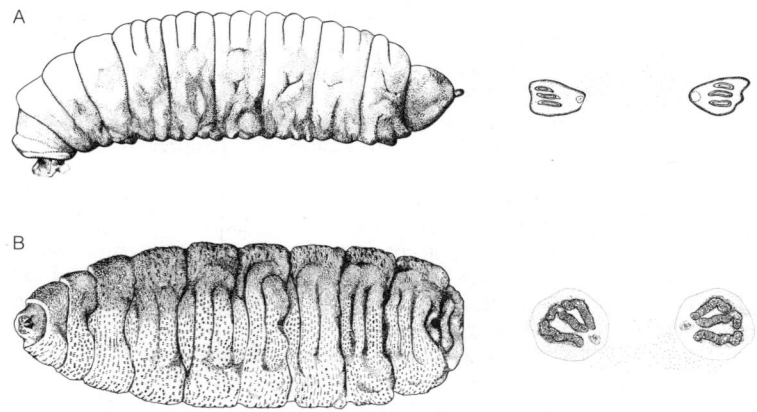

Fig. III.60 Third instar larva and posterior spiracles of *Auchmeromyia luteola* (A) and *Cordylobia anthropophaga* (B). (From Smith;[112] courtesy British Museum (Natural History) London.)

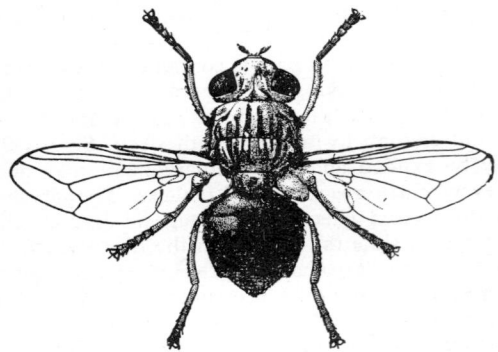

Fig. III.61 Female *Dermatobia hominis*. Twice natural size.

particularly hilly areas of secondary forest between 160 and 3000 m.

This species is remarkable for the unique manner in which it delivers its eggs to a new host, by using other insects as carriers or porters. The adult female *Dermatobia* catches and firmly holds the carrier insect, usually day-flying mosquitoes or other muscoid flies and attaches between six and 30 eggs on to its abdomen (Fig. III.62). The larva is very sensitive to temperature changes and remains in the egg shell until it senses its proximity to a warm-blooded host, whereupon it rapidly 'hatches' and penetrates the host's skin in 5–10 minutes, remaining at the site of penetration. Each larva penetrates individually and a small nodule develops around it with a central pore through which the larva breathes. Close examination of a lesion containing a larva will reveal its posterior end bearing two small dark brown spots which are the spiracles.

The first instar is sub-cylindrical with circlets of small spines. The second stage (Fig. III.63) is pyriform, with stronger, stout spines on the globular

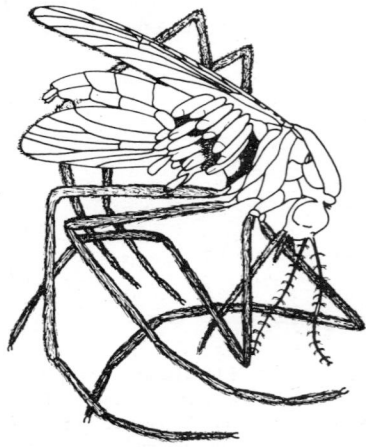

Fig. III.62 *Psorophora (Janthinosoma) lutzi* carrying eggs of *Dermatobium hominis*.

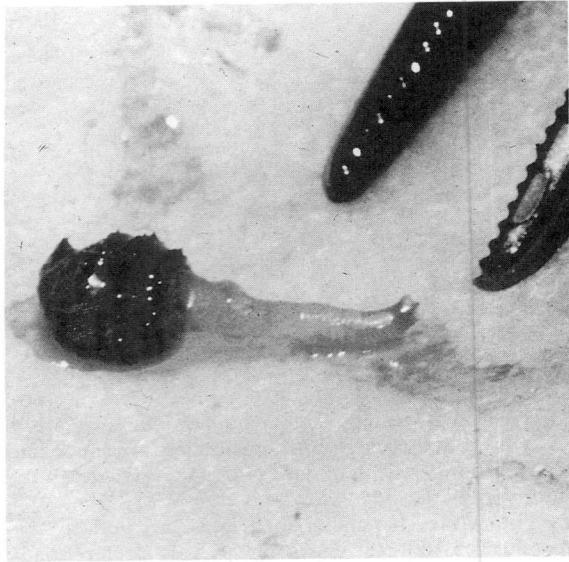

Fig. III.63 Second stage instar of *Dermatobia hominis*.

portion and no spines on the narrow posterior part which acts like a respiratory siphon. At this stage the larva is difficult to dislodge by virtue of its shape and the numerous concentric rows of backward projecting spines.

During larval life the wound continually oozes serous fluid or pus but bacteriostatic activity in the gut of the larva seems to prevent undesirable overgrowth of pyogenic bacteria in its environment[113] although in some cases secondary infection does occur.

The duration of larval development is a matter of some controversy, but probably lasts from six to 12 weeks in man, during which it grows slowly, feeding on tissue exudate. The mature larva (Fig. III.64) leaves the host and burrows into the soil to pupate, emerging after four to 11 weeks. The adults live 8–9 days, never feed and are sexually mature about 3 hours after emergence.

Cutaneous swellings harbouring larvae usually occur on exposed areas, although larvae can penetrate clothing and therefore can be found on any part of the body. They are often single, although 12 have been reported on one individual. It is a common cause of ocular myiasis in Colombia (Chapter 70). Rarely, serious complications occur, such as fatal cerebral myiasis in children. Most infestations by *Dermatobia* are painful and consequently larvae are removed in the first or second stages. Occasionally first instar larvae may be removed by the methods described for *Cordylobia,* but usually they and second instar larvae are best removed surgically, via a cruciate incision. Care must be taken not to course the central hole as this may result in damage to the larva, portions of which are then left in the wound. A prophylactic anti-

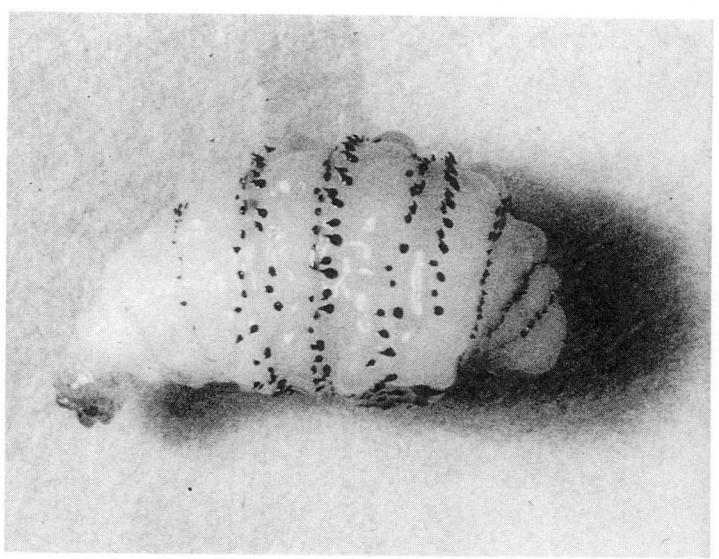

Fig. III.64 Third stage instar of *Dermatobia hominis*.

biotic is probably not necessary in developed countries. The long period of development means that cases may appear in any part of the world.

2   *Creeping myiasis and roving swellings* (Chapter 51)

Species causing this syndrome are usually specialized endoparasites of other animals which are unable to develop fully in man. It is important to distinguish them from *Ancylostoma* (nematodes) which produce similar effects.

Hypoderma bovis and *H. lineatum* cause creeping swellings and eruptions, especially in persons associated with cattle. On hatching, the larvae penetrate into the subcutaneous tissues, more deeply than *Gastrophilus*, producing an inflamed swelling resembling a boil, which is painful. They migrate sometimes for considerable distances and have been reported to invade the nervous system. The larva can be extracted through a cruciform incision.

Gastrophilus species are common parasites of horses and occasionally affect man. The larvae may rarely penetrate the skin but do not develop beyond the first instar, causing a swelling and a wandering tunnel in the lower epidermis, in which they may progress for long periods.

3   *Larvae attacking wounds and sores* (Chapter 51)

This includes myiasis produced by obligate and facultative parasites. Larvae of several groups of flies usually associated with carrion have been found in wounds and gangrenous tissue, where they act as facultative parasites feeding on necrotic tissue and occasionally they may attack healthy tissue: *Calliphora, Lucilia, Phormia, Musca, Fannia* (Fig. III.65). Occasionally, larvae are found living in soiled folds of the skin. Species which are usually found infesting soiled areas around the anus or genitalia may exceptionally enter the rectum or vagina to become internal parasites. At one time it was practice to use larvae of carefully cultivated *Lucilia* to clean septic wounds by removal of infected tissue but the practice has now been abandoned.

Cochliomyia (= *Callitroga*) *hominivorax* (screwworm fly) is an obligate parasite from the New World, which may produce serious cases of myiasis. Only clean wounds are attacked, which may be very small; even a scratch or stubbed toenail could become affected. Additionally, eggs may be deposited in the ears, and nasal passages and even in the vulva and vagina. The fly lays eggs on dry skin and the larvae subsequently invade the wound and feed rapaciously on healthy tissue, usually in groups to produce characteristic pocket-like injuries. They grow rapidly and reach maturity in 4–8 days. A case mortality rate of 8% has been reported, and people in close contact with infested cattle are particularly at risk. This species gained notoriety for its efficient control by the release of radiation-sterilized males. A related species, *C. macellaria*, is a facultative parasite responsible for the secondary invasion of wounds as well as scavenging on dead tissues.

Wohlfahrtia magnifica (Old World flesh fly, sheep maggot) occurs in the warmer parts of the Europe and the USSR; it deposits its larvae in skin lesions, nasal sinuses, ears, sore eyes and vagina, producing serious disfigurement. Like the larvae of *W. vigil* and *Chrysomya bezziana*, these larvae rely on living tissue for development and do not feed on carrion or excreta.

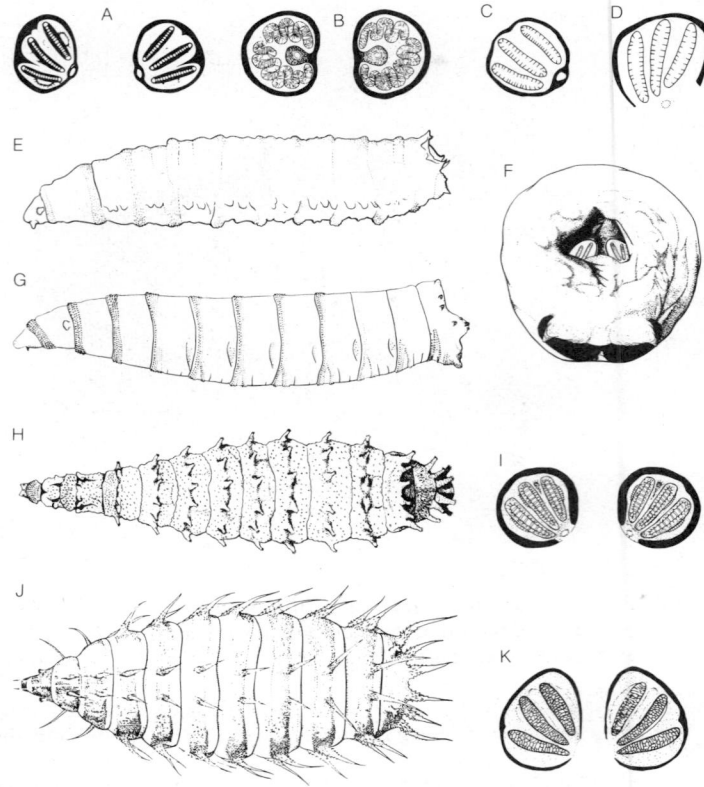

Fig. III.65 General views of mature, third instar larvae to show range in form and posterior spiracles used in identification. A, *Lucilia serricata*. B, *Musca domestica*. C, *Calliphora* sp. D, *Wohlfahrtia* sp. E and F, *Sarcophaga* sp. G and I, *Callitroga macellaria*. H and K, *Chrysomyia albiceps*. J, *Fannia* sp. (From Smith,[112] courtesy British Museum (Natural History) London.)

Wohlfahrtia vigil (Nearctic flesh fly) deposits its larvae in lesions of the skin or mucous membranes, or even on uninjured skin. It is attracted by foul odours from secretions of the ear, eye or nose and possibly from the soiled nappies of babies. Young children are particularly attractive to the flies. The flies do not enter houses. Other species of *Wohlfahrtia* have been incriminated.

4 *Sanguinivorous larvae* (Chapter 51)

The larvae of several genera are obligatory parasites living free in nests of birds and mammals, feeding on the blood of their hosts, but only one, *Auchmeromyia luteola* (Fig. III.66) (the Congo floor-maggot) has been reported attacking man. This species is widely distributed from Nigeria to Natal in wet and dry climates. The larva is dirty white, about 15 mm long and has three short, fleshy lobes bearing spines on the posterior portion of each segment. The spiracles are distinctive. After feeding with its mouth-hooks, the conspicuously red larva (Fig. III.60A) retreats to cracks in the floor. Larvae are frequently found under sleeping mats and in the earth to a depth of 7.5 cm. They feed mainly at night and drop off immediately if disturbed. The yellowish adults can be found resting in dark areas of huts.

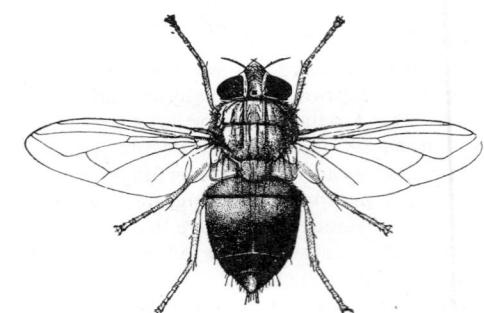

Fig. III.66 Female *Auchmeromyia luteola*. Twice natural size.

Myiasis of body cavities (Chapter 51)

Several species which attack wounds and sores (discussed above) are also involved with myiasis of the eye, orbit, nasal cavities and ear canal. In nasal myiasis the initial symptoms are tickling pain and nasal obstruction. Epistaxis is common, but the discharge soon becomes purulent and fetid. Inhalation of chloroform or packing with chloroform gauze, or the careful local use of weak carbolic acid and turpentine have been advocated but the nasal sinuses may need to be opened.

Chrysomya bezziana (Old World screw worm) is a large metallic-blue fly with a bright green thorax. It is found throughout Asia and Africa south of the Sahara and, unlike other species in this genus, is an obligatory parasite. Myiasis due to *C. bezziana* is much rarer in Africa than Asia. The females lay numerous eggs in the nasal cavities, especially where there is chronic nasal discharge, or in ulcers or skin wounds (for instance in leprosy), or even in the gums, conjunctiva, ears or vagina. The larvae require living tissue in which to develop, they hatch in a few hours and burrow into the tissues, even to the bones of the nose, producing foul, infected, discharging and disfiguring lesions. These can be treated with a douche of 15% chloroform in light vegetable oil. A few drops of the mixture applied to an infested wound will cause the larvae to appear, and they can be removed with sinus forceps.

Several other species of this genus have been incriminated as facultative myiasis agents, usually in wounds, but their identification in both the larval and adult stage is difficult.

Ophthalmomyiasis is the presence of larvae in the orbit, and accessory glands of eye and eyeball. Infections may be quite common (10 per 100 000 population[114]) in some parts of the world (asiatic USSR, North Africa). Both obligatory and facultative parasites are involved. The commonest cause of ophthalmomyiasis is first stage larvae of the sheep nasal bot fly (*Oestrus ovis*) (Fig. III.67) which drop their eggs

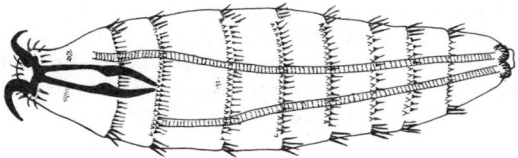

Fig. III.67 First instar larva of *Oestrus ovis* – a common cause of ophthalmomyiasis in North Africa.

into the orbit, rarely the mouth or outer ear. Typically patients report being struck in the eye by an insect or foreign object. Within a few hours a painful inflammation occurs, which may last for a few days as the larvae cannot develop any further in man. Occasionally larvae reach the nasal cavities (its natural habitat in sheep and goats) where they cause swelling and pain as well as frontal headache but do not live longer than 10 days. Other obligatory parasites of domestic animals, such as the horse bot fly (*Rhinoestrus purpureus* in southern and eastern Europe, Near East and North Africa), cattle warble flies (*Hypoderma*) and in parts of tropical Africa *Gedoelstia*, may affect man by invading the orbit and (especially in *Hypoderma*) penetrating the eyeball. Rarely, carcase breeding species such as *Lucilia serricata* cause myiasis of the

eye, but only when a pre-existing putrefying wound exists near the orbit, and this is therefore typical wound myiasis.

Myiasis of organ systems (Chapter 51)

In the majority of cases this is due to accidental 'parasitism'.

Intestinal myiasis

This type of myiasis is usually diagnosed from the presence of larvae in vomit or stools. Obligatory gut parasites of animals will not develop in man and therefore species which cause intestinal myiasis are facultative or accidental parasites. About fifty species have been recorded, but many cases of suspected gut myiasis have in fact been subsequent contamination of samples after collection, as some species (e.g. *Sarcophaga* spp.) can develop to the third larval stage in 24 hours, and others will lay larvae (larviposition) on faeces as they are being deposited. Occasionally previously contaminated collection vessels have been responsible for mistaken reports.

Larvae may be swallowed in contaminated food and pass through the gut unaffected by the extreme environment, e.g. *Piophila* (cheese skipper). However, this is unusual as most ingested larvae die and may be passed dead or, exceptionally, live if there is a concurrent gut infection. Even under these circumstances, larvae may cause intestinal lesions, damage to mucous membranes or haemorrhagic infiltrations, demonstrated by severe gastrointestinal disturbances (vomiting, diarrhoea, nausea). Reports that larvae develop in the anterior and median gut in man, and even become paedogenic, are highly doubtful.[115]

Flies which are normally attracted to faeces may, under particularly poor standards of hygiene, deposit their eggs on or near the anus and the larvae then penetrate into the posterior part of the rectum. Several authentic cases caused by *Eristalis* (Syrphidae), which commonly lives in sewage, have been reported.

Urogenital myiasis

There are no obligatory species, but facultative parasites may be excreted in the urine or found in the vagina. A mistaken diagnosis of urinary myiasis due to a larva from a contaminated vessel in which urine has been collected, or introduced into the urine after it has been passed, is not uncommon, but there have been cases in which the larvae have been undoubtedly passed via the urethra from the bladder. If the vulva or vagina is infested there are obvious opportunities for larvae to enter the bladder. The flies concerned are usually of the families Psychodidae, Muscidae, Calliphoridae and Sarcophagidae.

Collection and preservation of larvae

After removal of the larvae from the host by irrigation, manipulation or surgery the larvae should be killed in hot water to retain their overall shape. The posterior respiratory spiracles are an important means of identification. The spiracles can be seen under a high-power dissecting microscope, but it may be necessary to remove, macerate and slide mount them for detailed examination. Larvae should be preserved in 80%

alcohol. Identification of accidental or facultative parasites is often difficult, as many species can be involved. In contrast, the identification of obligate parasites is easier as fewer species are involved, although the superficial similarity of flies of widely separated genera makes it necessary to submit specimens for identification by a specialist whenever a precise identification is required. Identification is greatly eased if larvae are reared to adults on small pieces of meat. Smith[112] gives details for identification.

LICE

G. B. *White*

SUPERORDER: PHTHIRAPTERA

The Phthiraptera[116,117] are comprised of two orders: the Anoplura ('sucking lice') and the Mallophaga ('chewing lice'). Anoplura are parasitic only on mammals and feed on blood, whilst Mallophaga are found both on birds and mammals (though not on man) and feed on ectodermal detritus or blood.

Lice are obligate ectoparasites, requiring the environment of the host skin and underfur at all stages of the life-cycle. Though the insects may survive for a period if separated from the host (*Pediculus humanus* has been kept in vitro without food for 12 hours at 40°C and 10 days at 5°C) they rapidly become weakened and unable to establish on a fresh host. Infestation of host animals takes place during contact between host individuals.

The temperature requirements of lice keep them within a few millimetres of the skin of the host and hair further out from the skin is not utilized. The insulating properties of human clothing extend the region habitable by lice away from the body, which has enabled *Pediculus humanus* to become adapted in some ways to living on clothing.

The majority of lice are strictly host-specific and it is uncommon to find a species of louse parasitizing more than a single host species. As a consequence, though lice from domestic animals may be found on man, such infestations are unlikely to persist.

ORDER: ANOPLURA

The Anoplura ('sucking lice') are dorsoventrally compressed insects, generally under 5 mm in length. The species found on man, because of their lack of strongly sclerotized abdominal plates, are brownish-red or greyish in colour, with dark brown claws, thorax and head. The mouthparts are adapted for piercing and sucking; no jaws are present. The antennae are as long as or longer than the head and clearly visible. The legs are modified for grasping hair (Fig. III.68) and have only a single tarsal claw; the insects are capable of rapid movement through hair or over rough fabric, but are unable to move with ease on smooth surfaces.

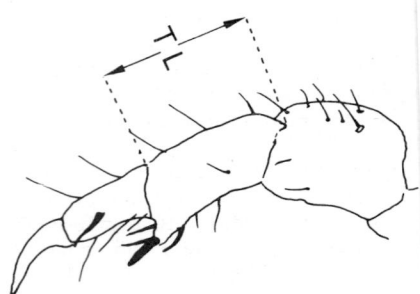

Fig. III.68   The second leg of *Pediculus*, showing the length of the tibia (TL). In *P. capitis*, TL = approx. 0.3 mm and in *P. humanus* TL = approx. 0.4 mm.

Wings are absent. The abdomen is divided into nine apparent segments, which in many species have undergone some fusion. In the lice found on man segmentation is not apparent because of the absence of tergal and sternal plates. Spiracles are mounted on prominent pleurites.

The eggs ('nits') are cemented to the hairs of the host by the female; almost invariably the egg is attached to a single hair, the only exception being *Pediculus humanus*, which may cement the egg to one or more fibres of clothing.

The eggs hatch to nymphs similar in appearance to the adults, which then undergo several moults to reach the adult stage; there is no resting (pupal) stage.

Three species of Anoplura are found on man: the body louse (*Pediculus humanus* Linnaeus),* the head louse (*Pediculus capitis* DeGeer)† and the crab or pubic louse (*Pthirus pubis* Linnaeus).‡ None of these has any other known host.

---

* Synonyms of *P. humanus* are: *P. albidior, P. chinensis, P. corporis, P. marginatus, P. nitritarum, P. nigrescens, P. tabescentium, P. vestementi.*
† Synonyms of *P. capitis* are: *P. americanus, P. angustus, P. cervicalis, P. humanus capitis, P. maculatus, P. pubescens.*
‡ Synonyms of *Pthirus pubis* are: *Pediculus pubis, Phthirus pubis, Pthirus inguinalis.*

Infestation by any of these species is a hygienic nuisance and may lead to medical conditions of greater or lesser severity. Irritation caused by bites may lead to scratching which in turn enlarges the wounds and increases the chance of fungal or bacterial infection of the skin; impetigo or a dermatitis may result. In laboratory experiments all three species have been demonstrated as potential vectors of rickettsial fevers and the two *Pediculus* species as potential vectors of relapsing fevers. Only *Pediculus humanus* has been incriminated as a vector in natural conditions.

FAMILY: PEDICULIDAE

GENUS: *Pediculus*

Species of *Pediculus* are parasitic on a number of primates; two very closely-related species are found on man. *Pediculus humanus* lives on the body, body hairs and clothes, *P. capitis* on the scalp and among scalp hairs.

Behavioural differences lead them to stay in their separate habitats, though occasionally accidental transfer may occur. The two species are morphologically similar (Fig. III.69); the head is round, with antennae of length equal to head width; the body is elongate-oval (though shape varies with states of nutrition and female reproduction) with no clear demarcation between thorax and abdomen; the head, thorax and pleura may be lightly or heavily sclerotized. The legs are all of similar size, each terminating in a long slender claw. The most reliable morphological distinction between the two species is in the tibial length of the middle (second) leg. This reflects a general difference in body size, the tibial length averaging about 0.30 mm in the smaller *P. capitis* compared with 0.40 mm in the larger *P. humanus* (Fig. III.68). Interbreeding of the two species is experimentally possible, but the infrequency of intermediate forms in natural populations indicates that hybridization does not often happen.

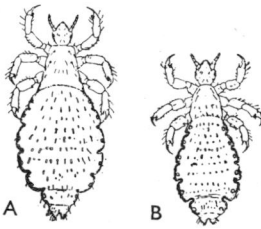

Fig. III.69 A, Female *Pediculus humanus*. B, Female *Pediculus capitis*.

P. capitis females cement the eggs to the bases of head hairs; growth of the hair may eventually bring the empty shells into view after the eggs have hatched. *P. humanus* females sometimes attach their eggs to human body hair, but more often the eggs are cemented to clothing fibres, usually along seams or folds in garments.

Reproduction and development are similar in the two species. The female lice produce an average of four or five eggs per day throughout their laying life, which may last up to a month; eggs are generally not laid on the first two or the last day of the female's adult life. The nymphs hatch in 8 days (at 32°C) and undergo three moults to become adult in a period of about 18 days. Nymphs and adult lice take blood meals two to five times per day throughout their lives.

Pediculus infestations are usually acquired through close contact with lousy persons, shared clothing or bedding. Lice tend to leave patients with fever or sweating, thus promoting spread of disease, and will leave a corpse as it becomes cold; lice also avoid light.

P. capitis is principally a hygienic nuisance, but occasionally infests in such numbers that severe dermatitis can result from scratching, treatment being rendered more difficult by the mass of dried blood and pus from the wounds. *P. humanus* is the vector of exanthematic typhus (*Rickettsia prowazeki*), trench fever (*R. quintana*) and European relapsing fever (*Spirochaeta* (= *Borrelia*) *recurrentis*). In addition, it can act as a vector of murine typhus (*R. prowazeki mooseri*) from man to man, and of relapsing fever (*Borrelia duttoni*).

FAMILY: PTHIRIDAE

GENUS: *Pthirus*

The third type of louse found exclusively on man is the crab or pubic louse, *Pthirus pubis* (Linnaeus) (Fig. III.70). This species is most commonly found in the genital and inguinal regions, but may be found on any of the body hair (not usually on the scalp), including beards, chest hair, eyelashes etc. *Pthirus* is shorter and broader than *Pediculus* and has massive claws on the second and third legs, by which it clings to hairs. Less is known of its biology than that of the other two human lice. The eggs are attached to hairs, never to clothing. The nymphs hatch in 7–8 days and after a period of about 13 days they become adult, having undergone three moults. The adult life-span is about a month. Crab lice are unable to survive off the host for more than about 24 hours. Transmission is usually

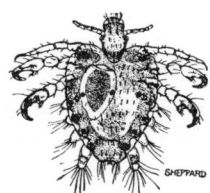

Fig. III.70 Female *Pthirus pubis*, showing the contained ovum. × 12.

through sexual or other close personal contact, but may occur through shared clothing. Infestation is normally noticed by irritation caused by the bites; sometimes a characteristic small 'blue spot' (2 or 3 mm across) may result from the bite, different from the red spot usually caused by the bites of pediculid lice. Crab lice are cosmopolitan in distribution, but are not known to transmit any disease.

FAMILY: HAEMATOPINIDAE

GENUS: *Haematopinus*

Haematopinus suis, the sucking louse of pigs, has been recorded as living on man, but such an infestation is unlikely to persist and has no medical significance.

FAMILY: POLYPLACIDAE

GENUS: *Polyplax*

Polyplax spinulosa, the sucking louse of rats, may act as a vector of murine typhus (*Rickettsia prowazeki mooseri*) between rats. This parasite is frequently found on laboratory animals.

ORDER: MALLOPHAGA

The Mallophaga ('chewing lice') are dorsoventrally compressed insects generally under 5 mm in length. Sclerotized abdominal plates give the lice a brownish coloration. The mouthparts are adapted for biting and chewing; jaws are present on the ventral surface of the head. The antennae are short and carried close to the head. The legs are modified for grasping hair or feathers; mammal lice have a single tarsal claw on each leg, bird lice two. Wings are absent. Only a single species, *Trichodectes canis*, is thought to have any medical significance.

FAMILY: TRICHODECTIDAE

GENUS: *Trichodectes*

Trichodectes canis, the chewing louse of dogs, acts as one of the larval hosts of the dog tapeworm, *Dipylidium caninum*, and may be responsible for occasional transmission to humans (although *T. canis* cannot live on man).

CONTROL OF LICE AND THE TREATMENT OF LOUSY PATIENTS

Pediculus. Destruction of the lice and eggs on clothes is most efficiently achieved by heating to 60°C for 30–40 minutes. For practical purposes, 70°C for 30 minutes is recommended. Particular attention should be paid to folds and pleats and the application of a hot iron to these is useful. Head lice may be treated by cutting the hair short and combing with a fine louse-comb, used with soft soap to remove nits. The most efficient comb of this type (Sacker patent) is now in short supply, but others are available, though for best effect they should be used in conjunction with chemical treatments. Chemical methods of control (both species) include applications of DDT or permethrin dusts, or malathion and other insecticides prepared as suitable lotions or shampoos that are commercially available. As insecticide resistance is becoming a problem in many areas, susceptibility tests should be made before widespread application of an insecticide. Such tests should be made on the target species. Resistance in one of the pediculids in a given area does not imply similar resistance in the other.

Pthirus. Chemical methods, as outlined above, are normally used for this species. Resistance to insecticides is not widespread.

CIMICID AND TRIATOMINE BUGS

D. M. Minter

ORDER: HEMIPTERA
SUBORDER: HETEROPTERA
FAMILY: CIMICIDAE

GENUS: *Cimex*

Bed bugs (*Cimex*) have a worldwide distribution with well over 70 species; all are wingless and dorsoventrally flattened. The species parasitic on man are *Cimex lectularius* (Fig. III.71), the cosmopolitan bed bug, and *C. hemipterus* (= *rotundatus*), the common bed bug of the tropics, which is distinguished by its elongated narrow abdomen and the shape and proportion of the thorax (Fig. III.71). In West Africa a species of another genus, *Leptocimex boueti*, attacks man. The body of *C. lectularius* is broad and flat, the head short and broad, attached to the thorax, the antennae four-jointed and the eyes present but

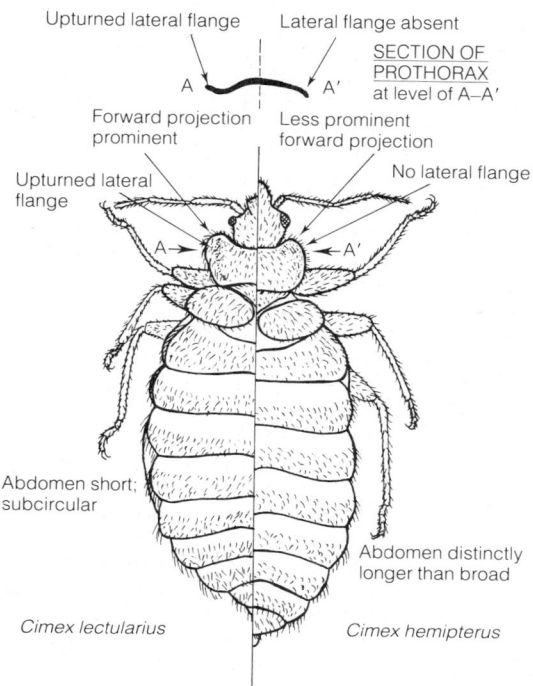

Upturned lateral flange
Lateral flange absent

SECTION OF
PROTHORAX
at level of A–A'

A ⎰ A'

Forward projection
prominent
Less prominent
forward projection

Upturned lateral
flange
No lateral flange

A→ ←A'

Abdomen short;
subcircular
Abdomen distinctly
longer than broad

Cimex lectularius
Cimex hemipterus

Fig. III.71 Comparison between *Cimex lectularius* (the common bed bug) (left) and *C. hemipterus* (the tropical bed bug) (right) when viewed from above.

reduced in size. The mouthparts consist externally of a segmented rostrum (proboscis) and are normally folded back under the head. The maxillae are serrated at the tip. On the thorax of the adults are short pad-like hemielytra, which are vestigial forewings. Both sexes of *Cimex* feed only on blood and can resist starvation well. The labium does not pierce the skin, but buckles up during feeding like that of a mosquito. The bodies of bugs give out a nasty pungent odour. Bed bugs are nocturnal in their feeding habits, hiding in crevices during the daytime. The eggs are ovoid and operculated and are cemented on to the surfaces of the crevices of woodwork in houses, beds, mattresses, behind pictures and in nail holes. Aggregations of bugs can be located by finding the black faeces round holes.

The females deposit eggs in daily batches from 10 to 50, totalling 200–500. The eggs are large, about 1 mm in diameter, yellowish-white and easily visible to the naked eye. The five successive nymphal stages resemble adults, but have no hemielytra; they mature in about six weeks if fed at each stage, but can resist starvation for up to two months. Under less favourable conditions, development may be protracted for six months or more. Adults may live for many months. Bed bugs are sensitive to high temperatures: even 37.8°C with a fairly high humidity will kill many. A cheap and effective control method is fumigation with sulphur. The dosage necessary varies from 0.34 to 0.74 kg/28 m³, with an exposure of at least 6 hours. Sulphur dioxide is cheap and, owing to its smell, free from hazard. It kills the active stages of the bug, but a few eggs may escape, and complete combustion must be assured.

Hydrocyanic acid fumigation is very effective, but dangerous, and has been largely superseded by the use of insecticides. 5% DDT emulsion, 0.5% HCH, 2% malathion, 0.5% diazinon or 0.5% dichlorvos are effective, particularly when combined with 0.1–0.2% pyrethrin (or synthetic pyrethroids, e.g. biores-methrin), which act as an irritant and cause bugs to leave their hiding places.

Though bed bugs can cause a great deal of irritation by their bites, it has not actually been proved that they disseminate disease, with the possible exception of viral hepatitis.

FAMILY: REDUVIIDAE
SUBFAMILY: TRIATOMINAE

Triatomine bugs are also known as 'cone-nose', 'kissing' or, erroneously, 'assassin' bugs; they have many local names in South America, including chipo (Venezuela), barbeiro (Brazil) and vinchuca (Argentina). The group includes more than 100 species, divided into five tribes and 14 genera (see Table III.12). Both sexes and the five nymphal stages feed solely on vertebrate blood. The triatomine bugs are one of more than 20 subfamilies of the family Reduviidae; all the

Table III.12 Haematophagous reduviidae: tribes and genera of the subfamily Triatominae (Jeannel, 1919), with numbers of the 114 species in each genus: the most important genera are shown in bold.

Tribe	Genus	Number of species	Tribe	Genus	Number of species
Alberproseniini:	*Alberprosenia*	1	Rhodniini:	*Psammolestes*	3
				Rhodnius	**12**
Bolboderini:	*Belminus*	4			
	Bolbodera	1	triatomini:	*Dipetalogaster*	1
	Parabelminus	2		*Eratyrus*	2
	Microtriatoma	2		*Linshcosteus*	5
				Panstrongylus	**13**
Cavernicolini:	*Cavernicola*	1		*Paratriatoma*	1
				Triatoma	**66**

other subfamilies are predators of other insects and are the true 'assassin' bugs. Many species of the predatory Reduviidae are, however, capable of inflicting a painful bite, usually in self-defence, but do not feed on blood. Many superficially resemble the haematophagous Triatominae but can be distinguished by the presence of a rostrum that is frequently curved and is always rigid and inflexible. The triatomines have a three-segmented rostrum that is always both straight and flexible; at rest it lies closely applied to the ventral aspect of the head and more or less parallel to it. Its extreme tip normally lies in a finely ridged stridulatory groove in the anteroventral part of the thorax. (The triatomine genera *Linshcosteus*, and *Cavernicola* are unusual in that they lack this sound-producing stridulatory mechanism, in which the tip of the rostrum acts as a plectrum.)

The outer and visible part of the rostrum is the modified labium, which forms a protective sheath for the paired stylet-like mandibles and maxillae. During the act of feeding the rostrum is swung forward (about 120°) in front of the head and is neither flexed nor telescoped; the tip of the labium rests on the surface of the skin and the apically serrate mandibles penetrate the epidermis and anchor the mouthparts in place. The smooth lanceolate maxillary stylets then penetrate deeply and perforate small blood capillaries. The maxillae enclose the salivary duct and the food canal and form the functional mouth. The bite of triatomines is generally painless but by no means always. This explains why sleeping people are seldom awoken by the bite of bugs and can be bitten repeatedly in the course of the night.

In common with other Heteroptera, the adult triatomines have two pairs of functional wings; the forewings are hardened basally (the corium and clavus) and membranous distally. Thus they are referred to as hemielytra. The posterior wings are membranous throughout and lie beneath the hemielytra at rest. The wings are folded scissor-like over the back of the bug and the lateral margins of the abdominal tergites are visible; these are often colour-banded and are a useful taxonomic feature. Female bugs, viewed from above have a broad ovate abdomen which is generally pointed posteriorly; males have a more slender abdomen with a fully rounded posterior end. The plate-like male external genitalia can easily be seen in lateral and ventral view. Female bugs are generally rather larger than males.

The visible dorsal part of the thorax consists of a large trapezoidal pronotum, usually rigid and provided with tubercles. Behind the pronotum and visible between the sclerotized bases of the hemielytra, is a triangular scutellum, strongly pointed posteriorly. The ground colour of the triatomines is usually brownish or black, often relieved with flashes of colour (mainly shades of red, yellow or orange) on thorax and abdomen. Eyes are usually black, but white- or pink-eyed mutants are not uncommon. Adults, unlike all nymphal stages, have paired dorsal ocelli posterior to the prominent compound eyes.

The proportions of the head in lateral view are useful to separate the three genera of main medical importance (Fig. III.72). The head of *Rhodnius* is elongated with long four-jointed antennae arising close to its apical portion. In *Triatoma* the head is

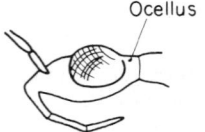

Ocellus

Insect-predatory reduviid
Proboscis curved (mainly)
and rigid

Haematophagous members (Triatominae):
Proboscis straight and flexible

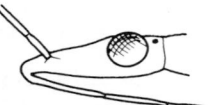

Rhodnius
Head long
Antennae forward
Examples: *R. prolixus,*
          R. pallescens

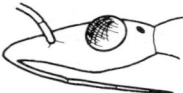

Triatoma
Head medium length
Antennae median
Examples: *T. infestans,*
          T. dimidiata

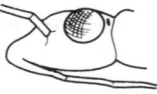

Panstrongylus
Head short
Antennae close to eye
Example: *P. megistus*

Fig. III.72   Lateral view of the head of an insect-predatory reduviid (top) with usually *curved* and always *inflexible* proboscis which serves to distinguish it from the haematophagous genera of the subfamily Triatominae, all of which have a proboscis which is *straight* and *flexible* (bottom row). The proportions of the head and the site of insertion of the antennae serve to separate members of the triatomine genera *Rhodnius*, *Triatoma* and *Panstrongylus*.

shorter and the antennae are inserted midway between the eye and the forward tip of the head. In the genus *Panstrongylus* the head is stouter and shorter, with the antennae arising close to the eye. See also Figs. III.73–75.

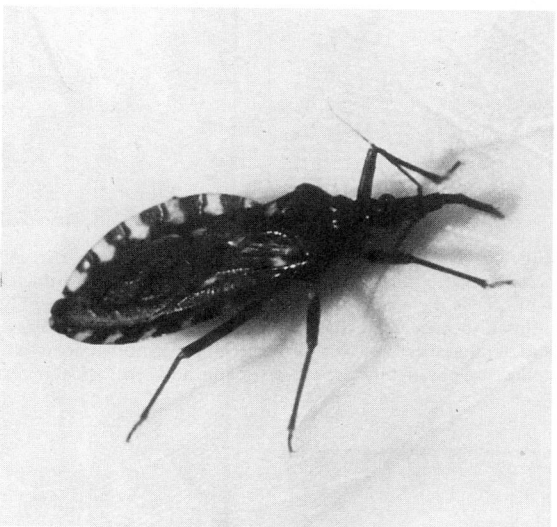

Fig. III.73 Genus *Triatoma*. Head of intermediate length, with antennae set midway between eyes and front of head. The specimen illustrated is a female *Triatoma infestans*, with its proboscis directed forwards whilst feeding. The ground colour is black with yellowish markings on the lateral edges of the abdomen, legs and hemielytra. Males are 21–26 mm long; females 26–29 mm. Nymphal stages lack the coloration seen in the adults. (Courtesy Dr T.V. Barrett.)

The five nymphal stages are essentially miniatures of the adult but lack wings; in the fifth nymphal stage the 'wing pads' are prominent on either side of the scutellum. Triatomines are generally quite large insects, usually between 20 and 28 mm long in the adult female. Some genera contain species that are only about 5 mm long as adults and the Mexican *Dipetalogaster maxima* is the giant of the triatomines, attaining a length of nearly 4.5 cm. Lent and Wygodzinsky[118] give comprehensive keys to genera and species.

Reproduction and life-cycle

Female triatomines commence laying eggs 10–30 days after copulation; eggs are laid singly or in small groups, either unattached or cemented to the substrate, depending on species. The ovoid, operculate fresh eggs are whitish; in some species they later turn through pink to cherry-red; in other species the original colour is maintained. The number of eggs laid by a female in her life depends upon species and external factors but about 500 is normal and 1000 not uncom-

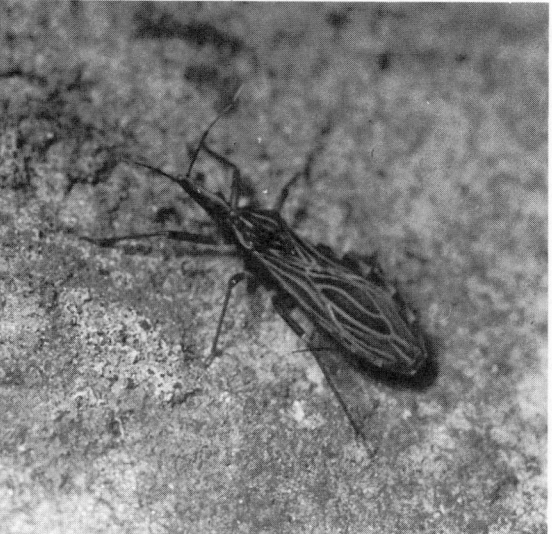

Fig. III.74 Genus *Rhodnius*. Head long, antennae set well forward. The specimen shown is an adult male *Rhodnius prolixus;* males are generally less than 20 mm in length, females up to 21.5 mm. General colour pale brown; lighter markings on thorax and forewings give the overall impression of longitudinal stripes. Nymphal stages have less obvious 'pepper and salt' markings. (Courtesy C.J. Webb.)

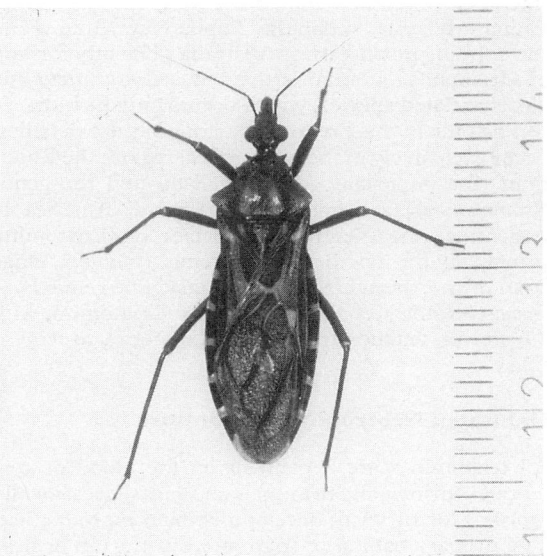

Fig. III.75 Genus *Panstrongylus*. Head short, with antennae set close to the eye. The male *Panstrongylus megistus* illustrated is black in overall colour with red, or reddish-brown, markings on the lateral margins of the abdomen, the thoracic pronotum, and scutellum and the hemielytra (forewings). The nymphal stages lack the prominent coloration of the adults. The specimen shown measures 25 mm; females are slightly larger.

mon. Virgin females will also lay eggs but these are few in number and infertile. Eggs hatch after 10–30 days; the emerging first stage nymph is at first pink and soft-bodied but hardens sufficiently to take its first blood meal within 48–72 hours of leaving the egg. At least one full blood meal is required by each nymphal stage, sometimes more, before the moult to the next stage can be initiated.

All triatomines have a long life-cycle, even in hot climates; the average is about 300 days from egg to adult, though some species may take up to two years. *Rhodnius* spp. develop more rapidly than *Triatoma* and *Panstrongylus* and can reach maturity in three to four months.

Geographical distribution

The five tribes occur in tropical and subtropical areas of the Neotropical region. Members of one tribe, the Triatomini, have species which are also found in the Oriental region. The Triatomini also marginally enter the Australasian region. The subfamily is entirely absent from the Palaearctic and Afrotropical (= Ethiopian) regions but *T. rubrofasciata* has been spread to all the major tropical ports by human agency. This species is always closely associated with *Rattus* spp., among which it transmits the rat trypanosome *Trypanosoma (Megatrypanum) conorhini*. Other endemic, and purely sylvatic, species of the tribe Triatomini (members of the *T. rubrofasciata* group) occur in south China, Malaysia, Indonesia, Papua New Guinea and the extreme north-east of Australia. The other group of Oriental Triatomini is the genus *Linshcosteus* (six closely related species) which occurs only in India.

The bulk of the Triatominae (four of the five tribes) occur exclusively in the Neotropical region: the Rhodniini (the important genus *Rhodnius* and the genus *Psammolestes*) are found from Central America to Argentina; the Neotropical species of Triatomini, principally the members of the genus *Triatoma*, range from the northern USA to Patagonia. The genus *Panstrongylus*, the second largest in the Triatomini, with 13 species, extends from Central America to Argentina.

Habitat of Neotropical triatomines

All triatomines are dependent on the blood of vertebrates (principally mammals and birds, occasionally reptiles) for survival, development and reproduction. The primary habitat of triatomines is thus in or near the shelters, roosts, burrows and nests of a variety of wild animals, prominent among which are marsupials (e.g. *Didelphis* (Fig. III.76), *Marmosa*), edentates (e.g. *Dasypus*), rodents (*Rattus*, *Neotoma*), carnivores, bats and birds. Many of the animals and birds find their main shelter in palm fronds or in arboreal epiphytic bromeliads (Fig. III.77), under fallen logs or in hollow trees. Triatomines also occur under rocks, under loose

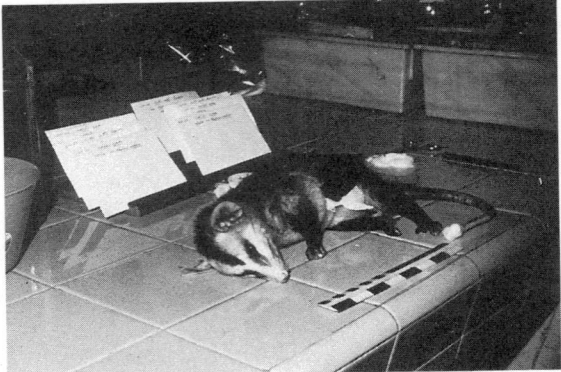

Fig. III.76 The common opossum, *Didelphis* sp., the cat-sized sylvatic marsupial most frequently naturally infected with *Trypanosoma cruzi* throughout the Americas. The animal shown is *D. albiventris* (= *D. azarae*) from Brazil and is anaesthetized whilst undergoing xenodiagnosis and collection of tail-blood for microscopic and serological investigation.

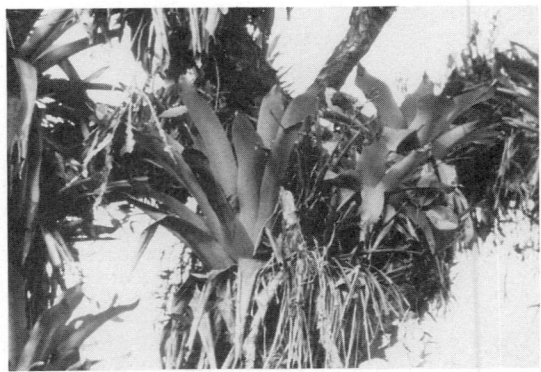

Fig. III.77 Arboreal epiphytic bromeliads (commonly species of the genera *Aechmea* and *Holmbergia*) are frequently the nesting habitat of marsupials, rodents and birds and are thus also a natural biotope of many sylvatic triatomine species.

bark and in stone walls and feed on the local rodents or lizards.

A number of triatomine species have the ability to colonize the artificial habitats created by man. Some species seldom penetrate further than the peridomestic area: stables, cattle enclosures, chicken houses, pig sties, etc., which provide a rich food source. A relatively few species are able to colonize the extensive crevice habitat which is provided by the simple homes of the Latin American peasant majority. These houses are usually constructed of mud and wattle or unplastered adobe brick and roofed with palm fronds (Fig. III.78). More sophisticated houses with smooth plastered walls and roofs of tile or corrugated sheet are less readily and heavily colonized,

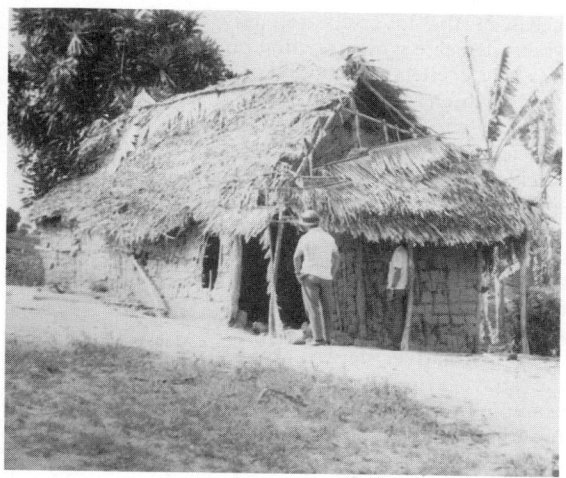

Fig. III.78 A characteristic palm-thatched, mud-and-wattle Latin American peasant house of the type often infested with domiciliary triatomine species. The deep cracks in the mud walls provide ideal harbourage for large populations of *Rhodnius*, *Triatoma* or *Panstrongylus*.

often being very lightly infested or not at all. The more traditional and basic peasant house, made of local materials, may support a triatomine population that can run into thousands, particularly of *Rhodnius prolixus* or *Triatoma infestans*.

Although probably all triatomines will support the development of *Trypanosoma cruzi* (well over half the species have been found infected in the wild), it is only the relatively few species that have the capacity to colonize human dwellings which are of overriding medical importance as the domiciliary vectors of Chagas' disease to man. By virtue of their wide geographical distribution and large domiciliary populations, together with the large human population in the areas they occupy, the three species *Rhodnius prolixus*, *Triatoma infestans* and *Panstrongylus megistus* are of prime importance. Other species of the same three genera (particularly *Triatoma* spp. and especially *T. dimidiata*) are of considerable importance on a lesser geographical scale (e.g. *T. dimidiata*, *T. barberi*, *T. brasiliensis*, *T. pallidipennis*, *T. phyllosoma*, *R. pallescens* and *R. ecuadorensis*).

It is possible to divide the triatomines into convenient groups based on their association, or lack of it, with human dwellings.

Most species are fully sylvatic: a few species as flying adults are attracted by light and enter houses (when they may occasionally bite) but seem unable to colonize: an example is the geographically widespread *Panstrongylus geniculatus*, normally closely associated with the burrows of its usual host, the armadillo (*Dasypus* spp.). Others, such as *Triatoma brasiliensis*, are attracted by lights into houses and may establish small domiciliary or peridomestic populations.

Species such as the Central American *Triatoma dimidiata* live normally in hollow trees but are often passively transported to houses (in firewood) and form large colonies. *Triatoma sordida* is found naturally in a variety of habitats in the central and southern parts of South America, including crevices among tree bark; it readily adapts to fence-posts and timber outbuildings but never forms large domiciliary populations. This may be because it is regularly found in houses together with heavy infestations of *Triatoma infestans;* in Venezuela and elsewhere in northern South America, *T. maculata* is in a somewhat similar situation when small populations are established in houses among heavy infestations of *R. prolixus*. Both *T. sordida* and *T. maculata* may have the potential to form epidemiologically significant domiciliary populations if and when the major domiciliary species are controlled or eradicated by insecticidal treatment. Much the same happened in southern Brazil when *T. infestans* was controlled by insecticides and within a few years large numbers of *Panstrongylus megistus* (until then a purely sylvatic species in that area) had replaced it as the domiciliary vector of *Trypanosoma cruzi*.

Within human habitations, triatomines prefer to hide during the day in dark and moist places; the extensive crevice habitat provided by unplastered cracked walls of mud or mud-brick can support large populations. Smaller numbers are found among furniture, boxes and, particularly, beds and bedding. Others occur among clothes hanging from pegs in the walls, or behind pictures (Fig. III.79). Some species also readily colonize palm roofs (e.g. *R. prolixus*). Other species are rarely found in the roof (e.g. *P. megistus*).

Most frequently, bugs are found by day close to the areas in which they will encounter sleeping hosts at night—bedrooms are normally the most heavily

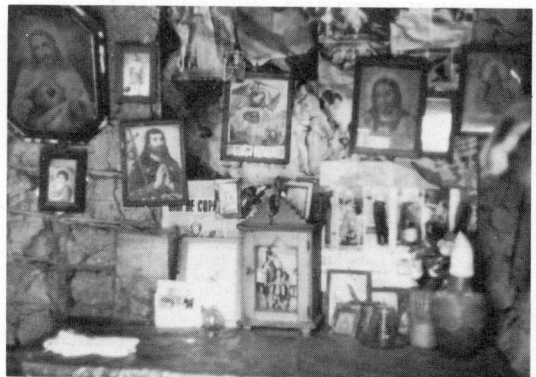

Fig. III.79 Many peasant homes incorporate a domestic shrine such as that shown here; a central case houses the family saints and the walls nearby are covered with pictures both sacred and profane. Sites such as these are often the principal hiding place for bugs not located in the bedroom walls and furniture.

infested parts of the house. As a rule, feeding behaviour of domiciliary triatomines is governed more by proximity to a suitable host than by specific host preference.

Some entirely or essentially sylvatic species, however, are normally associated with particular hosts: *Cavernicola pilosa* is always associated with bats and all three species of *Psammolestes*, *T. platensis* and *T. delpontei* are found only in the nests of birds. *P. geniculatus* has a close link with burrows of armadillos: *Paratriatoma hirsuta* and species of the *T. protracta* group prey exclusively on *Neotoma* spp., the wood rat (although adults not infrequently fly into houses, attracted by lights, they never colonize; perhaps this is in some way connected with their dependence on wood rats).

All stages of triatomines, in particular the larger nymphal stages, have a remarkable ability to endure long periods of starvation (up to several months). The adults are in general poor fliers and probably take flight only when their nutritional status is poor and their weight lowest, to disperse at random to seek new habitats with new hosts on which to feed. For domiciliary species in particular, passive transport by human agency is probably responsible for nearly all house-to-house dispersal, on or in domestic goods including furniture and clothes. Triatomines of various species have been recovered from the baggage of passengers on long-distance buses and lorries and occasionally even in aircraft. Some species of *Rhodnius* may be transported long distances as young nymphs, or as eggs, in the feathers of large migratory birds (*Jabiru mycteria* (jabiru) and *Mycteria americana* (American Wood Ibis)) when these leave their nests, in which bugs live and breed, on seasonal migration.

The role of triatomines as vectors of *Trypanosoma cruzi* and *Trypanosoma rangeli*

Other blood-sucking arthropods can be experimentally infected with *Trypanosoma cruzi* but only triatomines are important in the epizootiology and epidemiology of Chagas' disease (and of the less important apathogenic trypanosome affecting man in the Neotropical regions, *Trypanosoma* (*Herpetosoma*) *rangeli*). Chagas' disease is a zoonosis and probably all triatomines are potential vectors of *Trypanosoma cruzi*, but *Trypanosoma rangeli* is naturally infective only to species of the genus *Rhodnius* (mainly *R. prolixus*, but also *R. pallescens* and *R. ecuadorensis*); although species of *Triatoma* can be experimentally infected with *Trypanosoma rangeli*, they are rarely infected in the wild. So far as the importance of triatomine species in transmission of *Trypanosoma cruzi* to man is concerned, only a relatively few species of bugs are actual and effective vectors.

Because of the contaminative (and hence inefficient) method of transmission of *Trypanosoma cruzi* in the faeces of the invertebrate, only those bug species which defecate whilst feeding on the human host are able to be effective vectors. Further, only in those species which are capable of colonizing houses in large numbers and feeding predominantly from man, and to a lesser extent his household animals (cats, dogs, chickens, etc.), is contaminative transmission sufficiently intense to lead to a high probability of successful infection among householders, given a high infection rate among the triatomine population. For a domiciliary vector to be of major epidemiological importance, it is also necessary for it to have a wide geographical range.

Of the relatively few triatomine species which fulfil the above criteria, *T. infestans* is the outstanding example in view of its wide occurrence in South America (from 10° north to 40° south and from Atlantic to Pacific coasts). In this extensive area it is almost exclusively a domiciliary species and the geographical range has often been extended by passive movement due to human agency. It is an aggressive and active species with a relatively short life-cycle, which helps it to compete successfully with other longer-lived species (such as *P. megistus*) that are also domicilary and which *T. infestans* tends to displace if accidentally introduced.

There are no domiciliary triatomine species in the broad expanse of the Amazon basin but to the north of this area *Rhodnius prolixus* is the main species of epidemiological importance; it is found predominantly from about 3° north (Colombia, Venezuela, the Guyanas) from sea level to an altitude of over 2000 m, and ranges to about 20° north in Mexico. It is the major domiciliary vector of Chagas' disease in Colombia and Venezuela and is one of several important species in Central America. Throughout its range it is also the main vector of *Trypanosoma rangeli* to wild and domestic animals as well as to man. Unlike *T. infestans*, it has an extensive extradomiciliary biotope; particularly important is its frequent occurrence in species of palm trees (where it is found in the nests of mammals and birds) that are frequently used as roofing materials for houses. Among the palms infested the genera *Attalea* and *Acrocomia* are widespread and numerous (Fig. IIII.80). *R. prolixus* also occurs in the palms *Copernica* and *Leopoldina*.

In the densely populated areas of the eastern seaboard of Brazil, *Panstrongylus megistus* is the important domiciliary triatomine; in the southern part of its range it also occurs in sylvatic foci, but further north it is confined to houses, perhaps because the almost total destruction of the original coastal forest vegetation in this area, over the past four centuries, has rendered conditions unsuitable for its survival in the wild. Alternatively, *P. megistus* may have been passively transported from south to north by human agency, but for various reasons this explanation seems less likely.

T. dimidiata is a highly variable species in color-

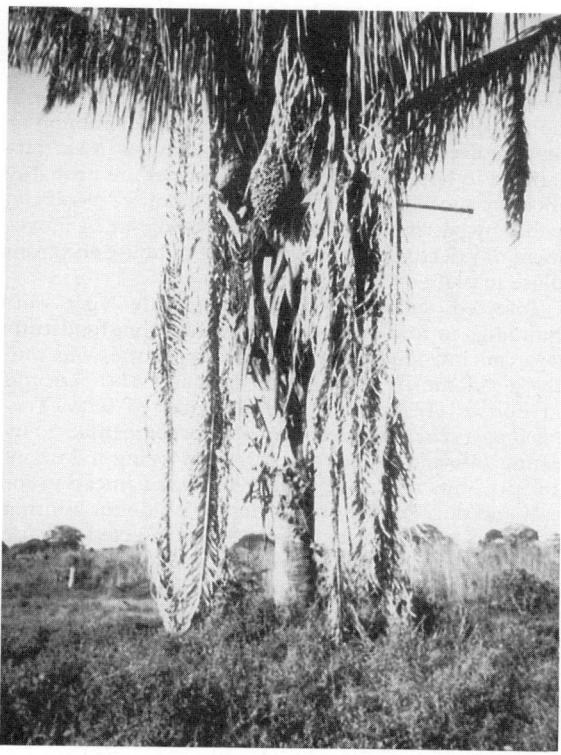

Fig. III.80 Palm tree (*Attalea humboldtiana*), sylvatic habitat of *Rhodnius prolixus* in Venezuela. Several genera and species of palm trees are a principal habitat of many triatomine species throughout Latin America, associated with the nests of various mammals and birds which inhabit the crowns and dependent fronds.

ation, etc. and was until recently divided into three subspecies (*T. d. dimidiata*, *T. d. maculipennis* and *T. d. capitata*) which are no longer recognized. The species is an important domiciliary vector in Ecuador, Peru and Central America as far as 22° north in Mexico.

The northern limit of domiciliated triatomines, and hence essentially that of human Chagas' disease, is to all intents and purposes the tropic of Cancer: isolated cases have occurred in Texas and elsewhere in the southern USA, but none of the several sylvatic triatomines present have become domiciliated, although some are natural vectors of *Trypanosoma cruzi* in wood rat colonies. Housing standards in the areas of the USA where bugs naturally occur are such that colonization by triatomines is in any event unlikely.

Feeding behaviour of triatomines

All triatomines take large blood meals relative to their own body weight; the actual quantity varies greatly from stage to stage and from species to species; the larger bugs obviously take larger quantities.

The first stage nymphs at their first feed take up ten times their own body weight; successive stages take progressively less in terms of body weight, but more in actual quantity. In volumetric terms the fifth stage nymphs take the largest feed; this represents about three to four times their body weight. Adult bugs of both sexes take less blood than the fifth stage, but feed more often; on each occasion about two or three times their own body weight.

Blood meal identifications have been made by precipitin tests and other methods for many species of bugs in different geographical areas and variously from sylvatic, peridomestic and domestic ecotopes. In general terms, the results show that sylvatic species in the wild feed primarily on marsupials (especially the common opossums, *Didelphis* spp.), rodents, birds and edentates (e.g. armadillos, *Dasypus* sp.), bats and occasionally reptiles and amphibians.

Domiciliary bug populations, however, always feed predominantly upon man. Often, the domestic host fed upon most frequently after man is the epidemiologically unimportant chicken (birds are not susceptible to *Trypanosoma cruzi* infection).

Different species of important domiciliary vectors may either feed frequently on cats and/or dogs (e.g. *T. infestans*, *T. dimidiata*) or feed infrequently from these hosts (e.g. *R. prolixus*, *P. megistus*). In the case of *T. infestans* and *T. dimidiata*, cats and/or dogs are important domestic reservoirs for Chagas' disease, since infected animals are a perpetual source of *Trypanosoma cruzi* and bugs become infected by feeding on them. Neither *R. prolixus* nor *P. megistus* in houses feed on cats or dogs to any significant extent and these animals, even if infected, thus provide little or no feedback of trypanosomes into the domestic bug population and are thus an epidemiological dead end.

The species of domiciliary bugs so far investigated differ in the frequency with which blood from different hosts can be detected in the same individual triatomine. Since blood proteins are detectable in bugs for up to 100–120 days, the occurrence of many individual meals of mixed origin in a bug population suggests that the bugs are frequently changing from one type of host to the other; a low frequency of multiple blood meals indicates that individuals are feeding repeatedly from the same host species. A high rate of feeds on man, combined with a low rate of feeds from other sources, especially of mixed feeds, clearly indicates that bug-mediated transmission occurs from man to man, rather than from animals to man. This is the situation found with domiciliary *R. prolixus* and *P. megistus*, in Venezuela and Brazil respectively. Domestic populations of *T. maculata* (in Venezuela) and *T. sordida* (in Brazil) feed predominantly from the uninfectable chicken; these species are therefore of very little epidemiological importance in the domestic transmission cycle.

Triatomines can become infected with *Trypanosoma cruzi* (and/or *Trypanosoma rangeli*) at any stage in their life from their first feed onward. Once infected with *Trypanosoma cruzi*, the infection probably almost always persists for life; infection rates found in different stages rise from a small percentage in the first stage nymphs to levels approaching or exceeding 90% among fifth stage nymphs and adults. Bugs appear in no way adversely affected by infection with *Trypanosoma cruzi*. Unlike *Trypanosoma cruzi*, however, *Trypanosoma rangeli* is pathogenic to its invertebrate hosts and causes a disturbance in the moulting mechanism, such that the moult is delayed and mortality during moulting is significantly increased. In adult bugs infected with *Trypanosoma rangeli*, there is also a reduction in the number of eggs laid by females and a decrease in egg viability.

Since, particularly where *R. prolixus* is the domiciliary vector, mixed infections of bugs, animals and man by *Trypanosoma cruzi* and *Trypanosoma rangeli* are common, it is frequently necessary to distinguish the two parasites, in both vertebrate and invertebrate hosts. The bloodstream stages are easily separable by their distinctive morphology; the stages in the bug can be less readily distinguished, except when trypomastigotes occur in the haemolymph and salivary glands (always *Trypanosoma rangeli*). Infective forms of *Trypanosoma rangeli* and *Trypanosoma cruzi* in the recta of bugs are difficult to separate without recourse to animal inoculation and study of the bloodstream stages. *Trypanosoma rangeli* can certainly be transmitted to vertebrates and man by the inoculative route when trypomastigotes occur in the salivary glands. There is controversy, however, as to whether contaminative infection by *Trypanosoma rangeli* (via trypomastigote forms shed in the faeces) occurs to any significant extent, or at all (see also Appendix I, p. 1292).

Transmission cycles of *Trypanosoma cruzi*

The possible cycles and their interrelationship, in bug-mediated *Trypanosoma cruzi* infections of animals and man are summarized in Fig. III.81. Zoonotic cycles involve the majority of the 114 triatomine species currently recognized and some 120 species and subspecies of mammals. Foremost among the mammal hosts closely associated with sylvatic triatomines, and therefore frequently infected with *Trypanosoma cruzi*, are the marsupials of several genera, particularly *Didelphis* spp., which occupy a range that is more than coextensive with that of *Trypanosoma cruzi*. *Didelphis* spp. play a role in the epizootiology and epidemiology of *Trypanosoma cruzi* that is in some respects reminiscent of that of the bushbuck in the case of *Trypanozoon* trypanosomes in eastern Africa. The cat-sized *Didelphis* (Fig. III.76) are carnivorous and nocturnal and are among the last wild animals to be disturbed by human activities. They frequently enter houses and outbuildings to search for food, steal eggs, etc. and often roost in the roofs of houses or in trees

near by. They are thus well placed to introduce sylvatic *Trypanosoma cruzi* strains into the peridomestic and domestic environments. Sylvatic triatomines, already infected with *Trypanosoma cruzi*, may fly into houses or be carried in on palm fronds for roofing or among firewood. Strains of *Trypanosoma cruzi* circulated in houses by domiciliary species are probably most frequently transferred between houses passively, either by passive transfer of infected bugs or by movement of infected people from house to house and from place to place.

Infected sylvatic rodents frequently visit outbuildings to feed on stored grain and other foodstuffs and can introduce new parasites from the wild into the peridomestic area. *Rattus* spp. and *Mus musculus* in houses are not infrequently infected with *Trypanosoma cruzi*, but they probably become infected by eating infected bugs, rather than by being fed upon. In turn, rats and mice form a source of infection for cats and dogs by the oral route and no doubt hunting dogs and foraging cats frequently eat infected sylvatic animals. It should again be emphasized, however, that neither sylvatic nor domestic birds are ever a source of *Trypanosoma cruzi*, since they are totally insusceptible to infection, possibly owing in part to their higher body temperature, among other factors. The role of cats and dogs within the domestic cycle has been discussed earlier in relation to the feeding behaviour of domiciliary triatomines. The role of infected rats and mice in houses can be assessed in a similar way and, from available evidence, it would seem that they are rarely of direct importance in the household epidemiology of Chagas' disease. Although the larger domestic animals, such as pigs, are susceptible to *Trypanosoma cruzi* and are sometimes fed upon by peridomestic/domestic triatomines (e.g. *T. infestans, P. megistus, T. dimidiata*), it is noteworthy that natural infections have been found only very rarely in pigs, rabbits or other larger domestic animals, which thus appear to play no significant role in the transmission of the parasite or in its transfer from sylvatic to peridomestic circumstances.

Once domiciliary transmission is established in the presence of large bug populations, transmission of *Trypanosoma cruzi* is chiefly man-bug-man and new human infections can occur among uninfected family members at a relatively high rate; among two families (20 persons) living in bug-infected premises in Brazil which were followed by serology and xenodiagnosis for four years, four new parasitologically confirmed infections occurred (a rate of 4% per annum); if two individuals with conversion to positive serology (but negative to xenodiagnosis on a single occasion) were included, the annual rate of new infections was 7.5%.

Because the contaminative method of transmission of *Trypanosoma cruzi* by bugs is inherently an inefficient mechanism, a heavy trypanosome challenge over a long period from biting and defaecating bugs is probably necessary for infection to occur. This is

TRANSMISSION CYCLES OF TRYPANOSOMA CRUZI

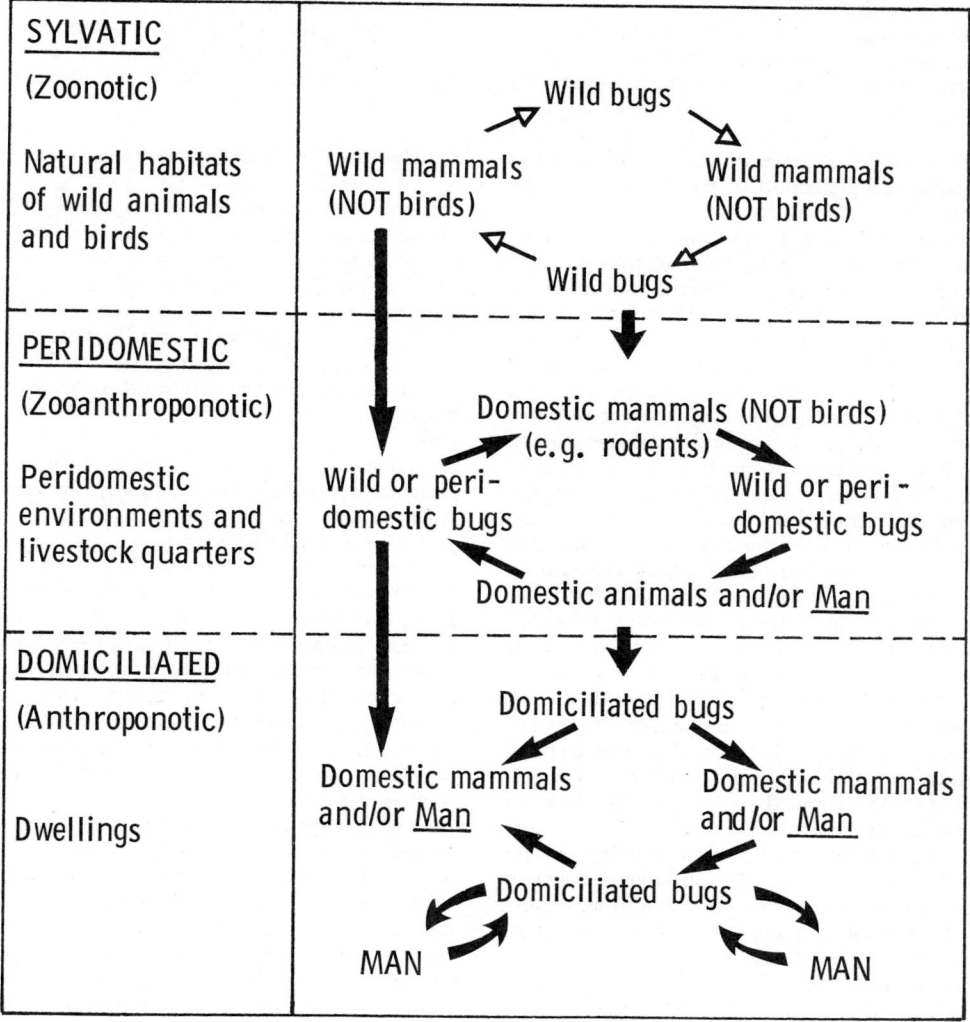

Fig. III.81 Transmission cycles of bug-mediated *Trypanosoma cruzi* infections.

probably linked with the fact that young children are seldom infected (except congenitally or via the maternal milk) until they are between two and three years of age, even under conditions of heavy challenge. Rates of infection among children are already high, however, among five- to 10-year-olds and rise further in later age groups.

Xenodiagnosis

The parasitological diagnosis of *Trypanosoma cruzi* infection suggestive of present or future chagasic symptomatology can be made by conventional blood film microscopy only in the initial febrile stage of acute onset, which many infected individuals fail to experience. In the later chronic indeterminate stage of the disease, parasitological diagnosis becomes increasingly difficult, since the parasitaemia falls below the level at which it can be detected by routine methods, including standard concentration techniques. It has been shown that haemoculture is a sensitive diagnostic technique but since only immotile amastigote stages may develop in cultures initially, much skill and experience are required to detect positive cultures in the first weeks, sometimes months, for which they need to be examined until the motile stages appear in sufficient number. The method of haemoculture is also difficult to use in the field.

If triatomine bugs are grown in laboratory culture under conditions which preclude the possibility of their infection with pathogenic organisms (in Latin America this is usually ensured by feeding them on pigeons or chickens), then allowed to feed in sufficient numbers on individuals suspected to be infected with *Trypanosoma cruzi*, kept for several weeks (usually about four) and then examined for the presence of *Trypanosoma cruzi* in their recta, this will often result in the unequivocal detection of parasites and is the process termed xenodiagnosis; the triatomines act as a 'living culture' for the trypanosomes. This technique is expensive, unaesthetic and time-consuming, but it is effective and has the great advantage that it can be used under field conditions. Technical details (number of bugs, species and stage) vary from one laboratory or hospital to another, as does the method of examination of the bugs used (expression of a faecal drop, dissection and examination of the entire rectal contents of the individual or pooling and maceration of batches of bugs) and there is much need for increased standardization. There is clear evidence from several sources that local 'strains' of vectors are generally most susceptible to infection by the local parasite and that microscopical examination of the rectal contents of individual bugs is more sensitive than the expressed faecal drop or pooling methods; the latter, however, are often adopted for routine purposes because they save time and effort. Whenever possible it is advantageous to use fifth stage nymphs in xenodiagnosis, since these take the largest feed and increase the possibility that a low parasitaemia can be detected. In practice, a minimum number of bugs to use would be five fifth stage nymphs allowed to feed in the dark for about 30 minutes in a secure gauze-covered container; 10 or 20 bugs would be preferable but not always possible for logistic reasons. Repeated xenodiagnosis on several occasions also increases the number of successful diagnoses. On an experimental basis, the 'smaller' instars of the very large *Dipetalogaster maxima* gave results comparable with those with fifth stage nymphs of the main 'standard' xenodiagnosis species (*R. prolixus* and *T. infestans*), with a saving of time and expense on colony maintenance. Artificial xenodiagnosis' is now widely used in Venezuela, in which bugs feed through a membrane on venous blood drawn from the patient. This is claimed to be more acceptable and equally successful as conventional xenodiagnosis.

Xenodiagnosis clearly has many disadvantages and a better and more effective method of parasitological diagnosis is obviously desirable, as a back-up for the increasingly improved serological tests now available. Serological tests, by their nature, detect antibodies to parasite antigen rather than the parasites themselves.

Not only are triatomines the principal means by which people become infected with *Trypanosoma cruzi* (and *Trypanosoma rangeli*), but bugs build up large domiciliary populations and these are a significant source of blood loss in many households. Calculations show that, in houses in Venezuela with heavy infestations of *R. prolixus*, monthly blood loss was in the order of 100 cm³ per person per month. Occasionally individuals become sensitized to bug bites and may suffer severe allergic reactions as a result. This phenomenon may also be a complicating factor in xenodiagnosis.

Control of domiciliary triatomines

Roughly the same number of people, about 250 million in each case, live in countries affected by African trypanosomiasis and in areas of Latin America affected by Chagas' disease. In Africa there are often fewer than 5000 new (treatable) infections annually. In Latin America, for diagnostic and logistic reasons, the number of new (and essentially incurable) cases each year is unknown, but crude estimates suggest up to 850 000 new infections per annum. At any one time, about 24 million people are seropositive for *Trypanosoma cruzi* and a further 65 million at risk in endemic areas. Serological surveys in various countries indicate that between 5% and 10% of national populations are infected.

The magnitude of the problem which such figures indicate is immense. Unlike sleeping sickness, there is no safe and effective chemotherapy, and diagnosis of Chagas' disease is more difficult; early case detection and treatment are therefore of little value. Ultimately may come the development of an effective vaccine; meanwhile, improvements in standards of new and existing houses (in the latter case, particularly by individual or community-based self-help measures), and increased public health awareness in general, would help to diminish transmission levels to a considerable degree, but alone are probably insufficient to achieve interruption of disease transmission.

Only the larger and more affluent of the Latin American countries (notably Argentina, Venezuela and Brazil) have long recognized Chagas' disease as a public health problem and have resources sufficient to undertake extensive insecticidal vector control campaigns. Other countries (Mexico, Colombia and Bolivia are examples) have more recently realized the importance of Chagas' disease as a national public health problem, but as yet lack the means to tackle it adequately, if at all. In some countries the problem is not officially recognized and its importance has yet to be assessed.

Triatomines have many natural enemies (microorganisms, microhymenopteran egg parasites, ants and other predators such as spiders, lizards and chickens) and there are indications that some form of biological control may be a future possibility. For the present and in the foreseeable future, however, triatomine control on a large scale must rely on the use of insecticides (see Table III.13). These have inherent disadvantages in that they are expensive to buy and to apply, must be repeated regularly to be effective

Table III.13 Insecticides for triatomine control.

Organochlorines: [minimum of 2 applications per year]
    gamma-BHC (=HCH, Lindane, Gammexane etc)
        [usual application rate: 0.5–2 g/m²]
    dieldrin [usual application rate: 1 g/m²]

Organophosphates: [2 applications p.a.]
    malathion (like DDT, not very effective: not recommended)
    fenitrothion
    fenthion (high mammal toxicity: not recommended)
    chlorpyrifos
    iodofenphos
    pirimiphos-methyl

Carbamates: [2 applications p.a.]
    bendiocarb
    propoxur

Synthetic pyrethroids: [1 annual application only]
    permethrin   [application rate: 0.5 g/m²]
    deltamethrin [application rate: 0.1–1 g/m²[a]]

---

[a] 0.1 g/m² gives control for 10 months, 0.5 g/m² for 11 months, 1.0 g/m² for 17 months. *But* costs per kg are about 50 times that of BHC. *Annual cost per square metre treated*, however, is comparable to BHC.

(generally twice each year), and their effects often can be negated by active or passive reinvasion. Insecticide resistance has occurred (with dieldrin in Venezuela) but has not become a widespread or serious problem, although it everywhere remains a daunting threat. It is undoubtedly because of the long generation time of triatomines that resistance has yet to become a practical difficulty.

DDT was not effective in triatomine control and was soon replaced. The insecticides most widely used are gamma-benzene hexachloride (known also as HCH, gammexane and lindane) at 2 g/m² and dieldrin at 1 g/m². Malathion, other organophosphates and carbamates sometimes have been used, but have no inherent advantages over BHC or dieldrin. Two annual applications are necessary for effective control to be maintained (average annual costs exceed US$ 10 per house). Triatomine populations recover very rapidly after insecticide application; this may be due in part to reinvasion, but also because populations are regulated by density-dependent factors; population growth is therefore most rapid when numbers are least.

Improved cost-effectiveness of insecticidal treatments can be achieved with slow-release formulations (including paints and mastics applied to wall surfaces) and by use of synthetic pyrethroids, especially deltamethrin and permethrin, at dose rates of 0.1 g/m² and 0.5 g/m², respectively. Despite their high unit cost

(up to 50 times that of BHC), these compounds are competitive because of the very low doses required and because operational costs are significantly reduced since only one annual application is needed to maintain adequate control.

Other chemicals have been tested experimentally but are not in general use. Among these are the juvenile hormone mimics and the plant-derived precocens, which interfere in different ways with moulting and, indirectly, with reproduction. Chemosterilants have received little attention, however, largely because of the risks inherent in their use in houses. Genetic manipulation, by release of sterile males for example, is impracticable for several reasons; not least because males also feed on blood and transmit *Trypanosoma cruzi* to the same degree as females. Traps and attractants have been tried, but are not a practical method of control.

Simple and cheap methods to improve existing rural houses offer an attractive alternative to the regular use of insecticides, particularly if householders are encouraged, possibly even subsidized, to undertake the work themselves. The plastering of mud walls and/or the replacement of palm-thatch roofs by corrugated metal or plastic sheets, or locally made tiles, drastically reduces the crevice habitat available to the various domiciliary triatomine species, and hence the level of infestation. A durable and crack-resistant wall plaster can be made from sand, cattle-dung, earth and lime. Lime can often be prepared cheaply from local limestone, by firing it overnight in a suitable kiln fuelled by wood or charcoal.

The mud used to build new mud-and-wattle houses can be stabilized to resist erosion, shrinkage and cracks; this can be done by adding lime, cement or bitumen (to make 'asfadobe'). Hand-operated hydraulic and mechanical rams are available which make compressed, stabilized soil building blocks with properties similar to fired bricks. The initial capital investment is relatively high (about US$ 2000), but the machines are rugged and durable; each family which uses the press can produce enough blocks to build a house within a week, by their own unskilled labour and for the cost only of the small amount of lime or cement necessary to stabilize the local soil. The machines can be adapted readily to produce roof and floor tiles, or liners for pit-latrines. Allied with an energetic campaign of health education, and measures to encourage community participation, much could be achieved by the application of simple house improvement measures on a wide scale, particularly were this integrated with the use of insecticides, especially at the start.

In many Latin American countries serological screening of potential blood donors is recommended, but this and the sterilization of the stored blood with gentian violet (the latter both effective and a legal requirement) are largely flouted in practice. Transmission of *Trypanosoma cruzi* by blood transfusion is therefore frequent and this is undoubtedly the commonest mode of human infection after natural, bug-mediated transmission. In the modern towns and cities of the continent, blood transfusion is indeed the predominant, sometimes even the only, cause of Chagas' disease among urban residents.

FLEAS

G. B. White

ORDER: SIPHONAPTERA

Fleas are small (length 1–4 mm) and wingless, with laterally compressed bodies composed of a blunt head, compact thorax and a relatively large rounded abdomen (Fig. III.82). In colour they are usually dark brown as adults. Eyes and antennae are small, the latter being modified in males for clasping the female from below during copulation. When not extended, each antenna lies in a groove on the side of the head. This groove may be extended as a strengthening bar within the head from eye to eye (e.g. in *Pulex*). Ventrally the head bears a series of appendages for sensory and feeding functions: paired maxillary palps at the front, slender epipharynx and paired maxillary laciniae forming the proboscis, with basal stipes and paired labial palps posteriorly.

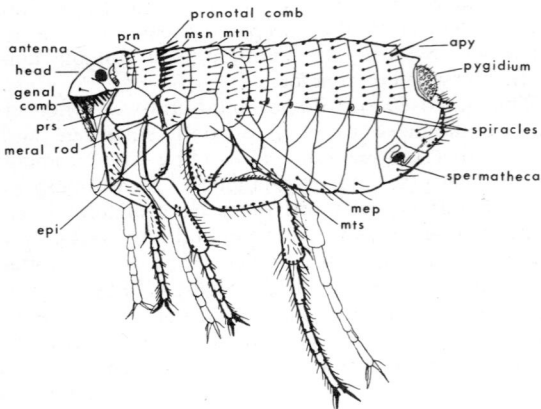

Fig. III.82 Lateral view of an adult female flea showing some of the principal taxonomic features. apy, antepygidial bristle; epi, episternum; prn, pronotum; prs, prosternum; mep, metepimeron; msn, mesonotum; mtn, metanotum; mts, metepisternum. The meral rod (mesopleural rod) or vertical bar is present in most genera but absent from *Pulex*, the human flea.

Within the thorax, the oesophagus leads to a crop or proventriculus with a constriction before the capacious stomach in the abdomen. Patches of strongly barbed spines protrude into the proventricular lumen so that blood corpuscles may be ruptured as they pass towards the stomach for digestion. Plague vectors, such as *Xenopsylla* spp., have large proventricular spines on which plague bacilli accumulate and multiply, tending to promote thrombus formation and blocking of the proventriculus. Bacilli may then be regurgitated when the flea next tries to feed, so that transmission to another host occurs.

The bodies of adult fleas bear many characteristic setae and spines. The lower margin (gena) of the head and the hind edge of the prothorax are sometimes modified to form cuticular teeth or combs (ctenidia). The sizes and positions of combs, spines and setae are important in relation to the taxonomy and identification of genera and species of fleas. All three pairs of legs are strongly developed, the hindlegs being longest and the forelegs shortest. At the base of each midleg the mesopleuron is usually strengthened with a vertical rod of cuticle internally. Many species of fleas can jump to a height of several metres for purposes of reaching hosts or escaping capture. Flea jumps are powered by a mechanism involving energy storage in the thoracic arch, which consists of cuticle impregnated with resilin, a rubbery protein. Tension is built up by the thoracic muscles and released to kick the hindlegs.[119] General information on the anatomy and biology of fleas is summarized by Smit[120] and by Traub and Starcke.[121]

Adult fleas of all species are obligate, temporary ectoparasites of birds (6%) or of mammals (94% of flea species). More than 2000 species of fleas have been described and are classified into some 200 genera. They are moderately host-specific, meaning that each kind of flea tends to infest only one or a few kinds of host. Man is frequently attacked by fleas from domestic or wild animals, as well as by the human flea *Pulex irritans*. Development takes place in the nests of particular hosts, including human dwellings. For some flea species (e.g. the European rabbit flea *Spilopsyllus cuniculi*, but not the human flea, cat flea or dog flea) host hormone levels may influence reproductive cycles of the associated fleas so that flea breeding coincides with host nesting.[119] The period of development from egg to pupa is two weeks or more, depending on temperature. The active white larvae (Fig. III.83B) have sparse hairs and a small but strong head capsule. Development takes place among dust and litter in the nest of the host, or indoors among fabrics or between floorboards. Larvae feed on organic debris and may require nutrient fragments of dried blood

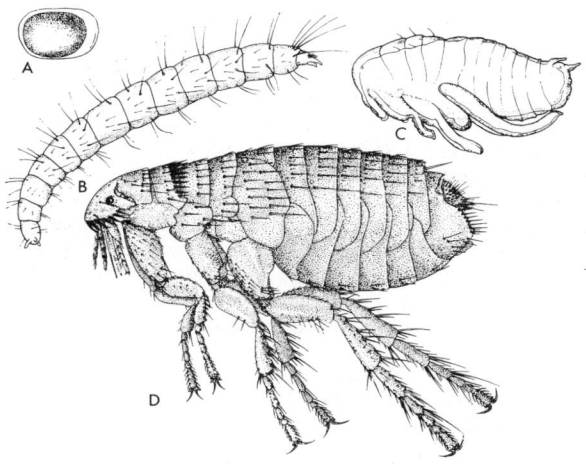

Fig. III.83 Life stages of a flea. A, Egg. B, Larva. C, Pupa. D, Adult female.

1 Head rounded; combs absent: *Pulex* or *Xenopsylla*. Mesopleural rod present: *Xenopsylla*; absent: *Pulex*. Cephalic bar present above eyes: *Pulex*; absent: *Xenopsylla*.

2 Head biangular anteriorly, combs absent: *Echidnophaga*.

3 Head sharply pointed anteriorly, combs absent, postabdomen with large spiracles: *Tunga*.

4 Head and prothorax with combs: *Ctenocephalides*.

5 Head without comb, prothorax with comb: *Nosopsyllus*.

6 Head with comb and with two spines anteriorly, eyes absent: *Leptopsylla*.

FAMILY: PULICIDAE

The members of this family, being fleas without ctenidia (combs), include several species of medical importance as pests and as disease vectors.

Pulex irritans, the human flea, is an ubiquitous pest of man, prevailing in many temperate and tropical situations. It is also commonly associated with various other coarse-coated mammals, both wild and domestic, especially dogs and pigs. Occasionally suspected of bubonic plague transmission from man to man, *P. irritans* is more certainly the vector responsible for vesicular and tonsillar plague outbreaks in Ecuador. Five other *Pulex* spp. are known, of which *P. simulans* also attacks man sometimes in North and South America and is distinguished by laciniae longer than those in *P. irritans*. Like many other fleas found in houses, *P. irritans* occasionally acts as an intermediate host of the dog tapeworm *Dipylidium caninum* which may infect man and is mostly transmitted via *Ctenocephalides* fleas.

Xenopsylla cheopis, the oriental or black rat flea, normally infests *Rattus rattus* in urban situations throughout the world, but is scarce in parts of the northern temperate zone. It frequently attacks man in rat-infested buildings, and is the classical vector of epidemic plague (*Yersinia pestis*) and of murine typhus (*Rickettsia mooseri*) from rat to rat and from rat to man. Other *Xenopsylla* spp. fulfil similar roles regionally, notably *X. brasiliensis* in tropical Africa where it thrives in wattle huts; the species has spread to parts of India and South America (hence its name). The equivalent endemic Indian flea is *X. astia*. Diagnostic differences between these three common species of *Xenopsylla* are depicted in Fig. III.84. The rat tapeworm *Hymenolepis diminuta* produces eggs which may be ingested by *Xenopsylla* larvae. Intestinal infection of rodents and sometimes children results from eating adult fleas in which cysticercoids have formed. Some strains of *H. nana*, the dwarf tapeworm of man, may also be transmitted from rat to rat via *Xenopsylla* spp.

Echidnophaga gallinacea, the sticktight flea of poultry, sometimes also infests dogs, cats, rabbits and other animals and can be a nuisance to people. Unlike most other fleas they stay attached to the host for

defaecated by adult fleas. There are two larval instars before the pupal stage.

Flea pupae are encased in a cocoon, loosely spun by the larva around itself. Hatching of the adult may be delayed for months until the proximity of a host (vibration, warmth) stimulates emergence. Adult fleas can survive actively and away from the host for many weeks, provided that the climate is not too harsh. In general fleas thrive at temperatures of 20–30°C and humidites of 60–90%. Host temperatures (i.e. 35–42°C) actually inhibit egg hatching and larval development, which is why breeding on the host does not normally occur. Below about 8°C development stops and adult fleas become lethargic.

Female fleas tend to be larger than males of the same species. Both sexes feed regularly on blood and so become liable to transmit pathogens from host to host. Recognition of the female depends on presence of the spermatheca within the posterior abdomen (Figs. III.82 and III.84), whereas the male abdomen includes a conspicuous, curved phallosome for eventration during copulation.

Relatively large, sticky white eggs are produced by female fleas at a rate of 10–25 per day, being dropped indiscriminately among host fur or feathers or on the floor. In warm situations the eggs hatch within 2 or 3 days.

Identification keys for important genera and species of fleas in all parts of the world have been provided by Smit.[120] Specimens for identification should first be soaked for one or two days in 10% caustic soda to clear them before being washed and slide-mounted. Non-specialists should be cautious in trying to identify fleas, since many species are confusingly alike. The following guidelines may help to distinguish the genera which attack man most frequently.

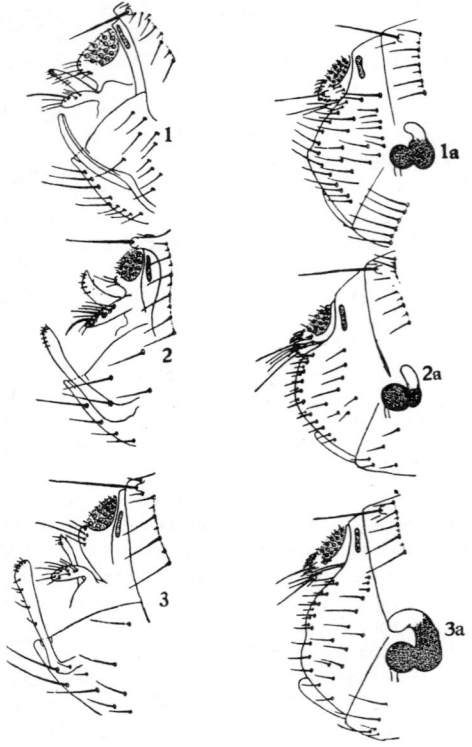

Fig. III.84 Diagnostic characters of the three widespread species of *Xenopsylla* rat fleas. 1, *X. astia*, male terminalia. 1a, *X. astia*, female terminalia with spermatheca. 2, *X. brasiliensis*, male terminalia. 2a, *X. brasiliensis*, female terminalia with spermatheca. 3, *X. cheopis*, male terminalia. 3a, *X. cheopis*, female terminalia with spermatheca. These species all possess the generic characteristics of a strong mesopleural rod, but no combs on head or pronotum.

prolonged periods and may copulate while feeding. *E. gallinacea* tends to cluster on the heads of chickens, which scratch and injure themselves to such an extent that blindness may ensue. Ulceration of the host is often caused by sticktight fleas and the females are said to oviposit deliberately into such wounds. Usually, however, development takes place in the litter of poultry-houses.

 Ctenocephalides is a small genus of nine species found mainly on carnivores in Africa and Eurasia, with two species that have become generally distributed: *C. canis* and *C. felis*, the dog and cat fleas respectively. Actually, each of these species infests both cats and dogs interchangeably and *C. felis* tends to be more often found on both kinds of hosts. In modern centrally heated homes in temperate countries. *C. canis* and *C. felis* often thrive, sometimes in the temporary absence of cats and dogs. Recurrent infestations of these species may be more of a nuisance to man than is *P. irritans*, especially in developed countries where

intermittent domestic control cannot eliminate *Ctenocephalides* spp. Cat and dog fleas are characterized by pronounced ctenidial combs on the gena (ventral edge of head) and posteriorly on the prothorax. Fig. III.85 shows how *C. felis* has a relatively longer head than *C. canis*. The dog tapeworm *Dipylidium caninum* produces eggs which may be ingested by *Ctenocephalides* larvae. Intestinal infection of cats, dogs and sometimes of man results from eating adult fleas carrying cysticercoids. A similar life-cycle involving *Ctenocephalides* is sometimes followed by strains of *Hymenolepis nana*, the human dwarf tapeworm, which usually does not have an intermediate host.

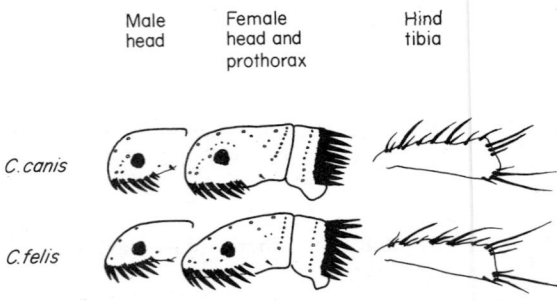

Fig. III.85 *Ctenocephalides* fleas possess rows of comb teeth (ctenidia) below the head and posteriorly on the prothorax. *C. felis*, the cat flea, has a relatively longer and more pointed head than *C. canis*, the dog flea. On the hind tibia, the number of posterior notches bearing strong setae is eight in *C. canis* and six in *C. felis*.

FAMILY: LEPTOPSYLLIDAE

Leptopsylla segnis, the European mouse flea, is frequently found indoors in various parts of the world. It also infests rats and sometimes transmits enzootic plague but seldom bites man.

FAMILY: CERATOPHYLLIDAE

Ceratophyllus gallinae, the European chicken flea, has spread to many parts of the world, has a wide range of bird hosts and occasionally invades houses and attacks people. It is a particularly large flea with a painful bite. Unlike *Echidnophaga*, it drops off the host directly after feeding. An equivalent North American species is *C. niger*, the western chicken flea. Numerous comb teeth on the pronotum facilitate the identification of *Ceratophyllus* spp.

 Nosopsyllus fasciatus, the brown rat flea, has also become widespread with its main host *Rattus norvegicus; is* also infests *R. rattus* and many other small mammals and often attacks man, but is seldom involved in plague transmission. Like *Ctenocephalides*, *N. fasciatus* serves as an intermediate host of the dog tapeworm *D. caninum* which may infect man if infective fleas are eaten.

FAMILY: TUNGIDAE

Tunga penetrans, the sand flea or jigger (chigoe, chique), has females adapted for intracutaneous permanent attachment on the host. *T. penetrans* regularly infects man, pigs, poultry and other creatures in Central America, West and East Africa and parts of the Indian subcontinent. As for other fleas, the larvae are free-living, dusty or sandy soil being best for *T. penetrans.* Adults are also free-living at first, when copulation occurs. The fertilized female then finds a suitable host and tries to penetrate crevices in the skin, such as cracks in the soles of the feet (Fig. 52.1, p. 920), between the toes and especially around the toenails. Any part of the human anatomy can be affected. By means of the mouthparts, the female *Tunga* becomes firmly attached and soon swells to the size and shape of a small white pea. Somehow the host skin envelops the jigger, which lies below the stratum corneum but above the stratum granulosum, leaving only the posterior spiracles exposed to the air. Only when the jigger is almost mature and distended, after 8 to 12 days, does the infection begin to irritate. Severe inflammation and ulceration ensues, so that scratching helps to expel large numbers of white eggs from the jigger. With skill and care it is possible to remove the whole insect, using a needle or forceps, but often the soft abdomen ruptures leaving the head attached in the lesion.

The jigger seldom attacks the leg above the dorsum of the foot, but no part of the body may escape. The soles (Fig. 52.2, p. 920), the skin between the toes and that at the roots of the nails are favourite situations. Usually only one or two jiggers are found at a time, but occasionally they are present in hundreds, the little pits left after extraction or expulsion being sometimes so closely set that parts of the surface may look like honeycomb. During her gestation the jigger causes a considerable amount of irritation. In consequence of this pus may form around her distended abdomen which now raises the integument into a pea-like elevation. After the eggs are laid the superjacent skin ulcerates and the jigger is expelled, leaving a small sore which may become infected sometimes causing phagedaena or even tetanus. Ulceration is common and may follow removal of the jigger or natural extrusion of the egg sac. The ulcer commences as a tiny pit and as it extends the sloping edge may develop into a septic ulcer. It remains more or less circular in outline, except under the nail or nail margin, where the outline is more irregular and a pocket of pus forms beneath it. Chronic absorption of pus may lead to thrombophlebitis.

MEDICAL IMPORTANCE AND CONTROL OF FLEAS

More than 50 genera and numerous species of fleas have been implicated as vectors of enzootic plague in various parts of the world (Table 27.1, p. 589), meaning that they maintain the transmission of *Yersinia pestis* bacilli among rodents. Man is seldom infected primarily through the bites of such zoophilic fleas, except when infected *Xenopsylla* move on to man after plague-stricken rats have died. Rarely are conditions conducive for man-to-man transmission by *Pulex* or *Ctenocephalides* to reach epidemic proportions. Overwintering of plague bacilli may occur in hibernating fleas.

Various flea species may also be involved in the transmission cycles of murine typhus, tularaemia, pseudotuberculosis, melioidosis, brucellosis, lymphocytic choriomeningitis and possibly other diseases.[122] Only the first depends on fleas, as well as parasitic mites and lice, as vectors. Thus the agent of murine typhus, *Rickettsia typhi* (= *R. mooseri*), is commonly transmitted by *X. brasiliensis, X. cheopis,* and possibly *N. fasciatus* or *L. segnis,* with a similar epidemiological picture to that of plague.[123]

As mentioned previously, some fleas serve as the intermediate hosts for tapeworms usually found in animals: *Dipylidium caninum* of dogs and cats; *Hymenolepis diminuta* of rodents; *H. nana* strains endemic in rodents. These occasionally cause diarrhoea in human beings, especially children who may happen to become infected by eating infective fleas.

People suffer localized dermal reactions to flea bites, which can be soothed with antihistamines. Generalized allergic sensitization is not uncommon and should be overcome by means of flea control in preference to desensitization treatment of the patient. The irritation and nuisance caused by fleas crawling on the human body and the pain of their frequent probing and biting always justify control measures.

Simple hygienic measures of keeping houses well swept and floors washed and clean are beneficial and the regular use of a vacuum suction cleaner is highly effective for gathering up fleas, their eggs and larvae. When flea-infested premises are re-entered after a period of disuse, newly emerged fleas may become activated and attack people in surprising numbers. Temporary relief may be gained through the use of insect repellent creams or lotions based on dimethyl phthallate, diethytoluamide, indalone and proprietary brands. Floors can be treated with a solution of naphthalene in benzene, or simply with detergents. Synthetic chemical insecticides should be sprayed or dusted into corners, cracks and fabrics where flea larvae may be expected to occur. The value of DDT for such purposes has become diminished by the problem of insecticide resistance in many areas. Various organophosphates, carbamates and pyrethroids are ample substitutes, but compounds with high mammalian toxicity should not be used indoors. Flea-ridden domestic animals themselves may be washed thoroughly with carbolic soap, dusted with pyrethroid powder, treated with insecticidal lotion or shampoo (e.g. malathion) or fitted with a 'flea-collar' made of plastic impregnated with dichlorvos which has a prolonged, localized vapour action within the fur. For direct killing of fleas it is convenient to employ spray-canisters giving aerosols of synergized pyrethrins or similar quick-acting insecticides.

The particular personal problems caused by sand fleas or jiggers (*T. penetrans*) have already been mentioned. Affected areas of soil may be burnt off in an effort to kill them, and their breeding on livestock and pets should not be allowed. Since female jiggers are not good jumpers, human infestation is normally confined to the feet. Daily inspection of the interdigital clefts, roots of nails and soles of feet should cause freshly burrowing female jiggers to be detected and removed before they have grown much. To prevent their attack, good shoes should be worn at all times. An old deterrent is to rub the feet with lysol or creosol in paraffin oil; modern repellents may be better.

In places where *T. penetrans* is common, the local people become quite skilful at removing them with sharp instruments. The characteristic, circular, open lesions should be dressed antiseptically and protected until healed. Often they become ulcerated and secondarily infected, with much pus produced, chronic absorption of which may lead to thrombophlebitis or gangrene. Timely use of antibiotics is therefore advisable and the affected limb should be rested.

REFERENCES

1 Kettle, D.S. (1984) *Medical and Veterinary Entomology*. London: Croom Helm.
2 Riley, J. (1986) *Adv. Parasit.* **15**, 46–128.
3 Khalil, G.M. (1972) *J. Egyption publ. Hlth Ass.* **47**, 363–369.
4 World Health Organization (1984) *Wld Hlth Org. tech. Rep. Ser.* **701**, 140.
5 Lanson, R. & Shaw, J.J. (1979) The role of animals in the epidemiology of South American leishmaniasis. In *Biology of the Kinetoplastida*, ed. W.H.R. Lumsden & D.A. Evans, vol. II, p.1. New York and London: Academic Press.
6 Peters, C.J. & LeDuc, J.W. (1985) Bunyaviruses, Phleboviruses and related viruses. In *Textbook of Human Virology*, ed. R.B. Belshe, pp. 547–598. Littleton, Mass.: PSG Publishing.
7 Lewis, D.J., Young, D.G., Fairchild, G.B. et al (1977) *Syst. Entomol.* **2**, 319–332.
8 Lane, R.P. (1986) *Insect Sci. Applic.* **7**, 225–230.
9 World Health Organization (1975) *Manual on Practical Entomology in Malaria*. Geneva: World Health Organization.
10 Knight, K.L. & Stone, A. (1977) *A Catalog of the Mosquitoes of the World*. The Thomas Say Foundation, Vol. VI. College Park: Entomological Society of America (Supplement 1978).
11 Dennis, P.T., Partomo, F., Durnomo, A.A. et al (1976) *Am. J. trop. Med. Hyg.* **25**, 797.
12 Reid, J.A. (1968) *Anopheline Mosquitoes of Malaya and Borneo*. Studies from the Institute for Medical Research, Malaysia, No. 31. Kuala Lumpur: Government of Malaysia.
13 White, G.B. (1978) *Mosquito System.* **10**, 13.
14 Carpenter, S.J. & La Casse, W.J. (1974) *Mosquitoes of North America*. Berkeley & Los Angeles: University of California Press.
15 Gillies, M.T. & de Meillon, B. (1968) *The Anophelinae of Africa South of the Sahara*. Johannesburg: South African Institute for Medical Research.
16 Garnham P.C.C. (1966) *Malaria Parasites and Other Haemosporidia*. Oxford: Blackwell Scientific Publications.
17 Kalra, S.L. (1978) *J. communic. Dis.* **10**, 1.
18 Webber, R.H. (1979) *Trans. R. Soc. trop. Med. Hyg.* **73**, 722.
19 White, G.B. (1974) *Trans. R. Soc. trop. Med. Hyg.* **68**, 278.
20 Zavortink, T.J. (1973) *Contr. Am. ent. Inst.* **9**, 1.
21 Faran, M.E. (1980) *Contr. Am. ent. Inst.* **15**, 1.
22 Le Duc, J.W. (1979) *J. med. Ent,* **16**, 1.
23 Dutary, B.E. & Le Duc, J.W. (1981) *Trans. R. Soc. Trop. Med. Hyg.* **75**, 128.
24 Belkin, J.N. (1962) *Mosquitoes of the South Pacific*. Berkeley & Los Angeles: California University Press.
25 Huang, Y.M. (1977) *Mosquito System,* **9**, 289 (also Document WHO/VBC/76. 654, WHO/FIL/76.143).
26 Huang, Y.M. & Hitchcock, J.C. (1980) *Contr. Am. ent. Inst.* **17**, 1.
27 MacDonald, W.W. (1976) Mosquito genetics in relation to filaria infections. *Symp. Br. Soc. Parasit.* **14**, 1.
28 Christophers, S.R. (1960) *Aedes aegypti (L.), the Yellow Fever Mosquito*. London: Cambridge University Press.
29 McClelland, G.A.H. (1974) *Trans. R. ent. Soc. Lond.* **126**, 239.
30 Powell, J.R., Tabachnik, W.J. & Arnold, J. (1980) *Science, N.Y.* **208**, 1385.
31 McIntosh, B.M. (1975) *Mosquitoes as Vectors of Viruses in Southern Africa*. Entomology Memoir No. 43, Pretoria: Department of Agricultural and Technical Services.
32 Arnell, J.H. (1973) *Contr. Am. ent. Inst.* **10**, 1.
33 Belkin, J.N., Heinemann, S.L. & Page, W.A. (1970) *Contr. Am. ent. Inst.* **6**, 1.
34 Bram, R.A. (1967) *Contr. Am. ent. Inst.* **2**, 1.
35 Sirivanakarn, S. (1976) *Contr. Am. ent. Inst.* **12**, 1.
36 Southgate, B.A. (1979) *Trop. Dis. Bull.* **76**, 1045.
37 Sasa, M. (1976) *Human Filariasis*. University of Tokyo Press.
38 Sirivanakarn, S. (1982) *Contr. Am. ent. Inst.*, in press.
39 Maslov, A.V. (1967) *Ent. Obozrenie* **43**, 193 (English trans. *Ent. Rev., Wash.,* **43**, 97.)
40 Wharton, R.H. (1962) *Bulletin No.11*. Institute for Medical Research, Federation of Malaya.
41 Bates, M. (1949) *The Natural History of Mosquitoes*. New York: Macmillan.
42 Gillett, J.D. (1971) *Mosquitoes*. London: Weidenfeld & Nicholson.
43 Harbach, R.E. & Knight, K.L. (1980) *Taxonomists' Glossary of Mosquito Anatomy*. Marlton, New Jersey: Plexus Publishing.
44 Harwood, R.T. & James, M.T. (1979) *Entomology in Human and Animal Health*. New York, Toronto & London: Macmillan.

45 Horsfall, W. R. (1955) *Mosquitoes—Their Bionomics and Relation to Disease.* New York: Ronald Press.

46 Mattingly, P. F. (1969) *The Biology of Mosquito-borne Disease.* Science of Biology Series, No. 1. London: Allen & Unwin.

47 Service, M. W. (1976) *Mosquito Ecology: Field Sampling Methods.* London: Applied Science Publishers.

48 Edwards, F. W. (1941) *Mosquitoes of the Ethiopian Region. III.—Culicine Adults and Pupae.* London: British Museum (Natural History).

49 Hopkins, G. H. E. (1952) *Mosquitoes of the Ethiopian Region. I.—Larval Bionomics of Mosquitoes and Taxonomy of Culicine Larvae.* London: British Museum (Natural History).

50 Mattingly, P. F. (1952–3) *Bull. Br. Mus. (Nat. Hist.)* (*B*), **2**, 233; **3**, 1.

51 Gerberg, E. J. & van Someren, E. C. C. (1970) Document WHO/VBC/70.236.

52 Cordellier, R., Germain, M., Hervy, J. P. et al (1977). *Guide Pratique pour L'Etude des Vecteurs de Fièvre Jaune en Afrique et Méthode de Lutte.* Initiations, Documentations Techniques, No. 33. Paris: Office de la Recherche Scientifique et Technique Outre-Mer.

53 Lane, J. (1953) *Neotropical Culicidae,* Vols. 1 and 2. University of São Paulo.

54 Forratini, O. P. (1962) *Entomologia Médica,* Vol. 1. *Anophelini.* E. Blucher and University of São Paulo.

55 Forratini, O. P. (1965) *Entomologia Médica,* Vol. 2. *Culicini: Culex, Aedes e Psorophora.* E. Blucher and University of São Paulo.

56 Wood, D. M., Dang, P. T. & Ellis, R. A. (1980) *The Mosquitoes of Canada. The Insects and Arachnids of Canada, Part 6.* Hull, Quebec: Agriculture Canada.

57 Darsie, R. F. & Ward, R. A. (1981) *Identification and Geographical Distribution of the Mosquitoes of North America.* Fresno, California: American Mosquito Control Association.

58 Mattingly, P. F. & Knight, K. L. (1956) *Bull. Br. Mus. (Nat. Hist.)* (*B*) **4**, 89.

59 Lee, D. J. (1944) *An Atlas of the Mosquito Larvae of the Australasian Region. Tribes Megorhinini and Culicini.* Australian Military Forces.

60 Lee, D. J. & Woodhill, A. R. (1944) *The Anopheline Mosquitoes of the Australasian Region.* Department of Zoology, University of Sydney, Monograph 2.

61 Dobrotworsky, N. V. (1965) *The Mosquitoes of Victoria.* Melbourne: Melbourne University Press.

62 Marks, E. N. (1973) *An Atlas of Common Queensland Mosquitoes.* St. Lucia: University of Queensland.

63 Ribeiro, H., Ramos, H. C., Capela, R. A. et al (1980) *Estudios, Ensaios e Documentos No. 135.* Lisbon: Junta de Investigacoes Cientificas do Ultramar.

64 Dahl, C. & White, G. B. (1978) *Limnofauna Europaea,* ed. J. Illies, pp. 390–395.

65 Christophers, S. R. (1933) *Fauna Br. India* 4, 1.

66 Bhatia, M. L., Kalra, N. L., Rao, V. V. et al (1961) *Vectors of Malaria in India.* Delhi: National Society of India for Malaria and Other Mosquito-Borne Diseases.

67 Barraud, P. J. (1934) *Fauna Br. India* **5**, 1.

68 Tanaka, K., Mizusawa, K. & Saugstad, E. S. (1979) *Contr. Am. ent. Inst* **16**, 987.

69 Grjebine, A. (1966) *Faune de Madagascar, XXII. Insectes Diptères Culicidae Anophelinae.* Paris: Lahure.

70 RavaonJanahary, C. (1978) *Trav. Doc. Off. Rech. sci. tech. Outre-Mer,* **87.**

71 Rioux, J. A. (1958) *Encycl. ent. B* **35**, 1.

72 Senevet, G. & Andarelli, L. (1959) *Encycl. ent. A,* **37,** 1.

73 Van den Assem, J. & Bonne-Wepster, J. (1964) *Zool. Bijdr.* **6,** 1.

74 Belkin, J. N. (1968) *Contr. Am. ent. Inst.* **3,** 1.

75 Bonne-Wepster, J. & Swellengrebel, N. H. (1953) *The Anopheline Mosquitoes of the Indo-Australian Region.* Amsterdam: de Bussy.

76 Harrison, B. A. & Scanlon, J. E. (1975) *Contr. Am. ent. Inst,* **12,** 1.

77 Mattingly, P. F. (1957–65) Part I (1957) *Ficalbia;* part II (1957) *Heizmannia;* part III *Aedes* (*Paraedes*) and (*Cancraedes*); part IV *Aedes* (*Skusea*), (*Diceromyia*) (*Geoskusea*) and (*Christophersiomyia*); part V *Aedes* (*Mucidus*), (*Ochlerotatus*), and (*Neomelaniconion*); part VI *Aedes* (*Stegomyia*). London: British Museum (Natural History).

78 Mattingly, P. F. (1970) *Contr. Am. ent. Inst.* **5,** 1.

79 Reinert, J. F. (1973) *Contr. Am. ent. Inst* **9,** 1.

80 Huang, Y. M. (1979) *Contr. Am. ent. Inst.* **15,** 1.

81 Delfinado, M. D. (1966) *Mem. Am. ent. Inst.* **7,** 1.

82 Basio, R. G. (1971) *Nat. Mus. Philipp. Monogr* **4.**

83 Gutsevich, A. V., Monchadsky, A. S. & Stackelberg, A. A. (1970) *Fauna SSSR.* VII (4). *Family Culicidae.* Leningrad: Akad, Nauk. SSSR Zool. Inst. (English translation (1974) Jerusalem: Keter Press).

84 Mattingly, P. F. & Brown, E. S. (1955) *Bull. ent. Res.* **46,** 69.

85 Foote, R. H. & Cook, D. R. (1959) *Mosquitoes of Medical Importance.* United States Department of Agriculture, Agricultural Handbook, **152,** 1–158.

86 Mattingly, P. F. (1971) *Contr. Am. ent. Inst.,* 7, 1. (Reproduced in Smith, K. G. V. (1973) *Insects and Other Arthropods of Medical Importance.* London: British Museum (Natural History).)

87 Laird, M. & Miles, J. W. (eds.) (1983, 1985). *Integrated Mosquito Control Methodologies,* 2 vols. London: Academic Press.

88 Reiter, P. (1980) *Ann. trop. Med. Parasit.* **74,** 541.

89 Detinova, T. S. (1962) *Age-grouping Methods in Diptera of Medical Importance.* WHO Monograph Series No. 417.

90 Clements, A. N. (1963) *The Physiology of Mosquitoes.* Oxford: Pergamon Press.

91 Linley, J. R., Hoch, A. L. & Pinheiro, F. P. (1983) *J. med. Ent.* **20,** 347–364.

92 Raccurt, C., Lowrie, R. C. & McNeeley, D. F. (1980) *Am. J. trop. Med Hyg.* **29,** 803–808.

93 Nathan, M. B. (1981) *Bull. ent. Res.* **71,** 97–105.

94 Linley, J. R. & Davies, J. B. (1971) *J. econ. Ent.* **64,** 264–278.

95 Stanek, G. (1985) *Microb. Sci.* **2,** 231–234.

96 Schmid, G. P. (1985) *Rev. infect Dis.* **7,** 41–50.

97 Magnarelli, L. A., Anderson, J. F. & Barbour, A. G. (1986) *J. infect. Dis.* **154,** 355–358.

98 Mulligan, H. W. (1970) *The African Trypanosomiases.* London: George Allen & Unwin.

99 Ford, J. (1971) *The Role of the Trypanosomiases in African Ecology: A Study of the Tsetse Fly Problem.* Oxford: Clarendon Press.

100 Potts.

101 Pollock, J. N. (1982) *Training Manual for Tsetse Control Personnel,* 3 vols. Rome: FAO.

102 Jackson, C. H. N. (1946) *Bull. ent. Res.* **37,** 291.

103 Saunders (1962).

104 Challier (1965).

105   Challier, A. (1982) *Insect Sci. Applic.* **3,** 97–143.
106   Molyneux, D. H. & Ashford, R. W. (1983) *The Biology of Trypansoma and Leishmania, Parasites of Man and Domestic Animals.* London: Taylor and Francis.
107   Molyneux, D. H. (1983) *Rev. infect. Dis.* **5,** 945–956.
108   Allsopp, R. (1984) *Bull. ent. Res,* **74,** 1–23.
109   Jordan, A. M. (1985) *Br. med. Bull.* **41,** 181–186.
110   Jordan, A. M. (1986) *Trypanosomiasis Control and African Rural Development.* Harlow (UK): Longman.

111   Zumpt, F. (1965) *Myiasis in Animals and Man in the Old World.* London.
112   Smith, K. G. V. (ed.) (1973) *Insects and Other Arthropods of Medical Importance.* London: British Museum (Natural History).
113   Landi (1960)
114   Dar, M. S., Ben Amer, M., Dar, E. K. et al (1980) *Trans. R. Soc. trop. Med. Hyg.* **74,** 303.

115   Zumpt, F. (1963) *S.A. med. J.* **37,** 305–307.
116   Clay, T. (1970) *Bull. Br. Mus. Nat. Hist. (Ent.),* **25,** 73.
117   Scholt, L. L. (1979) *The Epidemiology of Human Pediculosis,* p. 150. Florida: Navy Disease Vector Ecology and Control Centre.
118   Lent, H. & Wygodzinsky, P. (1979) *Bull. Am. Mus. Nat. Hist.* **163,** 123.
119   Rothschild, M. (1975) *A. Rev. Ent.* **20,** 241.
120   Smit, F. G. A. M. (1973) Siphonaptera (fleas). In *Insects and other Arthropods of Medical Importance,* ed. K. G. V. Smith, p. 325. London: British Museum (Natural History).
121   Traub, R. & Starcke, H. (1980) *Fleas.* Rotterdam: Balkema.
122   Bibikova, V. A. (1977) *A. Rev. Ent.* **22,** 1.
123   Traub, R., Wisseman, C. L. & Farhang-Azad, A. (1978) *Trop. Dis. Bull.* **75,** 237.

Appendix IV
Laboratory Diagnosis of Parasitic Disease

Wendi Bailey

When examining specimens for the presence of parasite cysts or ova it is often necessary to measure an object under investigation to see if it falls within a given size range. Before beginning any microscopy it is therefore necessary to calibrate a micrometer eyepiece with the microscope that you are going to use. For this purpose you will need access to a stage micrometer which has an engraved scale of 1 mm. Once your microscope has been calibrated for the × 10, × 40 and oil immersion objectives make a note on the eyepiece micrometer of divisions/micrometres.

Calibration of microscope using stage and eyepiece micrometers (Fig. IV. 1)

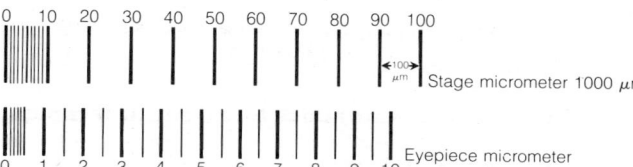

1 The stage micrometer is a glass slide in the centre of which is a scale with divisions from 0 to 100. The total scale measures 1 mm (1000 µm). Place the stage micrometer on your microscope and focus on this scale.

$$1\,mm = 100\ \text{divisions} = 1000\,\mu m$$
$$0.1\,mm = 10\ \text{divisions} = 100\,\mu m$$
$$0.01\,mm = 1\ \text{division} = 10\,\mu m$$

2 Using the × 10 microscope objective: remove one eyepiece from your microscope and replace it with the micrometer eyepiece. Turn this micrometer until both scales are parallel. Line up the eyepiece graticule until the zeros of both scales are together. Note the largest figure on the eyepiece graticule that corresponds to a whole division on the stage micrometer. From the readings obtained calculate the number of micrometres/eyepiece division e.g. 85 eyepiece divisions = 80 stage divisions;
therefore as each small stage division is 10 µm width

85 eyepiece divisions $= 80 \times 10$
$= 800\,\mu m$
1 eyepiece division $= \dfrac{800}{85}$
$= 9.4\,\mu m$

Calibrate the × 40 and the × 100 (oil immersion) objectives in the same way. Make a note of these calibrations for future reference.

Examination of stool

When a stool specimen is received it is important to make a note of the appearance of the specimen—colour, consistency, presence of blood and mucus. If a specimen cannot be examined immediately it should be placed out of direct sunlight, in the coolest area of the laboratory, until it can be examined. Try to find out how old the specimen is—if one is looking for trophozoites of *Entamoeba histolytica* it is pointless

Fig. IV.1 Calibration of microscope using (a) stage micrometer; (b) eyepiece micrometer.

examining an old specimen. In cases like this it is necessary to examine a 'hot' (freshly passed) stool otherwise the trophozoites will no longer be motile and therefore impossible to distinguish. The trophozoites of most protozoan parasites will not remain active for very long once the stool has been passed. Another problem is the presence of motile nematode species larvae. In a freshly passed specimen one might expect to see *Strongyloides stercoralis* larvae but, in a specimen which has been sitting around on a bench for a few hours in the heat it is possible for hookworm species ova to hatch out. Both these rhabditiform larvae look superficially very similar but they must obviously be distinguished from each other.

The first examination to be made on a stool specimen is a saline preparation. A drop of physiological (0.85%) saline is placed in the centre of a microscope slide. A wooden stick is used to remove a portion of faecal material—this is emulsified in the saline solution. If the smear is too thin then scanty parasites may be missed; if it is too thick then they may still be missed, because the smear does not allow anything to be seen properly! A rough guide is to make a smear and then look at a piece of printed paper through the smear. If you can just read the print then the smear is of the right thickness.

A coverslip should be placed on top of the smear and the slide examined microscopically using the × 10 objective. The whole area under the coverslip should be examined systematically—if you see anything suspicious then examine the object with the × 40 objective. It is important to get used to using the × 10 objective for scanning; using the × 40 routinely would take far too long and the smear would probably have dried up by the time you had finished.

If you see any objects that you think may be cysts then make another smear, this time using Lugol's iodine instead of saline. This will stain up cyst nuclei and any glycogen mass thus enabling a diagnosis to be made. Iodine preparations should be examined within 5 to 15 minutes of making the smear as iodine is a progressive stain and if left too long cysts will overstain.

Generally in a busy laboratory in the tropics it is only feasible to perform direct examinations on faecal specimens. However, it is sometimes necessary to use a concentration technique—for example to exclude the possibility of a patient harbouring *Schistosoma mansoni* ova. (These may be present in small numbers and be missed by direct examination.) One of the commonly used concentration techniques (formol ether concentration) is described below.

Lugol's iodine

Iodine	1.0 g
Potassium iodide	2.0 g
Distilled water	100 ml

Dissolve the potassium iodide in the water then add the iodine. Store in an amber glass bottle, out of direct sunlight.

10% Formol saline

Sodium chloride	8.5 g
Conc. formaldehyde (37–41% solution)	100 ml
Distilled water	900 ml

Dissolve sodium chloride in water. Add formaldehyde solution.

Formol ether concentration for ova and cysts

1 Pour about 12 ml of 10% formol saline into a clean bottle containing glass beads.
2 Add approximately 2 g faeces (with a wooden stick) to the bottle, place a lid on and shake the bottle well (the beads will break up the specimen).
3 Pass this solution through a plastic tea strainer into a 15 ml glass centrifuge tube to within 2 inches of the top of the tube.
4 Add about half an inch of ether to the centrifuge tube, place a gloved thumb on top of the tube and

shake the solution well for a couple of minutes. Invert the tube a few times during this procedure and gently release the pressure by removing your thumb.
5 Centrifuge the tube at 3000 r.p.m. for 5 minutes. (If there is not a centrifuge available leave to stand out of direct sunlight for 30 minutes.)
6 After centrifugation there will be a fatty plug at the top of the solution. Loosen this with a wooden stick and discard this and the supernatant fluid. The deposit should be resuspended with saline or iodine and examined for parasites (Fig. IV. 2).

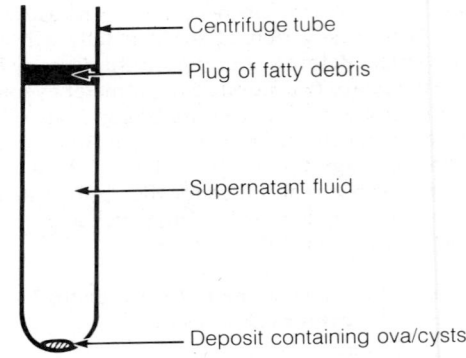

Fig. IV.2 Appearance of stool specimen after centrifugation.

Cellophane (Kato) thick faecal smear technique

1 Transfer 50 mg of faeces to a clean microscope slide using a wooden applicator stick. (If the sample contains large amounts of fibre then pass the sample through a 105 mesh metal or nylon sieve, scrape the sample from the underside of the mesh and transfer to microscope slide.)
2 Cover the sample with a previously soaked cellophane coverslip and press it against a piece of absorbent paper until the smear covers the area under the coverslip.
3 Leave the smear until it clears—about 60 minutes at room temperature. The clearing process may be slowed down by inverting the slide and placing on a piece of card or by placing at 4°C until convenient to examine.
4 Examine the whole area using the × 4 objective.
5 Hookworm ova are visible for up to 30 minutes after the preparation has been made. *Schistosoma* ova are best seen at about 24 hours after preparation. *Trichuris* and *Ascaris* ova can be seen at any time.

As the cellophane coverslips are soaked in a malachite green solution the background colour of the slides will be green. Schistosome and hookworm ova will appear colourless.

Cellophane. Water wettable cellophane supplied as rolls (22 mm width), for use cut into rectangles

22 × 30 mm (list of suppliers available from the World Health Organization).

Glycerin–malachite green solution. Mix 100 ml glycerol, 100 ml water and 1 ml of 3% aqueous malachite green solution. Place in a screw-topped jar and add the cellophane coverslips. Coverslips must be soaked in this solution for a minimum of 24 hours before use.

Faecal egg counts

There have been many methods described for counting helminth ova. The following technique is the modified Stoll method. As a very small amount of faeces is examined the method is not suitable where less than 200 ova are present per gram of faeces.

1 Place some glass balls in a screw-capped bottle and add 20 ml of formol saline solution.
2 Weigh out 2 g of faeces and add to the bottle.
3 Mix well by shaking until all the faecal material is well broken up.
4 Filter the liquid through a mesh sieve (100 mesh) or tea strainer if sieve not available. Collect filtrate.
5 Mix the filtrate well and remove 150 μl (0.15 ml) of the suspension on to a clean microscope slide. Use a larger coverslip than usual as this is a fairly large volume of fluid. Count all the ova on the slide, even those which may have been pushed out from under the coverslip, using the × 10 objective.
6 The total number of ova counted is multiplied by 70 to give number ova/g faeces.
NB The formol ether technique may be followed and the deposit fluid used to perform counts on; if this regime is followed then the faeces must be weighed out prior to placing it in formol saline.

Diagnostic features of some common protozoa

Entamoeba histolytica

Trophozoite. Must be motile and contain ingested erythrocytes (Fig. 17.8a).

Cyst. Refractile with × 10 objective if microscope light is correctly adjusted. Small, round cysts, from 10–15 μm in diameter, containing one, two or four nuclei. In fresh cysts two chromatoid bodies may be seen. With iodine the nuclei are much clearer, chromatoid bodies are not visible, and a glycogen mass can be seen (Fig. 17.8c).

Giardia lamblia

Trophozoite. Approximately 12 μm long × 7 μm wide. Characteristic 'pear' shape. Four pairs of flagellae, axonemes and two nuclei. The movement must be distinguished from that of *Trichomonas* and *Chilomastix.*

Some authors have likened the movement of *Giardia* trophozoites to that of a 'falling leaf' (Fig. 17.17).

Cyst. Oval, refractile, approximately 12 × 6 μm. Two or four nuclei, the remains of the flagellae and axonemes may be visible (Fig. 17.18).

Entamoeba coli

Trophozoite. Sluggish movement compared to *E. histolytica.* It may contain ingested particles but no erythrocytes (Fig. 17.8b).

Cyst. Large, round, cysts 15–20 μm diameter. Up to eight nuclei. Young cysts may contain a glycogen vacuole; this is large and dense in cysts containing no nuclei (Fig. 17.8d).

Trichomonas hominis

Trophozoite. Pear-shaped, with five flagellae, active with spinning motion.
   A cyst stage is not known.

Chilomastix mesnili

Trophozoite. Rounded body tapering to a point. Rotating movement.

Cyst. Small, 7–10 μm, lemon-shaped.

Nematode larvae in fresh stool specimens

Stool specimens may contain active larvae which must be identified. The most common larva to be found in stools is that of *Strongyloides stercoralis;* the ova are not normally found in faeces. In the tropics one may find that hookworm sp. ova have hatched so it is important to distinguish between these two types of larvae. On finding rhabditiform larvae in a faecal specimen one must examine the anterior end of the parasite in order to be able to identify it. If the larva is alive it will be moving too quickly for identification so it must be killed. The easiest way to do this is to add a drop of iodine to the side of the coverslip. Examine the larva using a × 40 objective—*Strongyloides* larvae have a short buccal cavity, hookworm sp., larvae have a long one (Figs. IV.3 and II.11).

It may be difficult to decide which type of larva you are looking at as it may already be dead. Alternatively you may have a negative stool sample but may wish to make sure that the patient is not harbouring *Strongyloides.* In these circumstances it is necessary to set up a stool culture. If there are any rhabditiform larvae present in a sample these will develop into filariform larvae under the right conditions. Filariform larvae of *Strongyloides* have a notched posterior end whereas filariform larvae of hookworm sp. have a pointed posterior end (Figs. IV.4 and II.11).

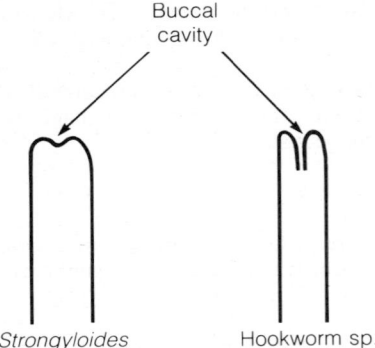

Fig. IV.3   Rhabditiform larvae—anterior end.

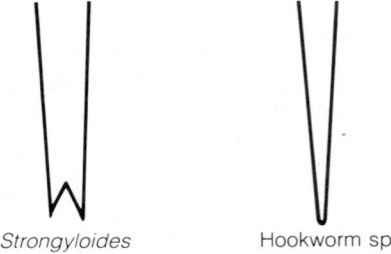

Fig. IV.4   Filariform larvae—posterior end.

Culture of stools for *Strongyloides* larvae

Charcoal cultures

1 Mix equal quantities of faeces with granular charcoal* in a 55 mm Petri dish. Moisten this with distilled, or boiled, cooled water so that a damp paste is formed.

2 Place this dish inside a 90 mm Petri dish and fill the large dish with distilled water to just below the level of the smaller dish. Place a cover on the large Petri dish (Fig. IV.5).

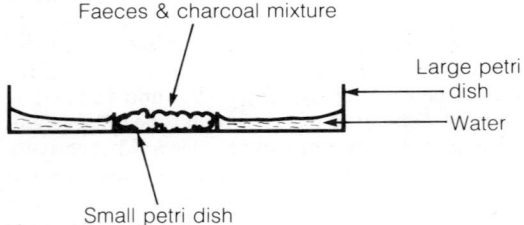

Fig. IV.5   Charcoal culture for *Strongyloides* larvae.

3 Leave the dish in an incubator at 26°C for 6 days. In the tropics the dish may be left on the bench out of direct sunlight.

4 Examine the water in the outer dish for the presence of filariform (L3) larvae. These will be actively swimming. If numerous larvae are present they may be seen as a white 'mass' visible to the naked eye. In lighter infections a hand lens or stereomicroscope will be needed to examine the culture. This technique will also work for hookworm sp. larvae so it is important to identify which L3 larvae you have grown. Remove larvae on to a microscope slide, kill with iodine and examine.

NB Take care as L3 (filariform) larvae are the infective stage.

*Charcoal, granular, 10–18 mesh (BDH Ltd, product No. 33034). If not available sterile soil will work just as well.

Filter paper culture (*modified Harada–Mori culture*) (Fig. IV.6)

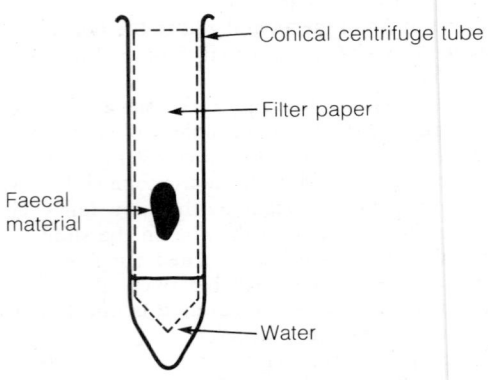

Fig. IV.6   Filter paper culture for *Strongyloides* larvae.

1 Spread faecal material on to a piece of filter paper.

2 Dampen paper with distilled water.

3 Place into a test-tube to within half an inch of the bottom of the tube.

4 Add water to the tube, to just below the level of the faecal smear.

5 Place tube in a rack, out of direct sunlight and examine after 6 days.

6 Larvae will be found in the water at the bottom of the tube.

Techniques for whole worms, proglottides, etc.

Tapeworms

Gravid segments (proglottides) may be found in a faecal specimen or may be brought in for examination. Most commonly these will be either *Taenia solium* or *Taenia saginata*.

A segment should be transferred on to a microscope slide, blotting off any faecal material with blotting paper. A second slide should be placed on top of the segment, the two pressed firmly together and held up to the light. It is then possible to see the shape and size of the uterus inside the gravid proglottid.

Taenia saginata (Figs. IV.7a and 23.4b): size of proglottid approximately 5 mm wide by up to 20 mm long. There are more than 12 side branches of the uterus (i.e. very difficult to count the number).

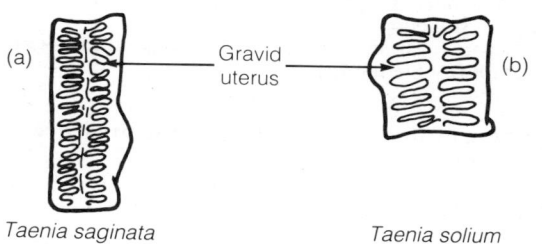

Taenia saginata   Taenia solium

Fig. IV.7   Proglottides of (a) *Taenia saginata*; (b) *T. solium*.

Taenia solium (Figs. IV.7b and 23.4a): size of proglottid approximately 8 mm wide by 12 mm long. There are up to 12 side branches to the uterus (able to count them).
NB Either wear gloves when handling the proglottides or kill the eggs by fixing in hot formol saline before handling.

If the branches of the uterus cannot be easily seen inject the proglottid with 'Indian ink' using a fine needle.

Enterobius vermicularis (Figs. 21.5 and 21.6)

Adult worms or ova may be found in the faeces but it is advisable to look for ova on the perianal skin.

Sellotape (Scotch tape) method

1 Use Sellotape slightly narrower than the width of a microscope slide (26 mm).
2 Wearing gloves, place the tape sticky side down on the anal skin and press with the thumb. Do this several times around the area.
3 Smooth the tape, sticky side down, on to a microscope slide, making it as flat as possible.
4 Examine the slide microscopically using the × 10 objective.

Cotton swab method

1 Soak a cotton swab in physiological saline and squeeze off excess liquid.
2 Pass the swab over and around the anal skin.
3 Either press the swab on to a microscope slide, cover with a coverslip and examine on a microscope using the × 10 objective, or place the swab in a tube, cover with saline and leave for several minutes.
4 Examine the fluid microscopically.

Examination of urine for *Schistosoma haematobium* ova (Figs. 22.21)

1 Test the urine for the presence of blood and albumin; these are usually present in a patient with schistosomiasis.
2 Mix the sample of urine well and pour into a centrifuge tube. Centrifuge at 5000 r.p.m. for about 5 minutes. Discard supernatant and examine deposit for ova.
NB In light infections there may only be one or two ova in the sample. It is therefore important to examine the whole of the deposit, not just one slide.

Filtration of urine for diagnosis of *Schistosoma haematobium* ova

1 Collect total urine between 11 a.m. and 2 p.m. on one day.
2 If there is a large volume of urine allow the sample to stand for about 30 minutes. This will ensure that any ova are at the bottom of the container.
3 Remove most of the urine by means of a suction pump and discard—take care not to disturb the bottom 20 ml or so of urine.
4 Mix the remaining urine well and by means of a syringe inject the sample through a Millipore* (Swinnex) filter holder containing a 12 µm Nuclepore† membrane.
5 After the urine has been completely expressed from the syringe, the syringe is removed, filled with air, and reinjected into the filter holder. This procedure is repeated twice to remove excess urine and to help any ova adhere to the surface of the membrane.
6 The filter holder is then opened and the membrane is removed with a pair of forceps and placed face upwards on a microscope slide.
7 Add one drop of saline to the top of the membrane and cover with a coverslip. Examine on a microscope using the × 10 objective and count the number of ova observed.
* Swinnex filter holder, 25 mm diameter—Cat. No. SX00 02500 Millipore Ltd.
† Nuclepore 12.0 µm pore size, 25 mm diameter—Cat. No. 110616 Sterilin Ltd.

Skin snips for *Onchocerca volvulus*

1 Remove a piece of skin using a fine scalpel blade or Walser punch forceps. (The usual sites are shoulder, iliac crest, thigh and calf.)
2 Place the piece of skin on a clean microscope slide, cover with 1 drop of physiological saline and examine microscopically after 30 minutes using a × 4 objective. Any microfilariae will be seen as motile, whitish-silver 'threads'.
3 If no microfilariae are visible then transfer the piece of skin to a plastic microtitre tray, cover with 3 drops of physiological saline* and cover the cells with a piece

of sticky tape to prevent evaporation. Incubate at 37°C for 24 hours.

4 After incubation the skin will have softened. Using a glass Pasteur pipette suck up the saline from the well, ensuring to agitate the tissue to remove any microfilariae.

5 Transfer this saline to a microscope slide. Do not spread the liquid out too much—there is no need for a coverslip; examine using a × 10 objective. Any microfilariae should still be active.

6 If the original skin snip was contaminated with blood it is advisable to stain the microfilariae to ensure that they are indeed *Onchocerca volvulus* and not other blood-inhabiting species (Figs. 20.18 and II.73,1).

* If required, collagenase (Sigma, Type II crystalline) at a concentration of 3 mg/ml in saline can be used instead of just saline. This will help to break down the tissue and release microfilariae.

Examination of blood for presence of microfilariae

1 Place a drop of fresh blood on a slide, cover with a coverslip and examine using the × 4 objective for the presence of motile microfilariae.

2 Make thick blood films and stain as described on the following page.

3 Knott's concentration technique:
   (a) Add 1 ml of anticoagulated blood to a tube containing about 12 ml of 1% formalin (in water) solution.
   (b) Centrifuge at 3000 r.p.m. for about 5 minutes.
   (c) Discard supernatant and examine deposit microscopically using a × 4 objective.

Filtration of blood for microfilariae

1 Collect blood in EDTA (sequestrene). If unable to perform filtration on the same day as the blood is collected microfilariae will survive at room temperature for 2 days.

2 Take up a maximum of 2.5 ml of blood in a syringe, plus about 3 ml of air.

3 Force the blood through a Swinnex* holder containing a 3 μm Nuclepore† membrane.

4 After the blood has been completely expressed from the syringe, push through another syringe, full of air to empty the holder completely of blood.

5 Using the same syringe, wash the membrane through in situ with approximately 20 ml of physiological saline.

6 Remove membrane from the holder and place face upwards on a microscope slide. Examine immediately for the presence of microfilariae (these should still be motile).

7 If a species identification is required leave the membrane to dry on the slide for about 1 hour. Fix with methanol for 30 seconds and dry slide upright.

8 Stain membrane by covering the slide with dilute Giemsa stain for 20 minutes.

9 Dehydrate the membrane through 70%, 90% and absolute alcohol for 2 minutes in each solution.

10 Clear membrane in xylene for 2 minutes.

11 Mount in immersion oil of a neutral mounting medium such as Xam.

* Swinnex filter holder, 25 mm diameter—Cat. No. SX00 02500—Millipore.

† Nuclepore 3.0 μm pore size. 25 mm diam.—Cat. No. 110612—Sterilin Ltd.

Staining of thick blood films for the presence of microfilariae

Mayer's haemalum

1 Make a thick blood film; this should be quite a large film using more blood than one would use for a malaria thick film.

2 Leave the blood on a bench to dry naturally for a few hours (overnight if possible), cover to prevent flies from eating the blood.

3 Dehaemoglobinize the film by placing it upright in a beaker of tap water, lift the slide gently in and out of the water until most of the haemoglobin has left the film.

4 Dry film upright.

5 Fix film for 30 seconds to 1 minute in methanol.

6 Cover the film with Mayer's haemalum; gently warm the underside of the film until the stain is steaming. Leave for about 5 minutes.

7 Wash off stain with tap water, leave the slide in running water to 'blue' the nuclei of the microfilariae. This may take from 2 minutes up to 15 minutes depending on the batch of stain used. Remove the slide from the water at intervals, dry the back and examine under the microscope until the colour of the nuclei is satisfactory.

8 Dry film upright and examine, using the × 4 or × 10 objective to locate the microfilariae and then the × 40 (or × 100) for identification.

NB When using the × 40 objective, a drop of xylene placed on the film and covered with a glass coverslip will make the microfilariae much clearer to see.

TO MAKE STAIN

Haematoxylin	1.0 g
Aluminium potassium sulphate	25 g
Absolute alcohol	10 ml
Distilled water	500 ml
Glacial acetic acid	10 ml
Sodium iodate	100 mg

Dissolve the haematoxylin in the alcohol. Dissolve the aluminium potassium sulphate in 400 ml of the water by warming. Allow to cool then mix the two solutions together. Dissolve the sodium iodate in the remaining 100 ml of distilled water and add to the stain solution. Add the glacial acetic acid. Store for one week before using.

Giemsa stain

1 Make thick film and air dry for several hours.
2 Dehaemoglobinize the film in tap water.
3 Air dry upright.
4 Fix film for 1 minute in methyl alcohol.
5 Make a 10% solution of Giemsa stain in buffered water pH 7.2.
6 Pour the stain in a trough, add film and leave to stain for 20–30 minutes.
7 Rinse slide in buffered water.
8 Air dry and examine as before.
NB The sheath of *Wucheraria bancrofti* will take up the stain but that of *Loa loa* will not.

Leishman's stain

1 Make thick film, dry and dehaemoglobinize as above.
2 No need to fix film as Leishman's stain is made up in methyl alcohol.
3 Cover film with stain; after 30 seconds add twice as much buffered water pH 7.2.
4 Leave to stain for 10 minutes.
5 Wash off stain with tap water and examine as previously mentioned.

Leishman's stain for thin blood films

1 Make a thin film and air dry rapidly.
2 Flood film with stain and leave for 30 seconds to 1 minute to fix the film.
3 Add twice as much buffered water pH 7.2 (preferably from a plastic 'wash' bottle as this allows better mixing of the two solutions), leave to stain for 10 minutes.
4 Wash off stain with tap water, wipe the back of the slide free from any unwanted stain before the slide is left to dry.
5 Dry upright.
6 Examine microscopically using the × 40 then the oil immersion (× 100) objective. (Scanty microfilariae or trypanosomes may be missed if × 100 objective is used initially.)
NB If using Leishman's stain for marrow smears for *Leishmania* amastigotes then leave the film to stain for 20 minutes.

To make stain

Leishman's powder	1.5 g
Methyl alcohol	500 ml

Add glass beads and stain powder to an amber glass bottle. Shake well and leave bottle on a rotary shaker for 1 day. Incubate at 37°C overnight. There is no need to filter the stain if care is taken not to disturb the deposit.

Buffered water

Potassium dihydrogen phosphate	700 mg
Disodium hydrogen phosphate	1.0 g

Dissolve in 1 litre of distilled water.

Field's stain for thick blood films

1 Make thick blood film and leave flat on the bench to air dry. (Care should be taken in the tropics to protect wet films from flies, etc.)
2 Dip film in stain 'A' for 5 seconds; drain.
3 Rinse gently in jar of tap water for 5 seconds; drain.
4 Dip film in stain 'B' for 3 seconds; drain.
5 Rinse gently in jar of tap water for 5 seconds; drain.
6 Dry films upright.
7 Examine when dry in a polychromatic area (where leukocyte nuclei are stained purple); in this area parasite nuclei will be red and cytoplasm blue.
8 Examine film with the × 40 objective before putting oil on the film. Trypanosomes and malaria gametocytes can be seen easily at this magnification.
NB Microfilariae may not stain with Field's stain.

To make stains

Field's A:

Methylene blue	0.8 g
Azure I	0.5 g
Disodium hydrogen phosphate (anhydrous)	5.0 g
Potassium hydrogen phosphate	6.25 g
Distilled water	500 ml

Field's B:

Eosin	1.0 g
Disodium hydrogen phosphate (anhydrous)	5.0 g
Potassium hydrogen phosphate	6.25 g
Distilled water	500 ml

Dissolve the phosphates in the water. Add the appropriate stain. Leave for 24 hours; filter.

Giemsa stain

For microfilariae, amastigotes and malaria parasites.
 Filter stain before use—use a 15% solution of stain in buffered water pH 7.2.

Thin film

1 Fix film in methyl alcohol for 1 minute.
2 Place stain in a trough, add slides and leave for 15 minutes to stain.
3 Remove slides from trough and wash with buffered distilled water.
4 Dry slides upright.

Thick films

1 Allow film to dry thoroughly.
2 Place in jar of stain (do not fix films) and leave for 15 minutes.
3 Wash and dry as above.

To make stain

Giemsa powder	3.8 g
Methyl alcohol	250 ml
Glycerol	250 ml

Add stain to an amber glass bottle containing glass beads. Add glycerol and alcohol, shake bottle vigorously and place at 37°C for 24 hours. Remove from incubator and place on a rotary shaker for several hours. The stain is ready for use; filter small amounts for use as required.

Staining of thick and thin blood films for parasites on one slide

1 Prepare a thick and thin blood film on a slide and allow to dry (Fig. IV.8).

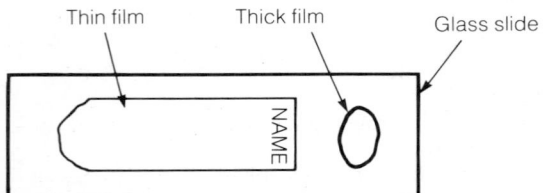

Fig. IV.8 Thick and thin blood films on one slide.

2 Label the thin smear, using a pencil, with the patient's name.
3 Place the films on a flat surface and cover to keep out flies. If the films will be stained within the next 48 hours no further treatment is necessary. If unable to stain within this period then the thick film must be dehaemoglobinized by placing it in a container of water then allowed to dry. The thin film should be fixed by dipping into a container of methanol for a few seconds and left to dry. Once dry store films out of direct sunlight.
  Do *not* fix thick film.

Staining

1 Once dry, fix the thin film for 30 seconds in methanol, drain off and allow to dry. (If the slide has been stored for some time and treated as in **3** above omit this step.)
2 Dilute Giemsa stain to 15% in buffered water pH 7.2 and place in a trough.
3 Place slides in the trough and stain for 15 minutes.

4 Wash off excess stain with tap water and dry films upright.
NB This stain can be used for any slides you wish to stain on the day that the stain was diluted. Fresh stain must be prepared daily.

Appearance of *Plasmodium* species in thin blood films

Plasmodium falciparum (Plate I.12–15)

1 Infected erythrocytes are normal sized.
2 Ring stage of the parasite most commonly seen (Plate I.12); later trophozoites and gametocytes also found, other stages not normally present in peripheral blood.
3 Rings may have one or two chromatin dots; acolé form common.
4 Multiple infection of erythrocytes common unless very light infection (Plate II.2).
5 If infection has progressed numbers of rings may be seen.
6 Infected erythrocyte may contain coarse dots—Maurer's clefts (Plate I.18).
7 Mature schizont contains 24 merozoites—not normally seen in peripheral blood (Plate I.13).
8 Crescent (sausage)-shaped gametocyte (Plate I.14 and 15).

Plasmodium vivax (Plate I.8–11)

1 Infected erythrocyte usually enlarged except very early on in the infection.
2 All stages of parasite may be seen in peripheral blood film.
3 Multiple infections of erythrocytes may rarely occur.
4 Double chromatin dot of ring stage may also rarely be seen.
5 Stippling of infected erythrocyte usually seen—Schüffner's dots (Plate I.16).
6 Amoeboid-trophozoite diagnostic (Plate I.9 and 10).
7 Rings generally larger than those of *P. falciparum* and not as delicate (Plate I.8).
8 Mature chizont contains 16 merozoites (Plate I.11).
9 Large, round, gametocyte (Plate II.1).

Plasmodium malariae (Plates I.5–7 and II.3)

1 Infected erythrocyte not enlarged—may appear smaller than usual.
2 Trophozoites very solid, compact and dense staining (Plate I.5 and Plate II.3).
3 Band form trophozoite often seen (Plate I.6).
4 No stippling of erythrocytes.
5 Mature schizont is like a 'flower head'; central portion of golden pigment surrounded by eight merozoites (Plate I.7).

6 All stages of parasite may be seen in peripheral blood.
7 Multiple infections of erythrocytes is exceptional.
8 Round gametocyte.

Plasmodium ovale (Plate I.1–4)

1 Up to one-third of infected erythrocytes may be slightly enlarged and oval-shaped with fimbriated ends (Plate I.1).
2 Stippling—Schüffner's dots—usually seen.
3 Trophozoites solid—'*P. vivax*-type erythrocytes containing *P. malariae*-type parasites' (Plate I.2).
4 Multiple infection of erythrocyte rarely seen.
5 All stages of parasite may be found in peripheral blood.
6 Round gametocyte.

Diagnosis of leishmaniasis

Cutaneous

1 Puncture the edge of the lesion (by the healing margin) and remove some of this material on to a clean microscope slide.
2 Make a smear and leave to air dry. Label the slide with a wax pencil or diamond marker.
3 Fix in methanol for 1 minute.
4 Stain with a 10% solution of Giemsa in buffered water pH 7.2 for 30 minutes or in Leishman's stain for 20 minutes.
5 Examine smear for amastigotes using oil immersion ($\times$ 100) objective.

Visceral

1 Obtain biopsy material marrow or spleen.
2 Make a thin smear and leave to air dry.
3 Fix and stain as above.
NB amastigotes may be found within macrophages or as extracellular bodies.

Blood collection for the identification of trypanosomes

1 Swab a fingertip with spirit and allow to dry.
2 Stab the digit using a sterile lancet, squeeze the finger gently and discard the first two drops of blood.
3 Using clean microscope slides:
  (a) Place one drop of blood in the centre of a slide and cover with a coverslip. Examine this preparation for motile parasites immediately.
  (b) Place two or three drops of blood on the middle of a slide, using the clean edge of another slide make a thick film, spreading the blood with a circular motion.
  (c) Place one drop of blood on the end of a slide and make a thin film.
  (d) Label the slides with the patient's identification.

4 Leave the thick blood film to dry out of direct sunlight.

Examination of blood

1 Whilst the thick film is drying examine the wet preparation, using a $\times$ 10 eyepiece and the $\times$ 40 objective.
2 Stain the thick film with Field's stain.
3 Examine film using the $\times$ 10 eyepiece and the $\times$ 40 objective; using this magnification the whole thick film can be examined in a short time. Trypanosomes can be confirmed by using the $\times$ 100 (oil immersion) objective.
  If your laboratory has a microhaematocrit centrifuge a sample of blood should be taken into a heparinized capillary tube at the time that the patient has a fingerprick done. If the wet preparation and the thick film are negative then this tube can be further processed for examination.
1 (a) Seal the microhaematocrit tube at one end.
  (b) Place in microhaematocrit and centrifuge the tube for 5 minutes.
  (c) Place the tube on a microscope slide and secure it with a piece of sticky tape.
  (d) Examine the 'buffy layer' on the microscope using the $\times$ 40 objective; motile trypanosomes if present will be found in this area.
2 Follow (a)–(c) above but cut the tube just below the level of the white cell layer; take care when breaking the tube to avoid infecting yourself. Transfer the buffy layer and a small amount of plasma to a slide, either examine as a wet preparation or spread to make a film staining when dry.
NB Capillary tubes should be examined as soon as they have been centrifuged (as trypanosomes may move up the tube and therefore not be seen).

Examination of cerebrospinal fluid (CSF) for the presence of trypanosomes

1 CSF should be examined as soon as the sample is received.
2 Record whether the sample is clear or cloudy.
3 Mix the sample of CSF and remove one drop on to a clean microscope slide. Place a coverslip on the slide and examine, using the $\times$ 40 objective, for the presence of motile trypanosomes.
4 Before beginning the microscopical examination the remainder of the CSF should be centrifuged at approximately 2000 r.p.m. for 10 minutes. (The slide can be examined whilst this is centrifuging.)
5 After centrifugation the CSF supernatant should be removed into a clean tube; a protein determination can be performed on this sample.
6 The deposit should be gently resuspended with a Pasteur pipette and a cell count performed using a Fuchs Rosenthal haemocytometer. Fill the chamber and perform a leukocyte count using the $\times$ 10 eyepiece

and the ×40 objective (at the same time looking for the presence of motile trypanosomes).

Counting

1 If there are not too many cells use undiluted CSF.
2 Count all the leukocytes seen in five large squares of the haemocytometer; the actual number of cells counted is reported as 'x' cells/mm³ (Fig. IV.9).

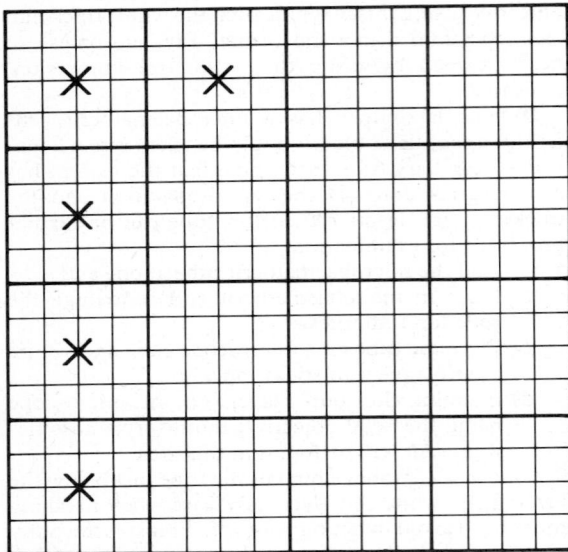

Fig. IV. 9   Fuchs Rosenthal chamber showing squares to be counted.

If there are so many cells that counting would be difficult then the sample should be reported as cells^{+++} (no need to try to count).
NB If the sample of CSF is bloody it should be discarded—cells or trypanosomes may have originated from the blood.

Mini anion exchange technique (Fig. IV.10)

This is a useful concentration technique where other investigations for trypanosomes in the blood have proved negative.
    Blood is passed through a column of cellulose. Erythrocytes are retained in the column and trypanosomes pass out into a collecting tube.
1 Place a piece of dry sponge into a 2 ml syringe barrel. (This is now termed the column.)
2 Add 4 drops of phosphate buffered saline (PBS) to dampen the sponge and allow to drain out of the column.
3 Shake the cellulose (DE52—diethylaminoethyl cellulose) thoroughly to resuspend and pour into the column up to the 2 ml mark. Allow to stand so that excess PBS will drain out.

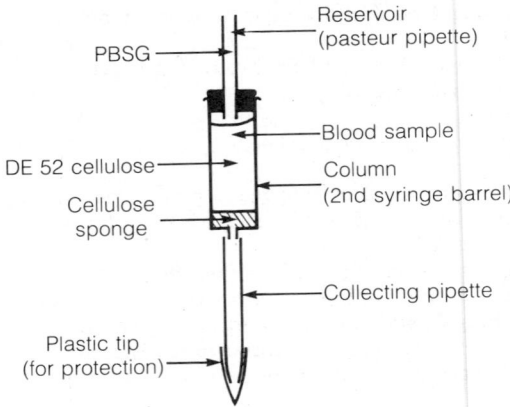

Fig. IV.10   Mini anion exchange technique.

4 Add a few ml of phosphate buffered saline plus glucose (PBSG) to the top of the column and allow it to drain through.
5 Take 150–200 μl of blood (from a finger prick) and drop on to the top of the column. Allow the blood to soak into the column. Attach a collecting pipette to the base of the column.
6 Pipette a few drops of PBSG on top of the blood and *immediately* attach the reservoir and fill with PBSG (approximately 1.5 ml). This will drip slowly on to the column.
7 Leave until all the PBSG has washed through the column. (This should take approximately 4 minutes.)
8 The collecting pipette will now be full of PBSG plus any trypanosomes that were present in the blood.
9 Centrifuge the collecting pipette (in its plastic cover) at 2000 r.p.m. for 10 minutes.
10 Place the pipette on a slide or viewing chamber and examine the tip of the pipette, using ×20 objective, within 20 minutes for motile trypanosomes.
    The buffers and DE 52 for use in this technique are described below.

Preparation of materials for use with mini anion columns

CELLULOSE (DE 52 WHATMAN LTD) PRODUCT NO. 4057–050
1 Weigh out 25 g of DE 52 and add 100 ml of working strength PBS.
2 Mix well and leave to stand. After 30 minutes remove any fine particles with a suction pump.
3 Add fresh buffer to the cellulose, mix, and leave to stand as in **2** Repeat this process four times.
4 Mix the solution well and adjust to pH 8.0 with 1/20 orthophosphoric acid.
5 Allow this solution to stand, discard most of the supernatant fluid, i.e. leave the cellulose as a wet slurry.

6 Transfer to a large bottle and autoclave at 5 lb/in², for 10 minutes.

7 Mix well and distribute as 20 ml aliquots into bottles. This will keep for several months stored at 4°C or room temperature (20°C).

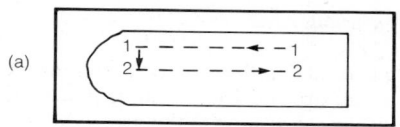

(a)

BUFFER CONCENTRATE (PBS)

Na$_2$HPO$_4$ (anhydrous)	27.00 g
NaH$_2$PO$_4$.2H$_2$O	1.55 g
NaCl	8.50 g
Distilled water	(to) 100 ml

Dissolve by warming. This is a concentrated solution, the working strength solution for human blood is further diluted with distilled water. If the solution is to be used immediately 3 ml of the concentrated solution is made up to 150 ml with distilled water.

If the solution is to be stored for future use then the concentrate should be placed in 3 ml aliquots in glass bottles. The liquid portion is evaporated off by placing these bottles (without lids) in a hot box at 80°C until dry. Remove from the hot box, place lids on and store at room temperature until needed. If stored in this manner the buffer will keep indefinitely with no deterioration of pH.

To use this dried buffer add 150 ml of distilled water to each aliquot.

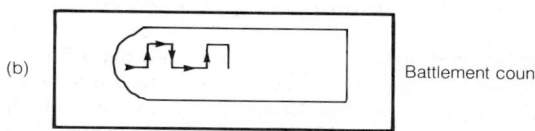

(b)   Battlement count

Fig. IV.11 Differential, leukocyte count (a) Counting in a strip; (b) 'battlement' count.

PBSG

The working strength PBS must have the appropriate amount of glucose added (for anion exchange purposes). For human blood this is 2.6% glucose

Add 3.9 g glucose to 150 ml of working strength PBS immediately before use.

NB Once the glucose has been added the solution should be discarded at the end of the day. PBS should be all right for a further day if kept at 4°C overnight.

I am grateful to Mr C.D. Kimber of the London School of Hygiene and Tropical Medicine for allowing me to reproduce details of the miniature anion exchange centrifugation technique.

Differential leukocyte count

Make a thin blood film, ensuring that it is not too thin. If the film is made too thinly the leukocytes tend to accumulate at the tail-end and edges of the film.

1 Stain film with Leishman's stain using buffered water pH 6.8 as a diluent. Stain for 10 minutes.

2 Clean the back of the slide after staining and leave to air dry.

Either:

3 a Using the oil immersion objective, count a total of 200 leukocytes in a strip, running down the length of the film. If insufficient cells are found then count an additional strip (Fig. IV.11a).

Or

3 b Perform a 'battlement' count until 200 cells have been counted (Fig. IV.11b).

4 Record the total number of each of the types of

leukocytes seen, divide these totals by two to give a percentage figure for each type.

NB Lymphocytes and monocytes: dark purple nuclei with blue cytoplasm. Neutrophils; purple nuclei, pale cytoplasm. Eosinophils; red granules in cytoplasm. Basophils: large dark blue granules in cytoplasm.

Other diagnostic techniques

1 *Skin scrapes for fungus*

Place skin scrapings on a clean microscope slide and cover with one or two drops of 10% aqueous potassium hydroxide solution. Add a glass coverslip and leave suspension on the bench for 15 minutes. Examine microscopically, using the ×10 and ×40 objectives for fungal hyphae. The hydroxide solution will have disrupted epithelial cells and thus made hyphae easier to detect.

2 *Sputum for Paragonimus ova* (Fig. 22.47)

Add sample of sputum to a test tube and overlay with 1 or 2 ml of 5% potassium hydroxide, mix with a wooden stick. Fill up the tube with distilled water, centrifuge at 3000 r.p.m. for 5 minutes. Examine deposit microscopically.

3 *Urine examination*

Sometimes a urine deposit may be difficult to focus due to the small number of cells, etc. in it. To make examination easier, routinely add one drop of 0.75% methylene blue (made up in physiological saline) to urine deposits. Epithelial cells will stain blue, erythrocytes pale pink, pus cells and mucus blue; the stain will not damage *Schistosoma* ova.

4 *Indian ink preparations*

Indian ink is often used for the negative staining of spirochaetes. A small drop of Indian ink is placed at one end of a microscope slide next to the drop of blood to be examined. Mix the two together and spread to make a thin film. Air dry and examine microscopically. Spirochaetes will appear white (unstained) against a black background.

Ziehl–Neelsen staining for mycobacteria

Hot, strong carbol fuchsin is used as the primary stain—this is capable of penetrating the thick waxy coat of all mycobacteria. Because of this waxy coat *M. tuberculosis* can resist decolorization by strong acid (up to 25% sulphuric acid). This strength of acid will decolorize *M. leprae* bacteria. In practice it is advisable to use 1% acid alcohol as a decolorizing agent when staining for tuberculosis or leprosy bacilli. (For leprosy make a slit skin smear, for tuberculosis use pus from sputum.)

1 Prepare a thin film and allow to dry thoroughly.
2 Heat fix film by passing through a flame several times.
3 Flood slide with strong carbol fuchsin. Heat slide gently until the stain begins to steam—do *not* boil. Stain for 5 minutes. Keep steaming during this period adding extra stain if necessary to prevent film from drying out.
4 Tip off stain and wash well with tap water until no more pink colour comes out of the film.
5 Place slide back on staining rack and cover with 1% acid alcohol, leave for a few seconds, tip off, water rinse. Repeat this process until the smear is colourless or a very pale pink.
6 Counterstain with aqueous 1% methylene blue or malachite green stain for 30 seconds.
7 Wash well in tap water, dry upright and examine microscopically using oil immersion objective.

Acid-fast bacilli will be stained red, about $3\,\mu m \times 0.3\,\mu m$.

Carbol fuchsin

Basic fuchsin	1 g
Absolute alcohol	10 ml
Phenol	5 g
Distilled water	100 ml

Dissolve the fuchsin in the alcohol. Dissolve phenol in the water. Mix the two solutions together and filter.

1% Acid alcohol

Hydrochloric acid	1 ml
70% Alcohol	99 ml

Safranin/methylene blue stain for *Cryptosporidium*

1 Make a thin smear of faeces in saline and allow to dry.
2 Pass the smear through a flame once and allow to cool.
3 Fix for 3 minutes with 3% hydrochloric acid in methanol.
4 Air dry.
5 Cover the smear with 1% aqueous safranin solution and heat the stain until it is just bubbling (about $1\frac{1}{2}$ minutes). Leave to stain for another 30 seconds.
6 Wash off stain with water and drain slide.
7 Stain smear with 1% aqueous methylene blue for 30 seconds.
8 Water wash and drain.
9 Air dry.
10 Mount smear with neutral mountant and examine with ×20 or ×40 objective.
11 *Cryptosporidium* appear as orange spheres, $3–5\,\mu m$ in diameter.
(This method has been reproduced by kind permission of Professor Hart, Department of Medical Microbiology, University of Liverpool.)

Index